W9-AVM-828

CURRENT
Diagnosis & Treatment
Pediatrics

NINETEENTH EDITION

Edited by

William W. Hay, Jr., MD
Professor, Department of Pediatrics
Section of Neonatology and the Division of Perinatal Medicine
University of Colorado School of Medicine and The Children's Hospital, Denver

Myron J. Levin, MD
Professor, Departments of Pediatrics and Medicine
Section of Pediatric Infectious Diseases
University of Colorado School of Medicine and The Children's Hospital, Denver

Judith M. Sondheimer, MD
Professor Emeritus, Department of Pediatrics
Section of Pediatric Gastroenterology, Hepatology, and Nutrition
University of Colorado School of Medicine and The Children's Hospital, Denver

Robin R. Deterding, MD
Professor, Department of Pediatrics
Section of Pediatric Pulmonary Medicine
University of Colorado School of Medicine and The Children's Hospital, Denver

and Associate Authors

The Department of Pediatrics at the University of Colorado School of Medicine
is affiliated with The Children's Hospital of Denver.

New York   Chicago   San Francisco   Lisbon   London   Madrid   Mexico City
Milan   New Delhi   San Juan   Seoul   Singapore   Sydney   Toronto

---

NOTICE

Medicine is an ever-changing science. As new research and clinical experience broaden our knowledge, changes in treatment and drug therapy are required. The authors and the publisher of this work have checked with sources believed to be reliable in their efforts to provide information that is complete and generally in accord with the standards accepted at the time of publication. However, in view of the possibility of human error or changes in medical sciences, neither the authors nor the publisher nor any other party who has been involved in the preparation or publication of this work warrants that the information contained herein is in every respect accurate or complete, and they disclaim all responsibility for any errors or omissions or for the results obtained from use of the information contained in this work. Readers are encouraged to confirm the information contained herein with other sources. For example and in particular, readers are advised to check the product information sheet included in the package of each drug they plan to administer to be certain that the information contained in this work is accurate and that changes have not been made in the recommended dose or in the contraindications for administration. This recommendation is of particular importance in connection with new or infrequently used drugs.

This book was set by Silverchair Science + Communications, Inc.
The editors were Anne M. Sydor and Harriet Lebowitz.
The production supervisor was Sherri Souffrance.
The index was prepared by PPA.
The cover designer Mary McKeon.
The book designer was Alan Barnett Design.
RR Donnelley was printer and binder.

This book is printed on acid-free paper.

Contents

Authors

Frank J. Accurso, MD
Professor, Department of Pediatrics, Head, Section of
Pediatric Pulmonary Medicine, University of Colorado
School of Medicine; The Children's Hospital, Denver,
Colorado
accurso.frank@tchden.org
Pediatric Laboratory Medicine and Reference Ranges

Daniel R. Ambruso, MD
Professor, Department of Pediatrics, Section of Pediatric
Hematology/Oncology/Bone Marrow Transplant,
Associate Medical Director, Belle Bonfils Blood Center,
University of Colorado School of Medicine; The
Children's Hospital, Denver, Colorado
daniel.ambruso@uchsc.edu
Hematologic Disorders

Marsha S. Anderson, MD
Associate Professor, Department of Pediatrics, Section of
Pediatric Infectious Diseases, University of Colorado
School of Medicine; The Children's Hospital, Denver,
Colorado
anderson.marsha@tchden.org
Infections: Bacterial & Spirochetal

Vivek Balasubramaniam, MD
Assistant Professor, Department of Pediatrics, Section of
Pediatric Pulmonary Medicine, University of Colorado
School of Medicine; The Children's Hospital, Denver,
Colorado
Vivek.Balasubramaniam@uchsc.edu
Respiratory Tract & Mediastinum

Timothy A. Benke, MD, PhD
Assistant Professor, Departments of Pediatrics, Neurology,
and Pharmacology, Director, Division of Child
Neurology Residency Training Program, University of
Colorado School of Medicine; The Children's Hospital,
Denver, Colorado
tim.benke@uchsc.edu
Neurologic & Muscular Disorders

Timothy J. Bernard, MD
Assistant Professor, Departments of Pediatrics and
Neurology, University of Colorado School of Medicine;
The Children's Hospital, Denver, Colorado
tim.bernard@hotmail.com
Neurologic & Muscular Disorders

Mark Boguniewicz, MD
Professor, Divisions of Pediatric Allergy-Immunology,
Department of Pediatrics, National Jewish Medical and
Research Center; University of Colorado School of
Medicine, Denver, Colorado
boguniewiczm@njc.org
Allergic Disorders

Rebecca Sands Braverman, MD
Assistant Professor, Department of Ophthalmology,
University of Colorado School of Medicine; Rocky
Mountain Lions Eye Institute, Denver, Colorado
rebecca.sands@uchsc.edu
Eye

Robert M. Brayden, MD
Associate Professor, Department of Pediatrics, Section of
General Academic Pediatrics, University of Colorado
School of Medicine; The Children's Hospital, Denver,
Colorado
brayden.robert@tchden.org
Ambulatory & Community Pediatrics

Jeffrey M. Brown, MD, MPH, CPE
Professor, Department of Pediatrics, University of Colorado
School of Medicine; Director, General Pediatrics
Division, Denver Health Medical Center, Denver,
Colorado
jeff.brown@dhha.org
Ambulatory & Community Pediatrics

Maya Bunik, MD, MSPH
Assistant Professor, Department of Pediatrics, University of
Colorado School of Medicine; The Children's Hospital,
Denver, Colorado
maya.bunik@uchsc.edu
Ambulatory & Community Pediatrics

Joanna M. Burch, MD
Assistant Professor, Departments of Dermatology and
Pediatrics, University of Colorado School of Medicine,
Denver, Colorado
joanna.burch@uchsc.edu
Skin

Todd C. Carpenter, MD

Associate Professor, Department of Pediatrics, Section of Pediatric Critical Care Medicine, University of Colorado School of Medicine; The Children's Hospital, Denver, Colorado
todd.carpenter@uchsc.edu
Critical Care

Keith L. Cavanaugh, MD

Assistant Professor, Department of Pediatrics, Section of Pediatric Pulmonary Medicine, University of Colorado School of Medicine; The Children's Hospital, Denver, Colorado
cavanaugh.keith@tchden.org
Respiratory Tract & Mediastinum

H. Peter Chase, MD

Professor, Department of Pediatrics, Clinical Director Emeritus, Barbara Davis Center for Childhood Diabetes, University of Colorado School of Medicine, Denver, Colorado
peter.chase@uchsc.edu
Diabetes Mellitus

Antonia Chiesa, MD

Senior Instructor, Department of Pediatrics, University of Colorado School of Medicine; Kempe Child Protection Team, The Children's Hospital and Kempe Center for the Prevention and Treatment of Child Abuse and Neglect, Denver, Colorado
chiesa.antonia@tchden.org
Child Abuse & Neglect

Gerald H. Clayton, PhD

Instructor, Department of Physical Medicine/Rehabilitation, University of Colorado School of Medicine; The Children's Hospital, Denver, Colorado
Rehabilitation Medicine

Ronina A. Covar, MD

Assistant Professor, Division of Pediatric Allergy-Immunology, Department of Pediatrics, National Jewish Medical and Research Center; University of Colorado School of Medicine, Denver, Colorado
covarr@njc.org
Allergic Disorders

Matthew F. Daley, MD

Assistant Professor, Department of Pediatrics, Section of General Academic Pediatrics, University of Colorado School of Medicine; The Children's Hospital, Denver, Colorado
daley.matthew@tchden.org
Ambulatory & Community Pediatrics
Immunization

Richard C. Dart, MD, PhD

Professor, Department of Surgery, University of Colorado School of Medicine, Director, Rocky Mountain Poison and Drug Center, Denver, Colorado
rdart@rmpdc.org
Poisoning

Jeffrey R. Darst, MD

Fellow, Pediatric Cardiology, University of Colorado School of Medicine; The Children's Hospital, Denver, Colorado
jeffrey.darst@uchsc.edu
Cardiovascular Diseases

Bert Dech, MD

Clinical Instructor, Department of Psychiatry, The Children's Hospital, Denver, Colorado
dech.bert@tchden.org
Child & Adolescent Psychiatric Disorders & Psychosocial Aspects of Pediatrics

Robin R. Deterding, MD

Professor, Department of Pediatrics, Section of Pediatric Pulmonary Medicine, University of Colorado School of Medicine; The Children's Hospital, Denver, Colorado
deterding.robin@tchden.org
Respiratory Tract & Mediastinum

Emily L. Dobyns, MD

Associate Professor, Department of Pediatrics, Section of Pediatric Critical Care Medicine, University of Colorado School of Medicine; The Children's Hospital, Denver, Colorado
dobyns.emily@tchden.org
Critical Care

Samuel R. Dominguez, MD, PhD

Assistant Professor, Department of Pediatrics, Section of Pediatric Infectious Diseases, University of Colorado School of Medicine; The Children's Hospital, Denver, Colorado
samuel.dominguez@uchsc.edu
Infections: Parasitic & Mycotic

Robert E. Eilert, MD

Clinical Professor, Department of Orthopedic Surgery, University of Colorado School of Medicine; Chairman, Department of Orthopedic Surgery, The Children's Hospital, Denver, Colorado
eilert.robert@tchden.org
Orthopedics

George S. Eisenbarth, MD, PhD
Professor, Department of Pediatrics, Executive Director, Barbara Davis Center for Childhood Diabetes, University of Colorado School of Medicine, Denver, Colorado
george.eisenbarth@uchsc.edu
Diabetes Mellitus

Ellen R. Elias, MD
Associate Professor, Departments of Pediatrics and Genetics, Section of Clinical Genetics and Metabolism, University of Colorado School of Medicine; Director, Special Care Clinic, The Children's Hospital, Denver, Colorado
elias.ellen@tchden.org
Genetics & Dysmorphology

Glenn Faries, MD
Assistant Professor, Department of Pediatrics, Co-Director, Core Clerkship Block in Urgent Care/ Emergency Medicine, University of Colorado School of Medicine; Medical Director, Continuing Medical Education, The Children's Hospital, Denver, Colorado
faries.glenn@tchden.org
Emergencies & Injuries

Monica J. Federico, MD
Assistant Professor, Department of Pediatrics, Section of Pediatric Pulmonary Medicine, University of Colorado School of Medicine; The Children's Hospital, Denver, Colorado
federico.monica@tchden.org
Respiratory Tract & Mediastinum

David M. Fleischer, MD
Assistant Professor, Division of Pediatric Allergy-Immunology, Department of Pediatrics National Jewish Medical and Research Center; University of Colorado School of Medicine, Denver, Colorado
fleischerd@njc.org
Allergic Disorders

Douglas M. Ford, MD
Professor, Department of Pediatrics, Section of Pediatric Renal Medicine, University of Colorado School of Medicine; The Children's Hospital, Denver, Colorado
ford.douglas@tchden.org
Fluid, Electrolyte, & Acid-Base Disorders & Therapy

Nicholas K. Foreman, MD
Professor, Department of Pediatrics, Section of Hematology/Oncology/Bone Marrow Transplant, University of Colorado School of Medicine; The Children's Hospital, Denver, Colorado
foreman.nicholas@tchden.org
Neoplastic Disease

Norman R. Friedman, MD
Professor Department of Otolaryngology, University of Colorado School of Medicine; The Children's Hospital, Denver, Colorado
friedman.norman@tchden.org
Ear, Nose, & Throat

Jeffrey L. Galinkin, MD, FAAP
Associate Professor of Anesthesiology, Director of Research, Department of Anesthesia, University of Colorado School of Medicine; The Children's Hospital, Denver, Colorado
jeffrey.galinkin@uchsc.edu
Pain Management & Palliative Care

Roger H. Giller, MD
Professor, Department of Pediatrics, Section of Pediatric Hematology/Oncology/Bone Marrow Transplant, Director, Pediatric BMT program, University of Colorado School of Medicine; The Children's Hospital, Denver, Colorado
giller.roger@tchden.org
Neoplastic Disease

Neil A. Goldenberg, MD
Assistant Professor, Departments of Pediatrics and Medicine, Center for Cancer and Blood Disorders; Associate Director, Mountain States Regional Hemophilia and Thrombosis Center, Aurora, Colorado; University of Colorado at Denver and Health Sciences Center; The Children's Hospital, Denver, Colorado
neil.goldenberg@uchsc.edu
Hematologic Disorders

Edward Goldson, MD
Professor, Department of Pediatrics, Child Development Unit, University of Colorado School of Medicine; The Children's Hospital, Denver, Colorado
goldson.edward@tchden.org
Child Development & Behavior

Doug K. Graham, MD, PhD
Assistant Professor, Department of Pediatrics, Section of Pediatric Hematology/Oncology/Bone Marrow Transplant, University of Colorado School of Medicine; The Children's Hospital, Denver, Colorado
doug.graham@uchsc.edu
Neoplastic Disease

Eva N. Grayck, MD
Associate Professor, Department of Pediatrics, Section of Pediatric Critical Care Medicine, University of Colorado School of Medicine; The Children's Hospital, Denver, Colorado
Eva.Grayck@uchsc.edu
Critical Care

Brian S. Greffe, MD

Associate Professor, Department of Pediatrics, Section of Pediatric Hematology/Oncology/Bone Marrow Transplant, University of Colorado School of Medicine; The Children's Hospital, Denver, Colorado
greffe.brian@tchden.org
Neoplastic Disease
Pain Management & Palliative Care

Jennifer Hagman, MD

Associate Professor, Department of Psychiatry, University of Colorado School of Medicine; Co-Director, Eating Disorders Treatment Program; The Children's Hospital, Denver, Colorado
hagman.jennifer@tchden.org
Child & Adolescent Psychiatric Disorders & Psychosocial Aspects of Pediatrics

Taru Hays, MD

Professor, Department of Pediatrics, Section of Pediatric Hematology/Oncology/Bone Marrow Transplant, University of Colorado School of Medicine; The Children's Hospital, Denver, Colorado
hays.taru@tchden.org
Hematologic Disorders

Francis Hoe, MD

Instructor, Department of Pediatrics, Section of Pediatric Endocrinology, University of Colorado School of Medicine; The Children's Hospital, Denver, Colorado
francis.hoe@uchsc.edu
Endocrine Disorders

J. Roger Hollister, MD

Professor, Departments of Pediatrics and Medicine, Head, Section of Pediatric Rheumatology, University of Colorado School of Medicine; The Children's Hospital; Senior Staff Physician, National Jewish Medical and Research Center, Denver, Colorado
hollister.roger@tchden.org
Rheumatic Diseases

Richard B. Johnston, Jr., MD

Professor of Pediatrics, Section of Immunology, Associate Dean for Research Development, Executive Vice President for Academic Affairs, National Jewish Medical and Research Center; University of Colorado School of Medicine, Denver, Colorado
richard.johnston@uchsc.edu
Immunodeficiency

David W. Kaplan, MD, MPH

Professor, Department of Pediatrics, Head, Section of Adolescent Medicine, University of Colorado School of Medicine; The Children's Hospital, Denver, Colorado
kaplan.david@tchden.org
Adolescence

Michael S. Kappy, MD, PhD

Professor, Department of Pediatrics, Head, Section of Pediatric Endocrinology, University of Colorado School of Medicine; The Children's Hospital, Denver, Colorado
kappy.michael@tchden.org
Endocrine Disorders

Paritosh Kaul, MD

Assistant Professor, Department of Pediatrics, Director, Denver School Based Health Centers, Section of Adolescent Medicine, University of Colorado School of Medicine; The Children's Hospital; Denver Health Medical Center, Denver, Colorado
paritosh.kaul@dhha.org
Adolescent Substance Abuse

Amy K. Keating, MD

Assistant Professor, Department of Pediatrics, Section of Pediatric Hematology/Oncology/Bone Marrow Transplant, Center for Cancer and Blood Disorders, University of Colorado School of Medicine; The Children's Hospital, Denver, Colorado
keating.amy@tchden.org
Neoplastic Disease

Peggy E. Kelley, MD

Associate Professor, Department of Otolaryngology, University of Colorado School of Medicine; The Children's Hospital, Denver, Colorado
kelley.peggy@tchden.org
Ear, Nose, & Throat

Gwendolyn S. Kerby, MD

Assistant Professor, Department of Pediatrics, Section of Pediatric Pulmonary Medicine, University of Colorado School of Medicine; The Children's Hospital, Denver, Colorado
kerby.gwendolyn@tchden.org
Respiratory Tract & Mediastinum

Nancy A. King, RN, MSN, CPNP

Senior Instructor, Department of Pediatrics, Section of Pediatric Hematology/Oncology/Bone Marrow Transplant, University of Colorado School of Medicine; The Children's Hospital, Denver, Colorado
king.nancy@tch.den.org
Pain Management & Palliative Care

Ulrich Klein, DMD, DDS, MS
Associate Professor & Chair, Pediatric Dentistry, Director of Postgraduate Program, The Children's Hospital, Denver, Colorado
klein.ulrich@tchden.org
Oral Medicine & Dentistry

Nancy F. Krebs, MD, MS
Professor, Department of Pediatrics, Head, Section of Nutrition, University of Colorado School of Medicine; The Children's Hospital, Denver, Colorado
nancy.krebs@uchsc.edu
Normal Childhood Nutrition & Its Disorders

Richard D. Krugman, MD
Professor, Department of Pediatrics, Dean, University of Colorado School of Medicine, Denver, Colorado
richard.krugman@uchsc.edu
Child Abuse & Neglect

Myron J. Levin, MD
Professor, Departments of Pediatrics and Medicine, Section of Pediatric Infectious Diseases, University of Colorado School of Medicine; The Children's Hospital, Denver, Colorado
myron.levin@uchsc.edu
Infections: Viral & Rickettsial
Infections: Parasitic & Mycotic

Paul Levisohn, MD
Assistant Professor, Department of Pediatric Neurology, University of Colorado School of Medicine; The Children's Hospital, Denver, Colorado
Neurologic & Muscular Disorders

Andrew H. Liu, MD
Associate Professor, Department of Pediatrics, Section of Allergy & Clinical Immunology, National Jewish Medical & Research Center; University of Colorado School of Medicine, Denver Colorado
liua@njc.org
Immunodeficiency

Kathryn A. Love-Osborne, MD
Assistant Professor, Department of Pediatrics, Section of Adolescent Medicine, University of Colorado School of Medicine; The Children's Hospital, Denver, Colorado
kathryn.love-osborne@dhha.org
Adolescence

Gary M. Lum, MD
Professor, Departments of Pediatrics and Medicine, Head, Section of Pediatric Renal Medicine, University of Colorado School of Medicine; The Children's Hospital, Denver, Colorado
lum.gary@tchden.org
Kidney & Urinary Tract

Kelly Maloney, MD
Associate Professor, Department of Pediatrics, Section of Pediatric Hematology/Oncology/Bone Marrow Transplant, University of Colorado School of Medicine; The Children's Hospital, Denver, Colorado
maloney.kelly@tchden.org
Neoplastic Disease

David K. Manchester, MD
Professor, Department of Pediatrics, Section of Clinical Genetics and Metabolism, University of Colorado School of Medicine; Co-Director, Division of Genetic Services, The Children's Hospital, Denver, Colorado
manchester.david@tchden.org
Genetics & Dysmorphology

Maria J. Mandt, MD
Assistant Professor, Department of Pediatrics, University of Colorado School of Medicine; Attending Physician, Emergency Department, The Children's Hospital, Denver, Colorado
mandt.maria@tchden.org
Emergencies & Injuries

Elizabeth J. McFarland, MD
Associate Professor, Department of Pediatrics, Section of Pediatric Infectious Diseases, University of Colorado School of Medicine; The Children's Hospital, Denver, Colorado
betsy.mcfarland@uchsc.edu
Human Immunodeficiency Virus Infection

Shelley D. Miyamoto, MD
Instructor, Department of Pediatrics, Section of Pediatric Cardiology, University of Colorado School of Medicine; The Children's Hospital, Denver, Colorado
miyamoto.shelley@tchden.org
Cardiovascular Diseases

Paul G. Moe, MD
Professor, Departments of Pediatrics and Neurology, Division of Child Neurology, University of Colorado School of Medicine; The Children's Hospital, Denver, Colorado
moe.paul@tchden.org
Neurologic & Muscular Disorders

Joseph G. Morelli, MD
Professor, Departments of Dermatology and Pediatrics, University of Colorado School of Medicine, Denver, Colorado
joseph.morelli@uchsc.edu
Skin

Peter M. Mourani, MD
Assistant Professor, Department of Pediatrics, Section of Pediatric Critical Care Medicine, University of Colorado School of Medicine; The Children's Hospital, Denver, Colorado
peter.mourani@uchsc.edu
Critical Care

Kristen Nadeau, MD
Assistant Professor, Department of Pediatrics Section of Pediatric Endocrinology, University of Colorado School of Medicine; The Children's Hospital, Denver, Colorado
kristen.nadeau@uchsc.edu
Endocrine Disorders

Michael R. Narkewicz, MD
Professor, Department of Pediatrics, Section of Pediatric Gastroenterology, Hepatology and Nutrition, The Pediatric Liver Center, University of Colorado School of Medicine; The Children's Hospital, Denver, Colorado
narkewicz.michael@tchden.org
Liver & Pancreas

Ann-Christine Nyquist, MD, MSPH
Associate Professor, Department of Pediatrics, Section of Pediatric Infectious Diseases, University of Colorado School of Medicine; The Children's Hospital, Denver, Colorado
nyquist.ann-christine@tchden.org
Immunization
Sexually Transmitted Infections

John W. Ogle, MD
Professor, Department of Pediatrics, Section of Pediatric Infectious Diseases, University of Colorado School of Medicine; The Children's Hospital; Director, Department of Pediatrics, Denver Health Medical Center, Denver, Colorado
jogle@dhha.org
Antimicrobial Therapy
Infections: Bacterial & Spirochetal

K. Brooke Pengel, MD
Assistant Professor, Department of Rehabilitation Medicine, University of Colorado School of Medicine; The Children's Hospital Rehabilitation Center, Denver, Colorado
pengel.kimberly@tchden.org
Sports Medicine

John D. Polousky, MD
Assistant Professor, Department of Orthopedic Surgery, University of Colorado School of Medicine; The Children's Hospital, Denver, Colorado
polousky.john@tchden.org
Orthopedics

Laura E. Primak, RD, CNSD, CSP
Professional Research Assistant, Nutritionist, Section of Nutrition, Department of Pediatrics, University of Colorado School of Medicine; The Children's Hospital, Denver, Colorado
laura.primak@uchsc.edu
Normal Childhood Nutrition & Its Disorders

Ralph R. Quinones, MD
Associate Professor, Department of Pediatrics, Section of Pediatric Hematology/Oncology/Bone Marrow Transplant, Director, Pediatric Blood and Marrow Processing Laboratory, University of Colorado School of Medicine; The Children's Hospital, Denver, Colorado
quinones.ralph@tchden.org
Neoplastic Disease

Ann Reynolds, MD
Assistant Professor, Department of Pediatrics, Section of Developmental and Behavioral Pediatrics, University of Colorado School of Medicine; The Children's Hospital, Denver, Colorado
reynolds.ann@tchden.org
Child Development & Behavior

Adam Rosenberg, MD
Professor, Department of Pediatrics, Section of Neonatology, Medical Director of the Newborn Service, University of Colorado Hospital; Director, Pediatric Residency Training Program, University of Colorado School of Medicine; The Children's Hospital, Denver, Colorado
adam.rosenberg@uchsc.edu
The Newborn Infant

Barry H. Rumack, MD
Clinical Professor, Department of Pediatrics, University of Colorado School of Medicine; Director Emeritus, Rocky Mountain Poison and Drug Center, Denver Health Authority, Denver, Colorado
barry@rumack.com
Poisoning

Scott D. Sagel, MD
Assistant Professor, Department of Pediatrics, Section of Pediatric Pulmonary Medicine, University of Colorado School of Medicine; The Children's Hospital, Denver, Colorado
sagel.scott@tchden.org
Respiratory Tract & Mediastinum

Elizabeth M. Shaffer, MD
Associate Professor, Department of Pediatrics, Section of Pediatric Cardiology, University of Colorado School of Medicine; The Children's Hospital, Denver, Colorado
shaffer.elizabeth@tchden.org
Cardiovascular Diseases

Eric J. Sigel, MD
Associate Professor, Department of Pediatrics, Section of Adolescent Medicine, University of Colorado School of Medicine; The Children's Hospital, Denver, Colorado
sigel.eric@tchden.org
Eating Disorders
Sexually Transmitted Infections

Eric A. F. Simoes, MB, BS, DCH, MD
Professor of Pediatrics, Department of Pediatrics, Section of Pediatric Infectious Diseases, University of Colorado School of Medicine; The Children's Hospital, Denver, Colorado
eric.simoes@UCDenver.edu
Immunization

Georgette Siparsky, PhD
Supervisor, Clinical Chemistry Laboratory, Department of Pathology, The Children's Hospital, Denver, Colorado
siparsky.georgette@tchden.org
Pediatric Laboratory Medicine and Reference Ranges

Andrew P. Sirotnak, MD
Associate Professor, Department of Pediatrics, University of Colorado School of Medicine; Director, Kempe Child Protection Team, The Children's Hospital and Kempe Children's Center for the Prevention and Treatment of Child Abuse, Denver, Colorado
sirotnak.andrew@tchden.org
Child Abuse & Neglect

Jennifer B. Soep, MD
Assistant Professor, Departments of Pediatrics and Medicine, Section of Pediatric Rheumatology, University of Colorado School of Medicine; The Children's Hospital, Denver, Colorado
soep.jennifer@tchden.org
Rheumatic Diseases

Ronald J. Sokol, MD
Professor and Vice-Chair Head, Department of Pediatrics, Section of Pediatric Gastroenterology, Hepatology and Nutrition, The Pediatric Liver Center; Director, Pediatric Clinical Translational Research Center, University of Colorado School of Medicine; The Children's Hospital, Denver, Colorado
sokol.ronald@tchden.org
Liver & Pancreas

Henry M. Sondheimer, MD
Senior Director, Student Affairs and Student Programs, Association of American Medical Colleges, Washington, D.C.; Professor Emeritus, University of Colorado Denver School of Medicine
hsondheimer@aamc.org
Cardiovascular Diseases

Judith M. Sondheimer, MD
Professor Emeritus, Department of Pediatrics, Section of Pediatric Gastroenterology, Hepatology and Nutrition, University of Colorado School of Medicine; The Children's Hospital, Denver, Colorado
judith.sondheimer@gmail.com
Gastrointestinal Tract

Brian Stafford, MD, MPH
Assistant Professor of Psychiatry and Pediatrics, Consult-Liaison Child Psychiatrist, The Children's Hospital; Medical Director, Postpartum Depression Intervention Program, The Kempe Center, Denver, Colorado
stafford.brian@tchden.org
Child & Adolescent Psychiatric Disorders & Psychosocial Aspects of Pediatrics

Kurt R. Stenmark, MD
Professor, Department of Pediatrics, Head, Section of Pediatric Critical Care Medicine, Director, Developmental Lung Biology Lab, University of Colorado School of Medicine; The Children's Hospital, Denver, Colorado
kurt.stenmark@uchsc.edu
Critical Care

Lora J. Stewart, MD
Associate Physician, Premier Allergy & Asthma, Department of Pediatrics, Section of Allergy & Clinical Immunology, National Jewish Medical & Research Center; University of Colorado School of Medicine, Denver, Colorado
lstewart@premierallergy.com
Immunodeficiency

Shikha Sundaram, MD, MSCI
Assistant Professor, Department of Pediatrics Section of Pediatric Gastroenterology, Hepatology and Nutrition, University of Colorado School of Medicine; The Children's Hospital, Denver, Colorado
sundaram.shikha@tchden.org
Gastrointestinal Tract

Elizabeth H. Thilo, MD
Associate Professor, Department of Pediatrics, Section of Neonatology, University of Colorado School of Medicine; The Children's Hospital, Denver, Colorado
thilo.elizabeth@tchden.org
The Newborn Infant

Janet A. Thomas, MD
Assistant Professor, Department of Pediatrics, Section of Clinical Genetics and Metabolism, University of Colorado School of Medicine; The Children's Hospital, Denver, Colorado
thomas.janet@tchden.org
Inborn Errors of Metabolism

Sharon H. Travers, MD
Associate Professor, Department of Pediatrics, Section of Pediatric Endocrinology, University of Colorado School of Medicine; The Children's Hospital, Denver, Colorado
travers.sharon@tchden.org
Endocrine Disorders

Anne Chun-Hui Tsai, MD, MSc
Associate Professor, Department of Pediatrics Section of Hematology/Oncology/Bone Marrow Transplant, University of Colorado School of Medicine; The Children's Hospital, Denver, Colorado
tsai.chun-hui@tchden.org
Genetics & Dysmorphology

Johan L. K. Van Hove, MD, PhD, MBA
Associate Professor, Department of Pediatrics, Section of Clinical Genetics and Metabolism, University of Colorado School of Medicine; The Children's Hospital, Denver, Colorado
vanhove.johan@tchden.org
Inborn Errors of Metabolism

Adriana Weinberg, MD
Professor, Departments of Pediatrics and Medicine, Director of Clinical Virology Laboratory, Section of Pediatric Infectious Diseases, University of Colorado School of Medicine; The Children's Hospital, Denver, Colorado
adriana.weinberg@uchsc.edu
Infections: Viral & Rickettsial
Infections: Parasitic & Mycotic

Pamela E. Wilson, MD
Assistant Professor, Department of Rehabilitation Medicine, University of Colorado School of Medicine; The Children's Hospital Rehabilitation Center, Denver, Colorado
wilson.pamela@tchden.org
Sports Medicine
Rehabilitation Medicine

Patricia J. Yoon, MD
Assistant Professor, Department of Otolaryngology, University of Colorado School of Medicine; The Children's Hospital, Denver, Colorado
yoon.patricia@tchden.org
Ear, Nose, & Throat

Philip S. Zeitler, MD, PhD
Professor, Department of Pediatrics, Section of Pediatric Endocrinology, University of Colorado School of Medicine; The Children's Hospital, Denver, Colorado
phil.zeitler@uchsc.edu
Endocrine Disorders

Preface

The 19th edition of *Current Diagnosis & Treatment: Pediatrics* (CDTP) features practical, up-to-date, well-referenced information on the care of children from birth through infancy and adolescence. CDTP emphasizes the clinical aspects of pediatric care while also covering important underlying principles. CDTP provides a guide to diagnosis, understanding, and treatment of the medical problems of all pediatric patients in an easy-to-use and readable format.

INTENDED AUDIENCE

Like all Lange medical books, CDTP provides a concise yet comprehensive source of current information. Students will find CDTP an authoritative introduction to pediatrics and an excellent source for reference and review. CDTP provides excellent coverage of The Council on Medical Student Education in Pediatrics (COMSEP) curriculum used in pediatric clerkships. Residents in pediatrics (and other specialties) will appreciate the detailed descriptions of diseases as well as diagnostic and therapeutic procedures. Pediatricians, family practitioners, nurses and nurse practitioners, and other health-care providers who work with infants and children will find CDTP a useful reference on management aspects of pediatric medicine.

COVERAGE

Forty-four chapters cover a wide range of topics, including neonatal medicine, child development and behavior, emergency and critical care medicine, and diagnosis and treatment of specific disorders according to major problems and organ systems. A wealth of tables and figures provides quick access to important information, such as acute and critical care procedures in the delivery room, the office, the emergency room, and the critical care unit; anti-infective agents; drug dosages; immunization schedules; differential diagnosis; and developmental screening tests. The final chapter is a handy guide to normal laboratory values.

NEW TO THIS EDITION

The 19th edition of CDTP has been revised comprehensively by the editors and contributing authors. New references as well as up-to-date and useful Web sites have been added, permitting the reader to consult original material and to go beyond the confines of the textbook. As editors and practicing pediatricians, we have tried to ensure that each chapter reflects the needs and realities of day-to-day practice.

CHAPTERS WITH MAJOR REVISIONS INCLUDE:

  1 The Newborn Infant
  9 Immunization
 12 Poisoning
 16 Oral Medicine & Dentistry
 19 Cardiovascular Diseases
 20 Gastrointestinal Tract
 40 Infections: Bacterial & Spirochetal
 41 Infections: Parasitic & Mycotic

NEW CHAPTERS INCLUDE:

  6 Child & Adolescent Psychiatric Disorders & Psychosocial Aspects of Pediatrics
 25 Sports Medicine
 26 Rehabilitation Medicine
 30 Pain Management & Palliative Care

CHAPTER REVISIONS

The eight chapters that have been extensively revised, with new authors added in several cases, reflect the substantially updated material in each of their areas of pediatric medicine. The Gastrointestinal Tract chapter, with contributions from a new author, has been thoroughly revised, particularly the sections on inflammatory bowel disease and gastroesophageal reflux, as well as new sections on cyclic vomiting syndrome and eosinophilic esophagitis. Especially important are updates to the chapters on Infectious Diseases, including information on methicillin-resistant staphylococcus and tropical diseases such as dengue and malaria. The Neonatology chapter includes a major revision on hyperbilirubinemia. The Poisoning chapter has been revised to include more references and guidelines. The Oral Medicine & Dentistry chapter has a new author and a focus on preventive dentistry. The Cardiovascular chapter has been streamlined and includes a thoroughly updated section on ultrasound and a new section on cardiac transplant and treatment of rejection. A new chapter on Pain Management & Palliative Care has been added. The Rehabilitation Medicine & Sports Medicine chapter has been separated into two chapters to clarify and emphasize the unique aspects of each. Child & Adolescent Psychiatric Disorders & Psychosocial Aspects of Pediatrics has been completely revised by two new authors.

All other chapters are substantially revised and references have been updated. Eighteen new authors have contributed to these revisions.

ACKNOWLEDGMENT

The Editors would like to thank Bonnie Savone for her expert assistance in managing the flow of manuscripts and materials among the chapter authors, editors, and publishers. Her attention to detail was enormously helpful.

William W. Hay, Jr., MD
Myron J. Levin, MD
Judith M. Sondheimer, MD
Robin R. Deterding, MD

Denver, Colorado
August, 2008

The Newborn Infant

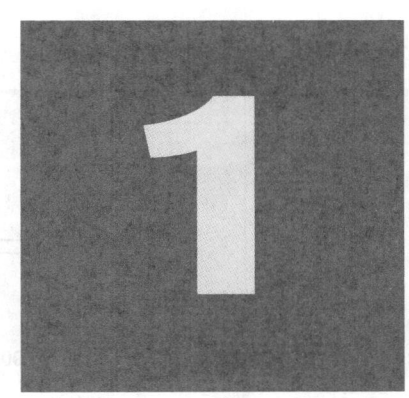

Elizabeth H. Thilo, MD

Adam A. Rosenberg, MD

The newborn period is defined as the first 28 days of life. In practice, however, sick or very immature infants may require neonatal care for many months. There are three levels of newborn care. Level 1 refers to basic care of well newborns, neonatal resuscitation, and stabilization prior to transport. Level 2 refers to specialty neonatal care of premature infants greater than 1500 g or more than 32 weeks' gestation. Level 3 is subspecialty care of higher complexity ranging from 3A to 3D based on newborn size and gestational age, availability of general surgery, cardiac surgery, and extracorporeal membrane oxygenation. Level 3 care is often part of a perinatal center offering critical care and transport to the high-risk mother and fetus as well as the newborn infant.

▼ THE NEONATAL HISTORY

The newborn medical history has three key components: (1) maternal and paternal medical and genetic history, (2) maternal past obstetric history, and (3) current antepartum and intrapartum obstetric history.

The mother's medical history includes chronic medical conditions, medications taken during pregnancy, unusual dietary habits, smoking history, occupational exposure to chemicals or infections of potential risk to the fetus, and any social history that might increase the risk for parenting problems and child abuse. Family illnesses with genetic implications should be sought. The past obstetric history includes maternal age, gravidity, parity, blood type, and pregnancy outcomes. The current obstetric history includes the results of procedures during the current pregnancy such as ultrasound, amniocentesis, screening tests (rubella antibody, hepatitis B surface antigen, serum quadruple screen for genetic disorders, HIV), and antepartum tests of fetal well-being (eg, biophysical profiles, nonstress tests, or Doppler assessment of fetal blood flow patterns). Pregnancy-related maternal complications such as urinary tract infection, pregnancy-induced hypertension, eclampsia, gestational diabetes, vaginal bleeding, and

preterm labor should be documented. Significant peripartum events include duration of ruptured membranes, maternal fever, fetal distress, meconium-stained amniotic fluid, type of delivery (vaginal or cesarean section), anesthesia and analgesia used, reason for operative or forceps delivery, infant status at birth, resuscitative measures, and Apgar scores.

ASSESSMENT OF GROWTH & GESTATIONAL AGE

It is important to know the infant's gestational age because normal behavior and possible medical problems can be predicted on this basis. The date of the last menstrual period is the best indicator of gestational age. Uterine fundal height and early fetal ultrasound provide supporting information. Postnatal physical characteristics and neurologic development are also clues to gestational age. Table 1–1 lists the physical and neurologic criteria of maturity used to estimate gestational age by the Ballard score method. Adding the scores assigned to each neonatal physical and neuromuscular sign yields a score corresponding to gestational age.

Disappearance of the anterior vascular capsule of the lens is also helpful in determining gestational age. Until 27–28 weeks' gestation, the lens capsule is covered by vessels; by 34 weeks, this vascular plexus is completely atrophied. Foot length, from the heel to the tip of the longest toe, also correlates with gestational age in appropriately grown infants. The foot measures 4.5 cm at 25 weeks' gestation and increases 0.25 cm per week until term.

If the physical examination indicates a gestational age within 2 weeks of that predicted by the obstetric dates, the gestational age is as assigned by the obstetric date. Birth weight and gestational age are plotted on standard grids (Figure 1–1) to determine whether the birth weight is appropriate for gestational age (AGA), small for gestational age (SGA) or large for gestational age (LGA). Another term for SGA is intrauterine growth restriction (IUGR). Birth weight for gestational age in normal neonates varies with

Table 1–1. New Ballard score for assessment of fetal maturation of newly born infants.[a]

Neuromuscular Maturity								
	Score							**Record Score Here**
Neuromuscular Maturity Sign	**−1**	**0**	**1**	**2**	**3**	**4**	**5**	
Posture								
Square window (wrist)	>90°	90°	60°	45°	30°	0°		
Arm recoil		180°	140° to 180°	110° to 140°	90° to 110°	<90°		
Popliteal angle	180°	160°	140°	120°	100°	90°	<90°	
Scarf sign								
Heel to ear								
							Total Neuromuscular Maturity Score	

Physical Maturity								
	Score							**Record Score Here**
Physical Maturity Sign	**−1**	**0**	**1**	**2**	**3**	**4**	**5**	
Skin	Sticky, friable, transparent	Gelatinous, red, translucent	Smooth, pink; visible veins	Superficial peeling &/or rash; few veins	Cracking, pale areas; rare veins	Parchment, deep cracking; no vessels	Leathery, cracked, wrinkled	
Lanugo	None	Sparse	Abundant	Thinning	Bald areas	Mostly bald		
Plantar surface	Heel toe 40–50 mm: −1 < 40 mm: −2	> 50 mm: no crease	Faint red marks	Anterior transverse crease only	Creases anterior 2/3	Creases over entire sole		
Breast	Imperceptible	Barely perceptible	Flat areola; no bud	Stippled areola; 1- to 2-mm bud	Raised areola; 3- to 4-mm bud	Full areola; 5- to 10-mm bud		
Eye/Ear	Lids fused loosely: −1 tightly: −2	Lids open; pinna flat; stays folded	Slightly curved pinna; soft; slow recoil	Well-curved pinna; soft but ready recoil	Formed & firm instant recoil	Thick cartilage; ear stiff		
Genitals (male)	Scrotum flat, smooth	Scrotum empty; faint rugae	Testes in upper canal; rare rugae	Testes descending; few rugae	Testes down; good rugae	Testes pendulous; deep rugae		
Genitals (female)	Clitoris prominent & labia flat	Prominent clitoris & small labia minora	Prominent clitoris & enlarging minora	Majora & minora equally prominent	Majora large; minora small	Majora cover clitoris & minora		
							Total Physical Maturity Score	

Maturity	Score	−10	−5	0	5	10	15	20	25	30	35	40	45	50
	Rating	Weeks	20	22	24	26	28	30	32	34	36	38	40	42	44

[a]See text for a description of the clinical gestational age examination.
Reproduced, with permission, from Ballard JL et al: New Ballard Score, expanded to include extremely premature infants. J Pediatr 1991;119:417.

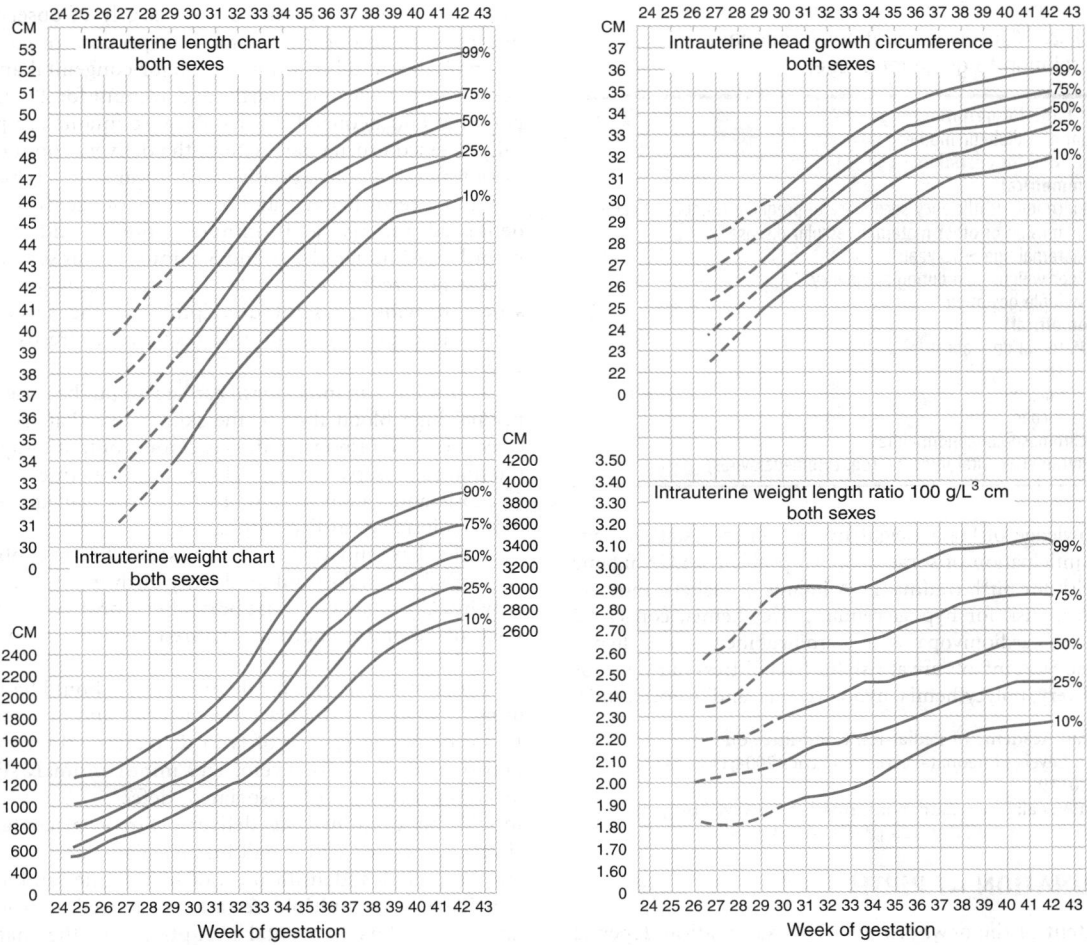

▲ **Figure 1–1.** Intrauterine growth curves for weight, length, and head circumference for singleton births in Colorado. (Reproduced, with permission, from Lubchenco LO et al: Intrauterine growth in length and head circumference as estimated from live births at gestational ages from 26 to 42 weeks. Pediatrics 1966;37:403.)

race, maternal nutrition, access to obstetric care, and environmental factors such as altitude, smoking, and drug and alcohol use. Whenever possible, standards for newborn weight and gestational age based on data derived from the local or regional population should be used. Birth weight related to gestational age is a screening tool that should be supplemented by clinical data when entertaining a diagnosis of IUGR or excessive fetal growth. These data include the infant's physical examination and other factors such as parental size and the birth weight–gestational age of siblings.

An important distinction, particularly in SGA infants, is whether a growth disorder is symmetrical (weight, length, and occipitofrontal circumference [OFC] all ≤ 10%) or asymmetrical (only weight ≤ 10%). Asymmetrical growth restric-

tion implies a problem late in pregnancy, such as pregnancy-induced hypertension or placental insufficiency. Symmetrical growth restriction implies an event of early pregnancy: chromosomal abnormality, drug or alcohol use, or congenital viral infections. In general, the outlook for normal growth and development is better in asymmetrically growth-restricted infants whose intrauterine brain growth has been spared (Table 1–2).

The fact that SGA infants have fewer problems (such as respiratory distress syndrome) than AGA infants of the same birth weight but a lower gestational age has led to the misconception that SGA infants have accelerated maturation. SGA infants, when compared with AGA infants of the same gestational age, actually have increased morbidity and mortality rates.

Table 1–2. Causes of variations in neonatal size in relation to gestational age.

Infants large for gestational age
Infant of a diabetic mother
Infants small for gestational age
Asymmetrical
Placental insufficiency secondary to pregnancy-induced hypertension or other maternal vascular disease
Maternal age > 35 years
Poor weight gain during pregnancy
Multiple gestation
Symmetrical
Maternal drug abuse
Narcotics
Cocaine
Alcohol
Chromosomal abnormalities
Intrauterine viral infection (eg, cytomegalovirus)

Knowledge of birth weight in relation to gestational age allows anticipation of some neonatal problems. LGA infants are at risk for birth trauma; LGA infants of diabetic mothers are also at risk for hypoglycemia, polycythemia, congenital anomalies, cardiomyopathy, hyperbilirubinemia, and hypocalcemia. SGA infants are at risk for fetal distress during labor and delivery, polycythemia, hypoglycemia, and hypocalcemia.

American Academy of Pediatrics: Committee on Fetus and Newborn: Levels of neonatal care. Pediatrics 2004;114:1341 [PMID: 15520119].

Leviton A et al: The wealth of information conveyed by gestational age. J Pediatr 2005;146:123 [PMID: 15644836].

EXAMINATION AT BIRTH

The extent of the newborn physical examination depends on the condition of the infant and the setting. Examination in the delivery room consists largely of observation plus auscultation of the chest and inspection for congenital anomalies and birth trauma. Major congenital anomalies occur in 1.5% of live births and account for 20–25% of perinatal and neonatal deaths. Because infants are physically stressed during parturition, the delivery room examination should not be extensive. The Apgar score (Table 1–3) should be recorded at 1 and 5 minutes of age. In severely depressed infants, a 10-minute score should also be recorded. Although the 1- and 5-minute Apgar scores have almost no predictive value for long-term outcome, serial scores provide a useful description of the severity of perinatal depression and the response to resuscitative efforts.

Skin color is an indicator of cardiac output because of the normal high blood flow to the skin. Stress that triggers a catecholamine response redirects cardiac output away from the skin to preserve oxygen delivery to more critical organs. Cyanosis and pallor are thus two signs of inadequate skin oxygenation and cardiac output.

Skeletal examination at delivery serves to detect obvious congenital anomalies and to identify birth trauma, particularly in LGA infants or those born after a protracted second stage of labor in whom a fractured clavicle or humerus might be found.

The number of umbilical cord vessels should be determined. Normally, there are two arteries and one vein. In 1% of deliveries (5–6% of twin deliveries), the cord has only one artery and one vein. This minor anomaly slightly increases the risk of associated defects. The placenta should be examined at delivery. Small placentas are always associated with small infants. The placental examination includes identification of membranes and vessels (particularly in multiple gestations) as well as placental infarcts or clots (placental abruption) on the maternal side.

Table 1–3. Infant evaluation at birth—Apgar score.[a]

	Score		
	0	**1**	**2**
Heart rate	Absent	Slow (< 100)	> 100
Respiratory effort	Absent	Slow, irregular	Good, crying
Muscle tone	Limp	Some flexion	Active motion
Response to catheter in nostril[b]	No response	Grimace	Cough or sneeze
Color	Blue or pale	Body pink; extremities blue	Completely pink

©1958 American Medical Association.

[a]One minute and 5 minutes after complete birth of the infant (disregarding the cord and the placenta), the following objective signs should be observed and recorded.

[b]Tested after the oropharynx is clear.

Reproduced, with permission, from Apgar V et al: Evaluation of the newborn infant—Second report. JAMA 1958;168:1985.

EXAMINATION IN THE NURSERY

The examiner should have warm hands and a gentle approach. Start with observation, then auscultation of the chest, and then palpation of the abdomen. Examination of the eyes, ears, throat, and hips should be performed last, as these maneuvers are most disturbing to the infant. The heart rate should range from 120–160 beats/min, and the respiratory rate from 30–60 breaths/min. Systolic blood pressure on day 1 ranges from 50–70 mm Hg and increases steadily during the first week of life. Blood pressure is influenced more significantly by perinatal asphyxia and mechanical ventilation than it is by gestational age. An irregularly irregular heart rate, usually caused by premature atrial contractions, is common, benign, and usually resolves in the first days of life.

Approximately 15–20% of healthy newborns have one minor anomaly. Those with a minor anomaly have a 3% risk of an associated major anomaly. Approximately 0.8% of newborns have two minor anomalies, and 0.5% have three or more, with a risk of 10% and 20%, respectively, of a major malformation. Common minor anomalies requiring no special investigation in healthy infants include preauricular pits, a single sacral dimple without other cutaneous abnormality within 2.5 cm of the anus, a single transverse palmar crease, and three or fewer café-au-lait spots in a white infant or five or fewer in an African-American infant.

Skin

Observe for bruising, petechiae (common over the presenting part), meconium staining, and jaundice. Peripheral cyanosis is commonly present when the extremities are cool or the infant is polycythemic. Generalized cyanosis merits immediate evaluation. Pallor may be caused by acute or chronic blood loss or by acidosis. In dark-skinned infants, pallor and cyanosis should be assessed in the lips, mouth, and nail beds. Plethora suggests polycythemia. Note vernix caseosa (a whitish, greasy material covering the body that decreases as term approaches) and lanugo (the fine hair covering the preterm infant's skin). Dry skin with cracking and peeling of the superficial layers is common in postterm infants. Edema may be generalized (hydrops) or localized (eg, on the dorsum of the feet in Turner syndrome). Check for birthmarks such as capillary hemangiomas (lower occiput, eyelids, and forehead) and mongolian spots (bluish-black pigmentation over the back and buttocks). Milia (small white keratogenous cysts) are common on the cheeks, forehead, nose, and nasolabial folds. Miliaria (blocked ducts of sweat glands) occurs in intertriginous areas and on the face or scalp. Milia can also appear as small vesicles (crystallina), small erythematous papules (rubra), or pustules. Erythema toxicum is a benign rash characterized by fleeting erythematous papules and pustules filled with eosinophils. Pustular melanosis leaves pigmented macules when the pustules rupture. The pustules are noninfectious but contain neutrophils. Jaundice in the first 24 hours is abnormal and should be evaluated.

Head

Check for cephalohematoma (a swelling over one or both parietal bones contained within suture lines) and caput succedaneum (edema over the presenting part that crosses suture lines). Subgaleal hemorrhages (beneath the scalp) are uncommon but can cause extensive blood loss into this large potential space with hypovolemic shock. Skull fractures may be linear or depressed and may be associated with cephalohematoma. Check for the presence and size of the fontanelles. The anterior fontanelle varies from 1–4 cm in any direction; the posterior fontanelle should be less than 1 cm. A third fontanelle is a bony defect along the sagittal suture in the parietal bones and may be seen in syndromes, such as trisomy 21. Sutures should be freely mobile, but are often overriding just after birth. Craniosynostosis, a prematurely fused suture, is more easily diagnosed a few days or more after birth.

Face

Odd facies may be associated with a specific syndrome. Bruising from birth trauma (especially with face presentation) and forceps application should be identified. Face presentation may cause soft tissue swelling around the nose and mouth and significant facial distortion. Facial nerve palsy is obvious during crying; the unaffected side of the mouth moves normally, giving a distorted grimace.

Eyes

Subconjunctival hemorrhages are a frequent result of birth trauma. Less commonly, a corneal tear may occur and present as a clouded cornea. Ophthalmologic consultation is indicated in such cases. Extraocular movements should be assessed. Occasional uncoordinated eye movements are common, but persistent irregular movements are abnormal. The iris should be inspected for abnormalities such as Brushfield spots (trisomy 21) and colobomas. Retinal red reflexes should be present and symmetrical. Dark spots, unilateral blunted red reflex, absent reflex, or a white reflex all require ophthalmologic evaluation. Leukokoria can be caused by glaucoma (cloudy cornea), cataract, or tumor (retinoblastoma). Infants with suspected or known congenital viral infection should have a retinoscopic examination with pupils dilated to look for chorioretinitis.

Nose

Examine the nose for size and shape. In utero compression can cause deformities. Because infants younger than 1 month of age are obligate nose breathers, any nasal obstruction (eg, bilateral choanal atresia or stenosis) can cause respiratory distress. Unilateral choanal atresia can be diagnosed by occluding each naris. Patency is best checked by holding a cold metal surface (eg, a chilled laryngoscope blade) under the nose, and observing the fog from both nares on the metal. Purulent nasal discharge at birth suggests congenital syphilis.

Ears

Malformed or malpositioned (low-set or posteriorly rotated) ears are often associated with other congenital anomalies. The tympanic membranes should be visualized. Preauricular pits and tags are common minor variants but may be associated with hearing loss.

Mouth

Epithelial (Epstein) pearls are retention cysts along the gum margins and at the junction of the hard and soft palates. Natal teeth may be present and sometimes must be removed to prevent their aspiration. Check the integrity and shape of the palate. A small mandible and tongue with cleft palate is seen with Pierre Robin syndrome and can result in respiratory difficulty, as the tongue occludes the airway. Prone positioning can be beneficial. A prominent tongue can be seen in trisomy 21 and Beckwith-Wiedemann syndrome. Excessive oral secretions suggest esophageal atresia or a swallowing disorder.

Neck

Redundant neck skin or webbing is seen in Turner syndrome. Cervical sinus tracts may be seen as remnants of branchial clefts. Check for masses: midline (thyroid), anterior to the sternocleidomastoid (branchial cleft cysts), within the sternocleidomastoid (hematoma and torticollis), and posterior to the sternocleidomastoid (cystic hygroma).

Chest & Lungs

Check for fractured clavicles (crepitus, bruising, and tenderness). Increased anteroposterior diameter (barrel chest) can be seen with aspiration syndromes. Check air entry bilaterally and the position of the mediastinum and heart tones. Decreased breath sounds with respiratory distress and a shift in the mediastinum suggests pneumothorax (tension) or a space-occupying lesion (eg, diaphragmatic hernia). Pneumomediastinum causes muffling of the heart sounds. Expiratory grunting and decreased air entry are observed in hyaline membrane disease. Rales are not of clinical significance at this age.

Heart

Cardiac murmurs are common in the first hours and are most often benign. Severe congenital heart disease in the newborn infant may be present with no murmur at all. The two most common presentations of heart disease in the new-

born infant are (1) cyanosis and (2) congestive heart failure with abnormalities of pulses. In hypoplastic left heart and critical aortic stenosis, pulses are diminished at all sites. In aortic coarctation and interrupted aortic arch, pulses are diminished in the lower extremities. Examination of the newborn heart is described in detail in Chapter 19.

Abdomen

Check for softness, distention, and bowel sounds. If polyhydramnios was present or excessive oral secretions are noted, pass a soft catheter into the stomach to rule out esophageal atresia. Most abdominal masses in the newborn infant are associated with kidney disorders (eg, multicystic or dysplastic, and hydronephrosis). When the abdomen is relaxed, normal kidneys may be felt but are not prominent. A markedly scaphoid abdomen plus respiratory distress suggests diaphragmatic hernia. Absence of abdominal musculature (prune belly syndrome) may occur in association with renal abnormalities. The liver and spleen are superficial in the neonate and discernible by light palpation. A distended bladder may be seen and palpated above the pubic symphysis.

Genitalia & Anus

Male and female genitals show characteristics according to gestational age (see Table 1–1). In the female infant during the first few days, a whitish vaginal discharge with or without blood is normal. Check the patency and location of the anus.

Skeleton

Check for obvious anomalies such as absence of a bone, clubfoot, fusion or webbing of digits, and extra digits. Examine for hip dislocation by attempting to dislocate the femur posteriorly and then abducting the legs to relocate the femur. Look for extremity fractures and for palsies (especially brachial plexus injuries). Rule out myelomeningocele and other spinal deformities (eg, scoliosis). Arthrogryposis (multiple joint contractures) results from chronic limitation of movement in utero that may result from lack of amniotic fluid or from congenital neuromuscular disease.

Neurologic Examination

Normal newborns have reflexes that facilitate survival (eg, rooting and sucking reflexes), and sensory abilities (eg, hearing and smell) that allow them to recognize their mother within a few weeks of birth. Although the retina is well developed at birth, visual acuity is poor (20/400) because of a relatively immobile lens. Acuity improves rapidly over the first 6 months, with fixation and tracking becoming well developed by 2 months.

Observe the newborn's resting tone. Normal term newborns should exhibit flexion of the upper and lower extremities and symmetrical spontaneous movements. Extension of the extremities should result in spontaneous recoil to the flexed position. Assess the character of the cry; a high-pitched cry may indicate disease of the central nervous system (CNS) such as hemorrhage. Hypotonia and a weak cry may indicate systemic disease or congenital neuromuscular disorder. Check the following newborn reflexes:

1. Sucking reflex in response to a nipple or the examiner's finger in the mouth. This reflex is observed by 14 weeks' gestation.
2. Rooting reflex: Head turns to the side of a facial stimulus. This reflex develops by 28 weeks' gestation.
3. Traction response: The infant is pulled by the arms to a sitting position. Initially, the head lags, then with active flexion, comes to the midline briefly before falling forward.
4. Palmar grasp with placement of the examiner's finger in the palm. This reflex develops by 28 weeks' gestation and disappears by age 4 months.
5. Deep tendon reflexes: Several beats of ankle clonus and an upgoing Babinski reflex may be normal.
6. Moro (startle) reflex: Hold the infant supine while supporting the head. Allow the head to drop 1–2 cm suddenly. The arms will abduct at the shoulder and extend at the elbow with spreading of the fingers. Adduction with flexion will follow. This reflex develops by 28 weeks' gestation (incomplete) and disappears by age 3 months.
7. Tonic neck reflex: Forcibly turn the infant's head to one side; the arm and leg on that side will extend while the opposite arm and leg flex ("fencing position"). This reflex disappears by age 8 months.

Adam M, Hudgins L: The importance of minor anomalies in the evaluation of the newborn. NeoReviews 2003;4:e99.
Hernandez JA, Morelli JG: Birthmarks of medical significance. NeoReviews 2003;4:e263.

CARE OF THE WELL NEONATE

The primary responsibility of the Level 1 nursery is care of the well neonate—promoting mother-infant bonding, establishing feeding, and teaching the basics of newborn care. Staff must monitor infants for signs and symptoms of illness, including temperature instability, change in activity, refusal to feed, pallor, cyanosis, early or excessive jaundice, tachypnea, respiratory distress, delayed (beyond 24 hours) first stool or first void, and bilious vomiting. Several preventive measures are routine in the normal newborn nursery.

Prophylactic erythromycin ointment is applied to the eyes within 1 hour of birth to prevent gonococcal ophthalmia. Vitamin K (1 mg) is given intramuscularly or subcutaneously within 4 hours of birth to prevent hemorrhagic disease of the newborn.

All infants should receive hepatitis B vaccine. Both hepatitis B vaccine and hepatitis B immune globulin (HBIG) are administered if the mother is positive for hepatitis B surface antigen (HBsAg). If maternal HBsAg status is unknown, vaccine should be given, maternal blood should be tested for HBsAg, and HBIG should be given to the neonate before 7 days of age if the test is positive.

Cord blood is collected from all infants at birth and used for blood typing and Coombs testing if the mother is type O or Rh-negative.

Rapid glucose testing should be performed in infants at risk for hypoglycemia (infants of diabetic mothers, preterm, SGA, LGA, or stressed infants). Values below 45 mg/dL should be confirmed by laboratory blood glucose testing and treated. Hematocrit should be measured at age 3–6 hours in infants at risk for or those who have symptoms of polycythemia or anemia.

State-sponsored newborn genetic screens (for inborn errors of metabolism such as phenylketonuria [PKU], galactosemia, sickle cell disease, hypothyroidism, and cystic fibrosis) are performed prior to discharge, after 24–48 hours of age if possible. In many states, a repeat test is required at 8–14 days of age because the PKU test may be falsely negative when obtained before 48 hours of age. Not all state-mandated screens include the same panel of diseases. The most recent addition in some states is a screen for congenital adrenal hyperplasia. In infants with prolonged postpartum hospitalization, genetic screening should be performed by 1 week of age. In addition to the state-mandated screen, some centers offer expanded newborn screening by tandem mass spectrometry to look for other inborn errors such as fatty acid oxidation defects.

Infants should routinely be positioned supine to minimize the risk of sudden infant death syndrome (SIDS). Prone positioning is contraindicated unless there are compelling clinical reasons for that position. Bed sharing with adults and prone positioning are associated with increased risk of SIDS.

FEEDING THE WELL NEONATE

A neonate is ready for feeding if he or she is (1) alert and vigorous, (2) has no abdominal distention, (3) has good bowel sounds, and (4) has a normal hunger cry. These signs usually occur within 6 hours after birth, but fetal distress or traumatic delivery may prolong this period. The healthy full-term infant should be allowed to feed every 2–5 hours on demand. The first breast feeding may occur in the delivery room. For formula-fed infants, the first feeding usually occurs by 3 hours of life. The feeding volume generally increases from 0.5–1 oz per feeding initially to 1.5–2 oz per feeding on day 3. By day 3, the average full-term newborn takes about 100 mL/kg/d of milk.

A wide range of infant formulas satisfy the nutritional needs of most neonates. Breast milk is the standard on which formulas are based (see Chapter 10). Despite low concentrations of several vitamins and minerals in breast milk, bioavailability is high. All the necessary nutrients, vitamins, minerals, and water are provided by human milk for the first 6 months of life except vitamin K (1 mg IM is administered at birth), vitamin D (200–300 IU/d is needed if minimal sunlight exposure), and vitamin B_{12} (0.3–0.5 mg/d if the mother is a strict vegetarian and takes no B_{12} supplement). Other advantages of breast milk include (1) immunologic, antimicrobial, and anti-inflammatory factors such as immunoglobulin A (IgA) and cellular, protein, and enzymatic components that decrease the incidence of upper respiratory and gastrointestinal infections; (2) possible decreased frequency and severity of childhood eczema and asthma; (3) improved mother-infant bonding; and (4) improved neurodevelopmental outcome.

Although about 70% of mothers in the United States start by breast feeding, only 33% continue to do so at 6 months. Hospital practices that facilitate successful initiation of breast feeding include rooming-in, nursing on demand, and avoiding unnecessary supplemental formula. Nursery staff must be trained to recognize problems associated with breast feeding and provide help and support for mothers in the hospital. An experienced professional should observe and assist with several feedings to document good latch-on. Good latch-on is important in preventing the common problems of sore nipples, unsatisfied infants, breast engorgement, poor milk supply, and hyperbilirubinemia.

Table 1–4 presents guidelines the nursing mother and health care provider can use to assess successful breast feeding.

American Academy of Pediatrics Committee on Fetus and Newborn: Controversies concerning vitamin K and the newborn. Pediatrics 2003;112:191 [PMID: 12837888].

American Academy of Pediatrics Section on Breastfeeding Policy Statement: Breastfeeding and the use of human milk. Pediatrics 2005;115:496 [PMID: 15687461].

Hunt CE, Hauck FR: Sudden infant death syndrome. CMAJ 2006;174:1861 [PMID: 16785462].

Ostrea EM et al: Drugs that affect the fetus and newborn via the placenta or breast milk. Pediatr Clin North Am 2004;51:539 [PMID: 15157585].

Watson MS: Current status of newborn screening: Decision-making about the conditions to include in screening programs. Ment Retard Dev Disabil Res Rev 2006;12:230 [PMID: 17183572].

EARLY DISCHARGE OF THE NEWBORN INFANT

Discharge at 24–36 hours of age is safe and appropriate for most newborns if there are no contraindications (Table 1–5) and if a follow-up visit within 48 hours is ensured. Most infants with cardiac, respiratory, or infectious disorders are identified in the first 12 hours of life. The exception may be the infant treated intrapartum with antibiotic prophylaxis for maternal group B streptococcal (GBS) colonization or infection. The Centers for Disease Control and Prevention (CDC) and the American Academy of Pediatrics (AAP) recommend that such infants be observed in hospital for 48 hours because of the possibility of "partial treatment" and delayed onset of symptomatic infection. Recent data show that maternal antibiotics during labor do not change the type or timing of symptoms related to GBS infection in full-term infants. Thus, hospital observation beyond 24 hours may not be necessary for the asymptomatic full-term infant who received intrapartum chemoprophylaxis. Other problems, such as jaundice and breast-feeding problems, typically occur after 48 hours and can usually be dealt with on an outpatient basis.

The AAP recommends a follow-up visit within 48 hours for all newborns discharged before 72 hours of age. Infants who are small or slightly premature—especially if breast feeding—are at particular risk for inadequate intake. Suggested guidelines for the follow-up interview and physical examination are presented in Table 1–6. The optimal timing of discharge must be determined in each case based on medical, social, and financial factors.

CIRCUMCISION

Circumcision is an elective procedure to be performed only in healthy, stable infants. The procedure has medical benefits, including prevention of phimosis, paraphimosis, balanoposthitis, and urinary tract infection. Important later benefits of circumcision include decreased incidence of penile cancer, decreased incidence of sexually transmitted diseases (including HIV), and decreased incidence of cervical cancer in female sexual partners. Most parental decisions regarding circumcision are religious and social, not medical. The risks of circumcision include local infection, bleeding, removal of too much skin, and urethral injury. The combined incidence of complications is less than 1%. Local anesthesia by dorsal penile nerve block or circumferential ring block using 1% lidocaine without epinephrine, or topical anesthetic cream are safe and effective methods that should always be used. Techniques allowing visualization of the glans throughout the procedure (Plastibell and Gomco clamp) are preferred to blind techniques (Mogen clamp) as occasional amputation of the glans occurs with the latter technique. Circumcision is contraindicated in infants with genital abnormalities (eg, hypospadias). A coagulation screen should be performed prior to the procedure in infants with a family history of serious bleeding disorders.

HEARING SCREENING

Normal hearing is critical to normal language development. Significant bilateral hearing loss is present in 1–3 infants per 1000 well neonates and in 2–4 per 100 neonates in the intensive care unit population. Infants should be screened for hearing loss by auditory brainstem evoked responses or

Table 1–4. Guidelines for successful breast feeding.

	First 8 Hours	First 8-24 Hours	Day 2	Day 3	Day 4	Day 5	Day 6 Onward
Milk supply	You may be able to express a few drops of milk.		Milk should come in between the second and fourth days.			Milk should be in. Breasts may be firm or leak milk.	Breasts should feel softer after feedings.
Baby's activity	Baby is usually wide-awake in the first hour of life. Put baby to breast within 30 min after birth.	Wake up your baby. Babies may not wake up on their own to feed.	Baby should be more cooperative and less sleepy.	Look for early feeding cues such as rooting, lip smacking, and hands to face.			Baby should appear satisfied after feedings.
Feeding routine	Baby may go into a deep sleep 2-4 h after birth.	Feed your baby every 1-4 h or as often as wanted—at least 8-12 times a day.	Use chart to write down time of each feeding.			May go one longer interval (up to 5 h between feeds) in a 24-h period.	
Breast feeding	Baby will wake up and be alert and responsive for several more hours after initial deep sleep.	As long as the mother is comfortable, nurse at both breasts as long as baby is actively sucking.	Try to nurse both sides each feeding, aiming at 10 min per side. Expect some nipple tenderness.	Consider hand expressing or pumping a few drops of milk to soften the nipple if the breast is too firm for the baby to latch on.	Nurse a minimum of 10-30 min per side every feeding for the first few weeks of life. Once milk supply is well established, allow baby to finish the first breast before offering the second.		Mother's nipple tenderness is improving or is gone.
Baby's urine output		Baby must have a minimum of one wet diaper in the first 24 h.	Baby must have at least one wet diaper every 8-11 h.	You should see an increase in wet diapers (up to four to six) in 24 h.	Baby's urine should be light yellow.	Baby should have six to eight wet diapers per day of colorless or light yellow urine.	
Baby's stool		Baby may have a second very dark (meconium) stool.	Baby may have a second very dark (meconium) stool.	Baby's stools should be in transition from black-green to yellow.	Baby should have three or four yellow, seedy stools a day.	The number of stools may decrease gradually after 4-6 weeks of life.	

Modified, with permission, from Gabrielski L: Lactation support services. The Children's Hospital, Denver, 1999.

Table 1–5. Contraindications to early newborn discharge.

Contraindications to early newborn discharge
1. Jaundice at ≤ 24 h
2. High risk for infection (eg, maternal chorioamnionitis); discharge allowed after 24 h with a normal transition
3. Known or suspected narcotic addiction or withdrawal
4. Physical defects requiring evaluation
5. Oral defects (clefts, micrognathia)
Relative contraindications to early newborn discharge (infants at high risk for feeding failure, excessive jaundice)
1. Prematurity or borderline prematurity (< 38 weeks' gestation)
2. Birth weight < 2700 g (6 lb)
3. Infant difficult to arouse for feeding; not demanding regularly in nursery
4. Medical or neurologic problems that interfere with feeding (Down syndrome, hypotonia, cardiac problems)
5. Twins or higher multiples
6. ABO blood group incompatibility or severe jaundice in previous child
7. Mother whose previous breast-fed infant gained weight poorly
8. Mother with breast surgery involving periareolar areas (if attempting to nurse)

evoked otoacoustic emissions as early as possible because up to 40% of hearing loss will be missed by risk analysis alone. Primary care providers and parents should be advised of the possibility of hearing loss and offered immediate referral in suspect cases. With the use of universal screening, the average age at which hearing loss is confirmed has dropped from 24–30 months to 2–3 months. If remediation is begun by 6 months, language and social development are commensurate with physical development.

American Academy of Pediatrics Committee on Fetus and Newborn Policy Statement: Hospital stay for healthy term newborns. Pediatrics 2004;113:1434 [PMID: 15121968].

Flynn P et al: Male circumcision for prevention of HIV and other sexually transmitted diseases. Pediatrics 2007;119:821 [PMID: 17403855].

Morton CC, Nance WE: Newborn hearing screening—a silent revolution. N Eng J Med 2006;354:2151 [PMID: 16707752].

COMMON PROBLEMS IN THE TERM NEWBORN

NEONATAL JAUNDICE

▶ General Considerations

Sixty-five percent of newborns develop visible jaundice with a total serum bilirubin (TSB) level higher than 6 mg/dL during the first week of life. The normal newborn is deficient in antioxidants such as vitamin E, catalase, and superoxide dismutase. Bilirubin is a potent antioxidant and peroxyl scavenger and may protect the newborn from oxygen toxicity in the first days of life. Approximately 8–10% of newborns develop excessive hyperbilirubinemia (TSB > 17 mg/dL), and 1–2% have TSB above 20 mg/dL. Extremely high and potentially dangerous TSB levels are rare. Approximately 1 in 700 infants have TSB higher than 25 mg/dL, and 1 in 10,000 have TSB above 30 mg/dL. Such high levels can cause kernicterus, characterized by injury to the basal ganglia and brainstem.

Kernicterus caused by hyperbilirubinemia was common in neonates with Rh-isoimmunization until the institution of exchange transfusion for affected infants and postpartum high-titer Rho (D) immune globulin treatment for sensitized mothers. For several decades after the introduction of exchange transfusion and phototherapy aimed at keeping the neonate's TSB below 20 mg/dL, there were no reported cases of kernicterus in the United States. Since the early 1990s, however, there has been a reappearance of kernicterus, with more than 120 cases reported to a voluntary registry. Common factors in the recent cases are newborn discharge before 48 hours (all but one), breast feeding (100%), delayed measurement of TSB, unrecognized hemolysis, lack of early postdischarge follow-up, and failure to recognize the early symptoms of encephalopathy.

Bilirubin is produced by the breakdown of heme (iron protoporphyrin) in the reticuloendothelial system and bone marrow. Heme is cleaved by heme oxygenase to iron, which is conserved; carbon monoxide, which is exhaled; and biliverdin, which is converted to bilirubin by bilirubin reductase. Each gram of hemoglobin yields 34 mg of bilirubin (1 mg/dL = 17.2 mmol/L of bilirubin). This unconjugated bilirubin is bound to albumin and carried to the liver, where it is taken up by hepatocytes. In the presence of the uridyldiphosphoglucuronyl transferase (UDPGT; glucuronyl transferase), bilirubin is conjugated to one or two glucu-

Table 1–6. Guidelines for early outpatient follow-up evaluation.

History
Rhythmic sucking and audible swallowing for at least 10 min total per feeding?
Infant wakes and demands to feed every 2–3 h (at least 8–10 feedings per 24 h)?
Do breasts feel full before feedings, and softer after?
Are there at least 6 noticeably wet diapers per 24 h?
Are there yellow bowel movements (no longer meconium)—at least 4 per 24 h?
Is infant still acting hungry after nursing (frequently sucks hands, rooting)?
Physical assessment
Weight, unclothed: should not be more than 8–10% below birth weight
Extent and severity of jaundice
Assessment of hydration, alertness, general well-being
Cardiovascular examination: murmurs, brachial and femoral pulses, respirations

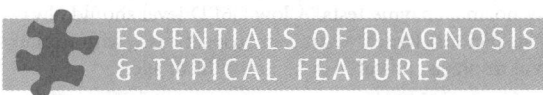

▲ Figure 1–2. Risk designation of full-term and near-term newborns based on their hour-specific bilirubin values. (Reproduced, with permission, from Bhutani VK et al: Predictive ability of a predischarge hour-specific serum bilirubin test for subsequent significant hyperbilirubinemia in healthy term and near-term newborns. Pediatrics 1999;103:6.)

ronide molecules. Conjugated bilirubin is then excreted through the bile to the intestine. In the presence of normal gut flora, conjugated bilirubin is metabolized to stercobilins and excreted in the stool. Absence of gut flora and slow gastrointestinal (GI) motility, both characteristic of the newborn, cause a build up of conjugated bilirubin in the intestinal lumen, where mucosal β-glucuronidase removes the glucuronide molecules and leaves unconjugated bilirubin to be reabsorbed (enterohepatic circulation).

Excess accumulation of bilirubin in blood depends on both the rate of bilirubin production and the rate of excretion. It is best determined by reference to an hour-specific TSB level above the 95th percentile for age in hours (Figure 1–2).

1. Physiologic Jaundice

ESSENTIALS OF DIAGNOSIS & TYPICAL FEATURES

▸ Visible jaundice appearing after 24 hours of age.
▸ Total bilirubin rises by < 5 mg/dL (86 mmol/L) per day.

▸ Peak bilirubin occurs at 3–5 days of age, with a total bilirubin of no more than 15 mg/dL (258 mmol/L).
▸ Visible jaundice resolves by 1 week in the full-term infant and by 2 weeks in the preterm infant.

Factors contributing to physiologic jaundice in neonates include low UDPGT activity, relatively high red cell mass, absence of intestinal flora, slow intestinal motility and increased enterohepatic circulation of bilirubin. Hyperbilirubinemia outside of the ranges noted in Figure 1–2 is not physiologic and requires further evaluation.

2. Pathologic Unconjugated Hyperbilirubinemia

Pathologic unconjugated hyperbilirubinemia can be grouped into two main categories: overproduction of bilirubin or decreased conjugation of bilirubin (Table 1–7). The TSB is a reflection of the balance between these processes. Visible jaundice with a TSB greater than 5 mg/dL before 24 hours of age is most commonly a result of significant hemolysis.

Table 1–7. Causes of pathologic unconjugated hyperbilirubinemia.

Overproduction of bilirubin
1. Hemolytic causes of increased bilirubin production (reticulocyte count elevated)
   a. Immune-mediated: positive direct antibody (DAT, Coombs) test
      • ABO blood group incompatibility, Rh incompatibility, minor blood group incompatibility
   b. Nonimmune: negative direct antibody (DAT, Coombs) test
      • Abnormal red cell shapes: spherocytosis, elliptocytosis, pyknocytosis, stomatocytosis
      • Red cell enzyme abnormalities: glucose-6-phosphate dehydrogenase deficiency, pyruvate kinase deficiency, hexokinase deficiency, other metabolic defects
   c. Patients with bacterial or viral sepsis
2. Nonhemolytic causes of increased bilirubin production (reticulocyte count normal)
   a. Extravascular hemorrhage: cephalohematoma, extensive bruising, intracranial hemorrhage
   b. Polycythemia
   c. Exaggerated enterohepatic circulation of bilirubin: bowel obstruction, functional ileus
   d. Breast milk-associated jaundice ("lack of breast milk jaundice")
Decreased rate of conjugation
1. Crigler-Najjar syndrome
   a. Type I glucuronyl transferase deficiency, autosomal-recessive
   b. Type II glucuronyl transferase deficiency, autosomal-dominant
2. Gilbert syndrome
3. ?Hypothyroidism

A. Increased Bilirubin Production

Increased bilirubin production may be caused by pathologic destruction of neonatal red blood cells. Destruction may be mediated by maternal antibodies (Coombs test–positive), abnormal red cell membranes (spherocytosis), or abnormal red cell enzymes (glucose-6-phosphate dehydrogenase [G6PD] deficiency) causing decreased red cell life span. Antibodies can be directed against the major blood group antigens (type A or type B infant of a type O mother) or the minor antigens of the Rh system (D, E, C, d, e, c, Kell, Duffy, and others).

1. Antibody-mediated hemolysis (Coombs test–positive)

A. ABO BLOOD GROUP INCOMPATIBILITY—This finding can accompany any pregnancy in a type O mother. Hemolysis is usually mild, but the severity is unpredictable because of variability in the amount of naturally occurring maternal anti-A or anti-B IgG antibodies. Although 20% of pregnancies are "set-ups" for ABO incompatibility (mother O, infant A or B), only 33% of infants in such cases have a positive direct Coombs test and only 20% of these develop jaundice that requires therapy. Persistent maternal antibodies may cause the newborn to gradually become anemic over the first few weeks of life, even to the point of requiring transfusion.

B. RH ISOIMMUNIZATION—This finding is less common than ABO incompatibility. It increases in severity with each immunized pregnancy because of increased maternal IgG antibody production. Most Rh disease can be prevented by giving high-titer Rho (D) immune globulin to the Rh-negative woman after invasive procedures during pregnancy or after miscarriage, abortion, or delivery of an Rh-positive infant. Neonates are often anemic at birth, and hemolysis rapidly causes hyperbilirubinemia and more severe anemia. The most severe form of Rh isoimmunization, erythroblastosis fetalis, is characterized by life-threatening anemia, generalized edema, and fetal or neonatal heart failure. Without antenatal intervention, fetal or neonatal death may result. The cornerstone of antenatal management is transfusion of the fetus with Rh-negative cells, either directly into the umbilical vein or into the fetal abdominal cavity. Phototherapy is usually started in these infants upon delivery, with exchange transfusion given if needed. Intravenous immune globulin (IVIG; 0.5–1 g/kg) given to the infant as soon as the diagnosis is made decreases the need for exchange transfusion. Ongoing hemolysis occurs until all maternal antibody is gone; therefore, these infants require monitoring for 2–3 months for anemia severe enough to require transfusion.

2. Nonimmune hemolysis (Coombs test–negative)

A. HEREDITARY SPHEROCYTOSIS—This condition is the most common of the red cell membrane defects and causes hemolysis by decreasing red cell deformability. Affected infants may have hyperbilirubinemia severe enough to require exchange transfusion. Splenomegaly may be present. Diagnosis is suspected by peripheral blood smear and family history. Because spherocytes are seen in any hemolytic process, confirmation of diagnosis by osmotic fragility testing is required after 2–3 months of age.

B. G6PD DEFICIENCY—This condition is the most common **red cell enzyme defect** causing hemolysis, especially in infants of African, Mediterranean, or Asian descent. Onset of jaundice is at about 7 days of age, which is later than in physiologic jaundice and isoimmune hemolytic disease. The role of G6PD deficiency in neonatal jaundice is probably underestimated as up to 10–13% of African Americans are G6PD-deficient. Although the disorder is X-linked, even female heterozygotes are at increased risk of hyperbilirubinemia. In most cases, no triggering agent for hemolysis is found. Some infants who develop severe jaundice with G6PD deficiency have been found to have concomitant Gilbert syndrome. Their bilirubin production is exaggerated by a decreased rate of bilirubin conjugation. G6PD enzyme activity is high in reticulocytes. Thus, neonates with a large number of reticulocytes may have falsely normal enzyme tests. A low G6PD level should always raise suspicions. Repeat testing in suspect cases with initially normal results is indicated at 2–3 months of age.

3. Nonhemolytic increased bilirubin production—
Enclosed hemorrhage, such as cephalohematoma, intracranial hemorrhage, or extensive bruising in the skin, can lead

to jaundice. **Polycythemia** leads to jaundice by increased red cell mass, with increased numbers of cells reaching senescence daily. **Ileus,** either paralytic or mechanical, related to bowel obstruction, leads to increased enterohepatic circulation.

B. Decreased Rate of Conjugation

1. UDPGT deficiency: Crigler-Najjar syndrome type I (complete deficiency, autosomal recessive) and type II (partial deficiency, autosomal dominant)—These two conditions result from mutations in the exon or encoding region of the UDPGT gene that cause complete or nearly complete absence of enzyme activity. Both are rare but can cause severe unconjugated hyperbilirubinemia, bilirubin encephalopathy, and death if untreated. In type II, the enzyme can be induced with phenobarbital, which may lower bilirubin levels by 30–80%. Liver transplantation is curative (see Chapter 21).

2. Gilbert syndrome—This is a mild autosomal dominant disorder characterized by decreased hepatic UDPGT activity caused by genetic polymorphism at the promoter region of the UDPGT gene. Approximately 9% of the population is homozygous, and 42% is heterozygous, with a gene frequency of 0.3. Affected individuals tend to develop hyperbilirubinemia in the presence of conditions that increase bilirubin load. They are also more likely to have prolonged neonatal jaundice and breast milk jaundice.

C. Hyperbilirubinemia Caused by Unknown or Multiple Factors

1. Racial differences—Asians (23%) are more likely than whites (10–13%) or African Americans (4%) to have a peak neonatal TSB greater than 12 mg/dL (206 mmol/L). Some of these differences result from racial variations in prevalence of UDPGT gene polymorphisms or associated G6PD deficiency.

2. Prematurity—Premature infants often have poor enteral intake, delayed stooling, and increased enterohepatic circulation. Red cell life span is shorter in premature infants. Infants at 35–36 weeks' gestation are 13 times more likely than term infants to be readmitted for hyperbilirubinemia. Even near-term infants (37 weeks' gestation) are four times more likely than term neonates to have TSB greater than 13 mg/dL (224 mmol/L).

3. Breast feeding and jaundice

A. Breast milk jaundice—Unconjugated hyperbilirubinemia lasting until 2–3 months of age is common in breast-fed infants. An increased prevalence of the Gilbert syndrome promoter genotype is likely involved. Moderate unconjugated hyperbilirubinemia for 6–12 weeks in a thriving breast-fed infant without evidence of hemolysis, hypothyroidism, or other disease strongly suggests this diagnosis.

Table 1–8. Signs of inadequate breast milk intake.

Weight loss of > 8-10% from birth
Fewer than six noticeably wet diapers per 24 h by day 3-4
Fewer than four stools per day, or still meconium, by day 3-4
Nursing fewer than eight times per 24 h, or for less than 10 min each feeding

B. Breast feeding–associated jaundice—This common entity is also called "lack-of-breast-milk jaundice." Breast-fed infants have a higher incidence (9%) of unconjugated serum bilirubin levels greater than 13 mg/dL (224 mmol/L) than do formula-fed infants (2%) and are more likely to have bilirubin greater than 15 mg/dL (258 mmol/L) than formula-fed infants (2% versus 0.3%). The pathogenesis is probably poor enteral intake and increased enterohepatic circulation. There is no apparent increase in bilirubin production as measured by carbon monoxide exhalation. Although rarely severe enough to cause bilirubin encephalopathy, nearly 100% of the infants with kernicterus reported to the registry were breast fed, and in 50%, breast feeding was the only known risk factor. Excessive jaundice should be considered a possible sign of failure to establish adequate milk supply and should prompt specific inquiries (Table 1–8). If intake is inadequate, the infant should receive supplemental formula and the mother should be instructed to nurse more frequently and to use an electric breast pump every 2 hours to enhance milk production. Consultation with a lactation specialist should be considered. Because hospital discharge of normal newborns occurs before the milk supply is established and before jaundice peaks, a follow-up visit 2 days after discharge is recommended by the AAP to evaluate adequacy of intake and jaundice.

3. Bilirubin Toxicity

Unconjugated bilirubin anion is the agent of bilirubin neurotoxicity. The anion binds to the phospholipids (gangliosides) of neuronal plasma membranes causing injury, which then allows more anion to enter the neuron. Intracellular bilirubin anion binds to the membrane phospholipids of subcellular organelles, causing impaired energy metabolism, altered excitatory amino acid homeostasis, excitotoxic neuronal injury, and cell death. The blood-brain barrier undoubtedly has a role in protecting the infant from brain damage, but its integrity is impossible to measure clinically. The amount of albumin available to bind the unconjugated bilirubin anion and the presence of other anions that may displace bilirubin from albumin binding sites are also important. It is unknown whether there is a fixed level of bilirubin above which brain damage always occurs. The term *kernicterus* describes the pathologic finding of staining of basal ganglia and brainstem nuclei, as well as the chronic brain injury. The term *acute bilirubin encephalopathy* describes the signs and symptoms of brain damage in the newborn.

Table 1–9. BIND scoring system.

	1 Point (Nonspecific, Subtle)	2 Points (Progressive Toxicity)	3 Points (Advanced Toxicity)
Mental status	Sleepy, poor feeding	Lethargy + irritability	Semi-coma, seizures, apnea
Muscle tone	Slight decrease	Hypertonia or hypotonia, depending on arousal state or Mild arching	Markedly increased (opisthotonus) or decreased or Bicycling
Cry	High-pitched	Shrill	Inconsolable

BIND, bilirubin-induced neurologic dysfunction.
Adapted, with permission, from Bhutani VK, Johnson LH, Keren R: Treating acute bilirubin encephalopathy—before it's too late. Contemp Pediatr 2005;22:57.

The risk of bilirubin encephalopathy is small in healthy, term neonates even at bilirubin levels of 25–30 mg/dL (430–516 mmol/L). Risk depends on the duration of hyperbilirubinemia, the concentration of serum albumin, associated illness, acidosis, and the concentrations of competing anions such as sulfisoxazole and ceftriaxone. Premature infants are at greater risk than term infants because of the greater frequency of associated illness affecting the integrity of the blood-brain barrier, reduced albumin levels, and decreased affinity of albumin binding sites. For these reasons, the "exchange level" in premature infants may be lower than that of a term infant.

Correlation between TSB and level of neurotoxicity is poor. Although 65% of cases reported to the registry had TSB levels above 35 mg/dL, 15% had levels below 30 mg/dL, and 8% were below 25 mg/dL. Measurement of free, unbound, unconjugated bilirubin (B_f) may be a more meaningful predictor of risk for brain injury, although this test is not widely available. Currently the best means of assessing neurotoxicity may be the auditory brainstem evoked response, which shows predictable, early effects of bilirubin toxicity.

4. Acute Bilirubin Encephalopathy

ESSENTIALS OF DIAGNOSIS & TYPICAL FEATURES

▶ Lethargy, poor feeding.

▶ Irritability, high-pitched cry.

▶ Arching of the neck (retrocollis) and trunk (opisthotonos).

▶ Apnea, seizures, coma (late).

Newborns infants may be described as "sleepy and not interested in feeding." Although these symptoms are nonspecific, they are also the earliest signs of acute bilirubin encephalopathy and should trigger detailed evaluation of the jaundiced infant's birth and postnatal history, feeding and elimination history, and perhaps an urgent assessment for signs of bilirubin-induced neurologic dysfunction (BIND). A scoring system has been proposed (Table 1–9) to monitor the severity and progression of bilirubin encephalopathy. A score of 4–6 indicates progressive encephalopathy likely to be reversible with aggressive treatment, whereas a score of 7–9 represents advanced and possibly irreversible damage.

5. Chronic Bilirubin Encephalopathy (Kernicterus)

ESSENTIALS OF DIAGNOSIS & TYPICAL FEATURES

▶ Extrapyramidal movement disorder (choreoathetoid cerebral palsy).

▶ Gaze abnormality, especially limitation of upward gaze.

▶ Auditory disturbances (deafness, failed auditory brainstem evoked response with normal evoked otoacoustic emissions, auditory neuropathy, auditory dyssynchrony).

▶ Dysplasia of the enamel of the deciduous teeth.

Kernicterus is an irreversible brain injury characterized by choreoathetoid cerebral palsy and hearing impairment. Intelligence is probably normal but may be difficult to assess because of associated hearing, communication, and coordination problems. The diagnosis is clinical but is strengthened if audiologic testing shows auditory neuropathy and auditory dyssynchrony in which the otoacoustic emission test is normal but the auditory brainstem response is absent. Infants with such findings are usually deaf. Infants with milder kernicterus may have normal audiograms but abnormal auditory processing and subsequent problems with speech comprehension. Magnetic resonance imaging (MRI) scanning of the brain is nearly diagnostic if it shows abnormalities isolated to the globus pallidus or the subthalamic nuclei, or both.

Evaluation of Hyperbilirubinemia

Because most newborns are discharged at 24–48 hours of age, before physiologic jaundice peaks and before maternal milk supply is established, a predischarge TSB or a transcutaneous bilirubin measurement (TcB) may help predict which infants are at risk for severe hyperbilirubinemia. In all infants, an assessment of risk for severe hyperbilirubinemia should be performed before discharge (Table 1–10). As recommended by the AAP, follow-up within 24–48 hours for all infants discharged before 72 hours of age (depending on the number of risk factors present) is imperative. Although jaundice is usually visible above a TSB level of 5 mg/dL (86 mmol/L), visual estimation of the bilirubin level is inaccurate. TSB should be measured and interpreted based on the age of the infant in hours at the time of sampling. Infants with a TSB level greater than the 95th percentile for age in hours have a 40% risk of developing significant hyperbilirubinemia (see Figure 1–2). Serial bilirubin levels should be obtained from a single laboratory whenever possible to make interpretation of serial measurements more meaningful.

Infants with visible jaundice on the first day of life or who develop excessive jaundice require further evaluation. The minimal evaluation consists of:

- Feeding and elimination history.
- Birth weight and daily weight change since birth.
- Examination for sources of excessive heme breakdown.
- Assessment of blood type, Coombs testing, complete blood count (CBC) with smear, serum albumin, and TSB.
- G6PD test if jaundice presents later than usual, and in African-American infants with severe jaundice.
- Fractionated bilirubin level in infants who appear ill, those with prolonged jaundice, acholic stool, or dark urine

Treatment of Indirect Hyperbilirubinemia

A. Protoporphyrins

Tin and zinc protoporphyrin or mesoporphyrin (Sn-PP, Zn-PP; Sn-MP, Zn-MP) are inhibitors of heme oxygenase, the enzyme that initiates the catabolism of heme (iron protoporphyrin). Studies are underway involving a single injection of these substances shortly after birth to prevent the formation of bilirubin. Although results are promising, these drugs are not yet approved for use in the United States.

B. Phototherapy

Phototherapy is the most common treatment for indirect hyperbilirubinemia. It is relatively noninvasive and safe. Light of wavelength 425–475 nm (blue-green spectrum) is absorbed by unconjugated bilirubin in the skin and converted to a water-soluble stereoisomer that can be excreted in bile without conjugation. The minimum effective light dose is

Table 1–10. Factors affecting the risk of severe hyperbilirubinemia in infants 35 or more weeks' gestation (in approximate order of importance).

Major risk factors
Predischarge TSB or TcB level in the high-risk zone (> 95th percentile; see Figure 1-2)
Jaundice observed in the first 24 h
Blood group incompatibility with positive direct Coombs test, other known hemolytic disease (eg, G6PD deficiency), or elevated ETCO
Gestational age 35-36 weeks
Previous sibling required phototherapy
Cephalohematoma or significant bruising
Exclusive breast feeding, particularly if weight loss is excessive
East Asian race[a]

Minor risk factors
Predischarge TSB or TcB level in the high-intermediate risk zone (75-95th percentile)
Gestational age 37-38 weeks
Jaundice observed before discharge
Previous sibling with jaundice
Macrosomic infant of a diabetic mother

Decreased risk (these factors are associated with decreased risk of significant jaundice, listed in order of decreasing importance)
TSB or TcB level in the low-risk zone (see Figure 1-2)
Gestational age ≥ 41 weeks
Exclusive bottle feeding
Black race[a]
Discharge from hospital after 72 h

[a]Race as defined by mother's description.
ETCO, end-tidal carbon monoxide; G6PD, glucose-6-phosphate dehydrogenase; TcB, transcutaneous bilirubin; TSB, total serum bilirubin.

10–14 μW/cm^2 irradiance. Intensive phototherapy employs irradiance of 30 μW/cm^2 or higher. Irradiance can be increased by increasing the exposed body surface area or by moving the light source closer to the infant. Special blue fluorescent tubes labeled F20 T12/BB or TL52/20W are most commonly used. Fiberoptic blankets are useful as adjuncts but are not adequate as sole therapy for term infants because they do not cover sufficient surface area. Intensive phototherapy should decrease TSB by 30–40% in the first 24 hours, most significantly in the first 4–6 hours. The infant's eyes should be shielded to prevent retinal damage. Diarrhea, which sometimes occurs during phototherapy, can be treated if necessary by feeding a non–lactose-containing formula.

Phototherapy is started electively when the TSB is approximately 5 mg/dL (86 mmol/L) lower than the exchange level for that infant (eg, at 15–18 mg/dL [258–310 mmol/L] for a full-term infant). AAP guidelines for phototherapy and exchange transfusion in infants of 35 or more weeks' gestation are shown in Figures 1–3 and 1–4. Hyperbilirubinemic infants should be fed by mouth if possible to decrease enterohepatic bilirubin circulation. Casein hydrolysate formula to supplement breast milk decreases enterohepatic circulation by inhibiting mucosal β-glucuronidase

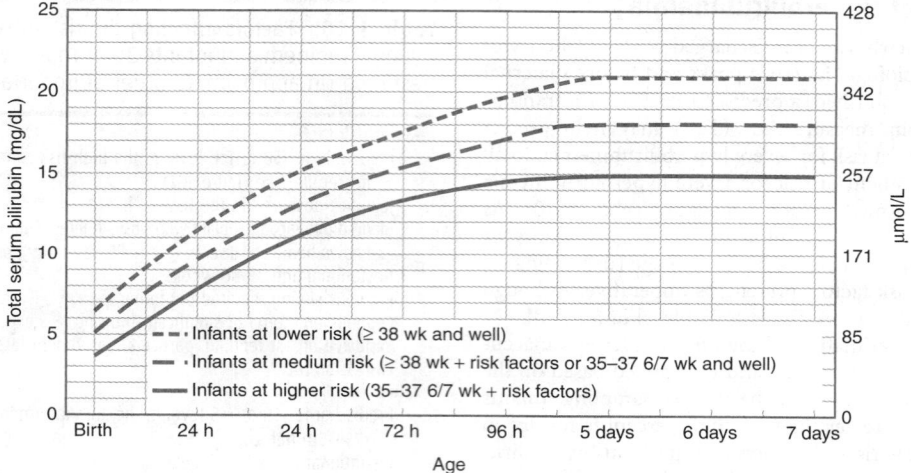

- Use total bilirubin, Do not subtract direct reacting of conjugated bilirubin.
- Risk factors = isoimmune hemolytic disease, G6PD deficiency, asphyxia, significant lethargy, temperature instability, sepsis, acidosis, or albumin < 3.0 g/dL (if measured).
- For well infants 35–37 6/7 wk can adjust TSB levels for intervention around the medium risk line. It is an option to intervene at lower TSB levels for infants closer to 35 wks and at higher TSB levels for those closer to 37 6/7 wk.
- It is an option to provide conventional phototherapy in hospital or at home at TSB levels 2–3 mg/dL (35–50 mmol/L) below those shown but home phototherapy should not be used in any infant with risk factors.

▲ **Figure 1–3.** Guidelines for phototherapy in hospitalized infants of 35 or more weeks' gestation. These guidelines are based on limited evidence and levels shown are approximations. The guidelines refer to the use of intensive phototherapy (at least 30 µW/cm^2 in the blue-green spectrum), which should be used when the total serum bilirubin (TSB) exceeds the line indicated for each category. If TSB approaches the exchange level, the sides of the incubator or bassinet should be lined with aluminum foil or white material. (Reproduced, with permission, from the AAP Subcommittee on Hyperbilirubinemia: Management of hyperbilirubinemia in the newborn infant 35 or more weeks of gestation. Pediatrics 2004;114:297.)

activity. IVIG (0.5–1.0 g/kg) in severe antibody-mediated hemolysis interrupts the hemolytic process. Although phototherapy has been shown to decrease the need for exchange transfusion, its long-term benefits, if any, in infants with less severe jaundice are unknown.

C. Exchange Transfusion

Although most infants with indirect hyperbilirubinemia can be treated with phototherapy, extreme indirect hyperbilirubinemia is a medical emergency. Infants should be admitted at once to a neonatal intensive care unit where exchange transfusion can be performed before irreversible neurologic damage occurs. Intensive phototherapy should be instituted immediately, during transport to the hospital if possible.

Double-volume exchange transfusion (approximately 160–200 mL/kg body weight) is most often used in infants with extreme hyperbilirubinemia secondary to Rh isoimmunization, ABO incompatibility, or hereditary spherocytosis. The procedure decreases serum bilirubin acutely by approximately 50% and removes about 80% of sensitized or abnormal red blood cells and offending antibody so that ongoing hemolysis is decreased. Exchange transfusion is also indicated in any infant with TSB above 30 mg/dL, in infants with signs of encephalopathy, or when intensive phototherapy has not lowered TSB by at least 0.5 mg/dL/h after 4 hours. The decision to perform exchange transfusion should be based on TSB, not on the indirect fraction of bilirubin.

As TSB nears the potentially toxic range, serum albumin should be determined. Albumin (1 g/kg) will aid in binding and removal of bilirubin during exchange transfusion. Table 1–11 illustrates the bilirubin/albumin ratios at which exchange transfusion should be considered.

Exchange transfusion is invasive, risky, and infrequently performed. It should therefore be performed at a referral center. Mortality is 1–5% and is greatest in the smallest, most immature, and unstable infants. Sudden death during the procedure can occur in any infant. There is a 5–10% risk of serious complications such as necrotizing enterocolitis (NEC), infection, electrolyte disturbances, or thrombocytopenia. Isovolemic exchange (withdrawal through an arterial

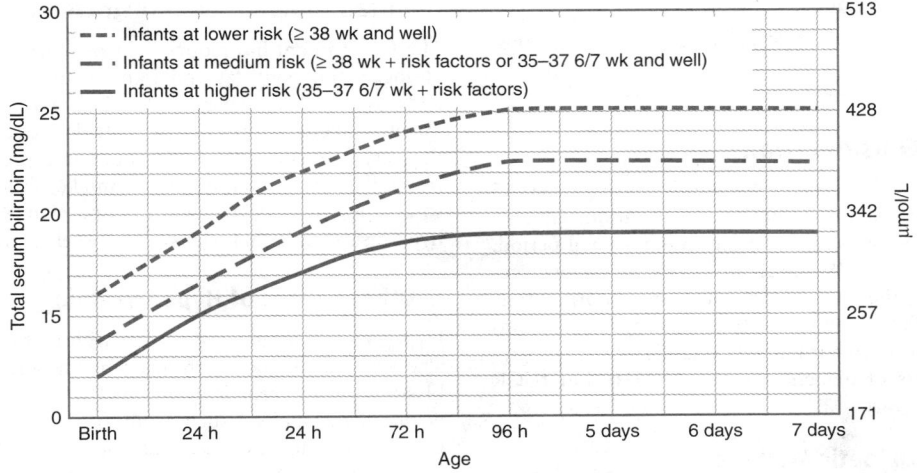

- The dashed lines for the first 24 hours indicate uncertainty due a wide range of clinical circumstances and a range of responses to phototherapy.
- Immediate exchange transfusion is recommended if infant shows signs of acute bilirubin encephalopathy (hypertonia, arching, retrocolitis, opisthotonos, fever, high pitched cry) or if TSB is ≥ 5 mg/dL (85 μmol/L) above these lines.
- Risk factors—isoimmune hemolytic disease, G6PD deficiency, asphyxia, significant lethargy, temperature instability, sepsis, acidosis.
- Measure serum albumin and calculate B/A ratio (see legend).
- Use total bilirubin. Do not subtract direct reading or conjugated bilirubin.
- If infant is well and 35–37 6/7 wk (median risk) can individualize TSB levels for exchange based on actual gestational age.

▲ **Figure 1-4.** Guidelines for exchange transfusion in infants of 35 or more weeks' gestation. These guidelines represent approximations for which an exchange transfusion is indicated in infants treated with intensive phototherapy. For readmitted infants, if the total serum bilirubin (TSB) level is above the exchange level, repeat TSB measurement every 2–3 hours and consider exchange if the TSB remains above the level after 6 hours of intensive phototherapy. The total serum bilirubin/albumin ratio (TSB [mg/dL]/Alb [g/dL]; 8.0 for infants at lower risk, 7.2 for medium risk, and 6.8 for higher risk) can be used together with, but not in lieu of the TSB level as an additional factor in determining the need for transfusion. If the TSB is at or approaching exchange level, send blood for an immediate type and crossmatch. (Reproduced, with permission, from the AAP Subcommittee on Hyperbilirubinemia: Management of hyperbilirubinemia in the newborn infant 35 or more weeks of gestation. Pediatrics 2004;114:297.)

line with infusion through a venous line) may decrease the risk of some complications.

American Academy of Pediatrics Subcommittee on Hyperbilirubinemia: Clinical practice guideline: Management of hyperbilirubinemia in the newborn infant 35 or more weeks of gestation. Pediatrics 2004;114:297 [PMID: 15231951].

De Almeida MF, Draque CM: Neonatal jaundice and breastfeeding. NeoReviews 2007;8:e282.

Keren R, Bhutani VK: Predischarge risk assessment for severe neonatal hyperbilirubinemia. NeoReviews 2007;8:e68.

Maisels MJ: Neonatal jaundice. Pediatr Rev 2006;27:443 [PMID: 17142466].

Shapiro SM et al: Hyperbilirubinemia and kernicterus. Clin Perinatol 2006;33:387 [PMID: 16765731].

Watchko JF: Hyperbilirubinemia and bilirubin toxicity in the late preterm infant. Clin Perinatol 2006;33:839 [PMID: 17148008].

Wennberg RP et al: Toward understanding kernicterus: A challenge to improve the management of jaundiced newborns. Pediatrics 2006;117:474 [PMID: 16452368].

HYPOGLYCEMIA

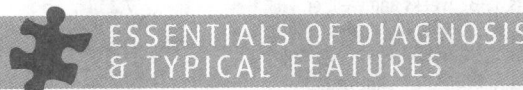

ESSENTIALS OF DIAGNOSIS & TYPICAL FEATURES

► Defined as blood glucose < 45 mg/dL.

► LGA, SGA, preterm, and stressed infants at risk.

▶ May be asymptomatic.

▶ Infants can present with lethargy, poor feeding, irritability, or seizures.

▶ General Considerations

Blood glucose concentration in the fetus is approximately 15 mg/dL less than maternal glucose concentration. Glucose concentration decreases in the immediate postnatal period. Concentrations below 45 mg/dL are considered hypoglycemic. By 3 hours, the glucose concentration in normal full-term infants stabilizes between 50 and 80 mg/dL. The two groups of full-term newborn infants at high risk for hypoglycemia are infants of diabetic mothers (IDMs) and IUGR infants.

A. Infants of Diabetic Mothers

The IDM has abundant glucose stores in the form of glycogen and fat but develops hypoglycemia because of hyperinsulinemia induced by maternal and fetal hyperglycemia. Increased energy supply to the fetus from the maternal circulation results in a macrosomic infant. The large infant is at increased risk for trauma during delivery. Some infants have cardiomyopathy (asymmetrical septal hypertrophy) which may present with murmur, respiratory distress or cardiac failure. Microcolon is occasionally present in IDMs and causes symptoms of low intestinal obstruction similar to Hirschsprung disease. Other neonatal problems include hypercoagulability and polycythemia, a combination that predisposes the infant to large vein thromboses (especially the renal vein). IDMs are often somewhat immature for their gestational age and are at increased risk for hyaline membrane disease, hypocalcemia, and hyperbilirubinemia. Infants of mothers who were diabetic at conception have a higher incidence of congenital anomalies, probably related to first-trimester glucose control.

Table 1–11. Additional guidelines for exchange transfusion: effects of albumin.

Risk Category	Bilirubin/Albumin Ratio at Which to Consider Exchange Transfusion (TSB [mg/dL]:Albumin [g/dL])
Infants > 38 weeks and well	8.0
Infants 35–38 weeks and well, or > 38 weeks with higher risk (hemolysis, G6PD, sepsis, acidosis)	7.2
Infants 35–38 weeks with higher risk, as above	6.8

G6PD, glucose-6-phosphate dehydrogenase; TSB, total serum bilirubin.

B. Intrauterine Growth-Restricted Infants

The IUGR infant has reduced glucose stores in the form of glycogen and body fat and is prone to hypoglycemia. In addition, marked hyperglycemia and a transient diabetes mellitus–like syndrome occasionally develop, particularly in the very premature IUGR infant. These problems usually respond to adjustment in glucose intake, although insulin is sometimes needed transiently. Some IUGR infants have hyperinsulinemia that persists for a week or more.

C. Other Causes of Hypoglycemia

Hypoglycemia occurs in disorders with islet cell hyperplasia. These include the Beckwith-Wiedemann syndrome, erythroblastosis fetalis, genetic forms of hyperinsulinism, inborn errors of metabolism such as glycogen storage disease and galactosemia, and endocrine disorders such as panhypopituitarism and counterregulatory hormone deficiency. Hypoglycemia also occurs, probably secondary to stress, in infants with birth asphyxia, hypoxia, and bacterial and viral sepsis. Premature infants are at risk for hypoglycemia because of decreased glycogen stores.

▶ Clinical Findings

The signs of hypoglycemia in the newborn infant may be nonspecific and subtle: lethargy, poor feeding, irritability, tremors, jitteriness, apnea, and seizures. Hypoglycemia due to increased insulin is the most severe and most resistant to treatment. Cardiac failure may occur in severe cases, particularly in IDMs with cardiomyopathy. Hypoglycemia in hyperinsulinemic states can develop within the first 30–60 minutes of life.

Blood glucose can be measured by heelstick using a bedside glucometer. All infants at risk should be screened, including IDMs, IUGR infants, premature infants, and any infant with suggestive symptoms. All low or borderline values should be confirmed by laboratory measurement of blood glucose concentration. It is important to continue surveillance of glucose concentration until the baby has been on full enteral feedings without intravenous supplementation for 24 hours. Relapse of hypoglycemia thereafter is unlikely.

Infants with hypoglycemia requiring IV glucose infusions for more than 5 days should be evaluated for less common disorders, including inborn errors of metabolism, hyperinsulinemic states, and deficiencies of counterregulatory hormones.

▶ Treatment

Therapy is based on the provision of enteral or parenteral glucose. Treatment guidelines are shown in Table 1–12. In hyperinsulinemic states, glucose boluses should be avoided and a higher glucose infusion rate used. After initial correction with a bolus of 10% dextrose in water ($D_{10}W$; 2 mL/kg),

Table 1–12. Hypoglycemia: suggested therapeutic regimens.

Screening Test[a]	Presence of Symptoms	Action
20–45 mg/dL	No symptoms of hypoglycemia	Draw blood glucose[b]; if the infant is alert and vigorous, feed; follow with frequent glucose monitoring.
		If the infant continues to have blood glucose < 40–45 mg/dL or is unable to feed, provide intravenous glucose at 6 mg/kg/min (D_{10}W at 3.6 mL/kg/h).
< 45 mg/dL	Symptoms of hypoglycemia present	Draw blood glucose[b]; provide bolus of D_{10}W (2 mL/kg) followed by an infusion of 6 mg/kg/min (3.6 mL/kg/h).
< 20 mg/dL	With or without symptoms of hypoglycemia	Draw blood glucose[b]; provide bolus of D_{10}W followed by an infusion of 6 mg/kg/min.
		If IV access cannot be obtained immediately, an umbilical vein line should be used.

[a]Rapid bedside determination.
[b]Laboratory confirmation.

glucose infusion should be increased gradually as needed from a starting rate of 6 mg/kg/ min. IDMs and IUGR infants with polycythemia are at greatest risk for symptomatic hypoglycemia. In such infants, hypoglycemia and polycythemia should be treated with IV glucose and partial exchange transfusion, respectively.

► Prognosis

The prognosis of hypoglycemia is good if therapy is prompt. CNS sequelae are more common in infants with hypoglycemic seizures and in neonates with persistent hyperinsulinemic hypoglycemia. Hypoglycemia may also potentiate brain injury after perinatal depression and should be avoided.

Boluyt N et al: Neurodevelopment after neonatal hypoglycemia: A systematic review and design of an optimal future study. Pediatrics 2006;117:2231 [PMID: 16740869].
Dekelbab BH, Sperling MA: Hypoglycemia in newborns and infants. Adv Pediatr 2006;53:5 [PMID: 17089861].
Fournier SH, Stanley CA: Genetic and nongenetic forms of hyperinsulinism in neonates. NeoReviews 2004;5:e370.
Garg M, Devaskar SU: Glucose metabolism in the late preterm infant. Clin Perinatol 2006;33:853 [PMID: 17148009].

Hussain K, Aynsley-Green A: The effect of prematurity and intrauterine growth restriction on glucose metabolism in the newborn. NeoReviews 2004;5:e365.
Kahler SG: Metabolic disorders associated with neonatal hypoglycemia. NeoReviews 2004;5:e377.
Nold JL, Georgieff MK: Infants of diabetic mothers. Pediatr Clin North Am 2004;51:619 [PMID: 15157588].
Rozance PJ, Hay W: Hypoglycemia in newborn infants: Features associated with adverse outcomes. Biol Neonate 2006;90:74 [PMID: 16534190].

RESPIRATORY DISTRESS IN THE TERM NEWBORN INFANT

ESSENTIALS OF DIAGNOSIS & TYPICAL FEATURES

► Tachypnea, respiratory rate > 60 breaths/min.
► Intercostal and sternal retractions.
► Expiratory grunting.
► Cyanosis in room air.

► General Considerations

Respiratory distress is one of the most common symptom complexes of the newborn. It may result from cardiopulmonary and noncardiopulmonary causes (Table 1–13). Chest radiography, arterial blood gases, and pulse oximetry are useful in assessing the cause and severity of the distress. It is important to consider the noncardiopulmonary causes (see Table 1–13), because the natural tendency is to focus on the heart and lungs. Most of the noncardiopulmonary causes can be ruled out by the history, physical examination, and a few simple laboratory tests. The most common pulmonary causes of respiratory distress in the full-term infant are transient tachypnea, aspiration syndromes, congenital pneumonia, and air leaks.

A. Transient Tachypnea (Retained Fetal Lung Fluid)

Respiratory distress is typically present at birth, usually associated with a mild to moderate oxygen requirement (25–50% O_2). The infant is usually full term or near term, nonasphyxiated, and born following a short labor or cesarean section without labor. The chest radiograph shows perihilar streaking and fluid in interlobar fissures. Resolution usually occurs within 12–24 hours.

B. Aspiration Syndromes

The infant is typically full-term or near-term with fetal distress prior to delivery or depression at delivery. Blood or meconium is often present in the amniotic fluid. Respiratory distress is present from birth, often manifested by a barrel chest appear-

Table 1–13. Causes of respiratory distress in the newborn.

Noncardiopulmonary
  Hypothermia or hyperthermia
  Hypoglycemia
  Polycythemia
  Metabolic acidosis
  Drug intoxications or withdrawal
  Insult to the central nervous system
    Asphyxia
    Hemorrhage
  Neuromuscular disease
  Phrenic nerve injury
  Skeletal dysplasia
Cardiovascular
  Left-sided outflow tract obstruction
    Hypoplastic left heart
    Aortic stenosis
    Coarctation of the aorta
  Cyanotic lesions
    Transposition of the great vessels
    Total anomalous pulmonary venous return
    Tricuspid atresia
    Right-sided outflow obstruction
Pulmonary
  Upper airway obstruction
    Choanal atresia
    Vocal cord paralysis
    Lingual thyroid
  Meconium aspiration
  Clear fluid aspiration
  Transient tachypnea
  Pneumonia
  Pulmonary hypoplasia
  Hyaline membrane disease
  Pneumothorax
  Pleural effusions
  Mass lesions
    Lobar emphysema
    Cystic adenomatoid malformation

Reproduced, with permission, from Rosenberg AA: Neonatal adaptation. In Gabbe SG et al (editors): *Obstetrics: Normal and Problem Pregnancies.* Churchill Livingstone, 1996.

ance and coarse breath sounds. Pneumonitis may cause an increasing O_2 need and may require intubation and ventilation. The chest radiograph shows coarse irregular infiltrates, hyperexpansion, and in the worst cases, lobar consolidation. In some cases, because of secondary surfactant deficiency, the radiograph shows a diffuse homogeneous infiltrate pattern.

When amniotic fluid contains meconium or blood, suctioning the infant's mouth and nose prior to delivery of the chest is not recommended as it may provoke aspiration. If the infant is not vigorous at birth, suctioning of the trachea under direct vision is recommended before commencing positive-pressure ventilation (PPV). Although tracheal suctioning is recommended, it does not prevent all cases of meconium or blood aspiration. Aspiration may have

occurred in utero as the stressed infant gasps. Infants who aspirate are at risk of pneumothorax because of uneven aeration with segmental overdistention and are at risk for persistent pulmonary hypertension (see section on Cardiac Problems in the Newborn Infant, later).

C. Congenital Pneumonia

Infants of any gestational age, with or without a history of prolonged rupture of membranes, chorioamnionitis, or maternal antibiotic administration, may be affected. Respiratory distress may begin at birth or may be delayed for several hours. The chest radiograph may resemble that of retained lung fluid or hyaline membrane disease. Rarely, there may be a lobar infiltrate.

The lungs are the most common site of infection in the neonate. Infections usually ascend from the genital tract before or during labor, with the vaginal or rectal flora the most likely agents (group B streptococci, *Escherichia coli,* and *Klebsiella*). Shock, poor perfusion, absolute neutropenia (< 2000/mL), and elevated C-reactive protein provide corroborating evidence for pneumonia. Gram stain of tracheal aspirate may be helpful. Because no signs or laboratory findings can confirm a diagnosis of pneumonia, all infants with respiratory distress should have a blood culture performed and should receive broad-spectrum antibiotic therapy (ampicillin, 100 mg/kg in two divided doses, and gentamicin, 4 mg/kg q24h or 2.5 mg/kg q12h) until the diagnosis of bacterial infection is ruled out.

D. Spontaneous Pneumothorax

Spontaneous pneumothorax occurs in 1% of all deliveries. Risk is increased by manipulations such as PPV in the delivery room. Respiratory distress (primarily tachypnea) is present from birth and typically is not severe. Breath sounds may be decreased on the affected side; heart tones may be shifted toward the opposite side and may be distant. The chest radiograph shows pneumothorax or pneumomediastinum.

Treatment usually consists of supplemental O_2 and watchful waiting. Breathing 100% O_2 for a few hours may accelerate reabsorption of extrapulmonary gas by creating a diffusion gradient for nitrogen across the surface of the lung (nitrogen washout technique). This is effective only if the infant was breathing room air or a small O_2 supplement at the time of the pneumothorax. Drainage by needle thoracentesis or tube thoracostomy is occasionally required. There is a slightly increased risk of renal abnormalities associated with spontaneous pneumothorax. Thus, careful physical examination of the kidneys and observation of urine output are indicated. If pulmonary hypoplasia with pneumothorax is suspected, renal ultrasound is also indicated.

E. Other Pulmonary Causes

Other pulmonary causes of respiratory distress are rare. Bilateral choanal atresia should be suspected if there is no air movement when the infant breathes through the nose. These infants have good color and heart rate while crying at delivery but become cyanotic and bradycardiac when they resume normal nasal breathing. Other causes of upper airway obstruction usually produce some degree of stridor or poor air movement despite good respiratory effort. Pleural effusion is likely in hydropic infants. Space-occupying lesions cause a shift of the mediastinum with asymmetrical breath sounds and are apparent on chest radiographs.

▶ **Treatment**

Whatever the cause, neonatal respiratory distress is treated with supplemental oxygen sufficient to maintain a PaO_2 of 60–70 mm Hg and an oxygen saturation by pulse oximetry (SpO_2) of 92–96%. PaO_2 less than 50 mm Hg is associated with pulmonary vasoconstriction, which can exacerbate hypoxemia. PaO_2 greater than 100 mm Hg may increase the risk of oxygen toxicity without additional benefit. Oxygen should be warmed, humidified, and delivered through an air blender. Concentration should be measured with a calibrated oxygen analyzer. An umbilical or peripheral arterial line should be inserted in infants requiring more than 45% FIO_2 by 4–6 hours of life to allow frequent blood gas determinations. Noninvasive monitoring with pulse oximetry should be used.

Other supportive treatment includes provision of IV glucose and water. Unless infection can be ruled out, blood cultures should be obtained and broad-spectrum antibiotics started. Volume expansion (normal saline) can be given in infusions of 10 mL/kg over 30 minutes for low blood pressure, poor perfusion, and metabolic acidosis. Sodium bicarbonate (1–2 mEq/kg) is given for metabolic acidosis unresponsive to initial oxygen, ventilation, and volume. Other specific testing should be done as indicated by the history and physical examination. In most cases, a chest radiograph, blood gas measurements, CBC, and blood glucose determination allow a diagnosis.

Intubation and ventilation should be undertaken if there is respiratory failure (PaO_2 < 60 mm Hg in 60–80% FIO_2, $PaCO_2$ greater than 60 mm Hg, or repeated apnea). Peak pressures should be adequate to produce chest wall expansion and audible breath sounds (usually 18–24 cm H_2O). Positive end-expiratory pressure (4–6 cm H_2O) should be used. Ventilation rates of 20–50 breaths/min are usually required. The goal is to maintain a PaO_2 of 60–70 mm Hg and a $PaCO_2$ of 45–55 mm Hg.

▶ **Prognosis**

Most respiratory conditions of the full-term infant are acute and resolve in the first several days. Meconium aspiration and congenital pneumonia carry a mortality rate of up to 10–20% and produce significant long-term pulmonary morbidity. Mortality has been reduced by use of high-frequency oscillatory ventilation, inhaled nitric oxide for pulmonary hypertension, and extracorporeal membrane oxygenation (ECMO).

Aly H: Respiratory disorders in the newborn: Identification and diagnosis. Pediatr Rev 2004;25:201 [PMID: 15173453].

Flidel-Raman O, Shinwell ES: Respiratory distress in the term and near-term infant. NeoReviews 2005;6:e289.

Hansen AK et al: Elective caesarean section and respiratory morbidity in the term and near-term neonate. Acta Obstet Gynecol Scand 2007;86:389 [PMID: 17486457].

Jain L, Eaton DC: Physiology of fetal lung fluid clearance and the effect of labor. Semin Perinatol 2006;30:34 [PMID: 16549212].

Ross MG: Meconium aspiration syndrome—more than intrapartum meconium. N Engl J Med 2005;353:946 [PMID: 16135842].

Sasidharan P: An approach to diagnosis and management of cyanosis and tachypnea in term infants. Pediatr Clin North Am 2004;51:999 [PMID: 15275985].

HEART MURMURS (SEE ALSO SECTION ON CARDIAC PROBLEMS IN THE NEWBORN INFANT)

Heart murmurs are common in the first days of life and do not usually signify structural heart problems. If a murmur is present at birth, it should be considered a valvular problem until proved otherwise because the common benign transitional murmurs (eg, patent ductus arteriosus) are not audible until minutes to hours after birth.

If an infant is pink, well-perfused, and in no respiratory distress, with palpable and symmetrical pulses (right brachial pulse no stronger than the femoral pulse), the murmur is most likely transitional. Transitional murmurs are soft (grade 1–3/6), heard at the left upper to midsternal border, and generally loudest during the first 24 hours. If the murmur persists beyond 24 hours of age, blood pressure in the right arm and a leg should be determined. If there is a difference of more than 15 mm Hg (arm > leg) or if the pulses in the lower extremities are difficult to palpate, a cardiologist should evaluate the infant for coarctation of the aorta. If there is no difference, the infant can be discharged home with follow-up in 2–3 days for auscultation and evaluation for signs of congestive failure. If signs of congestive failure or cyanosis are present, the infant should be referred for evaluation without delay. If the murmur persists without these signs, the infant can be referred for elective evaluation at age 2–4 weeks. Some centers now recommend routine pulse oximetry screening in the nursery to identify infants with congenital heart disease. Oxygen saturation less than 95% at sea level is evaluated by echocardiogram.

Frommelt MA: Differential diagnosis and approach to a heart murmur in term infants. Pediatr Clin North Am 2004;51:1023 [PMID: 15331284].

Valmari P: Should pulse oximetry be used to screen for congenital heart disease? Arch Dis Child Fetal Neonatal Ed 2007;92:F219 [PMID: 17449857].

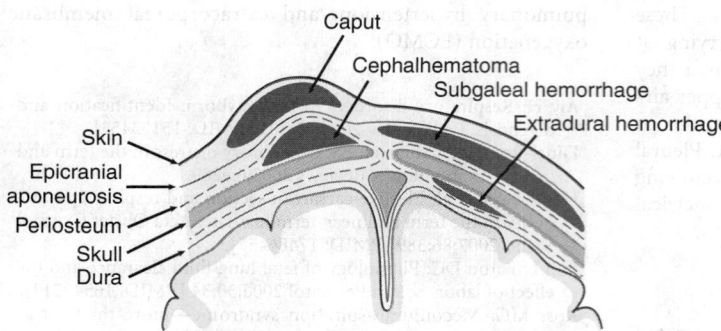

Caput
Cephalhematoma
Subgaleal hemorrhage
Extradural hemorrhage

Skin
Epicranial aponeurosis
Periosteum
Skull
Dura

▲ **Figure 1-5.** Sites of extracranial bleeding in the newborn. (Adapted and reproduced, with permission, from Pape KE, Wigglesworth JS: *Haemorrhage Ischemia and the Perinatal Brain.* JB Lippincott, 1979.)

BIRTH TRAUMA

Most birth trauma is associated with difficult delivery (eg, large fetus, abnormal presenting position, or fetal distress requiring rapid extraction). The most common injuries are soft tissue bruising, fractures (clavicle, humerus, or femur), and cervical plexus palsies. Skull fracture, intracranial hemorrhage (primarily subdural and subarachnoid), and cervical spinal cord injury can also occur.

Fractures are often diagnosed by the obstetrician, who may feel or hear a snap during delivery. Clavicular fractures may cause decreased spontaneous movement of the arm, with local tenderness and crepitus. Humeral or femoral fractures usually cause tenderness and swelling over the shaft with a diaphyseal fracture, and always cause limitation of movement. Epiphyseal fractures are harder to diagnose radiographically owing to the cartilaginous nature of the epiphysis. After 8–10 days, callus is visible on radiographs. Treatment in all cases is gentle handling, with immobilization for 8–10 days: the humerus against the chest with elbow flexed; the femur with a posterior splint from below the knee to the buttock.

Brachial plexus injuries may result from traction as the head is pulled away from the shoulder during delivery. Injury to the C5–C6 roots is most common (Erb-Duchenne palsy). The arm is limp, adducted, and internally rotated, extended and pronated at the elbow, and flexed at the wrist (so-called waiter's tip posture). Grasp is present. If the lower nerve roots (C8–T1) are injured (Klumpke palsy), the hand is flaccid. Isolated involvement of the cervical roots is rare. If the entire plexus is injured, the arm and hand are flaccid, with associated sensory deficit. Early treatment for brachial plexus injury is conservative, because function usually returns over several weeks. Referral should be made to a physical therapist so that parents can be instructed on range-of-motion exercises, splinting, and further evaluation if needed. Return of function begins in the deltoid and biceps, with recovery by 3 months in most cases.

Spinal cord injury can occur at birth, especially in difficult breech extractions with hyperextension of the neck, or in midforceps rotations when the body fails to turn with the head. Infants are flaccid, quadriplegic, and without respiratory effort at birth. Facial movements are preserved. The long-term outlook for such infants is poor.

Facial nerve palsy is sometimes associated with forceps use but more often results from in-utero pressure of the baby's head against the mother's sacrum. The infant has asymmetrical mouth movements and eye closure with poor facial movement on the affected side. Most cases resolve spontaneously in a few days to weeks.

Subgaleal hemorrhage into the large potential space under the scalp (Figure 1–5) is associated with difficult vaginal deliveries and repeated attempts at vacuum extraction. It can lead to hypovolemic shock and death from blood loss and coagulopathy triggered by consumption of clotting factors and release of thromboplastin from the injured brain. This is an emergency requiring rapid replacement of blood and clotting factors.

Noetzel MJ: Perinatal trauma and cerebral palsy: Is there a link. Clin Perinatol 2006;33:355 [PMID:16765729].

Rosenberg AA: Traumatic birth injuries. NeoReviews 2003;4:e270.

Sutcliffe TL: Brachial plexus injury in the newborn. NeoReviews 2007;8:e239.

Uhring MR: Management of birth injuries. Clin Perinatol 2005;32:19 [PMID: 15777819].

INFANTS OF MOTHERS WHO ABUSE DRUGS

Current studies estimate that up to 15% of women use alcohol and 5–15% use illicit drugs during pregnancy, depending on the population studied and the methods of ascertainment. Drugs most commonly used are tobacco, alcohol, marijuana, cocaine, and methamphetamine. Because mothers may abuse many drugs and give an unreliable history of drug usage, it is difficult to pinpoint which drug is causing the morbidity seen in a newborn infant. Early hospital discharge makes recognition of these infants based on physical findings and abnormal behavior difficult.

1. Cocaine & Methamphetamine

ESSENTIALS OF DIAGNOSIS & TYPICAL FEATURES

▶ Triad of no prenatal care, premature delivery, placental abruption.

▶ Possible intrauterine growth restriction.

▶ Irritability.

Cocaine and methamphetamine are currently the most common hard drugs used during pregnancy, often in association with other drugs such as tobacco, alcohol, and marijuana. These stimulants can cause maternal hypertension, decreased uterine blood flow, fetal hypoxemia, uterine contractions, and placental abruption. Rates of stillbirth, placental abruption, IUGR, and preterm delivery are increased two- to fourfold in users compared with nonusers. In the high-risk setting of no prenatal care, placental abruption, and preterm labor, urine toxicology screens should be performed on the mother and infant. Meconium should be sent for drug screening as it enhances diagnosis by indicating cumulative drug exposure from the first trimester forward. Although no specific malformation complex or withdrawal syndrome is described for cocaine and methamphetamine abuse, infants may show irritability and growth restriction.

Children of mothers who use methamphetamines are at particularly high risk for neglect and abuse. Social services evaluation is especially important to assess the home environment for these risks. The risk of SIDS is three to seven times higher in infants of users than in those of nonusers (0.5–1% of exposed infants). The risk may be lessened by environmental interventions such as avoidance of tobacco smoke and supine infant positioning.

2. Opioids

ESSENTIALS OF DIAGNOSIS & TYPICAL FEATURES

▶ CNS—irritability, hyperactivity, hypertonicity, incessant high-pitched cry, tremors, seizures.

▶ GI—vomiting, diarrhea, weight loss, poor feeding, incessant hunger, excessive salivation.

▶ Metabolic and respiratory—nasal stuffiness, sneezing, yawning, sweating, hyperthermia.

▶ Often IUGR.

▶ Clinical Findings

The withdrawal signs of infants born to heroin-addicted mothers or mothers who have been in methadone maintenance programs are similar. The symptoms in infants born to methadone-maintained mothers may be delayed in onset, more severe, and more prolonged than those seen with heroin addiction. Symptoms usually begin within 1–2 days of life. The clinical picture is typical enough to suggest a diagnosis even if a maternal history of narcotic abuse has not been obtained. Confirmation should be made with urine and meconium toxicology screening.

▶ Treatment

If opioid abuse or withdrawal is suspected, the infant is not a candidate for early discharge. Supportive treatment includes swaddling the infant and providing a quiet, dimly lit environment. Specific treatment should be avoided unless the infant has severe symptoms or excessive weight loss. No single drug has been identified as optimally effective. Phenobarbital is used at an initial loading dose of 10–20 mg/kg IM, followed by a maintenance dose of 5 mg/kg/d in two divided doses given orally. Opioids, diazepam, and clonidine have also been used, although the present authors prefer phenobarbital if irritability is the primary symptom because of its safety and predictability. If diarrhea and weight loss are prominent, or if adequate control of symptoms has not been achieved, tincture of opium (25-fold dilution to 0.4 mg/mL morphine equivalent; 0.1 mL/kg q4h to start) titrated to improve symptoms, or methadone (0.05–0.1 mg/kg q6h) are more beneficial than phenobarbital alone. Treatment can be tapered over several days to 2 weeks. Disturbing the infant by procedures should be minimized. It is also important to review maternal tests for HIV, hepatitis B, and hepatitis C, as all are common in intravenous drug users.

▶ Prognosis

These infants often have chronic neurobehavioral handicaps; however, it is difficult to distinguish the effects of in-utero drug exposure from those of the environment. Infants of opioid abusers have a four- to fivefold increased risk of SIDS.

3. Alcohol

Alcohol is the only recreational drug of abuse that is clearly teratogenic and is the most common preventable cause of mental retardation. Prevalence estimates of fetal alcohol syndrome (FAS) in the United States range from 0.5–2 per 1000 live births with up to 1 in 100 having lesser effects (fetal alcohol spectrum disorders). The effects of alcohol on the fetus and newborn are determined by the degree and timing of ethanol exposure and by the maternal, fetal, and placental metabolism of ethanol, which is likely genetically determined. Although there is no clear evidence that minimal amounts of alcohol are harmful, there is no established safe dose. Fetal growth and development are adversely affected if drinking continues throughout the pregnancy, and infants can occasionally experience withdrawal similar to that asso-

Table 1–14. Features observed in fetal alcohol syndrome in the newborn.

Craniofacial
  Short palpebral fissures
  Thin vermillion of upper lip
  Flattened philtrum
Growth
  Prenatal and postnatal growth deficiency (small for gestational age, failure to thrive)
Central nervous system
  Microcephaly
  Partial or complete agenesis of the corpus callosum
  Optic nerve hypoplasia
  Hypotonia, poor feeding

ciated with maternal opioid abuse. Clinical features of FAS that may be observed in the newborn period are listed in Table 1–14. This diagnosis is usually easier to recognize in older infants and children.

4. Tobacco Smoking

Smoking has a negative effect on fetal growth rate. The more the mother smokes, the greater is the degree of IUGR. There is a twofold increase in low birth weight even in light smokers (< 10 cigarettes per day). Smoking during pregnancy has been associated with mild neurodevelopmental handicaps. The possibility of multiple drug abuse also applies to smokers, and the potential interaction of multiple factors on fetal growth and development must be considered.

5. Toluene Embryopathy

Solvent toxicity may be intentional (paint, lacquer, or glue sniffing) or environmental (dry cleaning industry). The active organic solvent in these agents is toluene. Features attributable to in-utero toluene exposure are prematurity, IUGR, microcephaly, craniofacial abnormalities similar to those associated with in-utero alcohol exposure (see Table 1–14), large anterior fontanelle, hair patterning abnormalities, nail hypoplasia, and renal anomalies. Long-term effects include postnatal growth deficiency and developmental delay.

6. Marijuana

Marijuana is the most frequently used illegal drug. It does not appear to be teratogenic, and although a mild abstinence-type syndrome has been described, infants exposed to marijuana in utero rarely require treatment. Some long-term neurodevelopmental problems, particularly disordered sleep patterns, have been noted.

7. Other Drugs

Drugs with potential effects on the newborn fall in two categories. First are drugs to which the fetus is exposed because of therapy for maternal conditions. The human placenta is relatively permeable, particularly to lipophilic solutes. If possible, maternal drug therapy should be postponed until after the first trimester to avoid teratogenic effects. Drugs with potential fetal toxicity include antineoplastics, antithyroid agents, warfarin, lithium, and angiotensin-converting enzyme inhibitors (eg, captopril and enalapril). Anticonvulsants, especially high-dose or multiple drug therapy, may be associated with craniofacial abnormalities. The use of selective serotonin reuptake inhibitors, benzodiazepines, and antipsychotic medications appears to be generally safe, and risk should be balanced against the risk of untreated psychiatric conditions in the mother.

In the second category are drugs transmitted to the infant in breast milk. Most drugs taken by the mother achieve some concentration in breast milk, although they usually do not present a problem to the infant. If the drug is one that could have adverse effects on the infant, timing breast feeding to coincide with trough concentrations in the mother may be useful. The AAP (see below) has reviewed drugs contraindicated in the breast-feeding mother.

American Academy of Pediatrics Committee on Drugs: The transfer of drugs and other chemicals into human milk. Pediatrics 2001;108:776 [PMID: 11533352].

Austin MP: To treat or not to treat: Maternal depression, SSRI use in pregnancy and adverse neonatal effects. Psychol Med 2006;36:1663 [PMID: 16863595].

Crome IB, Kumar MT: Epidemiology of drug and alcohol use in young women. Semin Fet Neonat Med 2007;12:98 [PMID 17292681].

Kuschel C: Managing drug withdrawal in the newborn infant. Semin Fet Neonat Med 2007;12:127 [PMID: 17321815].

Manning MA, Hoyme HE: Fetal alcohol spectrum disorders: A practical clinical approach to diagnosis. Neurosci Biobehav Rev 2007;31:230 [PMID: 16962173].

MULTIPLE BIRTHS

 ESSENTIALS OF DIAGNOSIS & TYPICAL FEATURES

▶ Monochorial twins
  · Always monozygous and same sex.
  · Can be diamniotic or monoamniotic.
  · Risk for twin-to-twin transfusion and higher risk of congenital anomalies, neurodevelopmental problems, and cerebral palsy.
▶ Dichorial twins
  · Either dizygous or monozygous; same sex or different sex.
  · Can have growth restriction due to abnormal placental implantation.

- Not at risk for twin transfusion syndrome; less risk for anomalies and neurodevelopmental problems than monochorial twins.

Twinning historically occurred at a rate of 1 in 80 pregnancies (1.25%). The incidence of twinning and higher-order multiple births in the United States has increased because of in-vitro fertilization and other assisted reproductive technologies. In 2002, twins occurred in 1 in 32 live births in the United States, with multiple births accounting for 3.3% of all births.

A distinction should be made between dizygous (fraternal) and monozygous (identical) twins. Race, maternal parity, and maternal age affect the incidence of dizygous, but not monozygous, twinning. Drugs used to induce ovulation, such as clomiphene citrate and gonadotropins, increase the incidence of dizygotic or polyzygotic twinning. Monozygous twinning also seems to be more common after assisted reproduction. The incidence of malformations is also increased in identical twins and may affect only one of the twins. If a defect is found in one twin, the other should be examined carefully for lesser degrees of the same defect.

Early transvaginal ultrasound and examination of the placenta after birth can help establish the type of twinning: Two amnionic membranes and two chorionic membranes are found in all dizygous twins and in one third of monozygous twins even when the placental disks appear to be fused into one. A single chorionic membrane always indicates monozygous twins. The rare monochorial, monoamniotic situation (1% of twins) is especially dangerous, with a high risk of antenatal cord entanglement and death of one or both twins. Close fetal surveillance is indicated.

▶ Complications of Multiple Births

A. Intrauterine Growth Restriction

There is some degree of IUGR in most multiple pregnancies, especially after 32 weeks, although it is usually not clinically significant with two exceptions. First, in monochorial twin pregnancy an arteriovenous shunt may develop between the twins (twin-twin transfusion syndrome). The twin on the venous side (recipient) becomes plethoric and larger than the smaller anemic twin (donor), who may ultimately die or be severely growth restricted. The occurrence of polyhydramnios in the larger twin and oligohydramnios in the smaller may be the first sign of this problem. Second, discordance in size (birth weights that are significantly different) can also occur when separate placentas are present if one placenta develops poorly, because of a poor implantation site. In this instance, no fetal exchange of blood takes place but the growth rates of the two infants are different.

B. Preterm Delivery

Length of gestation tends to be inversely related to the number of fetuses. The mean age at delivery for singletons is 38.8 weeks, for twins 35.3 weeks, for triplets 32.2 weeks, and for quadruplets 29.9 weeks. The prematurity rate in multiple gestations is 5–10 times that of singletons, with 50% of twins and 90% of triplets born before 37 weeks. There is an increased incidence of cerebral palsy in multiple births, more so with monochorial than dichorial infants. Prematurity is the main cause of increased mortality and morbidity in twins, although in the case of monochorial twins, intravascular exchange through placental anastomoses, particularly after the death of one twin, also increases the risk substantially.

C. Obstetric Complications

Polyhydramnios, pregnancy-induced hypertension, premature rupture of membranes, abnormal fetal presentations, and prolapsed umbilical cord occur more frequently in women with multiple fetuses. Multiple pregnancy should always be identified prenatally with ultrasound examinations; doing so allows the obstetrician and pediatrician or neonatologist to plan management jointly. Because neonatal complications are usually related to prematurity, prolongation of pregnancy significantly reduces neonatal morbidity.

Lopriore E et al: Incidence, origin, and character of cerebral injury in twin-to-twin transfusion syndrome treated with fetoscopic laser surgery. Am J Obstet Gynecol 2006;194:1215 [PMID: 16647903].

Ong SSC et al: Prognosis for the co-twin following single-twin death: A systematic review. BJOG 2006;113:992 [PMID: 16903844].

Pharoah POD: Risk of cerebral palsy in multiple pregnancies. Clin Perinatol 2006;33:301 [PMID: 16765726].

Reddy UM et al: Infertility, assisted reproductive technology, and adverse pregnancy outcomes: Executive summary of a National Institute of Child Health and Human Development workshop. Obstet Gynecol 2007;109:967 [PMID: 17400861].

Yeast JD: Polyhydramnios/oligohydramnios in twin pregnancy. NeoReviews 2006;7:e305.

▼ NEONATAL INTENSIVE CARE

PERINATAL RESUSCITATION

Perinatal resuscitation refers to the steps taken by the obstetrician to support the infant during labor and delivery and the resuscitative steps taken by the pediatrician after delivery. Intrapartum support includes maintaining maternal blood pressure, maternal oxygen therapy, positioning the mother to improve placental perfusion, readjusting oxytocin infusions or administering a tocolytic if appropriate, minimizing trauma to the infant, obtaining all necessary cord blood samples, and completing an examination of the placenta. The pediatrician or neonatologist focuses on temperature support, initiation and maintenance of effective ventilation, maintenance of perfusion and hydration, and glucose regulation.

A number of conditions associated with pregnancy, labor, and delivery place the infant at risk for birth asphyxia: (1) maternal diseases such as diabetes, pregnancy-induced hypertension, heart and renal disease, and collagen-vascular disease; (2) fetal conditions such as prematurity, multiple births, growth restriction, and fetal anomalies; and (3) labor and delivery conditions, including fetal distress with or without meconium in the amniotic fluid, and administration of anesthetics and opioid analgesics.

Physiology of Birth Asphyxia

Birth asphyxia can be the result of: (1) acute interruption of umbilical blood flow (eg, prolapsed cord with cord compression), (2) premature placental separation, (3) maternal hypotension or hypoxia, (4) chronic placental insufficiency, and (5) failure to perform resuscitation properly.

The neonatal response to asphyxia follows a predictable pattern (Figure 1–6). The initial response to hypoxia is an increase in respiratory rate and a rise in heart rate and blood pressure. Respirations then cease (primary apnea) as heart rate and blood pressure begin to fall. The initial period of apnea lasts 30–60 seconds. Gasping respirations (3–6 per minute) then begin, while heart rate and blood pressure gradually decline. Secondary or terminal apnea then ensues, with further decline in heart rate and blood pressure. The longer the duration of secondary apnea, the greater is the risk for hypoxic organ injury. A cardinal feature of the defense against hypoxia is the underperfusion of certain tissue beds (eg, skin, muscle, kidneys, and GI tract), which allows maintenance of perfusion to core organs (ie, heart, brain, and adrenals).

Response to resuscitation also follows a predictable pattern. During the period of primary apnea, almost any physical stimulus causes the infant to initiate respirations. Infants in secondary apnea require PPV. The first sign of recovery is an increase in heart rate, followed by an increase in blood pressure with improved perfusion. The time required for rhythmic, spontaneous respirations to occur is related to the duration of the secondary apnea. As a rough rule, for each minute past the last gasp, 2 minutes of PPV is required before gasping begins, and 4 minutes is required to reach rhythmic breathing. Not until some time later do spinal and corneal reflexes return. Muscle tone gradually improves over the course of several hours.

Delivery Room Management

When asphyxia is anticipated, a resuscitation team of at least two persons should be present, one to manage the airway and one to monitor the heartbeat and provide assistance. The necessary equipment and drugs are listed in Table 1–15.

A. Steps in the Resuscitative Process (see Figure 1–7)

1. Dry the infant well, and place him or her under a radiant heat source. Do not allow the infant to become hyperthermic.
2. Position the infant to open the airway. Gently suction the mouth, then the nose.
3. Quickly assess the infant's condition. The best criteria are the infant's respiratory effort (apneic, gasping or, regular) and heart rate (> 100 or < 100 beats/min). A depressed heart rate—indicative of hypoxic myocardial depression—is the single most reliable indicator of the need for resuscitation.
4. Infants who are breathing and have heart rates above 100 beats/min usually require no further intervention other than supplemental oxygen if cyanotic. Infants with heart rates less than 100 beats/min and apnea or irregular respiratory efforts should be stimulated vigorously. The infant's back should be rubbed with a towel while oxygen is provided near the face.
5. If the infant fails to respond to tactile stimulation within a few seconds, begin bag and mask ventilation, using a soft mask that seals well around the mouth and nose. For the initial inflations, pressures of 30–40 cm H_2O may be necessary to overcome surface-active

▲ **Figure 1–6.** Schematic depiction of changes in rhesus monkeys during asphyxia and on resuscitation by positive-pressure ventilation. (Adapted and reproduced, with permission, from Dawes GS: *Fetal and Neonatal Physiology.* Year Book, 1968.)

Table 1–15. Equipment for neonatal resuscitation.

Clinical Needs	Equipment
Thermoregulation	Radiant heat source with platform, mattress covered with warm sterile blankets, servocontrol heating, temperature probe, occlusive skin cover (preterm)
Airway management	**Suction:** bulb suction, mechanical suction with sterile catheters (6F, 8F, 10F), meconium aspirator
	Ventilation: manual infant resuscitation bag connected to manometer or with a pressure-release valve capable of delivering 100% oxygen, appropriate masks for term and preterm infants, oral airways, stethoscope
	Intubation: neonatal laryngoscope with No. 0 and No. 1 blades; endotracheal tubes (2.5, 3.0, 3.5 mm outer diameter with stylet): extra bulbs and batteries for laryngoscope; scissors, adhesive tape, gloves, end-tidal CO_2 detection device
Gastric decompression	Nasogastric tube: 8F with 20-mL syringe
Administration of drugs and volume replacement	Sterile umbilical catheterization tray, umbilical catheters (3.5F and 5F), volume expanders, normal saline, drug box[a] with appropriate neonatal vials and dilutions, sterile syringes, needles, and alcohol sponges
Transport	Warmed transport isolette with oxygen source

[a]Epinephrine 1:10,000; naloxone hydrochloride 1 mg/mL; sodium bicarbonate 4.2% (5 mEq/10 mL); 10% dextrose.
Modified, with permission, from Rosenberg AA: Neonatal adaptation. In Gabbe SG et al (editors): *Obstetrics: Normal and Problem Pregnancies.* Churchill Livingstone, 1996.

forces in the lungs. Adequacy of ventilation is assessed by observing expansion of the infant's chest accompanied by an improvement in heart rate, perfusion, and color. After the first few breaths, lower the peak pressure to 15–20 cm H_2O. The chest movement should resemble that of an easy breath rather than a deep sigh. The rate of bagging should be 40–60 breaths/min.

6. Most neonates can be resuscitated effectively with a bag and mask. If the infant does not respond to bag and mask ventilation, reposition the head (slight extension), reapply the mask to achieve a good seal, consider suctioning the mouth and the oropharynx, and try ventilating with the mouth open. If the infant does not respond within 30 seconds, intubation is appropriate.

Failure to respond to intubation and ventilation can result from (1) mechanical difficulties (Table 1–16), (2) profound asphyxia with myocardial depression, and (3) inadequate circulating blood volume.

Quickly rule out the mechanical causes listed in Table 1–16. Check to ensure that the endotracheal tube passes through the vocal cords. A CO_2 detector placed between the endotracheal tube and the bag can be helpful as a rapid confirmation of proper tube position in the airway. Occlusion of the tube should be suspected when there is resistance to bagging and no chest wall movement. Very few neonates (approximately 0.1%) require either cardiac massage or drugs during resuscitation. Almost all newborns respond to ventilation if done effectively. Although current AAP Neonatal Resuscitation Program (NRP) guidelines recommend 100% oxygen for neonatal resuscitation when PPV is required, there is some evidence that this may increase the risk of postresuscitative oxidative injury. Resuscitation with room air or lower oxygen concentrations may be equally effective. At a minimum, when possible, blended oxygen should be available in the delivery room. Use of lower oxygen concentrations is further supported by review of oxygen saturations after birth in normal newborns. Oxygen saturation rises slowly and does not reach 90% for 5 minutes.

7. If mechanical causes are ruled out and the heart rate remains less than 60 beats/min after intubation and PPV for 30 seconds, cardiac compression should be initiated. Simultaneous delivery of chest compressions and PPV is likely to decrease the efficiency of ventilation. Therefore, chest compressions should be interspersed with ventilation at a 3:1 ratio (90 compressions and 30 breaths/min).

8. If drugs are needed, the drug and dose of choice is epinephrine 1:10,000 solution (0.1–0.3 mL/kg) given via the endotracheal tube or preferably through an umbilical venous line. If volume loss is suspected, 10 mL/kg of a volume expander (normal saline) should be administered through an umbilical vein line.

B. Continued Resuscitative Measures

The appropriateness of continued resuscitative efforts should be reevaluated in infants who do not respond to initial measures. In current practice, resuscitative efforts are made even in apparent stillbirths (ie, infants whose Apgar score at 1 minute is 0–1). Modern resuscitative techniques have led to improved survival in such infants, with 60% of survivors showing normal development. Although it is clear that resuscitation of these infants should be performed, subsequent continued support depends on the response to resuscitation. If the Apgar score does not improve markedly in the first 10 minutes of life, the mortality rate and the incidence of severe developmental handicaps among survivors are high.

C. Special Considerations

1. Preterm Infants

A. Minimizing heat loss improves survival. Prewarmed towels should be available. The environmental temperature of

Approximate Time

30 sec

BIRTH

- • Term gestation?
- • Amniotic fluid clear?
- • Breathing or crying?
- • Good muscle tone?

Yes →

Routine Care
- • Provide warmth
- • Clear airway if needed
- • Dry
- • Assess color

No ↓

A
- • Provide warmth
- • Position: clear airway* (as necessary)
- • Dry, stimulate, reposition

Evaluate respirations, heart rate, and color

Breathing, HR >100 & Pink → **Observational care**

Breathing, HR >100 but Cyanotic

Apneic or HR <100

30 sec

Give supplementry oxygen

Pink →

Persistent Cyanosis

Effective Ventilation, HR >100 & Pink →

B   Provide positive-pressure ventilation → **Postresuscitation Care**

HR <60   HR >60

30 sec

C
- • Provide positive-pressure ventilation*
- • Administer chest compressions

HR <60

D   Administer **epinephrine** and/or **volume***

*Endotracheal intubation may be considered at several steps

▲ **Figure 1–7.** Delivery room management. (Reproduced, with permission, from Kattwinkel J, et al: *Textbook of Neonatal Resuscitation*, 5th edition, American Heart Association and American Academy of Pediatrics, 2006.)

the delivery suite should be raised to more than 25°C (especially for infants weighing < 1500 g). A polyethylene occlusive skin cover should be used to minimize heat loss in the extremely low birth weight (< 1000 g) infant.

B. The lungs of preterm infants are especially prone to injury from PPV due to volutrauma. For this reason, if possible, ventilation efforts should be supported with nasal continuous positive airway pressure (CPAP) rather than PPV. If PPV is needed, a T-piece resuscitation device should be used to allow precise regulation of pressure delivery.

C. In the infant of extremely low gestational age (< 27 weeks), intubation for administration of surfactant should be considered.

D. Volume expanders should be infused slowly to minimize rapid swings in blood pressure.

2. Narcotic depression—In the case of opioid administration to the mother within 4 hours of delivery, perform the

Table 1–16. Mechanical causes of failed resuscitation.

Cause	Examples
Equipment failure	Malfunctioning bag, oxygen not connected or running
Endotracheal tube malposition	Esophagus, right main stem bronchus
Occluded endotracheal tube	
Insufficient inflation pressure to expand lungs	
Space-occupying lesions in the thorax	Pneumothorax, pleural effusions, diaphragmatic hernia
Pulmonary hypoplasia	Extreme prematurity, oligohydramnios

Reproduced, with permission, from Rosenberg AA: Neonatal adaptation. In Gabbe SG et al (editors): *Obstetrics: Normal and Problem Pregnancies.* Churchill Livingstone, 1996.

resuscitation as described earlier. When the baby is stable with good heart rate, color, and perfusion, but still has poor respiratory effort, a trial of naloxone (0.1 mg/kg IM, SC, IV, or IT) is indicated. Naloxone should not be administered in place of PPV. Naloxone should not be used in the infant of an opioid-addicted mother because it will precipitate withdrawal.

3. Meconium-stained amniotic fluid

A. The obstetrician performs routine suctioning of the mouth and nose after birth.

B. If the infant is active and breathing, requiring no resuscitation, the airway need not be inspected—only further suctioning of the mouth and nasopharynx is required.

C. The airway of any depressed infant requiring ventilation must be checked and cleared (by passage of a tube below the vocal cords) before PPV is instituted. Special adapters are available for use with regulated wall suction to allow suction to be applied directly to the endotracheal tube.

D. Because most severe cases of meconium aspiration syndrome with pulmonary hypertension likely have their origins in utero, resuscitative efforts should not be excessively delayed with attempts to clear the airway of meconium.

4. Universal precautions—In the delivery suite, universal precautions should always be observed.

Treatment of the Asphyxiated Infant

Asphyxia is manifested by multiorgan dysfunction, seizures, hypoxic-ischemic encephalopathy, and metabolic acidemia. The infant with significant perinatal hypoxia and ischemia is at risk for dysfunction of multiple end organs (Table 1– 17). The organ of greatest concern is the brain.

The features of hypoxic-ischemic encephalopathy are decreased level of consciousness, poor tone, decreased spontaneous movement, periodic breathing or apnea, and seizures. Brainstem signs (oculomotor and pupillary disturbances, absent gag reflex) may also be present. The severity and duration of clinical signs correlate with the severity of the insult. Other evaluations helpful in assessing severity in the full-term infant include electroencephalogram (EEG) and computed tomography (CT) scan. MRI, particularly diffusion-weighted imaging, is useful, especially in the early evaluation of infants with perinatal asphyxia.

A markedly abnormal EEG with voltage suppression and slowing evolving into a burst-suppression pattern is associated with severe clinical symptoms. Brain CT scan early in the course may demonstrate diffuse hypodensity and loss of gray/white matter tissue differentiation, whereas later scans may demonstrate brain atrophy and focal ischemic lesions. Management is directed at supportive care and treatment of specific abnormalities. Fluids should be restricted initially to 60–80 mL/kg/d; oxygenation should be maintained with mechanical ventilation if necessary; blood pressure should be

Table 1–17. Signs and symptoms caused by asphyxia.

Hypoxic-ischemic encephalopathy, seizures
Respiratory distress due to aspiration or secondary surfactant deficiency, pulmonary hemorrhage
Persistent pulmonary hypertension
Hypotension due to myocardial dysfunction
Transient tricuspid valve insufficiency
Anuria or oliguria due to acute tubular necrosis
Feeding intolerance; necrotizing enterocolitis
Elevated aminotransferases due to liver injury
Adrenal insufficiency due to hemorrhage
Disseminated intravascular coagulation
Hypocalcemia
Hypoglycemia
Persistent metabolic academia
Hyperkalemia

supported with judicious volume expansion (if hypovolemic) and pressors; and glucose should be in the normal range of 45–100 mg/dL. Hypocalcemia, coagulation abnormalities, and metabolic acidemia should be corrected and seizures treated with IV phenobarbital (20 mg/kg as loading dose, with total initial 24-hour dosing up to 40 mg/kg). Other anticonvulsants should be reserved for refractory seizures. Hypothermia, either selective head cooling with mild systemic hypothermia or whole body cooling, initiated within 6 hours of birth, has been shown to improve outcome at 18-month follow-up of infants with moderate neurologic symptoms and an abnormal 1-lead amplitude-integrated EEG. Efficacy has not been proved in the most severe cases of neonatal encephalopathy.

Birth Asphyxia: Long-Term Outcome

Fetal heart rate tracings, cord pH, and 1-minute Apgar scores are imprecise predictors of long-term outcome. Apgar scores of 0–3 at 5 minutes in full-term infants are associated with an 18–35% risk of death in the first year of life and an 8% risk of cerebral palsy among survivors. The risks of mortality and morbidity increase with more prolonged depression of the Apgar score. The single best predictor of outcome is the severity of clinical hypoxic-ischemic encephalopathy (severe symptomatology including coma carries a 75% chance of death and a 100% rate of neurologic sequelae among survivors). The major sequela of hypoxic-ischemic encephalopathy is cerebral palsy with or without mental retardation and epilepsy. Other prognostic features are prolonged seizures refractory to therapy, markedly abnormal EEG, and CT or MRI scan with evidence of major ischemic injury. Other clinical features required to support perinatal hypoxia as the cause of cerebral palsy include the presence of fetal distress prior to birth, a low arterial cord pH of less than 7.00, evidence of other end-organ dysfunction, and absence of a congenital brain malformation.

Aly H et al: Is it safer to intubate premature infants in the delivery room? Pediatrics 2005;115:1660 [PMID: 15930230].

American Heart Association and American Academy of Pediatrics: *Textbook of Neonatal Resuscitation*, 5th ed. American Heart Association/American Academy of Pediatrics, 2006.

Carlo WA, Schelonka R: The outcome of infants with an Apgar score of zero at 10 minutes: Past and future. Am J Obstet Gynecol 2007;196:422 [PMID: 17466692].

Fraser WD et al: Amnioinfusion for the prevention of the meconium aspiration syndrome. N Engl J Med 2005;353:909 [PMID: 16135835].

Gluckman PD et al: Selective head cooling with mild systemic hypothermia after neonatal encephalopathy: Multicentre randomized trial. Lancet 2005;365:663 [PMID: 15721471].

Harrington DJ et al: The long term outcome in surviving infants with Apgar zero at 10 minutes: A systematic review of the literature and hospital-based cohort. Am J Obstet Gynecol 2007;196:463.e1 [PMID: 17466703].

Mariani G et al: Pre-ductal and post-ductal O_2 saturation in healthy term neonates after birth. J Pediatr 2007;150:418 [PMID: 17382123].

Perlman JM: Intrapartum asphyxia and cerebral palsy: Is there a link? Clin Perinatol 2006;33:335 [PMID: 16765728].

Phelan JP et al: Birth asphyxia and cerebral palsy. Clin Perinatol 2005;32:61 [PMID: 15777821].

Richmond, S, Goldsmith JP: Air or 100% oxygen in neonatal resuscitation. Clin Perinatol 2006;33:11 [PMID: 16533630].

Speer M, Perlman JM: Modest hypothermia as a neuroprotective strategy in high risk term infants. Clin Perinatol 2006;33:169 [PMID: 16533643].

Thomson MA: Early nasal continuous positive airway pressure to minimize the need for endotracheal intubation and ventilation. NeoReviews 2005;6:e184.

Vain NE et al: Oropharyngeal and nasopharyngeal suctioning of meconium-stained neonates before delivery of their shoulders: Multicentre, randomized, controlled trial. Lancet 2004;364:597 [PMID: 15313360].

Velaphi S, Vidyasagar D: Intrapartum and post delivery management of infants born to mothers with meconium-stained amniotic fluid: Evidence based recommendations. Clin Perinatol 2006;33:29 [PMID: 16533631].

Vobra S et al: Heat loss prevention (HELP) in the delivery room: A randomized controlled trial of polyethylene occlusive skin wrapping in very preterm infants. J Pediatr 2004;145:750 [PMID: 15580195].

Wyckoff MH, Perlman JM: Use of high-dose epinephrine and sodium bicarbonate during neonatal resuscitation: Is there proven benefit? Clin Perinatol 2006;33:141 [PMID: 16533640].

THE PRETERM INFANT

Premature infants comprise the majority of high-risk newborns. The preterm infant faces a variety of physiologic handicaps:

1. The ability to coordinate sucking, swallowing, and breathing is not achieved until 34–36 weeks' gestation. Therefore, enteral feedings must be provided by gavage. Further, preterm infants often have gastroesophageal reflux and an immature gag reflex, which increases the risk of aspiration of feedings.

2. Lack of body fat stores causes decreased ability to maintain body temperature.

3. Pulmonary immaturity–surfactant deficiency is associated with structural immaturity in infants younger than 26 weeks' gestation. This condition is complicated by the combination of noncompliant lungs and extremely compliant chest wall, causing inefficient respiratory mechanics.

4. Immature respiratory control leads to apnea and bradycardia.

5. Persistent patency of the ductus arteriosus compromises pulmonary gas exchange because of overperfusion and edema of the lungs.

6. Immature cerebral vasculature and structure predisposes to subependymal or intraventricular hemorrhage and periventricular leukomalacia.

7. Impaired substrate absorption by the GI tract compromises nutritional management.

8. Immature renal function (including both filtration and tubular functions) complicates fluid and electrolyte management.

9. Increased susceptibility to infection.

10. Immaturity of metabolic processes predisposes to hypoglycemia and hypocalcemia.

1. Delivery Room Care

See section on Perinatal Resuscitation, earlier.

2. Care in the Nursery

A. Thermoregulation

Maintaining stable body temperature is a function of heat production and conservation balanced against heat loss. Heat production in response to cold stress occurs through voluntary muscle activity, involuntary muscle activity (shivering), and thermogenesis not caused by shivering. Newborns produce heat mainly through the last of these three mechanisms. This metabolic heat production depends on the quantity of brown fat, which is very limited in the preterm infant. Heat loss to the environment can occur through: (1) radiation—transfer of heat from a warmer to a cooler object not in contact; (2) convection—transfer of heat to the surrounding gaseous environment, influenced by air movement and temperature; (3) conduction—transfer of heat to a cooler object in contact; and (4) evaporation—cooling secondary to water loss through the skin. Heat loss in the preterm newborn is accelerated because of a high ratio of surface area to body mass, reduced insulation by subcutaneous tissue, and water loss through the immature skin.

The thermal environment of the preterm neonate must be regulated carefully. The infant can be kept warm in an isolette, in which the air is heated and convective heat loss is minimized. The infant can also be kept warm on an open bed with a radiant heat source. Although evaporative and convective heat losses are greater with radiant warmers, this

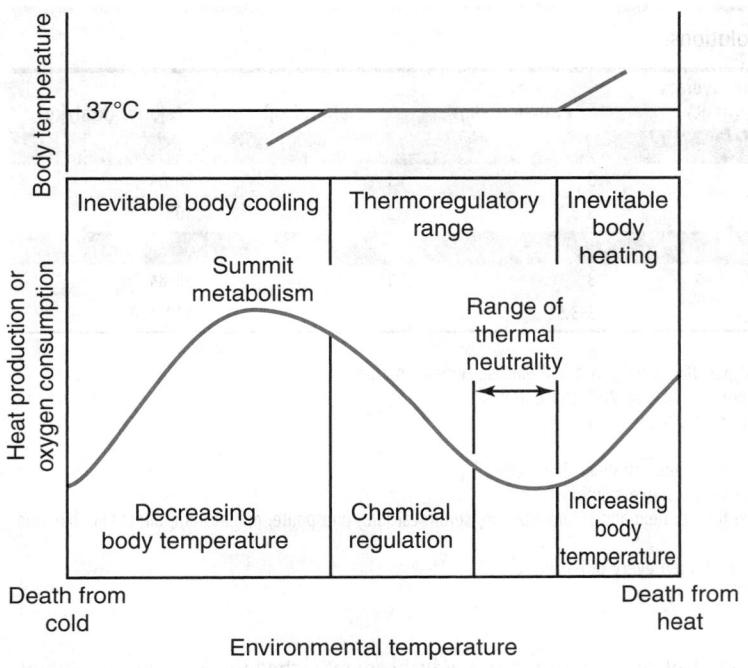

▲ **Figure 1–8.** Effect of environmental temperature on oxygen consumption and body temperature. (Adapted and reproduced, with permission, from Klaus MH, Fanaroff AA, Martin RJ: The physical environment. In: Klaus MH, Fanaroff AA [editors]: *Care of the High-Risk Neonate,* 5th ed. WB Saunders, 2001.)

system allows better access to an ill neonate. Ideally, the infant should be kept in a neutral thermal environment (Figure 1–8). The neutral thermal environment allows the infant to maintain a stable core body temperature with a minimum of metabolic heat production through oxygen consumption. The neutral thermal environment depends on the infant's size, gestational age, and postnatal age. The neutral thermal environment (for either isolette or radiant warmer care) can be obtained by maintaining an abdominal skin temperature of 36.5°C. Generally, when infants reach 1700–1800 g, they are able to maintain temperature while bundled in an open crib.

B. Monitoring the High-Risk Infant

At a minimum, equipment to monitor heart rate, respirations, and blood pressure should be available. Oxygen saturation can be assessed continuously using pulse oximetry, correlated with arterial oxygen tension (PaO_2) as needed. Transcutaneous PO_2 and PCO_2 can also be used to assess oxygenation and ventilation. Arterial blood gases, electrolytes, glucose, calcium, bilirubin, and other chemistries must be measured on small volumes of blood. Early in the care of a sick preterm infant, the most efficient way to sample blood for tests as well as to provide fluids and monitor blood pressure is through an umbilical arterial line. Once the infant is stable and the need for frequent blood samples is reduced (usually 4–7 days), the umbilical line should be removed. All indwelling lines are associated with morbidity from thrombosis or embolism, infection, and bleeding.

C. Fluid and Electrolyte Therapy

Fluid requirements in preterm infants are a function of (1) insensible losses (skin and respiratory tract), (2) urine output, (3) stool output (< 5% of total), and (4) others, such as nasogastric losses. In most circumstances, the fluid requirement is determined largely by insensible losses plus urine losses. The major contribution to insensible water loss is evaporative skin loss. The rate of water loss is a function of gestational age (body weight, skin thickness, and maturity), environment (losses are greater under a radiant warmer than in an isolette), and the use of phototherapy. Respiratory losses are minimal when humidified oxygen is used. The renal contribution to water requirement is influenced by the limited ability of the preterm neonate either to concentrate the urine and conserve water, or to excrete a water load.

Electrolyte requirements are minimal for the first 24–48 hours until there is significant urinary excretion. Basal requirements thereafter are as follows: sodium, 3 mEq/kg/d; potassium, 2 mEq/kg/d; chloride, 2–3 mEq/kg/d; and bicarbonate, 2–3 mEq/kg/d. In the infant younger than 30 weeks' gestation, sodium and bicarbonate losses in the urine are often elevated, thereby increasing the infant's requirements.

Initial fluid management after birth varies with the infant's size and gestation. Infants of more than 1500 g should start at 80–100 mL/kg/d of $D_{10}W$. Those weighing less should start at 100–120 mL/kg/d of either $D_{10}W$ or 5% dextrose in water (D_5W) (infants < 800 g and born before 26 weeks' gestation often become hyperglycemic on $D_{10}W$). The most critical issue in fluid management is monitoring. Mon-

Table 1–18. Use of parenteral alimentation solutions.

	Volume (mL/kg/d)	Carbohydrate (g/dL)	Protein (g/kg)	Lipid (g/kg)	Calories (kcal/kg)
Peripheral: short term (7–10 days)					
Starting solution	100–150	$D_{10}W$	3	1	56–84
Target solution	150	$D_{12.5}W$	3–3.5	3	108
Central: long term (> 10 days)					
Starting solution	100–150	$D_{10}W$	3	1	56–84
Target solution	130	D_{15}–$D_{20}W$	3–3.5	3	118–130

Notes:
1. Advance dextrose in central hyperalimentation as tolerated per day as long as blood glucose remains normal.
2. Advance lipids by 0.5–1.0 g/kg/d as long as triglycerides are normal. Use 20% concentration.
3. Total water should be 100–150 mL/kg/d, depending on the child's fluid needs.

Monitoring:
1. Blood glucose two or three times a day when changing dextrose concentration, then daily.
2. Electrolytes daily, then twice a week when the child is receiving a stable solution.
3. Every other week blood urea nitrogen and serum creatinine; total protein and serum albumin; serum calcium, phosphate, magnesium, direct bilirubin, and CBC with platelet counts.
4. Triglyceride level after 24 h at 2 g/kg/d and 24 h at 3 g/kg/d, then every other week.

itoring body weight, urine output, fluid and electrolyte intake, serum and urine electrolytes, and glucose allows fairly precise determination of the infant's water, glucose, and electrolyte needs. Parenteral nutrition should be started early and continued until an adequate enteral intake is achieved.

D. Nutritional Support

The average caloric requirement for the growing premature infant is 120 kcal/kg/d. Expected weight gain is 10–20 g/kg/d. Infants initially require IV glucose infusion to maintain blood glucose concentration in the range of 60–100 mg/dL. Infusions of 5–7 mg/kg/min (approximately 80–100 mL/kg/d of $D_{10}W$) are usually needed. Aggressive nutritional support in the very low birth weight infant should be started as soon as possible after birth, with parenteral alimentation solutions containing 3 g/kg/d of amino acids, given either peripherally or centrally via an umbilical vein line or percutaneous catheter (Table 1–18). Small-volume trophic feeds with breast milk or 20 kcal/oz premature formula should be started by gavage at 10% or less of the infant's nutritional needs (< 10 mL/kg/d) as soon as possible, generally within the first few days after birth. After several days of trophic feeds the infant can be slowly advanced to full caloric needs over 5–7 days. Even extremely small feedings can enhance intestinal readiness to accept larger feeding volumes. Intermittent bolus feedings are preferred because these appear to stimulate the release of gut-related hormones and may accelerate maturation of the GI tract, although in the extremely low birth weight infant (< 1000 g) or the postsurgical neonate, continuous-drip feeds are sometimes better tolerated. A more rapid advancement schedule is used for infants weighing more than 1500 g, and the slowest schedule for those weighing less than 1000 g.

In general, long-term nutritional support for infants of very low birth weight consists either of breast milk supplemented to increase protein, caloric density, and mineral content, or of infant formulas modified for preterm infants. In these formulas, protein concentrations (approximately 2 g/dL) and caloric concentrations (approximately 24 kcal/oz) are relatively high. In addition, premature formulas contain some medium-chain triglycerides—which do not require bile for emulsification—as an energy source. Increased calcium and phosphorus are provided to enhance bone mineralization. Formulas for both full-term and premature infants are enriched with long-chain polyunsaturated fatty acids in the hope of enhancing brain and retinal development. The infant should gradually be offered feedings of higher caloric density after a substantial volume (100–120 mL/kg/d) of either breast milk or formula (20 kcal/oz) is tolerated. Success of feedings is assessed by passage of feeds out of the stomach without emesis or large residual volumes, abdominal examination free of distention, and normal stool pattern.

When the preterm infant approaches term, the nutritional source for the bottle-fed infant can be changed to a transitional formula (22 kcal/oz) until age 6–9 months. Additional iron supplementation (2–4 mg/kg/d) is recommended for premature infants, beginning at about age 2 months. In some infants, iron supplementation may be indicated earlier. In particular, infants who are treated with erythropoietin (epoetin alfa) for prevention or treatment of anemia of prematurity require a higher dosage of 4–8 mg/kg/d.

Adamkin DH: Feeding problems in the late preterm infant. Clin Perinatol 2006;33:831 [PMID: 17148007].

Adamkin DH: Nutrition management of the very low-birthweight infant: I. Total parenteral nutrition and minimal enteral nutrition. NeoReviews 2006;7:e602.

Ehrenkranz RA: Early, aggressive nutritional management for very low birth weight infants: What is the evidence? Semin Perinatol 2007;31:48 [PMID: 17462488].

Heiman H, Schanler RJ: Enteral nutrition for premature infants: The role of human milk. Semin Fetal Neonat Med 2007;12:26 [PMID: 17185053].

Puntis JWL: Nutritional support in the premature newborn. Postgrad Med J 2006;82:192 [PMID: 16517801].

Te Braake FWJ et al: Parenteral amino acid and energy administration to premature infants in early life. Semin Fet Neonat Med 2007;12:11 [PMID: 17142119].

3. Apnea in the Preterm Infant

ESSENTIALS OF DIAGNOSIS & TYPICAL FEATURES

▸ Respiratory pause of sufficient duration to result in cyanosis or bradycardia.

▸ Most common in infants born before 34 weeks' gestation; onset before 2 weeks of age.

▸ Methylxanthines (eg, caffeine) provide effective treatment.

▶ General Considerations

Apnea is defined as a respiratory pause lasting more than 20 seconds—or any pause accompanied by cyanosis and bradycardia. Shorter respiratory pauses associated with cyanosis or bradycardia also qualify as significant apnea but must be differentiated from periodic breathing, which is common in full-term and preterm infants. Periodic breathing is defined as regularly recurring ventilatory cycles interrupted by short pauses not associated with bradycardia or color change. By definition, apnea of prematurity is not associated with a predisposing factor. However, a variety of processes may precipitate apnea (Table 1–19) and should be considered before a diagnosis of apnea of prematurity is established.

Apnea of prematurity is the most frequent cause of apnea. Most apnea of prematurity is mixed apnea characterized by a centrally (brainstem) mediated respiratory pause preceded or followed by airway obstruction. Less common is pure central or pure obstructive apnea. Apnea of prematurity is the result of immaturity of both the central respiratory regulatory centers and protective mechanisms that aid in maintaining airway patency.

▶ Clinical Findings

Onset is typically during the first 2 weeks of life. The frequency of spells gradually increases with time. Pathologic

Table 1–19. Causes of apnea in the preterm infant.

Temperature instability—both cold and heat stress
Response to passage of a feeding tube
Gastroesophageal reflux
Hypoxemia
Pulmonary parenchymal disease
Patent ductus arteriosus
?Anemia
Infection
Sepsis (viral or bacterial)
Necrotizing enterocolitis
Metabolic causes
Hypoglycemia
Intracranial hemorrhage
Posthemorrhagic hydrocephalus
Seizures
Drugs (eg, morphine)
Apnea of prematurity

apnea should be suspected if spells are sudden in onset, unusually frequent, or very severe. Apnea at birth or on the first day of life is unusual but can occur in the nonventilated preterm infant with respiratory distress syndrome. In the full-term or near-term infant, presentation at birth suggests neuromuscular abnormalities of an acute (asphyxia, birth trauma, or infection) or chronic (eg, congenital hypotonia or structural CNS lesion) nature.

All infants—regardless of the severity and frequency of apnea—require a minimum screening evaluation, including a general assessment of well-being (eg, tolerance of feedings, stable temperature, normal physical examination), a check of the association of spells with feeding, measurement of PaO_2 or SaO_2, blood glucose, hematocrit, and a review of the drug history. Infants with severe apnea of sudden onset require more extensive evaluation for primary causes, especially infection. Other specific tests are dictated by relevant signs, for example, evaluation for necrotizing enterocolitis (NEC) in an infant with apnea and abdominal distention or feeding intolerance.

▶ Treatment

Any underlying cause should be treated. If the apnea is due simply to prematurity, symptomatic treatment is dictated by the frequency and severity of apneic spells. Spells frequent enough to interfere with other aspects of care (eg, feeding), or severe enough to cause cyanosis or bradycardia necessitating bag and mask ventilation require treatment. First-line therapy is methylxanthines. Caffeine citrate (20 mg/kg as loading dose and then 5–10 mg/kg/d) is the drug of choice. Side effects of caffeine include tachycardia and feeding intolerance. The dose used should be the smallest dose necessary to decrease the frequency of apnea and eliminate severe spells. Target drug level is usually 10–20 mcg/mL. Nasal continuous positive airway pressure (CPAP), by treating the obstructive component of apnea, is effective in some infants. Intubation and ventilation can eliminate apneic spells but carry the risks associated with endotracheal intubation. Although many preterm infants are treated medically for possible reflux-associated apnea, there is little evidence to support this intervention.

Prognosis

In most premature infants, apneic and bradycardiac spells cease by 34–37 weeks postconception. Spells that require intervention cease prior to self-resolving episodes. In infants born at less than 28 weeks' gestation, episodes may continue past term. Apneic and bradycardiac episodes in the nursery are not predictors of later SIDS, although the incidence of SIDS is slightly increased in preterm infants. Thus, home monitoring in infants who experienced apnea in the nursery is rarely indicated.

4. Hyaline Membrane Disease

ESSENTIALS OF DIAGNOSIS & TYPICAL FEATURES

- ► Tachypnea, cyanosis, and expiratory grunting.
- ► Poor air movement despite increased work of breathing.
- ► Chest radiograph showing hypoexpansion and air bronchograms.

General Considerations

The most common cause of respiratory distress in the preterm infant is hyaline membrane disease. The incidence increases from 5% of infants born at 35–36 weeks' gestation to more than 50% of infants born at 26–28 weeks' gestation. This condition is caused by a deficiency of surfactant. Surfactant decreases surface tension in the alveolus during expiration, allowing the alveolus to remain partly expanded and maintain a functional residual capacity. The absence of surfactant results in poor lung compliance and atelectasis. The infant must expend a great deal of effort to expand the lungs with each breath, and respiratory failure ensues (Figure 1–9).

Clinical Findings

Infants with hyaline membrane disease show all the clinical signs of respiratory distress. On auscultation, air movement is diminished despite vigorous respiratory effort. The chest radiograph demonstrates diffuse bilateral atelectasis, causing a ground-glass appearance. Major airways are highlighted by the atelectatic air sacs, creating air bronchograms. In the unintubated child, doming of the diaphragm and underexpansion occur.

▲ **Figure 1–9.** Pressure–volume relationships for the inflation and deflation of surfactant-deficient and surfactant-treated preterm rabbit lungs. (Reproduced, with permission, from Jobe AH: The developmental biology of the lung. In: Fanaroff AA, Martin RJ [editors]: *Neonatal-Perinatal Medicine: Diseases of the Fetus and Infant,* 6th ed. Mosby, 1997.)

Treatment

Supplemental oxygen, nasal CPAP, early intubation for surfactant administration and ventilation, and placement of umbilical artery and vein lines are the initial interventions required. A ventilator that can deliver breaths synchronized with the infant's respiratory efforts (synchronized intermittent mandatory ventilation) should be used. High-frequency ventilators are available for rescue of infants doing poorly on conventional ventilation or who have air leak problems.

Surfactant replacement is used both in the delivery room as prophylaxis for infants born before 27 weeks' gestation and with established hyaline membrane disease as rescue, preferably within 2–4 hours of birth. Surfactant therapy decreases both the mortality rate in preterm infants and air leak complications of the disease. During the acute course, ventilator settings and oxygen requirements are significantly lower in surfactant-treated infants than in controls. The dose of the bovine-derived beractant (Survanta) is 4 mL/kg, the calf lung surfactant extract (Infasurf) is 3 mL/kg, and the porcine-derived poractant (Curosurf) is 1.25–2.5 mL/kg, given intratracheally. Repeat dosing is indicated in infants who remain on the ventilator in more than 30–40% oxygen. A total of two to three doses given 8–12 hours apart may be given. As the disease evolves, proteins that inhibit surfactant function leak into the air spaces, making surfactant replacement less effective. In stable infants, a trial of nasal CPAP at 5–6 cm H_2O pressure can be attempted prior to intubation and surfactant administration. For those who require mechanical ventilation, extubation to nasal CPAP should be done as early as possible to minimize lung injury and evolution of chronic lung disease. Antenatal administration of corticosteroids to the mother is an important strategy to accelerate lung maturation. Infants whose mothers were given corticosteroids more than 24 hours prior to preterm birth are less likely to have respiratory distress syndrome and have a lower mortality rate.

5. Chronic Lung Disease in the Premature Infant

▶ General Considerations

Chronic lung disease, defined as respiratory symptoms, oxygen requirement, and chest radiograph abnormalities at 36 weeks postconception, occurs in about 20% of preterm infants ventilated for surfactant deficiency. The incidence is higher at lower gestational ages and in infants exposed to chorioamnionitis prior to birth. The development of chronic lung disease is a function of lung immaturity at birth, inflammation, and exposure to high oxygen concentrations and ventilator volutrauma. Surfactant replacement therapy or early nasal CPAP has diminished the severity of chronic lung disease. The mortality rate from chronic lung disease is very low, but there is still significant morbidity secondary to reactive airway symptoms and hospital readmissions during the first 2 years of life for intercurrent respiratory infection.

▶ Treatment

Long-term supplemental oxygen, mechanical ventilation, and nasal CPAP are the primary therapies for chronic lung disease of the premature. Diuretics (furosemide, 1–2 mg/kg/d, or hydrochlorothiazide-spironolactone, 1–2 mg/kg/d), inhaled β_2-adrenergics, inhaled corticosteroids (fluticasone or budesonide), and systemic corticosteroids (dexamethasone, 0.2–0.5 mg/kg/d, or hydrocortisone, 1–3 mg/kg/d) are used as adjunctive therapy. The use of systemic corticosteroids remains controversial. Although a decrease in lung inflammation can aid infants in weaning from ventilator support, there are data associating dexamethasone use in the first several weeks of life with an increased incidence of cerebral palsy. This risk must be balanced against the higher risk of neurodevelopmental handicap in infants with severe chronic lung disease. There is likely a point in the course of these infants at which the benefit of using systemic corticosteroids for the shortest amount of time at the lowest dose possible outweighs the risk of continued mechanical ventilation. After hospital discharge, some of these infants will require oxygen at home. This can be monitored by pulse oximetry with a target SaO_2 of 94–96%. Some will continue to manifest pulmonary symptomatology into adolescence.

Ambalavanan N, Carlo WA: Ventilatory strategies in the prevention and management of bronchopulmonary dysplasia. Semin Perinatol 2006;30:192 [PMID: 16860159].

American Academy of Pediatrics Committee on Fetus and Newborn: Apnea, sudden infant death syndrome, and home monitoring. Pediatrics 2003;111:914 [PMID: 12671135].

Baveja R, Christou H: Pharmacologic strategies in the prevention and management of bronchopulmonary dysplasia. Semin Perinatol 2006;30:209 [PMID:16860161].

Chess PR et al: Pathogenesis of bronchopulmonary dysplasia. Semin Perinatol 2006;30:171 [PMID: 16860156].

DiFiore JM et al: Apnea is not prolonged by acid gastroesophageal reflux in preterm infants. Pediatrics 2005;116:1059 [PMID: 16263989].

Doyle LW et al: Bronchopulmonary dysplasia in very low birth weight subjects and lung function in late adolescence. Pediatrics 2006;118:108 [PMID: 16818555].

Doyle LW et al: Impact of postnatal systemic corticosteroids on mortality and cerebral palsy in preterm infants: Effect modification by risk for chronic lung disease. Pediatrics 2005;115:655 [PMID: 15741368].

Finer NN et al: Summary proceedings from the apnea-of-prematurity group. Pediatrics 2006;117:S47 [PMID: 16777822].

Jobe AH: The new BPD. NeoReviews 2006;7:e531.

Jobe AH: Why surfactant works for respiratory distress syndrome. NeoReviews 2006;7:e95.

Kinsella JP et al: Bronchopulmonary dysplasia. Lancet 2006;367:1421 [PMID: 16650652].

Martin RJ et al: Pathophysiologic mechanisms underlying apnea of prematurity. NeoReviews 2002;3:e59.

Speer CP et al: Pulmonary inflammation and bronchopulmonary dysplasia. J Perinatol 2006;26(Suppl 1):S57 [PMID: 16625227].

Stark AR: Risks and benefits of postnatal corticosteroids. NeoReviews 2005;6:e99.

Yeh TF et al: Outcomes at school age after postnatal dexamethasone therapy for lung disease of prematurity. N Engl J Med 2004;350:1304 [PMID: 15044641].

6. Patent Ductus Arteriosus

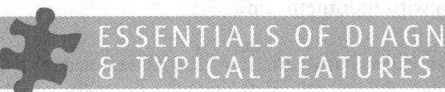

ESSENTIALS OF DIAGNOSIS & TYPICAL FEATURES

- ▶ Hyperdynamic precordium.
- ▶ Widened pulse pressure.
- ▶ Hypotension.
- ▶ Presence of a systolic heart murmur in many cases.

▶ General Considerations

Clinically significant patent ductus arteriosus usually presents on days 3–7 as the respiratory distress from hyaline membrane disease is improving. Presentation can be on days 1 or 2, especially in infants born before 28 weeks' gestation and in those who have received surfactant replacement therapy. The signs include a hyperdynamic precordium, increased peripheral pulses, and a widened pulse pressure with or without a systolic heart murmur. Early presentations are sometimes manifested by systemic hypotension without a murmur or hyperdynamic circulation. These signs are often accompanied by an increased need for respiratory support and metabolic acidemia. The presence of patent ductus arteriosus is confirmed by echocardiography.

▶ Treatment

Treatment of patent ductus arteriosus is by medical or surgical ligation. A clinically significant ductus can be closed with indomethacin (0.1–0.2 mg/kg IV q12–24h for three doses) in about two thirds of cases. If the ductus reopens or fails to close completely, a second course of drug may be used. If indomethacin fails to close the ductus or if a ductus reopens a second time, surgical ligation is appropriate. In some cases, a more prolonged course of indomethacin can be used to prevent recurrences. In addition, in the extremely low birth weight infant (< 1000 g) who is at very high risk of developing a symptomatic ductus, a prophylactic strategy of indomethacin (0.1 mg/kg q24h for 3–5 days) on the first day of life can be used. The major side effect of indomethacin is transient oliguria, which can be managed by fluid restriction until urine output improves. There may also be an increased incidence of NEC with prolonged therapy. Transient decrease in intestinal and cerebral blood flow caused by indomethacin can be ameliorated by giving the drug as a slow infusion over 1–2 hours. Indomethacin should not be used if the infant is hyperkalemic, if the creatinine is higher than 2 mg/dL, or if the platelet count is less than 50,000/mL. There is an increased incidence of intestinal perforation if used concomitantly with hydrocortisone in extremely low birth weight infants (9% versus 2% for either drug alone). Ibuprofen lysine can be used as an alternative to indomethacin given every 24 hours as an initial dose of 10 mg/kg and then 5 mg/kg for two doses. Oliguria is less severe and less frequent than with indomethacin.

Chorne N et al: Patent ductus arteriosus and its treatment as risk factors for neonatal and neurodevelopmental disability. Pediatrics 2007;119:1165 [PMID: 17545385].

Clyman RI, Chorne N: Patent ductus arteriosus: Evidence for and against treatment. J Pediatr 2007;150:216 [PMID: 17307530].

Hermes-DeSantis ER, Clyman RI: Patent ductus arteriosus: pathophysiology and management. J Perinatol 2006;26(Suppl 1):S14 [PMID:16625216].

Watterberg KL et al: Prophylaxis of early adrenal insufficiency to prevent bronchopulmonary dysplasia: A multicenter trial. Pediatrics 2004;114:1649 [PMID: 15574629].

7. Necrotizing Enterocolitis

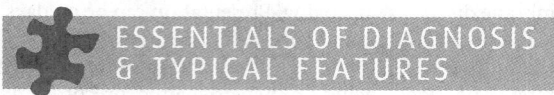

ESSENTIALS OF DIAGNOSIS & TYPICAL FEATURES

▶ Feeding intolerance with gastric residuals or vomiting.
▶ Bloody stools.
▶ Abdominal distention and tenderness.
▶ Pneumatosis intestinalis on abdominal radiograph.

General Considerations

NEC is the most common acquired GI emergency in the newborn. It is most common in preterm infants, with an incidence of 10% in infants less than 1500 g. In full-term infants, it occurs in association with polycythemia, congenital heart disease, and birth asphyxia. The pathogenesis of NEC is multifactorial. Previous intestinal ischemia, bacterial or viral infection, and immunologic immaturity of the gut are all thought to play a role. In up to 20% of affected infants, the only risk factor is prematurity. IUGR infants with a history of absent or reversed end-diastolic flow in the umbilical artery prior to delivery, have abnormalities of splanchnic flow after delivery and have an increased risk of NEC.

Clinical Findings

The most common presenting sign is abdominal distention. Other signs are vomiting, increased gastric residuals, heme-positive stools, abdominal tenderness, temperature instability, increased apnea and bradycardia, decreased urine output, and poor perfusion. There may be an increased white blood cell count with an increased band count or, as the disease progresses, absolute neutropenia. Thrombocytopenia often occurs along with stress-induced hyperglycemia and metabolic acidosis. Diagnosis is confirmed by the presence of pneumatosis intestinalis (air in the bowel wall) on a plain abdominal radiograph. There is a spectrum of disease, and milder cases may exhibit only distention of bowel loops with bowel wall edema.

Treatment

A. Medical Treatment

NEC is managed by nasogastric decompression of the gut, maintenance of oxygenation, mechanical ventilation if necessary, and IV fluids to replace third-space GI losses. Enough fluid should be given to restore good urine output. Other measures include broad-spectrum antibiotics (usually ampicillin, a third-generation cephalosporin or an aminoglycoside, and possibly additional anaerobic coverage), close monitoring of vital signs, serial physical examinations, and laboratory studies (blood gases, white blood cell count, platelet count, and radiographs). Although there are no proven strategies to prevent NEC, use of trophic feedings and cautious advancement of feeds, as well as probiotic agents in sick infants, may provide some protection.

B. Surgical Treatment

Indications for surgery are evidence of perforation (free air present on a left lateral decubitus or cross-table lateral film), a fixed dilated loop of bowel on serial radiographs, abdominal wall cellulitis, or deterioration despite maximal medical support. All of these signs are indicative of necrotic bowel. In the operating room, necrotic bowel is removed and ostomies are created. In extremely low birth weight infants, the initial surgical management may simply be the placement of peritoneal drains. Reanastomosis in infants with ostomies is performed after the disease resolves and the infant is bigger (usually > 2 kg and after 4–6 weeks).

Course & Prognosis

Infants treated medically or surgically should not be refed until the disease is resolved (normal abdominal examination and resolution of pneumatosis), usually in 10–14 days. Nutritional support during this time should be provided by total parenteral nutrition.

Death occurs in 10% of cases. Surgery is needed in fewer than 25% of cases. Long-term prognosis is determined by the amount of intestine lost. Infants with short bowel require long-term support with IV nutrition (see Chapter 20). Late strictures—about 3–6 weeks after initial diagnosis—occur in 8% of patients whether treated medically or surgically, and generally require operative management. Infants with surgically managed NEC have an increased risk of poor neurodevelopmental outcome.

Deshpande G et al: Probiotics for prevention of necrotizing enterocolitis in preterm neonates with very low birth weight: A systematic review of randomized controlled trials. Lancet 2007;369:1614 [PMID: 17499603].

Dorling J et al: Feeding growth restricted preterm infants with abnormal antenatal Doppler results. Arch Dis Child Fetal Neonatal Ed 2005;90:F359 [PMID: 16113150].

Jesse N, Neu J: NEC: Relationship to innate immunity, clinical features, and strategies for prevention. NeoReviews 2006;7:e143.

Lin PW, Stoll BJ: Necrotising enterocolitis. Lancet 2006;368:1271 [PMID: 17027734].

Moss RL et al: Laparotomy versus peritoneal drainage for necrotizing enterocolitis and perforation. N Engl J Med 2006;354:2225 [PMID: 16723614].

8. Anemia in the Premature Infant

General Considerations

In the premature infant, the hemoglobin concentration reaches its nadir at about 8–12 weeks and is 2–3 g/dL lower than that of the full-term infant. The lower nadir in premature infants appears to be the result of decreased erythropoietin response to the low red cell mass. Symptoms of anemia include poor feeding, lethargy, increased heart rate, poor weight gain, and perhaps periodic breathing.

Treatment

Transfusion is not indicated in an asymptomatic infant simply because of a low hematocrit. Most infants become symptomatic if the hematocrit drops below 20%. Infants on ventilators and supplemental oxygen are usually maintained with hematocrits above 30%. Alternatively, infants can be treated with erythropoietin (350 U/kg/d for 7–10 days for hematocrits < 28%). The therapeutic goal is to minimize blood draws and use conservative guidelines for transfusion.

Aher S, Ohlsson A: Late erythropoietin for preventing red blood cell transfusion in preterm and low birth weight infants. Cochrane Database Syst Rev 2006;(3):CD004868 [PMID: 16856064].

Murray NA, Roberts IAG: Neonatal transfusion practice. Arch Dis Child Fetal Neonatal Ed 2004;89:F101 [PMID: 14977890].

9. Intraventricular Hemorrhage

ESSENTIALS OF DIAGNOSIS & TYPICAL FEATURES

▶ Large bleeds cause hypotension, metabolic acidosis, and altered neurologic status; smaller bleeds can be asymptomatic.

▶ Routine cranial ultrasound scanning is essential for diagnosis in infants born before 32 weeks' gestation.

General Considerations

Periventricular–intraventricular hemorrhage occurs almost exclusively in premature infants. The incidence is 20–30% in infants born before 31 weeks' gestation and weighing less than 1500 g. The highest incidence occurs in infants of the lowest gestational age (< 26 weeks). Bleeding most commonly occurs in the subependymal germinal matrix (a region of undifferentiated cells adjacent to or lining the lateral ventricles). Bleeding can extend into the ventricular cavity. The proposed pathogenesis of bleeding is presented in Figure 1–10. The critical event is ischemia with reperfusion injury to the capillaries in the germinal matrix in the immediate perinatal period. The actual amount of bleeding is also influenced by a variety of factors that affect the pressure gradient across the injured capillary wall. This pathogenetic scheme applies also to intraparenchymal bleeding (venous infarction in a region rendered ischemic) and to periventricular leukomalacia (ischemic white matter injury in a watershed region of arterial supply). CNS complications in preterm infants are more frequent in infants exposed antenatally to intrauterine infection.

Clinical Findings

Up to 50% of hemorrhages occur before 24 hours of age, and virtually all occur by the fourth day. The clinical syndrome ranges from rapid deterioration (coma, hypoventilation, decerebrate posturing, fixed pupils, bulging anterior fontanelle, hypotension, acidosis, or acute drop in hematocrit), to a more gradual deterioration with more subtle neurologic changes, to absence of any specific physiologic or neurologic signs.

The diagnosis can be confirmed by real-time ultrasound scan. This is performed whenever bleeding is suspected. If symptoms are absent, routine scanning should be done at 10–14 days in all infants born before 29 weeks' gestation. Hemorrhages are graded as follows: grade I, germinal matrix hemorrhage only; grade II, intraventricular bleeding without ventricular enlargement; grade III, intraventricular bleeding with ventricular enlargement; or grade IV, any intraparenchymal bleeding. The amount of bleeding is minor (grade I or II) in 75% of infants and major in the remainder. Follow-

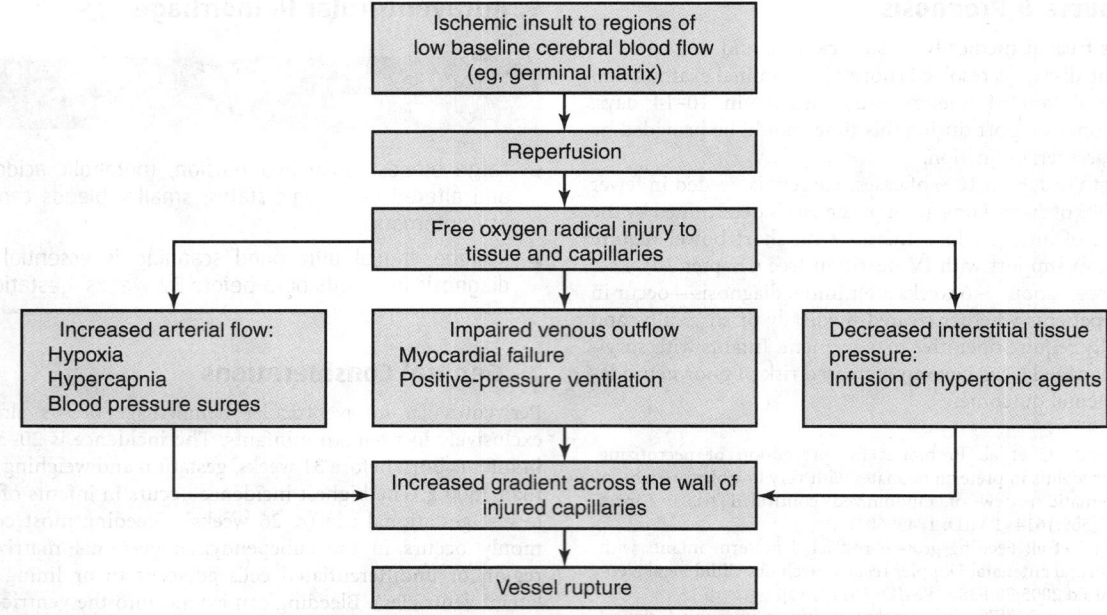

▲ Figure 1–10. Pathogenesis of periventricular and intraventricular hemorrhage.

up ultrasound examinations are scheduled based on the results of the initial scan. Infants with no bleeding or germinal matrix hemorrhage require only a single late scan at age 4–6 weeks to look for periventricular leukomalacia. An infant with blood in the ventricular system is at risk for posthemorrhagic ventriculomegaly. This is usually the result of impaired absorption of cerebrospinal fluid (CSF) but can also occur secondary to obstructive phenomena. An initial follow-up scan should be done 1–2 weeks after the initial scan. Infants with intraventricular bleeding and ventricular enlargement should be followed every 7–10 days until ventricular enlargement stabilizes or decreases.

▶ Treatment

During acute hemorrhage, supportive treatment (restoration of volume and hematocrit, oxygenation, and ventilation) should be provided to avoid further cerebral ischemia. Progressive posthemorrhagic hydrocephalus is treated initially with a subgaleal shunt. When the infant is large enough, this can be converted to a ventriculoperitoneal shunt.

Although the incidence and severity of intracranial bleeding in premature infants have decreased, strategies to prevent this complication are still needed. Maternal antenatal corticosteroids appear to decrease the risk of intracranial bleeding, and phenobarbital may have a role in the mother who has not been prepared with steroids and is delivering before 28 weeks' gestation. The route of delivery may be important as infants delivered by cesarean section have a decreased rate of intracranial bleed. Postnatal strategies are less effective. Early indomethacin administration may have some benefit in minimizing bleeding, especially in males, with unclear influence on long-term outcome.

▶ Prognosis

No deaths occur as a result of grade I and grade II hemorrhages. Grade III and grade IV hemorrhages carry a mortality rate of 10–20%. Posthemorrhagic ventricular enlargement is rarely seen with grade I hemorrhages but is seen in 54–87% of grade II–IV hemorrhages. Very few of these infants will require a ventriculoperitoneal shunt. Long-term neurologic sequelae are seen no more frequently in infants with grade I and grade II hemorrhages than in preterm infants without bleeding. In infants with grade III and grade IV hemorrhages, severe sequelae occur in 20–25% of cases, mild sequelae in 35% of cases, and no sequelae in 40% of cases. Severe periventricular leukomalacia, large parenchymal bleeds, and progressive ventriculomegaly greatly increase the risk of neurologic sequelae. It is important to note that extremely low birth weight infants without major ultrasound findings remain at increased risk for both cerebral palsy and cognitive delays. Recent reports using quantitative MRI scans demonstrate that subtle gray and white matter findings not seen with ultrasound are prevalent in preterm survivors and are predictive of neurodevelopmental handicap. This is especially true in infants born weighing less than 1000 g and before 28 weeks' gestation.

Dyet LE et al: Natural history of brain lesions in extremely preterm infants studied with serial magnetic imaging from birth and neurodevelopmental assessment. Pediatrics 2006;118:536 [PMID: 16882805].

Inder TE et al: Abnormal cerebral structure is present at term in premature infants. Pediatrics 2005;115:286 [PMID: 15687434].

Laptook AR et al: Adverse neurodevelopmental outcome among extremely low birth weight infants with normal head ultrasound: Prevalence and antecedents. Pediatrics 2005;115:673 [PMID: 15741371].

Volpe JJ: Encephalopathy of prematurity includes neuronal abnormalities. Pediatrics 2005;116:221 [PMID: 15995055].

10. Retinopathy of Prematurity

ESSENTIALS OF DIAGNOSIS & TYPICAL FEATURES

▶ Risk of severe retinopathy is greatest in the most preterm infants.

▶ Diagnosis depends on screening eye exams in at-risk preterm infants.

▶ Examination evaluates stage of abnormal retinal vascular development, extent of retinal detachment, and distribution and amount of retina involved.

Retinopathy of prematurity occurs only in the incompletely vascularized premature retina. The incidence of retinopathy in infants weighing less than 1250 g is 66%, but only 6% have retinopathy severe enough to warrant intervention. The incidence is highest in infants of the lowest gestational age. The condition appears to be triggered by an initial injury to the developing retinal vessels. Hypoxia, shock, asphyxia, vitamin E deficiency, and light exposure have been associated with this initial injury. After the initial injury, normal vessel development may follow or abnormal vascularization may occur, with ridge formation on the retina. The process can regress at this point or may continue, with growth of fibrovascular tissue into the vitreous associated with inflammation, scarring, and retinal folds or detachment. The disease is graded by stages of abnormal vascular development and retinal detachment (I–V), by the zone of the eye involved (1–3, with zone 1 being the posterior region around the macula), and by the amount of the retina involved, in "clock hours" (eg, a detachment in the upper, outer quadrant of the left eye would be defined as affecting the left retina from 12 to 3 o'clock).

Initial eye examination should be performed at 4–6 weeks of age in infants with a birth weight less than 1500 g or in those born before 28 weeks' gestation, as well as in infants weighing more than 1500 g with an unstable clinical course. Follow-up occurs at 1- to 2-week intervals until the retina is fully vascularized. Laser therapy is used in infants with progressive disease at risk for retinal detachment. Although this treatment does not always prevent retinal detachment, it reduces the incidence of poor outcomes based on visual acuity and retinal anatomy.

American Academy of Pediatrics Section on Ophthalmology, American Academy of Ophthalmology and Association for Pediatric Ophthalmology and Strabismus: Screening examination of premature infants for retinopathy of prematurity. Pediatrics 2006;117:572 [PMID: 16452383].

Drack A: Retinopathy of prematurity. Adv Pediatr 2006;53:211 [PMID: 17089868].

Early Treatment for Retinopathy of Prematurity Cooperative Group: The incidence and course of retinopathy of prematurity: Findings from the early treatment for retinopathy of prematurity study. Pediatrics 2005;116:15 [PMID: 15995025].

11. Discharge & Follow-Up of the Premature Infant

A. Hospital Discharge

Criteria for discharge of the premature infant include maintaining normal temperature in an open crib, nippling all feeds, gaining weight, and absence of apnea and bradycardia spells requiring intervention. Infants going home on supplemental oxygen should not desaturate below 80% in room air or should demonstrate the ability to arouse in response to hypoxia. Factors such as support for the mother at home and the stability of the family situation play a role in the timing of discharge. Home nursing visits and early physician follow-up can be used to hasten discharge.

B. Follow-Up

With advances in obstetric and maternal care, survival of infants born after 28 weeks' gestation or weighing as little as 1000 g at birth is now better than 90%. Seventy to 80% survive at 26–27 weeks' gestation and birth weights of 800–1000 g. Survival at gestational age 25 weeks and birth weight 700–800 g is 50–70%, with a considerable drop-off below this level (Figure 1–11).

These high rates of survival come with some morbidity. Major neurologic sequelae, including cerebral palsy, cognitive delay, and hydrocephalus, occur in 10–25% of survivors of birth weight less than 1500 g. The rate of these sequelae tends to be higher in infants with lower birth weights. Infants with birth weights less than 1000 g also have an increased rate of lesser disabilities, including learning, behavioral, and psychiatric problems. Risk factors for neurologic sequelae include seizures, grade III or IV intracranial hemorrhage, periventricular leukomalacia, ventricular dilation, white matter abnormalities on term-equivalent MRI examinations, severe IUGR, poor early head growth, need for mechanical ventilation, chronic lung disease, NEC, and low socioeconomic class. Maternal fever and chorioamnionitis are associated with an increased risk of cerebral palsy. Other morbidities include chronic lung disease and reactive airway disease, resulting in increased severity of respiratory infections and hospital readmissions in the first 2 years; retinopathy of prematurity with

Mortality by birth weight
Vermont Oxford Network 2004

▲ **Figure 1–11.** Mortality rates before discharge by 100-g birth weight subgroups in 2004. (Reproduced, with permission, from the Vermont Oxford Network, 2005.)

associated loss of visual acuity and strabismus; hearing loss; and growth failure. All of these issues require close multidisciplinary outpatient follow-up. Infants with residual lung disease are candidates for monthly palivizumab (Synagis) injections during their first winter after hospital discharge to prevent infection with respiratory syncytial virus. Routine immunizations should be given at the appropriate chronologic age and should not be age-corrected for prematurity.

American Academy of Pediatrics, Committee on Infectious Diseases and Committee on Fetus and Newborn: Revised indications for the use of palivizumab and respiratory syncytial virus immune globulin intravenous for the prevention of respiratory syncytial virus infection. Pediatrics 2003;112:1442 [PMID: 14654628].

Ehrenkranz, RA et al: Growth in the neonatal intensive care unit influences neurodevelopment and growth outcomes of extremely low birth weight infants. Pediatrics 2006;117:1253 [PMID: 16585322].

Hack M et al: Behavioral outcomes and evidence of psychopathology among very low birth weight infants at age 20 years. Pediatrics 2004;114:932 [PMID: 15466087].

Hack M et al: Chronic conditions, functional limitations, and special healthcare needs of school-aged children born with extremely low-birth-weight in the 1990's. JAMA 2005;294:318 [PMID: 16030276].

Ho S, Saigal S: Current survival and early outcomes of infants of borderline viability. NeoReviews 2005;6:e123.

Marlow N et al: Neurologic and developmental disability at six years of age after extremely preterm birth. N Engl J Med 2005;352:9 [PMID: 15635108].

Saigal S et al: Transition of extremely low-birth-weight infants from adolescence to young adulthood. Comparison with normal birth-weight controls. JAMA 2006;295:667 [PMID: 16467235].

Wilson-Costello D et al: Improved neurodevelopmental outcome for extremely low birth weight infants in 2000-2002. Pediatrics 2007;119:37 [PMID: 17200269].

Woodward LJ et al: Neonatal MRI to predict neurodevelopmental outcomes in preterm infants. N Engl J Med 2006;355–385 [PMID: 16914704].

THE LATE PRETERM INFANT

The rate of preterm births in the United States has increased 31% since 1981. The largest contribution to this increase is from births between 34 and 36 completed weeks of gestation, which now represent 70% of preterm births in the United States. Compared with term infants, late preterm infants have higher frequencies of respiratory distress, temperature instability, hypoglycemia, kernicterus, apnea, seizures, feeding problems, and rehospitalization after hospital discharge. The respiratory issues are caused by lack of clearance of lung fluid or relative deficiency of pulmonary surfactant, or both. Feeding issues are caused by lack of coordination of suck and swallow, which can interfere with bottle feeding and delay successful breast feeding, putting the infant at risk for poor weight gain and dehydration. Related both to feeding issues and immaturity, these infants have an eightfold increased risk of developing a TSB level above 20 mg/dL when compared with infants born after 40 completed weeks. As a consequence, late preterm infants are overrepresented in the kernicterus registry. Rehospitalizations due to jaundice, proven or suspected infection, feeding difficulties, and failure to thrive are much more common than in term infants. Late preterm infants should be considered preterm rather than near term and require close in-hospital monitoring after birth for complications. After nursery discharge, close outpatient follow-up is indicated, especially if they are sent home within 48–72 hours after birth.

Adamkin DH: Feeding problems in the late preterm infant. Clin Perinatol 2006;33:831 [PMID: 17148007].

Raju TNK et al: Optimizing care and outcome for late-preterm (near-term) infants: A summary of the workshop sponsored by the National Institute of Child Health and Human Development. Pediatrics 2006;118:1207 [PMID: 16951017].

Watchko JF: Hyperbilirubinemia and bilirubin toxicity in the late preterm infant. Clin Perinatol 2006;33:839 [PMID: 17148008].

Young PC et al: Mortality of late-preterm (near-term) newborns in Utah. Pediatrics 2007;119:e659 [PMID: 17332185].

CARDIAC PROBLEMS IN THE NEWBORN INFANT

STRUCTURAL HEART DISEASE

1. Cyanotic Presentations

ESSENTIALS OF DIAGNOSIS & TYPICAL FEATURES

► Cyanosis, initially without associated respiratory distress.
► Failure to increase PaO_2 with supplemental oxygen.
► Chest radiograph with decreased lung markings suggests right heart obstruction, while increased lung markings suggest transposition or pulmonary venous obstruction.

▶ General Considerations

The causes of cyanotic heart disease in the newborn are transposition of the great vessels, total anomalous pulmo-nary venous return, truncus arteriosus (some types), tricuspid atresia, and pulmonary atresia or critical pulmonary stenosis.

▶ Clinical Findings

Infants with these disorders present with early cyanosis. The hallmark of many of these lesions is cyanosis without associated respiratory distress. In most of these infants, tachypnea develops over time either because of increased pulmonary blood flow or secondary to metabolic acidemia from progressive hypoxemia. Diagnostic aids include comparing the blood gas or oxygen saturation in room air to that in 100% FIO_2. Failure of PaO_2 or SaO_2 to increase suggests cyanotic heart disease. *Note:* A PaO_2, if feasible, is the preferred measure. Saturation in the newborn may be misleadingly high despite pathologically low PaO_2 due to the left-shifted oxyhemoglobin dissociation curve seen with fetal hemoglobin. Other useful aids are chest radiography, electrocardiography, and echocardiography.

Transposition of the great vessels is the most common form of cyanotic heart disease presenting in the newborn. Examination generally reveals a systolic murmur and single S_2. Chest radiograph shows a generous heart size and a narrow mediastinum with normal or increased lung markings. There is little change in PaO_2 or SaO_2 with supplemental oxygen. Total anomalous pulmonary venous return, in which venous return is obstructed, presents early with severe cyanosis and tachypnea because the pulmonary venous return is obstructed, resulting in pulmonary edema. The chest radiograph typically shows a small to normal heart size with marked pulmonary edema. Infants with right heart obstruction (pulmonary and tricuspid atresia, critical pulmonary stenosis, and some forms of truncus arteriosus) have decreased lung markings on chest radiographs and, depending on the severity of hypoxia, may develop metabolic acidemia. Those lesions with an underdeveloped right heart will have left-sided predominance on electrocardiography. Although tetralogy of Fallot is the most common form of cyanotic heart disease, the obstruction at the pulmonary valve is often not severe enough to result in cyanosis in the newborn. In all cases, diagnosis can be confirmed by echocardiography.

2. Acyanotic Presentations

ESSENTIALS OF DIAGNOSIS & TYPICAL FEATURES

► Most newborns with acyanotic heart disease have left-sided outflow obstruction.
► Differentially diminished pulses (coarctation) or decreased pulses throughout (aortic atresia).
► Metabolic acidemia.

▶ Chest radiograph showing large heart and pulmonary edema.

General Considerations

Newborn infants who present with serious acyanotic heart disease usually have congestive heart failure secondary to left-sided outflow tract obstruction. Infants with left-to-right shunt lesions (eg, ventricular septal defect) may have murmurs in the newborn period, but clinical symptoms do not occur until pulmonary vascular resistance drops enough to cause significant shunting and subsequent congestive heart failure (usually at 3–4 weeks of age).

Clinical Findings

Infants with left-sided outflow obstruction generally do well the first day or so until the ductus arteriosus—the source of all or some of the systemic flow—narrows. Tachypnea, tachycardia, congestive heart failure, and metabolic acidosis develop. On examination, all of these infants have abnormalities of the pulses. In aortic atresia (hypoplastic left heart syndrome) and stenosis, pulses are all diminished, whereas in coarctation syndromes, differential pulses (diminished or absent in the lower extremities) are evident. Chest radiographic films in these infants show a large heart and pulmonary edema. Diagnosis is confirmed with echocardiography.

3. Treatment of Cyanotic & Acyanotic Lesions

Early stabilization includes supportive therapy as needed (eg, IV glucose, oxygen, ventilation for respiratory failure, and pressor support). Specific therapy includes infusions of prostaglandin E_1 (0.025–0.1 µg/kg/min) to maintain ductal patency. In some cyanotic lesions (eg, pulmonary atresia, tricuspid atresia, and critical pulmonary stenosis) in which lung blood flow is ductus-dependent, this improves pulmonary blood flow and PaO_2 by allowing shunting through the ductus to the pulmonary artery. In left-sided outflow tract obstruction, systemic blood flow is ductus-dependent; prostaglandins improve systemic perfusion and resolve the acidosis. Further specific management—including palliative surgical and cardiac catheterization procedures—is discussed in Chapter 19. Neurodevelopmental outcome with congenital heart disease depends on the lesion, severity of neonatal presentation, and complications related to palliative and corrective surgery.

PERSISTENT PULMONARY HYPERTENSION

ESSENTIALS OF DIAGNOSIS & TYPICAL FEATURES

▶ Onset of symptoms on day 1 of life.

▶ Hypoxia with poor response to high concentrations of inspired oxygen.

▶ Right-to-left shunts through the foramen ovale, ductus arteriosus, or both.

▶ Most often associated with parenchymal lung disease.

General Considerations

Persistent pulmonary hypertension of the newborn (PPHN) results when the normal decrease in pulmonary vascular resistance after birth does not occur. Most affected infants are full term or postterm, and many have experienced perinatal asphyxia. Other clinical associations include hypothermia, meconium aspiration syndrome, hyaline membrane disease, polycythemia, neonatal sepsis, chronic intrauterine hypoxia, and pulmonary hypoplasia.

There are three underlying pathophysiologic mechanisms of PPHN: (1) vasoconstriction due to perinatal hypoxia related to an acute event such as sepsis or asphyxia; (2) prenatal increase in pulmonary vascular smooth muscle development, often associated with meconium aspiration syndrome; and (3) decreased cross-sectional area of the pulmonary vascular bed associated with lung hypoplasia (eg, diaphragmatic hernia).

Clinical Findings

Clinically, the syndrome is characterized by onset on the first day of life, usually from birth. Respiratory distress is prominent, and PaO_2 is usually poorly responsive to high concentrations of inspired oxygen. Many infants have associated myocardial depression with systemic hypotension. Echocardiography reveals right-to-left shunting at the level of the ductus arteriosus or foramen ovale, or both. The chest radiograph usually shows lung infiltrates related to associated pulmonary pathology (eg, meconium aspiration and hyaline membrane disease). If the majority of right-to-left shunting is at the ductal level, pre- and postductal differences in PaO_2 and SaO_2 will be observed.

Treatment

Therapy for PPHN involves treatment of other postasphyxia problems such as seizures, renal failure, hypoglycemia, and infection. Specific therapy is aimed at both increasing systemic arterial pressure and decreasing pulmonary arterial pressure to reverse the right-to-left shunting through fetal pathways. First-line therapy includes oxygen and ventilation (to reduce pulmonary vascular resistance) and crystalloid infusions (10 mL/kg, up to 30 mL/kg) to improve systemic pressure. Ideally, systolic pressure should be greater than 50 mm Hg. With compromised cardiac function, systemic pressors can be used as second-line therapy (eg, dopamine, 5–20 mcg/kg/min; dobutamine, 5–20 mcg/kg/ min; or both). Metabolic acidemia should be corrected because acidemia exacerbates pulmonary vasoconstriction. In some cases, a mild respiratory alkalosis may improve oxygenation. Pulmonary vasodilation can be enhanced using inhaled nitric oxide, which is identical or very similar to endogenous endothelium-derived relaxing factor, at doses of 5–20 ppm. High-frequency oscillatory ventilation has proved effective in many of these infants, particularly those with severe associated lung disease. Infants for whom conventional therapy is failing (poor oxygenation despite maximum support) may require extracorporeal membrane oxygenation (ECMO). The lungs are essentially at rest during ECMO, and with resolution of pulmonary hypertension infants are weaned from ECMO back to ventilator therapy. Approximately 10–15% of survivors of PPHN have significant neurologic sequelae, with cerebral palsy or cognitive delays. Other sequelae such as chronic lung disease, sensorineural hearing loss, and feeding problems have also been reported.

ARRHYTHMIAS

Irregularly irregular heart rates, commonly associated with premature atrial contractions and less commonly with premature ventricular contractions, are common in the first days of life in well newborns. These arrhythmias are benign. Clinically significant bradyarrhythmias are seen in association with congenital heart block. Heart block can be seen in an otherwise structurally normal heart (associated with maternal lupus) or with structural cardiac abnormalities. In the absence of fetal hydrops, the bradyarrhythmia is often well tolerated. Cardiac pacing may be required if there are symptoms of inadequate cardiac output.

On ECG, tachyarrhythmias can be either wide complex (ventricular tachycardia) or narrow complex (supraventricular tachycardia). Supraventricular tachycardia is the most common neonatal tachyarrhythmia and may be a sign of structural heart disease, myocarditis, left atrial enlargement, and aberrant conduction pathways. Acute treatment is ice to the face, and if unsuccessful, IV adenosine (50–200 mcg/kg). If there is no response, the dose can be increased to 300 mcg/kg. Long-term therapy is with digoxin or propranolol. Digoxin should not be used in infants with Wolff-Parkinson-White syndrome. Cardioversion is rarely needed for supraventricular tachycardia but is needed acutely for hemodynamically unstable ventricular tachycardia.

Kothari DS, Skinner JR: Neonatal tachycardias: An update. Arch Dis Child Fetal Neonatal Ed 2006;91:F136 [PMID: 16492952].

Larmay HJ, Strasburger JF: Differential diagnosis and management of the fetus and newborn with an irregular or abnormal heart rate. Pediatr Clin North Am 2004;51:1033 [PMID: 15275987].

Silberbach M, Hannan D: Presentation of congenital heart disease in the neonate and young infant. Pediatr Rev 2007;28:123 [PMID: 17400823].

Steinhorn RH, Farrow KN: Pulmonary hypertension in the neonate. NeoReviews 2007;8:e14.

GASTROINTESTINAL & ABDOMINAL SURGICAL CONDITIONS IN THE NEWBORN INFANT (SEE ALSO CHAPTER 20)

ESOPHAGEAL ATRESIA & TRACHEOESOPHAGEAL FISTULA

ESSENTIALS OF DIAGNOSIS & TYPICAL FEATURES

▶ Polyhydramnios.

▶ Excessive drooling and secretions; choking with attempted feeding.

▶ Unable to pass an orogastric tube to the stomach.

General Considerations

Esophageal atresia is characterized by a blind esophageal pouch with or without a fistulous connection between the proximal or distal esophagus (or both) and the airway. In 85% of infants, the fistula is between the distal esophagus and the airway. Polyhydramnios is common because of high GI obstruction. Incidence is approximately 1 in 3000 births.

Clinical Findings

Infants present in the first hours of life with copious secretions, choking, cyanosis, and respiratory distress. Diagnosis is confirmed with chest radiograph after careful placement of a nasogastric (NG) tube to the point at which resistance is met. The tube will be seen radiographically in the blind pouch. If a tracheoesophageal fistula is present to the distal esophagus, gas will be present in the bowel. In esophageal atresia without tracheoesophageal fistula, there is no gas in the bowel.

Treatment

The NG tube in the proximal pouch should be placed on low intermittent suction to drain secretions and prevent aspiration. The head of the bed should be elevated to prevent reflux of gastric contents through the distal fistula into the lungs. IV glucose and fluids should be provided and oxygen administered as needed. Definitive treatment is surgical, and the technique used depends on the distance between the segments of esophagus. If the distance is not too great, the fistula can be ligated and the ends of the esophagus anastomosed. If the ends of the esophagus cannot be brought together, the initial surgery is fistula ligation and a feeding gastrostomy. Echocardiography should be performed prior to surgery to rule out a right-sided aortic arch (for which a left-sided thoracotomy would be preferred).

Prognosis

Prognosis is determined primarily by the presence or absence of associated anomalies. Vertebral, anal, cardiac, renal, and limb anomalies are the most likely to be observed (VACTERL association). Evaluation for associated anomalies should be initiated early.

INTESTINAL OBSTRUCTION

ESSENTIALS OF DIAGNOSIS & TYPICAL FEATURES

▶ Infants with high intestinal obstruction present soon after birth with emesis.

▶ Bilious emesis suggests intestinal malrotation with midgut volvulus until proved otherwise.

▶ Low intestinal obstruction is characterized by abdominal distention and late onset of emesis.

▶ General Considerations

A history of polyhydramnios is common, and the fluid, if bile-stained, can easily be confused with thin meconium staining. The higher the location of the obstruction in the intestine, the earlier the infant will develop vomiting and the less prominent the distention will be. The opposite is true for lower intestinal obstructions. Most obstructions are bowel atresias, believed to be caused by an ischemic event during development. Approximately 30% of cases of duodenal atresia are associated with Down syndrome. Meconium ileus is a distal small bowel obstruction caused by the viscous meconium produced in utero by infants with pancreatic insufficiency secondary to cystic fibrosis. Hirschsprung disease is caused by a failure of neuronal migration to the myenteric

plexus of the distal bowel. The distal bowel lacks ganglion cells, causing a lack of peristalsis in that region with a functional obstruction.

Malrotation with midgut volvulus is a surgical emergency that appears in the first days to weeks as bilious vomiting without distention or tenderness. If malrotation is not treated promptly, torsion of the intestine around the superior mesenteric artery will lead to necrosis of the small bowel. For this reason, bilious vomiting in the neonate always demands immediate attention and evaluation.

▶ Clinical Findings

Diagnosis of intestinal obstructions depends on plain abdominal radiographs with either upper GI series (high obstruction suspected) or contrast enema (lower obstruction apparent) to define the area of obstruction. Table 1–20 summarizes the findings expected.

Infants with meconium ileus are presumed to have cystic fibrosis. Infants with pancolonic Hirschsprung disease, colon pseudo-obstruction syndrome, or colonic dysgenesis or atresia may also present with meconium impacted in the distal ileum. Definitive diagnosis of cystic fibrosis is by the sweat chloride test (Na^+ and Cl^- concentration > 60 mEq/L) or by genetic testing. Approximately 10–20% of infants with cystic fibrosis have meconium ileus. Infants with cystic fibrosis and meconium ileus generally have a normal immunoreactive trypsinogen on their newborn screen because of the associated severe exocrine pancreatic insufficiency in utero.

Intestinal perforation in utero results in meconium peritonitis with residual intra-abdominal calcifications. Many perforations are completely healed at birth. If the infant has no signs of obstruction, no immediate evaluation is needed.

Table 1–20. Intestinal obstruction.

Site of Obstruction	Clinical Findings	Plain Radiographs	Contrast Study
Duodenal atresia	Down syndrome (30–50%); early vomiting, sometimes bilious	"Double bubble" (dilated stomach and proximal duodenum, no air distal)	Not needed
Malrotation and volvulus	Bilious vomiting with onset anytime in the first few weeks	Dilated stomach and proximal duodenum; paucity of air distally (may be normal gas pattern)	UGI shows displaced duodenojejunal junction with "corkscrew" deformity of twisted bowel
Jejunoileal atresia, meconium ileus	Bilious gastric contents > 25 mL at birth; progressive distention and bilious vomiting	Multiple dilated loops of bowel; intra-abdominal calcifications if in-utero perforation occurred (meconium peritonitis)	Barium or osmotic contrast enema shows microcolon; contrast refluxed into distal ileum may demonstrate and relieve meconium obstruction (successful in about 50% of cases)
Meconium plug syndrome; Hirschsprung disease	Distention, delayed stooling (> 24 h)	Diffuse bowel distention	Barium or osmotic contrast enema outlines and relieves plug; may show transition zone in Hirschsprung disease; delayed emptying (> 24 h) suggests Hirschsprung disease

UGI, upper gastrointestinal contrast study.

A sweat test to rule out cystic fibrosis should be done at a later date.

Low intestinal obstruction may present with delayed stooling (> 24 hours in term infants is abnormal) with mild distention. Radiographic findings of gaseous distention should prompt contrast enema to diagnose (and treat) meconium plug syndrome. If no plug is found, the diagnosis may be small left colon syndrome (occurring in IDMs) or Hirschsprung disease. Rectal biopsy will be required to clarify these two diagnoses. Imperforate anus is generally apparent on physical examination, although a rectovaginal fistula with a mildly abnormal–appearing anus can occasionally be confused with normal. High imperforate anus in males may be associated with rectourethral or rectovesical fistula.

▶ Treatment

NG suction to decompress the bowel, IV glucose, fluid and electrolyte replacement, and respiratory support as necessary should be instituted. Antibiotics are usually indicated due to the bowel distention and possibility of translocation of bacteria. The definitive treatment for these conditions (with the exception of meconium plug syndrome, small left colon syndrome, and some cases of meconium ileus) is surgical.

▶ Prognosis

Up to 10% of infants with meconium plug syndrome are subsequently found to have cystic fibrosis or Hirschsprung disease. For this reason, it is appropriate to obtain a sweat chloride test and rectal biopsy in all of these infants before discharge. The infant with meconium plug syndrome who is still symptomatic after contrast enema should have a rectal biopsy.

In duodenal atresia associated with Down syndrome, the prognosis depends on associated anomalies (eg, heart defects) and the severity of prestenotic duodenal dilation and subsequent duodenal dysmotility. Otherwise, these conditions usually carry an excellent prognosis after surgical repair.

ABDOMINAL WALL DEFECTS

1. Omphalocele

Omphalocele is a membrane-covered herniation of abdominal contents into the base of the umbilical cord. There is a high incidence of associated anomalies (cardiac, GI, and chromosomal—eg, trisomy 13). The sac may contain liver and spleen as well as intestine.

At delivery, the omphalocele is covered with a sterile dressing soaked with warm saline to prevent fluid loss. NG decompression is performed, and IV fluids, glucose, and antibiotics are given. If the contents of the omphalocele will fit into the abdomen and can be covered with skin, muscle, or both, primary surgical closure is done. If not, staged closure is performed, with placement of a Gore-Tex patch over the exposed contents, and gradual coverage of the patch by skin over days to weeks. A large ventral hernia is left, which is repaired in the future.

2. Gastroschisis

In gastroschisis, the uncovered intestine extrudes through a small abdominal wall defect lateral to the umbilical cord. There is no membrane or sac and no liver or spleen outside the abdomen. Gastroschisis is associated with intestinal atresia in approximately 10% of infants. The evisceration is thought to be related to abnormal involution of the right umbilical vein, although the exact cause is unknown. The prevalence of gastroschisis has been increasing over the past 20 years, from 0.03% to 0.1%. Environmental factors, including use of drugs such as methamphetamine and cocaine, may be involved.

Therapy initially involves placing the bowel of the infant into a silastic bowel bag to decrease fluid and electrolyte losses as well as to conserve heat. IV fluids, antibiotics, and low intermittent gastric suction are required. The infant is placed right side down to preserve bowel perfusion. Subsequent therapy involves replacement of the bowel into the abdominal cavity. This is done as a single primary procedure if the amount of bowel to be replaced is small. If the amount of bowel is large, staged closure with placement of a silastic silo and gradual reduction of the bowel into the underdeveloped abdominal cavity over several days is the preferred method of treatment. Postoperatively, third-space fluid losses may be extensive; fluid and electrolyte therapy, therefore, must be monitored carefully. Bowel motility, especially duodenal, may be slow to return if the bowel was dilated, thickened, matted together, and covered with a fibrinous "peel" at delivery. Prolonged intravenous nutrition may be required.

DIAPHRAGMATIC HERNIA

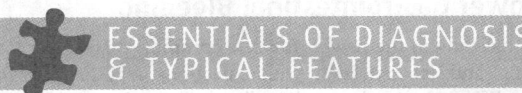

ESSENTIALS OF DIAGNOSIS & TYPICAL FEATURES

- ▶ Respiratory distress from birth.
- ▶ Poor breath sounds; flat or scaphoid abdomen.
- ▶ Bowel loops seen in the chest with mediastinal shift to opposite side on chest radiograph.

This congenital malformation consists of herniation of abdominal organs into the hemithorax (usually left-sided) through a posterolateral defect in the diaphragm. It presents in the delivery room as severe respiratory distress in an infant with poor breath sounds and scaphoid abdomen. The rapidity and severity of presentation depend on several factors: the degree of pulmonary hypoplasia resulting from lung compression by the intrathoracic abdominal contents in utero; degree of associated pulmonary hypertension; and associated anomalies, especially chromosomal abnormalities and congenital cardiac defects. Affected infants are prone to development of pneumothorax during attempts at ventilation of the hypoplastic lungs.

Treatment includes intubation, mechanical ventilation, and decompression of the GI tract with an NG tube. An IV infusion of glucose and fluid should be started. A chest radiograph confirms the diagnosis. Surgery to reduce the abdominal contents from the thorax and close the diaphragmatic defect is delayed until after the infant is stabilized and pulmonary hypertension and compliance have improved, usually after 24–48 hours. Both pre- and postoperatively, pulmonary hypertension may require therapy with high-frequency oscillatory ventilation, inhaled nitric oxide, or ECMO. The survival rate for infants with this condition is improving, and now approaches 80–90%, with survival dependent on the degree of pulmonary hypoplasia and presence of congenital heart disease or chromosomal abnormalities. Use of a gentle ventilation style and permissive hypercarbia is recommended to avoid barotrauma and further lung injury.

GASTROINTESTINAL BLEEDING

▶ Upper Gastrointestinal Bleeding

Upper GI bleeding sometimes occurs in the newborn nursery, but is rarely severe. Old blood ("coffee-grounds" material) in the stomach of the newborn may be either swallowed maternal blood or infant blood from gastritis or stress ulcer. Bright red blood from the stomach is most likely from acute bleeding, again due to gastritis. Treatment generally consists of gastric lavage (a sample can be sent for Apt testing or blood typing to determine if it is mother's or baby's blood) and antacid medication. If the volume of bleeding is large, intensive monitoring, fluid and blood replacement, and endoscopy are indicated. Coagulation studies should also be sent. (See Chapter 20.)

▶ Lower Gastrointestinal Bleeding

Rectal bleeding in the newborn is less common than upper GI bleeding and is associated with infections (eg, *Salmonella* acquired from the mother perinatally), milk intolerance (blood streaks with diarrhea), or, in ill infants, NEC. An abdominal radiograph should be obtained to rule out pneumatosis intestinalis or other abnormalities in gas pattern suggesting inflammation, infection, or obstruction. If the radiograph is negative and the examination is benign, a protein hydrolysate or predigested formula (eg, Nutramigen or Pregestimil) should be tried. The nursing mother should be instructed to avoid all dairy products in her diet. If the amount of rectal bleeding is large or persistent, endoscopy may be needed.

GASTROESOPHAGEAL REFLUX (SEE ALSO CHAPTER 20)

Physiologic regurgitation is common in infants. Reflux is pathologic and should be treated when it results in failure to thrive owing to excessive regurgitation, poor intake due to

dysphagia and irritability, apnea or cyanotic episodes, or chronic respiratory symptoms of wheezing and recurrent pneumonias. Diagnosis is clinical, with confirmation by pH probe or impedance study. Barium radiography is helpful to rule out anatomic abnormalities but is not diagnostic of pathologic reflux.

Initial steps in treatment include thickened feeds (rice cereal, 1 tbsp/oz of formula) for those with frequent regurgitation and poor weight gain. Gastric acid suppressants such as ranitidine (2 mg/kg bid) or lansoprazole (1.5 mg/kg/d) can also be used, especially if there is associated irritability. Prokinetic agents such as metoclopramide are of little benefit and have significant side effects. Because most infants improve by 12–15 months of age, surgery is reserved for the most severe cases, especially those with chronic neurologic or respiratory conditions that exacerbate reflux, and those who have life-threatening events caused by reflux.

Chabra S: Management of gastroschisis: Prenatal, perinatal, and neonatal. NeoReviews 2006;7:e419.

De la Hunt MN: The acute abdomen in the newborn. Semin Fet Neonat Med 2006;11:191 [PMID: 16616711].

Eggink BH et al: Outcome of gastroschisis: A 20-year case review of infants with gastroschisis born in Galveston, Texas. J Pediatr Surg 2006;41:1103 [PMID: 16769342].

Goyal A et al: Oesophageal atresia and tracheo-oesophageal fistula. Arch Dis Child Fetal Neonatal Ed 2006;91:F381 [PMID: 16923940].

Kays DW: Congenital diaphragmatic hernia: Real improvements in survival. NeoReviews 2006;7:e428.

Kays DW: Congenital diaphragmatic hernia and neonatal lung lesions. Surg Clin North Am 2006;86:329 [PMID: 16580927].

Keckler SJ et al: VACTERL anomalies in patients with esophageal atresia: An updated delineation of the spectrum and review of the literature. Pediatr Surg Int 2007;23:309 [PMID: 17377826].

Vandenplas Y et al: Will esophageal impedance replace pH monitoring? Pediatrics 2007;119:118 [PMID: 17200278].

▼ INFECTIONS IN THE NEWBORN INFANT

The fetus and the newborn are susceptible to infections. There are three major routes of perinatal infection: (1) blood-borne transplacental infection of the fetus (eg, cytomegalovirus, rubella, and syphilis); (2) ascending infection with disruption of the barrier provided by the amniotic membranes (eg, bacterial infections after 12–18 hours of ruptured membranes); and (3) infection on passage through an infected birth canal or exposure to infected blood at delivery (eg, herpes simplex, hepatitis B, HIV, and bacterial infections).

Susceptibility of the newborn infant to infection is related to immaturity of both the cellular and humoral immune systems at birth. This feature is particularly evident in the preterm neonate. Passive protection against some organisms is provided by transfer of IgG across the placenta during the third trimester of pregnancy. Preterm infants, especially those born before 30 weeks' gestation, do not have the full amount of passively acquired antibody.

BACTERIAL INFECTIONS

1. Bacterial Sepsis

ESSENTIALS OF DIAGNOSIS & TYPICAL FEATURES

▸ Most infants with early-onset sepsis present at < 24 hours of age.

▸ Respiratory distress is the most common presenting symptom.

▸ Hypotension, acidemia, and neutropenia are associated clinical findings.

▸ The presentation of late-onset sepsis is more subtle.

▸ General Considerations

The incidence of early-onset (< 5 days) neonatal bacterial infection is 4–5 in 1000 live births. If rupture of the membranes occurs more than 24 hours prior to delivery, the infection rate increases to 1 in 100 live births. If early rupture of membranes with chorioamnionitis occurs, the infection rate increases further to 1 in 10 live births. Regardless of membrane rupture, infection rates are five times higher in preterm than in full-term infants.

▸ Clinical Findings

Early-onset bacterial infections appear most commonly on day 1 of life, and the majority appear at less than 12 hours. Respiratory distress due to pneumonia is the most common presenting sign. Other features include unexplained low Apgar scores without fetal distress, poor perfusion, and hypotension. Late-onset bacterial infection (> 5 days of age) presents in a more subtle manner, with poor feeding, lethargy, hypotonia, temperature instability, altered perfusion, new or increased oxygen requirement, and apnea. Late-onset bacterial sepsis is more often associated with meningitis or other localized infections.

Low total white count, absolute neutropenia (< 1000/mL), and elevated ratio of immature to mature neutrophils all suggest neonatal bacterial infection. Thrombocytopenia is also a common feature. Other laboratory signs are hypoglycemia or hyperglycemia with no change in glucose administration, unexplained metabolic acidosis, and elevated C-reactive protein. In early-onset bacterial infection, pneumonia is invariably present; chest radiography shows infiltrates, but these infiltrates cannot be distinguished from those resulting from other causes of neonatal lung disease. Presence of a pleural effusion makes a diagnosis of pneumonia more likely. Definitive diagnosis is made by positive cultures from blood, CSF, and the like.

Early-onset infection is most often caused by group B β-hemolytic streptococci (GBS) and gram-negative enteric pathogens (most commonly *Escherichia coli*). Other organ-isms to consider are *Haemophilus influenzae* and *Listeria monocytogenes*. Late-onset sepsis is caused by coagulase-negative staphylococci (most common in infants with indwelling central venous lines), *Staphylococcus aureus*, GBS, *Enterococcus*, and gram-negative organisms.

▸ Treatment

A high index of suspicion is important in diagnosis and treatment of neonatal infection. Table 1–21 presents guidelines for the evaluation and treatment of full-term infants with risk factors or clinical signs of infection. Because the risk of infection is greater in the preterm infant and because respiratory disease is a common sign of infection, any preterm infant with respiratory disease requires blood cultures and broad-spectrum antibiotic therapy for 48–72 hours pending the results of cultures. Early-onset sepsis is usually caused by GBS or gram-negative enteric organisms; broad-spectrum coverage, therefore, should include ampicillin plus an aminoglycoside or third-generation cephalosporin—for example, ampicillin, 100–150 mg/kg/d divided q12h, and gentamicin, 2.5 mg/kg per dose q12–24h (depending on gestational age), or cefotaxime, 100 mg/kg/d divided q12h. In infants older than 34 weeks' gestation, gentamicin can also be given at a dosage of 4 mg/kg q24h. Late-onset infections can also be caused by the same organisms, but coverage may need

Table 1–21. Guidelines for evaluation of neonatal bacterial infection in the full-term infant.

Risk Factor	Clinical Signs of Infection	Evaluation and Treatment
Delivery 12–18 h after rupture of membranes	None	Observation
Delivery > 12–18 h after rupture of membranes, chorioamnionitis	None	CBC, blood culture, broad-spectrum antibiotics for 48–72 h[a]
Delivery > 12–18 h after rupture of membranes, chorioamnionitis, maternal antibiotics[b]	None	CBC, blood culture, broad-spectrum antibiotics for 48–72 h[a]
With or without risk factors	Present	CBC, blood and CSF cultures, perhaps urine culture (see below); broad-spectrum antibiotics[c]

[a]If clinical signs are absent, close observation without treatment may be sufficient.
[b]Minimum of 24 h of observation is indicated if no treatment is given.
[c]Irrespective of age at presentation, any infant who appears infected by clinical criteria should undergo CSF examination. Urine culture is indicated in the evaluation of infants who were initially well but have developed symptoms after 2–3 days of age.
CBC, complete blood count; CSF, cerebrospinal fluid.

Vaginal and Rectal GBS Cultures at 35–37 Weeks' Gestation for ALL Pregnant Women[a]

IAP INDICATED	

• Previous infant with invasive GBS disease
• GBS bacteriuria during current pregnancy
• Positive GBS screening culture during current pregnancy (*unless* a planned cesarean delivery is performed in the absence of labor or membrane rupture)
• Unknown GBS status *AND* any of the following:
  • Delivery at <37 weeks' gestation
  • Membranes ruptured for ≥18 hours
  • Intrapartum fever (temperature ≥ 38.0°C [>100.4°F])[b]
	• Previous pregnancy with a positive GBS screening culture (unless a culture also was positive during the current pregnancy or previous infant with invasive GBS disease)
	• Planned cesarean delivery performed in the absence of labor or membrane rupture (regardless of GBS culture status)
	• Negative vaginal and rectal GBS screening culture in late gestation, regardless of intrapartum risk factors

[a] Exceptions: women with GBS bacteriuria during the pregnancy or a women with a previous infant with invasive GBS disease.

[b] If chorioamnionitis is suspected, broad-spectrum antimicrobial therapy that includes an agent known to be active against GBS should replace GBS IAP. GBS = group B streptococcus, IAP = intrapartum antimicrobial prophylaxis.

▲ **Figure 1–12.** Indications for intrapartum antimicrobial prophylaxis to prevent early-onset group B streptococcal (GBS) disease using a universal prenatal culture screening strategy at 35–37 weeks' gestation for all pregnant women. (Reproduced, with permission, from the American Academy of Pediatrics: Red Book 2003 Report of the Committee on Infectious Disease, 2003.)

to be expanded to include staphylococci. In particular, the preterm infant with an indwelling line is at risk for infection with coagulase-negative staphylococci, for which vancomycin is the drug of choice at a dosage of 10–15 mg/kg q8–24h, depending on gestational and postnatal ages. Initial broad-spectrum coverage should also include a third-generation cephalosporin (cefotaxime or ceftazidime, 100 mg/kg/d divided q12h, when *Pseudomonas aeruginosa* is strongly suspected). To prevent the development of vancomycin-resistant organisms, vancomycin should be stopped as soon as cultures and sensitivities indicate that it is not needed. Other supportive therapy includes IVIG (500–750 mg/kg) in infants with overwhelming infection. The duration of treatment for proved sepsis is 10–14 days of IV antibiotics. In sick infants, the essentials of good supportive therapy should be provided: IV glucose and nutritional support, volume expansion, use of pressors as needed, and oxygen and ventilator support.

Prevention of neonatal GBS infection has been achieved with intrapartum administration of penicillin given more than 4 hours prior to delivery. The current guideline (Figure 1–12) is to perform a vaginal and rectal GBS culture at 35–37 weeks' gestation in all pregnant women. Prophylaxis with penicillin is given to GBS-positive women and to those who have unknown GBS status at delivery with risk factors for infection. Figure 1–13 presents a suggested strategy for the infant born to a mother who received intrapartum prophylaxis for prevention of early-onset GBS or for suspected chorioamnionitis. Some authors also recommend selective neonatal prophylaxis with 50,000 U/kg

of penicillin G given IM if adequate intrapartum treatment has not been given.

2. Meningitis

Any newborn with bacterial sepsis is at risk for meningitis. The incidence is low in infants with early-onset sepsis and much higher in infants with late-onset infection. The workup for any newborn with possible signs of CNS infection should include a lumbar puncture because blood cultures can be negative in neonates with meningitis. Diagnosis is suggested by a CSF protein level higher than 150 mg/dL, glucose less than 30 mg/dL, leukocytes of more than 25/μL, and a positive Gram stain. The diagnosis is confirmed by culture. The most common organisms are GBS and gram-negative enteric bacteria. Although sepsis can be treated with antibiotics for 10–14 days, meningitis often requires 21 days. The mortality rate of neonatal meningitis is approximately 10%, with significant neurologic morbidity present in one third of the survivors.

3. Pneumonia

The respiratory system can be infected in utero or on passage through the birth canal. Early-onset neonatal infection is usually associated with pneumonia. Pneumonia should also be suspected in older neonates with a recent onset of tachypnea, retractions, and cyanosis. In infants already receiving respiratory support, an increase in the requirement for oxygen or ventilator support may indicate pneumonia. Not

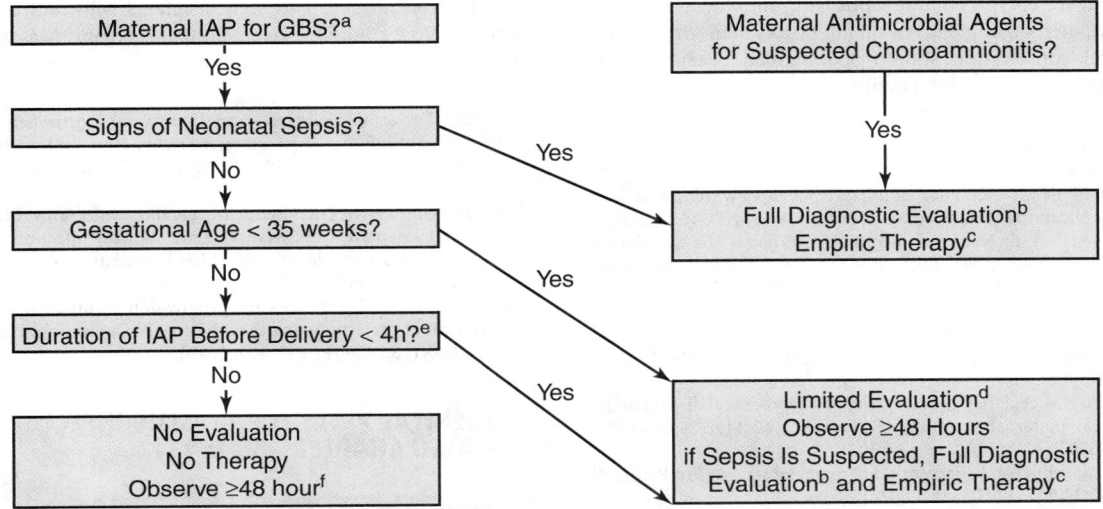

▲ Figure 1–13. Empiric management of a neonate born to a mother who received intrapartum antimicrobial prophylaxis (IAP) for prevention of early-onset group B streptococcal (GBS) disease or chorioamnionitis. (Reproduced, with permission, from the American Academy of Pediatrics: Red Book 2003 Report of the Committee on Infectious Disease, 2003.)

only common bacteria but also viruses (cytomegalovirus, respiratory syncytial virus, adenovirus, influenza, herpes simplex, parainfluenza) and *Chlamydia* can cause the disease. In infants with preexisting respiratory disease, intercurrent pulmonary infections may contribute to the ultimate severity of chronic lung disease.

4. Urinary Tract Infection

Infection of the urine is uncommon in the first days of life. Urinary tract infection in the newborn can occur in association with genitourinary anomalies and is caused by gram-negative enteric pathogens, *Enterococcus*, or other organisms. Urine should always be evaluated as part of the workup for late-onset infection. Culture should be obtained either by suprapubic aspiration or bladder catheterization. Antibiotic IV therapy is continued for 7–10 days if the blood culture is negative and clinical signs resolve quickly. Evaluation for genitourinary anomalies, starting with an ultra-

sound examination and a voiding cystourethrogram, should be done subsequently.

5. Omphalitis

A normal umbilical cord stump atrophies and separates at the skin level. A small amount of purulent material at the base of the cord is common and can be minimized by keeping the cord open to air and cleaning the base with alcohol several times a day. The cord can become colonized with streptococci, staphylococci, or gram-negative organisms that can cause local infection. Infections are more common in cords manipulated for venous or arterial lines. Omphalitis is diagnosed when redness and edema develop in the soft tissues around the stump. Local and systemic cultures should be obtained. Treatment is with broad-spectrum IV antibiotics (usually nafcillin, 50–75 mg/kg/d divided q8–12h, or vancomycin and a third-generation cephalosporin). Complications are determined by the degree of infection of the cord vessels and include septic thrombophlebitis, hepatic abscess, necrotizing fasciitis, and portal vein thrombosis. Surgical consultation should be obtained because of the potential for necrotizing fasciitis.

Bratcher D: Methicillin-resistant staphylococcus aureus in nurseries. NeoReviews 2005;6:e424.

Fraser N et al: Neonatal omphalitis. A review of its serious complications. Acta Paediatr 2006;95:519 [PMID: 16825129].

Garges HP et al: Neonatal meninigitis: What is the correlation among cerebrospinal fluid cultures, blood cultures, and cerebrospinal fluid parameters? Pediatrics 2006;117:1094 [PMID: 16585303].

Gerdes JS: Diagnosis and management of bacterial infections in the neonate. Pediatr Clin North Am 2004;51:939 [PMID: 15275982].

Puopolo KM et al: Early-onset group B streptococcal disease in the era of maternal screening. Pediatrics 2005;115:1240 [PMID: 15867030].

Schrag S, Schuchat A: Prevention of neonatal sepsis. Clin Perinatol 2005;32:601 [PMID: 16085022].

FUNGAL SEPSIS

ESSENTIALS OF DIAGNOSIS & TYPICAL FEATURES

► Risk factors include low birth weight, indwelling central lines, and multiple antibiotic exposures.

► Colonization with *Candida* species is common; systemic infection occurs in 2–5% of infants.

► Presents with often subtle clinical deterioration, thrombocytopenia, and hyperglycemia.

With the survival of smaller, sicker infants, infection with *Candida* species has become more common. Infants of low birth weight with central lines who have had repeated exposures to broad-spectrum antibiotics are at highest risk. For infants of birth weight less than 1500 g, colonization rates of 27–64% have been demonstrated. Many of these infants develop cutaneous lesions, although the GI tract appears to be the initial site of colonization. A much smaller percentage (2–5%) develops systemic disease.

Clinical features of fungal sepsis can be indistinguishable from those of late-onset bacterial sepsis but may be more subtle. Thrombocytopenia may be the earliest and only sign. Deep organ involvement (renal, eye, or endocarditis) is commonly associated with systemic candidiasis. Treatment is with amphotericin B (0.5–1.5 mg/kg/d). In severe infections, flucytosine (50–150 mg/kg/d) can be added for synergistic coverage. (See Chapter 41.) Fluconazole can also be considered as an alternative treatment. Prophylaxis with oral nystatin at 0.5–1 mL PO qid or fluconazole at 3–6 mg/kg/d as a single dose diminishes intestinal colonization with yeast and decreases the frequency of systemic disease.

Malassezia furfur is also seen in infants with central lines receiving IV fat emulsion. To eradicate this organism, as well as *Candida* species, it is necessary to remove the indwelling line.

Benjamin DK et al: Neonatal candidiasis among extremely low birth weight infants: Risk factors, mortality rates, and neurodevelopmental outcomes at 18–22 months. Pediatrics 2006;117:84 [PMID: 16396864].

Long SS, Stevenson DK: Reducing candida infections during neonatal intensive care: Management choices, infection control, and fluconazole prophylaxis. J Pediatr 2005;147:135 [PMID: 16126036].

Manzoni P et al: Risk factors for progression to invasive fungal infection in preterm neonates with fungal colonization. Pediatrics 2006;118:2359 [PMID: 17142519].

CONGENITAL VIRAL & PARASITIC INFECTIONS (SEE ALSO CHAPTERS 38 & 41)

ESSENTIALS OF DIAGNOSIS & TYPICAL FEATURES

► Can be acquired in utero, perinatally, and postnatally.

► Can be asymptomatic in the newborn period.

► Clinical symptom complexes include IUGR, chorioretinitis, cataracts, cholestatic jaundice, thrombocytopenia, skin rash, and brain calcifications.

► Diagnosis can be confirmed using polymerase chain reaction (PCR) testing, antigen and antibody studies, and culture.

1. Cytomegalovirus Infection

Cytomegalovirus (CMV) is the most common virus transmitted in utero. The incidence of congenital infection ranges from 0.2–2.2% of live births. Transmission of CMV can occur during either primary or reactivated maternal infection. Children, especially in the day care setting, are an important source of infection. The incidence of primary infection in pregnancy is 1–4%, with a 40% transplacental transmission rate. Of these infants, 85–90% are asymptomatic at birth, while 10–15% have clinically apparent disease—hepatosplenomegaly, petechiae, small size for gestational age, microcephaly, direct hyperbilirubinemia, thrombocytopenia, intracranial calcifications, and chorioretinitis. The risk of neonatal disease is higher when the mother acquires the infection in the first half of pregnancy. The incidence of reactivated infection in pregnancy is less than 1%, with an incidence of clinically apparent disease of 0–1%. Diagnosis in the neonate should be confirmed by culture of the virus from urine. Rapid diagnosis is possible with antigen detection techniques and PCR testing. Diagnosis can also be confirmed in utero from an amniocentesis specimen. Although not routinely recommended, ganciclovir therapy has been used in some severely ill neonates.

The mortality rate in patients with symptomatic congenital CMV may be as high as 20%. Sequelae such as hearing loss, mental retardation, delayed motor development, chorioretinitis and optic atrophy, seizures, language delays, and learning disability occur in 90% of symptomatic survivors. The incidence of complications is 5–15% in asymptomatic infants; the most frequent complication is hearing loss, which can be progressive.

Perinatal infection can also occur when virus is acquired around the time of delivery. These infections generally cause no symptoms or sequelae. Hepatitis, pneumonitis, and neurologic illness may occur in compromised seronegative premature infants. The virus can be acquired postnatally through blood transfusion or ingestion of CMV-infected breast milk. Transfusion risk can be minimized by using frozen, washed red blood cells or CMV antibody–negative donors.

2. Rubella

Congenital rubella infection occurs as a result of maternal rubella infection during pregnancy. The frequency of fetal infection and damage to the fetus is as high as 80% in mothers infected during the first trimester. Fetal infection rates decline in the second trimester before increasing again in the third trimester. Fetal damage generally does not occur in infections acquired after 18 weeks' gestation. Features of congenital rubella include adenopathy, bone radiolucencies, encephalitis, cardiac defects (pulmonary arterial hypoplasia and patent ductus arteriosus), cataracts, retinopathy, growth restriction, hepatosplenomegaly, thrombocytopenia, and purpura. Affected infants can be asymptomatic at birth but develop clinical sequelae during the first year of life. The diagnosis should be suspected in cases of a characteristic clinical illness in the mother (rash, adenopathy, and arthritis) confirmed by serologic testing. Diagnosis can be confirmed by an increase in serum rubella-specific IgM or culture of pharyngeal secretions in the infant. Congenital rubella is now rare because of widespread immunization.

3. Varicella

Congenital varicella infection is rare (< 5% after infection acquired during the first or second trimester) but may cause a constellation of findings, including limb hypoplasia, cutaneous scars, microcephaly, cortical atrophy, chorioretinitis, and cataracts. Perinatal exposure (5 days before to 2 days after delivery) can cause severe to fatal disseminated varicella in the infant. If maternal varicella infection develops within this perinatal risk period, 1 vial of varicella immune globulin should be given to the newborn. If varicella immune globulin is not available, IVIG can be used instead. If this has not been done, the illness can be treated with IV acyclovir (30 mg/kg/d divided q8h).

Hospitalized premature infants of at least 28 weeks' gestation whose mothers have no history of chickenpox— and all infants younger than 28 weeks' gestational age—

should receive varicella immune globulin following any postnatal exposure. Susceptible women of childbearing age should be immunized with varicella vaccine.

4. Toxoplasmosis

Toxoplasmosis is caused by the protozoan *Toxoplasma gondii*. Maternal infection occurs in 0.1–0.5% of pregnancies and is usually asymptomatic. When primary infection occurs during pregnancy, up to 40% of the fetuses become infected, of whom 15% have severe damage. The sources of transmission include exposure to cat feces and ingestion of raw or undercooked meat. Although the risk of transmission increases to 90% near term, fetal damage is most likely to occur when maternal infection occurs in the second to sixth month of gestation.

Clinical findings include growth restriction, chorioretinitis, seizures, jaundice, hydrocephalus, microcephaly, cerebral calcifications, hepatosplenomegaly, adenopathy, cataracts, maculopapular rash, thrombocytopenia, and pneumonia. The majority of affected infants are asymptomatic at birth but show evidence of damage (chorioretinitis, blindness, low IQ, and hearing loss) at a later time. The serologic diagnosis is based on a positive IgA or IgM in the first 6 months of life or a persistent IgG beyond 12 months. Infants with suspected infection should have eye and auditory examinations and a CT scan of the brain. Organism isolation from placenta or cord blood and PCR tests are also available for diagnosis in the neonate and from amniocentesis specimens.

Spiramycin treatment of primary maternal infection is used to try to reduce transmission to the fetus. Neonatal treatment using pyrimethamine and sulfadiazine with folinic acid can improve long-term outcome. (See Chapter 41.)

PERINATALLY ACQUIRED VIRAL INFECTIONS

1. Herpes Simplex (See also Chapter 38)

Herpes simplex virus infection is usually acquired at the birth during transit through an infected birth canal. The mother may have either primary or reactivated secondary infection. Primary maternal infection, because of the high titer of organisms and the absence of antibodies, poses the greatest risk to the infant. The risk of neonatal infection with vaginal delivery in this setting is 33–50%. Seventy percent of mothers with primary herpes at the time of delivery are asymptomatic. The risk to an infant born to a mother with recurrent herpes simplex is much lower (< 0–5%). Time of presentation of localized (skin, eye, or mouth) or disseminated disease (pneumonia, shock, or hepatitis) in the infant is usually 5–14 days of age. CNS disease usually presents at 14–28 days with lethargy and seizures. In about 10% of cases, presentation is as early as day 1 of life, suggesting in-utero infection. In about one third of patients, localized skin, eye, and mouth disease is the first indication of infection. In another third, disseminated or CNS disease precedes skin, eye, and mouth findings, whereas the remaining third have disseminated or CNS disease in the absence of skin, eye, and mouth disease. Preliminary diagnosis can be made by scraping the base of a vesicle and finding multinucleated giant cells. Viral culture from vesicles, usually positive in 24–72 hours, makes the definitive diagnosis. PCR technology can assist in diagnosis but may be falsely negative in the CSF early in the course. If a lumbar puncture performed shortly after the onset of symptoms is negative, a repeat test should be performed if herpes simplex virus disease is considered a strong possibility.

Acyclovir (60 mg/kg/d given q8h) is the drug of choice for neonatal herpes infection. Localized disease is treated for 14 days, and a 21-day course is used for disseminated or CNS disease. Treatment improves survival of neonates with CNS and disseminated disease and prevents the spread of localized disease. Prevention is possible by not allowing delivery through an infected birth canal (eg, by cesarean section within 6 hours after rupture of the membranes). However, antepartum cervical cultures are poor predictors of the presence of virus at the time of delivery. Furthermore, given the low incidence of infection in the newborn from secondary maternal infection, cesarean delivery is not indicated for asymptomatic mothers with a history of herpes. Cesarean deliveries are performed in mothers with active lesions (either primary or secondary) at the time of delivery. Infants born to mothers with a history of herpes simplex virus infection but no active lesions can be observed closely after birth. Cultures should be obtained and acyclovir treatment initiated only for clinical signs of herpes virus infection. In infants born to mothers with active lesions—regardless of the route of delivery—cultures of the eye, oropharynx, umbilicus, and rectum should be performed 24 hours after delivery. If the infant is colonized (positive cultures) or if symptoms consistent with herpes infection develop, treatment with acyclovir should be started. In cases of maternal primary infection at the time of vaginal delivery, infant specimens should be obtained and acyclovir started pending the results of cultures. The major problem facing perinatologists is the high percentage of asymptomatic primary maternal infection. In these cases, infection in the neonate is not preventable. Therefore, cultures should be obtained and acyclovir started, pending the results of those cultures, in any infant who presents at the right age with symptoms consistent with neonatal herpes.

The prognosis is good for localized skin and mucosal disease that does not progress. The mortality rate for disseminated and CNS herpes is high, with significant morbidity among survivors despite treatment. Recurrences are common, and examination of the CSF should occur each time.

2. Hepatitis B & C (See also Chapter 21)

Infants can be infected with hepatitis B at the time of birth. Clinical illness is rare in the neonatal period, but infants exposed in utero are at high risk of becoming chronic hepatitis B surface antigen (HBsAg) carriers and developing chronic active hepatitis, and later hepatocellular carcinoma. The pres-

ence of HBsAg should be determined in all pregnant women. If the result is positive, the infant should receive hepatitis B immune globulin (HBIG) and hepatitis B vaccine as soon as possible after birth, followed by two subsequent vaccine doses at 1 and 6 months of age. If HBsAg has not been tested prior to birth in a mother at risk, the test should be run after delivery and hepatitis B vaccine given within 12 hours after birth. If the mother is subsequently found to be positive, HBIG should be given as soon as possible (preferably within 48 hours, but not later than 1 week after birth). Subsequent vaccine doses should be given at 1 and 6 months of age. In premature infants born to HBsAg-positive mothers, vaccine and HBIG should be given at birth, but a three-vaccine hepatitis B series should be given after a weight of 2000 g is attained.

Perinatal transmission of hepatitis C occurs in about 5% of infants born to mothers who carry the virus. At present, no prevention strategies exist. Up to 12 months of age, the only reliable screen for hepatitis C infection is PCR. After that time, the presence of hepatitis C antibodies in the infant strongly suggests that infection has occurred.

3. Enteroviral Infection

Enteroviral infections occurs most frequently in the late summer and early fall. Infection is usually acquired in the perinatal period. There is often a history of maternal fever, diarrhea, and rash in the week prior to delivery. The illness appears in the infant in the first 2 weeks of life and is most commonly characterized by fever, lethargy, irritability, diarrhea, and rash. More severe forms occasionally occur, especially if infection occurs before 1 week of age, including meningoencephalitis, myocarditis, hepatitis, pneumonia, shock, and disseminated intravascular coagulation. Diagnosis can be confirmed by culture (rectum, CSF, or blood) or by PCR techniques.

No therapy has proved efficacy. The prognosis is good for all symptom complexes except severe disseminated disease, which carries a high mortality rate.

4. HIV Infection (See also Chapter 39)

Human immunodeficiency virus (HIV) can be acquired in utero or at the time of delivery, or can be transmitted postpartum via breast milk. Transmission of virus occurs in 13–39% of births to infected mothers. Treating the mother with zidovudine starting at 14–34 weeks' gestation and intrapartum, and the infant for the first 6 weeks of life (2 mg/kg PO qid) decreases vertical transmission to 7%. Shorter courses of zidovudine and cesarean delivery are also associated with decreased disease transmission. The combination of zidovudine treatment and cesarean delivery can lower transmission to 2%. The addition of other anti-HIV therapy may further reduce the risk of ante- and intrapartum transmission. Current guidelines for antiretroviral drugs in pregnant HIV-infected women are similar to those for nonpregnant patients (eg, highly active antiretroviral combination therapy). In cases of unknown HIV status at presentation in labor, rapid HIV testing and intrapartum treatment should be offered. The risk of transmission is increased in mothers with advanced disease, high viral loads, low CD4 counts, and intrapartum events such as chorioamnionitis and prolonged membrane rupture that increase exposure of the fetus to maternal blood.

Newborns with congenitally acquired HIV are often asymptomatic. Jaundice, giant cell hepatitis, and thrombocytopenia have been reported at birth. Failure to thrive, lymphadenopathy, hepatosplenomegaly, oral thrush, chronic diarrhea, bacterial infections with common organisms, and an increased incidence of upper and lower respiratory diseases, including lymphoid interstitial pneumonitis, may appear early or may be delayed for months to years.

Infants of HIV-infected women should be tested by HIV DNA PCR at less than 48 hours, at 1–2 months, and at 2–4 months. If an infant aged 4 months has a negative PCR result, infection can be reasonably excluded. HIV-positive mothers should be counseled not to breast feed their infants.

Protection of health workers caring for infected mothers and infants is important. Testing should be performed in all pregnant women. Because such testing fails to identify some infected patients, universal precautions should always be used. Gloves should be worn during all procedures involving blood and blood-contaminated fluids, intubation, and procedures using needles. When a splash exposure is possible, mask and eye covers should be used.

OTHER INFECTIONS

1. Congenital Syphilis

The infant is usually infected in utero by transplacental passage of *Treponema pallidum*. Active primary and secondary maternal syphilis leads to fetal infection in nearly 100% of infants, latent disease in 40%, and late disease in 10%. Fetal infection is rare before 18 weeks' gestation. Fetal infection can result in stillbirth or prematurity. Findings of early congenital syphilis (presentation before age 2 years) include mucocutaneous lesions, lymphadenopathy, hepatosplenomegaly, bony changes, and hydrops. Later manifestations (beyond age 2 years) include Hutchinson teeth and mulberry molars, keratitis, chorioretinitis, glaucoma, hearing loss, saddle nose, saber shins, and mental retardation. Newborn infants are often asymptomatic. An infant should be evaluated for congenital syphilis if he or she has proven or probable congenital syphilis, as defined in Table 1–22, or was

Table 1–22. Recommended treatment of neonates (≤ 4 weeks of age) with proven or possible congenital syphilis.

Clinical Status	Antimicrobial Therapy[a]
Proven or highly probable disease[b]	Aqueous crystalline penicillin G, 100,000–150,000 U/kg/d, administered as 50,000 U/kg per dose IV q12h during the first 7 days of life and q8h thereafter for a total of 10 days **or** Penicillin G procaine,[c] 50,000 U/kg/d, IM in a single dose for 10 days
Normal physical exam and serum quantitative nontreponemal titer the same or less than fourfold the maternal titer:	
1. (a) No penicillin treatment or inadequate or no documentation of penicillin treatment[d]; (b) mother was treated with erythromycin or other nonpenicillin regimen; (c) mother received treatment ≤ 4 wk before delivery	Aqueous crystalline penicillin G IV for 10 days[d] **or** Penicillin G procaine,[c] 50,000 U/kg/d, IM in a single dose for 10 days[d] **or** Clinical, serologic follow-up, and penicillin G benzathine,[c] 50,000 U/kg, IM in a single dose[d]
2. (a) Adequate therapy given > 1 month before delivery; (b) mother has no evidence of reinfection or relapse	Clinical, serologic follow-up, and penicillin G benzathine, 50,000 U/kg, IM in a single dose[e]
3. Adequate therapy before pregnancy and mother's nontreponemal serologic titer remained low and stable during pregnancy and at delivery	None[f]

[a]If more than 1 day of therapy is missed, restart the entire course.
[b]Abnormal PE, serum quantitative nontreponemal titer more than fourfold the mother's, or positive darkfield or fluorescent antibody test of body fluids.
[c]Penicillin G benzathine and penicillin G procaine are approved for IM administration *only*.
[d]A complete evaluation (CSF analysis, CBC and bone radiography) is not needed if administering 10 days of IV therapy, but may be done to support a diagnosis of congenital syphilis. If a single dose is used, evaluation must be done and be normal and follow up must be certain.
[e]Some experts would not treat the infant but would provide close serologic follow-up.
[f]Some experts would treat with a single IM benzathine penicillin dose if follow-up is uncertain.
CBC, complete blood count; CSF, cerebrospinal fluid; IM, intramuscularly; IV, intravenously.
Reprinted, with permission, from the American Academy of Pediatrics: Red Book 2006 Report of the Committee on Infectious Diseases, 2006.

born to a mother with positive nontreponemal tests confirmed by a positive treponemal test but without documented adequate treatment (parenteral penicillin G), including the expected fourfold decrease in nontreponemal antibody titer. Infants of mothers treated less than 1 month before delivery also require evaluation. Evaluation should include physical examination, a quantitative nontreponemal serologic test for syphilis, CBC, CSF examination for cell count and protein, Venereal Disease Research Laboratory testing, and long bone radiographs. Guidelines for therapy are presented in Table 1–22.

2. Tuberculosis (See also Chapter 40)

Congenital tuberculosis (TB) is rare but may occur in the infant of a mother with hematogenously spread TB or by aspiration of infected amniotic fluid in cases of tuberculous endometritis. Women with pulmonary TB are not likely to infect the fetus until after delivery. Postnatal acquisition is the most common mechanism of neonatal infection. Management in these cases is based on the mother's evaluation.

1. Mother or other household contact with a positive skin test and negative chest radiograph, or mother with an abnormal chest radiograph but no evidence of tuberculous disease after clinical evaluation: Investigate family contacts. Treat the mother or household contact for tuberculosis.

2. Mother has an abnormal chest radiograph consistent with tuberculous disease: Mother and infant should be separated until the mother is evaluated for active TB. Investigate family contacts.

3. Mother with clinical or radiographic evidence of acute and possibly contagious TB: Evaluate the infant for congenital TB (skin test, chest radiograph, lumbar puncture, and cultures) and the mother for HIV. Treat the mother and infant. If the infant is receiving isoniazid and the mother has no risks for multidrug-resistant TB, separation is not necessary.

If congenital TB is suspected, multidrug therapy should be initiated.

3. Conjunctivitis

Neisseria gonorrhoeae may colonize an infant during passage through an infected birth canal. Gonococcal ophthalmitis presents at 3–7 days with copious purulent conjunctivitis. The diagnosis can be suspected when gram-negative intracellular diplococci are seen on a Gram-stained smear and confirmed by culture. Treatment is with IV or IM ceftriaxone, 25–50 mg/kg (not to exceed 125 mg) given once. Prophylaxis at birth is with 0.5% erythromycin ointment. Infants born to mothers with known gonococcal disease should also receive a single dose of ceftriaxone.

Chlamydia trachomatis is another important cause of conjunctivitis, appearing at 5 days to several weeks of age with congestion, edema, and minimal discharge. The organism is acquired at birth after passage through an infected birth canal. Acquisition occurs in 50% of infants born to infected women, with a 25–50% risk of conjunctivitis. Prevalence in pregnancy is over 10% in some populations. Diagnosis is by isolation of the organism or by rapid antigen detection tests. Treatment is with oral erythromycin (30 mg/kg/d in divided doses q8–12h) for 14 days. Topical treatment alone will not eradicate nasopharyngeal carriage, leaving the infant at risk for the development of pneumonitis.

4. Parvovirus B19 Infection

Parvovirus B19 is a small, nonenveloped, single-stranded DNA virus that causes erythema infectiosum (fifth disease) in children, with a peak incidence at ages 6–7 years. Transmission to the mother is primarily by respiratory secretions. The virus replicates initially in erythroid progenitor cells and induces cell-cycle arrest, resulting in severe anemia, myocarditis, and nonimmune hydrops in approximately 3% and fetal death in up to 10% of fetuses infected in the second trimester. Resolution of the hydrops may occur in utero, either spontaneously or after fetal transfusion. Mothers who have been exposed may have specific serologic testing for antibody response, and serial ultrasound, Doppler exams, and percutaneous umbilical cord blood sampling of the fetus for anemia. If the fetus survives, the long-term outcome is good with no late effects from the infection.

Adler SP, Marshall B: Cytomegalovirus infections. Pediatr Rev 2007;28:92 [PMID: 17332168].

American Academy of Pediatrics and Canadian Paediatric Society Clinical Report: Evaluation and treatment of the human immunodeficiency virus-1-exposed infant. Pediatrics 2004;114: 497 [PMID: 15286240].

American Academy of Pediatrics Committee on Infectious Diseases: *Report of the Committee on Infectious Diseases*, 27th ed. Red Book 2006. American Academy of Pediatrics, 2006.

Brown ZA et al: Genital herpes complicating pregnancy. Obstet Gynecol 2005;106:845 [PMID: 16199646].

Frenkel LM: Challenges in the diagnosis and management of neonatal herpes simplex virus encephalitis. Pediatrics 2005;115:795 [PMID: 15741389].

Gras L et al: Association between prenatal treatment and clinical manifestations of congenital toxoplasmosis in infancy: A cohort study in 13 European centres. Acta Paediatr 2005;94:1721 [PMID: 16421031].

Goldschmidt RH, Fogler JA: Opportunities to prevent HIV transmission to newborns. Pediatrics 2006;117:208 [PMID: 16396878].

Hill J, Roberts S: Herpes simplex virus in pregnancy: New concepts in prevention and management. Clin Perinatol 2005;32:657 [PMID: 16085025].

Hollier LM, Grissom H: Human herpes viruses in pregnancy: Cytomegalovirus, Epstein-Barr virus, and varicella zoster virus. Clin Perinatol 2005;32:671 [PMID: 16085026].

Kumar ML, Abughali NF: Perinatal parvovirus B19 infection. NeoReviews 2005;6:e32.

Ross SA et al: Hearing loss in children with congenital cytomegalovirus infection born to mothers with preexisting immunity. J Pediatr 2006;148:332 [PMID: 16615962].

Shetty AK, Maldonado Y: Advances in the prevention of perinatal HIV-1 transmission. NeoReviews 2005;6:e12.

Stehel EK, Sanchez PJ: Cytomegalovirus infection in the fetus and neonate. NeoReviews 2005;6:e38.

▼ HEMATOLOGIC DISORDERS IN THE NEWBORN INFANT

BLEEDING DISORDERS

Neonatal coagulation is discussed in Chapter 28. Bleeding in the newborn infant may result from inherited clotting deficiencies (eg, factor VIII deficiency) or acquired disorders—hemorrhagic disease of the newborn, disseminated intravascular coagulation, liver failure, and isolated thrombocytopenia.

1. Vitamin K Deficiency Bleeding of the Newborn

ESSENTIALS OF DIAGNOSIS & TYPICAL FEATURES

▶ Frequently exclusively breast fed, otherwise clinically well infant.

▶ Bleeding from mucous membranes, GI tract, skin, or internal (intracranial).

▶ Prolonged prothrombin time (PT), relatively normal partial thromboplastin time (PTT), normal fibrinogen and platelet count.

Vitamin K deficiency bleeding is caused by the deficiency of the vitamin K–dependent clotting factors (II, VII, IX, and X). Bleeding occurs in 0.25–1.7% of newborns who do not receive vitamin K prophylaxis after birth, generally in the first 5 days to 2 weeks, but as late as 12 weeks in an otherwise well infant. There is an increased risk in infants of mothers receiving therapy with anticonvulsants that interfere with vitamin K metabolism. Early vitamin K deficiency bleeding (0–2 weeks) can be prevented by either parenteral or oral vitamin K administration, whereas late disease is most effectively prevented by administering parenteral vitamin K. Sites of ecchymoses and surface bleeding include the GI tract, umbilical cord, circumcision site, and nose, although devastating intracranial hemorrhage can occur. Bleeding from vitamin K deficiency is more likely to occur in exclusively breast-fed infants because of very low amounts of vitamin K in breast milk, with slower and more restricted intestinal colonization. Differential diagnosis includes disseminated intravascular coagulation and hepatic failure (Table 1–23).

Treatment consists of 1 mg of vitamin K SC or IV. IM injections should be avoided in infants who are actively bleeding. Such infants may also require factor replacement in addition to vitamin K administration.

2. Thrombocytopenia

ESSENTIALS OF DIAGNOSIS & TYPICAL FEATURES

▶ Generalized petechiae; oozing at cord or puncture sites.

▶ Thrombocytopenia, often marked (platelets < 10,000–20,000/mL).

▶ In an otherwise well infant, suspect isoimmune thrombocytopenia.

▶ In a sick or asphyxiated infant, suspect disseminated intravascular coagulation.

Table 1–23. Features of infants bleeding from vitamin K deficiency (VKDB), disseminated intravascular coagulation (DIC), or liver failure.

	VKDB	DIC	Liver Failure
Clinical	Well infant; no prophylactic vitamin K	Sick infant; hypoxia, sepsis, etc	Sick infant; hepatitis, inborn errors of metabolism, shock liver
Bleeding	GI tract, umbilical cord, circumcision, nose	Generalized	Generalized
Onset	2–3 days to 2 weeks	Any time	Any time
Platelet count	Normal	Decreased	Normal or decreased
Prothrombin time	Prolonged	Prolonged	Prolonged
Partial thromboplastin time	Normal or prolonged	Prolonged	Prolonged
Fibrinogen	Normal	Decreased	Decreased
Factor V	Normal	Decreased	Decreased

GI, gastrointestinal.

Infants with thrombocytopenia have generalized petechiae (not just on the presenting part) and platelet counts less than 150,000/mL (usually < 50,000/mL; may be < 10,000/mL). Neonatal thrombocytopenia can be isolated in a seemingly well infant or may occur in association with a deficiency of other clotting factors in a sick infant. The differential diagnosis for thrombocytopenia is presented in Table 1–24. Treatment of neonatal thrombocytopenia is transfusion of platelets (10 mL/kg of platelets increases the platelet count by approximately 70,000/mL). Indications for transfusion in the full-term infant are clinical bleeding or a total platelet count less than 20,000–30,000/mL. In the preterm infant at risk for intraventricular hemorrhage, transfusion is indicated for counts less than 40,000–50,000/mL.

Isoimmune (alloimmune) thrombocytopenia is analogous to Rh isoimmunization, with a human platelet antigen [HPA]-1a (in 80%) or HPA-5b (in 15%)–negative mother and an HPA-1a or HPA-5b–positive fetus. Transplacental passage of IgG antibody leads to platelet destruction. If platelet transfusion is required for acute bleeding, washed maternal platelets may be the most readily available antigen-negative platelet source, because 98% of the general population will also be HPA-1a or HPA-5b–positive. Treatment with steroids has been disappointing. Treatment with IVIG infusion, 1 g/kg/d for 2–3 days, until the platelet count has doubled or is over 50,000/mL, is potentially beneficial. Twenty to 30% of infants with isoimmune thrombocytopenia will experience intracranial hemorrhage, half of them before birth. Antenatal therapy of the mother with IVIG with or without steroids may reduce this risk.

Infants born to mothers with idiopathic thrombocytopenic purpura are at low risk for serious hemorrhage despite the thrombocytopenia, and treatment is usually unnecessary. If bleeding does occur, IVIG can be used.

ANEMIA

ESSENTIALS OF DIAGNOSIS & TYPICAL FEATURES

▶ Hematocrit < 45% at term birth.
▶ Acute blood loss–signs of hypovolemia, normal reticulocyte count.
▶ Chronic blood loss—pallor without hypovolemia, elevated reticulocyte count.
▶ Hemolytic anemia—accompanied by excessive hyperbilirubinemia.

The newborn infant with anemia from acute blood loss presents with signs of hypovolemia (tachycardia, poor perfusion, and hypotension), with an initially normal hematocrit that falls after volume replacement. Anemia from chronic blood loss is evidenced by pallor without signs of hypovolemia, with an initially low hematocrit and reticulocytosis.

Anemia can be caused by hemorrhage, hemolysis, or failure to produce red blood cells. Anemia occurring in the first 24–48 hours of life is the result of hemorrhage or hemolysis. Hemorrhage can occur in utero (fetoplacental, fetomaternal, or twin-to-twin), perinatally (cord rupture, placenta previa, placental abruption, or incision through the placenta at cesarean section), or internally (intracranial hemorrhage, cephalohematoma, or ruptured liver or spleen). Hemolysis is caused by blood group incompatibilities, enzyme or membrane abnormalities, infection, and disseminated intravascular coagulation, and is accompanied by significant hyperbilirubinemia.

Initial evaluation should include a review of the perinatal history, assessment of the infant's volume status, and a complete physical examination. A Kleihauer-Betke test for fetal cells in the mother's circulation should be done. A CBC, blood smear, reticulocyte count, and direct and indirect Coombs tests should be performed. This simple evaluation should suggest a diagnosis in most infants. Most infants tolerate anemia quite well due to the increased oxygen

Table 1–24. Differential diagnosis of neonatal thrombocytopenia.

Disorder	Clinical Tips
Immune	
Passively acquired antibody; idiopathic thrombocytopenic purpura, systemic lupus erythematosus, drug-induced	Proper history, maternal thrombocytopenia
Isoimmune sensitization to HPA-1a antigen	No rise in platelet count from random donor platelet transfusion. Positive antiplatelet antibodies in baby's serum, sustained rise in platelets by transfusion of mother's platelets
Infections Bacterial infections Congenital viral infections	Sick infants with other signs consistent with infection
Syndromes Absent radii Fanconi anemia	Congenital anomalies, associated pancytopenia
Disseminated intravascular coagulation (DIC)	Sick infants, abnormalities of clotting factors
Giant hemangioma	
Thrombosis	Hyperviscous infants, vascular catheters
High-risk infant with respiratory distress syndrome, pulmonary hypertension, etc	Isolated decrease in platelets is not uncommon in sick infants even in the absence of DIC (? localized trapping)

HPA, human platelet antigen.

availability in the extrauterine environment; however, treatment with erythropoietin or transfusion might be needed if the infant fails to thrive or develops signs of cardiopulmonary compromise. Additionally, if blood loss is the cause of the anemia, early supplementation with iron will be needed. It is important to remember that hemolysis related to blood group incompatibility can continue for weeks after birth. Serial hematocrits should be followed, because late transfusion may be needed.

POLYCYTHEMIA

ESSENTIALS OF DIAGNOSIS & TYPICAL FEATURES

▶ Hematocrit > 65% (venous) at term.

▶ Plethora, tachypnea, retractions.

▶ Hypoglycemia, irritability, lethargy, poor feeding.

Polycythemia in the newborn is manifested by plethora, cyanosis, respiratory distress with tachypnea and oxygen need, hypoglycemia, poor feeding, emesis, irritability, and lethargy. Hyperbilirubinemia is expected. The consequence of polycythemia is hyperviscosity with decreased perfusion of the capillary beds. Clinical symptomatology can affect several organ systems (Table 1–25). Renal vein, other deep vein, or artery thrombosis is a severe complication. Screening can be done by measuring a capillary (heelstick) hematocrit. If the value is greater than 68%, a peripheral venous hematocrit should be measured. Values greater than 65% should be considered consistent with hyperviscosity. The diagnosis of polycythemia should not be based solely on a capillary hematocrit.

Elevated hematocrits occur in 2–5% of live births. Delayed cord clamping is the most common cause of benign neonatal polycythemia. Although 50% of polycythemic infants are AGA, the prevalence of polycythemia is greater in the SGA and LGA populations. Other causes of increased hematocrit include (1) twin-twin transfusion, (2) maternal-fetal transfusion, and (3) chronic intrauterine hypoxia (SGA infants and LGA infants of diabetic mothers).

Treatment is recommended for symptomatic infants. Treatment for asymptomatic infants based strictly on hematocrit is controversial. Definitive treatment is isovolemic partial exchange transfusion with normal saline, effectively decreasing the hematocrit. The amount to exchange (in milliliters) is calculated using the following formula:

$$\text{Number of Milliliters to exchange} = (PVH - DH)/PVH \times BV(mL/kg) \times Wt(kg)$$

where PVH is peripheral venous hematocrit, DH is desired hematocrit, BV is blood volume in mL/kg, and Wt is weight in kilograms.

Blood is withdrawn at a steady rate from an umbilical venous line while the replacement solution is infused at the same rate through a peripheral IV line over 15–30 minutes. The desired hematocrit value is 50–55%; the assumed blood volume is 80 mL/kg.

American Academy of Pediatrics Committee on the Fetus and Newborn: Controversies concerning vitamin K and the newborn. Pediatrics 2003;122:191 [PMID: 12837888].

Anderson D et al: Guidelines on the use of intravenous immune globulin for hematologic conditions. Transfus Med Rev 2007;21:S9 [PMID: 17397769].

Bizzarro MJ et al: Differential diagnosis and management of anemia in the newborn. Pediatr Clin North Am 2004;51:1087 [PMID: 15275990].

Chalmers EA: Neonatal coagulation problems. Arch Dis Child Fetal Neonatal Ed 2004;89:F475 [PMID: 15499133].

Dempsey EM, Barrington K: Short and long term outcomes following partial exchange transfusion in the polycythaemic newborn: A systematic review. Arch Dis Child Fetal Neonatal Ed 2006;91:F2 [PMID: 16174666].

Hutton EK, Hassan ES: Late vs early clamping of the umbilical cord in full-term neonates. JAMA 2007;297:1241 [PMID: 17374818].

Kates EH, Kates JS: Anemia and polycythemia in the newborn. Pediatr Rev 2007;28:33 [PMID: 17197458].

Pappas A, Delaney-Black V: Differential diagnosis and management of polycythemia. Pediatr Clin North Am 2004;51:1063 [PMID: 15275989].

Wong W, Glader B: Approach to the newborn who has thrombocytopenia. NeoReviews 2004;5:444.

RENAL DISORDERS IN THE NEWBORN INFANT (SEE ALSO CHAPTER 22)

Renal function depends on postconceptional age. The glomerular filtration rate is 20 mL/min/1.73 m² in full-term neonates and 10–13 mL/min/1.73 m² in infants born at 28–30 weeks' gestation. The speed of maturation after birth also depends on postconceptional age. Creatinine can be used as a clinical marker of glomerular filtration rate. Values in the first month of life are shown in Table 1–26. Creatinine at birth reflects the maternal level and should decrease slowly

Table 1–25. Organ-related symptoms of hyperviscosity.

Central nervous system	Irritability, jitteriness, seizures, lethargy
Cardiopulmonary	Respiratory distress, secondary to congestive heart failure, or persistent pulmonary hypertension
Gastrointestinal	Vomiting, heme-positive stools, distention, necrotizing enterocolitis
Renal	Decreased urinary output, renal vein thrombosis
Metabolic	Hypoglycemia
Hematologic	Hyperbilirubinemia, thrombocytopenia

Table 1–26. Normal values of serum creatinine (mg/dL).

Gestational Age at Birth (weeks)	Postnatal Age (days)	
	0–2	28
< 28	1.2	0.7
29–32	1.1	0.6
33–36	1.1	0.45
36–42	0.8	0.3

over the first 3–4 weeks. An increasing serum creatinine is never normal.

The ability to concentrate urine and retain sodium also depends on gestational age. Infants born before 28–30 weeks' gestation are compromised in this respect and can easily become dehydrated and hyponatremic. Preterm infants also have an increased bicarbonate excretion and a low tubular maximum for glucose (approximately 120 mg/dL).

RENAL FAILURE

ESSENTIALS OF DIAGNOSIS & TYPICAL FEATURES

▶ Clinical setting—birth depression, hypovolemia, hypotension, shock.
▶ Low or delayed urine output (< 1 mL/kg/h).
▶ Rising serum creatinine; hyperkalemia; metabolic acidosis; fluid overload.

Renal failure is most commonly seen in the setting of birth asphyxia, hypovolemia, or shock from any cause. The normal rate of urine flow is 1–3 mL/kg/h. After a hypoxic or ischemic insult, acute tubular necrosis may ensue. Typically, 2–3 days of anuria or oliguria is associated with hematuria, proteinuria, and a rise in serum creatinine. The period of anuria or oliguria is followed by a period of polyuria and then gradual recovery. During the polyuric phase, excessive urine sodium and bicarbonate losses may be seen.

The initial management is restoration of the infant's volume status. Thereafter, restriction of fluids to insensible water loss (40–60 mL/kg/d) without added electrolytes, plus milliliter-for-milliliter urine replacement, should be instituted. Serum and urine electrolytes and body weights should be followed frequently. These measures should be continued through the polyuric phase. After urine output has been reestablished, urine replacement should be decreased to between 0.5 and 0.75 mL for each milliliter of urine output to see if the infant has regained normal function. If that is the case, the infant can be returned to maintenance fluids.

Finally, many of these infants experience fluid overload and should be allowed to lose enough water through urination to return to birth weight. Hyperkalemia, which may become life-threatening, may occur in this situation despite the lack of added IV potassium. If the serum potassium reaches 7–7.5 mEq/L, therapy should be started with glucose and insulin infusion, giving 1 unit of insulin for every 3 g of glucose administered, in addition to binding resins per rectum. Calcium chloride (20 mg/kg bolus) and correction of metabolic acidosis with bicarbonate are also helpful for arrhythmia resulting from hyperkalemia.

Peritoneal dialysis is occasionally needed for the management of neonatal acute renal failure, for removal of waste products and excess fluid. Hemodialysis, although possible, is difficult due to the small blood volume of the infant and problems with vascular access. Although most acute renal failure in the newborn resolves, ischemic injury severe enough to result in acute cortical necrosis and chronic renal failure can occur.

URINARY TRACT ANOMALIES

Abdominal masses in the newborn are most frequently caused by renal enlargement. Most common is a multicystic or dysplastic kidney; congenital hydronephrosis is second in frequency. Chromosomal abnormalities and syndromes with multiple anomalies frequently include renal abnormalities. An ultrasound examination is the first step in diagnosis. In pregnancies complicated by oligohydramnios, renal agenesis or obstruction secondary to posterior urethral valves should be considered.

Only bilateral disease or disease in a solitary kidney is associated with oligohydramnios, significant morbidity, and death. Such infants will generally also have pulmonary hypoplasia, and die from pulmonary rather than renal insufficiency.

Ultrasonography identifies many infants with renal anomalies (most often hydronephrosis) prior to birth. Postnatal evaluation of infants with hydronephrosis should include renal ultrasound and a voiding cystourethrogram at about 1week of age, depending on the severity of the antenatal findings. Earlier postnatal ultrasound might underestimate the severity of the hydronephrosis due to low glomerular filtration rates in the first days of life, although cases in which oligohydramnios or severe renal abnormality are suspected will be accurately diagnosed even on the first day of life. Until the presence and severity of vesicoureteral reflux is evaluated, these infants should receive antibiotic prophylaxis with low-dose penicillin or amoxicillin.

RENAL VEIN THROMBOSIS

ESSENTIALS OF DIAGNOSIS & TYPICAL FEATURES

▶ History of IDM, birth depression, dehydration.
▶ Hematuria, oliguria.
▶ Thrombocytopenia, polycythemia.
▶ Renal enlargement on exam.

Renal vein thrombosis occurs most often in dehydrated polycythemic newborns. At particular risk is the IDM with polycythemia. If fetal distress is superimposed on polycythemia and dehydration, prompt reduction in blood viscosity is indicated. Thrombosis usually begins in intrarenal venules and can extend into larger veins. Hematuria, oliguria, thrombocytopenia, and possibly an enlarged kidney raise suspicion for this diagnosis. With bilateral renal vein thrombosis, anuria ensues. Diagnosis can be confirmed with an ultrasound examination that includes Doppler flow studies of the kidneys. Treatment involves correcting the predisposing condition and systemic heparinization for the thrombosis. Use of thrombolytics for this condition is controversial. Prognosis for a full recovery is uncertain. Some infants will develop significant atrophy of the affected kidney and systemic hypertension.

Chua AN, Sarwal MM: Acute renal failure management in the neonate. NeoReviews 2005;6:e369.

Hubert KC, Palmer JS: Current diagnosis and management of fetal genitourinary abnormalities. Urol Clin N Am 2007;34:89 [PMID: 17145364].

Moghal NE, Embleton ND: Management of acute renal failure in the newborn. Semin Fet Neonat Med 2006;11:207 [PMID: 16584932].

NEUROLOGIC PROBLEMS IN THE NEWBORN INFANT

SEIZURES

ESSENTIALS OF DIAGNOSIS & TYPICAL FEATURES

▸ Usual onset at 12–48 hours.

▸ Most common seizure type is characterized by a constellation of findings.

▸ Most common causes include hypoxic-ischemic encephalopathy, intracranial bleeds, and infection.

Newborns rarely have well-organized tonic-clonic seizures because of their incomplete cortical organization and a preponderance of inhibitory synapses. The most common type of seizure is characterized by a constellation of findings, including horizontal deviation of the eyes with or without jerking; eyelid blinking or fluttering; sucking, smacking, drooling, and other oral-buccal movements; swimming, rowing, or paddling movements; and apneic spells. Strictly tonic or multifocal clonic episodes are also seen.

▸ Clinical Findings

The differential diagnosis of neonatal seizures is presented in Table 1–27. Most neonatal seizures occur between 12 and 48 hours of age. Later-onset seizures suggest meningitis, benign familial seizures, or hypocalcemia. Information regarding ante-

Table 1–27. Differential diagnosis of neonatal seizures.

Diagnosis	Comment
Hypoxic-ischemic encephalopathy	Most common cause (60%), onset in first 24 h
Intracranial hemorrhage	Up to 15% of cases, periventricular-intraventricular hemorrhage, subdural or subarachnoid bleeding, stroke
Infection	12% of cases
Hypoglycemia	Small for gestational age, infant of a diabetic mother (IDM)
Hypocalcemia, hypomagnesemia	Infant of low birth weight, IDM
Hyponatremia	Rare, seen with syndrome of inappropriate secretion of antidiuretic hormone (SIADH)
Disorders of amino and organic acid metabolism, hyperammonemia	Associated acidosis, altered level of consciousness
Pyridoxine dependency	Seizures refractory to routine therapy; cessation of seizures after administration of pyridoxine
Developmental defects	Other anomalies, chromosomal syndromes
Drug withdrawal	
No cause found	10% of cases
Benign familial neonatal seizures	

natal drug use, the presence of birth asphyxia or trauma, and family history (regarding inherited disorders) should be obtained. Physical examination focuses on neurologic features, other signs of drug withdrawal, concurrent signs of infection, dysmorphic features, and intrauterine growth. Screening workup should include blood glucose, ionized calcium, and electrolytes in all cases. Further workup depends on diagnoses suggested by the history and physical examination. If there is any suspicion of infection, a lumbar puncture should be done. Hemorrhages and structural disease of the CNS can be addressed with ultrasound, CT, and MRI scans. Metabolic workup should be pursued when appropriate. EEG should be done; the presence of spike discharges must be noted and the background wave pattern evaluated. At times correlation between EEG changes and clinical seizure activity is absent.

▸ Treatment

Adequate ventilation and perfusion should be ensured. Hypoglycemia should be treated immediately with a 2-mL/kg infusion of $D_{10}W$ followed by 6 mg/kg/min of $D_{10}W$ (100 mL/kg/d). Other treatments such as calcium or magnesium infusion and antibiotics are indicated to treat hypocalcemia, hypomagnesemia, and suspected infection. Electrolyte abnormalities should be corrected. Phenobarbital (20 mg/kg IV) should be administered to stop seizures. Supplemental doses of 5 mg/kg can be used if seizures persist, up to a total of 40 mg/kg. In most cases, phenobarbital controls seizures.

If seizures continue, therapy with fosphenytoin, sodium valproate, or lorazepam may be indicated. For refractory seizures, a trial of pyridoxine is indicated.

▶ Prognosis

Outcome is related to the underlying cause of the seizure. The outcomes for hypoxic-ischemic encephalopathy and intraventricular hemorrhage have been discussed earlier in this chapter. In these settings, seizures that are difficult to control carry a poor prognosis for normal development. Seizures resulting from hypoglycemia, infection of the CNS, some inborn errors of metabolism, and developmental defects also have a high rate of poor outcome. Seizures caused by hypocalcemia or isolated subarachnoid hemorrhage generally resolve without sequelae.

HYPOTONIA

One should be alert to the diagnosis of congenital hypotonia when a mother has polyhydramnios and a history of poor fetal movement. The newborn may present with poor respiratory effort and birth asphyxia. For a discussion of causes and evaluation, see Chapter 23.

INTRACRANIAL HEMORRHAGE[1]

1. Subdural Hemorrhage

Subdural hemorrhage is related to birth trauma; the bleeding is caused by tears in the veins that bridge the subdural space. Prospective studies relating incidence to specific obstetric complications are not available.

The most common site of subdural bleeding is in ruptured superficial cerebral veins with blood over the cerebral convexities. These hemorrhages can be asymptomatic or may cause seizures, with onset on days 2–3 of life, vomiting, irritability, and lethargy. Associated findings include retinal hemorrhages and a full fontanelle. The diagnosis is confirmed by CT scan.

Specific treatment entailing needle drainage of the subdural space is rarely necessary. Most infants survive; 75% are normal on follow-up.

2. Primary Subarachnoid Hemorrhage

Primary subarachnoid hemorrhage is the most common type of neonatal intracranial hemorrhage. In the full-term infant, it can be related to trauma of delivery, whereas subarachnoid hemorrhage in the preterm infant is seen in association with germinal matrix hemorrhage. Clinically, these hemorrhages can be asymptomatic or can present with seizures and irritability on day 2, or rarely, a massive hemorrhage with a rapid downhill course. The seizures associated with subarachnoid hemorrhage are very characteristic—usually brief, with a normal examination interictally. Diagnosis can be suspected on lumbar puncture and confirmed with CT scan. Long-term follow-up is uniformly good.

3. Neonatal Stroke

Focal cerebral ischemic injury can occur in the context of intraventricular hemorrhage in the premature infant and hypoxic-ischemic encephalopathy. Neonatal stroke has also been described in the context of underlying disorders of thrombolysis, maternal drug use (cocaine), a history of infertility, preeclampsia, prolonged membrane rupture, and chorioamnionitis. In some cases, the origin is unclear. The injury often occurs antenatally. The most common clinical presentation of an isolated cerebral infarct is with seizures, and diagnosis can be confirmed acutely with diffusion-weighted MRI scan. The most frequently described distribution is that of the middle cerebral artery.

Treatment is directed at controlling seizures. Long-term outcome is variable, ranging from near-normal to hemiplegias and cognitive deficits.

Chalmers EA: Perinatal stroke—risk factors and management. Br J Haematol 2005;130:333 [PMID: 16042683].

Lee J et al: Maternal and infant characteristics associated with perinatal arterial stroke in the infant. JAMA 2005;293:723 [PMID: 15701914].

Mercuri E et al: Neonatal cerebral infarction and neuromotor outcome at school age. Pediatrics 2004;113:95 [PMID: 14702455].

Tekgul H et al: The current etiologic profile and neurodevelopmental outcome of seizures in term newborn infants. Pediatrics 2006;117:1270 [PMID: 16585324].

Zupanc ML: Neonatal seizures. Pediatr Clin North Am 2004;51:961 [PMID: 15275983].

METABOLIC DISORDERS IN THE NEWBORN INFANT[2]

HYPERGLYCEMIA

Hyperglycemia may develop in preterm infants, particularly those of extremely low birth weight who are also SGA. Glucose concentrations may exceed 200–250 mg/dL, particularly in the first few days of life. This transient diabetes-like syndrome usually lasts approximately 1 week.

[1]Intraventricular hemorrhage is discussed earlier, in the section on the Preterm Infant.

[2]Hypoglycemia is discussed earlier, in the section on Common Problems in the Term Newborn.

Management may include simply reducing glucose intake while continuing to supply IV amino acids to prevent protein catabolism with resultant gluconeogenesis and worsened hyperglycemia. Intravenous insulin infusions will be needed in infants who remain hyperglycemic despite glucose infusion rates of only 5–6 mg/kg/min or less.

HYPOCALCEMIA (SEE ALSO CHAPTER 32)

ESSENTIALS OF DIAGNOSIS & TYPICAL FEATURES

▶ Irritability, jitteriness, seizures.

▶ Normal blood glucose.

▶ Possible dysmorphic features, congenital heart disease (DiGeorge syndrome).

Calcium concentration in the immediate newborn period decreases in all infants. The concentration in fetal plasma is higher than that of the neonate or adult. Hypocalcemia is usually defined as a total serum concentration less than 7 mg/dL (equivalent to a calcium activity of 3.5 mEq/L), although the physiologically active fraction, ionized calcium, should be measured whenever possible. Ionized calcium is usually normal even when total calcium is as low as 6–7 mg/dL. An ionized calcium level above 0.9 mmol/L (1.8 mEq/L; 3.6 mg/dL) is not likely to be detrimental.

▶ Clinical Findings

The clinical signs of hypocalcemia and hypocalcemic tetany include a high-pitched cry, jitteriness, tremulousness, and seizures.

Hypocalcemia tends to occur at two different times in the neonatal period. Early-onset hypocalcemia occurs in the first 2 days of life and has been associated with prematurity, maternal diabetes, asphyxia, and rarely, maternal hypoparathyroidism. Late-onset hypocalcemia occurs at approximately 7–10 days and is observed in infants receiving modified cow's milk rather than infant formula (high phosphorus intake) or in infants with hypoparathyroidism (DiGeorge syndrome, 22q11 deletion). Mothers in underdeveloped countries may have vitamin D deficiency, which can also contribute to late-onset hypocalcemia. Hypomagnesemia should be sought and treated in cases of hypocalcemia that are resistant to treatment.

▶ Treatment

A. Oral Calcium Therapy

The oral administration of calcium salts, often along with vitamin D, is the preferred method of treatment for chronic forms of hypocalcemia resulting from hypoparathyroidism. (See Chapter 32.)

B. Intravenous Calcium Therapy

IV calcium therapy is usually needed for infants with symptomatic hypocalcemia or an ionized calcium level less than 0.9 mmol/L. A number of precautions must be observed when calcium is given intravenously. The infusion must be given slowly so that there is no sudden increase in calcium concentration of blood entering the right atrium, which could cause severe bradycardia and even cardiac arrest. Furthermore, the infusion must be observed carefully, because an IV infiltrate containing calcium can cause full-thickness skin necrosis requiring grafting. For these reasons, IV calcium therapy should be given judiciously and through a central venous line if possible. IV administration of 10% calcium gluconate is usually given as a bolus of 100–200 mg/kg (1–2 mL/kg) over approximately 10–20 minutes, followed by a continuous infusion (0.5–1 g/kg/d) over 1–2 days. Ten percent calcium chloride (20 mg/kg or 0.2 mL/kg per dose) may result in a larger increment in ionized calcium and greater improvement in mean arterial blood pressure in sick hypocalcemic infants and thus may have a role in the newborn. *Note:* Calcium salts cannot be added to IV solutions that contain sodium bicarbonate because they precipitate as calcium carbonate.

▶ Prognosis

The prognosis is good for neonatal seizures entirely caused by hypocalcemia that is promptly treated.

INBORN ERRORS OF METABOLISM (SEE ALSO CHAPTER 34)

ESSENTIALS OF DIAGNOSIS & TYPICAL FEATURES

▶ Altered level of consciousness (poor feeding, lethargy, seizures) in a previously well-appearing infant.

▶ Tachypnea without hypoxemia or distress.

▶ Hypoglycemia, respiratory alkalosis, metabolic acidosis.

▶ Recurrent "sepsis" without proven infection.

Each individual inborn error of metabolism is rare, but collectively they have an incidence of 1 in 1000 live births. Expanded newborn genetic screening will undoubtedly aid in the diagnosis of these disorders; however, many infants will present prior to these results being available. The diseases are considered in detail in Chapter 34. These diagnoses should be entertained when infants who were initially well present with sepsis-like syndromes, recurrent hypoglycemia, neurologic syndromes (seizures or altered levels of consciousness), or unexplained acidosis (suggestive of organic acidemias).

In the immediate neonatal period, urea cycle disorders present as an altered level of consciousness secondary to hyperammonemia. A clinical clue that supports this diagnosis is hyperventilation with primary respiratory alkalosis, along with a lower-than-expected blood urea nitrogen. The other major diagnostic category to consider consists of infants with severe acidemia secondary to organic acidemias.

Cowan TM: Neonatal screening by tandem mass spectrometry. NeoReviews 2005;6:e539.

Enns GM: Inborn errors of metabolism masquerading as hypoxic-ischemic encephalopathy. NeoReviews 2005;6;e549.

Filiano JJ: Neurometabolic diseases in the newborn. Clin Perinatol 2006;33:411 [PMID: 16765732].

Marsden D, Larson C, Levy HL: Newborn screening for metabolic disorders. J Pediatr 2006;148:577 [PMID: 16737864].

Raghuveer TS et al: Inborn errors of metabolism in infancy and early childhood: An update. Am Fam Physician 2006;73:1981 [PMID: 16770930].

REFERENCES

Print Resources

Fanaroff AA, Martin RJ (editors): *Neonatal-Perinatal Medicine. Diseases of the Fetus and Infant,* 8th ed. Elsevier Mosby, 2005.

Jones KL (editor): *Smith's Recognizable Patterns of Human Malformation,* 6th ed. Elsevier Saunders, 2005.

Thureen PJ et al (editors): *Assessment and Care of the Well Newborn,* 2nd ed. Elsevier Saunders, 2005.

Web Resources

Cochrane neonatal database: http://www.nichd.nih.gov/cochraneneonatal/

Neonatal resuscitation program: http://www.aap.org/profed/nrp/nrpmain.html

NeoReviews : http://neoreviews.aapjournals.org/

Child Development & Behavior

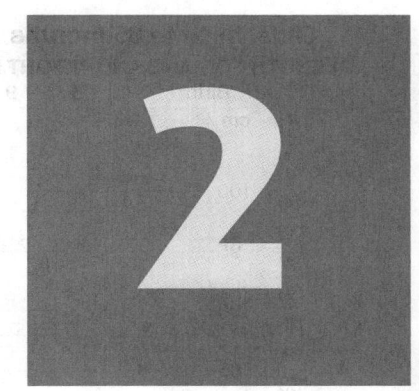

Edward Goldson, MD

Ann Reynolds, MD

The field of developmental and behavioral pediatrics has emerged as a subspecialty that addresses not only typical development but also the diagnosis and evaluation of atypical behavior and development. This chapter provides an overview of typical development, identifies developmental variations, and discusses several developmental disabilities. First, it discusses normal development, but does not cover the newborn period or adolescence (see Chapters 1 and 3, respectively). Second, it addresses behavioral variations, emphasizing that these variations reflect the spectrum of normal development and not pathology. Third, it deals with developmental and behavioral disorders and their treatment. The developmental principle, that is, the concept of ongoing change and maturation, is integral to the daily practice of pediatrics. For example, we recognize that a 3-month-old infant is very different from a 3-year-old and from a 13-year-old adolescent, not only with respect to what the child can do, but also in terms of the kind of illness he or she might have. From the perspective of the general pediatrician all of these areas should be viewed in the context of a "medical home." The medical home is defined as the setting that provides consistent, continuous, culturally competent, comprehensive and sensitive care to children and their families. It is a setting that advocates for all children, whether they are typical or have developmental challenges or disabilities. By incorporating the principles of child development—the concept that children are constantly changing—the medical home is the optimum setting to understand and enhance typical development and to address variations, delays, and deviations as they may occur in the life-trajectory of the child and family.

NORMAL DEVELOPMENT

Typical children follow a trajectory of increasing physical size (Figures 2–1 through 2–10) and increasing complexity of function (Figures 2–7 and 2–8 and Tables 2–1 and 2–2).

Table 2–3 provides the theoretical perspectives of human behavior, taking into consideration the work of Freud, Erikson, and Piaget.

The first 5 years of life are a period of extraordinary physical growth and increasing complexity of function. The child triples his or her birth weight within the first year and achieves two thirds of his or her brain size by age $2^{1}/_{2}$–3 years. The child progresses from a totally dependent infant at birth to a mobile, verbal person who is able to express his or her needs and desires by age 2–3 years. In the ensuing 3 years the child further develops the capacity to interact with peers and adults, achieves considerable verbal and physical prowess, and becomes ready to enter the academic world of learning and socialization.

It is critical for the clinician to identify disturbances in development during these early years because there may be windows of time or sensitive periods when appropriate interventions may be instituted to effectively address developmental issues.

THE FIRST 2 YEARS

From a motor perspective, children develop in a cephalocaudal direction. They can lift their heads with good control at 3 months, sit independently at 6 months, crawl at 9 months, walk at 1 year, and run by 18 months. The child learning to walk has a wide-based gait at first. Next, he or she walks with legs closer together, the arms move medially, a heel-toe gait develops, and the arms swing symmetrically by 18–24 months.

Clinicians often focus on gross motor development, but an appreciation of fine motor development and dexterity, particularly the grasp, can be instructive not only in monitoring normal development but also in identifying deviations in development. The grasp begins as a raking motion involving the ulnar aspect of the hand at age 3–4 months. The thumb is added to this motion at about age 5 months as the focus of the movement shifts to the radial side of the

▲ **Figure 2–1.** Percentile standards for length for age and weight for age in girls, birth to age 36 months. (Centers for Disease Control and Prevention.)

▲ **Figure 2–2.** Percentile standards for head circumference for age and weight for length in girls, birth to age 36 months. (Centers for Disease Control and Prevention.)

Boys, birth to 36 months
LENGTH FOR AGE AND WEIGHT FOR AGE PERCENTILES

Name _____

Record # _____

▲ **Figure 2–3.** Percentile standards for length for age and weight for age in boys, birth to age 36 months. (Centers for Disease Control and Prevention.)

▲ **Figure 2–4.** Percentile standards for head circumference for age and weight for length in boys, birth to age 36 months. (Centers for Disease Control and Prevention.)

Figure 2–5. Percentile standards for stature for age and weight for age in girls, 2–20 years. (Centers for Disease Control and Prevention.)

▲ **Figure 2–6.** Percentile standards for body mass index for age in girls, 2–20 years. (Centers for Disease Control and Prevention.)

Boys, 2 to 20 years

STATURE FOR AGE AND WEIGHT FOR AGE PERCENTILES

Name _____

Record # _____

▲ **Figure 2–7.** Percentile standards for stature for age and weight for age in boys, 2–20 years. (Centers for Disease Control and Prevention.)

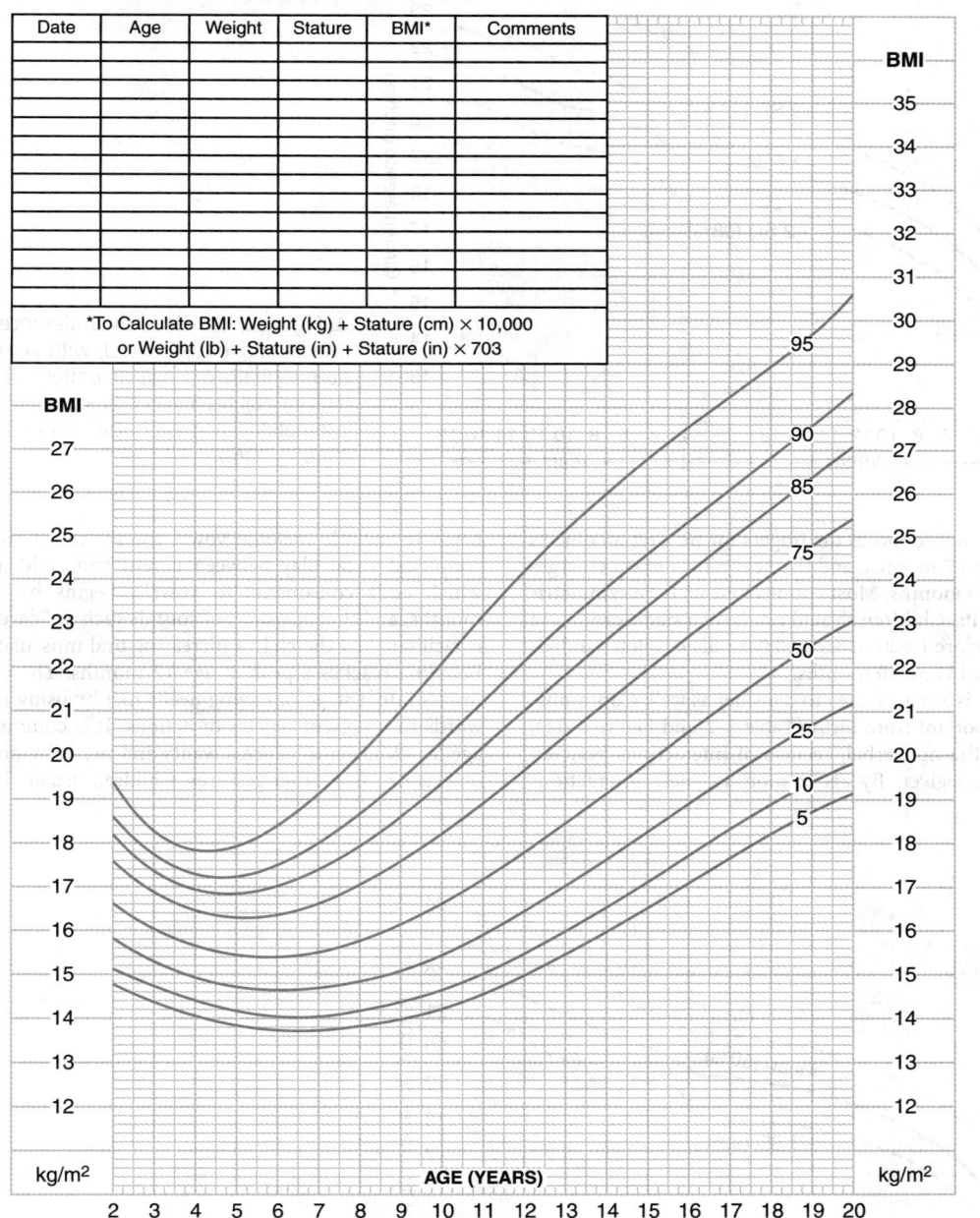

▲ Figure 2–8. Percentile standards for body mass index for age in boys, 2–20 years. (Centers for Disease Control and Prevention.)

▲ **Figure 2-9.** Head circumference of girls. (Modified and reproduced, with permission, from Nelhaus G: Head circumference from birth to eighteen years. Practical composite international and interracial graphs. Pediatrics 1968;41:106.)

hand. The thumb opposes the fingers for picking up objects just before age 7 months, and the neat pincer grasp emerges at about age 9 months. Most young children have symmetrical movements. Children should not have a significant hand preference before 1 year of age and typically develop handedness between 18 and 30 months.

Language is a critical area to consider as well. Communication is important from birth (Table 2–2 and Figure 2–11), particularly the nonverbal, reciprocal interactions between infant and caregiver. By age 2 months, these interactions

begin to include melodic vowel sounds called cooing and reciprocal vocal play between parent and child. Babbling, which adds consonants to vowels, begins by age 6–10 months, and the repetition of sounds such as "da-da-da-da" is facilitated by the child's increasing oral muscular control. Babbling reaches a peak at age 12 months. The child then moves into a stage of having needs met by using individual words to represent objects or actions. It is common at this age for children to express wants and needs by pointing to objects or using other gestures. Children usually have 5–10

▲ **Figure 2-10.** Head circumference of boys. (Modified and reproduced, with permission, from Nelhaus G: Head circumference from birth to eighteen years. Practical composite international and interracial graphs. Pediatrics 1968;41:106.)

Table 2–1. Developmental charts.

1–2 months

Activities to be observed:
Holds head erect and lifts head.
Turns from side to back.
Regards faces and follows objects through visual field.
Drops toys.
Becomes alert in response to voice.

Activities related by parent:
Recognizes parents.
Engages in vocalizations.
Smiles spontaneously.

3–5 months

Activities to be observed:
Grasps cube—first ulnar then later thumb opposition.
Reaches for and brings objects to mouth.
Makes "raspberry" sound.
Sits with support.

Activities related by parent:
Laughs.
Anticipates food on sight.
Turns from back to side.

6–8 months

Activities to be observed:
Sits alone for a short period.
Reaches with one hand.
First scoops up a pellet then grasps it using thumb opposition.
Imitates "bye-bye."
Passes object from hand to hand in midline.
Babbles.

Activities related by parent:
Rolls from back to stomach.
Is inhibited by the word *no*.

9–11 months

Activities to be observed:
Stands alone.
Imitates pat-a-cake and peek-a-boo.
Uses thumb and index finger to pick up pellet.

Activities related by parent:
Walks by supporting self on furniture.
Follows one-step verbal commands, eg, "Come here," "Give it to me."

1 year

Activities to be observed:
Walks independently.
Says "mama" and "dada" with meaning.
Can use a neat pincer grasp to pick up a pellet.
Releases cube into cup after demonstration.

Gives toys on request.
Tries to build a tower of 2 cubes.

Activities related by parent:
Points to desired objects.
Says 1 or 2 other words.

18 months

Activities to be observed:
Builds tower of 3–4 cubes.
Throws ball.
Seats self in chair.
Dumps pellet from bottle.

Activities related by parent:
Walks up and down stairs with help.
Says 4–20 words.
Understands a 2-step command.
Carries and hugs doll.
Feeds self.

24 months

Activities to be observed:
Speaks short phrases, 2 words or more.
Kicks ball on request.
Builds tower of 6–7 cubes.
Points to named objects or pictures.
Jumps off floor with both feet.
Stands on either foot alone.
Uses pronouns.

Activities related by parent:
Verbalizes toilet needs.
Pulls on simple garment.
Turns pages of book singly.
Plays with domestic mimicry.

30 months

Activities to be observed:
Walks backward.
Begins to hop on one foot.
Uses prepositions.
Copies a crude circle.
Points to objects described by use.
Refers to self as I.
Holds crayon in fist.

Activities related by parent:
Helps put things away.
Carries on a conversation.

3 years

Activities to be observed:
Holds crayon with fingers.
Builds tower of 9–10 cubes.

(continued)

Table 2–1. Developmental charts. *(Continued)*

Imitates 3-cube bridge.
Copies circle.
Gives first and last name.

Activities related by parent:
Rides tricycle using pedals.
Dresses with supervision.

3–4 years

Activities to be observed:
Climbs stairs with alternating feet.
Begins to button and unbutton.
"What do you like to do that's fun?" (Answers using plurals, personal pronouns, and verbs.)
Responds to command to place toy *in, on,* or *under* table.
Draws a circle when asked to draw a person.
Knows own sex. ("Are you a boy or a girl?")
Gives full name.
Copies a circle already drawn. ("Can you make one like this?")

Activities related by parent:
Feeds self at mealtime.
Takes off shoes and jacket.

4–5 years

Activities to be observed:
Runs and turns without losing balance.
May stand on one leg for at least 10 seconds.
Buttons clothes and laces shoes. (Does not tie.)
Counts to 4 by rote.
"Give me 2 sticks." (Able to do so from pile of 4 tongue depressors.)
Draws a person. (Head, 2 appendages, and possibly 2 eyes. No torso yet.)
Knows the days of the week. ("What day comes after Tuesday?")
Gives appropriate answers to: "What must you do if you are sleepy? Hungry? Cold?"
Copies + in imitation.

Activities related by parent:
Self-care at toilet. (May need help with wiping.)
Plays outside for at least 30 minutes.
Dresses self except for tying.

5–6 years

Activities to be observed:
Can catch ball.
Skips smoothly.
Copies a + already drawn.
Tells age.
Concept of 10 (eg, counts 10 tongue depressors). May recite to higher number by rote.

Knows right and left hand.
Draws recognizable person with at least 8 details.
Can describe favorite television program in some detail.

Activities related by parent:
Does simple chores at home (eg, taking out garbage, drying silverware).
Goes to school unattended or meets school bus.
Good motor ability but little awareness of dangers.

6–7 years

Activities to be observed:
Copies a Δ.
Defines words by use. ("What is an orange?" "To eat.")
Knows if morning or afternoon.
Draws a person with 12 details.
Reads several one-syllable printed words. (My, dog, see, boy.)

7–8 years

Activities to be observed:
Counts by 2s and 5s.
Ties shoes.
Copies a ◊
Knows what day of the week it is. (Not date or year.)
No evidence of sound substitution in speech (eg, *fr* for *thr*).
Draws a man with 16 details.
Reads paragraph #1 Durrell:

Reading:
Muff is a little yellow kitten. She drinks milk. She sleeps on a chair. She does not like to get wet.

Corresponding arithmetic:

$$
\begin{array}{cccc}
7 & 6 & 6 & 8 \\
+4 & +7 & -4 & -3 \\
\hline
\end{array}
$$

Adds and subtracts one-digit numbers.

8–9 years

Activities to be observed:
Defines words better than by use. ("What is an orange?" "A fruit.")
Can give an appropriate answer to the following: "What is the thing for you to do if . . .
   —you've broken something that belongs to someone else?"
   —a playmate hits you without meaning to do so?"
Reads paragraph #2 Durrell:

Reading:
A little black dog ran away from home. He played with two big dogs. They ran away from him. It began to rain. He went under a tree. He wanted to go home, but he did not know the way. He saw a boy he knew. The boy took him home.

(continued)

Table 2–1. Developmental charts. *(Continued)*

Corresponding arithmetic:

67	45	14	84
+4	16	−8	−36
	+27		

Is learning borrowing and carrying processes in addition and subtraction.

9–10 years

Activities to be observed:
Knows the month, day, and year.
Names the months in order. (15 seconds, 1 error.)
Makes a sentence with these 3 words in it: (1 or 2. Can use words orally in proper context.)

   1. work . . . money . . . men
   2. boy . . . river . . . ball

Reads paragraph #3 Durrell:

Reading:
Six boys put up a tent by the side of a river. They took things to eat with them. When the sun went down, they went into the tent to sleep. In the night, a cow came and began to eat grass around the tent. The boys were afraid. They thought it was a bear.

Should comprehend and answer the question: "What was the cow doing?"

Corresponding arithmetic:

5204	23	837
−530	×3	×7

Learning simple multiplication.

10–12 years

Activities to be observed:
Should read and comprehend paragraph #5 Durrell:

Reading:
In 1807, Robert Fulton took the first long trip in a steamboat. He went one hundred and fifty miles up the Hudson River. The boat went five miles an hour. This was faster than a steamboat had ever gone before. Crowds gathered on both banks of the river to see this new kind of boat. They were afraid that its noise and splashing would drive away all the fish.

Answer: "What river was the trip made on?"
Ask to write the sentence: "The fishermen did not like the boat."

Corresponding arithmetic:

420	9)72	31)62
×29		

Should do multiplication and simple division.

12–15 years

Activities to be observed:
Reads paragraph #7 Durrell:

Reading:
Golf originated in Holland as a game played on ice. The game in its present form first appeared in Scotland. It became unusually popular and kings found it so enjoyable that it was known as "the royal game." James IV, however, thought that people neglected their work to indulge in this fascinating sport so that it was forbidden in 1457. James relented when he found how attractive the game was, and it immediately regained its former popularity. Golf spread gradually to other countries, being introduced in America in 1890. It has grown in favor until there is hardly a town that does not boast of a private or public course.

Ask to write a sentence: "Golf originated in Holland as a game played on ice."

Answers questions:
"Why was golf forbidden by James IV?"
"Why did he change his mind?"

Corresponding arithmetic:

536)4762	$\frac{1}{3}$	$7\frac{1}{6}$
	$+\frac{1}{3}$	$-\frac{3}{4}$

Reduce fractions to lowest forms.
Does long division, adds and subtracts fractions.

Modified from Leavitt SR, Goodman H, Harvin D: Use of developmental charts in teaching well child care. Pediatrics 1963;31:499.

comprehensible words by 12–18 months; by age 2 years they are putting 2–3 words into phrases, 50% of which their caregivers can understand (see Tables 2–1 and 2–2 and Figure 2–11). The acquisition of expressive vocabulary varies greatly between 12 and 24 months of age. As a group, males and children who are bilingual tend to develop expressive language more slowly during that time. It is important to note, however, that for each individual, milestones should still fall within the expected range. Gender and exposure to two languages should never be used as an excuse for failing to refer a child who has significant delay in the acquisition of speech and language for further evaluation. It is also important to note that most children are not truly bilingual. Most children have one primary language, and any other languages are secondary.

Receptive language usually develops more rapidly than expressive language. Word comprehension begins to increase at age 9 months, and by age 13 months the child's receptive vocabulary may be as large as 20–100 words. After age 18 months, expressive and receptive vocabularies increase dramatically, and by the end of the second year there is typically a quantum leap in language development. The child begins to put together words and phrases and begins to use language to represent a new world, the symbolic world. Children begin to put verbs into phrases and focus much of their language on describing their new abili-

Table 2–2. Normal speech and language development.

Age	Speech	Language	Articulation
1 month	Throaty sounds		Vowels: \ah\, \uh\, \ee\
2 months	Vowel sounds ("eh"), coos		
2½ months	Squeals		
3 months	Babbles, initial vowels		
4 months	Guttural sounds ("ah," "go")		Consonants: m, p, b
5 months			Vowels: \o\, \u\
7 months	Imitates speech sounds		
8 months			Syllables: da, ba, ka
10 months		"Dada" or "mama" nonspecifically	Approximates names: baba/bottle
12 months	Jargon begins (own language)	One word other than "mama" or "dada"	Understandable: 2–3 words
13 months		Three words	
16 months		Six words	Consonants: t, d, w, n, h
18–24 months		Two-word phrases	Understandable 2-word phrases
24–30 months		Three-word phrases	Understandable 3-word phrases
2 years	Vowels uttered correctly	Approximately 270 words; uses pronouns	Approximately 270 words; uses phrases
3 years	Some degree of hesitancy and uncertainty common	Approximately 900 words; intelligible 4-word phrases	Approximately 900 words; intelligible 4-word phrases
4 years		Approximately 1540 words; intelligible 5-word phrases or sentences	Approximately 1540 words; intelligible 5-word phrases
6 years		Approximately 2560 words; intelligible 6- or 7-word sentences	Approximately 2560 words; intelligible 6- or 7-word sentences
7–8 years	Adult proficiency		

Data on articulation from Berry MF: *Language Disorders of Children.* Appleton-Century-Crofts, 1969; and from Bzoch K, League R: *Receptive-Expressive Emergent Language Scale.* University Park Press, 1970.

ties, for example, "I go out." They begin to incorporate prepositions, such as "I" and "you" into speech and ask "why?" and "what?" questions more frequently. They also begin to appreciate time factors and to understand and use this concept in their speech (see Table 2–1).

The Early Language Milestone Scale (see Figure 2–11) is a simple tool for assessing early language development in the pediatric office setting. It is scored in the same way as the Denver II (Figure 2–12) but tests receptive and expressive language areas in greater depth.

One may easily memorize the developmental milestones that characterize the trajectory of the typical child; however, these milestones become more meaningful and clinically useful if placed in empirical and theoretical contexts. The work of Piaget and others is quite instructive and provides some insight into behavioral and affective development (see Table 2–3). Piaget described the first 2 years of life as the sensorimotor period, during which infants learn with increasing sophistication how to link sensory input from the environment with a motor response. Infants build on prim-

itive reflex patterns of behavior (termed schemata; sucking is an example) and constantly incorporate or assimilate new experiences. The schemata evolve over time as infants accommodate new experiences and as new levels of cognitive ability unfold in an orderly sequence. Enhancement of neural networks through dendritic branching and pruning (apoptosis) occurs.

In the first year of life, the infant's perception of reality revolves around itself and what it can see or touch. The infant follows the trajectory of an object through the field of vision, but before age 6 months the object ceases to exist once it leaves the infant's field of vision. At age 9–12 months, the infant gradually develops the concept of object permanence, or the realization that objects exist even when not seen. The development of object permanence correlates with enhanced frontal activity on the electroencephalogram. The concept attaches first to the image of the mother or primary caregiver because of his or her emotional importance and is a critical part of attachment behavior (discussed later). In the second year, children extend their ability to manipulate

Table 2–3. Perspectives of human behavior.

Age	Theories of Development			Skill Areas		
	Freud	Erikson	Piaget	Language	Motor	Psychopathology
Birth to 18 months	Oral	Basic trust versus mistrust	Sensorimotor	Body actions; crying; naming; pointing	Reflex sitting, reaching, grasping, walking	Autism; anaclitic depression, colic; disorders of attachment; feeding, sleeping problems
18 months–3 years	Anal	Autonomy versus shame, doubt	Symbolic (pre-operational)	Sentences; telegraph jargon	Climbing, running	Separation issues; negativism; fearfulness; constipation; shyness, withdrawal
3–6 years	Oedipal	Initiative versus guilt	Intuition (pre-operational)	Connective words; can be readily understood	Increased coordination; tricycle; jumping	Enuresis; encopresis; anxiety; aggressive acting out; phobias; nightmares
6–11 years	Latency	Industry versus inferiority	Concrete operational	Subordinate sentences; reading and writing; language reasoning	Increased skills; sports, recreational cooperative games	School phobias; obsessive reactions; conversion reactions; depressive equivalents
12–17 years	Adolescence (genital)	Identity versus role confusion	Formal operational	Reason abstract; using language; abstract manipulation	Refinement of skills	Delinquency; promiscuity; schizophrenia; anorexia nervosa; suicide

Adapted and reproduced, with permission, from Dixon S: Setting the stage: Theories and concepts of child development. In Dixon S, Stein M (editors): *Encounters with Children,* 2nd ed. Year Book, 1992.

objects by using instruments, first by imitation and later by trial and error.

Freud described the first year of life as the oral stage because so many of the infant's needs are fulfilled by oral means. Nutrition is obtained through sucking on the breast or bottle, and self-soothing occurs through sucking on fingers or a pacifier. During this stage of symbiosis with the mother, the boundaries between mother and infant are blurred. The infant's needs are totally met by the mother, and the mother has been described as manifesting "narcissistic possessiveness" of the infant. This is a very positive interaction in the bidirectional attachment process called bonding. The parents learn to be aware of and to interpret the infant's cues, which reflect its needs. A more sensitive emotional interaction process develops that can be seen in the mirroring of facial expressions by the primary caregiver and infant and in their mutual engagement in cycles of attention and inattention, which further develop into social play. A parent who is depressed or cannot respond to the infant's expressions and cues can have a profoundly adverse effect on the child's future development. Erikson's terms of basic trust versus mistrust are another way of describing the reciprocal interaction that characterizes this stage. Turn-taking games, which occur between ages 3 and 6 months, are a pleasure for both the parents and the infant and are an extension of mirroring behavior. They also represent an early form of imitative behavior, which is important in later social and cognitive development. More sophisticated games, such as peek-a-boo, occur at approximately age 9 months. The infant's thrill at the reappearance of the face that vanished momentarily demonstrates the emerging understanding of object permanence. Age 8–9 months is also a critical time in the attachment process because this is when separation anxiety and stranger anxiety become marked. The infant at this stage is able to appreciate discrepant events that do not match previously known schemata. These new events cause uncertainty and subsequently fear and anxiety. The infant must be able to retrieve previous schemata and incorporate new information over an extended time. These abilities are developed by age 8 months and give rise to the fears that may subsequently develop: stranger anxiety and separation anxiety. In stranger anxiety, the infant analyzes the face of a stranger, detects the mismatch with previous schemata or what is familiar, and responds with fear or anxiety, leading to crying. In separation anxiety, the child perceives the difference between the primary caregiver's presence and his or her absence by remembering the schema of the caregiver's presence. Perceiving the inconsistency, the child first becomes uncertain and then anxious and fearful. This begins at age 8 months, reaches a peak at 15 months, and disappears by the end of 2 years in a relatively orderly progression as central nervous system (CNS) maturation facilitates the development of new skills. A parent can put the child's understanding of object permanence to good use by placing a picture of the mother (or father) near the child or by leaving an object (eg, her sweater) where the child can see it during her

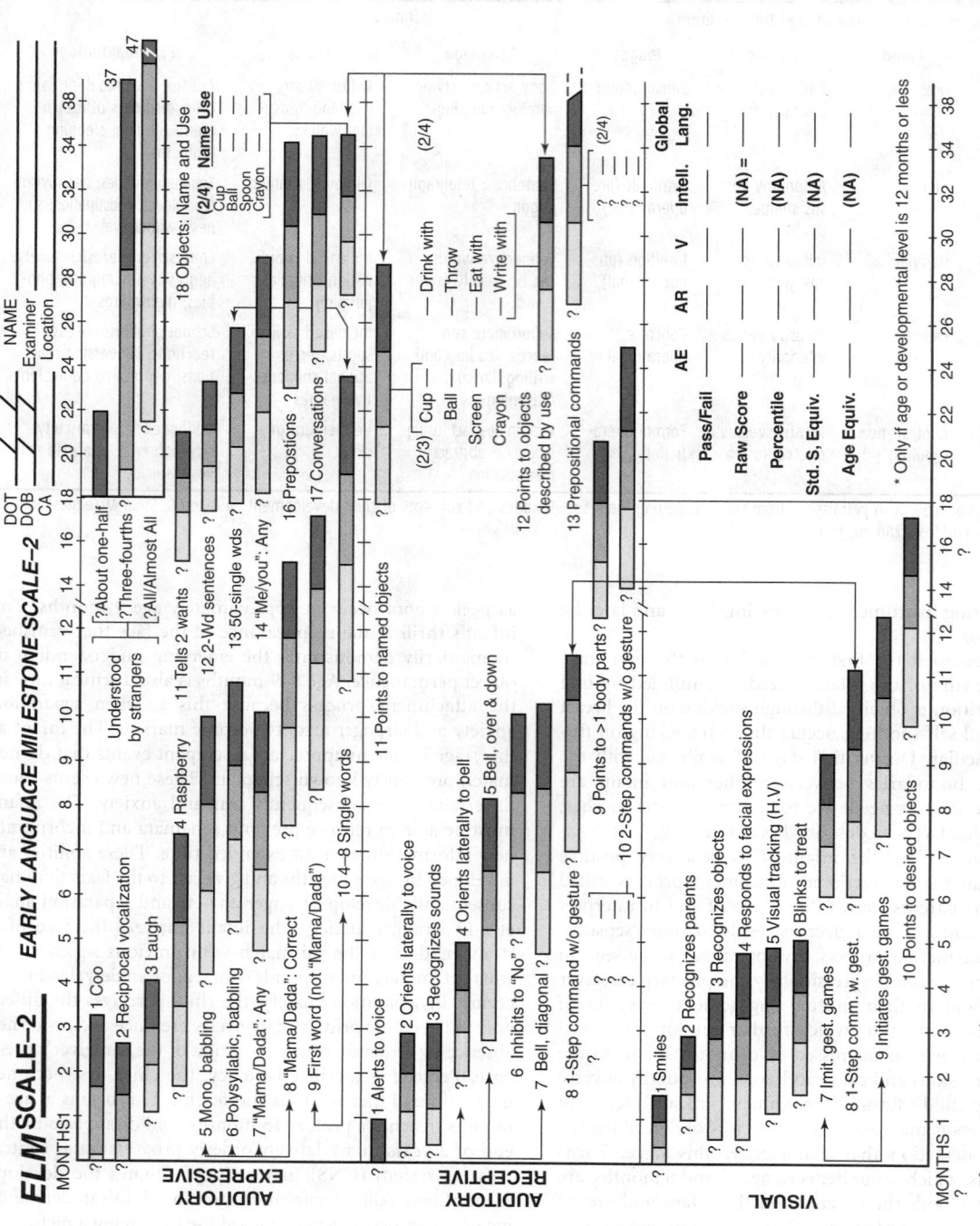

▲ **Figure 2-11.** Early Language Milestone Scale-2. (Reproduced, with permission, from Coplan J: *Early Language Milestone Scale*. Pro Ed, 1993.)

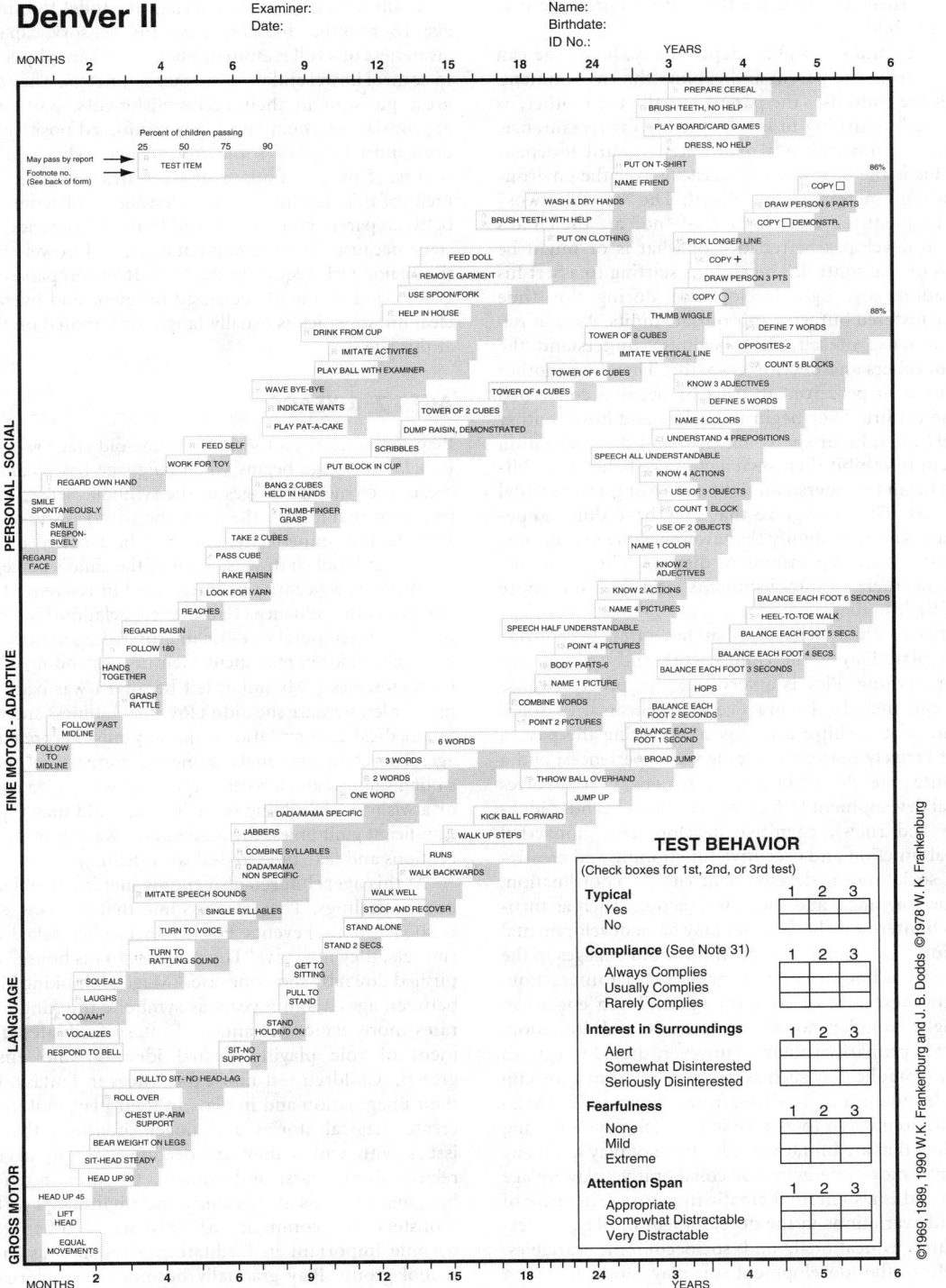

▲ **Figure 2–12.** Denver II. (Copyright © 1969, 1989, 1990 WK Frankenburg and JB Dodds. © 1978 WK Frankenberg.)

absence. A visual substitute for the mother's presence may comfort the child.

Once the child can walk independently, he or she can move away from the parent and explore the environment. Although the child uses the parent, usually the mother, as "home base," returning to her frequently for reassurance, he or she has now taken a major step toward independence. This is the beginning of mastery over the environment and an emerging sense of self. The "terrible twos" and the frequent self-asserting use of "no" are the child's attempt to develop a better idea of what is or might be under his or her control. The child is starting to assert his or her autonomy. Ego development during this time should be fostered but with appropriate limits. As children develop a sense of self, they begin to understand the feelings of others and develop empathy. They hug another child who is perceived distress or become concerned when one is hurt. They begin to understand how another child feels when he or she is harmed, and this realization helps them to inhibit their own aggressive behavior. Children also begin to understand right and wrong and parental expectations. They recognize that they have done something "bad" and may signify that awareness by saying "uh-oh" or with other expressions of distress. They also take pleasure in their accomplishments and become more aware of their bodies.

An area of child behavior that has often been overlooked is play. Play is the child's work and a significant means of learning. Play is a very complex process whose purpose can include the practice and rehearsal of roles, skills, and relationships; a means of revisiting the past; a means of actively mastering a range of experiences; and a way to integrate the child's life experiences. It involves emotional development (affect regulation and gender identification and roles), cognitive development (nonverbal and verbal function and executive functioning and creativity), and social/motor development (motor coordination, frustration tolerance, and social interactions such as turn-taking). Of interest is the fact that play has a developmental progression. The typical 6- to 12-month-old engages in the game of peek-a-boo, which is a form of social interaction. During the next year or so, although children engage in increasingly complex social interactions and imitation, their play is primarily solitary. However, they do begin to engage in symbolic play such as by drinking from a toy cup and then by giving a doll a drink from a toy cup. By age 2–3 years children begin to engage in parallel play (engaging in behaviors that are imitative). This form of play gradually evolves into more interactive or collaborative play by age 3–4 years and is also more thematic in nature. There are of course wide variations in the development of play, reflecting cultural, educational, and socioeconomic variables. Nevertheless, the development of play does follow a sequence that can be assessed and can be very informative in the evaluation of the child.

Brain maturation sets the stage for toilet training. After age 18 months, toddlers have the sensory capacity for awareness of a full rectum or bladder and are physically able to control bowel and urinary tract sphincters. They also take great pleasure in their accomplishments, particularly in appropriate elimination, if it is reinforced positively. Children must be given some control over when elimination occurs. If parents impose severe restrictions, the achievement of this developmental milestone can become a battle between parent and child. Freud termed this period the anal stage because the developmental issue of bowel control is the major task requiring mastery. It encompasses a more generalized theme of socialized behavior and overall body cleanliness, which is usually taught or imposed on the child at this age.

AGES 2–4 YEARS

Piaget characterized the 2- to 6-year-old stage as preoperational. This stage begins when language has facilitated the creation of mental images in the symbolic sense. The child begins to manipulate the symbolic world; sorts out reality from fantasy imperfectly; and may be terrified of dreams, wishes, and foolish threats. Most of the child's perception of the world is egocentric or interpreted in reference to his or her needs or influence. Cause-effect relationships are confused with temporal ones or interpreted egocentrically. For example, children may focus their understanding of divorce on themselves ("My father left because I was bad" or "My mother left because she didn't love me"). Illness and the need for medical care are also commonly misinterpreted at this age. The child may make a mental connection between a sibling's illness and a recent argument, a negative comment, or a wish for the sibling to be ill. The child may experience significant guilt unless the parents are aware of these misperceptions and take time to deal with them.

At this age, children also endow inanimate objects with human feelings. They also assume that humans cause or create all natural events. For instance, when asked why the sun sets, they may say, "The sun goes to his house" or "It is pushed down by someone else." Magical thinking blossoms between ages 3 and 5 years as symbolic thinking incorporates more elaborate fantasy. Fantasy facilitates development of role playing, sexual identity, and emotional growth. Children test new experiences in fantasy, both in their imagination and in play. In their play, children often create magical stories and novel situations that reflect issues with which they are dealing, such as aggression, relationships, fears, and control. Children often invent imaginary friends at this time, and nightmares or fears of monsters are common. At this stage, other children become important in facilitating play, such as in a preschool group. Play gradually becomes more cooperative; shared fantasy leads to game playing. Freud described the oedipal phase between ages 3 and 6 years, when there is strong attachment to the parent of the opposite sex. The child's fantasies may focus on play-acting the adult role with that parent, although by age 6 years oedipal issues are usually resolved and attachment is redirected to the parent of the same sex.

EARLY SCHOOL YEARS: AGES 5–7 YEARS

Attendance at kindergarten at age 5 years marks an acceleration in the separation-individuation theme initiated in the preschool years. The child is ready to relate to peers in a more interactive manner. The brain has reached 90% of its adult weight. Sensorimotor coordination abilities are maturing and facilitating pencil-and-paper tasks and sports, both part of the school experience. Cognitive abilities are still at the preoperational stage, and children focus on one variable in a problem at a time. However, most children have mastered conservation of length by age $5^1/_2$ years, conservation of mass and weight by $6^1/_2$ years, and conservation of volume by 8 years.

By first grade, there is more pressure on the child to master academic tasks—recognizing numbers, letters, and words and learning to write. Piaget described the stage of concrete operations beginning after age 6 years, when the child is able to perform mental operations concerning concrete objects that involve manipulation of more than one variable. The child is able to order, number, and classify because these activities are related to concrete objects in the environment and because these activities are stressed in early schooling. Magical thinking diminishes greatly at this time, and the reality of cause-effect relationships is better understood. Fantasy and imagination are still strong and are reflected in themes of play.

MIDDLE CHILDHOOD: AGES 7–11 YEARS

Freud characterized ages 7–11 years as the latency years, during which children are not bothered by significant aggressive or sexual drives but instead devote most of their energies to school and peer group interactions. In reality, throughout this period there is a gradual increase in sex drive, manifested by increasingly aggressive play and interactions with the opposite sex. Fantasy still has an active role in dealing with sexuality before adolescence, and fantasies often focus on movie and music stars. Organized sports, clubs, and other activities are other modalities that permit preadolescent children to display socially acceptable forms of aggression and sexual interest.

For the 7-year-old child, the major developmental tasks are achievement in school and acceptance by peers. Academic expectations intensify and require the child to concentrate on, attend to, and process increasingly complex auditory and visual information. Children with significant learning disabilities or problems with attention, organization, and impulsivity may have difficulty with academic tasks and subsequently may receive negative reinforcement

from teachers, peers, and even parents. Such children may develop a poor self-image manifested as behavioral difficulties. The pediatrician must evaluate potential learning disabilities in any child who is not developing adequately at this stage or who presents with emotional or behavioral problems. The developmental status of school-aged children is not documented as easily as that of younger children because of the complexity of the milestones. In the school-aged child, the quality of the response, the attentional abilities, and the child's emotional approach to the task can make a dramatic difference in success at school. The clinician must consider all of these aspects in the differential diagnosis of learning disabilities and behavioral disorders.

Bjorklund FP: *Children's Thinking.* Brooks/Cole, 1995.

Dixon SD, Stein MT: *Encounters with Children: Pediatric Behavior and Development,* 4th ed. Mosby-Year Book, 2006.

Feldman HM: Evaluation and management of language and speech disorders in preschool children. Pediatr Rev 2005;26:131 [PMID: 15805236].

Frankenberg WK et al: The Denver II: A major revision and restandardization of the Denver Developmental Screening Test. Pediatrics 1992;89:91 [PMID: 1370185].

Glascoe FP, Dworkin PH: The role of parents in the detection of developmental and behavioral problems. Pediatrics 1995; 95:829 [PMID: 7539122].

Green M, Palfrey JS (editors): *Bright Futures: Guidelines for Health Supervision of Infants, Children, and Adolescents,* 2nd ed revised. National Center for Education in Maternal and Child Health Georgetown University, 2002.

BEHAVIORAL & DEVELOPMENTAL VARIATIONS

Behavioral and developmental variations and disorders encompass a wide range of issues of importance to pediatricians. Practitioners will be familiar with most of the problems discussed in this chapter; however, with increasing knowledge of the factors controlling normal neurologic and behavioral development in childhood, new perspectives on these disorders and novel approaches to their diagnosis and management are emerging.

Variations in children's behavior reflect a blend of intrinsic biologic characteristics and the environments with which the children interact. The next section focuses on some of the more common complaints about behavior encountered by those who care for children. These behavioral complaints are by and large normal variations in behavior, a reflection of each child's individual biologic and temperament traits and the parents' responses. There are no cures for these behaviors, but management strategies are available that can enhance the parents' understanding of the child and the child's relationship to the environment. These strategies also facilitate the parents' care of the growing infant and child.

The last section of this chapter discusses developmental disorders of cognitive and social competence. Diagnosis and management of these conditions requires a comprehensive and often multidisciplinary approach. The health care provider can play a major role in diagnosis, in coordinating the child's evaluation, in interpreting the results to the family, and in providing reassurance and support.

Capute AJ, Accardo PJ (editors): *Developmental Disabilities in Infancy and Childhood*, 2nd ed. Vol. 1, *Neurodevelopmental Diagnosis and Treatment*. Vol. 2, *The Spectrum of Developmental Disabilities*. Brookes/Cole, 1996.

Levine MD et al (editors): *Developmental-Behavioral Pediatrics*, 3rd ed. WB Saunders, 1999.

Medical Home Initiatives for Children with Special Needs Project Advisory Committee, American Academy of Pediatrics: The medical home. Pediatrics 2002;110:184 [PMID: 12093969].

Wolraich ML et al: *The Classification of Child and Adolescent Mental Diagnoses in Primary Care: Diagnostic and Statistical Manual for Primary Care (DSM-PC) Child and Adolescent Version*. American Academy of Pediatrics, 1996.

NORMALITY & TEMPERAMENT

The physician confronted by a disturbance in physiologic function rarely has doubts about what is abnormal. Variations in temperament and behavior are not as straightforward. Labeling such variations as disorders implies that a disease entity exists.

The behaviors described in this section are viewed as part of a continuum of responses by the child to a variety of internal and external experiences. Variations in temperament have been of interest to philosophers and writers since ancient times. The Greeks believed there were four temperament types: choleric, sanguine, melancholic, and phlegmatic. In more recent times, folk wisdom has defined temperament as a genetically influenced behavioral disposition that is stable over time. Although a number of models of temperament have been proposed, the one usually used by pediatricians in clinical practice is that of Thomas and Chess, who describe temperament as being the "how" of behavior as distinguished from the "why" (motivation) and the "what" (ability). Temperament is an independent psychological attribute that is expressed as a response to an external stimulus. The influence of temperament is bidirectional: The effect of a particular experience will be influenced by the child's temperament, and the child's temperament will influence the responses of others in the child's environment. Temperament is the style with which the child interacts with the environment.

The perceptions and expectations of parents must be considered when a child's behavior is evaluated. A child that one parent might describe as hyperactive might not be characterized as such by the other parent. This truism can be expanded to include all the dimensions of temperament. Thus, the concept of "goodness of fit" comes into play. For example, if the parents want and expect their child to be

Table 2–4. Theories of temperament.

Thomas and Chess	Temperament is an independent psychologic attribute, biologically determined, which is expressed as a response to an external stimulus. It is the child's behavioral style: an interactive model.
Rothbart	Temperament is a function of biologically based individual differences in reactivity and self-regulation. It is subsumed under the concept of "personality" and goes beyond mere "behavioral style."
Buss and Plomin	Temperament is a set of genetically determined personality traits that appear early in life and are different from other inherited and acquired personality traits.
Goldsmith and Campos	Temperament is the individual's differences in the probability of experiencing emotions and arousal.

predictable but that is not the child's behavioral style, the parents may perceive the child as being bad or having a behavioral disorder rather than as having a developmental variation. An appreciation of this phenomenon is important because the physician may be able to enhance the parents' understanding of the child and influence their responses to the child's behavior. When there is goodness of fit, there will be more harmony and a greater potential for healthy development not only of the child but also of the family. When goodness of fit is not present, tension and stress can result in parental anger, disappointment, frustration, and conflict with the child.

Other models of temperament include those of Rothbart, Buss and Plomin, and Goldsmith and Campos (Table 2–4). All models seek to identify intrinsic behavioral characteristics that lead the child to respond to the world in particular ways. One child may be highly emotional and another less so (ie, calmer) in response to a variety of experiences, stressful or pleasant. The clinician must recognize that each child brings some intrinsic, biologically based traits to its environment and that such characteristics are neither good nor bad, right nor wrong, normal nor abnormal; they are simply part of the child. Thus, as one looks at variations in development, one should abandon the illness model and consider this construct as an aid to understanding the nature of the child's behavior and its influence on the parent-child relationship.

Barr RG: Normality: A clinically useless concept: The case of infant crying and colic. J Dev Behav Pediatr 1993;14:264 [PMID: 8408670].

Goldsmith HH et al: Roundtable: What is temperament? Four approaches. Child Dev 1987;58:505 [PMID: 3829791].

Prior M: Childhood temperament. J Child Psychol Psychiatr 1992;33:249 [PMID: 1737829].

Thomas A, Chess S: *Temperament and Development*. Brunner/Mazel, 1977.

COMMON DEVELOPMENTAL CONCERNS

COLIC

 ESSENTIALS OF DIAGNOSIS & TYPICAL FEATURES

▶ An otherwise healthy infant aged 2–3 months seems to be in pain, cries for > 3 hours a day, for > 3 days a week, for > 3 weeks ("rule of threes").

Infant colic is characterized by severe and paroxysmal crying that occurs mainly in the late afternoon. The infant's knees are drawn up and its fists are clenched, flatus is expelled, the facies is pained, and there is minimal response to attempts at soothing. Studies in the United States have shown that among middle-class infants, crying occupies about 2 hours per day at 2 weeks of age, about 3 hours per day by 6 weeks, and gradually decreases to about 1 hour per day by 3 months. The word "colic" is derived from Greek *kolikos* ("pertaining to the colon"). Although colic has traditionally been attributed to gastrointestinal disturbances, this has never been proved. Colic is a behavioral sign or symptom that begins in the first few weeks of life and peaks at age 2–3 months. In about 30–40% of cases, colic continues into the fourth and fifth months.

A colicky infant, as defined by Wessel, is one who is healthy and well fed but cries for more than 3 hours a day, for more than 3 days a week, and for more than 3 weeks—commonly referred to as the rule of threes. The important word in this definition is "healthy." Thus, before the diagnosis of colic can be made, the pediatrician must rule out diseases that might cause crying. With the exception of the few infants who respond to elimination of cow's milk from its own or the mother's diet, there has been little firm evidence of an association of colic with allergic disorders. Gastroesophageal reflux is often suspected as a cause of colicky crying in young infants. Undetected corneal abrasion, urinary tract infection, and unrecognized traumatic injuries, including child abuse, must be among the physical causes of crying considered in evaluating these infants. Some attempts have been made to eliminate gas with simethicone and to slow gut motility with dicyclomine. Simethicone has not been shown to ameliorate colic. Dicyclomine has been associated with apnea in infants and is contraindicated.

This then leaves characteristics intrinsic to the child (ie, temperament) and parental caretaking patterns as contributing to colic. Behavioral states have three features: (1) they are self-organizing—that is, they are maintained until it is necessary to shift to another one; (2) they are stable over several minutes; and (3) the same stimulus elicits a state-specific response that is different from other states. The behavioral states are (among others) a crying state, a quiet alert state, an active alert state, a transitional state, and a state of deep sleep.

The states of importance with respect to colic are the crying state and the transitional state. During transition from one state to another, infant behavior may be more easily influenced. Once an infant is in a stable state (eg, crying), it becomes more difficult to bring about a change (eg, to soothe). How these transitions are accomplished is probably influenced by the infant's temperament and neurologic maturity. Some infants move from one state to another easily and can be diverted easily; other infants sustain a particular state and are resistant to change.

The other component to be considered in evaluating the colicky infant is the feeding and handling behavior of the caregiver. Colic is a behavioral phenomenon that involves interaction between the infant and the caregiver. Different caregivers perceive and respond to crying behavior differently. If the caregiver perceives the crying infant as being spoiled and demanding and is not sensitive to or knowledgeable about the infant's cues and rhythms—or is hurried and "rough" with the infant—the infant's ability to organize and soothe him- or herself or respond to the caregiver's attempts at soothing may be compromised. Alternatively, if the temperament of an infant with colic is understood and the rhythms and cues deciphered, crying can be anticipated and the caregiver can intervene before the behavior becomes "organized" in the crying state and more difficult to extinguish.

▶ Management

Several approaches can be taken to the management of colic.

1. Parents may need to be educated about the developmental characteristics of crying behavior and made aware that crying increases normally into the second month and abates by the third to fourth month.

2. Parents may need reassurance, based on a complete history and physical examination, that the infant is not sick. Although these behaviors are stressful, they are a normal variant and are usually self-limited. This discussion can be facilitated by having the parent keep a diary of crying and weight gain. If there is a diurnal pattern and adequate weight gain, an underlying disease process is less likely to be present. Parental anxiety must be relieved, because it may be contributing to the problem.

3. For parents to effectively soothe and comfort the infant, they need to understand the infant's cues. The pediatrician can help by observing the infant's behavior and devising interventions aimed at calming both the infant and the parents. One can encourage a quiet environment without excessive handling. Rhythmic stimulation such as gentle swinging or rocking, soft music, drives in the car, or walks in the stroller may be helpful, especially if the parents are able to anticipate the onset of crying. Another approach is to change the feeding habits so that the infant is not rushed, has ample opportunity to burp, and if necessary can be fed more frequently so as to

decrease gastric distention if that seems to be contributing to the problem.

4. Medications such as phenobarbital elixir and dicyclomine have been found to be somewhat helpful, but their use is to be discouraged because of the risk of adverse reactions and overdosage. A trial of ranitidine hydrochloride might be of help if gastroesophageal reflux is contributing to the child's discomfort.

5. For colic that is refractory to behavioral management, a trial of changing the feedings, and eliminating cow's milk from the formula or from the mother's diet if she is nursing, may be indicated.

Barr RG: Colic and crying syndromes in infants. Pediatrics 1998;102:1282 [PMID: 9794970].

Barr RG et al (editors): *Crying as a Sign, a Symptom, and a Signal: Clinical, Emotional, and Developmental Aspects of Infant and Toddler Crying.* MacKeith Press, 2000.

Barr RG, Geertsma MA: Colic: The pain perplex. In: Schechter NL et al (editors): *Pain in Infants, Children and Adolescents.* Williams & Wilkins, 1993.

Dihigo SK: New strategies for the treatment of colic: Modifying the parent-infant interaction. J Pediatr Health Care 1998;12: 256 [PMID: 9987256].

Lucassen PL et al: Effectiveness of treatments for infantile colic: A systematic review. Br Med J 1998;316:1563 [PMID: 1945549].

Miller AR, Barr RG: Infantile colic: Is it a gut issue? Pediatr Clin North Am 1991;38:1407.

Treem WR: Infant colic: A pediatric gastroenterologist's perspective. Pediatr Clin North Am 1994;41:1121 [PMID: 7936776].

Turner JL, Palamountain S: Clinical features and etiology of colic. In: Rose BD (editor): *UpToDate.* UpToDate, 2005.

Turner JL, Palamountain S: Evaluation and management of colic. In: Rose BD (editor): *UpToDate.* UpToDate, 2005.

FEEDING DISORDERS IN INFANTS & YOUNG CHILDREN

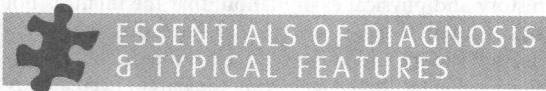

ESSENTIALS OF DIAGNOSIS & TYPICAL FEATURES

▶ Inadequate or disordered intake of food due to any of the following conditions:

- Poor oral motor coordination.
- Fatigue resulting from a chronic disease.
- Lack of appetite.
- Behavioral issues relating to parent-child interaction.
- Pain associated with feeding.

Children have feeding problems for various reasons including oral motor dysfunction, cardiopulmonary disorders leading to fatigue, gastrointestinal disturbances causing pain, social or emotional issues, and problems with regulation. The common denominator, however, is usually food refusal. Infants and young children may refuse to eat if they find eating painful or frightening. They may have had unpleasant experiences (emotional or physiologic) associated with eating, they may be depressed, or they may be engaged in a developmental conflict with the caregiver that is being played out in the arena of feeding. The infant may refuse to eat if the rhythm of the feeding experience with the caregiver is not harmonious. The child who has had an esophageal atresia repair and has a stricture may find eating uncomfortable. The very young infant with severe oral candidiasis may refuse to eat because of pain. The child who has had a choking experience associated with feeding may be terrified to eat (oral motor dysfunction or aspiration). The child who is forced to eat by a maltreating parent or an overzealous caregiver may refuse feeds. Children who have required nasogastric feedings or who have required periods of fasting and intravenous nutrition in the first 1–2 months of life are more likely to display food refusal behavior upon introduction of oral feedings.

Depression in children may be expressed through food refusal. Food refusal may develop when the infant's cues around feeding are not interpreted correctly by the parent. The infant who needs to burp more frequently or who needs time between bites but instead is rushed will often passively refuse to eat. Some will be more active refusers, turning their heads away to avoid the feeder, spitting out food, or pushing away food.

Chatoor and coworkers have proposed a developmental and interactive construct of the feeding experience. The stages through which the child normally progresses are establishment of homeostasis (0–2 months), attachment (2–6 months), and separation and individuation (6 months to 3 years). During the first stage, feeding can be accomplished most easily when the parent allows the infant to determine the timing, amount, pacing, and preference of food intake. During the attachment phase, allowing the infant to control the feeding permits the parent to engage the infant in a positive manner. This paves the way for the separation and individuation phase. When a disturbance occurs in the parent-child relationship at any of these developmental levels, difficulty in feeding may ensue, with both the parent and the child contributing to the dysfunctional interaction. One of the most striking manifestations of food refusal occurs during the stage of separation and individuation. Conflict may arise if the parent seeks to dominate the child by intrusive and controlling feeding behavior at the same time the child is striving to achieve autonomy. The scenario then observed is of the parent forcing food on the child while the child refuses to eat. This often leads to extreme parental frustration and anger, and the child may be inadequately nourished and developmentally and emotionally thwarted.

When the pediatrician is attempting to sort out the factors contributing to food refusal, it is essential first to obtain a complete history, including a social history. This should include information concerning the parents' perception of the child's behavior and their expectations of the child. Second, a complete physical examination should be performed, with emphasis on oral-motor behavior and other clues suggesting neurologic, anatomic, or physiologic abnormalities that could make feeding difficult. The child's emotional state and developmental level must be determined. This is particularly important if there is concern about depression or a history of developmental delays. If evidence of oral-motor difficulty is suspected, evaluation by an occupational therapist is warranted. Third, the feeding interaction needs to be observed live, if possible. Finally, the physician needs to help the parents understand that infants and children may have different styles of eating and different food preferences and may refuse foods they do not like. This is not necessarily abnormal but reflects temperamental differences and variations in the child's way of processing olfactory, gustatory, and tactile stimuli.

▶ **Management**

The goal of intervention is to identify factors contributing to the disturbance and to work to overcome them. The parents may be encouraged to view the child's behavior differently and try not to impose their expectations and desires. Alternatively, the child's behavior may need to be modified so that the parents can provide adequate nurturing.

When the chief complaint is failure to gain weight, a different approach is required. The differential diagnosis should include not only food refusal but also medical disorders and maltreatment. The most common reason for failure to gain weight is inadequate caloric intake. Excessive weight loss may be due to vomiting or diarrhea, to malabsorption, or to a combination of these factors. In this situation more extensive diagnostic evaluation may be needed. Laboratory studies may include a complete blood count; erythrocyte sedimentation rate; urinalysis and urine culture; blood urea nitrogen; serum electrolytes and creatinine; and stool examination for fat, occult blood, and ova and parasites. Some practitioners also include liver and thyroid profiles. Occasionally an assessment of swallowing function or evaluation for the presence of gastroesophageal reflux may be indicated. Because of the complexity of the problem, a team approach to the diagnosis and treatment of failure to thrive, or poor weight gain, may be most appropriate. The team should include a physician, nurse, social worker, and dietitian. Occupational and physical therapists, developmentalists, and psychologists may be required.

The goals of treatment of the child with poor weight gain are to establish a normal pattern of weight gain and to establish better family functioning. Guidelines to accomplishing these goals include the following: (1) establish a comprehensive diagnosis that considers all factors contributing to poor weight gain; (2) monitor the feeding interaction and ensure appropriate weight gain; (3) monitor the developmental progress of the child and the changes in the family dynamics that facilitate optimal weight gain and psychoso-

cial development; and (4) provide support to the family as they seek to help the child.

Benoit D: Phenomenology and treatment of failure to thrive. Child Adolesc Psychiatr Clin North Am 1993;2:61.

Chatoor I et al: Failure to thrive and cognitive development in toddlers with infantile anorexia. Pediatrics 2004;113:e440 [PMID: 15121987].

Krugman SD, Dubowitz H: Failure to thrive. Am Fam Physician 2003;68:879 [PMID: 13678136].

Macht J: *Poor Eaters*. Plenum, 1990.

Reilly SM et al: Oral-motor dysfunction in children who fail to thrive: Organic or non-organic? Dev Med Child Neurol 1999;41:115 [PMID: 10075097].

Skuse D: Epidemiologic and definitional issues in failure to thrive. Child Adolesc Psychiatr Clin North Am 1993;2:37.

SLEEP DISORDERS

ESSENTIALS OF DIAGNOSIS & TYPICAL FEATURES

▶ Children younger than age 12 years:

- Difficulty initiating or maintaining sleep that is viewed as a problem by the child or caregiver.
- May be characterized by its severity, chronicity, frequency, *and* associated impairment in daytime function in the child *or* family.
- May be due to a primary sleep disorder or occur in association with other sleep, medical, or psychiatric disorders.

▶ Adolescents—difficulty initiating or maintaining sleep, or early morning awakening, or nonrestorative sleep, or a combination of these problems.

Sleep is a complex physiologic process influenced by intrinsic biologic properties, temperament, cultural norms and expectations, and environmental conditions. Between 20% and 30% of children experience sleep disturbances at some point in the first 4 years of life. The percentage decreases to 10–12% in school-aged children. Sleep disorders fall into two categories. **Dyssomnias** refer to problems with initiating and maintaining sleep or to excessive sleepiness. **Parasomnias** refer to abnormalities of arousal, partial arousal, and transitions between stages of sleep.

Sleep is controlled by two different biologic clocks. The first is a circadian rhythm–daily sleep-wake cycle. The second is an ultradian rhythm that occurs several times per night—the stages of sleep. Sleep stages cycle every 50–60 minutes in infants to every 90 minutes in adolescents. The circadian clock is longer than 24 hours. Environmental cues entrain the sleep-wake cycle into a 24-hour cycle. The cues are light-dark, ambient temperature, core body temperature, noise, social interaction, hunger, pain, and hormone production. Without the ability to perceive these cues (ie, blindness or autism) a child might have difficulty entraining a 24-hour sleep-wake cycle.

Two major sleep stages have been identified clinically and with the use of polysomnography (electroencephalography, electro-oculography, and electromyelography): rapid eye movement (REM) and nonrapid eye movement (NREM) sleep. In REM sleep, muscle tone is relaxed, the sleeper may twitch and grimace, and the eyes move erratically beneath closed lids. In adults and children, REM sleep occurs throughout the night but is increased during the latter half of the night. NREM sleep is divided into four stages. In the process of falling asleep, the individual enters stage 1, light sleep, characterized by reduced bodily movements, slow eye rolling, and sometimes opening and closing of the eyelids. Stage 2 sleep is characterized by slowing of eye movements, slowing of respirations and heart rate, and relaxation of the muscles but with repositioning of the body. Most mature individuals spend about half of their sleep time in this stage. Stages 3 and 4 (also called delta or slow-wave sleep) are the deepest NREM sleep stages, during which the body is relaxed, breathing is slow and shallow, and the heart rate is slow. The deepest NREM sleep occurs during the first 1–3 hours after going to sleep. Most parasomnias occur early in the night during deep NREM sleep. Dreams and nightmares that occur later in the night occur during REM sleep.

Sleep is clearly a developmental phenomenon. Infants are not born with a sleep-wake cycle. REM sleep is more common than NREM sleep in newborns and decreases by 3–6 months of age. Sleep spindles and vertex waves are usually not seen until 9 weeks of age. By 3–6 months, stage 1 through 4 NREM sleep can be seen. By 6–12 months an infant's electroencephalogram (EEG) can be read using adult criteria. Infants also do not make melatonin until 9–12 weeks of age. Melatonin is a hormone that decreases core body temperature, which appears to play a role in sleep onset and sleep maintenance. This hormone is sensitive to light. It crosses the placenta and is present in breast milk.

Like the sleep EEG, sleep patterns slowly mature throughout infancy, childhood, and adolescence until they become adultlike. Newborns sleep 16–20 hours per day in 2- to 5-hour blocks. Over the first year of life the infant slowly consolidates sleep at night into a 9- to 12-hour block and naps gradually decrease to one per day by about 12 months. Most children stop napping between 3 and 5 years of age. School-aged children typically sleep 10–11 hours per night without a nap. Adolescents need 9–9$\frac{1}{2}$ hours per night but often only get 7–7$\frac{1}{4}$ hours per night. This is complicated by an approximate 2-hour sleep phase delay in adolescence that is due to physiologic changes in hormonal regulation of the circadian system. Often adolescents are not tired until 2 hours after their typical bedtime but still must get up at the same time in the morning. Some school districts have implemented later start times for high-school students because of this phenomenon.

1. Parasomnias

Parasomnias, consisting of arousal from deep NREM sleep, are probably the most frightening for parents. They include night terrors, sleeptalking, and sleepwalking (somnambulism).

A. Night Terrors and Sleepwalking

Night terrors commonly occur within 2 hours after falling asleep, during the deepest stage of NREM sleep, and are often associated with sleepwalking. They occur in about 3% of children. During a night terror, the child may sit up in bed screaming, thrashing about, and exhibiting rapid breathing, tachycardia, and sweating. The child is often incoherent and unresponsive to comforting. The episode may last up to half an hour, after which the child goes back to sleep and has no memory of the event the next day. The parents must be reassured that the child is not in pain and that they should let the episode run its course.

Management of night terrors is by reassurance of the parents plus measures to avoid stress, irregular sleep schedule, or sleep deprivation which prolongs deep sleep when night terrors occur. Scheduled awakening (awakening the child 30–45 minutes before the time the night terrors usually occur) can be used in children with nightly or frequent night terrors.

Sleepwalking also occurs during slow-wave sleep and is common between 4 and 8 years of age. It is typically benign except that injuries can occur while the child is walking around. Steps should be taken to ensure that the environment is free of obstacles and that doors to the outside are locked. Parents may also wish to put a bell on their child's door to alert them that the child is out of bed. As with night terrors, steps should be taken to avoid stress and sleep deprivation. Scheduled awakenings may also be used if the child sleep walks frequently and at a predictable time.

B. Nightmares

Nightmares are frightening dreams that occur during REM sleep, typically followed by awakening, which usually occurs in the latter part of the night. The peak occurrence is between ages 3 and 5 years, with an incidence between 25% and 50%. A child who awakens during these episodes is usually alert. He or she can often describe the frightening images, recall the dream, and talk about it during the day. The child seeks and will respond positively to parental reassurance. The child will often have difficulty going back to sleep and will want to stay with the parents. Nightmares are usually self-limited and need little treatment. They can be associated with stress, trauma, anxiety, sleep deprivation that can cause a rebound in REM sleep, and medications that increase REM sleep.

2. Dyssomnias

The dyssomnias comprise problems with going to sleep and maintaining sleep, and nighttime awakenings. Although parasomnias are frightening, dyssomnias are frustrating. They can result in daytime fatigue for both the parents and the child, parental discord about management, and family disruption.

Several factors contribute to these disturbances. The quantity and timing of feeds in the first years of life will influence nighttime awakening. Most infants beyond age 6 months can go through the night without being fed. Thus, under normal circumstances, night waking for feeds is probably a learned behavior and is a function of the child's arousal and the parents' response to that arousal.

Bedtime habits can influence settling in for the night as well as nighttime awakening. If the child learns that going to sleep is associated with pleasant parental behavior such as rocking, singing, reading, or nursing, going back to sleep after nighttime arousal without these pleasant parental attentions may be difficult. This is called a sleep onset association disorder and usually is the reason for night waking. Every time that the child gets to the light sleep portion of the sleep-wake cycle he or she may wake up. This is usually brief and not remembered the next morning, but for the child who does not have strategies for getting to sleep, getting back to sleep may require the same interventions needed to get to sleep initially, such as rocking, patting, and drinking or sucking. Most of these interventions require a parent. Night waking occurs in 40–60% of infants and young children. Parents need to set limits for the child while acknowledging the child's individual biologic rhythms. They should resist the child's attempts to put off bedtime or to engage them during nighttime awakenings. The goal is to establish clear bedtime rituals, to put the child to bed while still awake, and to create a quiet, secure bedtime environment.

The child's temperament is another factor contributing to sleep. It has been reported that children with low sensory thresholds and less rhythmicity (regulatory disorder) are more prone to night waking. Night waking often starts at about 9 months as separation anxiety is beginning. Parents should receive anticipatory guidance prior to that time so that they know to reassure their child without making the interaction prolonged or pleasurable.

Finally, psychosocial stressors and changes in routine can play a role in night waking.

3. Sleep-Disordered Breathing

Sleep-disordered breathing or obstructive sleep apnea is characterized by obstructed breathing during sleep accompanied by loud snoring, chest retractions, morning headaches and dry mouth, and daytime sleepiness. Obstructive sleep apnea occurs in 1–3% of preschoolers. It has its highest peak in childhood between the ages of 2 and 6 years, which corresponds with the peak in adenotonsillar hypertrophy. It has been associated with daytime behavioral disorders, including attention-deficit/hyperactivity disorder. A thorough physical examination is important to look for ade-

notonsillar hypertrophy, hypotonia, and facial anomalies that may predispose the child to obstruction during sleep. Lateral neck films may be helpful. The gold standard for diagnosis is polysomnography. (See also Chapter 17.)

4. Restless Legs Syndrome & Periodic Limb Movement Disorder

Restless legs syndrome and periodic limb movement disorder are common disorders in adults and frequently occur together. The frequency of these disorders in children is unknown. Restless legs syndrome is associated with an uncomfortable sensation in the lower extremities that occurs at night when trying to fall asleep, is relieved by movement, and is sometimes described by children as "creepy-crawly" or "itchy bones." Periodic limb movement disorder is stereotyped, repetitive limb movements often associated with a partial arousal or awakening. The etiology of these disorders is unknown but there has been some association with iron deficiency. A diagnosis of restless legs syndrome is generally made by history and a diagnosis of periodic limb movement disorder can be made with a sleep study.

A complete medical and psychosocial history should be obtained and a physical examination performed. A detailed sleep history and diary should be maintained to which both parents contribute. Lateral neck films and polysomnography may be indicated to complete the evaluation, especially if sleep-disordered breathing is suspected. It is important to consider disorders such as gastroesophageal reflux, which may cause discomfort or pain when recumbent.

Management of Sleep Disorders

The key to treatment of children who have difficulty going to sleep or who awaken during the night and disturb others is to recognize that both the child and the parents play significant roles in initiating and sustaining what may be an undesirable behavior. Thus, it becomes important for the physician and parents to understand normal sleep patterns, the parents' responses that inadvertently reinforce undesirable sleep behavior, and the child's individual temperament traits. It is also important to remember that individual circadian rhythms do not change immediately; they require consistency and regularity over a period of time before change will occur. Keeping sleep logs or diaries and patience are essential. There is currently little evidence base for pharmacologic management of sleep disorders. It is important to review adequate sleep hygiene and underlying causes such as sleep-disordered breathing, acute or chronic pain, allergies, and developmental or psychiatric disorders before considering any type of pharmacologic management.

Chervin RD et al: Inattention, hyperactivity, and symptoms of sleep-disordered breathing. Pediatrics 2002;109:449 [PMID: 11875140].

Ferber R: Clinical assessment of child and adolescent sleep disorders. Child Adolesc Psychiatr Clin North Am 1996;5:569.

France KG et al: Fact, act, and tact: A three-stage approach to treating the sleep problems of infants and young children. Child Adolesc Psychiatr Clin North Am 1996;5:581.

Grigg-Damberger M: Neurologic disorders masquerading as pediatric sleep problems. Pediatr Clin North Am 2004;51:89 [ISBN: 15008584].

Mindel JA, Owens JA: *A Clinical Guide to Pediatric Sleep: Diagnosis and Management of Sleep Problems*. Lippincott Williams & Wilkins, 2003.

Owens JA et al: The use of pharmacotherapy in the treatment of pediatric insomnia in primary care: Rational approaches. A consensus meeting summary. J Clin Sleep Med 2005;1:49 [PMID: 17561616].

Rhode Island Hospital–sponsored site on sleep and sleep disorders in children: http://www.kidzzzsleep.org

TEMPER TANTRUMS & BREATH-HOLDING SPELLS

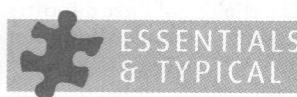

ESSENTIALS OF DIAGNOSIS & TYPICAL FEATURES

▶ Behavioral responses to stress, frustration, and loss of control.

▶ Tantrum—child may throw him- or herself on the ground, kick, scream, or strike out at others.

▶ Breath-holding spell—child engages in a prolonged expiration that is reflexive and may become pale or cyanotic.

▶ Rule out underlying organic disease in children with breath-holding spells (eg, CNS abnormalities, Rett syndrome, seizures).

1. Temper Tantrums

Temper tantrums are common between ages 12 months and 4 years, occurring about once a week in 50–80% of children in this age group. The child may throw him- or herself down, kick and scream, strike out at people or objects in the room, and hold his or her breath. These behaviors may be considered normal as the young child seeks to achieve autonomy and mastery over the environment. They are often a reflection of immaturity as the child strives to accomplish age-appropriate developmental tasks and meets with difficulty because of inadequate motor and language skills, impulsiveness, or parental restrictions. In the home, these behaviors may be annoying. In public, they are embarrassing.

Some children tolerate frustration well, are able to persevere at tasks, and cope easily with difficulties; others have a much greater problem dealing with experiences beyond their developmental level. Parents can minimize tantrums by understanding the child's temperament and what he or she is trying to communicate. Parents must also be committed to supporting the child's drive to master his or her feelings.

▶ Management

Appropriate intervention can provide an opportunity for enhancing the child's growth. The tantrum is a loss of control on the child's part that may be a frightening event and a blow to the child's self-image. The parents and the physician need to view these behaviors within the child's developmental context rather than from a negative, adversarial, angry perspective.

Several suggestions can be offered to parents and physicians to help manage tantrums:

1. Minimize the need to say "no" by "child-proofing" the environment so that fewer restrictions need to be enforced.

2. Use distraction when frustration increases; direct the child to other, less frustrating activities; and reward the positive response.

3. Present options within the child's capabilities so that he or she can achieve mastery and autonomy.

4. Fight only those battles that need to be won, and avoid those that arouse unnecessary conflict.

5. Do not abandon the preschool child when a tantrum occurs. Stay nearby during the episode without intruding. A small child may need to be restrained. An older child can be asked to go to his or her room. Threats serve no purpose and should not be used.

6. Do not use negative terms when the tantrum is occurring. Instead, point out that the child is out of control and give praise when he or she regains control.

7. Never let a child hurt him- or herself or others.

8. Do not "hold a grudge" after the tantrum is over, but do not grant the child's demands that led to the tantrum.

9. Seek to maintain an environment that provides positive reinforcement for desired behavior. Do not overreact to undesired behavior, but set reasonable limits and provide responsible direction for the child.

10. Approximately 5–20% of young children have severe temper tantrums that are frequent and disruptive. Such tantrums may result from a disturbance in the parent-child interaction, poor parenting skills, lack of limit-setting, and permissiveness. They may be part of a larger behavioral or developmental disorder or may emerge under adverse socioeconomic conditions, in circumstances of maternal depression and family dysfunction, or when the child is in poor health. Referral to a psychologist or psychiatrist is appropriate while the pediatrician continues to support and work with the family.

2. Breath-Holding Spells

Whereas temper tantrums can be frustrating to parents, breath-holding spells can be terrifying. The name for this behavior may be a misnomer in that it connotes prolonged inspiration. In fact, breath-holding occurs during expiration and is reflexive—not volitional—in nature. It is a paroxysmal event occurring in 0.1–5% of healthy children from age 6 months to 6 years. The spells usually start during the first year of life, often in response to anger or a mild injury. The child is provoked or surprised, starts to cry—briefly or for a considerable time—and then falls silent in the expiratory phase of respiration. This is followed by a color change. Spells have been described as either pallid (acyanotic) or cyanotic, with the latter usually associated with anger and the former with an injury such as a fall. The spell may resolve spontaneously, or the child may lose consciousness. In severe cases, the child may become limp and progress to opisthotonos, body jerks, and urinary incontinence. Only rarely does a spell proceed to asystole or a seizure.

▶ Management

For the child with frequent spells, underlying disorders such as seizures, orthostatic hypotension, obstructive sleep apnea, abnormalities of the CNS, tumors, familial dysautonomia, and Rett syndrome need to be considered. An association exists among breath-holding spells, pica, and iron-deficiency anemia. These conditions can be ruled out on the basis of the history, physical examination, and laboratory studies. Once it has been determined that the child is healthy, the focus of treatment is behavioral. Parents should be taught to handle the spells in a matter-of-fact manner and monitor the child for any untoward events. The reality is that parents cannot completely protect the child from upsetting and frustrating experiences and probably should not try to do so. Just as in temper tantrums, parents need to help the child control his or her responses to frustration. Parents need to be careful not to be too permissive and submit to the child's every whim for fear the child might have a spell.

If loss of consciousness occurs, the child should be placed on his or her side to protect against head injury and aspiration. Maintaining a patent oral airway is essential, but cardiopulmonary resuscitation should be avoided. There are no prophylactic medications. Atropine, 0.01 mg/kg given subcutaneously, has been used with some benefit in spells accompanied by bradycardia or asystole.

Breningstall GN: Breath holding spells. Pediatr Neurol 1996;14:91 [PMID: 8703234].

DiMario FJ Jr: Breath-holding spells in childhood. Am J Dis Child 1992;146:125 [PMID: 1736640].

Greene RW: *The Explosive Child*. Quill, 2001.

Needleman R et al: Psychosocial correlates of severe temper tantrums. J Dev Behav Pediatr 1991;12:77.

Needleman R et al: Temper tantrums: When to worry. Contemp Pediatr 1989;6:12.

▼ WELL CHILD SURVEILLANCE & SCREENING

The American Academy of Pediatrics (AAP) recently published guidelines for surveillance and screening at well child visits. Surveillance is a procedure for recognizing children at risk for a developmental disorder and involves asking parents if they have concerns about their child's development. The PEDS (Pediatric Evaluation of Developmental Status) can be used for this purpose. Screening involves use of a standardized tool to clarify identified risk. An evaluation would be done by a specialist and would involve a more definitive evaluation of a child's development.

Surveillance should occur at all well child visits. Screening of development should occur at 9, 18, and 30 months. Because a 30-month visit is not part of the standard well child visit schedule and may not be reimbursed, screening may occur at 24 months instead. It is also recommended that autism-specific screening should occur at the 18-month visit. Clinicians should keep in mind that if they are administering a screen because they are concerned and the child passes the screen, they should still schedule an early follow-up visit to ensure that appropriate progress has been made and that there are no further concerns.

Although an autism-specific screen was only recommended at the 18-month visit in the AAP guidelines, the Autism Workgroup of the AAP has recommended a second autism-specific screen at 24–30 months in order to pick up children missed at the 18-month screen. Because the average age of regression is 20 months, some children may be missed by a single screen at 18 months. Screening for autism earlier than 14 months, with the tools that are currently available, yields too many false-positive results. Development of screening tools for children younger than 18 months are ongoing.

Implementation of screening requires planning for timing of screening administration during office visits, defining the process for referral, and designing handouts prior to beginning screening. Aside from the important process of seeking to optimize the child's development with the use of these screenings they also demonstrate to the parent the interest their caretaker has not only for the child's physical wellbeing but also for the child's developmental and psychosocial wellbeing. Parents of children who received a developmental assessment expressed greater satisfaction with their care provider.

American Academy of Pediatrics: Identifying infants and young children with developmental disorders in the medical home: An algorithm for developmental surveillance and screening. Pediatrics 2006;118:405 [PMID: 1681859].

Dietz C et al: Screening for autistic spectrum disorder in children aged 14–15 months. II. Population screening with the Early Screening of Autism Traits Questionnaire (ESAT). Design and general findings. J Autism Dev Disord 2006;36:713 [PMID: 16644887].

Gupta VB et al: Identifying children with autism early? Pediatrics 2007;119:152 [PMID: 17200280].

Halfon N et al: Satisfaction with health care for young children. Pediatrics 2004;113:1926 [PMID: 15173468].

Luyster R et al: Early regression in social communication in autism spectrum disorders: A CPEA study. Dev Neuropsychol 2005;27:311 [PMID: 15843100].

Pinto-Martin JA et al: Developmental stages of developmental screening: Steps to implementation of a successful program. Am J Pub Health 2005;95:1928 [PMID: 16195523].

Reznick JS et al: A parent-report instrument for identifying one-year-olds at risk for an eventual diagnosis of autism: The first year inventory. J Autism Dev Disord 2007;37:1691 [PMID: 17180716].

DEVELOPMENTAL DISORDERS

Developmental disorders include abnormalities in one or more aspects of development, such as verbal, motor, visual-spatial, attentional, and social abilities. These problems are diagnosed by comparing the child's performance level with norms accumulated from observation and testing of children of the same age. Problems with development are often noted by parents when a child does not meet typical motor and language milestones. Developmental disorders may also include difficulties with behavior or attention. Attention-deficit/hyperactivity disorder (ADHD) is the most common neurodevelopmental disorder. ADHD occurs in 2–10% of school-aged children and may occur in combination with a variety of other learning or developmental issues. Mild developmental disorders are often not noted until the child is of school age.

Many biologic and psychosocial factors may influence a child's performance on developmental tests. In the assessment of the child, it is important to document adverse psychosocial factors, such as neglect or poverty, which can negatively influence developmental progress. Many of the biologic factors that influence development are genetic and are discussed throughout this section.

Evaluation

The neurodevelopmental evaluation must focus on (1) defining the child's level of developmental abilities in a variety of domains, including language, motor, visual-spatial, attentional, and social abilities; (2) attempting to determine the etiology for the child's developmental delays; and (3) planning a treatment program. These objectives are best achieved by a multidisciplinary team that includes the physician, a psychologist, a speech or language therapist, an occupational therapist, and an educational specialist. The psychologist will usually carry out standardized testing of intellectual ability appropriate to the child's age. The motor and language specialists will also carry out clinical testing to document the deficits in their areas and to organize a treatment program. The educational specialist will usually carry out academic testing for the school-aged child and plan a course of special education support through the school. The physician is usually the integrator of the information from the team and must also obtain a detailed medical and developmental history and conduct the physical and neurologic examinations.

Medical & Neurodevelopmental Examination

The medical history should begin with pregnancy, labor, and delivery to identify conditions that might compromise the child's CNS function. The physician must ask the child's parents about prenatal exposures to toxins, medications, alcohol, drugs, smoking, and infections; maternal chronic illness; complications of pregnancy or delivery and neonatal course. Problems such as failure to thrive, chronic illnesses, hospitalizations, and abuse can interfere significantly with normal development. Major illnesses or hospitalizations should be discussed. Any CNS problems, such as trauma, infection, or encephalitis should be documented. The presence of metabolic diseases, such as diabetes or phenylketonuria, and exposure to environmental toxins such as lead should be determined. Chronic diseases such as chronic otitis media, hyper- or hypothyroidism, and chronic renal failure can interfere with normal development. The presence of motor or vocal tics, seizures, or sleep disturbances should be documented. In addition, parents should be questioned about any motor, cognitive, or behavioral regression.

The physician should review and document the child's temperament, difficulties with feeding, and subsequent developmental milestones. The child's difficulties with tantrums, poor attention, impulsivity, hyperactivity, or aggression should be documented.

A detailed history of school-related events should be recorded, including previous special education support, evaluations through the school, history of repeating grades, difficulties with specific academic areas, problems with peers, and the teacher's impressions of the child's difficulties, particularly related to attentional problems, impulsivity, or hyperactivity. Input from teachers can be invaluable and should be sought prior to the evaluation.

Perhaps the most important aspect of the medical history is a detailed family history of learning strengths and weaknesses, emotional or behavioral problems, learning disabilities, mental retardation, or psychiatric disorders. Parental learning strengths and weaknesses, temperament difficulties, or attentional problems may be passed on to the child. For instance, dyslexia (deficits in decoding skills that result in reading difficulties) is often inherited.

The neurodevelopmental examination should include a careful assessment of dysmorphic features such as epicanthal folds, palpebral fissure size, shape of the philtrum, low-set or posteriorly rotated ears, prominent ear pinnae, unusual dermatoglyphics (eg, a single palmar crease), hyperextensibility of the joints, syndactyly, clinodactyly, or other unusual features. A detailed physical and neurologic examination needs to be carried out with an emphasis on both soft and hard neurologic findings. Soft signs can include motor incoordination, which can relate to handwriting problems and academic delays in written language or drawing. Visual motor coordination abilities can be assessed by having the child write, copy designs, or draw a person.

The child's growth parameters, including height, weight, and head circumference, need to be assessed, along with hearing and visual acuity. Cranial nerve abnormalities and oral-motor coordination problems need to be noted. The examiner should watch closely for motor or vocal tics. Both fine and gross motor abilities should be assessed. Dyspraxia (motor planning difficulties or imitating complex motor movements) and disorders of fine motor coordination are fairly common. Tandem walking, one-foot balancing, and coordinating a skip may often show surprising abnormalities. Tremors can be noted when watching a child stack blocks or draw.

The developmental aspects of the examination can include an assessment of auditory processing and perceptual ability with simple tasks, such as twofold to fivefold directions, assessing right and left directionality, memory for a series of spoken words or digit span, and comprehension of a graded paragraph. In assessing expressive language abilities, the examiner should look for difficulties with word retrieval, formulation, and articulation, and adequacy of vocabulary. Visual-perceptual abilities can be assessed by simple visual memory tasks, puzzles, or object assembly, and evaluating the child's ability to decode words or organize math problems. Visual-motor integration and coordination can be assessed again with handwriting, design copying, and drawing a person. Throughout the assessment the clinician should pay special attention to the child's ability to focus attention and concentrate, and to other aspects of behavior such as evidence of depression or anxiety.

Additional questionnaires and checklists—such as the Child Behavior Checklist by Achenbach; ADHD scales such as the Conners' Parent/Teacher Rating Scale; and the Swanson, Nolan and Pelham Questionnaire-IV, which includes the *Diagnostic and Statistical Manual of Mental Disorders, Fourth Edition, Text Revision* (DSM-IV-TR) criteria for ADHD—can be used to help with this assessment.

Referral of family to community resources is critical, as is a medical home (described earlier in the chapter).

American Academy of Pediatrics Council on Children with Disabilities: Care coordination in the medical home: Integrating health and related systems of care for children with special health care needs. Pediatrics 2005;116:1238 [PMID: 16264016].
Medical Home Initiatives for Children with Special Needs Project Advisory Committee, American Academy of Pediatrics: The medical home. Pediatrics 2002;110:184 [PMID: 12093969].
Reynolds CR, Mayfield JW: Neuropsychological assessment in genetically linked neurodevelopmental disorders. In Goldstein S, Reynolds CR (editors): *Handbook of Developmental and Genetic Disorders in Children*. Guilford, 1999.

ATTENTION-DEFICIT/ HYPERACTIVITY DISORDER

Attention-deficit/hyperactivity disorder (ADHD) is a common neurodevelopmental disorder that may affect 2–10% of school-aged children and may persist into adolescence and adulthood. It is associated with a triad of symptoms: impulsivity, inattention, and hyperactivity. DSM-IV-TR has described three ADHD subtypes: hyperactive-impulsive, inattentive, and combined. To be classified according to

Table 2–5. Attention-deficit/hyperactivity disorder subtypes.

Subtype	Symptoms[a]
Hyperactive-impulsive	Fidgetiness Difficulty remaining seated in the class Excessive running or climbing Difficulty in engaging in quiet activities Excessive talking and blurting out answers before questions have been completed Difficulty awaiting turns Interrupting and intruding on others
Inattentive	Failure to give close attention to detail Difficulty sustaining intention in task Failure to listen when spoken to directly Failure to follow instructions Difficulty organizing tasks and activities Reluctance to engage in tasks Losing utensils necessary for tasks or activities Easy distractibility Forgetfulness in daily activities

[a]The child must exhibit six or more of these symptoms.
Adapted, with permission, from American Psychiatric Association: *Diagnostic and Statistical Manual of Mental Disorders,* 4th ed. American Psychiatric Association, 1994.

either subtype, the child must exhibit six or more of the symptoms listed in Table 2–5.

The majority of children with ADHD have a combined type with symptoms of inattention as well as hyperactivity and impulsivity. Although symptoms begin in early childhood, they can diminish between ages 10 and 25 years. Hyperactivity declines more quickly, and impulsivity and inattentiveness often persist into adolescence and adulthood. ADHD may be combined with other psychiatric conditions, such as mood disorder in approximately 20% of patients, conduct disorders in 20%, and oppositional defiant disorder in up to 40%. Up to 25% of children with ADHD seen in a referral clinic have tics or Tourette syndrome. Conversely, well over 50% of individuals with Tourette syndrome also have ADHD.

ADHD has a substantial genetic component. Several candidate genes have been identified, although there is strong evidence that ADHD is a disorder involving multiple genes. ADHD is also associated with a variety of genetic disorders related to developmental disorders, including fragile X syndrome, Williams syndrome, Angelman syndrome, XXY syndrome (Klinefelter syndrome), and Turner syndrome. Fetal alcohol syndrome (FAS) is also strongly associated with ADHD. CNS trauma, CNS infections, prematurity, and a difficult neonatal course with brain injury can also be associated with later ADHD. Metabolic problems such as hyperthyroidism can sometimes cause ADHD. These organic causes of ADHD should be considered in the evaluation of any child presenting with attentional problems, hyperactivity, or impulsivity. However, in the majority of children who have ADHD the cause remains unknown.

▶ Management

The treatment of ADHD varies depending on the complexity of the individual case, including comorbid disorders such as anxiety and learning disabilities. It is important to educate the family regarding the symptoms of ADHD and to clarify that it is a neurologic disorder that at times is difficult for the child to control. Behavior modification techniques usually help these children and should include structure with consistency in daily routine, positive reinforcement whenever possible, and time out for negative behaviors. It is important to try to boost the child's self-esteem because psychological complications are common in ADHD. A variety of educational interventions can be helpful, including preferential seating in the classroom, a system of consistent positive behavior reinforcement, consistent structure, the repetition of information when needed, and the use of instruction that incorporates both visual and auditory modalities. Many children with ADHD have significant social difficulties, and social skills training can be helpful. Individual counseling is beneficial in alleviating poor self-esteem, oppositional behavior, and conduct problems.

The National Institute of Mental Health Collaborative Multisite Multimodal Treatment Study of Children With Attention-Deficit/Hyperactivity Disorder (MTA) evaluated 579 children with ADHD who were randomly assigned to four treatment groups: state-of-the-art medication management, intensive behavioral intervention, a combination of medication and behavior management, and a community treatment control group. This study found that children treated with state-of-the art medication management, which included blinded placebo-controlled dosage adjustment, monthly visits, and parent and teacher questionnaires, had better outcomes than children in the other groups. All groups improved over the course of the study, with those receiving intensive medication management and combined therapy doing better than children receiving behavioral intervention alone and community management. Combined therapy was not significantly better than intensive medication management alone for core ADHD symptoms. However, only the combined group showed significant improvement over the controls in other symptoms such as parent-child interaction, aggression, and social skills.

Stimulant medications (methylphenidate and dextroamphetamine) are available in short- and long-acting preparations. A newer medication, atomoxetine, has been found to be effective in some children with ADHD as a second-line drug. Alternative medications for the treatment of ADHD include clonidine or guanfacine, which are α_2-adrenergic presynaptic agonists that decrease norepinephrine levels.

They are particularly helpful for individuals who are hyperreactive to stimuli and may decrease motor tics in patients who have Tourette syndrome.

It is most important that, no matter what medication is used, the diagnosis is correct and the correct dosage is prescribed. A recent study has demonstrated that one of the major factors contributing to treatment failure is inadequate dosing or the failure to recognize the presence of comorbid conditions such as learning disability, anxiety disorders, and depression.

Seventy to 90% of children with normal intellectual abilities respond well to stimulant medications. Stimulants enhance both dopamine and norepinephrine neurotransmission, which seems to improve impulse control, attention, and hyperactivity. The main side effects of methylphenidate and dextroamphetamine include appetite suppression and resulting weight loss, as well as sleep disturbances. Atomoxetine is a selective inhibitor of the presynaptic norepinephrine transporter, which increases norepinephrine and dopamine, and has a similar side-effect profile to the stimulants. Cardiovascular effects of stimulant medications have undergone significant scrutiny over the past 2 years. It is unclear whether stimulants increase the risk of sudden death over the risk in the general population, especially in children without any underlying risk. Prior to beginning a stimulant medication, it is recommended that clinicians obtain any history of syncope, palpitations, chest pain, and family history of sudden death prior to age 30 that may predispose a child to sudden death. Some individuals experience increased anxiety, particularly with higher doses of stimulant medications. Stimulants may exacerbate psychotic symptoms. They may also exacerbate motor tics in 30% of patients, but in 10% motor tics may be improved.

Long-acting and short-acting forms of stimulant medications are available. The initial dose of methylphenidate can be 5, 10, 15, or 20 mg daily divided two or three times a day. Adderall, a stimulant that combines four dextro- and levo-amphetamine salts, is a more long-acting medication, and often a single morning dose suffices for the day. Starting doses can be 5, 7.5, 10, 12.5, or 15 mg, although higher doses may also be used.

Alternative medications for the treatment of ADHD include clonidine or guanfacine, which are α_2-adrenergic presynaptic agonists that decrease norepinephrine levels. They are particularly helpful for individuals who are hyperreactive to stimuli and may be helpful in decreasing motor tics in patients who have Tourette syndrome. Tricyclic antidepressant medications such as imipramine may also be effective treatment for ADHD, but the cardiovascular side effects at high dosages can include severe arrhythmias. Bupropion is an antidepressant medication that can also be effective for treatment of ADHD symptoms. Its use is contraindicated in patients with a history of seizures, because it will lower the seizure threshold. It has also been known to cause seizures in individuals who have anorexia or bulimia. It is used more commonly in adolescents and adults with ADHD than in children with the disorder.

American Academy of Pediatrics: Clinical practice guideline: Treatment of the school-aged child with attention-deficit/hyperactivity disorder. Pediatrics 2001;108:1033 [PMID: 11581465].

Brown RT et al; American Academy of Pediatrics Committee on Quality Improvement; American Academy of Pediatrics Subcommittee on Attention-Deficit/Hyperactivity Disorder: Treatment of attention-deficit/hyperactivity disorder: Overview of the evidence. Pediatrics 2005;115:e749 [PMID: 15930203].

Elia J et al: Treatment of attention deficit hyperactivity disorder. N Engl J Med 1999;340:780 [PMID: 1007214].

Goldman LS et al: Diagnosis and treatment of attention deficit hyperactivity disorder in children and adults. JAMA 1998;79:1100 [PMID: 9546570].

Jensen PS et al: Findings from the NIMS Multimodal Treatment Study of ADHD (MTA): Implications and applications for primary care providers. J Develop Behav Pediatr 2001;22:60 [PMID: 11265923].

Krull KA: Evaluation and diagnosis of attention deficit hyperactivity disorders in children. In Rose BD (editor): UpToDate. UpToDate, 2005.

Krull KA: Treatment and prognosis of attention deficit hyperactivity disorders in children. In Rose BD (editor): UpToDate. UpToDate, 2005.

Reiff MI: *ADHD: A Compete Authoritative Guide.* American Academy of Pediatrics, 2004.

Attention Deficit Disorder Association: http://www.add.org

Children and Adults with Attention Deficit/Hyperactivity Disorder: http://www.chadd.org

Questions and Answers: Safety of Pills For Treating ADHD: http://www.aap.org/healthtopics/adhd.cfm

AUTISM SPECTRUM DISORDERS

 ESSENTIALS OF DIAGNOSIS & TYPICAL FEATURES

▶ Three core deficits:
  - Qualitative impairments in communication
  - Qualitative impairments in reciprocal social interaction
  - Presence of stereotypic, restrictive, and repetitive patterns of behavior, interests, and activities.

Autism is a neurologic disorder characterized by (1) qualitative impairments in social interaction; (2) qualitative impairments in communication; and (3) restricted repetitive and stereotyped patterns of behavior, interests, and activities. Autism is currently grouped under the Pervasive Developmental Disorders in the DSM-IV with Asperger Disorder, Pervasive Developmental Disorder Not Otherwise Specified, Childhood Disintegrative Disorder, and Rett Syndrome. Asperger disorder is characterized by impairment in social interaction and restricted interest/repetitive behaviors. Individuals with Asperger disorder should not have significant delays in cognitive, language, or self-help skills. Pervasive developmental disorder not otherwise specified is characterized by impairment in reciprocal social interaction along with impairment in communication skills, or restricted interest or repetitive behaviors. Children with pervasive developmental disorder not otherwise specified do not meet full criteria for autism due to mild or atypical symptoms. Childhood disintegrative disorder is characterized by typical development for at least 2 years followed by a regression in at least two of the following three areas: social interaction, communication, and behavior (characterized by restricted interests or repetitive behaviors.) Rett syndrome is a genetic syndrome caused by a mutation on the X chromosome that is characterized by regression in skills in the first year of life. Table 2–6 lists the DSM-IV-TR criteria for diagnosis of an autism spectrum disorder.

Autism spectrum disorders are relatively common, occurring in approximately 1 in 150 children. Males are overrepresented 3–4:1, with reports as high as 9.5:1 (especially when higher functioning individuals are included). No known etiology can be found in 80–90% of cases. A genetic syndrome such as fragile X syndrome or chromosome 15q duplication is found in 10–20% of cases. There is a strong familial component. Parents of one child with autism of unknown etiology have a 2–9% chance of having a second child with autism. The concordance rate among monozygotic twins is high, and there is an increased incidence of speech, language, reading, attention, and affective disorders in family members of children with autism.

▶ Evaluation & Management

Children with autism are often not diagnosed until age 3–4 years, when their disturbances in reciprocal social interaction

Table 2–6. Criteria for diagnosis of an autism spectrum disorder.

Qualitative impairment in social interaction (at least 2)
Impairment in nonverbal behaviors such as eye contact
Failure to develop peer relationships
Lack of seeking to share enjoyment or interests
Lack of social or emotional reciprocity
Qualitative impairment in communication (at least 1)
Delay in or lack of spoken language
If speech is present, lack of ability to initiate or sustain conversation
Stereotyped and repetitive/idiosyncratic language
Lack of pretend/social imitative play
Restricted interests/repetitive behavior (at least 1)
Preoccupation with restricted interest
Inflexible adherence to nonfunctional routines or rituals
Stereotyped and repetitive motor mannerisms (hand flapping)
Persistent preoccupation with parts of objects

Reprinted, with permission, from American Psychiatric Association: *Diagnostic and Statistical Manual of Mental Disorders,* 4th ed, text revision. American Psychiatric Association, 2000.

and communication become more apparent. However, impairments in communication and behavior can often be recognized in the first 12–18 months of life. The most common characteristics during the first year are a consistent failure to orient to one's name, regard people directly, use gestures, and to develop speech. Even if one of these skills is present, it is often diminished in frequency, inconsistent, or fleeting. On the contrary, for all children every interaction should be an opportunity to engage. Sharing affect or enjoyment is an important precursor to social interaction. By 18 months a child should have "joint attention," which occurs when two people attend to the same thing at the same time. This is usually accomplished by shifting eye gaze, pointing, or saying "look." Toddlers should point to get needs met ("I want that") and to show ("look at that") by 1 year of age and they should do it regularly. By 18 months a toddler should be able to follow a point, imitate others, and engage in functional play (using toys in the way that they are intended to be used, such as rolling a car, throwing a ball, or holding a baby doll). Restricted interests and repetitive behaviors sometimes do not emerge until after age 2, but usually are present before age 2.

There is mounting evidence that a diagnosis of autism spectrum disorder can be made reliably by age 2 years and is stable over time. Because there is evidence that early intervention is particularly important for children with autism, great interest has arisen in developing a screening instrument that can be used in very young children. The Modified Checklist for Autism in Toddlers (M-CHAT) is designed for children 16–30 months of age. It is a parent report measure with 23 yes/no questions. This test is still undergoing study to determine sensitivity and specificity but preliminary outcomes show good sensitivity and specificity. Specificity is greater if parents of children who screen positive on the M-CHAT receive a follow-up phone call asking for specific examples of failed items to confirm accuracy. The M-CHAT has also been evaluated in both low-risk and high-risk groups.

An autism-specific screen is recommended at 18 months. A second autism-specific screen has been recommended at 24–30 months. The second screen was recommended because some of the symptoms may be more obvious in an older child, and because about 30% of children with autism spectrum disorders experience a regression in skills, on average at 20 months. Screening at 18 months would miss many of these children.

When behaviors raising concern for autism are noted, the child should be referred to a team of specialists experienced in the assessment of autism spectrum disorders. The child should also be referred to a local early intervention program and to a speech and language pathologist to begin therapy as soon as possible. All children with autism should have a formal audiology evaluation. Laboratory tests such as high-resolution chromosome analysis, DNA for fragile X syndrome, and fluorescence in situ hybridization (FISH) for 15q duplication should be considered. Metabolic screening, lead level, thyroid studies, and a Wood lamp test for tuberous sclerosis may also be done if indicated by findings in the history and physical examination. Neuroimaging is not routinely indicated even in the presence of macrocephaly because children with autism often have relatively large heads. Neuroimaging should be done if microcephaly or focal neurologic signs are noted.

Approximately 15–30% of children with autism demonstrate plateauing or loss of skills (usually language and social skills only) between 12 and 24 months of age. The loss is usually gradual. It can co-occur with atypical development and can be fluctuating. It usually occurs before the child attains a vocabulary of 10 words. If a child presents with regression, he or she should be referred to a child neurologist. A sleep-deprived EEG or an overnight EEG should be considered when there is a history of regression. The EEG must have adequate sampling of slow-wave sleep to rule out epileptiform discharges during slow-wave sleep. It should be noted that the recommendations for treatment of that type of EEG abnormality are still being debated.

According to the National Research Council, "A substantial subset of children with autistic spectrum disorders are able to make marked progress during the period that they receive intensive early intervention, and nearly all children with autistic spectrum disorders appear to show some benefit. Children with ASD who begin treatment before age 3 to $3^1/2$ years make the greatest gains with intervention." As with any child, treatment should be based on the individual needs of the child. It is clear, however, that intervention must begin early and must be comprehensive and intensive. Many specialists advocate 20–25 hours or more per week of structured behavioral treatments such as applied behavioral analysis, that target development of social attention, peer interactions, functional language, and appropriate play. There are many models for this type of intervention and much variability in what is available in different areas of the country. Families should be encouraged to find a model that best suits the needs of the child and the family.

Many complementary and alternative treatments for autism have been proposed. Research is currently underway to evaluate some of these treatments.

Autism and Developmental Disorders Monitoring Network Surveillance Year 2002 Principal Investigators; Centers for Disease Control and Prevention: Prevalence of autism spectrum disorders—Autism and Developmental Disabilities Monitoring Network, 14 Sites, United States, 2002. MMWR Surveill Summ 2007;56:12 [PMID: 17287715].

Baird G et al: A screening instrument for autism at 18 months of age: A 6-year follow-up study. J Am Acad Child Adolesc Psychiatr 2000;39:694 [PMID: 108946303].

Baird G et al: Current topic: Screening and surveillance for autism and pervasive developmental disorders. Arch Dis Child 2001;84:468 [PMID: 11369559].

Cohen DJ, Volkman FR (editors): Handbook of Autism and Pervasive Developmental Disorders, 2nd ed. John Wiley & Sons, 1997.

Commission on Behavioral and Social Sciences and Education: Educating Children with Autism. National Academies Press, 2001.

Dumont-Mathieu T, Fein D: Screening for autism in young children: The Modified Checklist for Autism in Toddlers (M-CHAT) and other measures. Ment Retard Dev Disabil Res Rev 2005;11:253.

Filipek PA et al: Practice parameter: Screening and diagnosis of autism: Report of the Quality Standards Subcommittee of the American Academy of Neurology and Child Neurology Society. Neurology 2000;55:468 [PMID: 10953176].

Gabriels RL, Hill DE (editors): *Autism: From Research to Individualized Practice*. Jessica Kingsley Publishers, 2002.

Gabriels RL, Hill DE (editors): *Growing Up with Autism: Working with School-Age Children and Adolescents*. Guildford, 2007.

Gilberg C, Coleman M (editors): *The Biology of the Autistic Syndromes*. MacKeith, 2000.

Goldson E: Autism spectrum disorders: An overview. Adv Pediatr 2004,51:63-109 [PMID: 15366771].

Harris SL, Handleman JS: Age and IQ at intake as predictors of placement for young children with autism: A four- to six-year follow-up. J Autism Dev Disord 2000;30:137 [PMID: 10832778].

Landa RJ et al: Social and communication development in toddlers with early and later diagnosis of autism spectrum disorders. Arch Gen Psychiatry 2007;64:853 [PMID: 17606819].

Lord C, McGee JP (editors): *Educating Children with Autism*. National Academy of Sciences Press, 2001.

Ozonoff S et al (editors): *Autism Spectrum Disorders: A Research Review for Practitioners*. American Psychiatric Publishing, 2003.

Rogers SJ: Empirically supported comprehensive treatments for young children with autism. J Clin Child Psychol 1998;27:168 [PMID: 9648034].

Autism Society of America: http://www.autism-society.org

Autism Speaks: http://www.autismspeaks.org

Division TEACCH (Treatment and Education of Autistic and Related Communication-handicapped Children): http://teacch.com

Family Voices (information on children with special health needs): http://www.familyvoices.org

First Signs (educational site on autism): http://firstsigns.org

Hanen Centre (information on family-focused early intervention programs): http://www.hanen.org

National Center on Birth Defects and Developmental Disabilities home page: http://www.cdc.gov/ncbddd/autism/actearly/

INTELLECTUAL DISABILITY/ MENTAL RETARDATION

The field of developmental disabilities has been evolving and redefining the constructs of disability and intellectual disability and thereby using new terms to reflect that evolution. The term *retardation* was first used in an educational context to describe educationally compromised students. Indeed, during the early 20th century, educators and psychologists struggled to identify the causes of the problems these students encountered. Interestingly, their "differential diagnoses" included biologic, environmental, and emotional etiologies, not dissimilar to those we deal with in the 21st century. In addition, it was—and continues to be—acknowledged that the term *mental retardation* and earlier terms such as *idiocy, feeblemindedness,* and *mental deficiency* are pejorative, demeaning, and dehumanizing.

Recently, a rethinking of the construct of disability has emerged that shifts the focus from limitations in intellectual functioning and adaptive capability (a person-centered trait) to a human phenomenon with its source in biologic or social factors and contexts. The current view is a social-ecological conception of disability that articulates the role of disease or disorder leading to impairments in structure and function, limitations in activities, and restriction in participation in personal and environmental interactions. The term *intellectual disability*, which is consistent with this broader view, is increasingly being used and reflects an appreciation of the humanness and potential of the individual. The diagnostic criteria currently remain the same; however, the construct and context has changed.

Having noted this, it is important to acknowledge that significant delays in the development of language, motor skills, attention, abstract reasoning, visual-spatial skills, and academic or vocational achievements are associated with intellectual disability/mental retardation (ID/MR). Deficits on standardized testing in cognitive and adaptive functioning greater than two standard deviations below the mean for the population are considered to fall in the range of ID/MR (Table 2–7). The most common way of reporting the results of these tests is by using an intelligence quotient. The intelligence quotient is a statistically derived number reflecting the ratio of age-appropriate cognitive function and the child's actual level of cognitive function. A number of accepted standardized measurement tools, such as the Wechsler Intelligence Scale for Children, third edition, can be used to assess these capacities. To receive a diagnosis of ID/MR a child must not only have an intelligence quotient of less than 70, but also must demonstrate adaptive skills more than two standard deviations below the mean. Adaptive function refers to the child's ability to function in his or her environment and can be measured by a parent or teacher interview recorded using an instrument such as the Vineland Adaptive Behavior Scales.

The prevalence of ID/MR is approximately 3% in the general population, although some states have reported a prevalence of less than 2%. Mild levels of ID/MR are more common and more likely to have a sociocultural cause than are more severe levels. Poverty, deprivation, or a lack of exposure to a stimulating environment can contribute to developmental delays and poor performance on standardized tests. In addition, physical problems such as hearing loss, blindness, and brain trauma can lead to developmental delays

Table 2–7. Categories of intellectual disability/mental retardation (ID/MR).

Mental ID/MR Range	Intelligence Quotient (IQ)
Mild ID/MR	50–69
Moderate ID/MR	35–49
Severe ID/MR	20–34
Profound ID/MR	< 20

Table 2–8. Causes of intellectual disability/mental retardation (ID/MR).

Cause	Percentage of Cases
Chromosomal abnormalities	4–28
Fragile X syndrome	2–5
Monogenetic conditions	4–14
Structural CNS abnormalities	7–17
Complications of prematurity	2–10
Environmental or teratogenic causes	5–13
"Cultural-familial" ID/MR	3–12
Metabolic or endocrine causes	1–5
Unknown	30–50

Adapted from Curry CJ et al: Evaluation of mental retardation: Recommendations of a consensus conference. Am J Med Genet 1997;72:468.

and low intelligence quotient test scores. Great strides in our identification of genetic causes of ID/MR have been made since the 1990s because of the Human Genome Project. More than 750 genetic disorders have been associated with ID/MR, and over 200 of those disorders are carried on the X chromosome alone. In approximately 60% of cases, the cause of the mental retardation can be identified. Table 2–8 summarizes the findings of several studies examining the causes of mental retardation.

▶ Evaluation

Children who present with developmental delays should be evaluated by a team of professionals as described at the beginning of this section. For children 0–3¹⁄₂ years of age, the Bayley Scales of Infant Development, second edition, is a well-standardized developmental test. For children older than 3 years of age standardized cognitive testing, such as the Wechsler Preschool and Primary Scale of Intelligence-Revised; the Wechsler Intelligence Scale for Children, third edition; the Stanford-Binet IV; or the Kaufman Assessment Battery for Children should be administered to assess cognitive function over a broad range of abilities, including verbal and nonverbal scales. For the nonverbal patient, a scale such as the Leiter-R will assess skills that do not involve language.

A full psychological evaluation in school-aged children should include an emotional assessment if psychiatric or emotional problems are suspected. Such problems are common in children with developmental delays or ID/MR. A hearing test and a vision screening or ophthalmologic evaluation are important to determine whether hearing and vision are normal.

Diagnostic testing should be carried out in an effort to find the cause of ID/MR. Because chromosomal abnormalities occur in 4–28% of patients with ID/MR, cytogenetic testing is important in cases without a known cause. A consensus panel has recommended a high-resolution karyotype so that small deletions or duplications can be visualized. In addition, FISH studies are available. These studies use a fluorescent DNA probe that hybridizes to a region of DNA where a deletion or duplication is suspected. Microdeletion syndromes—such as Prader-Willi syndrome or Angelman syndrome, caused by a deletion at 15q; velocardiofacial syndrome, caused by a deletion at 22q; Smith-Magenis syndrome, caused by a deletion at 17p; and Williams syndrome, caused by a 7p deletion—can be assessed with FISH studies. Sometimes the deletion is so small that it may not be visualized through the microscope even with high-resolution cytogenetic studies. If clinical features consistent with any of the microdeletion syndromes are present, then FISH studies should be ordered to look for a small deletion in a specific region. In addition, duplications may be present. For example, duplication at 15q has been associated with pervasive developmental disorder or autistic spectrum disorders and with ID/MR. This duplication can be identified by FISH testing.

Structural abnormalities of the brain can occur in many individuals with ID/MR. Magnetic resonance imaging is superior to computed tomography in identifying structural and myelination abnormalities. Computed tomography is the study of choice in evaluation of intracranial calcifications, such as those seen in congenital infections or tuberous sclerosis. The value of computed tomography and magnetic resonance imaging studies in a child with a normal-sized head and no focal neurologic signs is unclear, and they are not routinely carried out. Neuroimaging is important in patients with microcephaly, macrocephaly, seizures, loss of psychomotor skills, or specific neurologic signs such as spasticity, dystonia, ataxia, or abnormal reflexes. Neuroimaging is not routinely carried out in children with known genetic disorders such as Down syndrome, fragile X syndrome, or microdeletion syndromes because the CNS abnormalities have been well described and documentation of the abnormalities usually does not affect management.

Metabolic screening has a relatively low yield (0–5%) in children who present with developmental delay or ID/MR. Many patients with metabolic disorders such as hypothyroidism, phenylketonuria, and galactosemia are identified through newborn screening. Most patients with metabolic problems will present with specific indications for more focused testing, such as failure to thrive, recurrent unexplained illnesses, plateauing or loss of developmental skills, coarse facial features, cataracts, recurrent coma, abnormal sexual differentiation, arachnodactyly, hepatosplenomegaly, deafness, structural hair abnormalities, muscle tone changes, and skin abnormalities. Thyroid function studies should be carried out in any patient who has a palpably abnormal thyroid or exhibits clinical features associated with hypothyroidism. Serum amino acids, urine organic acid, and mucopolysaccharide screens should be considered in children with developmental delays and a suggestive history. Preliminary laboratory findings such as lactic acidosis, hyperuricemia, hyperammonemia, or a low or high cholesterol level require additional metabolic workup.

Serial follow-up of patients is important as the physical and behavioral phenotype changes over time and diagnostic testing improves with time. Although cytogenetic testing may have been negative 10 years earlier, advances in high-resolution techniques, FISH testing, and fragile X DNA testing may now reveal an abnormality that was not identified previously. A stepwise approach to diagnostic testing may also be more cost-effective, so that the test most likely to be positive is done first.

▶ Management

Once a diagnosis of ID/MR is made, treatment should include a combination of individual therapies, such as speech and language therapy, occupational therapy or physical therapy, special education support, behavioral therapy or counseling, and medical intervention, which may include psychopharmacology. To illustrate how these interventions work together, three disorders are described in detail in the next section.

Burack JA et al (editors): *Handbook of Mental Retardation and Development.* Cambridge University Press, 1999.

Curry CJ et al: Evaluation of mental retardation: Recommendations of a consensus conference. Am J Med Genet 1997;72:468 [PMID: 9375733].

Hagerman RJ: *Neurodevelopmental Disorders: Diagnosis and Treatment.* Oxford University Press, 1999.

Schalock RL et al: The renaming of *mental retardation*: Understanding the change to the term *intellectual disability.* Intellect Dev Disab 2007;45:116 [PMID: 17428134].

Smith JD, Smallwood G: From whence came mental retardation? Asking why while saying goodbye. Intellect Dev Disab 2007;45:132 [PMID: 17428137].

The Arc of the United States (grassroots advocacy organization for people with disabilities): http://www.thearc.org

SPECIFIC FORMS OF INTELLECTUAL DISABILITY & ASSOCIATED TREATMENT ISSUES

1. Fragile X Syndrome

The most common inherited cause of mental retardation is fragile X syndrome, which is caused by a trinucleotide expansion (CGG repeated sequence) within the fragile X mental retardation I (*FMR1*) gene. Individuals with mental retardation of unknown origin should receive *FMR1* DNA testing to see if they have an expansion of the CGG repeat causing dysfunction of this gene. The CGG sequence at *FMR1* in the normal population includes 5–50 repeats. Carriers of the premutation have 54–200 repeats, and have been considered unaffected. However, there is mounting evidence for a specific phenotype in these individuals. Women with the premutation have a higher incidence of premature ovarian failure, anxiety, and mild

facial dysmorphisms. Individuals with the premutation have normal levels of FMR1 protein but increased levels of mRNA. It should be noted that seemingly unaffected females can pass an expansion of the CGG repeat to the next generation. Approximately 1 in 250 women and 1 in 700 men in the general population are premutation carriers. When a premutation of more than 90 repeats is passed on by a female to her offspring, it will expand to a full mutation (more than 200 repeats) 100% of the time, which usually causes mental retardation or learning disabilities. The full mutation is associated with methylation of the gene, which turns off transcription, resulting in a deficiency in the FMR1 protein product. These deficiencies result in mental retardation or significant learning and emotional problems.

Fragile X syndrome includes a broad range of symptoms. Patients can present with shyness, social anxiety, and learning problems, or they can present with mental retardation. Girls are usually less affected by the syndrome because they have a second X chromosome that is producing FMR1 protein. Approximately 70% of girls with the full mutation have cognitive deficits in addition to emotional problems, such as mood lability, ADHD, anxiety, and shyness. Approximately 85% of males with the syndrome have mental retardation and autistic-like features, such as poor eye contact, hand flapping, hand biting, and tactile defensiveness. About 20% of fragile X males meet the criteria for autism.

Children with fragile X syndrome usually present with language delays, hyperactivity, and tantrum behavior in early childhood. Although prominent ears and hyperextensible finger joints are common, approximately 30% of children with the syndrome may not have these features, and the diagnosis must be suspected because of behavioral problems and developmental delays alone. As the boys move into puberty, macroorchidism develops with an average adult volume of 50 mL, or twice the normal volume. The child's face may become longer during puberty, and the majority of these children continue to have prominent ears.

▶ Management

All young children with fragile X syndrome benefit from language and motor therapy because delays in these areas are universal. Because approximately 10% of boys with the syndrome will be nonverbal at age 5 years, the use of augmentative communication techniques—such as signing; the use of pictures to represent food, toys, or activities; or the use of computers that can be programmed for communication—are helpful. Tantrums and hyperarousal to stimuli, along with hyperactivity, are common. Sensory integrative occupational therapy can be helpful in calming hyperarousal to stimuli and in improving the child's fine and gross motor coordination and motor planning. Speech and language therapy can decrease oral hypersensitivity, improve articulation, enhance verbal output and comprehension, and stimulate abstract reasoning skills.

If the behavioral problems are severe, it can be helpful to involve a behavioral psychologist who emphasizes positive reinforcement, time outs, consistency in routine, and the use of both auditory and visual modalities, such as a picture sequence, to help with difficult transition times and new situations.

Psychopharmacology can also be useful to treat ADHD, aggression, anxiety, or severe mood instability. Clonidine or guanfacine may be helpful in low doses, beginning in the preschool period to treat hyperarousal, tantrums, or severe hyperactivity. Stimulant medications such as methylphenidate, dextroamphetamine, and Adderall are usually beneficial by age 5 years and occasionally earlier. Relatively low doses are used (eg, 0.2–0.3 mg/kg per dose of methylphenidate) because irritability is often a problem with higher doses.

Shyness and social anxiety combined with mild ADHD are commonly seen in girls who have fragile X syndrome. The social anxiety is sometimes so severe that selective mutism (refusal to speak in some environments, especially school) is seen in girls who have the full mutation. The treatment for selective mutism includes fluoxetine, language therapy, and counseling.

Anxiety may also be a significant problem for boys with fragile X syndrome, and the use of a selective serotonin reuptake inhibitor (SSRI) such as fluoxetine, sertraline, fluvoxamine, or paroxetine is often helpful. SSRIs may also decrease aggression or moodiness, although in approximately 25% of cases, an increase in agitation or even hypomania may occur. The use of a more limited serotonin agent, buspirone, may also be helpful for anxiety, particularly if the patient cannot tolerate SSRIs.

Anticonvulsants such as carbamazepine, valproic acid, and gabapentin can be used to treat seizures, which occur in 20% of children with fragile X syndrome. They can also be helpful in treating more severe mood instability that does not improve with an SSRI, clonidine, or a stimulant medication. The use of carbamazepine and valproic acid requires careful monitoring of blood levels, liver function studies, electrolytes, blood count, and platelet level.

Aggression may become a significant problem in childhood or adolescence for boys with fragile X syndrome. Counseling can often be helpful, although medication may be needed. Stimulants, clonidine, and an SSRI may decrease aggression, although sometimes an atypical antipsychotic may be needed. If psychotic features are present, such as paranoia, delusions, or hallucinations, or if thinking is severely disorganized, then an atypical antipsychotic is usually helpful. Risperidone has been used most frequently in pediatrics and has a low risk for extrapyramidal symptoms. Side effects include sedation, excessive appetite and subsequent weight gain, and an increase in prolactin, which can cause breast tenderness and gynecomastia in boys. Usually a low dose of risperidone is well tolerated, and 0.5–2 mg at bedtime usually improves aggression, decreases hyperactivity, and stabilizes mood.

An important component of treatment is genetic counseling. Parents should meet with a genetic counselor after the diagnosis of fragile X syndrome is made because there is a high risk that other family members are carriers or may be affected by the syndrome. A detailed family history is essential, and all siblings of the proband should have *FMR1* DNA testing. If the mother received the gene from her father, then all of her sisters are obligate carriers, and their children are at 50% risk of having the fragile X mutation.

It is also helpful to link up a newly diagnosed family to a parent support group. Educational materials and parent support information may be obtained by calling the National Fragile X Foundation at 1-800-688-8765.

Hagerman RJ, Cronister AC (editors): *Fragile X Syndrome: Diagnosis, Treatment, and Research,* 3rd ed. Johns Hopkins University Press, 2001.
Fragile X Research Foundation: http://www.fraxa.org
National Fragile X Foundation: http://www.FragileX.org

2. Fetal Alcohol Spectrum Disorders

Alcohol exposure in utero is associated with a broad spectrum of developmental problems, ranging from learning disabilities to severe mental retardation. Fetal alcohol spectrum disorders (FASD) is an umbrella term describing the range of effects that can occur in an individual exposed to alcohol prenatally. The Institute of Medicine in 1996 defined the diagnostic categories in individuals with documented prenatal maternal alcohol exposure as follows.

A. Fetal Alcohol Syndrome

Fetal alcohol syndrome (FAS) refers to the full syndrome associated with prenatal alcohol exposure. The diagnosis of FAS requires the presence of a characteristic pattern of facial abnormalities (short palpebral fissures, thin upper lip, and indistinct or smooth philtrum, for which there are standard measurements), growth deficiency, and evidence of CNS damage and neurodevelopmental abnormalities.

B. Partial Fetal Alcohol Syndrome

The diagnosis of partial fetal alcohol syndrome requires the presence of some but not all components of the facial anomalies as well as growth retardation, CNS neurodevelopmental abnormalities, or behavioral or cognitive abnormalities that are inconsistent with the child's developmental level and cannot be explained by familial background or environment.

Partial fetal alcohol syndrome is a category that has been controversial, and some clinicians feel that the criteria are too vague and imprecise to be of clinical help. What is most important, if the child does not have all of the criteria for FAS, is the documentation of prenatal alcohol exposure and the presence of neurodevelopmental dysfunction (encephalopathy).

C. Alcohol-Related Neurodevelopmental Disorder

Alcohol-related neurodevelopmental disorder does not require the presence of dysmorphic facial features, but it does require the presence of neurodevelopmental abnormalities or evidence of a pattern of behavioral or cognitive abnormalities. These abnormalities may include learning disabilities; poor impulse control; and problems in memory, attention, and judgment.

D. Alcohol-Related Birth Defects

The diagnosis of alcohol-related birth defects requires the presence of congenital anomalies, including malformations and dysplasias in cardiac, skeletal, renal, ocular, or auditory areas (ie, sensorineural hearing loss).

Animal and human data support these diagnostic categories, including the controversial alcohol-related neurodevelopmental disorder diagnosis, which does not include dysmorphic features. The prevalence of FAS, partial fetal alcohol syndrome, and alcohol-related neurodevelopmental disorder combined is approximately 1 per 100 in the general population. These are common problems. Thus, the physician should always ask about alcohol (and other drug) intake during pregnancy. This is particularly true when evaluating a child presenting with developmental disturbances. The exact amount of alcohol consumption that leads to teratogenesis remains unclear. However, there is strong evidence that binge drinking during the first trimester, the critical period of embryogenesis, leads to FASD.

▶ Evaluation & Management

Essential to the evaluation of a child with FASD, or one suspected of having FASD, is an assessment by a multidisciplinary team. Growth deficiency, facial features, brain dysfunction, and the documentation of prenatal alcohol exposure are the most significant areas to be assessed.

The majority of children with alcohol-related syndromes present with ADHD symptoms, with or without significant developmental delays. To adequately assess involvement in other organs the following tests are recommended: an ophthalmologic examination, a hearing test, and a careful cardiac examination, with ultrasonography if abnormalities are detected. A careful examination for dysmorphic features and bony abnormalities is necessary. Renal function studies (ie, creatinine) should be conducted and a renal ultrasound obtained. Mental health problems are observed in over 90% of children and adolescents affected by alcohol in utero. Depression, panic attacks, anxiety, and mood instability are common. Because psychotic ideation is present in 20–40% of individuals with alcohol-related syndromes, a thorough emotional or psychiatric evaluation is essential. Long-term therapy and special education services are usually needed, and psychopharmacologic intervention may be helpful.

For treatment of ADHD symptoms, a dextroamphetamine preparation should be tried initially, although methylphenidate may also be helpful. SSRIs can help relieve anxiety, panic attacks, and depression, although mania or hypomanias, a side effect, may occur in 25–50% of patients. Mood instability may be severe, although it usually responds to a mood stabilizer such as valproate or carbamazepine. One should be cautious with lithium because kidney dysfunction, secondary to malformations or hypoplasia, occasionally occurs. Psychotic features can be treated with an atypical or typical antipsychotic agent. However, consultation with a psychiatrist is advised under these circumstances. A speech and language evaluation and an occupational therapy evaluation in childhood usually lead to documentation of problems, and ongoing therapy is usually helpful. The most significant problem in FASD is the high rate of legal problems, incarceration, and alcohol or drug abuse in adolescence and adulthood. A coordinated intensive treatment program must be put in place early on if the outcome for these children is to be improved. Long-term counseling and advocacy, along with intensive job training can be of help in preventing social and legal problems for children with FASD.

American Academy of Pediatrics, Committee on Substance Abuse and Committee on Child with Disabilities: Fetal alcohol syndrome and alcohol-related neurodevelopmental disorders. Pediatrics 2000;106:358 [PIMD: 10920168].

Claren SK: Fetal alcohol syndrome. In Wolraich ML (editor): *Disorders of Development and Learning*, 3rd ed. BC Decker, 2003.

Hagerman RJ: *Fetal Alcohol Syndrome in Neurodevelopmental Disorders: Diagnosis and Treatment*. Oxford University Press, 1999.

Mattson SN, Schoenfeld AM, Riley, EP: Teratogenic effects of alcohol on brain and behavior. Alcohol Res Health 2001;25:185 [PIMD: 11810956].

Streissguth AP: *Fetal Alcohol Syndrome: A Guide for Families and Communities*. Brookes/Cole, 1997.

National Organization on Fetal Alcohol Syndrome: http://www.nofas.org

REFERENCES

Print Resources

Levine MD, Carey WB, Crocker AC (editors): *Developmental-Behavioral Pediatrics*, 3rd ed. WB Saunders, 1999.

Parker S, Zuckerman B (editors): *Behavioral and Developmental Pediatrics: A Handbook for Primary Care*. Lippincott Williams & Wilkins, 2005.

Wolraich ML et al: *Developmental-Behavioral Pediatrics: Evidence and Practice*. Mosby Elsevier, 2008.

Wolraich ML (editor): *Disorders of Development and Learning: A Practical Guide to Assessment and Management*, 3rd ed. BC Decker, 2003.

Web Resources

The Arc of the United States (grassroots advocacy organization for people with disabilities): http://www.thearc.org

American with Disabilities Act Information: National Access for Public Schools Project: http://www.adaptenv.org

Family Voices (web site devoted to children and youth with special health care needs): http://www.familyvoices.org

The Hanen Centre (information on family-focused early intervention programs): http://www.hanen.org

National Association of Developmental Disabilities Councils: http://www.naddc.org

National Dissemination Center for Children with Disabilities: http://www.nichcy.org

Parent Training and Information Centers: Alliance Coordinating Office: http://www.taalliance.org

Title V Program Information: Institute for Child Health Policy: http://www.ichp.edu

Adolescence

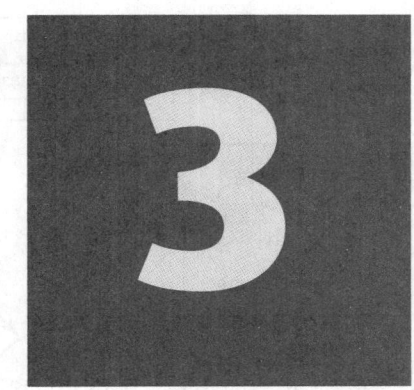

David W. Kaplan, MD, MPH
Kathryn A. Love-Osborne, MD

Adolescence is a period of rapid physical, emotional, cognitive, and social growth and development. Generally, adolescence begins at age 11–12 years and ends between ages 18 and 21. Most teenagers complete puberty by age 16–18 years; in western society, however, for educational and cultural reasons, the adolescent period is prolonged to allow for further psychosocial development before the individual assumes adult responsibilities.

The developmental passage from childhood to adulthood encompasses the following steps: (1) completing puberty and somatic growth; (2) developing socially, emotionally, and cognitively, and moving from concrete to abstract thinking; (3) establishing an independent identity and separating from the family; and (4) preparing for a career or vocation.

DEMOGRAPHY

In the United States in 2006, there were 21.3 million adolescents aged 15–19 years and 21.1 million aged 20–24 years. Adolescents and young adults (ages 15–24 years) constitute 14% of the U.S. population. In the next several decades, the proportion of racial and ethnic minority adolescents is expected to increase. It is projected that by 2040 the percentage of non-Hispanic whites will drop below 50%. Hispanics are becoming the second most populous racial and ethnic group.

MORTALITY DATA

In adolescents, cultural and environmental rather than organic factors pose the greatest threats to life. The three leading causes of death in the adolescents aged 15–19 years in 2004 were unintentional injury (50.0%), homicides (14.1%), and suicides (12.4%). These three causes of violent death accounted for 76.5% of all adolescent deaths. Although deaths from automobile crashes have decreased in the past decade, alcohol use remains the underlying cause of most teenage motor vehicle

deaths. Almost two thirds of motor vehicle deaths involving young drinking drivers occur on Friday, Saturday, or Sunday, and 70% occur between 8:00 PM and 4:00 AM.

There is continued concern with the problem of youth violence in the United States. The concern is stimulated by the high rate of homicides involving handguns among young males, the number of firearm-related suicides, and school shootings. Youths 12–17 years old are twice as likely as adults to be victims of serious violent crimes, including aggravated assault, rape, robbery, and homicide. Violent crimes committed by juveniles constitute about 25% of all violent crimes. Nationally, 18.5% of high-school students reported carrying a weapon at least once in the preceding 30 days. Violent crime victimization among adolescents has declined substantially since the early 1990s. In 2005, adolescents aged 12–19 were victimized at an all time low rate of 44.0 per 1000. This rate is less than half that reported for 1994. Adolescents who have been violently victimized are more likely to have physical and mental health problems, substance abuse problems, and problems at school.

MORBIDITY DATA

Demographic and economic changes in the American family have had a profound effect on children and adolescents. Between 1955 and 1990, the divorce rate rose from about 400,000 to nearly 1.2 million per year. Between 1960 and 1990, the number of children involved in divorce increased from 460,000 to 1.1 million per year. The percentage of children and adolescents living in two-parent households has decreased significantly, from 79% in 1980 to 68% in 2004. After peaking at 22% in 1992, the percentage of children living in families whose income was below the official poverty threshold fell during the late 1990s to 17%. However, the rate of poverty differs significantly by race and family structure. In 2005, 34% of black children and 28% of Hispanic children lived in families with incomes below the official poverty threshold. In 2005, 43% of children living in

▲ **Figure 3–1.** Interrelation of high-risk adolescent behavior.

single-mother families were poor, compared with 9% of children living in married-couple families.

The major causes of morbidity during adolescence are psychosocial and often correlated with poverty: unintended pregnancy, sexually transmitted infections (STIs), substance abuse, smoking, dropping out of school, depression, running away from home, physical violence, and juvenile delinquency. High-risk behavior in one area is frequently associated with problems in another (Figure 3–1). For example, teenagers who live in a dysfunctional family (eg, problems related to drinking or physical or sexual abuse) are much more likely than other teenagers to be depressed. A depressed teenager is at greater risk for drug and alcohol abuse, academic failure, inappropriate sexual activity, STIs, pregnancy, and suicide.

Early identification of the teenager at risk for these problems is important in preventing immediate complications and future associated problems. Early indicators for problems related to depression include the following:

1. Decline in school performance.
2. Excessive school absences or cutting class.
3. Frequent or persistent psychosomatic complaints.
4. Changes in sleeping or eating habits.
5. Difficulty in concentrating or persistent boredom.
6. Signs or symptoms of depression, extreme stress, or anxiety.

7. Withdrawal from friends or family, or change to a new group of friends.
8. Unusually severe violent or rebellious behavior, or radical personality change.
9. Conflict with parents.
10. Sexual acting-out.
11. Conflicts with the law.
12. Suicidal thoughts or preoccupation with themes of death.
13. Drug and alcohol abuse.
14. Running away from home.

Centers for Disease Control and Prevention: Web-based Injury Statistics Query and Reporting System (WISQARS). Atlanta: U.S. Department of Health and Human Services, CDC; 2007. Available at: http://www.cdc.gov/ncipc/wisqars/default.htm.

Chen LH et al: Graduated driver licensing programs and fatal crashes of 16-year-old drivers: A national evaluation. Pediatrics 2006;118:56 [PMID: 16818549]

Eaton DK et al: Youth risk behavior surveillance—United States, 2005. MMWR Surveill Summ 2006;55(SS-5):1 [PMID: 16760893]. Available at: http://www.cdc.gov/mmwr/preview/mmwrhtml/ss5505a1.htm.

Healthy People 2010: National Health Promotion and Disease Prevention Objectives. Washington, DC: U.S. Government Printing Office, 2000.

National Center for Health Statistics: Multiple Cause-of-Death Public-Use Data Files, 1990 through 2004. Hyattsville, MD: U.S. Department of Health and Human Services, CDC, National Center for Health Statistics; 2007.

Park MJ et al: The health status of young adults in the United States. J Adolesc Health 2006;39:305 [PMID: 16919791].

Steinberg L: Gallagher lecture. The family at adolescence: Transition and transformation. J Adolesc Health 2000;27:170 [PMID: 10960215].

Suicide trends among youths and young adults aged 10–24 years—United States, 1990–2004. MMWR Morb Mortal Wkly Rep 2007;56:905 [PMID: 17805220].

DELIVERY OF HEALTH SERVICES

How, where, why, and when adolescents seek health care depends on ability to pay, distance to health care facilities, availability of transportation, accessibility of services, time away from school, and privacy. Many common teenage health problems, such as unintended pregnancy and the need for contraception; STIs; and substance abuse, depression, and other emotional problems, have moral, ethical, and legal implications. Teenagers are often reluctant to confide in their parents for fear of punishment or disapproval. Recognizing this reality, health care providers have established specialized programs such as teenage family planning clinics, drop-in centers, STI clinics, hotlines, and adolescent clinics. Establishing a trusting and confidential relationship with adolescents is basic to meeting their health care needs. Patients who sense that the physician will inform their parents about a confidential problem may lie or fail to disclose information essential for proper diagnosis and treatment.

▼ GUIDELINES FOR ADOLESCENT PREVENTIVE SERVICES

The American Medical Association guidelines for adolescent preventive services and the American Academy of Pediatrics' *Bright Futures: Guidelines for Health Supervision of Infants, Children, and Adolescents* cover health screening and guidance, immunization, and health care delivery. The goals of these guidelines are (1) to deter adolescents from participating in behaviors that jeopardize health; (2) to detect physical, emotional, and behavioral problems early and intervene promptly; (3) to reinforce and encourage behaviors that promote healthful living; and (4) to provide immunization against infectious diseases. The guidelines recommend that adolescents between ages 11 and 21 years have annual routine health visits. Health services should be developmentally appropriate and culturally sensitive, and confidentiality between patient and physician should be ensured.

RELATING TO THE ADOLESCENT PATIENT

Adolescence is one of the physically healthiest periods in life. The challenge of caring for adolescents lies not in managing complex organic disease, but in accommodating the cognitive, emotional, and psychosocial growth that influences health behavior. How the physician initially approaches the adolescent may determine the success or failure of the visit. The physician should behave simply and honestly, without an authoritarian or excessively professional manner. Because the self-esteem of many young adolescents is fragile, the physician must be careful not to overpower and intimidate the patient. To establish a comfortable and trusting relationship, the physician should strive to present the image of an ordinary person who has special training and skills.

Because individuals vary in the onset and termination of puberty, chronologic age may be a poor indicator of physical, physiologic, and emotional development. In communicating with an adolescent, the physician must be sensitive to the patient's developmental level, recognizing that outward appearance and chronologic age may not give an accurate assessment of cognitive development.

Working with teenagers can be emotionally draining. Adolescents have a unique ability to identify hidden emotional vulnerabilities. The physician who has a personal need to control patients or foster dependency may be disappointed in caring for teenagers. Because teenagers are consumed with their own emotional needs, they rarely provide the physician with the ego rewards that younger or older patients do.

The physician should be sensitive to the issue of countertransference, the emotional reaction elicited in the physician by the adolescent. How the physician relates to the adolescent patient often depends on the physician's personal characteristics. This is especially true of physicians who treat families that are experiencing parent-adolescent conflicts. It is common for young physicians to overidentify with the teenage patient and for older physicians to see the conflict from the parents' perspective.

Overidentification with the parents is readily sensed by the teenager, who is likely to view the physician as just another authority figure who cannot understand the problems of being a teenager. Assuming a parental-authoritarian role may jeopardize the establishment of a working relationship with the patient. In the case of the young physician, overidentification with the teenager may cause the parents to become defensive about their parenting role and discount the physician's experience and ability.

THE SETTING

Adolescents respond positively to settings and services that communicate sensitivity to their age. A pediatrician's waiting room with toddlers' toys and infant-sized examination tables makes adolescent patients feel they have outgrown the practice. A waiting room filled with geriatric or pregnant patients can also make a teenager feel out of place.

It is not uncommon to see a teenage patient who has been brought to the office against his or her wishes, especially for evaluations of drug and alcohol use, parent-child conflict, school failure, depression, or a suspected eating disorder.

Even in cases of acute physical illness, the adolescent may feel anxiety about having a physical examination. If future visits are to be successful, the physician must spend time on the first visit to foster a sense of trust and an opportunity to feel comfortable.

CONFIDENTIALITY

It is helpful at the beginning of the visit to talk with the adolescent and the parents about what to expect. The physician should address the issue of confidentiality, telling the parents that two meetings, one with the teenager alone and one with only the parents, will take place. Adequate time must be spent with both the patient and the parents, or important information may be missed. At the beginning of the interview with the patient, it is useful to say, "I am likely to ask you some personal questions. This is not because I am trying to pry into your personal affairs, but because these questions may be important to your health. I want to assure you that what we talk about is confidential, just between the two of us. If there is something I feel we should discuss with your parents, I will ask your permission first unless I feel it is life-threatening."

THE STRUCTURE OF THE VISIT

Caring for adolescents is time-intensive. In many adolescent practices, a 40–50% no-show rate is not unusual. The stated chief complaint often conceals the patient's real concern. For example, a 15-year-old girl may say she has a sore throat but actually may be worried about being pregnant.

By age 11 or 12 years, patients should be seen alone. This gives them an opportunity to ask questions they may be embarrassed to ask in front of a parent. Because of the physical changes that take place in early puberty, some adolescents are too self-conscious to undress in front of a parent. If an adolescent comes in willingly, for an acute illness or for a routine physical examination, it may be helpful to meet with the adolescent and parent together to obtain the history. In angry adolescents brought in against their will, it is useful to meet with the parents and patient for 3–5 minutes to allow the parents to describe the conflict and voice their concerns. The adolescent should then be seen alone. This approach conveys that the physician is primarily interested in the adolescent patient, yet gives the physician an opportunity to acknowledge the parents' concerns.

The Interview

The first few minutes may dictate whether or not a trusting relationship can be established. A few minutes just getting to know the patient is time well spent. For example, immediately asking "Do you smoke marijuana?" when a teenager is brought in for suspected marijuana use confirms the adolescent's negative preconceptions about the physician and the purpose of the visit. It is preferable to spend a few minutes asking nonthreatening questions, such as "Tell me a little bit about yourself so I can get to know you," "What do you like to do most?" "Least?" and "What are your friends like?" Neutral questions help defuse some of the patient's anger and anxiety. Toward the end of the interview, the physician can ask more directed questions about psychosocial concerns.

Medical history questionnaires for the patient and the parents are useful in collecting historical data (Figure 3–2). The history should include an assessment of progress with psychodevelopmental tasks and of behaviors potentially detrimental to health. The review of systems should include questions about the following:

1. Nutrition: number and balance of meals; calcium, iron, and cholesterol intake; body image.
2. Sleep: number of hours, problems with insomnia or frequent waking.
3. Seat belt or helmet: regularity of use.
4. Self-care: knowledge of testicular or breast self-examination, dental hygiene, and exercise.
5. Family relationships: parents, siblings, relatives.
6. Peers: best friend, involvement in group activities, gangs, boyfriends, girlfriends.
7. School: attendance, grades, activities.
8. Educational and vocational interests: college, career, short-term and long-term vocational plans.
9. Tobacco: use of cigarettes, snuff, chewing tobacco.
10. Substance abuse: frequency, extent, and history of alcohol and drug use.
11. Sexuality: sexual activity, contraceptive use, pregnancies, history of STI, number of sexual partners, risk for HIV infection.
12. Emotional health: signs of depression and excessive stress.

The physician's personal attention and interest is likely to be a new experience for the teenager, who has probably received medical care only through a parent. The teenager should leave the visit with a sense of having a personal physician.

Physical Examination

During early adolescence, many teenagers may be shy and modest, especially with a physician of the opposite sex. The examiner should address this concern directly, because it can be allayed by acknowledging the uneasiness verbally and by explaining the purpose of the examination, for example, "Many boys that I see who are your age are embarrassed to have their penis and testes examined. This is an important part of the examination for a couple of reasons. First, I want to make sure that there aren't any physical problems, and second, it helps me determine if your development is proceeding normally." This also introduces the subject of sexual development for discussion.

A pictorial chart of sexual development is useful for showing the patient how development is proceeding and

TEEN HEALTH HISTORY

This information is *strictly confidential*. Its purpose is to help your caregiver give you better care. We request that you fill out the form completely, but you make skip any question that you do not wish to answer.

NAME _____ Date _____
            FIRST   MIDDLE INITIAL   LAST

BIRTHDATE _____ AGE _____ GRADE _____ Name that you like to be called _____

1. Why did you come to the clinic today?   _____

_____

_____

Medical History   **STRICTLY CONFIDENTIAL**

2. Are you allergic to any medicines?   –   YES NO
   Name of medicines _____
3. Are you taking any medicines now?   –   YES NO
   Name of medicines _____
4. Do you have any long-term health conditions?   –   YES NO
   Condition _____
5. Date or age at your last tetanus (or dT) shot _____

School Information

6. What grade do you usually make in English? _____
    (Example: A, B, C, D, E, F)
7. What grade do you usually make in Math? _____
8. How many days were you absent from school semester _____
9. How many days were you absent last semester because of illness?_____
10. How do you get along at school? _____

1	2	3	4	5	6	7
TEARRIBLE						GREAT

11. Have you ever been suspended? –   YES NO
12. Have you ever dropped out of school?–   YES NO
13. Do you plan to graduate from high school –   YES NO

Job/Career Information

14. Are you working? –   YES NO
    If YES, What is your job? _____
    How many hours do you work par week? _____
15. What are your future plans or career goals? _____

Family Information

16. Who do you live with? (Check all apply.)
    _____ Both natural parents   _____ Stepmother   _____ Brother(s)-ages:
    _____ Mother   _____ Stepfather   _____ Sister(s)-ages: _____
    _____ Father   _____ Guardian   _____ Other: Explain _____
    _____ Adoptive parents   _____ Alone   _____

17. Have there been any changes in your family? Check all that apply.
    _____ a. Marriage   _____ d. Serious illness   _____ g. Births
    _____ b. Separation   _____ e. Loss of job   _____ h. Deaths
    _____ c. Divorce   _____ f. Move to new home   _____ i. Other

18. Father's/stepfather's occupation or job:_____

    Mother's/stepmother's occupation or job: _____

▲ **Figure 3–2.** Adolescent medical history questionnaire. *(continued)*

STRICTLY CONFIDENTIAL

19. How do you get along at home?

1	2	3	4	5	6	7
TERRIBLE						GREAT

20. Have you ever run away from home? – YES NO
21. Have you ever lived in foster care or an institution? – – – – – – – – – – – – – – – – – – YES NO

Self Information

22. On the whole, how do you like yourself?

1	2	3	4	5	6	7
NOT VERY MUCH						A LOT

23. What do you do best? ————————————————————————
24. If you could, what would you like to change about yourself? ————————

25. List any habits you would like to break, ————————————————

26. Do you feel people expect too much from you? – YES NO
27. How do you get along with your friends/peers?

1	2	3	4	5	6	7
TERRIBLE						GREAT

28. Do you feel you have friends you can count on? – YES NO
29. Have you ever felt really sad or depressed for more than 3 days in a row? – – – – – – – – – YES NO
30. Have you ever thought of suicide as a solution to your problems? – – – – – – – – – – – – YES NO
31. Have you gotten into any trouble because of your anger/temper? – – – – – – – – – – – YES NO

Health Concern

32. On a scale of 1–7, how would you rate your general health?

1	2	3	4	5	6	7
TERRIBLE						GREAT

33. Do you have any questions or concerns about any of the following? (Check those that apply.)

—— Height/weight	—— Skin acne	—— Family violence/physical
—— Blood pressure	—— Arms, legs/muscle or	abuse
—— Head/headaches	joint pain	—— Feeling down or depressed
—— Dizziness/passing out	—— Frequent or painful	—— Dating
—— Eyes/vision	urination	—— Sex
—— Ears/hearing/earaches	—— Wetting the bed	—— Worried about VD/STD
—— Nose/frequent colds	—— Sexual organs/genitals	—— Masturbation
—— Mouth/teeth	—— Trouble sleeping	—— Sexual abuse/rape
—— Neck/back	—— Tiredness	—— Having children/parenting/
—— Chest/breathing/coughing	—— Diet food/appetite	adoption
—— Breasts	—— Eating disorder	—— Cancer/or dying
—— Heart	—— Smoking/drugs/alcohol	—— Other (explain) ——
—— Stomach/pain/vomiting	—— Future plans/jobs	
—— Diarrhea/constipation	—— Worried about parents	

Health Behavior Information

34. Have you lost or gained any weight in the last year? – – – – – – – – – – – – – – – – – – – YES NO
    Gained ( ) How much? ————————————————————
    Lost ( ) How much? ————————————————————
35. In the past year, have you tried to lose weight or control your weight by vomiting,
    taking diet pills or laxatives, or starving yourself? – – – – – – – – – – – – – – – – – – – YES NO
36. Do you ever drive after drinking or when high? – – – – – – – – – – – – – – – – – – – YES NO
37. Do you ever smoke cigarettes or use snuff or chewing tobacco? – – – – – – – – – – – YES NO
38. Do you ever smoke marijuana? – YES NO
39. Do you ever drink alcoholic beverages? – YES NO
40. Do you ever use street drugs (speed, cocaine, acid, crack, etc.)? – – – – – – – – – – – YES NO
41. Does anyone in your household smoke? – YES NO
42. Does anyone in your family have a problem with drugs or alcohol? – – – – – – – – – – – YES NO

▲ **Figure 3–2.** *(Continued)*

STRICTLY CONFIDENTIAL

43. Have you ever been in trouble with the police or the law? _____ YES NO
44. Have you begun dating? _____ YES NO
45. Do you currently have a boyfriend or girlfriend? _____ YES NO
    If YES, how old is he/she? _____
46. Do you think you might be gay/lesbian/homosexual? _____ YES NO
47. Have you ever had sex (sexual intercourse)? _____ YES NO
48. Are you interested in receiving information on preventing pregnancy? _____ YES NO
49. If you have had sex, are you (or your partner) using any kind of birth control? _____. YES NO
50. If you have had sex, have you ever been treated for gonorrhea or chlamydia
    or any other sexually transmitted disease? ---------------------------- YES NO

For males only

51. Have you been taught how to use a condom correctly? --------------------- YES NO
52. If you have had sex, do you use a condom every time or almost every time? --------- YES NO
53. Have you ever fathered a child? --------------------------------- YES NO

For females only

54. How old were you when your periods began? --------------------------- _____
55. What date did your last period start? ----------------------------- _____
56. Are your periods regular (once a month)? --------------------------- YES NO
57. Do you have painful or excessively heavy periods? ----------------------- YES NO
58. Have you ever had a vaginal infection or been treated for a female disorder? --------- YES NO
59. Do you think you might be pregnant? ------------------------------- YES NO
60. Have you ever been pregnant?------------------------------------ YES NO

Everyone

61. Do you have any other problems you would like to discuss with the caregiver? -------- YES NO

Past Medical History

62. Were you born prematurely or did you have any serious problems as an infant? ------- YES NO
63. Are you allergic to any medicines? ------------------------------- YES NO
    If YES, what? _____
    _____

64. List any medications that you are taking, and the problems for which the medication was
    given:

MEDICATION	REASON	HOW LONG

65. Have you ever been hospitalized?   ------------------------------- YES NO
    If Yes, describe your problem and your age at the time.

AGE	PROBLEM

66. Have you had any injuries? ----------------------------------- YES NO
    If YES, describe the injury and your age when it occurred.

AGE	KIND OF INJURY

67. Have you had any serious illnesses? ------------------------------- YES NO
    If YES, state the kind of illness and your age when it started.

AGE	ILLNESS

▲ **Figure 3–2.** *(Continued)*

STRICTLY CONFIDENTIAL

Family History

Have any members of your family, alive or dead (parents, grandparents, uncles, aunts, brothers, or sisters), had any of the following problems? If YES, please state the age of the person when the condition occurred and the person's relationship to you.

PROBLEM	YES	NO	DON'T KNOW	AGE	RELATIONSHIP
A. Seizure disorder Epilepsy					
B. Mental retardation Birth detects.					
C. Migraine headaches					
D. High blood pressure High cholesterol					
E. Heart attack or stroke at less than age 60					
F. Lung disease Tuberculosis					
G. Liver or intestinal disease					
H. Kidney disease					
I. Allergies Asthma Eczema					
J. Arthritis					
K. Diabetes					
L. Endocrine problems Other glandular problems					
M. Obesity Eating disorder					
N. Cancer					
O. Blood disorders Sickle cell anemia					
P. Emotional problems Suicide					
Q. Alcoholism Drug problems					

▲ **Figure 3-2.** *(Continued)*

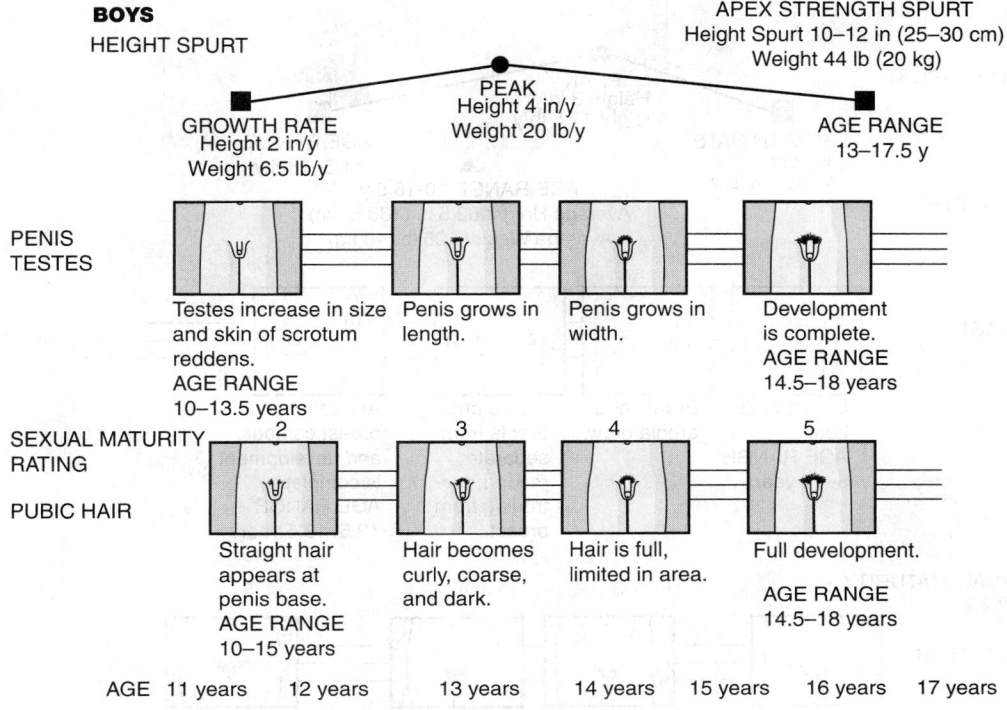

▲ Figure 3-3. Adolescent male sexual maturation and growth.

what changes to expect. Figure 3–3 shows the relationship between height, penis and testes development, and pubic hair growth in the male, and Figure 3–4 shows the relationship between height, breast development, menstruation, and pubic hair growth in the female. Although teenagers may not admit that they are interested in this subject, they are usually attentive when it is raised. This discussion is particularly useful in counseling teenagers who lag behind their peers in physical development.

Because teenagers are sensitive about their changing bodies, it is useful to comment during the examination: "Your heart sounds fine. I feel a small lump under your right breast. This is very common during puberty in boys. It is called gynecomastia and should disappear in 6 months to a year. Don't worry, you are not turning into a girl."

If a teenage girl has not been sexually active and has no gynecologic complaints or abnormalities, a pelvic examination is usually not necessary until about age 18 years. The following are indications for a pelvic examination in a younger teenage girl:

1. A history of sexual intercourse. (The pelvic examination should be done for purposes of contraceptive counseling and to rule out STI.)
2. Abnormal vaginal discharge.
3. Menstrual irregularities.
4. Suspicion of anatomic abnormalities, such as imperforate hymen.
5. Pelvic pain.
6. Patient request for an examination.

Bright Futures: Guidelines for Health Supervision of Infants, Children, and Adolescents. Elk Grove Village, IL: American Academy of Pediatrics, 2007.

Ford C, English A, Sigman G: Confidential Health Care for Adolescents: Position paper for the Society for Adolescent Medicine. J Adolesc Health 2004;35:160 [PMID: 15298005].

▼ GROWTH & DEVELOPMENT

PUBERTY

Pubertal growth and physical development are a result of activation of the hypothalamic-pituitary-gonadal axis in late childhood. Before puberty, pituitary and gonadal hormone levels are low. At onset of puberty, the inhibition of gonadotropin-releasing hormone in the hypothalamus is removed, allowing pulsatile production and release of the gonadotropins: luteinizing hormone (LH) and follicle-stimulating hor-

GIRLS

HEIGHT SPURT

PEAK
Height 3 in/y
Weight 17.5 lb/y

GROWTH RATE
Height 2 in/y
Weight 6 lb/y

AGE RANGE
11.5–16.5 y

MENARCHE

AGE RANGE 10-16.5 y
Average Height 62.5 in (158.5 cm)
Average Weight 106 lb (48 kg)

BREAST

Breast buds begin.
AGE RANGE 8–13 years

Breast and areola grow.

Nipple and areola from separate mound, protruding from breast.

Areola rejoins breast contour and development is complete.
AGE RANGE 12.5–18.5 years

SEXUAL MATURITY RATING   2   3   4   5

PUBIC HAIR

Initial hair is straight and fine.
AGE RANGE 8–14 years

Pubic hair becomes coarse, darkens, and spreads.

Hair looks like an adult's but limited in area.

Inverted triangular pattern is established
AGE RANGE 12.5–16.5 years

AGE   11 years   12 years   13 years   14 years   15 years

▲ **Figure 3–4.** Adolescent female sexual maturation and growth.

mone (FSH). In early to middle adolescence, pulse frequency and amplitude of LH and FSH secretion increase, stimulating the gonads to produce estrogen or testosterone. In females, FSH stimulates ovarian maturation, granulosa cell function, and estradiol secretion. LH is important in ovulation and also is involved in corpus luteum formation and progesterone secretion. Initially, estradiol inhibits the release of LH and FSH. Eventually, estradiol becomes stimulatory, and the secretion of LH and FSH becomes cyclic. Estradiol levels progressively increase, resulting in maturation of the female genital tract and breast development.

In males, LH stimulates the interstitial cells of the testes to produce testosterone. FSH stimulates the production of spermatocytes in the presence of testosterone. The testes also produce inhibin, a Sertoli cell protein that inhibits the secretion of FSH. During puberty, circulating testosterone levels increase more than 20-fold. Levels of testosterone correlate with the physical stages of puberty and the degree of skeletal maturation.

PHYSICAL GROWTH

A teenager's weight almost doubles in adolescence, and height increases by 15–20%. During puberty, major organs double in size, except for lymphoid tissue, which decreases in mass. Before puberty, there is little difference in the muscular strength of boys and girls. The body's musculature increases both in size and in strength during puberty, with maximal strength lagging behind the increase in size by many months. Boys attain greater strength and mass, and strength continues to increase into late puberty. Although motor coordination lags behind growth in stature and musculature, it continues to improve as strength increases.

The pubertal growth spurt begins nearly 2 years earlier in girls than in boys. Girls reach peak height velocity between ages $11\frac{1}{2}$ and 12 years, and boys, between ages $13\frac{1}{2}$ and 14 years. Linear growth at peak velocity is 9.5 cm/y ± 1.5 cm in boys and 8.3 cm/y ± 1.2 cm in girls. Pubertal growth lasts about 2–4 years and continues longer in boys than in girls. By age 11 years in girls and age 12 years in boys, 83–89% of ultimate height is attained. An additional 18–23 cm in females and 25–30 cm in males is achieved during late pubertal growth. Following menarche, growth is rarely more than 5–7.5 cm.

In boys, the quantity of body fat increases before onset of the height spurt, continues until the growth spurt has finished, and then gradually increases. Muscle mass doubles between 10 and 17 years. Girls, by contrast, store fat gradually from about 6 years of age and do not decrease the quantity of fat, although its location changes. There is an increase in subcutaneous fat in the pelvis, breasts, and upper back.

SEXUAL MATURATION

Sexual maturity rating (SMR) is useful for categorizing genital development. SMR staging includes age ranges of normal development and specific descriptions for each stage of pubic hair growth, penis and testis development in boys, and breast maturation in girls. Figures 3–3 and 3–4 show this chronologic development. SMR 1 is prepuberty and SMR 5 is adult maturity. In SMR 2 the pubic hair is sparse, fine, nonpigmented, and downy; in SMR 3, the hair becomes pigmented and curly and increases in amount; and in SMR 4, the hair is adult in texture but limited in area. The appearance of pubic hair precedes axillary hair by more than 1 year. Male genital development begins with SMR 2, in which the testes become larger and the scrotal skin reddens and coarsens. In SMR 3, the penis lengthens; and in SMR 4, the penis enlarges in overall size and the scrotal skin becomes pigmented.

Female breast development follows a predictable sequence. Small, raised breast buds appear in SMR 2. In SMR 3, the breast and areolar tissue generally enlarge and become elevated. The areola and nipple form a separate mound from the breast in SMR 4, and in SMR 5 the areola assumes the same contour as the breast.

There is great variability in the timing and onset of puberty and growth, and psychosocial development does not always parallel physical changes. Chronologic age, therefore, may be a poor indicator of physiologic and psychosocial development. Skeletal maturation correlates well with growth and pubertal development.

Teenagers began entering puberty at earlier ages in the last century because of better nutrition and socioeconomic conditions. In the United States, the average age at menarche is 12.16 years in African-American girls and 12.88 in white girls. Among girls reaching menarche, the average weight is 48 kg, and the average height is 158.5 cm. Menarche may be delayed until age 16 years or may begin as early as age 10. Although the first measurable sign of puberty in girls is the beginning of the height spurt, the first conspicuous sign usually is development of breast buds between 8 and 11 years. Although breast development usually precedes the growth of pubic hair, the sequence may be reversed. A common concern for girls at this time is whether the breasts will be of the right size and shape, especially because initial breast growth is often asymmetrical. The growth spurt starts at about age 9 years in girls and peaks at age 11$^{1}/_{2}$, usually at SMR 3–4 breast development and stage 3 pubic hair development. The spurt usually ends by age 14 years. Girls who mature early will reach peak height velocity sooner and attain their final height earlier. Girls who mature late will attain a greater final height because of the longer period of growth before the growth spurt. Final height is related to skeletal age at onset of puberty as well as genetic factors. The height spurt correlates more closely with breast developmental stages than with pubic hair stages.

The first sign of puberty in the male, usually between ages 10 and 12 years, is scrotal and testicular growth. Pubic hair usually appears early in puberty but may do so any time between ages 10 and 15 years. The penis begins to grow significantly a year or so after the onset of testicular and pubic hair development, usually between ages 10 and 13$^{1}/_{2}$. The first ejaculation usually occurs about 1 year after initiation of testicular growth, but its timing is highly variable. About 90% of boys have this experience between ages 11 and 15 years. Gynecomastia, a hard nodule under the nipple, occurs in a majority of boys, with a peak incidence between ages 14 and 15 years. Gynecomastia usually disappears within 6 months to 2 years. The height spurt begins at age 11 years but increases rapidly between ages 12 and 13, with the peak height velocity reached at age 13$^{1}/_{2}$ years. The period of pubertal development lasts much longer in boys and may not be completed until age 18 years. The height velocity is higher in males (8–11 cm/y) than in females (6.5–9.5 cm/y). The development of axillary hair, deepening of the voice, and the development of chest hair in boys usually occur in midpuberty, about 2 years after onset of growth of pubic hair. Facial and body hair begin to increase at age 16–17 years.

Biro FM et al: Pubertal maturation in girls and the relationship to anthropometric changes: Pathways through puberty. J Pediatr 2003;142:643 [PMID: 12838192].

Chumlea WC et al: Age at menarche and racial comparisons in US girls. Pediatrics 2003;111:110 [PMID: 12509562].

Herman-Giddens ME et al: Navigating the recent articles on girls' puberty in Pediatrics: What do we know and where do we go from here? Pediatrics 2004;113:911 [PMID: 15060243].

Rogol AD et al: Growth at puberty. J Adolesc Health 2002; 31(Suppl):192 [PMID: 12470915].

Rosen DS: Physiologic growth and development during adolescence. Pediatr Rev 2004;25:194 [PMID: 15173452].

Tanner JM, Davies PW: Clinical longitudinal standards for height and height velocity for North American children. J Pediatr 1985;107:317 [PMID: 3875704].

PSYCHOSOCIAL DEVELOPMENT

Adolescence is a period of progressive individuation and separation from the family. Adolescents must learn who they are, decide what they want to do, and identify their personal strengths and weaknesses. Because of the rapidity of physical, emotional, cognitive, and social growth during adolescence, it is useful to divide it into three phases. Early adolescence is roughly from 10 to 13 years of age; middle adolescence, from 14 to 16 years; and late adolescence, 17 years and later.

Early Adolescence

Early adolescence is characterized by rapid growth and development of secondary sex characteristics. Body image, self-concept, and self-esteem fluctuate dramatically. Concerns about how personal growth and development deviate from that of peers may be a great worry, especially short stature in boys and delayed breast development or delayed menarche in girls. Although there is a certain curiosity about sexuality, young adolescents generally feel more comfortable with members of the same sex. Peer relationships become increasingly important. Young teenagers still think concretely and cannot easily conceptualize about the future. They may have vague and unrealistic professional goals, such as becoming a movie star or a lead singer in a rock group.

Middle Adolescence

During middle adolescence as rapid pubertal development subsides, teenagers become more comfortable with their new bodies. Intense emotions and wide swings in mood are typical. Although some teenagers go through this experience relatively peacefully, others struggle. Cognitively, the midadolescent moves from concrete thinking to formal operations and abstract thinking. With this new mental power comes a sense of omnipotence and a belief that the world can be changed by merely thinking about it. Sexually active teenagers may believe they do not need to worry about using contraception because they can't get pregnant ("it won't happen to me"). Sixteen-year-old drivers believe they are the best drivers in the world and think the insurance industry is conspiring against them by charging high rates for automobile insurance. With the onset of abstract thinking, teenagers begin to see themselves as others see them and may become extremely self-centered. Because they are establishing their own identities, relationships with other people, including peers, are narcissistic. Experimenting with different images is common. As sexuality increases in importance, adolescents may begin dating and experimenting with sex. Relationships tend to be one-sided and narcissistic. Peers determine the standards for identification, behavior, activities, and fashion and provide emotional support, intimacy, empathy, and the sharing of guilt and anxiety during the struggle for autonomy. The struggle for independence and autonomy is often a stressful period for both teenagers and parents.

Late Adolescence

During late adolescence, the young person generally becomes less self-centered and more caring of others. Social relationships shift from the peer group to the individual. Dating becomes much more intimate. By 10th grade, 43% of adolescents have had sexual intercourse, and by 12th grade, 63%. Abstract thinking allows older adolescents to think more realistically about their plans for the future. Older adolescents have rigid concepts of what is right or wrong. This is a period of idealism.

Sexual Orientation

Sexual orientation develops during early childhood. One's gender identity is established by age 2 years, and a sense of masculinity or femininity usually solidifies by age 5 or 6 years. Homosexual adults describe homosexual feelings during late childhood and early adolescence, years before engaging in overt homosexual acts.

Although only 5–10% of American young people acknowledge having had homosexual experiences and only 5% feel that they are or could be gay, homosexual experimentation is common, especially during early and middle adolescence. Experimentation may include mutual masturbation and fondling the genitals and does not by itself cause or lead to adult homosexuality. Theories about the causes of homosexuality include genetic, hormonal, environmental, and psychological models.

The development of homosexual identity in adolescence commonly progresses through two stages. The adolescent feels different, develops a crush on a person of the same sex without clear self-awareness of a gay identity, and then goes through a coming-out phase in which the homosexual identity is defined for the individual and revealed to others. The coming-out phase may be a difficult period for the young person and the family. The young adolescent is afraid of society's bias and seeks to reject homosexual feelings. This struggle with identity may include episodes of both homosexual and heterosexual promiscuity, STIs, depression, substance abuse, attempted suicide, school avoidance and failure, running away from home, and other crises.

In a clinical setting, the issue of homosexual identity most often surfaces when the teenager is seen for an STI, family conflict, school problem, attempted suicide, or substance abuse rather than as a result of a consultation about sexual orientation. Pediatricians should be aware of the psychosocial and medical implications of homosexual identity and be sensitive to the possibility of these problems in gay adolescents. Successful management depends on the physician's ability to gain the trust of the gay adolescent and on the physician's knowledge of the wide range of medical and psychological problems for which gay adolescents are at risk. Pediatricians must be nonjudgmental in posing sexual questions if they are to be effective in encouraging the teenager to share concerns. Physicians who for religious or other personal reasons cannot be objective must refer the homosexual patient to another professional for treatment and counseling.

Eisenberg ME, Resnick MD: Suicidality among gay, lesbian and bisexual youth: The role of protective factors. J Adolesc Health 2006;39:662 [PMID: 17046502].

Frankowski BL: American Academy of Pediatrics Committee on Adolescence. Sexual orientation and adolescents. Pediatrics 2004;113:1827 [PMID: 15173519].

Gutgesell ME, Payne N: Issues of adolescent psychological development in the 21st century. Pediatr Rev 2004;25:79 [PMID: 14993515].

Russell ST, Joyner K: Adolescent sexual orientation and suicide risk: Evidence from a national study. Am J Public Health 2001;91:1276 [PMID: 11499118].

Ryan C, Futterman D: Caring for gay and lesbian teens. Contemp Pediatr 1998;15:107.

BEHAVIOR & PSYCHOLOGICAL HEALTH

It is not unusual for adolescents to seek medical attention for seemingly minor complaints. In early adolescence, teenagers may worry about normal developmental changes such as gynecomastia. They may present with vague symptoms, but have a hidden agenda of concerns about pregnancy or an STI. Adolescents with emotional disorders often present with somatic symptoms such as abdominal pain, headaches, dizziness, syncope, fatigue, sleep problems, and chest pain that appear to have no biologic cause. The emotional basis of such complaints may be varied: somatoform disorder, depression, or stress and anxiety.

PSYCHOPHYSIOLOGIC SYMPTOMS & CONVERSION REACTIONS

The most common somatoform disorder of adolescence is conversion disorder or conversion reaction. (A conversion reaction is a psychophysiologic process in which unpleasant feelings, especially anxiety, depression, and guilt, are communicated through a physical symptom.) Psychophysiologic symptoms result when anxiety activates the autonomic nervous system, causing tachycardia, hyperventilation, and vasoconstriction. The emotional feeling may be threatening or unacceptable to the individual, who expresses it as a physical symptom rather than verbally. The process is unconscious, and the anxiety or unpleasant feeling is dissipated by the somatic symptom. The degree to which the conversion symptom lessens anxiety, depression, or the unpleasant feeling is referred to as primary gain. Conversion symptoms not only diminish unpleasant feelings but also release the adolescent from conflict or an uncomfortable situation. This is called secondary gain. Secondary gain may intensify the symptoms, especially with increased attention from concerned parents and friends. Adolescents with conversion symptoms tend to have overprotective parents and become increasingly dependent on their parents as the symptom becomes a major focus of concern in the family.

▶ Clinical Findings

Symptoms may appear at times of stress. Nervous, gastrointestinal, and cardiovascular symptoms are common and include paresthesias, anesthesia, paralysis, dizziness, syncope, hyperventilation, abdominal pain, nausea, and vomiting. Specific symptoms may reflect existing or previous illness (eg, pseudoseizures in adolescents with epilepsy) or modeling of a close relative's symptom (eg, chest pain in a boy whose grandfather died of a heart attack).

Conversion symptoms are more common in girls than in boys. Although they occur in patients from all socioeconomic levels, the complexity of the symptom may vary with the sophistication and cognitive level of the patient.

▶ Differential Diagnosis

History and physical findings are usually inconsistent with a physical cause of symptoms. Conversion symptoms occur most frequently during stress and in the presence of individuals meaningful to the patient. The common personality traits of these patients include egocentricity, emotional lability, and dramatic and attention-seeking behaviors.

Conversion reactions must be differentiated from hypochondriasis, which is a preoccupation with developing or having a serious illness despite medical reassurance that there is no evidence of disease. Over time, the fear of one disease may give way to concern about another. In contrast to patients with conversion symptoms, who seem relieved if an organic cause is considered, patients with hypochondriasis become more anxious when such a cause is considered.

Malingering is uncommon during adolescence. The malingering patient consciously and intentionally fabricates false or exaggerated physical or psychological symptoms. Such patients are motivated by external incentives such as avoiding work, evading criminal prosecution, obtaining drugs, or obtaining financial compensation. These patients may be hostile and aloof. Parents of patients with conversion disorders and malingering have a similar reaction to illness. They have an unconscious psychological need to have sick children and reinforce their child's behavior.

Somatic delusions are physical symptoms, often bizarre, that accompany other signs of mental illness. Examples are visual or auditory hallucinations, delusions, incoherence or loosening of associations, rapid shifts of affect, and confusion.

▶ Treatment

The physician must emphasize from the outset that both physical and emotional causes of the symptom will be considered. The relationship between physical causes of emotional pain and emotional causes of physical pain should be described to the family, using examples such as stress causing an ulcer or making a severe headache worse. The patient should be encouraged to understand that the symptom may persist and that at least a short-term goal is to continue normal daily activities. Medication is rarely helpful. If the family will accept it, psychological referral is often the best initial step toward psychotherapy. If the family resists psychiatric or psychological referral, the pediatrician may need to begin to deal with some of the emotional factors responsible for the symptom while building rapport with the patient and family. Regular appointments should be scheduled. During visits, the teenager should be seen first and encouraged to talk about school, friends, the relationship with the parents, and the stresses of life. Discussion of the symptom itself should be minimized; however, the physician should be supportive and must never suggest that the pain is not real. As parents gain insight into the cause of the symptom, they will become less indulgent and facilitate resumption of normal activities. If management is successful, the adolescent will gain coping skills and become more independent, while decreasing secondary gain.

If the symptom continues to interfere with daily activities and if the patient and parents feel that no progress is being made, psychological referral is indicated. A psychotherapist experienced in treating adolescents with conversion reactions is in the best position to establish a strong therapeutic relationship with the patient and family. After referral is made, the pediatrician should continue to follow the patient to ensure compliance with psychotherapy.

American Psychiatric Association: *Diagnostic and Statistical Manual of Mental Disorders,* 4th ed, text revision. American Psychiatric Press, 2000.

Kreipe RE: The biopsychosocial approach to adolescents with somatoform disorders. Adolesc Med Clin 2006;17:1 [PMID: 16473291].

Silber TJ, Pao M: Somatization disorders in children and adolescents. Pediatr Rev 2003;24:255 [PMID: 12897265].

DEPRESSION (SEE ALSO CHAPTER 6)

Symptoms of clinical depression (lethargy, loss of interest, sleep disturbances, decreased energy, feelings of worthlessness, and difficulty concentrating) are common during adolescence. The intensity of feelings, often in response to seemingly trivial events such as a poor grade on an examination or not being invited to a party, makes it difficult to differentiate severe depression from normal sadness or dejection. In less severe depression, sadness or unhappiness associated with problems of everyday life is generally short-lived. The symptoms usually result in only minor impairment in school performance, social activities, and relationships with others. Symptoms respond to support and reassurance.

▶ Clinical Findings

The presentation of serious depression in adolescence may be similar to that in adults, with vegetative signs such as depressed mood, crying spells or inability to cry, discouragement, irritability, a sense of emptiness and meaninglessness, negative expectations of oneself and the environment, low self-esteem, isolation, helplessness, diminished interest or pleasure in activities, weight loss or weight gain, insomnia or hypersomnia, fatigue or loss of energy, feelings of worthlessness, and diminished ability to think or concentrate. However, it is not unusual

for a serious depression to be masked because the teenager cannot tolerate the severe feelings of sadness. Such a teenager may present with recurrent or persistent psychosomatic complaints, such as abdominal pain, chest pain, headache, lethargy, weight loss, dizziness, syncope, or other nonspecific symptoms. Other behavioral manifestations of masked depression include truancy, running away from home, defiance of authorities, self-destructive behavior, vandalism, drug and alcohol abuse, sexual acting out, and delinquency.

▶ Differential Diagnosis

A complete history and physical examination, including a careful review of the patient's medical and psychosocial history, should be performed. The family history should be explored for psychiatric problems.

The teenager should be questioned about the previously listed symptoms of depression, and specifically about suicidal ideation or preoccupation with thoughts of death. The history should include an assessment of school performance, looking for signs of academic deterioration, excessive absence or cutting class, changes in work or other outside activities, and changes in the family (eg, separation, divorce, serious illness, loss of employment by a parent, a recent move to a new school, increasing quarrels or fights with parents, or the death of a close relative). The teenager may have withdrawn from friends or family or switched allegiance to a new group of friends. The physician should inquire about possible physical and sexual abuse, drug and alcohol abuse, conflicts with the police, sexual acting out, running away from home, unusually violent or rebellious behavior, or radical personality changes. Patients with vague somatic complaints or concerns about having a fatal illness may have an underlying affective disorder.

Adolescents presenting with symptoms of depression require a thorough medical evaluation to rule out any contributing or underlying medical illness. Among the medical conditions associated with affective disorders are eating disorders, organic central nervous system disorders (tumors, vascular lesions, closed head trauma, and subdural hematomas), metabolic and endocrinologic disorders (systemic lupus erythematosus, hypothyroidism, hyperthyroidism, Wilson disease, hyperparathyroidism, Cushing syndrome, Addison disease, or premenstrual syndrome), infections (infectious mononucleosis or syphilis), and mitral valve prolapse. Marijuana use, phencyclidine abuse, amphetamine withdrawal, and excessive caffeine intake can cause symptoms of depression. Common prescription and over-the-counter medications, including birth control pills, anticonvulsants, and β-blockers, may cause depressive symptoms.

Some routine laboratory studies are indicated to rule out organic disease: a complete blood count and erythrocyte sedimentation rate, urinalysis, serum electrolytes, blood urea nitrogen, serum calcium, thyroxine and thyroid-stimulating hormone (TSH), Venereal Disease Research Laboratory or rapid plasma reagin, and liver enzymes. Although metabolic markers such as abnormal secretion of cortisol, growth hormone, and thyrotropin-releasing hormone have been useful in confirming major depression in adults, these neurobiologic markers are less reliable in adolescents.

The risk of depression appears to be greatest in families with a history of early-onset and chronic depression. Depression of early onset and bipolar illness are more likely to occur in families with a multigenerational history of depression. The lifetime risk of depressive illness in first-degree relatives of adult depressed patients is between 18% and 30%.

▶ Treatment

The primary care physician may be able to counsel adolescents and parents if depression is mild or is the result of an acute personal loss or frustration and if the patient is not contemplating suicide or other life-threatening behaviors. If there is evidence of a long-standing depressive disorder, suicidal thoughts, or psychotic thinking, or if the physician does not feel prepared to counsel the patient, psychological referral should be made.

Counseling involves establishing and maintaining a positive supportive relationship; following the patient at least weekly; remaining accessible to the patient at all times; encouraging the patient to express emotions openly, defining the problem, and clarifying negative feelings, thoughts, and expectations; setting realistic goals; helping to negotiate interpersonal crises; teaching assertiveness and social skills; reassessing the depression as it is expressed; and staying alert to the possibility of suicide.

Patients with bipolar disease or those with significant depression that is unresponsive to supportive counseling should be referred to a psychiatrist for evaluation and antidepressant medication. The Food and Drug Administration has issued a "black box warning" alerting providers that using antidepressants in children and adolescents may increase the risk of suicidal thoughts and behavior. Adolescents taking these medications should be monitored closely.

Belmaker RH: Bipolar disorder. N Engl J Med 2004;351:476 [PMID: 15282355].

Brent DA, Birmaher B: Clinical practice. Adolescent depression. N Engl J Med 2002;347:667 [PMID: 12200555].

Mann JJ: The medical management of depression. N Engl J Med 2005;353:1819 [PMID: 16251538].

March J et al: Fluoxetine, cognitive-behavioral therapy, and their combination for adolescents with depression: Treatment for Adolescents with Depression Study (TADS) randomized controlled trial. JAMA 2004;292:807 [PMID: 15315995].

Simon GE: The antidepressant quandary—considering suicide risk when treating adolescent depression. N Engl J Med 2006;355:2722 [PMID: 17192536].

ADOLESCENT SUICIDE (SEE ALSO CHAPTER 6)

In 2004, 4316 adolescents and young adults 15–24 years committed suicide. There were 1700 suicides among those aged 15–19 years, and 2616 among those aged 20–24 years. In the younger group, males had a suicide rate five times higher than females, and white males had the highest rate, 15.5 per 100,000. The incidence of unsuccessful suicide attempts is three times higher in females than in males. The estimated ratio of attempted suicides to actual suicides is estimated to be 100:1–50:1. Firearms account for 50% of suicide deaths in both males and females.

Mood swings are common in adolescence. Short periods of depression are common and may be accompanied by thoughts of suicide. Normal adolescent mood swings rarely interfere with sleeping, eating, or normal activities. Acute depressive reactions (transient grief responses) to the loss of a family member or friend may cause depression lasting for weeks or even months. An adolescent who is unable to work through this grief can become increasingly depressed. A teenager who is unable to keep up with schoolwork, does not participate in normal social activities, withdraws socially, has sleep and appetite disturbances, and has feelings of hopelessness and helplessness should be considered at increased risk for suicide.

Angry teenagers attempting to influence others by their actions may be suicidal. They may be only mildly depressed and may not have any long-standing wish to die. Teenagers in this group, usually females, may attempt suicide or make an impulsive suicidal gesture as a way of getting back at someone or gaining attention by frightening another person. Adolescents with serious psychiatric disease such as acute schizophrenia or psychotic depressive disorder are also at risk for suicide.

▶ Risk Assessment

The physician must determine the extent of the teenager's depression and the risk that he or she might inflict self-injury. Evaluation should include interviews with both the teenager and the family. The history should include the medical, social, emotional, and academic background. The physician should inquire about:

1. Common signs of depression
2. Recent events that could be the cause of an underlying depression
3. Evidence of long-standing problems in the home, at school, or with peers
4. Drug or substance use and abuse
5. Signs of psychotic thinking, such as delusions or hallucinations
6. Evidence of masked depression, such as rebellious behavior, running away from home, reckless driving, or other acting-out behavior

The physician should always ask depressed patients about thoughts of suicide, for example by asking, "Are things ever so bad that life doesn't seem worth living?" If the response is affirmative, a more specific question should be asked, for example, "Have you thought of taking your life?" If the patient has thoughts of suicide, the immediacy of risk can be assessed by determining if the patient has a concrete, feasible plan. Although patients who are at greatest risk have a concrete plan that can be carried out in the near future, especially if they have rehearsed the plan, the physician should not dismiss the potential risk of suicide in the adolescent who does not describe a specific plan. The physician should pay attention to his or her own instincts. Subtle nonverbal signs may indicate that the patient is at greater risk than may be apparent.

Treatment

The primary care physician is often in a unique position to identify an adolescent at risk for suicide, because many teenagers who attempt suicide seek medical attention in the weeks preceding the attempt. These visits are often for vague somatic complaints. If the patient shows evidence of depression, the physician must assess the severity of the depression and suicidal risk. The pediatrician should always seek emergency psychological consultation for any teenager who is severely depressed, psychotic, or acutely suicidal. It is the psychologist's or psychiatrist's responsibility to assess the seriousness of suicidal ideation and decide whether hospitalization or outpatient treatment is most appropriate. Adolescents with mild depression and low risk for suicide should be followed closely, and the extent of the depression should be assessed on an ongoing basis. If it appears that the patient is worsening or is not responding to supportive counseling, referral should be made.

American Academy of Child and Adolescent Psychiatry: Summary of the practice parameters for the assessment and treatment of children and adolescents with suicidal behavior. J Am Acad Child Adolesc Psychiatry 2001;40:495 [PMID: 11314578].

American Academy of Pediatrics Committee on Adolescence: Suicide and suicide attempts in adolescents. Pediatrics 2000;105:871 [PMID: 10742349].

Hatcher-Kay C, King CA: Depression and suicide. Pediatr Rev 2003;24:363 [PMID: 14595033].

Zametkin AJ et al: Suicide in teenagers: Assessment, management, and prevention. JAMA 2001;286:3120 [PMID: 11754678].

SUBSTANCE ABUSE

Substance abuse is a complex problem for adolescents and the broader society. See Chapter 4 for an in-depth look at this issue.

EATING DISORDERS (SEE CHAPTER 5)

OVERWEIGHT (SEE ALSO CHAPTER 10)

Obesity is defined as body mass index (BMI) greater than the 95th percentile for age. Overweight is defined as BMI greater than the 85th percentile for age. (Growth charts are available at the Centers for Disease Control and Prevention web site, http://www.cdc.gov/growthcharts; see also Chapter 2). These definitions have changed to reflect adult obesity definitions. It is important to note that mean BMI changes with age. For a 13-year-old, a BMI above 25 constitutes obesity, whereas in adolescents older than 18 years, BMI above 30 defines obesity.

Background

The National Health and Nutrition Examination Survey reported an increase in overweight among adolescents aged 12–19 from 5% in 1966–1970 to 17% in 2003–2004. The changes in BMI during and after adolescence are important predictors of adult adiposity. Generally, the longer a child remains overweight, the more likely obesity will persist into adulthood. The medical risks associated with obesity are discussed in Chapter 10. The psychosocial hazards of overweight are great in adolescence, causing alienation, distorted peer relations, poor self-esteem, guilt, depression, or altered body image.

Diagnosis

BMI should be recorded for all adolescents at the time of their annual physical examination. When overweight or obesity is diagnosed, additional information should be documented: blood pressure; condition of the skin, thyroid, heart, and abdomen. In patients with BMI in the 85–95% range, waist circumference at the umbilicus should be measured. Athletes with increased muscle mass may have elevated BMI but normal waist circumference, indicating that their weight may be normal for their muscular build. Acanthosis nigricans is a cutaneous finding characterized by velvety hyperpigmentation, most prominent behind the neck, in the axilla, and in the groin. Acanthosis nigricans is more common in dark-skinned persons and is a marker for insulin resistance. Endocrine causes of obesity, such as hypothyroidism and Cushing disease, can generally be excluded by the history and physical examination. If an adolescent is healthy and has no delay of growth or sexual maturation, an underlying endocrinologic, neurologic, or genetic cause is unlikely. Laboratory evaluation should include fasting lipids, glucose, and liver function tests to assess for nonalcoholic fatty liver disease.

Treatment

Poorly motivated adolescents may be alienated by an aggressive discussion of weight loss. Instead, providers may give basic information about healthy diet and regular exercise and be available for future visits if patients become interested in weight loss. For the highly motivated patient, treatment should be appropriate to age and developmental level. The adolescent should be taught appropriate eating and exercise habits to maintain weight reduction yet meet nutritional needs for growth and development. Providers are more likely to engage the adolescents by helping them to choose concrete, attainable goals (decreasing soda or other sugared drinks from three to two per day, decreasing portion sizes, or moderate exercise for 30 minutes 3 days a week). If patients are successful with these goals, they may be more likely to continue positive lifestyle changes. Appetite-suppressing drugs such as sibutramine have been used in older adolescents but are expensive and not usually covered by insurance. Bypass surgery has been used in some centers when the overweight adolescent has severe comorbidities of obesity. An age-appropriate behavior modification program incorporating dietary counseling and exercise is optimal, although a report from the U.S. Preventive Services Task Force did not find sufficient evidence that behavioral counseling is effective. In fact some studies indicate that increased activity is more important than dietary changes in long-term weight management. Lifestyle activity recommendations, such as walking and taking the stairs, may be more effective in the long run than regimented exercise programs. Avoiding labeling any food as "forbidden" improves long-term success with healthful eating behaviors. Behavioral treatment involving parents improves long-term maintenance of weight loss in children; parental involvement in adolescent weight loss programs has produced mixed results. In general, the most important factor in successful weight loss and weight maintenance is motivation. Monthly follow-up visits may help to maintain motivation, especially initially. Unfortunately, no program has been proven effective for long-term weight reduction.

Fernandez J et al: Waist circumference percentiles in nationally representative samples of African-American, European-American, and Mexican-American children and adolescents. J Pediatr 2004;145:439 [PMID: 15480363].

National Center for Health Statistics: Prevalence of overweight among children and adolescence: United States, 2002–2004. Available at: http://www.cdc.gov/nchs/products/pubs/pubd/hestats/overweight/overwght_child_03.htm.

U.S. Preventive Services Task Force: Screening and Interventions for overweight in children and adolescents: Recommendation statement. Pediatrics 2005;116:205 [PMID: 15995054].

SCHOOL AVOIDANCE

A teenager who has missed more than 1 week of school for a physical illness or symptom, and whose clinical picture is inconsistent with serious illness, should be suspected of having primary or secondary emotional factors that contribute to the absence. Investigation of absences may show a pattern, such as missing morning classes or missing the same days at the beginning or end of the week.

School avoidance should be suspected in children who are consistently absent in spite of parents' and professionals' attempts to encourage school attendance. Adolescents with school avoidance often have a history of excessive school absences or separation difficulties as a younger child. They may have a record of recurrent somatic complaints. Parents of a school avoider often feel helpless to compel their adolescent to attend school, may lack the sophistication to distinguish malingering from illness, or may have an underlying need to keep the teenager at home.

A complete history and physical examination should be performed, reviewing the patient's medical, educational, and psychiatric history. Signs of emotional problems should be explored. After obtaining permission from the patient and parents, the physician may find it helpful to speak directly with school officials and some key teachers. The adolescent may be having problems with particular teachers or subjects or experiencing adversity at school (eg, schoolyard bullying or an intimidating instructor). Some students get so far behind academically that they see no way of catching up and feel overwhelmed. Separation anxiety, sometimes of long duration, may be manifested in subconscious worries that something may happen to the mother while the teenager is at school.

The school nurse may give useful information, including the number of visits to the nurse during the last school year. An important part of the history is how the parents respond to the absences and somatic complaints. The parent(s) may be making a subconscious attempt to keep the adolescent at home, which may be coupled with secondary gains for the patient, such as increased parental attention.

► Treatment

The importance of returning to school quickly after a period of avoidance needs to be emphasized. The pediatrician should facilitate this process by offering to speak with school officials to excuse missed examinations, homework, and papers. The pediatrician should speak directly with teachers who are punitive with the objective of making the transition back to school as easy as possible. The longer adolescents stay out of school, the more anxious they may become about returning and the more difficult the return becomes. If an illness or symptom becomes so severe that an adolescent cannot go to school, the patient and the parents must be informed that a visit to a medical office is necessary. The physician focuses visits on the parents as much as on the adolescent to alleviate parental guilt about sending the child to school. If the adolescent cannot stay in school, hospitalization should be recommended for in-depth medical and psychiatric evaluation. Parents should be cautioned about the possibility of relapse after school holidays, summer vacation, or an acute illness.

Hanna GL et al: Separation anxiety disorder and school refusal in children and adolescents. Pediatr Rev 2006;27:56 [PMID: 16452275].

Suveg C et al: Separation anxiety disorder, panic disorder, and school refusal. Child Adolesc Psychiatr Clin N Am 2005;14:773 [PMID: 16171702].

SCHOOL FAILURE

The amount and complexity of course work increase significantly in middle school, at about the same time as the rapid physical, social, and emotional changes of puberty. To perform well academically, young adolescents must have the necessary cognitive capacity, study habits, concentration, motivation, interest, and emotional focus. Academic failure presenting at adolescence has a broad differential:

1. Limited intellectual abilities
2. Specific learning disabilities
3. Depression or emotional problems
4. Physical causes such as visual or hearing problems
5. Excessive school absenteeism secondary to chronic disease such as asthma or neurologic dysfunction
6. Lack of ability to concentrate
7. Attention-deficit/hyperactivity disorder
8. Lack of motivation
9. Drug and alcohol problems

Each of these causes must be explored. Evaluation requires a careful history, physical examination, and appropriate laboratory tests, as well as standardized educational and psychological testing.

Treatment

Management must be individualized to address specific needs, foster strengths, and implement a feasible program. For children with specific learning disabilities, an individual prescription for regular and special education courses, teachers, and extracurricular activities is important. Counseling helps these adolescents gain coping skills, raise self-esteem, and develop socialization skills. If the patient has hyperactivity or attention-deficit disorder along with poor ability to concentrate, a trial of stimulant medication (eg, methylphenidate or dextroamphetamine) may be useful. If the teenager appears depressed or if other serious emotional problems are uncovered, psychological evaluation should be recommended.

Wilens TE et al: Attention-deficit/hyperactivity disorder in adults. JAMA 2004;292:619 [PMID: 15292088].
Wolraich ML et al: Attention-deficit/hyperactivity disorder among adolescents: A review of the diagnosis, treatment, and clinical implications. Pediatrics 2005;115:1734 [PMID: 15930238].

BREAST DISORDERS

The breast examination should become part of the routine physical examination in girls as soon as breast budding occurs. The preadolescent thus comes to accept breast examination as a routine part of health care, and the procedure serves as an opportunity to offer reassurance about patient concerns. The breast examination begins with inspection of the breasts for symmetry and Tanner or sexual maturity rating (SMR) stage. Asymmetrical breast development is common in young adolescents, and is generally transient, although 25% of women may continue to have some degree of asymmetry into adulthood. Organic causes of breast asymmetry include unilateral breast hypoplasia, amastia, absence of the pectoralis major muscle, and unilateral virginal hypertrophy (massive enlargement of the breast during puberty).

Palpation of the breasts is performed with the patient supine and the ipsilateral arm placed behind the head. The examiner palpates the breast tissue with the flat of the fingers in concentric circles from the sternum, clavicle, and axilla in to the areola. The areola should be compressed gently to check for discharge.

Instructions for breast self-examination and its purpose can be given to older adolescents during this portion of the physical examination, and the patient older than 18 years should be encouraged to begin monthly self-examination after each menstrual flow. Because the vast majority of breast lesions in teens are benign, teaching younger adolescents breast self-examination may lead to unnecessary anxiety and overconcern with normal variants.

BREAST MASSES

Most breast masses in adolescents are benign (Table 3–1). Rare malignancies of adolescent girls include hemangiosarcoma, rhabdomyosarcoma, ductal carcinoma, cystosarcoma phyllodes, and metastatic tumor.

Table 3–1. Breast masses in adolescent females.

Common
Fibroadenoma
Fibrocystic changes
Breast cysts (including retroareolar cysts)
Breast abscess or mastitis
Fat necrosis (after trauma)
Less common or rare (benign)
Lymphangioma
Hemangioma
Juvenile papillomatosis
Giant fibroadenoma
Neurofibromatosis
Nipple adenoma or keratoma
Mammary duct ectasia
Intramammary lymph node
Lipoma
Hematoma
Hamartoma
Galactocele
Rare (malignant potential)
Adenocarcinoma
Juvenile secretory carcinoma
Fibrosarcoma
Fibrous histiocytoma
Cystosarcoma phyllodes
Intraductal carcinoma
Rhabdomyosarcoma, lymphoma, neuroblastoma
Lymphosarcoma, hemangiosarcoma
Metastatic cancer

1. Fibroadenoma

Fibroadenoma accounts for about two thirds of all breast masses in adolescents. It presents as a rubbery, well-demarcated, slowly growing, nontender mass in any quadrant, but is most common in the upper outer quadrant. The natural history of fibroadenomas is growth over 6–12 months followed by stabilization. The average size is 2–3 cm in diameter. In 10–25% of cases, multiple or recurrent lesions occur.

2. Cysts

Breast cysts are generally tender and spongy, with exacerbation of symptoms premenstrually and improvement after menses. Often they are multiple. Spontaneous regression occurs over two or three menstrual cycles in about 50% of cases.

It is reasonable to follow suspected fibroadenoma or cyst in adolescents for two or three menstrual cycles. About 25% of fibroadenomas become smaller, and about 50% of cysts resolve. If a presumed fibroadenoma does not change after two to three cycles, ultrasound will differentiate a solid tumor from a cyst. Patients with solid tumors larger than 2.5 cm in diameter should be referred for fine-needle aspiration or excisional biopsy. Those with tumors less than 2.5 cm in diameter may be followed every 3–6 months, because many of these tumors will shrink or remain the same. Persistent cystic lesions may be drained by needle aspiration. Patients with suspicious lesions should be referred immediately to a breast surgeon (Table 3–2).

3. Fibrocystic Breasts

Fibrocystic breast disease sometimes occurs in older adolescents and becomes more common with age. It is characterized by cyclic tenderness and nodularity bilaterally and is believed to be influenced by the estrogen-progesterone balance. Reassuring the young woman about the benign nature of the process and emphasizing the importance of breast self-examination as she becomes an adult may be all that is needed. Support bras may provide symptomatic relief. Oral contraceptive pills (OCPs) often improve symptoms. Studies have shown no association between methylxanthines and fibrocystic breasts; however, some women report reduced symptoms when they discontinue caffeine. The efficacy of vitamins E, B_1, and A is unknown. Evening primrose oil was beneficial in 44% of patients in one study. A trial of 1000 mg three times a day for 3 months may be helpful.

4. Breast Abscess

The female with a breast abscess usually complains of unilateral breast pain, and examination reveals overlying inflammatory changes. The examination may be misleading in that the infection may extend much deeper than suspected. A palpable mass is found only late in the course. Although breast feeding is the most common cause of mastitis, trauma and eczema involving the areola are factors in teenagers. *Staphylococcus aureus* is the most common pathogen. Other

Table 3–2. Breast lesions.

Fibroadenoma	Rubbery, well demarcated, nontender, slowly growing; most commonly found in the upper outer quadrant of the breast. Usually < 5 cm.
Adenocarcinoma	Hard, nonmobile, well-circumscribed, painless mass; generally indolent clinical course; occurs also in males but less frequently.
Cystosarcoma phyllodes	Firm, rubbery mass that may suddenly enlarge; associated with skin necrosis; most often benign.
Giant juvenile fibroadenoma	Remarkable large fibroadenoma with overlying dilated superficial veins; accounts for 5–10% of fibroadenomas in adolescents; benign but requires excision to prevent breast atrophy and for cosmetic reasons.
Intraductal papilloma	A cylindric tumor arising from the ductal epithelium; often subareolar but may be in the periphery of the breast in adolescents, with associated nipple discharge. Most are benign but require excision for cytologic diagnosis.
Fat necrosis	Localized inflammatory process in one breast; follows trauma in about half of cases. Subsequent scarring may be confused with cancer.
Virginal or juvenile hypertrophy	Massive enlargement of both breasts or, less often, one breast; attributed to end-organ hypersensitivity to normal hormonal levels just before or within a few years after menarche.
Miscellaneous	Fibroma, galactocele, hemangioma, intraductal granuloma, interstitial fibrosis, keratoma, lipoma, granular cell myoblastoma, papilloma, sclerosing adenosis.

aerobic and anaerobic organisms have also been implicated. Fluctuant abscesses should be surgically incised and drained. Fluid should be sent for culture. Oral antibiotics with appropriate coverage for methicillin-resistant *S aureus* should be given for 2–4 weeks. Ice packs for the first 24 hours and heat thereafter may relieve symptoms.

Cyclic mastodynia, fibrocystic disease, or chest wall pain may also be causes of breast pain, but no associated inflammatory signs are present in these conditions.

GALACTORRHEA

In teenagers, nipple discharge can be white, clear, red, brown, yellow, or green. Galactorrhea is most often benign; however, a careful history and workup are necessary. The most common causes of galactorrhea are medications, stimulation or irritation of the nipple, or pregnancy. Prolactinomas are the most common pathologic cause of galactorrhea in adolescents of both sexes and generally present as amenorrhea or failure of sexual maturation. Hypothyroidism is the second most common cause in adolescence but has been

Table 3–3. Medications and herbs associated with galactorrhea.

Amphetamines
Antidepressants (selective serotonin reuptake inhibitors, tricyclic anti-
   depressants)
Antihypertensives
Antipsychotics
Anxiolytics
Dihydroergotamine
Herbs (eg, anise, blessed thistle, fennel, fenugreek seed, nettle)
Histamine receptor blockers (eg, cimetidine)
Hormonal contraceptives
Isoniazid (INH)
Marijuana
Metoclopramide
Muscle relaxants (eg, cyclobenzaprine)
Opiates
Rimantadine
Sumatriptan
Valproic acid

reported only in girls, usually prepubertally. Ductal ectasia, with dilation of the mammary ducts, fibrosis, and inflammation, is benign and can present with bloody or brown nipple discharge. Bloody discharge with a mass can also result from papillomatosis, which has malignant potential.

Galactorrhea may be present postpartum and after spontaneous or induced abortions. Numerous prescribed and illicit drugs are possible causes (Table 3–3). Stimulation of the intercostal nerves (following surgery or due to herpes zoster infection), stimulation of the nipples, central nervous system disorders (hypothalamic injury), or emotional distress may produce galactorrhea.

► Clinical Findings

TSH and serum prolactin levels should be determined. Elevated TSH confirms the diagnosis of hypothyroidism. Elevated prolactin and normal TSH, often accompanied by amenorrhea, in the absence of medications suggest a hypothalamic or pituitary tumor, and a magnetic resonance imaging scan is indicated. When the prolactin level is normal, uncommon causes such as adrenal, renal, or ovarian tumors should be considered. Males with a negative workup and normal puberty need to be followed intensively. Males with elevated prolactin levels require a magnetic resonance imaging scan every 12–18 months even if the galactorrhea resolves, because of the significant risk of a small pituitary adenoma that may become apparent with serial examinations.

► Treatment

Treatment depends on the underlying cause. Prolactinomas may be removed surgically or suppressed with dopamine agonists such as bromocriptine. Bromocriptine may also be beneficial to some amenorrheic females with normal serum

prolactin levels. The female with a negative workup and persistent galactorrhea may be followed with menstrual history and serum prolactin level every 6–12 months. In many cases, symptoms resolve spontaneously and no diagnosis is made. The female with an elevated serum prolactin concentration but negative prolactinoma workup may be treated with bromocriptine if her symptoms are bothersome or may be observed with a magnetic resonance imaging scan every 1–2 years for several years.

GYNECOMASTIA

Gynecomastia is a common concern of male adolescents, 60–70% of whom have transient subareolar breast tissue during SMR stages 2 and 3. Causes include testosterone-estrogen imbalance, increased serum prolactin level, and abnormal serum protein binding levels.

► Clinical Findings

In type I idiopathic gynecomastia, the adolescent has a unilateral (20% bilateral) tender, firm mass beneath the areola. Generalized breast enlargement is classified as type II. Pseudogynecomastia refers to excessive fat tissue or prominent pectoralis muscles.

► Differential Diagnosis

Gynecomastia may be drug-induced (Table 3–4). Testicular, adrenal, or pituitary tumors, Klinefelter syndrome, primary hypogonadism, thyroid or hepatic dysfunction, or malnutrition may also be associated with gynecomastia (Table 3–5). Onset of gynecomastia in late (rather than early or middle) adolescence is more likely to be indicative of organic disease.

► Treatment

If gynecomastia is idiopathic, reassurance about the common and benign nature of the process can be given. Resolution may take up to 2 years. Surgery is reserved for those with significant psychological trauma or severe breast enlargement.

ACOG Committee Opinion: Breast concerns in the adolescent. Obstet Gynecol 2006;108:1329 [PMID: 17077268].
Arca MJ, Caniano DA: Breast disorders in the adolescent patient. Adolesc Med Clin 2004;15:473 [PMID: 15625988].
De Silva et al: Disorders of the breast in children and adolescents, part 2: Breast masses. J Pediatr Adolesc Gynecol 2006;19:415 [PMID: 17174833].

▼ GYNECOLOGIC DISORDERS IN ADOLESCENCE

PHYSIOLOGY OF MENSTRUATION

The ovulatory menstrual cycle is divided into three consecutive phases: follicular (the first 14 days), ovulatory (midcycle), and

Table 3–4. Drugs associated with gynecomastia.

Antibiotics
Isoniazid
Ketoconazole
Metronidazole
Anti-ulcer drugs
Cimetidine
Omeprazole
Ranitidine
Cardiovascular drugs
Captopril
Digoxin
Enalapril
Methyldopa
Reserpine
Verapamil
Chemotherapeutic drugs
Busulfan
Vincristine
Drugs and substances of abuse
Alcohol
Amphetamines
Marijuana
Opiates
Hormones or related agents
Anabolic steroids
Estrogens
Chorionic gonadotropin
Psychoactive medications
Tricyclic antidepressants, eg, amitriptyline
Antipsychotics, eg, chlorpromazine, fluphenazine, haloperidol
Anxiolytics, eg, chlordiazepoxide, diazepam

luteal (days 16–28). During the follicular phase, pulsatile gonadotropin-releasing hormone from the hypothalamus stimulates anterior pituitary secretion of FSH and LH. Under the influence of FSH and LH, a dominant ovarian follicle emerges by days 5–7 of the menstrual cycle, and the other follicles become atretic. Rising estradiol levels produced by the maturing

Table 3–5. Disorders associated with gynecomastia.

Klinefelter syndrome
Traumatic paraplegia
Male pseudohermaphroditism
Testicular feminization syndrome
Reifenstein syndrome
17-Ketosteroid reductase deficiency
Endocrine tumors (seminoma, Leydig cell tumor, teratoma, feminizing
   adrenal tumor, hepatoma, leukemia, hemophilia, bronchogenic
   carcinoma, leprosy, etc)
Hypothyroidism
Hyperthyroidism
Cirrhosis
Herpes zoster
Friedreich ataxia

follicle cause proliferation of the endometrium. By the midfollicular phase, FSH is beginning to decline secondary to estradiol-mediated negative feedback, whereas LH continues to rise as a result of estradiol-mediated positive feedback.

The rising LH initiates progesterone secretion and luteinization of the granulosa cells of the follicle. Progesterone in turn further stimulates LH and FSH. This leads to the LH surge, which causes the follicle to rupture and expel the oocyte.

During the luteal phase, LH and FSH gradually decline. The corpus luteum secretes progesterones. The endometrium enters the secretory phase in response to rising levels of estrogen and progesterone, with maturation 8–9 days after ovulation. If no pregnancy occurs or placental human chorionic gonadotropin is released, luteolysis begins; estrogen and progesterone levels decline; and the endometrial lining is shed as menstrual flow approximately 14 days after ovulation.

During the first 2 years after menarche, the majority of cycles are anovulatory (50–80%). Between 10% and 20% of cycles remain anovulatory for up to 5 years after menarche.

PELVIC EXAMINATION

A pelvic examination may be indicated to evaluate abdominal pain or menstrual disorders or to detect a suspected STI in the sexually active adolescent. Urine STI screening can be utilized in asymptomatic patients. The first Papanicolaou (Pap) smear should be performed within 3 years of the initiation of sexual activity or age 21 years, whichever comes first. Pap smears should be performed earlier in adolescents with a history of sexual abuse with penile penetration. The adolescent may be apprehensive about the first examination. It should not be rushed, and an explanation of the procedure and its purpose should precede it. The patient can be encouraged to relax by slow, deep breathing and by relaxation of her lower abdominal and inner thigh muscles. A young adolescent may wish to have her mother present during the examination, but the history should be taken privately. A female chaperone should be present with male examiners.

The pelvic examination begins by placing the patient in the dorsal lithotomy position after equipment and supplies are ready (Table 3–6). The examiner inspects the external genitalia, noting the pubic hair maturity rating, the size of the clitoris (2–5 mm is normal), Skene glands just inside the urethral meatus, and Bartholin glands at 4 o'clock and 8 o'clock outside the hymenal ring. In cases of alleged sexual abuse or assault, the presence of any lacerations, bruises, scarring, or synechiae about the hymen, vulva, or anus should be noted.

A vaginal speculum is then inserted at a 45-degree twist and angled 45 degrees downward. (A medium Pedersen speculum is most often used in sexually experienced patients; a narrow Huffman is used for virginal patients.) The vaginal walls are inspected for estrogen effects, inflammation, or lesions. The cervix should be dull pink. Cervical ectropion is commonly observed in adolescents; the columnar epithelium

Table 3–6. Items for pelvic exam tray.

Medium and virginal speculums (use warm water before exam)
Gloves
Applicator sticks, sterile
Large swabs to remove excess discharge
Cervical spatulas and brushes and available PAP media or slides
Microscope slides and cover slips if provider is to perform tests
Test tube (if swab is to be placed in saline and prepared elsewhere)
NaCl and KOH if provider is to perform tests
Gonorrhea test media
Chlamydia test media
Lubricant
Facial tissue

extends outside the cervical os onto the face of the cervix until later adolescence, when it recedes.

Specimens are obtained, including a wet preparation for leukocytes, trichomonads, and clue cells (vaginal epithelial cells stippled with adherent bacteria); potassium hydroxide preparation for yeast and whiff test; cervical swab for gonorrhea and *Chlamydia;* and endocervical and cervical samples for Pap smear testing if indicated. A cervical brush and spatula are typically used together. Pap smears should be interpreted by a cytopathologist at a laboratory using the Bethesda system of classification. Liquid-based Pap testing is often used with reflex human papillomavirus testing if the Pap result is atypical squamous cells of uncertain etiology.

The speculum is then removed, and bimanual examination is performed to assess uterine size and position, adnexal enlargement or tenderness, or cervical motion tenderness. Bimanual examination may reveal beading in the adnexa secondary to endometriosis.

MENSTRUAL DISORDERS

1. Amenorrhea

Amenorrhea is the absence of menarche when normally anticipated. Primary amenorrhea is defined as no menstrual periods or secondary sex characteristics by age 14 years or no menses in the presence of secondary sex characteristics by age 15 years. Constitutional delay is normal pubertal progression at a delayed onset or rate. Secondary amenorrhea is the absence of menses for at least three cycles after regular cycles have been present. In some instances, evaluation should begin immediately, without waiting for the specified age or duration of lapsed periods, such as in patients with suspected pregnancy, short stature with the stigmata of Turner syndrome, or an anatomic defect.

A. Evaluation for Primary Amenorrhea

Primary amenorrhea may be the result of anatomic abnormalities, chromosomal deviations, or physiologic delay (Table 3–7).

Table 3–7. Causes of amenorrhea.

Hypothalamic-pituitary axis
  Hypothalamic suppression
    Emotional stress
    Depression
    Chronic disease
    Weight loss
    Obesity
    Severe dieting
    Strenuous athletics
    Drugs (post-birth control pills, phenothiazines)
  Central nervous system lesion
    Pituitary lesion: adenoma, prolactinoma
    Craniopharyngioma, brainstem, or parasellar tumors
    Head injury with hypothalamic contusion
    Infiltrative process (sarcoidosis)
    Vascular disease (hypothalamic vasculitis)
  Congenital conditions[a]
    Kallmann syndrome
Ovaries
  Gonadal dysgenesis[a]
    Turner syndrome (XO)
    Mosaic (XX/XO)
  Injury to ovary
    Autoimmune disease
    Infection (mumps, oophoritis)
    Toxins (alkylating chemotherapeutic agents)
    Irradiation
    Trauma, torsion (rare)
  Polycystic ovary syndrome
  Ovarian failure
    Premature menopause
    Resistant ovary
Uterovaginal outflow tract
  Müllerian dysgenesis[a]
    Congenital deformity or absence of uterus, uterine tubes, or vagina
  Imperforate hymen, transverse vaginal septum, vaginal agenesis, agenesis of the cervix[a]
  Testicular feminization (absent uterus)[a]
  Uterine lining defect
    Asherman syndrome (intrauterine synechiae postcurettage or endometritis)
    Tuberculosis, brucellosis
Defect in hormone synthesis or action (virilization may be present)
  Adrenal hyperplasia[a]
  Cushing disease
  Adrenal tumor
  Ovarian tumor (rare)
  Drugs (steroids, ACTH)

[a]Indicates condition that usually presents as primary amenorrhea.
ACTH, adrenocorticotropic hormone.

The history should include whether puberty has commenced, level of exercise, nutritional intake, presence of stressors, and the age at menarche for female relatives. Adrenal androgens are largely responsible for axillary and pubic hair; estrogen is responsible for breast development, maturation of the external genitalia, vagina, and uterus, and menstruation.

A careful physical examination should be done, noting the percentage of ideal body weight for height and age, SMR stage, vaginal patency, presence of the uterus (assessed through rectoabdominal examination or ultrasonography if pelvic examination is not appropriate), signs of virilization (acne, clitoromegaly of > 5 mm, or hirsutism), or stigmata of Turner syndrome (< 152 cm tall, shieldlike chest, widely spaced nipples, increased carrying angle of the arms, and webbed neck). If pelvic examination reveals normal female external genitalia and pelvic organs, the patient should be given a challenge of medroxyprogesterone, 10 mg orally twice daily for 5 days (or 10 mg/d for 7–10 days) (Figure 3–5). If withdrawal bleeding occurs within 7 days after administration of medroxyprogesterone, normal anatomy and adequate estrogen effect are implied. If physical examination reveals an absent uterus (Figure 3–6), karyotyping should be performed to differentiate testicular feminization from müllerian duct defect, because these two entities are managed differently.

Laboratory studies should include complete blood count, erythrocyte sedimentation rate, and TSH. If systemic illness is suspected, a urinalysis and a chemistry panel (including renal and liver function tests) should be obtained. If short stature is present, a bone age should be done. If the diagnosis remains unclear after preliminary evaluation, or if no withdrawal bleeding occurs after a medroxyprogesterone challenge, FSH, LH, and prolactin levels should be obtained. Low levels of gonadotropins indicate a more severe hypothalamic suppression, caused by anorexia nervosa, chronic disease, or a central nervous system tumor. Involvement of a gynecologist or endocrinologist is helpful at this point. If gonadotropin levels are high, ovarian failure or gonadal dysgenesis is implied, and a karyotype should be obtained.

B. Evaluation and Treatment of Secondary Amenorrhea

Secondary amenorrhea results when estrogen stimulation is unopposed, maintaining the endometrium in the proliferative phase. The most common causes are pregnancy, stress, and polycystic ovary syndrome (PCOS). Ovarian failure can also present as secondary amenorrhea, caused by mosaic Turner syndrome or autoimmune oophoritis.

The history should focus on issues of stress, chronic illness, drugs, weight change, strenuous exercise, sexual activity, and contraceptive use. A review of systems should include questions about headaches, visual changes, hirsutism, constipation, cold intolerance, and galactorrhea.

Physical examination should include ophthalmoscopic and visual field examination, palpation of the thyroid, determination of blood pressure and heart rate, compression of the areola to check for galactorrhea, and a search for signs of androgen excess (eg, hirsutism, clitoromegaly, severe acne, or ovarian enlargement).

The first laboratory study obtained is a pregnancy test, even if the patient denies sexual activity. If the teenager is not pregnant, a progesterone challenge (medroxyprogesterone, 10 mg orally bid for 5 days or 10 mg/d for 7–10 days) should be done to determine whether the uterus is primed with estrogen (Figure 3–7).

Most patients who have withdrawal flow after progesterone challenge have mild hypothalamic suppression due to weight change, athletics, stress, or illness; however, disorders such as PCOS, adrenal disorders, ovarian tumors, thyroid disease, and diabetes mellitus should be excluded by history and physical examination and appropriate laboratory studies. (See Primary Amenorrhea, earlier, and Figure 3–6.)

If withdrawal flow occurs after the progesterone challenge (see Figure 3–5), but the adolescent continues to have problems with amenorrhea, serum levels of estradiol, FSH, LH, and prolactin should be checked. An elevated FSH level accompanied by a low estrogen level implies ovarian failure, in which case blood for karyotype and antiovarian antibodies (if the karyotype is normal) should be obtained and laparoscopy considered. If gonadotropin levels are low or normal and the estradiol level is low, hypothalamic amenorrhea is likely; however, one must consider the possibilities of a central nervous system tumor (prolactinoma or craniopharyngioma), pituitary infarction from postpartum hemorrhage or sickle cell anemia, uterine synechiae, or chronic disease. Further evaluation may be necessary.

If signs of virilization are present (see Figure 3–6), determining levels of free testosterone, 17-hydroxyprogesterone, and dehydroepiandrosterone sulfate will help to distinguish PCOS from adrenal causes of virilization and amenorrhea. Although elevation of testosterone and dehydroepiandrosterone sulfate may occur in patients with PCOS, the elevation is not as dramatic as with androgen-producing adrenal or ovarian tumors, adrenal hyperplasia, or Cushing syndrome. Endocrinologic consultation will assist in differentiating the cause of significantly elevated androgens.

PCOS is a spectrum of disorders accompanied by symptoms of obesity, insulin resistance, hirsutism, acne, oligomenorrhea, and infertility. PCOS is very common, with a prevalence estimated at 5–10%. Although a classic LH:FSH ratio of more than 2.5:1 is described in PCOS, up to 40% of patients do not have elevated LH levels. Because of insufficient FSH, androstenedione cannot be converted to estradiol in the ovarian follicle, and anovulation and production of excess androgens result. OCPs containing a low androgenic progestin (desogestrel or norgestimate) help to regulate menses and improve acne and hirsutism. Patients who do not wish to take an OCP can be given progesterone (10 mg daily) for the first 10 days of each month to allow withdrawal flow; however, this treatment does not suppress ovarian androgen production. Hirsute patients should have a lipid profile checked, because PCOS patients have an increased risk of dyslipidemias. OCPs may reduce terminal hair growth, but antiandrogens such as spironolactone reduce the growth and diameter of terminal hair and may be useful for more severe hirsutism. Weight loss in obese patients helps to suppress ovarian androgen production. Insulin-sensitizing medications,

Figure 3–5. Evaluation of primary amenorrhea in a normal female. CNS, central nervous system; FSH, follicle-stimulating hormone; hCG, human chorionic gonadotropin; IBW, ideal body weight; LH, luteinizing hormone.

▲ **Figure 3–6.** Evaluation of primary amenorrhea in a female without a uterus or with virilization. ACTH, adrenocortico-tropic hormone; DHEAS, dehydroepiandrosterone sulfate; FSH, follicle-stimulating hormone; IVP, intravenous pyelogram; LH, luteinizing hormone.

such as metformin, have been shown to improve menstrual regularities in adolescents with PCOS.

2. Dysmenorrhea

Dysmenorrhea is the most common gynecologic complaint of adolescent girls, with an incidence of about 80% by age 18 years. Yet many teenage girls do not seek help from a physician, relying instead on female relatives, friends, and the media for advice. Therefore, the physician should ask about menstrual cramps when taking a review of systems.

Dysmenorrhea can be divided into primary and secondary dysmenorrhea on the basis of whether underlying pelvic disease exists (Table 3–8). Primary dysmenorrhea accounts for 80% of cases of adolescent dysmenorrhea and most often affects women younger than age 25 years.

Pelvic examination is normal in females with primary dysmenorrhea. The pelvic examination has diagnostic benefits and provides an opportunity to educate and reassure the patient about her normal reproductive function. However, if the patient has never been sexually active and the history is consis-

tent with primary dysmenorrhea, a trial of a nonsteroidal anti-inflammatory drug is justified. Patients should be instructed to begin nonsteroidal anti-inflammatory drugs at the first sign of menses or dysmenorrhea and continue them for 2–3 days. Recommended doses are ibuprofen, 400–800 mg every 6 hours, or naproxen, 220–550 mg twice a day. If the patient does not respond to nonsteroidal anti-inflammatory drugs, OCPs are an effective treatment for primary dysmenorrhea. If patients do not respond to either of these treatments, secondary dysmenorrhea is more likely and a pelvic examination is indicated.

Secondary dysmenorrhea is menstrual pain due to an underlying pelvic lesion (see Table 3–8). Although uncommon in adolescents, when present it is most often due to infection or endometriosis. In one study of adolescent females with chronic pelvic pain, more than 40% who had not received a definitive diagnosis by the third visit were found to have endometriosis.

The clinician evaluating a patient with secondary dysmenorrhea should take a sexual history and conduct a pelvic examination even if the patient is not sexually active. Testing for gonorrhea and *Chlamydia*, a complete blood count and

▲ **Figure 3–7.** Evaluation of secondary amenorrhea. CBC, complete blood count; CT, computed tomography; DHEAS, dehydroepiandrosterone sulfate; FSH, follicle-stimulating hormone; LH, luteinizing hormone; MRI, magnetic resonance imaging scan; 17-OH-P, 17-hydroxyprogesterone; T_4, thyroxine.

erythrocyte sedimentation rate, and a pregnancy test should be done. Gynecologic consultation is indicated to look for endometriosis or congenital problems by ultrasonography or laparoscopy. Treatment depends on the cause (see Table 3–8).

3. Dysfunctional Uterine Bleeding

Dysfunctional uterine bleeding may consist of menorrhagia (normal intervals with excessive flow) or metrorrhagia (irregular intervals with excessive flow). It results when an endometrium that has proliferated under unopposed estro-

gen stimulation finally begins to slough, but does so incompletely, causing irregular, painless bleeding. The unopposed estrogen stimulation occurs during anovulatory cycles, common in younger adolescents who have not been menstruating for long. Anovulation may also occur in older adolescents during times of stress or illness (Figure 3–8).

▶ **Clinical Findings**

Typically, the adolescent has had several years of regular cycles and then begins to have menses every 2 weeks, or

Table 3–8. Dysmenorrhea in the adolescent.

	Etiology	Onset and Duration	Symptoms	Pelvic Exam	Treatment
Primary Dysmenorrhea[a]					
Primary	Excessive amount of prostaglandin F$_2\alpha$, which attaches to myometrium, causing uterine contractions, hypoxia, and ischemia. Also, directly sensitizes pain receptors.	Begins with onset of flow or just prior and lasts 1–2 d. Does not start until 6–18 mo after menarche, when cycles become ovulatory.	Lower abdominal cramps radiating to lower back and thighs. Associated nausea, vomiting, diarrhea, and urinary frequency also due to excess prostaglandins.	Normal. May wait to examine if never sexually active and history is consistent with primary dysmenorrhea.	Mild—heating pad, warm baths, NSAIDs. Moderate to severe—NSAIDs at onset of flow or pain. Consider OCPs.
Secondary Dysmenorrhea[b]					
Infection	Most often due to an STI such as chlamydia or gonorrhea.	Recent onset of pelvic cramps.	Pelvic cramps, excessive bleeding, intermenstrual spotting or vaginal discharge.	Mucopurulent or purulent discharge from cervical os, cervical friability, cervical motion tenderness, adnexal tenderness, positive test for STI.	Appropriate antibiotics.
Endometriosis	Aberrant implants of endometrial tissue in pelvis or abdomen; may result from reflux.	Generally starts more than 2 y after menarche.	Pelvic pain, may occur intermenstrually.	Two thirds are tender on exam, especially during late luteal phase.	Hormonal suppression by OCPs, DMPA or danazol. Surgery may be necessary for extensive disease.
Complication of pregnancy	Spontaneous abortion, ectopic pregnancy.	Acute onset.	Pelvic cramps associated with a delay in menses.	Positive hCG, enlarged uterus or adnexal mass.	Immediate gynecologic consult.
Congenital anomalies	Transverse vaginal septum, septate uterus, or cervical stenosis.	Onset at menarche.	Pelvic cramps.	Underlying congenital anomaly may be apparent. May require exam under anesthesia.	Gynecologic consult for ultrasound, hysteroscopy, or laparoscopy.
IUD	Increased uterine contractions, or increased risk for pelvic infection.	Onset after placement of IUD or acutely if due to infection.	Pelvic cramps, heavy menstrual bleeding, may have vaginal discharge.	Normal, or see infection above.	NSAIDs or mefenamic acid may be drug of choice because they also reduce flow. Appropriate antibiotics and consider removal of IUD if infection is present.
Pelvic adhesions	Previous abdominal surgery or pelvic inflammatory disease.	Delayed onset after surgery or PID.	Abdominal pain, may or may not be associated with menstrual cycles; possible alteration in bowel pattern.	Variable.	Surgery. Consider a trial of tricyclic antidepressants.

[a]No pelvic pathology.
[b]Underlying pathology present. (Always perform pelvic exam if secondary dysmenorrhea suspected or patient is sexually active. Tests for *Chlamydia* and gonorrhea, complete blood test, and erythrocyte sedimentation rate should be obtained.)
DMPA, depot medroxyprogesterone acetate; hCG, human chorionic gonadotropin; IUD, intrauterine device; NSAID, nonsteroidal anti-inflammatory drug; OCP, oral contraceptive pill; PID, pelvic inflammatory disease; STI, sexually transmitted infection.

complains of bleeding for 2–3 weeks after 2–3 months of amenorrhea. A history of painless, irregular periods at intervals of less than 3 weeks may also be elicited. Bleeding for more than 10 days should be considered abnormal. Dysfunctional uterine bleeding must be considered a diagnosis of exclusion (Table 3–9).

Patient with DYSFUNCTIONAL UTERINE BLEEDING

▲ **Figure 3–8.** Evaluation of dysfunctional uterine bleeding. CBC, complete blood count; Hgb, hemoglobin, OCP, oral contraceptive pills.

Table 3–9. Differential diagnosis of dysfunctional uterine bleeding in adolescents.

Anovulation
Sexually transmitted infections
   Cervicitis
   Pelvic inflammatory disease
Pregnancy complications
   Ectopic pregnancy
   Spontaneous abortion
Bleeding disorders
   von Willebrand disease
   Thrombocytopenia
   Coagulopathy
Endocrine disorders
   Hypothyroidism
   Hyperprolactinemia
   Adrenal hyperplasia
   Polycystic ovary syndrome
Anatomic abnormalities
Uterine fibroids
Trauma
Foreign body
Chronic illness
Malignancy
   Leukemia
   Carcinoma
Drugs
   Oral contraceptive pills
   DMPA

DMPA, depot medroxyprogesterone acetate.

▶ Treatment

A pregnancy test and pelvic examination with appropriate tests for sexually transmitted infections should be performed in sexually active patients. A complete blood count, including a platelet count, should be obtained. The history and physical findings may suggest the need for additional coagulation or hormonal studies. Coagulation studies should be done if the patient presents with severe anemia, especially within 1 year after menarche. Management depends on the severity of the problem (Table 3–10). It is important to treat for a minimum of 3–4 months to progressively reduce the endometrium to baseline thickness.

4. Mittelschmerz

Mittelschmerz is midcycle pain caused by irritation of the peritoneum due to spillage of fluid from the ruptured follicular cyst at the time of ovulation. The patient presents with a history of midcycle, unilateral dull or aching abdominal pain lasting a few minutes to as long as 8 hours. This pain rarely mimics the abdominal findings of acute appendicitis, torsion or rupture of an ovarian cyst, or ectopic pregnancy. The patient should be reassured and treated symptomatically. If the findings are severe enough to warrant consideration of the previously mentioned diagnoses, laparoscopy may be done.

5. Premenstrual Syndrome

Premenstrual syndrome (PMS) is a cluster of physical and psychological symptoms temporally related to the luteal phase of the menstrual cycle and alleviated by the onset of menses. PMS should be distinguished from major depression, idiopathic cyclic edema, fibromyalgia, chronic fatigue syndrome, and psychosomatic disorders. This may be difficult because of the diversity of symptoms ascribed to PMS and the variability from month to month in the same patient. Premenstrual behavioral symptoms include emotional lability, anxiety, depression, irritability, impulsivity, hostility, and impaired social function. Physical symptoms include bloating, breast tenderness, fatigue, and appetite changes. Previously thought to be a disorder limited to adult women, studies indicate that adolescents also experience premenstrual symptoms. Although several causes have been proposed (progesterone deficiency, hyperprolactinemia, estrogen excess or imbalance of the estrogen-progesterone ratio, vitamin B_{12} deficiency, fluid retention, low levels of endorphins and prostaglandins, hypoglycemia, and psychosomatic factors), none has been proved. Hormones may play a role; women who have undergone hysterectomy but not oophorectomy may have cyclic symptoms resembling PMS, whereas postmenopausal women have no such symptoms.

Several treatments have been advocated but are without consistent benefits. OCPs or nonsteroidal anti-inflammatory drugs may be beneficial for some women. Sertraline (50–100 mg) has been shown to be significantly better than placebo for treatment of premenstrual dysphoria.

6. Ovarian Cysts

Functional cysts account for 20–50% of ovarian tumors in adolescents and are a result of the normal physiologic process of ovulation. They may be asymptomatic or may cause menstrual irregularity, constipation, or urinary frequency. Functional cysts, unless large, rarely cause abdominal pain; however, torsion or hemorrhage of an ovarian cyst may present as an acute abdomen. Follicular cysts account for the majority of ovarian cysts. They are produced every cycle but occasionally are not resorbed. Follicular cysts are unilateral, usually not larger than 4 cm in diameter, and resolve spontaneously. If the patient is asymptomatic, she can be reexamined monthly. The patient should be referred to a gynecologist for laparoscopy if she is premenarcheal, if the cyst has a solid component or is larger than 5 cm by ultrasonography, if she has symptoms or signs suggestive of hemorrhage or torsion, or if the cyst fails to regress within 2 months. Luteal cysts occur less commonly and may be 5–10 cm in diameter. The patient may have associated amenorrhea, or as the cyst becomes atretic, heavy vaginal bleeding. The patient may be monitored for 3 months but should have a laparoscopy if the cyst is larger than 5 cm, does not resolve within 2 months, or if there is pain or bleeding from the cyst.

Table 3–10. Management of dysfunctional uterine bleeding.[a]

	Mild	Moderate	Severe
Hemoglobin (Hgb) value	Hgb > 12 g/dL	Hgb 9–12 g/dL	Hgb < 9 g/dL (or dropping); orthostatic symptoms and signs
Acute treatment	Menstrual calendar; iron supplementation. NSAID with menses may help reduce flow. Consider OCPs if patient is sexually active and desires contraception.	Monophasic OCPs, up to four pills per day, and taper over 2–3 wk; may need antiemetic. Bleeding should stop in a few days. Begin tapering dose 2–3 d after bleeding stops. Expect withdrawal flow a few days after last dose.	Fluids, blood transfusion as needed, admit to hospital if Hgb < 7 g/dL or patient is hemodynamically unstable. For hemostasis, consider: conjugated estrogens, 25 mg IV every 4–6 h for 24 h or until bleeding stops. Provide antiemetic medication. Then, OCPs: 4 pills/d for 4 d 3 pills/d for 4 d 2 pills/d for 17 d withdrawal bleeding for 7 d[b]
Long-term management	Monitor menstrual calendar and Hgb. Follow-up in 2–3 mo.	Cycle with either: (1) Provera,[c] 10 mg PO daily for 10 d starting on day 14 of each cycle for 3–6 mo, or (2) OCPs for 3–6 mo beginning the Sunday after withdrawal bleeding starts. Provide iron supplementation. Monitor Hgb. Follow-up within 2–3 wk and every 3 mo.	Next: OCPs cycle (using 28-d packs) for 3 mo. Begin the Sunday after withdrawal bleeding begins. Length of use depends on resolution of anemia. Monitor Hgb. Follow-up within 2–3 wk and every 3 mo.

[a]Diagnosis: Prolonged (> 8 d) painless menses; heavy flow (> 6 tampons/pads per day); short cycles (< 21 d); no cause found.
[b]This schedule will use three 21-d packages.
[c]Provera = medroxyprogesterone acetate.
NSAID, nonsteroidal anti-inflammatory drug; OCP, oral contraceptive pill; PO, by mouth.
Modified, with permission, from Blythe M: Common menstrual problems. Part 3. Abnormal uterine bleeding. Adolesc Health Update 1992;4:1.

Dickerson LM et al: Premenstrual syndrome. Am Fam Physician 2003;67:1743 [PMID: 12725453].

Slap GB: Menstrual disorders in adolescence. Best Pract Res Clin Obstet Gynaecol 2003;17:75 [PMID: 12758227].

CONTRACEPTION

According to the Youth Risk Behavior Survey of high school students in 2005, 46.8% have had sexual intercourse; 62.8% reported they used a condom at last intercourse. According to the 2002 National Survey of Family Growth, teens were more likely to use contraception when they began having intercourse; 79% in 1999–2002, up from 61% in the 1980s. Teens were also more likely to have used contraception at their most recent intercourse in 2002 (83% in 2002 compared with 71% in 1995). Still, many adolescent pregnancies occur within the first 6 months of initiation of sexual activity. Adolescents often delay seeing a clinician for prescription contraceptives after initiating sexual activity.

Abstinence & Decision Making

Many adolescents have given little thought to their developing sexuality or how they will handle sexual situations. Talking with teenagers about sexual intercourse and its implications, and alternatives to intercourse, can help teens make informed decisions before they find themselves with an unplanned pregnancy or an STI.

If an adolescent chooses to remain abstinent, the clinician should reinforce that decision. Encouraging adolescents to use contraception when they do engage in sexual intercourse does not lead to higher rates of sexual activity. Another approach to decreasing teen pregnancy is to educate adolescent males on the importance of hormonal contraception and emergency contraception for their partners, in addition to condom use. The teen pregnancy, birth, and abortion rates are higher in the United States than in any other developed country, despite similar rates of sexual experience.

Emergency Contraception

A discussion of emergency contraception (EC), which could potentially prevent 50–90% of unintended pregnancies and elective abortions, should be part of anticipatory guidance given to both female and male teenagers. Indications for EC include unprotected intercourse within the past 120 hours (5 days), condom breakage, more than two missed OCPs, or more than 14 weeks since the last depot medroxyprogesterone acetate (DMPA) injection. The pregnancy rate after EC is 1.8%, compared with 6.8% without such intervention. (See Table 3–11 for dosages.) EC works best within 24 hours of intercourse but can be taken up to 120 hours afterward. It

Table 3–11. Emergency postcoital contraception regimens.

Pill	Dosage	Each Dose Achieves:
Plan B[a]	Two tablets orally	Levonorgestrel, 1.5 mg
Nordette[b]	Four tablets orally and repeat in 12 h	Levonorgestrel, 0.6 mg
Lo-Ovral[b]	Four tablets orally and repeat in 12 h	Norgestrel, 1.2 mg
Alesse[b]	Five pink pills orally and repeat in 12 h	Levonorgestrel, 0.5 mg
Triphasil[b]	Four yellow pills orally and repeat in 12 h	Levonorgestrel, 0.5 mg

[a]Both doses can be given at the same time.
[b]An antiemetic drug taken 30 minutes before the dose may help reduce nausea.

should be verified that other instances of unprotected intercourse beyond 120 hours have not occurred. The only contraindication to the use of EC is pregnancy. Plan B is a progestin-only method that causes significantly less nausea and vomiting than combined estrogen-progesterone methods. It is available over the counter for patients older than age 18. The two pills can be given at the same time if there is a single episode of unprotected intercourse; patients with multiple episodes of unprotected intercourse should receive the doses 12 hours apart. If this method is not available, certain combined OCPs can be used for EC. It is important to note that some progestin-containing contraceptives are *not* approved for EC. A follow-up appointment should be held in 2–3 weeks, to test for pregnancy if menses have not occurred, to screen for STIs if indicated, and to counsel regarding contraceptive use.

Condoms & Spermicides

Condoms have been used more widely in the last several decades as a result of educational and marketing efforts driven by the AIDS epidemic. Regardless of whether another method is used, all sexually active adolescents should be counseled to use condoms. Condoms offer protection against STIs by decreasing (but not eliminating) the transmission of gonorrhea, *Chlamydia,* syphilis, herpes simplex, hepatitis, and HIV. Spermicides containing nonoxynol-9 are no longer recommended, as evidence suggests that repeated use of spermicide increases transmission of HIV. Aside from the diaphragm and cervical cap, barrier methods do not require a medical visit or prescription and are widely available. The polyurethane vaginal pouch, or female condom, is also available. Although it has pregnancy and STI prevention properties similar to those of the male condom, its higher cost and greater difficulty of insertion make it less appealing to adolescents.

Oral & Cutaneous Contraceptives

OCPs have a three-pronged mechanism of action: (1) suppression of ovulation; (2) thickening of the cervical mucus, thereby making sperm penetration more difficult; and (3) atrophy of the endometrium, which diminishes the chance of implantation. The latter two actions are progestin effects.

Combination OCPs contain both estrogen and progestin. Ethinyl estradiol is the estrogen currently used in nearly all OCPs in the United States. A number of progestins are used in OCPs and differ in their estrogenic, antiestrogenic, and androgenic effects. As estrogen doses decreased in OCPs, the androgenic side effects of progestins became more apparent, leading to the development of two progestins (desogestrel and norgestimate) with lower androgenic potential. All of the lower androgenic pills improve acne and may especially benefit patients with polycystic ovary syndrome. Reports of increased risk of thromboembolism associated with the newer progestins are likely related to an excess of first-time users among desogestrel patients. Factor V Leiden has been identified as a risk factor for venous thrombosis; 5% of patients of European ancestry are carriers of factor V Leiden. Carriers have a 30-to 50-fold increased risk for thrombosis. Testing family members with a history of venous thrombosis for factor V Leiden and other conditions such as the prothrombin gene mutation, proteins C and S, and antithrombin III before prescribing estrogen-containing OCPs to the adolescent may prevent these complications. OCPs have many noncontraceptive benefits, including improvement of dysmenorrhea, menorrhagia, acne, and PMS; suppression of ovarian and breast cysts; and lower risk of anemia, pelvic inflammatory disease, and ectopic pregnancy. A pill containing 30–35 mg of ethinyl estradiol with norgestimate, desogestrel, or 0.5 mg norethindrone is recommended for most adolescents beginning OCPs.

Ortho Evra is a combined estrogen-progesterone patch, which is worn 3 weeks out of every 4. It releases 150 mcg of norelgestromin and 20 mcg of ethinyl estradiol per day. Side effects are similar to those of combined OCPs. Reports of increased thrombotic events reinforce the importance of screening patients for risk factors for thrombosis (personal or family history of thrombosis) prior to prescription of the patch. Five percent of patients report having a patch come off. Two percent report skin irritation. Efficacy may be reduced in patients weighing more than 200 pounds. The patch is an attractive alternative to OCPs for adolescents who have difficulty remembering to take a pill every day, as compliance is increased. The failure rate for the patch is reported to be 1%.

Progestin-only pills contain no estrogen. Their chief use is in women who experience unacceptable estrogen-related side effects with combination OCPs or who have a contraindication to estrogen-containing pills. Their lack of estrogen, however, is also responsible for the main side effect, less predictable menstrual patterns. For this reason, progestin-only pills are not often desirable for adolescents. Their mechanism of action relies on the progestin-mediated actions, and ovulation is suppressed in only 15–40% of cycles.

A. Indications and Contraindications

Combined OCPs may be the method of choice for sexually active adolescents who frequently have unplanned intercourse; however, the patient must be able to comply with a daily dosing regimen. Most states allow OCPs to be prescribed to minors confidentially. Ideally, it is best to wait until 6–12 regular menstrual cycles have occurred before beginning hormonal contraception; however, if the teenager is already sexually active, the medical and social risks of pregnancy outweigh the risks of hormonal contraception.

OCPs or the contraceptive patch may also be used to treat dysmenorrhea, menorrhagia, dysfunctional uterine bleeding, and acne (see previous discussion).

Contraindications to combined OCPs or the contraceptive patch can be categorized as absolute and relative (Table 3–12). When use of estrogenic agents is contraindicated, progestin-only pills and DMPA are alternatives.

B. Beginning Oral Contraceptive Pills or the Contraceptive Patch and Follow-up

Before a patient begins taking OCPs or the patch, a careful menstrual history, medical history, and family medical history should be taken. In addition, baseline weight and blood pressure should be established. If time constraints are present and a patient has no symptoms suggesting an STI, OCPs or the patch may be started and a follow-up appointment for STI screening can be scheduled as soon as possible.

If the teen has no contraindications (see Table 3–12), she may begin her first pack of pills or the patch with her next menstrual period (either the first Sunday after flow begins or

Table 3–12. Contraindications to combined birth control pills.

Absolute contraindications
Pregnancy
Lactation (first 6 wk postpartum to allow milk supply to become established)
History of thrombophlebitis, thromboembolic disorder, cerebrovascular disease, or ischemic heart disease
Structural heart disease with endocarditis, atrial fibrillation, or pulmonary hypertension
Breast cancer
Migraine headaches with neurologic changes (numbness or unilateral weakness)
History of active liver disease or tumor
Hypertension SBP > 160 mm Hg or DBP > 100 mm Hg
Prolonged immobilization after surgery on legs or pelvis
Relative contraindications
First 3 wk postpartum due to increased risk of thromboembolism
Lactation (6 wk–6 mo)
Active gallbladder disease
Use of drugs that affect liver enzymes (rifampin, griseofulvin, phenytoin, carbamazepine, barbiturates)

DBP, diastolic blood pressure; SBP, systolic blood pressure.

Table 3–13. Noncontraceptive health benefits of oral contraceptive pills.

Protection against life-threatening conditions
Ovarian cancer
Endometrial cancer
Pelvic inflammatory disease
Ectopic pregnancy
Morbidity and mortality due to unintended pregnancies
Alleviate conditions affecting quality of life
Iron-deficiency anemia
Benign breast disease
Dysmenorrhea
Irregular cycles
Functional ovarian cysts
Premenstrual syndrome
Acne
Mounting evidence
Improved bone density

the first day of flow, depending on the brand). An alternate approach, termed "quick start," allows adolescents to begin their contraception on the day of the appointment. This approach may lead to increased adherence with the method of choice. A low-dose monophasic combined oral contraceptive or a triphasic pill of low androgenic profile is used for those without contraindications to use of estrogen. The patient should be instructed on the use of her pills and on the possible risks and side effects and their warning signs. In addition, the patient should be advised to use condoms at every intercourse to prevent STIs. A follow-up visit every 3 months for the first year may improve adherence, because teenagers often discontinue birth control pills because of nonmedical reasons or minor side effects. Teenagers may need reassurance about the safety of birth control pills and their added benefits (Table 3–13).

C. Management of Side Effects

A different type of combined oral contraceptive should be tried if a patient has a persistent minor side effect for more than the first 2–3 months. Adjustments should be made on the basis of hormonal effects desired (Table 3–14). Changes are most often made for persistent breakthrough bleeding not related to missed pills.

Injectable Hormonal Contraceptives

The depot form of medroxyprogesterone acetate (DMPA), or Depo-Provera, is a long-acting injectable progestational contraceptive. It is given as a deep intramuscular injection of 150 mg into the gluteal or deltoid muscle every 13 weeks. The first injection should be given within the first 5 days of the menstrual cycle to ensure immediate contraceptive protection. The quick-start method may also be used with DMPA. Adolescents who have been sexually active within the previous 2 weeks should be informed of the chance of pregnancy and instructed

Table 3–14. Estrogenic, progestogenic, and androgenic effects of oral contraceptive pills.

Estrogenic Effects	Progestogenic Effects	Androgenic Effects
Nausea	Breast tenderness	Decreased production of testosterone, improved acne, less oily skin, and improved hirsutism. The progestin component may have androgenic as well as progestational effects:
Increased breast size (ductal and fatty tissue)	Headaches	Increased appetite and weight gain
Cyclic weight gain due to fluid retention	Hypertension	Depression, fatigue
Leukorrhea	Myocardial infarction (rare)	Decreased libido
Cervical eversion or ectopy		Increased breast tenderness or breast size
Hypertension		Increased LDL cholesterol levels
Telangiectasia		Decreased HDL cholesterol levels
Thromboembolic complications, including pulmonary emboli (rare), deep venous thrombosis, cerebrovascular accident, or myocardial infarction (rare)		Decreased carbohydrate tolerance; increased insulin resistance Pruritus

HDL, high density lipoprotein; LDL, low-density lipoprotein.
Adapted, with permission, from Hatcher RA et al: *Contraceptive Technology,* 17th ed. Ardent Media, 1998.

to return for a repeat pregnancy test 2 weeks after initiating DMPA. DMPA works chiefly by blocking the LH surge, thereby suppressing ovulation, but it also thickens cervical mucus and alters the endometrium to inhibit implantation. With a failure rate of less than 0.3%, minimal compliance issues, long-acting nature, reversibility, lack of interference with intercourse, and lack of estrogen-related side effects, it may be an attractive contraceptive for many adolescents. Patients should be warned about unpredictable menstrual patterns, the possibility of weight gain or mood changes, and the potential for decreased bone density. The Food and Drug Administration has issued a black box warning about decreased bone density with DMPA. Whether this decrease in bone density is reversible remains under investigation. Current recommendations are for adolescents to consider another method of contraception after 2 years of DMPA. Providers must take into consideration the risk of pregnancy, including deleterious effects on bone density with pregnancy. DMPA may reduce intravascular sickling and increase hemoglobin and red cell survival in patients with sickle cell disease. Moreover, DMPA may be the preferred method for patients with seizure disorders, because it has been found to reduce the number of seizures in some patients. DMPA may also be helpful for adolescents with von Willebrand disease, since amenorrhea (which decreases blood loss) is a common effect of DMPA. Studies have shown no increased risk of liver cancer, breast cancer, or invasive squamous cell cervical cancer among users of DMPA, and the risk of endometrial and ovarian cancers is also reduced.

Implantable Contraceptive Methods

Implanon is a single implant, effective for 3 years. It contains etonogestrel. It has a failure rate approaching 0%. Side effects include irregular bleeding, headache, nausea, breast pain, and depression. Return to fertility is rapid following removal. Insertion and removal are reportedly significantly easier than with Norplant. The implantable contraceptives do not lead to decreased bone density, likely due to lower levels of progestins. Providers must complete formal training in order to be able to insert Implanon.

Contraceptive Vaginal Ring

The NuvaRing is a vaginal ring that releases 15 mcg of ethinyl estradiol and 120 mcg of etonogestrel per day. The ring is placed inside the vagina for 3 weeks, followed by 1 week without the ring to allow for withdrawal bleeding. A new ring is inserted each month. The failure rate is 1%. Side effects include vaginitis in 5%, headache in 6%, and foreign body sensation in 2.5%. The vaginal ring is easier to insert correctly than the diaphragm. However, like the diaphragm, adolescents are often reluctant to use contraception requiring insertion into the vagina.

Contraceptive Methods Not Usually Recommended for Teenagers

Adolescents should understand the menstrual cycle and be taught that ovulation typically occurs 2 weeks before the next menstrual period and may be difficult to predict. Because teenagers frequently have irregular cycles, the rhythm, or calendar, method is not effective. Adolescents also need to be taught that withdrawal is not a reliable method of contraception. Diaphragms and cervical caps require professional fitting and skill with insertion and are not popular among teenagers. Adolescents who have never been pregnant or who engage in behaviors that carry a risk of STIs should not use an intrauterine device.

Eaton DK et al: Youth risk behavior surveillance—United States, 2005. MMWR Surveill Summ 2006;55(SS-5):1 [PMID: 16760893]. Available at: http://www.cdc.gov/mmwr/preview/mmwrhtml/ss5505a1.htm.

Gallo MF et al: Skin patch and vaginal ring versus combined oral contraceptives for contraception. Cochrane Database Syst Rev 2003;(1):CD003552 [PMID: 12535478].

Meirik O et al: Implantable contraceptives for women. Hum Reprod Update 2003;9:49 [PMID: 12638781].

Petitti DB: Clinical practice: Combination estrogen-progestin oral contraceptives. N Engl J Med 2003;349:1443 [PMID: 14534338].

Westhoff C et al: Initiation of oral contraceptives using a quick start compared with a conventional start: A randomized controlled trial. Obstet Gynecol 2007;109:1270 [PMID: 17540797].

PREGNANCY

Approximately 750,000 adolescents younger than age 19 become pregnant every year. The birth rate fell to 40.4 births per 1000 females 15–19 years of age in 2005. The decline in the birth rate for younger teens, 15–17 years of age, fell to 21.4 births per 1000 females in 2005, dropping 45% since 1991.

Abortions in adolescents have also decreased over the past decade, down to 215,000 in 2002. Despite decreasing rates, the United States still has the highest adolescent pregnancy rate of any developed country. Lower socioeconomic status and lower maternal education are risk factors for teen pregnancy regardless of racial or ethnic group.

Presentation

Adolescents report delayed or missed menses or may request a pregnancy test, but often they present with an unrelated concern. The level of denial is high. The complaint may be abdominal pain, urinary frequency, dizziness, or other nonspecific symptoms, and the adolescent may not have considered the possibility of pregnancy. A history of weight gain, nausea, painful or engorged breasts, an unusually light or mistimed period, or urinary frequency may be present. Denial contributes to delay in seeking prenatal care. Clinicians need to have a low threshold for suspecting pregnancy. If any suspicion exists, a urine pregnancy test should be obtained.

Diagnosis

The history and physical examination assists in making the diagnosis. Bluish coloring and softening of the cervix appear on speculum examination. The uterine fundus may be palpable on abdominal examination after about 14 weeks' gestation. If uterine size on bimanual examination does not correspond to dates, one must consider ectopic pregnancy, incomplete or missed abortion, twin gestation, or inaccurate dates.

Enzyme-linked immunosorbent assay test kits specific for the β-human chorionic gonadotropin subunit and sensitive to less than 50 mIU/mL of human chorionic gonadotropin can be performed on urine (preferably the first morning-voided specimen, because it is more concentrated) in less than 5 minutes and are accurate by the expected date of the missed period in almost all patients. Serum radioimmunoassay is also specific for the β subunit, is accurate within 7 days after conception, and is helpful in ruling out ectopic pregnancy or threatened abortion.

The timing of pregnancy tests is important, because human chorionic gonadotropin levels rise initially after conception, peak at about 60–70 days, then drop to levels not detected by routine office slide tests after 16–20 weeks.

Management

A. Counseling at the Time of Pregnancy Testing

When an adolescent presents for pregnancy testing, it is helpful, before performing the test, to find out what she hopes the result will be and what she thinks she will do if the test is positive. If she wants to be pregnant and the test is negative, further counseling about the implications of teen pregnancy should be offered. Prenatal vitamins should be prescribed. For those who do not wish to be pregnant, contraception should be discussed, because teens with a negative pregnancy test have a high risk of pregnancy within the next 2 years.

If the adolescent is pregnant, the physician must discuss her support systems and her options with her (abortion, adoption, or raising the infant). If providers are not comfortable discussing the option of abortion, the adolescent should be referred to a provider comfortable with options counseling. Many teenagers need help in telling and involving their parents. It is important to be available for further assistance with decision making. Patients should be informed of the gestational age and time frames required for the different options. If the patient knows what she wants to do, she should be referred to the appropriate resources. If a teenager is ambivalent about her plans, it is helpful to follow up in 1 week to be certain that a decision has been made. Avoiding a decision reduces the adolescent's options and may result in poor pregnancy outcomes. Providers can help ensure that the patient obtains prenatal care if she has chosen to continue the pregnancy. In addition, brief counseling about healthful diet; folic acid supplementation (400 mcg/d); and avoiding alcohol, tobacco, and other drugs is important.

B. Fathers of Infants Born to Adolescent Mothers

Statistics regarding the age of fathers of infants born to adolescent mothers are limited due to fear of statutory rape prosecution and also the inclusion of 18- and 19-year-old women in statistics of teen pregnancy. Data have shown that adult males impregnated 27–40% of 15–17-year-old adolescent mothers. These data vary by race and ethnicity, with larger age differences typical in Hispanic and Asian couples. Regardless of age, fathers of children born to adolescent mothers have lower academic achievement, lower income, and higher rates of substance abuse and involvement with the law than fathers of children born to adult women. The majority of these fathers do not provide long-term support for their children. Most do not continue a romantic relationship with the adolescent mother.

C. Pregnancy Outcomes

Young maternal age, low maternal prepregnancy weight, poor weight gain, delay in prenatal care, maternal depression, and low socioeconomic status contribute to low birth weight and poor fetal outcome. The poor nutritional status of some teenagers, substance abuse, and high incidence of STIs also play a role. Teenagers are at greater risk than adult women for preeclampsia, eclampsia, iron-deficiency anemia, cephalopelvic disproportion, prolonged labor, premature labor, and maternal death.

Maternal risk factors are linked to adverse neonatal outcome, including higher rates of low birth weight babies (< 2500 g) and neonatal mortality. Specific risk factors leading to adverse outcomes include poverty, maternal depression, exposure to domestic violence, and inadequate support. Good family support, early prenatal care, and good nutrition can make a difference with several of these problems. The psychosocial consequences for the teenage mother and her infant are listed in Table 3–15. Teenagers who are pregnant require additional support from their caregivers. Multidisciplinary clinics for young mothers, if available, may be the best providers for pregnant adolescents.

Adolescent mothers tend to be more negative and authoritative when disciplining their children. They may have inadequate knowledge of normal behavior and development. Providers can help by educating the adolescent mother during routine visits regarding appropriate discipline and expectations of her child's behavior.

Postpartum contraceptive counseling and follow-up may help prevent additional pregnancies. In untreated girls, the risk of a second unintended pregnancy within the next 2 years is approximately 30%. Combined OCPs, the vaginal ring, or the contraceptive patch can be started 6 weeks after delivery in non–breast-feeding adolescents; progestin-only methods can be started immediately postpartum, even in breast-feeding adolescents.

Ectopic Pregnancy

In the United States, approximately 2% of pregnancies are ectopic. Adolescents have the highest mortality rate from ectopic pregnancy, most likely related to delayed entry into health care. Risk factors include history of pelvic inflammatory disease or STIs. Repeat infections with *Chlamydia* increase risk for ectopic pregnancy, as does cigarette smoking. Conception while on progestin-only methods of contraception also increases the risk of ectopic pregnancy, because of the progestin-mediated decrease in tubal motility. Providers should have a high level of suspicion when any adolescent presents with vaginal bleeding and abdominal pain. Patients typically present 6–8 weeks after their last menstrual period. Urine pregnancy test is usually positive by the time of presentation. Patients should be referred urgently to a gynecologist. Diagno-

Table 3–15. Psychosocial consequences of pregnancy for the adolescent mother and her infant.

Mother	Infant
Increased morbidity related to pregnancy	**Greater health risks**
Greater risk of eclampsia, anemia, prolonged labor, premature labor	Increased chance of low birth weight or prematurity
Increased chance of miscarriages, stillbirths	Increased risk of infant death
Increased chance of maternal mortality	Increased risk of injury and hospitalization by age 5 y
Decreased educational attainment	**Decreased academic achievement**
Less likely to get high school diploma, go to college, or graduate	Lower cognitive scores
	Decreased development
	Greater chance of being behind grade or needing remedial help
Delayed education (average 2 y)	Lower chance of advanced academics
Lower occupational attainment and prestige	Lower academic aptitude as a teenager and perhaps a higher probability of dropping out of school
Less chance of stable employment (some resolution over time)	
Lower job satisfaction	**Psychosocial consequences**
Lower income and wages	Greater risk of behavior problems
Greater dependence on public assistance	Poverty
Less stable marital relationships	Higher probability of living in a nonintact home while in high school
Higher rates of single parenthood	
Earlier marriage (though less common than in the past)	Greater risk of adolescent pregnancy
Accelerated pace of marriage, separation, divorce, and remarriage	
Faster pace of subsequent childbearing	
High rate of repeat unintended pregnancy	
More births out of marriage	
Closer spacing of births	
Larger families	

sis is based on serial serum quantitative human chorionic gonadotropin levels and transvaginal ultrasound.

Abma JC et al: Teenagers in the United States: Sexual activity, contraceptive use, and childbearing, 2002. Vital Health Stat 2004;24:1 [PMID: 15648540].

Elfenbein DS et al: Adolescent pregnancy. Pediatr Clin North Am 2003;50:781, viii [PMID: 12964694].

Klein DJ: Adolescent pregnancy: Current trends and issues. Pediatrics 2005;116:281 [PMID: 15995071].

Markovitz BP et al: Socioeconomic factors and adolescent pregnancy outcomes: Distinctions between neonatal and post-neonatal deaths? BMC Public Health 2005, 5:79 [PMID: 16042801].

National Center for Health Statistics birth data. Available at: http://www.cdc.gov/nchs/products/pubs/pubd/hestats/prelimbirths05/prelimbirths05.htm.

Seeber B, Barnhart K: Suspected ectopic pregnancy. Obstet Gynecol 2006;107:399 [PMID: 16449130].

VULVOVAGINITIS

Vaginitis may be due to pathogens or to indigenous flora after a change in milieu of the vagina. Candidal vulvovaginitis and bacterial vaginosis (formerly called *Gardnerella, Haemophilus,* or nonspecific vaginitis) may occur in patients who are not sexually active. These are examples of indigenous flora that may cause symptoms. Bacterial vaginosis, however, is more prevalent in those who are sexually active. In sexually active patients, *Trichomonas* infection or cervicitis due to sexually transmitted pathogens must be considered (see Chapter 42). For this reason, appropriate specimens should be obtained from sexually active patients or suspected victims of sexual abuse in order to detect STIs, even if yeast forms are present or bacterial vaginosis is identified.

1. Physiologic Leukorrhea

Leukorrhea is the normal vaginal discharge that begins around the time of menarche. The discharge is typically clear or white, and its consistency may vary according to cyclic hormonal influences. There should be no odor. Girls in early adolescence may have concerns about such a discharge and need reassurance that it is normal. This may be a good time to tell girls that there is no need for douching. If a vaginal wet preparation is examined, a few squamous epithelial cells may be revealed, but there should be fewer than five polymorphonuclear cells per high-power field.

2. Candidal Vulvovaginitis

Candidal vulvovaginitis is caused by yeast (*Candida albicans* or less commonly *C glabrata* or *tropicalis*). It may occur following a course of antibiotics, after which the normal perineal flora are altered and yeast is allowed to proliferate. Diabetic patients, those with compromised immune systems, and those who are pregnant or receiving OCPs are more prone to develop candidal infections. *Candida* are normal flora; therefore, only symptomatic patients should be treated.

▷ Clinical Findings

The patient usually complains of vulvar pruritus and a thick vaginal discharge, frequently beginning the week before menses. Dysuria or dyspareunia may also be present. Examination of the vulva reveals erythematous mucosa, sometimes with excoriation, and a thick, white, cheesy discharge. The discharge may be adherent to the walls of the vagina. Leukocytes may be seen on a wet preparation, and a potassium hydroxide preparation may reveal budding yeast or mycelia. The vaginal preparations are often not helpful, and the patient should be treated on the basis of the clinical examination.

▷ Treatment

Clotrimazole, miconazole, terconazole, or tioconazole vaginal creams or suppositories designed for seven nightly doses are effective in most patients. Patients with recurrent infections may benefit from 10–14 days of treatment. Fluconazole (150 mg once orally) is also effective and may be beneficial in virginal adolescents. Patients with recurrent episodes may be given prophylactic treatment whenever they take antibiotics. It may be helpful to simultaneously treat the partners of sexually active patients with recurrent candidal infections.

3. Bacterial Vaginosis

Bacterial vaginosis may be caused by any of the indigenous vaginal flora, such as *Gardnerella, Bacteroides, Peptococcus, Mycoplasma hominis,* lactobacilli, or other anaerobes.

▷ Clinical Findings

The patient generally complains of a malodorous discharge or wetness. On examination, a thin, homogeneous, grayish-white discharge is found adhering to the vaginal wall. A whiff test, in which a drop of potassium hydroxide is added to a smear of the discharge on a slide, results in the release of amines, causing a fishy odor. Wet preparation reveals more than 20% of epithelial cells as clue cells and small pleomorphic rods.

▷ Treatment

Treatment for bacterial vaginosis should be reserved for symptomatic patients. First-line treatment is with metronidazole (500 mg orally twice daily for 7 days), which results in 95% cure, or clindamycin (300 mg orally twice daily for 7 days). Patients who are prescribed metronidazole should be warned that a disulfiram-type reaction of nausea and vomiting may occur when alcohol is consumed. Topical metronidazole or clindamycin may also be effective. Ampicillin (500 mg orally 4 times daily for 7 days) is the alternative for pregnant patients.

4. Other Causes of Vulvovaginitis

A. Sexually Transmitted Infections

STIs are a common cause of vaginal discharge in adolescents (see Chapter 42). *Chlamydia* and gonorrhea testing should be done whenever a sexually active adolescent complains of vaginal discharge even when the cervix appears normal.

B. Foreign Body Vaginitis

Foreign bodies (most commonly retained tampons or condoms) cause extremely malodorous vaginal discharges. Treatment consists of removal, for which ring forceps may be useful. Further treatment is generally not necessary.

C. Allergic or Contact Vaginitis

Bubble baths, feminine hygiene sprays, or vaginal contraceptive foams or suppositories may cause chemical irritation of the vaginal mucosa. Discontinuing use of the offending agent is indicated.

Freeto J et al: "What's really going on down there?": A practical approach to the adolescent who has gynecologic complaints. Pediatr Clin North Am 2006; 53:529 [PMID: 16716795].

Adolescent Substance Abuse

Paritosh Kaul, MD

The use and abuse of mood-altering substances—alcohol, marijuana, opioids, cocaine, amphetamines, sedative-hypnotics, hallucinogens, inhalants, nicotine, anabolic steroids, γ-hydroxybutyrate (GHB), methylenedioxymethamphetamine (ecstasy), and recently, prescription drugs—is a serious public health problem. The short- and long-term health, social, emotional, legal, and behavioral consequences of substance abuse are particularly damaging during childhood and adolescence. Not only does early substance use portend chronic, severe polysubstance abuse later in life, but substance use may also compromise physical, cognitive, and psychosocial aspects of adolescent development if this maladaptive behavior becomes the preferred response to environmental stressors.

Substance abuse tends to be a chronic, progressive disease. The first or initiation stage—from nonuser to user—is such a common feature of becoming an American adult that many authorities call it normative behavior. At this stage, substance use is typically limited to experimentation with tobacco or alcohol (so-called gateway substances). During adolescence, young people are expected to establish an independent, autonomous identity. They try out a variety of behaviors within the safety of their family circles and peer groups. This process often involves experimentation with psychoactive substances, usually in culturally acceptable circumstances. Progression to the second or continuation stage of substance abuse is a nonnormative risk behavior with the potential to compromise adolescent development. The American Psychiatric Association has outlined criteria that can be used to judge the severity of substance use that progresses beyond the experimentation stage to substance abuse or substance dependency (the former being more severe). Maintenance and progression within a class of substances (eg, from beer to liquor) and progression across classes of substances (eg, from alcohol to marijuana) represent the third and fourth stages of substance abuse. Individuals at these stages are polysubstance abusers, and most manifest one or more of the symptoms of dependency such as tolerance or withdrawal. The transition from one stage to the next is typically a cyclic process of regression, cessation, and relapse. Common symptoms and physiologic effects of intoxication (which can occur at any stage) and withdrawal (a symptom of dependency) for the major classes of substances are presented in Tables 4–1 and 4–2.

American Psychiatric Association: *Diagnostic and Statistical Manual of Mental Disorders,* 4th ed. Text Revision. American Psychiatric Association, 2000.

Greydanus DE, Patel DR: Substance abuse in adolescents: A complex conundrum for the clinician. Pediatr Clin North Am 2003;50:1179 [PMID: 14558685].

U.S. Department of Health and Human Services: *Healthy People 2010,* 2nd ed, with *Understanding and Improving Health and Objectives for Improving Health* (2 vols.). U.S. Government Printing Office, 2000.

SCOPE OF THE PROBLEM

The best source of information about the prevalence of substance abuse among American children and adolescents is the annual Monitoring the Future Study, which tracks health-related behaviors in a sample of 50,000 8th, 10th, and 12th graders in more than 400 schools across the United States. This study probably understates the magnitude of the problem of substance abuse because it excludes two high-risk adolescent groups—school dropouts and runaways. Although the exclusion of these youngsters may minimize prevalence estimates only moderately for the entire population, errors in estimating drug use among subgroups with high rates of school dropout (eg, urban minority youths) are thought to be substantial. Data from this survey and others show that alcohol is the most frequently abused substance in our society. Experimentation with alcohol typically begins in or before middle school; is more common among boys than girls; and is most common among whites, less common among Hispanics and Native Americans, and least common

Table 4–1. Physiologic effects of commonly abused mood-altering substances.

EYES/PUPILS	
Mydriasis	Amphetamines, MDMA, or other stimulants; cocaine; glutethimide; jimson weed; LSD. Withdrawal from alcohol and opioids
Miosis	Alcohol, barbiturates, benzodiazepines, opioids, PCP
Nystagmus	Alcohol, barbiturates, benzodiazepines, inhalants, PCP
Conjunctival injection	LSD, marijuana
Lacrimation	Inhalants, LSD. Withdrawal from opioids
CARDIOVASCULAR	
Tachycardia	Amphetamines, MDMA, or other stimulants; cocaine; LSD; marijuana; PCP. Withdrawal from alcohol, barbiturates, benzodiazepines
Hypertension	Amphetamines, MDMA, or other stimulants; cocaine; LSD; marijuana; PCP. Withdrawal from alcohol, barbiturates, benzodiazepines
Hypotension	Barbiturates, opioids. Orthostatic: marijuana. Withdrawal from depressants
Arrhythmia	Amphetamines, MDMA, or other stimulants; cocaine; inhalants; opioids; PCP
RESPIRATORY	
Depression	Opioids, depressants, GHB
Pulmonary edema	Opioids, stimulants
CORE BODY TEMPERATURE	
Elevated	Amphetamines, MDMA, or other stimulants; cocaine; PCP. Withdrawal from alcohol, barbiturates, benzodiazepines, opioids
Decreased	Alcohol, barbiturates, benzodiazepines, opioids, GHB
PERIPHERAL NERVOUS SYSTEM RESPONSE	
Hyperreflexia	Amphetamines, MDMA, or other stimulants; cocaine; LSD; marijuana; methaqualone; PCP. Withdrawal from alcohol, barbiturates, benzodiazepines
Hyporeflexia	Alcohol, barbiturates, benzodiazepines, inhalants, opioids
Tremor	Amphetamines or other stimulants, cocaine, LSD. Withdrawal from alcohol, barbiturates, benzodiazepines, cocaine
Ataxia	Alcohol, amphetamines, MDMA, or other stimulants; barbiturates; benzodiazepines; inhalants; LSD; PCP; GHB
CENTRAL NERVOUS SYSTEM RESPONSE	
Hyperalertness	Amphetamines, MDMA, or other stimulants; cocaine
Sedation, somnolence	Alcohol, barbiturates, benzodiazepines, inhalants, marijuana, opioids, GHB
Seizures	Alcohol, amphetamines, MDMA, or other stimulants; cocaine; inhalants; methaqualone; opioids (particularly meperidine, propoxyphene). Withdrawal from alcohol, barbiturates, benzodiazepines
Hallucinations	Amphetamines, MDMA, or other stimulants; cocaine; inhalants; LSD; marijuana; PCP. Withdrawal from alcohol, barbiturates, benzodiazepines
GASTROINTESTINAL	
Nausea, vomiting	Alcohol, amphetamines or other stimulants, cocaine, inhalants, LSD, opioids, peyote, GHB. Withdrawal from alcohol, barbiturates, benzodiazepines, cocaine, opioids

GHB, γ-hydroxybutyrate; LSD, lysergic acid diethylamide; MDMA, methylenedioxymethamphetamine (ecstasy); PCP, phencyclidine hydrochloride.
Adapted, with permission, from Schwartz B, Alderman EM: Substance abuse. Pediatr Rev 1997;18:215.

among blacks and Asians. Over 50% of children consume alcohol before high school, and over 90% do so before graduation. Over 25% of eighth graders and over 50% of high-school students seen in an average American pediatric practice have used alcohol within the last 30 days, and half have consumed five or more drinks on at least one occasion. Use of tobacco, marijuana, and other mood-altering substances is less common. Marijuana is the most commonly used illicit drug in the United States. First experiences with marijuana and the substances listed in Table 4–2 typically occur during middle school and early high school. Initiation of substance abuse is rare after age 20 years.

The level of substance abuse among American youth rose in the 1960s and 1970s, declined in the 1980s, rose again in the early 1990s, and has declined somewhat since then. Between 1999 and 2006, substance use initiation

Table 4–2. Effects of commonly abused mood-altering substances.

Substance	Pharmacology	Intoxication	Withdrawal	Chronic Use
Alcohol (ethanol)	Depressant; 10 g/drink Drink: 12 oz beer, 4 oz wine, 1^1/$_2$ oz liquor; one drink increases blood level by approximately 0.025 g/dL (varies by weight)	Legal: 0.05–0.1 g/dL (varies by state) Mild (< 0.1 g/dL): disinhibition, euphoria, mild sedation and impaired coordination Moderate (0.1–0.2 g/dL): impaired mentation and judgment, slurred speech, ataxia Severe: > 0.3 g/dL: confusion, stupor > 0.4 g/dL: coma, depressed respiration	Mild: headache, tremors, nausea and vomiting ("hangover") Severe: fever, sweaty, seizure, agitation, hallucination, hypertension, tachycardia Delirium tremens (chronic use)	Hepatitis, cirrhosis, cardiac disease, Wernicke encephalopathy, Korsakoff syndrome
Marijuana (cannabis)	δ-9-Tetrahydrocannabinol (THC); 4–6% in marijuana; 20–30% in hashish	Low: euphoria, relaxation, impaired thinking High: mood changes, depersonalization, hallucinations Toxic: panic, delusions, paranoia, psychosis	Irritability, disturbed sleep, tremor, nystagmus, anorexia, diarrhea, vomiting	Cough, gynecomastia, low sperm count, infertility, amotivational syndrome, apathy
Cocaine	Stimulant; releases biogenic amines; concentration varies with preparation and route of administration	Hyperalert, increased energy, confident, insomnia, anxiety, paranoia, dilated pupils, tremors, seizures, hypertension, arrhythmia, tachycardia, fever, dry mouth Toxic: coma, psychosis, seizure, myocardial infarction, stroke, hyperthermia, rhabdomyolysis	Drug craving, depression, dysphoria, irritability, lethargy, tremors, nausea, hunger	Nasal septum ulceration, epistaxis, lung damage, intravenous drug use
Opioids (heroin, morphine, codeine, methadone, opium, fentanyl, meperidine, propoxyphene)	Depressant; binds central opioid receptor; variable concentrations with substance	Euphoria, sedation, impaired thinking, low blood pressure, pinpoint pupil, urinary retention Toxic: hypotension, arrhythmia, depressed respiration, stupor, coma, seizure, death	Only after > 3 weeks of regular use: drug craving, rhinorrhea, lacrimation, muscle aches, diarrhea, anxiety, tremors, hypertension, tachycardia	Intravenous drug use: cellulitis, endocarditis, embolisms, HIV
Amphetamines	Stimulant; sympathomimetic	Euphoria, hyperalert state, hyperactive, hypertension, arrhythmia, fever, flushing, dilated pupils, tremor, ataxia, dry mouth	Lethargy, fatigue, depression, anxiety, nightmares, muscle cramps, abdominal pain, hunger	Paranoia, psychosis
MDMA (ecstasy)	Stimulant, psychedelic; releases serotonin, dopamine, and norepinephrine; inhibits reuptake of neurotransmitters; increases dopamine synthesis; inhibits MAO	Enhanced empathy, euphoria, increased energy and self-esteem, tachycardia, hypertension, increased pyschomotor drive, sensory enhancement, illusions, difficulty concentrating and retaining information, headaches, palpitations, flushing, hyperthermia	None	Paranoid psychosis

(continued)

Table 4–2. Effects of commonly abused mood-altering substances. *(Continued)*

Substance	Pharmacology	Intoxication	Withdrawal	Chronic Use
		Toxic: frank psychosis, coma, seizures, intracranial hemorrhage, cerebral infarction, asystole, pulmonary edema, multisystem organ failure, acute renal or hepatic failure, ARDS, DIC, SIADH, death		
GHB (liquid ecstasy)	Depressant, endogenous CNS transmitter; influences dopaminergic activity, higher levels of GABA-B activity	10 mg/kg: sleep 30 mg/kg: memory loss 50 mg/kg: general anesthesia Toxic: CNS and respiratory depression, aggressiveness, seizures, bradycardia, apnea	Only after chronic use with dosing every 3 h Early: mild tremor, tachycardia, hypertension, diaphoresis, moderate anxiety, insomnia, nausea, vomiting Progressive: confusion, delirium, hallucinations, autonomic instability, death	Wernicke-Korsakoff syndrome
Sedative-hypnotics (barbiturates, benzodiazepines, methaqualone)	Depressant	Sedation, lethargy, slurred speech, pinpoint pupils, hypotension, psychosis, seizures Toxic: stupor, coma, cardiac arrest, seizure, pulmonary edema, death	Only after weeks of use: agitation, delirium, psychosis, hallucinations, fever, flushing, hyper- or hypotension, death	Paranoia
Hallucinogens (LSD, peyote, mescaline, mushrooms, nutmeg, jimson weed)	Inhibition of serotonin release	Illusions, depersonalization, hallucination, anxiety, paranoia, ataxia, dilated pupils, hypertension, dry mouth Toxic: coma, terror, panic, "crazy feeling"	None	Flashbacks
Phencyclidine	Dissociative anesthetic	Low dose (< 5 mg): illusions, hallucinations, ataxia, hypertension, flushing Moderate dose (5–10 mg): hyperthermia, salivation, myoclonus High dose: (> 10 mg): rigidity, seizure, arrhythmia, coma, death	None	Flashbacks
Inhalants (toluene, benzene, hydrocarbons and fluorocarbons)	Stimulation progressing to depression	Euphoria, giddiness, impaired judgment, ataxia, rhinorrhea, salivation, hallucination Toxic: respiratory depression, arrhythmia, coma, stupor, delirium, sudden death	None	Permanent damage to nerves, liver, heart, kidney, brain
Nicotine	Releases dopamine, 1 mg nicotine per cigarette	Relaxation, tachycardia, vertigo, anorexia	Drug craving, irritability, anxiety, hunger, impaired concentration	Permanent damage to lung, heart, cardiovascular system

(continued)

Table 4–2. Effects of commonly abused mood-altering substances. *(Continued)*

Substance	Pharmacology	Intoxication	Withdrawal	Chronic Use
Anabolic steroids[a]	Bind steroid receptor Stacking: use many types simultaneously; pyramiding: increase dosage	Increased muscle bulk, strength, endurance, increased drive, hypogonadism, low sperm count, gynecomastia, decreased libido, virilization, irregular menses, hepatitis, early epiphysial closure, aggressiveness	Drug craving, dysphoria, irritability, depression	Tendon rupture, cardiomyopathy, atherosclerosis, peliosis hepatis (orally active C17 derivatives of testosterone are especially hepatotoxic)

[a]Despite conventional assumptions, scientific studies show that anabolic steroids do not improve aerobic athletic performance and improve strength only in athletes trained in weight lifting before they begin using steroids who continue to train and consume a high-protein diet.
ARDS, acute respiratory distress syndrome; CNS, central nervous system; DIC, disseminated intravascular coagulation; GABA, γ-aminobutyric acid; GHB, γ-hydroxybutyrate; HIV, human immunodeficiency virus; LSD, lysergic acid diethylamide; MAO, monoamine oxidase; MDMA, methylenedioxymethamphetamine; SIADH, syndrome of inappropriate secretion of antidiuretic hormone.

among adolescents has decreased. Despite the overall decline, there is still a significant pattern of drug use among adolescents. The use of alcohol, tobacco, and illicit drugs doubles from 8th grade to 12th grade. The rate of alcohol and cigarette use more than triples from adolescence (12–17 years) to young adulthood (18–25 years). The prevalence of marijuana use among 12th graders in 2006 was 32%. In the past decade, LSD, ecstasy, and methamphetamine use decreased but cocaine use increased. The most disturbing trend among adolescents is the recreational use of prescription medications, particularly psychotherapeutic agents. Studies indicate that the rise and fall in use of a substance is heralded by changes in the perceived risks and benefits of using the substance. The use of inhalants had been rising until 2006, when both experience and educational efforts resulted in a perception of these substances as being "dangerous."

Becker CE et al: Glue sniffing polyneuropathy: An under recognized aspect of a public health hazard. J Adolesc Health 2004;34:94 [PMID: 14706411].

Camenga DR et al: The changing risk profile of the American adolescent smoker: Implications for prevention programs and tobacco interventions. J Adolesc Health 2006;39:120.e1 [PMID: 16781972].

Cance JD et al: Unhealthy weight control behaviors and MDMA (ecstasy) use among adolescent females. J Adolesc Health 2005;37:409 [PMID: 16227128].

Friedman RA: The changing face of teenage drug abuse—the trend toward prescription drugs. N Engl J Med 2006;354:1448 [PMID: 16598042].

Halpern-Felsher BL, Cornell JL: Preventing underage alcohol use: Where do we go from here? J Adolesc Health 2005;37:1 [PMID: 15963895].

Johnston LD et al: *The Monitoring the Future National Survey Results on Adolescent Drug Use: Overview of Key Findings.* National Institute on Drug Abuse, US Department of Health and Human Services, 2007 (NIH Publication No. 07–6202). Available at: http://www.monitoringthefuture.org.

Substance Abuse and Mental Health Services Administration: *Results from the 2006 National Survey of Drug Use and Health: National Findings* (DHHS Publication No. SMA 07-4293). National Institute on Drug Abuse, 2007. Available at: http:oas.samhsa.gov/NSDUH.htm.

Sung HE et al: Nonmedical use of prescription opioids among teenagers in the United States: Trends and correlates. J Adolesc Health 2005;37:44 [PMID: 15963906].

Williams JF, Storck M; American Academy of Pediatrics Committee on Substance Abuse; American Academy of Pediatrics Committee on Native American Child Health: Inhalant abuse. Pediatrics 2007;119:1009 [PMID: 17473104].

Zamboanga BL et al: Subjective evaluations of alcohol expectancies and their relevance to drinking game involvement in female college students. J Adolesc Health 2005;37:77 [PMID: 15963914].

MORBIDITY DATA

Use and abuse of alcohol or other mood-altering substances is tightly linked with the leading causes of death among adolescents in the United States (ie, motor vehicle accidents, unintentional injury, homicide, and suicide). Substance abuse is also associated with physical and sexual abuse. Up to two thirds of sexual assaults and acquaintance or date rapes are linked to alcohol or other drug use. Drug use and abuse also contribute to other high-risk behaviors, such as unsafe sexual activity, unintended pregnancy, and sexually transmitted diseases. The use of drugs during periods of low self-esteem and depression increases the risk of suicide. Adolescents are also involved with selling of drugs.

The risks associated with tobacco, alcohol, and cocaine are listed in Table 4–2. Less well known are the long- and short-term adolescent morbidities connected with the currently most popular illicit drugs, marijuana and ecstasy. The active ingredient in marijuana, δ-9-tetrahydrocannabinol (THC), transiently causes tachycardia, mild hypertension, and bronchodilation. Regular use can cause lung changes similar to those seen in tobacco smokers. Heavy use decreases fertility in both sexes and immunocompetence. It is also associated with damage to the hippocampus and basal ganglia, which causes abnormalities of cognition, learning, coordination, and memory. It is possible that heavy marijuana use is the cause of the so-called amotivational syndrome, characterized by inattention to environmental stimuli and impaired goal-directed thinking and behavior. Analysis of confiscated marijuana has shown increasing THC concentration and adulteration with other substances.

Ecstasy is gaining in both popularity and accessibility among adolescents. Chronic use destroys the serotonin system of the brain and is associated with progressive decline of immediate and delayed memory and with alterations in mood, sleep, and appetite that may be permanent. Even first-time users may develop frank psychosis indistinguishable from schizophrenia. Irreversible cardiomyopathy, noncardiogenic pulmonary edema, and pulmonary hypertension may occur with long-term use. Acute overdose can cause hyperthermia and multiorgan system failure.

A growing problem is the abuse of prescribed and over-the-counter (OTC) medications by adolescents. Medication used in the medical management of chronic pain, depression, anxiety, and attention-deficit/hyperactivity disorder can be drugs of abuse either by the patients or by those they supply with the drug.

Environmental and prenatal exposure to abused substances carries health risks. Parental tobacco smoking is associated with low birth weight in newborns, sudden infant death syndrome, bronchiolitis, asthma, otitis media, and fire-related injuries. Paternal use of marijuana during pregnancy is associated with an increased risk of sudden infant death syndrome. In utero exposure to cocaine and alcohol may produce fetal malformations, intrauterine growth restriction, and brain injury.

American Academy of Pediatrics Committee on Substance Abuse: Tobacco's toll: Implications for the pediatrician. Pediatrics 2001;107:794 [PMID: 11335763].

Bailey SL et al: Diary study of substance use and unsafe sex among adolescents with substance use disorders. J Adolesc Health 2006;38:297.e13 [PMID: 16488830].

Burd L, Wilson H: Fetal, infant, and child mortality in a context of alcohol use. Am J Med Genet C Semin Med Genet 2004;15;127:51 [PMID: 15095472].

Hertz JA, Knight JR: Prescription drug misuse: A growing national problem. Adolesc Med Clin 2006;17:751 [PMID: 17030290].

Klonoff-Cohen H, Lam-Kruglick P: Maternal and paternal recreational drug use and sudden infant death syndrome. Arch Pediatr Adolesc Med 2001;155:765 [PMID: 11434841].

Knishkowy B, Amitai Y: Water-pipe (narghile) smoking: An emerging health risk behavior. Pediatrics 2005;116:e113 [PMID: 15995011].

Kulig JW; American Academy of Pediatrics Committee on Substance Abuse: Tobacco, alcohol, and other drugs: The role of the pediatrician in prevention, identification, and management of substance abuse. Pediatrics 2005;115:816 [PMID: 15741395].

Ownby DR et al: Passive cigarette smoke exposure in infants. Arch Pediatr Adolesc Med 2000;154:1237 [PMID: 11115309].

Steinman KJ: Drug selling among high school students: Related risk behaviors and psychosocial characteristics. J Adolesc Health 2005;36:71.e1 [PMID: 15661603].

Tapert SF et al: Adolescent substance use and sexual risk-taking behavior. J Adolesc Health 2001;28:181 [PMID: 11226840].

Tschann JM et al: Emotional distress, alcohol use, and peer violence among Mexican-American and European-American adolescents. J Adolesc Health 2005;37:11 [PMID: 15963902].

Van Beurden E et al: Heavy episodic drinking and sensation seeking in adolescents as predictors of harmful driving and celebrating behaviors: Implications for prevention. J Adolesc Health 2005;37:37 [PMID: 15963905].

Williams JF, Kokotailo PK: Abuse of proprietary (over-the-counter) drugs. Adolesc Med Clin 2006;17:733 [PMID: 17030289].

Wu LT et al: Use of nitrite inhalants ("poppers") among American youth. J Adolesc Health 2005;37:52 [PMID: 15963907].

SUPPLEMENT USE & ABUSE

Use of supplements or special diets to enhance athletic performance dates to antiquity. Today, many elite and casual athletes use ergogenic supplements in an attempt to improve performance. The most popular products used by adolescents are protein supplements, creatine, and the prohormones. Strength athletes (ie, weight lifters) use protein powders and shakes to enhance muscle repair and mass. The amount of protein consumed by athletes often greatly exceeds the recommended daily allowance for weight lifters and other resistance-training athletes (1.6–1.7 g/kg/d). The American Academy of Pediatrics (AAP) condemns the use of performance-enhancing substances. Excess consumption of protein provides no added strength or muscle mass and can provoke renal failure in teens with underlying renal dysfunction.

Sales of creatine supplements are over $400 million (U.S.) per year. Creatine—a combination of glycine, arginine, and methionine that is produced naturally in the liver, kidneys, and pancreas—facilitates production of adenosine triphosphate and increases free energy for muscle contraction. It maximizes power during short-duration, intense exercise and improves baseline strength in adults. Creatine does not improve performance in longer-duration, aerobic exercise nor has its effectiveness been analyzed in children. Although the American College of Sports Medicine discourages its use by people younger than 18 years of age, recent studies show that creatine is extensively used by athletes in grades 6–12. Side effects include weight gain, headache, abdominal pain, diarrhea, and increased muscle strain. There are conflicting reports about the risk of renal damage.

There has been a disturbing increase in the availability and use of prohormones, specifically dehydroepiandrosterone (DHEA) and androstenedione. Sold as dietary supplements, these precursors to testosterone and other sex hormones are sold without federal regulation. Endogenous DHEA is produced in the adrenal cortex as a precursor of gonadal hormones. Putative benefits of DHEA are increased fat catabolism; increased muscle mass; increased libido; "improved" immune function; and decreased memory loss, heart disease, cancer, type 2 diabetes mellitus, and Alzheimer and Parkinson disease. Although its effects on strength and performance in athletes remain unstudied and unproven, the advertised benefits are attractive to many athletes. Its effect on young, healthy individuals (ie, those with higher baseline DHEA levels) has not been studied. In adults, two studies have shown that doses of 50–100 mg/d cause increased androgenic steroid plasma levels and increased subjective perception of physical and psychological well-being. Users of DHEA report few adverse effects.

Androstenedione, which is banned by the International Olympic Committee, National Collegiate Athletic Association, and National Football League, is converted to testosterone in the liver. A recent study of young athletes concluded that oral androstenedione does not increase plasma testosterone concentration. In young eugonadal men it has no anabolic effect on muscle protein metabolism. Other studies have shown increased biologically active estrogen levels. No long-term studies have been conducted. Its side effects are believed to be similar to those of other anabolic and androgenic agents. Most side effects are secondary to androgen excess—hyperlipidemia, hypertension, insulin resistance, hyperinsulinism, depression, aggression, paranoia, acne, male pattern baldness, alopecia, and priapism. Most effects are reversible with cessation of use. Irreversible side effects include virilization in females (hair loss, clitoromegaly, hirsutism, and voice-deepening) and gynecomastia in males.

As the use of supplements and herbs increases, it will be increasingly important for pediatric care providers to be familiar with their common side effects. The Internet has become a source for information about and distribution of these products. The easy accessibility, perceived low risk, and low cost of these products significantly increase the likelihood that they will become substances of abuse by the pediatric population.

Calfee R, Fadale P: Popular ergogenic drugs and supplements in young athletes. Pediatrics 2006;117:e577 [PMID: 16510635].

Casavant MJ et al: Consequences of use of anabolic androgenic steroids. Pediatr Clin North Am 2007;54:677 [PMID: 17723870].

Dodge TL, Jaccard JJ: The effect of high school sports participation on the use of performance-enhancing substances in young adulthood. J Adolesc Health 2006;39:367 [PMID: 16919798].

Gomez J: American Academy of Pediatrics Committee on Sports Medicine and Fitness: Use of performance-enhancing substances. Pediatrics 2005;115:1103 [PMID: 15805399].

Gregory AJM, Fitch RW: Sports medicine: Performance-enhancing drugs. Pediatr Clin North Am 2007;54:797 [PMID: 17723878].

Holland-Hall C: Performance-enhancing substances: Is your adolescent patient using? Pediatr Clin North Am 2007;54:651 [PMID: 17723868].

Kerr JM, Congeni JA: Anabolic-androgenic steroids: Use and abuse in pediatric patients. Pediatr Clin North Am 2007;54:771 [PMID: 17723876].

Moore MJ, Werch CE: Sport and physical activity participation and substance use among adolescents. J Adolesc Health 2005;36:486 [PMID: 15901513].

VandenBerg P et al: Steroid use among adolescents: Longitudinal findings from Project EAT. Pediatrics 2007;119:476 [PMID: 17332200].

RESPONSE TO THE PROBLEM

Federal, state, and local governments attempt to control the damage caused by substance abuse by prohibiting use and by legislating against associated high-risk behaviors (eg, enacting drunk-driving laws and nighttime curfews). However, neither these legal actions nor the large sums of money spent on school- and community-based drug abuse prevention and treatment programs have curbed the problem. Hence, the AAP recommends that pediatricians become knowledgeable about the extent and nature of drugs used in their community, provide anticipatory guidance to parents starting with the first prenatal visit, and be aware of community referral and treatment resources.

The Internet has made the task of limiting drug use more difficult. For example, poor methods for age verification make it easy for minors to purchase tobacco products online. The media also glamorize use of tobacco and alcohol. Pro-tobacco marketing and media stimulate tobacco use among youth while recent state budget crises have cut anti-tobacco advertising. Exposure to tobacco company youth-targeted smoking prevention advertising generally has had no beneficial outcomes for youths.

Emery S et al: Televised state-sponsored antitobacco advertising and youth smoking beliefs and behavior in the United States, 1999–2000. Arch Pediatr Adolesc Med 2005;159:639 [PMID: 15996997].

Gruber EL et al: Alcohol, tobacco and illicit substances in music videos: A content analysis of prevalence and genre. J Adolesc Health 2005;37:81 [PMID: 15963915].

Kodjo CM, Klein JD: Prevention and risk of adolescent substance abuse. The role of adolescents, families, and communities. Pediatr Clin North Am 2002;49:257 [PMID: 11993282].

Kulig JW; American Academy of Pediatrics Committee on Substance Abuse: Tobacco, alcohol, and other drugs: The role of the pediatrician in prevention, identification, and management of substance abuse. Pediatrics 2005;115:816 [PMID: 15741395].

Ribisl KM et al: Internet sales of cigarettes to minors. JAMA 2003;290:1356 [PMID: 12966128].

Strasburger VC: Risky business: What primary care practitioners need to know about the influence of the media on adolescents. Prim Care 2006;33:317 [PMID: 16713765].

Wakefield M et al: Effect of televised, tobacco company-funded smoking prevention advertising on youth smoking-related beliefs, intentions, and behavior. Am J Public Health 2006;96:2154 [PMID: 17077405].

Wellman RJ et al: The extent to which tobacco marketing and tobacco use in films contribute to children's use of tobacco: A meta-analysis. Arch Pediatr Adolesc Med 2006;160:1285 [PMID: 17146027].

PREDICTING THE PROGRESSION FROM USE TO ABUSE

Most adolescents use mood-altering substances intermittently or experimentally at the start. The challenge to pediatric health care providers is to recognize the warning signs, identify potential abusers early, and intervene in an effective and timely fashion before acute or chronic use results in morbidity. The

Table 4–3. Factors that influence the progression from substance use to substance abuse.

Enabling Risk Factors	Potentially Protective Factors
SOCIETAL AND COMMUNITY	
Experimentation encouraged by media Illicit substances available Extreme economic deprivation Neighborhood disorganization, crowding Tolerance of licit and illicit substance use	Regular involvement in church activities Support for norms and values of society Strict enforcement of laws prohibiting substance use among minors and abuse among adults Neighborhood resources, supportive adults
SCHOOL	
Lack of commitment to school or education Truancy Academic failure Early, persistent behavior problems	Strong commitment to school or education Future-oriented goals Achievement oriented
FAMILY	
Models of substance abuse and other unconventional behavior Dysfunctional parenting styles; excessive authority or permissiveness High family conflict; low bonding	Models of conventional behavior Attachment to parents Cohesive family Nurturing parenting styles
PEERS	
Peer rejection in elementary grades Substance use prevalent among peers Peer attitudes favorable to substance abuse and unconventional behavior	Popular with peers Abstinent friends Peer attitudes favor conventional behavior
INDIVIDUAL	
Genetic predisposition Psychological diagnoses (attention-deficit/hyperactivity disorder; antisocial personality) Depression and low self-esteem Alienation and rebelliousness Sexual or physical abuse Early onset of deviant behavior or delinquency Early onset of sexual behavior Aggressive	Positive self-concept, good self-esteem Intolerance of deviance Internally motivated, takes charge of problems

best predictors of ethanol and drug abuse are male sex, young age at first use, and associating with drug-using peers. It is still unclear why only a minority of the young people exhibiting the high-risk characteristics listed in Table 4–3 go on to abuse substances. Substance abuse is a symptom of personal and social maladjustment as often as it is a cause. Because there is a direct relationship between the number of risk factors listed in Table 4–3 and the frequency of substance abuse, a combination of risk factors is the best indicator of risk. Even so, most teenagers with multiple risk characteristics never develop a substance abuse problem, presumably because the protective factors listed in Table 4–3 give them enough resilience to cope with stress in more socially adaptive ways. Being aware of the risk domains in Table 4–3 will help physicians identify youngsters most apt to need counseling about substance abuse.

Brown RT: Risk factors for substance abuse in adolescents. Pediatr Clin North Am 2002;49:247 [PMID: 11993281].

Hill KG et al: Family influences on the risk of daily smoking initiation. J Adolesc Health 2005;37:202 [PMID: 16109339].
Nash SG et al: Pathways to adolescent alcohol use: Family environment, peer influence, and parental expectations. J Adolesc Health 2005;37:19 [PMID: 15963903].

MANAGEMENT OF SUBSTANCE ABUSE

Office Screening

The AAP Committee on Substance Abuse recommends that pediatricians include discussions of substance abuse as part of their anticipatory care, starting with parents at the first prenatal visit. Given the high incidence of substance abuse and the subtlety of its early signs and symptoms, a general psychosocial assessment is the best way to screen for substance abuse among adolescents. Interviewing and counseling techniques and methods for taking a psychosocial history are discussed in

Chapter 3. In an atmosphere of trust and confidentiality, physicians must ask routine screening questions of all patients and be alert for addictive diseases, recognizing the high level of denial often present in addicted patients. The universal screening approach outlined in the American Medical Association (AMA) Guidelines for Adolescent Preventive Services (GAPS) is a good guide for routine screening and diagnosis. Clues to possible substance abuse include truancy, failing grades, problems with interpersonal relationships, delinquency, depressive affect, chronic fatigue, recurrent abdominal pains, chest pains or palpitations, headache, chronic cough, persistent nasal discharge, and recurrent complaints of sore throat. Substance abuse should be included in the differential diagnosis of all behavioral, family, psychosocial, and medical problems. Pediatricians seeing patients in emergency departments, trauma units, or prison must have an especially high index of suspicion. A family history of drug addiction or abuse should raise the level of concern about drug abuse in the pediatric patient. Possession of promotional products such as T-shirts and caps with cigarette or alcohol logos should also be a red flag because teenagers who own these items are more likely to use the products they advertise.

Briones DF et al: Risk factors and prevention in adolescent substance abuse: A biopsychosocial approach. Adolesc Med Clin 2006;17:335 [PMID: 16814697].

Collins RL et al: Saturated in beer: Awareness of beer advertising in late childhood and adolescence. J Adolesc Health 2005;37:29 [PMID: 15963904].

Dias PJ: Adolescent substance abuse. Assessment in the office. Pediatr Clin North Am 2002;49:269 [PMID: 11993283].

Gruber EL et al: Alcohol, tobacco and illicit substances in music videos: A content analysis of prevalence and genre. J Adolesc Health 2005;37:81 [PMID: 15963915].

Levy S et al: Office-based intervention for adolescent substance abuse. Pediatr Clin North Am 2002;49:329 [PMID: 11993286].

Schydlower M (editor): Substance Abuse: A Guide for Health Professionals, 2nd ed. American Academy of Pediatrics, 2002

Weddle M, Kokotailo P: Adolescent substance abuse. Confidentiality and consent. Pediatr Clin North Am 2002;49:301 [PMID: 11993284].

Diagnosis

Although few children and adolescents will have been abusing substances long enough to have developed overt signs and symptoms, it is important to look for them on physical examination. Positive physical findings can be a tool to penetrate a patient's denial and convince him or her of the significance of the alcohol or drug use.

When the psychosocial history suggests the possibility of substance use, the primary tasks of the diagnostic interview are the same as for the evaluation of other medical problems (Table 4–4).

First, specific information about the extent of the problem must be gathered. Eliciting multiple-choice answers is a useful technique. For example, "Has anything really good ever happened to you when you are high?" or "Some of my

Table 4–4. Causes of false-positive drug screens.

I. Define the extent of the problem by determining:
Age at onset of substance use
Which substances are being used
Circumstances of use
Where?
When?
With whom?
To what extent substances are being used
How frequently?
How much (quantity)?
With what associated symptoms (eg, tolerance, withdrawal)?
With what result?
What does the patient gain from becoming high?
Does the patient get into risky situations while high?
Does the patient engage in behaviors while high that are later regretted?
II. Define the cause of the problem by developing a differential diagnosis

patients like to get high because they feel good; others find it helps them relax and be sociable with friends; and some find it helps them forget their problems. Are any of these things true for you?"

Second, the provider needs to determine why the patient has progressed from initiation to the continuation or maintenance phase of substance abuse. The cause may be different at different periods of development. Although peer group characteristics are one of the best predictors of substance use among early and middle adolescents, this is not so among older adolescents and young adults.

In the primary care setting, insufficient time and lack of training in management of positive screens are the greatest barriers to screening adolescents for substance abuse. Brief questionnaires can be used if time does not allow for more detailed investigation. A screening instrument that has been rigorously studied in primary care settings is the CAGE questionnaire. CAGE is a mnemonic derived from the first four questions listed in Table 4–5. A score of 2 or more is highly suggestive of substance abuse.

Although constructed as a screening tool for alcohol abuse in adults, the CAGE questionnaire can be adapted to elicit similar information about use of other mood-altering substances by pediatric patients and by their close contacts (eg, parents and older siblings). Finally, clinicians may find it helpful to use such questionnaires to stimulate discussion of the patient's self-perception of his or her substance use. For example, if an adolescent admits to a previous attempt to cut down on drinking, this provides an opportunity to inquire about events that may have led to the attempt.

Knight JR et al: Motivational interviewing for adolescent substance use: a pilot study. J Adolesc Health 2005;37:167 [PMID: 16026730].

Table 4–5. CAGE questionnaire.

CUT DOWN: Have you ever felt you ought to cut down on your drinking (drug use)?

ANNOYED: Have people annoyed you by criticizing your drinking (drug use)?

GUILTY: Have you ever felt bad about your drinking (drug use)?

EYE OPENER: Have you ever had a drink (used drugs) to steady your nerves in the morning?

(Score 1 point for each positive answer; refer if total points ≥ 2)

Used, with permission, from Ewing JE: Detecting alcoholism: The CAGE questionnaire. JAMA 1984;252:1905.

Knight JR et al: Validity of brief alcohol screening tests among adolescents: A comparison of the AUDIT, POSIT, CAGE, and CRAFFT. Alcohol Clin Exp Res 2003;27:67 [PMID: 12544008].

Knight JR et al: Validity of the CRAFFT substance abuse screening test among adolescent clinic patients. Arch Pediatr Adolesc Med 2002;156:607 [PMID: 12038895].

Van Hook S et al. The "Six T's": Barriers to screening teens for substance abuse in primary care. J Adolesc Health 2007;40:456 [PMID: 17448404].

Comorbidity

There are often numerous comorbidities among substance-abusing patients. Substance abusers are more likely to have another psychiatric disorder. Affective disorder, anxiety disorder, and mania are most strongly associated with alcohol and drug dependence. Adolescents with depression are likely to use drugs in an attempt to feel pleasure, but this type of self-medication may exacerbate their condition. Attention-deficit/hyperactivity has been closely linked with adolescent substance abuse. In addition to identifying psychiatric comorbidities, it is imperative that providers look for medical conditions that mimic symptoms of drug withdrawal or intoxication. Patients with significant primary medical conditions may use illicit substances to relieve symptoms (severe pain or chemotherapeutic side effects). Although it is often difficult to determine which diagnosis is primary, it is important for pediatric health care providers to recognize the possibility of a comorbid condition and provide appropriate treatment.

Barkley RA et al: Does the treatment of attention-deficit/hyperactivity disorder with stimulants contribute to drug use/abuse? A 13-year prospective study. Pediatrics 2003;111:97 [PMID: 12509561].

Ernst M et al: Behavioral predictors of substance-use initiation in adolescents with and without attention-deficit/hyperactivity disorder. Pediatrics 2006;117:2030 [PMID: 16740845].

Mertens JR et at: Medical conditions of adolescents in alcohol and drug treatment: Comparison with matched controls. J Adolesc Health 2007;40:173 [PMID: 17259058].

Pilowsky DJ, Wu LT: Psychiatric symptoms and substance use disorders in a nationally representative sample of American adolescents involved with foster care. J Adolesc Health 2006;38:351 [PMID: 16549295].

Shrier LA et al: Substance use problems and associated psychiatric symptoms among adolescents in primary care. Pediatrics 2003;111(6 Pt 1):e699 [PMID: 12777588].

Pharmacologic Screening

The use of urine and blood testing for detecting substance abuse is controversial. The consensus is that pharmacologic screening should be reserved for situations in which behavioral dysfunction is of sufficient concern to outweigh the practical and ethical drawbacks of testing. The AAP recommends screening under certain circumstances (eg, an inexplicably obtunded patient in the emergency department) but discourages routine screening for the following reasons: (1) Voluntary screening programs are rarely truly voluntary owing to the negative consequences for those who decline to participate; (2) infrequent users or individuals who have not used substances recently may be missed; (3) confronting substance-abusing individuals with objective evidence of their use has little or no effect on their behavior; (4) the AAP reminds providers that their role is counseling and treatment, not law enforcement, so drug testing should not be done for the purpose of detecting illegal use. If testing is to be performed, the provider should discuss the plan for screening with the patient, explain the reasons for it, and obtain informed consent. The AAP does not consider parental request and permission sufficient justification for involuntary screening of mentally competent minors.

Beyond the ethical concerns, there are also practical concerns. If testing is to be performed, it is imperative that it be done accurately and that the limitations of testing be understood by all parties. Tests range from inexpensive, chromatographic spot tests, which can be performed in the office, to gas chromatography and mass spectrometry, which require specialized laboratory equipment and are usually reserved for forensic investigations. Most commercial medical laboratories use the enzyme multiplication immunoassay technique, in which a sample of the fluid to be tested is added to a test reagent containing a known quantity of the radiolabeled index drug under question. If the index drug is also present in the patient's urine or serum, it competes with the radiolabeled drug for binding sites on the test kit antibody. The unbound or excess drug can then be quantified with a spectrophotometer. Most of the commonly abused mood-altering substances, with the exception of solvents and inhalants, can be detected by this method.

Interpretation of results is complicated by false-positives resulting from antibody cross-reactions with some medications and substances (Table 4–6) or from a patient's passive exposure to illicit substances. The most common cause of false-negative tests is infrequent use. Table 4–7 shows the duration of detectability in the urine after last use by class of substance and duration of use. Detectability ranges from a few hours for alcohol to several weeks for regular marijuana use. False-negative results can occur if the patient alters or adulterates the specimen. Some of the commercial products

Table 4–6. Causes of false-positive drug screens.

Opioids
Poppy seeds
Dextromethorphan
Chlorpromazine
Diphenoxylate
Amphetamines
Ephedrine
Phenylephrine
Pseudoephedrine
N-acetylprocainamide
Chloroquine
Procainamide
Phencyclidines
Dextromethorphan
Diphenhydramine
Chlorpromazine
Doxylamine
Thioridazine

used to adulterate samples include glutaraldehyde, nitrite, pyridinium chlorochromate, peroxidate, and peroxide (stealth). Household products such as bleach, vinegar, Visine eye drops (for marijuana), strong alkali drain cleaners, and detergents are also used. (Teenagers should be advised that despite street lore, ingesting these compounds is an ineffec-

Table 4–7. Duration of urine positivity for selected drugs.

Drug Class	Detection Time
Amphetamines	< 48 h
Barbiturates	Short-acting: 1 d Long-acting: 2–3 wk
Benzodiazepines	Single dose: 3 d Habitual use: 4–6 wk
Cocaine metabolites	Acute use: 2–4 d Habitual use: 2 wk
Ethanol	2–14 h
Methadone	Up to 3 d
Opioids	Up to 2 d
Propoxyphene	6–48 h
Cannabinoids	Moderate use: 5 d Habitual use: 10–20 d
Methaqualone	2 wk
Phencyclidine	Acute use: 1 wk Habitual use: 3 wk
Anabolic steroids	Days to weeks

Reprinted, with permission, from Woolf A, Shannon M: Clinical toxicology for the pediatrician. Pediatr Clin North Am 1995;42:317.

tive and potentially dangerous way to prevent drug detection in the urine.) Close observation during collection and pre-testing the temperature, specific gravity, and pH of urine samples may detect attempts at deception.

Internet-based home drug-testing products are available for parents; however, these products have limitations and potential risks. The AAP recommends that home and school-based drug testing not be implemented until the safety and efficacy of these procedures can be established. It further recommends that parents be encouraged to consult the adolescent's primary care provider rather than relying on home drug-testing products.

American Academy of Pediatrics Committee on Substance Abuse: Testing for drugs of abuse in children and adolescents. Pediatrics 1996;98:305 [PMID: 8692638].

Committee on Substance Abuse, American Academy of Pediatrics; Council on School Health, American Academy of Pediatrics, Knight JR, Mears CJ: Testing for drugs of abuse in children and adolescents: Addendum—testing in schools and at home. Pediatrics 2007;119:627 [PMID: 17332219].

Jaffee WB et al: Is this urine really negative? A systematic review of tampering methods in urine drug screening and testing. J Subst Abuse Treat 2007;33:33 [PMID: 17588487].

Knight J, Levy S: The national debate on drug testing in schools. J Adolesc Health 2007;41:419 [PMID: 17950160].

Levy S et al: Drug testing of adolescents in ambulatory medicine: Physician practices and knowledge. Arch Pediatr Adolesc Med 2006;160:146 [PMID: 16461869].

Levy S et al: Drug testing of adolescents in general medical clinics, in school and at home: Physician attitudes and practices. J Adolesc Health 2006;38:336 [PMID: 16549293].

Levy S et al: Results of random drug testing in an adolescent substance abuse program. Pediatrics 2007;119:e843 [PMID: 17403828].

Levy S, Van Hook S, Knight J: A review of Internet-based home drug-testing products for parents. Pediatrics 2004;113:720 [PMID15060218].

TREATMENT & REFERRAL

Office-Based Treatment

The AMA and the AAP recommend that all children and adolescents receive counseling about the dangers of substance use and abuse from their primary care providers. By offering confidential health care services and routinely counseling about the risks associated with drug abuse, primary care providers can help most patients avoid the adverse consequences of experimentation with mood-altering substances. However, more intervention is required for youngsters in environments where substance abuse is regarded as acceptable recreational behavior. Counseling strategies appropriate for patients who wish to change their behavior may be ineffective for patients who do not consider use of mood-altering substances to be a problem. It may therefore be preferable to begin discussions about treatment by helping youngsters consider alternative ways of meeting the needs that substance use is currently providing. The clinician may in this way help the patient devise alternatives that are more attractive than substance use. Realistically, few substance-abusing teenagers will choose to quit because of a single conversation even with a highly respected health care provider. The message is most effective when offered repeatedly from many sources—family, peers, guidance counselors, and teachers. Brief interventions for adolescents have shown some improvement among high-risk youth. Motivational interviewing for substance-abusing teens has shown some promise.

Assessment of the patient's readiness to change is the critical first step in office-based intervention. Clinicians should consider the construct presented in Table 4–8. In theory, individuals pass through this series of stages in the course of changing problem behaviors. Thus, to be maximally effective, providers should tailor their counseling messages to the patient's stage of readiness to change.

Once it has been established that a patient is prepared to act on information about treatment, the next step is to select the program that best fits his or her individual needs. Most drug treatment programs are not designed to recognize and act on the individual vulnerabilities that have predisposed the patient to substance abuse. When programs are individualized, even brief (5- to 10-minute) counseling sessions may promote reductions in cigarette smoking and drinking. This strategy appears to be most effective when the health care provider's message is part of an office-wide program so that the entire staff reinforces the cessation message with every patient.

Table 4–8. Stages of change and intervention tasks.

Patient Stage	Motivation Tasks
Precontemplation	Create doubt, increase the patient's awareness of risks and problems with current patterns of substance use
Contemplation	Help the patient weigh the relative risks and benefits of changing substance use; evoke reasons to change and risks of not changing; strengthen the patient's self-efficacy for changing current use
Determination	Help the patient determine the best course of action to change substance use from among available alternatives
Action	Help the patient establish a clear plan of action toward changing substance use
Maintenance	Help the patient identify and use strategies to prevent relapse
Relapse	Help the patient renew the process of change starting at contemplation

Reprinted, with permission, from Werner MJ: Principles of brief intervention for adolescent alcohol, tobacco, and other drug use. Pediatr Clin North Am 1995;42:341.

Grenard JL et al: Brief intervention for substance use among at-risk adolescents: A pilot study. J Adolesc Health 2007;40:188 [PMID: 17259065].

Grenard JL et al: Motivational interviewing with adolescents and young adults for drug-related problems. Int J Adolesc Med Health 2006;18:53 [PMID: 16639859].

Knight JR et al: Motivational interviewing for adolescent substance use: a pilot study. J Adolesc Health 2005;37:167 [PMID: 16026730].

Smoking Cessation in Pediatrics

Although more than half of adolescents who smoke regularly say they want to quit and have tried to quit, only a minority report that they have been advised or helped to do so by a health care provider. Practitioners unfamiliar with approaches to smoking cessation may feel that smoking cessation interventions are time-consuming, nonreimbursable, and impractical in a busy office. An easy guideline for health care providers is the "Five As" for tobacco cessation (Table 4–9), published by the Public Health Service and endorsed by the AAP.

Smoking cessation is a process that takes time. Relapse must be regarded as a normal part of quitting rather than evidence of personal failure or a reason to forgo further attempts. Patients can actually benefit from relapses if they are helped to identify the circumstances that led to the relapse and to devise strategies to prevent subsequent relapses or respond to them in a different manner.

Nicotine is a physically and psychologically addictive substance. Replacement therapy improves smoking cessation rates and may relieve withdrawal symptoms. Two types of nicotine replacement therapies are available. Nicotine gum and transdermal nicotine patches are recommended for teens.

Providers should be aware that adolescents may not exhibit the same symptoms of nicotine dependence as adults, and that dependence may be established within as little as 4 weeks. Those who are not comfortable prescribing and monitoring nicotine replacement therapies should limit their involvement with patients who smoke to those who do not exhibit signs of nicotine dependency (eg, patients who smoke less than a pack of cigarettes a day or do not feel a

Table 4–9. "Five As" for tobacco cessation.

Ask about tobacco use from all patients
Advise all tobacco users to quit
Assess willingness and motivation for tobacco user to make a quit attempt
Assist in the quit attempt
Arrange for follow-up

Adapted from Fiore MC et al: *Treating Tobacco Use and Dependence. Clinical Practice Guidelines*. U.S. Department of Health and Human Services, Public Health Service, 2000.

craving to smoke their first cigarette within 30 minutes after waking). In addition to nicotine replacement therapies, sustained-release forms of the antidepressants bupropion, clonidine, and nortriptyline have been shown in randomized trials to help smokers quit and to decrease relapse rates fivefold.

Adelman WP: Tobacco use cessation for adolescents. Adolesc Med Clin 2006;17:697 [PMID: 1703028].

American Academy of Pediatrics Committee on Substance Abuse: Tobacco's toll: Implications for the pediatrician. Pediatrics 2001;107:794 [PMID: 11335763].

Bagot KS et al: Tobacco craving predicts lapse to smoking among adolescent smokers in cessation treatment. Nicotine Tob Res 2007;9:647 [PMID: 17558821].

Fagan P et al: Addressing tobacco-related health disparities. Addiction 2007;102(Suppl 2):30 [PMID: 17850612].

Fiore MC et al: *Treating Tobacco Use and Dependence. Clinical Practice Guidelines.* U.S. Department of Health and Human Services, Public Health Service, 2000.

Irwin CE Jr: Tobacco use during adolescence and young adulthood: The battle is not over. J Adolesc Health 2004;35:169 [PMID: 15313497].

Prokhorov AV et al: Tobacco Consortium, American Academy of Pediatrics Center for Child Health Research: Youth tobacco use: A global perspective for child health care clinicians. Pediatrics 2006;118:e890 [PMID: 16950972].

VA/DoD clinical practice guideline for the management of tobacco use. Department of Veteran Affairs, 2004.

Wheeler KC et al: Screening adolescents for nicotine dependence: The Hooked On Nicotine Checklist. J Adolesc Health 2004;35:225 [PMID: 15313504].

Ziedonis D at al: Adolescent tobacco use and dependence: Assessment and treatment strategies. Adolesc Med Clin 2006;17:381 [PMID: 16814699].

Referral

There is no consensus about which substance-abusing patients can be adequately treated in the office, which require referral, and which require hospitalization. Factors to be considered are summarized in Table 4–10. When doubt exists about the seriousness of the problem or the advisability of office management, consultation with a specialist should be sought.

Although most primary pediatric providers will not assume responsibility for the treatment of substance-abusing youngsters, clinicians can be instrumental in motivating their patients to seek treatment and in guiding them to appropriate treatment resources. Substance-abusing teenagers must be treated in teen-oriented treatment facilities. Despite the similarities between adult and adolescent substance abuse, adult programs are usually developmentally inappropriate and ineffective for adolescents. As discussed in Chapter 3, many adolescents are concrete thinkers. Their inability to reason deductively, especially about emotionally charged issues, makes it difficult for them to understand the abstract concepts (such as denial) that are an integral component of most adult-oriented programs. This invariably

Table 4–10. Factors to consider prior to referral for substance abuse.

Duration and frequency of substance use
The type of substances being used
Presence of other psychological disorders
Attention-deficit/hyperactivity disorder
Depression
Antisocial personality disorder
Presence of other social morbidities
School failure
Delinquency
Homelessness
Ongoing or past physical or sexual abuse
Program evaluation
View on substance abuse as primary disorder vs symptom
Offers comprehensive evaluation of patient and can manage associated problems identified in initial assessment (eg, comorbid conditions)
Adherence to abstinence philosophy
Patient-to-staff ratios
Separate adolescent and adult treatment programs
Follow-up and continuing care

frustrates counselors who misinterpret lack of comprehension as resistance to therapy, and concrete responses as evidence of deceit.

Treatment programs range from low-intensity, outpatient, school-based student assistance programs, which rely heavily on peers and nonprofessionals, to residential, hospital-based programs staffed by psychiatrists and other professionals. Outpatient counseling programs are most appropriate for motivated patients who do not have significant mental health or behavioral problems and are not at risk for withdrawal. Some investigators have raised the concern that in pediatric settings, low-problem users may actually experience a strengthening of the drug subculture by associating with high-problem users in group therapy. More intensive day treatment programs are available for those who require a structured environment. Inpatient treatment should be considered for patients who need medical care and detoxification in addition to counseling, education, and family therapy.

Finally, special dual-diagnosis facilities are available for substance-abusing patients who also have other psychological conditions. These patients are difficult to diagnose and treat because it is often unclear whether their symptoms are a consequence of substance use or a symptom of a comorbid psychological disorder. Recognition of such disorders is critical because they must be treated in programs that include psychiatric expertise.

Approaches to the treatment of substance abuse in children and adolescents are typically modeled after adult treatment programs. Key elements of an effective adolescent drug treatment program include: assessment and treatment matching, comprehensive, integrated treatment approach, family involvement, developmentally appropriate program, engaging and retaining teens, qualified staff, gender and cultural competence, continuing care, and treatment outcomes. Several studies of adolescent substance abuse treatment programs have shown that many do not adequately address all of the important components of therapy.

Anton RF, Swift RM: Current pharmacotherapies of alcoholism: A U.S. perspective. Am J Addict 2003;12:S53 [PMID: 14972780].

Bertholet N et al: Reduction of alcohol consumption by brief alcohol intervention in primary care: systematic review and meta-analysis. Arch Intern Med 2005;165:986 [PMID: 15883236].

Brannigan R et al: The quality of highly regarded adolescent substance abuse treatment programs: Results of an in-depth national survey. Arch Pediatr Adolesc Med 2004;158:904 [PMID: 15351757].

Cox LS et al: Efficacy of bupropion for relapse prevention in smokers with and without a past history of major depression. J Gen Intern Med 2004;19:828 [PMID: 15242467].

Horigian VE et al: Cultural differences in adolescent drug abuse. Adolesc Med Clin 2006;17:469 [PMID: 16814703].

Mark TL et al: Characterizing substance abuse programs that treat adolescents. J Subst Abuse Treat 2006;31:59 [PMID: 16814011].

PREVENTION

Prevention of substance abuse has been a public health priority since the 1980s. Pediatric health care providers are important as advocates and educators of the community and government on developmentally appropriate programs. *Primary level* programs focus on preventing the initiation of substance use. The Drug Awareness and Resistance Education (D.A.R.E.) program is a familiar example of a primary prevention program that attempts to educate elementary and middle school students about the adverse consequences of substance abuse and enable them to resist peer pressures.

Secondary level programs target populations at increased risk for substance use. The aim is to prevent progression from initiation to continuance and maintenance, relying on individualized intervention to reduce the risk and enhance the protective factors listed in Table 4–3. This approach enables the provider to focus scarce resources on those who are most likely to benefit from them. Alateen, which supports the children of alcoholic parents, typifies secondary level prevention.

Tertiary level prevention programs target young people who have been identified as substance abusers. The aim is to prevent the morbid consequences of substance use. One example is identifying adolescents who misuse alcohol and drugs at parties and providing them with a safe ride home. Because prevention is more effective when targeted at reducing the initiation of substance use than at decreasing use, tertiary prevention is the least effective approach.

Very few population-based programs undergo rigorous scientific evaluation. It is the consensus among drug educators that primary prevention programs, such as D.A.R.E., have minimal effect in decreasing the use of illicit substances.

During the 1990s, when these programs were most popular, a smaller proportion of middle- and high-school students perceived illicit drug and alcohol use as dangerous, and substance use actually increased. Even when knowledge- and resistance-based programs do increase student understanding of adverse consequences, there is no evidence that they change attitudes or abuse rates.

The failure of resistance education programs has fostered interest in a potentially more effective type of program, exemplified by the Adolescents Training and Learning to Avoid Steroids program. This program, a same-sex, peer-educator program designed to simultaneously reduce the use of steroids and improve dietary and exercise habits of teen athletes has proven effective in randomized controlled trials. Pediatric health care providers should promote developmentally appropriate prevention programs like this one that address the social and psychological problems predisposing youngsters to substance abuse and provide realistic alternative solutions.

Parents and others should understand that most adolescents who abuse alcohol and drugs do not do so just for the high. Rather, these behaviors are often purposeful, developmentally appropriate coping strategies. To the extent that these behaviors meet young peoples' developmental needs, they are not apt to be abandoned unless equally attractive alternatives are available. For example, even though many teenagers cite stress and anxiety as reasons for smoking, teen-oriented smoking cessation programs rarely address the young smoker's need for alternative coping strategies by offering stress management training. Similarly, for the youngster growing up in an impoverished urban environment, the real costs of substance abuse may be too low and the rewards too high to be influenced by talk and knowledge alone. It is unreasonable to expect a talk-based intervention to change attitudes and behaviors in a direction that is opposite to that of the child's own social milieu. The efficacy of the most promising prevention models and interventions is apt to decay over time unless changes in the social environment provide substance-abusing children and adolescents with realistic alternative ways to meet their developmental needs.

Goldberg L et al: Drug testing athletes to prevent substance abuse: background and pilot study results of the SATURN (Student Athlete Testing Using Random Notification) study. J Adolesc Health 2003;32:16 [PMID: 12507797].

Perry CL et al: A randomized controlled trial of the middle and junior high school D.A.R.E. and D.A.R.E. Plus programs. Arch Pediatr Adolesc Med 2003;157:178 [PMID: 12580689].

REFERENCES

Web Resources

American Lung Association (site for and by teens): http://www.lungusa.org/smokefreeclass

Monitoring the Future Study (detailed information and longitudinal data): http://www.monitoringthefuture.org

National Clearinghouse Drug and Alcohol Abuse (information and resources, including free publications for providers, parents, and adolescents): http://www.health.org

National Institute on Drug Abuse: http://www.nida.nih.gov

Substance Use and Mental Health Services Administration (SAMSA; resources for both substance use and mental health services): http://www.samhsa.gov

I would like to dedicate this chapter to Catherine Stevens Simon for her heart and nurturing soul. —PK

Eating Disorders

Eric J. Sigel, MD

Teenagers and younger children continue to develop eating disorders at a significant rate. The spectrum of eating disorders includes anorexia nervosa (AN), bulimia nervosa (BN), eating disorders not otherwise specified (EDNOS), and binge-eating disorder. The relationship between genetics and environment in the development of eating disorders is complex. These disorders are best defined in a biopsychosocial context.

ETIOLOGY

A genetic susceptibility to develop eating disorders probably exists. The incidence of AN is 7% in first-degree relatives of anorexic patients compared with 1–2% in the general population. The concordance rate in monozygotic twins is 55%, compared with 7% in dizygotic twins. Twin studies estimate the heritability of AN as 33–84%, and BN as 28–83%. First-degree female relatives of males with AN have a 20-fold relative risk of AN. Most studies have found a higher incidence of eating disorders among first-degree relatives of bulimic patients as well. Genomic regions on chromosome 1 (for AN) and chromosome 10 (for BN) appear to harbor susceptibility genes.

Abnormalities of leptin, a hormone secreted by adipocytes that regulates energy homeostasis and satiety signaling, do not appear to cause AN primarily, but may mediate energy changes that affect the hypothalamic-pituitary axis and play a role in perpetuating AN. Leptin physiology is deranged in patients with AN. Leptin levels increase to excessive levels as individuals regain weight. The idiosyncratic higher levels of leptin may contribute to the difficulty AN patients have when trying to regain weight, as higher leptin levels signal the body to decrease energy intake. Leptin also plays a significant role in some of the sequelae of AN, with low levels signaling the hypothalamus to inhibit reproductive hormone production.

There is evidence of persistently altered serotonergic and [do]minergic function in AN. Other alterations in neu-

ropeptides and gut peptides are found both in AN and BN. Adiponectin appears elevated in AN, although it is unclear whether this is due to the malnourished state, or elevated independently of malnutrition. Cholecystokinin is decreased in BN, perhaps contributing to the lack of postingestion satiety that perpetuates a binge. An alteration in dopamine has also been recognized, although its significance is not clear. Ghrelin, a gut peptide, is elevated in patients with AN and does not decrease in the normal fashion after a meal in these patients.

Despite significant research into the neurobiology of eating disorders, it remains unclear whether alterations contribute to the development of eating disorders or are present as a consequence of the physiologic changes associated with the disorders. Patients with BN or binge-eating disorder appear to have a blunted serotonin response to eating and satiety. With a decreased satiety response, patients continue to eat, leading to a binge. Treatment with selective serotonin reuptake inhibitors (SSRIs) tends to equilibrate satiety regulation. More research is needed to determine which factors are causative and which are results of the eating disorder.

Traditional psychological theory has suggested many environmental factors that might promote the development of eating disorders. Enmeshment of mother with daughter to the point that the teenager cannot develop her own identity (a key developmental marker of adolescence) may be a predisposing factor. The teenager may cope by asserting control over food, as she senses her lack of control in the developmental realm. A second theory involves father-daughter distancing. As puberty progresses and a girl's sexuality blossoms, a father may experience difficulty in dealing with his daughter as a sexual being and may respond by withdrawing both emotionally and physically. The teenage girl may intuitively recognize this and subconsciously decrease her food intake in order to become prepubertal again. A third theory is related to puberty itself. Some teenagers may fear or dislike their changing bodies. By restricting food intake they lose weight, stop menstruating, and effectively reverse pubertal development.

Society has provided the message that being thin or muscular is necessary for attractiveness and success. The ease of access to diet products—foods and diet pills—as well as internet instructions (pro-anorexia sites) makes it simple for adolescents to embark on a quest for thinness or muscularity.

Genetic predisposition, psychological factors, and environmental factors combine to create a milieu that promotes adolescent eating disorders.

Bailer UF, Kaye WH: A review of neuropeptide and neuroendocrine dysregulation in anorexia and bulimia nervosa. Curr Drug Target CNS Neurol Disord 2003;2:53 [PMID: 12769812].

Bosanac P et al: Serotonergic and dopaminergic systems in anorexia nervosa: A role for atypical antipsychotics? Aust N Z J Psychiatry 2005;39:146 [PMID: 15701063].

Bulik CM, Tozzi F: Genetics in eating disorders: State of the science. CNS Spectrums 2005;9:511 [PMID: 15208510].

Chan JL, Manzoros CS: Role of leptin in energy deprived states: Normal human physiology and clinical implications for hypothalamic amenorrhea and anorexia nervosa. Lancet 2005;366:74 [PMID: 15993236].

Modin-Moses D et al: Modulation of adiponectin and leptin during refeeding of female anorexia nervosa patients. J Clin Endo Metab 2007;92:1843 [PMID: 17327386].

Strober M et al: Males with anorexia nervosa: A controlled study of eating disorders in first-degree relatives. Int J Eat Disord 2001;29:263 [PMID: 11262504].

Tolle V et al: Balance in ghrelin and leptin plasma levels in anorexia nervosa patients and constitutionally thin women. J Clin Endocrinol Metab 2003;88:109 [PMID: 12519838].

INCIDENCE

AN is the third most common chronic illness of teenaged girls in the United States. The incidence has been increasing steadily in the United States since the 1930s. Although ascertaining exact incidence is difficult, most studies show that 1–2% of teenagers develop AN and 2–4% develop BN. Adolescents outnumber adults 5 to 1, although the number of adults with eating disorders is rising. Incidence is also increasing among younger children. Prepubertal patients often have significant associated psychiatric diagnoses. Males comprise about 10% of the patients with eating disorders, and this prevalence appears to be increasing. Prevalence of full or partial syndrome BN is 1.1% in males and 3.2% in females (1:2.9 male-to-female ratio). Prevalence of full or partial syndrome AN is 0.9% in males and 1.8% in females (1:2 ratio). The increasing number of males with eating disorders correlates with the increased media emphasis on muscular, chiseled appearance as the male ideal.

Recent literature on preadolescents with eating disorders suggests that patients younger than 13 years are more likely to be male and more likely to have EDNOS. Younger patients are less likely to engage in behaviors characteristic of BN. They present with more rapid weight loss and lower percentile body weight than adolescents.

Many youth engage in some eating disorder behaviors. In the most recent Youth Risk Behavior Survey of U.S. teenagers published by the Centers for Disease Control and Prevention (Eaton et al, 2005), 62% of females and 30% of males had attempted to lose weight during the 30 days preceding the survey. Twelve percent had fasted for more than 24 hours to lose weight, and 6.1% had used diet pills, powders, or liquids to lose weight (8.1% of girls and 4.6% of boys). Self-induced vomiting or laxative use was common; 6.2% of females and 2.8% of males used one or the other. Forty-six percent of females and 30% of males reported at least one bingeing episode during their lifetime. Although the number of youth with full-blown eating disorders is low, it is alarming that so many youth experiment with unhealthy weight control habits. These signs may be precursors to the development of eating disorders, and clinicians should explore these practices with all of their adolescent patients.

Eaton DK et al: Youth Risk Behavior Surveillance—United States 2005. MMWR Surveill Summ 2006;55(SS05):1 [PMID: 16760893]. Available at: http://www.cdc.gov/mmwr/preview/mmwrhtml/ss5505a1.htm.

Peebles R et al: How do children with eating disorders differ from adolescents with eating disorders at initial evaluation? J Adolesc Health 2006;39:800 [PMID: 17116508].

Woodside DB et al: Comparisons of men with full or partial eating disorders, men without eating disorders, and women with eating disorders in the community. Am J Psychol 2001;158:570 [PMID: 11282690]

PREDISPOSING FACTORS

In the past, the typical anorexic patient was described as a high-achieving, athletic, straight-A student from a middle-class family. Demographics have changed, and eating disorders now occur across all racial and ethnic groups. There is no difference among blacks, Asians, Hispanics, and whites in the frequency of eating disorder symptoms or eating disorder risk factors. Children involved in gymnastics, figure skating, and ballet—activities that emphasize (and in which coaches often require) thin bodies—are at higher risk for anorexia than are children in sports that do not emphasize body image. Adolescents who believe that being thin represents the ideal frame for a female, those who are dissatisfied with their bodies, and those with a history of dieting are at increased risk for eating disorders. Sudden changes in dietary habits, such as becoming vegetarian, may be a first sign of anorexia, especially if the change is abrupt and without good reason.

The typical bulimic patient is more impulsive, tending engage in risk-taking behavior such as alcohol use, drug and sexual experimentation. Bulimic patients are of appropriate weight for height or slightly overweis' have average academic performance. Some stv that 50% of bulimic patients have been sex Youth with diabetes have an increased risk ' wrestling predisposes to BN, and homose associated with binge eating.

Shaw H et al: Body image and eating disturbances across ethnic groups: More similarities than differences. Psychol Addict Behav 2004;18:8 [PMID: 15008651].

Striegel-Moore RH, Bulik CM: Risk factors for eating disorders. Am Psychol 2007;62:181 [PMID: 17469897].

ANOREXIA NERVOSA

Table 5–1 lists the diagnostic criteria for AN, according to the *Diagnostic and Statistical Manual of Mental Disorders, Fourth Edition, Text Revision* (DSM-IV-TR). There are two forms of AN. In the restricting type, patients do not regularly engage in binge eating or purging. In the purging type, classic AN is combined with binge eating or purging behavior, or both. Distinguishing between the two is important as they carry different implications for prognosis and treatment. There is ongoing debate about the criteria for AN. Some experts suggest eliminating amenorrhea as a specific criterion. Though patients may not demonstrate all features of AN, they may still exhibit the deleterious symptoms associated with AN.

▶ Clinical Findings

A. Symptoms and Signs

Clinicians should recognize the early symptoms and signs of AN because early intervention may prevent the full-blown syndrome from developing. Patients may show some of the behaviors and psychology of AN, such as reduction in dietary fat and intense concern with body image, even before weight loss or amenorrhea occurs.

Making the diagnosis of AN can be challenging because adolescents may try to conceal their illness. Assessing the patient's body image is essential to determining the diagnosis. Table 5–2 lists screening questions that help tease out a teenager's perceptions of body image. Other diagnostic screening tools (eg, Eating Attitudes Test) assess a range of eating and dieting behaviors. Parental observations are critical in determining whether a patient has expressed dissatisfaction over body habitus and determining which weight loss techniques the child has used. If the teenager is unwilling to share his or her concerns about body image, the clinician may find clues to the diagnosis by carefully considering other presenting symptoms. Weight loss from a baseline of normal body weight is an obvious red flag and should raise the clinical suspicion for the presence of an eating disorder. Additionally, AN should be considered in any girl with secondary amenorrhea who has lost weight.

Physical symptoms are usually secondary to weight loss and proportional to the degree of malnutrition. The body effectively goes into hibernation, becoming functionally hypothyroid (euthyroid sick) to save energy. Body temperature decreases, and patients report being colder than normal. Patients become bradycardic, especially in the supine position. Dizziness, lightheadedness, and syncope may occur as a result of orthostasis and hypotension secondary to impaired cardiac function. Left ventricular mass is decreased (as is the mass of all striated muscle), stroke volume is compromised, and peripheral resistance is increased, contributing to left ventricular systolic dysfunction. Patients can develop prolonged QTc syndrome and increased QT dispersion, putting them at risk for cardiac arrhythmias. Peripheral circulation is reduced. Hands and feet may be blue and cool. Hair thins, nails become brittle, and skin becomes dry. Lanugo develops as a primitive response to starvation. The gastrointestinal (GI) tract may be affected. Inability to take in normal quantities of food, early satiety, and gastroesophageal reflux can develop as the body adapts to reduced intake. The normal gastrocolic reflex may be lost due to lack of stimulation by food, causing bloating and constipation. One study

Table 5–1. Diagnostic criteria for anorexia nervosa.

A. Refusal to maintain body weight at or above a minimally normal weight for age and height (eg, weight loss leading to maintenance of body weight less than 85% of that expected; or failure to make expected weight gain during a period of growth, leading to body weight less than 85% of that expected).
B. Intense fear of gaining weight or becoming fat, even though underweight.
C. Disturbance in the way in which one's body weight or shape is experienced, undue influence of body weight or shape on self-evaluation, or denial of the seriousness of the current low body weight.
D. In postmenarchal females, amenorrhea, ie, the absence of at least three menstrual cycles. (A woman is considered to have amenorrhea if her periods occur only following hormone, eg, estrogen, administration.)

Reprinted, with permission, from the *Diagnostic and Statistical Manual of Mental Disorders,* 4th ed, text revision. Copyright 2000. American Psychiatric Association.

Table 5–2. Screening questions to help diagnose anorexia and bulimia nervosa.

How do you feel about your body?
Are there parts of your body you might change?
When you look at yourself in the mirror, do you see yourself as overweight, underweight, or satisfactory?
If overweight, how much do you want to weigh?
If your weight is satisfactory, has there been a time that you were worried about being overweight?
If overweight [underweight], what would you change?
Have you ever been on a diet?
What have you done to help yourself lose weight?
Do you count calories or fat grams?
Do you keep your intake to a certain number of calories?
Have you ever used nutritional supplements, diet pills, or laxatives to help you lose weight?
Have you ever made yourself vomit to get rid of food or lose weight?

showed that delayed gastric emptying is present in restricting type and purging type AN. Long-term physical rehabilitation improves gastric emptying and dyspeptic symptoms in AN restricting type, but not inpurgers.

Neurologically, patients may experience decreased cognition, inability to concentrate, increased irritability, and depression, which may be related to structural brain changes and decreased cerebral blood flow.

A combination of malnutrition and stress causes hypothalamic hypogonadism. The hypothalamic-pituitary-gonadal axis shuts down as the body struggles to survive, directing finite energy resources to vital functions. This may be mediated by the effect of low serum leptin on the hypothalamic-pituitary axis. Both males and females experience decreased libido and interruption of pubertal development, depending on the timing of the illness. Skeletal growth may be interrupted.

Nutritional assessment is vital. Often patients eliminate fat from their diets and may eat as few as 100–200 kcal/d. A gown-only weight after urination is the most accurate way to assess weight. Patients tend to wear bulky clothes and may hide weights in their pockets or drink excessive fluid (water-loading) to trick the practitioner. Calculating body mass index (BMI)—weight in kilograms divided by height in meters squared—is an efficient way to interpret degree of malnutrition. BMI below the 25th percentile indicates risk for malnutrition, and one below the fifth percentile significant malnutrition. Ideal body weight (IBW) for height should be calculated, using the 50th percentile of BMI for age. A weight less than 85% IBW is one of the diagnostic criteria for AN.

A hallmark physical sign of girls with AN is amenorrhea, which occurs for two reasons. The hypothalamic-pituitary-ovarian axis shuts down under stress, causing hypothalamic amenorrhea. Additionally, adipose tissue is needed to convert estrogen to its activated form. When weight loss is significant, adipose tissue is lost and there is not enough substrate to activate estrogen. Resumption of normal menses occurs only when both body weight and body fat increase. Approximately 73% of postmenarchal girls will resume menstruating if they reach 90% of IBW. An adolescent female needs about 17% body fat to restart menses and 22% body fat if she has primary amenorrhea. One study demonstrated that target weight gain for return of menses is approximately 1 kg higher than the weight at which menses ceased.

B. Laboratory Findings

Most organ systems can suffer some degree of damage in the anorexic patient, related both to severity and duration of illness (Table 5–3). Initial screening should include complete blood count with differential; serum levels of electrolytes, blood urea nitrogen, creatinine, phosphorus, calcium, magnesium, and thyroid-stimulating hormone; liver function tests; and urinalysis. An electrocardiogram should be performed, because significant electrocardiographic abnormalities may be present, most importantly prolonged QTc syn-

Table 5–3. Laboratory findings: anorexia nervosa.

Increased blood urea nitrogen and creatinine secondary to renal insufficiency
Decreased white blood cells, platelets, and less commonly red blood cells and hematocrit secondary to bone marrow suppression or fat atrophy of the bone marrow
Increased AST and ALT secondary to malnutrition
Increased cholesterol, thought to be related to fatty acid metabolism
Decreased alkaline phosphatase secondary to zinc deficiency
Low to low-normal thyroid-stimulating hormone and thyroxine
Decreased follicle-stimulating hormone, luteinizing hormone, estradiol, and testosterone secondary to shutdown of hypothalamic-pituitary-gonadal axis
Abnormal electrolytes related to hydration status
Decreased phosphorus
Decreased insulin-like growth factor
Increased cortisol
Decreased urine specific gravity in cases of intentional water intoxication

ALT, alanine aminotransferase; AST, aspartate aminotransferase.

drome. Bone densitometry should be done if amenorrhea has persisted for 6 months, as patients begin to accumulate risk for osteoporosis.

Differential Diagnosis

If the diagnosis is unclear (ie, the patient has lost a significant amount of weight but does not have typical body image distortion or fat phobia), then the clinician must consider the differential diagnosis for weight loss in adolescents. This includes inflammatory bowel disease, diabetes, hyperthyroidism, malignancy, and depression. Less common diagnoses include adrenal insufficiency and malabsorption syndromes such as celiac disease. The history and physical examination should direct specific laboratory and radiologic evaluation.

Complications (Table 5–4)

A. Short-Term Complications

1. Early satiety—Patients may have significant difficulty tolerating even modest quantities of food as their bodies adapt to increased caloric intake. Gastric emptying is poor. Pancreatic and biliary secretion is diminished. Patients may benefit from a gastric-emptying agent such as metoclopramide. This complication usually resolves after a patient has become used to larger meals.

2. Superior mesenteric artery syndrome—As patient become malnourished, the fat pad between the super mesenteric artery and the duodenum may shrink, com ing the transverse duodenum and causing vomit intolerance of oral intake, especially solids. D made by an upper GI series showing to and fro barium in the descending and transverse du mal to the obstruction. Treatment involve.

Table 5-4. Complications of anorexia and bulimia nervosa.

Cardiovascular
  Bradycardia
  Postural hypotension
  Arrhythmia, sudden death
  Congestive heart failure (during refeeding)
  Pericardial effusion
  Mitral valve prolapse
  ECG abnormalities (prolonged QT, low voltage, T-wave abnormalities, conduction defects)
Endocrine
  ↑ LH, FSH
  ↓ T_3, ↑ rT_3; ↓ T_4, TSH
  Irregular menses
  Amenorrhea
  Hypercortisolism
  Growth retardation
  Delayed puberty
Gastrointestinal
  Dental erosion
  Parotid swelling
  Esophagitis, esophageal tears
  Delayed gastric emptying
  Gastric dilation (rarely rupture)
  Pancreatitis
  Constipation
  Diarrhea (laxative abuse)
  Superior mesenteric artery syndrome
  Hypercholesterolemia
  ↑ Liver function tests (fatty infiltration of the liver)
	Hematologic
	  Leukopenia
	  Anemia
	  Thrombocytopenia
	  ↓ ESR
	  Impaired cell-mediated immunity
	Metabolic
	  Dehydration
	  Acidosis
	  Hypokalemia
	  Hyponatremia
	  Hypochloremia
	  Hypochloremic alkalosis
	  Hypocalcemia
	  Hypophosphatemia
	  Hypomagnesemia
	  Hypercarotenemia
	Neurologic
	  Cortical atrophy
	  Peripheral neuropathy
	  Seizures
	  Thermoregulatory abnormalities
	  ↓ REM and slow-wave sleep
	Renal
	  Hematuria
	  Proteinuria
	  ↓ Renal concentrating ability
	Skeletal
	  Osteopenia
	  Fractures

ECG, electrocardiogram; ESR, erythrocyte sedimentation rate; FSH, follicle-stimulating hormone; LH, luteinizing hormone; REM, rapid eye movement; rT_3, resin triiodothyronine uptake; T_3, triiodothyronine; T_4, thyroxine; TSH, thyroid-stimulating hormone.

nasoduodenal feedings until restoration of the fat pad has occurred, coincident with weight gain.

3. Constipation—Patients may have prolonged constipation, often not having a bowel movement for several weeks. Two mechanisms contribute: loss of the gastrocolic reflex and loss of colonic muscle tone. Typically stool softeners are not effective because the colon has decreased peristaltic amplitude. Agents that induce peristalsis, such as bisacodyl, as well as osmotic agents, such as polyethylene glycol–electrolyte solution (MiraLax), are helpful. Constipation can persist for up to 6–8 weeks after refeeding. Occasionally enemas are required.

4. Refeeding syndrome—This is described in the Treatment section.

B. Long-Term Complications

1. Osteoporosis—Approximately 50% of females with AN have reduced bone mass at one or more sites. The causes of osteopenia and osteoporosis are multiple. Estrogen and testosterone are essential to potentiate bone development. Higher

ghrelin level is an independent predicator of bone density in healthy adolescents; however, it does not appear to contribute to bone loss in patients with AN. Teenagers are particularly at risk as they accrue 40% of their bone mineral during adolescence. Low body weight is most predictive of bone loss. Amenorrhea, an indicator of estrogen deficiency and hypothalamic amenorrhea, is highly correlated with osteoporosis. Bone minerals begin to resorb without estrogen. Elevated cortisol levels and decreased insulin-like growth factor-1 also contribute to bone resorption. Studies show that as few as 6 months of amenorrhea can lead to osteopenia or osteoporosis. In one study, 44% of adolescents with anorexia had osteopenia of the lumbar spine. Males also can develop osteoporosis due to decreased testosterone and elevated cortisol.

A recent finding has shown that depression in adolescent females with AN is associated with a higher risk of osteoporosis, compared with AN alone. The reason for this association is unknown.

The only proven treatment for osteoporosis in girls with AN is regaining sufficient weight and body fat to restart the menstrual cycle. Most studies do not support use of hormone replacement therapy to improve bone recovery; however, some evidence indicates that use of hormone replacement therapy may stop further bone loss and may be of particular benefit for patients with extremely low body weight (< 70% IBW). Some practitioners use hormone replacement therapy if amenorrhea has been present for more than 1 year and the patient is not able to achieve normal body weight. Bisphosphonates used to treat postmenopausal osteoporosis are currently being studied in adolescents. Two small randomized controlled trials have shown small positive effects on bone density with alendronate and risedronate, although clinical effectiveness has not yet been determined. Newer treatments with possible effectiveness, including recombinant insulin-like growth factor-1 injection and dehydroepiandrosterone, are still under investigation.

2. Brain changes—As malnutrition becomes more pronounced, brain tissue—both white and gray matter—is lost, with a compensatory increase in cerebrospinal fluid in the sulci and ventricles. Follow-up studies of weight-recovered anorexic patients show a persistent loss of gray matter, although white matter returns to normal. Functionally there does not seem to be a direct relationship between cognition and brain tissue loss, although studies have shown a decrease in cognitive ability and decreased cerebral blood flow in very malnourished patients. Making patients and family aware that brain tissue can be lost may improve their perception of the seriousness of this disorder.

Asiero D, Frishman WH: Cardiovascular complications of eating disorders. Cardiol Rev 2006;14:227 [PMID: 16924163].

Castro J et al: Bone mineral density in male adolescents with anorexia nervosa. J Am Acad Child Adolesc Psychiatry 2002; 41:613 [PMID: 12014794].

Golden NH et al: Alendronate for the treatment of osteopenia in anorexia nervosa: A randomized, double-blind, placebo-controlled trial. J Clin Endocrinol Metab 2005;90:3179 [PMID: 15784715].

Golden NH: Osteopenia and osteoporosis in anorexia nervosa. Adolesc Med State Art Rev 2003;14:97 [PMID: 12529194].

Yager J, Anderson AA: Anorexia nervosa. N Engl J Med 2005;353:1481 [PMID:16207850].

Kerem NC, Katzman DK: Brain structure and function in adolescents with anorexia nervosa. Adolesc Med State Art Rev 2003;14:109 [PMID: 12529195].

Konstantynowicz J et al: Depression in anorexia nervosa: A risk factor for osteoporosis. J Clin Endocrinol Metab 2005;90:5382 [PMID: 15941868].

C. Mortality

Patients with eating disorders are at a higher risk of death than the general population. Meta-analysis shows that the risk of dying is 5.9% in such patients. Mortality estimates vary between 0% and 18%, depending on the patient population and the duration of follow-up. One study showed the risk of dying to be 0.56% per year. Death in anorexic patients is due to suicide, abnormal electrolytes, and cardiac arrhythmias.

Herzog DB et al: Mortality in eating disorders: A descriptive study. Int J Eat Disord 2000;28:20 [PMID: 10800010].

Treatment

A. General Approach

Factors that determine treatment interventions are severity of illness, duration of illness, specific manifestations of disease, previous treatment approaches and outcomes, program availability, financial resources, and insurance coverage. Treatment options include outpatient management, day treatment hospitalization, and inpatient medical or psychiatric hospitalization. Residential treatment is most often used when outpatient management or short-term hospitalization fails and the eating disorder becomes chronic. Residential treatment usually lasts 2–6 months. Day treatment programs are a good intervention for patients who do not yet need inpatient care but who are not improving with outpatient management. Treatment is costly. Many patients do not have insurance benefits that adequately cover the cost of treatment, leaving parents and practitioners with profound dilemmas as to how to best provide treatment in the face of financial constraints.

Regardless of the treatment program, a multidisciplinary approach is most effective and should include medical monitoring, nutrition therapy, and individual and family psychotherapy by experienced practitioners. Family therapy is especially helpful with younger teenagers, whereas older teenagers tend to benefit more from individual therapy. Family therapy is an important means of helping families understand the development of the disease and addressing issues that may be barriers to recovery. Both types of therapy are encouraged in most treatment programs, and recovery without psychotherapy is unusual. The average length of therapy is roughly 6–9 months, although some individuals continue therapy for extended periods. Adjunctive modalities include art and horticulture therapy, therapeutic recreation, and massage therapy.

A newer family therapy approach, manualized family therapy, developed in Britain by Maudsley and adapted by Lock and LeGrange, has shifted the therapeutic approach to adolescents with AN. Traditional therapy allowed the adolescent to control his or her eating, and the parents to remain uninvolved with the food-portion of recovery. The manualized approach gives power and control back to parents. Treatment is prescribed for 20 weekly sessions. The first 10 weeks are devoted to empowering parents, putting them in control of their child's nutrition and exercise. Parents are educated about the dangers of malnutrition and are instructed to supervise each meal. The next phase—sessions 11–16—returns control over eating to the adolescent once he or she accepts the demands of the parents. The last phase of treatment, sessions 17–20, occurs when the patient is maintaining a healthy weight, and shifts the focus away from eating disorder, examining instead the impact that disorder has had on establishing a healthy adolescent identity. This approach is reported to result in good immediate outcomes in 90% of treated adolescents

Careful instruction in nutrition helps the teenager and family dispel misconceptions about nutrition, identify realistic nutritional goals, and normalize eating. Initially, nutrition education may be the most important intervention as the teenager slowly works through his or her fears of fat-containing foods and weight gain. The teenager begins to trust the nutrition therapist and restore body weight, eventually eating in a well-balanced, healthy manner.

The key to determining level of intervention is the degree of malnutrition, the rapidity of weight loss, the degree of medical compromise, and the presence of life-threatening electrolyte abnormalities. No absolute criteria determine level of intervention. The practitioner must examine the degree of medical compromise and consider immediate risks and the potential for an individual to reverse the situation on his or her own.

B. Inpatient Treatment

Table 5–5 lists the criteria for hospital admission generally used in the medical community. It is usually quite difficult for a patient who is losing weight rapidly (> 2 lb/wk) to reverse the weight loss because the body is in a catabolic state.

Goals of hospitalization include arresting weight loss and stabilizing hemodynamics. Nutrition is the most vital inpatient medicine. Clinicians can safely begin with a meal plan containing approximately 250 kcal more than the patient has been routinely eating, which can usually be accomplished orally. Ideally, with the help of a nutritionist, patients should start with a well-balanced meal plan, with appropriate proportions of carbohydrate, protein, and fat. Usually patients tolerate oral meals. If the patient resists, nasogastric or intravenous alimentation can be used for a short time. Aside from caloric needs, the clinician needs to consider the patient's hydration and include the appropriate amount of fluid with the meal plan. Dehydration should be corrected slowly. The oral route is usually adequate. Aggressive intravenous fluid administration should be avoided because left ventricular mass is compromised and a rapid increase in volume may not be tolerated. Regulating fluid intake is important, because water intoxication can contribute to abnormal electrolytes and falsified weights.

During the initial introduction of food, the clinician should monitor the patient for refeeding syndrome, a phenomenon that occurs if caloric intake is increased too rapidly. Signs of refeeding syndrome are decreased serum phosphorus (as the body resumes synthesis of adenosine triphosphate), decreased serum potassium (as increased insulin causes K^+ to shift from extracellular fluid into K^+-depleted cells), and rarely, edema related to fluid shifts or congestive heart failure.

Although specific guidelines do not exist, many practitioners begin phosphorus supplementation if patients are severely malnourished (< 70% IBW) or their intake has been consistently less than 500 kcal/d.

Caloric intake can be increased 250 kcal/d as long as refeeding syndrome does not occur. Weight goals vary depending on programmatic approach. Typically intake is adjusted to reach a goal of 0.1–0.25 kg/d weight gain.

Overnight monitoring for bradycardia is helpful in assessing degree of metabolic compromise. Usually the more rapid and severe the weight loss is, the worse the bradycardia. Improving bradycardia correlates with weight recovery. Orthostatic hypotension is most severe around hospital day 4, improving steadily and correcting by the third week of nutritional rehabilitation. An electrocardiogram should be obtained because the patient is at risk for prolonged QTc syndrome and junctional arrhythmias related to the severity of bradycardia.

It usually takes 2–3 weeks to reach the initial goals of hospitalization—steady weight gain, toleration of oral diet without signs of refeeding syndrome, corrected bradycardia (heart rate > 45 beats/min for three consecutive nights), and correction of orthostasis. Specific weight criteria are used by many programs when considering discharge. This depends partly on admission weight. Ideally a patient gains at least 5% of his or her ideal weight. Some programs set discharge at 80%, 85%, or 90% IBW. Patient outcomes are improved with discharge at a higher body weight. One study has shown that patients do better if discharged at 95% IBW. Frequently, insurance companies do not pay for hospital stays beyond strict medical stabilization (normal vital signs and normal electrolytes). In many practitioners' experience, relapse rate is high if patients are discharged at less than 75% IBW.

Extremely malnourished patients may not benefit from individual psychotherapy or nutritional instruction initially because of their cognitive impairment. Beginning family psychotherapy at first, with the addition of individual psychotherapy after the first week of refeeding, may be more effective.

C. Pharmacotherapy

Use of psychotropic medications is common in treatment of AN, despite lack of solid proof of efficacy. The most promising class of medication is the atypical antipsychotics. Several open label trials support the use of atypical antipsychotics (risperidone olanzapine, quetiapine), which target specifically the body image distortion of these patients. One review found that olanzapine (2.5–15 mg/d) was associated with improved

Table 5–5. Criteria for inpatient treatment of anorexia nervosa.

Body weight < 75% of ideal body weight
Supine heart rate < 45/min
Symptomatic hypotension or syncope
Hypokalemia: K^+ < 2.5 mEq/L
Rapid weight loss that cannot be interrupted as outpatient
Failure of outpatient management
Acute food refusal

body weight, decreased delusional thinking, improvement in body image, and decreased agitation and premeal anxiety. There have not yet been any published randomized placebo-controlled trials of the atypical antipsychotics, although several are pending.

SSRIs repeatedly have been shown to not be helpful in the initial therapy of AN. However, once the patient has achieved approximately 85% IBW, then SSRIs (fluoxetine, citalopram, or sertraline) may help prevent relapse.

Zinc deficiency is common in AN, and several studies support its use as a supplement during the initial phases of treatment. Because zinc deficiency adversely affects neurotransmitters, administering zinc helps restore neurotransmitter action to baseline. Additionally zinc may restore appetite and improve depressive mood. Zinc should be administered for approximately 2 months from the beginning of therapy, with at least 14 mg of elemental zinc daily.

Due to global nutritional deficits, a multivitamin with iron is also recommended daily. Symptomatic treatment for disturbances in the GI system should be used appropriately until symptoms resolve.

D. Outpatient Treatment

Not all patients with AN need inpatient treatment, especially if parents and clinicians recognize the warning signs early. These patients can receive treatment as outpatients, employing the same multidisciplinary team approach. Manualized family-based treatment, described earlier under General Approach, is ideal for the outpatient setting, if a trained therapist is available. Appropriate nutrition counseling is vital in guiding a patient and family through the initial stages of recovery. As the nutrition therapist is working at increasing the patient's caloric intake, a practitioner needs to monitor the patient's weight and vital signs. Often activity level needs to be decreased to help reverse the catabolic state. A reasonable weight gain goal may be 0.2–0.5 kg/wk. If weight loss persists, careful monitoring of vital signs, including supine heart rate, is important in determining whether an increased level of care is needed. Concomitantly, the patient should be referred to a psychotherapist, and if indicated, assessed by a psychiatrist.

Birmingham CL, Gritzner S: How does zinc supplementation benefit anorexia nervosa? Eat Weight Disord 2006;11:e109 [PMID:17272939].

Claudino AM et al: Antidepressants for anorexia nervosa. Cochrane Database Systematic Rev 2006;(1):CD004365 [PMID: 16437485].

Dunican KC, DelDotto D: The role of olanzapine in the treatment of anorexia nervosa. Ann Pharmacother 2007;41:111 [PMID: 17190846].

LeGrange D et al: Manualized family-based treatment for anorexia nervosa: A case series. J Am Acad Child Adolesc Psychiatry 2005;44:41 [PMID: 15608542].

Miller KK et al: Medical findings in outpatients with anorexia nervosa. Arch Intern Med 2005;165:561 [PMID: 15767533].

Mondraty N et al: Randomized controlled trial of olanzapine in the treatment of cognitions in anorexia nervosa. Australas Psychiatry 2005;13:72 [PMID: 15777417].

Swenne I: Weight requirements for return of menstruations in teenage girls with eating disorders, weight loss, and secondary amenorrhea. Acta Paediatr 2004;93:1449 [PMID: 08035253].

BULIMIA NERVOSA

Table 5–6 lists the diagnostic criteria for BN. Binge eating is either eating excessive amounts of food during a normal mealtime or having a meal that lasts longer than usual. Bulimic individuals feel out of control while eating, unable or unwilling to recognize satiety signals. Any type of food may be eaten in a binge, although typically it is either carbohydrates or junk food. Extreme guilt is often associated with the episode. At some point, either prior to or during a binge, bulimic individuals often decide to purge as a means of preventing weight gain. The most common ways to purge are self-induced vomiting, exercise, and laxative use. Some individuals will vomit multiple times during a purge episode, after using large amounts of water to cleanse their system. This can induce significant electrolyte abnormalities such as hyponatremia and hypokalemia, which may put the patient at acute risk for arrhythmia or seizure. Other methods of purging include diuretics, diet pills, cathartics, and nutritional supplements, including Metabolife.

Diagnosing BN can be difficult unless the teenager is forthcoming or parents or caregivers can supply direct observations. Bulimic patients are usually average or slightly above average in body weight and have no physical abnormalities. Screening all teenagers for body image concerns is crucial. If the teenager

Table 5–6. Diagnostic criteria for bulimia nervosa.

A. Recurrent episodes of binge eating. An episode of binge eating is characterized by both of the following:
  (1) eating, in a discrete period of time (eg, within any 2-hour period), an amount of food that is definitely larger than most people would eat during a similar period of time and under similar circumstances.
  (2) a sense of lack of control over eating during the episodes (eg, a feeling that one cannot stop eating or control what or how much one is eating).
B. Recurrent inappropriate compensatory behavior in order to prevent weight gain, such as self-induced vomiting; misuse of laxatives, diuretics, enemas, or other medications; fasting; or excessive exercise.
C. The binge eating and inappropriate compensatory behaviors both occur, on average, at least twice a week for 3 months.
D. Self-evaluation is unduly influenced by body shape and weight.
E. The disturbance does not occur exclusively during episodes of anorexia nervosa.

expresses concern about being overweight, then the clinician needs to screen the patient about dieting methods. Asking whether patients have binged, feel out of control while eating, or whether they cannot stop eating can clarify the diagnosis. Parents may report that significant amounts of food are missing or disappearing more quickly than normal. If the physician is suspicious, direct questioning about all the ways to purge should follow. Indicating first that the behavior is not unusual can make questioning less threatening and more likely to elicit a truthful response. For example, the clinician might say, "Some teenagers who try to lose weight make themselves vomit after eating. Have you ever considered or done that yourself?" (See Table 5–2 for additional screening questions.)

► Clinical Findings

A. Symptoms and Signs

Symptoms are related to the mechanism of purging. GI problems are most prominent. Abdominal pain is common. This can be due to gastroesophageal reflux, as the lower esophageal sphincter is compromised due to repetitive vomiting. Frequent vomiting may result in esophagitis or gastritis, as the mucosa is irritated from increased acid exposure. Early satiety, involuntary vomiting, and complaints of food "coming up" on its own are frequent. Less common but more serious is hematemesis or esophageal rupture. Patients may report diarrhea or constipation, especially if laxatives have been used. Sialadenitis (parotid pain and enlargement) may be caused by frequent vomiting. Erosion of dental enamel results from increased oral acid exposure during vomiting. Because comorbid depression is common in BN, patients may report difficulty sleeping, decreased energy, decreased motivation, and headaches. Lightheadedness or syncope may develop secondary to dehydration.

It is important to note that most purging methods are ineffective. When patients binge, they may consume thousands of calories. Digestion begins rapidly. Although the patient may be able to vomit some of the food, much is actually digested and absorbed. Laxatives work in the large intestine, leading to fluid and electrolyte loss. Consumed calories are still absorbed from the small intestine. Use of diuretics may result in decreased fluid weight and electrolyte imbalance.

On physical examination, bulimic patients may be dehydrated and have orthostatic hypotension. Sialadenitis, tooth enamel loss, dental caries, and abdominal tenderness are the most common findings. Abrasion of the proximal interphalangeal joints may occur secondary to scraping the fingers against teeth while inducing vomiting. Rarely a heart murmur is heard. Irreversible cardiomyopathy can develop secondary to ipecac use. Tachycardia and hypertension may occur secondary to caffeine and diet pill use.

B. Laboratory Findings

Electrolyte disturbances are common in bulimic patients. The method of purging results in specific abnormalities.

Vomiting causes metabolic alkalosis, hypokalemia, and hypochloremia. If laxatives are used, then a metabolic acidosis develops with hypokalemia and hypochloremia. Amylase may be increased secondary to chronic parotid stimulation.

► Complications

A. Short-Term Complications

Complications in normal-weight bulimic patients are related to the mechanisms of purging, and many of these complications are listed under Symptoms and Signs, earlier. If the bulimic patient is significantly malnourished, complications may be the same as those encountered in the anorexic patient. Other complications of bulimia include esophageal rupture, acute or chronic esophagitis, and rarely, Barrett syndrome. Chronic vomiting can lead to metabolic alkalosis, and laxative abuse may cause metabolic acidosis. Patients may develop aspiration pneumonia from vomiting. Diet pill use can cause insomnia, hypertension, tachycardia, palpitations, seizures, and sudden death.

Patients who stop taking laxatives can have severe constipation. Treating constipation can be difficult psychologically, because the practitioner may need to prescribe agents similar to the drugs of abuse used during the eating disorder.

B. Mortality

The mortality rate in bulimic patients is similar to that in anorexic patients. Death usually results from suicide or electrolyte derangements.

► Treatment

Treatment of BN depends on the frequency of bingeing and purging and the severity of biochemical and psychiatric derangement. If K^+ is less than 3.0 mEq/L, inpatient medical admission is warranted. Typically extracellular K^+ is spared at the expense of intracellular K^+, so a patient may become hypokalemic several days after the serum K^+ concentration appears to be corrected. Usually cessation of purging is sufficient to correct K^+ concentration and is the recommended intervention for K^+ above 3.0 mEq/L. If K^+ is 2.5–2.9 mEq/L, oral supplementation is suggested. If K^+ is less than 2.5 mEq/L, then intravenous therapy is recommended. Supplements can be stopped once K^+ levels are more than 3.5 mEq/L. Total body K^+ can be assumed to be normal when serum K^+ corrects and remains normal 2 days after supplements are stopped. Continued hospitalization depends on the patient's psychological status.

Many bulimic patients abuse laxatives and may be chronically dehydrated. The renin-angiotensin-aldosterone axis and the antidiuretic hormone level may be elevated to compensate. These systems do not shut down automatically when laxatives are stopped, and fluid retention of up to 10 kg/wk may result. This puts patients at risk for congestive heart failure and can scare them as their weight increases dramatically. Diuresis often occurs after 7–10 days. Parents and patients should be advised of this possible complication of initial therapy to help maintain their confidence in the care plan.

Another reason to hospitalize bulimic patients is failure of outpatient management. The binge-purge cycle is addictive and can be difficult for patients to interrupt on their own. Hospitalization can offer a forced break from the cycle, allowing patients to normalize their eating, interrupt the addictive behavior, and regain the ability to recognize satiety signals.

Outpatient management can be pursued if patients are medically stable. Cognitive-behavioral therapy is crucial to help bulimic patients understand their disease and to offer suggestions for decreasing bingeing and purging. Nutrition therapy offers patients ways to regulate eating patterns so that they can avoid the need to binge. Medical monitoring should be done to check electrolytes periodically, depending on the purging method used.

SSRIs are generally helpful in treating the binge-purge cycle. Fluoxetine has been studied most extensively; a dose of 60 mg/d is most efficacious in teenagers. Other SSRIs appear to be effective as well and may be used in patients experiencing side effects of fluoxetine. Treatment for gastroesophageal reflux and gastritis should be used when appropriate. The pain and swelling of enlarged parotid glands can be helped by sucking on tart candy and by the application of heat.

American Psychiatric Association: *Diagnostic and Statistical Manual of Mental Disorders*, 4th ed, text revision. American Psychiatric Association, 2000.

Bacaltchuk J et al: Antidepressant versus placebo for the treatment of bulimia nervosa: A systematic review. Aust N Z J Psychiatry 2000;34:310 [PMID: 10789536].

Benini LT et al: Gastric emptying in patients with restricting and binge/purging subtypes of anorexia nervosa. Am J Gastroenterol 2004;99:1448 [PMID: 15307858].

Mehler P: Bulimia nervosa. N Engl J Med 2003;349:875 [PMID: 12944574].

Panagiotopoulos C et al: Electrocardiographic findings in adolescents with eating disorders. Pediatrics 2000;105:1100 [PMID: 10790469].

BINGE-EATING DISORDER

The diagnostic category of binge-eating disorder was created in DSM-IV. Officially, it is still considered a research diagnosis. Studies show that most adults who have binge-eating disorder (a prevalence of 2–4%) develop symptoms during adolescence. Table 5–7 lists the diagnostic criteria.

▶ Clinical Findings

A. Symptoms and Signs

Binge-eating disorder most often occurs in overweight or obese individuals. Eighteen percent of such patients report bingeing at least once in the past year. Patients with binge-eating disorder have an increased incidence of depression

Table 5–7. Diagnostic criteria for binge-eating disorder.

A. Recurrent episodes of binge eating. An episode of binge eating is characterized by both of the following:
  (1) eating, in a discrete period of time (eg, within any 2-hour period), an amount of food that is definitely larger than most people would eat in a similar period of time under similar circumstances.
  (2) a sense of lack of control over eating during the episode (eg, a feeling that one cannot stop eating or control what or how much one is eating).
B. The binge-eating episodes are associated with three (or more) of the following:
  (1) eating much more rapidly than normal
  (2) eating until feeling uncomfortably full
  (3) eating large amounts of food when not feeling physically hungry
  (4) eating alone because of being embarrassed by how much one is eating
  (5) feeling disgusted with oneself, depressed, or very guilty after overeating
C. Marked distress regarding binge eating at present.
D. The binge eating occurs, on average, at least 2 days a week for 6 months.
E. The binge eating is not associated with regular use of inappropriate compensatory behaviors (eg, purging, fasting, excessive exercise) and does not occur exclusively during the course of anorexia nervosa or bulimia nervosa.

and substance abuse. Using the DSM-IV-TR diagnostic criteria as a guide for evaluation, the possibility of binge-eating disorder should be raised for any significantly overweight patient. Specific questionnaires are available for evaluating patients suspected of binge-eating disorder.

B. Laboratory Findings

The clinician should assess causes and complications of obesity, and laboratory evaluation should include thyroid function tests and measurement of cholesterol and triglyceride levels.

Fairburn CG et al: The natural course of bulimia nervosa and binge eating disorder in young women. Arch Gen Psychiatry 2000;57:659 [PMID: 10891036].

Johnson WG et al: Measuring binge eating in adolescents: Adolescent and parent versions of the questionnaire of eating and weight patterns. Int J Eat Disord 1999;26:301 [PMID: 10441246].

Schneider M: Bulimia nervosa and binge eating disorder in adolescents. Adolesc Med State Art Rev 2003;14:119 [PMID: 12529196].

▶ Treatment

A combination of cognitive-behavioral therapy and pressant medication has been helpful in treati eating disorder in adults. Use of SSRIs for disorder in adolescents has not been studied, but in adults, fluoxetine and citalopram help decrease binge episodes, improve depressive symptoms, and possibly decrease appetite. This evidence suggests that SSRIs in adolescents with binge-eating disorder may be helpful as well.

McElroy SL et al: Citalopram in the treatment of binge-eating disorder: A placebo-controlled trial. J Clin Psychiatry 2003;64:807 [PMID: 12934982].

EATING DISORDER NOT OTHERWISE SPECIFIED

An additional DSM-IV-TR diagnostic category is eating disorder not otherwise specified (EDNOS). Patients do not meet all the criteria for either AN or BN, but have features of either or both. Table 5–8 lists the diagnostic criteria. This has become a "catch-all" category and some researchers describe this as an atypical eating disorder or partial syndrome eating disorder. EDNOS is estimated to affect 0.5–14% of the general adolescent population. Careful attention by clinicians to patient concerns about body weight and dieting behavior can provide clues to the diagnosis. Symptoms and sequelae depend on patient behaviors. Some patients with EDNOS will go on to develop full-blown AN or BN, and early recognition and treatment may decrease further complications.

Chamay-Weber C et al: Partial eating disorders among adolescents: A review. J Adolesc Health 2005;37:417 [PMID: 16227132].

PROGNOSIS

Outcome in eating disorders, especially AN, has been studied extensively. Unfortunately, most studies have focused on specific inpatient treatment programs, and few have evaluated the less ill patients who do not need hospitalization. About 40–50% of patients receiving treatment recover; 20–30% have intermittent relapses; and 20% have chronic, unremitting illness. As time from initial onset lengthens, the recovery rate decreases and mortality associated with AN and BN increases.

The course of AN often includes significant weight fluctuations over time, and it may be a matter of years until recovery is certain. The course of BN often includes relapses of bingeing and purging, although bulimic patients initially recover faster than do anorexic patients. Up to 50% of anorexic patients may develop bulimia, as well as major psychological complications, including depression, anxiety, and substance abuse disorders. Bulimic patients also develop similar psychological illness but rarely develop anorexia. Long-term medical sequelae, aside from low body weight and amenorrhea, have not been studied in an outcome format, although AN is known to have multiple medical consequences, including osteoporosis and structural brain changes.

It is unclear whether age at onset affects outcome, but shorter length of time between symptom onset and ther-

Table 5–8. Diagnostic criteria for eating disorder not otherwise specified.

The eating disorder not otherwise specified category is for disorders of eating that do not meet the criteria for any specific eating disorder. Examples include
1. For females, all of the criteria for anorexia nervosa are met except that the individual has regular menses.
2. All of the criteria for anorexia nervosa are met except that, despite significant weight loss, the individual's current weight is in the normal range.
3. All of the criteria for bulimia nervosa are met except that the binge eating and inappropriate compensatory mechanisms occur at a frequency of less than twice a week or for a duration of less than 3 months.
4. The regular use of inappropriate compensatory behavior by an individual of normal body weight after eating small amounts of food (eg, self-induced vomiting after the consumption of two cookies).
5. Repeatedly chewing and spitting out, but not swallowing, large amounts of food.

Reprinted, with permission, from the *Diagnostic and Statistical Manual of Mental Disorders*, 4th ed, text revision. Copyright 2000. American Psychiatric Association.

apy tends to improve outcome. Various treatment modalities can be equally effective. Favorable outcomes have been found with brief medical hospitalization and long psychiatric or residential hospitalization. Higher discharge weight seems to improve the initial outcome. It is difficult to compare treatment regimens, because the numbers are small and the type of patient and illness varies between studies. No existing studies compare outpatient to inpatient treatment or the effects of day treatment on recovery.

Binge-eating disorder has been recognized only recently, and outcomes have not been studied. Intervention with an SSRI appears to help the bingeing, but little is known regarding long-term prognosis.

Fichter MM et al: Twelve-year course and outcome predictors of anorexia nervosa. Int J Eat Disord 2006;39:87 [PMID: 16231345].
Fisher M: The course and outcome of eating disorders in adults and in adolescents: A review. Adolesc Med State Art Rev 2003;14:149 [PMID: 12529198].
Strober M et al: The long-term course of severe anorexia nervosa in adolescents: Survival analysis of recovery, relapse, and outcome predictors of 10–15 years in a prospective study. Int J Eat Disord 1997;22:339 [PMID: 9356884].

REFERENCES

Kreipe RE, Birndorf SA: Eating disorders in adolescents and young adults. Med Clin North Am 2000;84:1027 [PMID: 10928200].
Rome E et al: Children and adolescents with eating disorders: State of the art. Pediatrics 2003;111:e98 [PMID: 12509603].

Child & Adolescent Psychiatric Disorders & Psychosocial Aspects of Pediatrics

Brian Stafford, MD, MPH

Jennifer Hagman, MD

Bert Dech, MD

Mental illness affects between 14% and 20% of children and adolescents. The prevalence is higher for those juveniles living in poor socioeconomic circumstances. Unfortunately, the shortage of mental health providers, stigma attached to receiving mental health services, chronic underfunding, institutional barriers of the public mental health system, and disparate insurance benefits have contributed to the fact that only 2% of these children are actually seen by mental health specialists. About 75% of children with psychiatric disturbances are seen in primary care settings, and half of all pediatric office visits involve behavioral, psychosocial, or educational concerns. Parents and children often prefer discussing these issues with someone they already know and trust. As a result, primary care physicians are compelled to play an important role in the identification, initiation, management, and coordination of mental health care in children and adolescents.

Despite being strategically positioned as the gatekeeper for identifying these concerns, primary care physicians identify fewer than 20% of children with emotional and behavioral problems during health supervision visits when these concerns are also present. In addition, these problems are not identified when they begin (and are more readily amenable to treatment). This gatekeeper role has become more important over the past decade as advances in mental health awareness and treatment have improved opportunities for early identification and intervention. This role is especially critical since child psychiatry remains an underserved medical specialty, with only 7000 board-certified child and adolescent psychiatrists in the United States. In contrast, the more than 50,000 board-certified pediatricians in the United States are in a unique position to identify issues affecting the emotional health of children and to initiate treatment or referrals to other providers.

Emotional problems that develop during childhood and adolescence can have a significant impact on development and may continue into adulthood; in fact, most "adult" psychiatric disorders have their onset during childhood.

Most disorders do not present as an "all-or-none" phenomenon; rather, they progress from adjustment concerns to perturbations in functioning to significant disturbances and severe disorders. Pediatricians have the capacity to manage emotional problems and behavioral conditions early on, when improvement can be achieved with less intensive interventions. If pediatricians and schools do not appropriately identify mental health problems, provide education about the benefits of intervention, and encourage and initiate intervention, childhood-onset disorders are more likely to persist, cause worsening impairment, and lead to a downward spiral of school and social difficulties, poor employment opportunities, and poverty in adulthood.

Pediatricians and other primary care providers may be the first or sometimes only medical professional in a position to identify a mental health problem. This chapter reviews prevention, surveillance, and screening for mental illness; situations that may arise in the context of such assessments; illnesses that are often diagnosed during childhood or adolescence; current recommendations for interventions and use of psychotropic medications; and indications for referral to mental health professionals.

Costello EJ et al: 10-year research update review: The epidemiology of child and adolescent psychiatric disorders: I. Methods and public health burden. J Am Acad Child Adolesc Psychiatry 2005;44:972 [PMID: 16175102].

DeAngelis C et al: Final report of the FOPE II pediatric workforce workgroup. Pediatrics 2000;106:1245 [PMID: 11073554].

MODELS OF CARE ENCOMPASSING MENTAL HEALTH IN THE PRIMARY CARE SETTING

Given the many barriers to receiving mental health care, new approaches to providing mental health professional servic have been recently explored.

Usual or typical pediatric care of emotional and b ioral problems is related to the comfort level of the ; ual pediatric provider and available resources. The ʳ surveillance in the form of developmentally appropriate anticipatory guidance and counseling is variable; the average time spent is 2.5 minutes. However, as stated earlier, the majority of emotional and behavioral problems are not identified in this model of care. In addition, when they are identified, the logistics of referral can be problematic. Although pediatricians often refer to mental health providers, only 50% of families will actually attend an appointment and the average number of appointments attended is only slightly greater than one. Based on level of comfort and training, the primary clinician in this model is more likely to be responsible for psychiatric medications if prescribed.

Among the technological interventions that can enhance identification of problems and target specific symptoms for assessment is the **Child Health and Interactive Developmental System (CHADIS)** (http://www.childhealthcare.org). In this system, parents use a computer kiosk to note their level of concern about various behaviors, which triggers algorithmic interviews for each concern based on psychiatric diagnostic criteria. The CHADIS system provides an electronic worksheet of analyzed results, school communication tools, as well as other resources.

Enhanced care is a model of care in which a pediatric developmental or behavioral specialist is embedded in the clinic, thus making for improved referral and communication and management. This "co-location" creates easier access for patients and improved communication with mental health professionals.

Collaborative care provides high-quality, multidisciplinary and collaborative care through the co-location of educators, consultants, or direct service providers in the clinic. Successful collaborative care results in greater specialist involvement by negating identification and referral and other system-of-care barriers. Successful components include a leadership team, primary clinicians, mental health and developmental specialists, administrators, clinical informatics specialists, and care managers. Collaborative care implies that nearly all visits are done jointly and that mental health professionals are always available for consultation, in contrast to the approach in the enhanced care model, which requires the scheduling of an appointment with a mental health specialist in the practice. These interventions can be accomplished through collaboration among mental health and primary care providers, mental health systems and primary care practices, and in academic settings with interdepartmental collaboration. Typically, philanthropic or other foundation grants are necessary to start a collaborative program so that reimbursement and sustainability concerns can be identified and remedied.

Connor DF et al: Targeted child psychiatric services: A new model of pediatric primary clinician—child psychiatry collaborative care. Clin Pediatr 2005;45:423 [PMID: 16891275].

Kelleher KJ et al: Management of pediatric mental disorders in primary care: Where are we now and where are we going? Curr Opin Pediatr 2006;18:649 [PMID: 17099365].

Williams J et al: Co-location of mental health professionals in primary care settings: Three North Carolina models. Clin Pediatr (Phila) 2006;45;537 [PMID: 16893859].

EARLY IDENTIFICATION & PREVENTION OF DEVELOPMENTAL & SOCIOEMOTIONAL PROBLEMS

The role of the primary care pediatrician continues to expand to include public health, mental health, and community concerns. The American Academy of Pediatrics (AAP) Policy Statement on Community Pediatrics addresses the fact that today's children and families live in a period of rapid social change. In addition, the economic organization of the health care and social service systems in the United States is undergoing profound changes. For many pediatricians, efforts to promote the health of children have been directed at attending to the needs of particular children in a practice setting, on an individual basis, and providing them with a medical home. This approach, in combination with pediatricians' own personal community interests and commitments, has been dramatically successful. Increasingly, however, the major threats to the health of U.S. children—the new morbidity—arise from problems that cannot be adequately addressed by the practice model alone. These problems include unacceptably high infant mortality rates in certain communities, extraordinary levels of intentional and unintentional injuries, chemical dependency, behavioral and developmental consequences of inappropriate care and experience, family dysfunction, sexually transmitted diseases, unplanned pregnancies and out-of-wedlock births, and lack of a medical home. The Policy Statement concludes that "We must become partners with others, or we will become increasingly irrelevant to the health of children."

Today's community pediatrician seeks to provide a far more realistic and complete clinical picture by taking responsibility for all children in a community, providing preventive and curative services, and understanding the determinants and consequences of child health and illness, as well as the effectiveness of services provided.

Bright Futures

The Bright Futures Task Force, a partnership initiated by the Maternal and Child Health Bureau (MCHB) over a decade ago, is a philosophy and approach that is dedicated to the principle that every child deserves to be healthy, and that optimal health involves a trusting relationship between the health professional, the child, the family, and the community. As part of this initiative, *Bright Futures: Guidelines for Health Supervision of Infants, Children, and Adolescents* was developed to provide comprehensive health supervision guidelines, including recommendations on immunizations, routine health screenings, and anticipatory guidance. In addition, Bright Futures for Mental Health provides numerous guidelines, tools, and strategies for improving mental health identification, assessment, initiation, management, and coordination.

Surgeon General's National Action Plan

The U.S. Surgeon General also recommends that pediatrics continue to evolve and include lifestyle, health system, and other psychosocial areas. The U.S. Surgeon General's National Action Agenda on Mental Health includes several calls to primary care pediatricians, including the following: engage other professional organizations in educating new frontline providers in various systems (eg, teachers, physicians, nurses, hospital emergency personnel, day care providers, probation officers, and other child health care providers) in child development; equip them with skills to address and enhance children's mental health; and train them to recognize early symptoms of emotional or behavioral problems for proactive intervention. Such training must focus on developmental and cultural differences in cognitive, social, emotional, and behavioral functioning, and understanding these issues in familial and ecological context.

Rushton FE Jr: American Academy of Pediatrics Committee on Community Health Services: The pediatrician's role in community pediatrics. Pediatrics 2005;115:1092 [PMID: 15805396].

Bright Futures Task Force: http://www.brightfutures.org/mentalhealth/index.html

U.S Surgeon General's National Action Agenda: http://www.surgeongeneral.govlcmh/childreport.htm

Summary of the Pediatrician's Role

Given these calls for a new pediatric role as the gatekeeper for socioemotional health, the expanding role of the primary care pediatric provider encompasses the following broad categories: identification, assessment, initiation, management, coordination, and collaboration (Table 6–1).

IDENTIFICATION & ASSESSMENT DURING HEALTH MAINTENANCE VISITS

Most families seek help from their primary care providers when they are concerned about a child's health, growth, or development. Historically, the most efficient indicator in eliciting psychosocial problems is the history provided by parents or guardians, and interview and observation of the child. The possible approaches to identification of problems include surveillance, screening, and assessment

Surveillance consists of the following elements: checking in, eliciting concerns, asking open-ended questions, watching and waiting, listening for red flags, identifying risk factors, and monitoring closely over time. Like vital signs, which represent an essential component of the physical evaluation, the essential components of the primary care surveillance for mental health concerns should generally include a review of the youth's general functioning in different aspects of their life. Five questions forming the mnemonic **PSYCH** can be addressed to parents and youth as a surveillance means of uncovering areas of concern.

1. **Parent-child interaction:** How are things going with you and your parents? Or you and your infant (or toddler)?

Table 6–1. The pediatric primary care provider's role in mental health.

Role	Specific Activities
Identification	Shared family concern Surveillance Screening
Assessment	Interview Assessment tools Comorbid conditions
Initiation	Psychoeducation about condition and treatment options • Wait and watch • Refer to mental health for further evaluation • Refer for therapy • Start medication
Management	Monitor condition for improvement Monitor for side effects
Coordination	With social work, therapist, psychologist, or psychiatrist
Collaboration	With mental health service providers With child protection With local schools

2. **School:** How are things going in school (or day care)? (academically and behaviorally)

3. **Youth:** How are things going with peer relationships?

4. **Casa:** How are things going at home? (including siblings, family stresses, and relationship with parents)

5. **Happiness:** How would you describe your mood?

Many pediatric practices are strapped by lack of continuity and not enough time to do in-depth surveillance. In addition, surveillance is notoriously tied to office and provider characteristics. Given current time constraints for current pediatric visits, and the fact that only 18% of parents reporting elevated behavior problems in children actually told their providers about it, surveillance is currently considered nonoptimal. Although part of the clinical interview with families, surveillance is not, under current Medicaid and insurance reimbursement plans, a separate and billable service, whereas formal screening is.

Screening is the process of using standardized instruments to determine the existence of a problem. Newborn, hearing, vision, and developmental screenings are common in today's pediatric practice. However, the morbidity associated with developmental, emotional, and psychosocial problems requires that socioemotional screening to identify presence of symptoms of emotional, behavioral, or relationship disorders be performed, as well. Screening to brief, easy to use, and can be administered as a ques-

or using an interview format. A positive screen warrants a more complete assessment. The use of screening tools can also lead to early identification and interrupt the adjustment-perturbation-disturbance-disorder pathway. Newer methods of eliciting socioemotional and behavior concerns have been developed (see next sections). Helpful information can also be obtained from broad screening checklists and symptom-specific questionnaires (such as depression or anxiety self-report inventories). Questions can be incorporated into the general pediatric office screening forms, or specific questionnaires can be used.

Tools for Mental Health Screening in the Office Setting

Given the low rates of identification of psychosocial problems by pediatric surveillance, the use of standardized screening tools has become standard practice. Typically, broad screeners that elicit information from multiple domains are employed first and are followed by targeted screens to address symptomatology, severity, impairment, and context.

A. General or Broad Screening Tools

1. Strengths and Difficulties Questionnaires (SDQ)—
The SDQ are brief behavioral screening questionnaires targeting patients 3–16 years old. They exist in several versions to meet the needs of researchers, clinicians, and educators. They have been well validated and are available on the Internet without cost. The findings can then influence how the assessment is carried out and which professionals may need to be involved in that assessment. The SDQ are available in over 40 languages. For further information, refer to the following web site: http://sdquinfo.com.

Muris P et al: The Strengths and Difficulties Questionnaire (SDQ)—further evidence for its reliability and validity in a community sample of Dutch children and adolescents. Eur Child Adolesc Psychiatry 2003;12:1 [PMID: 12601558].

2. Pediatric Symptoms Checklist (PSC)—The PSC is a one-page questionnaire listing a broad range of children's emotional and behavioral problems that reflects parents' impressions of their children's psychosocial functioning. An adolescent self-report version is also available for children older than age 11 years. The PSC was developed initially for children older than age 5, but cutoff scores for preschool and school-aged children indicating clinical levels of dysfunction have been empirically derived. The questionnaire is easy to score, is free of charge, and is available in English and Spanish from the following web sites: http://brightfutures.org/mentalhealth/pdf/professionals/ped_symptom_chklst.pdf; http://psc.partners.org/psc_order.htm.

Reijneveld SA et al: Use of the Pediatric Symptom Checklist for the detection of psychosocial problems in preventive child healthcare. BMC Public Health 2006;6:197 [PMID: 16872535].

3. Parents Evaluation of Developmental Status (PEDS)—
The PEDS is a valid screener for socioemotional, developmental, and behavioral issues in children aged 1 month to 8 years. It requires more time to score than other general screening tools and must be purchased. Its benefits include extensive validity data and useful pathways for level of concern and referral. It is available in English, Vietnamese, and Spanish. For further information, see the following web site: http://www.pedstest.com.

Brothers KT et al: PEDS: Developmental milestones—an accurate brief tool for surveillance and screening. Clin Pediatr (Phila.)2007; Dec 5 [Epub ahead of print] [PMID: 18057141].

4. Ages and Stages, Socio-Emotional (SE)—The Ages and Stages, SE is a companion to the Ages and Stages Developmental Screen. It is an easy-to-use tool with a deep, exclusive focus on infant, toddlers, and younger children's social and emotional behavior and is cost-effective, photocopiable, and culturally sensitive for use in pediatric clinics. Screens are available for the 6, 12, 18, 24, 36, 48, and 60 month visits, and in English, French, Spanish, and Korean.

Squires J et al: Revision of a parent-completed developmental screening tool: Ages and Stages Questionnaires. J Pediatr Psychol 1997;22:313 [PMID: 9212550].
Ages and Stages, SE (technical data): http://www.brookespublishing.com/store/books/bricker-asq/asq-technical.pdf

Assessment of Behavioral & Emotional Signs & Symptoms

When an emotional problem or mental illness is mentioned by the patient or parents, elicited by an interview, or identified by a screening instrument, a thorough evaluation is indicated. At least 30 minutes should be scheduled, and additional appointments may be necessary to gather information or perform tests to clarify a diagnosis. Examples of more thorough questions and observation are given in Table 6–2. Targeted assessment screening tools are also useful in determining severity, comorbidity, and context of impairment.

It is useful to see both parents and the child first together, then the parents alone, and then the child alone. This sequence enables the physician to observe interactions among family members and gives the parents and the child an opportunity to talk confidentially about their concerns. Parents and children often feel shame and guilt about some personal inadequacy they perceive to be causing the problem. The physician can facilitate the assessment by acknowledging that the family is trying to cope and that the ultimate task of assessment is to seek solutions and not to assign blame. An attitude of nonjudgmental inquiry can be communicated with supportive statements such as, "Let's see if we can figure out what might be happening here and find some ways to make things better."

Table 6–2. Assessment of psychosocial problems.

Developmental history	**Observation of the parents**
1. Review the landmarks of psychosocial development	1. Do they agree on the existence of the problem or concern?
2. Summarize the child's temperamental traits	2. Are they uncooperative or antagonistic about the evaluation?
3. Review stressful life events and the child's reactions to them	3. Do the parents appear depressed or overwhelmed?
a. Separations	4. Can the parents present a coherent picture of the problem and
b. Losses	their family life?
c. Marital conflict	5. Do the parents accept some responsibility for the child's
d. Illnesses, injuries, and hospitalizations	problems, or do they blame forces outside the family and beyond
4. Obtain details of past mental health problems and their treatment	their control?
Family history	6. Do they appear burdened with guilt about the child's problem?
1. Marital/Relationship history	**Observation of the child**
a. Overall satisfaction with the marriage/partnership	1. Does the child acknowledge the existence of a problem or
b. Conflicts or disagreements within the relationship	concern?
c. Quantity and quality of time together away from children	2. Does the child want help?
d. Whether the child comes between or is a source of conflict	3. Is the child uncooperative or antagonistic about the assessment?
between the parents	4. What is the child's predominant mood or attitude?
e. Marital history prior to having children	5. What does the child wish could be different (eg, "three
2. Parenting history	wishes")?
a. Feelings about parenthood	6. Does the child display unusual behavior (activity level, manner-
b. Whether parents feel united in dealing with the child	isms, fearfulness)?
c. "Division of labor" in parenting	7. What is the child's apparent cognitive level?
d. Parental energy or stress level	**Observation of parent-child interaction**
e. Sleeping arrangements	1. Do the parents show concern about the child's feelings?
f. Privacy	2. Does the child control or disrupt the joint interview?
g. Attitudes about discipline	3. Does the child respond to parental limits and control?
h. Interference with discipline from outside the family	4. Do the parents inappropriately answer questions addressed to
(eg, ex-spouses, grandparents)	the child?
3. Stresses on the family	5. Is there obvious tension between family members?
a. Problems with employment	**Data from other sources**
b. Financial problems	1. Waiting room observations by office staff
c. Changes of residence	2. School (teacher, nurse, social worker, counselor, day-care
d. Illness, injuries, and deaths	provider)
4. Family history of mental health problems	3. Department of social services
a. Depression? Who?	4. Other caregivers: grandparents, etc
b. Suicide attempts? Who?	
c. Psychiatric hospitalizations? Who?	
d. "Nervous breakdowns"? Who?	
e. Substance abuse or problems? Who?	
f. Nervousness or anxiety? Who?	

A. History of the Presenting Problem

First, obtain a detailed description of the problem.

- When did it start?
- Were there unusual stresses at that time?
- How are the child's life and the family's functioning affected?
- What does the child say about the problem?
- What attempts have been made to alleviate the problem?
- Do the parents have any opinions about the cause of the problem?

B. Techniques for Interviewing Children and Adolescents

1. Interviewing the preschool child—Preschool children should be interviewed with their parents. As the parents

discuss their concerns, the physician can observe the child's behavior, including their activity level and any unusual behaviors or symptoms. It is helpful to have toy human figures, animals, or puppets, and crayons and paper available that the child can use to express him- or herself. After hearing the history from the parents and observing and talking with the child, the physician can begin to develop an impression about the problem and formulate a treatment plan to discuss with the family.

2. Interviewing the school-aged child—Most school-aged children have mastered separation anxiety sufficientl' to tolerate at least a brief interview alone with the physic In addition, they may have important information to ' about their own worries. The child should be told ' hand by the parents or physician (or both) that th will want to talk to the child about his or her feelin' aged children understand and even appreciate parental concern about unhappiness, worries, and difficulty in getting along with people. At the outset, it is useful to explore the child's thoughts about certain issues raised by the parents and ask whether the child thinks that a problem exists (eg, unhappiness, anxiety, or sleep disturbance) and any other concerns the child may have. The physician should ask the child to describe the problem in his or her own words and ask what he or she thinks is causing the problem. It is important to ask the child how the problem affects the child and the family. At the end of the interview with the child, it is important to share or reiterate the central points derived from the interview and to state that the next step is to talk with the parents about ways to make things better for the child. At that time, it is good to discuss any concerns or misgivings the child might have about sharing information with parents so that the child's right to privacy is not arbitrarily violated. Most children want to make things better and thus will allow the physician to share appropriate concerns with the parents.

3. Interviewing the adolescent—The physician usually begins by meeting briefly with the parents and adolescent together to define the concerns. Because the central developmental task of adolescence is to create an identity separate from that of the parents, the physician must show respect for the teen's point of view. The physician should then meet alone with the adolescent. After the physician has interviewed the adolescent and talked further with the parents, he or she should formulate thoughts and recommendations. Whenever possible, it is helpful to discuss these with the adolescent before presenting them to the parents and teen together. The issue of confidentiality must be discussed early in the interview: "What we talk about today is between you and me unless we decide together that someone should know or unless it appears to me that you might be in a potentially dangerous situation."

The interview with the adolescent alone might start with a restatement of the parents' concerns. The teen should be encouraged to describe the situation in his or her own words and say what he or she would like to be different. The physician should ask questions about the adolescent's primary concerns, predominant mood state, relationships with family members, level of satisfaction with school and peer relationships, plans for the future, drug and alcohol use, and sexual activity.

In concluding the interview, the physician should summarize his or her thoughts and develop a plan with the teenager to present to the parents. If teenagers participate in the solution, they are more likely to work with the family to improve the situation. This should include a plan either for further investigation or for ways of dealing with the problem and arranging subsequent appointments with the physician or an appropriate referral to a mental health care provider.

C. Targeted Screening Tools and Assessment Measures

As with broad screening tools, targeted screening tools or assessment instruments can be very valuable in the clinic since they are standardized and allow for the assessment of current symptoms and severity. They can also be useful for following or reassessing a patient's progress after initiation of treatment.

1. Vanderbilt Assessment Scales for Attention-Deficit/ Hyperactivity Disorder—These scales are included in the American Academy of Pediatrics/National Initiative for Children's Health Quality (AAP/NICHQ) Attention-Deficit/Hyperactivity Disorder Practitioner's Toolkit, available at: http://www.nichq.org/resources/toolkit/ or http://www.schoolpsychiatry.org.

2. Center for Epidemiologic Scales Depression Scale for Children (CESD-C)—Available at: http://www.brightfutures.org/mentalhealth/pdf/tools.html.

3. Self-Report for Childhood Anxiety Related Emotional Disorders (SCARED)—Available at: http://www.wpic.pitt.edu/research/.

4. Other tools

A. BRIGHT FUTURES—The Bright Futures Tool Kit has numerous guidelines, tools, and other resources for identifying mental health concerns. Available at: http://www.brightfutures.org/mentalhealth/pdf/tools.html.

B. CHADDIS—See earlier discussion of models of health care.

C. DISORDER-SPECIFIC SCREENING TOOLS—Useful tools for evaluating other mental health concerns, such as obsessive-compulsive disorder (OCD), post-traumatic stress disorder (PTSD), and pervasive developmental disorder (PDD), can be found at the following web site: http://www.schoolpsychiatry.org.

Diagnostic Formulation & Interpretation of Findings

Diagnosis, the final product of the assessment, starts with a description of the presenting problem, which is then evaluated within the context of the child's age, developmental needs, the stresses and strains on the child and the family, and the functioning of the family system.

The physician's first task is to decide whether a problem exists. For example, how hyperactive must a 5-year-old child be before he or she is too hyperactive? When a child's functioning is impaired in major domains of life, such as learning, peer relationships, family relationships, authority relationships, and recreation, or when a substantial deviation from the trajectory of normal developmental tasks occurs, a differential diagnosis should be sought based on the symptom profile. The physician then develops an etiologic hypothesis based on the information gathered:

1. The behavior falls within the range of normal given the child's developmental level.
2. The behavior is a temperamental variation.
3. The behavior is related to central nervous system impairment (eg, prematurity, exposure to toxins in utero, seizure disorder, or genetic disorders).
4. The behavior is a normal reaction to stressful circumstances (eg, medical illness, change in family structure, or loss of a loved one).
5. The problem is primarily a reflection of family dysfunction (eg, the child is the symptom bearer, scapegoat, or the identified patient for the family).
6. The problem indicates a possible psychiatric disorder.
7. The problem is complicated by an underlying medical condition.
8. Some combination of the above.

Sharing of the diagnosis is also the beginning of initiating treatment. The physician's interpretation of the complaint and diagnosis is then presented to the family. The interpretive process includes the following components:

1. Psychoeducation: an explanation of how the presenting problem or symptom is a reflection of a suspected cause and typical outcomes both with and without intervention.
2. A discussion of possible interventions, including the following options:
   a. Close monitoring.
   b. Counseling provided by the primary care provider.
   c. Referral to a mental health professional.
   d. Initiation of medication.
   e. Some combination of the above.
3. A discussion of the parent's and adolescent's response to the diagnosis and potential interventions.

A joint plan involving the physician, parents, and child is then negotiated to address the child's symptoms and developmental needs in light of the family structure and stresses. If an appropriate plan cannot be developed, or if the physician feels that further diagnostic assessment is required, referral to a mental health practitioner should be recommended.

Fritz G: Promoting effective collaboration between pediatricians and child and adolescent psychiatrists. Pediatr Ann 2003;32:387 [PMID: 12846016].
Gardner W et al: Primary care clinicians' use of standardized tools to assess child psychosocial problems. Ambul Pediatr 2003; 3:191 [PMID: 12882596].
Glazebrook C et al: Detecting emotional and behavioural problems in paediatric clinics. Child Care Health Dev 2003;29:141 [PMID: 12603359].
Kelleher KJ et al: Management of pediatric mental disorders in primary care: Where are we now and where are we going? Curr Opin Pediatr 2006;18:649 [PMID: 17099365].

Richardson LP, Katzenellenbogen R: Childhood and adolescent depression: The role of primary care providers in diagnosis and treatment. Curr Probl Pediatr Adolesc Health Care 2005;35:6 [PMID: 15611721].
Williams J et al: Diagnosis and treatment of behavioral health disorders in pediatric practice. Pediatrics 2004;114:601 [PMID: 15342827].

Situations Requiring Emergent or More Extensive Psychiatric Assessment

If there is any concern about the child's safety the provider must also evaluate the risk of danger to self (suicidal attempts or ideation), danger to others (assault, aggression, or homicidal ideation), and screen for other factors that could heighten the risk of danger to self or others, such as physical or sexual abuse or illicit substance use or abuse. The presence of drug or alcohol abuse in adolescent patients may require referral to community resources specializing in the treatment of these addictive disorders.

The following questions should be asked of the youth. The parents should be asked similar questions about what they have observed. Specific details about the circumstances should be asked if any question below is answered with "yes."

1. Have you ever been sad for more than a few days at a time such that it affected your sleep or appetite?
2. Have you ever been so sad that you wished you weren't alive?
3. Have you ever thought of ways of killing yourself or made a suicide attempt?
4. Have you ever thought about killing someone else, or tried to kill someone?
5. Has anyone ever hit you and left marks? (If yes, ask who, when, and under what circumstances, and if it was reported.)
6. Has anyone ever touched your private areas when they weren't supposed to, or in a way that made you feel uncomfortable? (If yes, ask who, when, and under what circumstances, and if it was reported.)
7. Do you use alcohol, tobacco, or illicit drugs? (If yes, ask what, when, with whom, and how much.)

A. Civil Commitment and Involuntary Mental Health "Holds"

If further assessment indicates a need for inpatient hospitalization, it is optimal if the patient and guardian give consent for this care. In a situation in which the guardian is unwilling or unable to give consent for emergency department–based assessment or inpatient hospitalization of a child or adolescent, an involuntary mental health "hold" may become necessary.

The term involuntary mental health "hold" refers to a legal process that can be initiated by physicians, police officers, ar certified mental health professionals, that allows the indi ual to be prevented from leaving the emergency depar or hospital for up to 72 hours. This allows the phys establish a safe environment and prevent the individual from harming themselves or others, and allows sufficient time to determine if the individual is a risk to him- or herself or others due to mental illness. Each state has laws specifying rules and regulations that must be followed as part of this process. A specific form must be completed and the patient and family informed of their rights. As this involves revoking the civil rights of a patient or their guardian, it is critical to implement the procedure correctly. All physicians should be familiar with their state laws regulating this process.

Although the precise wording and conditions of involuntary mental health holds may vary slightly from state to state, they are generally quite similar. A 72-hour involuntary mental health hold is obtained for the purpose of acute evaluation and determination of the patient's safety when the evaluator elicits sufficient information to confirm a significant risk exists of danger to self or others. Additional criteria for involuntary psychiatric admission include a determination that the patient is "gravely disabled" by virtue of impaired judgment, which renders the patient unable to provide food, clothing, or shelter for him- or herself, or in the case of a child or adolescent, that he or she is unable to eat and perform normal activities of daily living.

B. Circumstances Under Which a Mental Health Hold May Be Discontinued

At any time after a patient's acute admission but within 72 hours, one of three possibilities must be chosen by the physician or psychiatric treatment team.

1. The clinician may determine that the patient is safe for further treatment in a less restrictive setting and may decide to end the 72-hour mental health hold and discharge the patient from the emergency department or the inpatient psychiatric setting. This requires assessment and documentation that the patient is now safe and a physician signature on an order form to discontinue the hold.

2. The patient or his or her guardian may agree to inpatient psychiatric treatment and offer to remain in the hospital as a voluntary psychiatric inpatient. In this case, the mental health hold is discontinued and the patient and guardian sign a request for voluntary mental health treatment.

3. Finally, the clinician and patient or guardian may continue to disagree about the need for inpatient psychiatric treatment. In this case, when the psychiatrist believes the patient continues to be a risk to him- or herself or others or is gravely disabled, the psychiatrist may petition the mental health court to place the patient on a "short term certification" (this is the term in use in Colorado, but other states have different terms and processes) for continued involuntary mental health treatment on an inpatient psychiatric unit by completing the appropriate evaluation and paperwork. In Colorado a short term

certification can remain in effect for up to 90 days or be discontinued at any time at the clinician's discretion or by a judge. Short term certification also mandates that a patient has access to legal representation in the form of his or her own lawyer or, if the patient is unable to afford legal council, a court-appointed attorney. Patients have the right to contest their involuntary commitment in front of a mental health judge. If the case goes to court, the health care providers must also be present at the hearing. It is always preferable to work with the guardian and the patient to obtain informed consent for treatment and to minimize the need for legal proceedings. Figure 6–1 outlines the steps in identifying the need for involuntary mental health treatment.

C. Mandatory Reporting of Abuse or Neglect or Threat to Others

Mandatory reporting by a physician of suspicion of physical or sexual abuse or neglect to the local human services agency is discussed in greater detail in Chapter 7. The "Tarasoff Rule" refers to a California legal case that led to a "duty to warn": Physicians are mandated to warn potential victims of harm when plans are disclosed to them about serious threats to harm specific individuals. Documentation of a phone call and registered letter to the individual being threatened are mandated. Under such circumstances, arrangement for the involuntary civil commitment of the potential perpetrator of harm is likely to be in order as well.

D. Referral of Patients to Mental Health Care Professionals

Primary care physicians often refer patients to a child and adolescent psychiatrist or other qualified child mental health professional when the diagnosis or treatment plan is uncertain, or when medication is indicated and the pediatrician prefers that a specialist initiate or manage treatment of the mental illness (Table 6–3). For academic difficulties not associated with behavioral difficulties, a child or educational psychologist may be most helpful in assessing patients for learning disorders and potential remediation. For cognitive difficulties associated with head trauma, epilepsy, or brain tumors, a referral to a pediatric neuropsychologist may be indicated.

Patients with private mental health insurance need to contact their insurance company for a list of local mental health professionals trained in the assessment and treatment of children and adolescents who are on their insurance panel. Patients with Medicaid or without mental health insurance coverage can usually be assessed and treated at their local mental health care center. The referring pediatrician or staff should assist the family by providing information to put them in touch with the appropriate services. Personal relationships with community mental health administrators and clinicians improve the success of referrals. Additionally, new delivery systems in which mental

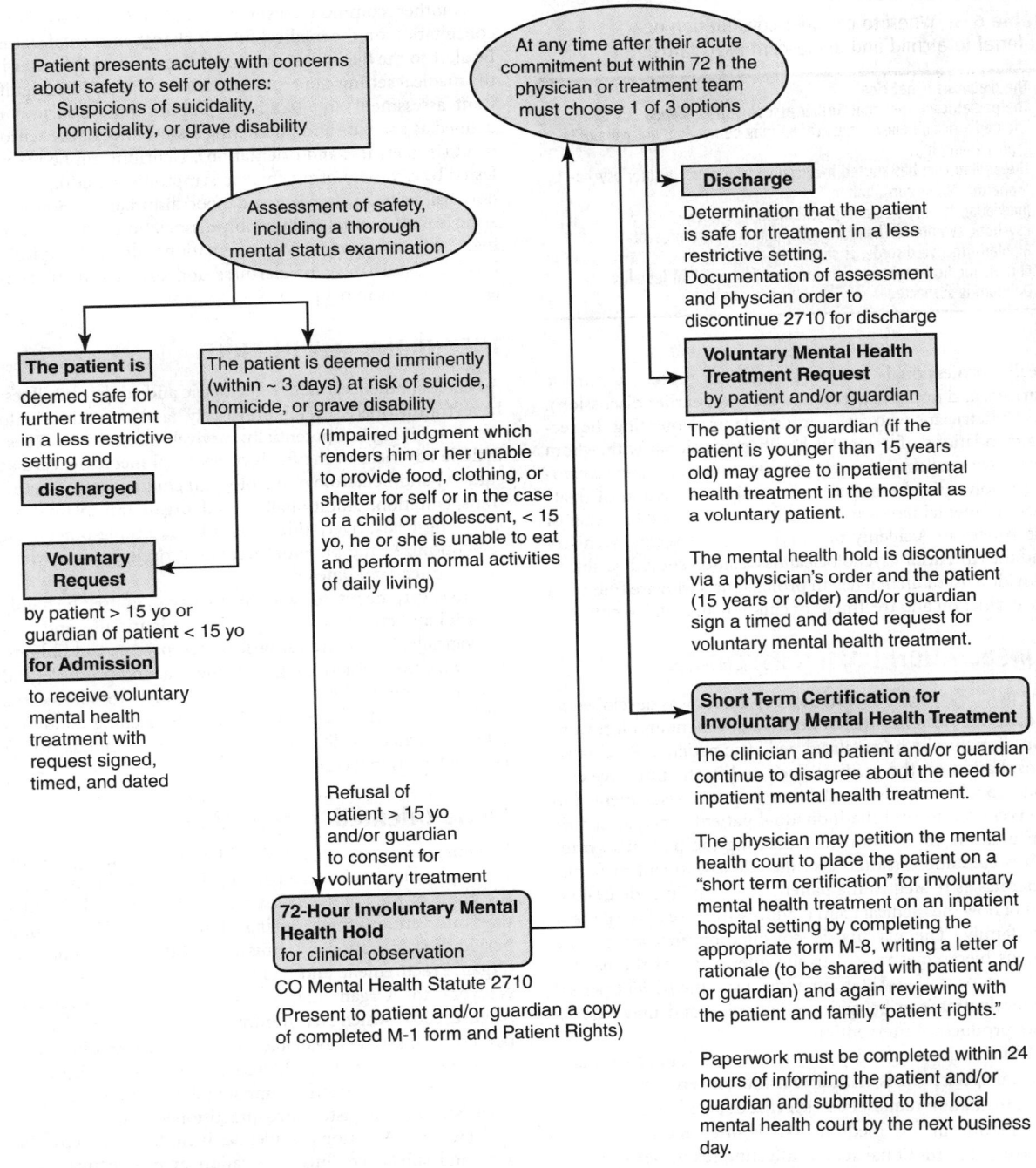

Patient presents acutely with concerns about safety to self or others: Suspicions of suicidality, homicidality, or grave disability

Assessment of safety, including a thorough mental status examination

At any time after their acute commitment but within 72 h the physician or treatment team must choose 1 of 3 options

The patient is deemed safe for further treatment in a less restrictive setting and **discharged**

The patient is deemed imminently (within ~ 3 days) at risk of suicide, homicide, or grave disability

(Impaired judgment which renders him or her unable to provide food, clothing, or shelter for self or in the case of a child or adolescent, < 15 yo, he or she is unable to eat and perform normal activities of daily living)

Discharge
Determination that the patient is safe for treatment in a less restrictive setting. Documentation of assessment and physcian order to discontinue 2710 for discharge

Voluntary Mental Health Treatment Request by patient and/or guardian

The patient or guardian (if the patient is younger than 15 years old) may agree to inpatient mental health treatment in the hospital as a voluntary patient.

The mental health hold is discontinued via a physician's order and the patient (15 years or older) and/or guardian sign a timed and dated request for voluntary mental health treatment.

Voluntary Request by patient > 15 yo or guardian of patient < 15 yo

for Admission to receive voluntary mental health treatment with request signed, timed, and dated

Refusal of patient > 15 yo and/or guardian to consent for voluntary treatment

72-Hour Involuntary Mental Health Hold for clinical observation

CO Mental Health Statute 2710

(Present to patient and/or guardian a copy of completed M-1 form and Patient Rights)

Short Term Certification for Involuntary Mental Health Treatment

The clinician and patient and/or guardian continue to disagree about the need for inpatient mental health treatment.

The physician may petition the mental health court to place the patient on a "short term certification" for involuntary mental health treatment on an inpatient hospital setting by completing the appropriate form M-8, writing a letter of rationale (to be shared with patient and/or guardian) and again reviewing with the patient and family "patient rights."

Paperwork must be completed within 24 hours of informing the patient and/or guardian and submitted to the local mental health court by the next business day.

▲ **Figure 6–1.** Steps in the process of civil commitment and involuntary mental health treatment in Colorado.

Table 6–3. When to consider consultation or referral to a child and adolescent psychiatrist.

The diagnosis is not clear
The pediatrician feels that further assessment is needed
The pediatrician believes medication may be needed, but will not be prescribing it
The pediatrician has started medications and needs further psychopharmacologic consultation
Individual, family, or group psychotherapy is needed
Psychotic symptoms (hallucinations, paranoia) are present
Bipolar affective disorder is suspected
Chronic medical regimen nonadherence has a risk of lethality
Delirium is suspected

health professionals are "co-located" in the clinic remove barriers and improve access and care (see earlier discussion).

Pediatricians who feel comfortable implementing the recommendations of a mental health professional with whom they have a collaborative relationship should consider remaining involved in the management and coordination of treatment of mental illness in their patients. The local branches of the American Academy of Child and Adolescent Psychiatry and the American Psychological Association should be able to provide a list of mental health professionals who are trained in the evaluation and treatment of children and adolescents.

CONSULTATION-LIAISON PSYCHIATRY

The field of consultation-liaison psychiatry was developed to address the need for mental health assessment and intervention of medically hospitalized pediatric patients. Psychiatric consultation on the medical floor and in the intensive care units can be complex and often requires assessment and intervention beyond the individual patient. The psychiatric consultation, in addition to evaluating the patient's symptom presentation, should also include assessment of family dynamics as related to the patient, and may include evaluation of how the medical team is addressing care of the patient and family. The psychiatric consultation focuses on the various hierarchies related to the interaction of the patient and staff, or staff and staff, in addition to the patient per se; this evaluation can be quite enlightening and may lead to more productive interventions.

When requesting a psychiatric consultation, as with any medical specialty it is critical that the concern and focus of the consultation request be as specific as possible. Psychiatric consultation on the medical floor is often requested when the patient's emotional state is affecting his or her response to medical care, or when an underlying mental illness may be contributing to the presenting symptoms. Patients admitted to the intensive care unit or a medical floor after a suicide attempt or supposed unintentional overdose should be evaluated by a psychiatric consultant before discharge.

Another common reason for requesting a psychiatric consultation on the medical floor is change in mental status. Be alert to the likelihood that acute mental status changes in the medical setting can represent delirium, as this has significant assessment and treatment implications. Delirium is defined as an acute and fluctuating disturbance of the sensorium (ie, alertness and orientation). Delirium can be manifested by a variety of psychiatric symptoms including paranoia, hallucinations, anxiety, and mood disturbances. However, aside from dementia and possibly dissociation and malingering, primary psychiatric presentations do not typically involve disturbances of alertness and orientation that are always present in delirium.

THE CHRONICALLY ILL CHILD

Advances in the treatment of pediatric and adolescent illness have transformed several previously fatal conditions into life-threatening but potentially survivable conditions. These include advances in the fields of neonatal medicine, cardiac surgery, and hematology-oncology, including bone marrow transplantation. Additionally, solid organ transplantation, including heart, liver, kidney, and lung, among others, has revolutionized the potential treatment options for a whole host of once-fatal illnesses.

However, the intensity of treatment can in itself be highly stressful and even traumatic physically, financially, and psychologically, for children as well as their parents and siblings. Survivors are at risk of long-term medical and psychological sequelae. Those who are fortunate enough to survive the initial treatment of a potentially life-threatening condition often exchange a life-threatening biologic illness for a chronic emotional condition.

Phase-Oriented Intervention

Psychosocial interventions should vary depending on the developmental level of the patient, siblings, and family, and the phase of the illness. A first crisis is dealt with differently than interventions made during a long course of illness, or a period of stabilization or remission. With this in mind, the Organ Procurement and Transplantation Network/United Network for Organ Sharing established new by-laws in August 2004 which set minimum requirements for the psychosocial services available as part of an accredited solid organ transplant program. Included in these guidelines is the establishment of a team comprising a transplantation psychiatrist, psychologist, nurse practitioner, and psychiatric social worker. Additional guidelines include a formal psychiatric and substance abuse evaluation of prospective transplantation candidates as well as evaluation of any potential renal or hepatic living donors. These guidelines include the availability of individual supportive counseling, crisis intervention, support groups, and death, dying, and bereavement counseling to transplantation patients and their families.

Reactions to Chronic Physical or Mental Illness & Disability

Between 5% and 10% of individuals experience a prolonged period of medical illness or disability during childhood and another 5–10% experience the onset of mental illness in childhood. The psychosocial effects for the child and the family are often profound. Although the specific effect of illness on children and their families depends on the characteristics of the illness, the age of the child, and premorbid functioning, it can be expected that both the child and the parents will go through stages toward eventual acceptance of the disease state. It may take months for a family to accept the diagnosis, to cope with the stresses, and to resume normal life to the extent possible. These stages resemble those that follow the loss of a loved one. If anxiety and guilt remain prominent within the family, a pattern of overprotection can evolve. Likewise, when the illness is not accepted as a reality to be dealt with, a pattern of denial may become prominent. The clinical manifestations of these patterns of behavior are presented in Table 6–4.

Children are very observant and intuitive when it comes to understanding their illness and its general prognosis. At the same time, their primary concerns usually are the effects of the illness on everyday life, feeling sick, and limitations on normal activities. Children are also keenly aware of the family's reactions and may be reluctant to bring up issues they know are upsetting to their parents. Whenever possible, parents should be encouraged to discuss the child's illness and to answer questions openly and honestly, including exploration of the child's fears and fantasies. Such interactions promote closeness and relieve the child's sense of isolation. Even with these active attempts to promote effective sharing between the child and the family, ill children frequently experience fear, anxiety, irritability, and anger over their illness, and guilt over causing family distress. Sleep disturbances, tears, and clinging, dependent behavior are not infrequent or abnormal. Parents frequently need support in an individual or group format to help them cope with the diagnosis and stress caused by the disease, its treatments, and its affect on the afflicted child and other family members.

The Vicious Cycle of Disease Empowerment

Submission to the power of illness, resulting, for example, in staying in bed longer than strictly necessary or withdrawing from friends and family, reduces a variety of opportunities to experience normal life. When reinforced by further relapses, increased helplessness and apprehension about symptoms raise the idea that symptoms and relapse strike unpredictably and cannot be influenced by the patient. Consequently, the patient experiences an increase in fear of illness and a reduction of activity because it can be interrupted at any time by unpredictable relapse. This submission to fear of illness by waiting for relapse reinforces the status of the

Table 6–4. Patterns of coping with chronic illness.

Overprotection
- Persistent anxiety or guilt
- Few friends and peer activities
- Poor school attendance
- Overconcern with somatic symptoms
- Secondary gain from the illness

Effective coping
- Realistic acceptance of limits imposed by illness
- Normalization of daily activities with peers, play, and school

Denial
- Lack of acceptance of the illness
- Poor medical compliance
- Risk-taking behaviors
- Lack of parental follow-through with medical instructions
- General pattern of acting-out behavior

chronically ill with increased helplessness. Both cycles result in lowering of self-esteem and disempowerment.

Families of chronically ill patients sometimes continue to use the same behavior and strategies, favoring rigidity and predictable long-standing habits. Although such rigidity is constraining, families often consider change as being unsafe. Past, present, and future collapse into a timeless dimension under the tyranny of illness. Rituals and metaphors serve the purpose of introducing distinctions in time. Rituals have always been used to demarcate different phases in life and to celebrate significant moments. Introducing different rituals that are consistent with family growth and helping the family to seek out their developmental priorities can represent an important intervention.

Discussions and interventions that take into account both emotional and medical symptoms will help the child and family better understand their experiences and attitude toward illness and life. The family and child will benefit from discussions about such questions as "What is the real nature of this illness? Why has it affected us? What will be our future? What does the treatment do to me?" Such discussions can be quite enlightening and empowering, as they encourage open discussion for the child and parents and an active role in treatment.

Patient-reported and parent-reported outcome tools, known either as Health Status or Health Related Quality of Life (HRQOL) measures, can also be routinely used in pediatric specialty clinics. These measures adopt the World Health Organization's definition of health as "a state of complete physical, mental, and social well-being and not merely the absence of disease." Health-related quality of life refers to the subjective and objective impact of dysfunction associated with an illness or injury and is multidimensional, including four core domains: disease state and physical symptoms, functional status, psychological functioning, and social functioning. A team approach is often necessary when providing care to complex and chronically ill children. Including these measures during annual visits and in rating a mental health professional on the team can improve overall adjustment and quality of care.

THE TERMINALLY ILL CHILD

The diagnosis of a potentially fatal illness in a child is a severe blow even to families who have reason to suspect that outcome. The discussion with parents and the child about terminal illness is one of the most difficult tasks for a physician working with children and adolescents. Although parents want and need to know the truth, they are best told in stepwise fashion beginning with temporizing phrases such as "The news is not good" and "This is a life-threatening illness." The parents' reactions and questions can then be observed for clues about how much they want to be told at any one time. The physician must also attempt to gauge how much of the information the parents are able to comprehend during the initial discussion and consider involvement of appropriate support services. Some parents may dissociate during the sharing of frightening and overwhelming news, and crucial information may need to be addressed again when the parents are in a less-traumatized and more receptive state. Parents' reactions may proceed in a grief sequence, including initial shock and disbelief lasting days to weeks, followed by anger, despair, and guilt over weeks to months, and ending in acceptance of the reality of the situation. These responses vary in their expression, intensity, and duration for each member of the family. Even when the illness is cured, some parents may continue to suffer from post-traumatic stress symptoms related to the diagnosis and treatment.

Developmental and phase-oriented perspectives of patients, siblings, parents, and caretakers are reviewed in Table 6–5. Although most children do not fully understand the permanency of death until about age 8, most ill children experience a sense of danger and doom that is associated with death before that age. Even so, the question of whether to tell a child about the fatal nature of a disease should in most cases be answered in the affirmative unless the parents object. When the parents object, this should alert the physician to involve the unit social worker, who can work with the family to ensure their decision is in the best interest of the child. Refusal of the adults to tell the child, especially when the adults themselves are very sad, leads to a conspiracy of silence that increases fear of the unknown in the child and leads to feelings of loneliness and isolation at the time of greatest need. In fact, children who are able to discuss their illness with family members are less depressed, have fewer behavior problems, have higher self-esteem, feel closer to their families, and adapt better to the challenges of their disease and its treatment.

The siblings of dying children are also significantly affected. They may feel neglected and deprived because of the time their parents must spend with the sick child. Anger and jealousy may then give rise to feelings of guilt over having such feelings about their sick sibling. Awareness of the emotional responses, coping abilities, and available resources for support of other family members can diminish these feelings and make a significant difference in the family's overall ability to cope with the illness.

After the child dies, the period of bereavement may last for years. Family members may need outside help in dealing with their grief through supportive counseling services or peer-support groups. Bereavement usually does not substantially interfere with overall life functioning for more than 2–3 months. Most parents and siblings are able to return to work and school within a month, although their emotional state and thoughts may continue to be dominated by the loss for some time. When the individual is unable to function in his or her societal and family role beyond this time frame, a diagnosis of complicated bereavement, major depression, post-traumatic stress disorder (PTSD), or adjustment disorder should be considered and appropriate interventions recommended, such as referral for counseling or psychotherapy and possibly antidepressant medication.

Long-Term Coping

The process of coping with a chronic or terminal illness is complex and varies with the dynamics of each individual child and family. Each change in the illness course and each new developmental stage present different challenges for the child and family. It is important for health care providers to continually assess the family's and child's needs and coping abilities over time and to provide appropriate support, information, and access to interventions.

Assistance from Health Care Providers

A. Educate the Patient and Family

Children and their families should be given information about the illness, including its course and treatment, at frequent intervals. Factual, open discussions minimize anxieties. The explanation should be comprehensible to all, and time should be set aside for questions and answers. The setting can be created with an invitation such as "Let's take some time together to review the situation again."

B. Prepare the Child for Changes and Procedures

The physician should explain, in an age-appropriate manner, what is expected with a new turn in the illness or with upcoming medical procedures. This explanation enables the child to anticipate and in turn to master the new development and promotes trust between the patient and the health care providers.

C. Encourage Normal Activities

The child should attend school and play with peers as much as the illness allows. Individual education plans should be requested from the school if accommodation beyond the regular classroom is necessary. At the same time, parents should be encouraged to apply the same rules of discipline and behavior to the ill child as to the siblings.

Table 6–5. Death and childhood.

	Before — Developmental Concerns			During			After		
				Sudden	Acute	Chronic			
Child									
0–5 y	Ideas on death; Abandonment; punishment	Death and stage anxieties; Fear of loss of love			Avoidance of pain; need for love	Withdrawal; separation anxiety			
5–10 y	Concepts of inevitability; confusion	Castration anxiety			Guilt (bad), regression, denial	Guilt (religious), regression, denial			
10–15 y	Reality	Control of body and other developmental tasks			Depression; despair for future	Depression; despair, anxiety, anger			
	Sudden	Acute	Chronic				Sudden	Acute	Chronic
Parents		Anxiety; concern; hopefulness	Premature mourning, guilt, anticipatory grief, reaction formation and displacements, need for information	Disbelief; displaced rage; accelerated grief; prolonged numbness	Desperate concern; denial; guilt	Denial; remorse; resurgence of love	Guilt; mourning	Anger at doctors; need for follow-up, over-idealizing, fantasy loss	Remorse; relief and guilt
Siblings									
0–5 y	Reactions to changes in parents (sense of loss of love and withdrawal)						1. Respond to reaction of parents		
5–10 y	Concern about their implications; fearful for themselves						2. Survivor guilt		
10–15 y	Generally supportive								
Staff	Anxiety; conspiracy of silence			Reaction: withdraw Tasks: 1. Correct distortions (e.g., "Am I safe?"; "Will someone be with me?"; "Will I be helped to feel better?") 2. Comfort parents 3. Allow hope and promote feeling of actively coping 4. Protect dignity of patient			Need for aftercare of survivors; autopsy request tactful; accurate information regarding disposal of body; delay billing		

Adapted, with permission, from Lewis M: *Clinical Aspects of Child Development*, 2nd ed. Lea & Febiger, 1982.

D. Encourage Compensatory Activities, Interests, and Skill Development

Children who experience disability or interruption of their usual activities and interests should be encouraged to explore new interests, and the family should be supported in adapting the child's interests for their situation, and in presenting new opportunities.

E. Promote Self-Reliance

Children often feel helpless when others must do things for them, or assist with their daily needs. The health care provider should guide and encourage parents in helping ;' children assume responsibility for some aspects of tł medical care and continue to experience age-appror independence and skills whenever possible.

F. Periodically Review Family Coping

Families are often so immersed in the crisis of their child's illness that they neglect their own needs or the needs of other family members. From time to time, the physician should ask "How is everyone doing?" The feelings of the patient, the parents, and other children in the family are explored. Parents should be encouraged to stay in touch with people in their support system, and to encourage their children in such efforts as well. Feelings of fear, guilt, anger, and grief should be monitored and discussed as normal reactions to difficult circumstances. If these experiences are interfering with the family's functioning, involvement of the pediatric social worker or a therapist can be helpful.

Appropriate lay support groups for the patient and family should be recommended. Many hospitals have such groups, and hospital social workers can facilitate participation for the patient and family.

Browning D: To show our humanness—Relational and communicative competence in pediatric palliative care. Bioethics Forum 2002;18:23 [PMID: 12744267].

Christian B: Growing up with chronic illness: Psychosocial adjustment of children and adolescents with cystic fibrosis. Annu Rev Nurs Res 2003;21:151 [PMID: 12858696].

Feudtner C et al: Spiritual care needs of hospitalized children and their families: A national survey of pastoral care providers' perceptions. Pediatrics 2003;111:e67 [PMID: 12509597].

Freeman K et al: Childhood brain tumors: Children's and siblings' concerns regarding the diagnosis and phase of illness. J Pediatr Oncol Nurs 2003;20:133 [PMID: 12776261].

Freeman K et al: Childhood brain tumors: Parental concerns and stressors by phase of illness. J Pediatr Oncol Nurs 2004;21:87 [PMID: 15125552].

Geist R et al: Psychosocial issues in the child with chronic conditions. Best Pract Res Clin Gastroenterol 2003;17:141 [PMID: 12676111].

Haase JE: The adolescent resilience model as a guide to interventions. J Pediatr Oncol Nurse 2004;21:289 [PMID: 15381798].

Kübler-Ross E: On Children and Death. Collier Books, Macmillan Publishing, 1983.

Laws T: Fathers struggling for relevance in the care of their terminally ill child. Contemp Nurse 2004;18:34 [PMID: 15729796].

Lewis M, Vitulano LA: Biopsychosocial issues and risk factors in the family when the child has a chronic illness. Child Adolesc Psychiatr Clin N Am 2003;12:389 [PMID: 12910814].

Meyer EC et al: Parental perspective on end-of-life care in the pediatric intensive care unit. Crit Care Med 2002;30:226 [PMID: 11902266].

Oliver RC et al: Beneficial effects of a hospital bereavement intervention program after traumatic childhood death. J Trauma 2001;50:440 [PMID: 11265051].

Stewart JL: Children living with chronic illness: An examination of their stressors, coping responses and health outcomes. Annu Rev Nurs Res 2003;21:203 [PMID: 12858698].

Suris JC: Chronic conditions and adolescence. J Pediatr Endocrinol Metab 2003;16(Suppl)2:247 [PMID: 12729399].

Van Riper M: The sibling experience of living with childhood chronic illness and disability. Annu Rev Nurs Res 2003;21:279 [PMID: 12858700].

Waugh S: Parental views on disclosure of diagnosis to their HIV-positive children. AIDS Care 2003;15:169 [PMID: 12856338].

PSYCHIATRIC DISORDERS OF CHILDHOOD & ADOLESCENCE

A psychiatric disorder is defined as a characteristic cluster of signs and symptoms (emotions, behaviors, thought patterns, and mood states) that are associated with subjective distress or maladaptive behavior. This definition presumes that the individual's symptoms are of such intensity, persistence, and duration that the ability to adapt to life's challenges is compromised.

Psychiatric disorders have their origins in neurobiologic, genetic, psychological (life experience), or environmental sources. The neurobiology of childhood disorders is one of the most active areas of investigation in child and adolescent psychiatry. Although much remains to be clarified, data from genetic studies point to heritable transmission of attention-deficit/hyperactivity disorder (ADHD), schizophrenia, mood and anxiety disorders, eating disorders, pervasive developmental disorders, learning disorders, and tic disorders, among others. About 3–5% of children and 10–15% of adolescents will experience psychiatric disorders.

The *Diagnostic and Statistical Manual of Mental Disorders, Fourth Edition, Text Revision* (DSM-IV-TR) is the formal reference text for psychiatric disorders and includes the criteria for each of the mental illnesses, including those that begin in childhood and adolescence. Psychiatric diagnoses are given on five axes to allow the physician to address the developmental, medical, psychosocial, and overall adaptive issues that contribute to the primary diagnosis on axis I or II.

Axis I: Clinical disorders

Axis II: Personality disorders, mental retardation, learning disabilities

Axis III: General medical conditions

Axis IV: Psychosocial and environmental problems

Axis V: Global assessment of functioning (on a scale of 0–100, with 100% being the highest level of functioning)

Unfortunately, available mental health classification systems are infrequently used in pediatric primary care settings since they address the more severe and extensive conditions. As previously stated, primary care providers frequently see a spectrum of disturbances in their clinical practice, many not achieving full DSM-IV-TR criteria. In order to combat the fact that current nosologies do not provide enough detail about common problems and situations that primary care pediatric providers come across, the AAP and the American Psychiatric Association (APA) collaboratively developed the DSM-IV Primary Care (DSM-PC), including a child and adolescent version. The key assumptions of the DSM-PC (C&A) are based on the fact that children's environments have an impact on their mental health, and that children demonstrate a continuum of symptoms from normality to severe disorders. The DSM-PC is compatible with the DSM-IV-TR, is clear and concise, and is available for research testing and subsequent refinement. It is organized into sections covering environmental situations, child manifestations, and severity (Table 6–6). Categories of the major environmental factors that may affect a child, ranging from economic issues to family violence, are described and given V codes. Specific behavioral manifestations are listed under broad groupings and include complaints, definitions, symptoms, differential diagnosis, developmental variation, and etiology. Severity, in the DSM-PC, has several dimensions including symptoms, functioning, burden of suffering, and risk and protective factors. The DSM-PC has a great deal of promise, not only as a mechanism to classify the complexities of children's behavior problems, but also as a mechanism for the future to facilitate financial reimbursement for early identification of and intervention for children's behavioral problems. Pediatricians should find this manual to be a valuable tool in the care of children and their families.

The descriptions of disorders in this chapter follow the DSM-IV-TR nosology rather than the DSM-PC criteria. Pediatricians are encouraged to become familiar with the DSM-PC, perhaps mastering one section at a time. A revised DSM-PC is being developed.

American Psychiatric Association: *Diagnostic and Statistical Manual of Mental Disorders*, 4th edition, text revision. American Psychiatric Association, 2000.

American Academy of Pediatrics: *Diagnostic and Statistical Manual for Primary Care (DSM-PC), Child and Adolescent Version*. American Academy of Pediatrics, 1996.

PERVASIVE DEVELOPMENTAL DISORDERS & AUTISM

Pervasive developmental disorders (PDDs) and childhood autism are early-onset, severe neuropsychiatric disorders that were once referred to as childhood psychoses. PDDs (including autistic disorder) are now distinguished from childhood schizophrenia on the basis of clinical differences and family histories. The term *pervasive developmental disorder* denotes a group of disorders with the common findings of impairment of socialization skills and characteristic behavioral abnormalities (Table 6–7). Speech and language deficits are common as well.

1. Autistic Disorder

ESSENTIALS OF DIAGNOSIS & TYPICAL FEATURES

▶ Severe deficits in social responsiveness and interpersonal relationships.

▶ Abnormal speech and language development.

▶ Behavioral peculiarities such as ritualized, repetitive, or stereotyped behaviors; rigidity; and poverty of age-typical interests and activities.

▶ Onset in infancy or early childhood (before age 3 years).

Table 6–6. Areas of focus in the Diagnostic and Statistical Manual, Primary Care (DSM-PC).

DSM-PC Section	Area of Focus
Environmental situations	Challenges to primary support group
	Changes in caregiving
	Community or social changes
	Educational challenges
	Parent or adolescent occupational challenges
	Housing challenges
	Economic challenges
	Inadequate access to health or mental health services
	Legal system or crime problem
	Other environmental situations
	Health-related situations
Child manifestations	Developmental competencies
	Impulsive, hyperactive, and inattentive behaviors
	Negative and antisocial behaviors
	Substance use and abuse
	Emotions and moods, and emotional behaviors
	Somatic behaviors
	Feeding, eating, and elimination
	Illness-related behaviors
	Sexual behaviors
	Atypical behaviors
Severity of disorder	
Mild	Unlikely to cause serious developmental difficulties or impairment in functioning
Moderate	May cause, or is causing, some developmental difficulties or impairment. Further evaluation and intervention planning are warranted.
Severe	Is causing serious developmental difficulties and dysfunction in one or more key areas of the child's life. Mental health referral and comprehensive treatment planning are often indicated, possibly on an urgent basis.

▶ General Considerations

Improved identification of autistic disorder has led to earlier interventions as well as confusion about etiology and fear about supposed rising incidence. Autism is more common than was once thought, with an incidence of approximately 16–40 cases per 10,000 school-aged children. More boys than girls are affected (3–4:1). Although the cause of autism is unknown, central nervous system dysfunction is suggested by its higher incidence in populations affected by perinatal disorders: rubella, phenylketonuria, tuberous sclerosis, infantile spasms, encephalitis, and fragile X syndrome. Studies of twins reveal over 90% concordance for autistic disorder

Table 6–7. Characteristics of pervasive developmental disorders.

Disorder	Age at Onset	Clinical Features
Asperger syndrome	Early childhood	"Odd" individuals (probably more common in males) with normal intelligence, motor clumsiness, eccentric interests, and a limited ability to appreciate social nuances
Childhood disintegrative disorder	3–4 y	Profound deterioration to severe autistic disorder
Pervasive developmental disorder	Early childhood	Two to three times more common than autistic disorder, with similar but less severe symptoms
Rett syndrome	5 mo–4 y	Females with reduced head circumference and loss of social relatedness who develop stereotyped hand movements and have impaired language and mental functioning
Autistic disorder	Before age 1 y	Severe deficit in social interaction, poor language development, abnormal eating and sleeping patterns.

monozygotic twins compared with 24% in dizygotic twins. Twenty-five percent of families with an autistic child have other family members with language-related disorders. Although there has been much debate over the past decade about a possible link between vaccines or dietary factors and the onset of autism spectrum disorders, research studies have not supported these as causal factors.

Rutter M: Incidence of autism spectrum disorders: Changes over time and their meaning. Acta Paediatrica 2005;94:2 [PMID: 15858952].

Minshew N, Williams DL: The new neurobiology of autism: Cortex, connectivity, and neuronal organization. Arch Neurol: 2007;64:945 [PMID: 17620483].

▶ **Clinical Findings**

Severe deficits in reciprocal social interaction (eg, delayed or absent social smile, failure to anticipate interaction with caregivers, and a lack of attention to a primary caregiver's face) are often evident even in the first year of life. In toddlers, findings include deficiencies in imitative play and a relative lack of interest in interactions with others. Language development is often quite delayed. In fact, children are often first referred for audiologic evaluation because of failure to respond as expected to sounds. When speech does begin to develop, it may be echolalic or nonsensical. Children with autism often display peculiar interests; bizarre responses to sensory stimuli; repetitive, stereotypical motor behaviors (eg, twirling and hand-flapping); odd posturing; self-injurious behavior; abnormal patterns of eating and sleeping; and unpredictable mood changes. Thematic pretend play is often impaired. An intense preoccupation with an age-unusual interest (eg, power poles) may replace the usual broad range of interests of the child's age-mates. About 40–60% of children with autism have intelligence quotients (IQs) below 70.

▶ **Differential Diagnosis**

A hearing or visual impairment must be ruled out with appropriate screening. Children with developmental speech and language disorders typically show better interpersonal interactions than children with autism. Evaluation should include investigations for metabolic disorders and fragile X syndrome. As stated, early identification usually predicts a better response to treatment. Use of the Ages and Stages and the Ages and Stages-SE will likely improve detection of early language or socioemotional disturbance. A formal screen with the Modified Checklist for Autism in Toddlers (M-CHAT) may help further guide the pediatric provider in making an early referral to appropriate early childhood evaluation services. (See also Chapter 2.)

▶ **Complications**

Approximately 30% of individuals with autism develop a seizure disorder, with the onset often occurring during puberty. The onset of puberty can also be associated with worsening of aggression, hyperactivity and self-destructive behaviors. These symptoms, along with the development of a seizure disorder, are more common in individuals who have a low IQ associated with their autism diagnosis. Comorbid psychiatric disorders should be screened for if significant changes in mood and behavior occur. Some adolescents with autism who have higher cognitive skills become distressed and possibly depressed as their awareness of their differences from their peers increases.

▶ **Treatment**

Parents and families need strong support as well as education in caring for a child with autism. Early interventions to facilitate the development of reciprocal interactions, language, and social skills are critical. Occupational therapy for sensory integration is also an integral component of the comprehensive assessment. Sensory integration interventions help the family better support the child and adapt the environment to their specific needs.

Behaviorally oriented special education classes or day treatment programs are vital in supporting the development of more appropriate social, linguistic, self-care, and cognitive skills.

No specific medications are available to treat the core symptoms of autistic disorder. Pharmacotherapy is aimed at reducing specific target symptoms and must be continually assessed and reevaluated for efficacy and side effects. Coexisting diagnoses must be carefully considered. Antipsychotic medications (eg, risperidone, olanzapine, and haloperidol) may modify a variety of disruptive symptoms, including hyperactivity and aggressiveness. Stimulants may improve inattentive or hyperactive symptoms but can sometimes worsen behavior or mood. Antidepressants—especially the selective serotonin reuptake inhibitors (SSRIs)—may benefit both mood symptoms and symptoms of excessive rigidity or obsessive behavior. Mood stabilizers may diminish irritability, mood swings, or episodic dyscontrol. Naltrexone may help control severe self-injurious behavior or stereotypes. Controlled studies do not support the use of secretin or chelation therapy for autism.

Prognosis

Autism is a lifelong disorder. The best prognosis is for children who have normal intelligence and have developed symbolic language skills by age 5 years. Individuals with autism may not be able to live independently and may require significant support and supervision throughout their lives. Approximately one-sixth of children with autism become gainfully employed as adults, and another one-sixth are able to function in sheltered workshops or special work and school environments. Placement in specialized residential homes or programs may be necessary for some individuals whose guardians are unable to meet their special needs or provide a secure and safe home environment.

Chakrabarti S, Fombonne E: Pervasive developmental disorders in preschool children. JAMA 2002;285:3093 [PMID: 11427137].

Dunn-Geier J et al: Effect of secretin on children with autism: A randomized controlled trial. Dev Med Child Neurol 2000;42:796 [PMID: 11132252].

Findling RL: Pharmacologic treatment of behavioral symptoms in autism and pervasive developmental disorders. J Clin Psychiatry 2005;66(Suppl 10):26 [PMID: 16401147].

King BH, Bostic JQ: An update on pharmacologic treatments for autism spectrum disorders. Child Adolesc Psychiatr Clin N Am 2006;15:161 [PMID: 16321729].

McDougle CJ et al: Research Units on Pediatric Psychopharmacology (RUPP) Autism Network: Background and rationale for an initial controlled study of risperidone. Child Adolesc Psychiatr Clin North Am 2000;9:201 [PMID: 10674197].

Posey DJ et al: The use of selective serotonin reuptake inhibitors in autism and related disorders. J Child Adolesc Psychopharmacol 2006;16:181 [PMID: 16553558].

Volkmar F et al: Practice parameters for the assessment and treatment of children, adolescents and adults with autism and other pervasive developmental disorders. J Am Acad Child Adolesc Psychiatry 1999;38(Suppl):32S [PMID: 10624084].

2. Nonautistic Pervasive Developmental Disorders

These disorders comprise Asperger syndrome, childhood disintegrative disorder, pervasive developmental disorder not otherwise specified (PDD-NOS), and Rett syndrome (see Table 6–7).

ESSENTIALS OF DIAGNOSIS & TYPICAL FEATURES

▶ Substantial social impairment, either primary or representing a loss of previously acquired social skills.

▶ Abnormalities in speech and language development or behavior resembling autistic disorder.

▶ Onset by early childhood (may be as late as age 9 years in childhood disintegrative disorder).

General Considerations

Children with nonautistic PDDs display a wide range of deficits in social, language, and behavioral skills that are similar to those in children with autistic disorder. However, these children deviate from the clinical profile for autistic disorder by failing to meet all the necessary diagnostic criteria, by failing to fulfill the severity threshold (ie, milder functional impairment), by manifesting atypical symptomatology (eg, the characteristic hand-wringing or gender distribution [female] in Rett syndrome), or by experiencing onset at a later age. In the past, many of these children would have been classified in the group manifesting so-called atypical development. Children with nonautistic PDDs probably outnumber autistic children by as much as 2–3:1. The majority of Rett syndrome cases are now known to be due to a mutation in the *MECP2*, an X-linked gene.

Differential Diagnosis

Specific developmental speech and language disorders should be distinguished. Hearing impairment should be ruled out with appropriate screening.

Treatment

The backbone of treatment for Asperger syndrome and PDD-NOS is a cognitive-behavioral approach aimed at teaching and reinforcing more appropriate social and language skills and behaviors. Rett syndrome and childhood disintegrative disorder have much worse prognoses and call for multidisciplinary, often milieu-based interventions (as for autistic disorder). Occupational therapy for sensory integration interventions may be helpful. In all cases, family education and support are important.

Children should be screened for the presence of other psychiatric conditions, including mood disorders, obsessive-compulsive disorder (OCD), ADHD, and anxiety disorders, and appropriate interventions should be initiated. Medications may be helpful for treating specific target symptoms described for autistic disorder.

Prognosis

These are lifelong disorders. The prognosis is variable depending on the severity of social and language deficits and response to treatment interventions.

Starr E et al: Stability and change among high-functioning children with pervasive developmental disorders: A 2-year outcome study. J Autism Dev Disord 2003;33:15 [PMID: 12708576].

Tanguay P: Pervasive developmental disorders: A 10 year review. J Am Acad Child Adolesc Psychiatry 2000;39:1079 [PMID: 10986804].

Tidmarsh L, Volkmar FR: Diagnosis and epidemiology of autism spectrum disorders. Can J Psychiatry 2003;48:517 [PMID: 14574827].

MOOD DISORDERS

1. Depression in Children & Adolescents

ESSENTIALS OF DIAGNOSIS & TYPICAL FEATURES

► Dysphoric mood, mood lability, irritability or depressed appearance, persisting for days to months at a time.
► Characteristic neurovegetative signs and symptoms (changes in sleep, appetite, concentration, and activity levels).
► Suicidal ideation, feeling of hopelessness.

General Considerations

The incidence of depression in children increases with age, from 1–3% before puberty to around 8% for adolescents. The rate of depression in females approaches adult levels by age 15. The lifetime risk of depression ranges from 10–25% for women and 5–12% for men. The incidence of depression in children is higher when other family members have been affected by depressive disorders. The sex incidence is equal in childhood, but with the onset of puberty the rates of depression for females begin to exceed those for males by 5:1.

Clinical Findings

Clinical depression can be defined as a persistent state of unhappiness or misery that interferes with pleasure or productivity. The symptom of depression in children and adolescents is as likely to be an irritable mood state accompanied by tantrums or verbal outbursts as it is to be a sad mood. Typically, a child or adolescent with depression begins to look unhappy and may make comments such as "I have no friends," "Life is boring," "There is nothing I can do to make things better," or "I wish I were dead." A change in behavior patterns usually takes place that includes social isolation, deterioration in schoolwork, loss of interest in usual activities, anger, and irritability. Sleep and appetite patterns commonly change, and the child may complain of tiredness and nonspecific pain such as headaches or stomach aches (Table 6–8).

Table 6–8. Clinical manifestations of depression in children and adolescents.

Depressive Symptom	Clinical Manifestations
Anhedonia	Loss of interest and enthusiasm in play, socializing, school, and usual activities; boredom; loss of pleasure
Dysphoric mood	Tearfulness; sad, downturned expression; unhappiness; slumped posture; quick temper; irritability; anger
Fatigability	Lethargy and tiredness; no play after school
Morbid ideation	Self-deprecating thoughts, statements; thoughts of disaster, abandonment, death, suicide, or hopelessness
Somatic symptoms	Changes in sleep or appetite patterns; difficulty in concentrating; bodily complaints, particularly headache and stomach ache

Differential Diagnosis

Clinical depression can usually be identified simply by asking about the symptoms. Children are often more accurate than their caregivers in describing their own mood state. When several depressive symptoms cluster together over time, are persistent (2 weeks or more) and cause impairment, a major depressive disorder may be present. When depressive symptoms are of lesser severity but have persisted for 1 year or more, a diagnosis of dysthymic disorder should be considered. Milder symptoms of short duration in response to some stressful life event may be consistent with a diagnosis of adjustment disorder with depressed mood.

The Center for Epidemiologic Study of Depression–Child Version (CESD-C), Child Depression Inventory (CDI), Beck Depression Rating Scale, and Reynolds Adolescent Depression Scale are self-report rating scales that are easily used in primary care to assist in assessment and monitoring response to treatment.

Depression often coexists with other mental illnesses such as ADHD, conduct disorders, anxiety disorders, eating disorders, and substance abuse disorders. Medically ill patients also have an increased incidence of depression. Every child and adolescent with a depressed mood state should be asked directly about suicidal ideation and physical and sexual abuse. Depressed adolescents should also be screened for hypothyroidism and substance abuse.

Complications

The risk of suicide is the most significant risk associated with depressive episodes. In addition, adolescents are likely to self-medicate their feelings through substance abuse, or indulge in self-injurious behaviors such as cutting or burning themselves (without suicidal intent). School performance usually suffers during a depressive episode, as children are unable to concentrate or motivate themselves to complete homework or projects. The irritability, isolation, and withdrawal that often result from the depressive episode can lead to loss of peer relationships and tense dynamics within the family.

Treatment

Treatment includes developing a comprehensive plan to treat the depressive episode and help the family to respond more effectively to the patient's emotional needs. Referrals should always be made for individual and family therapy. Cognitive-behavioral therapy has been shown to effectively improve depressive symptoms in children and adolescents. Cognitive-behavioral therapy includes a focus on building coping skills to change negative thought patterns that predominate in depressive conditions. It also helps the young person to identify, label, and verbalize feelings and misperceptions. In therapy, efforts are also made to resolve conflicts between family members and improve communication skills within the family.

When the symptoms of depression are moderate to severe and persistent, and have begun to interfere with relationships and school performance, antidepressant medications may be indicated (Table 6–9). Mild depressive symptoms often do not require antidepressant medications and may improve with psychotherapy alone. A positive family history of depression increases the risk of early-onset depression in children and adolescents and the chances of a positive response to antidepressant medication. Depression in toddlers and young children is best approached with parent-child relational therapies.

Controversy continues regarding the efficacy and safety of antidepressants in children and adolescents. (See Psychopharmacology section, later.) Following the addition of a "black box warning" for all antidepressants in October 2005, a 20% decrease in prescriptions for those under age 20 was noted with a corresponding 18% increase in suicides. Also supporting treatment is the finding that suicide rates in children and adolescents were lowest in areas of the country that had had the highest rate of SSRI prescriptions. These debates will continue, but best practice is to educate the family and monitor carefully, especially in the first 4 weeks and subsequent 3 months, watching carefully for any increase in suicidal ideation or self-injurious urges, as well as improvement in target symptoms of depression.

Prognosis

A comprehensive treatment intervention, including psychoeducation for the family, individual and family psychotherapy, medication assessment, and evaluation of school and home environments, often leads to complete remission of depressive symptoms over a 1- to 2-month period. If medications are started and prove effective, they must be continued for 6–9 months after remission of symptoms to prevent relapse. Early-onset depression (before age 15) is associated

Table 6–9. Interventions for the treatment of depression.

Disorder	Interventions	
Adjustment disorder with depressed mood	Refer for psychotherapy	Medications usually not needed
Mild depression	Refer for psychotherapy	Medications may not be needed
Moderate depression	Refer for psychotherapy	Consider antidepressant medication
Severe depression	Refer for psychotherapy	Strongly encourage antidepressant medication

with increased risk of recurrent episodes and the potential need for longer term treatment with antidepressants. Education of the family and child (or adolescent) will help them identify depressive symptoms sooner and limit the severity of future episodes with earlier interventions. Some studies suggest that up to 30% of preadolescents with major depression manifest bipolar disorder at 2-year follow-up. It is important to reassess the child or adolescent with depressive symptoms regularly for at least 6 months and to maintain awareness of the depressive episode in the course of well-child care.

American Academy of Child and Adolescent Psychiatry: Practice parameters for the assessment and treatment of children and adolescents with depressive disorders. J Am Acad Child Adolesc Psychiatry 1998;37(Suppl):63S [PMID: 9785729].

Birmaher B et al: Course and outcome of child and adolescent major depressive disorder. Child Adolesc Psychiatr Clin North Am 2002;11:619 [PMID: 12222086].

Cheung A: Review: 3 of 4 RCTs on the treatment of adolescent depression in primary care have positive results. Evid Based Med 2007;12:27 [PMDI: 17264275].

Compton SN et al: Cognitive-behavioral psychotherapy for anxiety and depressive disorders in children and adolescents; an evidence-based medicine review. J Am Acad Child Adolesc Psychiatry 2004;43:930 [PMID: 15266189].

Emslie GJ et al: Fluoxetine for acute treatment of depression in children and adolescents: A placebo-controlled randomized clinical trial. J Am Acad Child Adolesc Psychiatry 2002;41:1205 [PMID: 12364842].

Emslie GJ et al: Predictors of response to treatment in children and adolescents with mood disorders. Psychiatr Clin North Am 2003;26:435 [PMID: 12778842].

Hughes CW et al: Texas Children's Medication Algorithm Project: Update from Texas Consensus Conference Panel on Medication Treatment of Childhood Major Depressive Disorder. J Am Acad Child Adolesc Psychiatry 2007;46:667 [PMDI: 17513980].

Jackson B, Lurie S: Adolescent depression: Challenges and opportunities: A review and current recommendations for clinical practice. Adv Pediatr 2006;53:111 [PMID: 17089865].

Louters LL: Don't overlook childhood depression. JAAPA 2004; 17:18 [PMID: 15500189].

Olsen AL et al: Primary care pediatrician's roles and perceived responsibility in the identification and management of depression in children and adolescents. Ambulatory Pediatr 2001 [PMID: 11888379].

Treatment for Adolescents with Depression Study (TADS) Team: The Treatment for Adolescents with Depression Study (TADS): Demographic and clinical characteristics. J Am Acad Child Adolesc Psychiatry 2005;44:28 [PMID: 15608541].

Wong IC et al: Use of selective serotonin reuptake inhibitors in children and adolescents. Drug Saf 2004;27:991 [PMID: 15471506].

2. Bipolar Affective Disorder

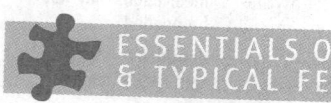

ESSENTIALS OF DIAGNOSIS & TYPICAL FEATURES

▶ Periods of abnormally and persistently elevated, expansive, or irritable mood, and heightened levels of energy and activity.

▶ Associated symptoms: grandiosity, diminished need for sleep, pressured speech, racing thoughts, impaired judgment.

▶ Not caused by prescribed or illicit drugs.

▶ General Considerations

Bipolar affective disorder (previously referred to as manic-depressive disorder) is an episodic mood disorder manifested by alternating periods of mania and major depressive episodes or, less commonly, manic episodes alone. Children and adolescents often exhibit a variable course of mood instability combined with aggressive behavior and impulsivity. At least 20% of bipolar adults experience onset of symptoms before age 20 years. Onset of bipolar disorder before puberty is uncommon; however, symptoms often begin to develop and may be initially diagnosed as ADHD or other disruptive behavior disorders. The lifetime prevalence of bipolar disorder in middle to late adolescence approaches 1%.

▶ Clinical Findings

In about 70% of patients, the first symptoms are primarily those of depression; in the remainder, manic, hypomanic, or mixed states dominate the presentation. Patients with mania display a variable pattern of elevated, expansive, or irritable mood along with rapid speech, high energy levels, difficulty in sustaining concentration, and a decreased need for sleep. The child or adolescent may also have hypersexual behavior, usually in the absence of a history or sexual abuse. (It is critical to rule out abuse, or be aware of abuse factors contributing to the clinical presentation.) Patients often do not acknowledge any problem with their mood or behavior. The clinical picture can be quite dramatic, with florid psychotic symptoms of delusions and hallucinations accompanying extreme hyperactivity and impulsivity. Other illnesses on the bipolar spectrum are bipolar type II, which is characterized by recurrent major depressive episodes alternating with hypomanic episodes (lower intensity manic episodes that do not cause social impairment and do not typically last as long as manic episodes) and cyclothymic

disorder, which is diagnosed when the child or adolescent has had 1 year of hypomanic symptoms alternating with depressive symptoms that do not meet criteria for major depression.

It is also common for individuals diagnosed with bipolar spectrum disorders to have a history of attentional and hyperactivity problems in childhood, and some will have a diagnosis of ADHD as well. ADHD and bipolar disorder are highly comorbid; however, it is also felt that attentional and hyperactivity problems accompanied by mood swings can be an early sign of bipolar disorder before full criteria for the disorder have emerged and clustered together in a specific pattern.

▶ Differential Diagnosis

Differentiating ADHD, bipolar disorder, and major depressive disorder can be a challenge even for the seasoned clinician, and confusion about the validity of the disorder in younger children still exists. The situation is further complicated by the potential for the coexistence of ADHD and mood disorders in the same patient.

A history of the temporal course of symptoms can be most helpful. ADHD is typically a chronic disorder of lifelong duration. However, it may not be a problem until the patient enters the classroom setting. Mood disorders are typically characterized by a normal baseline followed by an acute onset of symptoms usually associated with acute sleep, appetite, and behavior changes. If inattentive, hyperactive, or impulsive behavior was not a problem a year ago, it is unlikely to be ADHD. Typically, all of these disorders are quite heritable, so a positive family history for other affected individuals can be enlightening. Successful treatment of relatives can offer guidance for appropriate treatment.

In prepubescent children, mania may be difficult to differentiate from ADHD and other disruptive behavior disorders. In both children and adolescents, preoccupation with violence, decreased need for sleep, impulsivity, poor judgment, intense and prolonged rages or dysphoria, hypersexuality, and some cycling of symptoms suggest bipolar disorder. Table 6–10 further defines points of differentiation between ADHD, conduct disorder, and bipolar disorder.

Physical or sexual abuse and exposure to domestic violence can also cause children to appear mood labile, hyperactive, and aggressive, and PTSD should be considered by reviewing the history for traumatic life events in children with these symptoms. Diagnostic considerations should also include substance abuse disorders, and an acute organic process, especially if the change in personality has been relatively sudden, or is accompanied by other neurologic changes. Individuals with manic psychosis may resemble those with schizophrenia. Psychotic symptoms associated with bipolar disorder should clear with resolution of the mood symptoms, which should also be prominent. Hyperthyroidism should be ruled out. The Young Mania Rating Scale and The Child Mania Rating Scale may be helpful in eliciting concerning symptoms and educating families and patients, and in aiding timely referral to local mental health resources.

Table 6–10. Differentiating behavior disorders.

	ADHD	Conduct Disorder	Bipolar Disorder
School problems	Yes	Yes	Yes
Behavior problems	Yes	Yes	Yes
Defiant attitude	Occasional	Constant	Episodic
Motor restlessness	Constant	May be present	May wax and wane
Impulsivity	Constant	May be present	May wax and wane
Distractibility	Constant	May be present	May wax and wane
Anger expression	Short-lived (minutes)	Plans revenge	Intense rages (minutes to hours)
Thought content	May be immature	Blames others	Morbid or grandiose ideas
Sleep disturbance	May be present	No	May wax and wane
Self-deprecation	Briefly, with criticism	No	Prolonged, with or without suicidal ideation
Obsessed with ideas	No	No	Yes
Hallucinations	No	No	Diagnostic, if present
Family history	May be a history of school problems	May be a history of antisocial behavior	May be a history of mood disorders

ADHD, attention-deficit/hyperactivity disorder.

▶ Complications

Children and adolescents with bipolar disorder are more likely to be inappropriate or aggressive toward peers and family members. Their symptoms almost always create significant interference with academic learning and peer relationships. The poor judgment associated with manic episodes predisposes to dangerous, impulsive, and sometimes criminal activity. Legal difficulties can arise from impulsive acts, such as excessive spending, and acts of vandalism, theft, or aggression, that are associated with grandiose thoughts. Affective disorders are associated with a 30-fold greater incidence of successful suicide. Substance abuse may be a further complication, often representing an attempt at self-medication for the mood problem.

▶ Treatment & Prognosis

Most patients with bipolar disorder respond to pharmacotherapy with mood stabilizers, such as lithium, or atypical antipsychotics. The recent data on the mood stabilizers carbamazepine and valproate have been less promising. The atypical neuroleptics are increasingly being used as primary mood stabilizers to treat bipolar disorder as primary agents, and olanzapine, risperidone, quetiapine, aripiprazole, and ziprasidone have been approved by the Food and Drug Administration (FDA) for the treatment of bipolar affective disorder in adults. If the individual is being treated primarily for manic episodes with a non-antipsychotic mood stabilizer (such as lithium) the addition of a neuroleptic medication may be necessary if psychotic symptoms (hallucinations, paranoia, or delusions) or significant aggression is also present. In cases of severe impairment, hospitalization is required to maintain safety and initiate treatment. Dual use of mood stabilizers and antipsychotics is still used in most settings, although the only approved medication for treatment of acute mania in youth aged 12 and older is lithium. It is often possible to discontinue the antipsychotic after remission of psychotic symptoms, it is usually necessary to continue treatment with a mood stabilizer for at least a year, and longer if the individual has had recurrent episodes. It is not uncommon for the patient to need lifelong medication. Supportive psychotherapy for the patient and family and education about the recurrent nature of the illness are critical. Family therapy should also include improving skills for conflict management and appropriate expression of emotion.

In its adult form, bipolar disorder is an illness with a remitting course of alternating depressive and manic episodes. The time span between episodes can be years or months depending on the severity of illness and ability to comply with medication interventions. In childhood, the symptoms may be more pervasive and not fall into the intermittent episodic pattern until after puberty.

Blumberg HP et al: Significance of adolescent neurodevelopment for the neural circuitry of bipolar disorder. Ann NY Acad Sci 2004;1021:376 [PMID: 1521913].

Carlson GA: Early onset bipolar disorder: Clinical and research consideration. J Clin Child Adolesc Psychol 2005;34:333 [PMID: 15901234].

Kent L, Craddock N: Is there a relationship between attention deficit hyperactivity disorder and bipolar disorder? J Affect Disord 2003;73:211 [PMID: 12547289].

Kowatch RA et al: Treatment guidelines for children and adolescents with bipolar disorder. J Am Acad Child Adolesc Psych try 2005;44:213 [PMID: 15725966].

Lofthouse N, Fristad MA: Psychosocial interventions for children with early-onset bipolar spectrum disorder. Clin Child Fam Psychol Rev 2004;7:71 [PMID: 15255173].

McClellan J et al: Work Group on Quality Issues: Practice parameter for the assessment and treatment of children and adolescents with bipolar disorder. J Am Acad Child Adolesc Psychiatry 2007;46:107 [PMID: 17195735].

McElroy SL: Diagnosing and treating comorbid (complicated) bipolar disorder. J Clin Psychiatry 2004;65(Suppl 15):35 [PMID: 15554795].

Pavuluri MN et al: Pediatric bipolar disorder: A review of the past 10 years. J Am Acad Child Adolesc Psychiatr 2005;44:846 [PMID: 16113615].

Quinn CA, Fristad MA: Defining and identifying early onset bipolar spectrum disorder. Curr Psychiatry Rep 2004;6:101 [PMID: 15038912].

Youngstrom EA, Youngstrom JK: Clinician's guide to evidence based practice: Assessment of pediatric bipolar disorder. J Am Acad Child Adolesc Psychaitr 2005;44:823 [PMID: 16034285].

SUICIDE IN CHILDREN & ADOLESCENTS

The suicide rate in young people has remained high for several decades. In 2007, suicide was the third leading cause of death among children and adolescents aged 10–24 years in the United States. The suicide rate among adolescents aged 15–19 years quadrupled from approximately 2.7 to 11.3 per 100,000 since the 1960s. It is estimated that each year, approximately 2 million U.S. adolescents attempt suicide, yet only 700,000 receive medical attention for their attempt. Suicide and homicide rates for children in the United States are two to five times higher than those for the other 25 industrialized countries combined, primarily due to the prevalence of firearms in the United States. For children younger than 10 years old, the rate of completed suicide is low, but from 1980 to 1992 it increased by 120%, from 0.8 to 1.7 per 100,000.

Adolescent girls make three to four times as many suicide attempts as boys of the same age, but the number of completed suicides is three to four times greater in boys. Firearms are the most commonly used method in successful suicides, accounting for 40–60% of cases; hanging, carbon monoxide poisoning, and drug overdoses each account for approximately 10–15% of cases.

Suicide is almost always associated with a psychiatric disorder and should not be viewed as a philosophic choice about life or death or as a predictable response to overwhelming stress. Most commonly it is associated with a mood disorder and the hopelessness that accompanies a severe depressive episode. Suicide rates are higher for Native American and Native Alaskan populations than for white, black, and Latinos/Hispanic populations. Although suicide attempts are more common in individuals with a history of behavior problems and academic difficulties, other suicide victims are high achievers who are temperamentally anxious and perfectionistic and who commit suicide impulsively after a failure or rejection, either real or perceived. Mood disorders (in both sexes, but especially in females), substance abuse disorders (especially in males), and conduct disorders are commonly diagnosed at psychological autopsy in adolescent suicide victims. Some adolescent suicides reflect an underlying psychotic disorder, with the young person usually committing suicide in response to auditory hallucinations or psychotic delusions.

The vast majority of young people who attempt suicide give some clue to their distress or their tentative plans to commit suicide. Most show signs of dysphoric mood (anger, irritability, anxiety, or depression). Over 60% make comments such as "I wish I were dead" or "I just can't deal with this any longer" within the 24 hours prior to death. In one study, nearly 70% of subjects experienced a crisis event such as a loss (eg, rejection by a girlfriend or boyfriend), a failure, or an arrest prior to completed suicide.

Assessment of Suicide Risk

Any clinical assessment for depression must include direct questions about suicidal ideation. If a child or adolescent expresses suicidal thinking, the physician must ask if he or she has an active plan. Suicidal ideation accompanied by any plan warrants immediate referral for a psychiatric crisis assessment. This can usually be accomplished at the nearest emergency department.

Assessment of suicide risk calls for a high index of suspicion and a direct interview with the patient and his or her parents or guardians. The highest risk of suicide is among white adolescent boys. High-risk factors include previous suicide attempts, a suicide note, and a viable plan for suicide with the availability of lethal means, close personal exposure to suicide, conduct disorder, and substance abuse. Other risk factors are signs and symptoms of major depression or dysthymia, a family history of suicide, a recent death in the family, and a view of death as a relief from the pain in the patient's life.

Intervention

Suicidal ideation and any suicide attempt must be considered a serious matter. The patient should not be left alone, and the physician should express concern and convey a desire to help. The physician should meet with the patient and the family, both alone and together, and listen carefully to their problems and perceptions. It should be made clear that with the assistance of mental health professionals, solutions can be found.

The majority of patients who express suicidal ideation and all who have made a suicide attempt should be referred for psychiatric evaluation and possible hospitalization. Most providers feel uncomfortable and have little experience in evaluating suicidality and risk. In addition, this evaluation frequently takes considerable time and requires contact with multiple informants. **The physician should err on the side of caution as referral for further assessment is always appropriate when there is concern about suicidal thinking and behavior.**

An evaluation in a psychiatrist's office or the emergency department will help determine level of risk and disposition. If the patient has suicidal ideation without a plan, has a therapist he or she can see the next day, is able to "contract for safety," and the family is able to provide supervision and support, then the evaluating physician can consider sending the patient and family home that day from the office or emergency department without need for hospitalization. If there appears to be potential for suicide as determined by suicidal ideation with a plan, there are no available resources for therapy, and the patient is not able to cooperate with a plan to ensure safety; if the patient is severely depressed or intoxicated; if the family does not appear to be appropriately concerned; or if there are practical limitations on providing supervision and support to ensure safety, the individual should be hospitalized on an inpatient psychiatric unit. **Any decision to send the patient home from the emergency department without hospitalization should be made only after consultation with a mental health expert.** The decision should be based on lessening of the risk of suicide and assurance of the family's ability to follow through with outpatient therapy and provide appropriate support and supervision. Guns, knives, and razor blades should be removed from the home, and as much as possible, access to them outside the home must be denied. Medications and over-the-counter drugs should be kept locked in a safe place with all efforts made to minimize the risk of the patient having access (eg, key kept with a parent, or use of combination lock on the medicine chest). The patient should be restricted from driving for at least the first 24 hours to lessen the chance of impulsive motor vehicle crashes. Instructions and phone numbers for crisis services should be given, and the family must be committed to a plan for mental health treatment.

Suicide prevention efforts include heightened awareness in the community and schools to promote identification of at-risk individuals and increasing access to services, including hotlines and counseling services. Restricting young people's access to firearms is also a critical factor, as firearms are responsible for 85% of deaths due to suicide or homicide in youth in the United States.

Finally, the physician should be aware of his or her own emotional reactions to dealing with suicidal adolescents and their families. Because the assessment can require considerable time and energy, the physician should be on guard against becoming tired, irritable, or angry. The physician should not be afraid of precipitating suicide by direct and frank discussions of suicidal risk. Reviewing difficult cases with colleagues, developing formal or informal relationships with psychiatrists, and attending workshops on assessment and management of depression and suicidal ideation can decrease the anxiety and improve competence for primary care providers.

American Academy of Child and Adolescent Psychiatry: Practice parameters for the assessment and treatment of children and adolescents with suicidal behavior. J Am Acad Child Adolesc Psychiatry 2001;40(Suppl):24S [PMID: 11314578].

Borowsky IW et al: Adolescent suicide attempts: Risks and protectors. Pediatrics 2001;107:485 [PMID: 11230587].

Borowsky IW: The role of the pediatrician in preventing suicidal behavior. Minerva Pediatr 2002;54:41 [PMID: 11862165].

Gould MS et al: Youth suicide risk and prevention interventions: A review of the past 10 years. J Am Acad Child Adolesc Psychiatry 2003;42:386 [PMID: 12649626].

Kennedy SP et al: Emergency department management of suicidal adolescents. Ann Emerg Med 2004;43:452 [PMID: 15039687].

Pelkonen M, Marttunen M: Child and adolescent suicide: Epidemiology, risk factors and approaches to prevention. Paediatr Drugs 2003;5:243 [PMID: 12662120].

Schmidt P et al: Suicide in children, adolescents, and young adults. Forensic Sci Int 2002;127:161 [PMID: 12175945].

Spirito A, Overholser J: The suicidal child: assessment and management of adolescents after a suicide attempt. Child Adolesc Psychiatr Clin N Am 2003;12:649 [PMID: 14579644].

Weller EB et al: Overview and assessment of the suicidal child. Depress Anxiety 2001;14:157 [PMID: 11747125].

ADJUSTMENT DISORDERS

The most frequent and most disturbing stresses for children and adolescents are marital discord, separation and divorce, family illness, the loss of a loved one, a change of residence, and for adolescents, peer relationship problems. When faced with stress, children can experience many different symptoms, including changes in mood, changes in behavior, anxiety symptoms, and physical complaints. Key findings for the diagnosis of an adjustment disorder include the following:

- The precipitating event or circumstance is identifiable.
- The symptoms have appeared within 3 months after the occurrence of the stressful event.
- Although the child experiences distress or some functional impairment, the reaction is not severe or disabling.
- The reaction does not persist more than 6 months after the stressor has terminated.

▶ Differential Diagnosis

When symptoms are a reaction to an identifiable stressor but are severe, persistent, or disabling, depressive disorder, anxiety disorder, and conduct disorders must be considered.

▶ Treatment

The mainstay of treatment is the physician's genuine empathy and assurance to the parents and the patient that the emotional or behavioral change is a predictable consequence of the stressful event. This validates the child's reaction and encourages the child to talk about the stressful occurrence and its aftermath. Parents are encouraged to help the child with appropriate verbal expression of feelings, while defining boundaries for behavior that prevent the child from feeling out of control.

▶ Prognosis

The duration of symptoms in adjustment reactions depends on the severity of the stress; the child's personal sensitivity to stress and vulnerability to anxiety, depression, and other psychiatric disorders; and the available support system.

SCHIZOPHRENIA

The incidence of schizophrenia is about 1 per 10,000 per year. The onset of schizophrenia is typically between the middle to late teens and early 30s, with onset before puberty being relatively rare. Symptoms usually begin after puberty, although a full "psychotic break" may not occur until the young adult years. Childhood onset (before puberty) of psychotic symptoms due to schizophrenia is uncommon and usually indicates a more severe form of the spectrum of schizophrenic disorders. Childhood-onset schizophrenia is more likely to be found in boys.

Schizophrenia is a biologically based disease with a strong genetic component. Other psychotic disorders that may be encountered in childhood or adolescence include schizoaffective disorder and psychosis not otherwise specified (psychosis NOS). Psychosis NOS may be used as a differential diagnosis when psychotic symptoms are present, but the cluster of symptoms is not consistent with a schizophrenia diagnosis.

ESSENTIALS OF DIAGNOSIS & TYPICAL FEATURES

▶ Delusional thoughts.

▶ Disorganized speech (rambling or illogical speech patterns).

▶ Disorganized or bizarre behavior.

▶ Hallucinations (auditory, visual, tactile, olfactory).

▶ Paranoia, ideas of reference.

▶ Negative symptoms (ie, flat affect, avolition, alogia).

▶ Clinical Findings

Children and adolescents display many of the symptoms of adult schizophrenia. Hallucinations or delusions, bizarre and morbid thought content, and rambling and illogical speech are typical. Affected individuals tend to withdraw into an internal world of fantasy and may then equate fantasy with external reality. They generally have difficulty with schoolwork and with peer relationships. Adolescents may have a prodromal period of depression prior to the onset of psychotic symptoms. The majority of patients with childhood-onset schizophrenia have had nonspecific psychiatric symptoms or symptoms of delayed development for months or years prior to the onset of their overtly psychotic symptoms.

▶ Differential Diagnosis

Obtaining the family history of mental illness is critical when assessing children and adolescents with psychotic symptoms.

Psychological testing is often helpful in identifying or ruling out psychotic thought processes. Psychotic symptoms in children younger than age 8 years must be differentiated from manifestations of normal vivid fantasy life or abuse-related symptoms. Children with psychotic disorders often have learning disabilities and attention difficulties in addition to disorganized thoughts, delusions, and hallucinations. In psychotic adolescents, mania is differentiated by high levels of energy, excitement, and irritability. Any child or adolescent exhibiting new psychotic symptoms requires a medical evaluation that includes physical and neurologic examinations (including consideration of magnetic resonance imaging and electroencephalogram), drug screening, and metabolic screening for endocrinopathies, Wilson disease, and delirium.

▶ Treatment

The treatment of childhood and adolescent schizophrenia focuses on four main areas: (1) decreasing active psychotic symptoms, (2) supporting development of social and cognitive skills, (3) reducing the risk of relapse of psychotic symptoms, and (4) providing support and education to parents and family members. Antipsychotic medications (neuroleptics) are the primary psychopharmacologic intervention. In addition, a supportive, reality-oriented focus in relationships can help to reduce hallucinations, delusions, and frightening thoughts. A special school or day treatment environment may be necessary depending on the child's or adolescent's ability to tolerate the school day and classroom activities. Support for the family emphasizes the importance of clear, focused communication and an emotionally calm climate in preventing recurrences of overtly psychotic symptoms.

▶ Prognosis

Schizophrenia is a chronic disorder with exacerbations and remissions of psychotic symptoms. It is generally believed that earlier onset (prior to age 13 years), poor premorbid functioning (oddness or eccentricity), and predominance of negative symptoms (withdrawal, apathy, or flat affect) over positive symptoms (hallucinations or paranoia) predict more severe disability, while later age of onset, normal social and school functioning prior to onset, and predominance of positive symptoms are generally associated with better outcomes and life adjustment to the illness.

American Academy of Child and Adolescent Psychiatry: Practice parameters for the assessment and treatment of children and adolescents with schizophrenia. J Am Acad Child Adolesc Psychiatry 2001;40(Suppl):4S [PMID: 11434484].

Arango C et al: Clinical effectiveness of new generation antipsychotics in adolescent patients. Eur Neuropsychopharmacol 2004;14(Suppl 4):S471 [PMID: 15572266].

Calderoni D et al: Differentiating childhood-onset schizophrenia from psychotic mood disorders. J Am Acad Child Adolesc Psychiatry 2001;40:1190 [PMID: 11589532].

Masi G et al: Children with schizophrenia: Clinical picture and pharmacological treatment. CNS Drugs 2006;20:841 [PMID: 16999454].

Shaeffer JL, Ross RG: Childhood onset schizophrenia: Premorbid and prodromal diagnostic and treatment histories. J Am Acad Child Adolesc Psychiatry 2002;41:538 [PMID: 12014786].

Toren P et al: Benefit-risk assessment of atypical antipsychotics in the treatment of schizophrenia and comorbid disorders in children and adolescents. Drug Saf 2004;27:1135 [PMID: 15554747].

CONDUCT DISORDERS

ESSENTIALS OF DIAGNOSIS & TYPICAL FEATURES

▶ A persistent pattern of behavior that includes the following:
  · Defiance of authority.
  · Violating the rights of others or society's norms.
  · Aggressive behavior toward persons, animals, or property.

General Considerations

Disorders of conduct affect approximately 9% of males and 2% of females younger than 18 years. This is a very heterogeneous population, and overlap occurs with ADHD, substance abuse, learning disabilities, neuropsychiatric disorders, mood disorders, and family dysfunction. Many of these individuals come from homes where domestic violence, child abuse, drug abuse, shifting parental figures, and poverty are environmental risk factors. Although social learning partly explains this correlation, the genetic heritability of aggressive conduct and antisocial behaviors is currently under investigation.

Clinical Findings

The typical child with conduct disorder is a boy with a turbulent home life and academic difficulties. Defiance of authority, fighting, tantrums, running away, school failure, and destruction of property are common symptoms. With increasing age, fire-setting and theft may occur, followed in adolescence by truancy, vandalism, and substance abuse. Sexual promiscuity, sexual perpetration, and other criminal behaviors may develop. Hyperactive, aggressive, and uncooperative behavior patterns in the preschool and early school years tend to predict conduct disorder in adolescence with a high degree of accuracy, especially when ADHD goes untreated. A history of reactive attachment disorder is an additional childhood risk factor. The risk for conduct disorder increases with inconsistent and severe parental disciplinary techniques, parental alcoholism, and parental antisocial behavior.

Differential Diagnosis

Young people with conduct disorders, especially those with more violent histories, have an increased incidence of neurologic signs and symptoms, psychomotor seizures, psychotic symptoms, mood disorders, ADHD, and learning disabilities. Efforts should be made to identify these associated disorders (see Table 6–10) because they may suggest specific therapeutic interventions. Conduct disorder is best conceptualized as a final common pathway emerging from a variety of underlying psychosocial, genetic, environmental, and neuropsychiatric conditions.

Treatment

Effective treatment can be complicated by the psychosocial problems often found in the lives of children and adolescents with conduct disorders, and the related difficulty achieving compliance with treatment recommendations. Efforts should be made to stabilize the environment and improve functioning within the home, particularly as it relates to parental functioning and disciplinary techniques. Identification of learning disabilities and placement in an optimal school environment is also critical. Any associated neurologic and psychiatric disorders should be addressed.

Residential treatment may be needed for some individuals whose symptoms do not respond to lower level interventions, or whose environment is not able to meet their needs for supervision and structure. It is not unusual for the juvenile justice system to be involved when conduct disorder behaviors lead to illegal activities, theft, or assault.

Medications such as mood stabilizers, neuroleptics, stimulants, and antidepressants have all been studied in youth with conduct disorders, yet none has been found to be consistently effective in this population. Early involvement in programs such as Big Brothers, Big Sisters, scouts, and team sports in which consistent adult mentors and role models interact with youth decreases the chances that the youth with conduct disorders will develop antisocial personality disorder. Multisystemic therapy (MST) is being used increasingly as an intervention for youth with conduct disorders and involvement with the legal system. Multisystemic therapy is an intensive home-based model of care that seeks to stabilize and improve the home environment and to strengthen the support system and coping skills of the individual and family.

Prognosis

The prognosis is based on the ability of the child's support system to mount an effective treatment intervention consistently over time. The prognosis is generally worse for children in whom the disorder presents before age 10 years; those who display a diversity of antisocial behaviors across multiple settings; and those who are raised in an environment characterized by parental antisocial behavior, alcoholism or other substance abuse, and conflict. Nearly half individuals with a childhood diagnosis of conduct disorder develop antisocial personality disorder as adults.

1. Oppositional Defiant Disorder

ESSENTIALS OF DIAGNOSIS
& TYPICAL FEATURES

▶ A pattern of negativistic, hostile, and defiant behavior lasting at least 6 months.

▶ Loses temper, argues with adults, defies rules.

▶ Blames others for own mistakes and misbehavior.

▶ Angry, easily annoyed, vindictive.

▶ Does not meet criteria for conduct disorder.

Oppositional defiant disorder usually is evident before 8 years of age and may be an antecedent to the development of conduct disorder. The symptoms usually first emerge at home, but then extend to school and peer relationships. The disruptive behaviors of oppositional defiant disorder are generally less severe than those associated with conduct disorder and do not include hurting other individuals or animals, destruction of property, or theft.

Oppositional defiant disorder is more common in families in whom caregiver dysfunction is present, and in children with a history of multiple changes in caregivers; inconsistent, harsh, or neglectful parenting; or serious marital discord.

Interventions include careful assessment of the psychosocial situation and recommendations to support parenting skills and optimal caregiver functioning. Assessment for comorbid psychiatric diagnoses such as learning disabilities, depression, and ADHD should be pursued and appropriate interventions recommended.

American Academy of Child and Adolescent Psychiatry: Practice parameters for the assessment and treatment of children and adolescents with conduct disorder. J Am Acad Child Adolesc Psychiatry 1997;36(Suppl):122S [PMID: 9334568].

Burke JH et al: Oppositional defiant disorder and conduct disorder: Review of the past 10 years, part II. J Am Acad Child Adolesc Psychiatry 2002;41:1275 [PMID: 12410070].

Farmer EM et al: Review of the evidence base for treatment of childhood psychopathology: Externalizing disorders. J Consult Clin Psychol 2002;70:1267 [PMID: 12472301].

Flory K et al: Relation between childhood disruptive behavior disorders and substance use and dependence in young adulthood. Psychol Addictive Behav 2003;17:151 [PMID: 12814279].

Henggeler SW et al: One-year follow-up of multisystemic therapy as an alternative to the hospitalization of youths in psychiatric crisis. J Am Acad Child Adolesc Psychiatry 2003;42:543 [PMID: 12707558].

Kutcher S et al: International consensus statement on attention-deficit/hyperactivity disorder (ADHD) and disruptive behavior disorders (DBDs): Clinical implications and treatment practice suggestions. Eur Neuropsychopharmacol 2004;14:11 [PMID: 14659983].

Loeber R et al: Oppositional defiant and conduct disorder: A review of the past 10 years. Part 1. J Am Acad Child Adolesc Psychiatry 2000;39:1468 [PMID: 11128323].

Steiner H, Remsing L: Work Group on Quality Issues. Practice parameter for the assessment and treatment of children and adolescents with oppositional defiant disorder. J Am Acad Child Adolesc Psychiatry 2007;46:126 [PMID: 17195736].

2. Violent Behavior in Youth

Of particular concern to physicians today, as well as to society at large, is the tragic increase in teen violence, including school shootings. There is strong evidence that screening and initiation of interventions by primary care providers can make a significant difference in violent behavior in youth. Although the prediction of violent behavior remains a difficult and imprecise endeavor, physicians can support and encourage several important prevention efforts.

- The vast majority of the increase in youth violence including suicides and homicides involves the use of firearms. Thus the presence of firearms in the home, the method of storage and safety measures taken when present, and access to firearms outside the home should be explored regularly with all adolescents as part of their routine medical care.

- Violent behavior is often associated with suicidal impulses. In the process of screening for violent behavior, suicidal ideation should not be overlooked. In general, the suicidal youth is somewhat easier to identify than the homicidal youth, and in many cases may be one and the same (see the section on Suicide in Children and Adolescents, earlier). Any comment about wishes to be dead or hopelessness should be taken seriously and help sought.

- Parents and guardians should be aware of their child's school attendance and performance and peer groups. They should know their children's friends and be aware of who they are going out with, where they will be, what they will be doing, and when they will be home. Any concerns should be discussed with the teen and interventions sought if necessary.

- Most students involved in school violence could have benefited from earlier interventions to address problems in social and educational functioning in the school environment. Many communities and school districts have increased their efforts to identify and intervene with students whom teachers, peers, or parents recognize as having difficulty.

Birnbaum AS et al: School functioning and violent behavior among young adolescents: A contextual analysis. Health Educ Res 2003;18:389 [PMID: 12828239].

Borowsky IW et al: Effects of a primary care based intervention on behavior and injury in children. Pediatrics 2004;4:e392 [PMID: 15466063].

Denninghoff KR et al: Emergency medicine: Competencies for youth violence prevention and control. Acad Emerg Med 2002;9:947 [PMID: 12208685].

Fergus S, Zimmerman MA: Adolescent resilience: a framework for understanding healthy development in the face of risk. Annual Rev Public Health 2005;26:399 [PMID: 15760295].

Grant KE et al: Stressors and child and adolescent psychopathology: Moving from markers to mechanisms of risk. Psychol Bull 2003;129:447 [PMID: 12784938].

Johnson SB et al: Urban youths' perspective on violence and the necessity of fighting. Inj Prev 2004;10:287 [PMID: 15470008].

Pontin LE: *The Romance of Risk, Why Teenagers Do the Things They Do.* Basic Books, 1997.

Rappaport N, Thomas C: Recent research findings on aggressive and violent behavior in youth: Implications for clinical assessment and intervention. J Adolesc Health 2004;35:260 [PMID: 15450540].

Tremblay RE et al: Physical aggression during early childhood: trajectories and predictors. Pediatrics 2004;114:e43 [PMID: 15231972].

ANXIETY DISORDERS

1. Anxiety-Based School Refusal (School Avoidance)

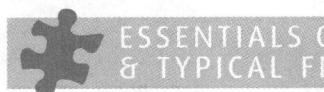

ESSENTIALS OF DIAGNOSIS & TYPICAL FEATURES

▸ A persistent pattern of school avoidance related to symptoms of anxiety.

▸ Somatic symptoms on school mornings, with symptoms resolving if the child is allowed to remain at home.

▸ No organic medical disorder that accounts for the symptoms.

▸ High levels of parental anxiety are commonly observed.

General Considerations

Anxiety-based school refusal should be considered if a child presents with a medically unexplained absence from school for more than 2 weeks. Anxiety-based school refusal is a persistent behavioral symptom rather than a diagnostic entity. It refers to a pattern of school nonattendance resulting from anxiety, which may be related to a dread of leaving home (separation anxiety), a fear of some aspect of school, or a fear of feeling exposed or embarrassed at school (social phobia). In all cases, a realistic cause of the fear (eg, an intimidating teacher or a playground bully) should be ruled out. In most cases, anxiety-based school refusal is related to developmentally inappropriate separation anxiety. The incidence between males and females is about equal, and there are peaks of incidence at ages 6–7 years, again at ages 10–11 years, and in early adolescence.

Clinical Findings

In the preadolescent years, school refusal often begins after some precipitating stress in the family. The child's anxiety is then manifested either as somatic symptoms or in displacement of anxiety onto some aspect of the school environment. The somatic manifestations of anxiety include dizziness, nausea, and stomach distress. Characteristically, the symptoms become more severe as the time to leave for school approaches and then remit if the child is allowed to remain at home for the day. In older children, the onset is more insidious and often associated with social withdrawal and depression. The incidence of anxiety and mood disorders is increased in these families.

Differential Diagnosis

The differential diagnosis of school nonattendance is presented in Table 6–11. Medical disorders that may be causing the somatic symptoms must be ruled out. Children with learning disorders may wish to stay home to avoid the sense of failure they experience at school. Children may also have transient episodes of wanting to stay at home during times of significant family stress or loss. The onset of school avoidance in middle or late adolescence may be related to the onset of schizophrenia. Children who are avoiding school for reasons related to oppositional defiant disorder or conduct disorder can be differentiated on the basis of their chronic noncompliance with adult authority and their preference for being with peers rather than at home.

Complications

The longer a child remains out of school, the more difficult it is to return and the more strained the relationship between

Table 6–11. Differential diagnosis of school nonattendance.[a]

I. Emotional or anxiety-based refusal[b]
A. Separation anxiety disorder (50–80% of anxious refusers)
B. Generalized anxiety disorder
C. Mood or depressive disorder (with or without combined anxiety)
D. Social phobia
E. Specific phobia
F. Panic disorder
G. Psychosis
II. Truancy[c] **behavior disorders**
A. Oppositional defiant disorder, conduct disorder
B. Substance abuse disorders
III. Situation-specific school refusal
A. Learning disability, unaddressed or undetected
B. Bullying or gang threat
C. Psychologically abusive teacher
D. Family-sanctioned nonattendance
1. For companionship
2. For child care
3. To care for the parent (role-reversal)
4. To supplement family income
E. Socioculturally sanctioned nonattendance (school is not valued)
F. Gender concerns
IV. Undiagnosed medical condition (including pregnancy)

[a]Medically unexplained absence of more than 2 weeks.
[b]Subjectively distressed child who generally stays at home.
[c]Nonsubjectively distressed and not at home.

child and parent becomes. Many parents of nonattending children feel tyrannized by their defiant, clinging child. Children often feel accused of making up their symptoms, leading to further antagonism between the child, parents, and medical caregivers.

► Treatment

Once the comorbid diagnoses and situations related to school avoidance or refusal have been identified and interventions begun (ie, educational assessment if learning disabilities are suspected, medication if necessary for depression or anxiety, or addressing problems in the home), the goal of treatment is to help the child confront anxiety and overcome it by returning to school. This requires a strong alliance between the parents and the health care provider. The parent must understand that no underlying medical disorder exists, that the child's symptoms are a manifestation of anxiety, and that the basic problem is anxiety that must be faced to be overcome. Parents must be reminded that being good parents in this case means helping a child cope with a distressing experience. Children must be reassured that their symptoms are caused by worry and that they will be overcome on return to school.

A plan for returning the child to school is then developed with parents and school personnel. Firm insistence on full compliance with this plan is essential. The child is brought to school by someone not likely to give in, such as the father or an older sibling. If symptoms develop at school, the child should be checked by the school nurse and then returned to class after a brief rest. The parents must be reassured that school staff will handle the situation at school and that school personnel can reach the primary health care provider if any questions arise.

If these interventions are ineffective, increased involvement of a therapist and consideration of a day treatment program may be necessary. For children with persistent symptoms of separation that do not improve with behavioral interventions, medications such as SSRIs should be considered. Comorbid diagnoses of panic disorder, generalized anxiety disorder, or major depression should be carefully screened for, and if identified, treated appropriately.

► Prognosis

The vast majority of preadolescent children improve significantly with behavioral interventions and return to school. The prognosis is worsened by the length of time the child remains out of school. Long-term outcomes are influenced by comorbid diagnoses and responsiveness to behavioral or medication interventions. A history of school refusal is more common in adults with panic and anxiety disorders and agoraphobia than in the general population.

Connolly SD, Bernstein GA; Work Group on Quality Issues: Practice parameter for the assessment and treatment of children and adolescents with anxiety disorders. J Am Acad Child Adolesc Psychiatry 2007;46:267 [PMID: 17242630].

Table 6–12. Signs and symptoms of anxiety in children.

Psychological
Fears and worries
Increased dependence on home and parents
Avoidance of anxiety-producing stimuli
Decreased school performance
Increased self-doubt and irritability
Frightening themes in play and fantasy
Psychomotor
Motoric restlessness and hyperactivity
Sleep disturbances
Decreased concentration
Ritualistic behaviors (eg, washing, counting)
Psychophysiologic
Autonomic hyperarousal
Dizziness and lightheadedness
Palpitations
Shortness of breath
Flushing, sweating, dry mouth
Nausea and vomiting
Panic
Headaches and stomach aches

Egger HL et al: School refusal and psychiatric disorders: A community study. J Am Acad Child Adolesc Psychiatry 2003;42:797 [PMID: 12819439].

King NJ, Bernstein GA: School refusal in children and adolescents: A review of the past 10 years. J Am Acad Child Adolesc Psychiatry 2001;40:197 [PMID: 11211368].

Masi G et al: Separation anxiety disorder in children and adolescents: Epidemiology, diagnosis, and management. CNS Drugs 2001;15:93 [PMID: 11460893].

2. Generalized Anxiety Disorder & Panic Disorder

Anxiety can be manifested either directly or indirectly, as shown in Table 6–12. The characteristics of anxiety disorders in childhood are listed in Table 6–13. Community-based studies of school-aged children and adolescents suggest that nearly 10% of children have some type of anxiety disorder. The differential diagnosis of symptoms of anxiety is presented in Table 6–14.

The evaluation of anxiety symptoms in children must consider the age of the child, the developmental fears that can normally be expected at that age, the form of the symptoms and their duration, and the degree to which the symptoms disrupt the child's life. The family and school environment should be evaluated for potential stressors, marital discord, family violence, harsh or inappropriate disciplinary methods, sexual abuse, neglect, and emotional overstimulation. The child's experience of anxiety and its relationship to life events should be explored, and therapy to incorporate specific cognitive and behavioral techniques to diminish the anxiety should be recommended. Finally, when panic attacks or anxiety symptoms do not remit with cognitive, behavioral, and environmental interventions, and they significantly affect life functioning, psychopharmacologic agents may be helpful. SSRIs may be effective across a broad spectrum of anxiety symptoms.

Table 6–13. Anxiety disorders in children and adolescents.

Disorder	Major Clinical Manifestations
Generalized anxiety disorder	Intense, disproportionate or irrational worry, often about future events
Panic disorder	Unprovoked, intense fear with sympathetic hyperarousal, and often palpitations or hyperventilation
Post-traumatic stress disorder	Fear of a recurrence of an intense, anxiety-provoking traumatic experience, causing sympathetic hyperarousal, avoidance of reminders, and the reexperiencing of aspects of the traumatic event
Separation anxiety disorder	Developmentally inappropriate wish to maintain proximity with caregivers; morbid worry of threats to family integrity or integrity of self upon separation; intense homesickness
Social phobia	Painful shyness or self-consciousness; fear of humiliation with public scrutiny
Specific phobia	Avoidance of specific feared stimuli

Table 6–14. Differential diagnosis of symptoms of anxiety.

I. Normal developmental anxiety
  A. Stranger anxiety (5 mo–2$^{1}/_{2}$ years, with a peak at 6–12 mo)
  B. Separation anxiety (7 mo–4 y, with a peak at 18–36 mo)
  C. The child is fearful or even phobic of the dark and monsters (3–6 y)
II. "Appropriate" anxiety
  A. Anticipating a painful or frightening experience
  B. Avoidance of a reminder of a painful or frightening experience
  C. Child abuse
III. Anxiety disorder (see Table 6–13), with or without other comorbid psychiatric disorders
IV. Substance abuse
V. Medications and recreational drugs
  A. Caffeinism (including colas and chocolate)
  B. Sympathomimetic agents
  C. Idiosyncratic drug reactions
VI. Hypermetabolic or hyperarousal states
  A. Hyperthyroidism
  B. Pheochromocytoma
  C. Anemia
  D. Hypoglycemia
  E. Hypoxemia
VII. Cardiac abnormality
  A. Dysrhythmia
  B. High-output state
  C. Mitral valve prolapse

▶ Prognosis

There is continuity between high levels of childhood anxiety and anxiety disorders in adulthood. Anxiety disorders are thus likely to be lifelong conditions, yet with effective interventions, individuals can minimize their influence on overall life functioning.

Arnold P et al: Childhood anxiety disorders and developmental issues in anxiety. Curr Psychiatry Rep 2003;5:252 [PMID: 12857528].

Arnold PD et al: Genetics of anxiety disorders. Curr Psychiatry Rep 2004;6:243 [PMID: 15260939].

Connolly SD, Bernstein GA; Work Group on Quality Issues: Practice parameter for the assessment and treatment of children and adolescents with anxiety disorders. J Am Acad Child Adolesc Psychiatry 2007;46:267 [PMID: 17242630].

Blanco C et al: Pharmacotherapy of social anxiety disorder. Biol Psychiatry 2002;51:1098 [PMID: 11801236].

Chavira DA et al: Comorbidity of generalized social anxiety disorder and depression in a pediatric primary care sample. J Affect Disord 2004;80:163 [PMID: 15207929].

Compton SN et al: Cognitive-behavioral psychotherapy for anxiety and depressive disorders in children and adolescents: an evidence based medicine review. J Am Acad Child Adolesc Psychiatr 2004;43:930 [PMID: 15266189].

Hudson JL et al: Nature, assessment and treatment of generalized anxiety disorder in children. Pediatr Ann 2005;34:97 [PMID: 15768686].

Kelly MN: Recognizing and treating anxiety disorder in children. Pediat Ann 2005;34:147 [PMID: 15768691].

Ginsburg GS, Grover RL: Assessing and treating social phobia in children and adolescents. Pediatr Ann 2005;34:119 [PMID: 15768688].

Jursbergs N, Ledley DR: Separation anxiety disorder. Pediatr Ann 2005;34:108 [PMID: 15768687].

Scott RW et al: An overview of controlled studies of anxiety disorders treatment in children and adolescents. J Natl Med Assoc 2005;97:13 [PMID: 15710867].

Reinblatt SP, Riddle MA: The pharmacological management of childhood anxiety disorders: A review. Psychopharmacology (Berl) 2007;191:67 [PMID: 17205317].

Wren FJ et al: Screening for childhood anxiety symptoms in primary care: integrating child and parent reports. J Am Acad Child Adolesc Psychiatry 2004;43:1364 [PMID: 15502595].

OBSESSIVE-COMPULSIVE DISORDER

ESSENTIALS OF DIAGNOSIS
& TYPICAL FEATURES

▶ Recurrent obsessive thoughts, impulses, or images that are not simply excessive worries about real-life problems.

▶ Obsessions and compulsions cause marked distress, are time-consuming, and interfere with normal routines.

▶ Repetitive compulsive behaviors or mental acts are performed to prevent or reduce distress stemming from obsessive thoughts.

Obsessive-compulsive disorder (OCD) is an anxiety disorder that often begins in early childhood but may not be diagnosed until the teen or even young adult years. The essential features of OCD are recurrent obsessions or compulsions that are severe enough to be time-consuming or cause marked distress and functional impairment. Obsessions are persistent ideas, thoughts, or impulses that are intrusive and often inappropriate. Children may have obsessions about contamination or cleanliness; ordering and compulsive behaviors will follow, such as frequent hand-washing, counting, or ordering objects. The goal of the compulsive behavior for the individual with OCD is to reduce anxiety and distress. There may be significant avoidance of situations due to obsessive thoughts or fears of contamination. OCD is often associated with major depressive disorder. OCD is a biologically based disease and has a strong genetic/familial component. Pediatric autoimmune disorders associated with group B streptococci have also been implicated in the development of OCD for some children. The prevalence of OCD is estimated to be around 2%, and the rates are equal between males and females.

Trichotillomania, while technically classified as an impulse disorder, is also thought to be related to OCD. It involves the recurrent pulling out of hair, often to the point of bald patches, and can also involve pulling out eyelashes, eyebrows, and hair from any part of the body. Trichotillomania should be considered in the differential diagnosis for any patient with alopecia. Treatment often includes the same medications used to treat OCD, and behavior therapy to decrease hair-pulling and restore normal social functioning.

▶ Treatment

OCD is best treated with a combination of cognitive-behavioral therapy specific to OCD and medications in more severe cases. SSRIs are effective in diminishing OCD symptoms. Fluvoxamine and sertraline have FDA approval for the treatment of pediatric OCD. The tricyclic antidepressant (TCA) clomipramine has FDA approval for the treatment of OCD in adults.

▶ Prognosis

Although OCD is usually a lifelong condition, most individuals can achieve significant remission of symptoms with the combination of cognitive-behavioral therapy and medications. A minority of individuals with OCD are completely disabled by their symptoms.

Comer JS et al: Obsessing/worrying about the overlap between obsessive-compulsive disorder and generalized anxiety disorder in youth. Clin Psychol Rev 2004;24:663 [PMID: 15385093].

Connolly SD, Bernstein GA; Work Group on Quality Issues: Practice parameter for the assessment and treatment of children and adolescents with anxiety disorders. J Am Acad Child Adolesc Psychiatry 2007;46:267 [PMID: 17242630].

Cook EH et al: Long-term sertraline treatment of children and adolescents with obsessive-compulsive disorder. J Am Acad Child Adolesc Psychiatry 2001;40:1175 [PMID: 11589530].

Freeman JB et al: Family based treatment of early onset obsessive-compulsive disorder. J Child Adolesc Psychopharmacol 2004;13(Suppl 1):S71 [PMID: 12880502].

Geller DA et al: Fluoxetine treatment for OCD in children and adolescents: A placebo controlled trial. J Am Acad Child Adolesc Psychiatry 2001;40:773 [PMID: 11437015].

Kaplan A, Hollander D: A review of pharmacologic treatment for obsessive-compulsive disorder. Psychiatr Serv 2003;54:1111 [PMID: 12883138].

March JS: Cognitive-behavioral psychotherapy for children and adolescents with OCD: A review and recommendations for treatment. J Am Acad Child Adolesc Psychiatry 1995;34:7.

March JS et al: Cognitive-behavioral psychotherapy for pediatric obsessive-compulsive disorder. J Clin Child Psychol 2001;30:8 [PMID: 11294080].

Snider LA, Swedo SE: PANDAS: Current status and directions for research. Mol Psychiatry 2004;9:900 [PMID: 1521433].

Stewart SE et al: Long-term outcome of pediatric obsessive-compulsive disorder: A meta-analysis and qualitative review of the literature. Acad Psychiatr Scand 2004;110:4 [PMID: 15180774].

Tay YK, Levy ML, Metry DW: Trichotillomania in childhood: Case series and review. Pediatrics 2004;113:e494 [PMID: 15121993].

Waters TL et al: Cognitive-behavioral family treatment of childhood obsessive-compulsive disorder: Preliminary findings. Am J Psychother 2001;55:372 [PMID: 11641879].

POST-TRAUMATIC STRESS DISORDER

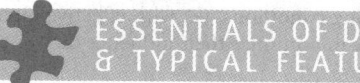

ESSENTIALS OF DIAGNOSIS & TYPICAL FEATURES

▶ Signs and symptoms of autonomic hyperarousal such as easy startle, increased heart rate, and hypervigilance.

▶ Avoidant behaviors and numbing of responsiveness.

▶ Flashbacks to a traumatic event, such as nightmares and intrusive thoughts.

▶ Follows traumatic events such as exposure to violence, physical or sexual abuse, natural disasters, car accidents, dog bites, and unexpected personal tragedies.

▶ General Considerations

Factors that predispose individuals to the development of post-traumatic stress disorder (PTSD) include proximity to the traumatic event or loss, a history of exposure to trauma, preexisting depression or anxiety disorder, and lack of an adequate support system. PTSD can develop in response to natural disasters, terrorism, motor vehicle crashes, and significant personal injury, in addition to physical, sexual, and emotional abuse. Natural disasters such as hurricanes, fires, flooding, and earthquakes, for example, can create situations in which large numbers of affected individuals are at heightened risk for PTSD. Individuals who have a previous history of trauma, or an unstable social situation are at greatest risk of PTSD.

Long overdue, attention is now being paid to the substantial effects of family and community violence on the psychological development of children and adolescents. Abused children are most likely to develop PTSD and to suffer wide-ranging symptoms and impaired functioning. As many as 25% of young people exposed to violence develop symptoms of PTSD.

Heightened concern about terrorism in the United States has created increased awareness of PTSD and community-based interventions to decrease the risk of PTSD. Studies after the terrorist attacks of September 11, 2001, and the Oklahoma City bombing reported up to 40% of children and adolescents experienced PTSD symptoms. Studies after the Space Shuttle *Challenger* explosion and the Oklahoma City bombing strongly suggested that overexposure to media coverage of these tragic events also led to symptoms of PTSD for some children and adults.

▶ Clinical Findings

Children and adolescents with PTSD show persistent evidence of fear and anxiety and are hypervigilant to the possibility of repetition. They may regress developmentally and experience fears of strangers, of the dark, and of being alone, and avoid reminders of the traumatic event. Children also frequently reexperience elements of the events in nightmares and flashbacks. In their symbolic play, one can often notice a monotonous repetition of some aspect of the traumatic event. Children with a history of traumatic experiences or neglect in infancy and early childhood are likely to show signs of reactive attachment disorder and have difficulty forming relationships with caregivers.

▶ Treatment

The cornerstone of treatment for PTSD is education of the child and family regarding the nature of the disorder so that the child's emotional reactions and regressive behavior are not mistakenly viewed as crazy or manipulative. Support, reassurance, and repeated explanations and understanding are needed. It is critical that the child be living in a safe environment, and if caregivers have been abusive, concerns must be reported to social services. Efforts should be made to establish or maintain daily routines as much as possible, especially after a trauma or disaster that interrupts the family's environment. In the case of media coverage of a disaster or event, children's viewing should be avoided or limited. Interventions to maintain safety of the child are imperative. Individual and family psychotherapy are central features of treatment interventions. Specific fears usually wane with time, and behavioral desensitization may help. Cognitive-behavioral therapy is considered first-line treatment for PTSD, and there is some preliminary evidence eye movement desensitization and reprocessing (EMDR) may also be useful.

A supportive relationship with a caregiving adult is essential. Frequently caregivers also have PTSD and need referral for treatment so that they can also assist in their child's recovery.

For children with more severe and persistent symptoms, assessment for treatment with medication is indicated. Sertraline has approval for the treatment of PTSD in adults. Target symptoms (eg, anxiety, depression, nightmares, and aggression) should be clearly identified and appropriate medication trials initiated with close monitoring. Some of the medications used to treat children with PTSD include clonidine or guanfacine (Tenex), mood stabilizers, antidepressants, and neuroleptics. Children who have lived for an extended time in abusive environments or who have been exposed to multiple traumas are more likely to require treatment with medications. Occupational therapy for sensory integration can also be effective in decreasing reactivity to stimuli and helping the child and caregivers develop and implement self-soothing skills. Individuals who have suffered single-episode traumas usually benefit significantly from psychotherapy and may require limited treatment with medication to address symptoms of anxiety, nightmares, and sleep disturbance.

▶ Prognosis

At 4- to 5-year follow-up investigations, many children who have been through a traumatic life experience continue to have vivid and frightening memories and dreams and a pessimistic view of the future. The effects of traumatic experiences can be far-reaching. The ability of caregivers to provide a safe, supportive, stable, empathic environment enhances the prognosis for individuals with PTSD. Timely access to therapy and use of therapy over time to work through symptoms also enhance prognosis. Evidence is growing to support a connection between victimization in childhood and unstable personality and mood disorders in later life.

American Academy of Child and Adolescent Psychiatry: Practice parameters for the assessment and treatment of children and adolescents with posttraumatic stress disorder. J Am Acad Child Adolesc Psychiatry 1998;37(Suppl):4S [PMID: 9785726].

Brown DJ: Clinical characteristics and efficacious treatment of posttraumatic stress disorder in children and adolescents. Pediatr Ann 2005;34:138 [PMID: 15768690].

Carr A: Interventions for post-traumatic stress disorder in children and adolescents. Pediatr Rehabil 2004;7:231 [PMID: 15513767].

De Bellis MD, Van Dillen T: Childhood post-traumatic stress disorder: An overview. Child Adolesc Psychiatr Clin N Am 2005;14:745 [PMID: 16171701].

Fremont WP: Childhood reactions to terrorism-induced trauma: a review of the past 10 years. J Am Acad Child Adolesc Psychiatry 2004;43:381 [PMID: 15187798].

Margolin G: Children's exposure to violence: Exploring developmental pathways to diverse outcomes. J Interpers Violence 2005;20:72 [PMID: 15618563].

Pine DS: Developmental psychobiology and response to threats: Relevance to trauma in children and adolescents. Biol Psychiatry 2003;53:796 [PMID: 12725972].

Scheeringa MS et al: New findings on alternative criteria for PTSD in preschool children. J Am Acad Child Adolesc Psychiatry 2003;42:561 [PMID: 12707560].

Stallard P: Psychological interventions for post-traumatic reactions in children and young people: a review of randomised controlled trials. Clin Psychol Rev 2006;26:895 [PMID: 16481081].

Strand VC et al: Assessment and screening tools for trauma in children and adolescents. Trauma Violence Abuse 2005;6:55 [PMID: 15574673].

SOMATOFORM DISORDERS

ESSENTIALS OF DIAGNOSIS & TYPICAL FEATURES

▶ A symptom suggesting physical dysfunction.

▶ No physical disorder accounting for the symptom.

▶ Symptoms causing distress, dysfunction, or both.

▶ Symptoms not voluntarily created or maintained, as in malingering.

Clinical Findings

Hypochondriasis, somatization, and conversion disorders involve an unhealthy overemphasis and preoccupation with somatic experiences and symptoms. Somatoform disorders are defined by the presence of physical illness or disability for which no organic cause can be identified, although neither the patient nor the caregiver is consciously fabricating the symptoms. The category includes body dysmorphic disorder, conversion disorder, hypochondriasis, somatization disorder, and somatoform pain disorder (Table 6–15).

Conversion symptoms most often occur in school-aged children and adolescents. The exact incidence is unclear, but in pediatric practice they are probably seen more often as transient symptoms than as chronic disorders requiring help from mental health practitioners. A conversion symptom is thought to be an expression of underlying psychological conflict. The specific symptom may be symbolically determined by the underlying conflict; the symptom may resolve the dilemma created by the underlying wish or fear (eg, a seemingly paralyzed child need not fear expressing his underlying rage or aggressive retaliatory impulses). Although children can present with a variety of symptoms, the most common include neurologic and gastrointestinal complaints. Children with conversion disorder may be surprisingly unconcerned about the substantial disability deriving from their symptoms. Symptoms include unusual sensory phenomena, paralysis, vomiting, abdominal pain, intractable headaches, and movement or seizure-like disorders.

Table 6–15. Somatoform disorders in children and adolescents.

Disorder	Major Clinical Manifestations
Body dysmorphic disorder	Preoccupation with an imagined defect in personal appearance
Conversion disorder	Symptom onset follows psychologically stressful event; symptoms express unconscious feelings and result in secondary gain
Hypochondriasis	Preoccupation with worry that physical symptoms manifest unrecognized and threatening condition; medical assurance does not provide relief from worry
Somatization disorder	Long-standing preoccupation with multiple somatic symptoms
Somatoform pain disorder	Preoccupation with pain that results in distress or impairment beyond what would be expected from physical findings

In the classic case of conversion disorder, the child's symptoms and examination findings are not consistent with the clinical manifestations of any organic disease process. The physical symptoms often begin within the context of a family experiencing stress, such as serious illness, a death, or family discord. On closer examination, the child's symptoms are often found to resemble symptoms present in other family members. Children with conversion disorder may have some secondary gain associated with their symptoms. Several reports have pointed to the increased association of conversion disorder with sexual overstimulation or sexual abuse. As with other emotional and behavioral problems, health care providers should always screen for physical and sexual abuse.

Differential Diagnosis

It is sometimes not possible to rule out medical disease as a source of the symptoms. Medical follow-up is required to monitor for changes in symptoms and response to recommended interventions.

Somatic symptoms are often associated with anxiety and depressive disorders (see Tables 6–8 and 6–12). Occasionally, psychotic children have somatic preoccupations and even somatic delusions.

Treatment & Prognosis

In most cases, conversion symptoms resolve quickly when the child and family are reassured that the symptom is a way of reacting to stress. The child is encouraged to continue with normal daily activities, knowing that the symptom will abate when the stress is resolved. Treatment of conversion disorders includes acknowledging the symptom rather than telling the child that the symptom is not medically justified and responding with noninvasive interventions such as physical therapy while continuing to encourage normalization of the symptoms. If the symptom does not resolve with reassurance, further investigation by a mental health professional is indicated. Comorbid diagnoses such as depression and anxiety disorders should be addressed, and treatment with psychopharmacologic agents may be helpful.

Patients presenting with somatoform disorders are often resistant to mental health treatment, in part fearing that any distraction from their vigilance will put them at greater risk of succumbing to a medical illness. Psychiatric consultation is often helpful and for severely incapacitated patients, referral psychiatric consultation is always indicated.

Somatoform disorder is not associated with the increased morbidity and mortality associated with other psychiatric disorders such as mood disorders or psychotic illness. Somatoform patients are best treated with regular, short, scheduled medical appointments to address the complaints at hand. In this way they do not need to precipitate emergencies to elicit medical attention. Avoid invasive procedures unless clearly indicated and offer sincere concern and reassurance. Avoid telling the patient "it's all in your head" and do not abandon or avoid the patient, as somatoform patients are at great risk of seeking multiple alternative treatment providers and potentially unnecessary treatments.

Campo JV et al: Recurrent abdominal pain, anxiety and depression in primary care. Pediatrics 2004;113:817 [PMID: 15060233].

Campo JV, Fritz G: A management model for pediatric somatization. Psychosomatics 2001;42:467 [PMID: 11815681].

Dhossche D et al: Somatoform disorders in children and adolescents: A comparison with other internalizing disorders. Ann Clin Psychiatry 2002;14:23 [PMID: 12046637].

Fritz GK et al: Somatoform disorders in children and adolescents: A review of the past 10 years. J Am Acad Child Adolesc Psychiatry 1997;36:1329 [PMID: 9334545].

Silber TJ, Pao M: Somatization disorders in children and adolescents. Pediatr Rev 2003;24:255 [PMID: 12897265].

ELIMINATION DISORDERS

Elimination disorders are defined as problems with age-appropriate bowel and bladder control. These disorders are often identified and addressed by primary care providers. Enuresis and encopresis are not always associated with mental health problems and can simply be due to delayed development of consistent bowel and bladder control, or parental difficulty in managing this developmental stage. Elimination disorders may also be treated by child psychiatrists when they are found to be comorbid with other mental health problems, such as PTSD, anxiety disorders, and developmental disabilities.

1. Enuresis

It is important for the primary care provider to carefully assess the developmental age of the child and the situation in which enuresis is occurring, and to screen for medical concerns before deciding that the enuresis or encopresis is

attributable to a behavioral or emotional disorder. It is not uncommon for parents to have unrealistic expectations about toilet training young children. In many cases of enuresis, the child is simply not developmentally ready or sometimes is unable to remain dry at night. Most children with enuresis are able to remain dry by age 9 years.

ESSENTIALS OF DIAGNOSIS & TYPICAL FEATURES

► Urinary incontinence in a child age 5 years (or developmental equivalent) or older.

► Not due to medication or a medical disorder.

General Considerations

Enuresis is the passage of urine into bedclothes or undergarments, whether involuntary or intentional. At least 90% of enuretic children have primary nocturnal enuresis—that is, they wet only at night during sleep and have never had a sustained period of dryness. Diurnal enuresis (daytime wetting) is much less common, as is secondary enuresis, which develops after a child has had a sustained period of bladder control. The latter two varieties are much more commonly associated with emotional stress, anxiety, and psychiatric disorders. Primary nocturnal enuresis is most often a parasomnia, a deep-sleep (stage 3 or stage 4) event. Etiologically, it is generally viewed as a developmental disorder or maturational lag that children will outgrow. Only infrequently is it associated with a serious psychopathologic disorder.

Clinical Findings

Primary nocturnal enuresis is common (Table 6–16). The incidence is three times higher in boys than in girls. Most children with enuresis become continent by adolescence or earlier. The family history in such cases frequently reveals other members, especially fathers, who have had prolonged nighttime bedwetting problems. Although the cause of primary nocturnal enuresis is not established, it appears to be related to maturational delay of sleep and arousal mechanisms or to delay in development of increased bladder capacity.

Daytime wetting most often occurs in timid and shy children or in children with ADHD. It occurs with about equal frequency in boys and girls, and 60–80% of daytime wetters also wet at night. Secondary enuresis typically follows a stressful event, such as the birth of a sibling, a loss, or discord within the family. The symptom can be seen as the result of regression in response to stress or as a more symbolic expression of the child's feelings.

Differential Diagnosis

The differential diagnosis includes urinary tract infections, neurologic diseases, seizure disorders, diabetes mellitus, and

Table 6–16. Incidence of enuresis in children.

Age (y)	Primary Nocturnal Enuresis (%)	Occasional Daytime Enuresis (%)[a]
5	15	8
7–8	7	—
10	3–5	—
12	2–3	1
14	1	—

[a]Diurnal (daytime) enuresis tends to resolve by developmental age 6 y, with a slight recurrence around age 12 y in early adolescence.

structural abnormalities of the urinary tract. Urinalysis and urine culture and observing the child's urinary stream can rule out the majority of organic causes of enuresis.

Complications

The most common complication of enuresis is low self-esteem in response to criticism from caregivers and embarrassment if peers are aware of the problem. Older children with enuresis may be reluctant to attend sleep-overs and be self-conscious with peers.

Treatment

Treatment should emphasize that the symptom of nocturnal enuresis is a developmental lag and often will be outgrown even without treatment. Even with these interventions, many children will have difficulty remaining dry. If the child chooses to pursue treatment, a program of bladder exercises can be prescribed: fluids should be limited after dinner; the child should attempt to hold urine as long as possible during the day and then start and stop the stream at the toilet bowl; the child is instructed to practice getting up from bed and going to the bathroom at bedtime before sleep. These procedures are helpful in perhaps 30–40% of children with nighttime wetting. Another option is a "potty pager." This is a beeper-like object that attaches to the child's underwear and vibrates when the child is wet in an attempt to rouse the child into a wakeful state and increase awareness of the need to urinate.

Desmopressin acetate (DDAVP), administered intranasally at bedtime, can result in complete remission of nocturnal enuresis in 50% of children as long as they continue the treatment. DDAVP is expensive, but can be useful until the child develops the ability to hold urine through the night or awaken to use the bathroom. For others, a trial of the TCA imipramine is worthwhile, at dosages of 25–50 mg at bedtime for children younger than age 12 years and 50–75 mg for older children. Because many patients relapse once the drug is stopped, its primary use is for camp attendance or overnight visits. Mental health treatment is more often needed for children with daytime wetting or secondary

enuresis. The focus is on the verbal expression of feelings that may be associated with perpetuation of the symptom and behavioral interventions to work toward dryness and cope with episodes of wetting.

Cedron M: Removing the stigma: Helping reduce the psychosocial impact of bedwetting. Urol Nurs 2002;22:286 [PMID: 12242905].

Fritz G, Rockney R: Summary of the practice parameter for the assessment and treatment of children and adolescents with enuresis. J Am Acad Child Adolesc Psychiatry 2004;43:23 [PMID: 14691370].

Gottsegen DN: Curing bedwetting on the spot: A review of one-session cures. Clin Pediatr 2003;42:273 [PMID: 12739927].

Mercer R: Dry at night. Treating nocturnal enuresis. Adv Nurs Pract 2003;11:26 [PMID: 12640815].

Thiedke CC: Nocturnal enuresis. Am Fam Physician 2003;67:1499 [PMID: 12722850].

2. Encopresis

 ESSENTIALS OF DIAGNOSIS & TYPICAL FEATURES

▶ Fecal incontinence in a child age 4 years (or developmental equivalent) or older.

▶ Not due to medication or a medical disorder.

General Considerations

Functional encopresis is defined as the repeated passage of feces in inappropriate places by a child of at least the developmental equivalent of age 4 years. It may be either involuntary or intentional, although most often it is involuntary. It affects approximately 1–1.5% of school-aged children, boys four times more often than girls. Functional fecal incontinence is rare in adolescence.

Clinical Findings

Functional encopresis can be divided into four types: retentive, continuous, discontinuous, and toilet phobia.

A. Retentive Encopresis

In retentive encopresis, also called psychogenic megacolon, the child withholds bowel movements, leading to the development of constipation, fecal impaction, and the seepage of soft or liquid feces around the margins of the impaction into the underclothing. Marked constipation and painful defecation often contribute to a vicious cycle of withholding, thus creating larger impaction and further seepage. These children often have a history of crossing their legs to resist the urge to defecate and of infrequent bowel movements large enough to stop up the toilet, and they are found on examination to have large fecal masses in their rectal vaults. The soiling that occurs distresses most of these children.

B. Continuous Encopresis

Children with continuous encopresis have never gained primary control of bowel function. The bowel movement is usually randomly deposited in underclothing without regard to social norms. Typically, the family structure does not encourage organization and skill training, and for that reason the child has never had adequate bowel training. These children and their parents are more apt to be socially or intellectually disadvantaged.

C. Discontinuous Encopresis

Children with discontinuous encopresis have a history of normal bowel control for an extended period. Loss of control often occurs in response to a stressful event, such as the birth of a sibling, a separation, family illness, or marital disharmony. These children may soil their pants or on occasion defecate on the floor or smear feces as an expression of anger or of a wish to be perceived as younger. They typically display relative indifference to the symptom.

D. Toilet Phobia

In the infrequent case of toilet phobia, a young child views the toilet as a frightening structure to be avoided. These children may view the bowel movement as an extension of themselves, which is then swept away in a frightening manner. They may think that they, too, may be swept away down the toilet.

Differential Diagnosis

Differential diagnosis includes the medical causes of constipation and retentive encopresis. Hirschsprung disease can be ruled out with reasonable certainty by the history of passing large-caliber bowel movements in the past and by the presence of palpable stool in the rectal vault. Neurologic disorders, hypothyroidism, hypercalcemia, and diseases of smooth muscle must be considered as well. The child should be examined for anal fissures, which tend to encourage the withholding of bowel movements.

Treatment

Identifying the type of encopresis is important in treatment planning. Another important variable is the child's own concern about the symptom. Encopresis in children who display denial or indifference is much harder to treat. Children with coexisting illnesses need to receive treatment for those conditions before focusing treatment on soiling. Parents should be given guidance on responding calmly and firmly to this behavior.

With the most common type of encopresis, the retentive type, efforts are made to soften stool so that constipation and painful defecation do not perpetuate the behavior. These children are then taught to adopt a regular schedule of sitting on the toilet after meals. A system of positive reinforcement can be added in which the child is rewarded for each day with no soiled underclothes. The responsibility for rinsing soiled clothing and depositing it in the appropriate receptacle rests with the child. In the case of continuous encopresis, the family is taught to train the child. For toilet phobia, a progressive series of rewarded desensitization steps is necessary. Children with discontinuous encopresis that persists over several weeks often need psychotherapy to help them recognize and verbally express their anger and wish to be dependent, rather than express themselves through fecal soiling.

Prognosis

Although the ultimate prognosis is excellent, parental distress and parent-child conflict may be substantial prior to the cessation of symptoms. The natural history of soiling is that it resolves by adolescence in all but the most severely disturbed teenagers.

Bonner L, Dobson P: Children who soil: Guidelines for good practice. J Fam Health Care 2003;13:32 [PMID: 12793299].

Borowitz SM et al: Treatment of childhood encopresis: A randomized trial comparing three treatment protocols. J Pediatr Gastroenterol Nutr 2002;34:378 [PMID: 11930093].

Cox DF et al: Psychological differences between children with and without chronic encopresis. J Pediatr Psychol 2002;27:585 [PMID: 12228330].

Fishman L et al: Trends in referral to a single encopresis clinic over 20 years. Pediatrics 2003;111(5 pt 1):e604 [PMID: 12728118].

Mikkelson EJ: Enuresis and encopresis: Ten years of progress. Am J Child Adolesc Psychiatr 2001;40:1146 [PMID: 11589527].

Van Ginkel R et al: Childhood constipation: Longitudinal follow-up beyond puberty. Gastroenterology 2003;125:357 [PMID: 12891536].

OTHER PSYCHIATRIC CONDTIONS

Several psychiatric conditions are covered elsewhere in this book. Refer to the following chapters for detailed discussion:

- Attention-deficit/hyperactivity disorder (ADHD): see Chapter 2.
- Eating disorders: see Chapter 5.
- Intellectual disability/mental retardation: see Chapter 2.
- Substance abuse: see Chapter 4.
- Sleep disorders: see Chapter 2.
- Tourette syndrome: see Chapter 23.

OVERVIEW OF PEDIATRIC PSYCHOPHARMACOLOGY

Pediatric psychopharmacology has improved significantly over the past decade with increasing study of the effect of psychoactive medications on mental illness in childhood and adolescence. Although relatively few medications are approved for use in children, many of the same psychopharmacologic agents used in adults are used in children and adolescents.

As with any medication, the risks as well as the benefits of administering psychoactive medications must be discussed with the child's parent or guardian and with the child or adolescent, as is age-appropriate. A recommendation for medication is warranted if the symptoms observed and reported by the child and family are associated with a psychiatric diagnosis known to respond to a particular medication or class of medications. Medication is more likely to be recommended if the disorder is interfering with psychosocial development, interpersonal relationships, daily functioning, or the patient's sense of personal well-being, and if there is significant potential for benefit with the medication and relatively low risk of harm. Informed consent should be given by the parent or guardian and noted in the record. The recommendation and target symptoms for medication should be discussed with both children and adolescents, and adolescents should also provide informed consent for treatment. In some states adolescents aged 15 and older must give informed consent. Informed consent includes a discussion of the diagnosis, target symptoms, possible common side effects, any side effects that should be closely monitored, potential benefits associated with the medication, and documentation of informed consent in the medical record. Psychopharmacologic agents are seldom the only treatment for a psychiatric disorder. They are best used in combination with other interventions such as individual therapy, family psychotherapy, and other psychosocial interventions, including assessment of school functioning and special needs.

When considering the use of psychoactive medications, specific target symptoms of the medication should be identified and followed to evaluate the efficacy of treatment. These symptoms should be also measured either by self-report rating scales (child, family, or both) and clinician-rated scales. When initiating treatment, start with low doses and increase slowly (in divided doses, if indicated) while monitoring for side effects along with therapeutic effects. When a medication is discontinued, it should usually be tapered over 2–4 weeks to minimize withdrawal effects. When multiple choices exist, one should select the medication that has a pediatric FDA approval (Table 6–17), or has been studied for the specific indication for which it is being prescribed, ideally in the age range of the patient. The side-effect profile of each option should be carefully considered, and the medication selected with the fewest and least serious risks and side effects. Polypharmacy should be avoided by choosing one drug that might diminish most or all of the target symptoms before considering the simultaneous administration of two or more agents. General guidelines regarding comfort level for pediatric providers in initiating and managing psychotropic classes of medications are outlined in Table 6–18.

In the text that follows, the major classes of psychopharmacologic agents with clinical indications in child and adolescent psychiatry are represented. The more commonly prescribed drugs from each class are reviewed with reference

Table 6–17. Psychoactive medications approved by the FDA for use in children and adolescents.[a]

Drug	Indication	Age for Which Approved (y)
Mixed amphetamine salts (Adderall)	ADHD	3 and older
Dextroamphetamine (Dexedrine, Dextrostat)	ADHD	3 and older
Methylphenidate (Concerta, Ritalin, others)	ADHD	6 and older
Clomipramine (Anafranil)	OCD	10 and older
Fluvoxamine (Luvox)	OCD	8 and older
Sertraline (Zoloft)	OCD	6 and older
Risperidone (Risperdal)	Aggression and autism	5 and older
	Schizophrenia and mania	10 and older
Pimozide (Orap)[b]	Tourette syndrome	12 and older
Lithium (Eskalith, Lithobid, Lithotabs)	Bipolar disorder	12 and older
Fluoxetine (Prozac)	Depression	12 and older
	OCD	6 and older
Imipramine (Norpramin)	Enuresis	6 and older

[a]Haloperidol and chlorpromazine have an indication for use in psychotic disorders. Their use in children, however, is not currently recommended.
[b]Use of pimozide in the treatment of extrapyramidal disorders is discussed in Chapter 23.
ADHD, attention-deficit/hyperactivity disorder; FDA, Food and Drug Administration; OCD, obsessive-compulsive disorder.

to indications, relative contraindications, initial medical screening procedures (in addition to a general pediatric examination), dosage, adverse effects, drug interactions, and medical follow-up recommendations. This is meant to be a brief reference guide, and the physician should consult a child and adolescent psychopharmacology textbook for additional information on specific medications.

MEDICATIONS FOR ATTENTION-DEFICIT/ HYPERACTIVITY DISORDER

Dextroamphetamine (Dexedrine, Dextrostat)
Mixed amphetamine salts (Adderall, Adderall XR)
Methylphenidate (Concerta, Metadate, Methylin, Ritalin, Ritalin LA, Ritalin SR, Daytrana, Transdermal)
Dexmethylphenidate (Focalin, Focalin XR)
Clonidine (Catapres); guanfacine (Tenex)
Atomoxetine (Strattera)
Lisdexamfetamine (Vyvanse)

Table 6–18. Guidelines for management of psychiatric medications by the pediatrician.

Drug or Class	Comfort Initiating	Comfort Managing
Stimulants	+++	+++
Alpha agonists	++	+++
Antidepressants	+/–	++
Atypical antipsychotics	Recommend psychiatrist involvement	++
Typical antipsychotics	Requires psychiatrist involvement	+/–
Clozapine (Clozaril)	Requires psychiatrist involvement	Requires psychiatrist involvement
Mood stabilizers	Recommend psychiatrist involvement	+
Lamotrigine (Lamictal)	Requires psychiatrist involvement	++
Sleep medicines	+	++
Tricyclic antidepressants	+	++

Symbols: +++, high comfort; ++, comfort; +, mild caution; +/–, caution required.

1. Indications—Approximately 75% of children with ADHD experience improved attention span, decreased hyperactivity, and decreased impulsivity when given stimulant medications. Children with ADHD who do not respond favorably to one stimulant may respond well to another. Children and adolescents with ADHD without prominent hyperactivity (ADHD, predominantly inattentive type) are also likely to be responsive to stimulant medications. Atomoxetine (Strattera) and bupropion (Wellbutrin) are nonstimulant medications used to treat ADHD. Atomoxetine has FDA approval for the treatment of ADHD and is a selective noradrenergic reuptake inhibitor. Bupropion is primarily used as an antidepressant, and blocks serotonin, dopamine, and norepinephrine reuptake.

2. Contraindications—Although there has been much debate about stimulants causing sudden death in children, the FDA reviewed the literature and found no risk, except in cases of an underlying cardiac conduction or structural abnormality. Stimulants should also be used cautiously in individuals with a personal or family history of motor tics or Tourette syndrome, as these medications may cause or worsen motor tics. Caution should also be taken if there is a personal or family history of substance abuse or addictive disorders, as these medications can be abused or sold as drugs of abuse. Stimulants are also contraindicated for individuals with psychotic disorders, as they can significantly worsen psychotic symptoms. Stimulants should be used with

caution in individuals with comorbid bipolar affective disorder and ADHD and consideration of concurrent mood stabilization is critical.

3. Initial medical screening—The child should be observed for involuntary movements. Height, weight, pulse, and blood pressure should be recorded. (See also Chapter 2.)

4. Adverse effects—These are often dose-related and time-limited.

A. COMMON ADVERSE EFFECTS—Anorexia, weight loss, abdominal distress, headache, insomnia, dysphoria and tearfulness, irritability, lethargy, mild tachycardia, and mild elevation in blood pressure.

B. LESS COMMON EFFECTS—Interdose rebound of ADHD symptoms, emergence of motor tics or Tourette syndrome, behavioral stereotypy, tachycardia or hypertension, depression, mania, and psychotic symptoms. Reduced growth velocity occurs only during active administration. Growth rebound occurs during periods of discontinuation. Ultimate height is not usually noticeably compromised. Treatment with stimulant medications does not predispose to future substance abuse.

5. Drug interactions—Additive stimulant effects are seen with sympathomimetic amines (ephedrine and pseudoephedrine).

6. Medical follow-up—Pulse, blood pressure, height, and weight should be recorded every 3–4 months and at times of dosage increases. Assess for abnormal movements such as motor tics at each visit.

7. Dosage

A. METHYLPHENIDATE—The usual starting dose is 5 mg once or twice a day, before school and at noon (or 2.5 mg twice a day for children aged 4–6 years), gradually increasing as clinically indicated. The maximum daily dose should not exceed 60 mg, and a single dose should not exceed 0.7 mg/kg. Administration on weekends and during vacations is determined by the need at those times. The duration of action is approximately 3–4 hours. Extended-release forms can prevent the need for taking medication at school. Dexmethylphenidate (Focalin) is typically administered at a dose of 2.5 mg twice a day (8 AM and noon, for example), to a maximum of 20 mg.

B. DEXTROAMPHETAMINE SULFATE—The dose is 2.5–10 mg twice daily, before school and at noon, with or without another dose at 4 PM. A sustained-release preparation may have clinical effects for up to 8 hours. There is also an extended-release form.

C. PEMOLINE—Pemoline is generally not recommended for the treatment of ADHD due to a significant risk of liver failure.

D. ATOMOXETINE HYDROCHLORIDE—The starting dose for children and adolescents up to 70 kg is 0.5 mg/kg, with titration to a maximum dose of 1.2 mg/kg, in single or divided dosing.

ANTIDEPRESSANTS

The "black box warning" that was issued in October 2005 for all antidepressants has had a significant impact on prescription of these medications for children. The black box warning reads "Pooled analysis of short term (4–16 weeks) placebo-controlled trials of antidepressant drugs (SSRIs and others) in children and adolescents with Major Depressive Disorder (MDD), Obsessive-Compulsive Disorder (OCD) and other psychiatric disorders (a total of 24 trials involving more than 4400 patients) has revealed a greater risk of adverse events representing suicidal thinking or behavior (suicidality) during the first few months of treatment in those receiving antidepressants. The average risk of such events was 4%, twice the placebo risk of 2%. No suicides occurred in these trials."

The "medication guide" created for consumers along with the black box warning that now appears in all antidepressant packaging recommends the following monitoring schedule for health care providers when starting an antidepressant:

- Once every week for the first 4 weeks
- Every 2 weeks for the next 4 weeks
- After taking the antidepressant for 12 weeks
- After 12 weeks, follow your health care provider's advice on how often to come back.

The Treatment of Adolescent Depression Study found that cognitive-behavioral therapy combined with fluoxetine led to the best outcomes in the treatment of pediatric depression.

It is important to be cognizant of evidence-based medical practice when prescribing for any indication. Target symptoms should be carefully monitored for improvement or worsening, and it is important to ask and document the responses about any suicidal thinking and self-injurious behaviors. When recommending an antidepressant, the physician should also firmly recommend cognitive-behavioral therapy and discuss the options for medication treatment, including which medications have FDA approval for pediatric indications (see Table 6–17). Recent findings suggest that fluoxetine has the best evidence for improvement in depressive symptoms.

1. Selective Serotonin Reuptake Inhibitors

Citalopram, escitalopram (Celexa, Lexapro)
Fluvoxamine (Luvox)
Paroxetine (Paxil)
Sertraline (Zoloft)

1. Indications—The SSRIs have become the agents of first choice for the treatment of depression and anxiety. Fluvoxamine and sertraline both have approval from the FDA for treatment of pediatric OCD and fluoxetine has approval for pediatric depression. Although no other SSRIs have FDA approval for pediatric indications, some published studies support the efficacy of SSRIs for the treatment of depression, anxiety, and OCD in pediatric populations. Each SSRI has different FDA indications. However, once an indication is obtained for one SSRI, it is widely believed that other SSRIs are likely to be effective as well for the same indication. The FDA-approved indications for SSRIs are the following:

Major depression: fluoxetine (age 6 years and older); citalopram, escitalopram, paroxetine, sertraline (18 and older).

Panic disorder: sertraline (18 and older), paroxetine (18 and older).

OCD: fluvoxamine (6 and older), sertraline (6 and older).

Bulimia: fluoxetine (18 and older).

PTSD: sertraline (18 and older).

Premenstrual dysphoric disorder: fluoxetine (18 and older).

2. Contraindications—Caution should be used in cases of known liver disease or chronic or severe illness where multiple medications may be prescribed, because all SSRIs are metabolized in the liver. Caution should be used when prescribing for an individual with a family history of bipolar disorder, or when the differential diagnosis includes bipolar disorder, because antidepressants can induce manic or hypomanic symptoms.

3. Initial medical screening—General medical examination.

4. Adverse effects—Often dose-related and time-limited: gastrointestinal (GI) distress and nausea (can be minimized by taking medication with food), headache, tremulousness, decreased appetite, weight loss, insomnia, sedation (10%), sexual dysfunction (25%). Irritability, social disinhibition, restlessness, and emotional excitability can occur in approximately 20% of children taking SSRIs. Monitor for improvement and onset or worsening of suicidal or self-injurious thinking, in addition to other target symptoms.

5. Drug interactions—All SSRIs inhibit the efficiency of the hepatic microsomal enzyme system. The order of inhibition is: fluoxetine > fluvoxamine > paroxetine > sertraline > citalopram > escitalopram. This can lead to higher-than-expected blood levels of other drugs, including antidepressants, antiarrhythmics, antipsychotics, β-blockers, opioids, and antihistamines. Taking tryptophan while on an SSRI may result in a serotonergic syndrome of psychomotor agitation and GI distress. A potentially fatal interaction that clinically resembles neuroleptic malignant syndrome may occur when SSRIs are administered concomitantly with monoamine oxidase inhibitors. Fluoxetine has the longest half-life of the SSRIs and should not be initiated within 14 days of the discontinuation of a monoamine oxidase inhibitor, or a monoamine oxidase inhibitor initiated within at least 5 weeks of the discontinuation of fluoxetine.

Table 6–19. Medications used to treat depression in adolescents.

Generic	Trade Name	Adolescent Starting Dose	Target Dose (Average Effective Dose)	Maximum Dose
Selective serotonin reuptake inhibitors				
Citalopram	Celexa	20 mg q AM	20 mg q AM	40–60 mg q AM
Escitalopram	Lexapro	10 mg	10 mg	30 mg
Fluoxetine[a]	Prozac	10 mg q AM	20 mg q AM	60 mg q AM
Fluvoxamine	Luvox	50 mg qhs	100–150 mg qd	100 mg bid
Paroxetine	Paxil	10 mg q AM	20 mg q AM	60 mg q AM
Paroxetine CR	Paxil CR	25 mg	25 mg	50 mg
Sertraline	Zoloft	25 mg q AM	50 mg q AM	150 mg q AM
Other antidepressants				
Bupropion	Wellbutrin	75 mg q AM	150 mg bid	200 mg bid
Bupropion SR	Wellbutrin SR	100 mg q AM	100 mg bid	150 mg bid
Duloxetine	Cymbalta	20 mg bid	20 mg bid	60 mg qd
Mirtazapine	Remeron	7.5 mg qhs	15 mg qhs	30 mg qhs
Venlafaxine	Effexor	37.5 mg q AM	75 mg bid	150 mg bid
Venlafaxine XR	Effexor XR	37.5 mg q AM	150 mg qd	225 mg qd

[a]FDA approved for depression in children older than age 12 y.
bid, twice a day; q AM, every morning; qd, every day; qhs, every night at bedtime.

6. Dosage (Table 6–19)—Therapeutic response should be expected 4–6 weeks after a therapeutic dose has been reached. The starting dose for a child younger than 12 years old is generally half the starting dose for an adolescent.

A. SSRIs—The SSRIs are usually given once a day, in the morning with breakfast. One in ten individuals may experience sedation and prefer to take the medication at bedtime. Fluoxetine is the only SSRI with FDA approval and replicable efficacy.

B. Alternative antidepressants and fluvoxamine—The alternative antidepressants (see below) and fluvoxamine are usually given in twice-daily dosing. Paroxetine, bupropion, and venlafaxine are now available in a sustained- and extended-release form.

2. Other Antidepressants

Bupropion (Wellbutrin), bupropion SR (sustained-release), bupropion XL (extended-release)

Duloxetine (Cymbalta)

Mirtazapine (Remeron)

Venlafaxine (Effexor), venlafaxine XR (extended-release)

A. Bupropion

1. Indications—Bupropion is an antidepressant that inhibits reuptake of primarily serotonin, but also norepinephrine

and dopamine. It is approved for treatment of major depression in adults, but is receiving favorable attention for its therapeutic effects in adolescents with major depressive disorder and in children and adolescents with ADHD. Like the SSRIs, bupropion has very few anticholinergic or cardiotoxic effects.

2. Contraindications—History of seizure disorder or bulimia nervosa.

3. Initial medical screening and follow-up—General medical examination.

4. Adverse effects—Psychomotor activation (agitation or restlessness), headache, GI distress, nausea, anorexia with weight loss, insomnia, tremulousness, precipitation of mania, and induction of seizures with doses above 450 mg/d.

B. Venlafaxine

Venlafaxine is an antidepressant that primarily inhibits reuptake of serotonin and norepinephrine.

1. Indications—It is approved for the treatment of major depression in adults.

2. Contraindications—Hypertension.

3. Initial medical screening and follow-up—General medical examination.

4. Adverse effects—The most common adverse effects are nausea, nervousness, and sweating. Hypertension is likely with doses over 300 mg or over 225 mg of the extended-release version. Venlafaxine must be discontinued slowly to minimize withdrawal symptoms: severe headaches, dizziness, and significant flulike symptoms. It is also available in an extended-release form.

C. Mirtazapine

Mirtazapine is an α_2-antagonist that enhances central noradrenergic and serotonergic activity.

1. Indications—It is approved for the treatment of major depression in adults.

2. Contraindications—Mirtazapine should not be given in combination with monoamine oxidase inhibitors. Very rare side effects are acute liver failure (1 case per 250,000–300,000), neutropenia, and agranulocytosis.

3. Initial medical screening and follow-up—General medical examination.

4. Adverse effects—Dry mouth, increased appetite, constipation, weight gain.

D. Duloxetine

Duloxetine is a selective serotonin and norepinephrine reuptake inhibitor.

1. Indications—It is approved for the treatment of major depression, generalized anxiety disorder, and diabetic peripheral neuropathic pain in adults.

2. Contraindications—Duloxetine should not be given in combination with monoamine oxidase inhibitors. Very rare side effects are orthostatic hypotension and liver toxicity.

3. Initial medical screening and follow-up—General medical examination.

4. Adverse effects—Nausea, dizziness, dry mouth, and fatigue.

3. Tricyclic Antidepressants

    Imipramine
    Desipramine
    Clomipramine
    Nortriptyline
    Amitriptyline

With the introduction of the SSRIs and alternative antidepressants, use of the TCAs has become uncommon for the treatment of depression and anxiety disorders. The TCAs have more significant side-effect profiles, require more substantial medical monitoring, and are quite cardiotoxic in overdose. For these reasons, in general, SSRIs or alternative antidepressants should be considered before recommending a TCA. In some countries, where access to newer and more costly medications is difficult, TCAs are still frequently employed for certain behavioral, emotional, and functional conditions.

1. Indications—TCAs have been prescribed for chronic pain syndromes, migraines, headache, depression, anxiety, enuresis, bulimia nervosa, OCD, and PTSD in children and adolescents. Imipramine and desipramine have FDA approval for the treatment of major depression in adults and for enuresis for children age 6 years and older. Some published studies have demonstrated clinical efficacy in the treatment of ADHD, panic disorder, anxiety-based school refusal, separation anxiety disorder, bulimia, night terrors, and sleepwalking. But as yet, the FDA has not approved their use for these indications. **Studies have not supported efficacy in major depression in children and adolescents.** Nortriptyline has FDA approval for the treatment of major depression in adults. Clomipramine has FDA approval for the treatment of depression and OCD in adults and may be helpful for obsessive symptoms in autism.

2. Contraindications—Known cardiac disease or arrhythmia, undiagnosed syncope, known seizure disorder, family history of sudden cardiac death or cardiomyopathy, known electrolyte abnormality (with bingeing and purging).

3. Initial medical screening—The family history should be examined for sudden cardiac death; the patient's history for cardiac disease, arrhythmias, syncope, seizure disorder, or congenital hearing loss (associated with prolonged QT interval). Other screening procedures include serum electrolytes and blood urea nitrogen in patients who have eating disorders, cardiac examination, and a baseline electrocardiogram (ECG).

4. Medical follow-up—Measure pulse and blood pressure (monitor for tachycardia and orthostatic hypotension) with each dosage increase, and obtain an ECG to monitor for arteriovenous block with each dosage increase; after reaching steady state, record pulse, blood pressure, and ECG every 3–4 months.

5. Adverse effects

A. CARDIOTOXIC EFFECTS—The cardiotoxic effects of TCAs appear to be more common in children and adolescents than in adults. In addition to anticholinergic effects, TCAs have quinidine-like effects that result in slowing of cardiac conduction. Increased plasma levels appear to be weakly associated with an increased risk of cardiac conduction abnormalities. Steady-state plasma levels of desipramine or of desipramine plus imipramine should therefore not exceed 300 ng/mL. In addition, for each dosage increase above 3 mg/kg/d, pulse and blood pressure must be carefully checked, and repeated ECGs obtained to monitor for arteriovenous block. Upper limits for cardiovascular parameters when administering TCAs to children and adolescents are listed in Table 6–20.

Table 6–20. Upper limits of cardiovascular parameters with tricyclic antidepressants.

Heart rate	130/min
Systolic blood pressure	130 mm Hg
Diastolic blood pressure	85 mm Hg
PR interval	0.2 s
QRS interval	0.12 s, or no more than 30% over baseline
QT corrected	0.45 s

B. ANTICHOLINERGIC EFFECTS—Tachycardia, dry mouth, stuffy nose, blurred vision, constipation, sweating, vasomotor instability, withdrawal syndrome (GI distress and psychomotor activation).

C. OTHER EFFECTS—Orthostatic hypotension and dizziness, lowered seizure threshold, increased appetite and weight gain, sedation, irritability and psychomotor agitation, rash (often associated with yellow dye No. 5), headache, abdominal complaints, sleep disturbance and nightmares, mania.

6. Drug interactions—TCAs may potentiate the effects of central nervous system depressants and stimulants; barbiturates and cigarette smoking may decrease plasma levels; phenothiazines, methylphenidate, and oral contraceptives may increase plasma levels; SSRIs given in combination with TCAs will result in higher TCA blood levels due to inhibition of TCA metabolism by liver enzymes (eg, cytochrome P-450 isoenzymes).

7. Dosage—Refer to a pediatric psychopharmacology text for dosages. Daily dosage requirements vary considerably with different clinical disorders.

MOOD STABILIZERS AND ATYPICAL ANTIPSYCHOTICS

▶ Mood Stabilizers

Carbamazepine (Tegretol), oxycarbamazepine (Trileptal)

Gabapentin (Neurontin)

Lamotrigine (Lamictal)

Lithium carbonate (Eskalith, Eskalith CR, Lithobid, Lithotabs)

Valproic acid (Depakote, Depakote ER)

▶ Atypical Antipsychotics

Aripiprazole (Abilify)

Olanzapine (Zyprexa)

Risperidone (Risperdal)

Quetiapine (Seroquel)

Ziprasidone (Geodon)

Lithium and antiepileptic medications have historically been the drugs of choice for mood stabilization in bipolar mood disorder. New research also finds that the atypical antipsychotic medications are also effective. Lithium, valproic acid, olanzapine, risperidone, aripiprazole, and ziprasidone are FDA approved for the treatment of adult bipolar disorder. Carbamazepine and oxcarbazepine, although not FDA approved for treatment of bipolar disorder, may also be effective and carry less risk of weight gain. Lamotrigine (Lamictal) was recently approved for the treatment of bipolar depression in adults. Other antiepileptic medications, such as gabapentin and topiramate, have also been used with varying efficacy. Medications that are effective as mood stabilizers may be helpful also in the treatment of severe aggressive symptoms.

A. Lithium

1. Indications—Lithium remains a front-line drug in the treatment of bipolar disorder and has been shown to have an augmenting effect when combined with SSRIs for treatment-resistant depression and OCD.

2. Contraindications—Lithium is contraindicated in patients with known renal, thyroid, or cardiac disease; those at high risk for dehydration and electrolyte imbalance (eg, vomiting and purging); and those who may become pregnant (teratogenic effects).

3. Initial medical screening—General medical screening with pulse, blood pressure, height, and weight; complete blood cell count (CBC); serum electrolytes, blood urea nitrogen, and creatinine; and thyroid function tests, including thyroid-stimulating hormone levels.

4. Dosage—For children the starting dose is usually 150 mg once or twice a day, with titration in 150- to 300-mg increments. (Dose may vary with the brand of lithium used; consult a psychopharmacology textbook for medication-specific information.) Oral doses of lithium should be titrated to maintain therapeutic blood levels of 0.8–1.2 mEq/L. The drug is generally given in two doses. Blood samples should be drawn 12 hours after the last dose.

5. Adverse effects

A. LITHIUM TOXICITY—Lithium has a narrow therapeutic index. Blood levels required for therapeutic effects are close to those associated with toxic symptoms. Mild toxicity may be indicated by increased tremor, GI distress, neuromuscular irritability, and altered mental status (confusion), and can occur when blood levels exceed 1.5 mEq/L. Moderate to severe symptoms of lithium toxicity are associated with blood levels above 2 mEq/L. Acute renal failure can occur at levels over 2.5–3 mEq/L.

B. SIDE EFFECTS—Lithium side effects include intention tremor, GI distress (including nausea and vomiting and sometimes diarrhea), hypothyroidism, polyuria and polydipsia, drowsiness, malaise, weight gain, acne, and granulocytosis.

6. Drug interactions—Excessive salt intake and salt restriction should be avoided. Thiazide diuretics and nonsteroidal anti-inflammatory agents (except aspirin and acetaminophen) can lead to increased lithium levels. Ibuprofen should be avoided by individuals who take lithium due to combined renal toxicity. Precautions against dehydration are required in hot weather and during vigorous exercise.

7. Medical follow-up—Serum lithium levels should be measured 5–7 days following a change in dosage and then quarterly at steady state; serum creatinine and thyroid-stimulating hormone concentrations should be determined every 3–4 months.

B. Valproic Acid

1. Indications—Valproate has FDA approval for the treatment of bipolar disorder in adults. Its efficacy in acute mania equals that of lithium, but it is generally better tolerated. Valproate is more effective than lithium in patients with rapid-cycling bipolar disorder (more than four cycles per year) and in patients with mixed states (coexisting symptoms of depression and mania). Valproate may be more effective than lithium in adolescents with bipolar disorder because they often have rapid cycling and mixed states.

2. Contraindications—Liver dysfunction.

3. Initial medical screening—CBC and liver function tests (LFTs).

4. Dosage—The starting dose is usually 15 mg/kg/d. This is increased in increments of 5–10 mg/kg/d every 1–2 weeks to a range of 500–1500 mg/d in two or three divided doses. Trough levels in the range of 80–120 mg/mL are thought to be therapeutic.

5. Adverse effects—Between 10% and 20% of patients experience sedation or anorexia, especially early in treatment or if the dose is increased too rapidly. GI upset occurs in 25% of patients, and when severe, can usually be treated with cimetidine. Increased appetite and weight gain can be troublesome for children and adolescents. Blurred vision, headache, hair loss, and tremor occur occasionally. Slight elevations in aminotransferases are frequent. Severe idiosyncratic hepatitis, pancreatitis, thrombocytopenia, and agranulocytosis occur only rarely.

6. Medical follow-up—LFTs should be checked monthly for 3–4 months; subsequently, LFTs, a CBC, and trough valproate levels should be obtained every 3–4 months.

C. Carbamazepine

1. Indications—Similarly to lithium and valproate, carbamazepine may be effective for treating bipolar disorder or for the target symptoms of mood instability, irritability, or behavioral dyscontrol. Some data suggest that it is more effective than valproate for the depressive phases of bipolar disorder. A new form of carbamazepine—oxcarbazepine (Trileptal)—is also rarely being used for pediatric mood disorders; however, its efficacy has not been established. Reportedly, it does not have the worrisome side effects of bone marrow suppression and liver enzyme induction. Blood levels cannot be monitored, and the dose range is similar to that of carbamazepine.

2. Contraindications—History of previous bone marrow depression or adverse hematologic reaction to another drug; history of sensitivity to a TCA.

3. Initial medical screening—Obtain a CBC with platelets, reticulocytes, serum iron, and blood urea nitrogen; LFTs; urinalysis.

4. Dosage—The drug is usually started at 10–20 mg/kg/d, in two divided doses, in children younger than 6 years; 100 mg twice daily in children aged 6–12 years; and 200 mg twice daily in children older than 12 years. Doses may be increased weekly until there is effective symptom control. Total daily doses should not exceed 35 mg/kg/d in children younger than 6 years; 1000 mg/d in children aged 6–15 years; and 1200 mg/d in adolescents older than 15 years. Plasma levels in the range of 4–12 mg/mL are thought to be therapeutic.

5. Adverse effects—Nausea, dizziness, sedation, headache, dry mouth, diplopia, and constipation reflect the drug's mild anticholinergic properties. Rashes are more common with carbamazepine than with other mood stabilizers. Aplastic anemia and agranulocytosis are rare. Leukopenia and thrombocytopenia are more common, and if present, should be monitored closely for evidence of bone marrow depression. These effects usually occur early and transiently and then spontaneously revert toward normal. Liver enzyme induction may significantly change the efficacy of medications given concurrently.

6. Medical follow-up—Hematologic, hepatic, and renal parameters should be followed at least every 3 months for the first year. White blood cell counts below 3000/mL and absolute neutrophil counts below 1000/mL call for discontinuation of the drug and referral for hematology consultation.

D. Lamotrigine

Lamotrigine is approved for the treatment of bipolar depression in adults. The most concerning side effects of this medication are serious rashes that can require hospitalization and can include Stevens-Johnson syndrome (0.8% incidence). Lamotrigine should be used very carefully. The starting dose is 25 mg, with a slow titration of increasing the dose by 25 mg per week to a target dose (as clinically indicated) of 300 mg/d.

E. Gabapentin

Like valproate and carbamazepine, gabapentin is an anticonvulsant that has been used as a mood stabilizer in some adult populations. It may be used along with either valproate or carbamazepine in individuals with treatment-resistant disorders. The usual adult dose range for seizure disorders is 900–1800 mg/d in three divided doses and may need to be adjusted downward in individuals with renal impairment. Although its use among adolescents and even children is increasing, gabapentin is not approved for this indication, and reports of its efficacy remain largely anecdotal. Some reports suggest it may worsen behavioral parameters in children with underlying ADHD.

ANTIPSYCHOTICS

▶ Atypical Antipsychotics

Aripiprazole (Abilify)
Clozapine (Clozaril)
Olanzapine (Zyprexa)
Risperidone (Risperdal)
Quetiapine (Seroquel)
Ziprasidone (Geodon)

▶ Conventional Neuroleptics

Chlorpromazine
Haloperidol
Molindone
Perphenazine
Thioridazine
Thiothixene
Trifluoperazine

The antipsychotics, formerly known as neuroleptics, are indicated for psychotic symptoms in patients with schizophrenia. Some now have an FDA-approved indication for bipolar affective disorder in adults (risperidone and olanzapine). They are also used for acute mania and as adjuncts to antidepressants in the treatment of psychotic depression (with delusions or hallucinations). The antipsychotics may be used cautiously in refractory PTSD, in refractory OCD, and in individuals with markedly aggressive behavioral problems unresponsive to other interventions. They may also be useful for the body image distortion and irrational fears about food and weight gain associated with anorexia nervosa.

The "atypical antipsychotics" differ from conventional antipsychotics in their receptor specificity and effect on serotonin receptors. Conventional antipsychotics are associated with a higher incidence of movement disorders and extrapyramidal symptoms (EPS) due to their wider effect on dopamine receptors. The introduction of the atypical antipsychotics has significantly changed neuroleptic prescribing patterns. The atypical antipsychotics have a better side-effect profile for most individuals and comparable efficacy for the treatment of psychotic symptoms and aggression. Atypical antipsychotics have a decreased incidence of EPS and tardive dyskinesia (TD). Significant side effects can include substantial weight gain and sedation. Because of their increased use over conventional antipsychotics, this section focuses primarily on the atypical antipsychotics.

A. Aripiprazole

Aripiprazole (Abilify) is the newest atypical neuroleptic and is indicated for the treatment of adults with schizophrenia and bipolar disorder. It is a partial dopamine blocker and a serotonin agonist. Side effects include nausea and vomiting and fatigue. It is associated with minimal weight gain. Doses over 30 mg are more likely to be associated with EPS. The dose range is 5–30 mg, and pills can be split.

B. Olanzapine

The FDA has approved this agent for the treatment of schizophrenia and bipolar disorder in adults. Olanzapine (Zyprexa) has greater affinity for type 2 serotonin receptors than dopamine-2 receptors and also has an effect on muscarinic, histaminic, and α-adrenergic receptors. As with the other atypical antipsychotics, it may be more helpful for treating the negative symptoms of schizophrenia (flat affect, isolation and withdrawal, and apathy) than conventional antipsychotics. Anecdotal and case report data support its utility in child and adolescent psychotic disorders. The adult dose range of 5–15 mg/d administered in a single bedtime dose is probably applicable to adolescents as well. Weight gain can be a significant side effect. The starting dose for children is usually 1.25 mg.

C. Quetiapine

Quetiapine (Seroquel) is an antagonist at multiple receptor sites, including serotonin (5-HT_{1A} and 5-HT_2), dopamine (D_1 and D_2), histamine, and adrenergic receptors. Quetiapine is given in 25- to 50-mg increments up to 800 mg for the treatment of psychotic symptoms. It is thought to be a weight-neutral medication, and the primary side effect is sedation.

D. Risperidone

Risperidone (Risperdal) blocks type 2 dopamine receptors (similarly to haloperidol) and type 2 serotonin receptors. It is approved for the treatment of schizophrenia and bipolar affective disorder in adults. Risperidone has also demonstrated clinical efficacy in the treatment of Tourette syndrome. The initial dose is 1–2 mg/d. It is typically titrated up in 0.5–1 mg increments to a maximum dose of 4–10 mg for psychotic disorders. Side effects include weight gain and sedation.

E. Ziprasidone

Ziprasidone (Geodon) has affinity for multiple serotonin receptors (5-HT_2, 5-HT_{1A}, 5-HT_{1D}, and 5-HT_{2C}) and dopamine-2 receptors, and it moderately inhibits norepinephrine and serotonin reuptake. It also has moderate affinity for H_1 and α_1 receptors. Ziprasidone has a greater effect on cardiac QT intervals and requires a baseline ECG and ECG monitoring when a dose of 80 mg is reached and with each dose change above 80 mg to monitor for QT prolongation. Ziprasidone is reported to cause minimal weight gain. The initial dose is 20 mg, with dose changes in 20-mg increments to a total daily dose of 140 mg for the treatment of psychotic symptoms in adults. There are no studies of ziprasidone in children and adolescents at this time.

F. Clozapine

Clozapine (Clozaril) is usually reserved for individuals who have not responded to multiple other antipsychotics due to its side effect of agranulocytosis. Clozapine blocks type 2 dopamine receptors weakly and is virtually free of EPS, apparently including TD. It was very effective in about 40% of adult patients with chronic schizophrenia who did not respond to conventional antipsychotics.

Non–dose-related agranulocytosis occurs in 0.5–2% of subjects. Some case reports note benefit from clozapine in child and adolescent schizophrenic patients who were resistant to other treatment. Contraindications are concurrent treatment with carbamazepine and any history of leukopenia. Initial medical screening should include a CBC and LFTs. The daily dose is 200–600 mg in two divided doses. Because of the risk of neutropenia, patients taking clozapine must be registered with the Clozapine Registry and a white blood cell count must be obtained biweekly before a 2-week supply of the drug is dispensed. If the white count falls below 3000/mL, clozapine is usually discontinued. Other side effects include sedation, weight gain, and increased salivation. The incidence of seizures increases with doses above 600 mg/d.

General Antipsychotic Information

The following adverse effects of antipsychotics apply to both typical and atypical antipsychotics, but are thought to have a significantly lower incidence with the atypical antipsychotics.

1. Initial medical screening—One should observe and examine for tremors and other abnormal involuntary movements and establish baseline values for CBC and LFTs. An ECG should be obtained if there is a history of cardiac disease or arrhythmia, and to establish a baseline QT interval (cardiac repolarization) prior to initiation of the antipsychotics that have a greater effect on the QT interval (eg, ziprasidone and thioridazine). Antipsychotics can cause QT prolongation leading to ventricular arrhythmias, such as torsades de pointes. Medications that affect the cytochrome P-450 isoenzyme pathway (including SSRIs) may increase the neuroleptic plasma concentration and increase risk of QTc prolongation.

2. Adverse effects—The most troublesome adverse effects of the atypical antipsychotics are cognitive slowing, sedation,

orthostasis, and weight gain. The conventional antipsychotics have an increased incidence of EPS and TD. Sedation, cognitive slowing, and EPS all tend to be dose-related. Because of the risk of side effects, neuroleptic medications should be used with caution and monitored regularly. The risk-benefit ratio of the medication for the identified target symptom should be carefully considered and reviewed with the parent or guardian.

A. EXTRAPYRAMIDAL SIDE EFFECTS—EPS and acute dystonic reactions are tonic muscle spasms, often of the tongue, jaw, or neck. EPS symptoms can be mildly uncomfortable or may result in such dramatically distressing symptoms as oculogyric crisis, torticollis, and even opisthotonos. Onset is usually within days after a dosage change and symptoms may occur in up to 25% of children treated with conventional antipsychotics. Acute neuroleptic-induced dystonias are quickly relieved by anticholinergics such as benztropine (Cogentin) and diphenhydramine.

B. TARDIVE DYSKINESIAS—TDs are involuntary movement disorders that are often irreversible and may appear after long-term use of neuroleptic medications. Choreoathetoid movements of the tongue and mouth are most common, but the extremities and trunk may also be involved. The risk of TD is small in patients on atypical antipsychotics, and those on conventional antipsychotics for less than 6 months. There is no universally effective treatment.

C. PSEUDOPARKINSONISM—Pseudoparkinsonism is usually manifested 1–4 weeks after the start of treatment. It presents as muscle stiffness, cogwheel rigidity, masklike facial expression, bradykinesia, drooling, and occasionally pill-rolling tremor. Anticholinergic medications or dosage reductions are helpful.

D. AKATHISIA—Akathisia is usually manifested after 1–6 weeks of treatment. It presents as an unpleasant feeling of driven motor restlessness that ranges from vague muscular discomfort to a markedly dysphoric agitation with frantic pacing. Anticholinergic agents or β-blockers are sometimes helpful.

E. NEUROLEPTIC MALIGNANT SYNDROME—Neuroleptic malignant syndrome is a very rare medical emergency associated primarily with the conventional antipsychotics, although it has also been reported with atypical antipsychotics. It is manifested by severe muscular rigidity, mental status changes, fever, autonomic lability, and myoglobinemia. Neuroleptic malignant syndrome can occur without muscle rigidity in patients taking atypical antipsychotics and should be considered in the differential diagnosis of any patient on antipsychotics who presents with high fever and altered mental status. Mortality as high as 30% has been reported. Treatment includes immediate medical assessment, withdrawal of the neuroleptic, and may require transfer to an intensive cares unit.

F. WITHDRAWAL DYSKINESIAS—Withdrawal dyskinesias are reversible movement disorders that appear following withdrawal of neuroleptic medications. Dyskinetic movements develop within 1–4 weeks after withdrawal of the drug and may persist for months.

G. OTHER ADVERSE EFFECTS—These include cardiac arrhythmias, irregular menses, gynecomastia and galactorrhea due to increased prolactin, sexual dysfunction, photosensitivity, rashes, lowered seizure threshold, hepatic dysfunction, and blood dyscrasias.

3. Drug interactions—Potentiation of central nervous system depressant effects or the anticholinergic effects of other drugs may occur, as well as increased plasma levels of antidepressants.

4. Medical follow-up—The patient should be examined at least every 3 months for signs of the side effects listed. An Abnormal Involuntary Movement Scale can be used to monitor for TD in patients taking antipsychotics. Most antipsychotic treatments seem to be associated with relevant weight gain, which increases the risk of the development of metabolic syndrome and future cardiovascular morbidity and mortality. New recommendations include quarterly monitoring of blood pressure, weight gain, abdominal circumference, dietary and exercise habits, and, if indicated, fasting blood glucose and lipid panels. In cases of significant weight gain or abnormal laboratory values, patients should either be switched to an agent with a decreased risk for these adverse events or should receive additional treatments to reduce specific adverse events in cases in which discontinuation of the offending agent is clinically contraindicated or unfeasible.

ADRENERGIC AGONISTS

Clonidine (Catapres) & Guanfacine (Tenex)

1. Indications—Clonidine is a nonselective α-adrenergic agonist that is clinically useful in decreasing states of hyperarousal seen in children and adolescents with PTSD and ADHD. Guanfacine is a selective agonist for α_2-adrenergic receptors with advantages over the nonselective agonist clonidine. Guanfacine is less sedating and less hypotensive than clonidine and has a longer half-life, allowing for twice-daily dosing. Case reports find guanfacine effective in ADHD and in Tourette syndrome with comorbid ADHD. Bedtime doses of adrenergic agonists can be helpful for the delayed onset of sleep and nightmares that can occur with PTSD, for the difficulty settling for sleep seen in ADHD, or for ameliorating the side effects of stimulant medications. These agents are also effective in the treatment of tics in Tourette syndrome

2. Contraindications—Adrenergic agonists are contraindicated in patients with known renal or cardiovascular disease and in those with a family or personal history of depression.

3. Initial medical screening—The pulse and blood pressure should be recorded prior to starting an adrenergic agonist.

4. Dosage—The initial dosage of clonidine is usually 0.025–0.05 mg at bedtime. The dosage can be increased after 3–5 days by giving 0.05 mg in the morning. Further dosage increases are made by adding 0.05 mg first in the morning, then at noon, and then in the evening every 3–5 days to a maximum total daily dose of 0.3 mg in three or four divided doses per day. The half-life of clonidine is in the range of 3–4 hours. Although a clinical response generally becomes apparent by about 4 weeks, treatment effects may increase over 2–3 months. Therapeutic doses of methylphenidate can frequently be decreased by 30–50% when used in conjunction with clonidine. Transdermal administration of clonidine using a skin patch can be quite effective but may result in skin irritation in 40% of patients. Patches are generally changed every 5 days.

The starting dosage of guanfacine is usually 0.5–1 mg once a day, increasing as clinically indicated after 3–5 days to 2–4 mg/d in two or three divided doses per day. Adverse effects include transient headaches and stomach aches in 25% of patients. Sedation and hypertension are mild. For medical follow-up, pulse and blood pressure should be checked every 1–2 weeks for 2 months and then at 3-month intervals.

5. Adverse effects—Sedation can be prominent. Side effects include fatigability, dizziness associated with hypotension, increased appetite and weight gain, headache, sleep disturbance, GI distress, skin irritation with transdermal clonidine administration, and rebound hypertension with abrupt withdrawal. Bradycardia can occasionally be marked.

6. Drug interactions—Increased sedation with central nervous system depressants; possible increased anticholinergic toxicity. Several case reports have mentioned cardiac toxicity with clonidine when combined with methylphenidate, although other medications and clinical factors were present in each case.

7. Medical follow-up—Pulse and blood pressure should be recorded every 2 weeks for 2 months and then every 3 months. The discontinuation of clonidine or guanfacine should occur gradually, with stepwise dosage decreases every 3–5 days to avoid rebound hypertension. Blood pressure should be monitored during withdrawal.

Baumgartner JL et al: Citalopram in children and adolescents with depression or anxiety. Ann Pharmacother 2002;36:1692 [PMID: 12398561].

Biederman J: Attention-deficit/hyperactivity disorder: A selective overview. Biol Psychiatry 2005;57:1215 [PMID: 15949990].

Birmaher B et al: Fluoxetine for the treatment of childhood anxiety disorders. J Am Acad Child Adolesc Psychiatry 2003;42:415 [PMID: 12649628].

Compton SN et al: Sertraline in children and adolescents with social anxiety disorder: An open trial. J Am Acad Child Adolesc Psychiatry 2001;40:564 [PMID: 11349701].

Courtney DB: Selective serotonin reuptake inhibitor and venlafaxine use in children and adolescents with major depressive disorder: A systematic review of published randomized controlled trials. Can J Psychiatry 2004;49:557 [PMID: 1543105].

DelBello M, Greevich S: Phenomenology and epidemiology of childhood psychiatric disorders that may necessitate treatment with atypical antipsychotics. J Clin Psychiatry 2004;65(Suppl 6):12 [PMID: 15104522].

Emslie GJ et al: Fluoxetine for acute treatment of depression in children and adolescents; a placebo-controlled randomized clinical trial. J Am Acad Child Adolesc Psychiatry 2002;41:1205 [PMID: 12364842].

Emslie GJ et al: Predictors of response to treatment in children and adolescents with mood disorders. Psychiatr Clin North Am 2003;26:435 [PMID: 12778842].

Galanter CA et al: Response to methylphenidate in children with ADHD and manic symptoms in the multimodal treatment study of children with ADHD titration trial. J Child Adolesc Psychopharmacol 2003;13:123 [PMID: 12880507].

Gleason MM et al: Psychopharmacological treatment for very young children: Contexts and guidelines. J Am Acad Child Adolesc Psychiatry 2007;46:1532 [PMID: 18030077].

Greenhill LL et al: Developing methodologies for monitoring long-term safety of psychotropic medications: Report on the NIMH conference, Sept. 25, 2000. J Am Acad Child Adolesc Psychiatry 2003;42:651 [PMID: 12921472].

Green WH: *Child and Adolescent Psychopharmacology*, 3rd ed. Lippincott Williams & Wilkins, 2001.

Hellings JA et al: Weight gain in a controlled study of risperidone in children, adolescents and adults with mental retardation and autism. J Child Adolesc Psychopharmacol 2001;11:229 [PMID: 11642473].

Kaftantaris V et al: Lithium treatment of acute mania in adolescents: A large open trial. J Am Acad Child Adolesc Psychiatry 2003;42:1038 [PMID: 12960703].

Keller MB et al: Efficacy of paroxetine in the treatment of adolescent major depression: A randomized controlled trial. J Am Acad Child Adolesc Psychiatry 2001;40:762 [PMID: 11437014].

Kowatch RA, Delbello MP: The use of mood stabilizers and atypical antipsychotics in children and adolescents with bipolar disorders. CNS Spectr 2003;8:273 [PMID: 12679742].

Kowatch RA et al: Combination pharmacotherapy in children and adolescents with bipolar disorder. Biol Psychiatry 2003;53:978 [PMID: 12788243].

Kowatch RA et al: Effect size of lithium, divalproex sodium and carbamazepine in children and adolescents with bipolar disor-der. J Am Acad Child Adolesc Psychiatry 2000;39:713 [PMID: 10846305].

Kratochvil CJ et al: Pharmacotherapy of childhood anxiety disorders. Curr Psychiatry Rep 2002;4:264 [PMID: 12126594].

Labellarte MJ et al: The relevance of prolonged QTc measurement to pediatric psychopharmacology. J Am Acad Child Adolesc Psychiatry 2003;42:642 [PMID: 12921471].

March JS, Vitiello B: Advances in paediatric neuropsychopharmacology: An overview. Int J Neuropsychopharmacol 2001;4:141 [PMID: 11466164].

McClellan JM, Werry JS: Evidence-based treatments in child and adolescent psychiatry. J Am Acad Child Adolesc Psychiatry 2003;42:1388 [PMID: 14627873].

Pliszka SR et al: A feasibility study of the children's medication algorithm project (CMAP) for the treatment of ADHD. J Am Acad Child Adolesc Psychiatry 2003;42:279 [PMID: 12595780].

Plizka SR: Non-stimulant treatment of attention-deficit/hyperactivity disorder. CNS Spectr 2003;8:253 [PMID: 12679740].

Ryan ND: Child and adolescent depression: Short-term treatment effectiveness and long-term opportunities. Int J Methods Psychiatr Res 2003;12:44 [PMID: 12830309].

Ryan ND: Medication treatment for depression in children and adolescents. CNS Spectr 2003;8:283 [PMID: 12679743].

Scahill L et al: Lithium in children and adolescents. J Child Adolesc Psychiatr Nurs 2001;14:89 [PMID: 11883628].

Simeon J et al: A retrospective chart review of risperidone use in treatment-resistant children and adolescents with psychiatric disorders. Prog Neuropsychopharmacol Biol Psychiatry 2002;26:267 [PMID: 11817503].

Steiner H et al: Psychopharmacologic strategies for the treatment of aggression in juveniles. CNS Spectr 2003;8:298 [PMID: 12679744].

Wagner KD: Pharmacotherapy for major depression in children and adolescents. Prog Neuropsychopharmacol Biol Psychiatry 2005;29:819 [PMID: 15908090].

Walkup J et al: Treatment of pediatric anxiety disorders: An open-label extension of the research units pediatric psychopharmacology anxiety study. J Child Adolesc Psychopharmacol 2002;12:175 [PMID: 12427292].

Whittington CJ et al: Selective serotonin reuptake inhibitors in childhood depression: systematic review of published vs. unpublished data. Lancet 2004;363:1341 [PMID: 15110490].

Child Abuse & Neglect

Andrew P. Sirotnak, MD

Richard D. Krugman, MD

Antonia Chiesa, MD

The problem of child abuse and neglect, barely recognized as a significant problem in the early editions of this textbook, has grown to such serious proportions that in 1990 the U.S. Advisory Board on Child Abuse and Neglect called the present state of the nation's ability to protect children a "national emergency." Over a decade later and into the 21st century, the emergency is still with us. What Dr. Henry Kempe and his colleagues first called battered child syndrome was thought to affect 749 children in the United States in 1960. In 2005 an estimated 3.3 million referrals were made to child protective service agencies involving the alleged maltreatment of approximately 6 million children. This translates to an approximate national referral rate of 43.9 referrals per 1000 children. Just under 900,000 of these cases were substantiated by child protective services in 2005, yielding an abuse victimization rate of 12.1 per 1000 American children. At least 1500 children are victims of fatal child abuse each year, and in 2005 the rate of child abuse death was 1.96 per 100,000 children. This dramatic increase in cases has resulted from increased recognition of the problem by professionals, partly in response to statutory reporting mandates, a broadening of the definitions of abuse and neglect from the original battered child concept, and changes in the demography and social structure of families and neighborhoods over the past several decades. Substance abuse, poverty and economic strains, parental capacity and skills, and domestic violence are cited as the most common presenting problems in abusive families.

Abuse and neglect of children are best considered in an ecological perspective, which recognizes the individual, family, social, and psychological influences that come together to contribute to the problem. Kempe and Helfer termed this the *abusive pattern,* in which the child, the crisis, and the caregiver's potential to abuse are components in the event of maltreatment. For most pediatric health care professionals, however, their involvement will be limited to individual cases. This chapter focuses on the knowledge necessary for the recognition, intervention, and follow-up of the more common forms of child maltreatment and highlights the role of pediatric professionals in prevention.

FORMS OF CHILD MALTREATMENT

Child maltreatment may occur either within or outside the family. The proportion of intrafamilial to extrafamilial cases varies with the type of abuse as well as the gender and age of the child. Each of the following conditions may exist as separate or concurrent diagnoses. Neglect is the most commonly reported and substantiated form of child maltreatment annually.

Physical Abuse

Physical abuse of children is most often inflicted by a caregiver or family member but occasionally by a stranger. The most common manifestations include bruises, burns, fractures, head trauma, and abdominal injuries. A small but significant number of unexpected pediatric deaths, particularly in infants and very young children (eg, sudden unexpected infant death), are related to physical abuse.

Sexual Abuse

Sexual abuse is defined as the engaging of dependent, developmentally immature children in sexual activities that they do not fully comprehend and to which they cannot give consent, or activities that violate the laws and taboos of a society. It includes all forms of incest, sexual assault or rape, and pedophilia. This includes fondling, oral-genital-anal contact, all forms of intercourse or penetration, exhibitionism, voyeurism, exploitation or prostitution, and the involvement of children in the production of pornography. Although over the past decade there has been a small downward trend in total reports of sexual abuse cases, exploitation and enticement of children and adolescents via the Internet remains a growing trend.

Emotional Abuse & Neglect

Emotional or psychological abuse has been defined as the rejection, ignoring, criticizing, isolation, or terrorizing of children, all of which have the effect of eroding their self-esteem. The most common form is verbal abuse or denigration. Children who witness domestic violence should be considered emotionally abused. The most common feature of emotional neglect is the absence of normal parent-child attachment and a subsequent inability to recognize and respond to an infant's or child's needs. A common manifestation of emotional neglect in infancy is nutritional (nonorganic) failure to thrive.

Physical Neglect

Physical neglect is the failure to provide the necessary food, clothing, and shelter and a safe environment in which children can grow and develop. Although often associated with poverty or ignorance, physical neglect involves a more serious problem than just lack of resources. There is often a component of emotional neglect and either a failure or an inability, intentionally or otherwise, to recognize and respond to the needs of the child.

Medical Care Neglect

Medical care neglect is failure to provide the needed treatment to infants or children with life-threatening illness or other serious or chronic medical conditions.

Münchausen Syndrome by Proxy

Münchausen syndrome by proxy is a relatively unusual disorder in which a caregiver, usually the mother, either simulates or creates the symptoms or signs of illness in a child. The disorder has recently been termed *factitious disorder by proxy*. The child can present with a long list of medical problems or often bizarre, recurrent complaints. Persistent doctor shopping and enforced invalidism (eg, not accepting that the child is healthy and reinforcing that the child is somehow ill) are also described in the original definition of Münchausen syndrome by proxy. Fatal cases have been reported.

RECOGNITION OF ABUSE & NEGLECT

The most common features suggesting a diagnosis of child abuse are summarized in Tables 7–1 and 7–2. Obvious signs of injury, sexual abuse, or neglect may be present. Classic radiographic and laboratory findings are discussed later in this chapter. Psychosocial factors may indicate risk for or confirm child maltreatment.

Recognition of any form of abuse and neglect of children can occur only if child abuse is considered in the differential diagnosis of the child's presenting medical condition. The approach to the family should be supportive, nonaccusatory, and empathetic. The individual who brings the child in for care may not have any involvement in the abuse. Approximately one third of child abuse incidents occur in extrafamilial settings. Neverthe-

Table 7–1. Common historical features in child abuse cases.

Discrepant, evolving, or absent history
Delay in seeking care
Event or behavior by child that triggers a loss of control of caregiver
History of abuse in the caregiver's childhood
Inappropriate affect of the caregiver
Pattern of increasing severity or number of injuries if no intervention
Social or physical isolation of the child or the caregiver
Stress or crisis in the family or the caregiver
Unrealistic expectations of caregiver for the child

less, the assumption that the caregiver is "nice," combined with the failure to consider the possibility of abuse, can be costly and even fatal. Raising the possibility that a child has been abused is not the same as accusing the caregiver of being the abuser. The health professional who is examining the child can explain to the family that several possibilities might explain the child's injuries or abuse-related symptoms. If the family or presenting caregiver is not involved in the child's maltreatment, they may actually welcome the necessary report and investigation.

History

In all cases of abuse and neglect, a detailed psychosocial history is important. This should include information on who lives in the home, other caregivers, domestic violence, substance abuse, and prior family history of physical or sexual abuse. Inquiring about any previous involvement with social services or law enforcement can help to determine risk.

Table 7–2. Presentations of sexual abuse.

General or direct statements about sexual abuse
Sexualized knowledge, play, or behavior in developmentally immature children
Sexual abuse of other children by the victim
Behavioral changes
Sleep disturbances (eg, nightmares and night terrors)
Appetite disturbances (eg, anorexia, bulimia)
Depression, social withdrawal, anxiety
Aggression, temper tantrums, impulsiveness
Neurotic or conduct disorders, phobias or avoidant behaviors
Guilt, low self-esteem, mistrust, feelings of helplessness
Hysterical or conversion reactions
Suicidal, runaway threats or behavior
Excessive masturbation
Medical conditions
Recurrent abdominal pain or frequent somatic complaints
Genital, anal, or urethral trauma
Recurrent complaints of genital or anal pain, discharge, bleeding
Enuresis or encopresis
Sexually transmitted infections
Pregnancy
Promiscuity or prostitution, sexual dysfunction, fear of intimacy
School problems or truancy
Substance abuse

A. Physical Abuse

The medical diagnosis of physical abuse is based on the presence of a discrepant history, in which the history offered by the caregiver is not consistent with the clinical findings. The discrepancy may exist because the history is absent, partial, changing over time, or simply illogical or improbable. The presence of a discrepant history should prompt a request for consultation with a multidisciplinary child protection team or a report to the child protective services agency. This agency is mandated by state law to investigate reports of suspected child abuse and neglect. Investigation by social services and possibly law enforcement officers, as well as a home visit, may be required to sort out the circumstances of the child's injuries. Other common historical features in child abuse cases are listed in Table 7–1.

B. Sexual Abuse

Sexual abuse may come to the clinician's attention in different ways: (1) The child may be brought in for routine care or for an acute problem, and sexual abuse may be suspected by the medical professional as a result of the history or the physical examination. (2) The parent or caregiver, suspecting that the child may have been sexually abused, may bring the child to the health care provider and request an examination to rule in or rule out abuse. (3) The child may be referred by child protective services or the police for an evidentiary examination following either disclosure of sexual abuse by the child or an allegation of abuse by a parent or third party. Table 7–2 lists the presentations of child sexual abuse. It should be emphasized that with the exception of acute trauma, certain sexually transmitted infections (STIs), or forensic laboratory evidence, none of these presentations is specific. The presentations listed should arouse suspicion of the possibility of sexual abuse and lead the practitioner to ask the appropriate questions—again, in a compassionate and nonaccusatory manner. Asking the child nonleading, age-appropriate questions is important and is often best handled by the most experienced interviewer after a report is made. Community agency protocols may exist for child advocacy centers that help in the investigation of these reports. Concerns expressed about sexual abuse in the context of divorce and custody disputes should be handled in the same manner, with the same objective, nonjudgmental documentation. The American Academy of Pediatrics has published guidelines for the evaluation of child sexual abuse as well as other guidelines relating to child maltreatment.

C. Emotional Abuse

Emotional abuse may cause nonspecific symptoms in children. Loss of self-esteem or self-confidence, sleep disturbances, somatic symptoms (eg, headaches and stomach aches), hypervigilance, or avoidant or phobic behaviors (eg, school refusal or running away) may be presenting complaints. These complaints may also be seen in children who experience domestic violence. Emotional abuse can occur in the home or day care, school, sports team, or other settings.

D. Neglect

Even though in 2005 there were three times as many reports of neglect of children as of physical abuse, neglect is not easily documented on history. Physical neglect—which must be differentiated from the deprivations of poverty—will be present even after adequate social services have been provided to families in need. Emotionally neglectful parents appear to have an inability to recognize the physical or emotional states of their children. For example, an emotionally neglectful parent may ignore an infant's cry if the cry is perceived incorrectly as an expression of anger. This misinterpretation leads to inadequate nutrition and failure to thrive. The clinician must evaluate the psychosocial history and family dynamics when neglect is a consideration, and a careful social services investigation of the home and entire family may be required.

E. Failure to Thrive

The history offered in cases of growth failure (failure to thrive) is often discrepant with the physical findings. Infants who have experienced a significant deceleration in growth are probably not receiving adequate amounts or appropriate types of food despite the dietary history provided. Medical conditions causing poor growth in infancy and early childhood can be ruled out with a detailed history and physical examination with minimal laboratory tests. A psychosocial history may reveal maternal depression, family chaos or dysfunction, or other previously unknown social risk factors (eg, substance abuse, violence, poverty, or psychiatric illness). Placement of the child with another caregiver is usually followed by a dramatic weight gain. Hospitalization of the severely malnourished patient is sometimes required, but most cases are managed on an outpatient basis.

Physical Findings

A. Physical Abuse

The findings on examination of physically abused children may include abrasions, alopecia, bites, bruises, burns, dental trauma, fractures, lacerations, ligature marks, or scars. Injuries may be in multiple stages of healing. Bruises in physically abused children are sometimes patterned (eg, belt marks, looped cord marks, or grab or pinch marks) and are typically found over the soft tissue areas of the body. Toddlers or older children typically sustain accidental bruises over bony prominences such as shins and elbows. Any bruise in an infant not developmentally mobile should be viewed with concern. (Other child abuse emergencies are listed in Table 7–3.) Lacerations of the frenulum or tongue and bruising of the lips may be associated with force feeding. Pathognomonic burn pat-

Table 7–3. Potential child abuse medical emergencies.

Any infant with bruises (especially head, facial, or abdominal), burns, or fractures
Any infant or child younger than age 2 years with a history of suspected "shaken baby" head trauma or other inflicted head injury
Any child who has sustained suspicious or known inflicted abdominal trauma
Any child with burns in stocking or glove distribution or in other unusual patterns, burns to the genitalia, and any unexplained burn injury
Any child with disclosure or sign of sexual assault within 48–72 h after the alleged event if the possibility of acute injury is present or if forensic evidence exists

terns include stocking or glove distribution; immersion burns of the buttocks, sometimes with a "doughnut hole" area of sparing; and branding burns such as with cigarettes or hot objects (eg, grill, curling iron, or lighter). The absence of splash marks or a pattern consistent with spillage may be helpful in differentiating accidental from nonaccidental scald burns.

Head and abdominal trauma may present with signs and symptoms consistent with those injuries. Inflicted head trauma (eg, shaken baby syndrome) and abdominal injuries may have no visible findings on examination. Symptoms can be subtle and may mimic other conditions such as gastroenteritis. Studies have documented that cases of inflicted head injury will be missed when practitioners fail to consider the diagnosis. The finding of retinal hemorrhages in an infant without an appropriate medical condition (eg, leukemia, congenital infection, or clotting disorder) should arouse concern about possible inflicted head trauma. Retinal hemorrhages are not commonly seen after cardiopulmonary resuscitation in either infants or children.

B. Sexual Abuse

The genital and anal findings of sexually abused children, as well as the normal developmental changes and variations in prepubertal female hymens, have been described in journal articles and visual diagnosis guides. To maintain a sense of comfort and routine for the patient, the genital examination should be conducted in the context of a full body checkup. For non–sexually active, prepubertal girls, an internal speculum examination is rarely necessary unless there is suspicion of internal injury; the external female genital structures can be well visualized using labial separation and traction with the child in the supine frog leg or knee-chest position. The majority of victims of sexual abuse exhibit no physical findings. The reasons for this include delay in disclosure by the child, abuse that may cause no physical trauma (eg, fondling, oral-genital contact, or exploitation by pornographic photography), or rapid healing of minor injuries such as labial, hymenal, or anal abrasions, contusions, or lacerations. Nonspecific abnormalities of the genital and rectal regions such as erythema, rashes, and irritation may not suggest sexual abuse in the absence of a corroborating history, disclosure, or behavioral changes. Finally, some medical conditions may be misdiagnosed as sexual abuse (eg, vulvovaginitis, lichen sclerosus, dermatitis, labial adhesions, congenital urethral or vulvar disorders, Crohn's disease, and accidental straddle injuries to the labia) and can be ruled out by careful history and examination.

Certain STIs should strongly suggest sexual abuse. *Neisseria gonorrhoeae* infection or syphilis beyond the perinatal period is diagnostic of sexual abuse. *Chlamydia trachomatis*, herpes simplex virus, trichomoniasis, and human papillomavirus are all sexually transmitted, although the course of these perinatally acquired infections may be protracted. In the case of human papillomavirus, an initial appearance of venereal warts beyond the toddler age should prompt a discussion regarding concerns of sexual abuse. Human papillomavirus is a ubiquitous virus and can be spread innocently by caregivers with hand lesions; biopsy and viral typing is rarely indicated and often of limited availability. Finally, sexual abuse must be considered with the diagnosis of HIV infection when other modes of transmission (eg, transfusion or perinatal acquisition) have been ruled out. Postexposure prophylaxis medications for HIV in cases of acute sexual assault should be considered only after assessment of risk of transmission and consultation with an infectious disease expert.

Although sensitivity and specificity of nonculture tests such as nucleic acid amplification tests (NAATs) have improved, they have not yet been approved for the screening of STIs in sexual abuse victims or for children younger than 12 years of age. If an NAAT is positive, a confirmatory test is needed. Specimens from symptomatic patients should still be cultured. Finally, the Centers for Disease Control and Prevention and many sexual abuse atlases list guidelines for the screening and treatment of STIs in the context of sexual abuse.

C. Neglect and Nonorganic Failure to Thrive

Infants and children with nonorganic failure to thrive have a relative absence of subcutaneous fat in the cheeks, buttocks, and extremities. Other conditions associated with poor nutrient and vitamin intake may be present. If the condition has persisted for some time, these patients may also appear and act depressed. Older children who have been chronically emotionally neglected may also have short stature (ie, deprivation dwarfism). The head circumference is usually normal in cases of nonorganic failure to thrive. Microcephaly may signify a prenatal condition, congenital disease, or chronic nutritional deprivation and increases the likelihood of more serious and possibly permanent developmental delay.

D. Münchausen Syndrome by Proxy

Children with Münchausen syndrome by proxy may present with the signs and symptoms of whatever illness is factitiously produced or simulated. They may be actually ill or, more often, are reported to be ill and have a normal clinical appearance. Among the most common reported presentations are recurrent apnea, dehydration from induced vomiting or diarrhea, sepsis when contaminants are injected into a child, change in mental status, fever, gastrointestinal bleeding, and seizures.

Radiologic & Laboratory Findings

A. Physical Abuse

Certain radiologic findings are strong indicators of physical abuse. Examples are metaphyseal "corner" or "bucket handle" fractures of the long bones in infants, spiral fracture of the extremities in nonambulatory infants, rib fractures, spinous process fractures, and fractures in multiple stages of healing. Skeletal surveys in children aged 3 years or younger should be performed when a suspicious fracture is diagnosed. Computed tomography or magnetic resonance imaging findings of subdural hemorrhage in infants—in the absence of a clear accidental history—are highly correlated with abusive head trauma, especially after the advent of infant seat restraint laws that have reduced the incidence of head trauma in infants. Abdominal computed tomography is the preferred test in suspected abdominal trauma. Any infant or very young child with suspected abuse-related head or abdominal trauma should be evaluated immediately by an emergency physician or trauma surgeon.

Coagulation studies and a complete blood cell count with platelets are useful in children who present with multiple or severe bruising in different stages of healing. Coagulopathy conditions may confuse the diagnostic picture but can be excluded with a careful history, examination, laboratory screens, and hematologic consultation if necessary.

The differential diagnosis of all forms of physical abuse can be considered in the context of a detailed trauma history, family medical history, radiographic findings, and laboratory testing. The diagnosis of osteogenesis imperfecta or other collagen disorders, for example, may be considered in the child with skin and joint findings or multiple fractures with or without the classic radiographic presentation and is best made in consultation with a geneticist, an orthopedic surgeon, and a radiologist. Trauma—accidental or inflicted—leads the differential diagnosis list for subdural hematomas. Coagulopathy; disorders of copper, amino acid, or organic acid metabolism (eg, Menkes syndrome and glutaric acidemia type 1); chronic or previous central nervous system infection; birth trauma; or congenital central nervous system malformation (eg, arteriovenous malformations or cerebrospinal fluid collections) may need to be ruled out in some cases. It should be recognized, however, that children with these rare disorders can also be victims of abuse or neglect.

B. Sexual Abuse

The forensic evaluation of sexually abused children should be performed in a setting that prevents further emotional distress. If the history indicates that the child may have had contact with the ejaculate of a perpetrator within 72 hours, an examination to look for semen or its markers (eg, acid phosphatase) should be performed according to established protocols. This should occur in an emergency department or clinic where chain of custody for specimens can be assured. More important, if there is a history of possible sexual abuse within the past 48–72 hours, and the child reports a physical complaint or a sign is observed (eg, genital or anal bleeding or discharge), the child should be examined for signs of trauma. The most experienced examiner (pediatrician, nurse examiner, or child advocacy center) is preferable. The laboratory and serologic evaluation of STIs should be guided by the type of contact reported and the epidemiology of these infections in the community.

C. Neglect and Growth Failure

Children with failure to thrive or malnutrition may not require an extensive workup. Assessment of the patient's growth curve, as well as careful plotting of subsequent growth parameters after treatment, is critical. Complete blood cell count, urinalysis, electrolyte panel, and thyroid and liver function tests are sufficient screening. Newborn screening should be documented as usual. Other tests should be guided by any aspect of the clinical history that points to a previously undiagnosed condition. A skeletal survey and head computed tomography scan may be helpful if concurrent physical abuse is suspected. The best screening method, however, is placement in a setting in which the child can be fed and monitored. Hospital or foster care placement may be required. Weight gain may not occur for several days to a week in severe cases.

D. Münchausen Syndrome by Proxy

Recurrent polymicrobial sepsis (especially in children with indwelling catheters), recurrent apnea, chronic dehydration of unknown cause, or other highly unusual unexplained laboratory findings should raise the suspicion of Münchausen syndrome by proxy.

MANAGEMENT & REPORTING

Physical abuse injuries, STIs, and medical sequelae of neglect should be treated immediately. Children with failure to thrive related to emotional and physical neglect need to be placed in a setting in which they can be fed and cared for. Likewise, the child in danger of recurrent abuse or neglect needs to be placed in a safe environment.

In the United States, clinicians and many other professionals who come in contact with or care for children are mandated reporters. If abuse or neglect is suspected, a report must be made to the local or state agency designated to investigate such matters. In most cases, this will be the child protective services agency. Law enforcement agencies may also receive such reports. The purpose of the report is to permit professionals to gather the information needed to determine whether the child's environment (eg, home, school, day care setting, or foster home) is safe. Recent backlash against physicians in Great Britain involved in high-profile child abuse cases should not deter anyone in the United States from following the state-specific child abuse reporting laws. Many hospitals and communities make child protection teams or consultants available when there are questions about the diagnosis and management in a child abuse case. A listing of pediatric consultants in child abuse is available from the American Academy of Pediatrics.

Except in extreme cases, the reporting of emotional abuse is not likely to generate an immediate response from child protection agencies. This should not deter reporting, especially if there is also concern for domestic violence or other forms of abuse or neglect. Practitioners can encourage parents to become involved with parent effectiveness training programs (eg, Healthy Families America or Parents Anonymous) or to seek mental health consultation. Support for the child may also include mental health counseling or age-appropriate peer and mentoring activities in school or the community. Finally, communication with social services, case management, and careful follow-up by primary care providers is crucial to ensuring ongoing safety of child.

PREVENTION

Physical abuse is preventable in many cases. Extensive experience with and evaluation of high-risk families have shown that the provision of home visitor services to families at risk can prevent abuse and neglect of children. These services can be provided by public health nurses or trained paraprofessionals, although more data are available describing public health nurse intervention. The availability of these services could make it as easy for a family to pick up the telephone and ask for help before they abuse a child as it is for a neighbor or physician to report an episode of abuse after it has occurred. Parent education and anticipatory guidance are also helpful, with attention to handling situations that stress parents (eg, colic, crying behavior, and toilet training), age-appropriate discipline, and general developmental issues. Prevention of abusive injuries perpetrated by nonparent caregivers (eg, babysitters, nannies, and unrelated adults in the home) may be addressed by education and counseling of mothers about safe child care arrangements and advocating for affordable day care for all families. Promising new data suggest the efficacy of hospital-based programs that teach parents about the dangers of shaking an infant and how to respond to a crying infant.

The prevention of sexual abuse is more difficult. Most efforts in this area involve teaching children to protect themselves and their "private parts" from harm or interference. The age of toilet training is a good time to provide anticipatory guidance to encourage parents to consider this

discussion. The most rational approach is to place the burden of responsibility of prevention on the adults who supervise the child and the medical providers rather than on the children themselves. Knowing the parents' own history of any victimization is important, as the ability to engage in this anticipatory guidance discussion with a provider and their child may be affected by that history. Promoting Internet safety and limiting exposure to sexualized materials and media should be part of this anticipatory guidance. Finally, many resource books on this topic for parents can be found in the parenting and health sections of most bookstores.

Efforts to prevent emotional abuse of children have been undertaken through extensive media campaigns. No data are available to assess the effectiveness of this approach. The primary care physician can promote positive, nurturing, and nonviolent behavior in parents. The message that they are role models for a child's behavior is important. Screening for domestic violence during anticipatory guidance discussions on discipline, home, and safety can be effective in identifying parents and children at risk.

REFERENCES

2006 Guidelines for the treatment of sexually transmitted diseases. MMWR Recomm Rep 2006;55(RR-11). Available at: http://www.cdc.gov/std/treatment/2006/rr5511.pdf.

Adams JA et al: Guidelines for medical care of children who may have been sexually abused. J Pediatr Adolesc Gynecol 2007;20:163 [PMID: 17561184].

American Academy of Pediatrics, Hymel KP; Committee on Child Abuse and Neglect; National Association of Medical Examiners: Distinguishing sudden infant death syndrome from child abuse fatalities. Pediatrics 2006;118:421 [PMID: 16818592].

American Academy of Pediatrics, Hymel KP; Committee on Child Abuse and Neglect: When is lack of supervision neglect? Pediatrics 2006;118:1296 [PMID: 16951030].

American Academy of Pediatrics: Clinical report: The evaluation of sexual abuse of children. Pediatrics 2005;116:506 [PMID: 16061610].

American Academy of Pediatrics: Diagnostic imaging of child abuse. Pediatrics 2000;105:1345 [PMID:10835079].

American Academy of Pediatrics: Visual Diagnosis of Child Abuse. [CD ROM], 2nd ed. American Academy of Pediatrics, 2008 (forthcoming).

Augustyn M, McAlister B: If we don't ask, they aren't going to tell: Screening for domestic violence. Contemp Pediatr 2005; 22:43.

Berkowitz CD: Recognizing and responding to domestic violence. Pediatr Ann 2005;34:395 [PMID: 15948350].

DeBellis MD: The psychobiology of neglect. Child Maltreat 2005;10:150 [PMID: 15798010].

Dias MS et al: Preventing abusive head trauma among infants and young children: A hospital-based, parent education program. Pediatrics 2005;115:e470 [PMID: 15805350].

Giardino AP, Finkel MA: Evaluating child sexual abuse. Pediatr Ann 2005;34:382 [PMID: 15948349].

Giardino AP, Monteleone JA. Child Maltreatment: Training Modules and Visuals. GW Medical Publishing, 2000.

Horner G: Domestic violence and children. J Pediatr Health Care 2005;19:206 [PMID: 16010259].

Johnson CF: Child sexual abuse. Lancet 2004;364:462 [PMID: 15288746].

Krous HF et al: Sudden infant death syndrome and unclassified sudden infant deaths: A definitional and diagnostic approach. Pediatrics 2004;114:234 [PMID: 15231934].

McCann J et al: Healing of hymenal injuries in prepubertal and adolescent girls: A descriptive study. Pediatrics 2007;119:e1094. [PMID: 17420260].

Malloy MH, MacDorman M: Changes in the classification of sudden infant deaths: United States 1992–2001. Pediatrics 2005;115:1247 [PMID: 15867031].

Mears DP, Visher CA: Trends in understanding and addressing domestic violence. J Interpers Violence 2005;20:204 [PMID: 15601793].

Olds DL et al: Effects of home visits by paraprofessionals and by nurses: Age 4 follow-up results of a randomized trial. Pediatrics 2004; 114:1560 [PMID: 15574615].

Olds DL et al: Programs for parents of infants and toddlers: Recent evidence from randomized trials. J Child Psychol Psychiatry 2007;48:355 [PMID: 17355402].

Schreier H: Münchausen syndrome by proxy. Current Probl Pediatr Adolesc Health Care 2004;34:126 [PMID: 15039661].

Sirotnak AP et al: Physical abuse of children. Pediatr Rev 2004; 25:264 [PMID: 15286272].

Thompson S: Accidental or inflicted? Pediatr Ann 2005;34:372 [PMID: 15948348].

U.S. Department of Health and Human Services: Administration for Children, Youth, and Families. Child Maltreatment 2005. Available at: http://www.acf.hhs.gov/programs/cb/pubs/cm05/index.htm

Wheeler PL: Shaken baby syndrome—an introduction to the literature. Child Abuse Rev 2003;12:401. Available at: www3.interscience.wiley.com/cgi-bin/abstract/107612477.

Zenzel JA (guest editor): Child abuse and victimization: Guidelines for identifying abuse and protecting your patients. Pediatr Ann 2005;34:338–420.

Ambulatory & Community Pediatrics

Robert M. Brayden, MD

Maya Bunik, MD, MSPH

Jeffrey M. Brown, MD, MPH, CPE

Matthew F. Daley, MD

Pediatric ambulatory outpatient services provide children and adolescents with preventive health care and acute and chronic care management services and consultations. In this chapter, special attention is given to the pediatric history and physical examination, normal developmental stages, office telephone management, and community pediatrics.

The development of a physician–patient–parent relationship is crucially important if the patient and parent are to effectively confide their concerns. This relationship develops over time, with increasing numbers of visits, and is facilitated by the continuity of clinicians and other staff members. This clinical relationship is based on trust that develops as a result of several experiences in the context of the office visit. Perhaps the greatest factor facilitating the relationship is for patients or parents to experience advice as valid and effective. Important skills include choosing vocabulary that communicates understanding and competence, demonstrating commitment of time and attention to the concern, and showing respect for areas that the patient or parent does not wish to address (assuming there are no concerns relating to physical or sexual abuse or neglect). Parents and patients expect that their concerns will be managed confidentially and that the clinician understands and sympathizes with those concerns. The effective physician–patient–parent relationship is one of the most satisfying aspects of ambulatory pediatrics.

PEDIATRIC HISTORY

A unique feature of pediatrics is that the history represents an amalgam of parents' objective reporting of facts (eg, fever for 4 days), parents' subjective interpretation of their child's symptoms (eg, infant crying interpreted by parents as abdominal pain), and for older children their own history of events. Parents and patients may provide a specific and detailed history, or a vague history that necessitates more focused probing. Parents may or may not be able to distinguish whether symptoms are caused by organic illness or a psycho-

logical concern. It is often helpful to ask what problems the parents specifically wish to address in order to determine what really prompted the office visit. Some visits are occasioned by problems at school, such as low grades or troublesome peer relationships. Understanding the family and its hopes for and concerns about the child can help in the process of distinguishing organic illness from emotional or behavioral conditions, thus minimizing unnecessary testing and intervention.

Although the parents' concerns need to be understood, it is essential also to obtain as much of the history as possible directly from the patient. Direct histories not only provide firsthand information but also give the child a degree of control over a potentially threatening situation and may reveal important information about the family.

Obtaining a comprehensive pediatric history is time-consuming. Many offices provide questionnaires for parents to complete before the clinician sees the child. Data from questionnaires can make an outpatient visit more productive, allowing the physician to address problems in detail while more quickly reviewing areas that are not of concern. Questionnaires may be more productive than face-to-face interviews in revealing sensitive parts of the history. However, failure to review and assimilate this information prior to the interview may cause a parent or patient to feel that the time and effort have been wasted.

Elements of the history that will be useful over time should be readily accessible in the medical record. Such information can be accumulated on a summary sheet, as illustrated in Figure 8–1. Demographic data; a problem list; information about chronic medications, allergies, and previous hospitalizations; and the names of other physicians providing care for the patient are commonly included. Documentation of immunizations, including all data required by the National Childhood Vaccine Injury Act, should be kept on a second page.

The components of a comprehensive pediatric history are listed in Table 8–1. The information should, ideally, be obtained at the first office visit. The first seven items may be included on a summary sheet at the front of the medical

Name _____ Nickname _____ D.O.B _____
Mother _____ Father _____ Sibs _____
S.S# _____ Insurance _____

Problems			Chronic Medications		
Date of onset	Description	Date resolved	Start date		Stop date
			Allergies		
			Date		
Date	**Hospitalizations/Injuries/Procedures**		Date	**Consultants**	

▲ **Figure 8–1.** Use of a summary sheet such as this at the front of the record facilitates reorienting the caregiver and his or her partners to the patient. Some practices keep track of health supervision visits on this sheet to tell the physician whether the child is likely to have received the appropriate preventive services. A second page documenting immunizations should record data required by the National Childhood Vaccine Injury Act. When an allergy with potential for anaphylaxis is identified, the patient should wear a medical alert bracelet and obtain an epinephrine kit, if appropriate.

record. Items 8 and 9, and a focused review of systems, are dealt with at each acute or chronic care visit. The entire list should be reviewed and augmented with relevant updates at each health supervision visit.

PEDIATRIC PHYSICAL EXAMINATION

During the pediatric physical examination, time must be taken to allow the patient to become familiar with the examiner. Interactions and instructions help the child under-stand what is occurring and what is expected. A gentle, friendly manner and a quiet voice help establish a setting that yields a nonthreatening physical examination. The examiner should take into consideration the need for a quiet child, the extent of trust established, and the possibility of an emotional response (crying!) when deciding the order in which the child's organ systems are examined. Painful or unpleasant procedures (eg, otoscopic examinations) should be deferred until the end of the examination. Whether or not the physician can establish rapport with the child, the process should proceed efficiently and systematically.

Table 8–1. Components of the pediatric historical database.[a]

1. Demographic data	Patient's name and nickname, date of birth, social security number, sex, race, parents' names (first and last), siblings' names, and payment mechanism.
2. Problem list	Major or significant problems, including dates of onset and resolution.
3. Allergies	Triggering allergen, nature of the reaction, treatment needed, and date allergy diagnosed.
4. Chronic medications	Name, concentration, dose, and frequency of chronically used medications.
5. Birth history	Maternal health during pregnancy, medications, street drugs used, complications of pregnancy; duration and ease of labor; form of delivery; analgesics and anesthetics used; need for monitoring; and labor complications. Infant's birth weight, gestational age, Apgar scores, and problems in the neonatal period.
6. Screening procedures	Results of newborn screening, vision and hearing screening, any health screen, or screening laboratory tests. (Developmental screening results are maintained in the development section; see item 14, below.)
7. Immunizations	Date of each immunization administered, vaccine manufacturer and lot number, and name and title of the person administering the vaccine; previous reaction and contraindication to immunization (eg, immunodeficiency or an evolving neurologic problem).
8. Reasons for visit	The patient's or parents' concerns, stated in their own words, serve as the focus for the visit.
9. Present illness	A concise chronologic summary of the problems necessitating a visit, including the duration, progression, exacerbating factors, ameliorating interventions, and associations.
10. Medical history	A statement regarding the child's functionality and general well-being, including a summary record of significant illnesses, injuries, hospitalizations, and procedures.
11. Diet	Eating patterns, likes and dislikes, use of vitamins, and relative amounts of carbohydrates, fat, and protein in the diet.
12. Family history	Information about the illnesses of relatives, preferably in the form of a family tree.
13. Social history	Family constellation, relationships, parents' educational background, religious preference, and the role of the child in the family; socioeconomic profile of the family to identify resources available to the child, access to services that may be needed, and anticipated stressors.
14. Development	(1) Attainment of developmental milestones (including developmental testing results); (2) social habits and milestones (toilet habits, play, major activities, sleep patterns, discipline, peer relationships); (3) school progress and documentation of specific achievements and grades.
15. Sexual history	Family's sexual attitudes, sex education, sexual development and activity, sexually transmitted diseases, and birth control measures.
16. Review of systems (ROS)	This area tends to be overlooked because of the work required to obtain a complete ROS and integrate data into the patient's problems list and care plan. A focused ROS is essential if any problem is to be addressed adequately.

[a]The components of this table should be included in a child's medical record and structured to allow easy review and modification. The practice name and address should appear on all pages.

Because young children may fear the examination and become fussy, simple inspection is important. For example, during an acute-care visit for fever, the examiner should observe the child's skin color and work of breathing prior to beginning the examination. During a health supervision visit, observation will provide the examiner with an opportunity to assess parent–child interactions.

Clothing should be removed slowly and gently to avoid threatening the child. A parent or the child is usually the best person to do this. Modesty should always be respected, and gown or drapes should be provided. Examinations of adolescents should be chaperoned whenever a pelvic examination or a stressful or painful procedure is performed.

Examination tables are convenient, but a parent's lap is a comfortable location for a young child. For most purposes,

an adequate examination can be conducted on a "table" formed by the parent's and examiner's legs as they sit facing each other.

Although a thorough physical examination is important at every age, at some ages the examination tends to focus on specific issues and concerns. At any age, an astute clinician can detect signs of important clinical conditions in an asymptomatic child. In infancy, for example, physical examination can reveal the presence of craniosynostosis, congenital heart disease, or developmental dysplasia of the hip. Similarly, examination of a toddler may reveal pallor (possible iron-deficiency anemia) or strabismus. The routine examination of an adolescent may reveal scoliosis or acanthosis nigricans (a finding associated with insulin resistance).

HEALTH SUPERVISION VISITS

One of several timetables for recommended health supervision visits is illustrated in Figure 8–2. (**Note:** A PDF printable format of this figure is available from the American Academy of Pediatrics [AAP].) The federal Maternal and Child Health Bureau has developed comprehensive health supervision guidelines through their Bright Futures program. In areas where evidence-based information is lacking, expert opinion has been used as the basis for these plans. For example, immunizations are proven to be effective and necessary (Centers for Disease Control and Prevention [CDC]), whereas there is disagreement about whether screening for certain metabolic diseases is universally warranted. Practitioners should remember that guidelines are not meant to be rigid; services should be individualized according to the child's needs.

During health supervision visits, the practitioner should review child development and acute and chronic problems, conduct a complete physical examination, order appropriate screening tests, and anticipate future developments. New historical information should be elicited through an interval history. Development should be assessed by parental report and clinician observation at each visit. Developmental surveillance is augmented with systematic use of parent-directed questionnaires or screening tests. Growth is carefully recorded, and the growth chart is brought up to date (see Chapter 2). Vision and hearing should be assessed subjectively at each visit, with objective assessments at intervals beginning after the child is old enough to cooperate with the screening test, usually at age 3 or 4 years. Various laboratory screening tests may also be part of the visit.

Because fewer than 4% of asymptomatic children have physical findings on routine health maintenance visits, a major portion of the health supervision visit is devoted to anticipatory guidance. This portion of the visit enables the health care provider to address behavioral, developmental, injury prevention, and nutritional issues; school problems; and other age-appropriate issues that will arise before the next well-child visit.

American Academy of Pediatrics Committee on Practice and Ambulatory Medicine: Recommendations for preventive pediatric health care. Pediatrics 2000;105:645.

Dinkevich E, Ozuah PO: Well-child care: Effectiveness of current recommendations. Clin Pediatr 2002;41:211 [PMID: 12041716].

DEVELOPMENTAL & BEHAVIORAL ASSESSMENT

Addressing developmental and behavioral problems is one of the central features of pediatric primary care. The term *developmental delay* refers to the circumstance in which a child has not demonstrated a developmental skill (such as walking independently) by an age at which the vast majority of normally developing children have accomplished this task. Developmental delays are, in fact, quite common:

approximately 18% of children younger than age 18 years either have developmental delays or have conditions that place them at risk of developmental delays.

Pediatric practitioners are in a unique position to assess the development of their patients. This developmental assessment should ideally take the form of *developmental surveillance*, in which a skilled individual monitors development over time as part of providing routine care. Developmental surveillance includes several key elements: listening to parent concerns; obtaining a developmental history; making careful observations during office visits; periodically screening all infants and children for delays using validated screening tools; recognizing conditions and circumstances that place children at increased risk of delays; and referring children who fail screening tests for further evaluation and intervention.

The prompt recognition of children with developmental delays is important for several reasons. The presence of delays may lead practitioners to diagnose unsuspected but important conditions, such as genetic syndromes or metabolic disorders. Children with delays can be referred for a wide range of developmental therapies, such as those provided by physical therapists and speech/language therapists. Importantly, children with delays, regardless of the cause, make better developmental progress if they receive appropriate developmental therapies than if they do not. Finally, many infants and toddlers younger than age 3 years with developmental delays are eligible to receive a range of therapies and other services, often provided in the home, at no cost to families. Children aged 3 years and older with delays are also eligible for developmental services, at no cost, through the local school system.

Although the benefits of early detection of developmental delays are clear, it is often difficult to incorporate developmental surveillance into busy outpatient practice. Only 30% of pediatricians routinely use formal screening tests; most rely on clinical judgment alone. However, when screening tests are not used, delays are often not detected until school age, particularly when the delays are not severe. There are several practical barriers to performing routine surveillance using standardized screening tools: perceived lack of time to screen all children at every well child visit; lack of familiarity with the various screening tools; not wanting to concern parents by identifying a possible delay; and not knowing where in the community to refer patients with suspected delays. There are some solutions to these barriers, such as using parent developmental questionnaires rather than provider-administered tests to save time, become familiar with one or two screening tests, and making use of Internet-based resources. For example, the National Information Center for Children and Youth with Disabilities maintains a web site with links to a wide variety of resources in each state (http://www.nichcy.org).

Several parent-administered and physician-administered developmental screening tools are available. The Parents' Evaluation of Developmental Status, the Ages and Stages Questionnaires, and the Child Development Inventories are

Each child and family is unique; therefore, these **Recommendations for Preventive Pediatric Health Care** are designed for the care of children who are receiving competent parenting, have no manifestations of any important health problems, and are growing and developing in satisfactory fashion. **Additional visits may become necessary** if circumstances suggest variations from normal.

Recommendations for Preventive Pediatric Health Care

Developmental, psychosocial, and chronic disease issues for children and adolescents, may require frequent counseling and treatment visits separate from preventive care visits.

These guidelines represent a consensus by the American Academy of Pediatrics (AAP) and Bright Futures. The AAP continues to emphasize the great importance of **continuity of care** in comprehensive health supervision and the need to avoid **fragmentation of care.**

The recommendations in this statement do not indicate an exclusive course of treatment or standard of medical care. Variations, taking into account individual circumstances, may be appropriate.

Copyright © 2008 by the American Academy of Pediatrics.

Age[a]	INFANCY											EARLY CHILDHOOD				MIDDLE CHILDHOOD						ADOLESCENCE											
	Prenatal[b]	Newborn[c]	3–5 d[d]	By 1 mo	2 mo	4 mo	6 mo	9 mo	12 m	15 m	18 mo	24 mo	30 mo	3 y	4 y	5 y	6 y	7 y	8 y	9 y	10 y	11 y	12 y	13 y	14 y	15 y	16 y	17 y	18 y	19 y	20 y	21 y
HISTORY																																
Initial/interval	•	•	•	•	•	•	•	•	•	•	•	•	•	•	•	•	•	•	•	•	•	•	•	•	•	•	•	•	•	•	•	•
MEASUREMENTS																																
Length/height and weight		•	•	•	•	•	•	•	•	•	•	•	•	•	•	•	•	•	•	•	•	•	•	•	•	•	•	•	•	•	•	•
Head circumference		•	•	•	•	•	•	•	•	•	•	•																				
Weight for length		•	•	•	•	•	•	•	•	•	•																					
Body mass index												•	•	•	•	•	•	•	•	•	•	•	•	•	•	•	•	•	•	•	•	•
Blood pressure[e]		★	★	★	★	★	★	★	★	★	★	★	★	•	•	•	•	•	•	•	•	•	•	•	•	•	•	•	•	•	•	•
SENSORY SCREENING																																
Vision		★	★	★	★	★	★	★	★	★	★	★	★	•	•	•	•	★	•	★	•	★	•	★	★	•	★	★	•	★	★	★
Hearing[g]		•[g]	★	★	★	★	★	★	★	★	★	★	★	★	•	•	•	★	•	★	•	★	★	★	★	★	★	★	★	★	•	★
DEVELOPMENTAL/BEHAVIORAL ASSESSMENT																																
Developmental screening[h]								•			•		•																			
Autism screening[i]											•	•																				
Developmental surveillance[h]		•	•	•	•	•	•		•	•		•		•	•	•	•	•	•	•	•	•	•	•	•	•	•	•	•	•	•	•
Psychosocial/behavioral assessment[h]		•	•	•	•	•	•	•	•	•	•	•	•	•	•	•	•	•	•	•	•	•	•	•	•	•	•	•	•	•	•	•
Alcohol and drug use assessment																						★	★	★	★	★	★	★	★	★	★	★
PHYSICAL EXAMINATION[j]		•	•	•	•	•	•	•	•	•	•	•	•	•	•	•	•	•	•	•	•	•	•	•	•	•	•	•	•	•	•	•
PROCEDURES[k]																																
Newborn metabolic/hemoglobin screening[l]		•																														
Immunization[m]		•	•	•	•	•	•	•	•	•	•	•	•	•	•	•	•	•	•	•	•	•	•	•	•	•	•	•	•	•	•	•
Hematocrit or hemoglobin[n]						★			•or★[p]		★	★	★	★	★	★	★	★	★	★	★	★	★	★	★	★	★	★	★	★	★	★
Lead screening[o]							★	★	•or★[p]		★	•or★[p]	★	★	★	★	★															
Tuberculin test[q]				★			★		★			★		★		★	★		★		★	★	★	★	★	★	★	★	★	★	★	★
Dyslipidemia screening[r]												★			★		★		★	•	★	•	★	★	★	★	★	★	•	★	•	★
STI screening[s]																						★	★	★	★	★	★	★	★	★	★	★
Cervical dysplasia screening[t]																						★	★	★	★	★	★	★	★	★	★	•[v]
ORAL HEALTH[u]							•or★[u]	•or★[u]	•[v]		•[v]		•[v]	•[v]			•[v]															
ANTICIPATORY GUIDANCE[w]	•	•	•	•	•	•	•	•	•	•	•	•	•	•	•	•	•	•	•	•	•	•	•	•	•	•	•	•	•	•	•	•

● = to be performed   ★ = risk assessment to be performed, with appropriate action to follow, if positive   ◄——●——► = range during which a service may be provided, with the symbol indicating the preferred age

a   If a child comes under care for the first time at any point on the schedule, or if any items are not accomplished at the suggested age, the schedule should be brought up to date at the earliest possible time.

b   A prenatal visit is recommended for parents who are at high risk, for first-time parents, and for those who request a conference. The prenatal visit should include anticipatory guidance, pertinent medical history, and a discussion of benefits of breastfeeding and planned method of feeding per AAP statement "The Prenatal Visit" (2001) [URL:http://aappolicy.aappublications.org/cgi/content/full/pediatrics; 107/6/1456].

c   Every infant should have a newborn evaluation after birth, breastfeeding encouraged, and instruction and support offered.

d   Every infant should have an evaluation within 3 to 5 days of birth and within 48 to 72 hours after discharge from the hospital, to include evaluation for feeding and jaundice. Breastfeeding infants should receive formal breastfeeding evaluation, encouragement, and instruction as recommended in AAP statement "Breastfeeding and the Use of Human Milk" (2005) [URL:http://aappolicy.aappublications.org/cgi/content/full/pediatrics;115/2/496]. For newborns discharged in less than 48 hours after delivery, the infant must be examined within 48 hours of discharge per AAP statement "Hospital Stay for Healthy Term Newborns" (2004) [URL: http://aappolicy.aappublications.org/cgi/content/full/pediatrics;113/5/1434].

e   Blood pressure measurement in infants and children with specific risk conditions should be performed at visits before age 3 years.

f   If the patient is uncooperative, rescreen within 6 months per AAP statement "Eye Examination and Vision Screening in Infants, Children, and Young Adults" (1996) [URL:http://aappolicy.aappublications.org/cgi/reprint/pediatrics; 98/1/153.pdf].

g   All newborns should be screened per AAP statement "Year 2000 Position Statement: Principles and Guidelines for Early Hearing Detection and Intervention Programs" (2000) [URL:

http://aappolicy.aappublications.org/cgi/content/full/pediatrics;106/4/798]. Joint Committee on Infant Hearing. Year 2007 position statement: principles and guidelines for early hearing detection and intervention programs. *Pediatrics.* 2007;120:898–921.

h   AAP Council on Children With Disabilities, AAP Section on Developmental Behavioral Pediatrics, AAP Bright Futures Steering Committee. AAP Medical Home Initiatives for Children With Special Needs Project Advisory Committee. Identifying infants and young children with developmental disorders in the medical home: an algorithm for developmental surveillance and screening. *Pediatrics.* 2006;118:405–420 [URL:http://aappolicy.aappublications. org/cgi/content/full/pediatrics;118/1/405].

i   Gupta VB, Hyman SL, Johnson CP, et al. Identifying children with autism early? *Pediatrics,* 2007;119:152 –153 [URL:http://pediatrics. aappublications.org/cgi/content/full/119/1/152].

j   At each visit, age-appropriate physical examination is essential, with infant totally unclothed, older child undressed and suitably draped.

k   These may be modified, depending on entry point into schedule and individual need.

l   Newborn metabolic and hemoglobinopathy screening should be done according to state law. Results should be reviewed at visits and appropriate retesting or referral done as needed.

m   Schedules per the Committee on Infectious Diseases, published annually in the January issue of *Pediatrics.* Every visit should be an opportunity to update and complete a child's immunizations.

n   See AAP *Pediatric Nutrition Handbook,* 5th Edition (2003) for a discussion of universal and selective screening options. See also Recommendations to prevent and control iron deficiency in the United States. *MMWR Recomm Rep.* 1998; 47(RR-3):1–36.

o   For children at risk of lead exposure, consult the AAP statement "Lead Exposure in Children: Prevention, Detection, and Management" (2005) [URL:http://

aappolicy.aappublications.org/cgi/content/full/pediatrics; 116/4/1036]. Additionally, screening should be done in accordance with state law where applicable.

p   Perform risk assessments or screens as appropriate, based on universal screening requirements for patients with Medicaid or high prevalence areas.

q   Tuberculosis testing per recommendations of the Committee on Infectious Diseases, published in the current edition of *Red Book: Report of the Committee on Infectious Diseases.* Testing should be done in recognition of high-risk factors.

r   "Third Report of the National Cholesterol Education Program (NCEP) Expert Panel on Detection, Evaluation, and Treatment of High Blood Cholesterol in Adults (Adult Treatment Panel III) Final Report" (2002) [URL:http://circ. ahajournals.org/cgi/content/full/106/25/3143] and "The Expert Committee Recommendations on the Assessment, Prevention, and Treatment of Child and Adolescent Overweight and Obesity." Supplement to *Pediatrics.* In press.

s   All sexually active patients should be screened for sexually transmitted infections (STIs).

t   All sexually active girls should have screening for cervical dysplasia as part of a pelvic examination beginning within 3 years of onset of sexual activity or age 21 (whichever comes first).

u   Referral to dental home, if available. Otherwise, administer oral health risk assessment. If the primary water source is deficient in fluoride, consider oral fluoride supplementation.

v   At the visits for 3 years and 6 years of age, it should be determined whether the patient has a dental home. If the patient does not have a dental home, a referral should be made to one. If the primary water source is deficient in fluoride, consider oral fluoride supplementation.

w   Refer to the specific guidance by age as listed in Bright Futures Guidelines. (Hagen JF, Shaw JS, Duncan PM, eds. *Bright Futures: Guidelines for Health Supervision of Infants, Children, and Adolescents,* 3rd ed. Elk Grove Village, IL: American Academy of Pediatrics: 2008.)

▲ **Figure 8–2.** Recommendations for preventive health care. (Hagen JF, Shaw JS, Duncan PM, eds. *Bright Futures: Guidelines for Health Supervision of Infants, Children, and Adolescents.* 3rd ed. American Academy of Pediatrics, 2008.)

screening tests that rely on parent report. The Denver II screening test (reproduced in Chapter 2, Figure 2–12), the Early Language Milestone Scale (see Chapter 2, Figure 2–11), and the Bayley Infant Neurodevelopmental Screener all involve the direct observation of a child's skills by a care provider. All developmental screening tests have their strengths and weaknesses. The Denver II is familiar to many pediatric providers and is widely used. However, whereas the Denver II has relatively high sensitivity for detecting possible developmental delays, the specificity is poorer, and this may lead to the over-referral of normal children for further developmental testing.

Regardless of the approach taken to developmental screening, there are number of important considerations: (1) the range of normal childhood development is broad, and therefore a child with a single missing skill in a single developmental area is less likely to have a significant developmental problem than a child showing multiple delays in several developmental areas (eg, gross motor *and* language delays); (2) continuity of care is important, because development is best assessed over time; (3) it is beneficial to routinely use formal screening tests to assess development; (4) if developmental delays are detected in primary care, these patients need referral for further testing and likely will benefit from receiving developmentally focused therapies; (5) parents appreciate when attention is paid to their child's development, and generally react positively to referrals for appropriate developmental therapies.

Several developmental charts with age-based expectations for normal development are presented in Chapter 2 (see Tables 2–1, 2–2, and 2–3), as well as a discussion of the recommended medical and neurodevelopmental evaluation of a child with a suspected developmental disorder.

In addition to developmental issues, pediatric providers are an important source of information and counseling for parents regarding a broad range of behavioral issues. The nature of the behavioral problems, of course, varies with the child's age. Some common issues raised by parents, discussed in detail in Chapter 2, include colic, feeding disorders, sleep problems, temper tantrums, breath-holding spells, and noncompliance. Behavioral issues in adolescents are discussed in Chapter 3.

Albrecht SJ et al: Common behavioral dilemmas of the school-aged child. Pediatr Clin North Am 2003;50:841 [PMID: 12964697].
King TM, Glascoe FP: Developmental surveillance of infants and young children in pediatric primary care. Curr Opin Pediatr 2003;15:624 [PMID: 14631210].
Rydz D et al: Developmental screening. J Child Neurol 2005;20:4 [PMID: 15791916].

GROWTH PARAMETERS

Monitoring appropriate growth is pivotal in ambulatory pediatric practice. Pediatric growth charts are based on a broad sampling of the U.S. population, with representation of young infants, breast-fed infants, and certain ethnic minorities. The 2- to 18-year growth charts include a chart of body mass index (BMI) for age. The BMI is calculated as the weight (in kilograms) divided by the squared height (in meters). The BMI is useful for determining obesity (BMI ≥ 95th percentile for age) and underweight status (BMI ≤ 5th percentile for age). The BMI is highly correlated with secondary complications of obesity.

Height, weight, and head circumference are carefully measured and plotted at each visit during the first 3 years (see growth charts in Chapter 2). For children older than 3 years, height and weight should be measured at each well child examination. To ensure accurate weight measurements for longitudinal comparisons, infants should be undressed completely, and young children should be wearing underpants only. Recumbent length is plotted on the chart from birth to 3 years (see Figures 2–1 and 2–3). When the child is old enough to be measured upright, height should be plotted on the charts for ages 2–18 years (see Figures 2–5 and 2–7). If circumferential head growth has been steady for the first 2 years, routine measurements may be suspended. However, if a central nervous system problem exists or develops, or if the child has growth deficiency, this measurement continues to be useful. Tracking the growth velocity for each of these parameters allows early recognition of deviations from normal.

Kuczmarski RJ et al: *CDC Growth Charts: United States. Advance Data from Vital and Health Statistics,* No. 314. National Center for Health Statistics, 2000. Available at: http://www.cdc.gov/growthcharts/default.htm.

BLOOD PRESSURE

Blood pressure screening at well-child visits starts at age 3 years. If the child has a renal or cardiovascular abnormality, a blood pressure reading should be obtained at each visit regardless of age. Accurate determination of blood pressure requires proper equipment (stethoscope, manometer and inflation cuff, or an automated system) and a cooperative, seated subject in a quiet room. Although automated blood pressure instruments are widely available and easy to use, blood pressure readings from these devices are typically 5 mm Hg higher for diastolic and 10 mm Hg higher for systolic blood pressure compared with auscultatory techniques. Therefore, the diagnosis of hypertension should not be made on the basis of automated readings alone. Additionally, blood pressure varies somewhat by the height and weight of the individual. Consequently, hypertension is diagnosed as a systolic or diastolic blood pressure greater than the 95th percentile based on the age and height (or weight) percentile of the patient.

The width of the inflatable portion of the cuff should be 40–50% of the circumference of the limb. Obese children need a larger cuff size to avoid a falsely elevated blood pressure reading. Cuffs that are too narrow will overestimate and those that are too wide will underestimate the true blood pressure. Repeated measurements at different visits over time should be tracked using flow charts in an electronic medical record or equivalent in a paper chart. Blood pressure norms are provided in Chapter 19.

Norwood VF: Hypertension. Pediatr Rev 2002;23:197 [PMID: 12042594].

National High Blood Pressure Education Program Working Group in High Blood Pressure in Children and Adolescents: The fourth report on diagnosis, evaluation and treatment of high blood pressure in children and adolescents. Pediatrics 2004;114:555 [PMID: 15286277].

Park MK et al: Comparison of auscultatory and oscillometric blood pressures. Arch Pediatr Adolesc Med 2001;155:50 [PMID: 11177062].

VISION & HEARING SCREENING

Examination of the eyes and an assessment of vision should be performed at every health supervision visit. Parents should be queried about any concerns regarding vision, eye alignment, or any other eye problems. For example, parental observation of photophobia or excessive tearing may be suggestive of glaucoma.

In children from birth to 3 years of age, the eyes and eyelids should be inspected, the movement and alignment of the eyes assessed, and the pupils and red reflexes examined. The red reflex, performed on each pupil individually and then on both eyes simultaneously, is used to detect eye opacities (eg, cataracts or corneal clouding) and retinal abnormalities (eg, retinal detachment or retinoblastoma). In children younger than 3 years of age or in nonverbal children of any age, vision can be assessed by testing a child's ability to fixate on and follow an object.

In children aged 3 years and older, in addition to the eye evaluations, formal testing of visual acuity should be done. This can be performed in the office with a variety of tests, including the tumbling E chart or picture tests such as Allen cards. Each eye is tested separately, with the nontested eye completely covered. Credit is given for any line on which the child gets more than 50% correct. Children 4 years of age and older who are unable to cooperate should be retested, ideally within 1 month, and those who cannot cooperate with repeated attempts should be referred to an ophthalmologist. Because visual acuity improves with age, results of the test are interpreted using the cutoff values in Table 8–2. However, any two-line discrepancy between the two eyes, even within the passing range (eg, 20/20 in one eye, 20/30 in the other in a child aged 6 years or older) should be referred to an ophthalmologist. Throughout childhood and adolescence, clinicians should screen for undetected strabismus (ocular misalignment) and decreased visual acuity. The random dot E test is recommended for detecting strabismus. The corneal light reflex test, the cover test, and visual acuity tests are described further in Chapter 15.

Table 8–2. Age-appropriate visual acuity.[a]

Age (years)	Minimal Acceptable Acuity
3–5	20/40
6 and older	20/30

[a]Refer to an ophthalmologist if minimal acuity is not met at a given age or if there is a difference in scores of two or more lines between the eyes.

Hearing loss, if undetected, can lead to substantial impairments in speech, language, and cognitive development. Because significant bilateral hearing loss is one of the more common major anomalies found at birth, and early detection and intervention of hearing loss leads to better outcomes for children, universal hearing screening of all infants is required in many parts of the United States. Hearing in infants is assessed using either auditory brainstem evoked responses or evoked otoacoustic emissions. Because universal newborn hearing screening will inevitably be associated with some false-positive test results, confirmatory audiology testing is required for all abnormal tests.

Informal behavioral testing of hearing, such as observing an infant's response to a shaken rattle, may be unreliable. In fact, parental concerns about hearing are of greater predictive value than the results of informal tests, and such concerns should be taken seriously. Pure tone audiometry in the office is feasible beginning at age 3 years. Any evidence of hearing loss should be substantiated by repeated testing, and if still abnormal, a referral for a formal hearing evaluation should be made. A number of inherited or acquired conditions increase the risk of hearing loss. Children with any risk factors for hearing loss should be closely followed and periodically screened. Additional details regarding hearing assessment are provided in Chapter 17.

American Academy of Pediatrics et al: Eye examination in infants, children, and young adults by pediatricians. Pediatrics 2003; 111:902 [PMID: 12671132].

Cunningham M et al: Hearing assessment in infants and children: Recommendations beyond neonatal screening. Pediatrics 2003; 111:436 [PMID: 12563074].

Elden LM et al: Screening and prevention of hearing loss in children. Curr Opin Pediatr 2002;14:723 [PMID: 12436045].

LABORATORY SCREENING

Newborn Screening

Newborn screening involves population-wide testing for metabolic and genetic diseases. Blood samples are collected by heelstick from newborns before hospital discharge, and results are usually available within 1 week. Some states routinely repeat blood testing between 7 and 14 days of life, while others recommend it if the child is discharged in less than 24 hours. Repeat testing may be necessary to detect diseases of protein (eg, phenylketonuria [PKU]) or sugar metabolism (eg, galactosemia), which may not be discovered if the first newborn blood screen is performed before the child has had substantial milk intake.

All state newborn screening programs include tests for PKU and congenital hypothyroidism. If undiagnosed, both diseases result in severe mental retardation. Early treatment maintains cognitive function in the normal range. All states also test for classical galactosemia and sickle cell disease. Additional diseases screened for in the majority of states include congenital adrenal hyperplasia, homocystinuria, maple syrup urine disease, and biotinidase deficiency. Tests for tyrosinemia, cystic fibrosis, toxoplasmosis, and HIV are conducted in some states.

Infants with a positive screening result should receive close follow-up, with additional confirmatory studies performed at a center with experience in doing these tests. Screening tests are usually accurate, but the sensitivity and specificity of a particular screening test must be carefully considered. If symptoms of a disease are present despite a negative result on a screening test, the infant should be tested further. Once a diagnosis is confirmed, the infant will need further evaluation and treatment.

Advances in science and technology, such as tandem mass spectroscopy and the Human Genome Project, have created the potential to test for numerous additional inherited diseases. Treatments for these additional diseases vary from highly effective to ineffective. The risks and benefits of early detection of these conditions have been little studied but widely speculated upon. Preliminary results suggest that the early identification of rare metabolic diseases by screening leads to improved child health outcomes and reduced parent stress. The long-term effect of false-positive screens on parents is unknown.

Lead Screening

The developing infant and child are at risk of lead poisoning or toxicity because of their propensity to place objects in the mouth and their efficient absorption of the metal. High blood levels (> 70 mcg/dL) can cause severe health problems such as seizures and coma. Numerous neuropsychological deficits have been associated with increased lead levels. Blood lead levels less than 10 mcg/dL have been correlated with lower intelligence quotients. The primary source of lead exposure in this country remains lead-based paint, even though most of its uses have been banned since 1977. Lead levels have declined nationally from a mean of 16 mcg/dL in 1976 to 2 mcg/dL in 2001. However, considerable variation in lead levels exists in different regions of the United States, and a majority of children at risk of lead toxicity are not currently screened. To eliminate childhood lead poisoning by 2010 (one of the Healthy People 2010 national health objectives), health care providers need to be vigilant about this environmental health threat.

Despite the wide variation in the prevalence of lead toxicity, the CDC recommends universal lead screening for children at ages 1 and 2 and targeted screening for older children living in communities with a high percentage of old housing (> 27% of houses built before 1950) or a high percentage of children with elevated blood lead levels (> 12% of children with levels above 10 mcg/dL).

Communities with inadequate data regarding local blood lead levels should also undergo universal screening. Medicaid requires that all children aged 1–5 years be screened twice. Caregivers of children between 6 months and 6 years of age may be interviewed by questionnaire about environmental risk factors for lead exposure (Table 8–3), although the data to support the use of this screening are inconclusive. If risk factors are present, a blood lead level should be obtained.

A venous blood sample is preferred over a capillary specimen. An elevated capillary (fingerstick) blood sample should always be confirmed by a venous sample. No action is required for blood lead levels less than 10 mcg/dL. The cognitive development of children with confirmed blood levels higher than 14 mcg/dL should be evaluated and attempts made to identify the environmental source. Iron deficiency should be treated if present. Chelation of lead is indicated for levels of 45 mcg/dL and higher and is urgently required for levels above 70 mcg/dL. All families should receive education to decrease the risk of lead exposure. With any elevated lead level (> 10 mcg/dL) rescreening should be performed at recommended intervals.

Iron Deficiency

Iron deficiency is the most common nutritional deficiency in the United States. Severe iron deficiency causes anemia,

Table 8–3. Elements of a lead risk questionnaire.

Recommended questions
1. Does your child live in or regularly visit a house built before 1950? This could include a day care center, preschool, the home of a baby-sitter or relative, and so on.
2. Does your child live in or regularly visit a house built before 1978 with recent, ongoing, or planned renovation or remodeling?
3. Does your child have a sister or brother, housemate, or playmate being followed for lead poisoning?
Questions that may be considered by region or locality
1. Does your child live with an adult whose job (eg, at a brass/copper foundry, firing range, automotive or boat repair shop, or furniture refinishing shop) or hobby (eg, electronics, fishing, stained-glass-making, pottery-making) involves exposure to lead?
2. Does your child live near a work or industrial site (eg, smelter, battery recycling plant) that involves the use of lead?
3. Does your child use pottery or ingest medications that are suspected of having a high lead content?
4. Does your child have exposure to burning lead-painted wood?

behavioral problems, and cognitive effects, but recent evidence suggests that even iron deficiency without anemia may cause behavioral and cognitive difficulties. Furthermore, the developmental effects of iron deficiency may persist for 10 years, even if iron deficiency is corrected in infancy. Risk factors for iron deficiency include preterm or low birth weight births, multiple pregnancy, iron deficiency in the mother, use of nonfortified formula or cow's milk before age 12 months, and an infant diet that is low in iron-containing foods. Infants and toddlers consuming more than 24 oz/d of cow's milk are at risk, as are children with chronic illness, restricted diet, or extensive blood loss.

Primary prevention of iron deficiency should be achieved through dietary means, including feeding infants iron-containing cereals by age 6 months, avoiding low-iron formula during infancy, and limiting cow's milk to 24 oz/d in children aged 1–5 years. Selective early screening for iron deficiency should be considered with the presence of any of the preceding risk factors. A screening hemoglobin or hematocrit should be obtained for high-risk children between ages 9 and 12 months and again at 15–18 months, and it should be considered annually through age 5 years. Premature and low birth weight infants may need testing before 6 months of age. Universal anemia screening at 9 and 15 months of age is appropriate for children in communities or patient populations in which anemia is found in 5% or more of those tested. Biochemical tests of iron deficiency, including ferritin (low in the absence of inflammation), transferrin saturation (low), and erythrocyte protoporphyrin (elevated), are sensitive measures. Lead poisoning can cause iron-deficiency anemia and should be explored as a cause for at-risk infants and children. A screening hematocrit is recommended for pregnant teenagers.

Hypercholesterolemia & Hyperlipidemia

The benefits of screening and treatment for hypercholesterolemia and hyperlipidemia in children are not fully known. However, the AAP and the American Heart Association recommend obtaining a total cholesterol measurement in children older than 2 years who have a parent with elevated cholesterol (> 240 mg/dL). If there is a family history of cardiovascular disease before age 55 years, a complete lipoprotein analysis (fasting cholesterol, high-density lipoproteins, low-density lipoproteins, triglycerides) is recommended. For all children, a prudent diet is advised (see section on Nutrition Counseling, later).

Tuberculosis

According to the CDC, 13,779 cases of tuberculosis were reported in the United States in 2006. Risk of tuberculosis should be assessed at well-child visits, and screening should be based on high-risk status. High risk is defined as contact with a person with known or suspected tuberculosis; having symptoms or radiographic findings suggesting tuberculosis; birth, residence, or travel to a region with high tuberculosis prevalence (Asia, Middle East, Africa, Latin America); contact with a person with AIDS or HIV; or contact with a prisoner, migrant farm worker, illicit drug user, or a person who is or has been recently homeless. The Mantoux test (5 tuberculin units of purified protein derivative) is the only recommended screening test. It can be done as early as 3 months of age and should be repeated annually if the risk persists. The tine test should not be used. Previous vaccination with bacille Calmette-Guérin (BCG) is not a contraindication to tuberculosis skin testing.

Screening of Adolescent Patients

Screening adolescents for blood cholesterol, tuberculosis, and HIV should be offered based on high-risk criteria outlined in this chapter and in Chapter 39. Females with heavy menses, weight loss, poor nutrition, or athletic activity should have a screening hematocrit. During routine visits, adolescents should be questioned sensitively about risk factors (eg, multiple partners; early onset of sexual activity, including child sexual abuse) and symptoms (eg, genital discharge, infectious lesions, pelvic pain) of sexually transmitted diseases (STDs). A dipstick urinalysis for leukocytes is generally recommended for sexually active adolescents. Teenage girls who are sexually active and all girls aged 18 years and older, regardless of sexual experience, should have a pelvic examination with Papanicolaou (Pap) smear. A Pap smear should be performed at least every 3 years thereafter and more frequently in patients with STD risk factors. Because females with STDs are often not symptomatic, gonococcal and chlamydial cultures and screening tests for syphilis and trichomoniasis are appropriate at the time of each pelvic examination.

American Academy of Pediatrics: Tuberculosis. In Pickering LK (editor): *2006 Red Book: Report of the Committee on Infectious Diseases,* 27th ed. American Academy of Pediatrics 2006:678.

American Academy of Pediatrics, Committee on Environmental Health: Lead exposure in children: Prevention, detection, and management. Pediatrics 2005;116:1036 [PMID: 16199720].

Brotanek J et al: Iron deficiency in early childhood in the United States: Risk factors and racial/ethnic disparities. Pediatrics 2007;120:568 [PMID: 17766530].

Haney EM et al: Screening and treatment for lipid disorders in children and adolescents: Systematic evidence for the US Preventive Services Task Force. Pediatrics 2007;120:e189 [PMID: 17606543].

Centers for Disease Control and Prevention lead fact sheet. Available at: http://www.cdc.gov/lead/factsheets.htm.

Centers for Disease Control and Prevention, National Center for HIV, STD and TB Prevention: Tuberculosis Surveillance Reports. Available at: http://www.cdc.gov/tb/surv/surv2006/default.htm.

National Newborn Screening Status Report, updated September 2005. Available at: http://genes-r-us.uthscsa.edu.

ANTICIPATORY GUIDANCE

An essential part of the health supervision visit is anticipatory guidance. During this counseling, the clinician directs the parent's or the older child's attention to issues that may arise in the future. Guidance must be appropriate to age, focus on concerns expressed by the parent and patient, and address issues in depth rather than run through a number of issues superficially. Both oral and printed materials are used. Handouts can be an important supplement to anticipatory guidance. When selecting written materials, providers should be sensitive to issues of literacy and primary language spoken by the family members. A routine schedule for preventive handouts is shown in Table 8–4. Areas of concern include diet, injury prevention, developmental and behavioral issues, and health promotion. Injury prevention is discussed in the next section; other topics are found in other chapters of this book.

Injury Prevention

Injuries are the leading cause of death in children and adolescents after the first year of life (Figure 8–3). For young people aged 15–19 years, injuries are responsible for more than half of all deaths. Each year, 16 million visits to emergency departments are occasioned by injuries to children and adolescents, and more than 500,000 of these patients are hospitalized. In the case of physical injury to a young child, the physician must recognize that some injuries may be intentional or the result of parental neglect (see Chapter 7).

Injury prevention counseling is an important component of each health supervision visit and can be reinforced during all visits. Counseling should focus on problems that are frequent and age appropriate. Passive strategies of prevention should be emphasized, because these are more effective than active strategies; for example, placing chemicals out of reach in high, locked cupboards to prevent poisoning will be more effective than instructing parents to watch their children closely.

Informational handouts about home safety, such as The Injury Prevention Program (TIPP; available from the AAP), can be provided in the waiting room. Advice can then be tailored to the specific needs of each family, with reinforcement from age-specific TIPP handouts.

The pediatrician's influence can extend beyond the office to advocate for safer communities. For example, a community program in Seattle, Washington, to promote the use of bicycle helmets has increased helmet use from 2% to more than 60% through a combination of office education, low-cost helmets, and legislative advocacy. The primary care provider is in an ideal position to identify high-risk situations and intervene before injury occurs. For example, if a teenager has emotional problems (eg, depression) and a history of driving violations, the clinician should recommend a mental health referral; this, in turn, could prevent a motor vehicle accident.

A. Motor Vehicle Injuries

The primary cause of death of children in the United States is motor vehicle injuries. In 1998, about 57% of children aged 15 years or younger who were killed in motor vehicle accidents were unrestrained. Car safety seats for children are

Table 8–4. Preventive handouts for health supervision visits.

Age	Suggested Topics
2 wk	Breast feeding
2 mo	Attachment
4 mo	Language and motor development
6 mo	Nutrition
12 mo	Safe and constructive family relationships
18 mo	Toilet training basics
2 y	Time-out technique
3 y	Chores and social competence
4 y	Sexuality education across the ages
5 y	Media and child health
6 y	School work: Encouraging success
8 y	Sibling rivalry
10 y	Social competence
12 y	Adolescents: Promoting responsibility

required in all U.S. states, and their proper use could reduce vehicle-associated fatalities and hospitalizations by at least 50%. The type of safety seat to be used depends on the child's weight and age: rear-facing infant seat for a child under 20 lb and 1 year of age; forward-facing car seat for a child 20–40 lb and older than 1 year; and belt-positioning booster seat for a child who has outgrown the safety seat but is under 60 lb. When children have grown enough to properly fit the vehicle seat belts (usually when 4 feet tall), they should use a combination lap and shoulder belt. A rear-facing car seat should never be used in a seat with a passenger air bag. A car seat should never be used if the child has outgrown the seat—for example, ears above the back of the seat or shoulders above the seat strap slots.

Up-to-date information on car seats is available through the AAP (at http://www.aap.org/family/carseatguide.htm).

When a child is a passenger in a car crash, the case fatality rate is 1%; for children hit by cars, the risk of fatality increases threefold. Pedestrian safety skills should be taught to children early in childhood; however, parental supervision of children near roadways continues to be required for many years. A final motor vehicle risk for health involves the use of portable electronic devices. Using a cellular telephone while driving is associated with a fourfold increase in motor vehicle accidents. Parents and teenage drivers should avoid this risk.

B. Bicycle Injuries

In 2001, over 400,000 Americans sustained a bicycle-related injury, and two thirds of these injuries involved children or adolescents. Head trauma accounts for three fourths of all

Children 1 – 4 years

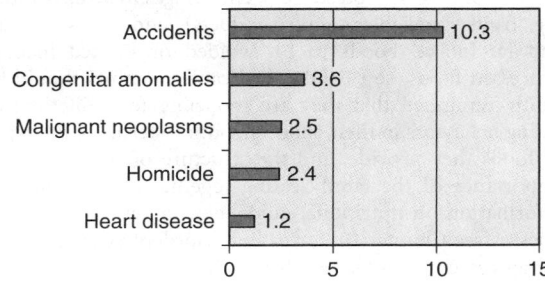

Children 5 – 9 years

Older children 10 – 14 years

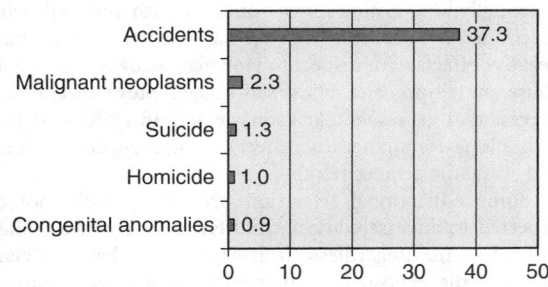

Young adults 15 – 19 years

▲ **Figure 8–3.** Leading causes of death in children at 1–4 years, 5–9 years, 10–14 years, and 15–19 years (the 2004 rate per 100,000 population). (National Center for Health Statistics, 2007.)

bicycle-related fatalities. More than 85% of brain injuries can be prevented through the use of bicycle helmets, and due to a recent increase in use of helmets, the rate of fatality to bicyclists is dropping. Bike riders—parents and children alike—should wear a helmet every time they ride. Unfortunately, low bicycle helmet use rates are still common in some communities.

C. Injuries and Violence Prevention

The United States has a higher rate of firearm-related death than any other industrialized country. Injuries from firearms are more frequent among young people aged 15–24 years than among any other age group, and black males are especially vulnerable. Some gun deaths may be accidental, but most are the result of homicide or suicide. A gun in the home doubles the likelihood of a lethal suicide attempt. Although handguns are often kept in homes for protection, a gun is more likely to kill a family member or a friend than an intruder. The most effective way to prevent firearm injuries is to remove guns from the home and community. Families who keep firearms at home should lock them in a cabinet or drawer and store ammunition in a separate locked location.

A nonviolent environment should be provided to all children. Secure parent–infant attachments, social and conflict-resolution skills, and the avoidance of violence (on television or actual) all have a role in promoting nonviolence.

D. Drowning and Near Drowning

Drowning is the second leading cause of injury-related death in children, and those aged 1–3 years have the highest rate of drowning. For every death by drowning, six children are hospitalized for near drowning, and up to 10% of survivors experience severe brain damage. Children younger than 1 year of age are most likely to drown in the bathtub. Buckets filled with water also present a risk of drowning to the older infant or toddler. For children aged 1–4 years, drowning or near drowning occurs most often in home swimming pools; and for school-aged children and teens, drowning occurs most often in large bodies of water (eg, swimming pools or open water). After the age of 5 years, the risk of drowning in a swimming pool is much greater for black males than white males. School-aged children should be taught to swim, and recreational swimming should always be supervised. Home pools must be fenced securely, and parents should know how to perform cardiopulmonary resuscitation.

E. Fire and Burn Injuries

Fires and burns are the leading cause of injury-related deaths in the home. Categories of burn injury include smoke inhalation; flame contact; scalding; and electrical, chemical, and ultraviolet burns. Scalding is the most common type of burn in children. Most scalds involve foods and beverages, but nearly one fourth of scalds are with tap water, and for that reason it is recommended that hot water heaters be set to less than 54°C (130°F). Most fire-related deaths result from smoke inhalation. Smoke detectors can prevent 85% of the injuries and deaths caused by fires in the home. Families should discuss a fire plan with children and practice emergency evacuation from the home.

Sunburn is a common thermal injury, perhaps because symptoms of excessive sun exposure do not begin until after the skin has been damaged. Sunburn and excessive sun exposure are associated with skin cancers. Prevention of sunburn is best achieved by sun avoidance, particularly during the midday hours of 10 AM to 3 PM. Sunscreen using a sun protection factor (SPF) of 15–30 extends the duration of time that a child can spend in the sun without sunburn. It should be applied liberally (15 mL for a 7-year-old) and reapplied every 2 hours even if designated as waterproof. Hats, sunglasses, and special precautions for fair-skinned individuals and infants are also important aspects of safe sun exposure. The safety of sunscreen is not established for infants younger than 6 months; thus sun avoidance, appropriate clothing, and hats are recommended for this age group. Lightweight fabric wetsuits with long sleeves are now made for children and offer more protection from the sun than a traditional swimsuit.

American Academy of Pediatrics, Committee on Injury and Poison Prevention: Bicycle helmets. Pediatrics 2001;108:1030 [PMID: 11581464].

American Academy of Pediatrics, Committee on Injury and Poison Prevention: Firearm-related injuries affecting the pediatric population. Pediatrics 2000;105:888 [PMID: 10742344].

American Academy of Pediatrics, Committee on Injury and Poison Prevention: Reducing the number of deaths and injuries from residential fires. Pediatrics 2000;105:1355 [PMID: 10835082].

Brenner RA et al: Where children drown, United States, 1995. Pediatrics 2001;108:85 [PMID: 11433058].

NUTRITION COUNSELING

Screening for nutritional problems and guidance for age-appropriate dietary choices should be part of every health supervision visit. Overnutrition, undernutrition, and eating disorders can be detected by a careful analysis of dietary and activity patterns interpreted in the context of a child's growth pattern. When obtaining a dietary history, it is helpful to assess the following: who purchases and prepares food; who feeds the child; whether meals and snacks occur at consistent times and in a consistent setting; whether children are allowed to snack or "graze" between meals; the types and portion sizes of food and drinks provided; the frequency of eating meals in restaurants or eating take-out food; and whether the child eats while watching television.

Iron-fortified formula or breast milk should be used for the first year of life, after which whole cow's milk can be given. Because of continued rapid growth and high energy needs, children should continue to drink whole milk until age 2 years. Baby foods are generally introduced at about 4–6 months of age.

For children 2 years of age and older, a prudent diet consists of diverse food sources, encourages high-fiber foods (eg, fruits, vegetables, grain products), and limits sodium and fat intake. Foods to be avoided or limited include processed foods, soft drinks, and candy. Parents should be gently reminded that they are modeling for a lifetime of eating behaviors in their children, both in terms of the types of foods they provide, and the structure of meals (eg, the importance of the family eating together). For additional information on nutritional guidelines, undernutrition, and obesity, see Chapter 10; for eating disorders, see Chapter 5; for adolescent obesity, see Chapter 3.

American Academy of Pediatrics, Committee on Nutrition: Prevention of pediatric overweight and obesity. Pediatrics 2003;112:424 [PMID: 12897303].

COUNSELING ABOUT TELEVISION & OTHER MEDIA

The average child in the United States watches approximately 3 hours of television per day, and this does not include time spent watching videotapes or DVDs, playing video games, or playing on computers. Having a television set in the bedroom is associated with watching more television, and 32% of 2- to 7-year-olds and 65% of 8- to 18-year-olds have a bedroom television set.

The excessive watching of television has a negative and potentially long-lasting impact on the health and well-being of children. Television viewing has been shown to have negative effects with respect to violence, sexuality, substance abuse, nutrition, and body self-image. More recent data suggest that excessive television viewing in childhood may have a long-lasting negative effect on cognitive development and academic achievement.

Some educational television programs would not be expected to adversely affect children and may in fact have some benefit. Regardless, it is important that clinicians assess media exposure in their patients, and offer parents concrete advice. The AAP recommends that children younger than 2 years of age should not watch any television, and that children 2 years and older be limited to 2 hours total time each day for all media. Additionally, parents should monitor what their children watch, remove television sets from their children's bedrooms, and encourage alternative activities.

Borzekowski DLG, Robinson TN: The remote, the mouse, and the No. 2 pencil—the household media environment and academic achievement among third grade students. Arch Pediatr Adolesc Med 2005;159:607 [PMID: 15996991].

Hancox RJ et al: Association of television viewing during childhood with poor educational achievement. Arch Pediatr Adolesc Med 2005;159:614 [PMID: 15996992].

Jordan A: The role of media in children's development: an ecological perspective. J Dev Behav Pediatr 2004;25:196 [PMID: 15194905].

IMMUNIZATIONS

A child's immunization status should be assessed at every clinic visit and every opportunity should be taken to vaccinate. Even though parents may keep an immunization record, it is critical that providers also keep an accurate record of a child's immunizations. This information should be written in a prominent location in the paper or electronic chart or kept in an immunization registry.

Despite high overall national immunization coverage levels, areas of underimmunization continue to exist in the United States. An understanding of true contraindications (versus "false contraindications") and a "no missed opportunities" approach to immunization delivery has been shown to successfully increase immunization levels. Therefore, it is important that clinicians screen records and administer required immunizations at all types of visits, and administer all needed vaccinations simultaneously. Additionally, clinicians should operate reminder/recall systems, in which parents of underimmunized children are prompted by mail or telephone to visit the clinic for immunization. The assessment of clinic-wide immunization levels and feedback of these data to providers have also been shown to increase immunization rates.

Immunization schedules and other details of specific vaccines are presented in Chapter 9. A wealth of information for parents and providers about immunizations is also available at the National Immunization Program's web site (http://www.cdc.gov/vaccines).

Santoli JM et al: Immunization pockets of need: Science and practice. Am J Prev Med 2000;19(1S):89 [PMID: 11024333].

Task Force on Community Preventive Services: Recommendations regarding interventions to improve vaccination coverage in children, adolescents, and adults. Am J Prev Med 2000;18 (1S):92 [PMID: 10806981].

OTHER TYPES OF GENERAL PEDIATRIC SERVICES

ACUTE-CARE VISITS

Acute-care visits account for 30% or more of the general pediatrician's office visits. These visits are conducted in an efficient, structured way. Office personnel should determine the reason for the visit and whether it is an emergent situation, obtain a brief synopsis of the child's symptoms, carefully document vital signs, and list known drug allergies. The pediatric clinician should document the events related to the presenting problem and carefully describe them in the medical record. The record should include supporting laboratory data and a diagnosis. Treatments and follow-up instructions must be recorded, including when to return to the office if the problem is not ameliorated. Immunization status should be screened, as previously discussed. Depend-ing on the severity of illness, this may also be an opportunity for age-appropriate health maintenance screenings and anticipatory guidance. This may be particularly true with older school-aged children or adolescents who may be seen more rarely for routine health maintenance visits.

PRENATAL VISITS

Ideally, a couple's first trip to a physician's office should take place before the birth of their baby. A prenatal visit goes a long way toward establishing trust and enables a pediatric provider to learn about a family's expectations, concerns, and fears regarding the anticipated birth. If the infant develops a problem during the newborn period, a provider who has already met the family is in a better position to maintain rapport and communication with the new parents.

In addition to helping establish a relationship between parents and pediatric providers, the prenatal visit can be used to gather information about the parents and the pregnancy, provide information and advice, and identify high-risk situations. A range of information can be provided to parents regarding feeding choices and the benefits of breast feeding; injury prevention, including sleeping position and the appropriate use of car seats; and techniques for managing colic. Potential high-risk situations that may be identified include mental health issues in the parents, a history of domestic violence, or maternal medical problems that may affect the infant.

Serwint JR: The prenatal pediatric visit. Pediatr Rev 2003;24:31 [PMID: 12509543].

SPORTS PHYSICALS

The purpose of the preparticipation health evaluation is to determine whether a child can safely participate in organized sports activity. Attention should be directed toward those parts of the body that are most vulnerable to the stresses of sports. The history and physical examination should focus on the following systems: cardiovascular (stenotic lesions, hypertension, surgery), respiratory (asthma), vision, genitourinary (absence or loss of function of one testicle), gastrointestinal (hepatosplenomegaly, hernia), skin (infection), musculoskeletal (inflammation, dysfunction), and neurologic (concussions, uncontrolled seizures). The sports physical should include counseling about medication usage, protective equipment, proper supervision and instruction, injury management, and the emotional aspects of competition and teamwork. Information about certain sports should be included. For example, protective eyewear, mouth guards, padded goalposts, and efforts to minimize heading the ball should be discussed with a soccer player and his or her parent. The physician should suggest sports that will be compatible with the child's size, strength, endurance, agility, and history of chronic illness. The potential for mild menstrual irregularities should be explained to the adolescent female athlete. The athlete with moderate to severe menstrual irregularities should be referred for endocrinologic evaluation. Anticipatory guidance should address nutritional needs to maintain growth, cessation of activity when pain occurs, and fluid and electrolyte availability to avoid dehydration. (See Chapter 25 for a more detailed discussion of sports medicine.)

Injuries in youth soccer: A subject review. American Academy of Pediatrics. Committee on Sports Medicine and Fitness. Pediatrics 2000;105:659 [PMID: 10699129].

CHRONIC DISEASE MANAGEMENT

Chronic disease in pediatrics is defined as illness that has been present for more than 3 months. Twenty-five percent of children and 35% of adolescents have illnesses that meet the definition of a chronic illness. The most common chronic illnesses in pediatric practice include asthma, otitis media with effusion, skin disorders, attention-deficit/hyperactivity disorder, and allergic diseases.

The goal of chronic disease management is to optimize quality of life while minimizing the side effects of treatment interventions. The child and family's emotional responses to chronic illness should be addressed, and referrals to counselors should be offered if needed. Pediatric subspecialty referrals need to be arranged and monitored and results recorded in the chart in an organized manner. Chronic problems often mean chronic use of medications and the need to monitor their use. Documentation should be made in the medical record whenever a prescription is refilled. A medication summary page in the chart allows easy access to the drug history and is a convenient place to make notes (Figure 8–4).

Nutrition and the management of medical devices (eg catheters, gastrostomy tubes) may need to be addressed.

Ludder-Jackson P, Vessey JA: *Primary Care of the Child with a Chronic Condition*, 3rd ed. Mosby-Year Book, 2000.

COUNSELING

Topics amenable to office counseling include behavioral issues such as negativism and noncompliance, temper tantrums, oppositional behavior, and biting; childhood fears and feeding disorders; school problems; family upheavals such as separation, divorce, or remarriage; attention-deficit/hyperactivity disorder; and deaths of family members or close friends. Forty-five minutes is usually enough time for the therapeutic process to evolve, and this time should be protected from interruption. The young child is usually interviewed with the parent; school-aged children and adolescents benefit from time alone with the physician. After assessing the situation in one or two sessions, the primary care physician must decide whether the child's and family's needs are within his or her area of expertise or whether referral to another professional such as a psychologist or an education specialist would be appropriate. The pediatrician should know the warning signs of childhood depression and bipolar disorder and have a low threshold for referral of these concerns to the appropriate mental health professional.

CONSULTATIONS

Physicians, other professionals, and parents may initiate consultations with a general pediatrician. Parents, subspecialists,

Medication: _____

Date: Visit (V) or Phone Call (PC)	Tablet Size or Liquid Concentration	Sig.	Disp.	Number of Refills	Approved by	Called by	Pharmacy and Phone No.

Notes (eg, levels): _____

▲ **Figure 8–4.** Medication summary sheet.

family physicians, or professionals such as school officials, psychologists, or social workers may all seek medical consultation. Finally, an insurance company representative may want a second opinion before authorizing a set of services.

Consultations usually require one or two 45- to 60-minute appointments. When the patient is referred to a pediatric consultant, the number of visits and the extent of service should be specified. A screening questionnaire, completed in advance by a parent, should delineate the patient's physical, behavioral, and developmental (or school) problems and serve as an initial database.

The types of consultations the general pediatrician may be asked to do include an evaluation only, an evaluation and interpretation, or an evaluation and treatment of an isolated problem. The type of consultation being requested should be clearly determined at the time of referral of the patient. This understanding should be clarified with the patient's insurance company so that appropriate authorization and reimbursement for the visit can occur.

Communication with the Referring Source

Communication is the key to a satisfactory referral process. The pediatric consultant frequently sends the referral source a brief letter acknowledging the referral and requesting additional information. The final consultation report should be sent promptly, with content appropriate for the referring source. School officials will want to know whether the patient is physically healthy or, if not, to receive a summary of their health care responsibilities. A referring physician expects a full report, and a copy is usually sent to the patient's parents. Recommendations should be specific (eg, drugs, dosages, other forms of therapy, duration of therapy, specific laboratory tests). A copy of or reference to a recent review article on the subject will also be appreciated.

A medical evaluation should contain a factual summary of the history, physical examination, and laboratory and radiologic findings. Families are grateful if a copy is sent to them for their information and records. At the end of the consultation, the parents should be told when the patient should see the primary physician—usually in 1–2 weeks. Positive comments about the referring physician's competence and judgment serve to support the primary physician–patient relationship. The parents must feel confident that the primary physician can provide the necessary follow-up care. If the referring physician had tentatively made the correct diagnosis prior to referral, the consultant's corroboration should be made clear to the parents and included in the consultation report.

TELEPHONE MANAGEMENT & WEB-BASED INFORMATION

Providing appropriate, efficient, and timely clinical advice over the telephone is a critical element of pediatric primary care in the office setting. An estimated 20–30% of all clinical care delivered by general pediatric offices is provided by telephone. Telephone calls to and from patients occur both during regular office hours and after the office has closed (termed after-hours), and the personnel and systems in place to handle office-hours versus before- and after-hours calls may differ. In either circumstance, several principles are important: (1) advice is given only by clinicians or other staff with formal medical education (eg, nurse, medical assistant), (2) staff is given additional training in providing telephone care, (3) documentation is made of all pertinent information from calls, (4) standardized protocols covering the most common pediatric symptoms are used, and (5) a physician is always available to handle urgent or difficult calls.

During routine office hours, approximately 20–25% of all telephone calls to pediatric offices involve clinical matters. Many of these calls, however, are routine in nature, and an experienced nurse within the office can screen calls and provide appropriate advice by telephone. Calls from inexperienced or anxious parents about simple concerns should be answered with understanding and respect. Certain types of calls received during office hours should be promptly transferred to a physician: (1) true emergencies, (2) calls regarding hospitalized patients, (3) calls from other medical professionals, and (4) calls from parents who demand to speak with a physician. Nurses should also seek help from a clinician whenever they are uncertain about how to handle a particular call. When in doubt about the diagnosis or necessary treatment, nurses giving telephone advice should err on the side of having the patient seen in the office.

Several different options are available for handling after-hours pediatric telephone care. Clinicians may choose to take all calls from their patients, may rely on "advice" nurses without specific pediatric protocols or training, or may use a system specifically designed for pediatric telephone care, called a pediatric after-hours call center. Pediatric call centers, although not available in all communities, have certain benefits. Calls are managed using standardized protocols, the call centers are typically staffed by nurses with abundant pediatric experience, the calls are well-documented, and call centers often perform ongoing quality assurance. Extensive research on pediatric call centers has revealed a high degree of appropriate referrals to emergency departments, safety in terms of outcomes, parent satisfaction with the process, and savings to the health care system.

In general, after-hours pediatric telephone calls tend to be more serious than calls made during regular office hours. Deciding which patients need to be seen, and how urgently, are the most important aspects of these after-hours telephone "encounters." Several factors influence this final patient disposition: (1) the age of the patient, (2) the duration and type of symptom, (3) the presence of any underlying chronic condition, (4) whether the child appears "very sick" to the caller, and (5) the anxiety level of the caller. Once all the pertinent medical information is gathered, a decision is made about whether the child should be seen immediately (by ambulance versus car), seen in the office later (today versus tomorrow), or whether the illness can be safely cared for at home. At the end of the call, it should be confirmed that parents understand and feel comfortable with the plan for their child.

The use of the World Wide Web (Internet) has become common in the pediatric office setting. Many practices routinely use the Internet to give information about the practice, the care of common minor problems, scheduling of appointments, insurance issues, and so on. With time, the Internet is sure to become a larger part of the ambulatory pediatric practice.

Bunik M et al: Pediatric telephone call centers—how do they affect health care utilization and costs? Pediatrics 2007;119:e1 [PMID: 17272593].

Kempe A et al: Delivery of pediatric after-hours care by call centers: A multicenter study of parental perceptions and compliance. Pediatrics 2001;108:e111 [PMID: 11731638].

Kempe A et al: How safe is triage by an after-hours telephone call center? Pediatrics 2006;118:457 [PMID: 16882795].

Liederman EM, Morefield CS: Web messaging: A new tool for patient-physician communication. J Am Med Inform Assoc 2003;10:260 [PMID: 12626378].

Luberti AA: After-hours telephone care: Options for the pediatrician. Pediatr Ann 2001;30:249 [PMID: 11383464].

Poole SR: Creating an after-hours telephone triage system for office practice. Pediatr Ann 2001;30:268 [PMID: 11383466].

COMMUNITY PEDIATRICS

According to the AAP, community pediatrics is "a perspective that enlarges the pediatrician's focus from one child to all children in the community." Pediatricians have historically been very involved in supporting and developing services for vulnerable children in their communities. As a group, pediatricians recognize that communities are integral determinants of a child's health and that the synthesis of public health and personal health principles and practices is important in the practice of community pediatrics. As well, pediatricians have long been committed to working with other professionals in the community and advocating for the needs of all children. For example, pediatricians have been instrumental in the passage of laws requiring protective fencing around swimming pools.

Pediatricians in practice are frequently instrumental in referring children and families to valuable services and resources. For example, uninsured children can be enrolled in either their state Medicaid program or State Children's Health Insurance Program (SCHIP). Children with special health care needs may be eligible for services typically funded through state health departments and through programs such as those provided based on the Individuals with Disabilities Education Act (IDEA). A variety of community-based immunization programs can provide access to needed immunizations for eligible children. Food and nutrition programs such as the federally funded Women, Infants, and Children (WIC) program provide sources of food at no cost to eligible fami-

lies. Finally, subsidized preschool and child care services such as the federally funded Head Start program provide needed preschool programs. Pediatricians are in a unique position to make referrals to these important services.

American Academy of Pediatrics: The pediatrician's role in community pediatrics. Pediatrics 2005;115:1092 [PMID: 15805396].

Duggan A et al: The essential role of research in community pediatrics. Pediatrics 2005;115(Suppl):1195 [PMID: 15821310].

Satcher D et al: The expanding role of the pediatrician in improving child health in the 21st century. Pediatrics 2005;115(Suppl):1124 [PMID: 15821293].

▼ COMMON GENERAL PEDIATRIC ISSUES

FEVER

▶ General Considerations

Fever is one of the most common reasons for pediatric office visits, emergency department encounters, and after-hours telephone calls. Several different definitions of fever exist, but most experts define fever as a rectal temperature of 38°C or above. Temperature in pediatric patients can be measured in a variety of manners: rectal (using a mercury or digital thermometer), oral (mercury or digital), axillary (mercury, digital, or liquid crystal strip), forehead (liquid crystal strip), or tympanic (using a device that measures thermal infrared energy from the tympanic membrane). Tympanic measurement of temperature is quick and requires little patient cooperation. Several cautions apply to the use of this technique: tympanic temperatures have been shown to be less accurate in infants younger than 3 months of age and are subject to false readings if the instrument is not positioned properly or the external ear canal is occluded by wax.

▶ Causes

Fever occurs when there is a rise in the hypothalamic set-point in response to endogenously produced pyrogens. Among the broad range of conditions that cause fever are infections, malignancies, autoimmune diseases, metabolic diseases, chronic inflammatory conditions, medications (including immunizations), central nervous system abnormalities, and exposure to excessive environmental heat. In most settings, the majority of fevers in pediatric patients are caused by self-limiting viral infections. Teething does not cause fever over 38.4°C.

▶ Clinical Findings

A. Initial Evaluation

When evaluating a child with fever, one should elicit from the parents information about the duration of fever, how the temperature was taken, the maximum height of fever documented at home, all associated symptoms, any chronic medical conditions, any medications taken, medication allergies, fluid intake, urine output, exposures and travel, and any additional features of the illness that concern the parents (Table 8–5). In the office, temperature, heart rate, respiratory rate, and blood pressure should be documented, as well as an oxygen saturation if the child has any increased work of breathing. A complete physical examination, including a neurologic examination, should then be performed, with particular attention paid to the child's degree of toxicity and hydration status. A well-appearing, well-hydrated child with evidence of a routine viral infection can be safely sent home with symptomatic treatment and careful return precautions.

Depending on patient age, presence of underlying conditions, type of infection, and the provider's assessment of toxicity and hydration, many children with focal bacterial infections can also be treated as outpatients, with appropriate oral antibiotics as discussed in Chapter 40.

B. Fever without a Focus of Infection

Children who present with fever but without any symptoms or signs of a focal infection are often a diagnostic and management challenge. When assessing a child with fever but no apparent source of infection on examination, the provider needs to carefully consider the likelihood of a serious but "hidden" or occult bacterial infection. With the widespread use of effective vaccines against *Haemophilus influenzae* type b and *Streptococcus pneumoniae*, two of the most common causes of invasive bacterial infections in unimmunized children, the incidence of occult bacterial infections has declined. However, vaccines are not 100% effective, and other organisms cause serious occult infections in children; therefore, febrile children will always demand careful evaluation and observation. Appropriate choices for empiric antibiotic therapy of children with fever without focus are discussed in Chapter 37.

Febrile infants 28 days old or younger, because of their likelihood of serious disease including sepsis, should always be treated conservatively. Hospitalization and parenteral antibiotics should be strongly considered in all circumstances. An initial diagnostic evaluation should include complete blood count; blood culture; urinalysis; urine culture; and Gram stain, protein and glucose tests, and culture of cerebrospinal fluid. Consideration should also be given to the possibility of a perinatal herpes simplex virus infection (neonatal herpes is described in more detail in Chapter 38). A chest radiograph should be obtained for any infant with increased work of breathing.

Infants aged 29–90 days are at risk of developing a variety of invasive bacterial infections, including perinatally acquired organisms (eg, group B streptococci) or infections acquired in the household (eg, pneumococci or meningococci). Febrile infants without a focus of infection can be divided into those who appear toxic versus nontoxic, and those at low risk versus higher risk of invasive bacterial disease. As with febrile

Table 8–5. Guidelines for evaluating children with fever.

A. See immediately if:
1. Child is younger than age 3 months.
2. Fever is >40.6°C.
3. Child is crying inconsolably or whimpering.
4. Child is crying when moved or even touched.
5. Child is difficult to awaken.
6. Child's neck is stiff.
7. Purple spots or dots are present on the skin.
8. Child's breathing is difficult, and not better after nasal passages are cleared.
9. Child is drooling saliva and is unable to swallow anything.
10. A convulsion has occurred.
11. Child acts or looks "very sick."

B. See within 24 hours if:
1. Child is 3–6 months old (unless fever occurs within 48 h after a diphtheria-tetanus-pertussis vaccination and infant has no other serious symptoms).
2. Fever exceeds 40°C (especially if child is younger than age 3 years).
3. Burning or pain occurs with urination.
4. Fever has been present for more than 24 h without an obvious cause or identified site of infection.
5. Fever has subsided for more than 24 h and then returned.
6. Fever has been present > 72 h.

neonates, toxic children in this age group should be admitted to the hospital for parenteral antibiotics and close observation. In nontoxic infants, low risk has been defined as previously healthy; no focal infection on examination; white blood cell (WBC) count between 5000 and 15,000/mm^3; band cells less than 1500/mm^3; normal urinalysis; and, when diarrhea is present, less than 5 WBCs per high-power field. Nontoxic low-risk infants in this age group are typically treated as outpatients with close follow-up. Clinicians should be confident that lumbar puncture is unnecessary if they decide not to perform this procedure.

In an era of increasing immunization coverage against the most commonly invasive pneumococcal serotypes, it is difficult to estimate the risk of occult bacteremia in febrile 3–36-month-olds with no focus of infection. Nevertheless, when assessing children aged 3–36 months with temperatures of 39°C or higher, urine cultures should be considered in all male children younger than 6 months of age and in all females younger than 2 years of age. Chest radiographs should be performed in any child with increased work of breathing and should also be considered in children with high (20,000/mm^3) WBC counts but no respiratory symptoms. Depending on the child's appearance, underlying medical condition, and height of fever, blood cultures should also be obtained. Empiric antibiotic therapy may be considered, particularly for children with temperature of 39°C and WBC count of 15,000/mm^3. However, in previously healthy, well-appearing, fully immunized children with reassuring laboratory studies, observation without antibiotics is appropriate.

▶ Treatment

Fever phobia is a term that describes parents' anxious response to the fevers that all children experience. In a recent study, 91% of caregivers thought that a fever could cause harmful effects. Seven percent of parents thought that if they did not treat the fever, it would keep going higher. Parents need to be reassured that fevers lower than 41.7°C do not cause brain damage. They should be counseled that, although fevers can occasionally cause seizures—in which case their child needs to be seen—febrile seizures are generally harmless and likewise do not cause brain damage.

Several safe and effective medications are available for the treatment of fever. Acetaminophen is indicated in children older than 2 months of age who have fever of 39°C or are uncomfortable. Acetaminophen is given in a dosage of 15 mg/kg of body weight per dose and can be given every 4–6 hours. The other widely used antipyretic is ibuprofen. Ibuprofen is given in a dosage of 10 mg/kg of body weight per dose and can be given every 6–8 hours. Ibuprofen and acetaminophen are similar in safety and their ability to reduce fever; however, ibuprofen is longer lasting. Aspirin should not be used for treating fever in any child or adolescent, because of its association with the development of Reye syndrome (particularly during infections with varicella and influenza). With all antipyretics, parents should be counseled to be very careful with dosing and frequency of administration as poisoning can be dangerous.

Crocetti M et al: Fever phobia revisited: Have parental misconceptions about fever changed in 20 years? Pediatrics 2001;107:1241 [PMID: 11389237].

Klein JO: Management of the febrile child without a focus of infection in the era of universal pneumococcal immunization. Pediatr Infect Dis J 2002;21:584 [PMID: 12182394].

McCarthy PL: Fever without apparent source on clinical examination. Curr Opin Pediatr 2002;14:103 [PMID: 11880744].

Rehm KP: Fever in infants and children. Curr Opin Pediatr 2001;13:83 [PMID: 11216593].

GROWTH DEFICIENCY

Growth deficiency—formerly termed failure to thrive—is deceleration of growth velocity resulting in crossing two major percentile lines on the growth chart. The diagnosis also is warranted if a child younger than age 6 months has not grown for 2 consecutive months or if a child older than age 6 months has not grown for 3 consecutive months. Growth deficiency occurs in about 8% of children.

Patterns of growth deficiency suggest, but are not specific for, different causes. In type I growth deficiency, the head circumference is preserved and the weight is depressed more than the height. This most common type results from inadequate caloric intake, excessive loss of calories, excessive intake of calories, or inability to use calories peripherally. Most such cases result from inadequate delivery of calories. This may be the result of poverty, lack of caregiver under-standing, poor caregiver-child interaction, abnormal feeding patterns, or a combination of factors. Type II growth deficiency, which is associated with genetically determined short stature, endocrinopathies, constitutional growth delay, heart or renal disease, or various forms of skeletal dysplasias, is characterized by normal head circumference and proportionate diminution of height and weight. In type III growth deficiency, all three parameters of growth—head circumference, weight, and height—are lower than normal. This pattern is associated with central nervous system abnormalities, chromosomal defects, and in utero or perinatal insults.

▶ Clinical Findings

A. Initial Evaluation

The history and physical examination will identify the cause of growth reduction in the vast majority of cases (Table 8–6). The physical examination should focus on signs of organic disease or evidence of abuse or neglect: dysmorphic features, skin lesions, neck masses, adventitial breath sounds, heart murmurs, abdominal masses, and neuromuscular tone and strength. Throughout the evaluation, the physician should observe the caregiver-child interaction and the level of family functioning. Developmental screening and laboratory screening tests (complete blood count, blood urea nitrogen, creatinine, electrolytes, urinalysis, and urine culture) complete the initial office evaluation.

B. Further Evaluation

A prospective 3-day diet record should be a standard part of the evaluation. Occasionally an infant or child may need to be hospitalized to obtain an accurate assessment of intake. This is useful in assessing undernutrition even when organic disease is present. The diet history is evaluated by a pediatric dietitian for calories, protein, and micronutrients as well as for the pattern of eating. Additional laboratory

Table 8–6. Components of initial evaluation for growth deficiency.

Birth history: newborn screening result; rule out intrauterine growth retardation, anoxia, congenital infections
Feeding and nutrition: difficulty sucking, chewing, swallowing
Feeding patterns: intake of formula, milk, juice, solids
Stooling and voiding of urine: diarrhea, constipation, vomiting, poor urine stream
Growth pattern: several points on the growth chart are crucial
Recurrent infections
Hospitalizations
HIV risk factors
Developmental history
Social and family factors: family composition, financial status, supports, stresses; heritable diseases, heights and weights of relatives
Review of systems

tests should be ordered based on the history and physical examination. For example, stool collection for fat determination is indicated if a history of diarrhea suggests malabsorption. Moderate or high amounts of proteinuria should prompt workup for nephrotic syndrome. Vomiting should suggest a gastrointestinal, metabolic, neurologic, infectious, or renal cause. The tempo of evaluation should be based on the severity of symptoms and the magnitude of growth failure.

Treatment

A successful treatment plan addresses the child's diet and eating patterns, the child's development, caregiver skills, and any organic disease. High-calorie diets in the form of higher calorie formula or liquid supplement and frequent monitoring (every 1 or 2 weeks initially) are essential. Acceptable weight gain varies by age (Table 8–7).

The child with growth deficiency may also be developmentally delayed because of living in an environment that fails to promote development or from the effect on the brain of nutrient deprivation. Restoring nutrition does not fully reverse the deficit but does reduce the long-term consequences.

Education in nutrition, child development, and behavioral management as well as psychosocial support of the primary caregiver is essential. If family dysfunction is mild, behavior modification and counseling will be useful. Day care may benefit the child by providing a structured environment for all activities, including eating. If family dysfunction is severe, the local department of social services can help provide structure and assistance to the family. Rarely, the child may need to be temporarily or permanently removed from the home. Hospitalization is reserved for management of dehydration, for cases in which home therapy has failed to

Table 8–7. Acceptable weight gain by age.

Age (months)	Weight Gain (g/d)
Birth to 3	20–30
3–6	15–20
6–9	10–15
9–12	6–11
12–18	5–8
18–24	3–7

result in expected growth, for children who show evidence of abuse or willful neglect, for management of an illness that compromises a child's ability to eat, or for care pending foster home placement.

Weston JA: Growth deficiency. In Berman S (editor): *Pediatric Decision Making*, 4th ed. Mosby-Year Book, 2003.

Web Resources

American Academy of Pediatrics: http://www.aap.org
American Heart Association: http://americanheart.org
Bright Futures national health promotion initiative: http://www.brightfutures.org
Centers for Disease Control and Prevention: vaccines and immunizations home page: http://www.cdc.gov/vaccines
Healthy People 2010: http://www.healthypeople.gov
National Information Center for Children and Youth with Disabilities: http://www.nichcy.org
National Newborn Screening Status Report (2005): http://genes-r-us.uthscsa.edu

Immunization

Matthew F. Daley, MD

Eric A. F. Simoes, MB, BS, DCH, MD

Ann-Christine Nyquist, MD, MSPH

Immunization has been widely recognized as one of the greatest public health achievements of the past century. Largely as a consequence of immunization, the annual incidences of diphtheria, paralytic polio, measles, mumps, rubella, and *Haemophilus influenzae* type b (Hib) in the United States have fallen by more than 99% compared with the average annual incidences of these diseases in the 20th century. Through routine vaccination, children and adolescents can now receive protection against at least 16 different diseases, and many new vaccines are under development.

Every year, roughly 4 million children are born in the United States, and successful immunization of each birth cohort requires the concerted effort of health care providers, public health officials, vaccine manufacturers, and the public. Public perceptions about immunizations, particularly routine childhood immunizations, are generally positive. However, parent concerns about the safety of vaccines have risen in recent years, in part fueled by unfounded speculation about an association between various vaccines or vaccine components and autism. Modern vaccines have a high degree of safety, and serious adverse events following vaccination are rare. Nonetheless, health care providers need to be prepared to discuss the benefits and risks of vaccination with uncertain parents, providing factual information in a clear and empathic fashion.

This chapter starts with general principles regarding immunizations and the recommended pediatric and adolescent vaccination schedules, followed by a discussion of vaccine safety. Descriptions of each routinely recommended vaccine are then presented, in roughly the chronologic order in which they are given. Vaccines that are only given in special circumstances are presented at the end of the chapter. Several abbreviations that are commonly used in this and other vaccine-related publications are summarized in the accompanying box.

Because the field of immunizations is rapidly changing, it is important for health care providers to seek the most up-to-date information available. The immunization recommendations outlined in this chapter are current but will change as technology evolves and our understanding of the epidemiology of vaccine-

preventable diseases changes. The most useful sources for regularly updated information about immunization are the following:

1. National Center for Immunization and Respiratory Diseases at the Centers for Disease Control and Prevention (CDC). Maintains a web site with extensive vaccine-related resources, including the immunization recommendations of the Advisory Committee on Immunization Practices (ACIP), vaccination schedules, Vaccine Information Statements, information for the public and providers, and links to other vaccine materials. Available at: http://www.cdc.gov/vaccines.
2. CDC Contact Center. The CDC-INFO contact center provides services to the public and health care professionals regarding a variety of health-related issues, including immunizations, 24 hours a day, 7 days a week, at 1-800-232-4636 (English and Spanish).
3. *The Red Book: Report of the Committee on Infectious Diseases.* Published at 2- to 3-year intervals by the American Academy of Pediatrics (AAP). The 2006 *Red Book* is available from the AAP. Updates are published in the journal *Pediatrics* and can also be accessed at http://aapredbook.aappublications.org.
4. Immunization Action Coalition. This nonprofit organization creates and distributes educational materials for health care providers and the public related to vaccines. All materials are provided free of charge and can be accessed at http://www.immunize.org.
5. *Morbidity and Mortality Weekly Report* (MMWR). Published weekly by CDC (Atlanta, GA, 30333). Available at: http://www.cdc.gov/mmwr.

STANDARDS FOR PEDIATRIC IMMUNIZATION PRACTICES

In the United States, every infant requires between 25 and 26 doses of vaccine by age 18 months to be protected against 14 childhood diseases. In 2006, the immunization rate for

VACCINE-RELATED ABBREVIATIONS

ACIP	Advisory Committee on Immunization Practices
BCG	Bacillus Calmette-Guérin vaccine against tuberculosis
DT	Pediatric diphtheria-tetanus toxoid
DTaP	Pediatric diphtheria and tetanus toxoids and acellular pertussis vaccine
DTP	Pediatric diphtheria and tetanus toxoids and whole-cell pertussis vaccine
HBIG	Hepatitis B immune globulin
HBsAg	Hepatitis B surface antigen
HepA	Hepatitis A vaccine
HepB	Hepatitis B vaccine
Hib	*Haemophilus influenzae* type b
HIV	Human immunodeficiency virus
HPV	Human papillomavirus
IPV	Inactivated poliovirus vaccine
LAIV	Live attenuated influenza vaccine
MCV4	Meningococcal conjugate vaccine
MMR	Measles-mumps-rubella vaccine
MMRV	Measles-mumps-rubella-varicella vaccine
MPSV	Meningococcal polysaccharide vaccine
OPV	Oral poliovirus vaccine
PCV7	Pneumococcal conjugate vaccine, 7-valent
PPV23	Pneumococcal polysaccharide vaccine, 23-valent
TB	Tuberculosis
Td	Adult tetanus and diphtheria toxoid
Tdap	Tetanus, reduced diphtheria, and acellular pertussis vaccine for adolescents and adults
TIV	Trivalent inactivated influenza vaccine
VAERS	Vaccine Adverse Events Reporting System
VAR	Varicella virus vaccine
VIS	Vaccine Information Statement
VSD	Vaccine Safety Datalink
VZIg	Varicella-zoster immune globulin
VZV	Varicella-zoster virus

children aged 19–35 months for the routine childhood immunization series was 77%, below the targeted rate of 80% set in the Healthy People 2010 national health goals. Additionally, data from the Vaccine Safety Datalink (VSD) project shows that only 36% of children younger than age 2 years were completely compliant with vaccination recommendations: 30% had a missed opportunity for immunization; 20% had an invalid immunization; and 12% received unnecessary immunization (costing an estimated $26.5 million). The AAP recommends the following specific proven practices to improve these defects: (1) sending caretakers reminder and recall notices, (2) using prompts during all visits, (3) periodic measurement of immunization rates, and (4) having standing orders for vaccines.

The National Childhood Vaccine Injury Act of 1986 requires that for each vaccine covered under the Vaccine Injury Compensation Program, caretakers should be advised about the risks and benefits of vaccination in a standard manner, using Vaccine Information Statements (VIS) produced by the CDC. Each time a Vaccine Injury Compensation Program–covered vaccine is administered, the current version of the VIS must be provided to the nonminor patient or legal caretaker. Documentation is required in the medical record, including the vaccine manufacturer, lot number, and date of administration and expiration. The name and address of the person administering the vaccine, VIS version and date, and site and route of administration should also be recorded.

Needles used for vaccination should be sterile and disposable to minimize the opportunity for contamination. A 70% solution of alcohol is appropriate for disinfection of the stopper of the vaccine container and of the skin at the injection site. A 5% topical emulsion of lidocaine-prilocaine applied to the site of vaccination for 30–60 minutes prior to the injection minimizes the pain, especially when multiple vaccines are administered.

Compliance with the manufacturer's recommendations for route and site of administration of injectable vaccines are critical for safety and efficacy. All vaccines containing an adjuvant must be administered intramuscularly to avoid granuloma formation or necrosis. With the exception of Bacillus Calmette-Guérin (BCG) vaccine, which is used rarely in the United States, all vaccines are given either intramuscularly or subcutaneously. Intramuscular injections are given at a 90-degree angle to the skin, using a needle that is sufficiently long to reach the muscle tissue, but not so long as to injure underlying nerves, blood vessels, or bones. The anterolateral thigh is the preferred site of vaccination in newborns and children up to 2 years of age, and the deltoid muscle of the arm is the preferred site for children aged 3–18 years. Needle length and location should be as follows: $5/8$ inch in newborn infants in the thigh; 1 inch in infants 1–12 months old (thigh), 1 inch to $1^1/4$ inches in 1–18 year olds (thigh), and $5/8$ inch to 1 inch in 1–18 year olds (deltoid). Subcutaneous injections should be administered at a 45-degree angle into the anterolateral aspect of the thigh (for infants younger than 12 months) or the upper outer triceps area (for children 12 months and older) using a 23- or 25-gauge $5/8$-inch needle. Pulling back on the syringe prior to vaccine injection (aspiration) is not required in CDC recommendations. A separate syringe and needle should be used for each vaccine.

Many combinations of vaccines can be administered simultaneously without increasing the risk of adverse effects or compromising response. Inactivated vaccines (with the exception of cholera and yellow fever) can be given simultaneously with, or at any time after, a different vaccine. Injectable or nasally given live-virus vaccines, if not administered on the same day, should be given at least 4 weeks apart (eg, measles-mumps-rubella [MMR] and varicella [VAR]). Lapses in the immunization schedule do not call for reinstitution of the series. Extra doses of hepatitis B (HepB), Hib, MMR, and VAR are not harmful, but repetitive exposure to tetanus vaccine beyond the recommended intervals can result in hypersensitivity reactions and should be avoided. If an immunoglobulin (Ig) or blood product has been administered, live-virus vaccination should be delayed 3–11 months, depending on the product, to avoid interference with the immune response (eg, 3 months for tetanus Ig, hepatitis A Ig, and hepatitis B Ig; 5–6 months for measles Ig or cytomegalovirus Ig; and 11 months for intravenous Ig for Kawasaki disease).

With the large number of vaccine preparations available, interchangeability of vaccines is an issue. All brands of Hib conjugate, HepB, and hepatitis A (HepA) vaccines are interchangeable. For vaccines containing acellular pertussis antigens, it is recommended that the same brand be used, but when the brand is unknown or the same brand is unavailable, any vaccine with diphtheria and tetanus toxoids and acellular pertussis should be used to continue vaccination. A longer than recommended interval between vaccinations does not reduce final antibody titers, and lapsed schedules do not require restarting the series.

Vaccines very rarely cause acute anaphylactic-type reactions. Nonetheless, all vaccine providers should have the equipment, medications, staff, and training to manage emergencies that may occur following vaccination.

CDC: General recommendations on immunization: recommendations of the Advisory Committee on Immunization Practices (ACIP). MMWR Recomm Rep 2006;55(RR-15):1 [PMID: 17136024].

CDC: National, state, and local area vaccination coverage among children aged 19–35 months—United States, 2006. MMWR Morb Mortal Wkly Rep 2007;56:880 [PMID: 17728693].

Mell LK et al: Compliance with national immunization guidelines for children younger than 2 years, 1996–1999. Pediatrics 2005;115:461 [PMID: 15687456].

ROUTINE CHILDHOOD & ADOLESCENT IMMUNIZATIONS

Each year, the CDC issues recommended immunization schedules for children and adolescents. While variation from these schedules may be necessitated by epidemiologic or individual clinical circumstances, these schedules serve as an important guide for vaccination providers. In the schedules, vaccines are roughly ordered by the age at which the vaccines

are first given. For example, HepB is given to newborn infants at birth, followed by rotavirus, diphtheria-tetanus-acellular pertussis (DTaP), Hib, pneumococcal conjugate 7-valent (PCV7) and inactivated poliovirus (IPV) vaccines beginning at 2 months of age. Table 9–1 sets forth a schedule of routine immunizations for normal infants and children from birth to 6 years. Table 9–2 presents a schedule of routine immunization for persons aged 7–18 years. Table 9–3 presents recommended schedules for children who did not start vaccination at the recommended time during the first year of life.

Combination vaccines help solve the problem of large numbers of injections during any single clinic visit. Currently available combination vaccines include MMR, measles-mumps-rubella-varicella (MMRV), and various combinations of Hib, HepB, IPV, and DTaP, including a DTaP-HepB-IPV combination vaccine. Additional combination vaccines, including some vaccines specifically for older children and adolescents, are in development. Separate vaccines should not be combined into one syringe by the provider unless approved by the Food and Drug Administration (FDA), because this could decrease the efficacy of each component vaccine.

SAFE HANDLING OF VACCINES

The numerous vaccines and other immunologic substances used by the practitioner vary in the storage temperatures required. The majority of vaccines should never be subjected to freezing temperatures. Vaccines that require routine freezing are MMRV, VAR, and herpes zoster vaccines. Yellow fever vaccine may also be stored frozen. Product package inserts should be consulted for detailed information on vaccine storage conditions and shelf life.

CDC: Recommended childhood and adolescent immunization schedule—United States, 2008. MMWR Morb Mortal Wkly Rep 2007;56:Q1–Q4.

SAFETY OF IMMUNIZATION

Although no vaccine is 100% safe and effective, after decades of experience and many millions of doses administered, vaccines have proven to be among the safest of medical interventions. However, as diseases such as measles and polio become exceedingly rare in the United States, the apparent risks of vaccination have taken a more prominent role in the public discourse. When vaccine-preventable diseases are perceived to be treatable or rare, the risks of vaccination may appear to outweigh the benefits, particularly to persons who misunderstand the actual risks from vaccines and the potential for resurgence of some diseases when the public is not adequately immunized. Decisions about vaccination, both at the individual and societal level, need to be made based on accurate and timely information. Parents with questions about vaccine safety should be directed to trusted web sites, such as those of the AAP, the American Academy of Family Physicians

Table 9-1. Recommended immunization schedule for children aged 0–6 years, United States, 2008.

Recommended Immunization Schedule for Persons Aged 0–6 Years — UNITED STATES • 2008

For those who fall behind or start late, see the catch-up schedule

Vaccine ▼ Age ▶	Birth	1 month	2 months	4 months	6 months	12 months	15 months	18 months	19–23 years	2–3 years	4–6 years
Hepatitis B [1]	HepB	HepB	see footnote 1		HepB						
Rotavirus [2]			Rota	Rota	Rota						
Diphtheria, Tetanus, Pertussis [3]			DTaP	DTaP	DTaP	see footnote 3	DTaP				DTaP
Haemophilus influenzae type b [4]			Hib	Hib	Hib [4]	Hib					
Pneumococcal [5]			PCV	PCV	PCV	PCV					PPV
Inactivated Poliovirus			IPV	IPV		IPV					IPV
Influenza [6]						Influenza (Yearly)					
Measles, Mumps, Rubella [7]						MMR					MMR
Varicella [8]						Varicella					Varicella
Hepatitis A [9]						HepA (2 doses)				HepA Series	
Meningococcal [10]										MCV4	

Range of recommended ages

Certain high-risk groups

This schedule indicates the recommended ages for routine administration of currently licensed childhood vaccines, as of December 1, 2007, for children aged 7–18 years. Additional information is available at www.cdc.gov/vaccines/recs/schedules. Any dose not administered at the recommended age should be administered at any subsequent visit, when indicated and feasible. Additional vaccines may be licensed and recommended during the year. Licensed combination vaccines may be used whenever any components of the combination are indicated and other components of the vaccine are not contraindicated and if approved by the Food and Drug Administration for that dose of the series. Providers should consult the respective Advisory Committee on Immunization Practices statement for detailed recommendations, including for high risk conditions: http://www.cdc.gov/vaccines/pubs/ACIP-list.htm. Clinically significant adverse events that follow immunization should be reported to the Vaccine Adverse Event Reporting System (VAERS). Guidance about how to obtain and complete a VAERS form is available at www.vaers.hhs.gov or by telephone, 800-822-7967.

1. Hepatitis B vaccine (HepB). *(Minimum age: birth)*

At birth:
- Administer monovalent HepB to all newborns prior to hospital discharge.
- If mother is hepatitis B surface antigen (HBsAg) positive, administer HepB and 0.5 mL of hepatitis B immune globulin (HBIG) within 12 hours of birth.
- If mother's HBsAg status is unknown, administer HepB within 12 hours of birth. Determine the HBsAg status as soon as possible and if HBsAg positive, administer HBIG (no later than age 1 week).
- If mother is HBsAg negative, the birth dose can be delayed, in rare cases, with a provider's order and a copy of the mother's negative HBsAg laboratory report in the infant's medical record.

After the birth dose:
- The HepB series should be completed with either monovalent HepB or a combination vaccine containing HepB. The second dose should be administered at age 1–2 months. The final dose should be administered no earlier than age 24 weeks. Infants born to HBsAg-positive mothers should be tested for HBsAg and antibody to HBsAg after completion of at least 3 doses of a licensed HepB series, at age 9–18 months (generally at the next well-child visit).

4-month dose:
- It is permissible to administer 4 doses of HepB when combination vaccines are administered after the birth dose. If monovalent HepB is used for doses after the birth dose, a dose at age 4 months is not needed.

2. Rotavirus vaccine (Rota). *(Minimum age: 6 weeks)*
- Administer the first dose at age 6–12 weeks.
- Do not start the series later than age 12 weeks.
- Administer the final dose in the series by age 32 weeks. Do not administer any dose later than age 32 weeks.
- Data on safety and efficacy outside of these age ranges are insufficient.

3. Diphtheria and tetanus toxoids and acellular pertussis vaccine (DTaP). *(Minimum age: 6 weeks)*
- The fourth dose of DTaP may be administered as early as age 12 months, provided 6 months have elapsed since the third dose.
- Administer the final dose in the series at age 4–6 years.

4. *Haemophilus influenzae* type b conjugate vaccine (Hib). *(Minimum age: 6 weeks)*
- If PRP-OMP (PedvaxHIB® or ComVax® [Merck]) is administered at ages 2 and 4 months, a dose at age 6 months is not required.
- TriHIBit® (DTaP/Hib) combination products should not be used for primary immunization but can be used as boosters following any Hib vaccine in children age 12 months or older.

5. Pneumococcal vaccine. *(Minimum age: 6 weeks for pneumococcal conjugate vaccine [PCV]; 2 years for pneumococcal polysaccharide vaccine [PPV])*
- Administer one dose of PCV to all healthy children aged 24–59 months having any incomplete schedule.
- Administer PPV to children aged 2 years and older with underlying medical conditions.

6. Influenza vaccine. *(Minimum age: 6 months for trivalent inactivated influenza vaccine [TIV]; 2 years for live, attenuated influenza vaccine [LAIV])*
- Administer annually to children aged 6–59 months and to all eligible close contacts of children aged 0–59 months.
- Administer annually to children 5 years of age and older with certain risk factors, to other persons (including household members) in close contact with persons in groups at higher risk, and to any child whose parents request vaccination.
- For healthy persons (those who do not have underlying medical conditions that predispose them to influenza complications) ages 2–49 years, either LAIV or TIV may be used.
- Children receiving TIV should receive 0.25 mL if age 6–35 months or 0.5 mL if age 3 years or older.
- Administer 2 doses (separated by 4 weeks or longer) to children younger than 9 years who are receiving influenza vaccine for the first time or who were vaccinated for the first time last season but only received one dose.

7. Measles, mumps, and rubella vaccine (MMR). *(Minimum age: 12 months)*
- Administer the second dose of MMR at age 4–6 years. MMR may be administered before age 4–6 years, provided 4 weeks or more have elapsed since the first dose.

8. Varicella vaccine. *(Minimum age: 12 months)*
- Administer second dose at age 4–6 years; may be administered 3 months or more after first dose.
- Do not repeat second dose if administered 28 days or more after first dose.

9. Hepatitis A vaccine (HepA). *(Minimum age: 12 months)*
- Administer to all children aged 1 year (i.e., aged 12–23 months). Administer the 2 doses in the series at least 6 months apart.
- Children not fully vaccinated by age 2 years can be vaccinated at subsequent visits.
- HepA is recommended for certain other groups of children, including in areas where vaccination programs target older children.

10. Meningococcal vaccine. *(Minimum age: 2 years for meningococcal conjugate vaccine (MCV4) or meningococcal polysaccharide vaccine (MPSV4))*
- Administer MCV4 to children aged 2–10 years with terminal complement deficiencies or anatomic or functional asplenia and certain other high-risk groups. MPSV4 is also acceptable.
- Administer MCV4 to persons who received MPSV4 3 or more years previously and remain at increased risk for meningococcal disease.

The Recommended Immunizations Schedules for Persons Aged 0–18 Years are approved by the Advisory Committee on Immunization Practices (www.cdc.gov/vaccines/recs/acip), The American Academy of Pediatrics (http://www.aap.org), and the American Academy of Family Physicians (http://www.aafp.org).

DEPARTMENT OF HEALTH AND HUMAN SERVICES • CENTERS FOR DISEASE CONTROL AND PREVENTION • SAFER · HEALTHIER · PEOPLE™

Reproduced, with permission, from CDC: Recommended childhood and adolescent immunization schedule—U.S., 2008. MMWR Morb Mortal Wkly Rep 2007;56:Q1-Q4.

Table 9–2. Recommended immunization schedule for persons aged 7–18 years, United States, 2008.

Recommended Immunization Schedule for Persons Aged 7–18 Years — UNITED STATES • 2008
For those who fall behind or start late, see the green bars and the catch-up schedule

Vaccine ▼ Age ▶	7–10 years	11–12 years	13–18 years	
Diphtheria, Tetanus, Pertussis [1]	see footnote 1	Tdap	Tdap	Range of recommended ages
Human Papillomavirus [2]	see footnote 2	HPV (3 doses)	HPV Series	
Meningococcal [3]	MCV4	MCV4	MCV4	
Pneumococcal [4]	PPV			Catch-up immunization
Influenza [5]	Influenza (Yearly)			
Hepatitis A [6]	HepA Series			
Hepatitis B [7]	HepB Series			Certain high-risk groups
Inactivated Poliovirus [8]	IPV Series			
Measles, Mumps, Rubella [9]	MMR Series			
Varicella [10]	Varicella Series			

This schedule indicates the recommended ages for routine administration of currently licensed childhood vaccines, as of December 1, 2007, for children aged 7–18 years. Additional information is available at www.cdc.gov/vaccines/recs/schedules. Any dose not administered at the recommended age should be administered at any subsequent visit, when indicated and feasible. Additional vaccines may be licensed and recommended during the year. Licensed combination vaccines may be used whenever any components of the combination are indicated and other components of the vaccine are not contraindicated and if approved by the Food and Drug Administration for that dose of the series. Providers should consult the respective Advisory Committee on Immunization Practices statement for detailed recommendations, including for high risk conditions: http://www.cdc.gov/vaccines/pubs/ACIP-list.htm. Clinically significant adverse events that follow immunization should be reported to the Vaccine Adverse Event Reporting System (VAERS). Guidance about how to obtain and complete a VAERS form is available at www.vaers.hhs.gov or by telephone, 800-822-7967.

1. Tetanus and diphtheria toxoids and acellular pertussis vaccine (Tdap). *(Minimum age: 10 years for BOOSTRIX ® and 11 years for ADACEL™)*
- Administer at age 11–12 years for those who have completed the recommended childhood DTP/DTaP vaccination series and have not received a tetanus and diphtheria toxoids (Td) booster dose.
- 13–18-year-olds who missed the 11–12 year Tdap or received Td only are encouraged to receive one dose of Tdap 5 years after the last Td/DTaP dose.

2. Human papillomavirus vaccine (HPV). *(Minimum age: 9 years)*
- Administer the first dose of the HPV vaccine series to females at age 11–12 years.
- Administer the second dose 2 months after the first dose and the third dose 6 months after the first dose.
- Administer the HPV vaccine series to females at age 13–18 years if not previously vaccinated.

3. Meningococcal vaccine.
- Administer MCV4 at age 11–12 years and at age 13–18 years if not previously vaccinated. MPSV4 is an acceptable alternative.
- Administer MCV4 to previously unvaccinated college freshmen living in dormitories.
- MCV4 is recommended for children aged 2–10 years with terminal complement deficiencies or anatomic or functional asplenia and certain other high-risk groups.
- Persons who received MPSV4 3 or more years previously and remain at increased risk for meningococcal disease should be vaccinated with MCV4.

4. Pneumococcal polysaccharide vaccine (PPV).
- Administer PPV to certain high-risk groups.

5. Influenza vaccine.
- Administer annually to all close contacts of children aged 0–59 months.
- Administer annually to persons with certain risk factors, health-care workers, and other persons (including household members) in close contact with persons in groups at higher risk.

- Administer 2 doses (separated by 4 weeks or longer) to children younger than 9 years who are receiving influenza vaccine for the first time or who were vaccinated for the first time last season but only received one dose.
- For healthy nonpregnant persons (those who do not have underlying medical conditions that predispose them to influenza complications) ages 2–49 years, either LAIV or TIV may be used.

6. Hepatitis A vaccine (HepA).
- Administer the 2 doses in the series at least 6 months apart.
- HepA is recommended for certain other groups of children, including in areas where vaccination programs target older children.

7. Hepatitis B vaccine (HepB).
- Administer the 3-dose series to those who were not previously vaccinated.
- A 2-dose series of Recombivax HB ® is licensed for children aged 11–15 years.

8. Inactivated poliovirus vaccine (IPV).
- For children who received an all-IPV or all-oral poliovirus (OPV) series, a fourth dose is not necessary if the third dose was administered at age 4 years or older.
- If both OPV and IPV were administered as part of a series, a total of 4 doses should be administered, regardless of the child's current age.

9. Measles, mumps, and rubella vaccine (MMR).
- If not previously vaccinated, administer 2 doses of MMR during any visit, with 4 or more weeks between the doses.

10. Varicella vaccine.
- Administer 2 doses of varicella vaccine to persons younger than 13 years of age at least 3 months apart. Do not repeat the second dose if administered 28 or more days following the first dose.
- Administer 2 doses of varicella vaccine to persons aged 13 years or older at least 4 weeks apart.

The Recommended Immunizations Schedules for Persons Aged 0–18 Years are approved by the Advisory Committee on Immunization Practices (www.cdc.gov/vaccines/recs/acip). The American Academy of Pediatrics (http://www.aap.org), and the American Academy of Family Physicians (http://www.aafp.org).

DEPARTMENT OF HEALTH AND HUMAN SERVICES • CENTERS FOR DISEASE CONTROL AND PREVENTION • SAFER · HEALTHIER · PEOPLE™

Reproduced, with permission, from CDC: Recommended childhood and adolescent immunization schedule—U.S., 2008. MMWR Morb Mortal Wkly Rep 2007;56:Q1–Q4.

Table 9–3. Recommended immunization schedule for children and adolescents who start late or who are more than 1 month behind: United States, 2008.

Catch-up Immunization Schedule

UNITED STATES • 2008

for Persons Aged 4 Months–18 Years Who Start Late or Who Are More Than 1 Month Behind

The table below provides catch-up schedules and minimum intervals between doses for children whose vaccinations have been delayed. A vaccine series does not need to be restarted, regardless of the time that has elapsed between doses. Use the section appropriate for the child's age.

		CATCH-UP SCHEDULE FOR PERSONS AGED 4 MONTHS–6 YEARS			
Vaccine	Minimum Age for Dose 1	**Minimum Interval Between Doses**			
		Dose 1 to Dose 2	Dose 2 to Dose 3	Dose 3 to Dose 4	Dose 4 to Dose 5
Hepatitis B [1]	Birth	4 weeks	**8 weeks** (and 16 weeks after first dose)		
Rotavirus [2]	6 wks	4 weeks	4 weeks		
Diphtheria, Tetanus, Pertussis [3]	6 wks	4 weeks	4 weeks	6 months	6 months [3]
Haemophilus influenzae type b [4]	6 wks	**4 weeks** if first dose administered at younger than 12 months of age / **8 weeks (as final dose)** if first dose administered at age 12-14 months / **No further doses needed** if first dose administered at 15 months of age or older	**4 weeks** [4] if current age is younger than 12 months / **8 weeks (as final dose)** [4] if current age is 12 months or older and second dose administered at younger than 15 months of age / **No further doses needed** if previous dose administered at age 15 months or older	**8 weeks (as final dose)** This dose only necessary for children aged 12 months–5 years who received 3 doses before age 12 months	
Pneumococcal [5]	6 wks	**4 weeks** if first dose administered at younger than 12 months of age / **8 weeks (as final dose)** if first dose administered at age 12 months or older or current age 24–59 months / **No further doses needed** for healthy children if first dose administered at age 24 months or older	**4 weeks** if current age is younger than 12 months / **8 weeks (as final dose)** if current age is 12 months or older / **No further doses needed** for healthy children if previous dose administered at age 24 months or older	**8 weeks (as final dose)** This dose only necessary for children aged 12 months–5 years who received 3 doses before age 12 months	
Inactivated Poliovirus [6]	6 wks	4 weeks	4 weeks	4 weeks [6]	
Measles, Mumps, Rubella [7]	12 mos	4 weeks			
Varicella [8]	12 mos	3 months			
Hepatitis A [9]	12 mos	6 months			
		CATCH-UP SCHEDULE FOR PERSONS AGED 7–18 YEARS			
Tetanus, Diphtheria/ Tetanus, Diphtheria, Pertussis [10]	7 yrs [10]	4 weeks	**4 weeks** if first dose administered at younger than 12 months of age / **6 months** if first dose administered at age 12 months or older	**6 months** if first dose administered at younger than 12 months of age	
Human Papillomavirus [11]	9 yrs	4 weeks	**12 weeks** (and 24 weeks after the first dose)		
Hepatitis A [9]	12 mos	6 months			
Hepatitis B [1]	Birth	4 weeks	**8 weeks** (and 16 weeks after first dose)		
Inactivated Poliovirus [6]	6 wks	4 weeks	4 weeks	4 weeks [6]	
Measles, Mumps, Rubella [7]	12 mos	4 weeks			
Varicella [8]	12 mos	**4 weeks** if first dose administered at age 13 years or older / **3 months** if first dose administered at younger than 13 years of age			

1. Hepatitis B vaccine (HepB).
- Administer the 3-dose series to those who were not previously vaccinated.
- A 2-dose series of Recombivax HB® is licensed for children aged 11–15 years.

2. Rotavirus vaccine (Rota).
- Do not start the series later than age 12 weeks.
- Administer the final dose in the series by age 32 weeks.
- Do not administer a dose later than age 32 weeks.
- Data on safety and efficacy outside of these age ranges are insufficient.

3. Diphtheria and tetanus toxoids and acellular pertussis vaccine (DTaP).
- The fifth dose is not necessary if the fourth dose was administered at age 4 years or older.
- DTaP is not indicated for persons aged 7 years or older.

4. *Haemophilus influenzae* type b conjugate vaccine (Hib).
- Vaccine is not generally recommended for children aged 5 years or older.
- If current age is younger than 12 months and the first 2 doses were PRP-OMP (PedvaxHIB ® or ComVax® [Merck]), the third (and final) dose should be administered at age 12–15 months and at least 8 weeks after the second dose.
- If first dose was administered at age 7–11 months, administer 2 doses separated by 4 weeks plus a booster at age 12–15 months.

5. Pneumococcal conjugate vaccine (PCV).
- Administer one dose of PCV to all healthy children aged 24–59 months having any incomplete schedule.
- For children with underlying medical conditions, administer 2 doses of PCV at least 8 weeks apart if previously received less than 3 doses, or 1 dose of PCV if previously received 3 doses.

6. Inactivated poliovirus vaccine (IPV).
- For children who received an all-IPV or all-oral poliovirus (OPV) series, a fourth dose is not necessary if third dose was administered at age 4 years or older.

- If both OPV and IPV were administered as part of a series, a total of 4 doses should be administered, regardless of the child's current age.
- IPV is not routinely recommended for persons aged 18 years and older.

7. Measles, mumps, and rubella vaccine (MMR).
- The second dose of MMR is recommended routinely at age 4–6 years but may be administered earlier if desired.
- If not previously vaccinated, administer 2 doses of MMR during any visit with 4 or more weeks between the doses.

8. Varicella vaccine.
- The second dose of varicella vaccine is recommended routinely at age 4–6 years but may be administered earlier if desired.
- Do not repeat the second dose in persons younger than 13 years of age if administered 28 or more days after the first dose.

9. Hepatitis A vaccine (HepA).
- HepA is recommended for certain groups of children, including in areas where vaccination programs target older children. See *MMWR* 2006;55(No. RR-7):1–23.

10. Tetanus and diphtheria toxoids vaccine (Td) and tetanus and diphtheria toxoids and acellular pertussis vaccine (Tdap).
- Tdap should be substituted for a single dose of Td in the primary catch-up series or as a booster if age appropriate; use Td for other doses.
- A 5-year interval from the last Td dose is encouraged when Tdap is used as a booster dose. A booster (fourth) dose is needed if any of the previous doses were administered at younger than 12 months of age. Refer to ACIP recommendations for further information. See *MMWR* 2006;55(No. RR-3).

11. Human papillomavirus vaccine (HPV).
- Administer the HPV vaccine series to females at age 13–18 years if not previously vaccinated.

Information about reporting reactions after immunization is available online at http://www.vaers.hhs.gov or by telephone via the 24-hour national toll-free information line 800-822-7967. Suspected cases of vaccine-preventable diseases should be reported to the state or local health department. Additional information, including precautions and contraindications for immunization, is available from the National Center for Immunization and Respiratory Diseases at http://www.cdc.gov/vaccines or telephone, 800-CDC-INFO (800-232-4636).

Reproduced, with permission, from CDC: Recommended childhood and adolescent immunization schedule—U.S., 2008. MMWR Morb Mortal Wkly Rep 2007;56:Q1-Q4.

(AAFP), the CDC (http://www.cdc.gov/vaccines), and the Immunization Action Coalition (http://www.immunize.org).

The safety standards for all vaccines licensed for use in the United States are established by the FDA and involve regular examination of manufacturing techniques as well as production lots of vaccine. No incidents of bacterial or viral contamination of vaccines at the factory level have been reported in the United States for decades.

All vaccines have certain contraindications and precautions that guide their administration. A contraindication indicates that the potential vaccine recipient is at increased risk of a serious adverse event. A vaccine should not be given when a contraindication to that vaccine is present, whereas a precaution indicates a circumstance that might increase the risk of adverse events or diminish the effectiveness of the vaccine. In the setting of precautions, the risks and benefits of vaccination must be carefully weighed prior to a decision regarding vaccination. Precautions are often temporary, in which case vaccination can resume once the precaution no longer applies. Contraindications and precautions are listed below with each vaccine. Additional, more detailed information is available from the CDC, in the AAP *Red Book,* and in vaccine package inserts.

Healthy Children

Minor acute illnesses, with or without low-grade fever, are not contraindications to vaccination, because there is no evidence that vaccination under these conditions increases the rate of adverse effects or decreases efficacy. A moderate to severe febrile illness may be a reason to postpone vaccination. Routine physical examination and temperature assessment are not necessary before vaccinating healthy infants and children.

Children with Chronic Illnesses

Most chronic diseases are not contraindications to vaccination; in fact, children with chronic diseases may be at greater risk of complications from vaccine-preventable diseases, such as influenzal and pneumococcal infections. Premature infants are a good example. They should be immunized according to their chronologic, not gestational, age. Vaccine doses should not be reduced for preterm or low-birth-weight infants. One exception to this rule is children with progressive central nervous system disorders. Vaccination with DTaP should be deferred until the child's neurologic status has been clarified and is more stable.

Immunodeficient Children

Congenitally immunodeficient children should not be immunized with live-virus (oral polio vaccine [OPV], MMR, VAR, MMRV, yellow fever, or live-attenuated influenza vaccine [LAIV]) or live-bacteria vaccines (BCG or live typhoid fever vaccine). Depending on the nature of the immunodeficiency, other vaccines are safe, but may fail to evoke an immune response. Children with cancer and children receiving high-dose corticosteroids or other immunosuppressive agents should not be vaccinated with live-virus or live-bacteria vaccines. This contraindication does not apply if the malignancy is in remission and chemotherapy has not been administered for at least 90 days. Live-virus vaccines may also be administered to previously healthy children receiving low to moderate doses of corticosteroids (defined as up to 2 mg/kg/d of prednisone or prednisone equivalent, with a 20 mg/d maximum) for less than 14 days; children receiving short-acting alternate-day corticosteroids; children being maintained on physiologic corticosteroid therapy without other immunodeficiency; and children receiving only topical, inhaled, or intraarticular corticosteroids.

Contraindication of live-pathogen vaccines also applies to children with HIV infection who are severely immunosuppressed. In general those who receive MMR should have at least 15% CD4 cells and a CD4 lymphocyte count equivalent to CDC immunologic class 2. MMR for these children is recommended at 12 months of age (after 6 months during an epidemic). The booster dose may be given as early as 1 month later, but doses given before 1 year of age should not be considered part of a complete series. VAR vaccination is also recommended for HIV-infected children with CD4 cells preserved as listed above. OPV, which is contraindicated, is no longer recommended in the United States. The ACIP recommends routine vaccination for all children only with IPV. Thus immunodeficient children should no longer be exposed to OPV through household contacts. MMR and VAR are not contraindicated in household contacts of immunocompromised children.

Allergic or Hypersensitive Children

Hypersensitivity reactions are rare following vaccination (1.53 cases/million doses). They are generally attributable to a trace component of the vaccine other than the antigen itself; for example, MMR, IPV, and VAR contain microgram quantities of neomycin, and IPV also contains trace amounts of streptomycin and polymyxin B. Children with known anaphylactic responses to these antibiotics should not be given these vaccines. Trace quantities of egg antigens may be present in both inactivated and live influenza and yellow fever vaccines. Children who have had anaphylactic reactions to eggs should not be given these vaccines; children with less serious reactions to eggs can generally be safely immunized. Some vaccines (MMR, MMRV, and VAR) contain gelatin, a substance to which persons with known food allergy may develop an anaphylactic reaction. For any persons with a known history of anaphylactic reaction to any component contained in a vaccine, the vaccine package insert should be reviewed and additional consultation sought, such as from a pediatric allergist.

Special Circumstances

Detailed recommendations for preterm low-birth-weight infants; pediatric transplant recipients; Alaskan Natives/

American Indians; children in residential institutions or military communities; or refugees, new immigrants, or travelers are available from the CDC (at http://www.cdc.gov/vaccines) and from the AAP *Red Book*.

Monitoring Vaccine Safety

Physicians administering vaccines are obliged to report serious adverse events following immunization to the Vaccine Adverse Events Reporting System (VAERS). This is a nationwide passive surveillance program for vaccine safety managed cooperatively by the CDC and the FDA. Reports of possible adverse events related to vaccination may be made via the Internet or by mail. VAERS can be reached at http://vaers.hhs.gov, or by telephone at 1-800-822-7967. The CDC also undertakes numerous studies using large linked databases of computerized vaccination and medical records. The VSD project, which is a network of health maintenance organizations that share information on immunizations, medical outcomes, and potential confounders, serves as a useful tool to accumulate and analyze data as new vaccine issues arise.

AAP: *Red Book: 2006 Report of the Committee on Infectious Diseases*, 27th ed. American Academy of Pediatrics, 2006.

Bohlke K et al: Risk of anaphylaxis after vaccination of children and adolescents. Pediatrics 2003;112:815 [PMID: 14523172].

CDC: General recommendations on immunization: Recommendations of the Advisory Committee on Immunization Practices (ACIP). MMWR Recomm Rep 2006;55(RR-15):1 [PMID: 17136024].

Davis RL et al: Active surveillance of vaccine safety: a system to detect early signs of adverse events. Epidemiology 2005;16:336 [PMID: 15824549].

Iskander JK et al: The role of the Vaccine Adverse Event Reporting system (VAERS) in monitoring vaccine safety. Pediatr Ann 2004;33:599 [PMID: 15462575].

HEPATITIS B VACCINATION

The incidence of reported cases of acute hepatitis B has declined dramatically in the United States, largely attributable to vaccination. Based on surveillance data from 2005, acute hepatitis B incidence has declined by 79% since 1990, to the lowest rate ever measured. The greatest declines have been seen in children younger than 15 years of age, in whom rates have decreased by 98%.

Successes in reducing the burden of hepatitis B are due, in large part, to a comprehensive hepatitis B prevention strategy initiated in 1991. The four central elements of this approach are (1) immunization of all infants beginning at birth; (2) routine screening of all pregnant women for hepatitis B infection, and provision of hepatitis B immune globulin (HBIg) to all infants born to infected mothers; (3) routine vaccination of previously unvaccinated children and adolescents; and (4) vaccination of adults at increased risk of hepatitis B infection.

While high immunization rates have been achieved in young children (more than 93% were fully immunized in 2006), the nation has been less successful at identifying

hepatitis B–infected mothers and at immunizing high-risk adults. Of the estimated 23,000 mothers who deliver each year who are hepatitis B surface antigen (HBsAg) positive, only 9000 are identified through prenatal screening. This circumstance represents a significant missed opportunity for prevention, given that administration of hepatitis B vaccine (HepB) in conjunction with HBIg is 95% effective at preventing mother-to-infant transmission of the virus. Similarly, while HepB alone is 90–95% effective at preventing hepatitis B infection, only 45% of high-risk adults have been vaccinated.

All pregnant women should be routinely screened for HBsAg. Infants born to HBsAg-positive mothers should receive both HepB and HBIg immediately after birth. Infants for whom the maternal HBsAg status is unknown should receive vaccine (but not HBIg) within 12 hours of birth. In such circumstances, the mother's HBsAg status should be determined as soon as possible during her hospitalization, and the infant given HBIg if the mother is found to be HBsAg-positive. For all infants, the hepatitis B immunization series should be started at birth, with the first dose given prior to discharge from the hospital. Given the importance of the birth dose of HepB in preventing perinatal infection, the ACIP has recommended that any decision to defer the birth dose require an explanation in the medical record, accompanied by a copy of the mother's negative HBsAg test during the current pregnancy.

Routine immunization with three doses of HepB is recommended for all infants and all previously unvaccinated children aged 0–18 years. A two-dose schedule is available for adolescents as well. In addition, persons 19 years and older with an increased risk of exposure to hepatitis B virus should be vaccinated. This includes men who have sex with men, persons with multiple sexual partners, intravenous and injection drug users, recipients of clotting factors concentrates, hemodialysis patients, household contacts and sexual contacts of persons with chronic hepatitis B infection, long-term international travelers to endemic areas, and all health care personnel. Screening for markers of past infection before vaccinating is generally not indicated for children and adolescents, but may be considered for high-risk adults. Because HepB vaccines consist of an inactivated subunit of the virus, the vaccines are not infectious and are not contraindicated in immunosuppressed individuals or pregnant women.

▶ Vaccines Available

1. Hepatitis B vaccine (Recombivax HB, Merck) contains recombinant HepB only.
2. Hepatitis B vaccine (Engerix-B, GlaxoSmithKline) contains recombinant HepB only.
3. Hepatitis B-Hib (Comvax, Merck) contains vaccines against hepatitis B and Hib.
4. DTaP-HepB-IPV (Pediarix, GlaxoSmithKline) contains vaccines against diphtheria, tetanus, pertussis, hepatitis B, and poliovirus.

Only the single-antigen vaccines (Recombivax HB and Engerix-B) can be given between birth and 6 weeks of age. Any single or combination vaccine listed above can be used to complete the hepatitis B vaccination series. Thimerosal has been removed from all pediatric HepB formulations. A combination vaccine against hepatitis A and hepatitis B (Twinrix, GlaxoSmithKline) is available, but is only licensed in the United States for persons 18 years and older.

▶ Dosage & Schedule of Administration

HepB is recommended for all infants and children in the United States. Table 9–4 presents the vaccination schedule for newborn infants, dependent on maternal HBsAg status. Infants born to mothers with positive or unknown HBsAg status should receive HepB vaccine within 12 hours of birth. Infants born to HBsAg-negative mothers should receive the vaccine prior to hospital discharge.

For children younger than 11 years of age not previously immunized, three intramuscular doses of HepB are needed. Adolescents aged 11–15 years have two options: the standard pediatric three-dose schedule or two doses of adult Recombivax HB (1.0-mL dose), with the second dose administered 4–6 months after the first dose. Simultaneous administration with other vaccines at different sites is safe and effective. The vaccine should be given intramuscularly in either the anterolateral thigh or deltoid, depending on the age and size of the patient.

Certain patients may have reduced immune response to HepB vaccination, including preterm infants weighing less than 2000 g at birth; immunosuppressed patients; and those receiving dialysis. Preterm infants whose mothers are HBsAg-positive or with unknown HBsAg status should receive both HepB and HBIg within 12 hours of birth. For preterm infants whose mothers are known to be HBsAg-negative, initiation of the vaccination series should be delayed until 30 days of chronologic age if the infant is medically stable or prior to

Table 9–4. Hepatitis B vaccine schedules for newborn infants, by maternal hepatitis B surface antigen (HBsAg) status.[a]

Maternal HBsAg Status	Single-Antigen Vaccine		Single Antigen + Combination Vaccine	
	Dose	Age	Dose	Age
Positive	1[b]	Birth (≤ 12 h)	1[b]	Birth (≤ 12 h)
	HBIg[c]	Birth (≤ 12 h)	HBIg	Birth (≤ 12 h)
	2	1–2 mo	2	2 mo
			3	4 mo
	3[d]	6 mo	4[d]	6 mo (Pediarix) or 12–15 mo (Comvax)
Unknown[e]	1[b]	Birth (≤ 12 h)	1[b]	Birth (≤ 12 h)
	2	1–2 mo	2	2 mo
			3	4 mo
	3[d]	6 mo	4[d]	6 mo (Pediarix) or 12–15 mo (Comvax)
Negative	1[b,f]	Birth (before discharge)	1[b,f]	Birth (before discharge)
	2	1–2 mo	2	2 mo
			3	4 mo
	3[d]	6–18 mo	4[d]	6 mo (Pediarix) or 12–15 mo (Comvax)

[a]See text for vaccination of preterm infants weighing < 2000 g.
[b]Recombivax HB or Engerix-B should be used for the birth dose. Comvax and Pediarix cannot be administered at birth or before age 6 weeks.
[c]Hepatitis B immune globulin (HBIg) (0.5 mL) administered intramuscularly in a separate site from vaccine.
[d]The final dose in the vaccine series should not be administered before age 24 weeks (164 days).
[e]Mothers should have blood drawn and tested for HBsAg as soon as possible after admission for delivery; if the mother is found to be HBsAg-positive, the infant should receive HBIg as soon as possible, but no later than age 7 days.
[f]On a case-by-case basis and only in rare circumstances, the first dose may be delayed until after hospital discharge for an infant who weighs ≥ 2000 g and whose mother is HBsAg-negative, but only if a physician's order to withhold the birth dose and a copy of the mother's original HBsAg-negative laboratory report are documented in the infant's medical record.
Reproduced, with permission, from CDC: A comprehensive immunization strategy to eliminate transmission of hepatitis B virus infection in the United States, part 1: Immunization of infants, children, and adolescents. MMWR Recomm Rep 2005;54(RR-16):1.

hospital discharge if the infant is discharged before 30 days of age. Hemodialysis patients and immunocompromised persons may require larger doses or an increased number of doses, with dose amounts and schedules available in the most recent CDC hepatitis B recommendations (see references).

Contraindications & Precautions

HepB vaccine should not be given to persons with a serious allergic reaction to yeast or to any vaccine components. Individuals with a history of serious adverse events, such as anaphylaxis, after receiving HepB should not receive additional doses. Vaccination is not contraindicated in persons with a history of Guillain-Barré syndrome, multiple sclerosis, autoimmune disease, or other chronic conditions. Pregnancy is also not a contraindication to vaccination.

Adverse Effects

The overall rate of adverse effects is low, with minor effects reported, including fever (1–6%) and pain at the injection site (3–29%). There is no evidence of an association between vaccination and sudden infant death syndrome, multiple sclerosis, autoimmune disease, or chronic fatigue syndrome.

Postexposure Prophylaxis

Postexposure prophylaxis is indicated for unvaccinated persons with perinatal, sexual, household, percutaneous, or mucosal exposure to hepatitis B. When prophylaxis is indicated, unvaccinated individuals should receive HBIg (0.06 mL/kg) and the first dose of HepB at a separate anatomic site. For sexual contact or household blood exposure to an acute case of hepatitis B, HBIg and HepB should be given. Sexual and household contacts of someone with chronic infection should receive HepB (but not HBIg). For individuals with percutaneous or permucosal exposure to blood, HepB should be given, and HBIg considered depending on the HBsAg status of the person who was the source of the blood and on the vaccination response status of the exposed person. All previously vaccinated persons exposed to hepatitis B should be retested for anti-HBs. If antibody levels are adequate (≥ 10 mIU/mL), no treatment is necessary. If levels are inadequate and the exposure was to HBsAg-positive blood, HBIg and vaccination are required.

Antibody Preparations

HBIg is prepared from HIV-negative and hepatitis C virus negative donors with high titers of hepatitis B surface antibody. The process used to prepare this product inactivates or eliminates any undetected HIV and hepatitis C virus. The uses of HBIg are described earlier in this section.

CDC: A comprehensive immunization strategy to eliminate transmission of hepatitis B virus infection in the United States, part 1: Immunization of infants, children, and adolescents. MMWR Recomm Rep 2005;54(RR-16):1 [PMID: 16371945].

Goldstein ST et al: A mathematical model to estimate global hepatitis B disease burden and vaccination impact. Int J Epidemiol 2005;34:1329 [PMID: 16249217].

Shepard CW et al: Epidemiology of hepatitis B and hepatitis B virus infection in United States children. Pediatr Infect Dis J 2005;24:755 [PMID: 16148839].

Shepard CW et al: Hepatitis B virus infection: Epidemiology and vaccination. Epidemiol Rev 2006;28:112 [PMID: 16754644].

Wasley A et al: Surveillance for acute viral hepatitis—United States, 2005. MMWR Surveill Summ 2007;56:1 [PMID: 17363893].

ROTAVIRUS VACCINATION

Rotavirus is the leading cause of hospitalization and death from acute gastroenteritis in young children worldwide. The burden of rotavirus is particularly severe in the developing world, where as many as 500,000 children die each year from rotavirus-associated dehydration and other complications. While deaths from rotavirus are uncommon in the United States (20–60 deaths per year), rotavirus infections cause substantial morbidity: annually, rotavirus causes an estimated 2.7 million diarrheal illnesses, 500,000 office visits, and 55,000–70,000 hospitalizations.

The first licensed rotavirus vaccine (RotaShield), was developed from virus strains isolated from rhesus monkeys. Shortly after its licensure in 1998, the vaccine was found to be associated with intussusception at an estimated rate of 1 case per 10,000 vaccine recipients. Because of this association, the vaccine was withdrawn from the U.S. market in October 1999. Using other parent rotavirus strains, substantial efforts continued to develop safe and effective rotavirus vaccines. In February 2006, a human-bovine reassortant rotavirus vaccine (RotaTeq) was licensed for use in the United States. Soon after licensure, the ACIP recommended the administration of rotavirus vaccine to all infants at 2, 4, and 6 months of age. The vaccine is highly effective, with the three-dose series demonstrating 98% efficacy at preventing severe rotavirus gastroenteritis and 74% at preventing any rotavirus gastroenteritis.

Prior to the licensure of RotaTeq, a large-scale randomized controlled trial of more than 70,000 infants was conducted specifically to evaluate the risk of intussusception following vaccination. The study had adequate statistical power to detect clinical events as uncommon as those seen after RotaShield vaccination. In this study, no increased risk of intussusception or other serious adverse events was seen in vaccine recipients compared with infants who received a placebo.

Concern has been expressed that some health care providers and parents may be reluctant to use the new rotavirus vaccine, either because of the withdrawal of the first rotavirus vaccine or because of the perception that the burden of rotavirus in the United States does not justify vaccination. Several important considerations should alleviate these concerns. Because RotaTeq was developed using fundamentally different techniques than the prior rotavirus vaccine, intussusception following vaccination should not be anticipated on theoretical grounds. The large size of prelicensure vaccine trials provides additional reassuring data about vaccine safety. Further, the safety of this vaccine is continuously monitored through a number of mechanisms such as the VSD project and VAERS. Finally, while rotavirus infection is an uncommon cause of death in the United States, thousands of hospitalizations could be prevented through vaccination.

Vaccine Available

There is currently a single rotavirus vaccine licensed in the United States, a human-bovine reassortant vaccine (RotaTeq, manufactured by Merck). The vaccine contains five reassorted virus types, each with human- and bovine-derived components, suspended in a buffered solution that does not contain thimerosal or other preservatives.

Dosage & Schedule of Administration

Rotavirus vaccine is a liquid vaccine given by mouth and should never be given by any other route of administration. Each 2-mL dose is dispensed in a squeezable plastic tube with a twist-off cap. Infants readily swallow the vaccine in most circumstances; however, if an infant spits up or vomits after a dose is administered, the dose should not be readministered; the infant can receive the remaining doses at the normal intervals.

Infants should be given rotavirus vaccine at approximately 2, 4, and 6 months of age. The first dose should be given between 6 and 12 weeks of age, subsequent doses should be given between 4 and 10 weeks after the preceding dose, and all three doses should be given by 32 weeks of age. The first dose should not be given to infants older than 12 weeks of age, and no doses should be given to infants older than 32 weeks of age. The vaccination schedule for rotavirus vaccine is more restrictive than for other routinely recommended vaccines for infants because some, although not all, studies of the prior rhesus-based vaccine suggested that the risk of intussusception following vaccination increased with increasing age.

Contraindications & Precautions

Rotavirus vaccine should not be given to infants with a severe hypersensitivity to any components of the vaccine, or to infants who had a serious allergic reaction to a previous dose of the vaccine. Theoretical concerns exist that giving rotavirus vaccine to infants with acute, moderate to severe gastroenteritis will reduce the immunogenicity of the vaccine. Vaccination should therefore be deferred in this circumstance until the gastroenteritis has improved. Limited data suggest that rotavirus vaccination is safe and effective in premature infants. However, vaccine safety and efficacy in infants with immunocompromising conditions, preexisting chronic gastrointestinal conditions (eg, Hirschsprung disease or short-gut syndrome), or a prior episode of intussus-

ception, has not been established. Clinicians should weigh the risks and benefits of vaccination in such circumstances. Infants living in households with pregnant women or immunocompromised persons can be vaccinated. To minimize the risk of vaccine virus transmission, good hand hygiene should be used when changing the vaccinated infant's diapers.

▶ Adverse Effects

In several large randomized controlled trials, no serious adverse events were associated with rotavirus vaccination, including no increase in rates of intussusception. Rates of vomiting and diarrhea were 1–3% higher in vaccine recipients than in placebo recipients. Rates of fever, irritability, and hematochezia were similar between vaccine and placebo recipients.

Any unexpected or clinically significant event occurring after rotavirus vaccination should be reported to VAERS (http://www.vaers.hhs.gov). There have been cases of intussusception reported to VAERS after rotavirus vaccination, but the rate of such cases was not increased above that expected by chance alone.

CDC: Postmarketing monitoring of intussusception after RotaTeq vaccination—United States, February 1, 2006–February 15, 2007. MMWR Morb Mortal Wkly Rep 2007;56:218 [PMID: 17363890]

CDC: Prevention of rotavirus gastroenteritis among infants and children. MMWR Recomm Rep 2006;55(RR-12):1 [PMID: 16902398].

Kempe A et al: Will pediatricians adopt the new rotavirus vaccine? Pediatrics 2007;119:1 [PMID: 17200265].

Tai JH et al: Rotavirus vaccination and intussusception: Can we decrease temporally associated background cases of intussusception by restricting the vaccination schedule? Pediatrics 2006;118:e258 [PMID: 16882770].

Vesikari T et al: Safety and efficacy of a pentavalent human-bovine (WC3) reassortant rotavirus vaccine. N Engl J Med 2006;354:23 [PMID: 16394299].

DIPHTHERIA-TETANUS-ACELLULAR PERTUSSIS VACCINATION

Diphtheria, tetanus, and pertussis vaccines (DTP vaccines) have been given together in a combined vaccine for many decades, and have led to dramatic reductions in each of these diseases. The efficacy of the combined vaccine is similar to that of individual preparations. For many decades the pertussis component of DTP vaccines contained a whole-cell pertussis vaccine, and this vaccine is still used widely in the world. DTP vaccine has been replaced in the United States entirely with DTaP vaccines, which are acellular pertussis vaccines made with purified, inactivated components of the bacterium.

Diphtheria is caused by a gram-positive bacillus, *Corynebacterium diphtheriae*. It is a toxin-mediated disease, with diphtheria toxin causing local tissue destruction, as in pharyngeal and tonsillar diphtheria, as well as systemic disease, particularly myocarditis and neuritis. The overall case fatality rate is between 5% and 10%, with higher death rates in persons younger than 5 years or older than 40 years of age. As many as 200,000 cases of diphtheria occurred each year in the 1920s in the United States. Largely because of successful vaccination programs, only 5 cases of diphtheria have been reported in the United States since 2000. In the last several decades, the majority of diphtheria cases in the United States have been in unimmunized or inadequately immunized persons. The clinical efficacy of diphtheria vaccine is not precisely known but has been estimated to be greater than 95%.

The anaerobic gram-positive rod *Clostridium tetani* causes tetanus, usually through infection of a contaminated wound. When *C tetani* colonizes devitalized tissue, the exotoxin tetanospasmin is disseminated to inhibitory motor neurons, resulting in generalized rigidity and spasms of skeletal muscles. Tetanus-prone wounds include (1) puncture wounds, including those acquired due to body piercing, tattooing, and intravenous drug abuse; (2) animal bites; (3) lacerations and abrasions; and (4) wounds resulting from nonsterile delivery and umbilical cord care (neonatal tetanus). In persons who have completed the primary vaccination series and have received a booster dose within the past 10 years, vaccination is virtually 100% protective. In 2005, the last year for which data are available, 27 cases of tetanus occurred in the United States, with no cases of neonatal tetanus.

Pertussis is also primarily a toxin-mediated disease. Called whooping cough because of the high-pitched inspiratory whoop that can follow intense paroxysms of cough, pertussis is caused by the bacterium *Bordetella pertussis*. Complications from pertussis include death, often from associated pneumonia, seizures, and encephalopathy. Sixty-six deaths from pertussis were reported to the CDC in 2004–2005; 85% were in children 3 months of age or younger. Prior to the widespread use of pertussis vaccines in the 1940s, roughly 1 million pertussis cases were reported over a 6-year period. Pertussis incidence in the United States declined dramatically between the 1940s and 1980s, but beginning in the early 1980s incidence has been slowly increasing, with adolescents and adults accounting for a greater proportion of reported cases. A single booster dose of a different formulation, Tdap, is now recommended for all adolescents and adults, as discussed in more detail later in this chapter. Providing a booster dose of pertussis-containing vaccine should prevent adolescent and adult pertussis cases, but also has the potential to reduce the spread of pertussis to infants, who are most susceptible to complications from the disease.

▶ Vaccines Available

Diphtheria, Tetanus, and Pertussis Combinations

1. DTaP (Daptacel, Sanofi Pasteur) contains tetanus toxoid, diphtheria toxoid, and acellular pertussis vaccine. This DTaP is licensed for ages 6 weeks through 6 years and can be used for doses 1–5.

2. DTaP (Infanrix, GlaxoSmithKline) contains tetanus toxoid, diphtheria toxoid, and acellular pertussis vaccine. This DTaP is licensed for ages 6 weeks through 6 years and can be used for doses 1–5.

3. DTaP (Tripedia, Sanofi Pasteur) contains tetanus toxoid, diphtheria toxoid, and acellular pertussis vaccine. This DTaP is licensed for ages 6 weeks through 6 years and can be used for doses 1–5.

4. Tdap (Boostrix, GlaxoSmithKline) is a tetanus-diphtheria-acellular pertussis vaccine formulated for adolescents aged 10–18 years.

5. Tdap (Adacel, Sanofi Pasteur) is a tetanus-diphtheria-acellular pertussis vaccine for persons aged 11–64 years.

DTaP Combined with Other Vaccines

1. DTaP-Hib (TriHIBit, Sanofi Pasteur) contains a Hib vaccine reconstituted with Tripedia. It is licensed for the fourth dose of the DTaP and Hib vaccination series, but not for doses 1–3.

2. DTaP-IPV-Hepatitis B (Pediarix, GlaxoSmithKline) contains DTaP combined with polio and HepB. It is approved for doses at 2, 4, and 6 months of age. Although it is approved for use through age 6 years, it is not licensed for booster doses. It cannot be used, for example, as the fourth dose of DTaP (the dose typically given at 15–18 months of age).

Diphtheria and Tetanus Combinations

1. DT (generic, Sanofi Pasteur) contains tetanus toxoid and diphtheria toxoid to be used only in children younger than age 7 years with a contraindication to pertussis vaccination.

2. Td (Decavac, Sanofi Pasteur) contains tetanus toxoid and a reduced quantity of diphtheria toxoid, which is typically used for adults requiring tetanus prophylaxis.

3. Td (generic, Massachusetts Biological Labs) contains tetanus toxoid and a reduced quantity of diphtheria toxoid, which is typically used for adults requiring tetanus prophylaxis.

Tetanus Only

TT (generic, Sanofi Pasteur) contains tetanus toxoid only, and can be used for adults or children.

▶ Dosage & Schedule of Administration

Although several different vaccines are available, a few general considerations can help guide their use in specific circumstances. DTaP (alone or combined with other vaccines) is used for infants and children between 6 weeks and 6 years of age. There is no pertussis-containing vaccine licensed for children aged 7–9 years, so Td is used for this age group when tetanus or diphtheria vaccination is needed. For adolescents and adults, a single dose of Tdap is used, followed by booster doses of Td every 10 years; a detailed description of its use is provided later in this chapter.

The primary series of DTaP vaccination should consist of four doses, given at 2, 4, 6, and 15–18 months of age. The fourth dose may be given as early as 12 months of age if 6 months have elapsed since the third dose. Giving the fourth dose between 12 and 15 months of age is indicated if the provider thinks the child is unlikely to return for a clinic visit between 15 and 18 months of age. Children should receive a fifth dose of DTaP at 4–6 years of age. However, a fifth dose of DTaP is not needed if the fourth dose was given after the child's fourth birthday. The same brand of DTaP should be used for all doses if feasible.

▶ Contraindications & Precautions

DTaP vaccines should not be used in individuals who have had an anaphylactic-type reaction to a previous vaccine dose or to a vaccine component. DTaP should not be given to children who developed encephalopathy not attributable to another identified cause within 7 days of a previous dose of DTaP or DTP. DTaP vaccination should also be deferred in individuals with progressive neurologic disorders, such as infantile spasms, uncontrolled epilepsy, or progressive encephalopathy, until their neurologic status is clarified and stabilized.

Precautions to DTaP vaccination include: high fever ($\geq 40.5°F$), persistent inconsolable crying, or shocklike state within 48 hours of a previous dose of DTP or DTaP; seizures within 3 days of a previous dose of DTP or DTaP; Guillain-Barré syndrome less than 6 weeks after a previous tetanus-containing vaccine; or moderate or severe acute illness with or without a fever.

▶ Adverse Effects

Local reactions, fever, and other mild systemic effects occur with one-fourth to two-thirds the frequency noted following whole-cell DTP vaccination. Moderate to severe systemic effects, including fever of 40.5°C, persistent inconsolable crying lasting 3 hours or more, and hypotonic-hyporesponsive episodes, are less frequent than with whole-cell DTP. These are without sequelae. Severe neurologic effects have not been temporally associated with DTaP vaccinations in use in the United States. A recent study from Canada showed no evidence of encephalopathy related to pertussis vaccine (< 1 case per 3 million doses of DTP and < 1 per 3.5 million doses of DTaP). Data are limited regarding differences in reactogenicity among currently licensed acellular pertussis vaccines. With all currently licensed DTaP vaccines, reports of the frequency and magnitude of substantial local reactions at injection sites have increased with increasing dose number (including swelling of the thigh or entire upper arm after receipt of the fourth and fifth doses).

▶ Diphtheria Antibody Preparations

Diphtheria antitoxin, manufactured in horses, is available for the treatment of diphtheria. Dosage depends on the size and location of the diphtheritic membrane and an estimate of the patient's level of intoxication. Sensitivity to diphtheria antitoxin must be tested before it is given. Consultation on the use of diphtheria antitoxin is available from the CDC's National Center for Immunization and Respiratory Diseases (formerly the National Immunization Program). Diphtheria antitoxin is not commercially available in the United States and must be obtained from the CDC.

▶ Tetanus Antibody Preparations

Human tetanus immune globulin (TIg) is indicated in the management of tetanus-prone wounds in individuals who have had an uncertain number or fewer than three tetanus immunizations. Persons fully immunized with at least three doses do not require TIg, regardless of the nature of their wounds (Table 9–5). The optimal dose of TIg has not been established, but some sources recommend 3000–5000 units as a single dose, with part of the dose infiltrated around the wound.

CDC: Diphtheria. In Atkinson J et al (editors): *Epidemiology and Prevention of Vaccine-Preventable Diseases,* 10th ed. Public Health Foundation, 2007:59.

CDC: Summary of notifiable diseases—United States, 2005. MMWR Morb Mortal Wkly Rep 2007;54:1 [PMID: 17392681].

CDC: Tetanus. In Atkinson J et al (editors): *Epidemiology and Prevention of Vaccine-Preventable Diseases,* 10th ed. Public Health Foundation, 2007:71.

Moore DL et al: Lack of evidence of encephalopathy related to pertussis vaccine: Active surveillance by IMPACT, Canada, 1993–2002. Pediatr Infect Dis J 2004;23:568 [PMID: 15194842].

Munoz FM. Pertussis in infants, children, and adolescents: Diagnosis, treatment, and prevention. Semin Pediatr Infect Dis 2006;17:14 [PMID: 16522501].

Pichichero ME et al: Immunogenicity and safety of a combination diphtheria, tetanus toxoid, acellular pertussis, hepatitis B, and inactivated poliovirus vaccine coadministered with a 7-valent pneumococcal conjugate vaccine and a Haemophilus influenzae type b conjugate vaccine. J Pediatr 2007;151:43 [PMID: 17586189].

HAEMOPHILUS INFLUENZAE TYPE B VACCINATION

H influenzae type b (Hib) causes a wide spectrum of serious bacterial illnesses, particularly in young children, including meningitis, epiglottitis, pneumonia, septic arthritis, and cellulitis. Before the introduction of effective vaccines, Hib was the leading cause of invasive bacterial disease in children younger than 5 years of age in the United States. Nearly all Hib disease occurred in this age group, and roughly two thirds of cases occurred in children younger than 18 months of age.

Hib bacteria are surrounded by a polysaccharide capsule (polyribosyl ribitol phosphate [PRP]) that contributes to virulence, and antibodies to this polysaccharide confer immunity to the disease. A polysaccharide-only Hib vaccine was first licensed in the United States in 1985, but the polysaccharide was not strongly immunogenic, did not

Table 9–5. Recommendations for the use of tetanus prophylaxis after a wound.

History of Tetanus Toxoid–containing Vaccine[a]	Clean, Minor Wounds		All Other Wounds	
	DT, Td, or Tdap[b]	TIg	DT, Td, or Tdap[b]	TIg
< 3 doses or unknown vaccine status[a]	Yes	No	Yes	Yes
≥ 3 doses and 5–9 y since last tetanus toxoid–containing vaccine[c]	No	No	Yes[d]	No
≥ 3 doses and > 10 y since last tetanus toxoid–containing vaccine[c]	Yes[c]	No	Yes[c]	No

[a]For infants younger than age 6 months who have not received 3 doses of tetanus-containing vaccine, use maternal tetanus immunization history at the time of delivery and apply the guidelines in the table above.
[b]Age-appropriate tetanus-containing vaccines should be given. Children younger than age 7 years should receive DTaP or DT. Tdap is preferred (over Td) for adolescents who have never previously received Tdap. Tdap is licensed for 1 dose only. In adolescents who have *previously* received a dose of Tdap and who need additional tetanus toxoid–containing vaccine, Td should be used.
[c]Persons who have received at least 3 doses of tetanus toxoid–containing vaccines but have not received a tetanus toxoid-containing vaccine for more than 10 years should receive an age-appropriate tetanus toxoid–containing vaccine regardless of the nature of the wound.
[d]Persons who received at least 3 doses of tetanus toxoid–containing vaccines but have not received a tetanus toxoid–containing vaccine for more than 5 years, should receive an age-appropriate tetanus toxoid–containing vaccine unless the wounds are clean and minor.
Recommendations based on American Academy of Pediatrics: Tetanus. In Pickering LK et al (editors): *Red Book, 2006 Report of the Committee on Infectious Diseases,* 27th ed. American Academy of Pediatrics, 2006:650.

induce long-term immune memory, and the vaccine was not effective in children younger than 18 months of age. However, when Hib polysaccharide was chemically bonded (conjugated) to certain protein carriers, the conjugate induced T-cell dependent immune memory and was highly effective in young children. All current Hib vaccines are based on this polysaccharide-protein conjugate technology.

Precisely describing the epidemiology of invasive Hib disease is difficult because bacterial serotyping is required to differentiate Hib-caused infections from those caused by other encapsulated and nonencapsulated *H influenzae* species. However, it has been estimated that roughly 20,000 cases of invasive Hib disease occurred each year in the United States in the early 1980s. Since the introduction of Hib vaccines, disease incidence has declined by more than 99%.

In the United States in 2005, the year from which most recent data are available, 9 cases of invasive Hib disease occurred in children younger than age 5 years. An additional 217 cases were caused by *H influenzae* species in which the serotype was not reported. In recent years, most cases of Hib disease occurred in unvaccinated or partially vaccinated children, including children younger than 6 months of age who were too young to have completed the primary vaccination series.

Vaccines Available

Four vaccines against Hib disease are available in the United States; two are Hib-only vaccines, and two are combination vaccines. Each vaccine contains Hib polysaccharide conju-

gated to a protein carrier, but different protein carriers are used. The Hib conjugate vaccine that uses a meningococcal outer membrane protein carrier is abbreviated PRP-OMP; and PRP-T vaccine uses a tetanus toxoid carrier.

1. Hib (PedvaxHIB, uses PRP-OMP, Merck).
2. Hib (ActHIB, uses PRP-T, Sanofi Pasteur).
3. DTaP-Hib (TriHIBit, uses PRP-T reconstituted with Tripedia brand of DTaP, Sanofi Pasteur).
4. Hepatitis B-Hib (Comvax, uses PRP-OMP, Merck).

Dosage & Schedule of Administration

Hib vaccination is routinely recommended for all infants in the United States. The vaccine dose is 0.5 mL given intramuscularly. As shown in Table 9–6, the vaccination schedule depends on which type of Hib vaccine is used. The recommended interval between doses in the primary series is 8 weeks, but a minimal interval of 4 weeks is permitted. For infants who missed the primary vaccination series, a catch-up schedule is used (see Table 9–3). Hib vaccine is not generally recommended for children 5 years of age or older.

Contraindications & Precautions

Hib vaccine should not be given to anyone who has had a severe allergic reaction to a prior vaccine dose or to any vaccine components. Hib vaccine should not be given to infants before 6 weeks of age, since they appeared to develop immune tolerance and did not mount appropriate immune responses to subsequent doses.

Table 9–6. Schedule for *Haemophilus influenzae* type b (Hib) vaccination depending on type of protein conjugate used.

Conjugate Type	Trade Name	Age			
		2 Months	4 Months	6 Months	12–15 Months
PRP-T[a]	ActHIB, TriHIBit	Dose 1	Dose 2	Dose 3	Booster dose
PRP-OMP[b]	PedvaxHIB, Comvax[c]	Dose 1	Dose 2		Booster dose

[a]Tetanus toxoid carrier.
[b]Meningococcal outer membrane protein.
[c]See Table 9-4 for the use of Comvax in infants born to mothers with positive or unknown hepatitis B surface antigen status.

▶ Adverse Effects

Adverse reactions following Hib vaccination are uncommon. Between 5% and 30% of vaccine recipients experience swelling, redness, or pain at the vaccination site. Systemic reactions such as fever and irritability are rare.

CDC: *Haemophilus influenzae* type b. In Atkinson W et al (editors): *Epidemiology and Prevention of Vaccine-Preventable Diseases,* 10th ed. Public Health Foundation, 2007:115.
CDC: Progress toward elimination of *Haemophilus influenzae* type b invasive disease among infants and children—United States, 1998–2000. MMWR Morb Mortal Wkly Rep 2002;51:234 [PMID: 11925021].
Kelly DF et al: *Haemophilus influenzae* type b conjugate vaccines. Immunology 2004;113:163 [PMID: 15379976].

PNEUMOCOCCAL VACCINATION

Streptococcus pneumoniae is the most common cause of invasive bacterial infection in children, with most invasive disease occurring in children younger than age 2 years. Two kinds of vaccines are available in the United States against pneumococci: a 23-valent polysaccharide vaccine (PPV23) and a 7-valent protein-conjugated polysaccharide vaccine (PCV7). Clinical trials with extended spectrum vaccines include a 9-valent vaccine (in South Africa and the Gambia), an 11-valent vaccine (Philippines), and a 13-valent vaccine (Israel). The serotypes represented in available vaccines were chosen for their frequency in disease among adults (PPV23) or children in industrialized countries (PCV7). Additional serotypes needed in developing countries are included in the 9-, 11- and 13-valent vaccines. As in Hib vaccine, the carrier protein may be CRM 197, protein D of *H influenzae*, tetanus and diphtheria toxoids, or meningococcal outer membrane protein. Prior to the year 2000, only PPV23 was available in the United States. The efficacy of this vaccine was 57%; it was not effective in children younger than 2 years; and it was only indicated for certain high-risk children age 2 years or older.

The 7- and 9-valent pneumococcal conjugate vaccines have been evaluated for efficacy against invasive pneumococcal disease in four trials (in the United States, South Africa, the Gambia, and the Navajo Indian Nation). The pooled efficacy estimate from the first three vaccine trials was 93% (95% confidence interval [CI] 81% and 98%) against invasive disease caused by serotypes in the vaccine. Four studies (in the United States, South Africa, the Gambia, and the Philippines) have evaluated the impact of the vaccine on pneumonia, documenting 20–37% reduction in radiographically confirmed pneumonia. Several trials have evaluated the efficacy of pneumococcal conjugate vaccines against otitis media. Although two trials in Finland using 7-valent vaccines showed significant reduction in culture-confirmed pneumococcal otitis media caused by vaccine serotypes, there was no net reduction of otitis media in the vaccinated children. This was the result of an increase in the rates of otitis media due to nonvaccine types of pneumococci, *H influenzae* and *Moraxella catarrhalis*. However, a trial in Northern California showed that PCV7 had a protective effect against frequent otitis media. There was a 10% reduction in patients with 3 otitis-related visits and a 26% reduction in patients with 10 otitis-related visits within a 6-month period. Furthermore, otitis requiring tympanostomy tube placement was reduced by 24%. A trial of an 11-valent vaccine in the Czech Republic showed a vaccine efficacy of 58% against acute otitis media caused by the vaccine serotypes and a 34% reduction in acute otitis media overall. However, a trial in 383 Dutch children with recurrent acute otitis media showed no efficacy in this population. Finally, in the Gambian vaccine trial, which was conducted in a rural area where access to round-the-clock medical care was difficult, there was a 16% reduction in mortality.

Since the introduction of routine PCV7 immunization in the United States in 2000, dramatic direct and indirect effects have been seen. By 2005, the incidence of invasive disease due to vaccine-related serotypes declined by 90%. Not only has invasive pneumococcal disease due to vaccine serotypes in children declined, but invasive disease in adults and especially the elderly has also declined, with reductions in mortality. There have been reductions in other diseases (eg, otitis media and pneumonia), and a reduced rate of infection and colonization by antibiotic-resistant strains.

An unanticipated effect of the reduction in infection and colonization by vaccine serotypes in both vaccinated children and adults has been an increased prevalence of colonization and disease caused by nonvaccine strains of pneumococci (bacterial replacement). Overall in the United States, despite the changing prevalence of colonizing strains by vaccine serotypes, the slight increase in invasive pneumococcal disease due to nonvaccine strains has been overshadowed by the dramatic decline in disease caused by vaccine serotypes. One of the most common nonvaccine serotypes causing infections is serotype 19A. A recent study from Alaska (not yet replicated in other indigenous populations, such as the Navajo or aboriginal Australians) showed a dramatic decline in overall invasive pneumococcal disease (67% in Alaska Native children younger than 2 years between the prevaccine period and the 3 years after introduction of the vaccine). Subsequent to that, between 2004 and 2006, there has been an 82% increase in invasive pneumococcal disease in this population, caused by nonvaccine serotypes. Serotype 19A accounted for almost one third of the invasive pneumococcal disease in these children.

Universal immunization of all infants with PCV7 is now recommended, with four doses given at 2, 4, 6, and 12–15 months of age. Children aged 24–59 months at high risk of invasive pneumococcal disease should receive both the conjugate and polysaccharide vaccines (PCV7 and PPV23). Although definitive data about using PCV7 and PPV23 in combination are not available for invasive disease, it did reduce acute otitis media in one study. It is also known that immunization with PCV7 induces immunologic memory that is boosted by some of the serotypes in PPV23. Additionally, PPV23 provides coverage against a broader range of serotypes than does PCV7. Recommendations for using PPV23 in children older than 24 months are found in Table 9–7. Children at high risk of invasive pneumococcal disease include those with chronic cardiovascular, pulmonary (including cystic fibrosis but not asthma), and liver diseases; and those with anatomic and functional asplenia (including sickle cell disease), nephrotic syndrome, chronic renal failure, diabetes mellitus, cerebrospinal fluid leak, or immunosuppression (including those with HIV infection, complement deficiencies, malignancies, prolonged use of steroids, and organ transplants). Penicillin prophylaxis of patients with sickle cell disease should be continued regardless of vaccination with PCV7 or PPV23. Insufficient data are available to provide definitive recommendations for pneumococcal vaccination for immunocompromised children 5 years and older, but two doses of PCV7 and one dose of PPV23 was immunogenic and safe in HIV-infected children aged 2–19 years receiving highly active antiretroviral therapy. For children who had received hematopoietic stem cell transplantation, three doses of PCV7 were safe and immunogenic. For children aged 5–9 years at increased risk of invasive pneumococcal disease, providers can consider giving one dose each of PCV7 and PPV23, with PCV7 administered first, followed

Table 9–7. Recommendations for PPV23 immunization in children 2 years and older who have previously received PCV7.

Population	Initial Vaccination with PPV23	Revaccination with PPV23
Healthy children	Not recommended[a]	Not recommended
Children with sickle cell disease or anatomic or functional asplenia; immunocompromised; or HIV-infected	1 dose of PPV23 at 24 months of age or older, given at least 2 months after last dose of PCV7	Recommended[b]
Persons with chronic illness	1 dose of PPV23 at 24 months of age or older, given at least 2 months after last dose of PCV7	Not recommended

[a]PPV23 should be considered in Alaskan Native and American Indian children.
[b]For patients 10 years or younger, revaccination with PPV23 should occur 3–5 years after previous dose of PPV23; for patients older than 10 years, revaccination should occur 5 years or more after previous dose of PPV23. Reproduced, with permission, from CDC: Preventing pneumococcal disease among infants and young children. Recommendations of the Advisory Committee on Immunization Practices (ACIP). MMWR 2000;49(RR-9):1.

by PPV23 at least 8 weeks later. An additional PPV23 booster should be given 3–5 years later.

▶ Vaccines Available

The currently available PCV7 vaccine (Prevnar, Wyeth) is composed of seven purified capsular polysaccharides, each coupled to a nontoxic modified diphtheria toxin. Serotypes included in the vaccine and potentially cross-reacting serotypes accounted for 86% of bacteremia, 83% of meningitis, and 65% of acute otitis media cases caused by pneumococcus in the prevaccine era. The vaccine is licensed for use in children aged 6 weeks to 9 years.

PPV23 (Pneumovax 23, Merck) is only for use in persons 2 years and older. It contains 25 μg of each purified capsular polysaccharide antigen of 23 serotypes of pneumococcus. These 23 types cause 88% of cases of pneumococcal bacteremia and meningitis in adults and nearly 100% of those in children in the United States. Cross-reactive antibody responses may protect against an additional 8% of bacteremic serotypes in adults.

▶ Dosage & Schedule of Administration

PCV7 is given as a 0.5-mL intramuscular dose. The first dose can be given as early as 6 weeks of life, with a recommended vaccination schedule of 2, 4, 6, and 12–15 months. Children who receive their first dose of PCV7 at 7–11 months of age should receive two doses separated by at least 8 weeks, followed by a booster dose at 12–15 months. Children who receive their first dose of PCV7 at 12–23 months require two doses total, separated by 8 weeks. PCV7 may be given concurrently with the other routinely recommended childhood immunizations.

Children older than 23 months at high risk of invasive pneumococcal disease should receive both PCV7 and PPV23, as outlined in Table 9–7. PCV7 and PPV23 should not be given simultaneously, and when both are indicated, they should be given 8 weeks apart. The dose of PPV23 is 0.5 mL given intramuscularly. If splenectomy or immunosuppression can be anticipated, vaccination should be done at least 2 weeks beforehand. Revaccination with PPV23 may be considered after 3–5 years in children at high risk of fatal pneumococcal infection.

Contraindications & Precautions

For both PCV7 and PPV23, vaccination is contraindicated in individuals who suffered a severe allergic reaction such as anaphylaxis after a previous vaccine dose or to a vaccine component. PCV7 and PPV23 vaccination should be deferred during moderate or severe acute illness, with or without fever. A history of invasive pneumococcal disease is not a contraindication to vaccination.

Adverse Effects

The most common adverse effects associated with PCV7 administration are fever, induration, and tenderness at the injection site. When it is given simultaneously with DTaP, no increase in febrile seizures has been seen when compared with administration of DTaP alone.

With PPV23, 50% of vaccine recipients develop pain and redness at the injection site. Fewer than 1% develop systemic side effects such as fever and myalgia. Anaphylaxis is rare. Vaccine safety has not been evaluated during pregnancy.

Abzug MJ et al: Immunogenicity, safety, and predictors of response after a pneumococcal conjugate and pneumococcal polysaccharide vaccine series in human immunodeficiency virus-infected children receiving highly active antiretroviral therapy. Pediatr Infect Dis J 2006;25:920 [PMID: 17006288].

Grijalva CG et al: Decline in pneumonia admissions after routine childhood immunization with pneumococcal conjugate vaccine in the USA: A time-series analysis. Lancet 2007;369:1179 [PMID: 17416262].

Poehling KA et al: Invasive pneumococcal disease among infants before and after introduction of pneumococcal conjugate vaccine. JAMA 2006;295:1668 [PMID: 16609088].

Singleton RJ et al: Invasive pneumococcal disease caused by nonvaccine serotypes among Alaska Native children with high levels of 7-valent pneumococcal conjugate vaccine coverage. JAMA 2007;297:1784 [PMID: 17456820].

POLIOMYELITIS VACCINATION

Vaccines directed against poliovirus infections have eliminated the naturally occurring disease in industrialized countries. In the United States, the number of reported cases of paralytic poliomyelitis has fallen from more than 18,000 in 1954. In September 2005, four infections with a type 1 vaccine-derived poliovirus were recorded in unvaccinated Amish children in Minnesota, the first report in the United States since 2000, when OPV use was discontinued. Vaccine-derived pathogenic polioviruses can emerge from OPV, and be spread because of continuous replication in immunodeficient persons such as the index case in this outbreak, or by circulation in populations with low vaccine coverage. As of November, 2007, 735 confirmed wild-type poliovirus cases and 50 vaccine-derived poliovirus cases had been reported worldwide since the beginning of the year. This was three times the number of cases in 2003. Poliomyelitis is now endemic in India, Pakistan, Afghanistan, and Nigeria. In 2007 outbreaks following importation occurred in Niger, Chad, the Democratic Republic of Congo, Sudan, Angola, Somalia, and Myanmar.

An injectable poliovirus vaccine of enhanced potency, which has a higher content of antigens than the old IPV, is the only vaccine against poliomyelitis available in the United States since 2000. IPV is incapable of causing poliomyelitis by virtue of being inactivated, whereas OPV can do so rarely.

Completely immunized adult visitors to areas of continuing wild-type poliovirus circulation should receive a booster dose of IPV. Unimmunized or incompletely immunized adults and children should have received two (preferably three) doses of the vaccine prior to travel to these and other areas with circulation of wild-type or vaccine-type virus.

Vaccines Available

1. IPV (IPOL, Sanofi Pasteur) contains antigens of types 1, 2, and 3 poliovirus.
2. DTaP-HepB-IPV (Pediarix, GlaxoSmithKline) contains diphtheria and tetanus toxoids and acellular pertussis adsorbed, hepatitis B, and inactivated poliovirus vaccine.

Dosage & Schedule of Administration

IPV is administered in a dose of 0.5 mL subcutaneously. The DTaP-HepB-IPV combination vaccine can be used in the primary series at 2, 4, and 6 months, and can be used to complete the primary series. It can be administered with Hib and PCV7 vaccines at separate sites but is not approved for the fourth dose of IPV or the fourth and fifth doses of DTaP.

Contraindications & Precautions

IPV vaccination is contraindicated in individuals who suffered a severe allergic reaction such as anaphylaxis after a previous vaccine dose or to a vaccine component. IPV vaccination should be deferred during moderate or severe acute illness with or without fever. Pregnancy is also a precaution to IPV vaccination. Receipt of previous doses of OPV is not a contraindication to IPV.

Adverse Effects

IPV has essentially no adverse effects associated with it other than possible rare hypersensitivity reactions to trace quantities of antibiotics. The DTaP-HepB-IPV combination has similar rates of local and systemic adverse responses to three components administered separately except for fever, which is higher in the combination-vaccinated children.

CDC: Update on vaccine-derived polioviruses—worldwide, January 2006–August 2007. MMWR Morb Mortal Wkly Rep 2007;56:996 [PMID: 17898693].

Lahariya C: Global eradication of polio: The case for "finishing the job". Bull World Health Organ 2007;85:487 [PMID: 17639247].

Thompson KM et al: Eradication versus control for poliomyelitis: An economic analysis. Lancet. 2007;369:1363 [PMID: 17448822].

INFLUENZA VACCINATION

Influenza occurs each winter and early spring, often associated with significant morbidity and mortality in certain high-risk persons. Up to 36,000 deaths per year in the United States are attributable to influenza, and global epidemics (pandemics) can occur. The current threat of a global pandemic with the avian influenza virus (H5N1 strain) is very real, with greater than 300 cases by mid-2007 and a case fatality rate of 60%. Currently there is one vaccine available for the H5N1 virus and more vaccines may become available. Each year, recommendations are formulated in the spring and summer regarding the constituents of influenza vaccine for the coming season. These recommendations are based on the results of surveillance in Asia and the southern hemisphere during the spring and summer. The vaccine each year is a trivalent vaccine containing antigens from two strains of influenza A and one strain of influenza B, which are chosen as being likely to circulate in the United States during the upcoming winter. Children at high risk of seasonal influenza-related complications include those with hemoglobinopathies or with chronic cardiac, pulmonary (including asthma), metabolic, renal, and immunosuppressive diseases (including immunosuppression caused by medications or by HIV); and those with any condition (eg, cognitive dysfunction, spinal cord injuries, seizure disorders, or other neuromuscular disorders) that can compromise respiratory function, or the handling of respiratory secretions, or that can increase the risk of aspiration. Children and adolescents receiving long-term aspirin therapy are also at risk of influenza-related Reye syndrome. Healthy children aged 6–23 months are at substantially increased risk of influenza-related hospitalizations, and children aged 24–59 months (ie, 2–4 years) are at increased risk of influenza-related clinic and emergency department visits.

Annual influenza vaccination is indicated for all children older than 6 months of age who have a chronic health condition that increases their risk of complications from influenza infection. Annual vaccination is now routinely recommended for all children aged 6–59 months. Members (including other children) of households with persons in high-risk groups and with children younger than age 5 years should also be immunized. Physicians should identify high-risk children in their practices and encourage parents to seek influenza vaccination for them as soon as influenza vaccine is available. In pandemic years, it may be important to advocate vaccination of all children regardless of their usual state of health and in particular school-aged children who are often the epicenter of outbreaks within the community. Influenza prevention may also help prevent lower respiratory tract disease or other secondary complications in high-risk groups, thereby decreasing hospitalizations and deaths.

Vaccines Available

The trivalent inactivated influenza vaccine virus (TIV) is grown in eggs, formalin-inactivated, and may contain trace quantities of thimerosal as a preservative. Only split-virus or purified surface antigen preparations are available in the United States. Several manufacturers produce similar vaccines each year. Fluzone split-virus (Sanofi Pasteur) is approved for children 6 months and older; Fluvirin (Chiron) is approved only for children 4 years and older. Additional manufacturers (GlaxoSmithKline, CSL Biotherapies, ID Biomedical Corporation) produce influenza vaccines approved for adults.

To eliminate the need for injections, and potentially to enhance mucosal and systemic immune response to vaccination, a live attenuated intranasal vaccine has been developed. This vaccine is cold-adapted, and temperature-sensitive. These viruses replicate poorly in the lower respiratory tract, but well in the nasal mucosa (thereby producing immunity). The intranasal trivalent live attenuated influenza virus vaccine (LAIV) (FluMist, MedImmune) is also produced in a trivalent formulation using the virus strains present in the inactivated vaccine. It is also made in eggs and comes in a single-use prefilled sprayer that should be stored refrigerated at 2–8°C.

Dosage & Schedule of Administration

A. Inactivated Influenza Virus Vaccine

Because influenza can circulate yearly from November through early March in the United States, the key time to initiate vaccination is as soon as vaccine is available in the early fall. However, providers should continue vaccinating individuals as long as vaccine is available and there is still influenza activity in the community. Children younger than age 6 months should not be immunized. Two doses are recommended for children younger than age 9 years who are receiving influenza vaccine for the first time; subsequent seasons require single doses. Older children receiving vaccine for the first time require only a single dose. The dose for children aged 6–35 months is 0.25 mL given intramuscularly; for older children the dose is 0.5 mL given intramuscularly. The recommended site of vaccination is the anterolateral aspect of the thigh for younger children and the deltoid for older children. Pregnancy is not a contraindication to use of inactivated vaccine, and vaccine is recommended for all pregnant women and those contemplating pregnancy during the influenza season. Simultaneous administration with other routine vaccinations is acceptable.

B. Live Attenuated Influenza Virus Vaccine

This vaccine is supplied in a prefilled single-use sprayer containing 0.2 mL of the vaccine, approximately half of which is sprayed into each nostril. A dose divider clip is provided to assist in dividing the dose. If the patient sneezes during administration, the dose should not be repeated. It can be administered to children with minor illnesses, but should not be given if significant nasal congestion is present. Because it is a live vaccine it should be administered 48 hours after cessation of therapy in children receiving anti-influenza antiviral drugs, and antivirals should not be given for 2 weeks after vaccination. Unvaccinated children aged 2–8 years should receive two doses of vaccine 4 weeks apart, and one dose is required for previously vaccinated children aged 2–8, or any older individuals 9–49 years of age.

► Contraindications & Precautions

A. Inactivated Influenza Virus Vaccine

TIV is contraindicated in individuals with history of hypersensitivity to eggs or egg proteins, or with life-threatening reactions to previous influenza vaccinations. For patients with anaphylactic egg allergies in whom influenza vaccination is indicated, a protocol for influenza vaccination is referenced later in this chapter.

B. Live Attenuated Influenza Virus Vaccine

LAIV is contraindicated in individuals with history of hypersensitivity to eggs, egg proteins, gentamicin, gelatin, or arginine, or with life-threatening reactions to previous influenza vaccinations, and in children and adolescents receiving concomitant aspirin or aspirin-containing therapy. LAIV should not be administered to the following persons: (1) children younger than 24 months of age, because of an increased risk of hospitalization and wheezing that was observed in clinical trials; (2) any individual with asthma or children younger than age 5 years with recurrent wheezing unless the potential benefit outweighs the potential risk; or (3) individuals with severe asthma or active wheezing.

► Adverse Effects

A. Inactivated Influenza Virus Vaccine

Injection site reactions are the most common adverse events after TIV administration. A small proportion of children will experience some systemic toxicity, consisting of fever, malaise, and myalgias. These symptoms generally begin 6–12 hours after vaccination and may last 24–48 hours. Cases of

Guillain-Barré syndrome followed the swine influenza vaccination program in 1976–1977, but careful study by the Institute of Medicine showed no association with that vaccine in children and young adults—nor in any age group that received vaccines in subsequent years.

B. Live Attenuated Influenza Virus Vaccine

The most common adverse reactions (occurring at ≥ 10% in individuals receiving LAIV and at least 5% greater than in placebo) are runny nose or nasal congestion in recipients of all ages and fever higher than 37.7°C in children 2–6 years of age. These reactions were reported more frequently with the first dose and were all self-limited. Antiviral therapy should not be administered until 2 weeks after LAIV unless medically necessary and health care providers should wait 48 hours after cessation of antiviral therapy before administering LAIV.

AAP Committee on Infectious Diseases: Prevention of influenza: Recommendations for influenza immunization of children, 2006–2007. Pediatrics 2007;119:846 [PMID:17403861].

Beigel JH et al: Avian influenza A (H5N1) infection in humans. N Engl J Med 2005;353:1374 [PMID: 16192482].

CDC: Prevention and control of influenza. Recommendations of the Advisory Committee on Immunization Practices (ACIP). MMWR Recomm Rep 2007;56(RR-6): 1 [PMID:17625497].

Jefferson T et al: Assessment of the efficacy and effectiveness of influenza vaccines in healthy children: systematic review. Lancet 2005;365:773 [PMID: 15733718].

Prosser LA et al: Health benefits, risks, and cost-effectiveness of influenza vaccination of children. Emerg Infect Dis 2006;12:1548 [PMID:17176570].

MEASLES, MUMPS, & RUBELLA VACCINATION

In the 20 years after the 1963 introduction of measles vaccination in the United States, the annual number of reported cases decreased from 500,000 to fewer than 1500. However, between 1989 and 1991 there was a resurgence of measles, with 50,000 cases reported. The major reasons for the increase in cases and the resulting deaths were failure to provide vaccine to preschool children aged 15 months or older, the presence in the community of susceptible children younger than age 15 months, and the growing number of appropriately vaccinated, but nonimmune individuals (2–10% primary vaccine failures) in schools and colleges. These reasons led to recommendations for a two-dose vaccination schedule at 12–15 months and at 4–6 years of age.

In the United States, after the introduction of mumps vaccine in 1967 and the recommendation for its use in 1977, there was a 99% decline in mumps from 185,691 cases reported in 1968 to fewer than 300 cases each year between 2001 and 2003. However, between 2005 and 2006, there was a large multistate outbreak of mumps with almost 6000 confirmed or probable mumps cases reported to the CDC. Six states—Iowa, Kansas, Wisconsin, Illinois, Nebraska, and South Dakota—recorded 85% of the cases. This outbreak occurred mostly on college campuses, but also involved high schools and middle schools. Several factors may have contributed to the outbreaks: conditions on college and high school campuses may be conducive to spread of respiratory infections; two doses of MMR vaccine may not be 100% effective in preventing mumps and even less effective in preventing asymptomatic infection; and waning immunity may have occurred in young adults who had last received mumps-containing vaccine 6–17 years earlier.

Although these outbreaks have not changed the recommendations for two doses of MMR vaccination for all children, in May 2006 the ACIP redefined evidence of immunity to mumps as follows: one dose of a live mumps virus vaccine for preschool children and adults not at high risk; and two doses for children in grades K–12 and adults at high risk (health care workers, international travelers, and students at post–high school level educational facilities). Other evidence of immunity is birth before 1957, documentation of physician-diagnosed mumps, or laboratory evidence of immunity. The ACIP recommended that health care facilities should consider recommending one dose of MMR vaccine to unvaccinated health workers born before 1957 who do not have other evidence of mumps immunity, and two doses of MMR during a mumps outbreak. The Iowa Department of Public Health curtailed the epidemic by successively introducing mumps vaccine into counties with the largest colleges and universities, expanding vaccination to the whole state, and finally vaccinating adults up to age 46 years.

The use of rubella vaccine is not intended to protect individuals from rubella infection, but rather to prevent the serious consequences of rubella infection during pregnancy: miscarriage, fetal demise, and congenital rubella syndrome. Congenital rubella syndrome is a group of birth defects including deafness, cataracts, heart defects, and mental retardation. In the United States and the United Kingdom, the approach has been to vaccinate young children. The intent is to reduce transmission to susceptible women of childbearing age via a herd immunity effect. Immunity lasts for at least 15 years. With the use of rubella vaccines since 1970, rubella incidence rates have declined more than 99%. However, approximately 10% of young adults are now susceptible to rubella. Rubella is rare in the United States. Currently most cases of rubella are seen in foreign-born adults, and outbreaks have occurred in poultry and meat processing plants that employ many foreign-born workers. Similarly, almost all infants with congenital rubella syndrome are born to foreign-born mothers.

Recently, reports in the medical and lay press have suggested a possible association between MMR vaccination, autism, and gastrointestinal inflammation. The initial reports have been refuted because of the limited number of patients studied, methods of case and control selection, the laboratory evaluations employed, and means of determining developmental regression. Several large epidemiologic studies subsequently found no association between MMR vaccination and either autism or bowel inflammation. Also, no evidence has been found to support the need for separate administration of measles, mumps, and rubella vaccines (as opposed to the MMR combination). However, the influence of the lay press in the United Kingdom may have contributed to low vaccination rates with measles vaccine, which has resulted in a resurgence of measles.

▶ Vaccines Available

1. Measles-only vaccine (Attenuvax, Merck): The Moraten strain is a live attenuated vaccine derived from the Edmonston B strain after multiple passages in chick embryo tissue culture.

2. Mumps-only vaccine (Mumpsvax, Merck): The Jeryl Lynn Strain is the only mumps vaccine available in the United States. It is prepared from a clinical isolate passaged in embryonated eggs and in chick embryo tissue culture.

3. Rubella-only vaccine (Meruvax II, Merck): The RA 27/3 strain is the only vaccine available in the United States. It is grown in human diploid cells. The RA 27/3 strain is available as a monovalent vaccine, in combined preparations with measles vaccine, or in measles and mumps vaccines. In most circumstances, MMR or MMRV vaccination is the recommended means of immunizing against rubella.

4. Measles-mumps-rubella (MMR II, Merck)

5. MMRV: In September 2005 the FDA licensed a combined live attenuated measles, mumps, rubella, and varicella vaccine (ProQuad, Merck) for use in children 1–12 years of age. It is identical in composition to MMR with the exception that the varicella component is five times more potent than in the varicella-only (VAR) vaccine. Concomitant administration of MMRV, DTaP, Hib, and HepB vaccines showed that the immune responses to all the antigens when administered simultaneously were comparable to sequential administration of MMRV and the other antigens.

▶ Dosage & Schedule of Administration

A. Routine Vaccination

Measles, mumps and rubella vaccinations should be given as MMRV or MMR at 12–15 months and again at 4–6 years of age. MMRV is the preferred vaccine if available. A dose of 0.5 mL should be given subcutaneously. The second dose of MMRV or MMR is recommended at school entry to help prevent school-based measles and mumps outbreaks. Children not reimmunized at school entry should receive their second dose by age 11– 12 years. If an infant receives the vaccine before 12 months of age, two doses are required to complete the series, the first after at least 12 months of age and the second at least 1 month later. Ig interferes with the immune response to the attenuated vaccine strains of MMR. Therefore, MMR immunization after Ig administration should be deferred by 3–11 months, depending on the type of Ig product received. Consult the AAP's 2006 *Red Book* for specific recommendations.

A person can be considered immune to rubella only with documentation of either serologic immunity to rubella or vaccination with at least one dose of rubella vaccine after age 1 year, or if born before 1957. A clinical diagnosis of rubella is unacceptable. Susceptible pubertal girls and postpubertal women identified by premarital or prenatal screening should also be immunized. Whenever rubella vaccination is offered to a woman of childbearing age, pregnancy should be ruled out and the woman advised to prevent conception for 3 months following vaccination. If a pregnant woman is vaccinated or becomes pregnant within 3 weeks of vaccination, she should be counseled regarding the risk to her fetus. No cases of rubella vaccine-related fetal anomalies have been reported, although theoretical risk of this exists. The risk of congenital rubella syndrome after wild-type maternal infection in the first trimester of pregnancy is 20–85%. All susceptible adults in institutional settings (including colleges), day care center personnel, military personnel, and hospital and health care personnel should be immunized.

B. Vaccination of Travelers

People traveling abroad should be immune to measles and mumps. In high-risk areas, age at primary vaccination should be as soon as possible after the first birthday (ie, at 12 months). However, younger infants 6–11 months of age traveling to high-risk areas should receive the monovalent measles vaccine followed by two subsequent doses of MMR or MMR followed by MMRV at 12–15 months given at least 4 weeks apart. MMR or MMRV at 4–6 years completes the series. Because maternal antibody to mumps is present in most infants, and the disease is not severe in infancy, infants younger than 12 months of age traveling to endemic countries need not routinely be given mumps vaccine.

C. Revaccination Under Other Circumstances

Persons entering college and other institutions for education beyond high school, medical personnel beginning employment, and persons traveling abroad should have documentation of immunity to measles and mumps, defined as receipt of two doses of measles vaccine after their first birthday, birth before 1957, or a documented measles or mumps history or immunity.

D. Outbreak Control of Measles

A community outbreak is defined as a single documented case of measles. Control depends on immediate protection of all susceptible persons (defined as persons who have no documented immunity to measles in the affected community). In the case of unvaccinated individuals, the following recommendations hold: (1) age 6–11 months, monovalent measles vaccine (or MMR) if cases are occurring in children younger than age 1 year, followed by two doses of MMR at age 12–15 months and again at age 4–6 years; and (2) age 12 months or older, MMR followed by revaccination at 4–6 years. A child

with an unclear or unknown vaccination history should be reimmunized with MMR. Anyone with a known exposure who is not certain of receiving two doses of MMR should receive an additional dose. Unimmunized persons who are not immunized within 72 hours of exposure should be excluded from contact with potentially infected persons until at least 2 weeks after the onset of rash of the last case of measles.

▶ Contraindications & Precautions

MMR vaccination is contraindicated in pregnant women, women intending to become pregnant within the next 28 days, immunocompromised persons (except those with asymptomatic HIV who have age-specific CD4+ lymphocytes counts > 15%), and persons with anaphylactic egg or neomycin allergy. It is also contraindicated in children receiving high-dose corticosteroid therapy ($\geq$ 2 mg/kg/d, or 20 mg/d total, for longer than 14 days) with the exception of those receiving physiologic replacement doses. In these patients, an interval of 1 month between cessation of steroid therapy and vaccination is sufficient. Leukemic patients who have been in remission and off chemotherapy for at least 3 months can receive MMR safely. Children with minor acute illnesses (including febrile illnesses), nonanaphylactic egg allergy, or a history of tuberculosis should be immunized. MMR may be safely administered simultaneously with other routine pediatric immunizations.

▶ Adverse Effects

Between 5% and 15% of vaccinees receiving MMR become febrile to 39.5°C or higher about 6–12 days following vaccination, lasting approximately 1–2 days, and 5% may develop a transient morbilliform rash. Transient thrombocytopenia occurs in 1:25,000–1:100,000 persons. Encephalitis and other central nervous system conditions, such as aseptic meningitis and Guillain-Barré syndrome, are reported to occur at a frequency of 1 case per 3 million doses in the United States. This rate is lower than the rate of these conditions in unvaccinated children, implying that the relationship between them and MMR vaccination is not causal. MMR vaccination is associated with an increased risk of febrile seizures 8–14 days after vaccination, but no subsequent long-term complications have been seen. A recent study found an increase in female mortality in Guinea Bissau after receiving a high-titered measles vaccine (not used in the United States) at less than 6 months of age. Reactions after mumps vaccination are rare and include parotitis, low-grade fever, and orchitis. In 1989, a nationwide surveillance of neurologic complications after a mumps vaccine was conducted in Japan. At least 311 cases of mild aseptic meningitis (96 had vaccine-type mumps virus in the cerebrospinal fluid) occurred among 630,157 recipients. However, this was not the strain used in the U.S. vaccine. There were no sequelae. A high rate of aseptic meningitis was also found in Brazil, but not in Germany, where different vaccine strains were used. In children, adverse effects from rubella vaccination are very unusual. Between 5% and 15% of vaccinees develop rash, fever, or lymphadenopathy 5–12 days after rubella vaccination. Rash also occurs alone or as a mild rubella illness in 2–4% of adults. Arthralgia and arthritis occur in 10–25% of adult vaccinees, as opposed to only 0–2% of 6- to 16-year-old vaccinees. Chronic arthritis, which may be causally related to rubella vaccination, occurs more often in women aged 45 or older, starting 10–11 days after vaccination and lasting for up to 1 year. Rare complications include peripheral neuritis and neuropathy, transverse myelitis, and diffuse myelitis.

▶ Antibody Preparations Against Measles

If a child is seen within 72 hours after exposure to measles, vaccination is the preferred method of postexposure protection. If vaccine is contraindicated, Ig, given intramuscularly at a dose of 0.25 mL/kg (0.5 mL/kg in immunocompromised patients; maximum dose in either circumstance is 15 mL), is effective in preventing or modifying measles if it is given within 6 days after exposure. MMR vaccine should be given 5 months later to children receiving the 0.25-mL/kg dose and 6 months later for the higher dose. For children receiving regular intravenous immune globulin, a dose of 100–400 mg/kg should be adequate for measles prophylaxis for exposures occurring within 3 weeks of the last dose.

Black SB et al: Immunogenicity and safety of measles-mumps-rubella, varicella and Haemophilus influenzae type b vaccines administered concurrently with a fourth dose of heptavalent pneumococcal conjugate vaccine compared with the vaccines administered without heptavalent pneumococcal conjugate vaccine. Pediatr Infect Dis J 2006;25:306 [PMID: 16567981].

Castillo-Solorzano C et al: New horizons in the control of rubella and prevention of congenital rubella syndrome in the Americas. J Infect Dis 2003;187:S146 [PMID: 12721906].

CDC: Progress in reducing measles mortality—worldwide, 1999–2003. MMWR Morb Mortal Wkly Rep 2005;54:2005 [PMID: 15744229].

CDC: Notice to readers: Updated recommendations of the Advisory Committee on Immunization Practices (ACIP) for the control and elimination of mumps. MMWR Morb Mortal Wkly Rep 2006;55:629 [PMID: 16761359].

Miller E et al: Risks of convulsion and aseptic meningitis following measles-mumps-rubella vaccination in the United Kingdom. Am J Epidemiol 2007;165:704 [PMID: 17204517].

VARICELLA VACCINATION

Prior to the availability of vaccine, about 4 million cases of varicella-zoster virus (VZV) infection occurred annually in the United States, mostly in children younger than 10 years old. This resulted in 11,000 hospitalizations and 100 deaths per year due to severe complications such as secondary bacterial infections, pneumonia, encephalitis, hepatitis, and Reye syndrome.

A live, attenuated varicella vaccine (VAR) has been licensed in the United States since 1995, and routine immu-

nization of children 12 months of age and older has been recommended since then. The vaccine has been shown to be more than 95% effective at preventing severe disease. The morbidity, mortality, and medical costs associated with varicella infection have significantly declined since VAR was first licensed in the United States. While there is no national system of surveillance for varicella disease in place, a variety of data sources have all shown a consistent pattern of more than 85% reduction in varicella-associated disease. Varicella-related deaths have decreased between 75% and 88% in recent years, and this was observed in all ages, races, and ethnic groups. In the decade since the routine use of VAR has been recommended, there have been reports of "breakthrough" (usually very mild) varicella occurring in immunized patients. Outbreaks of wild-type infectious VZV have been reported in schools with high one-dose VAR vaccination coverage (96–100%). The vaccine efficacy in those outbreaks was similar (72–85%) to that previously observed. Varicella attack rates among these children varied between 11% and 17% and thus, it was concluded that a single VAR dose could not prevent varicella outbreaks completely.

A second dose of VAR vaccine in children, when given 3 months or 4–6 years after the initial dose, greatly increases the anti-VZV antibody response, which is a correlate of vaccine efficacy. A combination MMRV vaccine has also been shown to be immunologically noninferior to the individual components administered compared with MMR and VAR vaccines administered concomitantly, either as primary immunization or as a booster administered to children age 4–6 years. Among persons older than age 13 years, a second dose results in 94–99% seroconversion with detectable antibody levels persisting for at least 5 years in 97% of them. In a randomized clinical trial of one dose of vaccine compared with two doses administered 3 months apart, the vaccine efficacy for two doses over a 10-year observation period was 98%, significantly higher than the vaccine efficacy for one dose (94%). The two-dose regimen was also 100% efficacious against severe varicella. These observations have led to the recent recommendations of the ACIP and the AAP of two doses of VAR vaccine for children older than 12 months of age, and for adolescents and adults without evidence of immunity.

Data from U.S. and Japanese studies suggest that the vaccine is also effective in preventing or modifying VZV severity in susceptible individuals exposed to VZV if used within 3 days of exposure. A study in the United States suggests that the efficacy of postexposure vaccination is 95% for prevention of any disease and 100% for prevention of moderate or severe disease. There is no evidence that postexposure prophylaxis will increase the risk of vaccine-related adverse events or interfere with development of immunity.

▶ Vaccines Available

1. A cell-free preparation of OKA strain VZV is produced and marketed in the United States as Varivax (Merck). Each dose of VAR contains not less than 1350 plaque-

forming units of VZV and trace amounts of neomycin, fetal bovine serum, and gelatin. Storage in a freezer at a temperature of −15°C or colder provides a shelf life of 15 months. VAR may be stored for 72 hours at refrigerator temperature in its lyophilized state, and it must be administered within 30 minutes after thawing and reconstitution.

2. The availability of MMRV (measles-mumps-rubella-varicella; ProQuad, Merck) for use in children 1–12 years of age simplifies the administration of these antigens. MMRV is well tolerated and provides adequate immune response to all of the antigens it contains. Concomitant administration of MMRV with DTaP, Hib, and HepB vaccines is acceptable. MMRV should be stored in a freezer at a temperature of −15°C or colder.

Dosage & Schedule of Administration

Two doses (0.5 mL) of VAR vaccine are recommended for immunization of all healthy children aged 12 months and older, and for adolescents and adults without evidence of immunity. For children aged 12 months to 12 years the immunization interval is 3 months, and for persons 13 years or older it is 4 weeks. MMRV is approved only for healthy children aged 12 months to 12 years. A second dose of catch-up vaccination is required for children, adolescents, and adults who previously received one dose of VAR vaccine. All children should have received two doses of vaccine before prekindergarten or school. Asymptomatic or mildly symptomatic HIV-infected children ($\geq$ 15% CD4$^+$ cells) should receive two doses of the single-antigen vaccine (with a 3-month interval between doses).

VAR may be given simultaneously with MMR at separate sites. If not given simultaneously, the interval between administration of VAR and MMR must be greater than 28 days. Simultaneous VAR administration does not appear to affect the immune response to other childhood vaccines. VAR should be delayed 5 months after receiving intravenous immune globulin, blood or plasma. In addition persons who received a VAR vaccine should not be administered an antibody-containing product for at least 2 weeks, and if needed in that interval, the individual may need to be tested for immunity or revaccinated.

Contraindications & Precautions

Contraindications to VAR vaccination include a severe allergic reaction after a previous vaccine dose or to a vaccine component. Because VAR and MMRV are live-virus vaccines, they are also contraindicated in children who have cellular immunodeficiencies, including those with leukemia, lymphoma, other malignancies affecting the bone marrow or lymphatic systems, and congenital T-cell abnormalities (although VAR vaccine administration to children with acute lymphocytic leukemia is under investigation). The exception to this rule is the recommendation that VAR be administered to HIV-infected children who are not severely immunosuppressed. Children receiving immunosuppressive therapy, including high-dose steroids, should not receive VAR or MMRV. Household contacts of immunodeficient patients should be immunized. VAR should not be given to pregnant women; however, the presence of a pregnant mother in the household is not a contraindication to immunization of a child within that household.

Adverse Events

Since the approval of VAR in 1995, more than 50 million doses have been distributed in the United States. The most commonly recognized adverse reactions, occurring in approximately 20% of vaccinees, are minor injection site reactions. Additionally, 3–5% of patients will develop a rash at the injection site, and an additional 3–5% will develop a sparse varicelliform rash outside of the injection site. These rashes typically consist of two to five lesions and may appear 5–26 days after immunization. The two-dose vaccine regimen is generally well tolerated with a safety profile comparable to that of the one-dose regimen. The incidence of fever and varicelliform rash is lower after the second dose than the first.

Studies comparing MMRV to MMR and VAR administered concomitantly showed more systemic adverse events following MMRV (fever 21.5% vs 14.9% and measles-like rash 3% vs 2.1% respectively). The combination vaccine, when given as a second dose following MMR, showed significantly greater proportions of subjects with local site reactions.

Transmission of vaccine virus from healthy patients to healthy recipients is very rare, has never occurred in the absence of a rash in the index case, and has only resulted in mild disease. One case involved transmission from a vaccinee to a susceptible pregnant female. The pregnancy was terminated, but polymerase chain reaction analysis of the fetus showed no evidence of VZV infection. Based on data from the VAERS, rates of serious adverse events following VAR are not increased compared with rates expected after natural infection or the background rates of similar events in the community. Herpes zoster infection has occurred in recipients of VAR in immunocompetent and immunocompromised persons within 25–722 days after immunization. Many of these cases were due to presumably unappreciated latent wild-type virus. Furthermore, based on preliminary data, the age-specific risk of herpes zoster infection seems to be lower in immunocompetent children following VAR immunization than after natural infection.

Antibody Preparations

Varicella-zoster immune globulin (VZIg) is prepared from plasma harvested from persons known to have high titers of anti-VZV antibody. It has been reliably used in high-risk susceptible persons who are exposed to VZV, such as immunocompromised individuals without a history of chickenpox, susceptible pregnant women, newborns whose mothers develop varicella 5 days prior to delivery or within 48 hours after delivery, hospitalized premature infants of 28 weeks' or more gestation (whose mother lacks a history of chickenpox or is seronegative), and hospitalized premature infants less than 28 weeks' gestation (regardless of maternal history or serostatus). Exposure is defined as a household contact or playmate contact (> 1 hour per day), hospital contact (in the same or contiguous room or ward), intimate contact with a person with zoster deemed contagious, or a newborn contact. Susceptibility is defined as the absence of a reliable history of varicella in persons born after 1966. Uncertainty in this diagnosis can be resolved with an appropriate test for anti-VZV antibody. VZIg should be given as soon as possible after exposure, and should be administered within 96 hours. Newborns should be given one vial (125 U) intramuscularly. The dose for all others is 125 U/10 kg body weight intramuscularly (maximum dose, 625 U). VZIg should be readministered following reexposure of susceptible persons if more than 3 weeks has elapsed since a prior dose of VZIg.

The availability of VZIg is limited as the sole U.S. manufacturer has stopped production. A Canadian preparation (Vari Zig, Cangene Corporation) is available under an Investigational New Drug application Expanded Access Protocol and can be obtained from FFF Enterprises, Temecula, CA (1-800-843-7477). If VZIg is not available, it is recommended that intravenous Ig be used in its place. The dose is 400 mg/kg administered once. A subsequent exposure does not require additional prophylaxis if this occurs within 3 weeks of intravenous Ig administration.

AAP Committee on Infectious Diseases: Prevention of varicella: Recommendations for use of varicella vaccines in children, including a recommendation for a routine 2-dose varicella immunization schedule. Pediatrics 2007;120;221 [PMID: 17606582].

CDC: Varicella-related deaths—United States, January 2003–June 2004. MMWR Morb Mortal Wkly Rep 2005;54:272 [PMID: 15788992].

CDC: Prevention of varicella: recommendations of the Advisory Committee on Immunization Practices (ACIP). MMWR Recomm Rep 2007;56(RR-4):1 [PMID: 17585291].

Levin MJ et al: Administration of live varicella vaccine to HIV-infected children with current or past significant depression of CD4(+) T cells. J Infect Dis. 2006;194:247 [PMID: 16779732].

Lopez AS et al: One dose of varicella vaccine does not prevent school outbreaks: Is it time for a second dose? Pediatrics 2006;117:e1070 [PMID: 16740809].

Reisinger KS et al: A combination measles, mumps, rubella, and varicella vaccine (ProQuad) given to 4- to 6-year-old healthy children vaccinated previously with M-M-RII and Varivax. Pediatrics 2006;117:265 [PMID: 16452343].

Shinefield H et al: Safety and immunogenicity of a measles, mumps, rubella and varicella vaccine given with combined Haemophilus influenzae type b conjugate/hepatitis B vaccines and combined diphtheria-tetanus-acellular pertussis vaccines. Pediatr Infect Dis J 2006;25:287 [PMID: 16567978].

HEPATITIS A VACCINATION

The incidence of hepatitis A in the United States has decreased dramatically in recent years. In 2003, annual reported hepatitis A cases had declined by 76% compared with annual cases during 1990–1997, and the 2003 rate was the lowest recorded in the 40 years since surveillance began. While hepatitis A rates naturally fluctuate in multiyear cycles, a novel vaccination strategy appears to be significantly contributing to declining hepatitis A rates.

HepA vaccines first became available in the United States in 1995. The following year, the ACIP recommended hepatitis A vaccination of certain high-risk groups, such as travelers, users of illegal drugs, and men who have sex with men. However, most hepatitis A infections occur in individuals without known risk factors for the disease. More than 50% of all infections are thought to occur in children. Children are more likely than adults to be asymptomatic while infected, and are often the mechanism by which hepatitis A is spread through households and communities.

In recognition of these epidemiologic features of hepatitis A, the ACIP in 1999 recommended vaccination for all children 24 months and older living in 11 states with more than twice the national average of hepatitis A cases, and vaccination was encouraged in an additional 6 states with disease rates exceeding (but less than twice) the national average. Despite only modest immunization coverage levels among children in targeted states, hepatitis A incidence rates have declined in both children and adults, suggesting that herd immunity had been achieved in many regions. The most recent recommendation to further reduce hepatitis A incidence in the United States is the routine administration of hepatitis A vaccine (HepA) to all children 12–23 months of age.

In addition HepA vaccination is indicated for the following groups: (1) travelers to countries with high rates of hepatitis A, (2) children with chronic hepatitis B or hepatitis C infections or other chronic liver disease, (3) children with clotting factor disorders, (4) adolescent and adult males who have sex with men, (5) persons with an occupational exposure to hepatitis A, and (6) illegal drug users.

HepA vaccines are considered very safe; tens of millions of doses have been administered, and no serious adverse events have definitively been caused by the vaccine. Vaccine efficacy is 94–100% against clinical hepatitis A.

▶ Vaccines Available

Two inactivated HepA vaccines are currently available for children: Havrix (GlaxoSmithKline) and Vaqta (Merck). Havrix contains a preservative (2-phenoxyethanol), but Vaqta does not. Both vaccines are approved for children 12 months and older. A combination vaccine against hepatitis A and hepatitis B (Twinrix, GlaxoSmithKline) is also available, but is only licensed in the United States for persons 18 years and older.

▶ Dosage & Schedule of Administration

Havrix is available in two formulations. For individuals between the ages of 1 and 18 years, 720 ELU (enzyme-linked immunosorbent assay [ELISA] units) per dose is administered intramuscularly in two doses of 0.5 mL, separated by 6–12 months. For persons older than 18 years, a higher dose (1440 ELU per dose) is recommended, also in two doses of 1 mL.

Vaqta also has two formulations. For persons aged 1–18 years, two doses of 25 U per dose (0.5 mL) are given, separated by 6–18 months. Individuals older than 17 years are given 50 U per dose (1.0 mL) in a two-dose schedule.

Both vaccines should be shipped and stored at 2–8°C and should not be frozen. HepA vaccines are given intramuscularly, and may be given simultaneously with other vaccines, including HepB.

Contraindications & Precautions

HepA should not be given to anyone with a prior severe allergic reaction such as anaphylaxis after a previous vaccine dose or to a vaccine component. Precautions to vaccination include pregnancy and moderate or severe acute illness with or without fever. The vaccine should not be administered to children with hypersensitivity to 2-phenoxyethanol (in the case of Havrix) or alum (for both preparations).

Adverse Effects

Adverse reactions are uncommon and mild consisting of pain, swelling, and induration at the injection site (10–15%), headache, and loss of appetite.

Antibody Preparations

For children younger than age 12 months at increased risk of hepatitis A infection (eg, those traveling to endemic areas or those with clotting factor disorders), immunoglobulin (Ig) should be used as preexposure prophylaxis. The recommended dosages are 0.02 mL/kg in a single intramuscular dose if the duration of exposure is likely to be less than 3 months and 0.06 mL/kg if exposure is likely to be more than 3 months. For long-term prophylaxis of persons not eligible for vaccination, prophylactic doses can be repeated every 5 months.

Postexposure prophylaxis of persons who recently have been exposed to hepatitis A and who previously have not received HepA vaccine should be administered a single dose of single-antigen vaccine or Ig (0.02 mL/kg) as soon as possible. If vaccine and Ig are given together they should be given simultaneously with Ig at a different anatomic injection site. When indicated, a single intramuscular dose of Ig (0.02 mL/kg) should be given as soon as possible, but not more than 2 weeks after the last exposure. Postexposure prophylaxis is recommended for household or sexual contacts of persons with serologically confirmed hepatitis A, and for day care staff and attendees in outbreak situations.

AAP Committee on Infectious Diseases: Hepatitis A recommendations. Pediatrics 2007;120:189 [PMID:17606579].
Advisory Committee on Immunization Practices (ACIP): Prevention of hepatitis A through active or passive immunization: Recommendations of the Advisory Committee on Immunization Practices (ACIP). MMWR Recomm Rep 2006;55 (RR-7):1 [PMID:16708058].
CDC: Hepatitis A vaccination coverage among children aged 24–35 months—United States, 2004–2005. MMWR Morb Mortal Wkly Rep 2007;56:678 [PMID:17625495].
CDC: Update: Prevention of hepatitis A after exposure to hepatitis A virus and in international travelers. Updated recommendations of the Advisory Committee on Immunization Practices (ACIP). MMWR Morb Mortal Wkly Rep 2007;56:1080 [PMID:17947967].
Craig AS, Schaffner W: Prevention of hepatitis A with the hepatitis A vaccine. N Engl J Med 2004;350:476 [PMID: 14749456].
Wasley A et al: Incidence of hepatitis A in the United States in the era of vaccination. JAMA 2005;294:194 [PMID: 16014593].
Zhou F et al. Impact of hepatitis A vaccination on health care utilization in the United States, 1996–2004. Vaccine 2007;25:3581 [PMID:17306908].
CDC: Hepatitis A vaccine information: http://www.cdc.gov/Ncidod/diseases/hepatitis/a/index.htm#vaccine

MENINGOCOCCAL VACCINATION

Building upon the technology used to develop conjugate *H influenzae* type b (Hib) and *S pneumoniae* vaccines, a tetravalent meningococcal polysaccharide-protein conjugate vaccine (MCV4) was licensed in 2005 and is indicated for use in persons 2–55 years of age. This vaccine, protecting against meningococcal serogroups A, C, Y, and W-135, is currently recommended for routine use in young adolescents (aged 11–12 years), those entering high school (at approximately 15 years of age), and college freshmen living in dormitories, as well as other groups at increased risk of meningococcal disease.

Infections with *Neisseria meningitidis* cause significant morbidity and mortality, with an estimated 1400–2800 cases of meningococcal disease occurring in the United States annually. Even with appropriate treatment, meningococcal disease has an estimated case-fatality rate of 10–14%, and up to 19% of survivors are left with serious disabilities, such as neurologic deficits, loss of limbs or limb function, or hearing loss. Five serogroups of meningococcus (A, B, C, W-135, and Y) cause the vast majority of disease worldwide. Serogroups B, C, and Y are the predominant causes of invasive meningococcal disease in the United States, while serogroups A and C cause most disease in developing countries. Intensive research efforts have been made to develop an effective vaccine against serogroup B, which causes more than 50% of cases among children younger than 1 year of age. However, the bacterial capsule proteins of serogroup B are poorly immunogenic in humans, presenting a significant obstacle to vaccine development.

It is important to highlight the characteristics of the new MCV4 vaccine compared with the only other meningococcal vaccine available in the United States, a tetravalent meningococcal polysaccharide vaccine (MPSV4), which was licensed in 1981. Both MCV4 and MPSV4 protect against the same four strains of meningococcus, and both are safe and immunogenic. MCV4 is licensed for use in persons 2–55 years old, while MPSV4 is licensed for persons 2 years and older. The bacterial polysaccharides used in MPSV4 produce B-cell immune stimulation but no T-cell response. Therefore, MPSV4 does not produce long-lasting immunity, nor does it produce an anamnestic response after a subsequent exposure to the same bacterial antigens. In the case of MCV4, bacterial polysaccharides are conjugated (linked) to a modified diphtheria toxoid, which leads to the stimulation of a T-cell–dependent immune response. MCV4 immunogenicity data, as well as the experience with Hib and pneumococcal conjugate vaccines, support the premise that MCV4 will produce longer-lasting immunity than MPSV4 and will produce an immune memory response, which does not occur with MPSV4.

Since the introduction of MCV4, 15 cases of Guillain-Barré syndrome have been reported in persons aged 11–19 years with onset within 6 weeks of MCV4 vaccination. Guillain-Barré syndrome is a rare illness, regardless of etiology; expected incidence rates for Guillain-Barré syndrome are not precisely known, and the available data cannot determine with certainty whether MCV4 increases the risk of Guillain-Barré syndrome. The CDC has recommended that the routine use of MCV4 continue, given the known morbidity and mortality caused by meningococcus and the insufficient evidence to date to conclude that MCV4 causes Guillain-Barré syndrome.

A single dose of MCV4 is recommended for young adolescents (aged 11–12 years) and for adolescents entering high school (approximately 15 years of age). Meningococcal vaccination is also recommended for certain groups at increased risk of invasive meningococcal disease, including (1) college freshmen living in dormitories, (2) persons living in or traveling to countries with endemic or hyperendemic meningococcal disease, (3) persons with complement deficiencies, (4) persons with functional or anatomic asplenia, (5) military recruits, and (6) microbiologists who work with N meningitidis. Whenever meningococcal vaccination is indicated, MCV4 is preferred for persons 2–55 years old, while MPSV4 should be used for persons older than 55 years. If MCV4 is not available, MPSV4 is an appropriate alternative for persons 2–55 years old.

Vaccines Available

1. MCV4 (Menactra, Sanofi Pasteur). A single 0.5-mL dose contains 4 mcg each of capsular polysaccharide from serogroups A, C, Y, and W-135 conjugated to 48 mcg of diphtheria toxoid. Available in single-dose vials only.
2. MPSV4 (Menomune-A/C/Y/W-135, Sanofi Pasteur). Each dose consists of 50 mcg each of the four bacterial capsular polysaccharides. Available in single-dose and 10-dose vials.

Dosage & Schedule of Administration

1. MCV4 is given as a single intramuscular dose of 0.5 mL.
2. MPSV4 is administered as a single subcutaneous dose of 0.5 mL.

MCV4 and MPSV4 can be given at the same time as other vaccines, at a different anatomic site. Protective antibody levels are typically achieved within 10 days of vaccination. Persons 2–55 years old who received MPSV4 more than 3–5 years previously, and who remain at increased risk of meningococcal disease, should be considered for an additional dose of MCV4 vaccination, although data are limited about the need and effectiveness of revaccination.

Contraindications & Precautions

MCV4 and MPSV4 are contraindicated in anyone with a known severe allergic reaction to any component of the vaccine, including diphtheria toxoid (for MCV4) and rubber latex. MCV4 vaccination is contraindicated in someone with a prior history of Guillain-Barré syndrome. Both MCV4 and MPSV4 can be given to individuals who are immunosuppressed. MPSV4 is thought to be safe during pregnancy; no information is available regarding the safety of MCV4 during pregnancy.

Adverse Effects

Both MCV4 and MPSV4 are generally well tolerated in adolescent patients. Local vaccination reactions (redness, swelling, or induration) occurred in 11–16% of persons 11–18 years old receiving MCV4 and 4–6% of persons the same age receiving MPSV4. The most common solicited complaints among children aged 2–10 years were injection site pain and irritability. More severe systemic reactions (presence of any of the following: fever of 39.5°C or above; headache, fatigue, malaise, chills, or arthralgias requiring bed rest; anorexia; multiple episodes of vomiting or diarrhea; rash; or seizures) occurred in 4.3% of MCV4 recipients and 2.6% of MPSV4 recipients.

Postexposure Prophylaxis

Close contacts of a patient with invasive meningococcal disease should receive antimicrobial prophylaxis to prevent the spread of disease. Because the rate of disease among close contacts is highest immediately after exposure, postexposure prophylaxis should be started as soon as possible, ideally within 24 hours of exposure. Close contacts are defined as (1) household members, (2) day care center contacts, and (3) anyone encountering an infected patient's secretions, such as through kissing, mouth-to-mouth resuscitation, or endotracheal intubation. Rifampin or ceftriaxone are used for chemoprophylaxis in children; rifampin, ceftriaxone, or ciprofloxacin may be used for adults.

AAP, Committee on Infectious Diseases: Prevention and control of meningococcal disease: Recommendations for use of meningococcal vaccines in pediatric patients. Pediatrics 2005;116:496 [PMID: 15995007].
Baltimore RS: Recent trends in meningococcal epidemiology and current vaccine recommendations. Curr Opin Pediatr 2006;18:58 [PMID:16470164].

CDC: Update: Guillain-Barré syndrome among recipients of Menactra meningococcal conjugate vaccine—United States, June 2005–September 2006. MMWR Morb Mortal Wkly Rep 2006;55:1120 [PMID:17060898].

CDC: Prevention and control of meningococcal disease—recommendations of the Advisory Committee on Immunization Practices (ACIP). MMWR Recomm Rep 2005;54(RR-7):1 [PMID: 15917737].

CDC: Revised recommendations of the Advisory Committee on Immunization Practices to vaccinate all persons aged 11–18 years with meningococcal conjugate vaccine. MMWR Morb Mortal Wkly Rep 2007;56:794 [PMID:17694617].

Pichichero ME: Meningococcal conjugate vaccine in adolescents and children. Clin Pediatr 2005;44:479 [PMID:16015394].

TETANUS-DIPHTHERIA-ACELLULAR PERTUSSIS VACCINATION (ADOLESCENTS & ADULTS)

Pertussis is increasingly recognized as a disease affecting older children and adults, including fully vaccinated persons with waning immunity. In the United States, the most dramatic increases in pertussis incidence are among adolescents and young adults, prompting development of booster pertussis vaccines for this population. FDA approval in 2005 of the tetanus-diphtheria-acellular pertussis (Tdap) vaccine was based on comparable seroresponse to pertussis antigens and a safety profile similar to control Td. Adolescent and young adult immunization not only has the capacity to protect adolescents from pertussis, but also should limit spread of pertussis from adults to infants and decrease overall pertussis endemicity.

▶ Vaccines Available

1. Tdap (Boostrix, GlaxoSmithKline) contains tetanus toxoid, diphtheria toxoid, and three acellular pertussis antigens (detoxified pertussis toxin [PT], filamentous hemagglutinin (FHA), and pertactin) and is licensed for use in adolescents aged 10–18 years.
2. Tdap (Adacel, Sanofi Pasteur) contains tetanus toxoid, diphtheria toxoid, and five acellular pertussis antigens (PT, FHA, pertactin, and fimbriae types 2 and 3) and is licensed for use in persons aged 11–64 years.

▶ Dosage & Schedule of Administration

Adolescents 11–18 years of age should receive a single 0.5-mL dose of Tdap intramuscularly in the deltoid, instead of the tetanus and diphtheria toxoids (Td) vaccine for booster immunization. The preferred age for Tdap immunization is 11–12 years. An interval of at least 5 years between last Td vaccine and Tdap is suggested in order to reduce the risk of local and systemic reactions. Tdap and MCV4 should be administered during the same visit if both vaccines are indicated. If not administered at the same time, a minimum interval of 1 month between vaccines is suggested.

▶ Contraindications & Precautions

Contraindications to Tdap include severe allergic reaction to any vaccine component and encephalopathy (eg, coma, pro-longed seizures) not attributable to an identifiable cause within 7 days of administration of a vaccine with pertussis components. Precautions for Tdap administration include Guillain-Barré syndrome occurring within 6 weeks of a previous dose of a tetanus toxoid–containing vaccine, a progressive neurologic disorder, uncontrolled epilepsy, or progressive encephalopathy until the condition has stabilized. Tdap vaccination should be deferred for at least 10 years if there is a history of a severe Arthus reaction after a tetanus toxoid–containing or diphtheria toxoid–containing vaccine.

▶ Adverse Effects

Pain at the injection site was the most frequently reported local adverse event among adolescents. Headache and fatigue were the most frequently reported systemic adverse events.

AAP, Committee on Infectious Diseases: Prevention of pertussis among adolescents: Recommendations for use of tetanus toxoid, reduced diphtheria toxoid, and acellular pertussis (Tdap). Pediatrics 2006;117;965 [PMID:16382131].

CDC: Recommendations of the Advisory Committee on Immunization Practices (ACIP): Preventing tetanus, diphtheria, and pertussis among adolescents: use of tetanus toxoid, reduced diphtheria toxoid and acellular pertussis vaccines. MMWR Recomm Rep 2006;55(RR-3):1 [PMID:16557217].

Halperin SA: Canadian experience with implementation of an acellular pertussis vaccine booster-dose program in adolescents: Implications for the United States. Pediatr Infect Dis J 2005;24:S141 [PMID:15931142].

Pichichero ME et al: Combined tetanus, diphtheria, and 5-component pertussis vaccine for use in adolescents and adults. JAMA 2005;293:3003 [PMID:15933223].

Ward JI et al: Efficacy of an acellular pertussis vaccine among adolescents and adults. N Engl J Med 2005;353:1555 [PMID: 16221778].

CDC: Diphtheria-tetanus-acellular pertussis vaccine information: http://www.cdc.gov/vaccines/vpd-vac/combo-vaccines/DTaP-Td-DT/tdap.htm

HUMAN PAPILLOMAVIRUS VACCINATION

Genital human papillomavirus (HPV) is the most common sexually transmitted infection in the United States. Most of the estimated 6.2 million persons newly infected every year have no symptoms. Over 40% of the 100 HPV types identified can infect the genital area. Approximately 70% of cervical cancers are caused by the high cancer risk types 16 and 18. Over 90% of genital warts are caused by low cancer risk types 6 and 11.

In June 2006, the quadrivalent HPV vaccine types 6, 11, 16, 18 (Gardasil, Merck) was licensed for use in females aged 9–26 years for the prevention of vaccine HPV-type-related cervical cancer, cervical cancer precursors, vaginal and vulvar cancer precursors, and anogenital warts. Routine vaccination of females aged 11–12 years is recommended, although the vaccine series can be started as young as age 9 years. Catch-up vaccination for females aged 13–26 years who were not previously vaccinated or have not completed the full vaccine series should ideally be administered before potential exposure to HPV through sexual contact. However, females who might have been exposed to HPV or who have an equivocal or abnormal Pap test, a positive hybrid capture II high-risk test, or genital warts can receive and are likely to benefit from the quadrivalent HPV vaccine.

Vaccine Available

Quadrivalent HPV vaccine (Gardasil, Merck) inactivated vaccine; a 0.5-mL dose contains 20 mcg HPV-6 L1 protein, 40 mcg HPV-11 L1 protein, 40 mcg HPV-16 L1 protein, and 20 mcg HPV-18 L1 protein. The vaccine does not contain thimerosal or antibiotics, but contains an aluminum-containing adjuvant.

Dosage & Schedule of Administration

HPV vaccine is administered intramuscularly as three separate 0.5-mL doses. The second dose should be administered 2 months after the first dose and the third dose 6 months after the first dose. The minimum interval between the first and second dose is 4 weeks; the minimum recommended interval between the second and third doses of vaccine is 12 weeks. HPV vaccine may be administered with other vaccines. Each vaccine should be administered using a separate syringe at a different anatomic site. If the vaccine schedule is interrupted the series does not need to be restarted.

Contraindications & Precautions

Quadrivalent HPV vaccine is contraindicated in persons with a history of anaphylaxis to yeast or to any vaccine component. HPV vaccine is not recommended for use in pregnancy. The vaccine can be administered to persons with minor acute illnesses and to immunocompromised persons.

Adverse Effects

Injection site pain (83.9%), and mild to moderate swelling and erythema, were the most common adverse events reported by vaccine recipients. Fever (10.3%), nausea (4.2%), and dizziness (2.8%) were reported as systemic adverse events. Postmarketing reports of syncope have been reported after vaccination with quadrivalent HPV vaccine and may follow any vaccination, so vaccine recipients should be observed for 15 minutes after vaccination.

Barr E, Tamms G: Quadrivalent human papillomavirus vaccine. Clin Infect Dis 2007;45:609 [PMID:17682997].
CDC: Quadrivalent human papillomavirus vaccine: Recommendations of the Advisory Committee on Immunization Practices (ACIP). MMWR Recomm Rep 2007;56(RR-2):1 [PMID: 17380109].
Dunne EF et al: Genital human papillomavirus infection. Clin Infect Dis 2006;43:624 [PMID:16886157].
Friedman LS et al: Human papillomavirus (HPV) vaccine: a position statement of the Society for Adolescent Medicine. J Adol Health 2006;39:620 [PMID:16982407].

VACCINATIONS FOR SPECIAL SITUATIONS

RABIES VACCINATION

After symptoms of infection develop, rabies is almost invariably fatal in humans. Only six persons are known to have recovered from rabies infection, five of whom had either been vaccinated prior to infection or received some form of postexposure prophylaxis. The incidence of human rabies in the United States is very low, with fewer than three cases per year nationwide. Of the 37 human cases of rabies reported in the United States from 1995–2006, bat exposure was suspected in 28 cases. However, there was a definite history of bite in only one or two of these cases. Although dogs represent the most important vector for human rabies worldwide, in the United States, because of widespread vaccination of dogs and cats, bats are the most important cause of human rabies. Rabies is also common in skunks, raccoons, and foxes; it is uncommon in rodents.

Human rabies is preventable with appropriate and timely postexposure prophylaxis. Postexposure care consists of local wound care, passive immunization, and active immunization. Immediately after an animal bite, all wounds should be flushed and aggressively cleaned with soap and water. If possible, the wound should not be sutured. Passive immunization after high-risk exposure consists of the injection of human rabies immune globulin (RIg) near the wound, as described below. Active immunization is accomplished by completing a schedule of immunization with one of the three rabies vaccines licensed in the United States. Because bites from bats are often unrecognized, prophylaxis should be given if a bat is found indoors even if there is no history of contact, especially if found in the same room with a sleeping or unattended child or with an intoxicated or otherwise incapacitated individual.

Local public health officials should be consulted before postexposure rabies prophylaxis is started to avoid unnecessary vaccination and to assist in the proper handling of the animal (if confinement or testing of the animal is appropriate). To facilitate consultation, the physician should know the species of animal, its availability for testing or confinement, the nature of the attack (provoked or unprovoked), and the nature of the exposure (bite, scratch, lick, or aerosol of saliva). Preexposure prophylaxis is indicated for veterinarians, animal handlers, and any persons whose work or home environment potentially places them in close contact with animal species in which rabies is endemic. Rabies immunization should also be considered for children traveling to countries where rabies is endemic; this is particularly important for travelers who will not have prompt access to medical care should an exposure occur.

Vaccines Available

Rabies vaccines stimulate immunity after 7–10 days, and the immunity persists for 2 years or more postvaccination. Two preparations are licensed in the United States.

1. Imovax Rabies (Sanofi Pasteur) human diploid cell vaccine (HDCV).
2. RabAvert (Chiron) purified chick embryo cell vaccine (PCEC).

Dosage & Schedule of Administration

The two rabies vaccines licensed in the United States are equally safe and efficacious for both preexposure and postexposure prophylaxis. For each vaccine, 1 mL is given intramuscularly in the deltoid (for adults and older children) or anterolateral thigh (for infants and young children). The volume of the dose is not reduced for children. Vaccine should not be given in the gluteal region.

A. Primary Preexposure Vaccination

Preexposure rabies immunization should be considered for individuals at high risk of exposure to rabies (eg, veterinarians, animal handlers, spelunkers, and people moving to or extensively traveling in areas with endemic rabies). Three intramuscular injections in the deltoid area of 1 mL of any vaccine are given on days 0, 7, and 21 or 28.

B. Postexposure Prophylaxis

After an individual has possibly been exposed to rabies, decisions about whether to initiate postexposure prophylaxis need to be made urgently, in consultation with local public health officials.

1. In previously unvaccinated individuals—After proper wound care has been provided, an individual exposed to rabies should receive rabies vaccination and RIg. Vaccination is given on the day of exposure and on days 3, 7, 14, and 28 following exposure. RIg should also be given as soon as possible after exposure, ideally on the day of exposure, in a recommended dose of 20 IU/kg. If anatomically possible, the entire dose of RIg should be infiltrated into and around the wound. Any remaining RIg should be administered intramuscularly at an anatomic site distant from the location used for rabies vaccination. If Rig was not administered when vaccination was begun, it can be administered up to 7 days after the first dose of vaccine. Postexposure failures have occurred only when some deviation from the approved protocol occurred (eg, no cleansing of the wound, less than usual amount of Rig, no RIg at the wound site, or vaccination in the gluteal area).

2. In previously vaccinated individuals—RIg should not be administered, and only two doses of vaccine on days 0 and 3 after exposure are needed.

C. Booster Vaccination

Previously vaccinated individuals with potential continued exposure to rabies should have a serum sample tested for rabies antibody every 2 years. If the titer is less than 1:5 for virus neutralization, a booster dose of rabies vaccine should be administered.

Adverse Effects

The rabies vaccines are relatively free of serious reactions. Approximately 30–74% of adults experience pain, swelling, induration, or erythema at the injection site; 5–25% may have mild systemic reactions such as headache, nausea, muscle aches, and dizziness. An immune complex–like reaction occurs in about 6% of persons 2–21 days after receiving booster doses of the rabies vaccine.

Travelers to countries where rabies is endemic may need immediate postexposure prophylaxis and may have to use locally available vaccines and RIg. In many developing countries, the only vaccines readily available may be nerve tissue vaccines derived from the brains of adult animals or suckling mice, and the RIg may be of equine origin. Although adverse reactions to RIg are uncommon and typically mild, the nervous tissue vaccines may induce neuroparalytic reactions in 1:200–1:8000 vaccinees; this is a significant risk and may justify preexposure vaccination prior to travel in circumstances in which exposure to potentially rabid animals is likely.

Antibody Preparations

In the United States, RIg is prepared from the plasma of human volunteers hyperimmunized with rabies vaccine. The recommended dose is 20 IU/kg body weight. The rabies-neutralizing antibody content is 150 IU/mL, supplied in 2-mL or 10-mL vials. It is very safe.

Dobardzic A et al: Safety review of the purified chick embryo cell rabies vaccine: Data from the Vaccine Adverse Event Reporting System (VAERS), 1997–2005. Vaccine 2007;25:4244 [PMID: 17382435].
Rupprecht CE et al: Clinical practice: Prophylaxis against rabies. N Engl J Med 2004;351:2626 [PMID: 15602023].
Wilde H et al: Rabies update for travel medicine advisors. Clin Infect Dis 2003;37:96 [PMID: 12830414].
CDC: Rabies information page: http://www.cdc.gov/rabies/.

TYPHOID FEVER VACCINATION

Globally, the burden of typhoid fever is substantial, causing an estimated 22 million illnesses and 200,000 deaths each year. In the United States, typhoid fever is relatively uncommon, with approximately 150–300 laboratory-confirmed cases each year, the majority acquired abroad. In a review of typhoid fever cases reported to the CDC, 74% of patients reported recent travel outside the United States, only 4% of whom had received typhoid vaccination in the preceding 5 years. Approximately 40% of cases were seen in patients younger than 18 years, and both short-term and long-term travel was associated with infection.

Two vaccines against *Salmonella enterica typhi*, the bacterium that causes typhoid fever, are currently available in the United States: a live attenuated vaccine given orally (Ty21a), and an inactivated vaccine composed of purified capsular polysaccharide (ViCPS) given parenterally. Both vaccines protect 50–80% of vaccine recipients. The oral vaccine is most commonly used because of its ease of administration. However, noncompliance with the oral vaccine dosing schedule occurs frequently, and correct usage should be stressed or the parenteral ViCPS vaccine used.

Routine typhoid vaccination is recommended only for children who are traveling to typhoid-endemic areas or who reside in households with a documented typhoid carrier. While current CDC recommendations emphasize typhoid vaccination for travelers expected to have long-term exposure to potentially contaminated food and drink, vaccination should also be considered for short-term travel to high-risk countries. Although typhoid fever occurs throughout the world, areas of highest incidence include southern Asia and southern Africa. Travelers should be advised that because the typhoid vaccines are not fully protective, and because of the potential for other food- and water-borne illnesses, careful selection of food and drink and appropriate hygiene remain necessary when traveling internationally.

Vaccines Available

1. Parenteral ViCPS (Typhim Vi, Sanofi Pasteur) is for intramuscular use.
2. Oral live attenuated Ty21a vaccine (Vivotif Berna Vaccine, Swiss Serum and Vaccine Institute) is supplied as enteric-coated capsules.

Dosage & Schedule of Administration

ViCPS is administered as a single intramuscular dose (0.5 mL) in the deltoid muscle, with boosters needed every 3 years if exposure continues. It is approved for children aged 2 years and older.

The dose of the oral preparation is one capsule every 2 days for a total of four capsules, taken 1 hour before meals. The capsules should be taken with cool liquids and should be kept refrigerated. All doses should be administered at least 1 week prior to potential exposure. A full course of four capsules is recommended every 5 years if exposure continues. Mefloquine and proguanil may decrease the effect of the live vaccine, and the vaccine should be given at least 1 day or 10 days after a dose of mefloquine or proguanil, respectively. This vaccine is not approved for children younger than age 6 years. As with all live attenuated vaccines, Ty21a should not be given to immunocompromised patients.

Adverse Reactions

Both the oral and parenteral vaccines are well tolerated, and adverse reactions are uncommon and usually self-limited. The oral vaccine may cause gastroenteritis-like illness, fatigue, and myalgia, whereas the parenteral vaccine may cause local and abdominal pain, dizziness, and pruritus.

Bhan MK et al: Typhoid and paratyphoid fever. Lancet 2005;366:749 [PMID: 16125594].

Fraser A et al: Vaccines for preventing typhoid fever. Cochrane Database Syst Rev 2007:CD001261 [PMID: 17636661].

CHOLERA VACCINATION

Cholera causes significant morbidity and mortality worldwide. It may present only as traveler's diarrhea. For travelers, the risk of developing cholera per month of stay in a developing country is low, ranging from 0.001% to approximately 0.01%. No cholera vaccines are available in the United States. Because the causative bacterium, *Vibrio cholerae*, is not invasive, and because secretory IgA is crucial, newer vaccines available in other countries are administered orally. An oral vaccine (consisting of live attenuated bacteria combined with the B subunit of cholera toxin wc/vBS, Dukoral, SBL Vaccine AB, Stockholm, Sweden) is safe and immunogenic. It is given as two doses 1 week apart, has an 85% vaccine efficacy against *V cholerae* in the first 6 months and greater than 50% cross-protection against enterotoxigenic *Escherichia coli* diarrhea. Cholera vaccination is no longer required for international travel or for entry into any country.

Hill DR et al: Oral cholera vaccines: Use in clinical practice. Lancet Infect Dis 2006:361 [PMID: 16728322].
Zuckerman JN et al: The true burden and risk of cholera: Implications for prevention and control. Lancet Infect Dis 2007;7:521 [PMID: 1758453].

TUBERCULOSIS VACCINATION

During 1993–2003 the incidence of tuberculosis (TB) in the United States decreased by 44%, setting the stage for possible elimination of the disease. However, nearly 40% of new cases of TB occur in persons born in other countries. Bacille Calmette-Guérin vaccine (BCG) consists of live attenuated *Mycobacterium bovis*. BCG is not currently indicated for mass use in the United States, chiefly because of doubts about its efficacy. BCG is the most widely used vaccine in the world and has been administered to over 3 billion people (71% of infants worldwide are vaccinated) with a low incidence of serious complications. It is inexpensive, can be given any time after birth, sensitizes the vaccinated individual for 5–50 years, and stimulates both B-cell and T-cell immune responses. BCG is useful in two circumstances in the United States: (1) in tuberculin-negative infants or older children residing in households with untreated or poorly treated individuals with active infection with isoniazid-and rifampin-resistant *Mycobacterium tuberculosis,* and (2) in infants or children found to live under constant exposure without the possibility of removal from continuous exposure or access to prophylaxis and treatment. BCG reduces the risk of tuberculous meningitis and disseminated TB in pediatric populations by 50–100% when administered in the first month of life. BCG appears to have had little epidemiologic effect on TB, despite a reported efficacy of 50% in a meta-analysis of 26 vaccine trials, with the greatest protection against pulmonary disease.

The two currently licensed BCG vaccines in the United States are produced by Organon Teknika Corporation (Tice BCG) and Eli Lilly (BCG Vaccine). They are given intradermally in a dose of 0.05 mL for newborns and 0.1 mL for all other children. Mantoux testing is advised 2–3 months later, and revaccination is advised if the Mantoux test is negative. Adverse effects occur in 1–10% of healthy individuals, including local ulceration, regional lymph node enlargement, and lupus vulgaris. The vaccine is contraindicated in pregnant women and in immunocompromised individuals, including those with HIV infection, because it has caused disseminated or fatal infection.

Factors associated with increased probability that a positive TB skin test is due to *M tuberculosis* infection include (1) larger reactions, (2) contact with an individual known to be infected, (3) family history of TB, (4) longer interval between BCG administration and skin testing, and (5) country of origin with increased incidence of endemic TB. The details and cutoff observations for TB skin testing are described in Chapter 40. To ensure that those infected with TB are evaluated, a 5-mm or greater cutoff for a positive Mantoux test is used in immunocompromised children. In immunocompetent persons, the cutoff is 10 mm or above, whereas it is 15 mm or above when no risk factors are present in the absence of clinical disease (eg, screening). In 2001 a new test (QuantiFeron TB) that measures the release of interferon-γ in whole blood in response to stimulation with purified protein derivative was approved by the FDA. This test is not recommended for persons with symptoms of active TB who are at increased risk of progression to active TB, but may be used instead of a TB skin test in those at increased or low risk of latent TB infection, including as screening for recent immigrants.

BCG almost invariably causes its recipients to be tuberculin-positive (5–7 mm), but the reaction often becomes negative after 3–5 years. Thus, a positive Mantoux test in a child with a history of BCG vaccination who is being investigated for TB as a case contact should be interpreted as indicating infection with *M tuberculosis*.

Andersen P et al: The success and failure of BCG—implications for a novel tuberculosis vaccine. Nat Rev Microbiol 2005;3:656 [PMID: 16012514].

CDC: Controlling tuberculosis in the United States of America. Recommendations from the American Thoracic Society, CDC and the Infectious Diseases Society of America. MMWR Recomm Rep 2005;54(RR-12):1 [PMID: 16267499].

Mazurek GH, Villarino ME; CDC: Guidelines for using the QuantiFeron-TB test for diagnosing latent *Mycobacterium tuberculosis* infection. MMWR Recomm Rep 2003;52(RR-2):15 [PMID: 12583541].

Skeiky YA et al: Advances in tuberculosis vaccine strategies. Nat Rev Microbiol 2006;4:469 [PMID: 16710326].

Trunz BB et al: Effect of BCG vaccination on childhood tuberculous meningitis and military tuberculosis worldwide: A meta-analysis and assessment of cost-effectiveness. Lancet 2006;367:1173 [PMID: 16616560].

Walker V et al: Does neonatal BCG vaccination protect against tuberculous meningitis? Arch Dis Child 2006;91:789 [PMID: 16923863].

YELLOW FEVER VACCINATION

Immunization against yellow fever is indicated for children as young as age 6 months traveling to endemic areas or to countries that require it for entry, but otherwise immunization should be delayed until age 9 months or older. Public health authorities maintain updated information on these requirements and must be consulted. Yellow fever vaccine is a live vaccine made from the 17D yellow fever attenuated virus strain grown in chick embryos. It is contraindicated in infants younger than age 6 months due to an increased susceptibility to vaccine-associated encephalitis, in persons with anaphylactic egg allergy, and in immunocompromised individuals or individuals with a history of thymus disease. It can only be administered at licensed yellow fever vaccination locations (usually public health departments). A single subcutaneous injection of 0.5 mL of reconstituted vaccine is administered. The International Health Regulations require revaccination at 10-year intervals, but immunity may be lifelong. Adverse reactions are generally mild—consisting of low-grade fever, mild headache, and myalgia 5–10 days after vaccination occurring in fewer than 25% of vaccinees. The risk of vaccine-associated neurotropic disease within 30 days following vaccination has been estimated to be 4–6 cases per 1 million doses. A serious adverse reaction syndrome, vaccine-associated viscerotropic disease, consists of severe multiple organ system failure and death within 1–2 weeks postvaccination, especially in adults older than 60 years of age. The estimated incidence of this complication among vaccine recipients in the United States is 1 case per 200,000–300,000 doses distributed. Health care providers should be careful to administer yellow fever vaccine only to persons truly at risk of exposure to yellow fever. There is no contraindication to giving other live-virus vaccines simultaneously with yellow fever vaccine or at intervals of a few days to a month.

Barnett ED: Yellow fever: Epidemiology and prevention. Clin Infect Dis 2007;44:850 [PMID:17304460].

CDC: Yellow fever vaccine: Recommendations of the Advisory Committee on Immunization Practices (ACIP), 2002. MMWR Recomm Rep 2002;51(RR-17):1 [PMID: 22324159].

Marfin AA et al: Yellow fever and Japanese encephalitis vaccines: Indications and complications. Infect Dis Clin North Am 2005;19:151 [PMID: 15701552].

CDC: Yellow fever information page: http://www.cdc.gov/travel/yellowBookCh4-YellowFever.aspx

PASSIVE PROPHYLAXIS

1. Intramuscular Immune Globulin

Ig may prevent or modify infection with hepatitis A virus if administered in a dose of 0.02 mL/kg within 14 days after exposure. Measles infection may be prevented or modified in a susceptible person if Ig is given in a dose of 0.25 mL/kg within 6 days after exposure. Special forms of Ig include tetanus Ig (TIg), hepatitis B Ig (HBIg), rabies Ig (RIg), vaccinia Ig, and varicella-zoster Ig (VZIg). These are obtained from donors known to have high titers of antibody against the organism in question. Ig must be given intramuscularly. The dose varies depending on the clinical indication. Adverse reactions include pain at the injection site, headache, chills, dyspnea, nausea, and anaphylaxis, although all but the first are rare.

Prophylaxis to prevent respiratory syncytial virus (RSV) in infants and children at increased risk of severe disease is available as an intramuscular immune globulin. Palivizumab (Synagis, MedImmune) is a humanized monoclonal antibody against RSV and is used to prevent RSV infection in high-risk populations with monthly doses during RSV season. Palivizumab should be considered for (1) infants and children younger than age 2 years with chronic lung disease who have required medical therapy (supplemental oxygen, bronchodilator, diuretic, or corticosteroid therapy) for their disease within 6 months before the anticipated RSV season; (2) infants born between 33 and 35 weeks' (32 weeks 1 day and 35 weeks 0 days) gestation or earlier without chronic lung disease with two or more risk factors (child care attendance, school-aged siblings, exposure to environmental air pollution, congenital airway abnormalities, or severe neuromuscular disease) up to age 6 months; (3) infants born at 29–32 weeks' gestation up to 6 months of age; (4) infants up to age 12 months born at 28 weeks' gestation or earlier; and (5) infants and children who are 24 months old or younger with hemodynamically significant cyanotic or acyanotic congenital heart disease. Those most likely to benefit from prophylaxis are infants (< 1 year of age) who are receiving medication to control congestive heart disease, with moderate to severe pulmonary hypertension and cyanotic heart disease. RSV prophylaxis should be initiated at the onset of the RSV season and continued until the end of the season, regardless of breakthrough RSV illness during that RSV season.

Palivizumab is administered in a dose of 15 mg/kg once a month and is packaged in 50- and 100-mg vials. Palivizumab does not interfere with response to routine childhood vaccinations.

2. Intravenous Immune Globulin

The primary indications for IVIg are for replacement therapy in antibody-deficient individuals; for the treatment of Kawasaki disease, idiopathic thrombocytopenic purpura, Guillain-Barré syndrome, and other autoimmune diseases; and replacement therapy in chronic B-cell lymphocytic leukemia. IVIg may be beneficial in some children with HIV infection, toxic shock syndrome, and for anemia caused by parvovirus B19.

Elhassan NO et al: Cost-effectiveness analysis of palivizumab in premature infants without chronic lung disease. Arch Pediatr Adolesc Med 2006;160:1070 [PMID: 17018467].

Feltes TF, Sondheimer HM: Palivizumab and the prevention of respiratory syncytial virus illness in pediatric patients with congenital heart disease. Expert Opin Biol Ther 2007;7:1471 [PMID: 17727335].

Grimaldi M et al: Palivizumab efficacy in preterm infants with gestational age < or = 30 weeks without bronchopulmonary dysplasia. Pediatr Pulmonol 2007;42:189 [PMID: 17243184].

Simoes EA et al: Palivizumab prophylaxis, respiratory syncytial virus, and subsequent recurrent wheezing. J Pediatr 2007;151:34 [PMID: 17586188].

Normal Childhood Nutrition & Its Disorders

Nancy F. Krebs, MD, MS

Laura E. Primak, RD, CNSD, CSP

▼ NUTRITIONAL REQUIREMENTS

NUTRITION & GROWTH

The nutrient requirements of children are influenced by (1) growth rate, (2) body composition, and (3) composition of new growth. These factors vary with age and are especially important during early postnatal life. Growth rates are higher in early infancy than at any other time, including the adolescent growth spurt (Table 10–1). Growth rates decline rapidly starting in the second month of postnatal life (proportionately later in the premature infant). Nutrient requirements also depend on body composition. In the adult, the brain, which accounts for only 2% of body weight, contributes 19% to the total basal energy expenditure. In contrast, in a full-term neonate, the brain accounts for 10% of body weight and for 44% of total energy needs under basal conditions. Thus, in the young infant, total basal energy expenditure and the energy requirement of the brain are relatively high.

Composition of new tissue is another factor influencing nutrient requirements. For example, fat accounts for about 40% of weight gain between birth and 4 months but for only 3% between 24 and 36 months. The corresponding figures for protein are 11% and 21%; for water, 45% and 68%. The high rate of fat deposition in early infancy has implications not only for energy requirements but also for the optimal composition of infant feedings. The high percentage of fat in human milk results in efficient fuel storage for the infant.

Because of the high nutrient requirements for growth and the body composition, the young infant is especially vulnerable to undernutrition. Slowed physical growth rate is an early and prominent sign of undernutrition in the young infant. The limited fat stores of the very young infant mean that energy reserves are unusually modest. The relatively large size and continued growth of the brain render the central nervous system especially vulnerable to the effects of malnutrition in early postnatal life.

▼ ENERGY

The major determinants of energy expenditure are (1) basal metabolism, (2) metabolic response to food, (3) physical activity, and (4) growth. The efficiency of energy use may be a significant factor, and thermoregulation may contribute in extremes of ambient temperature if the body is inadequately clothed. Because adequate data on requirements for physical activity in infants and children are unavailable and because individual growth requirements vary, recommendations have been based on calculations of actual intakes by healthy subjects. Suggested guidelines for energy intake of infants and young children are given in Table 10–2. Also included in this table are calculated energy intakes of infants who are exclusively breast fed, which have been verified in a number of centers. Growth velocity of breast-fed infants during the first 3 months equals and may exceed that of formula-fed infants, but from 6–12 months breast-fed infants typically weigh less than formula-fed infants and may show a decrease in growth velocity. The World Health Organization (WHO) has developed growth standards derived from an international sample of healthy breast-fed infants and young children raised in environments that do not constrain growth.

After the first 4 years, energy requirements expressed on a body weight basis decline progressively. The estimated daily energy requirement is about 40 kcal/kg/d at the end of adolescence. Approximate daily energy requirements can be calculated by adding 100 kcal per year to the base of 1000 kcal per day at age 1 year. Appetite and growth are reliable indices of caloric needs in most healthy children, but intake also depends to some extent on the energy density of the food offered. Individual energy requirements of healthy infants and children vary considerably, and malnutrition and disease increase the variability. Premature infant energy requirements can exceed 120 kcal/kg/d, especially during illness or when catch-up growth is desired.

One method of calculating requirements for malnourished patients is to base the calculations on the "ideal body weight" (ie, 50th percentile weight for the patient's length-

Table 10–1. Changes in growth rate, energy required for growth, and body composition in infants and young children.

Age (months)	Growth Rate (g/d)			Energy Requirements for Growth (kcal/kg/d)	Body Composition		
	Male	Both	Female		Water	Protein	Fat
0–0.25		0[a]			75	11.5	11
0.25–1	40		35	50			
1–2	35		30	25			
2–3	28		25	16			
3–6		20		10	60	11.5	26
6–9		15					
9–12		12					
12–18		8					
18–36		6		2	61	16	21

[a]Birth weight is regained by 7–10 d. Weight loss of > 10% of birth weight indicates dehydration or malnutrition; this applies to both formula-fed and breast-fed infants.
Data reprinted, with permission, from Fomon SJ (editor): *Infant Nutrition,* 2nd ed. WB Saunders, 1974.

age, 50th percentile weight-for-length, or weight determined from current height and the 50th percentile body mass index [BMI] for age), rather than on actual weight.

World Health Organization: Report of a Joint FAO/WHO/UNO Expert Consultation: Energy and Protein Requirements. WHO Tech Rep Ser No. 724, 1985;724.
WHO Multicentre Growth Reference Study Group: WHO Child Growth Standards based on length/height, weight and age. Acta Paediatr 2006;Suppl 450:76 [PMID: 16817681].

PROTEIN

Only amino acids and ammonium compounds are usable as sources of nitrogen in humans. Amino acids are provided through the digestion of dietary protein. Nitrogen is absorbed from the intestine as amino acids and short peptides. Absorption of nitrogen is more efficient from synthetic diets that contain peptides in addition to amino acids. Some intact proteins are absorbed in early postnatal life, a process that may be important in the development of protein tolerance or allergy.

Because there are no major stores of body protein, a regular dietary supply of protein is essential. In infants and children, optimal growth depends on an adequate dietary protein supply. Relatively subtle effects of protein deficiency are now recognized, especially those affecting tissues with rapid protein turnover rates, such as the immune system and the gastrointestinal (GI) mucosa.

Relative to body weight, rates of protein synthesis and turnover and accretion of body protein are exceptionally high in the infant, especially the premature infant. Eighty percent of the dietary protein requirement of a premature infant is used for growth, compared with only 20% in a 1-year-old child. Protein requirements per unit of body weight decline rapidly during infancy as growth velocity decreases. The recommendations in

Table 10–2 are derived chiefly from the Joint FAO/WHO/UNO Expert Committee and are similar to the Recommended Dietary Allowances. They recommend a protein intake above the quantity provided in breast milk. The protein intake required to achieve protein deposition equivalent to the in utero rate in very low birth weight infants is 3.5–4.0 g/kg/d simultaneously with adequate energy intake. Protein requirements increase in the presence of skin or gut losses, burns, trauma, and infection. Requirements also increase during times of catch-up growth accompanying recovery from malnutrition (approximately 0.2 g of protein per gram of new tissue deposited). Young infants experiencing rapid recovery may need as much as 1–2 g/kg/d of extra protein. By age 1 year, the extra protein requirement is unlikely to be more than 0.5 g/kg/d. Inadequate protein intake may occur in breast-fed infants fed low-protein supplements (eg, fruit juices), in infants with malabsorption (cystic fibrosis), or in infants fed low-protein weaning food (eg, cassava or dilute cereal gruels) as the dietary staple.

The quality of protein depends on its amino acid composition. Infants require 43% of protein as essential amino acids, and children require 36%. Adults cannot synthesize eight essential amino acids: isoleucine, leucine, lysine, methionine, phenylalanine, threonine, tryptophan, and valine. Histidine may be added to this list. Cysteine and tyrosine are considered partially essential because their rates of synthesis are limited and may be inadequate in certain circumstances. In young infants, synthetic rates for cysteine, tyrosine, and perhaps taurine are insufficient for needs. Taurine, an amino acid used to conjugate bile acids, may also be conditionally essential in infancy. Lack of an essential amino acid leads to weight loss within 1–2 weeks. Wheat and rice are deficient in lysine, and legumes are deficient in methionine. Appropriate mixtures of vegetable protein are therefore necessary to achieve high protein quality.

Table 10–2. Recommendations for energy and protein intake.

Age	Energy (kcal/kg/d)			Protein (g/kg/d)	
	Based on Measurements of Energy Expenditure	Intake from Human Milk	Guidelines for Average Requirements	Intake from Human Milk	Guidelines for Average Requirements
10 d to 1 mo	—	105	120	2.05	2.5
1–2 mo	110	110	115	1.75	2.25
2–3 mo	95	105	105	1.36	2.25
3–4 mo	95	75–85	95	1.20	2.0
4–6 mo	95	75–85	95	1.05	1.7
6–12 mo	85	70	90	—	1.5
1–2 y	85	—	90	—	1.2
2–3 y	85	—	90	—	1.1
3–5 y	—	—	90	—	1.1

Data reprinted, with permission, from Krebs NF et al: Growth and intakes of energy and zinc in infants fed human milk. J Pediatr 1994;124:32; and Garza C, Butte NF: Energy intakes of human milk-fed infants during the first year. J Pediatr 1990;117:(S)124.

Because the mechanisms for removal of excess nitrogen are efficient, moderate excesses of protein are not harmful and may help to ensure an adequate supply of certain micronutrients. Adverse effects of excessive protein intake may include increased calcium losses in urine and, over a life span, increased loss of renal mass. Excessive protein intake may also cause elevated blood urea nitrogen, acidosis, hyperammonemia, and, in the premature infant, failure to thrive, lethargy, and fever.

Thureen P, Heird WC: Protein and energy requirements of the preterm/low birth weight (LBW) infant. Pediatr Res 2005;57(5 Pt 2):95R [PMID: 15817496].

LIPIDS

Fats are the main dietary energy source for infants and account for up to 50% of the energy in human milk. Over 98% of breast milk fat is triglyceride, which has an energy density of 9 kcal/g. Fats can be stored efficiently in adipose tissue with a minimal energy cost of storage. This is especially important in the young infant. Fats are required for the absorption of fat-soluble vitamins and for myelination of the central nervous system. Fat also provides essential fatty acids (EFAs) necessary for brain development, for phospholipids in cell membranes, and for the synthesis of prostaglandins and leukotrienes. The EFAs are polyunsaturated fatty acids, linoleic acid (18:2ω6) and linolenic acid (18:3ω3). Arachidonic acid (ARA, 20:4ω6) is derived from dietary linoleic acid and is present primarily in membrane phospholipids. Important derivatives of linolenic acid are eicosapentaenoic acid (20:6ω3) and docosahexaenoic acid (DHA, 22:6ω3) found in human milk and brain lipids. Visual acuity and possibly psychomotor development of for-mula-fed premature infants is improved with use of formulas supplemented with DHA (22:6ω3) and ARA (20:4ω6). The benefits of supplementing long-chain fatty acids in healthy formula-fed term infants remain unclear (although safety has been established).

Clinical features of EFA ω6 deficiency include growth failure, erythematous and scaly dermatitis, capillary fragility, increased fragility of erythrocytes, thrombocytopenia, poor wound healing, and susceptibility to infection. The clinical features of deficiency of ω3 fatty acids are less well defined, but dermatitis and neurologic abnormalities, including blurred vision, peripheral neuropathy, and weakness, have been reported. Fatty fish are the best dietary source of ω3 fatty acids. A high intake of fatty fish is associated with decreased platelet adhesiveness and decreased inflammatory response.

Up to 5–10% of fatty acids in human milk are polyunsaturated, with the specific fatty acid profile reflective of maternal dietary intake. Most of these are 6 series with smaller amounts of long-chain ω3 fatty acids. About 40% of breast milk fatty acids are monounsaturates, primarily oleic acid (18:1), and up to 10% of total fatty acids are medium-chain triglycerides (MCTs) (C_8 and C_{10}) with a calorie density of 7.6 kcal/g. In general, the percentage of calories derived from fat is a little lower in infant formulas than in human milk. Infant formulas have traditionally contained a relatively high percentage of linoleic acid but minimal long-chain ω3 fatty acid.

The American Academy of Pediatrics (AAP) recommends that infants receive at least 30% of calories from fat, with at least 2.7% of total fat as linoleic acid, and 1.75% of total fatty acids as linolenic. It is appropriate that 40–50% of energy requirements be provided as fat during at least the first year of life. Children older than 2 years should be switched gradually to a diet containing approximately 30% of total calories from fat, with no more than 10% of calories either from saturated fats or polyunsaturated fats.

β-Oxidation of fatty acids occurs in the mitochondria of muscle and liver. Carnitine is necessary for oxidation of the fatty acids, which must cross the mitochondrial membranes as acylcarnitine. Carnitine is synthesized in the human liver and kidney from lysine and methionine. Carnitine needs of infants are met by breast milk or infant formulas. In the liver, substantial quantities of fatty acids are converted to ketone bodies, which are then released into the circulation as an important fuel for the brain of the young infant.

MCTs are sufficiently soluble that micelle formation is not required for transport across the intestinal mucosa. They are transported directly to the liver via the portal circulation. MCTs are rapidly metabolized in the liver, undergoing β-oxidation or ketogenesis. They do not require carnitine to enter the mitochondria. Ketones are formed from MCTs even when provided orally. MCTs are useful for patients with luminal phase defects, absorptive defects, and chronic inflammatory bowel disease. The potential side effects of MCT administration include diarrhea when given in large quantities; high octanoic acid levels in patients with cirrhosis; and, if they are the only source of lipids, deficiency of EFA.

Bouwstra H et al: Long-chain polyunsaturated fatty acids and neurological developmental outcome at 18 months in healthy term infants. Acta Paediatr 2005;94:26 [PMID: 15858956].

McCann JC, Ames BN: Is docosahexaenoic acid, an n-3 long chain polyunsaturated fatty acid, required for development of normal brain function? An overview of evidence from cognitive and behavioral tests in humans and animals. Am J Clin Nutr 2005;82:281 [PMID: 16087970].

CARBOHYDRATES

The energy density of carbohydrate is 4 kcal/g. Approximately 40% of caloric intake in human milk is in the form of lactose, or milk sugar. Lactose supplies 20% of the total energy in cow's milk. The percent of total energy in infant formulas from carbohydrate is similar to that of human milk.

After the first 2 years of life, 50–60% of energy requirements should be derived from carbohydrates, with no more than 10% from simple sugars. These dietary guidelines are, unfortunately, not reflected in the diets of North American children, who typically derive 25% of their energy intake from sucrose and less than 20% from complex carbohydrates.

The rate at which lactase hydrolyzes lactose to glucose and galactose in the intestinal brush border determines how quickly milk carbohydrates are absorbed. Lactase levels are highest in young infants, and decline with age depending on genetic factors. About 20% of nonwhite Hispanic and black children younger than 5 years of age have lactase deficiency. White children typically do not develop symptoms of lactose intolerance until they are at least 4 or 5 years of age, whereas nonwhite Hispanic, Asian-American, and black children may develop these symptoms by 2 or 3 years of age. Lactose-intolerant children have varying symptoms depending on the specific activity of their intestinal lactase and the amount of lactose consumed. Galactose is preferentially converted to glycogen in the liver prior to conversion to glucose for subsequent oxidation. Infants with galactosemia, an inborn meta-bolic disease caused by deficient galactose-1-phosphate uridyl-transferase, require a lactose-free diet starting in the neonatal period.

Children and adolescents in North America consume large quantities of sucrose and high-fructose corn syrup in soft drinks and other sweetened beverages, candy, syrups, and sweetened breakfast cereals. Added sugar intake has been reported to average approximately 15% of total energy intake in adolescents, far exceeding recommended intakes. A high intake of these sugars, especially in the form of sweetened beverages, may predispose to obesity and insulin resistance, and is a major risk factor for dental caries. Sucrase hydrolyzes sucrose to glucose and fructose in the brush border of the small intestine. Fructose is absorbed more slowly than and independent of glucose by facilitated diffusion. Fructose does not stimulate insulin secretion or enhance leptin production. Since both insulin and leptin play a role in regulation of food intake, consumption of fructose (eg, as high-fructose corn syrup) may contribute to increased energy intake and weight gain. Fructose is also easily converted to hepatic triglycerides, which may be undesirable in malnourished patients or in patients with insulin resistance or metabolic syndrome and cardiovascular disease risk.

Dietary fiber can be classified as two major types: nondigested carbohydrate (β1–4 linkages) and noncarbohydrate (lignin). Insoluble fibers (cellulose, hemicellulose, and lignin) increase stool bulk and water content and decrease gut transit time. They may impair mineral absorption. Soluble fibers (pectins, mucilages, oat bran) bind bile acids and reduce lipid and cholesterol absorption. Pectins also slow gastric emptying and the rate of nutrient absorption. Few data regarding the fiber needs of children are available. The Dietary Reference Intakes recommend 14 g of fiber per 1000 kcal consumed. The AAP recommends that children older than 2 years consume in grams per day an amount of fiber equal to 5 plus the age in years. Fiber intakes are often low in North America. Children who have higher dietary fiber intakes have been found to consume more nutrient-dense diets than children with low fiber intakes. In general, higher fiber diets are associated with lower risk of chronic diseases such as obesity, cardiovascular disease, and diabetes.

Bray GA et al: Consumption of high-fructose corn syrup in beverages may play a role in the epidemic of obesity. Am J Clin Nutr 2004;80:537 [PMID: 15051594].

Heyman MB, Committee on Nutrition: Lactose intolerance in infants, children, and adolescents. Pediatrics 2006;118:1279 [PMID: 16951027].

Kranz S et al: Dietary fiber intake by American preschoolers is associated with more nutrient-dense diets. J Am Diet Assoc 2005;105:221 [PMID: 15668678].

MAJOR MINERALS

Calcium, phosphorus, magnesium, sodium, and potassium are essential components of human nutrition. Dietary sources, absorption, metabolism, and deficiency of these minerals are summarized in Table 10–3. Recommended dietary intakes are provided in Table 10–4.

Table 10–3. Summary of major minerals.

Mineral	Absorption/Metabolism	Deficiency	
		Causes	Clinical Features
Calcium *Dietary sources:* dairy products, legumes, broccoli, green leafy vegetables.	20–30% from diet; 60% from human milk (HM). Enhanced by lactose, glucose, protein; impaired by phytate, fiber, oxalate, unabsorbed fat. Absorption is regulated by serum calcitriol, which increases when PTH is secreted in response to low plasma-ionized calcium. PTH also promotes release of calcium from bone. Renal excretion.	Can occur in premature infants without adequate supplementation and in lactating adolescents with limited calcium intake or in patients with steatorrhea.	Osteopenia or osteoporosis, tetany.
Phosphorus *Dietary sources:* meats, eggs, dairy products, grains, legumes, and nuts; high in processed foods and sodas.	80% from diet. PTH decreases tubular resorption of phosphorus in kidney; homeostasis is maintained by GI tract and kidneys.	Rare, but can occur in premature infants fed unfortified HM (results in osteoporosis and rickets, sometimes hypercalcemia). Also seen in patients with protein-energy malnutrition.	Muscle weakness, bone pain, rhabdomyolysis, osteomalacia, and respiratory insufficiency.
Magnesium *Dietary sources:* vegetables, cereals, nuts.	Kidney regulates homeostasis by decreasing excretion when intake is low.	Occurs as part of refeeding syndrome with protein-energy malnutrition. Renal disease, malabsorption, or magnesium wasting medications may lead to depletion. May cause secondary hypocalcemia.	Neuromuscular excitability, muscle fasciculation, neurologic abnormalities, ECG changes.
Sodium *Dietary sources:* processed foods, table salt.	Hyponatremic and hypernatremic dehydration are discussed in Chapter 43. Kidney is primary site of homeostatic regulation.	Results from excess losses associated with diarrhea and vomiting.	Anorexia, vomiting, hypotension and mental apathy. Severe malnutrition, stress, and hypermetabolism may lead to excess intracellular sodium, affecting cellular metabolism.
Chloride *Dietary sources:* table salt or sea salt, seaweed, many vegetables.	Homeostasis is closely linked to sodium. Plays an important role in physiologic mechanisms of kidney and gut.	Can occur in infants fed low chloride-containing diets, or in children with cystic fibrosis, vomiting, diarrhea, chronic diuretic therapy, or Bartter syndrome.	Associated with failure to thrive and especially poor head growth; anorexia, lethargy, muscle weakness, vomiting, dehydration, hypovolemia. *Laboratory findings:* may include hypochloremia, hypokalemia, metabolic alkalosis, hyperreninemia.
Potassium *Dietary sources:* nuts, whole grains, meats, fish, beans, fruits and vegetables, especially bananas, orange juice.	Kidneys control potassium homeostasis via the aldosterone-renin-angiotensin endocrine system. Amount of total body potassium depends on lean body mass.	Occurs in protein-energy malnutrition (eg, refeeding syndrome) and can cause cardiac failure and sudden death if not treated aggressively. With loss of lean body mass, excessive potassium is excreted in urine in any catabolic state. Can also occur during acidosis, from diarrhea, and from diuretic use. Hyperkalemia may result from renal insufficiency.	Muscle weakness, mental confusion, arrhythmias.

ECG, electrocardiogram; GI, gastrointestinal; PTH, parathyroid hormone.

Table 10–4. Recommended daily intake of select minerals.

Age	Calcium	Chloride	Copper	Iron	Magnesium	Potassium	Phosphorus	Selenium	Sodium	Zinc
0–6 mos	210 mg	180 mg*	200 mcg*	0.27 mg*	30 mg*	400 mg	100 mg	15 mcg*	120 mg	2 mg
7 mos–1 y	270 mg	570 mg*	220 mcg*	11 mg	75 mg*	700 mg	275 mg	20 mcg*	370 mg	3 mg
1–3 y	500 mg	1500 mg*	340 mcg	7 mg	80 mg	3000 mg	460 mg	20 mcg	1000 mg	3 mg
4–8 y	800 mg	1900 mg*	440 mcg	10 mg	130 mg	3800 mg	500 mg	30 mcg	1200 mg	5 mg
9–13 y	1300 mg	2300 mg*	700 mcg	8 mg	240 mg	4500 mg	1250 mg	40 mcg	1500 mg	8 mg
14–18 y	1300 mg	2300 mg*	890 mcg	11 mg	410 mg	4700 mg	700 mg	55 mcg	1500 mg	9 mg (girls) 11 mg (boys)

*Adequate intakes.

TRACE ELEMENTS

Trace elements with recognized roles in human nutrition are iron, iodine, zinc, copper, selenium, manganese, molybdenum, chromium, cobalt (as a component of vitamin B_{12}), and fluoride. Information on food sources, functions, and deficiencies of selected trace elements with the most clinical relevance is summarized in Table 10–5. Dietary requirements are summarized in Table 10–4. Iron deficiency is discussed in detail in Chapter 28.

Fluoride is usually provided as an additive in drinking water or in supplemental vitamin preparations for infants and children. Recommendations for supplemental fluoride appear in Table 10–6.

Andersson M et al: Current global iodine status and progress over the last decade towards the elimination of iodine deficiency. Bull World Health Org 2005;83:518 [PMID: 16175826].

Bader JD et al: Physicians' roles in preventing dental caries in preschool children: A summary of the evidence for the U.S. Preventive Services Task Force. Am J Prev Med 2004;26:315 [PMID: 15110059].

Bhutta ZA: The role of zinc in child health in developing countries: Taking the science where it matters. Indian Pediatr 2004;41:429 [PMID: 15181293].

Black RE: Zinc deficiency, infectious disease and mortality in the developing world. J Nutr 2003;133:1485S [PMID: 12730449].

Hurwitz M et al: Copper deficiency during parenteral nutrition: A report of four pediatric cases. Nutr Clin Pract 2004;19:305 [PMID: 16215119].

VITAMINS

1. Fat-Soluble Vitamins

Because they are insoluble in water, the fat-soluble vitamins require digestion and absorption of dietary fat and a carrier system for transport in the blood. Deficiencies in these vitamins develop more slowly than deficiencies in water-soluble vitamins because the body accumulates stores of fat-soluble vitamins, but prematurity and some childhood conditions can place infants and children at risk (Table 10–7). For the same reason, excessive intakes carry a considerable potential for toxicity (Table 10–8). Recommended intakes are listed in Table 10–9.

Information about the dietary sources of fat-soluble vitamins, absorption and metabolism, and causes and clinical features of deficiency is summarized in Table 10–10. Table 10–11 outlines the clinical evaluation and treatment of these deficiencies.

Ambalavanan N et al: Vitamin A supplementation for extremely low birth weight infants: Outcome at 18 to 22 months. Pediatrics 2005;115:e249 [PMID: 15713907].

Gartner LM, Greer FR, Section on Breastfeeding and Committee on Nutrition, American Academy of Pediatrics: Prevention of rickets and vitamin D deficiency: New guidelines for vitamin D intake. Pediatrics 2003;111:908 [PMID: 12671133].

Holick MF: Vitamin D deficiency. N Engl J Med 2007;357:266 [PMID: 17634462].

Miller CA, Committee on Fetus and Newborn, American Academy of Pediatrics: Controversies concerning vitamin K and the newborn. Pediatrics 2003;112:191 [PMID: 12837888].

Pettifor JM: Rickets and vitamin D deficiency in children and adolescents. Endocrinol Metab Clin North Am 2005;34:537 [PMID: 16085158].

2. Water-Soluble Vitamins

Deficiencies of water-soluble vitamins are uncommon in the United States because of the abundant food supply and fortification of prepared foods. Cases of deficiencies (eg, scurvy) in children with special needs have been reported in the context of sharply restricted diets. Most bread and wheat products are fortified with B vitamins, including the manda-

Table 10–5. Summary of trace elements.

Mineral	Deficiency		
	Causes	Clinical Features	Treatment
Zinc *Dietary sources:* human milk, meats, shellfish, legumes, nuts, and whole grain cereals. *Functions:* component of many enzymes and gene transcription factors; plays critical roles in nucleic acid metabolism, protein synthesis, and gene expression; supports membrane structure and function.	Diets low in available zinc (high phytate), unfortified synthetic diets; malabsorptive diseases (enteritis, celiac disease, cystic fibrosis); excessive losses (chronic diarrhea); inborn errors of zinc metabolism (acrodermatitis enteropathica, mammary gland zinc secretion defect). Inadequate intake in breast-fed infants after age 6 mo. Prematurity and low birth weight are risk factors.	Mild: impaired growth, poor appetite, impaired immunity. Moderate–severe: mood changes, irritability, lethargy, impaired immune function, increased susceptibility to infection; acro-orificial skin rash, diarrhea, alopecia. Response to zinc supplement is gold standard for diagnosis of deficiency; plasma zinc levels are lowered by acute phase response.	1 mg/kg/d of elemental zinc for 3 mo (eg, 4.5 mg of $ZnSO_4 + 7\ H_2O$/kg/d), given separately from meals and iron supplements. With acrodermatitis enteropathica, 30–50 mg Zn^{2+} per day (or more) sustains remission.
Copper *Dietary sources:* human milk, meats, shellfish, legumes, nuts, and whole grain cereals. *Functions:* vital component of several oxidative enzymes: cytochrome c oxidase (electron transport chain), cytosolic and mitochondrial superoxide dismutase (free radical defense), lysyl oxidase, (cross-linking of elastin and collagen), ferroxidase, (oxidation of ferrous storage iron prior to transport to bone marrow).	Generalized malnutrition, prolonged PN without supplemental copper, malabsorption, or prolonged diarrhea. Prematurity is a risk factor.	Osteoporosis, enlargement of costochondral cartilages, cupping and flaring of long bone metaphyses, spontaneous rib fractures. Neutropenia and hypochromic anemia resistant to iron therapy. Defect of copper metabolism (Menkes kinky hair syndrome) results in severe CNS disease. Low plasma levels help to confirm deficiency; levels are normally very low in young infants. Age-matched normal data are necessary for comparison. Plasma levels are raised by acute phase response.	1% copper sulfate solution (2 mg of salt) or 500 mcg/d elemental copper for infants.
Selenium *Dietary sources:* seafood, meats, garlic (geochemical distribution affects levels in foods). *Function:* essential component of glutathione peroxidase (reduction of hydrogen peroxide to water in the cell cytosol).	Inadequate dietary intake; can occur with selenium-deficient PN. Renal disease.	Skeletal muscle pain and tenderness, macrocytosis, loss of hair pigment. Keshan disease, an often fatal cardiomyopathy in infants and children.	Minimum recommended selenium content for full-term infant formulas is 1.5 mcg/100 kcal, and for preterm formulas, 1.8 mcg/100 kcal. PN should be supplemented.
Iodine *Dietary source:* iodized salt. *Functions:* essential component of thyroid hormones; regulates metabolism, growth, and neural development.	Inadequate dietary intake. Maternal iodine deficiency causes endemic neonatal hypothyroidism in 5–16% of neonates who may have goiter at birth.	Neurologic endemic cretinism (severe mental retardation, deaf-mutism, spastic diplegia, and strabismus) occurs with severe deficiency. Myxedematous endemic cretinism occurs in some central African countries where signs of congenital hypothyroidism are present.	Use of iodized salt is effective in preventing goiter. Injections of iodized oil can also be used for prevention.
Fluoride *Function:* incorporated into the hydroxyapatite matrix of dentin.	Inadequate intake (unfluoridated water supply).	Low intake increases incidence of dental caries.	See Table 10–6 for supplementation guidelines. Excess fluoride intake results in fluorosis.

CNS, central nervous system; PN, parenteral nutrition.

Table 10–6. Supplemental fluoride recommendations (mg/d).

Age	Concentration of Fluoride in Drinking Water		
	< 0.3 ppm	0.3–0.6 ppm	> 0.6 ppm
6 mo to 3 y	0.25	0	0
3–6 y	0.5	0.25	0
6–16 y	1	0.5	0

Reproduced, with permission, from Centers for Disease Control and Prevention: Recommendations for using fluoride to prevent and control dental caries in the United States. MMWR Recomm Rep 2001;50(RR-14):8.

tory addition of folic acid to enriched grain products since January 1998. There is conclusive evidence that folic acid supplements (400 mcg/d) during the periconceptional period protect against neural tube defects. Dietary intakes of folic acid from natural foods and enriched products also are protective. Biologic roles of water-soluble vitamins are listed in Table 10–12.

The risk of toxicity from water-soluble vitamins is not as great as that associated with fat-soluble vitamins because excesses are excreted in the urine (see Table 10–8). However, deficiencies of these vitamins develop more quickly than deficiencies in fat-soluble vitamins because of limited stores (see Table 10–7). Additional salient details are summarized in Table 10–13. Although dietary intake of the water-soluble vitamins on a daily basis is not necessary, these vitamins, with

Table 10–7. Circumstances associated with risk of vitamin deficiencies.

Circumstance	Possible Deficiency
Prematurity	All vitamins
Protein-energy malnutrition	B_1, B_2, folate, A
Synthetic diets without adequate fortification (including total parenteral nutrition)	All vitamins
Vitamin–drug interactions	Folate, B_{12}, D, B_6
Fat malabsorption syndromes	Fat-soluble vitamins
Breast feeding	B_1,[a] folate,[b] B_{12},[c] D,[d] K[e]
Periconceptional	Folate
Bariatric surgery (all types)	B vitamins

[a]Alcoholic or malnourished mother.
[b]Folate-deficient mother.
[c]Vegan mother or maternal pernicious anemia.
[d]Infant not exposed to sunlight and mother's vitamin D status suboptimal.
[e]Maternal status poor; neonatal prophylaxis omitted.

Table 10–8. Effects of vitamin toxicity.

Vitamin	Clinical Features of Toxicity
Pyridoxine	Sensory neuropathy at doses > 500 mg/d
Niacin	Histamine release → cutaneous vasodilation; cardiac arrhythmias; cholestatic jaundice; gastrointestinal disturbance; hyperuricemia; glucose intolerance
Folic acid	May mask B_{12} deficiency, hypersensitivity
Vitamin C	Diarrhea; increased oxalic acid excretion; renal stones
Vitamin A	(> 20,000 IU/d): vomiting, increased intracranial pressure (pseudotumor cerebri); irritability; headaches; insomnia; emotional lability; dry, desquamating skin; myalgia and arthralgia; abdominal pain; hepatosplenomegaly; cortical thickening of bones of hands and feet
Vitamin D	(> 50,000 IU/d): hypercalcemia; vomiting; constipation; nephrocalcinosis
Vitamin E	(> 25–100 mg/kg/d IV): necrotizing enterocolitis and liver toxicity (but probably due to polysorbate 80 used as a solubilizer)
Vitamin K	*Lipid-soluble vitamin K:* very low order of toxicity. *Water-soluble, synthetic vitamin K:* vomiting, porphyrinuria; albuminuria; hemolytic anemia; hemoglobinuria; hyperbilirubinemia (do not give to neonates)

the exception of vitamin B_{12}, are not stored in the body to significant levels. Recommended intakes appear in Table 10–9.

Carnitine is synthesized in the liver and kidneys from lysine and methionine. In certain circumstances (see Table 10–12) synthesis is inadequate, and carnitine can then be considered a vitamin. A dietary supply of other organic compounds, such as inositol, may also be required in certain circumstances.

Bryan J et al: Nutrients for cognitive development in school-aged children. Nutr Rev 2004;62:295 [PMID: 15478684].

INFANT FEEDING

BREAST FEEDING

Breast feeding provides optimal nutrition for the normal infant during the early months of life. WHO recommends exclusive breast feeding for approximately the first 6 months of life, with continued breast feeding along with appropriate complementary foods through the first 2 years of life. Numerous immunologic factors in breast milk (including secretory IgA, lysozyme, lactoferrin, bifidus factor, and macrophages) provide protection against GI and upper respiratory infections. In developing countries, lack of refrigeration and contaminated water supplies make formula feeding hazardous. Although formulas have improved progressively and are made to resemble breast milk as closely as possible, it is

Table 10–9. Recommended daily intake of select vitamins.

Vitamin	0–6 mos	7 mos–1 y	1–3 y	4–8 y	9–13 y	14–18 y girl	14–18 y boy
Biotin	5 mcg*	6 mcg*	8 mcg*	12 mcg*	20 mcg*	25 mcg*	25 mcg*
Cobalamin	0.4 mcg*	0.5 mcg*	0.9 mcg	1.2 mcg	1.8 mcg	2.4 mcg	2.4 mcg
Folic Acid	65 mcg*	80 mcg*	100 mcg	200 mcg	300 mcg	400 mcg	400 mcg
Niacin	2 mg*	4 mg*	6 mg	8 mg	12 mg	16 mg	16 mg
Pantothenic Acid	1.7 mg*	1.8 mg*	2 mg*	3 mg*	4 mg*	5 mg*	5 mg*
Pyridoxine	0.1 mg*	0.3 mg*	0.5 mg	0.6 mg	1.0 mg	1.2 mg	1.3 mg
Riboflavin	0.3 mg*	0.4 mg*	0.5 mg	0.6 mg	0.9 mg	1.0 mg	1.3 mg
Thiamin	0.2 mg*	0.3 mg*	0.5 mg	0.6 mg	0.9 mg	1.0 mg	1.2 mg
Vitamin A	400 mcg*	500 mcg*	300 mcg	400 mcg	600 mcg	700 mcg	900 mcg
Vitamin C	40 mg*	50 mg*	15 mg	25 mg	75 mg	75 mg	90 mg
Vitamin D	5 mcg	5 mcg	5 mcg	5 mcg	5 mcg	5 mcg	5 mcg
Vitamin E	4 mg	5 mg	6 mg	7 mg	11 mg	15 mg	15 mg
Vitamin K	2 mcg	2.5 mcg	30 mcg	55 mcg	65 mcg	75 mcg	75 mcg

*Adequate intakes.

impossible to replicate the nutritional or immune composition of human milk. Additional differences of physiologic importance between human milk and formula continue to be identified. Furthermore, the relationship developed through breast feeding can be an important part of early maternal interactions with the infant and provides a source of security and comfort to the infant.

Breast feeding has been reestablished as the predominant initial mode of feeding young infants in the United States. Unfortunately, breast-feeding rates remain low among several subpopulations, including low-income, minority, and young mothers. Many mothers face obstacles in maintaining lactation once they return to work, and rates of breast feeding at 6 months are considerably less than the goal of 50%. Skilled use of a breast pump, particularly an electric one, can help to maintain lactation in these circumstances.

Absolute contraindications to breast feeding are rare. They include tuberculosis (in the mother) and galactosemia (in the infant). Breast feeding is associated with maternal-to-child transmission of HIV, but the risk is influenced by duration and pattern of breast feeding and maternal factors, including immunologic status and presence of mastitis. Complete avoidance of breast feeding by HIV-infected women is presently the only mechanism to ensure prevention of maternal-infant transmission. Current recommendations are that HIV-infected mothers in developed countries refrain from breast feeding if safe alternatives are available. In developing countries, the benefits of breast feeding, especially the protection of the child against diarrheal illness and malnutrition, outweigh the risk of HIV infection via breast

milk. In such circumstances, mixed feeding should be avoided because of the apparent increased risk of HIV transmission with mixed feeds.

In newborns weighing less than 1500 g, human milk should be fortified to increase protein, calcium, phosphorus, and micronutrient content as well as caloric density. Infants with cystic fibrosis can be breast-fed successfully if exogenous pancreatic enzymes are provided. If normal growth rates are not achieved in breast-fed infants with cystic fibrosis, energy or specific macronutrient supplements may be necessary. All infants with cystic fibrosis should receive supplemental vitamins A, D, E, and K, and sodium chloride.

Coutsoudis A, Rollins N: Breast-feeding and HIV transmission: The jury is still out. J Pediatr Gastroenterol Nutr 2003;26:434 [PMID: 12658031].
Gartner LM et al: Breastfeeding and the use of human milk. Pediatrics 2005;115:496 [PMID: 15687461].

Management of Breast Feeding

In developed countries, health professionals are now playing roles of greater importance in supporting and promoting breast feeding. Organizations such as the AAP and La Leche League have initiated programs to promote breast feeding and provide education for health professionals and mothers.

Perinatal hospital routines and early pediatric care have a great influence on the successful initiation of breast feeding by promoting prenatal and postpartum education, frequent mother-infant contact after delivery, one-on-one advice about breast-feeding technique, demand feeding,

Table 10–10. Summary of fat-soluble vitamins.

Vitamin	Absorption/Metabolism	Deficiency	
		Causes	Clinical Features
Vitamin A *Dietary sources:* dairy products, eggs, liver, meats, fish oils. Precursor β-carotene is abundant in yellow and green vegetables. *Functions:* has critical role in vision, helping to form photosensitive pigment rhodopsin; modifies differentiation and proliferation of epithelial cells in respiratory tract; and is needed for glycoprotein synthesis.	Retinol is stored in liver and from there is exported, attached to retinol-binding protein (RBP) and prealbumin. RBP may be decreased in liver disease or in protein energy malnutrition. Circulating RBP may be increased in renal failure.	Occurs in premature infants, in association with inadequately supplemented PN; protein-energy malnutrition (deficiency worsened by measles); dietary insufficiency and fat malabsorption.	Night blindness, xerosis, xerophthalmia, Bitot spots, keratomalacia, ulceration and perforation of cornea, prolapse of lens and iris, and blindness; follicular hyperkeratosis; pruritus; growth retardation; increased susceptibility to infection.
Vitamin K *Dietary sources:* leafy vegetables, fruits, seeds; synthesized by intestinal bacteria. *Functions:* necessary for the maintenance of normal plasma levels of coagulation factors II, VII, IX, and X; essential for maintenance of normal levels of the anticoagulation protein C; essential for osteoblastic activity.	Absorbed in proximal small intestine in micelles with bile salts; circulates with very low density lipoproteins (VLDL).	Occurs in newborns, especially those who are breast fed and who have not received vitamin K prophylaxis at delivery; in fat malabsorption syndromes; and with use of unabsorbed antibiotics and anticoagulant drugs (warfarin).	Bruising or bleeding in GI tract, genitourinary tract, gingiva, lungs, joints, and brain.
Vitamin E *Dietary sources:* vegetable oils, some cereals, dairy, wheat germ, eggs. *Functions:* α-tocopherol has highest biologic activity; as a free-radical scavenger, stops oxidation reactions. Located at specific sites in cell membrane to protect polyunsaturated fatty acids in membrane from peroxidation and to protect thiol groups and nucleic acids; also acts as cell membrane stabilizer; may function in electron transport chain; may modulate chromosomal expression.	Emulsified in intestinal lumen with bile salts; absorbed via passive diffusion; transported by chylomicrons and VLDL.	May occur with prematurity, cholestatic liver disease, pancreatic insufficiency, abetalipoproteinemia, and short bowel syndrome. Isolated inborn error of vitamin E metabolism. May result from increased consumption during oxidant stress.	Hemolytic anemia; progressive neurologic disorder with loss of deep tendon reflexes, loss of coordination, vibratory and position sensation, nystagmus, weakness, scoliosis, and retinal degeneration.
Vitamin D *Dietary sources:* fortified milk and formulas, egg yolk, fatty fish. *Functions:* calcitriol, the biologically active form of vitamin D, stimulates intestinal absorption of calcium and phosphate, renal reabsorption of filtered calcium, and mobilization of calcium and phosphorus from bone.	Normally obtained primarily from cholecalciferol (D_3) produced by UV radiation of dehydrocholesterol in skin. Ergocalciferol (D_2) is derived from UV irradiation of ergosterol in skin. Vitamin D is transported from skin to liver, attached to a specific carrier protein.	Results from a combination of inadequate sunlight exposure, dark skin pigmentation, and low dietary intake. Breast-fed infants are at risk because of low vitamin D content of human milk. Cow's milk and infant formulas are routinely supplemented with vitamin D. Deficiency also occurs in fat malabsorption syndromes. Hydroxylated vitamin D may be decreased by CYP-450–stimulating drugs, hepatic or renal disease, and inborn errors of metabolism.	Osteomalacia (adults) or rickets (children), in which osteoid with reduced calcification accumulates in bone. *Clinical findings:* craniotabes, rachitic rosary, pigeon breast, bowed legs, delayed eruption of teeth and enamel defects, Harrison groove, scoliosis, kyphosis, dwarfism, painful bones, fractures, anorexia, and weakness. *Radiographic findings:* cupping, fraying, flaring of metaphyses.

CYP, cytochrome P; GI, gastrointestinal; PN, parenteral nutrition; PTH, parathyroid hormone; UV, ultraviolet.

Table 10–11. Evaluation and treatment of deficiencies of fat-soluble vitamins.

Vitamin Deficiency	Diagnostic Laboratory Findings and Treatment
Vitamin A	*Laboratory findings:* serum retinol < 20 mcg/dL; molar ratio of retinol:RBP < 0.7 is also diagnostic.
	Treatment: xerophthalmia requires 5000–10000 IU/kg/d for 5 days PO or IM; with fat malabsorption, standard dose is 2500–5000 IU.
	Toxicity effects are listed in Table 10-8.
Vitamin K	*Laboratory findings:* assess plasma levels of protein-induced vitamin K absence (PIVKA) or PT.
	Treatment: Oral: 2.5–5.0 mg/d or IM/IV: 1–2 mg/dose as single dose.
Vitamin E	*Laboratory findings:* normal serum level is 3–15 mg/mL for children. Ratio of serum vitamin E to total serum lipid is normally $\geq$ 0.8 mg/g.
	Treatment: large oral doses (up to 100 IU/kg/d) correct deficiency from malabsorption; for abetalipoproteinemia, 100–200 IU/kg/d are needed.
Vitamin D	*Laboratory findings:* low serum phosphorus and calcium, high alkaline phosphatase, high serum PTH, low 25-OH-cholecalciferol.
	American Academy of Pediatrics recommends supplementation, as follows: 200 IU/d for all breast-fed infants, beginning in first 2 months of life and continuing until infant is receiving $\geq$ 500 mL/d of vitamin D–fortified formula or cow's milk.
	Treatment: 1600–5000 IU/d of vitamin D_3 for rickets. If poorly absorbed, give 0.05–0.2 mcg/kg/d of calcitriol.

IM, intramuscular; IV, intravenous; PO, by mouth; PT, prothrombin time; RBP, retinol-binding protein.

Table 10–12. Biologic roles of water-soluble vitamins.

Vitamin	Role
B vitamins involved in production of energy	
Thiamin (B_1)	Thiamin pyrophosphate is a coenzyme in oxidative decarboxylation (pyruvate dehydrogenase, α-ketoglutarate dehydrogenase, and transketolase).
Riboflavin (B_2)	Coenzyme of several flavoproteins (eg, flavin mononucleotide [FMN] and flavin adenine dinucleotide [FAD]) involved in oxidative/electron transfer enzyme systems.
Niacin	Hydrogen-carrying coenzymes: nicotinamide-adenine dinucleotide (NAD), nicotinamide-adenine dinucleotide phosphate (NADP); decisive role in intermediary metabolism.
Pantothenic acid	Major component of coenzyme A.
Biotin	Component of several carboxylase enzymes involved in fat and carbohydrate metabolism.
Hematopoietic B vitamins	
Folic acid	Tetrahydrofolate has essential role in one-carbon transfers. Essential role in purine and pyrimidine synthesis; deficiency $\rightarrow$ arrest of cell division (especially bone marrow and intestine).
Cobalamin (B_{12})	Methyl cobalamin (cytoplasm): synthesis of methionine with simultaneous synthesis of tetrahydrofolate (reason for megaloblastic anemia in B_{12} deficiency). Adenosyl cobalamin (mitochondria) is coenzyme for mutases and dehydratases.
Other B vitamins	
Pyridoxine (B_6)	Prosthetic group of transaminases, etc, involved in amino acid interconversions; prostaglandin and heme synthesis; central nervous system function; carbohydrate metabolism; immune development.
Other water-soluble vitamins	
L-Ascorbic acid (C)	Strong reducing agent—probably involved in all hydroxylations. Roles include collagen synthesis; phenylalanine $\rightarrow$ tyrosine; tryptophan $\rightarrow$ 5-hydroxytryptophan; dopamine $\rightarrow$ norepinephrine; Fe^{3+}; folic acid $\rightarrow$ folinic acid; cholesterol $\rightarrow$ bile acids; leukocyte function; interferon production; carnitine synthesis. Copper metabolism; reduces oxidized vitamin E.

rooming-in, avoidance of bottle supplements, early follow-up after delivery, maternal confidence, family support, adequate maternity leave, and advice about common problems such as sore nipples. Breast feeding is undermined by mother-infant separations, bottle-feeding of infants in the nursery at night, routine supplemental bottle feedings, conflicting advice from staff, incorrect infant positioning and latch-on, scheduled feedings, lack of maternal support, delayed follow-up, early return to employment, and inaccurate advice for common breast-feeding difficulties.

Very few women are physiologically unable to nurse their infants. The newborn is generally fed ad libitum every 2–3 hours, with longer intervals (4–5 hours) at night. Thus a newborn infant nurses at least 8–10 times a day, so that a generous milk supply is stimulated. This frequency is not an indication of inadequate lactation. In neonates, a loose stool is often passed with each feeding; later (at age 3–4 months), there may be an interval of several days between stools. Failure to pass several stools a day in the early weeks of breast feeding suggests inadequate milk intake and supply.

Expressing milk may be indicated if the mother returns to work or if the infant is premature, cannot suck adequately, or is hospitalized. Electric breast pumps are very effective and can be borrowed or rented.

Table 10–13. Summary of water-soluble vitamins.

Vitamin	Deficiency	
	Causes	Clinical Features
Thiamin (B₁) *Dietary sources:* whole and enriched grains, lean pork, legumes.	Beriberi in infants breast fed by mothers with history of alcoholism or poor diet; has been described as a complication of PN; protein-energy malnutrition; following bariatric surgery of all types (reported in adults and adolescents).	"Dry" Beriberi (paralytic or nervous): peripheral neuropathy, with impairment of sensory, motor, and reflex functions. "Wet" Beriberi: high output congestive ± signs of dry beriberi. Cerebral Beriberi: triad of ophthalmoplegia, ataxia, and mental confusion.
Riboflavin (B₂) *Dietary sources:* dairy products, meat, poultry, wheat germ, leafy vegetables.	General undernutrition; inactivation in PN solutions exposed to light.	Cheilosis; angular stomatitis; glossitis; soreness and burning of lips and mouth; dermatitis of nasolabial fold and genitals; ± ocular signs (photophobia → indistinct vision).
Niacin (B₃) *Dietary sources:* meats, poultry, fish, legumes, wheat, all foods except fats; synthesized in body from tryptophan.	Maize- or millet-based diets (high leucine and low tryptophan intakes); carcinoid tumors.	Pellagra (dermatitis, especially on sun-exposed areas; diarrhea; dementia.
Pyridoxine (B₆) *Dietary sources:* animal products, vegetables, whole grains.	Prematurity (these infants may not convert pyridoxine to pyridoxal-5-P); B₆ dependency syndromes; drugs (isoniazid).	Listlessness; irritability; seizures; anemia; cheilosis; glossitis.
Biotin *Dietary sources:* yeast, liver, kidneys, legumes, nuts, egg yolks (synthesized by intestinal bacteria).	Suppressed intestinal flora and impaired intestinal absorption; regular intake of raw egg whites.	Scaly dermatitis; alopecia; irritability; lethargy.
Folic acid *Dietary sources:* leafy vegetables (easily destroyed in cooking), fruits, whole grains, wheat germ, beans, nuts.	Breast-fed infants whose mothers are folate-deficient; term infants fed unsupplemented processed cow's milk or goat's milk; kwashiorkor; chronic overcooking of food sources; malabsorption of folate because of a congenital defect; celiac disease; drugs (phenytoin). Increased requirements in chronic hemolytic anemias, diarrhea, malignancies, extensive skin disease, cirrhosis, pregnancy.	Megaloblastic anemia; neutropenia; growth retardation; delayed maturation of central nervous system in infants; diarrhea (mucosal ulcerations); glossitis; neural tube defects.
Cobalamin (B₁₂) *Dietary sources:* eggs, dairy products, liver, meats; *none in plants.*	Breast-fed infants of mothers with latent pernicious anemia or who are on an unsupplemented vegan diet; absence of luminal proteases; short gut syndrome (absence of stomach or ileum); congenital malabsorption of B₁₂.	Megaloblastic anemia; hypersegmented neutrophils; neurologic degeneration: paresthesias, gait problems, depression.
Vitamin C *Dietary sources:* fruits and vegetables.	Maternal megadoses during pregnancy → deficiency in infants (rebound); diet without fruits or vegetables; seen in infants fed formula based on pasteurized cow's milk (historical).	Irritability, apathy, pallor; increased susceptibility to infections; hemorrhages under skin, petechiae, in mucous membranes, in joints and under periosteum; long-bone tenderness; costochondral beading.
Carnitine *Dietary sources:* meats, dairy products; *none in plants.*	Premature infants fed unsupplemented formula or fed intravenously; dialysis; inherited deficits in carnitine synthesis; organic acidemias; valproic acid.	Increased serum triglycerides and free fatty acids; decreased ketones; fatty liver; hypoglycemia; progressive muscle weakness, cardiomyopathy, hypoglycemia.

PN, parenteral nutrition.

Technique of Breast Feeding

Breast feeding can be started after delivery as soon as both mother and infant are stable. Correct positioning and breast-feeding technique are necessary to ensure effective nipple stimulation and optimal breast emptying with minimal nipple discomfort.

If the mother wishes to nurse while sitting, the infant should be elevated to the height of the breast and turned completely to face the mother, so that their abdomens touch. The mother's arms supporting the infant should be held tightly at her side, bringing the infant's head in line with her breast. The breast should be supported by the lower fingers of her free hand, with the nipple compressed between the thumb and index fingers to make it more protractile. The infant's initial licking and mouthing of the nipple helps make it more erect. When the infant opens its mouth, the mother should rapidly insert as much nipple and areola as possible.

The most common early cause of poor weight gain in breast-fed infants is poorly managed mammary engorgement, which rapidly decreases milk supply. Unrelieved engorgement can result from inappropriately long intervals between feeding, improper infant suckling, an undemanding infant, sore nipples, maternal or infant illness, nursing from only one breast, and latching difficulties. Poor maternal feeding technique, inappropriate feeding routines, and inadequate amounts of fluid and rest all can be factors. Some infants are too sleepy to do well on an ad libitum regimen and may need waking to feed at night. Primary lactation failure occurs in fewer than 5% of women.

A sensible guideline for duration of feeding is 5 minutes per breast at each feeding the first day, 10 minutes on each side at each feeding the second day, and 10–15 minutes per side thereafter. A vigorous infant can obtain most of the available milk in 5–7 minutes, but additional sucking time ensures breast emptying, promotes milk production, and satisfies the infant's sucking urge. The side on which feeding is commenced should be alternated. The mother may break suction gently after nursing by inserting her finger between the infant's gums.

Follow-Up

Individualized assessment before discharge should identify mothers and infants needing additional support. All mother-infant pairs require early follow-up. The onset of copious milk secretion between the second and fourth postpartum days is a critical time in the establishment of lactation. Failure to empty the breasts during this time can cause engorgement, which quickly leads to diminished milk production.

Common Problems

Nipple tenderness requires attention to proper positioning of the infant and correct latch-on. Ancillary measures include nursing for shorter periods, beginning feedings on the less sore side, air drying the nipples well after nursing, and use of lanolin cream. Severe nipple pain and cracking usually indicate improper infant attachment. Temporary pumping may be needed.

Breast-feeding jaundice is exaggerated physiologic jaundice associated with inadequate intake of breast milk, infrequent stooling, and unsatisfactory weight gain. (See Chapter 1.) If possible, the jaundice should be managed by increasing the frequency of nursing and, if necessary, augmenting the infant's sucking with regular breast pumping. Supplemental feedings may be necessary, but care should be taken not to decrease breast milk production further.

In a small percentage of breast-fed infants, breast milk jaundice is caused by an unidentified property of the milk that inhibits conjugation of bilirubin. In severe cases, interruption of breast feeding for 24–36 hours may be necessary. The mother's breast should be emptied with an electric breast pump during this period.

The symptoms of mastitis include flulike symptoms with breast tenderness, firmness, and erythema. Antibiotic therapy covering β-lactamase–producing organisms should be given for 10 days. Analgesics may be necessary, but breast feeding should be continued. Breast pumping may be helpful adjunctive therapy.

American Academy of Pediatrics Subcommittee on Hyperbilirubinemia: Management of hyperbilirubinemia in the newborn infant 35 of more weeks of gestation. Pediatrics 2004;114:297 [PMID: 15231951]. Erratum: Pediatrics 2004;114:1138.

Dann MH: The lactation consult: Problem solving, teaching, and support for the breastfeeding family. J Pediatr Health Care 2005;19:12 [PMID: 15662357].

Maternal Drug Use

Factors playing a role in the transmission of drugs in breast milk include the route of administration, dosage, molecular weight, pH, and protein binding. Generally, any drug prescribed to a newborn can be consumed by the breast-feeding mother without ill effect. Very few drugs are absolutely contraindicated in breast-feeding mothers; these include radioactive compounds, antimetabolites, lithium, diazepam, chloramphenicol, antithyroid drugs, and tetracycline. For up-to-date information, a regional drug center should be consulted.

Maternal use of illicit or recreational drugs is a contraindication to breast feeding. Expression of milk for a feeding or two after use of a drug is not an acceptable compromise. The breast-fed infants of mothers taking methadone (but not alcohol or other drugs) as part of a treatment program have generally not experienced ill effects when the daily maternal methadone dose is less than 40 mg.

Hale TW: Maternal medications during breastfeeding. Clin Obstet Gynecol 2004;47:696 [PMID: 15326432].

Case Western Reserve University breast-feeding web site: http://www.breastfeedingbasics.org

Dr. Hale's breast-feeding pharmacology page: http://neonatal.ttuhsc.edu/lact/

Nutrient Composition

The nutrient composition of human milk is summarized and compared with that of cow's milk and formulas in Table 10–14. Outstanding characteristics include (1) relatively low but highly bioavailable protein content, which is adequate for the normal infant; (2) generous but not excessive quantity of essential fatty acids; (3) long-chain unsaturated ω3 fatty acids, of which DHA is thought to be especially important; (4) relatively low sodium and solute load; and (5) lower concentration of highly bioavailable minerals, which are adequate for the needs of normal breast-fed infants for approximately 6 months.

Table 10–14. Composition of human and cow's milk and typical infant formula (per 100 kcal).

Nutrient (unit)	Minimal Level Recommended[a]	Mature Human Milk	Typical Commercial Formula	Cow's Milk (mean)
Protein (g)	1.8[b]	1.3–1.6	2.3	5.1
Fat (g)	3.3[c]	5	5.3	5.7
Carbohydrate (g)	—	10.3	10.8	7.3
Linoleic acid (mg)	300	560	2300	125
Vitamin A (IU)	250	250	300	216
Vitamin D (IU)	40	3	63	3
Vitamin E (IU)	0.7/g linoleic acid	0.3	2	0.1
Vitamin K (mcg)	4	2	9	5
Vitamin C (mg)	8	7.8	8.1	2.3
Thiamin (mcg)	40	25	80	59
Riboflavin (mcg)	60	60	100	252
Niacin (mcg)	250	250	1200	131
Vitamin B_6 (mcg)	15 mcg of protein	15	63	66
Folic acid (mcg)	4	4	10	8
Pantothenic acid (mcg)	300	300	450	489
Vitamin B_{12} (mcg)	0.15	0.15	0.25	0.56
Biotin (mcg)	1.5	1	2.5	3.1
Inositol (mg)	4	20	5.5	20
Choline (mg)	7	13	10	23
Calcium (mg)	5	50	75	186
Phosphorus (mg)	25	25	65	145
Magnesium (mg)	6	6	8	20
Iron (mg)	1	0.1	1.5	0.08
Iodine (mcg)	5	4–9	10	7
Copper (mcg)	60	25–60	80	20
Zinc (mg)	0.5	0.1–0.5	0.65	0.6
Manganese (mcg)	5	1.5	5–160	3
Sodium (mEq)	0.9	1	1.7	3.3
Potassium (mEq)	2.1	2.1	2.7	6
Chloride (mEq)	1.6	1.6	2.3	4.6
Osmolarity (mOsm)	—	11.3	16–18.4	40

[a]Committee on Nutrition, American Academy of Pediatrics.
[b]Protein of nutritional quality equal to casein.
[c]Includes 300 mg of essential fatty acids.

Complementary Feeding

The AAP and WHO recommend the introduction of solid foods in normal infants at about 6 months of age. Gradual introduction of a variety of foods, including fortified cereals, fruits, vegetables, and meats, should complement the breast milk diet. Meats provide an important dietary source of iron and zinc, both of which are low in human milk by 6 months, and pureed meats may be introduced as an early complementary food. Single-ingredient complementary foods are introduced one at a time at weekly intervals before a new food is given. Fruit juice is not an essential part of an infant diet. Juice should not be introduced until after 6 months; should only be offered in a cup; and the amount should be limited to 4 oz/d. Breast feeding should ideally continue for at least 12 months, and thereafter for as long as mutually desired. Infants who are not breast fed should receive standard iron-fortified infant formula. Whole cow's milk can be introduced after the first year of life.

Kramer MS et al: Infant growth and health outcomes associated with 3 compared with 6 months of exclusive breastfeeding. Am J Clin Nutr 2003;78:291 [PMID: 12885711].
Krebs NF, Hambidge KM: Complementary feeding: Clinically relevant factors affecting timing and composition. Am J Clin Nutr 2007;85:639S [PMID: 17284770].

SPECIAL DIETARY PRODUCTS FOR INFANTS

Soy Protein Formulas

Historically, a common rationale for the use of soy protein formulas was the transient lactose intolerance after acute gastroenteritis. Lactose-free cow's milk protein–based formulas are also now available. These formulas are also useful for infants with galactosemia and hereditary lactase deficiency. Soy protein formulas are often used in cases of suspected intolerance to cow's milk protein. Although infants with true cow's milk protein intolerance may also be intolerant of soy protein, those with documented IgE-mediated allergy to cow's milk protein usually do well on soy formula.

Semi-Elemental & Elemental Formulas

Semi-elemental formulas include protein hydrolysate formulas. The major nitrogen source of most of these products is casein hydrolysate, supplemented with selected amino acids, but partial hydrolysates of whey are also available. These formulas contain an abundance of EFA from vegetable oil; certain brands also provide substantial amounts of MCTs. Elemental formulas are available with free amino acids and varying levels and types of fat components.

Semi-elemental and elemental formulas are invaluable for infants with a wide variety of malabsorption syndromes. They are also effective in infants who cannot tolerate cow's milk and soy protein. Controlled trials suggest that for infants with a family history of atopic disease, partial hydrolysate formulas

may delay or prevent atopic disease. For specific product information, consult standard pediatric reference texts, formula manufacturers, or a pediatric dietitian.

Hays T, Wood RA: A systematic review of the role of hydrolyzed infant formulas in allergy prevention. Arch Pediatr Adolesc Med 2005;159:810 [PMID: 15143739].
Hernell O, Lonnerdal B: Nutritional evaluation of protein hydrolysate formulas in healthy term infants: Plasma amino acids, hematology, and trace elements. Am J Clin Nutr 2003;78:296 [PMID: 12885712].

Formula Additives

Occasionally it may be necessary to increase the caloric density of an infant feeding to provide more calories or restrict fluid intake. Concentrating formula to 24–26 kcal/oz is usually well tolerated, delivers an acceptable renal solute load, and increases the density of all the nutrients. Beyond this, individual macronutrient additives (Table 10–15) are usually employed to achieve the desired caloric density (up to 30 kcal/oz) based on the infant's needs and underlying condition(s). A pediatric nutrition specialist can be helpful in formulating calorically dense infant formula feedings. The caloric density of breast milk can be increased by adding infant formula powder or any of the additives used with infant formula. Human milk fortifiers are generally used only for premature infants because of their specialized nutrient composition.

Special Formulas

Special formulas are those in which one component, often an amino acid, is reduced in concentration or removed for the dietary management of a specific inborn metabolic disease. Also included under this heading are formulas designed for the management of specific disease states, such as hepatic failure, pulmonary failure with chronic carbon dioxide retention, and renal failure. These condition-specific formulas were formulated primarily for critically ill adults and are even used sparingly in those populations; thus their use in pediatrics should only be undertaken with clear indication and caution.

Complete information regarding the composition of these special formulas, the standard infant formulas, specific metabolic disease formulas, and premature infant formulas can be found in standard reference texts and in the manufacturers' literature.

NUTRITION FOR THE OLDER CHILD

Because of the association of diet with the development of such chronic diseases as diabetes, obesity, and cardiovascular disease, learning a healthy eating behavior at a young age is an important preventative measure.

Salient features of the diet for children older than 2 years include the following:

Table 10–15. Common infant formula additives.

Additive	kcal/g	kcal/Tbsp	kcal/mL	Comments
Dry rice cereal	3.75	15	—	Thickens formula but not breast milk
Polycose (Abbott Nutrition)	3.8	23	.2	Glucose polymers
Moducal (Mead Johnson)	3.75	30	—	Maltodextrin
MCT oil (Novartis)	8.3	116	7.7	Not a source of essential fatty acids
Microlipid (Novartis)	9	68.5	4.5	Safflower oil emulsion with 0.4 g linoleic acid/mL
Vegetable oil	9	124	8.3	Does not mix well
Promod (Abbott Nutrition)	4.3	16.8 (3 g protein)	—	Whey protein concentrate
Casec (Mead Johnson)	3.8	16.7 (4 g protein)	—	Calcium caseinate
Duocal (SHS)	4.9	42	—	Protein-free mix of hydrolyzed corn starch (60% kcal) and fat (35% MCT)

MCT, medium-chain triglyceride.

1. Consumption of three regular meals per day, and two or three healthful snacks according to appetite, activity, and growth needs.
2. Inclusion of a variety of foods. Diet should be nutritionally complete and promote optimal growth and activity.
3. Fat should comprise less than 35% of total calories (Severe fat restriction may result in an energy deficit and growth failure). Saturated fats should provide less than 10% of total calories. Monounsaturated fats should provide 10% or more of caloric intake. Consumption of trans-fatty acids, found in stick margarine and shortening, and in many processed foods, should be kept as low as possible.
4. Cholesterol intake less than 100 mg/1000 kcal/d, to a maximum of 300 mg/d.
5. Carbohydrates should provide 45–65% of daily caloric intake, with no more than 10% in the form of simple sugars. A high-fiber, whole-grain-based diet is recommended.
6. Limitation of grazing behavior, eating while watching television, and the consumption of soft drinks and other sweetened beverages.
7. Limitation of sodium intake by choosing fresh over processed foods.

The consumption of lean cuts of meats, poultry, and fish should be encouraged. Skim or low-fat milk, soft margarine, and vegetable oils (especially canola or olive oil) should be used. Whole-grain bread and cereals and plentiful amounts of fruits and vegetables are recommended. The consumption of processed foods, soft drinks, desserts, and candy should be limited.

A prudent diet should be only one component of counseling on lifestyles for children. Other aspects are the maintenance of a desirable body weight; promotion of regular physical activity and limiting sedentary behaviors; avoidance of smoking; and screening for hypertension. Universal screening for total cholesterol is controversial. Current recommendations are to routinely screen those children who have a positive family history of premature cardiovascular disease, although this approach will identify only about 50% of those with significantly elevated cholesterol levels. If the result is high (≥ 200 mg/dL), a fasting lipoprotein analysis should be obtained.

Gidding SS et al: Dietary Recommendations for Children and Adolescents: A Guide for Practitioners, Consensus Statement from the American Heart Association. Circulation 2005;112:2061 [PMID: 16186441].

Kavey RE et al: American Heart Association guidelines for primary prevention of atherosclerotic cardiovascular disease beginning in childhood. J Pediatr 2003;142:368 [PMID: 12712052].

PEDIATRIC UNDER- & OVERNUTRITION

PEDIATRIC UNDERNUTRITION

ESSENTIALS OF DIAGNOSIS AND TYPICAL FEATURES

▸ Poor weight gain or weight loss.
▸ Loss of subcutaneous fat, temporal wasting.
▸ Most commonly related to inadequate caloric intake.
▸ Often associated with marginal or low iron and zinc status.

General Considerations

Pediatric undernutrition is usually multifactorial in origin, and successful treatment depends on accurate identification and management of those factors. The terms "organic" and "nonorganic" failure to thrive, though still used by many medical professionals, are not helpful because any systemic illness or chronic condition can cause growth impairment and yet may also be compounded by psychosocial or behavioral problems.

Clinical Findings

Failure to thrive is a term used to describe infants and young children whose weight curve has fallen by two major percentile channels from a previously established rate of growth. (See Chapter 2.) The acute loss of weight, or failure to gain weight at the expected rate, produces a condition of reduced weight for height known as *wasting*. The reduction in height for age, as is seen with more chronic malnutrition, is termed *stunting*.

The typical pattern for mild pediatric undernutrition is decreased weight, with normal height and head circumference. In more chronic malnutrition, height and eventually head circumference growth slow relative to the standard for age. Significant calorie deprivation produces severe wasting, called *marasmus*. Significant protein deprivation in the face of adequate energy intake, possibly with additional insults such as infection, may produce edematous malnutrition called *kwashiorkor*.

A discussion of the multiple medical conditions that can cause pediatric undernutrition is beyond the scope of this chapter. However, the most common cause is inadequate dietary intake. In young but otherwise healthy breast-fed or bottle-fed infants, a weak suck is often the causative factor. Inappropriate formula mixing or a family's dietary beliefs may lead to hypocaloric or unbalanced dietary intakes. Diets restricted because of suspected food allergies or intolerances may result in inadequate intake of calories, protein, or specific micronutrients. Iron and zinc are micronutrients that are often marginal in many young children with undernutrition. Cases of severe malnutrition and kwashiorkor have occurred in infants of well-intentioned parents who substitute "health food" milk alternatives (eg, rice milk or unfortified soy milk) for infant formula.

Treatment

Poor eating is often a learned behavior. Families should be counseled regarding choices of foods that are appropriate for the age and developmental level of the child. Children should have structured meal times (eg, three meals and two to three snacks during the day), ideally at the same time other family members eat. Consultation with a pediatric dietitian can be helpful for educating families. Poor feeding may be related to family dysfunction. Children whose households are chaotic and children who are abused, neglected, or exposed to poorly controlled mental illness may be described as poor eaters, and may fail to gain. Careful assessment of the social environment of such children is critical, and disposition options may include support services, close medical follow-up visits, family counseling, and even foster placement while a parent receives therapy.

Block RW, Krebs NF: Failure to thrive as a manifestation of child neglect. Pediatrics 2005;116:1234 [PMID: 16264015].

Emond A et al: Postnatal factors associated with failure to thrive in term infants in the Avon Longitudinal Study of Parents and Children. Arch Dis Child 2007;92:115 [PMID: 16905563].

PEDIATRIC OVERWEIGHT/OBESITY (SEE ALSO CHAPTER 3 FOR SPECIFICS OF ADOLESCENT OBESITY)

ESSENTIALS OF DIAGNOSIS AND TYPICAL FEATURES

▶ Excessive rate of weight gain; upward change in BMI percentiles.

▶ BMI between the 85th and 95th percentiles indicates overweight.

▶ BMI > 95th percentile indicates obesity and is associated with increased risk of secondary complications.

General Considerations

The prevalence of childhood and adolescent obesity has increased rapidly in the United States and many other parts of the world. Currently in the United States, approximately 17% of 6- to 19-year-olds are obese, with even higher rates among subpopulations of minority and economically disadvantaged children. The increasing incidence of childhood obesity is related to a complex combination of genetic, environmental, psychosocial, biologic, and socioeconomic factors.

Overweight status in the pediatric population is associated with significant comorbidities which, if untreated, are likely to persist into adulthood. The probability of obesity persisting into adulthood has been estimated to increase from 20% at 4 years to 80% by adolescence. Obesity is associated with cardiovascular and endocrine abnormalities (eg, dyslipidemia, insulin resistance, and type 2 diabetes), orthopedic problems, pulmonary complications (eg, obstructive sleep apnea), and mental health problems.

Clinical Findings

A. Definitions

BMI is the standard measure of obesity in adults. Its use in children provides a consistent measure across age groups. BMI is correlated with more accurate measures of body fatness and is calculated with readily available information: weight and height (kg ÷ m^2). Routine plotting of the BMI on age- and gender-appropriate charts (available at http://www.cdc.gov/growthcharts; see also Chapter 2) can identify those with excess weight gain relative to linear growth. New definitions were proposed in 2007 by an Expert Committee (http://www.ama-assn.org/ped_obesity_recs.pdf). BMI between the 85th and 95th percentile for age and sex identifies those who are overweight. Obesity is defined as BMI at or above 95% and is associated with increased risk of secondary complications. Severe obesity is characterized by BMI for age and sex at or above the 99th percentile. An upward change in BMI percentiles in any range should prompt an evaluation and possible treatment. Although the degree of change that indicates risk has not been defined, an annual increase of 3–4 BMI units is almost always an indicator of a rapid increase in body fat. For children younger than 2 years, weight for length greater than the 95th percentile indicates overweight and warrants further assessment, especially of energy intake and feeding behaviors.

B. Risk Factors

There are multiple risk factors for developing obesity, reflecting the complex relationships between genetic and environmental factors. Family history is a strong risk factor. If one parent is obese, the odds ratio is approximately 3 for obesity in adulthood, but if both parents are obese, the odds ratio increases to greater than 10.

Environmental risk factors offer potential areas to target for intervention. Excessive consumption of sugar-sweetened beverages, large portion sizes, frequent consumption of foods prepared outside the home, excessive television viewing, and sedentary lifestyle are all associated with a greater risk of excessive weight gain.

C. Assessment

Early recognition of high-risk patterns of weight gain or high-risk behaviors is essential, as it is likely that anticipatory guidance or intervention before weight gain becomes severe will be more successful. Routine evaluation at well-child visits should include:

1. Measurement of weight and height, calculation of BMI, and plotting all three parameters on age- and sex-appropriate growth charts. Evaluate for upward crossing of BMI percentile channels.

2. History regarding diet and activity patterns (Table 10–16); family history, and review of systems. Physical examination should include careful blood pressure measurement, distribution of adiposity (central vs generalized); markers of comorbidities, such as acanthosis nigricans, hirsutism, hepatomegaly, orthopedic abnormalities; physical stigmata of genetic syndrome (eg, Prader-Willi syndrome).

3. Laboratory studies are generally reserved for children with BMI in the obesity category (> 95th percentile) or those in the overweight category who have risk factors. Suggested laboratory tests include fasting lipid profile and glucose; and liver function tests (aspartate transaminase [AST] and alanine transaminase [ALT]). Other studies should be guided by historical and physical findings.

Table 10–16. Suggested areas for assessment of diet and activity patterns.

Diet
- Portion sizes: adult portions for young children
- Frequency of meals away from home (restaurants or take out)
- Frequency/amounts of sugar-sweetened beverages (soda, juice drinks)
- Meal and snack pattern: structured vs grazing, skipping meals
- Frequency of eating fruits and vegetables
- Frequency of family meals

Activity
- Time spent in sedentary activity: television, video games
- Time spent in vigorous activity: organized sports, physical education, free play
- Activities of daily living: walking to school, chores, yard work

▶ Treatment

Therapy should be based on risk factors, including age, severity of obesity, and comorbidities, as well as family history and support. For all children with uncomplicated obesity, the primary goal is to achieve healthy eating and activity patterns, not necessarily to achieve ideal body weight. For children with a secondary complication, improvement of the complication is an important goal. For children 2–7 years old with BMI at the 95th percentile or modestly above and without complications, the goal should generally be maintenance of baseline weight, allowing the child to "grow into" his or her height, with a gradual normalization of BMI. For children 2–7 years old with BMI at the 95th percentile or above and secondary complications, weight loss is indicated. For children older than 7 years with BMI between the 85th and 95th percentile, without complications, weight maintenance is an appropriate goal. If secondary complications are present, weight loss is recommended; an appropriate goal is 1 pound weight loss per month until a BMI less than 85% is achieved. Excessive acute weight loss should be avoided, as this may contribute to nutrient deficiencies and linear growth stunting.

There are few studies of the long-term effects of weight control programs for children. Treatment focused on behavior changes in the context of family involvement has been associated with sustained weight loss and decreases in BMI. Clinicians should assess the family's readiness to take action (transtheoretical model and motivational interviewing). Concurrent changes in dietary patterns and increasing physical activity are most likely to provide success. The whole family should be encouraged to adopt healthy eating patterns, with parents modeling healthy food choices, controlling foods brought into the home, and guiding appropriate portion sizes. Limiting sedentary activity has been found to be more effective than specifically promoting increased physical activity. The AAP recommends no television for children younger than 2 years old, and a maximum of 2 h/d of television and video games for older children.

A "staged approach" for treatment has been proposed, with different levels depending on the severity of overweight, the age of the child, the ability of the family to implement changes, the preferences of the parents and child, and the skills of the health care provider.

1. *Prevention plus:* Counseling regarding problem areas identified by screening questions (see Table 10–16); emphasis on lifestyle changes, including healthy eating and physical activity patterns. This is especially appropriate for preventing further weight gain or for mildly overweight children.

2. *Structured weight management:* Provision of a more specific and structured dietary pattern, such as meal planning, exercise prescription, and behavior change goals. This may be done in the primary care setting but generally requires ancillary health professionals, including a dietitian, behavior specialist, and physical therapist. Monitoring is monthly or tailored to the needs of the patient and family.

3. *Comprehensive multidisciplinary approach:* This level further increases the structure of therapeutic interventions and support, uses a multidisciplinary team, and may involve weekly group meetings.

4. *Tertiary care intervention:* This level is for patients who have not been successful at the other intervention levels or who are severely obese. Interventions are prescribed by a multidisciplinary team, and may include intensive behavior therapy, specialized diets, medications, and surgery.

No single prescription is effective for all patients. The physician's focus should be on assessing the severity of the problem, identifying treatment needs in the context of the family's preferences and abilities, and utilizing local resources, including availability of registered dietitians with expertise in pediatric weight management and behaviorists or family therapists.

Pharmacotherapy can be an adjunct to dietary, activity, and behavioral treatment, but by itself it is unlikely to result in significant or sustained weight loss. Two medications are approved for obesity treatment in adolescents: sibutramine, a selective serotonin reuptake inhibitor, is approved for patients older than 16 years; orlistat, a lipase inhibitor, is approved for patients older than 12 years. Bariatric surgery is being performed in some centers for severe obesity in adolescents, particularly those with comorbidities. Evidence is emerging that in carefully selected and closely monitored patients, surgery can result in significant weight loss with a reduction in comorbidities for those who are severely afflicted.

Barlow SE: Expert Committee recommendations regarding the prevention, assessment, and treatment of child and adolescent overweight and obesity: Summary report. Pediatrics 2007;120:S165 [PMID: 18055651].

Daniels SR et al: Overweight in children and adolescents. Pathophysiology, consequences, prevention, and treatment. Circulation 2005;111:1999 [PMID: 15837955].

Dietz WH, Robinson TN: Overweight children and adolescents. N Engl J Med 2005;353:2100 [PMID: 15901863].

Ogden CL et al: Prevalence of overweight and obesity in the United States, 1999-2004. JAMA 2006;295:1549 [PMID: 16595758].

Schwartz RP et al: Office-based motivational interviewing to prevent childhood obesity. Arch Pediatr Adolesc Med 2007;161:495 [PMID: 17485627].

▼ NUTRITION SUPPORT

ENTERAL NUTRITION

Indications

Enteral nutrition support is indicated when a patient cannot adequately meet nutritional needs by oral intake alone and has a functioning GI tract. This method of support can be used for short- and long-term delivery of nutrition. Even when the gut cannot absorb 100% of nutritional needs, some enteral feedings should be attempted. Enteral nutrition, full or partial, has many benefits, including:

1. Maintaining gut mucosal integrity
2. Preserving gut-associated lymphoid tissue
3. Stimulating gut hormones and bile flow

The nutritional needs of most patients requiring enteral nutrition can be met with standard enteral formulations. Specialized formulas are available for patients of all ages with severe milk protein allergy, single- or multiple-nutrient malabsorption, renal failure, and hepatic failure. The decision to use such specialized formulas must be made in the context of the patient's condition and nutritional needs.

Access Devices

Nasogastric feeding tubes can be used for supplemental enteral feedings, but generally are not used for more than 6 months because of the complications of otitis media and sinusitis. Initiation of nasogastric feeding usually requires a brief hospital stay, especially for infants younger than age 6 months, to ensure tolerance to feedings and to allow for parental instruction in tube placement and feeding administration.

If long-term feeding support is anticipated, a more permanent feeding device, such as a gastrostomy tube, may be considered. Unfortunately, many insurance carriers do not cover the cost of formula for tube feedings. Referral to a home care company is necessary for equipment and other services such as nursing visits and dietitian follow-up.

Table 10–17 suggests appropriate timing for initiation and advancement of drip and bolus feedings, according to a child's age. Clinical status and tolerance to feedings should ultimately guide their advancement.

Monitoring

Monitoring the adequacy of enteral feeding depends on nutritional goals. Growth should be frequently assessed,

Table 10–17. Guidelines for the initiation and advancement of tube feedings.

Age	Drip Feeds		Bolus Feeds	
	Initiation	Advancement	Initiation	Advancement
Preterm	1–2 mL/kg	1 mL as tolerated	5–20 mL	5–10 mL as tolerated
Birth–12 mo	5–10 mL/h	5–10 mL q 2–8 h	10–60 mL	20–40 mL q 3–4 h
1–6 y	10–15 mL/h	10–15 mL q 2–8 h	30–90 mL	30–60 mL q feed
6–14 y	15–20 mL/h	10–20 mL q 2–8 h	60–120 mL	60–90 mL q feed
> 14 y	20–30 mL/h	20–30 mL q 2–8 h	60–120 mL	60–120 mL q feed

especially for young infants and malnourished children. Hydration status should be monitored carefully at the initiation of enteral feeding. Either constipation or diarrhea can be problems, and attention to stool frequency, volume, and consistency can help guide management. When diarrhea occurs, factors such as infection, hypertonic enteral medications, antibiotic use, and alteration in normal gut flora should be addressed before making formula changes.

It is important to determine whether the feeding schedule is developmentally appropriate. This will not be possible for all patients, especially those who are critically ill. However, for children who are more stable, tube-feeding schedules should mimic as closely as possible an age-appropriate feeding schedule (eg, six small feedings per day for a toddler). When night drip feedings are used in conjunction with daytime feeds, it is suggested that less than 50% of goal calories be delivered at night so as to maintain a daytime sense of hunger and satiety. This is especially important once a transition to oral intake begins. Children who are satiated by tube feedings are less likely to take significant amounts of food by mouth, thus possibly delaying the transition from tube to oral nutrition.

PARENTERAL NUTRITION

Indications

A. Peripheral Parenteral Nutrition

Peripheral parenteral nutrition (PN) is indicated when complete enteral feeding is temporarily impossible or undesirable. Short-term partial intravenous (IV) nutrition via a peripheral vein is a preferred alternative to administration of dextrose and electrolyte solutions alone. Because of the osmolality of the solutions required, it is usually impossible to achieve total calorie and protein needs with PN via a peripheral vein.

B. Central Parenteral Nutrition

Provision of total nutritional needs by the parenteral route will require a centrally placed venous catheter. Total PN should be provided only when clearly indicated. Apart from the expense, numerous risks are associated with this method of feeding (see section on Complications, later). Even when

PN is indicated, every effort should be made to provide at least a minimum of nutrients enterally to help preserve the integrity of the GI mucosa and of GI function.

The primary indication for PN is the loss of function of the GI tract that prohibits the provision of more than a small proportion of required nutrients by the enteral route. Important examples include short bowel syndrome, some congenital defects of the GI tract, and prematurity.

Catheter Selection & Position

An indwelling central venous catheter is preferred for long-term PN. For periods of up to 3–4 weeks, a percutaneous central venous catheter threaded into the superior vena cava from a peripheral vein can be used. For the infusion of dextrose concentrations higher than 12.5%, the tip of the catheter should be located in the superior vena cava. Catheter positioning in the right atrium has been associated with complications, including arrhythmias and right atrial thrombus. After placement, a chest radiograph must be obtained to check catheter position. If the catheter is to be used for nutrition and medications, a double-lumen catheter is preferred.

Complications

A. Mechanical Complications

1. Related to catheter insertion or to erosion of catheter through a major blood vessel—Complications include trauma to adjacent tissues and organs, damage to the brachial plexus, hydrothorax, pneumothorax, hemothorax, and cerebrospinal fluid penetration. The catheter may slip during dressing or tubing changes, or the patient may manipulate the line.

Chaturvedi A et al: Catheter malplacement during central venous cannulation through arm veins in pediatric patients. J Neurosurg Anesthes 2003;15:170 [PMID: 12826963].

2. Clotting of the catheter—Addition of heparin (1000 U/L) to the solution is an effective means of preventing this complication. If an occluded catheter does not respond to heparin flushing, filling the catheter with recombinant tissue plasminogen activator or sterile 95% ethanol may be effective.

3. Related to composition of infusate—Calcium phosphate precipitation may occur if excess amounts of calcium or phosphorus are administered. Factors that increase the risk of calcium phosphate precipitation include increased pH and decreased concentrations of amino acids. Precipitation of medications incompatible with PN or lipids can also cause clotting.

Freytes CO: Thromboembolic complications related to indwelling central venous catheters in children. Curr Opin Oncol 2003;15:289 [PMID: 12874506].

B. Septic Complications

Septic complications are the most common cause of nonelective catheter removal, but strict use of aseptic technique and limiting entry into the catheter can reduce the rates of line sepsis.

Fever above 38–38.5°C in a patient with a central catheter should be considered a line infection until proved otherwise. Cultures should be obtained and IV antibiotics empirically initiated. Removing the catheter may be necessary with certain infections (eg, fungal), and catheter replacement may be deferred until infection is treated.

C. Metabolic Complications

Many of the metabolic complications of IV nutrition are related to deficiencies or excesses of nutrients in administered fluids. These complications are less common as a result of experience and improvements in nutrient solutions. However, specific deficiencies still occur, especially in premature infants. Avoidance of deficiencies and excesses and of metabolic disorders requires attention to the nutrient balance, electrolyte composition, and delivery rate of the infusate and careful monitoring, especially when the composition or delivery rate is changed.

Currently the most challenging metabolic complication is cholestasis, which is particularly common in premature infants of very low birth weight. The cause of cholestasis associated with TPN is unknown. Patient and medical risk factors include prematurity, sepsis, hypoxia, major surgery (especially GI surgery), absence of enteral feedings, and small bowel bacterial overgrowth. Risk factors related to IV nutrition include amino acid excess or imbalance and prolonged duration of administration. Amino acid solutions with added cysteine decrease cholestasis. Practices that may minimize cholestasis include initiating even minimal enteral feedings as soon as feasible, avoiding sepsis by meticulous line care, avoiding overfeeding, using cysteine- and taurine-containing amino acid formulations designed for infants, preventing or treating small bowel bacterial overgrowth, protecting TPN solutions from light, and avoiding hepatotoxic medications.

Forchielli ML, Walker WA: Nutritional factors contributing to the development of cholestasis during parenteral nutrition. Adv Pediatr 2003;50:245 [PMID: 14626490].

NUTRIENT REQUIREMENTS & DELIVERY

Energy

When patients are fed intravenously, no fat and carbohydrate intakes are unabsorbed, and no energy is used in nutrient absorption. These factors account for at least 7% of energy in the diet of the enterally fed patient. The intravenously fed patient usually expends less energy in physical activity because of the impediment to mobility. Average energy requirements may therefore be lower in children fed intravenously, and the decrease in activity probably increases this figure to a total reduction of 10–15%. Caloric guidelines for the IV feeding of infants and young children are outlined below.

Age	Requirements (kcal/kg/d)
0–1 mo	100–110
2–4 mo	90–100
5–60 mo	70–90
> 5 y	1500 kcal for first 20 kg + 25 kcal for each additional kg/d

The guidelines are averages, and individuals vary considerably. Factors significantly increasing the energy requirement estimates include exposure to cold environment, fever, sepsis, burns, trauma, cardiac or pulmonary disease, and catch-up growth after malnutrition.

With few exceptions, such as some cases of respiratory insufficiency, at least 50–60% of energy requirements are provided as glucose. Up to 40% of calories may be provided by IV fat emulsions.

Dextrose

The energy density of IV dextrose (monohydrate) is 3.4 kcal/g. Dextrose is the main exogenous energy source provided by total IV feeding. IV dextrose suppresses gluconeogenesis and provides a substrate that can be oxidized directly, especially by the brain, red and white blood cells, and wounds. Because of the high osmolality of dextrose solutions ($D_{10}W$ yields 505 mOsm/kg H_2O), concentrations greater than 10–12.5% cannot be delivered via a peripheral vein or improperly positioned central line.

Dosing guidelines: The standard initial quantity of dextrose administered will vary by age (Table 10–18). Tolerance to IV dextrose normally increases rapidly, due primarily to suppression of hepatic production of endogenous glucose. Dextrose can be increased by 2.5 g/kg/d; by 2.5–5% per day; or by 2–3 mg/kg/min per day if there is no glucosuria or hyperglycemia. Standard final infusate for infants via a

Table 10–18. Pediatric macronutrient guidelines for parenteral nutrition.

	Dextrose		Amino Acids	Lipid
	mg/kg/min	g/kg/d	g/kg/d	g/kg/d
Age	50–60% kcal		10–20% kcal	30–40% kcal
Preterm	Initial 5–8 Max 11–12.5	Initial 7–11 Max 16–18	Initial 1.5–2 Max 3–4	Initial 0.5–1 Max 2.5–3.5
Birth–12 mo	Initial 6–8 Max 11–15	Initial 9–11 Max 16–21.5	Initial 1.5–2 Max 3	Initial 1 Max 2.5–3.5
1–6 y	Initial 6–7 Max 10–12	Initial 8–10 Max 14–17	Initial 1–1.5 Max 2–2.5	Initial 1 Max 2.5–3.5
> 6 y	Initial 5–7 Max 9	Initial 8–10 Max 13	Initial 1 Max 1.5–2	Initial 1 Max 3
> 10 y	Initial 4–5 Max 6–7	Initial 5–7 Max 8–10	Initial 1 Max 1.5–2	Initial 1 Max 2–3
Adolescents	Initial 2–3 Max 5–6	Initial 3–4 Max 7–8	Initial 1 Max 1.5–2	Initial 0.5–1 Max 2

properly positioned central venous line usually ranges from 15–25% dextrose, although concentrations of up to 30% dextrose may be used at low flow rates. Tolerance to IV dextrose loads is markedly diminished in premature neonates and in hypermetabolic states.

Problems associated with IV dextrose administration include hyperglycemia, hyperosmolality, and glucosuria (with osmotic diuresis and dehydration). Possible causes of unexpected hyperglycemia include the following: (1) inadvertent infusion of higher glucose concentrations than ordered, (2) uneven flow rate, (3) sepsis, (4) a stress situation, and (5) pancreatitis. IV insulin reduces hyperglycemia but does not increase glucose oxidation rates; it may also decrease the oxidation of fatty acids, resulting in less energy for metabolism. Hence, insulin should be used very cautiously. A standard IV dose is 1 U/4 g of carbohydrate, but much smaller quantities may be adequate and, usually, one starts with 0.2–0.3 U/4 g of carbohydrate.

Hypoglycemia may occur after an abrupt decrease in or cessation of IV glucose. When cyclic IV nutrition is provided, the IV glucose load should be decreased steadily for 1–2 hours prior to discontinuing the infusate. If the central line must be removed, the IV dextrose should be tapered gradually over several hours.

Maximum oxidation rates for infused dextrose decrease with age. It is important to note that the ranges for dextrose administration provided in Table 10–18 are guidelines and that individual patient tolerance and clinical circumstances may warrant administration of either less or more dextrose. Quantities of exogenous dextrose in excess of maximal glucose oxidation rates are used initially to replace depleted glycogen stores; hepatic lipogenesis occurs thereafter. Excess hepatic lipogenesis may lead to a fatty liver. Lipogenesis results in release of carbon dioxide, which when added to the amount of carbon dioxide produced by glucose oxidation (which is 40% greater than that produced by lipid oxidation) may elevate the $PaCO_2$ and aggravate respiratory insufficiency or impede weaning from a respirator.

Lipids

The energy density of lipid emulsions (20%) is 10 kcal/g of lipid or 2 kcal/mL of infusate. The lipids are derived from either soybean or safflower oil. All consist of more than 50% linoleic acid and 4–9% linolenic acid. It is recognized that this high level of linoleic acid is not ideal, except when small quantities of lipid are being given to prevent an EFA deficiency. Ultimately, improved emulsions are anticipated. Because 10% and 20% lipid emulsions contain the same concentrations of phospholipids, a 10% solution delivers more phospholipid per gram of lipid than a 20% solution. Twenty percent lipid emulsions are preferred.

The level of lipoprotein lipase (LPL) activity is the rate-limiting factor in the metabolism and clearance of fat emulsions from the circulation. LPL activity is inhibited or decreased by malnutrition, leukotrienes, immaturity, growth hormone, hypercholesterolemia, hyperphospholipidemia, and theophylline. LPL activity is enhanced by glucose, insulin, lipid, catecholamines, and exercise. Heparin releases LPL from the endothelium into the circulation and enhances the rate of hydrolysis and clearance of triglycerides. In small premature infants, low-dose heparin infusions may increase tolerance to IV lipid emulsion.

The advantages of using fat emulsions to provide up to 40% of caloric intake include the following:

1. The high energy density allows more energy to be provided when fluid volume is restricted.
2. The low osmolality (280 mOsm/kg H_2O) is of special value when using a peripheral line.
3. EFA deficiencies can be prevented.
4. The production of CO_2 is 40% lower per unit of energy, an important consideration in cases of pulmonary insufficiency.
5. The energy cost of fat storage is negligible.
6. The risk of fatty liver is decreased because of decreased hepatic lipogenesis from dextrose.

Potential disadvantages of fat emulsions include the following:

1. Impairment of function of neutrophils, macrophages, and the reticuloendothelial system.
2. Coagulation defects, including thrombocytopenia, elevated prothrombin time, and partial thromboplastin time.
3. Decrease in pulmonary oxygen diffusion.
4. Competition by free fatty acids with bilirubin and drugs for albumin-binding sites.
5. Increase in low-density lipoprotein cholesterol.

In general, these adverse effects can be avoided by starting with modest quantities and advancing cautiously in light of results of triglyceride monitoring and clinical circumstances. In cases of severe sepsis, special caution is required to ensure that the lipid is metabolized effectively. Monitoring with long-term use is also essential.

Dosing guidelines: Check serum triglycerides before starting and after increasing the dose. Commence with 1 g/kg/d, given over 12–20 hours or 24 hours in small preterm infants. Advance by 0.5–1.0 g/kg/d, every 1–2 days, up to goal (see Table 10–18).

As a general rule, do not increase the dose if the serum triglyceride level is above 250 mg/dL during infusion (150 mg/dL in neonates) or if the level is greater than 150 mg/dL 6–12 hours after cessation of the lipid infusion.

Serum triglyceride levels above 400–600 mg/dL may precipitate pancreatitis. In patients for whom normal amounts of IV lipid are contraindicated, 4–8% of calories as IV lipid should be provided (300 mg linoleic acid/100 kcal) to prevent essential fatty acid deficiency. Neonates and malnourished pediatric patients receiving lipid-free PN are at high risk for EFA deficiency because of limited adipose stores.

Nitrogen

One gram of nitrogen is yielded by 6.25 g of protein (1 g of protein contains 16% nitrogen). Caloric density of protein is equal to 4 kcal/g.

A. Protein Requirement

Protein requirements for IV feeding are the same as those for normal oral feeding (see Table 10–2).

B. Protein-Energy Interactions

There are important interactions between protein and energy requirements. A positive nitrogen balance cannot be achieved on a hypocaloric diet, because protein will be catabolized for energy. When energy intake is low, the administration of some amino acid does, however, lessen the severity of the negative nitrogen balance. Conversely, when nitrogen intake is low, the provision of calories improves nitrogen balance to some extent. In infants, the energy necessary to minimize nitrogen loss associated with an amino acid–free diet is approximately 70 kcal/kg/d. At this level of energy intake, positive nitrogen balance depends on the level of nitrogen intake and is independent of further increase in energy intake.

In infants receiving about 50 kcal/kg/d, increasing protein intake up to 3 g/kg/d improves the nitrogen balance. In these circumstances, therefore, a ratio of grams of nitrogen per kilocalorie as low as 1:100 can be advantageous. However, at higher levels of energy intake, ratios of 1:250 to 1:150 or more are optimal. Although these ratios provide a useful crude check, they are not usually the best means of determining protein requirements.

C. Intravenous Amino Acid Solutions

Nitrogen requirements can be met by one of the commercially available amino acid solutions. For older children and adults, none of the standard preparations has a clear advantage over the others as a source of amino acids. For infants, however, including premature infants, accumulating evidence suggests that the use of TrophAmine (B. Braun Medical) is associated with a normal plasma amino acid profile, superior nitrogen retention, and a lower incidence of cholestasis. TrophAmine contains 60% essential amino acids, is relatively high in branched-chain amino acids, contains taurine, and is compatible with the addition of cysteine within 24–48 hours after administration. The dose of added cysteine is 40 mg/g of TrophAmine. The relatively low pH of TrophAmine is also advantageous for solubility of calcium and phosphorus.

D. Dosing Guidelines

Amino acids can be started at 1–2 g/kg/d in most patients (see Table 10–18). In severely malnourished infants, the initial amount should be 1 g/kg/d. Even in infants of very low birth weight, there is evidence that higher initial amounts of amino acids are tolerated with little indication of protein "toxicity." Larger quantities of amino acids in relation to calories can minimize the degree of negative nitrogen balance when the infusate is hypocaloric. Amino acid intake can be advanced by 0.5–1.0 g/kg/d toward the goal. Normally the final infusate will contain 2–3% amino acids, depending on the rate of infusion. Concentration should not be advanced beyond 2% in peripheral vein infusate due to osmolality.

E. Monitoring

Monitoring for tolerance of the IV amino acid solutions should include routine blood urea nitrogen. Serum alkaline phosphatase, γ-glutamyltransferase, and bilirubin should be monitored to detect the onset of cholestatic liver disease.

Minerals & Electrolytes

A. Calcium, Phosphorus, and Magnesium

Intravenously fed premature and full-term infants should be given relatively high amounts of calcium and phosphorus. Current recommendations are as follows: calcium, 500–600 mg/L; phosphorus, 400–450 mg/L; and magnesium, 50–70 mg/L. After 1 year of age, the recommendations are as follows: calcium, 200–400 mg/L; phosphorus, 150–300 mg/L; and magnesium, 20–40 mg/L. The ratio of calcium to phosphorous should be 1.3:1.0 by weight or 1:1 by molar ratio. These recommendations are deliberately presented as milligrams per liter of infusate to avoid inadvertent administration of concentrations of calcium and phosphorus that are high enough to precipitate in the tubing. During periods of fluid restriction, care must be taken not to inadvertently increase the concentration of calcium and phosphorus in the infusate. These recommendations assume an average fluid intake of 120–150 mL/kg/d and an infusate of 25 g of amino acid per liter. With lower amino acid concentrations, the concentrations of calcium and phosphorus should be decreased.

B. Electrolytes

Standard recommendations are given in Table 10–19. After chloride requirements are met, the remainder of the anion required to balance the cation should be given as acetate to avoid the possibility of acidosis resulting from excessive chloride. The required concentrations of electrolytes depend to some extent on the flow rate of the infusate and must be modified if flow rates are unusually low or high and if there are specific indications in individual patients. IV sodium should be administered sparingly in severely malnourished patients because of impaired membrane function and high intracellular sodium levels. Conversely, generous quantities of potassium are indicated. Replacement electrolytes and fluids should be delivered via a separate infusate.

C. Trace Elements

Recommended IV intakes of trace elements are as follows: zinc, 100 mcg/kg; copper, 20 mcg/kg; manganese, 1 mcg/kg; chromium, 0.2 mcg/kg; selenium, 2 mcg/kg; and iodide, 1 mcg/kg. Of note, IV zinc requirements may be as high as 400 mcg/kg for premature infants and can be up to 250 mcg/kg for infants with short bowel syndrome and significant GI losses of zinc. When IV nutrition is supplemental or limited to fewer than 2 weeks, and preexisting nutritional deficiencies are absent, only zinc need routinely be added.

IV copper requirements are relatively low in the young infant because of the presence of hepatic copper stores. These are significant even in the 28-week fetus. Circulating levels of copper and manganese should be monitored in the presence of cholestatic liver disease. If monitoring is not feasible, temporary withdrawal of added copper and manganese is advisable. Copper and manganese are excreted primarily in the bile, but selenium, chromium, and molybdenum are excreted primarily in the urine. These trace elements, therefore, should be administered with caution in the presence of renal failure.

Although low doses of iron are routinely added in some centers to the IV infusate for infants and children, no official recommendation has been made because of the lack of adequate published data regarding compatibility. Iron added to the infusate should be in a diluted form of iron dextran in a concentration of 1 mg/L. After age 2 months, maintenance IV iron requirements for the full-term infant are approximately 100 mcg/kg/d. After the first month, the premature infant requires up to 200 mcg/kg/d intravenously. Although overload is unlikely to occur during short-term PN, a surreptitious accumulation of extra iron could occur if PN is prolonged. This risk is enhanced if the patient has received blood transfusions. A second concern is that the potential for free iron is increased in malnourished infants with low transferrin levels. Excess iron is thought to enhance the risk of gram-negative septicemia. Iron has powerful oxidant properties and can enhance the demand for antioxidants, especially vitamin E. None of these concerns appears to preclude the routine use of iron supplements during IV nutrition, but they do emphasize the need for a conservative approach in determining dosage schedules.

Vitamins

Two vitamin formulations are available for use in pediatric PN: MVI Pediatric and MVI-12 (Astra-Zeneca). MVI Pediatric contains the following: vitamin A, 0.7 mg; vitamin D, 400 IU; vitamin E, 7 mg; vitamin K, 200 mcg; ascorbic acid, 80

Table 10–19. Electrolyte requirements for parenteral nutrition.

Electrolyte	Preterm Infant	Full-Term Infant	Child	Adolescent
Sodium	2–5 mEq/kg	2–3 mEq/kg	2–3 mEq/kg	60–150 mEq/d
Chloride	2–5 mEq/kg	2–3 mEq/kg	2–3 mEq/kg	60–150 mEq/d
Potassium	2–3 mEq/kg	2–3 mEq/kg	2–3 mEq/kg	70–180 mEq/d

mg; thiamin, 1.2 mg; riboflavin, 1.4 mg; niacinamide, 17 mg; pyridoxine, 1 mg; vitamin B_{12}, 1 mcg; folic acid, 140 mcg; pantothenate, 5 mg; and biotin, 20 mcg. This formulation is suboptimal, with too little vitamin A and excessive amounts of water-soluble vitamins, but it is the best one available. Recommended dosing is as follows: 5 mL for children weighing more than 3 kg, 3.25 mL for infants 1–3 kg, and 1.5 mL for infants weighing less than 1 kg. Children older than 11 years can receive 10 mL of the adult formulation, MVI-12, which contains the following: vitamin A, 1 mg; vitamin D, 200 IU; vitamin E, 10 mg; ascorbic acid, 100 mg; thiamin, 3 mg; riboflavin, 3.6 mg; niacinamide, 40 mg; pyridoxine, 4 mg; vitamin B_{12}, 5 mcg; folic acid, 400 mcg; pantothenate, 15 mg; and biotin, 60 mcg. MVI-12 contains no vitamin K.

IV lipid preparations contain enough tocopherol to affect total blood tocopherol levels. The majority of tocopherol in soybean oil emulsion is α-tocopherol, which has substantially less biologic activity than the α-tocopherol present in safflower oil emulsions.

A dose of 40 IU/kg/d of vitamin D (maximum 400 IU/d) is adequate for both full-term and preterm infants.

Fluid Requirements

The initial fluid volume and subsequent increments in flow rate are determined by basic fluid requirements, the patient's clinical status, and the extent to which additional fluid administration can be tolerated and may be required to achieve adequate nutrient intake. Calculation of initial fluid volumes to be administered should be based on standard pediatric practice. Tolerance of higher flow rates must be determined on an individual basis. If replacement fluids are required for ongoing abnormal losses, these should be administered via a separate line.

Monitoring

Vital signs should be checked on each shift. In a patient with a central catheter in situ, a fever of more than 38.5°C requires that peripheral and central-line blood cultures, urine culture, complete physical examination, and examination of the IV entry point be made. Instability of vital signs, elevated white blood cell count with left shift, and glycosuria suggest sepsis. Removal of the central venous catheter should be considered if the patient is toxic or unresponsive to antibiotics.

A. Physical Examination

Monitor especially for hepatomegaly (differential diagnoses include fluid overload, congestive heart failure, steatosis, and hepatitis) and edema (differential diagnoses include fluid overload, congestive heart failure, hypoalbuminemia, and thrombosis of superior vena cava).

Table 10–20. Routine parenteral nutrition monitoring summary.

Variables	Acute Stage	Long-Term[a]
Growth		
Weight	Daily	Weekly
Length	Weekly	
Head circumference	Weekly	
Urine		
Glucose (dipstick)	With each void	With changes in intake or status
Specific gravity	Void	
Volume	Daily	
Blood		
Glucose	4 hours after changes,[b] then daily × 2 days	Weekly
Na^+, K^+, Cl^-, CO_2, blood urea nitrogen	Daily for 2 days after changes,[b] then twice weekly	Weekly
Ca^{2+}, Mg^{2+}, P	Initially, then twice weekly	Weekly
Total protein, albumin, bilirubin, aspartate transaminase, and alkaline phosphatase	Initially, then weekly	Every other week
Zinc and copper	Initially according to clinical indications	Monthly
Triglycerides	Initially, 1 day after changes,[b] then weekly	Weekly
Compete blood count	Initially, then twice weekly; according to clinical indications (see text)	Twice weekly

[a]Long-term monitoring can be tapered to monthly or less often, depending on age, diagnosis, and clinical status of patient.
[b]Changes include alterations in concentration or flow rate.

B. Intake and Output Record

Calories and volume delivered should be calculated from the previous day's intake and output records (that which was delivered rather than that which was ordered). The following entries should be noted on flow sheets: IV, enteral, and total fluid (mL/kg/d); dextrose (g/kg/d or mg/kg/min); protein (g/kg/d); lipids (g/kg/d); energy (kcal/kg/d); and percent of energy from enteral nutrition.

C. Growth, Urine, and Blood

Routine monitoring guidelines are given in Table 10–20. These are minimum requirements, except in the very long-term stable patient. Individual variables should be moni-

tored more frequently as indicated, as should additional variables or clinical indications. For example, a blood ammonia analysis should be ordered for an infant with lethargy, pallor, poor growth, acidosis, azotemia, or abnormal liver test results.

Greene HL et al: Guidelines for the use of vitamins, trace elements, calcium, magnesium, and phosphorus in infants and children receiving total parenteral nutrition: Report of the Subcommittee on Pediatric Parenteral Nutrient Requirements from the Committee on Clinical Practice Issues of the American Society for Clinical Nutrition. Am J Clin Nutr 1988;48:1324 [PMID: 3142247].

Shulman RJ, Phillips S: Parenteral nutrition in infants and children. J Pediatr Gastroenterol Nutr 2003;36:587 [PMID: 12717082].

Emergencies & Injuries

Maria J. Mandt, MD
Glenn Faries, MD

Maria J. Mandt, MD
Glenn Faries, MD

ADVANCED LIFE SUPPORT FOR INFANTS & CHILDREN

When faced with a seriously ill or injured child, a systematic approach and rapid determination of the child's physiologic status with concurrent initiation of resuscitative measures is imperative. Initial management must be directed at correcting any physiologic derangement. Specifically, one must evaluate the airway for any obstruction, assess ventilatory status, and evaluate for shock. Intervention to correct any abnormalities in these three parameters must be undertaken immediately. Following this initial intervention the provider must then carefully consider the underlying cause, focusing on those that are treatable or reversible. Specific diagnoses can then be made, and targeted therapy (eg, intravenous [IV] glucose for hypoglycemia) can be initiated.

Pediatric cardiac arrest more frequently represents progressive respiratory deterioration or shock rather than primary cardiac etiologies. Unrecognized deterioration may lead to bradycardia, agonal breathing, and ultimately asystole. Resulting hypoxic and ischemic insult to the brain and other vital organs make neurologic recovery extremely unlikely, even in the doubtful event that the child survives the arrest. Children who respond to rapid intervention with ventilation and oxygenation alone or to less than 5 minutes of advanced life support are much more likely to survive neurologically intact. Therefore, it is essential to recognize the child who is at risk for progressing to cardiopulmonary arrest and to provide aggressive intervention before asystole occurs.

Note: Standard precautions (personal protective equipment) must be maintained during resuscitation efforts.

THE ABCS OF RESUSCITATION

Any severely ill child should be rapidly evaluated in a deliberate sequence of *a*irway patency, *b*reathing adequacy, and *c*irculation integrity. Derangement at each point must be corrected before proceeding. Thus, if a child's airway is obstructed, the airway must be opened (eg, by head positioning and the chin lift maneuver) before breathing and circulation are assessed.

Airway

Look, listen, and feel for upper airway patency: *Look* for chest or abdominal wall movement suggestive of breathing effort. *Listen* for adventitious breath sounds such as stridor, stertor, or gurgling. Placing a stethoscope at the mouth or over the trachea improves the ability to hear air entry. *Feel* for air movement with your face near the child's mouth and nose. Evidence of spontaneous breathing effort and increased work of breathing without air movement is suggestive of airway obstruction. Significant airway obstruction often is associated with altered level of consciousness, including agitation or lethargy.

The airway is managed initially by noninvasive means such as oxygen administration, chin lift, jaw thrust, suctioning, or bag–valve–mask ventilation. Invasive maneuvers such as endotracheal intubation, laryngeal mask insertion, or rarely, cricothyroidotomy are required if the aforementioned maneuvers are unsuccessful. If neck injury is suspected, the cervical spine must be immobilized and kept from extension or flexion. (See section on Approach to the Pediatric Trauma Patient, later.) The following discussion assumes that basic life support has been instituted.

Knowledge of pediatric anatomy is important for airway management. Children's tongues are large relative to their oral cavities, and the larynx is high and anteriorly located. Infants are obligate nasal breathers; therefore, secretions or blood in the nasopharynx can cause significant distress.

A. Place the head in the sniffing position. The neck should be slightly flexed and the head gently extended so as to bring the face forward. This position aligns the oral, pharyngeal, and tracheal planes. Reposition the head if airway obstruction persists after head tilt and jaw thrust. In infants and children younger than about 8 years of age, the

▲ **Figure 11–1.** Correct positioning of the child younger than age 8 years for optimal airway alignment: a folded sheet or towel is placed beneath the shoulders to accommodate the occiput and align the oral, pharyngeal, and tracheal airways.

relatively large occiput causes significant neck flexion and poor airway positioning. This is relieved by placing a towel roll under the shoulders, thus returning the child to a neutral position (Figure 11–1). In an older child, slightly more head extension is necessary. Avoid hyperextension of the neck, especially in infants.

B. Perform the chin lift or jaw thrust maneuver (Figure 11–2). Lift the chin upward while avoiding pressure on the submental triangle, or lift the jaw by traction upward on the angle of the jaw. **Head tilt must not be done if cervical spine injury is possible.**

C. Suction the mouth of any foreign material.

D. Remove visible foreign bodies, using fingers or a Magill forceps. Visualize by means of a laryngoscope if necessary. Blind finger sweeps should not be done.

E. Insert an oropharyngeal airway or a nasopharyngeal airway in the conscious patient (Figure 11–3) to relieve upper airway obstruction due to prolapse of the tongue into the posterior pharynx. This is the most common cause of airway obstruction in unconscious children. The correct size for an oropharyngeal airway is obtained by measuring from the upper central gumline to the angle of the jaw (Figure 11–4). Nasopharyngeal airways should fit snugly within the nares and should be equal in length to the distance from the nares to the tragus (Figure 11–5).

Breathing

Assessment of respiratory status is largely accomplished by inspection. *Look* for adequate and symmetrical chest rise and fall, rate and work of breathing (eg, retractions, flaring, and grunting), accessory muscle use, skin color, and tracheal deviation. Note the mental status. Pulse oximetry measurement and end-tidal CO_2 determination, if available, are highly desirable. *Listen* for adventitious breath sounds such as wheezing. Auscultate for air entry, symmetry of breath sounds, and rales. *Feel* for subcutaneous crepitus.

If spontaneous breathing is inadequate, initiate positive-pressure ventilation with bag–mask ventilation and 100% oxygen and coordinate bagging with the patient's efforts, if present. Ensure a proper seal by choosing a mask that encompasses the area from the bridge of the nose to the cleft

A

B

▲ **Figure 11–2.** **A:** Opening the airway with the head tilt and chin lift in patients without concern for spinal trauma: gently lift the chin with one hand and push down on the forehead with the other hand. **B:** Opening the airway with jaw thrust in patients with concern for spinal trauma: lift the angles of the mandible; this moves the jaw and tongue forward and opens the airway without bending the neck.

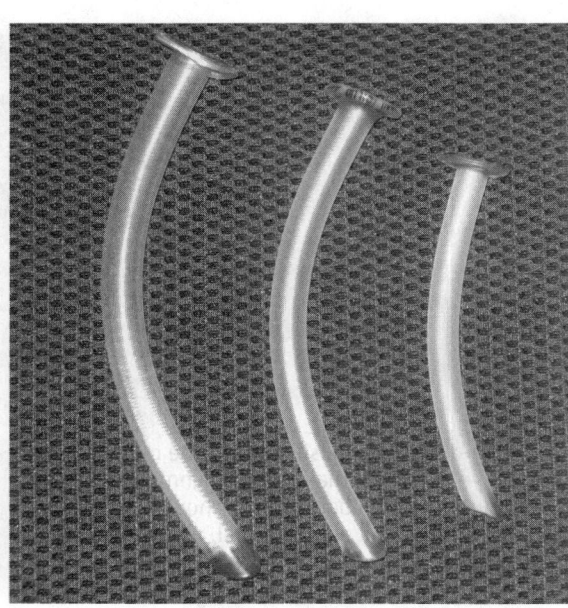

A

B

▲ **Figure 11–3.** **A:** Oropharyngeal airways of various sizes. **B:** Nasopharyngeal airways of different sizes.

of the chin. Form an E–C clamp around the mask to seal the mask tightly to the child's face. The thumb and index finger form the "C" surrounding the mask, while the middle, ring, and little fingers lift the jaw into the mask (Figure 11–6). Two-person ventilation using the technique is optimal. Adequacy of ventilation is reflected in adequate chest movement and auscultation of good air entry bilaterally. If the chest does not rise and fall easily with bagging, reposition the

airway as previously described. Perform airway foreign body extraction maneuvers if the airway remains obstructed, including visualizing the airway with a laryngoscope and using Magill forceps. The presence of asymmetrical breath sounds in a child in shock or in severe distress suggests pneumothorax and is an indication for needle thoracostomy. In small children, the transmission of breath sounds throughout the chest may impair the ability to auscultate the

▲ **Figure 11–4.** Size selection for the oropharyngeal airway: hold the airway next to the child's face and estimate proper size by measuring from the upper central gumline to the angle of the jaw.

▲ **Figure 11–5.** Size selection for the nasopharyngeal airway: hold the airway next to the child's face and estimate proper size by measuring from the nares to the tragus.

A

B

▲ **Figure 11–6.** **A:** Bag–valve–mask ventilation, one-person technique: the thumb and index finger form the "C" surrounding the mask, while the middle, ring, and little fingers lift the jaw into the mask. **B:** Bag–valve–mask ventilation, two-person technique: the first rescuer forms the "C" and "E" clamps with both hands; the second rescuer provides ventilation.

presence of a pneumothorax. Bag–mask ventilation is effective in the *vast* majority of cases.

Note: Effective oxygenation and ventilation are the keys to successful resuscitation.

Using cricoid pressure (Sellick maneuver) during all positive-pressure ventilation, intubate the trachea in patients who are unresponsive to bag–mask ventilation, those in coma, those who require airway protection, or those who will require prolonged ventilation. Cricothyroidotomy is rarely necessary. Advanced airway management techniques are described in the references accompanying this section. (See also section on Approach to the Pediatric Trauma Patient, later.)

Circulation

The diagnosis of shock can and should be made by clinical examination, and must be done rapidly. Clinical assessments A–F aid in assessing perfusion.

A. Pulses

Check adequacy of peripheral pulses. Pulses become weak and thready only with severe hypovolemia. Compare peripheral pulses with central pulses.

B. Heart Rate

Compare with age-specific norms. Tachycardia can be a nonspecific sign of distress; bradycardia for age is a prearrest sign and necessitates aggressive resuscitation.

C. Extremities

As shock progresses, extremities become cooler, from distal to proximal. A child whose extremities are cool distal to the elbows and knees is in severe shock.

D. Capillary Refill Time

This is an important indicator of perfusion; longer than 2 seconds is abnormal unless the child is cold.

E. Mental Status

Hypoxia, hypercapnia, or ischemia will result in altered mental status. Other important treatable conditions may also result in altered mental status, such as intracranial hemorrhage, meningitis, and hypoglycemia.

F. Skin Color

Pallor, gray, mottled, or ashen skin colors all indicate compromised circulatory status.

G. Blood Pressure

It is important to remember that shock (inadequate perfusion of vital organs) may be present before the blood pressure falls below the normal limits for age. As intravascular volume falls, peripheral vascular resistance increases. Blood pressure is maintained until there is 35–40% depletion of blood volume, followed by precipitous and often irreversible deterioration. Shock that occurs with any signs of decreased perfusion but normal blood pressure is **compensated** shock. When blood pressure also falls, **decompensated** shock is present. Blood pressure determination should be done manually, using an appropriately sized cuff, because automated machines can give erroneous readings in children.

MANAGEMENT OF SHOCK

IV access is essential but can be difficult to establish in children with shock. Peripheral access, especially via the antecubital veins, should be attempted first, but central cannulation should follow quickly if peripheral access is unsuccessful. Alternatives are percutaneous cannulation of femoral, subclavian, or internal or external jugular veins; cutdown at antecubital, femoral, or saphenous sites; or intraosseous (IO) lines (Figure 11–7). Consider IO needle placement in any severely ill child when venous access cannot be established rapidly. Decisions on more invasive access should be based on individual expertise as well as urgency of obtaining access. Use short, wide-bore catheters to allow maximal flow rates. Two IV lines should be started in severely ill children. In newborns, the umbilical veins may be cannulated. Consider arterial access if beat-to-beat monitoring or frequent laboratory tests will be needed.

Differentiation of Shock States & Initial Therapy

Therapy for inadequate circulation is determined by the cause of circulatory failure.

A. Hypovolemic Shock

The most common type of shock in the pediatric population is hypovolemia. Frequent causes include dehydration, diabetes, heat illness, hemorrhage, and burns. Normal saline or lactated Ringer solution (isotonic crystalloid) is given as initial therapy. Give 20 mL/kg body weight, repeated as necessary, with frequent reassessments, until perfusion normalizes. Children tolerate large volumes of fluid replacement. Typically, in hypovolemic shock, no more than 50 mL/kg is needed, but more may be required if ongoing losses are severe. Appropriate monitoring and reassessment will guide your therapy. Packed red blood cell transfusion is indicated in trauma patients not responding to two boluses of crystalloid solution. Pressors are not required in simple hypovolemic states.

▲ **Figure 11–7.** Interosseous (IO) cannulation technique. The IO line is inserted by grasping the needle hub firmly with the palm of the hand and angling the needle tip perpendicular to the anterior tibial surface approximately two fingerbreadths distal to the tibial plateau. With a firm, twisting motion, advance the needle until a sudden lessening of resistance is felt as the needle enters the marrow space. Aspiration of blood and marrow confirms IO placement.

B. Distributive Shock

Distributive shock results from increased vascular capacitance with normal circulating volume. Examples are sepsis, anaphylaxis, and spinal cord injury. Initial therapy is again isotonic volume replacement with crystalloid, but pressors may be required if perfusion does not normalize after delivery of two 20-mL/kg boluses of crystalloid. Children in distributive shock must be admitted to a pediatric intensive care unit.

C. Cardiogenic Shock

Cardiogenic shock can occur as a complication of congenital heart disease, myocarditis, dysrhythmias, ingestions (eg, clonidine, cyclic antidepressants), or as a complication of prolonged shock due to any cause. The diagnosis is suggested by any of the following signs: abnormal cardiac rhythm, distended neck veins, rales, abnormal heart sounds such as an S_3 or S_4, friction rub, narrow pulse pressure, or hepatomegaly. Chest radiographs may show cardiomegaly and pulmonary edema. An initial bolus of crystalloid may be given, but pressors, and possibly afterload reducers, are necessary to improve perfusion. Giving multiple boluses of fluid is deleterious. Comprehensive cardiopulmonary monitoring is essential. Children in cardiogenic shock must be admitted to a pediatric intensive care unit.

▶ Observation & Further Management

Clinically reassess physiologic response to each fluid bolus to determine additional needs. Serial central venous pressure determinations or a chest radiograph may help determine volume status. Place an indwelling urinary catheter to monitor urine output.

Caution must be exercised with volume replacement if intracranial pressure is potentially elevated, as in severe head injury, diabetic ketoacidosis, or meningitis. Even in such situations, however, normal intravascular volume must be restored in order to achieve adequate mean arterial pressure and, thus, cerebral perfusion pressure.

SUMMARY OF CARDIOPULMONARY RESUSCITATION

Assess the ABCs in sequential fashion and, before assessing the next system, immediately intervene if physiologic derangement is detected. It is essential that each system be reassessed after each intervention to ensure improvement and prevent failure to recognize clinical deterioration.

APLS: the pediatric emergency medicine resource: http://www.aplsonline.com

ECC Committee, Subcommittees and Task Forces of the American Heart Association: 2005 American Heart Association guidelines for Cardiopulmonary Resuscitation and Emergency Cardiovascular Care. Part 12: Pediatric Advanced Life Support. Circulation 2005;112(Suppl):IV167–IV187 [PMID: 16314375].

Goldstein B et al: International pediatric sepsis consensus conference: Definitions for sepsis and organ dysfunction in pediatrics. Pediatric Crit Care Med 2005;6:2 [PMID: 15636651].

Hazinski MF et al (editors): *PALS Provider Manual.* American Heart Association, 2006.

EMERGENCY PEDIATRIC DRUGS

Although careful attention to airway and breathing remains the mainstay of pediatric resuscitation, medications are often needed. Rapid delivery to the central circulation, which can be via peripheral IV catheter, is essential. Infuse medications close to the catheter's hub and flush in with saline to achieve the most rapid systemic effects. If no IV or IO access is achievable, some drugs may be given by endotracheal tube (Table 11–1). The use of length-based emergency measuring tapes that contain preprinted drug dos-

Table 11–1. Emergency drugs that can be given by endotracheal tube.

Lidocaine
Epinephrine
Atropine
Naloxone

ages, equipment sizes, and IV fluid amounts (Broselow tapes) or preprinted resuscitation drug charts is much more accurate than estimation formulas and helps minimize dosing errors. Selected emergency drugs used in pediatrics are summarized in Table 11–2.

▼ APPROACH TO THE SERIOUSLY ILL CHILD

An unstable patient may present with a known diagnosis (asthma with status asthmaticus and respiratory failure; complications of known congenital heart disease) or in cardiorespiratory failure of unknown cause. The initial approach must rapidly identify and reverse life-threatening conditions. Children with chronic disease may present with an acute exacerbation or secondary to a new, unrelated problem.

PREPARATION FOR EMERGENCY MANAGEMENT

Resuscitation occurs simultaneously at two levels: rapid cardiopulmonary assessment, with indicated stabilizing measures, while venous access is gained and cardiopulmonary monitoring initiated. The technique of accomplishing these concurrent goals is outlined as follows:

A. If advance notice of the patient's arrival has been received, prepare a resuscitation room and summon appropriate personnel as needed, such as a neurosurgeon for an unresponsive child after severe head injury or a radiology technician for imaging studies.

B. Assign team responsibilities, including a team leader plus others designated to manage the airway, perform chest compressions, achieve access, draw blood for laboratory studies, place monitors, gather additional historical data, and provide family support. The team approach is invaluable.

C. Age-appropriate equipment (including laryngoscope blade, endotracheal tubes, nasogastric or orogastric tubes, IV lines, and an indwelling urinary catheter) and monitors (cardiorespiratory monitor, pulse oximeter, and appropriate blood pressure cuff) should be assembled and readily available. Use a length-based emergency tape if available. See Table 11–3 for endotracheal tube sizes. Cuffed endotracheal tubes are acceptable during the inpatient setting for children and infants beyond the newborn period. Cuff inflation pressures must be carefully

Table 11–2. Emergency pediatric drugs.

Drug	Indications	Dosage and Route	Comment
Atropine	1. Bradycardia, especially cardiac in origin 2. Vagally mediated bradycardia, eg, during laryngoscopy and intubation 3. Anticholinesterase poisoning	0.01–0.02 mg/kg (minimum, 0.1 mg; maximum, 2 mg) IV, IO, ET. May repeat every 5 min.	Atropine may be useful in hemodynamically significant primary cardiac-based bradycardias. Because of paradoxic bradycardia sometimes seen in infants, a minimum dose of 0.1 mg is recommended by the American Heart Association. Epinephrine is the first-line drug in pediatrics for bradycardia caused by hypoxia or ischemia.
Bicarbonate	1. Documented metabolic acidosis 2. Hyperkalemia	1 mEq/kg IV or IO; by arterial blood gas: $0.3 \times kg \times$ base deficit. May repeat every 5 min.	Infuse slowly. Sodium bicarbonate will be effective only if the patient is adequately oxygenated, ventilated, and perfused. Some adverse side effects.
Calcium chloride 10%	1. Documented hypocalcemia 2. Calcium channel blocker overdose 3. Hyperkalemia, hypermagnesemia	10–30 mg/kg slowly IV, preferably centrally, or IO with caution.	Calcium is no longer indicated for asystole. Potent tissue necrosis results if infiltration occurs. Use with caution.
Epinephrine	1. Bradycardia, especially hypoxic-ischemic 2. Hypotension (by infusion) 3. Asystole 4. Fine ventricular fibrillation refractory to initial defibrillation 5. Pulseless electrical activity 6. Anaphylaxis	*Bradycardia and cardiac arrest:* IV/IO: 0.01 mg/kg of 1:10,000 solution. ET: 0.1 mg/kg of 1:1,000 solution. *Anaphylaxis:* SC/IM: 0.01 mg/kg of 1:1000 solution. Maximum dose: 0.3 mg. May repeat every 5–15 min. Constant infusion by IV drip: 0.1–1 mcg/kg/min	Epinephrine is the single most important drug in pediatric resuscitation. Recent pediatric studies have shown no added advantage to high-dose epinephrine in terms of survival to discharge or neurologic outcome. Because other studies have indicated adverse effects, including increased myocardial oxygen consumption during resuscitation and worsened postarrest myocardial dysfunction, high-dose epinephrine is no longer recommended.
Glucose	1. Hypoglycemia 2. Altered mental status (empirical) 3. With insulin, for hyperkalemia	0.25–0.5g/kg IV or IO. Continuous infusion may be necessary.	2-4 mL/kg D_{10}W, 1–2 mL/kg D_{25}W.
Naloxone	1. Opioid overdose 2. Altered mental status (empirical)	0.1 mg/kg IV, IO, or ET; maximum dose, 2 mg. May repeat as necessary.	Side effects are few. A dose of 2 mg may be given in young children. Repeat as necessary, or give as constant infusion in opioid overdoses.

D_5W, 5% glucose in water; ET, endotracheally; IO, intraosseously; IV, intravenously; SC, subcutaneously.

monitored and maintained below 20 cm H_2O. In certain circumstances, such as poor lung compliance or high airway resistance, the use of cuffed tubes may be preferable in controlled settings.

RECEPTION & ASSESSMENT

Upon patient arrival, the team leader begins a rapid assessment as team members perform their preassigned tasks. If the patient is received from prehospital care providers, careful attention must be paid to their report, which contains information that they alone have observed. Interventions and medications should be ordered only by the team leader to avoid confusion. The leader should refrain from personally performing procedures, which may distract him or her

from optimal direction of the resuscitation. A complete timed record should be kept of events, including medications, interventions, and response to intervention.

All Cases

In addition to cardiac compressions and ventilation, ensure that the following are instituted:

1. 100% high-flow oxygen.
2. Cardiorespiratory monitoring, pulse oximetry, and end-tidal CO_2 if the patient is intubated.
3. Vascular (peripheral, IO, or central) access; two lines preferred.
4. Blood drawn and sent. Bedside blood glucose determination is essential.

Table 11-3. Equipment sizes and estimated weight by age.

Age (years)	Weight (kg)	Endotracheal Tube Size (mm)[a,b]	Laryngoscope Blade (Size)	Chest Tube (Fr)	Foley (Fr)
Premature	1-2.5	2.5 (uncuffed only)	0	8	5
Term newborn	3	3.0 (uncuffed only)	0-1	10	8
1	10	3.5-4.0	1	18	8
2	12	4.5	1	18	10
3	14	4.5	1	20	10
4	16	5.0	2	22	10
5	18	5.0-5.5	2	24	10
6	20	5.5	2	26	12
7	22	5.5-6.0	2	26	12

Age (years)	Weight (kg)	Cuffed Endotracheal Tube Size (mm)[a,b]	Laryngoscope Blade (Size)	Chest Tube (Fr)	Foley (Fr)
8	24	6.0	2	28	14
10	32	6.0-6.5	2-3	30	14
Adolescent	50	7.0	3	36	14
Adult	70	8.0	3	40	14

[a]Internal diameter.
[b]Decrease tube size by 0.5 mm if using a cuffed tube.

5. Full vital signs.

6. Clothes removed.

7. Foley catheter and nasogastric or orogastric tube inserted.

8. Complete history.

9. Notification of needed consultants.

10. Family support.

11. Law enforcement or security activation and emergency unit lockdown for cases involving potential terrorism, gang violence, or threats to staff or family.

As Appropriate

1. Immobilize neck.

2. Obtain chest radiograph (line and tube placement).

3. Insert central venous pressure and arterial line.

Hammill WW, Butler J: Pediatric advanced life support update for emergency department physicians. Clin Ped Emerg Med 2005;6:207.

Ludwic S, Lavelle JM: Resuscitation—pediatric basic and advanced life support. In Fleisher GR et al (editors): *Textbook of Pediatric Emergency Medicine.* Lippincott Williams & Wilkins, 2006:3–33.

Weiss M, Gerber AC: Cuffed tracheal tubes in children—things have changed. Pediatric Anesthesia 2006;16:1005 [PMID: 16972827].

APPROACH TO THE PEDIATRIC TRAUMA PATIENT

Injuries, including motor vehicle crashes, falls, burns, and immersions, account for the greatest number of deaths among children older than age 1 year. All providers of pediatric care must be cognizant of this sobering statistic. Cooperative efforts between injury prevention specialists, prehospital providers, and emergency, critical care, and rehabilitation physicians and nurses will help reduce these terrible losses.

A team approach to the severely injured child, using assigned roles as outlined in the preceding section, will optimize outcomes. A calm atmosphere in the receiving area will contribute to thoughtful care. Conscious children are terribly frightened by serious injury; reassurance can help alleviate anxiety. Analgesia and sedation must be given to stable patients. It is unconscionable to let children suffer pain needlessly. Treat pain expeditiously using oral or parenteral analgesics with ongoing monitoring. Parents are often anxious, angry, or guilty, requiring ongoing support from staff, social workers, or child life workers (therapists knowledgeable about child development). To provide optimal multidisciplinary care, regional pediatric trauma centers provide dedicated teams of pediatric specialists in emergency pediatrics, trauma surgery, orthopedics, neurosurgery, and critical care. Most children with severe injuries are not seen in these centers. Primary care providers must be able to provide initial assessment and stabilization of the child with life-threatening injuries before transport to a verified pediatric trauma center.

MECHANISM OF INJURY

Document the time of occurrence, the type of energy transfer (eg, hit by a car, rapid deceleration), secondary impacts (if the child was thrown by the initial impact), appearance of the child at the scene, interventions performed, and clinical condition during transport. The report of emergency service personnel is invaluable. Forward all of this information with the patient to the referral facility if secondary transport occurs.

Trauma in children is predominantly blunt, with penetrating trauma occurring in 10% of cases. Head and abdominal injuries are particularly common and important.

INITIAL ASSESSMENT & MANAGEMENT

The vast majority of children who reach a hospital alive survive to discharge. As most deaths from trauma in children are due to head injuries, cerebral resuscitation must be the foremost consideration when treating children with serious injuries. The ultimate measure of outcome is the child's eventual level of functioning. Strict attention to the ABCs ensures optimal oxygenation, ventilation, and perfusion, and ultimately, cerebral perfusion.

The primary and secondary survey is a method for evaluating and treating injured patients in a systematic way that provides a rapid assessment and stabilization phase, followed by a head-to-toe examination and definitive care phase.

PRIMARY SURVEY

The primary survey is designed to immediately identify and treat all physiologic derangements resulting from trauma. It is the resuscitation phase. Priorities are still airway, breathing, and circulation, but with important further considerations in the trauma setting:

Airway, with cervical spine control

Breathing

Circulation, with hemorrhage control

Disability (neurologic deficit)

Exposure (maintain a warm Environment, undress the patient completely, and Examine)

Evaluation and treatment of the ABCs are discussed earlier in this chapter. Modifications in the trauma setting are added in the sections that follow.

Airway

Failure to manage the airway appropriately is the most common cause of **preventable** morbidity and death. Administer 100% high-flow oxygen to all patients. During assessment and management of the airway, provide cervical spine protection, initially by manual inline immobilization, not traction. A hard cervical spine collar is then applied. The head and body are secured to a backboard, surrounded by a lightweight means of cushioning (eg, rolled blankets) to further immobilize the head and body and allow log-rolling of the child in case of vomiting. Assess the airway for patency. Use jaw thrust rather than chin lift during intubation to avoid flexion or extension of the neck. Suction the mouth and pharynx free of blood, foreign material, or secretions, and remove loose teeth. Insert an oropharyngeal airway if upper airway noises are heard or obstruction from posterior prolapse of the tongue occurs. A child with a depressed level of consciousness (Glasgow Coma Scale score < 9), a need for prolonged ventilation or hyperventilation, severe head trauma, or an impending operative intervention requires endotracheal intubation after bag–mask preoxygenation. Orotracheal intubation is the route of choice and is possible without cervical spine manipulation. Nasotracheal intubation may be possible in children 12 years of age or older who have spontaneous respirations—if not contraindicated by midfacial injury with the possibility of cribriform plate disruption. Laryngeal mask airway (LMA) devices are being used with increasing frequency, in both the prehospital and hospital settings. The device consists of a flexible tube attached to an inflatable rubber mask (Figure 11–8). The LMA is inserted blindly into the hypopharynx and is seated over the larynx, occluding the esophagus. Advantages to its use include ease of insertion, lower potential for airway trauma, and higher success rates. Patients remain at higher risk for aspiration with LMA use compared with orotracheal intubation; therefore, the LMA should not be used for prolonged, definitive airway management. Rarely, if tracheal intubation cannot be accomplished—particularly in the setting of massive facial trauma—cricothyroidotomy may be necessary. Needle cricothyroidotomy using a large-bore catheter through the cricothyroid membrane is the procedure of choice in patients younger than age 12 years. Operative revision will be needed for formal controlled tracheostomy.

Breathing

Most ventilatory problems are resolved adequately by the airway maneuvers described earlier in this chapter and by positive-pressure ventilation. Breathing assessment is as described previously: Assess for an adequate rate and for symmetrical chest rise, work of breathing, color, tracheal deviation, crepitus, flail segments, deformity, or penetrating wounds. Sources of traumatic pulmonary compromise include pneumothorax, hemothorax, pulmonary contusion, flail chest, and central nervous system (CNS) depression. Asymmetrical breath sounds, particularly with concurrent tracheal deviation, cyanosis, or bradycardia, suggest pneumothorax, possibly under tension. To evacuate a tension pneumothorax, insert a large-bore catheter-over-needle assembly attached to a syringe through the second intercostal and urinalysis in all patients. Blood type and cross-match should be obtained in the hypotensive child unresponsive to isotonic fluid boluses or with known hemorrhage. Consider coagulation studies, chemistry panel, liver transaminases, amylase, and toxicologic screening as clinically indicated.

External hemorrhage can be controlled by direct pressure. To avoid damage to adjacent neurovascular structures, avoid placing hemostats on vessels, except in the scalp. Determination of the site of internal hemorrhage can be challenging. Sites include the chest, abdomen, retroperitoneum, pelvis, and thighs. Bleeding into the intracranial vault rarely causes shock in children except in infants. Evaluation by an experienced clinician with adjunctive computed tomography (CT) or ultrasound will localize the site of internal bleeding.

Suspect cardiac tamponade after penetrating or blunt injuries to the chest if shock, pulseless electrical activity, narrowed pulse pressure, distended neck veins, hepatomegaly, or muffled heart sounds are present. Ultrasound may be diagnostic if readily available. Diagnose and treat with pericardiocentesis and rapid volume infusion.

Trauma ultrasonography, or the focused assessment with sonography for trauma (FAST), is routinely used in the adult trauma population. The purpose of the four-view examination (Morison pouch, splenorenal pouch, pelvic retrovesical space, and subcostal view of the heart) is to detect free fluid or blood in dependent spaces. In adults, such detection indicates clinically significant injury likely to require surgery. Accuracy and indications in children are much less clear. Solid organ injuries are more frequently missed and much of the pediatric trauma management is nonoperative. As a result, detection of free fluid by ultrasound in children is less likely to lead to surgery or result in a change in management.

Treat signs of poor perfusion vigorously: A tachycardic child with a capillary refill time of 3 seconds, or other evidence of diminished perfusion, is in *shock* and is sustaining vital organ insults. Remember that hypotension is a late finding. Volume replacement is initially accomplished by rapid infusion of normal saline or lactated Ringer solution at 20 mL/kg of body weight, followed by 10 mL/kg of packed red blood cells if perfusion does not normalize after two crystalloid bolus infusions.

Rapid reassessment must follow each bolus. If clinical signs of perfusion have not normalized, repeat the bolus. Lack of response or later or recurring signs of hypovolemia suggest the need for blood transfusion and possible surgical exploration. For every milliliter of external blood loss, 3 mL of crystalloid solution should be administered.

A common problem is the brain-injured child who is at risk for intracranial hypertension and who is also hypovolemic. In such cases, circulating volume must be restored to ensure adequate cerebral perfusion; therefore, fluid replacement is required until perfusion normalizes. Thereafter provide maintenance fluids with careful serial reassessments. **Do not restrict fluids** for children with head injuries.

▲ **Figure 11–8.** Laryngeal mask airways of various sizes.

space in the midclavicular line into the pleural cavity and withdraw air. If a pneumothorax or hemothorax is present, place a chest tube in the fourth intercostal space in the anterior axillary line. Connect to water seal. Insertion should be over the rib to avoid the neurovascular bundle that runs below the rib margin. Open pneumothoraces can be treated temporarily by taping petrolatum-impregnated gauze on three sides over the wound, creating a flap valve.

Circulation

After airway and breathing interventions have begun, hemodynamic status should be addressed. In addition to the circulatory assessment previously discussed, evaluation for ongoing external or internal hemorrhage is also important in the trauma evaluation. Large-bore IV access should be obtained early during the assessment, preferably at two sites. If peripheral access is not readily available, a central line, cutdown, or IO line is established. A cardiorespiratory monitor and oximeter is applied, usually at patient arrival. Peripheral perfusion and blood pressure should be assessed and recorded at frequent intervals. Determine hematocrit

Table 11–4. AVPU system for evaluation of level of consciousness.

A Alert
V Responsive to Voice
P Responsive to Pain
U Unresponsive

Disability–Neurologic Deficit

Assess pupillary size and reaction to light and the level of consciousness. The level of consciousness can be reproducibly characterized by the AVPU system (Table 11–4). Pediatric Glasgow Coma Scale assessments can be done as part of the secondary survey (Table 11–5).

Exposure & Environment

Significant injuries can be missed unless the child is completely undressed and examined fully, front and back. Cutting away clothing can minimize movement. Because of their high ratio of surface area to body mass, infants and children cool rapidly. Hypothermia compromises outcome except with iso-

Table 11–5. Glasgow Coma Scale.[a]

Eye opening response	
Spontaneous	4
To speech	3
To pain	2
None	1
Verbal response: Child _(Infant modification)_[b]	
Oriented (_Coos, babbles_)	5
Confused conversation (_Irritable cry, consolable_)	4
Inappropriate words (_Cries to pain_)	3
Incomprehensible sounds (_Moans to pain_)	2
None	1
Best upper limb motor response: Child _(Infant modification)_[b]	
Obeys commands (_Normal movements_)	6
Localizes pain (_Withdraws to touch_)	5
Withdraws to pain	4
Flexion to pain	3
Extension to pain	2
None	1

[a]The appropriate number from each section is added to total between 3 and 15. A score < 8 usually indicates central nervous system depression requiring positive-pressure ventilation.
[b]If no modification is listed, the same response applies for both infants and children.

lated head injuries; therefore, continuously monitor the body temperature and use warming techniques as necessary. Hyperthermia can adversely affect outcomes in children with acute brain injuries, so maintain normal body temperatures.

Monitoring

Cardiopulmonary monitors, pulse oximetry, and end-tidal CO_2 monitors should be put in place immediately. At the completion of the primary survey, additional "tubes" should be placed.

A. Nasogastric or Orogastric Tube

Children's stomachs should be assumed to be full. Gastric distention from positive-pressure ventilation increases the chance of vomiting and aspiration. The nasogastric route should be avoided in patients with significant midface injuries, as its use increases the risk of intracranial placement.

B. Urinary Catheter

An indwelling urinary bladder catheter should be placed to monitor urine output. Contraindications are based on the risk of urethral transection; signs include blood at the meatus or in the scrotum or a displaced prostate detected on rectal examination. Urine should be tested for blood. After the initial flow of urine with catheter placement, the urine output should exceed 1 mL/kg/h.

SECONDARY SURVEY

After the resuscitation phase, a head-to-toe examination should be performed to reveal all injuries and determine priorities for definitive care.

Skin

Search for lacerations, hematomas, swelling, and abrasions. Remove foreign material, and cleanse as necessary. Cutaneous findings may indicate underlying pathology (eg, a flank hematoma overlying a renal contusion), although surface signs may be absent even with significant internal injury. Make certain the child's tetanus immunization status is current. Consider tetanus immune globulin for incompletely immunized children.

Head

Check for hemotympanum and for clear or bloody cerebrospinal fluid leak from the nares. Battle sign (hematoma over the mastoid) and raccoon eyes are late signs of basilar skull fracture. Explore wounds, evaluating for foreign bodies and defects in galea or skull. CT scan of the head is an integral part of evaluation for altered level of consciousness, post-traumatic seizure, or focal neurologic findings (see section on Head Injury, later). Pneumococcal vaccine is indicated for basilar skull fractures.

Spine

Cervical spine injury must be excluded in all children. This can be done clinically in children older than 4 or 5 years of age with normal neurologic findings on examination (including voluntary movement of all extremities) who are able to deny midline neck pain or midline tenderness on palpation of the neck and who have no other painful injuries that might obscure the pain of a cervical spine injury. If radiographs are indicated, a cross-table lateral neck view is obtained initially, followed by anteroposterior, odontoid, and in some cases oblique views. Normal studies do not exclude significant injury, either bony or ligamentous, or involving the spinal cord itself. Therefore, an obtunded child should be maintained in cervical spine immobilization until the child has awakened and an appropriate neurologic examination can be performed. The entire thoracolumbar spine must be palpated and areas of pain or tenderness examined by radiography.

Chest

Pneumothoraces are detected and decompressed during the primary survey. Hemothoraces can occur with rib fractures or with injury to intercostal vessels, large pulmonary vessels, or lung parenchyma. Tracheobronchial disruption is suggested by large continued air leak despite chest tube decompression. Pulmonary contusions may require ventilatory support. Myocardial contusions and aortic injuries are unusual in children.

Abdomen

Blunt abdominal injury is common in multisystem injuries. Significant injury may exist without cutaneous signs or instability of vital signs. Tenderness, guarding, distention, diminished or absent bowel sounds, or poor perfusion mandates immediate evaluation by a pediatric trauma surgeon. Injury to solid viscera frequently can be managed nonoperatively in stable patients; however, intestinal perforation or hypotension necessitates operative treatment. Serial examinations, ultrasound, and CT scan provide diagnostic help. Elevated liver function tests have good specificity but only fair sensitivity for hepatic injury. Coagulation studies are rarely beneficial if no concomitant closed head injury is present. Obtaining a serum amylase immediately postinjury is controversial, as recent studies have shown variable correlation between elevated levels and pancreatic injury.

Pelvis

Pelvic fractures are classically manifested by pain, crepitus, and abnormal motion. Pelvic fracture is a relative contraindication to urethral catheter insertion. Perform a rectal examination, noting tone, tenderness, and in boys, prostate position. Stool should be tested for blood.

Genitourinary System

If urethral transection is suspected (see earlier discussion), perform a urethrogram before catheter placement. Diagnostic imaging of the child with hematuria often includes CT scan or occasionally, IV urograms. Management of kidney injury is largely nonoperative except for renal pedicle injuries.

Extremities

Long bone fractures are common but rarely life-threatening. Test for pulses, perfusion, and sensation. Neurovascular compromise requires immediate orthopedic consultation. Delayed diagnosis of fracture may occur when children are comatose; reexamination is necessary to avoid overlooking previously missed fractures. Treatment of open fractures includes antibiotics, tetanus prophylaxis, and orthopedic consultation.

Central Nervous System

Most deaths in children with multisystem trauma are from head injuries, so optimal neurointensive care is important. Significant injuries include diffuse axonal injury; cerebral edema; subdural, subarachnoid, and epidural hematomas; and parenchymal hemorrhages. Spinal cord injury occurs less commonly. Level of consciousness by the AVPU system (see Table 11–4) or Glasgow Coma Scale (see Table 11–5) should be assessed serially. A full sensorimotor examination should be performed. Deficits require immediate neurosurgical consultation. Extensor or flexor posturing represents intracranial hypertension, not seizure activity, until proven otherwise. If accompanied by a fixed, dilated pupil, such posturing indicates that a herniation syndrome is present, and mannitol or 3% hypertonic saline should be given if perfusion is normal. Treatment goals include aggressively treating hypotension to optimize cerebral perfusion, providing supplemental oxygen to keep saturations above 90%, achieving eucapnia (end-tidal CO_2 35–40 mm Hg), avoiding hyperthermia, and minimizing painful stimuli. Early rapid sequence intubation, sedation, and paralysis should be considered. Mild prophylactic hyperventilation is no longer recommended, although brief periods of hyperventilation are still indicated in the setting of acute herniation. Seizure activity warrants exclusion of significant intracranial injury. In the trauma setting, seizures are frequently treated with fosphenytoin. Acute spinal cord injury may benefit from high-dose methylprednisolone therapy. Corticosteroids are not indicated for head trauma.

Advanced Trauma Life Support: http://www.facs.org/trauma/atls/information.html

Avarello JT, Cantor RM: Pediatric major trauma: An approach to evaluation and management. Emerg Med Clin North Am 2007;25:803 [PMID: 17826219].

Hegenbarth MA: Bedside ultrasound in the pediatric emergency department: Basic skill or passing fancy? Clin Ped Emerg Med 2004;5:201.

Kellogg ND, Committee on Child Abuse and Neglect: Evaluation of suspected child physical abuse. Pediatrics 2007;119:1232 [PMID: 17545397].

Orenstein JB: Prehospital pediatric airway management. Clin Ped Emerg Med 2006;7:31.

Platzer P et al: Cervical spine injuries in pediatric patients. J Trauma 2007;62:389 [PMID: 17297330].

Wegner S et al: Pediatric blunt abdominal trauma. Pediatr Clin North Am 2006;53:243 [PMID: 16574524].

▼ HEAD INJURY

Closed head injuries range in severity from minor asymptomatic trauma without sequelae, to those leading to death. Head injury, including the shaken-baby syndrome, is common in cases of child abuse. Even following minor closed head injury, neuropsychiatric sequelae can occur.

ASSESSMENT

The considerations discussed earlier in the Approach to the Pediatric Trauma Patient section apply here as well. The history should include the time, mechanism, and details of the injury. Distance of the fall, landing surface, level of consciousness at event, subsequent mental status and activity, amnesia, and vomiting are important details to obtain.

The physical examination, including a detailed neurologic examination, should be complete and mindful of the mechanism of injury. Look for associated injuries such as mandibular fracture, scalp or skull injury, or cervical spine injury. Cerebrospinal fluid leak from the ears or nose or the later appearance of periorbital hematomas (raccoon eyes) or Battle sign imply basilar skull fracture and indicate the need for pneumococcal vaccine. Obtain vital signs and assess the child's level of consciousness by the AVPU system (see Table 11–4) or Glasgow Coma Scale (see Table 11–5), noting irritability or lethargy; pupillary equality, size, and reaction to light; funduscopic examination; reflexes; body posture; and rectal tone. Always consider child abuse; the injuries observed should be consistent with the history and the child's developmental level.

Radiographic studies may be indicated. Plain films are useful only in cases of penetrating head trauma or for ruling out foreign bodies. Major morbidity does not result directly from skull fractures, but rather from the associated intracranial injury. CT scans should be performed based on clinical findings in the child with persistent vomiting or an abnormal or lateralizing neurologic examination, including an abnormal mental status that does not quickly return to normal. In infants, a normal neurologic examination does not exclude significant intracranial hemorrhage; in the setting of an appropriate mechanism, and if scalp findings such as large hematomas are found, consider performing CT.

CONCUSSION

A concussion injury is defined as a brief loss or alteration of consciousness followed by a return to normal. Brain tissue is not damaged, and there are no focal findings on detailed neurologic examination. There may be pallor, amnesia, or several episodes of vomiting. Disposition is based on the clinical course and suitability of follow-up. The patient may be discharged when neurologically normal after a period of observation. Parents should closely observe the child at home and return if the child exhibits altered level of consciousness, persistent vomiting, gait disturbances, unequal pupils, seizures, or increasing headache, or if the parents have any concerns.

CONTUSION

A bruise of the brain matter is a contusion. The child's level of consciousness decreases, and focal findings, if any, correspond to the area of the brain that is injured. These patients require CT scan, a period of observation, and consideration of neurorehabilitation follow-up for post-traumatic brain injury sequelae.

DIFFUSE AXONAL INJURY

Diffuse axonal injury is a potentially severe form of traumatic brain injury characterized by coma without focal signs on neurologic examination. No external signs of trauma may be apparent. The initial CT scan is normal or may demonstrate only scattered small areas of cerebral contusion and areas of low density. Prolonged disability may follow diffuse axonal injury.

ACUTE INTRACRANIAL HYPERTENSION

Close observation will detect early signs and symptoms of intracranial pressure elevation. Early recognition is essential to avoid disastrous outcomes. In addition to traumatic causes, intracranial pressure elevation with or without herniation syndromes may be seen in spontaneous intracranial hemorrhage, CNS infection, hydrocephalus, ruptured arteriovenous malformation, metabolic derangement (eg, diabetic ketoacidosis), ventriculoperitoneal shunt obstruction, or tumor. Symptoms include headache, vision changes, vomiting, gait difficulties, and a progressively decreasing level of consciousness. Other signs may include stiff neck, cranial nerve palsies, and progressive hemiparesis. Cushing triad (bradycardia, hypertension, and irregular respirations) is a late and ominous finding. Papilledema is also a late finding. Consider CT scan before lumbar puncture if there is concern about intracranial pressure elevation because of the risk of precipitating herniation. Lumbar puncture should be deferred if the patient is unstable.

► Treatment

Therapy for intracranial pressure elevation must be swift and aggressive. Strict attention to adequate oxygenation, ventilation, and perfusion is paramount. Controlled rapid sequence intubation with appropriate sedation, muscle relaxation, agents to reduce the intracranial pressure elevation that accompanies intubation, and avoidance of hypoperfusion and hypoxemia are all important aspects of treatment. Brief periods of hyperventilation are reserved for acute herniation. Mannitol (0.5 g/kg IV), an osmotic diuretic, will reduce brain water, as will furosemide (0.1–0.2 mg/kg IV). Hypertonic saline (3%) is also used for this purpose. These measures may acutely lower intracranial pressure. Fluid infusion and, ultimately, pressors should be used to maintain normal arterial blood pressure and peripheral perfusion, if necessary. Adjunctive measures include elevating the head of the bed 30 degrees, treating hyperpyrexia and pain, and maintaining the head in a midline position. Obtain immediate neurosurgical evaluation. Further details about management of intracranial hypertension (cerebral edema) are presented in Chapter 13.

DISPOSITION FOR CHILDREN WITH CLOSED HEAD INJURY

Patients with mild head injury may be discharged with detailed written instructions, if the examination remains normal after a period of observation and parental supervision and follow-up are appropriate. Children with persistent deficits require admission or prolonged observation. In patients whose mental status improves over time, observation may be done without further radiographic studies. If mental status deteriorates, however, CT scan and neurosurgical consultation are indicated. If the CT scan is normal and the neurologic findings normalize, these children may be discharged after a period of observation. Patients with severe head injury require cerebral resuscitation, evaluation by a neurosurgeon, and admission to hospital.

Dias MS: Traumatic brain and spinal cord injury. Pediatr Clin North Am 2004;51:271 [PMID: 15062672].
Pardes Berger R, Adelson PD: Evaluation and management of pediatric head trauma in the emergency department: Current concepts and state-of-the-art research. Clin Ped Emerg Med 2005;6:8.

BURNS

 ESSENTIALS OF DIAGNOSIS & TYPICAL FEATURES

▶ Burn classification depends on location and extent of injury.
▶ Burns of the hands, feet, face, eyes, ears, and perineum are always considered to be major burns.

Thermal injury is a major cause of accidental death and disfigurement in children. Pain, morbidity, the association with child abuse, and the preventable nature of burns constitute an area of major concern in pediatrics. Common causes include hot water or food, appliances, flames, grills, vehicle-related burns, and curling irons. Burns occur commonly in toddlers—in boys more frequently than in girls.

EVALUATION OF THE BURNED PATIENT

Classification

Burns are classified clinically according to the nature of the burn and the extent and thickness; associated injuries are ascertained in the initial evaluation.

Superficial burns are easily recognized and treated. They are painful, dry, red, and hypersensitive. Sunburn is a common example. Healing occurs with minimal damage to epidermis. Partial-thickness burns are subgrouped as superficial or deep, depending on appearance and healing time. Each subgroup is treated differently. Superficial partial-thickness burns are red and often blister. Deep partial-thickness burns are white and dry, blanch with pressure, and the involved skin has decreased sensitivity to pain. Full-thickness burns affect all epidermal and dermal elements, leaving devascularized skin. The wound is white or black, dry, depressed, leathery in appearance, and without sensation. Unless skin grafting is provided, the scar will be hard, uneven, and fibrotic. Deep full-thickness, or subdermal, burns are the most severe, extending through all layers of skin as well as into the underlying fascia, muscle, and possibly bone.

Management

Management also depends on the depth and extent of injury. Burn extent can be classified as major or minor. Minor burns are less than 10% of the body surface area for superficial and partial-thickness burns, or less than 2% for full-thickness burns. Partial- or full-thickness burns of the hands, feet, face, eyes, ears, and perineum are considered major.

A. Superficial and Partial-Thickness Burns

These injuries can generally be treated in the outpatient setting. It is *mandatory* that effective analgesia be rapidly provided, and redosed as indicated by the child. Oral codeine or parenteral narcotics are indicated. Superficial burns are treated with cool compresses and analgesia. Treatment of partial-thickness burns with blisters consists of antiseptic cleansing, topical antimicrobial coverage, and observation for infection. Blisters appear early in deeper partial-thickness burns and, if open, may be debrided. Alternatively, the blister may be used as a protective flap after cleaning and dressing. After debridement, the wound should be cleansed with dilute (1–5%) povidone-iodine solution, thoroughly washed with normal saline, and covered with topical antibiotic. The wound should be protected with a bulky dressing and reexamined within 24 hours and serially thereafter. Wounds with a potential to cause disfigurement or functional impairment—especially wounds of the hand or digits—should be referred promptly to a burn surgeon. Outpatient analgesia should be provided on discharge.

B. Full-Thickness, Deep or Extensive Partial-Thickness, and Subdermal Burns

Major burns require particular attention to the ABCs of trauma management. Early establishment of an artificial airway is critical with oral or nasal burns because of their association with inhalation injuries and critical airway narrowing.

The protocol for the primary survey should be followed (see earlier discussion). There may be inhalation injury from carbon monoxide, cyanide, or other toxic products. A naso-gastric tube and bladder catheter should be placed. The secondary survey should ascertain whether any other injuries are present, including those suggestive of abuse.

Fluid administration is based on several principles. Capillary permeability is markedly increased. Fluid needs are based on examination findings, percentage of body surface area burned, depth, and age. Maintaining normal intravascular pressure and replacing fluid losses are essential. Figure 11–9 shows percentages of body surface area by body part in infants and children. The Parkland formula for fluid therapy is 4 mL/kg/% body surface area burned for the first 24 hours, with half in the first 8 hours, **in addition to maintenance rates.** Acutely, however, fluid resuscitation should be based on clinical assessment of volume status.

Indications for admission include major burns as previously defined, uncertainty of follow-up, suspicion of abuse, presence of upper airway injury, explosion, inhalation, electrical or chemical burns, burns associated with fractures, or the need for parenteral pain control. Children with chronic metabolic or connective tissue diseases and infants deserve hospitalization. Children with subdermal burns require immediate hospitalization at a burn center under the care of a burn specialist, fluid resuscitation, debridement of the wound, and placement of temporary wound coverage.

ELECTRICAL BURNS

Even brief contact with a high-voltage source will result in a contact burn. When an infant or toddler bites an electric cord, burns to the commissure of the lips occur that appear gray and necrotic, with surrounding erythema. If an arc is created with passage of current through the body, the pattern of the thermal injury will depend on the path of the current; therefore, search for an exit wound and internal injuries. Extensive damage to deep tissues may occur. Current traversing the heart may cause nonperfusing arrhythmias. Neurologic effects of electrical burns can be immediate (eg, confusion, disorientation, peripheral nerve injury), delayed (eg, nerve damage in the thrombosed limb after compartment syndrome), or late (eg, impaired concentration or memory).

Duffy BJ et al: Assessment, triage, and early management of burns in children. Clin Ped Emerg Med 2006;7:82.

Infant Less Than One Year of Age

Name_____ Age_____ Ward_____

1st-degree erythema not to be included.

2nd-degree   3rd-degree

Variations From Adult Distribution in Infants and Children (in Percent).

	New-born	1 Year	5 Years	10 Years
Head	19	17	13	11
Both thighs	11	13	16	17
Both lower legs	10	10	11	12
Neck	2			
Anterior trunk	13			
Posterior trunk	13			
Both upper arms	8		These percentages	
Both lower arms	6		remain constant at	
Both hands	5		all ages	
Both buttocks	6			
Both feet	7			
Genitalia	1			
	100			

▲ **Figure 11–9.** Lund and Browder modification of Berkow scale for estimating extent of burns. (The table under the illustration is after Berkow.)

DISORDERS DUE TO ALTERED ENVIRONMENTAL TEMPERATURE

HEAT-RELATED ILLNESSES & HEAT STROKE

Compared with adults, children are at an increased risk of heat-related illnesses because of their unique response to heat stress. Related illnesses range from miliaria rubra (prickly heat) to heat cramps and exhaustion, to life-threatening heat stroke.

Miliaria rubra commonly occurs in infants and young children during hot weather and manifests as an erythematous, papular rash concentrated on the face, upper neck, and extremities. Superinfection may result in a pustular appearance to the rash. The condition results from the obstruction of immature sweat glands. Treatment includes dressing the child in loose-fitting clothing and avoiding oil-based topical lubricants.

Heat cramps are characterized by brief, severe cramping (not rigidity) of skeletal or abdominal muscles following exertion. Core body temperature is normal or slightly elevated. There may be associated hyponatremia, hypochloremia, and rarely, hypokalemia. Mild cases can be treated with oral salt-containing solutions; more severe cases require IV infusion of normal saline solution.

Heat exhaustion includes multiple and often vague constitutional symptoms manifesting after heat exposure. Patients continue to sweat and have varying proportions of salt and water depletion. Core temperatures should be monitored frequently and are often normal or slightly increased. Presenting symptoms and signs include weakness, fatigue, headache, disorientation, pallor, thirst, nausea and vomiting, and occasionally muscle cramps without CNS dysfunction. Shock may be present. Treat with IV fluids, guided by serum electrolyte levels. Both heat cramps and heat exhaustion can be prevented by acclimatization and liberal water and salt intake during exercise.

Heat stroke represents failure of thermoregulation and is life-threatening. Diagnosis is based on a rectal temperature above 40.6°C with associated neurologic signs in a patient with an exposure history. Lack of sweating is **not** a necessary criterion. Symptoms are similar to those of heat exhaustion, but CNS dysfunction is more prominent. Patients with heat stroke are often incoherent and combative. In more severe cases, vomiting, shivering, coma, seizures, nuchal rigidity, and posturing may be present. Cardiac output may be high, low, or normal. Cellular hypoxia, enzyme dysfunction, and disrupted cell membranes lead to global end-organ derangements: rhabdomyolysis, myocardial necrosis, electrolyte abnormalities, acute tubular necrosis and renal failure, hepatic degeneration, acute respiratory distress syndrome, and disseminated intravascular coagulation. Consider sepsis, malignant hyperthermia, and neuroleptic malignant syndrome in the differential diagnosis.

Heat Stroke Management

1. Address the ABCs (airway, breathing, circulation), and administer 100% oxygen.
2. Administer IV fluids: isotonic crystalloid for hypotension, 5% dextrose normal saline for maintenance. Consider central venous pressure monitoring.
3. Once resuscitative efforts have begun, cool the patient by removing clothing; misting with cool water; applying ice at neck, groin, and axilla; fanning; and other cooling devices.
4. Place monitors, check rectal temperatures continuously, and place a Foley catheter and nasogastric tube.
5. Order laboratory tests: complete blood count; electrolytes; glucose; creatinine; prothrombin time and partial thromboplastin time; creatine kinase; liver function tests; arterial blood gases; urinalysis; and serum calcium, magnesium, and phosphate.
6. Admit to the pediatric intensive care unit.

HYPOTHERMIA

Seriously ill children should have core temperature quickly determined. Hypothermia in children, defined as core body temperature less than 35°C, is frequently associated with cold water submersion incidents. Other disorders cause incidental hypothermia, including sepsis, metabolic derangements, ingestions, CNS disorders, and endocrinopathies. Neonates, trauma victims, intoxicated patients, and the chronically disabled are particularly at risk. Mortality rates are high and are related to the underlying disorder. Conversely, moderate therapeutic hypothermia (32–34°C) following hypoxic-ischemic CNS insult and isolated traumatic brain injury is now recommended as potentially beneficial for CNS recovery.

As core temperature falls, a variety of mechanisms begin to conserve and produce heat. Peripheral vasoconstriction allows optimal maintenance of core temperature. Heat production can be increased by a hypothalamic-mediated increase in muscle tone and metabolism. Shivering increases heat production to two to four times basal levels.

▶ Clinical Findings

Clinical manifestations of hypothermia vary with severity of body temperature depression. Severe cases (< 28°C) mimic death: patients are pale or cyanotic, pupils may be fixed and dilated, muscles are rigid, and there may be no palpable pulses. Heart rates as low as 4–6 beats/min may provide adequate perfusion, because of lowered metabolic needs in severe hypothermia. Because findings resulting from primary hypothermia may be easily confused with those of postmortem changes, death is not pronounced until the patient has been rewarmed and remains unresponsive to resuscitative efforts. Children with a core temperature as low as 19°C have survived neurologically intact.

▶ Treatment

A. General Supportive Measures

Management of hypothermia is largely supportive. Core body temperature must be continuously documented; monitor with a low-reading indwelling rectal thermometer. Patients must be handled gently, because the hypothermic myocardium is exquisitely sensitive and prone to arrhythmias. Ventricular fibrillation may occur spontaneously or as a result of minor handling or invasive procedures. If asystole or ventricular fibrillation is present on the cardiac monitor, perform chest compressions and use standard pediatric advanced life support techniques as indicated. Defibrillation and pharmacologic therapy should be initiated as appropriate but may not be successful until core rewarming has occurred. Spontaneous reversion to sinus rhythm at 28–30°C may take place as rewarming proceeds.

B. Rewarming

Remove wet clothing from all patients. Rewarming techniques are categorized as passive external, active external, or active core rewarming. The method chosen is based on the degree of hypothermia. Passive rewarming, such as covering with blankets, is appropriate only for mild cases (> 33°C). Active external rewarming methods include warming lights, thermal mattresses or electric warming blankets, immersion in warm baths, and hot water bottles or warmed bags of IV solutions. One must be aware of the potential for core temperature depression after rewarming has begun, as vasodilation allows cooler peripheral blood to be distributed to the core circulation.

Active core rewarming techniques are used alone or in combination with active external warming for moderate to severe hypothermia. The techniques include the delivery of warmed, humidified oxygen and the use of warmed (to 40°C) fluids for IV replacement, peritoneal dialysis, and mediastinal lavage. Bladder and bowel irrigation are not generally effective because of low surface areas for temperature exchange. Extracorporeal blood rewarming achieves controlled core rewarming, can stabilize volume and electrolyte disturbances, and is maximally effective (Table 11–6).

Grubenhoff JA et al: Heat-related illnesses. Clin Ped Emerg Med 2007;8:59.

Ulrich AS, Rathlev NK: Hypothermia and localized cold injuries. Emerg Med Clin North Am 2004;22:281 [PMID: 15163568].

SUBMERSION INJURIES

ESSENTIALS OF DIAGNOSIS & TYPICAL FEATURES

► CNS and pulmonary injuries account for major morbidity.

► Child may appear well at presentation, but late CNS and pulmonary changes can occur hours later.

► Minimum observation period is 8–12 hours.

Drowning is the second most common cause of death by unintentional injury among children. Water hazards are ubiquitous and include lakes and streams, swimming pools,

Table 11–6. Management of hypothermia.

General measures
Remove wet clothing.
Administer warmed and humidified 100% oxygen.
Monitor core temperature, heart and respiratory rates, and blood pressure continuously.
Consider central venous pressure determination for severe hypothermia.
Laboratory studies
Complete blood count and platelets
Serum electrolytes, glucose, creatinine, amylase
Prothrombin time, partial thromboplastin time
Arterial blood gases
Consider toxicology screen
Treatment
Correct hypoxemia, hypercapnia, pH < 7.2, clotting abnormalities, and glucose and electrolyte disturbances.
Start rewarming techniques: passive, active (core and external), depending on degree of hypothermia.
Replace intravascular volume with warmed intravenous crystalloid infusion at 42°C.
Treat asystole and ventricular fibrillation per PALS protocols. Continue cardiac massage at least until core temperature reaches 30°C, when defibrillation is more likely to be effective.

PALS, pediatric advanced life support.

bathtubs, and even toilets, buckets, and washing machines. Risk factors include epilepsy, alcohol, and lack of supervision. Males predominate in submersion deaths, as in most other nonintentional deaths. Prevention is paramount.

Major morbidity stems from CNS and pulmonary insult. Laryngospasm or breath-holding may lead to loss of consciousness and cardiovascular collapse before aspiration can occur (dry drowning). Anoxia from laryngospasm or aspiration leads to irreversible CNS damage after only 4–6 minutes. A child must fall through ice or directly into icy water for cerebral metabolism to be slowed sufficiently by hypothermia to provide protection from anoxic damage. Cardiovascular changes include myocardial depression and arrhythmias. Electrolyte alterations are generally slight. Unless hemolysis occurs, hemoglobin concentrations also change only slightly.

► Clinical Findings & Treatment

Depending on the duration of submersion and any protective hypothermia effects, children may appear clinically dead or completely normal. Observation over time assists with prognosis. The child who has been rewarmed to at least 33°C and is still apneic and pulseless will probably not survive to discharge or will be left with severe neurologic deficits. Until a determination of brain death can be made, however, aggressive resuscitation should be continued in a patient with return of circulation.

One should keep in mind possible associated injuries, including head or neck trauma. For children who appear well initially, observation for 8–12 hours will detect late pulmonary compromise or changes in neurologic status. Respiratory distress, an abnormal chest radiograph, abnormal arterial blood gases, or hypoxemia by pulse oximetry indicates the need for treatment with supplemental oxygen, cardiopulmonary monitoring, and frequent reassessment. Serially assess respiratory distress and mental status. Signs of pulmonary infection may appear many hours after the submersion event.

Patients who are in coma and who require mechanical ventilation have a high risk of anoxic encephalopathy. The value of therapy with hyperventilation, corticosteroids, intentional hypothermia, and barbiturates remains unproved.

Zuckerbraun NS, Saladino RA: Pediatric drowning: Current management strategies for immediate care. Clin Ped Emerg Med 2005;6:49.

ANIMAL & HUMAN BITES

Bites account for a large number of visits to the emergency department. Most fatalities are due to dog bites. However, human and cat bites cause the majority of infected bite wounds.

DOG BITES

Boys are bitten more frequently than girls, and the dog is known by the victim in most cases. Younger children have a higher incidence of head and neck wounds, whereas school-age children are bitten most often on the upper extremities.

Dog bites are treated similarly to other wounds: high-pressure, high-volume irrigation with normal saline, debridement of any devitalized tissue, removal of foreign matter, and tetanus prophylaxis. The risk of rabies from dogs is low in developed countries, but rabies prophylaxis should be considered when appropriate. Wounds should be sutured only if necessary for cosmetic reasons because wound closure increases the risk of infection. Prophylactic antibiotics have not been proven to decrease rates of infection in low-risk dog bite wounds not involving the hands or feet. If a bite involves a joint, periosteum, or neurovascular bundle, prompt orthopedic surgery consultation should be obtained.

Pathogens that infect dog bites include *Pasteurella canis* and *P multocida,* streptococci, staphylococci, and anaerobes. Infected dog bites can be treated with penicillin for *P multocida,* and broad-spectrum coverage can be provided by amoxicillin and clavulanic acid or cephalexin (see dose for cat bites in the next section). Complications of dog bites include scarring, CNS infections, septic arthritis, osteomyelitis, endocarditis, and sepsis.

CAT BITES

Cat-inflicted wounds occur more frequently in girls, and their principal complication is infection. The infection risk is higher in cat bites than dog bites because cat bites produce a puncture wound. Management is similar to that for dog bites. Cat wounds should *not* be sutured except when absolutely necessary for cosmetic reasons. *P multocida* is the most common pathogen. Cat bites create a puncture-wound inoculum, and prophylactic antibiotics (penicillin plus cephalexin, or amoxicillin and clavulanic acid) are recommended. The dose of amoxicillin trihydrate and clavulanic acid should be on the high side of recommended dosage in order to ensure adequate tissue penetration both in dog and cat bites. The dosage of the amoxicillin component should be 80 mg/kg/24 h in three divided doses. The maximum dosage is 2 g/24 h. Scratches or bites from cats may also result in cat scratch fever.

HUMAN BITES

Most human bites occur during fights. *P multocida* is not a known pathogen in human bites; cultures most commonly grow streptococci, staphylococci, anaerobes, and *Eikenella corrodens.* Hand wounds and deep wounds should be treated with antibiotic coverage against *E corrodens* and gram-positive pathogens by a penicillinase-resistant antibiotic. Wound management is the same as for dog bites. Only severe lacerations involving the face should be sutured. Other wounds can be managed by delayed primary closure or healing by secondary intention. A major complication of human bite wounds is infection of the metacarpophalangeal joints. A hand surgeon should evaluate clenched-fist injuries from human bites. Operative debridement is followed in many cases by IV antibiotics.

Younggren BN: Emergency management of difficulty wounds: Part I. Emerg Med Clin North Am 2007;25:101 [PMID: 17400075].

PROCEDURAL SEDATION & ANALGESIA (PSA)

Relief of pain and anxiety are paramount concepts in the provision of acute care pediatrics, and should be considered at all times. Many agents also have amnestic properties. Parenteral agents can be effective and safe and produce few side effects if used judiciously.

Conditions such as fracture reduction, laceration repair, burn care, sexual assault examinations, lumbar puncture, and diagnostic procedures such as CT and magnetic resonance imaging may all be performed more effectively and compassionately if effective sedation or analgesia is used. The clinician should decide whether procedures will require sedation, analgesia, or both, and then choose agents accordingly.

Safe and effective sedation requires thorough knowledge of the selected agent and its side effects, as well as suitable monitoring devices, resuscitative medications, equipment, and personnel. The decision to perform PSA must be patient-oriented and tailored to specific procedural needs, while ensuring the child's safety throughout the procedure.

In order to successfully complete this task, a thorough preprocedural assessment should be completed, including a directed history and physical examination. Risks, benefits, and limitations of the procedure should be discussed with the parent or guardian and informed, verbal consent must be obtained. PSA then proceeds as follows:

1. Choose the appropriate medication(s).
2. Ensure appropriate NPO (nothing-by-mouth) status for 2–6 hours, depending on age and type of intake. For certain emergency procedures, suboptimal NPO status may be allowed, with attendant risks identified.
3. Establish vascular access as required.
4. Ensure that resuscitative equipment and personnel are readily available. Attach appropriate monitoring devices, as indicated.
5. Give the agent selected, with continuous monitoring for side effects. A dedicated observer, usually a nurse, should monitor the patient at all times. Respiratory effort, perfusion, and mental status should be assessed and documented serially.
6. Titrate the medication to achieve the desired sedation level. The ideal level depends on sedation goals and procedure type. PSA goals in the emergency department setting usually involve minimal or moderate sedation. Minimal sedation is a state in which the patient's sensorium is dulled, but he is still responsive to verbal stimuli. Moderate sedation is a depression of consciousness in which the child responds to tactile stimuli. In both cases, airway reflexes are preserved. It is important to remember that sedation is a continuum and the child may drift to deeper, unintended levels of sedation.
7. Continue monitoring the patient after the procedure has finished and the child has returned to baseline mental status. Once a painful stimulus has been corrected, mental status can decrease.
8. Criteria for discharge include the child's ability to sit unassisted, take oral fluids, and answer verbal commands. A PSA discharge handout should be given, with precautions for close observation and avoidance of potentially dangerous activities.

The following are some commonly used sedatives and analgesics:

1. Midazolam—This agent has particular usefulness in pediatrics due to its safety, rapid onset, and short half-life. Administration may be oral, rectal, intranasal, intramuscular, or IV. When given slowly intranasally, the drug's kinetics are similar as when given intravenously, although many patients report a burning sensation with administration. Oral or rectal administration results in relatively delayed onset, and titration is difficult. Intramuscular injections can be combined with opioid analgesics if systemic analgesia is desired. IV administration allows optimal ability to titrate dosing to the desired sedation level. It is best to place an IV

for complicated or prolonged procedures to facilitate redosing, which also provides IV access if resuscitation becomes necessary. Potential side effects of midazolam include cardiorespiratory depression.

2. Barbiturates—This class of agents (eg, pentobarbital) has the benefit of minimizing movement during procedures, which makes them advantageous for diagnostic studies such as CT or magnetic resonance imaging. Rectal administration of thiopental is safe and effective. Onset of action with IV administration is rapid. Potential side effects, although uncommon, include cardiorespiratory depression and laryngospasm.

3. Narcotics—Agents such as fentanyl and morphine have powerful analgesic and sedative effects and can be combined with anxiolytics such as benzodiazepines. Desired and adverse effects, such as respiratory depression, are potentiated when benzodiazepines and narcotics or barbiturates are given together. Therefore, sedative doses should be reduced when sedatives and analgesics are given together.

4. Ketamine—A commonly used drug in the emergency department, ketamine provides analgesia, anxiolysis and amnesia while allowing the child to retain protective airway reflexes and cardiovascular stability. In addition to providing "dissociative sedation," this sympathomimetic drug also increases heart rate and blood pressure. Side effects include salivation (therefore, it is usually given with glycopyrrolate as an antisalivation agent), laryngospasm (rarely), nystagmus, emergence reactions, and vomiting. With comprehensive knowledge of this medication, its use can be a significant advantage to children.

5. Propofol—Propofol is a nonopioid, nonbarbiturate sedative that is highly effective. It is finding increased use as an adjunct to analgesia for painful procedures in the emergency department. Onset of action and recovery are rapid. Side effects include transient hypotension and dose-dependent respiratory depression or apnea. Careful monitoring is essential.

American Academy of Pediatrics; American Academy of Pediatric Dentistry; Coté CJ et al: Guidelines for monitoring and management of pediatric patients during and after sedation for diagnostic and therapeutic procedures: An update. Pediatrics 2006;18:2587 [PMID: 17142550].

Doyle L, Colletti JE: Pediatric procedural sedation and analgesia. Pediatr Clin North Am 2006;53:279 [PMID: 16574526].

Godwin SA et al: Clinical policy: procedural sedation and analgesia in the emergency department. Ann Emerg Med 2005;45:177 [PMID: 15671976].

Krauss B, Green SM: Procedural sedation and analgesia in children. Lancet 2006;367:766 [PMID: 16517277].

Meyer S et al: Sedation and analgesia for brief diagnostic and therapeutic procedures in children. Eur J Pediatr 2007;166:291 [PMID: 17205245].

Roback MG et al: Adverse events associated with procedural sedation and analgesia in a pediatric emergency department: A comparison of common parenteral drugs. Acad Emerg Med 2005;12:508 [PMID: 15930401].

Shankar V, Deshpande JK: Procedural sedation in the pediatric patient. Anesthesiol Clin North Am 2005;23:635 [PMID: 16310656].

Poisoning

Barry H. Rumack, MD
Richard C. Dart, MD, PhD

Accidental and intentional exposures to toxic substances occur in children of all ages. Children younger than age 6 years are primarily involved in accidental exposures, with the peak incidence in 2-year-olds. Of the more than 2.5 million exposures reported by the American Association of Poison Control Centers' National Poison Data System in 2006, 51% occurred in children aged 5 years and under, 6% in those aged 6–12 years, and 7% in those aged 13–19 years. Young children are occasionally exposed to intentional poisoning through the actions of parents or caregivers. Administration of agents such as diphenhydramine to induce sleep in a day-care setting, Münchausen syndrome by proxy to obtain parental secondary gain, or deliberate harm should be suspected when the history is not consistent. Involvement of child abuse specialists is very helpful in these cases. (See Chapter 7.) Adolescents are involved in intentional episodes when attempting suicide or experimenting with various drugs and agents. In some locales, small-scale industrial or manufacturing processes may be associated with homes and farms, and exposures to hazardous substances should be considered in the history.

Bronstein AC et al: 2006 Annual Report of the American Association of Poison Control Centers' National Poison Data System (NPDS). Clin Toxicol (Phila) 2007;45:815 [PMID: 18163234].

PHARMACOLOGIC PRINCIPLES OF TOXICOLOGY

In the evaluation of the poisoned patient, it is important to compare the anticipated pharmacologic or toxic effects with the patient's clinical presentation. If the history is that the patient ingested a tranquilizer 30 minutes ago, but the clinical examination reveals dilated pupils, tachycardia, dry mouth, absent bowel sounds, and active hallucinations—clearly anticholinergic toxicity—diagnosis and therapy should proceed accordingly.

LD$_{50}$

Estimates of the LD$_{50}$ (the amount per kilogram of body weight of a drug required to kill 50% of a group of experimental animals) or median lethal dose are of little clinical value in humans. It is usually impossible to determine with accuracy the amount swallowed or absorbed, the metabolic status of the patient, or in which patients the response to the agent will be atypical. Furthermore, these values are often not valid in humans even if the history is accurate.

Half-Life ($t_{1/2}$)

The $t_{1/2}$ of an agent must be interpreted carefully. Most published $t_{1/2}$ values are for therapeutic dosages. The $t_{1/2}$ may increase as the quantity of the ingested substance increases for many common intoxicants such as salicylates. One cannot rely on the published $t_{1/2}$ for salicylate (2 hours) to assume rapid elimination of the drug. In an acute salicylate overdose (150 mg/kg), the apparent $t_{1/2}$ is prolonged to 24–30 hours.

Volume of Distribution

The volume of distribution (Vd) of a drug is determined by dividing the amount of drug absorbed by the blood level. With theophylline, for example, the Vd is 0.46 L/kg body weight, or 32 L in an average adult. In contrast, digoxin distributes well beyond total body water. Because the calculation produces a volume above body weight this figure is referred to as an "apparent volume of distribution" (Table 12–1).

The Vd can be useful in predicting which drugs will be removed by dialysis or exchange transfusion. When a drug is differentially concentrated in body lipids or is heavily tissue or protein bound and has a high Vd, only a small proportion of the drug will be in the free form and thus accessible to diuresis, dialysis, or exchange transfusion. A drug that is water soluble, can be ionized, and has a low Vd may cross

Table 12–1. Some examples of pK$_a$ and Vd.[a]

Drug	pK$_a$	Diuresis	Dialysis	Apparent Vd
Amobarbital	7.9	No	No	200–300% body weight
Amphetamine	9.8	No	Yes	60% body weight
Aspirin	3.5	Alkaline	Yes	15–40% body weight
Chlorpromazine	9.3	No	No	40–50 L/kg (2800–3500% body weight)
Codeine	8.2	No	No	5–10 L/kg (350–700% body weight)
Desipramine	10.2	No	No	30–40 L/kg (2100–2800% body weight)
Ethchlorvynol	8.7	No	No	5–10 L/kg (350–700% body weight)
Glutethimide	4.5	No	No	10–20 L/kg (700–1400% body weight)
Isoniazid	3.5	Alkaline	Yes	61% body weight
Methadone	8.3	No	No	5–10 L/kg (350–700% body weight)
Methicillin	2.8	No	Yes	60% body weight
Phenobarbital	7.4	Alkaline	Yes	75% body weight
Phenytoin	8.3	No	No	60–80% body weight
Tetracycline	7.7	No	No	200–300% body weight

[a]Comprehensive listings of pharmacokinetic data for a large number of drugs are included just prior to the index in each edition of *Goodman & Gilman's The Pharmacological Basis of Therapeutics* (see reference list).

the dialysis membrane well and also respond to diuresis. In general, methods of extracorporeal elimination are not effective for toxic agents with a Vd greater than 1 L/kg.

Metabolism & Excretion

The route of excretion or detoxification is important for planning treatment. Methanol, for example, is metabolized to the toxic product, formic acid. This metabolic step may be blocked by the antidote fomepizole or ethanol.

Blood Levels

Care of the poisoned patient should never be guided solely by laboratory measurements. Treatment should be directed first by the clinical signs and symptoms, followed by more specific therapy based on laboratory determinations. Clinical information may speed the identification of a toxic agent by the laboratory.

PREVENTING CHILDHOOD POISONINGS

Inclusion of poison prevention as part of routine well child care should begin at the 6-month well baby visit. The poison prevention handout included as Table 12–2 may be copied and distributed to parents. It contains poison prevention information as well as first-aid actions that should be taken in the event of an exposure. All poison control centers in the United States can be reached by dialing 1-800-222-1222; the call will be automatically routed to the correct regional center.

GENERAL TREATMENT OF POISONING

The telephone is often the first contact in pediatric poisoning. Some patients may contact their pediatrician's office first. Proper telephone management can reduce morbidity and prevent unwarranted or excessive treatment. The decision to refer the patient is based on the identity and dose of the ingested agent, the age of the child, the time of day, the reliability of the parent, and whether child neglect or endangerment is suspected. Poison control centers are the source of expert telephone advice and have excellent follow-up programs to manage patients in the home as well as provide further poison prevention information.

INITIAL TELEPHONE CONTACT

Basic information obtained at the first telephone contact includes the patient's name, age, weight, address, and telephone number; the agent and amount of agent ingested; the patient's present condition; and the time elapsed since ingestion or other exposure. Use the history to evaluate the urgency of the situation and decide whether immediate emergency transportation to a health facility is indicated. An emergency exists if the ingestant is high risk (caustic solutions, hydrogen fluoride, drugs of abuse, or medications such as a calcium channel blocker, opioid, hypoglycemic agent, or antidepressant) or if the self-poisoning was intentional. If immediate danger does not exist, obtain more details about the suspected toxic agent. If the child requires transport to a health facility, instruct parents that everything in the vicinity of the child that may be a cause of poisoning should be brought to the health care facility.

It may be difficult to obtain an accurate history. Obtain names of drugs or ingredients, manufacturers, prescription numbers, names and phone numbers of prescribing physician and pharmacy and any other pertinent information. Find out whether the substance was shared among several children, whether it had been recently purchased, who had last used it, how full the bottle was, and how much was spilled. Determine if this occurred in the home, school or elsewhere. If unsure of the significance of an exposure, consult with a poison control center.

Each year, children are accidentally poisoned by medicines, polishes, insecticides, drain cleaners, bleaches, household chemicals, and materials commonly stored in the garage. It is the responsibility of adults to make sure that children are not exposed to potentially toxic substances.

Obtaining Information About Poisons

Current data on ingredients of commercial products and medications can be obtained from a certified regional poison center. It is important to have the actual container at hand when calling. *Caution:* Antidote information on labels of commercial products or in the *Physicians' Desk Reference* may be incorrect or inappropriate.

Follow-Up

In over 95% of cases of ingestion of potentially toxic substances by children, a trip to the hospital is not required. In these cases, it is important to call the parent at 1 and 4 hours after ingestion. If the child has ingested an additional unknown agent and develops symptoms, a change in management may be needed, including transportation to the hospital. An additional call should be made 24 hours after the ingestion to begin the process of poison prevention.

INITIAL EMERGENCY DEPARTMENT CONTACT

Make Certain the Patient Is Breathing

As in all emergencies, the principles of treatment are attention to airway, breathing, and circulation. These are sometimes overlooked under the stressful conditions of a pediatric poisoning.

Treat Shock

Initial therapy of the hypotensive patient should consist of laying the patient flat and administering intravenous (IV) isotonic solutions. Vasopressors should be reserved for poisoned patients in shock who do not respond to these standard measures.

Treat Burns & Skin Exposures

Burns may occur following exposure to strongly acidic or strongly alkaline agents or petroleum distillates. Burned areas should be decontaminated by flooding with sterile saline solution or water. A burn unit should be consulted if more than minimal burn damage has been sustained. Skin decontamination should be performed in a patient with cutaneous exposure. Emergency department personnel in contact with a patient who has been contaminated (with an organophosphate insecticide, for example) should themselves be decontaminated if their skin or clothing becomes contaminated.

Take a Pertinent History

The history should be taken from the parents and all individuals present at the scene. It may be crucial to determine all of the kinds of poisons in the home. These may include drugs used by family members, chemicals associated with the hobbies or occupations of family members, or the purity of the water supply. Unusual dietary or medication habits or other clues to the possible cause of poisoning should also be investigated.

DEFINITIVE THERAPY OF POISONING

Treatment of poisoning or potential poisoning has evolved over time, and general measures such as prevention of absorption and enhancement of excretion are only instituted when specifically indicated. Specific therapy is directed at each drug, chemical, or toxin as described in the management section that follows.

Prevention of Absorption

A. Emesis and Lavage

These measures are rarely used in pediatric patients and should be performed only in consultation with a poison center.

B. Charcoal

The dose of charcoal is 1–2 g/kg (maximum, 100 g) per dose. Repeating the dose of activated charcoal may be useful for those agents that slow passage through the gastrointestinal (GI) tract. When multiple doses of activated charcoal are given, repeated doses of sorbitol or saline cathartics must not be given. Repeated doses of cathartics may cause electrolyte imbalances and fluid loss. Charcoal dosing is repeated every 2–6 hours until charcoal is passed through the rectum.

C. Catharsis

Despite their widespread use, cathartics do not improve outcome. The use of cathartics should therefore be avoided.

Table 12–2. Poison prevention and emergency treatment handout.

POISON SAFETY TIPS

If you or your child has come in contact with poison, call the **Poison Control Center (1-800-222-1222).** Nurses and poison experts will answer your call. In most cases, they can help you take care of the problem right at home. When you need to get to the hospital, they will call ahead with detailed information to help doctors treat you or your child quickly and correctly.

How people get poisoned

People can breathe poison, eat or drink it, or get it on the skin or in the eyes. You probably know that antifreeze, bleach, and bug spray are poisonous. But did you know that vitamins, perfume, and makeup can be dangerous? Eating some plants can be toxic. Some spider bites can be dangerous. Taking medicine that is too old or not prescribed for you can make you sick. Also, mixing different kinds of medicine can be dangerous.

Poison safety "do's" and "don'ts"

DO:

1. Ask for "safety-lock" tops on all prescription drugs.

2. Keep cleaners, bug sprays, medicines, and other harmful products out of the reach and sight of children. If possible, keep the products locked up.

3. Store medicine in original containers.

4. Read the label before taking medicine; don't take medicine that doesn't have a label.

5. Follow the directions for all products.

DON'T:

1. Don't store food and household cleaners together.

2. Don't take medicine in front of children; children love to imitate "mommy" and "daddy."

3. Don't call medicine candy.

4. Don't take medicine that is not for you. Never take medicine in the dark.

5. Don't put gasoline, bug spray, antifreeze or cleaning supplies in soft-drink bottles, cups or bowls. Always keep them in their original containers.

Kids can get into things at any age!

Children aged 0–6 months

Learn to roll over and reach for things.

Learn about their environment by putting things in their mouths.

Children aged 7–12 months

Start to get curious and explore.

Learn to crawl, pull up to stand, and walk holding on.

Put everything in their mouths.

Pull things down.

Children aged 1–3 years

Have the highest accident rate of any group.

Begin to imitate parents and other adults.

Put things in their mouths.

Start to climb on things.

Different dangers at different times of the year

Spring and summer dangers

Pesticides

Fertilizers

Outdoor plants and mushrooms

Snake, spider, and other insect bites

Bee stings

Ticks

Charcoal lighter fluid

Fall and winter dangers

Antifreeze

Carbon monoxide

Black widow spider bites

Plants and autumn berries

Holly, mistletoe, and other holiday decorations

Follow this checklist to make sure your home is safe

Kitchen

__Remove products like detergent, drain cleaner, and dishwashing liquid from under the sink.

__Remove medicines from counters, tables, refrigerator top, or window sills.

__Put child safety latches on all drawers and cabinets that contain harmful products.

__Store harmful products away from food.

(continued)

Table 12–2. Poison prevention and emergency treatment handout. *(Continued)*

Bathroom

__Regularly clean out your medicine chest. Flush old medicine down the toilet.

__Keep all medicine in original safety-top containers.

__Keep medicine, hair spray, powder, makeup, fingernail polish, hair-care products, and mouthwash out of reach.

Bedroom

__Don't keep medicine in or on dresser or bedside table.

__Keep perfume, makeup, aftershave, and other products out of reach.

Laundry Area

__Keep bleach, soap, fabric softener, starch, and other supplies out of reach.

__Keep all products in their original containers.

Garage/Basement

__Keep bug spray, weed killers, gasoline, oil, paint, and other supplies in locked area.

__Keep all products in their original containers.

General Household

__Keep beer, wine, and liquor out of reach.

__Keep ashtrays clean and out of reach.

__Keep plants out of reach.

__Keep paint in good repair.

Emergency action in case your child...

Breathes Poison:

Get child to fresh air right away. Open doors and windows.

Gets Poison on the Skin:

Remove clothes that have poison on them. Rinse skin with lukewarm water for 10 minutes. Wash gently with soap and water and rinse.

Gets Poison in the Eye:

Gently pour lukewarm water over the eye from a large glass 2 or 3 inches from the eye. Repeat for 15 minutes. Have child blink as much as possible while pouring water in the eye. Do not force the eyelid open.

Swallows Poison:

Medicines: Do not give child **anything** until you talk with the poison center or your doctor.

Chemicals or household products: Unless your child has passed out or cannot swallow, give milk or water right away. Call the **Poison Control Center**.

Pediatrician: _____(Tel): _____

National Toll Free Number which connects with your local Poison Center: **1-800-222-1222**

Information adapted from, and used, courtesy of the Rocky Mountain Poison Center, Denver, CO.

D. Whole Gut Lavage

Whole bowel lavage uses an orally administered, nonabsorbable hypertonic solution such as CoLyte or GoLYTELY. The use of this procedure in poisoned patients remains controversial. Preliminary recommendations for use of whole bowel irrigation include poisoning with sustained-release preparations, mechanical movement of items through the bowel (eg, cocaine packets, iron tablets), and poisoning with substances that are poorly absorbed by charcoal (eg, lithium, iron). Underlying bowel pathology and intestinal obstruc-

tion are relative contraindications to its use. Consultation with a certified regional poison center is recommended.

American Academy of Clinical Toxicology, European Association of Poisons Centers and Clinical Toxicologists: Position paper: Ipecac syrup. J Toxicol Clin Toxicol 2004;42:133 [PMID: 15214617].

American Academy of Clinical Toxicology, European Association of Poisons Centers and Clinical Toxicologists: Position statement and practice guidelines on the use of multidose activated charcoal in the treatment of acute poisoning. J Toxicol Clin Toxicol 1999;37:731 [PMID: 10584586].

Gielen AC et al: Effects of improved access to safety counseling, products, and home visits on parents' safety practices: Results of a randomized trial. Arch Pediatr Adolesc Med 2002;156:33 [PMID: 11772188].

Thummel KE, Shen DD: Design and optimization of dosage regimens: Pharmacokinetic data. In Goodman LS et al (editors): *Goodman & Gilman's The Pharmacological Basis of Therapeutics.* McGraw-Hill, 2001:1917.

Enhancement of Excretion

Excretion of certain substances can be hastened by urinary alkalinization or dialysis. It is important to make certain that the patient is not volume depleted. Volume-depleted patients should receive a normal saline bolus of 10–20 mL/kg, followed by sufficient IV fluid administration to maintain urine output at 2–3 mL/kg/h.

A. Urinary Alkalinization

1. Alkaline diuresis—Urinary alkalinization should be chosen on the basis of the substance's pK_a, so that ionized drug will be trapped in the tubular lumen and not reabsorbed (see Table 12–1). Thus, if the pK_a is less than 7.5, urinary alkalinization is appropriate; if it is over 8.0, this technique is not usually beneficial. The pK_a is sometimes included along with general drug information. Urinary alkalinization is achieved with sodium bicarbonate. It is important to observe for hypokalemia, caused by the shift of potassium intracellularly. Follow serum K^+ and observe for electrocardiogram (ECG) evidence of hypokalemia. If complications such as renal failure or pulmonary edema are present, hemodialysis or hemoperfusion may be required.

B. Dialysis

Hemodialysis (or peritoneal dialysis if hemodialysis is unavailable) is useful in the poisonings listed below and in the general management of a critically ill patient. Dialysis should be considered part of supportive care if the patient satisfies any of the following criteria:

1. Clinical criteria

A. Potentially life-threatening toxicity that is caused by a dialyzable drug and cannot be treated by conservative means.

B. Hypotension threatening renal or hepatic function that cannot be corrected by adjusting circulating volume.

C. Marked hyperosmolality or severe acid–base or electrolyte disturbances not responding to therapy.

D. Marked hypothermia or hyperthermia not responding to therapy.

2. Immediate dialysis—Immediate dialysis should be considered in ethylene glycol and methanol poisoning only if acidosis is refractory, the patient does not respond to fomepizole treatment, or blood levels of ethanol of 100 mg/dL are consistently maintained. Refractory salicylate intoxication may benefit from dialysis.

MANAGEMENT OF SPECIFIC COMMON POISONINGS

ACETAMINOPHEN (PARACETAMOL)

Overdosage of acetaminophen is the most common pediatric poisoning and can produce severe hepatotoxicity. The incidence of hepatotoxicity in adults and adolescents has been reported to be 10 times higher than in children younger than age 5 years. In the latter group, fewer than 0.1% develop hepatotoxicity after acetaminophen overdose. In children, toxicity most commonly results from repeated overdosage arising from confusion about the age-appropriate dose, use of multiple products that contain acetaminophen, or use of adult suppositories.

Acetaminophen is normally metabolized in the liver. A small percentage of the drug goes through a pathway leading to a toxic metabolite. Normally, this electrophilic reactant is removed harmlessly by conjugation with glutathione. In overdosage, the supply of glutathione becomes exhausted, and the metabolite may bind covalently to components of liver cells to produce necrosis. Some authors have proposed that therapeutic doses of acetaminophen may be toxic to children with depleted glutathione stores. However, there is no evidence that administration of therapeutic doses can cause toxicity, and only a few inadequate case reports have been made in this regard.

▶ Treatment

Treatment is to administer acetylcysteine. It may be administered either orally or intravenously. Consultation on difficult cases may be obtained from your regional poison control center or the Rocky Mountain Poison and Drug Center (1-800-525-6115). Blood levels should be obtained 4 hours after ingestion or as soon as possible thereafter and plotted on Figure 12–1. The nomogram is used only for acute ingestion, not repeated supratherapeutic ingestions. If the patient has ingested acetaminophen in a liquid preparation, blood levels obtained 2 hours after ingestion will accurately reflect the toxicity to be expected relative to the standard nomogram (see Figure 12–1). Acetylcysteine is administered to patients whose acetaminophen levels plot in the toxic range on the nomogram. Acetylcysteine is effective even when given more than 24 hours after ingestion, although it is most effective when given within 8 hours postingestion.

The oral (PO) dose of acetylcysteine is 140 mg/kg, diluted to a 5% solution in sweet fruit juice or carbonated soft drink. The primary problems associated with administration are nausea and vomiting. After this loading dose, 70 mg/kg should be administered orally every 4 hours for 72 hours.

For children weighing 40 kg or more, IV acetylcysteine (Acetadote) should be administered as a loading dose of 150 mg/kg administered over 15–60 minutes; followed by a second infusion of 50 mg/kg over 4 hours, and then a third infusion of 100 mg/kg over 16 hours (a dosage calculator is available at http://www.acetadote.com) (Table 12–3).

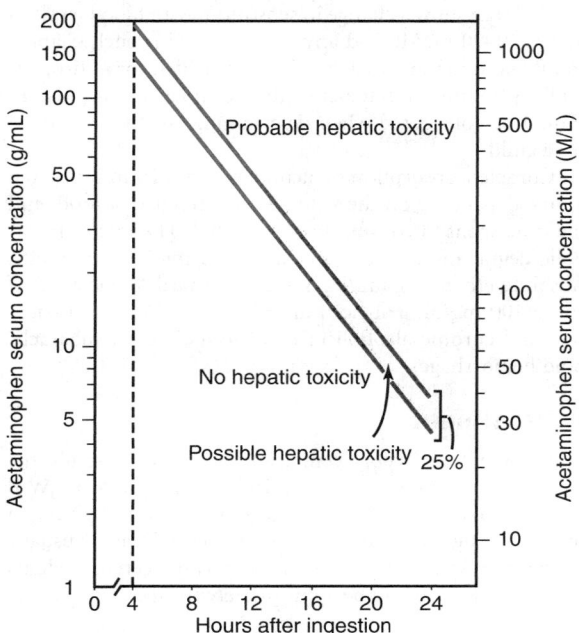

▲ **Figure 12–1.** Semi-logarithmic plot of plasma acetaminophen levels versus time. (Modified and reproduced, with permission, from Rumack BH, Matthew H: Acetaminophen poisoning and toxicity. Pediatrics 1975;55:871.)

For patients weighing less than 40 kg, IV acetylcysteine must have less dilution to avoid hyponatremia (Table 12–4).

Aspartate aminotransferase (AST–SGOT), alanine aminotransferase (ALT–SGPT), serum bilirubin, and plasma prothrombin time should be followed daily. Significant abnormalities of liver function may not peak until 72–96 hours after ingestion.

Repeated miscalculated overdoses given by parents to treat fever are the major source of toxicity in children younger than age 10 years, and parents are often unaware of the significance of symptoms of toxicity, thus delaying its prompt recognition and therapy.

Bond GR: Reduced toxicity of acetaminophen in children: It's the liver. J Toxicol Clin Toxicol 2004;42:149 [PMID: 15214619].

Marzullo L: An update of N-acetylcysteine treatment for acute acetaminophen toxicity in children. Curr Opin Pediatr 2005;17:239 [PMID: 15800420].

Rumack BH: Acetaminophen hepatotoxicity: The first 35 years. J Toxicol Clin Toxicol 2002;40:3 [PMID: 11990202].

ALCOHOL, ETHYL (ETHANOL)

Alcoholic beverages, tinctures, cosmetics, mouthwashes, and rubbing alcohol are common sources of poisoning in children. Concomitant exposure to other depressant drugs increases the seriousness of the intoxication. In most states, alcohol levels of 50–80 mg/dL are considered compatible with impaired faculties, and levels of 80–100 mg/dL are considered evidence of intoxication. (Blood levels cited here are for adults; comparable figures for children are not available.)

Recent erroneous information regarding hand sanitizers has indicated that a "lick" following application on the hand could cause toxicity in children. In fact this is not the case, but because these hand sanitizers contain 62% ethanol, toxicity following ingestion is very possible. Potential blood ethanol concentration following consumption of a 62% solution in a 10-kg child is calculated as follows:

$$1 \text{ oz} = 30 \text{ mL} \times 62\% = 18.6 \text{ mL of pure ethanol}$$

$$18.6 \text{ mL} \times 0.79 \text{ (the specific gravity)} = 14.7 \text{ g of ethanol, or } 14{,}700 \text{ mg}$$

Table 12–3. Intravenous acetylcysteine administration for children weighing 40 kg or more.

Body Weight		FIRST 150 mg/kg in 200 mL 5% Dextrose in 15 min	SECOND 50 mg/kg in 500 mL 5% Dextrose in 4 h	THIRD 100 mg/kg in 1000 mL 5% Dextrose in 16 h
(kg)	(lb)	Acetadote (mL)	Acetadote (mL)	Acetadote (mL)
100	220	75	25	50
90	198	67.5	22.5	45
80	176	60	20	40
70	154	52.5	17.5	35
60	132	45	15	30
50	110	37.5	12.5	25
40	88	30	10	20

In a patient weighing 10 kg, the distribution into total body water (Vd) will be 6 L—this is the amount of the body water into which the ethanol will be distributed.

$$14,700 \text{ mg} \div 6 \text{ L} = 2450 \text{ mg/L}$$

$$2450 \text{ mg/L} \div 10 = 245 \text{ mg/dL}$$

Based on these calculations, a 10-kg child consuming 0.5 oz would have a concentration of 122.5mg/dL; a 20-kg child consuming 1 oz would have a concentration of 122.5 mg/dL; a 30-kg child consuming 1 oz would have a concentration of 81.7 mg/dL; and a 70-kg adult consuming 1 oz would have a concentration of 35 mg/dL.

One "pump" from a hand sanitizer bottle dispenses approximately 2.5 mL of the product. If ingested, this amount (containing 62% ethanol) would create a blood ethanol concentration as follows:

1. In a 10-kg child: 23.1 mg/dL.
2. In a 20-kg child: 11.6 mg/dL.
3. In a 30-kg child: 7.7 mg/dL.

Children show a change in sensorium with blood levels as low as 10–20 mg/dL and any child displaying such changes should be seen immediately. Although a "lick" or a "drop" is unlikely to produce toxicity, the accuracy of the history should be considered when determining whether or not to see a child.

Complete absorption of alcohol requires 30 minutes to 6 hours, depending on the volume, the presence of food, and the time spent in consuming the alcohol. The rate of metabolic degradation is constant (about 20 mg/h in an adult). Absolute ethanol, 1 mL/kg, results in a peak blood level of about 100 mg/dL in 1 hour after ingestion. Acute intoxication and chronic alcoholism increase the risk of subarachnoid hemorrhage.

▶ Treatment

Management of hypoglycemia and acidosis is usually the only measure required. Start an IV drip of D_5W or $D_{10}W$ if blood glucose is less than 60 mg/dL. Fructose and glucagon have been suggested but are no longer used. Death is usually caused by respiratory failure. In severe cases, cerebral edema may occur and should be appropriately treated.

Table 12–4. Intravenous acetylcysteine administration for children weighing less than 40 kg.

Body Weight		Loading Infusion (15 min)—150 mg/kg		
(kg)	(lb)	NAC 20% (mL)	Diluent Volume D₅W (mL)	Final Volume (mL)
30	66	22.5	90	112.5
25	55	18.75	75	93.75
20	44	15	60	75
15	33	11.25	45	56.25
10	22	7.5	30	37.5
Body Weight		Second Infusion (4 h)—50 mg/kg		
(kg)	(lb)	NAC 20% (mL)	Diluent Volume D₅W (mL)	Final Volume (mL)
30	66	7.5	30	37.5
25	55	6.25	25	31.25
20	44	5	20	25
15	33	3.75	15	18.75
10	22	2.5	10	12.5
Body Weight		Third Infusion (16 h)—100 mg/kg		
(kg)	(lb)	NAC 20% (mL)	Diluent Volume D₅W (mL)	Final Volume (mL)
30	66	15	60	75
25	55	12.5	50	62.5
20	44	10	40	50
15	33	7.5	30	37.5
10	22	5	20	25

AMPHETAMINES & RELATED DRUGS (METHAMPHETAMINE)

▶ Clinical Presentation

A. Acute Poisoning

Amphetamine and methamphetamine poisoning is common because of the widespread availability of "diet pills" and the use of "speed," "crank," "crystal," and "ice" by adolescents. (Care must be taken in the interpretation of slang terms because they have multiple meanings.) A new cause of amphetamine poisoning is drugs for treating attention-deficit/hyperactivity disorder, such as methylphenidate. Symptoms include central nervous system (CNS) stimulation, anxiety, hyperactivity, hyperpyrexia, hypertension, abdominal cramps, nausea and vomiting, and inability to void urine. Severe cases often include rhabdomyolysis. A toxic psychosis indistinguishable from paranoid schizophrenia may occur. Methamphetamine laboratories in homes are a potential cause of childhood exposure to a variety of hazardous and toxic substances.

B. Chronic Poisoning

Chronic amphetamine users develop tolerance; more than 1500 mg of IV methamphetamine can be used daily. Hyperactivity, disorganization, and euphoria are followed by exhaustion, depression, and coma lasting 2–3 days. Heavy users, taking more than 100 mg/d, have restlessness, incoordination of thought, insomnia, nervousness, irritability, and visual hallucinations. Psychosis may be precipitated by the chronic administration of high doses. Depression, weakness, tremors, GI complaints, and suicidal thoughts occur frequently.

▶ Treatment

The treatment of choice is diazepam, titrated in small increments to effect. Very large total doses may be needed. In cases of extreme agitation or hallucinations, droperidol (0.1 mg/kg per dose) or haloperidol (up to 0.1 mg/kg) parenterally has been used. When combinations of amphetamines and barbiturates (diet pills) are used, the action of the amphetamines begins first, followed by a depression caused by the barbiturates. In these cases, treatment with additional barbiturates is contraindicated because of the risk of respiratory failure.

Chronic users may be withdrawn rapidly from amphetamines. If amphetamine–barbiturate combination tablets have been used, the barbiturates must be withdrawn gradually to prevent withdrawal seizures. Psychiatric treatment should be provided.

Schwartz RH, Miller NS: MDMA (ecstasy) and the rave: A review. Pediatrics 1997;100:705 [PMID: 9310529].

ANESTHETICS, LOCAL

Intoxication from local anesthetics may be associated with CNS stimulation, acidosis, delirium, ataxia, shock, convulsions, and death. Methemoglobinuria has been reported following local dental analgesia. The maximum recommended dose for subcutaneous (SQ) infiltration is 4.5 mg/kg. The temptation to exceed this dose in procedures lasting a long time is great and may result in inadvertent overdosage. PO application of viscous lidocaine may produce toxicity. Hypercapnia may lower the seizure threshold to locally injected anesthetics.

Local anesthetics used in obstetrics cross the placental barrier and are not efficiently metabolized by the fetal liver. Mepivacaine, lidocaine, and bupivacaine can cause fetal bradycardia, neonatal depression, and death. Prilocaine causes methemoglobinemia, which should be treated if levels in the blood exceed 40% or if the patient is symptomatic.

Accidental injection of mepivacaine into the head of the fetus during paracervical anesthesia has caused neonatal asphyxia, cyanosis, acidosis, bradycardia, convulsions, and death.

▶ Treatment

If the anesthetic has been ingested, mucous membranes should be cleansed carefully and activated charcoal may be administered. Oxygen administration is indicated, with assisted ventilation if necessary. Methemoglobinemia is treated with methylene blue, 1%, 0.2 mL/kg (1– 2 mg/kg per dose, IV) over 5–10 minutes; this should promptly relieve the cyanosis. Acidosis may be treated with sodium bicarbonate, seizures with diazepam, and bradycardia with atropine. Therapeutic levels of mepivacaine, lidocaine, and procaine are less than 5 mg/mL.

Spiller HA et al: Multi-center retrospective evaluation of oral benzocaine exposure in children. Vet Hum Toxicol 2000;42:228 [PMID: 10928690].

ANTIHISTAMINES

Although antihistamines typically cause CNS depression, children often react paradoxically with excitement, hallucinations, delirium, ataxia, tremors, and convulsions followed by CNS depression, respiratory failure, or cardiovascular collapse. Anticholinergic effects such as dry mouth, fixed dilated pupils, flushed face, fever, and hallucinations may be prominent.

Antihistamines are widely available in allergy, sleep, cold, and antiemetic preparations, and many are supplied in sustained-release forms, which increase the likelihood of dangerous overdoses. They are absorbed rapidly and metabolized by the liver, lungs, and kidneys. A potentially toxic dose is 10–50 mg/kg of the most commonly used antihistamines, but toxic reactions have occurred at much lower doses.

▶ Treatment

Activated charcoal should be used to reduce drug absorption. Whole bowel irrigation may be useful for sustained-release preparations. Physostigmine (0.5–2.0 mg IV, slowly administered) dramatically reverses the central and peripheral anticholinergic effects of antihistamines, but it should be used only for diagnostic purposes. Diazepam (0.1–0.2 mg/kg IV) can be used to control seizures. Forced diuresis is not helpful. Exchange transfusion was reported to be effective in one case.

Ten Eick AP et al: Safety of antihistamines in children. Drug Saf 2001;24:119 [PMID: 11235817].

ARSENIC

Arsenic is used in some insecticides (fruit tree or tobacco sprays), rodenticides, weed killers, and wood preservatives. It is well absorbed primarily through the GI and respiratory tracts, but skin absorption may occur. Arsenic can be found in the urine, hair, and nails by laboratory testing.

Highly toxic soluble derivatives of this compound, such as sodium arsenite, are frequently found in liquid preparations and can cause death in as many as 65% of victims. The organic arsenates found in persistent or preemergence weed killers are relatively less soluble and less toxic. Poisonings with a liquid arsenical preparation that does not contain alkyl methanearsonate compounds should be considered potentially lethal. Patients exhibiting clinical signs other than gastroenteritis should receive treatment until laboratory tests indicate that treatment is no longer necessary.

▶ Clinical Findings

A. Acute Poisoning

Abdominal pain, vomiting, watery and bloody diarrhea, cardiovascular collapse, paresthesias, neck pain, and garlic odor on the breath occur as the first signs of acute poisoning. Convulsions, coma, anuria, and exfoliative dermatitis are later signs. Inhalation may cause pulmonary edema. Death is the result of cardiovascular collapse.

B. Chronic Poisoning

Anorexia, generalized weakness, giddiness, colic, abdominal pain, polyneuritis, dermatitis, nail changes, alopecia, and anemia often develop.

▶ Treatment

In acute poisoning administer activated charcoal. Then immediately give dimercaprol (commonly known as BAL), 3–5 mg/kg intramuscularly (IM), and follow with 2 mg/kg IM every 4 hours. The dimercaprol–arsenic complex is dialyzable. A second choice is succimer. The initial dose is 10 mg/kg every 8 hours for 5 days. A third choice is penicillamine, 100 mg/kg PO to a maximum of 1 g/d in four divided doses.

Chronic arsenic intoxication should be treated with succimer or penicillamine. Collect a 24-hour baseline urine specimen and then begin chelation. If the 24-hour urine arsenic level is greater than 50 mg, continue chelation for 5 days. After 10 days, repeat the 5-day cycle once or twice, depending on how soon the urine arsenic level falls below 50 mg/24 h.

Abernathy CO et al: Arsenic: Health effects, mechanisms of actions, and research issues. Environ Health Perspect 1999;107:593 [PMID: 10379007].

BARBITURATES

The toxic effects of barbiturates include confusion, poor coordination, coma, miotic or fixed dilated pupils, and respiratory depression. Respiratory acidosis is commonly associated with pulmonary atelectasis, and hypotension occurs frequently in severely poisoned patients. Ingestion of more than 6 mg/kg of long-acting or 3 mg/kg of short-acting barbiturates is usually toxic.

▶ Treatment

Activated charcoal should be administered. Careful, conservative management with emphasis on maintaining a clear airway, adequate ventilation, and control of hypotension is critical. Urinary alkalinization and the use of multiple-dose charcoal may decrease the elimination half-life of phenobarbital but have not been shown to alter the clinical course. Hemodialysis is not useful in the treatment of poisoning with short-acting barbiturates. Analeptics are contraindicated.

Cote CJ et al: Adverse sedation events in pediatrics: Analysis of medications used for sedation. Pediatrics 2000;4:633 [PMID: 11015502].

BELLADONNA ALKALOIDS (ATROPINE, JIMSONWEED, POTATO LEAVES, SCOPOLAMINE, STRAMONIUM)

The effects of anticholinergic compounds include dry mouth; thirst; decreased sweating with hot, dry, red skin; high fever; and tachycardia that may be preceded by bradycardia. The pupils are dilated, and vision is blurred. Speech and swallowing may be impaired. Hallucinations, delirium, and coma are common. Leukocytosis may occur, confusing the diagnosis.

Atropinism has been caused by normal doses of atropine or homatropine eye drops, especially in children with Down syndrome. Many common plants and over-the-counter medications contain belladonna alkaloids.

▶ Treatment

If the patient is awake and showing no signs or symptoms, administer activated charcoal. Gastric emptying is slowed by anticholinergics, so that gastric decontamination may be useful even if delayed. Physostigmine (0.5–2.0 mg IV, administered slowly) dramatically reverses the central and peripheral signs of atropinism but should be used only as a diagnostic agent. High fever must be controlled. Catheterization may be needed if the patient cannot void.

Burns MJ et al: A comparison of physostigmine and benzodiazepines for the treatment of anticholinergic poisoning. Ann Emerg Med 2000;35:374 [PMID: 10736125].

CARBON MONOXIDE

The degree of toxicity correlates well with the carboxyhemoglobin level taken soon after acute exposure but not after oxygen has been given or when there has been some time since exposure. Onset of symptoms may be more rapid and more severe if the patient lives at a high altitude, has a high respiratory rate (ie, infants), is pregnant, or has myocardial insufficiency or lung disease. Normal blood may contain up to 5% carboxyhemoglobin (10% in smokers).

The most prominent early symptom is headache. Other effects include confusion, unsteadiness, and coma. Proteinuria, glycosuria, elevated serum aminotransferase levels, or ECG changes may be present in the acute phase. Permanent cardiac, liver, renal, or CNS damage occurs occasionally. The outcome of severe poisoning may be complete recovery, vegetative state, or any degree of mental injury between these extremes. The primary mental deficits are neuropsychiatric.

▶ Treatment

The biologic half-life of carbon monoxide on room air is approximately 200–300 minutes; on 100% oxygen, it is 60–90 minutes. Hyperbaric oxygen therapy at 2.0–2.5 atm of oxygen shortens the half-life to 30 minutes. After the level has been reduced to near zero, therapy is aimed at the nonspecific sequelae of anoxia. Dexamethasone (0.1 mg/kg IV or IM every 4–6 hours) should be added if cerebral edema develops.

Chou KJ: Characteristics and outcome of children with carbon monoxide poisoning with and without smoke exposure referred for hyperbaric oxygen therapy. Pediatr Emerg Care 2000;3:151 [PMID: 10888449].

CAUSTICS

1. Acids (Hydrochloric, Hydrofluoric, Nitric, & Sulfuric Acids; Sodium Bisulfate)

Strong acids are commonly found in metal and toilet bowl cleaners, batteries, and other products. Hydrofluoric acid is the most toxic and hydrochloric acid the least toxic of these household substances. However, even a few drops can be fatal if aspirated into the trachea.

Painful swallowing, mucous membrane burns, bloody emesis, abdominal pain, respiratory distress due to edema of the epiglottis, thirst, shock, and renal failure can occur. Coma and convulsions sometimes are seen terminally. Residual lesions include esophageal, gastric, and pyloric strictures as well as scars of the cornea, skin, and oropharynx.

Hydrofluoric acid is a particularly dangerous poison. Dermal exposure creates a penetrating burn that can progress for hours or days. Large dermal exposure or ingestion may produce life-threatening hypocalcemia abruptly as well as burn reactions.

▶ Treatment

Emetics and lavage are contraindicated. Water or milk (< 15 mL/kg) is used to dilute the acid, because a heat-producing chemical reaction does not occur. Take care not to induce emesis by excessive fluid administration. Alkalies should not be used. Burned areas of the skin, mucous membranes, or eyes should be washed with copious amounts of warm water. Opioids for pain may be needed. An endotracheal tube may be required to alleviate laryngeal edema. Esophagoscopy should be performed if the patient has significant burns or difficulty in swallowing. Acids are likely to produce gastric burns or esophageal burns. Evidence is not conclusive, but corticosteroids have not proved to be of use.

Hydrofluoric acid burns on skin are treated with 10% calcium gluconate gel or calcium gluconate infusion. Severe exposure may require large doses of IV calcium. Therapy should be guided by calcium levels, the ECG, and clinical signs.

2. Bases (Clinitest Tablets, Clorox, Drano, Liquid-Plumr, Purex, Sani-Clor—Examine the Label or Call a Poison Center to Determine Contents)

Alkalies produce more severe injuries than acids. Some substances, such as Clinitest tablets or Drano, are quite toxic, whereas the chlorinated bleaches (3–6% solutions of sodium hypochlorite) are usually not toxic. When sodium hypochlorite comes in contact with acid in the stomach, hypochlorous acid, which is very irritating to the mucous membranes and skin, is formed. Rapid inactivation of this substance prevents systemic toxicity. Chlorinated bleaches, when mixed with a strong acid (toilet bowl cleaners) or ammonia, may produce irritating chlorine or chloramine gas, which can cause serious lung injury if inhaled in a closed space (eg, bathroom).

Alkalies can burn the skin, mucous membranes, and eyes. Respiratory distress may be due to edema of the epiglottis, pulmonary edema resulting from inhalation of fumes, or pneumonia. Mediastinitis or other intercurrent infections or shock can occur. Perforation of the esophagus or stomach is rare.

▶ Treatment

The skin and mucous membranes should be cleansed with copious amounts of water. A local anesthetic can be instilled in the eye if necessary to alleviate blepharospasm. The eye should be irrigated for at least 20–30 minutes. Ophthalmologic consultation should be obtained for all alkaline eye burns.

Ingestions should be treated with water as a diluent. Routine esophagoscopy is no longer indicated to rule out burns of the esophagus due to chlorinated bleaches unless an unusually large amount has been ingested or the patient is symptomatic. The absence of oral lesions does not rule out the possibility of laryngeal or esophageal burns following granular alkali ingestion. The use of corticosteroids is controversial, but has not been shown to improve long-term outcome except possibly in partial-thickness esophageal burns. Antibiotics may be needed if mediastinitis is likely, but they should not be used prophylactically. (See Caustic Burns of the Esophagus section in Chapter 20.)

Hamza AF et al: Caustic esophageal strictures in children: 30 years' experience. J Pediatr Surg 2003;338:828 [PMID: 12778375].

Lovejoy FH Jr: Corrosive injury of the esophagus in children: Failure of corticosteroid treatment reemphasizes prevention. N Engl J Med 1990;323:668 [PMID: 2385270].

Tiryaki T et al: Early bougienage for relief of stricture formation following caustic esophageal burns. Pediatr Surg Intl 2005;21:78 [PMID: 15619090].

COCAINE

Cocaine is absorbed intranasally or via inhalation or ingestion. Effects are noted almost immediately when the drug is taken intravenously or smoked. Peak effects are delayed for about an hour when the drug is taken orally or nasally. Cocaine prevents the reuptake of endogenous catecholamines, thereby causing an initial sympathetic discharge, followed by catechol depletion after chronic abuse.

▶ Clinical Findings

A local anesthetic and vasoconstrictor, cocaine is also a potent stimulant to both the CNS and the cardiovascular system. The initial tachycardia, hyperpnea, hypertension, and stimulation of the CNS are often followed by coma, seizures, hypotension, and respiratory depression. In severe cases of overdose, various dysrhythmias may be seen, including sinus tachycardia, atrial arrhythmias, premature ventricular contractions, bigeminy, and ventricular fibrillation. If large doses are taken intravenously, cardiac failure, dysrhythmias, rhabdomyolysis, or hyperthermia may result in death.

In addition to those poisoned through recreational use of cocaine, others are at risk of overdose. A "body stuffer" is one who quickly ingests the drug, usually poorly wrapped, to avoid discovery. A "body packer" wraps the drug carefully for prolonged transport. A stuffer typically manifests toxicity within hours of ingestion; a packer is asymptomatic unless the package ruptures, usually days later.

▶ Treatment

Except in cases of body stuffers or body packers, decontamination is seldom possible. Activated charcoal should be administered, and whole bowel irrigation may be useful in selected cases. Testing for cocaine in blood or plasma is generally not clinically useful, but a qualitative analysis of the urine may aid in confirming the diagnosis. For severe cases, an ECG is indicated. In suspected cases of body packing, radiographs of the GI tract may show multiple packets. Radiographic films are usually not helpful for identifying stuffers. Seizures are treated with IV diazepam titrated to response. Hypotension is treated with standard agents.

Because cocaine abuse may deplete norepinephrine, an indirect agent such as dopamine may be less effective than a direct agent such as norepinephrine. Agitation is best treated with a benzodiazepine.

Delaney-Black V: Prenatal cocaine exposure as a risk factor for later developmental outcomes. JAMA 2001;286:46 [PMID: 11434823].

Qureshi AI et al: Cocaine use and the likelihood of nonfatal myocardial infarction and stroke: Data from the Third National Health and Nutrition Examination Survey. Circulation 2001;103:502 [PMID: 11157713].

CONTRACEPTIVE PILLS

The only known toxic effects following acute ingestion of oral contraceptive agents are nausea, vomiting, and vaginal bleeding in girls.

COSMETICS & RELATED PRODUCTS

The relative toxicities of commonly ingested products in this group are listed in Table 12–5. Permanent wave neutralizers may contain bromates, peroxides, or perborates. Bromates have been removed from most products because they can cause nausea, vomiting, abdominal pain, shock, hemolysis, renal failure, and convulsions.

Perborates can cause boric acid poisoning. Four grams of bromate salts is potentially lethal.

Poisoning is treated by gastric lavage with 1% sodium thiosulfate. Sodium bicarbonate, 2%, in the lavage fluid may reduce hydrobromic acid formation. Sodium thiosulfate, 25%, 1.65 mL/kg, can be given intravenously, but methylene blue should not be used to treat methemoglobinemia in this situation because it increases the toxicity of bromates. Dialysis is indicated in renal failure but does not enhance excretion of bromate.

Table 12–5. Relative toxicities of cosmetics and similar products.

High toxicity	Low toxicity
Permanent wave neutralizers	Perfume
Moderate toxicity	Hair removers
Fingernail polish	Deodorants
Fingernail polish remover	Bath salts
Metallic hair dyes	**No toxicity**
Home permanent wave lotion	Liquid makeup
Bath oil	Vegetable hair dye
Shaving lotion	Cleansing cream
Hair tonic (alcoholic)	Hair dressing (nonalcoholic)
Cologne, toilet water	Hand lotion or cream
	Lipstick

Fingernail polish removers used to contain toluene but now usually have an acetone base, which does not require specific treatment other than monitoring CNS status.

Cobalt, copper, cadmium, iron, lead, nickel, silver, bismuth, and tin are sometimes found in metallic hair dyes. In large amounts they can cause skin sensitization, urticaria, dermatitis, eye damage, vertigo, hypertension, asthma, methemoglobinemia, tremors, convulsions, and coma. Treatment for ingestions is to administer demulcents and, only with large amounts, the appropriate antidote for the heavy metal involved.

Home permanent wave lotions, hair straighteners, and hair removers usually contain thioglycolic acid salts, which cause alkaline irritation and perhaps CNS depression.

Shaving lotion, hair tonic, hair straighteners, cologne, and toilet water contain denatured alcohol, which can cause CNS depression and hypoglycemia.

Deodorants usually consist of an antibacterial agent in a cream base. Antiperspirants are aluminum salts, which frequently cause skin sensitization. Zirconium oxide can cause granulomas in the axilla with chronic use.

CYCLIC ANTIDEPRESSANTS

Cyclic antidepressants (eg, amitriptyline, imipramine) have a very low ratio of toxic to therapeutic doses, and even a moderate overdose can have serious effects.

Cyclic antidepressant overdosage causes dysrhythmias, coma, convulsions, hypertension followed by hypotension, and hallucinations. These effects may be life-threatening and require rapid intervention. One agent, amoxapine, differs in that it causes fewer cardiovascular complications, but it is associated with a higher incidence of seizures.

▶ Treatment

Decontamination should include administration of activated charcoal unless the patient is symptomatic.

An ECG should be obtained in all patients. A QRS interval greater than 100 ms specifically identifies patients at risk to develop dysrhythmias. If dysrhythmias are demonstrated, the patient should be admitted and monitored until free of irregularity for 24 hours. Another indication for monitoring is persistent tachycardia of more than 110 beats/min. The onset of dysrhythmias is rare beyond 24 hours after ingestion.

Alkalinization with sodium bicarbonate (0.5–1.0 mEq/kg IV) or hyperventilation may dramatically reverse ventricular dysrhythmias and narrow the QRS interval. Lidocaine may be added for treatment of arrhythmias. Bolus administration of sodium bicarbonate is recommended for all patients with QRS widening to above 120 ms and for those with significant dysrhythmias, to achieve a pH of 7.5–7.6. Forced diuresis is contraindicated. A benzodiazepine should be given for convulsions.

Hypotension is a major problem. Cyclic antidepressants block the reuptake of catecholamines, thereby producing initial hypertension followed by hypotension. Treatment with physostigmine is contraindicated. Vasopressors are generally effective. Dopamine is the agent of choice because it is readily available. If dopamine is ineffective, norepinephrine (0.1–1 µg/kg/min, titrated to response) should be added. Diuresis and hemodialysis are not effective.

Kerr GW et al: Tricyclic antidepressant overdose: A review. Emerg Med J 2001;18:236 [PMID: 11435353].

DIGITALIS & OTHER CARDIAC GLYCOSIDES

Toxicity is typically the result of incorrect dosing or unrecognized renal insufficiency. Clinical features include nausea, vomiting, diarrhea, headache, delirium, confusion, and, occasionally, coma. Cardiac dysrhythmias typically involve bradydysrhythmias, but every type of dysrhythmia has been reported in digitalis intoxication, including atrial fibrillation, paroxysmal atrial tachycardia, and atrial flutter. Death usually is the result of ventricular fibrillation. Transplacental intoxication by digitalis has been reported.

▶ Treatment

Administer activated charcoal. Potassium is contraindicated in acute overdosage unless there is laboratory evidence of hypokalemia. In acute overdosage, hyperkalemia is more common. Hypokalemia is common in chronic toxicity.

The patient must be monitored carefully for ECG changes. The correction of acidosis better demonstrates the degree of potassium deficiency present. Bradycardias have been treated with atropine. Phenytoin, lidocaine, magnesium salts (not in renal failure), amiodarone, and bretylium have been used to correct arrhythmias.

Definitive treatment is with digoxin immune Fab (ovine) (Digibind). Indications for its use include hypotension or any dysrhythmia, typically ventricular dysrhythmias and progressive bradydysrhythmias that produce clinical concern. Elevated T waves indicate high potassium and may be an indication for digoxin immune Fab (Digibind, DigiFab) use. Techniques of determining dosage and indications related to levels, when available are described in product literature.

Woolf AD et al: The use of digoxin-specific Fab fragments for severe digitalis intoxication in children. N Engl J Med 1992;326:1739 [PMID: 1997016].

DIPHENOXYLATE WITH ATROPINE (LOMOTIL) & LOPERAMIDE (IMODIUM)

Loperamide (Imodium) has largely replaced Lomotil and does not produce significant toxicity. Ingestions of up to 0.4 mg/kg can safely be managed at home.

Lomotil contains diphenoxylate hydrochloride, a synthetic narcotic, and atropine sulfate. Small amounts are potentially lethal in children; it is contraindicated in children younger than age 2 years. Early signs of intoxication with this preparation result from its anticholinergic effect and consist of fever, facial flushing, tachypnea, and lethargy. However, the miotic effect of the narcotic predominates. Later, hypothermia, increasing CNS depression, and loss of the facial flush occur. Seizures are probably secondary to hypoxia.

► Treatment

Prolonged monitoring (24 hours) with pulse oximetry and careful attention to airway is sufficient in most cases.

Naloxone hydrochloride (0.4–2.0 mg IV in children and adults) should be given. Repeated doses may be required because the duration of action of diphenoxylate is considerably longer than that of naloxone.

McCarron MM et al: Diphenoxylate-atropine (Lomotil) overdose in children: An update. Pediatrics 1991;87:694 [PMID: 2020516].

DISINFECTANTS & DEODORIZERS

1. Naphthalene

Naphthalene is commonly found in mothballs, disinfectants, and deodorizers. Naphthalene's toxicity is often not fully appreciated. It is absorbed not only when ingested but also through the skin and lungs. It is potentially hazardous to store baby clothes in naphthalene, because baby oil is an excellent solvent that may increase dermal absorption. **Note:** Most mothballs contain *para*-dichlorobenzene and not naphthalene (see next section). Metabolic products of naphthalene may cause severe hemolytic anemia, similar to that due to primaquine toxicity, 2–7 days after ingestion. Other physical findings include vomiting, diarrhea, jaundice, oliguria, anuria, coma, and convulsions. The urine may contain hemoglobin, protein, and casts.

► Treatment

Administer activated charcoal. Urinary alkalinization may prevent blocking of the renal tubules by acid hematin crystals. Anuria may persist for 1–2 weeks and still be completely reversible.

Siegel E, Wason S: Mothball toxicity. Pediatr Clin North Am 1986;33:369 [PMID: 3515301].

2. *P*-Dichlorobenzene, Phenolic Acids, & Others

Disinfectants and deodorizers containing *p*-dichlorobenzene or sodium sulfate are much less toxic than those containing naphthalene. Disinfectants containing phenolic acids are highly toxic, especially if they contain a borate ion. Phenol precipitates tissue proteins and causes respiratory alkalosis followed by metabolic acidosis. Some phenols cause methemoglobinemia.

Local gangrene occurs after prolonged contact with tissue. Phenol is readily absorbed from the GI tract, causing diffuse capillary damage and, in some cases, methemoglobinemia. Pentachlorophenol, which has been used in terminal rinsing of diapers, has caused infant fatalities.

The toxicity of alkalies, quaternary ammonium compounds, pine oil, and halogenated disinfectants varies with the concentration of active ingredients. Wick deodorizers are usually of moderate toxicity. Iodophor disinfectants are the safest. Spray deodorizers are not usually toxic, because a child is not likely to swallow a very large dose.

Signs and symptoms of acute quaternary ammonium compound ingestion include diaphoresis, strong irritation, thirst, vomiting, diarrhea, cyanosis, hyperactivity, coma, convulsions, hypotension, abdominal pain, and pulmonary edema. Acute liver or renal failure may develop later.

► Treatment

Activated charcoal may be used. Castor oil dissolves phenol and may retard its absorption. This property of castor oil, however, has not been proved clinically. Mineral oil and alcohol are contraindicated because they increase the gastric absorption of phenol. The metabolic acidosis must be managed carefully. Anticonvulsants or measures to treat shock may be needed.

Because phenols are absorbed through the skin, exposed areas should be irrigated copiously with water. Undiluted polyethylene glycol may be a useful solvent as well.

Van Berkel M, de Wolff FA: Survival after acute benzalkonium chloride poisoning. Hum Toxicol 1988;7:191 [PMID: 3378808].

DISK-SHAPED BATTERIES

Small, flat, smooth disk-shaped batteries measure between 10 and 25 mm in diameter. About 69% of them pass through the GI tract in 48 hours and 85% in 72 hours. Some may become entrapped. These batteries contain caustic materials and heavy metals.

Batteries impacted in the esophagus may cause symptoms of refusal to take food, increased salivation, vomiting with or without blood, and pain or discomfort. Aspiration into the trachea may also occur. Fatalities have been reported in association with esophageal perforation.

When a history of disk battery ingestion is obtained, radiographs of the entire respiratory tract and GI tract should be taken so that the battery can be located and the proper therapy determined.

► Treatment

If the disk battery is located in the esophagus, it must be removed immediately. If the battery has been in the esophagus for more than 24 hours, the risk of caustic burn is greater.

Location of the disk battery below the esophagus has been associated with tissue damage, but the course is benign in most cases. Perforated Meckel diverticulum has been the major complication. It may take as long as 7 days for spontaneous passage to occur, and lack of movement in the GI tract may not require removal in an asymptomatic patient.

Some researchers have suggested repeated radiographs and surgical intervention if passage of the battery pauses, but this approach may be excessive. Batteries that have opened in the GI tract have been associated with some toxicity due to mercury, but the patients have recovered.

Emesis is ineffective. Asymptomatic patients may simply be observed and stools examined for passage of the battery. If the battery has not passed within 7 days or if the patient becomes symptomatic, radiographs should be repeated. If the battery has come apart or appears not to be moving, a purgative, enema, or nonabsorbable intestinal lavage solution should be administered. If these methods are unsuccessful, surgical intervention may be required. Levels of heavy metals (mainly mercury) should be measured in patients in whom the battery has opened or symptoms have developed.

Dane S: A truly emergent problem: Button battery in the nose. Acad Emerg Med 2000;7:204 [PMID: 10691084].

Litovitz TL, Schmitz BF: Ingestion of cylindrical and button batteries: An analysis of 2382 cases. Pediatrics 1992;89:747 [PMID: 2304794].

ETHYLENE GLYCOL & METHANOL

Ethylene glycol and methanol are the toxic alcohols. The primary source of ethylene glycol is antifreeze, whereas methanol is present in windshield wiper fluid and also as an ethanol denaturant. Ethylene glycol causes severe metabolic acidosis and renal failure. Methanol causes metabolic acidosis and blindness. Onset of symptoms with both agents occurs within several hours after ingestion, longer if ethanol was ingested simultaneously.

▶ Treatment

The primary treatment is to block the enzyme alcohol dehydrogenase, which converts both agents to their toxic metabolites. This is accomplished with fomepizole (loading dose of 15 mg/kg) or ethanol. Fomepizole is preferred for children, due to its reduced side effects in this age group.

Barceloux DG et al: American Academy of Clinical Toxicology Practice Guidelines on the Treatment of Methanol Poisoning. J Toxicol Clin Toxicol 2002;40:415 [PMID: 12216995].

Brent J et al: Fomepizole for the treatment of ethylene glycol poisoning: Methylpyrazole for toxic alcohols study group. N Engl J Med 1999;40:832 [PMID: 10080845].

GAMMA-HYDROXYBUTYRATE, GAMMA-BUTYROLACTONE, & BUTANEDIOL

Gamma-hydroxybutyrate (GHB), γ-butyrolactone (GBL), and butanediol have become popular drugs of abuse in adolescents and adults. GHB is a CNS depressant that is structurally similar to the inhibitory neurotransmitter γ-aminobutyric acid. GBL and butanediol are converted in the body to GHB. These drugs cause deep but short-lived coma; the coma often lasts only 1–4 hours. Treatment consists of supportive care with close attention to airway and endotracheal intubation if respiratory depression or decreased gag reflex complicates the poisoning. Atropine has been used successfully for symptomatic bradycardia.

Withdrawal from GHB, GBL, or butanediol can cause several days of extreme agitation, hallucination, or tachycardia. Treatment with high doses of benzodiazepines or with butyrophenones (eg, haloperidol or droperidol) or secobarbital may be needed for several days.

Dyer JE et al: Gamma-hydroxybutyrate withdrawal syndrome. Ann Emerg Med 2001;37:147 [PMID: 11174231].

Sporer KA et al: Gamma-hydroxybutyrate serum levels and clinical syndrome after severe overdose. Ann Emerg Med 2003;42:3 [PMID: 12827115].

HYDROCARBONS (BENZENE, CHARCOAL LIGHTER FLUID, GASOLINE, KEROSENE, PETROLEUM DISTILLATES, TURPENTINE)

Ingestion of hydrocarbons may cause irritation of mucous membranes, vomiting, blood-tinged diarrhea, respiratory distress, cyanosis, tachycardia, and fever. Although a small amount (10 mL) of certain hydrocarbons is potentially fatal, patients have survived ingestion of several ounces of other petroleum distillates. The more aromatic a hydrocarbon is and the lower its viscosity rating, the more potentially toxic it is. Benzene, gasoline, kerosene, and red seal oil furniture polish are the most dangerous. A dose exceeding 1 mL/kg is likely to cause CNS depression. A history of coughing or choking, as well as vomiting, suggests aspiration with resulting hydrocarbon pneumonia. This is an acute hemorrhagic necrotizing disease that usually develops within 24 hours of the ingestion and resolves without sequelae in 3–5 days. However, several weeks may be required for full resolution of hydrocarbon pneumonia. Pneumonia may be caused by the aspiration of a few drops of petroleum distillate into the lung or by absorption from the circulatory system. Pulmonary edema and hemorrhage, cardiac dilation and dysrhythmias, hepatosplenomegaly, proteinuria, and hematuria can occur following large overdoses. Hypoglycemia is occasionally present. A chest radiograph may reveal pneumonia within hours after the ingestion. An abnormal urinalysis in a child with a previously normal urinary tract suggests a large overdose.

▶ Treatment

Both emetics and lavage should be avoided. Mineral oil should not be given, because it can cause a low-grade lipoid pneumonia.

Epinephrine should not be used with halogenated hydrocarbons because it may affect an already sensitized myocardium. The usefulness of corticosteroids is debated, and antibiotics should be reserved for patients with infections. Oxygen and mist are helpful. Extracorporeal membrane oxygenation has been successful in at least two cases of failure with standard therapy.

Lifshitz M et al: Hydrocarbon poisoning in children: A 5-year retrospective study. Wilderness Environ Med 2003;14:78 [PMID: 12825880].
Lorenc JD: Inhalant abuse in the pediatric populations: A persistent challenge. Curr Opin Pediatr 2003;15:204 [PMID: 12640280].

IBUPROFEN

Most exposures in children do not produce symptoms. In one study, for example, children ingesting up to 2.4 g remained asymptomatic. When symptoms occur, the most common are abdominal pain, vomiting, drowsiness, and lethargy. In rare cases, apnea (especially in young children), seizures, metabolic acidosis, and CNS depression leading to coma have occurred.

▶ **Treatment**

If a child has ingested less than 100 mg/kg, dilution with water or milk may be all that is necessary to minimize the GI upset. In children, the volume of liquid used for dilution should be less than 4 oz. When the ingested amount is more than 400 mg/kg, seizures or CNS depression may occur; therefore, gastric lavage may be preferred to emesis. Activated charcoal may also be of value. There is no specific antidote. Neither alkalinization of the urine nor hemodialysis is helpful.

Cuzzolin L et al: NSAID-induced nephrotoxicity from the fetus to the child. Drug Safety 2001;242:9 [PMID: 11219488].
Oker EE et al: Serious toxicity in a young child due to ibuprofen. Acad Emerg Med 2000;7:821 [PMID: 10917334].

INSECT STINGS (BEE, WASP, & HORNET)

Insect stings are painful but not usually dangerous; however, death from anaphylaxis may occur. Bee venom has hemolytic, neurotoxic, and histamine-like activities that can on rare occasion cause hemoglobinuria and severe anaphylactoid reactions. Massive envenomation from numerous stings may cause hemolysis, rhabdomyolysis, and shock leading to multiple organ failure.

▶ **Treatment**

The physician should remove the stinger, taking care not to squeeze the attached venom sac. For allergic reactions, epinephrine 1:1000 solution, 0.01 mL/kg, should be administered IV or SQ above the site of the sting. Three to four whiffs from an isoproterenol aerosol inhaler may be given at 3- to 4-minute intervals as needed. Corticosteroids (hydrocortisone; 100 mg IV) and diphenhydramine (1.5 mg/kg IV) are useful ancillary drugs but have no immediate effect. Ephedrine or antihistamines may be used for 2 or 3 days to prevent recurrence of symptoms.

A patient who has had a potentially life-threatening insect sting should be desensitized against the Hymenoptera group, because the honey bee, wasp, hornet, and yellow jacket have common antigens in their venom. For the more usual stings, cold compresses, aspirin, and diphenhydramine (1 mg/kg PO) are sufficient.

Ross RN et al: Effectiveness of specific immunotherapy in the treatment of hymenoptera venom hypersensitivity: A meta-analysis. Clin Ther 2000;22:351 [PMID: 10963289].
Vetter RS et al: Mass envenomations by honey bees and wasps. West J Med 1999;170:223 [PMID: 10344177].

INSECTICIDES

The petroleum distillates or other organic solvents used in these products are often as toxic as the insecticide itself. Decontamination may be performed by aspirating the stomach with a nasogastric tube.

1. Chlorinated Hydrocarbons (eg, Aldrin, Carbinol, Chlordane, DDT, Dieldrin, Endrin, Heptachlor, Lindane, Toxaphene)

Signs of intoxication include salivation, GI irritability, abdominal pain, vomiting, diarrhea, CNS depression, and convulsions. Inhalation exposure causes irritation of the eyes, nose, and throat; blurred vision; cough; and pulmonary edema.

Chlorinated hydrocarbons are absorbed through the skin, respiratory tract, and GI tract. Decontamination of skin with soap and evacuation of the stomach contents are critical. All contaminated clothing should be removed. Castor oil, milk, and other substances containing fats or oils should not be left in the stomach because they increase absorption of the chlorinated hydrocarbons. Convulsions should be treated with diazepam (0.1–0.3 mg/kg IV). Epinephrine should not be used because it may cause cardiac arrhythmias.

2. Organophosphate (Cholinesterase-Inhibiting) Insecticides (eg, Chlorothion, Co-Ral, DFP, Diazinon, Malathion, Paraoxon, Parathion, Phosdrin, TEPP, Thio-TEPP)

Dizziness, headache, blurred vision, miosis, tearing, salivation, nausea, vomiting, diarrhea, hyperglycemia, cyanosis, sense of constriction of the chest, dyspnea, sweating, weakness, muscular twitching, convulsions, loss of reflexes and sphincter control, and coma can occur.

The clinical findings are the result of cholinesterase inhibition, which causes an accumulation of acetylcholine.

The onset of symptoms occurs within 12 hours of the exposure. Red cell cholinesterase levels should be measured as soon as possible. (Some normal individuals have a low serum cholinesterase level.) Normal values vary in different laboratories. In general, a decrease of red cell cholinesterase to below 25% of normal indicates significant exposure.

Repeated low-grade exposure may result in sudden, acute toxic reactions. This syndrome usually occurs after repeated household spraying rather than agricultural exposure.

Although all organophosphates act by inhibiting cholinesterase activity, they vary greatly in their toxicity. Parathion, for example, is 100 times more toxic than Malathion. Toxicity is influenced by the specific compound, type of formulation (liquid or solid), vehicle, and route of absorption (lungs, skin, or GI tract).

▶ Treatment

Decontamination of skin, nails, hair, and clothing with soapy water is extremely important. Atropine plus a cholinesterase reactivator, pralidoxime, is an antidote for organophosphate insecticide poisoning. After assessment and management of the ABCs, atropine should be given and repeated every few minutes until airway secretions diminish. An appropriate starting dose of atropine is 2–4 mg IV in an adult and 0.05 mg/kg in a child. The patient should receive enough atropine to stop secretions (mydriasis in not an appropriate stopping point). Severe poisoning may require gram quantities of atropine administered over 24 hours.

Because atropine antagonizes the muscarinic parasympathetic effects of the organophosphates but does not affect the nicotinic receptor, it does not improve muscular weakness. Pralidoxime should also be given immediately in more severe cases and repeated every 6–12 hours as needed (25–50 mg/kg diluted to 5% and infused over 5–30 minutes at a rate of no more than 500 mg/min). Pralidoxime should be used in addition to—not in place of—atropine if red cell cholinesterase is less than 25% of normal. Pralidoxime is most useful within 48 hours after the exposure but has shown some effects 2–6 days later. Morphine, theophylline, aminophylline, succinylcholine, and tranquilizers of the reserpine and phenothiazine types are contraindicated. Hyperglycemia is common in severe poisonings.

Eisenstein EM, Amitai Y: Index of suspicion: Case 1. Organophosphate intoxication. Pediatr Rev 2000;21:205 [PMID: 10854316].

3. Carbamates (eg, Carbaryl, Sevin, Zectran)

Carbamate insecticides are reversible inhibitors of cholinesterase. The signs and symptoms of intoxication are similar to those associated with organophosphate poisoning but are generally less severe. Atropine titrated to effect is sufficient treatment. Pralidoxime should not be used with carbaryl poisoning but is of value with other carbamates. In combined exposures to organophosphates, give atropine but

reserve pralidoxime for cases in which the red cell cholinesterase is depressed below 25% of normal or marked effects of nicotinic receptor stimulation are present.

4. Botanical Insecticides (eg, Black Flag Bug Killer, Black Leaf CPR Insect Killer, Flit Aerosol House & Garden Insect Killer, French's Flea Powder, Raid)

Allergic reactions, asthma-like symptoms, coma, and convulsions have been reported. Pyrethrins, allethrin, and rotenone do not commonly cause signs of toxicity. Antihistamines, short-acting barbiturates, and atropine are helpful as symptomatic treatment.

IRON

Five stages of intoxication may occur in iron poisoning: (1) Hemorrhagic gastroenteritis, which occurs 30–60 minutes after ingestion and may be associated with shock, acidosis, coagulation defects, and coma. This phase usually lasts 4–6 hours. (2) Phase of improvement, lasting 2–12 hours, during which patient looks better. (3) Delayed shock, which may occur 12–48 hours after ingestion. Metabolic acidosis, fever, leukocytosis, and coma may also be present. (4) Liver damage with hepatic failure. (5) Residual pyloric stenosis, which may develop about 4 weeks after the ingestion.

Once iron is absorbed from the GI tract, it is not normally eliminated in feces but may be partially excreted in the urine, giving it a red color prior to chelation. A reddish discoloration of the urine suggests a serum iron level greater than 350 mg/dL.

▶ Treatment

GI decontamination is based on clinical assessment. The patient should be referred to a health care facility if symptomatic or if the history indicates toxic amounts. Gastric lavage and whole bowel irrigation should be considered in these patients.

Shock is treated in the usual manner. Sodium bicarbonate and Fleet Phospho-Soda left in the stomach to form the insoluble phosphate or carbonate have not shown clinical benefit and have caused lethal hypernatremia or hyperphosphatemia. Deferoxamine, a specific chelating agent for iron, is a useful adjunct in the treatment of severe iron poisoning. It forms a soluble complex that is excreted in the urine. It is contraindicated in patients with renal failure unless dialysis can be used. IV deferoxamine chelation therapy should be instituted if the patient is symptomatic and a serum iron determination cannot be obtained readily, or if the peak serum iron exceeds 400 mcg/dL (62.6 µmol/L) at 4–5 hours after ingestion.

Deferoxamine should not be delayed until serum iron levels are available in serious cases of poisoning. IV administration is indicated if the patient is in shock, in which case it should be given at a dosage of 15 mg/kg/h. Infusion rates up to 35 mg/kg/h have been used in life-threatening poisonings. Rapid IV administration can cause hypotension, facial flushing, urticaria, tachycardia, and shock. Deferoxamine, 90 mg/kg IM every 8 hours (maximum, 1 g), may be given if IV access cannot be established, but the procedure is painful. The indications for discontinuation of deferoxamine have not been clearly delineated. Generally, it can be stopped after 12–24 hours if the acidosis has resolved and the patient is improving.

Hemodialysis, peritoneal dialysis, or exchange transfusion can be used to increase the excretion of the dialyzable complex. Urine output should be monitored and urine sediment examined for evidence of renal tubular damage. Initial laboratory studies should include blood typing and cross-matching; total protein; serum iron, sodium, potassium, and chloride; P_{CO_2}; pH; and liver function tests. Serum iron levels fall rapidly even if deferoxamine is not given.

After the acute episode, liver function studies and an upper GI series are indicated to rule out residual damage.

Black J et al: Child abuse by intentional iron poisoning presenting as shock and persistent acidosis. Pediatrics 2003;111:197 [PMID: 12509576].

Juurlink DN et al: Iron poisoning in young children: Association with the birth of a sibling. CMAJ 2003;165:1539 [PMID: 12796332].

LEAD

Lead poisoning (plumbism) causes vague symptoms, including weakness, irritability, weight loss, vomiting, personality changes, ataxia, constipation, headache, and colicky abdominal pain. Late manifestations consist of retarded development, convulsions, and coma associated with increased intracranial pressure, which is a medical emergency.

Plumbism usually occurs insidiously in children younger than age 5 years. The most likely sources of lead include flaking leaded paint, artist's paints, fruit tree sprays, solder, brass alloys, home-glazed pottery, and fumes from burning batteries. Only paint containing less than 1% lead is safe for interior use (eg, furniture, toys). Repetitive ingestions of small amounts of lead are far more serious than a single massive exposure. Toxic effects are likely to occur if more than 0.5 mg of lead per day is absorbed.

Blood lead levels are used to assess the severity of exposure. A complete blood count and serum ferritin concentration should be obtained; iron-deficiency increases absorption of lead. Glycosuria, proteinuria, hematuria, and aminoaciduria occur frequently. Blood lead levels usually exceed 80 mcg/dL in symptomatic patients. Abnormal blood lead levels should be repeated in asymptomatic patients to rule out laboratory error. Specimens must be meticulously obtained in acid-washed containers. A normocytic, slightly hypochromic anemia with basophilic stippling of the red cells and reticulocytosis may be present in plumbism. Stippling of red blood cells is absent in cases involving only recent ingestion.

The cerebrospinal fluid (CSF) protein is elevated, and the white cell count usually is less than 100 cells/mL. CSF pressure may be elevated in patients with encephalopathy; lumbar punctures must be performed cautiously to prevent herniation.

▶ Treatment

Succimer is an orally administered chelator approved for use in children and reported to be as efficacious as calcium edetate. Treatment for blood lead levels of 20–45 mcg/dL in children has not been determined. Succimer should be initiated at blood lead levels over 45 mcg/dL. The initial dose is 10 mg/kg (350 mg/m²) every 8 hours for 5 days. The same dose is then given every 12 hours for 14 days. At least 2 weeks should elapse between courses. Blood lead levels increase somewhat (ie, rebound) after discontinuation of therapy. Courses of dimercaprol (4 mg/kg per dose) and calcium edetate may still be used but are no longer the preferred method, except in cases of lead encephalopathy.

Anticonvulsants may be needed. Mannitol or corticosteroids and volume restriction are indicated in patients with encephalopathy. A high-calcium, high-phosphorus diet and large doses of vitamin D may remove lead from the blood by depositing it in the bones. A public health team should evaluate the source of the lead. Necessary corrections should be completed before the child is returned home.

Markowitz M: Lead poisoning. Pediatr Rev 2000;21:327 [PMID: 11010979].

Rogan WJ et al: Treatment of Lead-Exposed Children Trial Group: The effect of chelation therapy with succimer on neuropsychological development in children exposed to lead. N Engl J Med 2001;344:1421 [PMID: 11346806].

MAGNETS

Although not strictly toxic, small magnets have been found to cause bowel obstructions in children. Recent cases have resulted in warnings and a recall by the Consumer Product Safety Commission following intestinal perforation and death in a 20-month-old child. Obstruction may occur following ingestion of as few as two magnets.

Alzahem AM et al: Ingested magnets and gastrointestinal complications. J Paediatr Child Health 2007;43:497 [PMID:17535185].

Consumer Product Safety Commission: http://www.cpsc.gov/CPSCPUB/PREREL/prhtml07/07163.html 2007

MUSHROOMS

Toxic mushrooms are often difficult to distinguish from edible varieties. Contact a poison control center to obtain identification assistance. Symptoms vary with the species ingested, time of year, stage of maturity, quantity eaten, method of preparation, and interval since ingestion. A mushroom that is toxic to one individual may not be toxic to another. Drinking alcohol and eating certain mushrooms may cause a reaction similar to that seen with disulfiram and alcohol. Cooking destroys some toxins but not the deadly one produced by *Amanita phalloides,* which is responsible for 90% of deaths due to mushroom poisoning. Mushroom toxins are absorbed relatively slowly. Onset of symptoms within 2 hours of ingestion suggests muscarinic toxin, whereas a delay of symptoms for 6–48 hours after ingestion strongly suggests *Amanita* (amanitin) poisoning. Patients who have ingested *A phalloides* may relapse and die of hepatic or renal failure following initial improvement.

Mushroom poisoning may produce muscarinic symptoms (salivation, vomiting, diarrhea, cramping abdominal pain, tenesmus, miosis, and dyspnea), coma, convulsions, hallucinations, hemolysis, and delayed hepatic and renal failure.

▶ Treatment

Administer activated charcoal. If the patient has muscarinic signs, give atropine, 0.05 mg/kg IM (0.02 mg/kg in toddlers), and repeat as needed (usually every 30 minutes) to keep the patient atropinized. Atropine, however, is used only when cholinergic effects are present and not for all mushrooms. Hypoglycemia is most likely to occur in patients with delayed onset of symptoms. Try to identify the mushroom if the patient is symptomatic. Consultation with a certified poison center is recommended. Local botanical gardens, university departments of botany, and societies of mycologists may be able to help. Supportive care is usually all that is needed; however, in the case of *A phalloides,* penicillin, silibinin, or hemodialysis may be indicated.

Lampe KF, McCann MA: Differential diagnosis of poisoning by North American mushrooms, with particular emphasis on *Amanita phalloides*-like intoxication. Ann Emerg Med 1987;16:956 [PMID: 3631682].

Pawlowska J et al: Liver transplantation in three family members after *Amanita phalloides* mushroom poisoning. Transplant Proc 2002;34:3313 [PMID: 12493457].

NITRITES, NITRATES, ANILINE, PENTACHLOROPHENOL, & DINITROPHENOL

Nausea, vertigo, vomiting, cyanosis (methemoglobinemia), cramping abdominal pain, tachycardia, cardiovascular collapse, tachypnea, coma, shock, convulsions, and death are possible manifestations of nitrite or nitrate poisoning.

Nitrite and nitrate compounds found in the home include amyl nitrite, butyl nitrates, isobutyl nitrates, nitroglycerin, pentaerythritol tetranitrate, sodium nitrite, nitrobenzene, and phenazopyridine. Pentachlorophenol and dinitrophenol, which are found in wood preservatives, produce methemoglobinemia and high fever because of uncoupling of oxidative phosphorylation. Headache, dizziness, and bradycardia have been reported. High concentrations of nitrites in well water or spinach have been the most common cause of nitrite-induced methemoglobinemia. Symptoms do not usually occur until 15–50% of the hemoglobin has been converted to methemoglobin. A rapid test is to compare a drop of normal blood with the patient's blood on a dry filter paper. Brown discoloration of the patient's blood indicates a methemoglobin level of more than 15%.

▶ Treatment

Administer activated charcoal. Decontaminate affected skin with soap and water. Oxygen and artificial respiration may be needed. If the blood methemoglobin level exceeds 30%, or if levels cannot be obtained and the patient is symptomatic, give a 1% solution of methylene blue (0.2 mL/kg IV) over 5–10 minutes. Avoid perivascular infiltration, because it causes necrosis of the skin and subcutaneous tissues. A dramatic change in the degree of cyanosis should occur. Transfusion is occasionally necessary. Epinephrine and other vasoconstrictors are contraindicated. If reflex bradycardia occurs, atropine should be used.

Kennedy N et al: Faulty sausage production causing methaemoglobinaemia. Arch Dis Child 1997;76:367 [PMID: 9166036].

OPIOIDS (CODEINE, HEROIN, METHADONE, MORPHINE, PROPOXYPHENE)

Opioid-related medical problems may include drug addiction, withdrawal in a newborn infant, and accidental overdoses. Unlike other narcotics, methadone is absorbed readily from the GI tract. Most opioids, including heroin, methadone, meperidine, morphine, and codeine, are excreted in the urine within 24 hours and can be detected readily.

Narcotic-addicted adolescents often have other medical problems, including cellulitis, abscesses, thrombophlebitis, tetanus, infective endocarditis, HIV infection, tuberculosis, hepatitis, malaria, foreign body emboli, thrombosis of pulmonary arterioles, diabetes mellitus, obstetric complications, nephropathy, and peptic ulcer.

▶ Treatment

A. Overdose

Opioids can cause respiratory depression, stridor, coma, increased oropharyngeal secretions, sinus bradycardia, and urinary retention. Pulmonary edema rarely occurs in children; deaths usually result from aspiration of gastric contents, respiratory arrest, and cerebral edema. Convulsions may occur with propoxyphene overdosage.

Although suggested doses for naloxone hydrochloride range from 0.01–0.1 mg/kg, it is generally unnecessary to calculate the dosage on this basis. This extremely safe antidote should be given in sufficient quantity to reverse opioid binding sites. For children younger than age 1 year, 1 ampoule (0.4 mg) should be given initially; if there is no response, five more ampoules (2 mg) should be given rapidly. Older children should be given 0.4–0.8 mg, followed by 2–4 mg if there is no response. An improvement in respiratory status may be followed by respiratory depression, because the antagonist's duration of action is less than 1 hour. Neonates poisoned in utero may require 10–30 mg/kg to reverse the effect.

B. Withdrawal in the Addict

Diazepam (10 mg every 6 hours PO) has been recommended for the treatment of mild narcotic withdrawal in ambulatory adolescents. Management of withdrawal in the confirmed addict may be accomplished with the administration of clonidine, by substitution with methadone, or with reintroduction of the original addicting agent, if available through a supervised drug withdrawal program. A tapered course over 3 weeks will accomplish this goal. Death rarely, if ever, occurs. The abrupt discontinuation of narcotics (cold turkey method) is not recommended and may cause severe physical withdrawal signs.

C. Withdrawal in the Newborn

A newborn infant in opioid withdrawal is usually small for gestational age and demonstrates yawning, sneezing, decreased Moro reflex, hunger but uncoordinated sucking action, jitteriness, tremor, constant movement, a shrill protracted cry, increased tendon reflexes, convulsions, vomiting, fever, watery diarrhea, cyanosis, dehydration, vasomotor instability, seizure, and collapse.

The onset of symptoms commonly begins in the first 48 hours but may be delayed as long as 8 days, depending on the timing of the mother's last fix and her predelivery medication. The diagnosis can be confirmed easily by identifying the narcotic in the urine of the mother and the newborn.

Several treatment methods have been suggested for narcotic withdrawal in the newborn. Phenobarbital (8 mg/kg/d IM or PO in 4 doses for 4 days and then reduced by one third every 2 days as signs decrease) may be continued for as long as 3 weeks. Methadone may be necessary in those infants with congenital methadone addiction who are not controlled in their withdrawal by large doses of phenobarbital. Dosage should be 0.5 mg/kg/d in two divided doses but can be increased gradually as needed. After control of the symptoms is achieved, the dose may be tapered over 4 weeks.

It is unclear whether prophylactic treatment with these drugs decreases the complication rate. The mortality rate of untreated narcotic withdrawal in the newborn may be as high as 45%.

Traub SJ et al: Pediatric "body packing". Arch Pediatr Adolesc Med 2003;157:174 [PMID: 12580688].

PHENOTHIAZINES (CHLORPROMAZINE, PROCHLORPERAZINE, TRIFLUOPERAZINE)

▶ Clinical Findings

A. Extrapyramidal Crisis

Episodes characterized by torticollis, stiffening of the body, spasticity, poor speech, catatonia, and inability to communicate although conscious are typical manifestations. These episodes usually last a few seconds to a few minutes but have rarely caused death. Extrapyramidal crises may represent idiosyncratic reactions and are aggravated by dehydration. The signs and symptoms occur most often in children who have received prochlorperazine. They are commonly mistaken for psychotic episodes.

B. Overdose

Lethargy and deep prolonged coma commonly occur. Promazine, chlorpromazine, and prochlorperazine are the drugs most likely to cause respiratory depression and precipitous drops in blood pressure. Occasionally, paradoxic hyperactivity and extrapyramidal signs as well as hyperglycemia and acetonemia are present. Seizures are uncommon.

C. Neuroleptic Malignant Syndrome

Neuroleptic malignant syndrome is a rare idiosyncratic complication of phenothiazine use that may be lethal. It is a syndrome involving mental status change (confusion, coma), motor abnormalities (lead pipe rigidity, clonus), and autonomic dysfunction (tachycardia, hyperpyrexia).

▶ Treatment

Extrapyramidal signs are alleviated within minutes by the slow IV administration of diphenhydramine, 1–2 mg/kg (maximum, 50 mg), or benztropine mesylate, 1– 2 mg IV (1 mg/min). No other treatment is usually indicated.

Patients with overdoses should receive conservative supportive care. Activated charcoal should be administered. Hypotension may be treated with standard agents, starting with isotonic saline administration. Agitation is best treated with diazepam. Neuroleptic malignant syndrome is treated by discontinuing the drug, giving aggressive supportive care, and administering dantrolene or bromocriptine.

O'Malley GF et al: Olanzapine overdose mimicking opioid intoxication. Ann Emerg Med 1999;34:279 [PMID: 10424936].

PLANTS

Many common ornamental, garden, and wild plants are potentially toxic. Only in a few cases will small amounts of a plant cause severe illness or death. Table 12–6 **lists the most toxic plants, symptoms and signs of poisoning, and treatment.** Contact your poison control center for assistance with identification.

PSYCHOTROPIC DRUGS

Psychotropic drugs consist of four general classes: stimulants (amphetamines, cocaine), depressants (eg, narcotics, barbiturates), antidepressants and tranquilizers, and hallucinogens (eg, LSD, PCP).

Table 12–6. Poisoning due to plants.[a]

	Symptoms and Signs	Treatment
Arum family: *Caladium, Dieffenbachia*, calla lily, dumbcane (oxalic acid)	Burning of mucous membranes and airway obstruction secondary to edema caused by calcium oxalate crystals.	Accessible areas should be thoroughly washed. Corticosteroids relieve airway obstruction. Apply cold packs to affected mucous membranes.
Castor bean plant (ricin—a toxalbumin) Jequinty bean (abrin—a toxalbumin)	Mucous membrane irritation, nausea, vomiting, bloody diarrhea, blurred vision, circulatory collapse, acute hemolytic anemia, convulsions, uremia.	Fluid and electrolyte monitoring. Saline cathartic. Forced alkaline diuresis will prevent complications due to hemagglutination and hemolysis.
Foxglove, lily of the valley, and oleander[b]	Nausea, diarrhea, visual disturbances, and cardiac irregularities (eg, heart block).	See treatment for digitalis drugs in text.
Jimsonweed: See Belladonna Alkaloids section in text	Mydriasis, dry mouth, tachycardia, and hallucinations.	Activated charcoal.
Larkspur (ajacine, *Delphinium*, delphinine)	Nausea and vomiting, irritability, muscular paralysis, and central nervous system depression.	Symptomatic. Atropine may be helpful.
Monkshood (aconite)	Numbness of mucous membranes, visual disturbances, tingling, dizziness, tinnitus, hypotension, bradycardia, and convulsions.	Activated charcoal, oxygen. Atropine is probably helpful.
Poison hemlock (coniine)	Mydriasis, trembling, dizziness, bradycardia. Central nervous system depression, muscular paralysis, and convulsions. Death is due to respiratory paralysis.	Symptomatic. Oxygen and cardiac monitoring equipment are desirable. Assisted respiration is often necessary. Give anticonvulsants if needed.
Rhododendron (grayanotoxin)	Abdominal cramps, vomiting, severe diarrhea, muscular paralysis. Central nervous system and circulatory depression. Hypertension with very large doses.	Atropine can prevent bradycardia. Epinephrine is contraindicated. Antihypertensives may be needed.
Yellow jessamine (active ingredient, geisemine, is related to strychnine)	Restlessness, convulsions, muscular paralysis, and respiratory depression.	Symptomatic. Because of the relation to strychnine, activated charcoal and diazepam for seizures are worth trying.

[a]Many other plants cause minor irritation but are not likely to cause serious problems unless large amounts are ingested. See Lampe KF, McCann MA: *AMA Handbook of Poisonous and Injurious Plants*. American Medical Association, 1985.
[b]Done AK: Ornamental and deadly. Emerg Med 1973;5:255.

▶ **Clinical Findings**

The following clinical findings are commonly seen in patients abusing drugs. See also other entries discussed in alphabetic order in this chapter.

A. Stimulants

Agitation, euphoria, grandiose feelings, tachycardia, fever, abdominal cramps, visual and auditory hallucinations, mydriasis, coma, convulsions, and respiratory depression.

B. Depressants

Emotional lability, ataxia, diplopia, nystagmus, vertigo, poor accommodation, respiratory depression, coma, apnea, and convulsions. Dilation of conjunctival blood vessels suggests marijuana ingestion. Narcotics cause miotic pupils and, occasionally, pulmonary edema.

C. Antidepressants and Tranquilizers

Hypotension, lethargy, respiratory depression, coma, and extrapyramidal reactions.

D. Hallucinogens and Psychoactive Drugs

Belladonna alkaloids cause mydriasis, dry mouth, nausea, vomiting, urinary retention, confusion, disorientation, paranoid delusions, hallucinations, fever, hypotension, aggressive behavior, convulsions, and coma. Psychoactive drugs such as LSD cause mydriasis, unexplained bizarre behavior, hallucinations, and generalized undifferentiated psychotic behavior.

▶ **Treatment**

Only a small percentage of the persons using drugs come to the attention of physicians; those who do are usually experiencing adverse reactions such as panic states, drug psychoses, homicidal or suicidal thoughts, or respiratory depression.

Even with cooperative patients, an accurate history is difficult to obtain. A drug history is most easily obtained in a quiet spot by a gentle, nonthreatening, honest examiner, and without the parents present. The user often does not really know what drug has been taken or how much. Street drugs are almost always adulterated with one or more other compounds. Multiple drugs are often taken together. Friends may be a useful source of information.

The patient's general appearance, skin, lymphatics, cardiorespiratory status, GI tract, and CNS should be focused on during the physical examination, because they often provide clues suggesting drug abuse.

Hallucinogens are not life-threatening unless the patient is frankly homicidal or suicidal. A specific diagnosis is usually not necessary for management; instead, the presenting signs and symptoms are treated. Does the patient appear intoxicated? In withdrawal? "Flashing back?" Is some illness or injury (eg, head trauma) being masked by a drug effect? (Remember that a known drug user may still have hallucinations from meningoencephalitis.)

The signs and symptoms in a given patient are a function not only of the drug and the dose but also of the level of acquired tolerance, the "setting," the patient's physical condition and personality traits, the potentiating effects of other drugs, and many other factors.

A common drug problem is the "bad trip," which is usually a panic reaction. This is best managed by "talking the patient down" and minimizing auditory and visual stimuli. Allowing the patient to sit with a friend while the drug effect dissipates may be the best treatment. This may take several hours. The physician's job is not to terminate the drug effect but to help the patient through the bad experience.

Drug therapy is often unnecessary and may complicate the clinical course of a drug-related panic reaction.

Although phenothiazines have been commonly used to treat bad trips, they should be avoided if the specific drug is unknown, because they may enhance toxicity or produce unwanted side effects. Diazepam is the drug of choice if a sedative effect is required. Physical restraints are rarely indicated and usually increase the patient's panic reaction.

For treatment of life-threatening drug abuse, consult the section on the specific drug elsewhere in this chapter and the section on general management at the beginning of the chapter.

After the acute episode, the physician must decide whether psychiatric referral is indicated; in general, patients who have made suicidal gestures or attempts and adolescents who are not communicating with their families should be referred.

Weir E: Raves: A review of the culture, the drugs and the prevention of harm. CMAJ 2000;162:1843 [PMID: 10906922].

SALICYLATES

The use of childproof containers and publicity regarding accidental poisoning have reduced the incidence of acute salicylate poisoning. Nevertheless, serious intoxication still occurs and must be regarded as an emergency. In recent years, the frequency of poisoning has begun to rise again.

Salicylates uncouple oxidative phosphorylation, leading to increased heat production, excessive sweating, and dehydration. They also interfere with glucose metabolism and may cause hypoglycemia or hyperglycemia. Respiratory center stimulation occurs early.

Patients usually have signs of hyperventilation, sweating, dehydration, and fever. Vomiting and diarrhea sometimes occur. In severe cases, disorientation, convulsions, and coma may develop.

The severity of acute intoxication can, in some measure, be judged by serum salicylate levels. High levels are always dangerous irrespective of clinical signs, and low levels may be misleading in chronic cases. Other laboratory values usually indicate metabolic acidosis despite hyperventilation, low serum K^+ values, and often abnormal serum glucose levels.

In mild and moderate poisoning, stimulation of the respiratory center produces respiratory alkalosis. In severe intoxication (occurring in severe acute ingestion with high salicylate levels and in chronic toxicity with lower levels), respiratory response is unable to overcome the metabolic overdose.

Once the urine becomes acidic, progressively smaller amounts of salicylate are excreted. Until this process is reversed, the half-life will remain prolonged, because metabolism contributes little to the removal of salicylate.

Chronic severe poisoning may occur as early as 3 days after a regimen of salicylate is begun. Findings usually include vomiting, diarrhea, and dehydration.

▶ Treatment

Charcoal binds salicylates well and should be given for acute ingestions. Mild poisoning may require only the administration of oral fluids and confirmation that the salicylate level is falling. Moderate poisoning involves moderate dehydration and depletion of potassium. Fluids must be administered at a rate of 2–3 mL/kg/h to correct dehydration and produce urine with a pH of greater than 7.0. Initial IV solutions should be isotonic, with sodium bicarbonate constituting half the electrolyte content. Once the patient is rehydrated, the solution can contain more free water and approximately 40 mEq/L of K^+.

Severe toxicity is marked by major dehydration. Symptoms may be confused with those of Reye syndrome, encephalopathy, and metabolic acidosis. Salicylate levels may even be in the therapeutic range. Major fluid correction of dehydration is required. Once this has been accomplished, hypokalemia must be corrected and sodium bicarbonate given. Usual requirements are sodium bicarbonate, 1–2 mEq/kg/h over the first 6–8 hours, and K$^+$, 20–40 mEq/L. A urine flow of 2–3 mL/kg/h should be established. Despite this treatment some patients will develop the paradoxical aciduria of salicylism. This is due to hypokalemia and the saving of K$^+$ and excretion of H$^+$ in the renal tubule. Correction of K$^+$ will allow the urine to become alkaline and ionize the salicylate, resulting in excretion rather than reabsorption of nonionized salicylate in acid urine.

Renal failure or pulmonary edema is an indication for dialysis. Hemodialysis is most effective and peritoneal dialysis is relatively ineffective. Hemodialysis should be used in all patients with altered mental status or deteriorating clinical status. Acetazolamide should not be used.

Yip L et al: Concepts and controversies in salicylate toxicity. Emerg Med Clin North Am 1994;12:351 [PMID: 8187688].

SCORPION STINGS

Scorpion stings are common in arid areas of the southwestern United States. Scorpion venom is more toxic than most snake venoms, but only minute amounts are injected. Although neurologic manifestations may last a week, most clinical signs subside within 24–48 hours.

The most common scorpions in the United States are *Vejovis, Hadrurus, Androctonus,* and *Centruroides* species. Stings by the first three produce edema and pain. Stings by *Centruroides* (the Bark scorpion) cause tingling or burning paresthesias that begin at the site of the sting; other findings include hypersalivation, restlessness, muscular fasciculation, abdominal cramps, opisthotonos, convulsions, urinary incontinence, and respiratory failure.

▶ Treatment

Sedation is the primary therapy. Antivenom is reserved for severe poisoning. In severe cases, the airway may become compromised by secretions and weakness of respiratory muscles. Endotracheal intubation may be required. Patients may require treatment for seizures, hypertension, or tachycardia.

The prognosis is good as long as the patient's airway is managed appropriately.

LoVecchio F et al: Incidence of immediate and delayed hypersensitivity to *Centruroides* antivenom. Ann Emerg Med 1999;34:615 [PMID: 10533009].

SEROTONIN REUPTAKE INHIBITORS

Fluoxetine (Prozac), paroxetine (Paxil), sertraline (Zoloft) and many other agents comprise this class of drugs. Adverse effects in therapeutic dosing include suicidal thoughts, aggressive behavior, extrapyramidal effects, and cardiac dysrhythmias, and in overdose may include vomiting, lethargy, seizures, hypertension, tachycardia, hyperthermia, and abdominal pain. The findings in overdose are included in the serotonin syndrome due to the action of these drugs, which results in an increase of serotonin (5-hydroxytryptamine [5-HT]). Despite the degree of toxicity these agents generally are not life–threatening and intervention usually is not necessary.

Emptying the stomach is not helpful, but activated charcoal may be useful. Laboratory measurements of the drugs are not of benefit other than to establish their presence.

Treatment with benzodiazepines is the most beneficial. Hypotension may be treated with fluids or norepinephrine. Cyproheptadine is an antagonist of serotonin, but its use has been limited. A dose of 0.25 mg/kg/d divided every 6 hours to a maximum of 12 mg/d may be useful in treating the serotonin syndrome. Adults and older adolescents have been treated with 12 mg initially followed by 2 mg every 2 hours to a maximum of 32 mg/d.

Boyer EW, Shannon M: The serotonin syndrome. N Engl J Med 2005;352:1112 [PMID: 15784664].

SNAKEBITE

Despite the lethal potential of venomous snakes, human morbidity and mortality rates are surprisingly low. The outcome depends on the size of the child, the site of the bite, the degree of envenomation, the type of snake, and the effectiveness of treatment.

Nearly all poisonous snakebites in the United States are caused by pit vipers (rattlesnakes, water moccasins, and copperheads). A few are caused by elapids (coral snakes), and occasional bites occur from cobras and other nonindigenous exotic snakes kept as pets. Snake venom is a complex mixture of enzymes, peptides, and proteins that may have predominantly cytotoxic, neurotoxic, hemotoxic, or cardiotoxic effects but other effects as well. Up to 25% of bites by pit vipers do not result in venom injection. Pit viper venom causes predominantly local injury with pain, discoloration, edema, and hemorrhage.

Swelling and pain occur soon after rattlesnake bite and are a certain indication that envenomation has occurred. During the first few hours, swelling and ecchymosis extend proximally from the bite. The bite is often obvious as a double puncture mark surrounded by ecchymosis. Hematemesis, melena, hemoptysis, and other manifestations of coagulopathy develop in severe cases. Respiratory difficulty and shock are the ultimate causes of death. Even in fatal rattlesnake bites, a period of 6–8 hours usually elapses between the bite and death; as a result, there is usually enough time to start effective treatment.

Coral snake envenomation causes little local pain, swelling, or necrosis; and systemic reactions are often delayed. The signs of coral snake envenomation include bulbar paralysis, dysphagia, and dysphoria; these signs may appear in 5–10 hours and may be followed by total peripheral paralysis and death in 24 hours.

▶ Treatment

Children in snake-infested areas should wear boots and long trousers, should not walk barefoot, and should be cautioned not to explore under ledges or in holes.

A. Emergency (First-Aid) Treatment

The most important first-aid measure is transportation to a medical facility. Splint the affected extremity and minimize the patient's motion. Tourniquets and ice packs are contraindicated. Incision and suction are not useful for either crotalid or elapid snake bite.

B. Definitive Medical Management

Blood should be drawn for hematocrit, clotting time and platelet function, and serum electrolyte determinations. Establish two secure IV sites for the administration of antivenom and other medications.

Specific antivenom is indicated when signs of progressive envenomation are present. Two antivenoms are available for treating pit viper envenomation: polyvalent pit viper antivenom and polyvalent Crotalidae Fab (CroFab). Both are effective, but their indications differ. For coral snake bites, an eastern coral snake antivenom (Wyeth Laboratories) is available. Patients with pit viper bites should receive antivenom if progressive local injury, coagulopathy, or systemic signs (eg, hypotension, confusion) are present. (Antivenom should not be given IM or SQ.) See package labeling or call your certified poison center for details of use. Hemorrhage, pain, and shock diminish rapidly with adequate amounts of antivenom. For coral snake bites, give three to five vials of antivenom in 250–500 mL of isotonic saline solution. An additional three to five vials may be required.

To control pain, administer a narcotic analgesic, such as meperidine (0.6–1.5 mg/kg per dose, given PO or IM). Cryotherapy is contraindicated because it commonly causes additional tissue damage. Early physiotherapy minimizes contractures. In rare cases, fasciotomy to relieve pressure within muscular compartments is required. The evaluation of function and of pulses will better predict the need for fasciotomy. Antihistamines and corticosteroids (hydrocortisone, 1 mg/kg, given PO for a week) are useful in the treatment of serum sickness or anaphylactic shock. Antibiotics are not needed unless clinical signs of infection occur. Tetanus status should be evaluated and the patient immunized, if needed.

Dart RC, McNally J: Efficacy, safety, and use of snake antivenoms in the United States. Ann Emerg Med 2001;37:181 [PMID: 11174237].

Offerman SR et al: Crotaline Fab antivenom for the treatment of children with rattle snake envenomation. Pediatrics 2002;110:968 [PMID: 12415038].

SOAPS & DETERGENTS

1. Soaps

Soap is made from salts of fatty acids. Some toilet soap bars contain both soap and detergent. Ingestion of soap bars may cause vomiting and diarrhea, but they have a low toxicity. Induced emesis is unnecessary.

2. Detergents

Detergents are nonsoap synthetic products used for cleaning purposes because of their surfactant properties. Commercial products include granules, powders, and liquids. Dishwasher detergents are very alkaline and can cause caustic burns. Low concentrations of bleaching and antibacterial agents as well as enzymes are found in many preparations. The pure compounds are moderately toxic, but the concentration used is too small to alter the product's toxicity significantly, although occasional primary or allergic irritative phenomena have been noted in persons who frequently use such products and in employees manufacturing these products.

A. Cationic Detergents (Ceepryn, Diaparene Cream, Phemerol, Zephiran)

Cationic detergents in dilute solutions (0.5%) cause mucosal irritation, but higher concentrations (10–15%) may cause caustic burns to mucosa. Clinical effects include nausea, vomiting, collapse, coma, and convulsions. As little as 2.25 g of some cationic agents have caused death in an adult. In four cases, 100–400 mg/kg of benzalkonium chloride caused death. Cationic detergents are rapidly inactivated by tissues and ordinary soap.

Because of the caustic potential and rapid onset of seizures, emesis is not recommended. Activated charcoal should be administered. Anticonvulsants may be needed.

B. Anionic Detergents

Most common household detergents are anionic. Laundry compounds have water softener (sodium phosphate) added, which is a strong irritant and may reduce ionized calcium. Anionic detergents irritate the skin by removing natural oils. Although ingestion causes diarrhea, intestinal distention, and vomiting, no fatalities have been reported.

The only treatment usually required is to discontinue use if skin irritation occurs and replace fluids and electrolytes. Induced vomiting is not indicated following ingestion of automatic dishwasher detergent, because of its alkalinity. Dilute with water or milk.

C. Nonionic Detergents (Brij Products; Tritons X-45, X-100, X-102, and X-144)

These compounds include lauryl, stearyl, and oleyl alcohols and octyl phenol. They have a minimal irritating effect on the skin and are almost always nontoxic when swallowed.

Klasaer AE et al: Marked hypocalcemia and ventricular fibrillation in two pediatric patients exposed to a fluoride-containing wheel cleaner. Ann Emerg Med 1996;28:713 [PMID: 8953969].

Vincent JC, Sheikh A: Phosphate poisoning by ingestion of clothes washing liquid and fabric conditioner. Anesthesiology 1998;53:1004 [PMID: 9893545].

SPIDER BITES

Most medically important bites in the United States are caused by the black widow spider (*Latrodectus mactans*) and the North American brown recluse (violin) spider (*Loxosceles reclusa*). Positive identification of the spider is helpful, because many spider bites may mimic those of the brown recluse spider.

1. Black Widow Spider

The black widow spider is endemic to nearly all areas of the United States. The initial bite causes sharp fleeting pain. Local and systemic muscular cramping, abdominal pain, nausea and vomiting, and shock can occur. Convulsions occur more commonly in small children than in older children. Systemic signs of black widow spider bite may be confused with other causes of acute abdomen. Although paresthesias, nervousness, and transient muscle spasms may persist for weeks in survivors, recovery from the acute phase is generally complete within 3 days. In contrast to popular opinion, death is extremely rare.

Most authors recommend calcium gluconate as initial therapy (50 mg/kg IV per dose, up to 250 mg/kg/24 h), although it is often not effective and the effects are of short duration. Methocarbamol (15 mg/kg PO) or diazepam titrated to effect is useful. Morphine or barbiturates may occasionally be needed for control of pain or restlessness, but they increase the possibility of respiratory depression. Antivenom is available but should be reserved for severe cases in which the previously mentioned therapies have failed. Local treatment of the bite is not helpful.

2. Brown Recluse Spider (Violin Spider)

The North American brown recluse spider is most commonly seen in the central and Midwestern areas of the United States. Its bite characteristically produces a localized reaction with progressively severe pain within 24 hours. The initial bleb on an erythematous ischemic base is replaced by a black eschar within 1 week. This eschar separates in 2–5 weeks, leaving an ulcer that heals slowly. Systemic signs include cyanosis, morbilliform rash, fever, chills, malaise, weakness, nausea and vomiting, joint pains, hemolytic reactions with hemoglobinuria, jaundice, and delirium. Fatalities are rare. Fatal disseminated intravascular coagulation has been reported.

Although of unproved efficacy, the following therapies have been used: dexamethasone, 4 mg IV four times a day, during the acute phase; polymorphonuclear leukocyte inhibitors, such as dapsone or colchicine, and oxygen applied to the bite site; and total excision of the lesion to the fascial level.

Clark RF et al: Clinical presentation and treatment of black widow spider envenomation: A review of 163 cases. Ann Emerg Med 1992;21:782 [PMID: 1351707].

Sams HH et al: Nineteen documented cases of *Loxosceles reclusa* envenomation. J Am Acad Dermatol 2001;44:603 [PMID: 11260528].

THYROID PREPARATIONS (THYROID DESICCATED, SODIUM LEVOTHYROXINE)

Ingestion of the equivalent of 50–150 g of desiccated thyroid can cause signs of hyperthyroidism, including irritability, mydriasis, hyperpyrexia, tachycardia, and diarrhea. Maximal clinical effect occurs about 9 days after ingestion—several days after the protein-bound iodine level has fallen dramatically.

Administer activated charcoal. If the patient develops clinical signs of toxicity, propranolol, 0.01–0.1 mg/kg (maximum, 1 mg), is useful because of its antiadrenergic activity.

Brown RS et al: Successful treatment of massive acute thyroid hormone poisoning with iopanoic acid. J Pediatr 1998;132:903 [PMID: 9602214].

VITAMINS

Accidental ingestion of excessive amounts of vitamins rarely causes significant problems. Occasional cases of hypervitaminosis A and D do occur, however, particularly in patients with poor hepatic or renal function. The fluoride contained in many multivitamin preparations is not a realistic hazard, because a 2- or 3-year-old child could eat 100 tablets, containing 1 mg of sodium fluoride per tablet, without experiencing serious symptoms. Iron poisoning has been reported with multivitamin tablets containing iron. Pyridoxine abuse has caused neuropathies; nicotinic acid has resulted in myopathy.

Dean BS, Krenzelok EP: Multiple vitamins and vitamins with iron: Accidental poisoning in children. Vet Hum Toxicol 1988;30:23 [PMID: 3354178].

Fraser DR: Vitamin D. Lancet 1995;345:104 [PMID: 7815853].

WARFARIN

Warfarin is used as a rodenticide. It causes hypoprothrombinemia and capillary injury. It is absorbed readily from the GI tract but is absorbed poorly through the skin. A dose of 0.5 mg/kg of warfarin may be toxic in a child. A prothrombin time is helpful in establishing the severity of the poisoning.

If bleeding occurs or the prothrombin time is prolonged, give 1–5 mg of vitamin K_1 (phytonadione) IM or SQ. For large ingestions with established toxicity, 0.6 mg/kg may be given.

Another group of long-acting anticoagulant rodenticides (brodifacoum, difenacoum, bromadoline, diphacinone, pinene, valone, and coumatetralyl) have been a more serious toxicologic problem than warfarin. They also cause hypo-prothrombinemia and a bleeding diathesis that responds to phytonadione, although the anticoagulant activity may persist for periods ranging from 6 weeks to several months. Treatment with vitamin K_1 may be needed for weeks.

Isbister GK, Whyte IM: Management of anticoagulant poisoning. Vet Hum Toxicol 2001;43:117 [PMID: 11308119].

Critical Care

Todd C. Carpenter, MD

Emily L. Dobyns, MD

Eva N. Grayck, MD

Peter M. Mourani, MD

Kurt R. Stenmark, MD

Caring for critically ill children remains one of the most demanding and challenging aspects of pediatrics. The care of patients with life-threatening conditions, from serious medical illness to traumatic injuries and recovery from major surgery, requires a detailed understanding of human physiology and the pathophysiology of major illnesses, as well as an understanding of and experience with the rapidly changing technologies available in a modern intensive care unit (ICU). In addition, the science of caring for the critically ill patient has evolved rapidly over the past decade, as the molecular mediators of illness have become better defined and new therapies have been devised based on those advances. As a result, critical care is more than ever a multidisciplinary field that requires a team-oriented approach, including critical care physicians and nursing staff, pharmacists, referring physicians, consulting specialists, and social services specialists.

The intensivist plays an essential role in coordinating and directing the care provided by the ICU team, and stands at the crossroads of the various participating disciplines. There are two primary models of ICU organization: "open" units, where primary responsibility for the patient remains with the referring physician and secondary responsibility lies with the intensivist as consultant; and "closed" units, where only the on-site intensivist is allowed to write orders directing the patient's care. Although the merits of these organizational approaches are debated, a substantial and growing body of evidence from studies conducted in adult medical, surgical, and pediatric ICUs suggests that the closed ICU model leads to significant reductions in ICU length of stay and resource use, and to reductions in mortality of as much as 15%.

An additional factor to consider in the provision of critical care services for children is the cost of those services in relation to the outcomes achieved. Critical care services in the United States are estimated to account for 30% of all acute-care hospital costs; some estimates run as high as 1% of the gross national product. One study examining the cost-effectiveness of pediatric ICU care, compared with adult ICU care, found that the short- and long-term mortality among pediatric patients was three times lower than it was among adult ICU patients, despite similar ICU costs and length of stay. These findings suggest that pediatric critical care services are relatively cost-effective.

Brilli RJ et al: Critical care delivery in the intensive care unit: Defining clinical roles and the best practice model. Crit Care Med 2001;29:2007 [PMID: 11588472].

Durbin CG Jr: Team model: Advocating for the optimal method of care delivery in the intensive care unit. Crit Care Med. 2006;34(Suppl):S12 [PMID: 16477198].

Epstein D, Brill JE: A history of pediatric critical care medicine. Pediatr Res 2005;58:987 [PMID: 16183804].

Pronovost PJ et al: Team care: Beyond open and closed intensive care units. Curr Opin Crit Care. 2006;12:604 [PMID: 17077695].

Seferian EG et al: Comparison of resource utilization and outcome between pediatric and adult intensive care unit patients. Pediatr Crit Care Med 2001;2:2 [PMID: 12797880].

ACUTE RESPIRATORY FAILURE

Acute respiratory failure, defined as the inability of the respiratory system to adequately deliver oxygen or remove carbon dioxide, contributes significantly to the morbidity and mortality of critically ill children. This condition accounts for approximately 50% of deaths in children younger than age 1 year. Anatomic and developmental differences place infants at higher risk than adults for respiratory failure. An infant's thoracic cage is more compliant than that of the adult or older child. The intercostal muscles are poorly developed and unable to achieve the "bucket-handle" motion characteristic of adult breathing. Furthermore, the diaphragm is shorter and relatively flat with fewer type I muscle fibers, and therefore less effective and more easily fatigued. The infant's airways are smaller in caliber than those in older children and adults, resulting in greater resistance to inspiratory and expiratory airflow and greater

Table 13–1. Types of respiratory failure.

Findings	Causes	Examples
Type I Hypoxia Decreased Pa_{O_2} Normal Pa_{CO_2}	Ventilation-perfusion defect	Positional (supine in bed), acute respiratory distress syndrome (ARDS), atelectasis, pneumonia, pulmonary embolus, bronchopulmonary dysplasia
	Diffusion impairment	Pulmonary edema, ARDS, interstitial pneumonia
	Shunt	Pulmonary arteriovenous malformation, congenital adenomatoid malformation
Type II Hypoxia Hypercapnia Decreased Pa_{O_2} Increased Pa_{CO_2}	Hypoventilation	Neuromuscular disease (polio, Guillain-Barré syndrome), head trauma, sedation, chest wall dysfunction (burns), kyphosis, severe reactive airways

susceptibility to occlusion by mucus plugging and mucosal edema. Compared with adults, the alveoli of children are smaller and have less collateral ventilation, resulting in a greater tendency to collapse and develop atelectasis. Finally, young infants may have an especially reactive pulmonary vascular bed, impaired immune system, or residual effects from prematurity, all of which increase the risk of respiratory failure.

Respiratory failure can be classified into two types, which usually coexist in variable proportion. The partial arterial oxygen pressure (Pa_{O_2}) is low in both, whereas the partial arterial carbon dioxide pressure (Pa_{CO_2}) is high only in patients with type II respiratory failure (Table 13–1). Type I respiratory failure is a failure of oxygenation and occurs in three situations: (1) **ventilation-perfusion mismatch,** or V/Q mismatch, which occurs when blood flows to parts of the lung that are inadequately ventilated, or when ventilated areas of the lung are inadequately perfused; (2) **diffusion defects,** caused by thickened alveolar membranes or excessive interstitial fluid at the alveolar-capillary junction; and (3) **intrapulmonary shunt,** which occurs when structural anomalies in the lung allow blood to flow through the lung without participating in gas exchange. Type II respiratory failure generally results from alveolar hypoventilation and is usually secondary to situations such as central nervous system (CNS) dysfunction, oversedation, or neuromuscular disorders (see Table 13–1).

▶ **Clinical Findings**

A. Symptoms and Signs

The clinical findings in respiratory failure are caused by the low Pa_{O_2}, high Pa_{CO_2}, and pH changes affecting the lungs, heart, kidneys, and brain. The clinical features of progressive respiratory failure are summarized in Table 13–2. Hypercapnia depresses the CNS, and also results in acidemia that depresses myocardial function. Patients in respiratory failure can exhibit significant changes in CNS and cardiac function. Features of respiratory failure are not always clinically evident, however, and some signs or symptoms may have nonrespiratory causes. Furthermore, a strictly clinical assessment of arterial hypoxemia or hypercapnia is not reliable. As a result, the precise assessment of the adequacy of oxygenation and ventilation must be based on both clinical and laboratory data.

B. Laboratory Findings

Laboratory findings are helpful in assessing the severity and acuity of respiratory failure and in determining specific treatment. Arterial oxygen saturation can be measured continuously and noninvasively by **pulse oximetry,** a technique that should be used in the assessment and treatment of all patients with suspected respiratory failure. **End-tidal CO_2** (ET_{CO_2}) **monitoring** provides a continuous noninvasive means of assessing arterial P_{CO_2}. Because carbon dioxide diffuses freely across the alveolar-capillary barrier, the ET_{CO_2} level approximates the alveolar P_{CO_2}, which should equal the arterial P_{CO_2}. Though useful for following trends in ventilation, this technique is susceptible to significant error, particularly with patients who have rapid, shallow breathing or increased dead space ventilation. **Arterial blood gas (ABG) analysis** remains the gold standard for assessment of acute respiratory failure. ABGs give information on the patient's acid-base status (with a measured pH and calculated bicarbonate level) as well as Pa_{O_2} and Pa_{CO_2} levels. The Pa_{O_2} is a

Table 13–2. Clinical features of respiratory failure.

Respiratory
Wheezing
Expiratory grunting
Decreased or absent breath sounds
Flaring of alae nasi
Retractions of chest wall
Tachypnea, bradypnea, or apnea
Cyanosis
Neurologic
Restlessness
Irritability
Headache
Confusion
Convulsions
Coma
Cardiac
Bradycardia or excessive tachycardia
Hypotension or hypertension
General
Fatigue
Sweating

▲ **Figure 13–1.** Relationship between alveolar ventilation, arterial oxygen saturation (Sa_{O_2}), and partial pressures of oxygen and CO_2 in the arterial blood (Pa_{O_2} and Pa_{CO_2}, respectively). (Reproduced, with permission, from Pagtakhan RD, Chernick V: Respiratory failure in the pediatric patient. Pediatr Rev 1982;3:244.)

Table 13–3. Key equations describing pulmonary function and oxygen delivery.

Pi_{O_2}	=	(barometric pressure – 47) × % inspired oxygen concentration
$A{-}aD_{O_2}$	=	$Pi_{O_2} - (Pa_{CO_2}/R) - Pa_{O_2}$ (normal = 5 – 15 mm Hg)
Ca_{O_2}	=	$(1.34 \times$ hemoglobin $\times Sa_{O_2}) + (0.003 \times Pa_{O_2})$
D_{O_2}	=	$Ca_{O_2} \times CI \times 10$ (normal 620 + 50 mL/min/m²)
Oxygen consumption (V_{O_2})	=	$(Ca_{O_2} - Cv_{O_2}) \times CI \times 10$ (normal 120–200 mL/min/m²)
$\dfrac{Qs}{Qt}$	=	$\dfrac{Cc_{O_2} - Ca_{O_2}}{Cc_{O_2} - Cv_{O_2}}$ (normal < 5%)
Vd	=	$\dfrac{(Pc_{O_2} - Pec_{O_2})}{Pc_{O_2}}$ (normal approximately 2 mL/kg)
Compliance	=	$\dfrac{\text{Volume (tidal volume)}}{\text{Pressure (PIP – PEEP)}}$ (normal varies with age)
$A{-}aD_{O_2}$	=	Alveolar-arterial oxygen difference (mm Hg)
Ca_{O_2}	=	Oxygen content of arterial blood (mL/dL)
Cc_{O_2}	=	Oxygen content of pulmonary capillary blood (mL/dL)
CI	=	Cardiac index (L/min)
C_{O_2}	=	Oxygen content of the blood (mL/dL)
Cv_{O_2}	=	Oxygen content of mixed venous blood (mL/dL)
D_{O_2}	=	Oxygen delivery (mL/min)
Pa_{CO_2}	=	Partial pressure of carbon dioxide in arterial blood (mm Hg)
Pa_{O_2}	=	Partial pressure of oxygen in arterial blood (mm Hg)
Pc_{CO_2}	=	Partial pressure of carbon dioxide in capillary blood (mm Hg)
Pe_{CO_2}	=	Partial pressure of carbon dioxide in expired air (mm Hg)
Pi_{O_2}	=	Partial pressure of oxygen in inspired air (mm Hg)
PIP	=	Peak inspiratory pressure
Qs/Qt	=	Intrapulmonary shunt (in patients without cardiac shunt) (%)
R	=	Respiratory quotient (usually 0.8)
Sa_{O_2}	=	Arterial oxygen saturation (fractional)
Vd	=	Physiologic dead space (anatomic dead space + alveolar dead space) (mL)
Ve	=	Expiratory minute volume (L/min)
V_{O_2}	=	Oxygen consumption per minute

critical determinant of oxygen delivery to the tissues, and the Pa_{CO_2} is a sensitive measure of ventilation related inversely to the minute ventilation (Figure 13–1). Although measurement of capillary or venous blood gases may provide some reassurance regarding ventilatory function when results are normal, they yield virtually no useful information regarding oxygenation and may generate highly misleading information about the ventilatory status of patients who have poor perfusion or who had difficult blood draws. As a result, ABG analysis is important for all patients with suspected respiratory failure, particularly those with abnormal venous or capillary gases.

Knowing the ABG values and the inspired oxygen concentration also enables one to calculate the difference between alveolar oxygen concentration and the arterial oxygen value, known as the **alveolar-arterial oxygen difference** ($A{-}aD_{O_2}$, or A–a gradient). The A–a gradient is less than 15 mm Hg under normal conditions, though it widens with increasing inspired oxygen concentrations to about 100 mm Hg in normal patients breathing 100% oxygen. This number has prognostic value in severe hypoxemic respiratory failure, with A–a gradients over 400 mm Hg being strongly associated with mortality. Diffusion impairment, shunts, and V/Q mismatch all increase the $A{-}aD_{O_2}$ (Table 13–3).

In addition to the calculation of the $A{-}aD_{O_2}$, assessment of intrapulmonary shunting (the percentage of pulmonary blood flow that passes through nonventilated areas of the lung) may be helpful. Normal individuals have less than a 5% physiologic shunt from bronchial, thebesian, and coronary circulations. Shunt fractions greater than 15% usually indicate the need for aggressive respiratory support. When intrapulmonary shunt reaches 50% of pulmonary blood flow, Pa_{O_2} does not increase regardless of the amount of supplemental oxygen used.

▶ Treatment

A. Oxygen Supplementation

Patients with hypoxemia induced by respiratory failure may respond to **supplemental oxygen** administration alone (Table 13–4). Those with hypoventilation and diffusion defects respond better than do patients with shunts or V/Q mismatch. Severe V/Q mismatch generally responds only to aggressive airway management and mechanical ventilation. Patients with severe hypoxemia, hypoventilation, or apnea require assistance with bag and mask ventilation until the airway is successfully intubated and controlled artificial ventilation can be provided. Ventilation may be maintained for some time with a mask of the proper size, but gastric distention, emesis, and inadequate tidal volumes are possible complications. An artificial airway may be lifesaving for patients who fail to respond to simple oxygen supplements.

B. Intubation

Intubation of the trachea in infants and children requires experienced personnel and the right equipment. A patient in respiratory failure whose airway must be stabilized should first be positioned properly to facilitate air exchange while supplemental oxygen is given. The sniffing position is used in infants. Head extension with jaw thrust is used in older children without neck injuries. If obstructed by secretions or vomitus, the airway must be cleared by suction. When not obstructed, the airway should open easily with proper positioning and placement of an oral or nasopharyngeal airway of the correct size. Patients with a normal airway may be intubated under intravenous (IV) anesthesia by experienced personnel (Table 13–5). Patients with obstructed upper airways (eg, patients with croup, epiglottitis, foreign bodies, or subglottic stenosis) should be awake when intubated unless trained airway specialists decide otherwise.

The size of the endotracheal tube is of critical importance in pediatrics (see Table 11–3 for sizes). An inappropriately large endotracheal tube can cause pressure necrosis of the tissues in the subglottic region, and can lead to scarring and stenosis of the subglottic region that requires surgical repair. An inappropriately small endotracheal tube can result in inadequate pulmonary toilet and excessive air leak around the endotracheal tube, making optimal ventilation and oxygenation difficult. Two useful methods for calculating the correct size of endotracheal tube for a child are (1) measuring the child's height with a Broselow tape and then reading the corresponding endotracheal tube size on the tape, or (2) in children older than age 2 years, choosing a tube size equal to the computation (16 + age in years) ÷ 4.

Correct placement of the endotracheal tube should be confirmed by auscultation for the presence of equal bilateral breath sounds and the use of a colorimetric filter (pH-sensitive indicator that changes from purple to yellow when exposed to carbon dioxide) by the detection of carbon dioxide. An assessment of air leakage around the endotracheal tube is also important. To do this, connect an anesthesia bag and pressure manometer to the endotracheal tube and allow it to inflate, creating positive pressure. Check for the leak by auscultating over the throat, noting the pressure at which air escapes around the endotracheal tube. Leaks at pressures of 15–20 cm H_2O are acceptable. Leaks at higher pressures are acceptable only in patients who have severe lung disease and poor compliance and thus require high pressures to ventilate and oxygenate. Leaks at lower pressures may lead to ineffective ventilation. The endotracheal tube should be up-sized or a cuffed endotracheal tube should be used if continued mechanical ventilation is needed. Special attention to the inflation pressure of the cuff endotracheal tube is required to avoid pressure necrosis of the airway. A chest radiograph is necessary for final assessment of endotracheal tube placement.

Table 13–4. Supplemental oxygen therapy.

Source	Maximum % O_2	Range of Rates	Advantages	Disadvantages
Nasal cannula	35–40%	0.125–4 L/min	Easily applied, relatively comfortable	Uncomfortable at higher flow rates, requires open nasal airways, easily dislodged, lower % O_2, nosebleeds
Simple mask	50–60%	5–10 L/min	Higher % O_2, good for mouth breathers	Uncomfortable, dangerous for patients with poor airway control and at risk for emesis, hard to give airway care, unsure of % O_2
Face tent	40–60%	8–10 L/min	Higher % O_2, good for mouth breathers, less restrictive	Uncomfortable, dangerous for patients with poor airway control and at risk for emesis, hard to give airway care, unsure of % O_2
Rebreathing mask	80–90%	5–10 L/min	Higher % O_2, good for mouth breathers, highest O_2 concentration	Uncomfortable, dangerous for patients with poor airway control and at risk for emesis, hard to give airway care, unsure of % O_2
Oxyhood	90–100%	5–10 L/min (mixed at wall)	Stable and accurate O_2 concentration	Difficult to maintain temperature, hard to give airway care

Table 13–5. Drugs commonly used for controlled intubation.

Drug	Class of Agent	Dose	Advantages	Disadvantages
Atropine	Anticholinergic	0.02 mg/kg, minimum of 0.1 mg	Prevents bradycardia, dries secretions	Tachycardia, fever; seizures and coma with high doses
Fentanyl	Narcotic (sedative)	1–3 mcg/kg IV	Rapid onset, hemodynamic stability	Respiratory depression, chest wall rigidity with rapid administration in neonates
Midazolam	Benzodiazepine (sedative)	0.1–0.2 mg/kg IV	Rapid onset, amnestic	Respiratory depression, hypotension
Thiopental	Barbiturate (anesthetic)	3–5 mg/kg IV	Rapid onset, lowers intracranial pressure (ICP)	Hypotension, decreased cardiac output, no analgesia provided
Ketamine	Dissociative anesthetic	1–2 mg/kg IV 2–4 mg/kg IM	Rapid onset, bronchodilator, hemodynamic stability	Increases oral and airway secretions, may increase ICP and pulmonary artery pressure
Rocuronium	Nondepolarizing muscle relaxant	1 mg/kg	Rapid onset, suitable for rapid sequence intubation, lasts 30 min	Requires refrigeration
Pancuronium	Nondepolarizing muscle relaxant	0.1 mg/kg	Longer duration of action (40–60 min)	Tachycardia, slow onset (2–3 min)

IV, intravenously, IM, intramuscularly.

Artigas A et al: The American-European Consensus Conference on ARDs, Part 2. Am J Respir Crit Care Med 1998;157:1332 [PMID: 9563759].

Bledsoe GH, Schexnayder SM: Pediatric rapid sequence intubation: A review. Pediatr Emerg Care 2004;20:339 [PMID: 15123910].

Caples SM, Hubmayr RD: Respiratory monitoring tools in the intensive care unit. Curr Opin Crit Care. 2003;9:230 [PMID: 12771676].

Green KE, Peters JI: Pathophysiology of acute respiratory failure. Clin Chest Med 1994;15:1 [PMID: 8200186].

Hedenstierna G, Lattuada M: Gas exchange in the ventilated patient. Curr Opin Crit Care 2002;8:39 [PMID: 12205405].

Isono S: Developmental changes of pharyngeal airway patency: Implications for pediatric anesthesia. Paediatr Anaesth 2006;16:109 [PMID: 16430405].

Mehta NM, Arnold JH: Mechanical ventilation in children with acute respiratory failure. Curr Opin Crit Care 2004;10:7 [PMID: 15166843].

Sagarin MJ et al; National Emergency Airway Registry (NEAR) investigators: Rapid sequence intubation for pediatric emergency airway management. Pediatr Emerg Care 2002;18:417 [PMID: 12488834].

Shapiro MB et al: Respiratory failure. Conventional and high-tech support. Surg Clin North Am 2000;80:871 [PMID: 10897266].

Sigillito RJ, DeBlieux PM: Evaluation and initial management of the patient in respiratory distress. Emerg Med Clin North Am 2003;21:239 [PMID: 12793613].

MECHANICAL VENTILATION

The increased compliance of an infant's chest wall, the relative alveolar hypoplasia in early childhood, the small caliber of the airways, and the small tidal volumes of young children make mechanical ventilation of the pediatric patient challenging. The goals of mechanical ventilation are to facilitate the movement of gas into and out of the lungs (ventilation) and to improve oxygen uptake into the bloodstream (oxygenation). Modern mechanical ventilators can accomplish these objectives in a variety of ways. Depending on the mode of ventilation selected, the ventilator can deliver a machine-controlled breath (control ventilation), or can assist the patient's own spontaneous respiratory efforts (support ventilation), or can do both (mixed mode ventilation). Additionally, ventilator breaths can be delivered as a targeted tidal volume (volume ventilation) or as a targeted airway pressure (pressure ventilation). This section describes the modes of mechanical ventilation most commonly used in pediatric intensive care units (PICUs).

Pressure Ventilation

In pressure-controlled modes of ventilation, air flow begins at the start of the inspiratory cycle and continues until a preset airway pressure is reached. That airway pressure is then maintained until, at the end of the set inspiratory time, the exhalation valve on the ventilator opens and gas exits into the machine. Because airway pressure is the controlling variable with this mode of ventilation, changes in the compliance of the respiratory system will lead to fluctuations in the actual tidal volume delivered to the patient. The advantage of pressure-controlled ventilation lies primarily in the avoidance of high airway pressures that might cause lung injury or barotrauma, particularly in patients with fragile lung parenchyma, such as premature infants. The main disadvantage of pressure-controlled ventilation is the possibility of delivering either inadequate or excessive tidal volumes during periods of changing lung compliance, as described earlier.

Volume Ventilation

Volume-controlled ventilation is the most commonly used mode of mechanical ventilation in most PICUs. Volume ventilation delivers a preset tidal volume. Changes in lung compliance will lead to fluctuations in the airway pressure generated by the tidal volume. The main advantage of volume ventilation is more reliable delivery of the desired tidal volume and thus better control of ventilation. More reliable tidal volume delivery may also help prevent atelectasis due to hypoventilation. Disadvantages of volume ventilation include the risk of barotrauma from excessive airway pressures and difficulties overcoming leaks in the ventilator circuit. Older volume ventilators also suffered from a lack of continuous gas flow through the circuit, thus increasing the patient's work of breathing on spontaneous breaths. Most modern machines provide a continuous flow through the circuit and have improved triggering mechanisms to deliver the breaths in synchrony with the patient's demands.

Modes of Ventilation

Most modern ventilators can deliver either a pressure-controlled or a volume-controlled breath in several manners. **Control** modes deliver breaths at a selected rate and duration (inspiratory time) and can be targeted for either volume or pressure set by the clinician (as opposed to the patient). Spontaneous breaths are not assisted, and the patient's own respiratory efforts are not considered. **Synchronized intermittent mandatory ventilation** is a mode in which the rate, inspiratory time, and volume or pressure settings are set by the clinician. But the ventilator allows a window of time around each breath in which it waits for the patient to make an inspiratory effort. The machine breath is then synchronized with the patient's effort, to improve the comfort for patients who are breathing spontaneously. In **pressure-support ventilation,** the patient's own efforts are assisted by the delivery of gas flow to achieve a certain airway pressure. This mode of ventilation allows the patient to determine the rate and inspiratory time of breaths, thus improving patient comfort and decreasing the work of breathing. Perhaps the most common mode of ventilation in PICUs is **synchronized intermittent mandatory ventilation with pressure support,** a mixed mode allowing pressure-supported breaths between the synchronized machine breaths. Whether such mixed modes of ventilation provide any measurable advantage over single modes remains unclear.

Setting the Ventilator

When initiating mechanical ventilation, the clinician will vary the parameters according to the mode of ventilation selected. Volume-controlled modes of ventilation generally require a set tidal volume, inspiratory time, rate, and level of positive end-expiratory pressure (PEEP). A typical initial tidal volume is 8–10 mL/kg, as long as that volume does not cause excessive airway pressures. The inspiratory time is typically set at 1 second or 33% of the respiratory cycle, whichever is shorter. Rate can be adjusted to patient comfort and blood gas measurements, but generally patients starting on mechanical ventilation require full support at least initially with a rate of 20–30 breaths/min.

Pressure-controlled ventilation is set up in a similar fashion, although the sufficiency of the inspiratory pressure to provide an adequate tidal volume is assessed by observing the patient's chest rise and by measuring the returned tidal volume. Typically, patients without lung disease require pressures of 15–20 cm H_2O, and patients with respiratory illnesses initially require 20–30 cm H_2O pressure to provide adequate ventilation.

Positive End-Expiratory Pressure

The PEEP level is the final major setting required to initiate mechanical ventilation. All mechanical ventilators open their expiratory limbs at the end of inspiration until a preset pressure is achieved; this is the PEEP value. During ventilation of normal lungs, physiologic PEEP is in the range of 2–4 cm H_2O pressure. This pressure helps to prevent the end-expiratory collapse of open lung units, thus preventing atelectasis and shunting. In disease states such as pulmonary edema, pneumonia, or acute respiratory distress syndrome (ARDS), a higher PEEP may increase the patient's functional residual capacity, help to keep open previously collapsed alveoli, increase mean airway pressure, and improve oxygenation. Conceptually, it is important to remember that PEEP is an expiratory pressure. As a result, high PEEP levels do not open lung units in and of themselves, but rather prevent the collapse of units opened during lung inflation. Indeed, some evidence suggests that elevated levels of PEEP are most effective at improving oxygenation when used together with specific lung recruiting maneuvers. High levels of PEEP, although often valuable in improving oxygenation, may also cause CO_2 retention, barotrauma with resultant air leaks, decreased central venous return and resulting decline in cardiac output, and increased intracranial pressure (ICP). In general, PEEP should be set at 3–5 cm H_2O initially and titrated up to maintain adequate oxygenation at an acceptable fractional inspiratory oxygen (F_{IO_2}), while watching carefully for the adverse effects listed earlier.

Monitoring the Ventilated Patient

Ventilated patients must be monitored carefully for respiratory rate and activity, chest wall movement, and quality of breath sounds. Oxygenation should be measured either by ABGs or by continuous pulse oximetry. Ventilation should be assessed by blood gas analysis or by noninvasive means, such as transcutaneous monitoring or end-tidal sampling. Transcutaneous P_{O_2} or P_{CO_2} measurements are most useful with younger patients who have good skin perfusion, but they become problematic with poorly perfused or obese patients. $ETCO_2$ monitoring is done by placing a gas-sampling port on the endotracheal tube and analyzing expired gas for CO_2. This technique is more valuable for patients with large tidal volumes, lower respiratory rates, and without leaks around the endotracheal tube. In practice, $ETCO_2$ values may differ significantly from measured Pa_{CO_2} values and thus are most useful for following relative fluctuations in ventilation. Frequent, preferably continuous, blood pressure monitoring is also necessary for patients receiving oxygen at a high PEEP, given the risk of adverse cardiovascular effects.

Adjusting the Ventilator

Mechanical ventilation can assist with both ventilation (P_{CO_2}) and oxygenation (P_{O_2}). Ventilation is most closely associated with the delivered minute volume, or the tidal volume multiplied by the respiratory rate. Abnormal P_{CO_2} values can be most effectively addressed by changes in the respiratory rate or the tidal volume. Increased rate or tidal volume should increase minute volume and thus decrease P_{CO_2} levels; decreases in rate or tidal volume should act in the opposite fashion. In some circumstances, additional adjustments may also be necessary. For example, for patients with disease characterized by extensive alveolar collapse, increasing PEEP may improve ventilation by helping to keep open previously collapsed lung units. Also, for patients with disease characterized by significant airway obstruction, decreases in respiratory rate may allow more time for exhalation and improve ventilation despite an apparent decrease in the minute volume provided.

The variables most closely associated with oxygenation are the inspired oxygen concentration and the mean airway pressure during the respiratory cycle. Increases in inspired oxygen concentration will generally increase arterial oxygenation, unless right-to-left intracardiac or intrapulmonary shunting is a significant component of the patient's illness. Concentrations of inspired oxygen above 60–65%, however, may lead to hyperoxic lung injury. Patients with hypoxemic respiratory failure requiring those levels of oxygen or higher to maintain adequate arterial saturations should have their hypoxemia addressed by increases in mean airway pressure.

Mean airway pressure is affected by PEEP, peak inspiratory pressure, and inspiratory time. Increases in any one of those factors will increase mean airway pressure and should improve arterial oxygenation. It is important to bear in mind, however, that increases in mean airway pressure may also lead to decreases in cardiac output. In this circumstance, raising mean airway pressure may increase arterial oxygenation but actually compromise oxygen delivery to the tissues. For patients with severe hypoxemic respiratory failure, these tradeoffs highlight the need for careful monitoring by experienced personnel.

High-frequency oscillatory ventilation (HFOV) is an alternate mode of mechanical ventilation in which the ventilator provides very small, very rapid tidal volumes. Respiratory rates used during oscillatory ventilation typically range from 5–10 Hz (rates of 300–600 breaths/min) in most PICU patients. This mode of ventilation has been used successfully for neonates, older pediatric patients, and adults; and for diseases as diverse as pneumonia, pulmonary contusion, ARDS, and asthma. HFOV is increasingly used as initial therapy in severe, diffuse lung diseases, such as ARDS, which require high mean airway pressures to maintain oxygenation. The advantage of HFOV is that these high levels of mean airway pressure can be achieved without high peak inspiratory pressures or large tidal volumes, thus theoretically protecting the lung from ventilator-induced lung injury. Disadvantages of HFOV include general poor tolerance by patients who are not heavily sedated or paralyzed, the risk of cardiovascular compromise due to high mean airway pressures, and the risk of barotrauma in patients with heterogeneous lung disease. Although HFOV clearly may be useful for selected patients, it remains unclear whether HFOV provides a benefit compared with carefully managed conventional modes of ventilation.

Managing the Ventilated Patient

Patients undergoing mechanical ventilation require the same meticulous supportive care given to all PICU patients. Since mechanical ventilation is often frightening and uncomfortable for patients, leading to dyssynchrony with the ventilator and impaired ventilation and oxygenation, careful attention must be directed toward optimizing comfort and decreasing anxiety. Sedative-anxiolytics are typically provided as intermittent doses of benzodiazepines, with or without opioids. Some patients respond better to the steady state of sedation provided by continuous infusion of these agents, although oversedation of the ventilated patient may lead to longer durations of ventilation and difficulties with weaning from the ventilator.

For a patient with severe respiratory illness, even small movements by the patient may compromise ventilation and oxygenation. In such cases, muscle paralysis may facilitate oxygenation and ventilation. Nondepolarizing neuromuscular blocking agents are most commonly used for this purpose, given as intermittent doses or as continuous infusions. When muscle relaxants are given, extra care must be taken to ensure that levels of sedation are adequate, as many of the usual signs of patient discomfort are masked by the paralytics.

Cheifetz IM: Invasive and noninvasive pediatric mechanical ventilation. Respir Care 2003;48:442 [PMID: 12667269].

Flaatten H et al: Outcome after acute respiratory failure is more dependent on dysfunction in other vital organs than on the severity of the respiratory failure. Crit Care 2003;7:R72 [PMID: 12930559].

Frank JA, Matthay MA: Science review: Mechanisms of ventilator-induced injury. Crit Care 2003;7:233 [PMID: 12793874].

Gattinoni L et al: Physiologic rationale for ventilator setting in acute lung injury/acute respiratory distress syndrome patients. Crit Care Med 2003;31:S300 [PMID: 12682456].

Marini JJ, Gattinoni L: Ventilatory management of acute respiratory distress syndrome: A consensus of two. Crit Care Med 2004;32:250 [PMID: 14707588].

ACUTE RESPIRATORY DISTRESS SYNDROME

ARDS is a syndrome of acute respiratory failure characterized by increased pulmonary capillary permeability and pulmonary edema that results in refractory hypoxemia, decreased lung compliance, and bilateral diffuse alveolar infiltrates on chest radiography. Statistics of ARDS reflect one of the true successes of current ICU management, as mortality has decreased over the past decade from approximately 50–60% to less than 40%.

An international consensus conference was convened in 1997 to establish the current guidelines defining four diagnostic criteria for ARDS: (1) an underlying illness or injury that predisposes to ARDS; (2) bilateral infiltrates on chest radiograph; (3) an absence of evidence of heart failure, and in particular left ventricular (LV) failure; and, most importantly, (4) severe hypoxemic respiratory failure. Hypoxemia is assessed using the ratio of the arterial oxygen level (Pa_{O_2}) to the inspired oxygen concentration (FI_{O_2}). When the Pa_{O_2}:FI_{O_2} ratio is less than 200, and the other criteria are met, the case is defined as ARDS. When the Pa_{O_2}:FI_{O_2} ratio is between 200 and 300, and the other criteria are met, the case is defined as acute lung injury. This definition is debated, however, particularly since the current criteria do not include any assessment of the airway pressure needed to oxygenate the patient. Numerous other diagnostic systems have been proposed.

In addition, because the clinical disorder or disorders that led to the development of acute lung injury clearly influence the patient's prognosis for recovery, precise definition of the underlying problem is important. Although the average mortality in this population is 40%, the rate is dependent on the associated clinical disorder. Mortality can be as high as 90% among adult ARDS patients with underlying liver failure, and less than 10% among pediatric ARDS associated with respiratory syncytial virus infection. The development of multisystem organ failure is a frequent complicating factor in the care of the patient with ARDS, and the failure of organs outside the lung has a large role in determining the prognosis. In fact, nonpulmonary organ failure is the leading cause of death in the most recent studies of adult or pediatric ARDS patients.

▶ Clinical Presentation & Pathophysiology

ARDS may be precipitated by a variety of insults (Table 13–6), of which infection is the most common. Despite the diversity of causes, the clinical presentation is remarkably similar in most cases. ARDS can be divided roughly into four clinical phases (Table 13–7). In the earliest phase, the patient may have dyspnea and tachypnea with a relatively normal P_{O_2} and hyperventilation-induced respiratory alkalosis. No significant abnormalities are noted on physical or radiologic examination of the chest. Experimental studies suggest that neutrophils accumulate in the lungs at this stage and that their products damage lung endothelium.

Over the next few hours, hypoxemia increases and respiratory distress becomes clinically apparent, with cyanosis, tachycardia, irritability, and dyspnea. Radiographic evidence of early parenchymal change is the appearance of "fluffy" alveolar infiltrates initially appearing in dependent lung fields, indicative of pulmonary edema. The edema fluid typically has

Table 13–6. Acute respiratory distress syndrome risk factors.

Direct Lung Injury	Indirect Lung Injury
Aspiration of gastric contents	Sepsis
Hydrocarbon ingestion or aspiration	Shock
	Pancreatitis
Inhalation injury (heat or toxin)	Burns
Pulmonary contusion	Trauma
Pneumonia	Fat embolism
Near-drowning	Drug overdoses (including aspirin, opioids, barbiturates, tricyclic antidepressants)
	Transfusion of blood products

a high concentration of protein (75–95% of plasma protein concentration), which is characteristic of an increased permeability-type edema and differentiates it from cardiogenic or hydrostatic pulmonary edema. Protein in the air spaces inactivates surfactant, which, combined with damage to type 2 alveolar pneumocytes, leads to a marked deficiency in surfactant content in the lung. As a result, the lung is particularly prone to collapse and to shearing injuries due to the high surface tension required to open collapsed alveoli.

Alveolar epithelial injury in ARDS lowers the threshold for alveolar edema formation and impairs gas exchange. The functional integrity of the alveolar epithelium, as measured by the ability of the alveoli to clear liquid out of the air spaces, has prognostic importance in ARDS. Those patients who still show evidence of functional alveolar liquid clearance mechanisms during the first day of their illness have a much higher survival rate than those with evidence of severe epithelial impairment.

Pulmonary hypertension, decrease in lung compliance, and increase in airway resistance are also commonly noted. Clinical studies suggest that airway resistance may be increased in 50% of patients with ARDS.

Computed tomography studies of adult patients in the acute phases of ARDS demonstrate heterogeneous collapse of the lung, with typical areas of dependent consolidation, overinflation in the upper zones, and relatively small areas of normally expanded lung. These findings suggest that the lung in ARDS is best viewed as "small" rather than stiff, prompting a shift toward ventilating these patients with smaller tidal volumes and a tolerance for the relative hypercarbia that may ensue. In addition, a large body of research has shown that ventilation with large tidal volumes and low PEEP levels allows a pattern of cyclic alveolar overdistention and collapse, which causes a lung injury histologically similar to ARDS, even in normal lungs. This phenomenon is now called ventilator-induced lung injury. Taken together, these findings have given rise to the view that the acute phase of ARDS can best be treated by rerecruiting those areas of dependent collapse and

Table 13–7. Pathophysiologic changes of modern acute respiratory distress syndrome (low-pressure pulmonary edema).

	Symptoms	Laboratory Findings	Pathophysiology
Phase 1 (early changes)			
Normal radiograph	Dyspnea, tachypnea, normal chest examination	Mild pulmonary hypertension, normoxemic or mild hypoxemia, hypercapnia.	Neutrophil sequestration, no clear tissue damage
Phase 2 (onset of parenchymal changes)[a]			
Patchy alveolar infiltrates beginning in dependent lung No perivascular cuffs (unless a component of high pressure edema is present) Normal heart size	Dyspnea, tachypnea, cyanosis, tachycardia, coarse rales	Pulmonary hypertension, normal wedge pressure, increased lung permeability, increased lung water, increasing shunt, progressive decrease in compliance, moderate to severe hypoxemia.	Neutrophil infiltration, vascular congestion, fibrin strands, platelet clumps, alveolar septal edema, intra-alveolar protein, white cells, type I epithelial damage
Phase 3 (acute respiratory failure with progression, 2–10 d)			
Diffuse alveolar infiltrates Air bronchograms Decreased lung volume No bronchovascular cuffs Normal heart	Tachypnea, tachycardia, hyperdynamic state, sepsis syndrome, signs of consolidation, diffuse rhonchi	Phase 2 changes persist. Progression of abnormalities, increasing shunt fraction, further decrease in compliance, increased minute ventilation, impaired oxygen extraction of hemoglobin.	Increased interstitial and alveolar inflammatory exudate with neutrophil and mononuclear cells, type II cell proliferation, beginning fibroblast proliferation, thromboembolic occlusion
Phase 4 (pulmonary fibrosis, pneumonia with progression, > 10 d)[b]			
Persistent diffuse infiltrates Superimposed new pneumonic infiltrates Recurrent pneumothorax Normal heart size Enlargement with cor pulmonale	Symptoms as above, recurrent sepsis, evidence of multiple organ system failure	Phase 3 changes persist. Recurrent pneumonia, progressive lung restriction, impaired tissue oxygenation, impaired oxygen extraction. Multiple organ system failure.	Type II cell hyperplasia, interstitial thickening; infiltration of lymphocytes, macrophages, fibroblasts; loculated pneumonia or interstitial fibrosis; medial thickening and remodeling of arterioles

[a]The process is readily reversible at this stage if the initiating factor is controlled.
[b]Multiple organ system failure is common. The mortality rate is greater than 80% at this stage, since resolution is more difficult.
Modified slightly and reproduced, with permission, from Demling RH: Adult respiratory distress syndrome: Current concepts. New Horizons 1993;1:388.

minimizing the stretch-induced injury, or volutrauma, in the nondependent areas of the lung. This approach has been termed the open-lung strategy and has been the subject of intense scrutiny in recent years (see below).

The subacute phase of ARDS (5–10 days after lung injury) is characterized by type 2 pneumocyte and fibroblast proliferation in the interstitium of the lung. This results in decreased lung volumes and signs of consolidation that are noted clinically and radiographically. Worsening of the hypoxemia with an increasing shunt fraction, as well as a further decrease in lung compliance, are noted. Some patients develop an accelerated fibrosing alveolitis in which fibroblasts and collagen formation in the interstitium are markedly increased. The mechanisms responsible for these changes are unclear. Current investigation centers on the role of growth and differentiation factors, such as transforming growth factor-β and platelet-derived growth factor released by resident and nonresident lung cells such as alveolar macrophages, mast cells, neutrophils, alveolar type 2 cells, and fibroblasts.

During the chronic phase of ARDS (10–14 days after lung injury), fibrosis, emphysema, and pulmonary vascular obliteration occur. During this phase of the illness, oxygenation defects generally improve, and the lung becomes more fragile and susceptible to barotrauma. Air leak is common among patients still ventilated with high levels of airway pressure at this late stage in their illness. Also, patients have increased amounts of dead space, and difficulties with ventilation are common. Airway compliance remains low, perhaps because of ongoing pulmonary fibrosis and insufficient surfactant production.

Secondary infections are common in the subacute and chronic phases of ARDS and significantly influence the outcome. The mechanisms responsible for increased host susceptibility to infection during this phase are not well understood.

Mortality in the late phase of ARDS exceeds 80%. Death is usually caused by multiorgan failure and systemic hemodynamic instability rather than by hypoxemia.

▶ Treatment

A. Monitoring

Multiorgan system monitoring is mandatory for patients with ARDS. ABG analysis is required for accurate assessment of oxygenation and ventilation and for the rational titration of ventilator strategies that may have profound adverse effects. Hemodynamic monitoring should include, at a minimum, central venous pressure (CVP) measurements to help determine the level of cardiac preload, and an indwelling arterial catheter for continuous blood pressure measurements and ABG sampling. For patients with severe disease or concurrent cardiac dysfunction, consideration can be given to pulmonary artery catheterization to help with fluid management and to allow assessment of mixed venous blood saturation as an index of overall tissue oxygenation. Obtaining chest films daily is important for patients receiving vigorous support because severe ARDS is associated with a 40–60% incidence of air leaks. Since secondary infections are common and increase mortality rates strikingly, surveillance for infection is important, requiring appropriate cultures and following the temperature curve and white blood cell count. Renal, liver, and gastrointestinal (GI) function should be watched closely because of the great likelihood of multiorgan dysfunction.

B. Fluid Management

Given the increases in pulmonary capillary permeability in ARDS, pulmonary edema accumulation is likely with any elevation in pulmonary hydrostatic pressures. In this setting, most clinicians reduce intravascular volume to the lowest level that is still compatible with an adequate cardiac output and adequate oxygen delivery to the tissues.

C. Hemodynamic Support

Hemodynamic support is directed toward increasing perfusion and oxygen delivery. In those circumstances when volume expansion is necessary to improve oxygen delivery, this can best be achieved by giving packed red blood cells to maintain the hematocrit between 35% and 40%, and by giving colloid or crystalloid solutions to nonanemic volume-depleted patients. Inotropes should be used as needed to optimize oxygen delivery to the tissues.

D. Ventilatory Support

In addition to the basic principles of ventilator management described earlier (see section on Adjusting the Ventilator), current ventilatory management of ARDS is directed at the rerecruitment of areas of dependent alveolar collapse and the protection of noncollapsed areas from overdistention. Since an FIO_2 greater than 60% over 24 hours can cause additional injury to the lung, mean airway pressure should be increased to provide an adequate PaO_2 (> 55 mm Hg) at an FIO_2 of 60% or less. In general, this can be accomplished by incremental increases in PEEP every 15–30 minutes until adequate oxygenation is achieved or until a limiting side effect of the PEEP is reached. Ventilation with high levels of PEEP acts by helping to prevent dependent collapse of edematous lung units. PEEP levels of 12–14 cm H_2O are not unusual, and levels as high as 20–25 cm H_2O have been used successfully in these patients. Before increasing PEEP significantly, the physician should optimize conditions by making sure that the patient's intravascular volume is appropriate, the endotracheal tube does not leak, and the patient is heavily sedated and paralyzed.

The actual mode of ventilation employed (volume or pressure) with an ARDS patient is probably unimportant. However, recent work from a large multicenter trial sponsored by the National Institutes of Health suggests that the tidal volumes used may be important. Using a PEEP strategy similar to that described in the preceding paragraph, the investigators compared the effects of a low (6 mL/kg) tidal volume versus a normal (12 mL/kg) tidal volume in 861 adult ARDS patients. Those patients ventilated with the lower tidal volume demonstrated fewer extrapulmonary organ failures and an overall 25% decrease in mortality. In keeping with these findings and with experimental data demonstrating ventilator-induced lung injury at alveolar pressures greater than 30 cm H_2O, we suggest that current practice for pediatric ARDS patients should consist of ventilation with tidal volumes in the 6- to 8-mL/kg range, or at least with tidal volumes small enough to keep alveolar pressures below 30–35 cm H_2O.

E. Other Therapies

As previously described, HFOV is an increasingly popular technique that has been used successfully in pediatric patients with ARDS. When used as part of a strategy of aggressive increases in mean airway pressure to rerecruit deflated areas of the lung and to prevent cyclic overdistention and collapse, HFOV is a physiologically rational approach to this illness. It has not yet been determined whether HFOV provides additional benefits compared with open-lung strategy ventilation using conventional ventilator modes.

Prone positioning is a technique of changing the patient's position in bed from supine to prone, with the goal of allowing postural drainage and improving ventilation of collapsed dependent lung units. This technique often dramatically improves oxygenation, particularly for patients early in the course of ARDS. The oxygenation improvements are often not sustained, however, necessitating repeated position changes to maintain the effect. Whether prone positioning contributes to improved outcomes for patients with ARDS remains uncertain.

Based on the ability of inhaled **nitric oxide** (iNO) to reduce pulmonary artery pressure and to improve the matching of ventilation with perfusion without producing systemic vasodilation, iNO has been proposed as a beneficial therapy for ARDS. Several recent multicenter trials of iNO in the treatment of ARDS, both in adults and in children, have shown acute improvements in oxygenation in subsets of patients but no significant improvement in overall survival. As a result, the current role of iNO in the treatment of ARDS remains unclear. Additional studies are now focusing on the anti-inflammatory role (by reducing neutrophil adhesion and activation) iNO may play in ARDS. Studies to evaluate the combined effects of several of these alternative therapies are also being planned.

Surfactant replacement therapy has been tried with some success in patients with ARDS. In some instances surfactant replacement improves lung compliance and oxygenation, and hastens weaning from mechanical ventilation. In randomized trials of surfactant replacement, there were no differences in outcome (death, length of ventilation, or hospitalization), but there was some evidence of decreased inflammation. A multicenter trial of surfactant treatment for pediatric ARDS is currently in progress.

The use of **corticosteroids** to modulate the inflammatory component of ARDS remains controversial, with many conflicting studies. Early trials demonstrated that, when administered at high dose to cure or to prevent ARDS, glucocorticoids provided no survival benefit and even may have favored life-threatening infections. More recent clinical data on low-dose, prolonged glucocorticoid treatment of ARDS have shown significant improvement in inflammation and lung physiology with a favorable benefit-risk profile A large multicenter trial of methylprednisolone in the late phase of ARDS (> 7 days after onset) in adults showed no difference in mortality rates compared with placebo, but an increased number of ventilator-free and shock-free days during the first 28 days, in association with improved oxygenation, respiratory-system compliance, and blood pressure with fewer days of vasopressor therapy. As compared with placebo, methylprednisolone did not increase the rate of infectious complications but was associated with a higher rate of neuromuscular weakness. In addition, starting steroids more than 2 weeks after the onset of ARDS was associated with an increased risk of death. A more recent multicenter trial of early and prolonged (2 weeks at full dose; then tapered off > 2 weeks) treatment with low-dose methylprednisolone (1 mg/kg/d) revealed that steroid treatment down-regulated systemic inflammation and was associated with significant improvement in pulmonary and extrapulmonary organ dysfunction, and with reduction in duration of mechanical ventilation and ICU length of stay. These recent studies suggest, with some exceptions, that early steroid treatment could be beneficial for ARDS patients; however, no definitive studies have been performed in the pediatric population.

Extracorporeal membrane oxygenation (ECMO) has been used in pediatric patients with severe ARDS. In older studies, patients who received ECMO had better survival rates than did control subjects. ECMO has not been studied in comparison with current conventional ventilation strategies. In addition, recent improvements in outcome for pediatric ARDS patients receiving conventional therapies have made the role of ECMO less clear and have made further prospective randomized studies of ECMO difficult to complete. For now, ECMO remains a rescue therapy for patients with severe ARDS unresponsive to other modalities.

F. Follow-Up

Information regarding the long-term outcome of pediatric patients with ARDS remains limited. One report of 10 children followed 1–4 years after severe ARDS showed three still symptomatic and seven with hypoxemia at rest. Until further information is available, all patients with a history of ARDS need close follow-up of pulmonary function.

Acute Respiratory Distress Syndrome Network: Ventilation with lower tidal volumes as compared with traditional tidal volumes for acute lung injury and the acute respiratory distress syndrome. N Engl J Med 2000;342:1301 [PMID: 10793162].

Anderson MR: Update on pediatric acute respiratory distress syndrome. Respir Care 2003;48:261 [PMID: 1266727].

Burns SM: Mechanical ventilation of patients with acute respiratory distress syndrome and patients requiring weaning; the evidence guiding practice. Crit Care Nurse 2005;25:14 [PMID: 16034030].

Calfee CS, Matthay MA: Recent advances in mechanical ventilation. Am J Med 2005;118:584 [PMID: 15922687].

Froese AB, Kinsella JP: High-frequency oscillatory ventilation: Lessons from the neonatal/pediatric experience. Crit Care Med. 2005;33(Suppl):S115 [PMID: 15753716].

Gattinoni L et al: Monitoring of pulmonary mechanics in acute respiratory distress syndrome to titrate therapy. Curr Opin Crit Care 2005;11:252 [PMID: 15928475].

Lewandowski K: Extracorporeal membrane oxygenation for severe acute respiratory failure. Crit Care 2000;4:156 [PMID: 11094500].

Matthay MA, Zimmerman GA: Acute lung injury and the acute respiratory distress syndrome: four decades of inquiry into pathogenesis and rational management. Am J Respir Cell Mol Biol 2005;33:319 [PMID: 16272252].

Meduri GU et al: Methylprednisolone infusion in early severe ARDS: Results of a randomized controlled trial. Chest. 2007;131:954 [PMID: 17426195].

Priestley MA, Helfaer MA: Approaches in the management of acute respiratory failure in children. Curr Opin Pediatr 2004;16:293 [PMID: 15167016].

Santos CC et al: Bench-to-bedside review: Biotrauma and modulation of the innate immune response. Crit Care 2005;9:280 [PMID: 15987418].

Shorr AF et al: D-Dimer correlates with proinflammatory cytokine levels and outcomes in critically ill patients. Chest 2002;121:1262 [PMID: 11948062].

Sokol J et al: Inhaled nitric oxide for acute hypoxemic respiratory failure in children and adults. Cochrane Database Syst Rev 2000;(4):CD002787 [PMID: 11914763].

Steinberg KP et al: Efficacy and safety of corticosteroids for persistent acute respiratory distress syndrome. N Engl J Med. 2006;354:1671 [PMID: 16625008].

Vincent JL: New management strategies in ARDS: Immunomodulation. Crit Care Clin 2002;18:69 [PMID: 11910733].

INDICATIONS FOR CENTRAL VENOUS & ARTERIAL CANNULATION

Placement of catheters into the central venous or arterial circulation may be justified for continuous assessment of intravascular volume or cardiac function; blood drawing for lab work; or administration of volume, drugs, or hyperalimentation. One should always weigh the risks of bleeding, infection, and clotting against the expected benefits before placing any indwelling catheter.

General Rules for Cannulation of the Venous System

1. Perform a "time-out" before beginning. Confirm out loud with the bedside nurse, the identity of the patient, the procedure needed, and the intended site for line placement.
2. Set up and examine all equipment needed before getting started. Use of a limited number of kits and equipment will provide greater consistency and success.
3. Properly position the patient.
4. Apply EMLA cream (eutectic mixture of local anesthetics, lidocaine 2.5% and prilocaine 2.5%) to the area of puncture (45 minutes before the procedure) or infiltrate with local anesthetic before prepping the skin. Sedation is often necessary but should be performed by a qualified person.
5. The remainder of the procedure should occur under aseptic technique (including gown, mask, and hair cover for operator and assistant).
6. Sterilize and drape the area around the point of entry.
7. When searching for the vessel, make straight passes while maintaining slight negative pressure. Advance and withdraw the needle at the same speed. Frequently, the blood return will occur during withdrawal.
8. Once there is free flow of venous blood into the syringe, remove the syringe without moving the needle, and if using the Seldinger technique, pass the J wire through the needle. When appropriate (subclavian and internal jugular vein cannulations), watch the electrocardiogram for arrhythmias, because they frequently occur when the J wire touches the right side of the heart.
9. Withdraw the needle over the J wire and clean the wire of blood.
10. If using a 5F or larger catheter, make a small nick with a No. 11 blade at the point where the J wire enters the skin. Dilate central veins by passing the dilator over the J wire into the vein. Remove the dilator (skip this step for arterial cannulation) and pass the intravascular catheter over the J wire. As you advance the catheter toward the entry site into the skin be sure the wire is always visible, or protrudes out the end of the catheter, to prevent the wire becoming lodged within the vessel.
11. With the catheters in place, remove the wire.
12. Check to make sure that blood can be drawn and flushed easily through each port of the new line. Withdraw blood through a syringe containing saline before flushing to prevent introduction of air bubbles.
13. Suture the line in place.
14. Verify the position of the line on radiograph.

Points of Entry for Venous Line Placement

A. External Jugular Vein

Place a soft cloth roll beneath the patient's shoulder and turn the head to the contralateral side (Figure 13–2). The Valsalva maneuver, Trendelenburg position, and occlusion of the vessel at the clavicular level are ways of temporarily increasing jugular distention and visibility.

To overcome the problems of this vessel's mobility and thick wall, apply cephalic retraction of the skin over the vessel superior to the point of needle entry. Maintain gentle negative pressure in the syringe attached to the needle as it is advanced toward the vessel. Needle entry into the vessel lumen is usually signaled by a change in resistance followed by appearance of venous blood in the hub of the needle. Remove the syringe without moving the needle and pass a soft J wire into the vessel lumen. Remove the needle and pass the central line over the J wire.

B. Internal Jugular Vein

Once the patient has been prepped, draped, and positioned as shown in Figure 13–3, feel for the trachea halfway between

External jugular vein
Sternocleidomastoid muscle

30°

▲ **Figure 13–2.** External jugular vein technique.

▲ **Figure 13–3.** **A:** The internal jugular vein and its relationship to the surrounding anatomy. **B:** Technique of anterior internal jugular cannulation.

the angle of the jaw and the suprasternal notch and then feel lateral to the trachea for the carotid pulse. Just lateral to the carotid pulse, at a 30-degree angle from horizontal, insert a finder needle (25-gauge), aiming between the ipsilateral nipple and shoulder. Once venous return is established, remove the finder needle and repeat the procedure with the appropriate-size larger needle.

C. Subclavian Vein

After the patient has been prepped, draped, and positioned (Figure 13–4), move the needle flat along the chest, enter-

ing along the inferior edge of the clavicle just lateral to the midclavicular line and aiming for the suprasternal notch. Once venous return is established, use the Seldinger technique.

D. Femoral Vein

With the patient's leg slightly abducted (Figure 13–5), find the femoral artery 3–4 cm below the inguinal ligament. The femoral vein is just medial and parallel to the femoral artery. Insert the needle at a 30- to 45-degree angle. Once venous return is established, use the Seldinger technique.

▲ **Figure 13–4.** Subclavian artery. **A:** Anatomy. **B:** Technique.

A

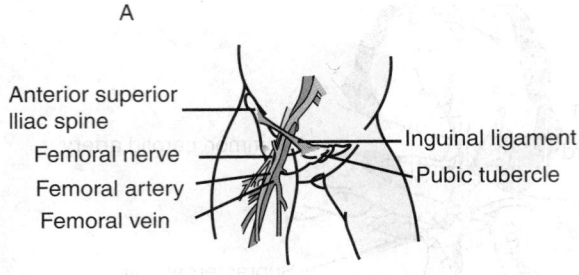

Anterior superior
Iliac spine
Femoral nerve
Femoral artery
Femoral vein

Inguinal ligament
Pubic tubercle

B

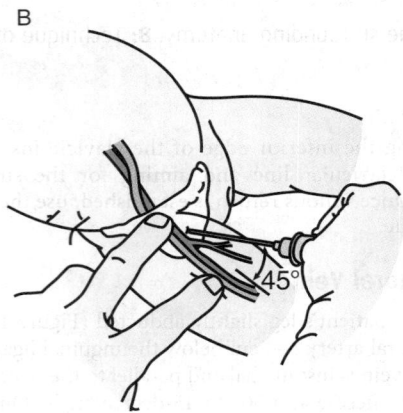

45°

▲ **Figure 13–5.** Femoral vein. **A:** Anatomy. **B:** Technique.

E. Antecubital Vein

Peripherally inserted catheter lines (2.8–4 F) are long, soft, Silastic, styletted catheters most commonly threaded from an antecubital vessel to the right atrium. These lines are not difficult to insert and are easy to dress and keep clean. They are suited for long-term use because they are tolerable for the patient, good for infusion of hyperalimentation and drugs, and less thrombogenic. In general, they are not suitable for obtaining blood for laboratory analysis.

General Rules for Cannulation of the Arterial System

The Seldinger technique can be applied for arterial tree cannulation as well. Most arteries can be cannulated percutaneously.

1. Puncture the skin at the insertion site to eliminate any drag or resistance on the catheter advancement.
2. Insert the cannula at a 30-degree angle to the skin surface, advancing at a slow rate toward the arterial pulse. Watch the hub of the cannula for a flash of arterial blood.

3. When arterial flash is seen, lower the catheter to a 10-degree angle with the surface of the skin and advance the catheter into the lumen of the artery. If successful, pulsatile arterial flow will continue into the catheter.
4. Hold the catheter while removing the needle stylet. Arterial blood will pulse out of the catheter if the tip is in the arterial lumen.
5. Advance the catheter into the lumen; attach a syringe containing normal saline with 1 U/mL of heparin; aspirate to make certain that there are no bubbles; and then gently flush the catheter.
6. If arterial flow into the needle stylet stops during catheter advancement, advance this unit an additional centimeter. Remove the needle stylet and place it on a sterile surface. Pull the catheter out slowly. When the tip of the catheter flips into the arterial lumen, the pulsatile arterial blood flow is seen. Rotate the catheter to ensure that the catheter is free within the vessel lumen, then advance the remainder of the catheter length into the vessel.
7. Suture the catheter in place while ensuring that the arterial trace is not damped.
8. Dress the insertion site with sterile gauze, and tape it to the skin.

Points of Entry for Arterial Line Placement

Always consider whether collateral arterial blood is flowing to the structures distal to the insertion point. The Allen test must be done prior to radial or ulnar artery cannulation.

Arterial sites, listed in order of preference, include:

1. Radial artery (nondominant arm first)
2. Femoral artery (morbidity is the same as for the radial artery beyond the newborn period)
3. Posterior tibial artery
4. Dorsalis pedis artery
5. Ulnar artery (if distal radial filling is present in that hand)
6. Axillary artery
7. Brachial artery (poor collateral flow, used only during cardiac surgery in newborn-sized patients with arterial access limitations)

Final Considerations

1. Patient benefit should outweigh any risks from central venous or arterial cannulation.
2. Coagulation status of the patient at the time of placement and throughout the time of use must be considered, because deep venous and arterial thrombus formation is partially related to the patient's coagulation status.
3. The incidence of catheter colonization and infection increases if central venous and arterial lines are left in for more than 6 days.

Chuan W et al: A randomized-controlled study of ultrasound prelocation vs anatomical landmark-guided cannulation of the internal jugular vein in infants and children. Paediatr Anaesth 2005;15:733 [PMID: 16101703].

Odetola FO et al: Nosocomial catheter-related bloodstream infections in a pediatric intensive care unit: Risk and rates associated with various intravascular technologies. Pediatr Crit Care Med 2003;4:432 [PMID: 14525637].

O'Grady NP et al: Guidelines for the prevention of intravascular catheter-related infections. The Hospital Infection Control Practices Advisory Committee, Center for Disease Control and Prevention, U.S. Pediatrics 2002;110:e51 [PMID: 12415057].

Stovroff M, Teague WG: Intravenous access in infants and children. Pediatr Clin North Am 1998;45:1373 [PMID: 9889758].

BRAIN INJURY & CEREBRAL EDEMA

Intracranial hypertension is a common feature of many illnesses treated in the PICU (Table 13–8). The early signs and symptoms of intracranial hypertension (Table 13–9) tend to be nonspecific. The classic Cushing triad of bradycardia, hypertension, and apnea occurs late and is often incomplete in children.

Accurate assessment and treatment of elevations in ICP requires an understanding of the basic pathophysiology of intracranial hypertension and of the current evidence supporting the various treatment options. Most of our understanding and approach to treatment is based on studies of patients with traumatic brain injuries. Whether those concepts are directly relevant to the pathophysiologic processes involved in more global CNS injuries, such as hypoxia and metabolic disorders, remains a matter of debate.

Table 13–8. Pediatric illnesses commonly associated with intracranial hypertension.

Diffuse processes
Trauma
Hypoxic-ischemic
Near-drowning
Cardiorespiratory arrest
Infectious
Encephalitis
Meningitis
Metabolic
Reye syndrome
Liver failure
Inborn error metabolism
Toxic
Lead
Vitamin A
Focal processes
Trauma
Hypoxic-ischemic
Trauma
Stroke
Infectious
Abscess
Mass lesions
Tumors
Hematomas

Within the constraints of a closed skull, an enlargement of brain tissue, an increased volume of cerebrospinal fluid (CSF), or an increased volume of blood (or the presence of a space-occupying lesion such as a tumor or an abscess) will reduce the size of the other compartments or increase pressure. The factors contributing to intracranial hypertension can be understood by considering each of these three primary compartments.

The brain occupies about 80% of the volume of the skull. Apart from solid tumors, increases in the brain compartment are generally a result of cerebral edema. Cerebral edema can be divided into three forms: vasogenic, hydrostatic, and cytotoxic. **Vasogenic** edema occurs in areas of inflamed tissue characterized by increased capillary permeability, and is most typical around CNS tumors, abscesses, and infarcts. This form of edema is thought to be at least partially responsive to corticosteroid therapy. **Hydrostatic,** or interstitial, edema is a result of elevated CSF hydrostatic pressures. It occurs primarily in lesions associated with obstruction to CSF flow, and in a typical periventricular distribution. This form of edema is best treated by CSF drainage. The third form of cerebral edema, **cytotoxic** edema, is the most common of the three forms seen in the PICU and is, unfortunately, the least easily treated. Cytotoxic edema occurs as a result of direct injury to brain cells, often leading to irreversible cell swelling and death. This form of cerebral edema is typical of traumatic brain injuries as well as hypoxic-ischemic injuries and metabolic disease.

CSF occupies an estimated 10% of the intracranial space. Intracranial hypertension due primarily to increases in CSF volume (eg, hydrocephalus, primary or secondary) is generally easily diagnosed by computed tomography scan and easily treated with appropriate drainage and shunting.

Cerebral blood volume comprises the final 10% of the intracranial space. Changes in cerebral blood volume generally result from alterations in vascular diameter in response to local metabolic demands or to local vascular pressures—

Table 13–9. Signs and symptoms of intracranial hypertension in children.

Early
Poor feeding, vomiting
Irritability, lethargy
Seizures
Hypertension
Late
Coma
Decerebrate responses
Cranial nerve palsies
Abnormal respirations
Bradycardia
Hypertension
Apnea

so-called metabolic and pressure autoregulation. These physiologic responses are the means by which the CNS circulation regulates and maintains adequate blood flow to the brain. Given the difficulty in effectively treating cytotoxic brain swelling and the relative rarity of uncomplicated CSF obstructive lesions in the PICU, most of the current therapies aimed at controlling intracranial hypertension rely on altering cerebral blood volume.

Several factors interact to control cerebral blood volume via the autoregulatory responses of the cerebral vasculature. The rate of cerebral metabolism is an important determinant of cerebral blood volume. High metabolic rates lead to vasodilation and increased blood volume, whereas low metabolic rates allow the vessels to constrict and reduce blood flow and blood volume. Partial pressure of carbon dioxide is another important determinant of cerebral blood volume, as elevations in blood Pco_2 lead to cerebral vasodilation and decreases in Pco_2 lead to vasoconstriction. Finally, cerebral blood volume is linked to cerebral blood flow through the phenomenon of pressure autoregulation. As shown in Figure 13–6, at low systolic blood pressures the cerebral vessels are maximally dilated and blood flow is only increased by increasing blood pressure. Within the range of autoregulation, the cerebral vessels attempt to maintain a constant flow rate over a range of blood pressures; increased blood pressure results in vasoconstriction, in turn reducing cerebral blood volume. Once the cerebral vessels are maximally constricted, continued increases in pressure may further increase cerebral blood flow and volume.

Treatments for intracranial hypertension are largely derived from experience with traumatic brain injury. An important concept in this regard is that of a "primary" as opposed to a "secondary" brain injury. In this context, primary injury refers to direct damage to brain tissue resulting from the original insult to the CNS, such as physical damage from trauma. This injury is complete before the patient reaches the health care system. As the injured brain swells due to cytotoxic edema, intracranial hypertension develops, potentially limiting cerebral blood flow to portions of the brain and leading to extension of the initial injury (ie, secondary injury). Medical treatment of the patient with intracranial hypertension aims to prevent or reduce secondary injuries.

The primary goal of treatment is to optimize perfusion of areas of the brain that are salvageable. This can be accomplished by reducing ICP and by ensuring adequate perfusion. Rational guidance of treatment requires invasive monitoring so that it can be effectively titrated. Although a complete discussion of the indications for ICP monitoring is beyond the scope of this chapter, the topic can be briefly summarized with the suggestion that an ICP monitor be used for patients at significant risk for intracranial hypertension, in whom the treatment of elevated CNS pressures is planned. Monitoring other parameters of CNS oxygen delivery (ie, blood pressure, ABGs, and intravascular volume) generally mandates the placement of arterial and central venous catheters. Little evidence exists to support the utility of ICP-directed therapies in conditions associated with global CNS injuries (eg, anoxic brain injuries).

Maintenance of adequate cardiac output and oxygen delivery to the CNS is critical in treating patients with intracranial hypertension. Studies in both adult and pediatric head injury patients show that even a single episode of hypotension or arterial hypoxemia is associated with a marked increase in mortality rates. Although studies have not delineated clear age-appropriate thresholds for blood pressure and PaO_2 in this setting, a rational starting point for therapy would seem to be maintenance of an adequate circulating blood volume, a blood pressure at least well within the normal range for age, and an PaO_2 of at least 60 mm Hg. Hypotension and hypoxemia should be treated urgently and aggressively.

In general, the threshold at which treatment for intracranial hypertension should be started is in the range of 15–20 cm H_2O pressure. Above this pressure, very minor increases in the volume of the intracranial contents lead to large increases in ICP (Figure 13–7). Initial therapy for intracranial hypertension should always consist of securing the airway and providing adequate sedation. Additional measures would include the removal of any mass lesions (eg, tumors, abscesses, and hematomas) and adequate ventricular drainage. Further efforts are then largely directed at reducing cerebral blood volume.

Osmotic diuretics such as mannitol or 3% normal saline are often used to treat intracranial hypertension. They are thought to act first by decreasing blood viscosity, allowing for increased flow and subsequent autoregulatory vasoconstriction. The osmotic effects on the cells and interstitium of the brain prolong the reduction in ICP. Although mannitol therapy has never been subjected to a placebo-controlled trial, it

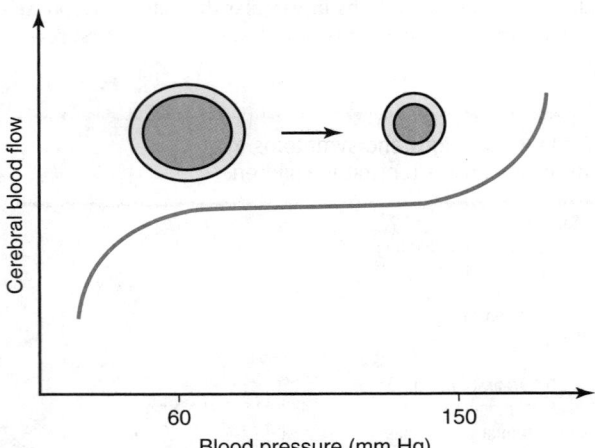

▲ **Figure 13–6.** Pressure autoregulation in the cerebral vasculature.

▲ **Figure 13–7.** Compliance curve of the skull with changing volume of intracranial contents.

leads to better outcomes than barbiturate therapy in patients with refractory ICP elevations. Current guidelines suggest the use of mannitol in doses of 0.25–0.5 g/kg for intracranial hypertension unresponsive to sedation. Renal failure due to acute tubular necrosis can be a treatment-limiting side effect, particularly if serum osmolarity is allowed to rise above 320 mmol and intravascular volume depletion occurs. Continuous infusion of 3% saline at 0.1–1 ml/kg/h can alternatively be used to increase osmolarity, using the minimum dose to achieve ICP of less than 20 mm Hg. Serum sodium and osmolarity should be followed and should generally not exceed sodium of 160 mEq/L or serum osmolarity of 360 mOsm/L.

Controlled ventilation is recommended for mild to moderate intracranial hypertension, maintaining P_{CO_2} of 30–35 mm Hg. Hyperventilation—long a mainstay in the treatment of intracranial hypertension—is controversial and only used in emergent situations involving patients with acute ICP elevations unresponsive to other measures, including sedation, paralysis, ventricular drainage, and osmotic diuretics. Although acutely effective in causing cerebral vasoconstriction, hyperventilation leads to much larger decreases in blood flow than in blood volume, such that hyperventilation to the point necessary to control ICP may actually compromise CNS perfusion and lead to worsened secondary injury. This concept has been confirmed by studies showing worse outcomes in head-injured patients consistently hyperventilated to a P_{CO_2} of 25 mm Hg or less. Due to the risks of worsened CNS ischemia, monitoring cerebral perfusion by blood flow studies or jugular bulb saturation is recommended for patients undergoing extreme hyperventilation.

The use of barbiturates in this setting is based on their suppression of cerebral metabolism and the subsequent metabolic autoregulatory effects on cerebral blood volume. Although effective in many instances for ICP elevations, these agents are potent cardiac depressants, and their use

often leads to hypotension, necessitating the use of a pressor to maintain perfusion. In addition, plasma barbiturate levels correlate poorly with effect on ICP, suggesting that monitoring of CNS electrical activity by electroencephalography is necessary to accurately titrate their use. Current guidelines suggest the use of barbiturates for treating intracranial hypertension refractory to sedation, paralysis, ventricular drainage, and osmotic diuretics.

Another important concept in the management of intracranial hypertension is that of the cerebral perfusion pressure. The cerebral perfusion pressure is the driving pressure across the cerebral circulation and is defined as mean arterial pressure minus CVP (or ICP, whichever is higher). Some authors have suggested that careful attention to maintenance of a supranormal cerebral perfusion pressure may lead to better outcomes for head-injured patients. Although there are no well-controlled trials to draw from (particularly for pediatric patients), current guidelines suggest that maintenance of a "normal" cerebral perfusion pressure for age (50–70 mm Hg) is a valid secondary goal of treatment, as long as it is included in a plan to use the other ICP-directed therapies discussed earlier.

A suggested treatment algorithm for patients with documented intracranial hypertension is presented in Figure 13–8. As mentioned earlier, this algorithm represents the current best evidence for the management of intracranial hypertension. The information is largely drawn from experience with traumatic brain injuries, and the direct applicability of these concepts to other illnesses associated with intracranial hypertension remains unclear.

Atabaki SM: Pediatric head injury. Pediatr Rev 2007;28:215 [PMID: 17545333].

Carney NA et al: Guidelines for the acute medical management of severe traumatic brain injury in infants, children, and adolescents. Pediatr Crit Care Med 2003;4:S1 [PMID: 12847355].

Gerber P, Coffman K: Nonaccidental head trauma in infants. Childs Nerv Syst 2007;23:499 [PMID: 17370080].

Giza CC et al: Pediatric traumatic brain injury: Not just little adults. Curr Opin Crit Care 2007;13:143 [PMID: 17327734].

Keenan HT, Bratton SL: Epidemiology and outcomes of pediatric traumatic brain injury. Dev Neurosci 2006;28:256 [PMID: 16943649].

Moppett IK: Traumatic brain injury: Assessment, resuscitation and early management. Br J Anaesth 2007;99:18 [PMID: 17545555].

ETHICAL DELIBERATION & END-OF-LIFE CARE IN THE PICU

Bioethics Consultation in the PICU

Advances in critical care medicine give PICU practitioners the ability to prolong life without being able to ensure a reasonable quality of life. Health care professionals in this setting are often called on to help patients and families wrestle with questions of medical futility. As conflict surrounding care and

Glasgow Coma Scale < 8

(and nonsurgical head injury)

Monitor ICP (consider placement of ventriculostomy at same time) and

If ICP remains elevated proceed through the following steps until there is a positive response.

FIRST TIER OF THERAPY:

1. Sedation, analgesia, elevate head of bed

2. Drain CSF via ventriculostomy if present

3. Neuromuscular blockade

4. Mannitol or 3% saline to maintain osmolarity > 320

5. Hyperventilation to P_{CO_2} of 30–35 mm Hg

If ICP remains elevated proceed to second-tier therapy (order nonspecified)

SECOND TIER OF THERAPY:

Decompressive craniectomy

Barbiturate therapy

Moderate hypothermia (32–34°C)

Place lumbar drain

Hyperventilation to P_{CO_2} < 30 mm Hg

▲ **Figure 13–8.** Proposed treatment algorithm for intracranial hypertension in head injury. CSF, cerebrospinal fluid; ICP, intracranial pressure; P_{CO_2}, partial pressure of arterial CO_2.

decision making has arisen, the introduction of ethics consultation in the ICU setting has served to improve the process by helping to identify, analyze, and resolve ethical problems. Ethics consultation can independently clarify views and allow the health care team, patient, and family to make decisions that respect patient autonomy and promote maximum benefit and minimal harm to the patient.

Managed Withdrawal of Treatment

With increasing frequency, PICU deaths are predictable and result from the withholding or withdrawing of life-sustaining medical therapy (LSMT). Discussions with patients and families regarding the decision to limit resuscitation or to withdraw LSMT should respect the following basic principles:

- Deliberations begin with a clear statement that the patient's good is the goal.
- With the assistance of the health care team, the patient and family can make reasonable decisions about limitation or withdrawal of LSMT based on goals of care for the patient.
- The burden of continued life (pain and suffering) should outweigh any potential benefit from continued therapy.
- Discussions with the patient and family are conducted by experienced personnel with the ability to communicate in a clear and compassionate manner at an appropriate time and place.
- It should be emphasized that decisions are not irrevocable; if at any time the family or health care providers wish to reconsider the decision, full medical therapy should be reinstituted until the situation is clarified.

Palliative Care

Helping a patient experience a dignified and pain-free death is one of the many unique challenges facing caregivers in the PICU. Pediatric death is characterized by its relative infrequency, by the prognostic uncertainties of many pediatric illnesses, and by the fine line between congenital disorder and incurable disease. When a predictable early death is likely, intensivists are often called on to care for the patient and family during the final days and hours of the patient's life.

In the past several years, palliative medicine has developed as a specialized field of practice to address the needs of dying children. The practice of providing supportive care at end of life in pediatrics is fundamentally different from that in adult medicine. In-hospital deaths in pediatrics encompass a more heterogeneous patient population with developmental issues and family dynamics that complicate the process.

Once the inclusive decision is made to limit or withdraw LSMT, a palliative care plan should be agreed on and instituted. The plan should address the following basic principles:

- Adequate pain control and sedation
- Provision of warmth and cleanliness
- Nutrition
- Ongoing patient and family support

The decision to withhold or withdraw LSMT from a pediatric patient does not suggest a plan to hasten the death. The goal of palliative care remains optimization of the patient's and family's experience prior to and following the death. (See also Chapter 30.)

Tissue & Organ Donation

Organ transplantation has become standard therapy. Although the demand for tissue and solid organs has increased, donations have not. The prospect of organ or tissue donation should be considered with all patients dying in the PICU. To be a solid organ donor, the patient must be clinically brain dead and have no conditions contraindicating donation. With patients from whom life-support must be withdrawn, tissue (heart valves, corneas, skin, and bone) can be obtained after cardiac death. The need for new donor organs has led to the reemergence of procuring organs from nonheartbeating (asystolic) donors. In these cases the family or patient has refused life-sustaining therapy and has chosen to have life-support withdrawn, and to donate organs after death.

Death is determined using "traditional" or "cardiopulmonary" criteria of (1) unresponsiveness, (2) apnea, and (3) absent circulation. A high level of scrutiny exists regarding nonheartbeating donors in pediatric patients, and before it has wide acceptance standards of practice need to be developed further. The Required Request Law mandates that health care professionals approach all donor-eligible families to inquire about organ procurement. The decision to donate must be made free of coercion, with informed consent, and without financial incentive.

Brain Death (See Chapter 23)

The development of criteria and expertise in the clinical brain death exam arose out of the demand for solid organs from patients still receiving LSMT. Currently, the diagnosis of brain death is based on national guidelines that render some clarity and standardization to this critical task.

Clinical Brain Death Examination

Establish the cause of the disease or injury and exclude potentially reversible syndromes that may produce signs similar to brain death. Also establish the following:

- Coexistence of coma and apnea[1] ("apnea test" ~3 minutes with $P_{CO_2} > 60$ mm Hg)
- Absence of brainstem function
- Normal blood pressure and temperature
- Flaccid muscle tone, no spontaneous movements
- Examination consistent throughout observation period

Recommended observation periods for children of the following ages:

- Seven days to 2 months old—Two examinations over 48 hours; with electroencephalography

- Two months to 1 year—Two examinations over 24 hours; with electroencephalography
- Over 1 year—Two examinations over 12–24 hours

Ethics Committee, American College of Critical Care Medicine; Society of Critical Care Medicine: Recommendations for non-heartbeating organ donation. A position paper of the Ethics Committee, American College of Critical Care Medicine, Society of Critical Care Medicine. Crit Care Med 2001;29:1826 [PMID: 11546995].

Deray M: Brain death and persistent vegetative state. International Pediatr 2005;20:113.

Goh AY, Mok Q: Clinical course and determination of brainstem death in a children's hospital. Acta Paediatr 2004;93:47 [PMID: 14989439].

Kopelman LM: Are the 21-year-old Baby Doe rules misunderstood or mistaken? Pediatrics 2005;116:797 [PMID: 15741390].

Solomon MZ et al: New and lingering controversies in pediatric end-of-life care. Pediatrics 2005;116:872 [PMID: 16999696].

Truog RD et al: Recommendations for end-of-life care in the intensive care unit: The Ethics Committee of the Society of Critical Care Medicine. Crit Care Med 2001;29:2332 [PMID: 11801837].

Shemie SD et al: Diagnosis of brain death in children. Lancet Neurol 2007;6:87 [PMID: 17166805].

NUTRITIONAL SUPPORT OF THE CRITICALLY ILL CHILD

Metabolic & Physiologic Responses

When severely ill pediatric patients are admitted to the PICU, the initial therapy is directed at the primary or underlying problem and at providing cardiorespiratory and hemodynamic support. Although this management is critical to sustaining life in these patients, provision of adequate nutritional support is often overlooked early in the course of therapy. As increasing evidence demonstrates that nutritional status and support affect the morbidity and mortality of critically ill patients, it is vital that this aspect of care be addressed early in the hospital course.

Trauma, surgery, burns, and sepsis impose metabolic and physiologic disturbances that vary in degree, but have many similarities. The insult triggers the afferent limb of the neurophysiologic reflex, which is composed of pain and neurosensory pathways. In response, the efferent limb consisting of neurologic and endocrine pathways, increases autonomic sympathetic activity with norepinephrine and epinephrine secretions and increases pituitary release of many hormones, including adrenocorticotropic hormone (ACTH), growth hormone, and antidiuretic hormone. Release of catecholamines inhibits insulin secretion and activity, and stimulates glucagon and ACTH production. ACTH and antidiuretic hormone increase corticosteroid release, inhibit insulin activity, and increase aldosterone. The overall effect is to direct an end-organ increase in metabolic rate and to provide increased substrate availability for energy use (Table 13–10). In addition, the body has a cellular response to tissue injury. Cells

---

[1]Cerebral angiography, radionuclide scanning, or transcranial Doppler ultrasonography can be used to assess brain function if apnea testing cannot be performed or if there is need for corroborative studies.

Table 13–10. Metabolic and physiologic responses to severe illness.

Physiologic
  Cardiovascular
    Increased cardiac output
    Peripheral vasodilatation and capillary leak
    Expansion of vascular compartment
  Pulmonary
    Increased minute ventilation
    Ventilation-perfusion mismatch
    Inefficient gas exchange
    Increased CO_2 responsiveness
  Skeletal muscle
    Easier fatigability
    Slower relaxation
    Altered force-frequency pattern
  Renal
    Salt and water retention
    Impaired concentrating ability
Metabolic
  Hormone and hormone-like levels
    Increased insulin
    Increased glucocorticoids
    Increased catecholamines
    Increased interleukin-1
    Increased tumor necrosis factor
  Carbohydrate metabolism
    Increased blood glucose
    Increased gluconeogenesis
    Increased glucose turnover
    Glucose intolerance
  Fat metabolism
    Increased lipid turnover and utilization
    Insuppressible lipolysis
    Decreased ketogenesis
  Protein metabolism
    Increased muscle protein catabolism
    Increased muscle branched-chain amino acid oxidation
    Increased serum amino acids
    Increased nitrogen losses

migrate to the damaged area to facilitate wound healing and aid in infection control with the release of inflammatory mediators. These cells are mainly dependent on glucose for their energy source, which is an important reason the hypermetabolic state is necessary. These events initiate a hypermetabolic response that influences the mobilization and use of nutrients as substrates. Although all substrates are increasingly used, the fraction of calories derived from glucose is reduced, and the fraction derived from protein and lipid breakdown is increased.

Hyperglycemia and glucose intolerance are characteristic traits of the hypermetabolic state. Although glucose use is increased, serum glucose levels are elevated, reflecting neuroendocrine stimulation of glycogenolysis and gluconeogenesis. Gluconeogenesis occurs primarily from lactate, alanine, glutamine, and other amino acids derived from muscle breakdown and from glycerol derived from lipolysis. The hepatic production of glucose is increased, and fails to respond to increased plasma concentrations of glucose or insulin when these substances are infused intravenously. Hyperglycemia and secondary hyperinsulinemia also inhibit ketosis despite the increased rate of lipolysis. The hyperglycemia does, however, maintain glucose supply to the brain. An elevated glucagon-insulin ratio and increased secretion and plasma concentrations of catecholamines produce relative peripheral insulin resistance. Inefficient glucose and fatty acid uptakes are inadequate to meet increased energy needs, leading to increased oxidation of branched-chain amino acids. Because branched-chain amino acids are essential amino acids, their oxidation depletes a valuable pool of precursors for protein synthesis. Administration of excess glucose can lead to hyperosmolar complications, excess energy expenditure, increased CO_2 production, cholestasis, and fatty infiltration of the liver.

Lipids are the major source of energy used during periods of stress starvation. Thus, lipolysis is increased and lipogenesis is decreased despite high levels of glucose and insulin. During stress starvation, peripheral tissues, such as skeletal muscle, myocardium, and respiratory muscles are able to use lipids as their primary energy source. Turnover of medium- and long-chain fatty acids is increased, although the clearance rate of long-chain fatty acids and triglycerides is reduced, primarily through a reduction in peripheral lipoprotein lipase activity that is inhibited by tumor necrosis factor-α (TNFα). If excess lipids are administered, complications such as hyperlipidemia, bacteremia, and suppression of in vitro tests of polymorphonuclear and lymphocyte function may occur.

Protein catabolism is the hallmark of the metabolic stress response. Although the rate of protein synthesis is actually increased in the hypermetabolic state, it is significantly inadequate compared with the rate of protein breakdown. Protein is broken down mainly to provide carbon skeletons for use in gluconeogenesis, but amino acids are also used to support the cellular inflammatory response, the hepatic synthesis of acute-phase reactant proteins, and wound healing. Thus, the contribution of protein to total caloric expenditure increases from 10% in normal children to 15–20% in critically ill children. The discrepancy between protein catabolism and synthesis leads to a negative nitrogen balance and loss of lean body mass. This condition can be reduced or even reversed with increased nonprotein calorie and protein nutrition. Increased nutrient intake appears to make a difference in the ability of the patient to tolerate stress.

Nutritional Assessment

The pediatric patient is at a marked disadvantage compared with adults during periods of stress starvation. The child is a growing organism with little metabolic reserve to compensate for the metabolic stresses created by surgery, trauma, and sepsis. Preexisting nutritional status and the degree of stress imposed by the disease process are important factors in

Table 13–11. Estimating needs for critically ill pediatric patients.[a]

	Age	Resting Energy Expenditure (REE) (kcal/kg)	Average Range of Energy Needs (kcal/kg)	Average Range of Protein Needs (g/kg)
Infants	0–6 mo	55	90–120	2–3.5
	6–12 mo	55	90–120	1.5–2.5
Children	1–3 y	55	75–100	1.5–2.5
	4–6 y	45	65–90	1.5–2.0
	7–10 y	40	55–70	1.0–2.0
Males	11–14 y	30	40–55	1.0–2.0
	15–18 y	30	40–45	1.0–1.5
	19–24 y	25	30–40	1.0–1.5
Females	11–14 y	30	40–55	1.0–2.0
	15–18 y	25	30–40	1.0–1.5
	19–24 y	25	30–40	1.0–1.5

[a]Based on World Health Organization formulas for protein and energy requirements.

estimating nutritional requirements of the critically ill patient. Accurate assessment of nutritional requirements is important as both overfeeding and underfeeding can increase morbidity. One way to estimate nutritional requirements is to apply U.S. recommended dietary allowances. However, because these recommendations are based on populations of normal healthy subjects, applying recommended dietary allowances to critically ill patients significantly overestimates their caloric requirements. Therefore, several equations have been formulated in an attempt to predict basal energy needs of the critically ill patient. Some of these formulas estimate the basal metabolic rate, which is the energy requirement for a fasting (10–12 hours) person who recently awoke from sleep and is at rest with a normal body temperature in the absence of any stress. Other formulas estimate the resting energy expenditure (REE), which is the energy expenditure of a person at rest with a normal body and ambient temperature, but not necessarily fasting. The basal metabolic rate and REE are similar, usually differing by less than 10%. Harris-Benedict and the World Health Organization have recommended formulas that are among the most commonly used (Table 13–11). Once the basal metabolic demand has been estimated, it is then multiplied by a stress factor correlated to the underlying disease process to determine the ultimate energy requirements for the patient (Table 13–12). Compared with recommended dietary allowances, these formulas better estimate energy requirements in sick patients. However, recent evidence suggests that even they may not be accurate enough to use in critically ill children.

Indirect calorimetry has been used to measure patients' REE and appears to reflect a more accurate method of determining nutritional requirements. Indeed, indirect calo-

rimetry measurements were used to derive the stress factors used with prediction formulas. Though this method was once used strictly for research, portable, accurate devices are available that can be used anywhere in the hospital. Indirect calorimetry measures the amount of oxygen absorbed across the lung. This value is assumed to be equal to the amount of oxygen consumed in metabolic processes. The metabolic rate determined in milliliters of oxygen consumed per minute can be converted to calories per hour, thereby providing a measure of REE. Carbon dioxide production is also meas-

Table 13–12. Activity and stress factors ($\times$ REE).

Condition	Factor
ICU on ventilation	Activity 1.0–1.15
Confined to bed	Activity 1.1–1.2
Light activity	Activity 1.2–1.3
Fever, per 1°C	Stress 1.12–1.13
Major surgery	Stress 1.2–1.3
Multiple fractures	Stress 1.2–1.35
Peritonitis	Stress 1.2–1.5
Cardiac failure	Stress 1.25–1.5
Head injury	Stress 1.3–1.4
Liver failure	Stress 1.4–1.5
Sepsis	Stress 1.4–1.5
Burns	Stress 1.5–2.0

ICU, intensive care unit; REE, resting energy expenditure.

ured. The ratio of CO_2 production to O_2 consumption yields the respiratory quotient, which is a measure of substrate use. Inefficiencies in substrate use can be discovered and corrected by modification of the respiratory quotient through alteration of energy substrates that are provided to the patient. A recent study compared the use of two well-known prediction formulas with indirect calorimetry in 55 critically ill children. The data suggest that prediction methods are unreliable for clinical use, and that indirect calorimetry is the only useful way of determining REE in sick children.

Provision of Nutrition

Once energy requirements are determined, the practitioner must decide whether to deliver nutritional support through the enteral or the parenteral route. Enteral feeding is preferred because it is more physiologic, associated with fewer complications, and in some cases the only way to safely deliver some nutrients. More knowledge exists about enteral feeding in relation to both energy requirements and utilization; and practically, it is less expensive than parental nutrition.

Patients should be screened shortly after admission for nutritional requirements and preferred route of administration. Over the years, many practice patterns have been developed that list specific conditions or therapies in which enteral feeding may not be well tolerated by patients. Recent studies are proving that these may not be based on true physiologic differences and that a majority of patients who are critically ill can tolerate enteral feedings. The list of absolute contraindications for enteral feeding is shrinking and now may be limited to diseases of the GI tract.

Because it provides for a more physiologic digestive process, direct gastric feeding is preferable to the intestinal route. Patients supported with gastric feeds can usually tolerate higher osmotic loads and larger volumes, and have a lower frequency of diarrhea. Gastric acid also has a bactericidal effect that may decrease a patient's susceptibility to infection. However, for severely ill patients who are sedated and on mechanical ventilation, the high risk of reflux and aspiration becomes an increasing concern with this manner of feeding. Therefore, transpyloric feeding has been instituted in these patients and in any patient at high risk for aspiration. Although transpyloric feeding may limit reflux and aspiration, it does not entirely eliminate it. A suggested enteral feeding algorithm for critically ill children is presented in Figure 13–9.

The choice of formulas must be based on age, GI function, history of feeding tolerance, nutrient requirements, and route of feeding. Osmolality, nutrient complexity, caloric density, and cost are all factors that should be taken into consideration. An increasing number of commercially made formulas and additives are now available to meet the nutritional needs of the critically ill patient (Table 13–13).

Parenteral nutrition is indicated for patients who are unable to meet nutritional needs with enteral feeds. It consists of the IV delivery of nutrients, fluid, carbohydrates, protein, fat, electrolytes, vitamins, minerals, and trace elements. The proportions of these elements are individualized to suit the patient's specific nutritional needs. Parenteral nutrition often requires central venous access, and thus this method also carries the risks associated with central venous catheters (infection, clots, and insertion-related complications).

Parenteral nutrition can be ordered in many ways, as nutrients can be ordered based on a child's weight or per liter, or a combination of both. Standard ranges and guidelines are usually provided on order forms. Parenteral energy needs can be approximately 10–15% lower than estimated enteral needs due to reduced energy required for digestion, absorption, and fecal losses. The percentage of protein, carbohydrate, and fat that contributes to ideal total energy intake varies with the individual and the disease condition. General guidelines for energy distribution are 8–15% protein, 45–60% carbohydrate, and 25–40% fat. Solutions should be instituted slowly and advanced gradually over several days as tolerated by the patient. Guidelines for the administration of a balanced parenteral diet are provided in Chapter 10. A constant flow rate is important to maintaining steady glucose delivery. If parenteral nutrition must be stopped abruptly, a 10% glucose solution should be started to prevent hypoglycemia. Administration of high glucose and amino acid concentrations in total parenteral nutrition requires central venous access.

Immunonutrition is an area of growing interest and research. The term describes a point of view that dietary factors can confer an advantage to the immune system or other adaptive functions in infants and children. The claims of health benefits ascribed to foods or dietary supplements are not new, but until recently these claims have not been supported by scientific review. Breast milk, the model for infant formula manufacturers, has long been recognized for its immunonutritive properties, containing such nutrients as secretory immunoglobulins, lysozymes, interferon, and growth factors. However, the contribution of specific components to a positive outcome has yet to be elucidated. Growing evidence supports the immunomodulatory effects of minerals (eg, iron, zinc, selenium, and vitamin A), amino acids (arginine and glutamine), and nucleotides. Evidence also points to the emergence of prebiotics, nondigestable food components that favor the colonization and growth of bacteria normally resident in the colon; and probiotics, live microbial feed supplements with beneficial effects to the host. Although some of these concepts hold promise, it is still too early to advocate any specific guidelines, because some of these nutrients used in high doses have been reported to produce possible harmful effects.

Briassoulis G et al: Early enteral administration of immunonutrition in critically ill children: Results of a blinded randomized controlled clinical trial. Nutrition 2005;21:799 [PMID: 15975487].

Coss-Bu JA et al: Energy metabolism, nitrogen balance and substrate utilization in critically ill children. Am J Clin Nutr 2001;74:664 [PMID: 11684536].

▲ **Figure 13–9.** Proposed enteral feeding algorithm for critically ill children. GERD, gastroesophageal reflux disease; GI, gastrointestinal; ICU, intensive care unit; NPO, nothing by mouth; p.o., orally; TPN, total parenteral nutrition.

Hulst JM et al: Causes and consequences of inadequate substrate supply to pediatric ICU patients. Curr Opin Clin Nutr Metab Care 2006;9:297 [PMID: 16607132].

King W et al: Enteral nutrition and cardiovascular medications in the pediatric intensive care unit. JPEN J Parenter Enteral Nutr 2004;28:334 [PMID: 15449573].

Lafeber HN: The art of using indirect calorimetry for nutritional assessment of sick infants and children. Nutrition 2005;21:280 [PMID: 15723759].

Suchner U et al: Immune-modulatory actions of arginine in the critically ill. Br J Nutr 2002;87:S121 [PMID: 11895148].

Wernerman J: Glutamine and acute illness. Curr Opin Crit Care 2003;9:279 [PMID: 12883282].

ASTHMA (LIFE-THREATENING)

Status asthmaticus may be defined as reversible small airway obstruction that is refractory to sympathomimetic and anti-inflammatory agents and that may progress to respiratory failure without prompt and aggressive intervention. Life-threatening asthma is caused by severe bronchospasm, excessive mucus secretion, inflammation, and edema of the airways (see Chapter 18). Reversal of these mechanisms is the key to successful treatment. Status asthmaticus remains a common diagnosis among children admitted to the PICU, and asthma is associated with surprisingly high mortality rates.

Table 13–13. Pediatric enteral formulas.

Formula Category	Formula Examples	Typical Uses
Standard, milk protein-based	PediaSure PediaSure with Fiber Kindercal (with/ without fiber) Nutren Junior	Nutritionally complete for ages 1-10 years. Can be used for tube feeds or oral supplements.
Food based	Compleat Pediatric	Made with beef protein, fruits, and vegetables—does contain lactose. Fortified with vitamins and minerals.
Semielemental	Peptamen Jr.	Indicated for impaired gut function with peptides as protein source, and high MCT content with lower total fat % than standard pediatric formulas.
Elemental	Pediatric Vivonex (24 kcal/oz) Elecare Neocate One Plus	Indicated for impaired gut function or protein allergy, and contains free amino acids and lower fat with majority as MCT.

MCT, medium-chain triglycerides.

The physical examination helps determine the severity of illness. Accessory muscle use (sternocleidomastoid) correlates well with a forced expiratory volume in 1 second and peak expiratory flow rates less than 50% of normal predicted values. A pulsus paradoxus of over 22 mm Hg has been correlated with elevated $PaCO_2$ levels. The absence of wheezing may be misleading because, in order to produce a wheezing sound, the patient must take in a certain amount of air. The ABG analysis remains the single most important laboratory determination in the evaluation of a child in severe status asthmaticus. Patients with severe respiratory distress, signs of exhaustion, alterations in consciousness, elevated $PaCO_2$, or acidosis should be admitted to the PICU.

▶ **Treatment**

Much of the morbidity associated with the treatment of severe asthma is related to the complications of mechanical ventilation that occur in patients with severe airflow obstruction. As a result, the goal of initial treatment of the patient with life-threatening status asthmaticus is to improve the patient's ability to ventilate without resorting to intubation and mechanical ventilation. The medical therapies described in the following discussion should be undertaken swiftly and aggressively with the goal of reversing the

bronchospasm before respiratory failure necessitates invasive ventilation.

Due to inadequate minute ventilation and V/Q mismatching, patients with severe asthma are almost always hypoxemic and should receive supplemental **humidified oxygen** immediately.

Inhaled β_2-agonist therapy with agents such as albuterol remains first-line therapy to reverse acute bronchoconstriction. If the patient is in severe distress and has poor inspiratory flow rates, thus preventing adequate delivery of nebulized medication, subcutaneous injection of epinephrine or terbutaline may be considered. The frequency of β_2-agonist administration varies according to the severity of the patient's symptoms and the occurrence of adverse side effects. Nebulized albuterol may be given intermittently at a dose of 0.1 mg/kg per nebulization up to 5.0 mg, or it can be administered continuously at a dose of 0.5 mg/kg/h to a maximum of 20 mg/h, usually without serious side effects. The heart rate and blood pressure should be monitored closely, because excessive tachycardia and ventricular ectopy may occur.

Systemic **corticosteroids** are the mainstay of therapy for the inflammatory component of asthma. Corticosteroids act by decreasing inflammation, stabilizing mast cells, and increasing β_2-receptor expression. These agents speed the resolution of asthma exacerbations and should be given to all patients admitted to the hospital with severe asthma. The anti-inflammatory effect is generally observed 6–12 hours after administration. It is preferable to administer the corticosteroid by the intravenous route due to the risk of vomiting or difficulty swallowing. A typical pediatric dose is 1 mg/kg of IV methylprednisolone every 6 hours, with the adult dose between 40 and 250 mg. The acute complications of corticosteroid use include GI bleeding, hyperglycemia, and hypertension.

Inhaled **anticholinergic bronchodilators** may also improve lung function when administered to patients with severe asthma along with albuterol. Nebulized ipratropium bromide is the drug of choice, and is given at a dose of 250–500 mcg per dose. Although it has variable effectiveness, ipratropium has fewer side effects and should be considered along with albuterol in patients with severe asthma, especially when they have chronic high use of β-agonists.

Intravenous β-agonists should be considered in patients with severe bronchospasm unresponsive to inhaled bronchodilators. The agent most commonly used in the United States is terbutaline, a relatively specific β_2-agonist, which can be given as a bolus dose or as a continuous infusion. Owing to its relative specificity for β_2-receptors, terbutaline has fewer cardiac side effects than previously available IV β-agonists such as isoproterenol. Terbutaline is given as a bolus or loading dose of 10 mcg/kg followed by a continuous infusion of 0.5–5 mcg/kg/min. In general, patients receiving IV β_2-agonist therapy should have indwelling arterial lines for continuous blood pressure and blood gas monitoring.

Theophylline is a methylxanthine that remains a controversial agent in the management of severe asthma. Clinical studies yield mixed results on its benefit when given with steroids and β_2-agonists for children with asthma. The theoretical advantage of this medication is that it relaxes airway smooth muscle by a separate mechanism from β_2-agonists by preventing degradation of cyclic guanosine monophosphate. Besides causing bronchodilation, this agent decreases mucociliary inflammatory mediators and reduces microvascular permeability. However, the pharmacokinetics of theophylline are erratic and therapeutic levels can be difficult to manage, and serious side effects, such as seizures and cardiac arrhythmias, can occur with high drug levels. Theophylline is given IV as aminophylline. Each 1 mg/kg of aminophylline given as a loading dose will increase the serum level by approximately 2 mg/dL. For a patient who has not previously received aminophylline or oral theophylline preparations, load with 7–8 mg/kg of aminophylline in an attempt to achieve a level of 10–15 mg/dL; then start a continuous infusion of aminophylline at a dosage of 0.8–1 mg/kg/h. A postbolus level and steady-state level should be drawn with the initiation of the medication. Watch closely for toxicity (gastric upset, tachycardia, and seizures) and continue to monitor steady-state serum levels closely, trying to maintain steady-state levels of 12–16 mg/dL.

Magnesium sulfate has been reported to be an effective bronchodilator in adult patients with severe status asthmaticus when given in conjunction with steroids and β_2-agonists, and may be considered for patients in danger of worsening respiratory failure. The mechanism of action of magnesium is unclear, but its smooth muscle relaxation properties are probably caused by interference with calcium flux in the bronchial smooth muscle cell. Magnesium sulfate is given IV at a dose of 25–50 mg/kg per dose. Although it is usually well tolerated, hypotension and flushing are side effects.

Heliox is a mixture of helium and oxygen that is less viscous than ambient air and can improve airway delivery of albuterol. A 2003 meta-analysis of heliox did not report a benefit in the initial treatment of acute asthma, although it may be considered in refractory asthma. The caveat for use of heliox is that it requires at least 60–70% helium to decrease airway resistance, limiting its use in patients requiring higher concentrations of supplemental oxygen.

While **leukotriene antagonists** are used for maintenance asthma therapy, their use in the intensive care setting has not been yet demonstrated.

If the previously described aggressive management fails to result in significant improvement, **mechanical ventilation** may be necessary. In general, if there is steady deterioration (increased acidosis and rising $PaCO_2$) despite intensive therapy for asthma, the patient should be intubated and ventilated mechanically. Mechanical ventilation for patients with asthma is difficult because the severe airflow obstruction often leads to very high airway pressures, air trapping, and resultant barotrauma. The goal of mechanical ventilation with an intubated asthmatic patient is to maintain adequate oxygenation and ventilation with the least amount of barotrauma until other therapies become effective. Worsening hypercarbia after intubation should be anticipated and aggressive efforts to normalize blood gases should be moderated, as such efforts may only lead to complications. Due to the severe airflow obstruction, these patients will require long inspiratory times to deliver a breath and long expiratory times to avoid air trapping. In general, the ventilator rate should be decreased until the expiratory time is long enough to allow emptying prior to the next machine breath. Ventilator rates of 8–12 breaths/min are typical initially. Either volume- or pressure-targeted modes of ventilation can be used effectively in these patients, although tidal volumes and pressure limits should be closely monitored. As a patient moves towards extubation, a support mode of ventilation is useful, as the patient can set his or her own inspiratory time and flow rate. Due to air trapping, patients can have significant auto-PEEP. The level of PEEP on the ventilator is usually set relatively low (3–5 cm H_2O) to minimize high peak pressures. Isolated reports have noted patients who respond to greater PEEP, but these cases are the exception. The acute ventilator strategies and the resulting hypercarbia typically are uncomfortable, requiring that patients be heavily sedated and often medically paralyzed. Fentanyl and midazolam are good choices for sedation. Ketamine, a dissociative anesthetic, should be considered for its sedative properties, although it also increases bronchial secretions, which can complicate management. Barbiturates should be avoided as well as morphine, which increases histamine release. Most patients, at least initially, will also require neuromuscular blockade to optimize ventilation and minimize airway pressures. In intubated patients who are not responding to the preceding strategies, **inhaled anesthetics,** such as isoflurane, can be considered. These agents can cause significant hypotension due to vasodilation.

▶ Monitoring

Severely asthmatic patients should be monitored for heart rate, blood pressure, O_2 saturation, and arterial pH and $PaCO_2$. Continuous blood pressure monitoring is necessary because air trapping can lead to increased levels of occult PEEP (auto-PEEP), an effect that can impair venous return and decrease cardiac output. Close ventilator monitoring is necessary because increases in inspiratory pressure or decreases in pulmonary compliance may signal worsening bronchoconstriction, mucus plugging, or an extrapleural air leak. Chest films of ventilated asthmatic patients should be obtained daily and immediately with sudden changes in patient condition, due to the risk of pneumothorax and pneumomediastinum. In addition, if the patient is receiving neuromuscular blocking agents, the degree of nerve block should be monitored closely because nondepolarizing agents such as pancuronium, when given with corticosteroids, can cause prolonged paralysis and muscle weakness.

Marcoux KK: Current management of status asthmaticus in the pediatric ICU. Crit Care Nurs Clin North Am 2005;17:463 [PMID: 16344215].

McFadden ER Jr: Acute severe asthma. Am J Respir Crit Care Med 2003;168:740 [PMID: 14522812].

Rodrigo GJ et al: Use of helium-oxygen mixtures in the treatment of acute asthma: A systematic review. Chest 2003;123:891 [PMID: 12628893].

Supplement to Circulation: Part 10.5 Near-fatal asthma. Circulation 2005;112:IV-139 to IV-142.

Walters EH et al: Long-acting beta2-agonists for chronic asthma in adults and children where background therapy contains varied or no inhaled corticosteroid. Cochrane Database Syst Rev 2007;(1):CD001385 [PMID: 17253458].

Werner HA: Status asthmaticus in children: A review. Chest 2001;119:1913 [PMID: 11399724].

SHOCK

Shock may be defined as failure of the cardiovascular system to deliver critical substrates (eg, oxygen) and remove toxic metabolites. This failure leads to anaerobic metabolism in cells and ultimately to irreversible cellular damage. Shock has been categorized into a series of recognizable stages: compensated, uncompensated, and irreversible.

Patients in compensated shock have relatively normal cardiac output and normal blood pressures, but have alterations in the microcirculation that increase flow to some organs and reduce flow to others. In infants, compensatory increase in cardiac output is achieved primarily by tachycardia rather than by increase in stroke volume. Heart rates of 190–210 beats/min are common in infants with compensated shock, but heart rates over 220 beats/min raise the possibility of supraventricular tachycardia. In older patients, cardiac contractility (stroke volume) and heart rate increase to improve cardiac output. Blood pressure remains normal initially because of peripheral vasoconstriction and increased systemic vascular resistance. Thus hypotension occurs late and is more characteristic of the uncompensated stage of shock. In the uncompensated stage, the oxygen and nutrient supply to the cells deteriorates further with subsequent cellular breakdown and release of toxic substances, causing further redistribution of flow. At this point, the patient is hypotensive, with poor cardiac output.

▶ Classification

Shock can be classified by mechanism into hypovolemic (including distributive), cardiogenic, and septic. Often, two or three of these occur together.

A. Hypovolemic Shock

Hypovolemic shock is caused by decreased circulating blood volume or preload. This may result from loss of whole blood or plasma or from fluid loss from the kidney or gut. These patients usually have intact compensatory mechanisms that maintain normal blood pressure by increasing cardiac out-

put and shunting blood away from certain organs. These responses protect blood flow to the heart and brain. Untreated, hypovolemic shock can progress to an irreversible stage. Additionally, a relative hypovolemia occurs when arterial and capillary shunting past tissue beds occurs with an increase in venous capacitance, causing blood to pool—so-called distributive shock. This results from anaphylaxis or vasodilating drugs.

B. Cardiogenic Shock/Failure

Age-dependent differences occur in myocardial physiology that are relevant to therapy. Neonatal myocardium has reduced systolic performance and contractility. The sarcolemma, sarcoplasmic reticulum, and T-tubules are less well developed, resulting in a greater dependency on trans-sarcolemma Ca^{2+} flux (ie, extracellular serum Ca^{2+}) for contraction. A high resting state of myocardial contractility occurs that limits the response to inotropic agents. Relatively minor increases in afterload can result in diminished stroke volume. Diastolic compliance is diminished, and small changes in volume result in large changes in ventricular wall tension. Consequently preload reserve is limited, and maximization of the Frank-Starling curve occurs relatively quickly (10–15 mm Hg in animal models). Aggressive volume resuscitation beyond this is often ineffective and not tolerated. Stroke volume is relatively fixed, and greater increases in cardiac output are seen through increased heart rate.

Central to the understanding of cardiogenic failure are the progressive nature of ventricular dysfunction and the compensatory mechanisms that occur in the presence of excessive hemodynamic demands. Inadequate cardiac output activates the renin-angiotensin system. The consequent sodium and water retention augments intravascular volume and increases cardiac output through increased preload. With progression, cardiac compliance is decreased and preload augmentation via the Frank-Starling mechanism is maximized. Subsequently, small changes in ventricular volume can lead to large increases in ventricular pressure, and therefore pulmonary venous pressure, with resultant pulmonary edema. Thus fluids should be cautiously administered in this setting and should possibly be guided by central venous pressure or left atrial/pulmonary artery capillary wedge pressure monitoring. The atrial distention that occurs in the failing heart leads to increased production and release of atrial natriuretic peptide, a vasodilator that augments sodium and water excretion.

Heart failure also induces autonomic nervous system changes, including increased activation of the adrenergic sympathetic system and decreased parasympathetic stimulation. Increased adrenergic tone is associated with elevated circulating norepinephrine levels and increased vasoconstriction and afterload. These combined factors in turn lead to a cycle of increased afterload, increased energy expenditure, decreased cardiac output, myocyte death, and progressive ventricular dysfunction. The cardiomyocyte effects of prolonged adrenergic stimulation include down-regulation of β-receptors, decreased norepinephrine stores, and therefore potentially decreased responses to sympathetic stimulation. Increased cellular concentrations of cyclic adenosine monophosphate and inositol triphosphate lead to increased inward Ca^{2+} flux and at least transient increases in contractility. Subsequently, sustained intracellular calcium impairs ventricular relaxation (lusiotropy) and augments the propensity for arrhythmias. Blood flow is redistributed away from the splanchnic system, skin, and muscles and toward the heart, brain, adrenal glands, and diaphragm. Endothelial dysfunction is common and contributes to the abnormal vascular tone. Endothelin-1 production is elevated in the lung and increases pulmonary vascular resistance and systemic vascular resistance (SVR). The release of endothelial-derived nitric oxide is also impaired. Circulating arginine vasopressin and TNFα levels are elevated. In the later stages of heart failure, cardiomyocyte hypertrophy, fibroblast hyperplasia, and increased production and accumulation of extracellular matrix proteins lead to impaired myocardial function.

Signs and symptoms of cardiac failure are produced by the body's attempts to compensate for the decreased pump function, including activating the sympathetic nervous and renin-angiotensin-aldosterone systems. The child in acute heart failure will present with hypotension and evidence of poor perfusion, such as metabolic acidosis and organ dysfunction. In response to the poor output, tachycardia and vasoconstriction will be manifest as cool and mottled extremities. Although the extremities are cool, the child's core temperature will be elevated. To improve cardiac output, the body will retain fluid and sodium, resulting in generalized edema. Pulmonary edema will cause tachypnea, and rales can be heard on auscultation. The pulmonary edema may be severe enough to compromise respiration and lead to hypoxemia and respiratory failure.

The workup can be performed at the same time treatment is initiated, and should include an echocardiogram to evaluate cardiac anatomy and function. Serial echocardiograms may also be helpful to specifically assess the improvement in function with treatment. A chest radiograph can reveal the amount of cardiomegaly, pulmonary edema, and the presence of any effusions. Laboratory tests should include electrolyte measurements and renal and liver function tests.

Management of cardiogenic failure in the pediatric patient is complicated by the varied underlying causes that often require disparate therapies. Cardiac output is a product of stroke volume and heart rate. The factors that influence cardiac output are preload, afterload, contractility, and cardiac rhythm. An analysis of a low cardiac output state should consider the specific cardiac lesion and should use these factors as a framework for therapy.

Cardiogenic failure results from an imbalance of systemic oxygen delivery and demand. Therapy is aimed at restoring oxygen delivery and reducing demand. Sedation, reduced environmental stress, temperature regulation, supplemental O_2, red cell transfusion, and augmentation of cardiac output all have roles. The overall goal of increasing cardiac output should include restoring an appropriate sinus rate and rhythm, optimizing preload, augmenting myocardial contractility with minimal increases in myocardial O_2 consumption, and maximizing afterload reduction. If bradycardia is excessive, temporary pacing with transthoracic, transesophageal, or intracardiac methods should be considered. Excessive tachycardia is to be avoided, as it shortens ventricular diastole, leading to a reduction in diastolic filling, shortened diastolic coronary perfusion, and increased myocardial O_2 consumption.

Cardiogenic failure is associated with elevated ventricular filling pressures (> 20 mm Hg). Thus, although increasing preload can result in augmented cardiac output (to a degree), volume should be administered cautiously—the Frank-Starling curve may remain flat with little further improvement possible, occurring at the expense of elevating pulmonary venous pressure with resultant pulmonary edema. Diuretics can be administered to reduce pulmonary edema and to improve pulmonary compliance, the work of breathing, and oxygenation. Contractility can be augmented through inotropic stimulation of myocardial $β_1$-receptors (Table 13–14). Dopamine is an α- and β-agonist that, at moderate doses (3–10 mcg/kg/min), improves myocontractility. Low doses (< 3 mcg/kg/min) may increase blood flow to the renal, coronary, and splanchnic beds, via D_1 receptors. Newer agents (eg, fenoldopam) are selective for the dopaminergic receptors and are being used to selectively improve renal blood flow and urine output. At higher doses (generally > 10 mcg/kg/min) the α-receptor effects predominate, with vasoconstriction increasing SVR and pulmonary vascular resistance. As a first-line pharmacotherapy single agent, low-dose dopamine is often beneficial by improving contractility without increasing afterload and by limiting chronotropic effect. Dobutamine is predominantly a β-agonist that additionally causes a dose-dependent vasodilation ($β_2$-receptor) and shifts the ventricular pressure-volume loop toward normal, reducing LV filling pressure and hence pulmonary venous pressure. Its use in infants may be limited by its chronotropic effects leading to impaired ventricular filling. Many institutes use dobutamine as an alternative first-line agent. Isoproterenol is a pure β-agonist that causes significant tachycardia, increased myocardial O_2 consumption, and systemic and pulmonary arterial vasodilation. Though limited by its tachycardic effects as an inotrope, it is useful in instances of associated bradycardia, such as occur in heart transplantation and heart block. Epinephrine is an α- and β-agonist that causes the greatest increase in myocardial O_2 consumption of all inotropes. At a low dose (< 0.05 mcg/kg/min) it increases heart rate and contractility and decreases SVR (β-receptor). At higher doses the α-receptor effects predominate, increasing SVR. Despite these drawbacks, epinephrine can be useful as a second-line agent in cases unresponsive to low-dose dopamine. A vasodilator is often

Table 13–14. Pharmacologic support of the shock patient.

Drug	Dose	Alpha-Adrenergic Effect[a]	Beta-Adrenergic Effect[a]	Vasodilator Effect	Actions and Advantages	Disadvantages
Dopamine	1–20 mcg/kg/min	+ to +++ (dose-related)	+ to +++ (dose-related)	At low doses, renal vasodilation occurs (dopaminergic receptors)	Moderate inotrope, wide and safe dosage range, short half-life.	May cause worsening of pulmonary vasoconstriction
Dobutamine	1–10 mcg/kg/min	0	+++		Moderate inotrope, less chronotropic, fewer dysrhythmias than with isoproterenol or epinephrine.	Marked variation among patients
Epinephrine	0.05–1 mcg/kg/min	++ to +++ (dose-related)	+++		Significant increases in inotropy, chronotropy, and SVR.	Tachycardia, dysrhythmias, renal ischemia, systemic and PVR
Isoproterenol	0.05–1 mcg/kg/min	0	+++	Peripheral vasodilation	Significant increase in inotropy and chronotropy. SVR can drop, and PVR should not increase and may decrease.	Significant myocardial oxygen consumption increases, tachycardia, dysrhythmias
Norepinephrine	0.05–1 mcg/kg/min	+++	+++		Powerful vasoconstrictor (systemic and pulmonary); rarely used except possibly in patients with very low SVR or in conjunction with vasodilator.	Reduced cardiac output if afterload is too high, renal ischemia
Nitroprusside	0.05–8 mcg/kg/min	0	0	Arterial and venous dilation (smooth muscle relaxation)	Decreases SVR and PVR, very short-acting. Blood pressure returns to previous levels within 1–10 min after infusion is stopped.	Toxicities (thiocyanates and cyanide), increased intracranial pressure and ventilation-perfusion mismatch, methemoglobinemia, increased intracranial pressure
Milrinone	0.25–0.75 mcg/kg/min	0	0		Phosphodiesterase III inhibition. Decreases SVR and PVR, increases myocardial contractility with only mild increase in myocardial O_2 consumption. Usually used with low-dose dopamine or dobutamine.	

[a]0, no effect; +, small effect; ++, moderate effect; +++, potent effect. PVR, pulmonary vascular resistance; SVR, systemic vascular resistance.

administered in combination with epinephrine to offset the drug's α-receptor effects. Milrinone (0.25–0.75 mcg/kg/min) is a useful phosphodiesterase inhibitor, preventing degradation of both cyclic guanosine monophosphate and cyclic adenosine monophosphate. Its beneficial effects include a limited increase in myocardial O_2 consumption, decreased SVR and pulmonary vascular resistance, increased contractility, and improved lusiotropy. It is frequently used as a first-line drug, often in combination with low-dose dopamine or epinephrine.

Afterload reduction is an important additional therapy that increases stroke volume and decreases myocardial O_2 consumption. Agents commonly used are nitroprusside, hydralazine, and the angiotensin-converting enzyme inhibitors. Nitroprusside is a rapid-acting IV agent that is readily titratable and causes venodilation and arteriolar dilation, resulting in decreased SVR and pulmonary vascular resistance. Venodilation can decrease preload, and volume may therefore need to be coadministered to restore an appropriate preload. It is limited by its toxic metabolite, cyanide, which will accumulate over days of treatment and inhibit mitochondrial function, leading to metabolic acidosis. Angiotensin-converting enzyme inhibitors are the agents of choice for oral afterload reduction and have been shown to improve survival and functional status in adults. Patients should be switched to angiotensin-converting enzyme inhibitors as soon as indicated. LV afterload is a function of systolic transmural pressure (aortic pressure/intrapleural pressure), and mechanical afterload reduction can be attained by delivering positive airway pressure through mechanical ventilation or through continuous or bilevel positive airway pressure. This must be taken into account when weaning a patient with significant LV dysfunction from mechanical ventilation. If cardiac output cannot be augmented sufficiently despite aggressive medical therapy, consideration should be given to mechanical circulatory support as a bridge to cardiac transplantation. Such support is provided by ECMO, a ventricular access device, or intraaortic balloon pump counterpulsation.

Congenital heart defects pose special concerns. **Aortic stenosis,** for instance, obstructs flow across the LV outflow tract, elevates intraventricular pressure, and increases systolic workload and LV hypertrophy. Due to the outflow tract gradient and hypertrophy, diastolic flow in the coronaries is decreased, which can result in subendocardial ischemia. Dopamine is indicated for inotropic support. Afterload reduction is relatively contraindicated, as it may further compromise coronary flow.

Hypertrophic cardiomyopathy is associated with a hypertrophied nondilated left ventricle, often with dynamic left or biventricular outflow tract obstruction. Coronary abnormalities with luminal compromise are frequent. Systolic function is elevated, ejection fraction is increased, and diastolic dysfunction is evident. Inotropes are avoided due to increased dynamic gradient, coronary compromise, and subendocardial ischemia. Cardiac output is optimized by providing sufficient preload and pharmacotherapy with β-blockers and calcium channel antagonists.

Aortic insufficiency is associated with retrograde flow into the left ventricle during diastole. The amount of regurgitation depends in part on the pressure gradient across the aortic valve and on the heart rate. With increasing heart rates, diastole is shortened and regurgitation limited. Therapy should include inotropic support to improve overall cardiac output and aggressive afterload reduction to reduce the regurgitant fraction. Heart rate can be increased with isoproterenol or transesophageal pacing.

In **mitral regurgitation,** blood is forced back into the low-pressure left atrium during systole. The regurgitant fraction depends partly on the relative resistance to flow across the mitral and aortic valves during systole. Therapy includes inotropic support to improve total cardiac output, and aggressive afterload reduction to improve antegrade aortic flow.

Patients with **anomalous left coronary artery** exhibit myocardial dysfunction secondary to myocardial ischemia. The anomalous coronary artery typically arises from the pulmonary artery. In this scenario, blood flow to the right coronary artery is diverted to the left coronary artery and into the pulmonary artery, resulting in a "steal" phenomenon in the left coronary distribution and ischemia. Medical therapy is futile, though dopamine and milrinone may be use to temporize the situation while awaiting urgent surgical correction. Prior to surgery, care must be exercised not to reduce pulmonary arterial pressure (and increase steal) or excessively increase myocardial O_2 consumption.

Cardiopulmonary bypass (high or low flow) and deep hypothermic circulatory arrest are frequently required to facilitate surgical correction of congenital defects. These techniques are associated with widespread organ system effects, including increased total body water, transient myocardial dysfunction, gas exchange abnormalities, coagulation abnormalities, and hormonal and stress responses. Impairment in myocardial contractility is predictable 6–12 hours following surgery. The myocardium can be supported with increased preload, inotropes, and afterload reduction. The use of perioperative steroids and modified ultrafiltration are tools that appear to limit post-bypass–induced myocardial and vascular dysfunction.

C. Septic Shock

Septic shock has components of both cardiogenic and hypovolemic shock. Septic shock is only indirectly caused by microorganisms. Rather, septic shock is the direct result of the production and secretion of inflammatory mediators. Proinflammatory mediators (TNFα, interleukin-1, interleukin-6, interleukin-8, and platelet-activating factor) are produced and released in excess of the anti-inflammatory mediators (interleukin-10, glucocorticoids, and catecholamines), resulting in a proinflammatory cascade that initiates a number of pathophysiologic responses.

Septic shock caused by gram-negative organisms appears to be mediated by endotoxins (lipopolysaccharides) and the subsequent release of cytokines (TNFα, interleukin-1, and interleukin-10), eicosanoid products, bradykinin, and endorphins. These agents can directly mediate many of the manifestations of septic shock and act to amplify the injury by attracting granulocytes and macrophages—cells that cause further cellular injury. Vasodilators (prostaglandin I_2 and endorphins) predominate early, causing a drop in systemic vascular resistance. Cardiac output generally is increased to compensate for the decreased systemic vascular resistance. This phase has been described as warm shock, because the skin remains well perfused and warm. As septic shock progresses, the heart is no longer able to maintain such a high output, and vasoconstrictors (thromboxane, leukotrienes, and endothelin) predominate, with resultant decreased peripheral perfusion. Extremities become cool, urine output decreases, and oxygen delivery falls.

Shock caused by gram-positive organisms is becoming more common in the PICU. This may be due to use of broad-spectrum empiric antibiotics, the increasing use of long-term intravascular catheters and other surgically implanted foreign bodies, the changing epidemiology of gram-positive pathogens, and antibiotic resistance among gram-positive organisms. The pathogenesis of gram-positive septic shock is different from that of gram-negative sepsis. Gram-positive infections most often arise from skin wounds, soft tissues, and catheter sites, rather than the GI and genitourinary sources associated with gram-negative infections. Gram-negative bacteria have an outer membrane composed of endotoxin that plays a key role in the pathogenesis of gram-negative infection, while the cell wall of gram-positive bacteria is embedded with molecules of lipoteichoic acid that are able to mimic some properties of endotoxin. Additionally, gram-positive bacteria make a range of soluble extracellular toxins, including the pyrogenic toxin superantigens of staphylococci and streptococci.

These superantigens are unusual because they do not require previous processing and specific presentation by antigen-presenting cells, and are able to bind and activate more lymphocytes than conventionally processed antigens. It is hypothesized that toxins are released in gram-positive septic shock, resulting in a massive lymphocyte activation with a release of T-cell cytokines, which are the proximate cause of cellular injury and organ failure.

The host response to gram-positive sepsis is also different from that of gram-negative sepsis. Gram-negative endotoxin induces a rapid (1–5 hours) release of proinflammatory cytokines. Gram-positive toxins induce a more delayed response (50–75 hours) dominated by TNFα and interferon-α.

D. Other Organ Involvement

Organ dysfunction is common during and after an episode of shock. Dysfunction most often affects the kidney, blood coagulation, the lungs, the CNS, the liver, and the GI tract. The kidney responds to hypotension by increasing plasma renin and angiotensin concentrations, thereby decreasing glomerular filtration rate and urine output. This can progress to damage of the energy-consuming renal parenchyma, causing acute tubular necrosis. Coagulopathies may exist in any type of shock, but are especially common in septic shock. They result from the release of mediators that activate the clotting cascade, leading ultimately to a consumptive coagulopathy (ie, disseminated intravascular coagulation). The

CNS dysfunction is related to decreased cerebral perfusion pressure and thus to decreased substrate delivery to the brain. Liver dysfunction commonly occurs after shock and may be manifested by increases in liver enzymes and decreased production of clotting factors leading to a bleeding diathesis. GI problems include ileus, bleeding (eg, gastritis and ulcers), and necrosis with sloughing of intestinal mucosa. Evaluation of multiorgan system dysfunction is mandatory in the workup of shock. Multiorgan system failure secondary to shock greatly increases the mortality of the disease.

▶ Monitoring

Both noninvasive and invasive monitoring of the patient in shock provides information on the severity, progression, and response to treatment. Extremely valuable information can be derived from examination of the cardiovascular, mucocutaneous, musculoskeletal, renal, and central nervous systems.

A. Clinical Findings

1. Cardiovascular system—Tachycardia is not always present, even when hypotension is profound. Hypotension occurs late in pediatric shock (median systolic blood pressure for a child older than age 2 years can be estimated by adding 90 mm Hg to twice the age in years). An important part of the cardiovascular examination is simultaneous palpation of distal and proximal pulses. An increase in the amplitude difference of pulses between proximal arteries (carotid, brachial, and femoral) and distal arteries (radial, posterior tibial, and dorsalis pedis) can be palpated in early shock and reflects increased systemic vascular resistance. Distal pulses may be thready or absent even in the presence of normal blood pressure because of poor stroke volume compensated by tachycardia and increased systemic vascular resistance. In uncompensated shock, hypotension is present and proximal pulses are also diminished. Early shock causes peripheral cutaneous vasoconstriction, which preserves flow to vital organs.

2. Skin—Because of peripheral vasoconstriction, the skin is gray or ashen in newborns and pale and cold in older patients. Capillary refilling after blanching is slow (> 3 seconds). Mottling of the skin may also be observed.

3. Musculoskeletal system—Decreased oxygen delivery to the musculoskeletal system produces hypotonia. Decreased spontaneous motor activity, flaccidity, and prostration are observed.

4. Urinary output—Urine output is directly proportionate to renal blood flow and the glomerular filtration rate and therefore is a good reflection of cardiac output. Catheterization of the bladder is necessary to give accurate and continuous information. (Normal urine output is > 1 mL/kg/h; output < 0.5 mL/kg/h is considered significantly decreased.)

5. Central nervous system—The level of consciousness reflects the adequacy of cortical perfusion. When cortical perfusion is severely impaired, the infant or child fails to respond first to verbal stimuli, then to light touch, and finally to pain. Lack of motor response and failure to cry in response to venipuncture or lumbar puncture should alert the clinician to the severity of the situation. In uncompensated shock in the presence of hypotension, brainstem perfusion may be decreased. Poor thalamic perfusion can result in loss of sympathetic tone. Finally, poor medullary flow produces irregular respirations followed by gasping, apnea, and respiratory arrest.

B. Invasive Monitoring

Patients with poor cardiac output who are hypovolemic often need invasive monitoring for diagnostic and therapeutic reasons. Arterial catheters give constant blood pressure readings, and to an experienced interpreter, the shape of the waveform is helpful in evaluating cardiac output. CVP monitoring gives useful information about relative changes in volume status as therapy is given. CVP monitoring does not provide information about absolute volume status, as decreased right ventricular compliance will produce a higher CVP for the same volume status as a normally compliant ventricle. Intravascular volume can be assessed more accurately by monitoring pulmonary capillary wedge pressure or left atrial pressure using a pulmonary artery catheter. The pulmonary artery catheter also provides valuable information on cardiac status and vascular resistance and enables calculations of oxygen delivery and consumption (Table 13–15), but is associated with a higher complication rate than CVP lines. Most patients can be managed using alternative strategies to monitor clinical status. Measurements of arterial and mixed venous oxygen saturations and arterial and central venous pressures, along with echocardiography, are useful in assessing cardiac function and oxygen consumption. Newer technologies are under investigation to monitor cardiac output via a peripheral artery.

▶ Treatment

Early stabilization of hemodynamics with fluid and inotropes is similar in either gram-positive or gram-negative sepsis.

A. Fluid Resuscitation

Fluid infusion should start with 20 mL/kg boluses titrated to clinical monitors of cardiac output, heart rate, urine output, capillary refill, and level of consciousness. Patients who do not respond rapidly to a 30- to 60 mL/kg fluid bolus should be monitored in an intensive care setting and considered for invasive hemodynamic monitoring (placement of a CVP monitor, arterial line, and occasionally pulmonary artery catheter).

Initially, most patients tolerate crystalloid (salt solution), which is readily available and inexpensive. However, 4 hours after a crystalloid infusion, only 20% of the solution remains in the intravascular space. Patients with serious capillary leaks and ongoing plasma losses (eg, burn cases) should initially receive crystalloid, because in these cases colloid (protein and salt solution) leaks into the interstitium. The protein draws intravascular fluid into the interstitium, thus increasing ongoing losses. Patients with hypoalbuminemia or those with intact capillaries who need to retain volume in the intravascular space (eg, patients at risk for cerebral edema) probably benefit from colloid infusions. Experience with dextran (a starch compound dissolved in salt solution) is limited. Patients with normal heart function tolerate increased volume better than those with poor function. Additionally, large volumes of fluid for acute stabilization in children with shock do not increase the incidence of ARDS or cerebral edema. Increased fluid requirements may persist for several days.

B. Pharmacotherapy

Empiric antibiotics are chosen according to the most likely cause of infection. Inotropic support should be considered

Table 13–15. Hemodynamic parameters.[a]

Parameter	Formula	Normal Values	Units
Cardiac output	$CO = HR \times SV$	Wide age-dependent range	L/min
Cardiac index	$CI = CO/BSA$	3.5–5.5	L/min/m^2
Stroke index	$SI = SV/BSA$	30–60	mL/m^2
Systemic vascular resistance	$SVR = 79.9 \dfrac{(MAP - CVP)}{CI}$	800–1600	dyne s/cm^{-5}/m^2
Pulmonary vascular resistance	$PVR = 79.9 \dfrac{(MPAP - PCWP)}{CI}$	80–240	dyne s/cm^{-5}/m^2

[a]Formulas and normal values from Katz RW, Pollack M, Weibley R: Pulmonary artery catheterization in pediatric intensive care. Adv Pediatr 1983;30:169. BSA, body surface area; CVP, central venous pressure; HR, heart rate; MAP, mean arterial pressure; MPAP, mean pulmonary artery pressure; PCWP, pulmonary capillary wedge pressure; SV, stroke volume.

for patients who continue to have clinical evidence of decreased cardiac output after receiving 60 mL/kg of fluid resuscitation. Dopamine remains the first-line vasopressor although there is ongoing interest in early use of norepinephrine in patients with low SVR and hypotension. Dopamine causes vasoconstriction by stimulating the release of norepinephrine from sympathetic nerves. Infants younger than 6 months of age may not have fully developed sympathetic vesicles and may therefore be resistant to dopamine and more responsive to norepinephrine. As discussed earlier with cardiogenic shock, dopamine can increase myocardial contractility and renal, coronary, and cerebral blood flow by its action on β-receptors and dopaminergic receptors. At higher doses (10–15 mg/kg/min), α-vasoconstrictor actions predominate. Dobutamine may be added to dopamine; however, children younger than 12 months of age may be less responsive. For septic patients with hypotension and low-output states, epinephrine is another front-line agent that can be used alone or in conjunction with dopamine (see Table 13–14). Hypocalcemia is often a contributor to cardiac dysfunction in shock. Calcium replacement should be given to normalize ionized calcium levels.

The role of inflammatory mediators in the pathogenesis of septic shock continues to be defined. Drugs that block some of these mediators appear to be beneficial when given early to animals. Human studies of these same blockers have failed to demonstrate a clear benefit. The differences in pathogenesis and host response to gram-positive or gram-negative sepsis may explain some of the differential responsiveness to anti-inflammatory agents seen in past clinical trials. Additionally, the discrepancies may result from low-affinity binding by these antibodies. The molecular mechanisms by which lipopolysaccharide activates cells are becoming better understood, which may assist in the development of more effective therapies. Modulation of T cells (with glucocorticoids, cyclosporine, and antibodies directed at cytokines) in models of superantigen-induced injury have proven beneficial, but remain experimental. Ibuprofen, because of its ability to block cyclooxygenase (cyclooxygenase metabolites are potent modulators of cell function), was also extensively studied in patients with septic shock, although the evidence does not support the use of ibuprofen for septic shock. Excess production of nitric oxide by the inducible isoform of nitric oxide synthase in inflammatory cells contributes to the hypotension and poor perfusion occurring in shock. Analogs of N-methyl-L-arginine, however, while useful in animal models of septic shock, worsened outcome in studies of adults with severe septic shock, presumably due to broad deleterious effects of total blockade of nitric oxide production.

Protein C is a primary regulator of coagulation, fibrinolysis, and coagulation-induced inflammation. Deficits in protein C activation correlate with morbidity and mortality in septic shock. Deficiencies of protein C have been found in children and adults with sepsis. Recombinant activated protein C reduced mortality rates in an animal model of sepsis. A large randomized, double-blind, placebo-controlled trial of recombinant activated protein C in adults with severe sepsis showed a significant reduction in mortality rates in treated patients. A similarly designed clinical trial of activated protein C in pediatric patients with severe sepsis was halted due to concern over hemorrhagic complications without an observed clear benefit.

Corticosteroids, by virtue of their action on many mediators, are thought to play a role in shock, and based on positive results in animal models of septic shock, have been advocated for treatment of shock in humans. Children with meningococcal meningitis and patients with AIDS who have *Pneumocystis carinii* pneumonia have shown improvement in oxygenation and a trend toward improved survival when treated with corticosteroids. The use of hydrocortisone in adults with relative adrenal insufficiency and septic shock improved short-term outcome. Importantly, a low aldosterone state may be more common in children with septic shock than was previously thought. Hydrocortisone (50 mg/kg) should be considered for children at risk for adrenal insufficiency—those with purpura fulminans or pituitary or adrenal abnormalities, those receiving steroids for chronic illness, and those with septic shock and multiorgan system dysfunction not responding well to traditional inotropic therapy. The studies do not currently support a definitive need for an adrenal stimulation test prior to initiating corticosteroid therapy due to the difficulty in interpreting the results.

Vasopressin is under investigation as an additional agent to treat refractory septic shock. Early studies indicate that it can improve organ perfusion and decrease the doses of epinephrine required to maintain organ perfusion.

ECMO has been considered in the treatment of shock in patients with recoverable cardiac and pulmonary function who require both pulmonary and cardiac support.

Annane D et al: Septic shock. Lancet 2005;365:63 [PMID: 15639681].

Carcillo JA: Pediatric septic shock and multiple organ failure. Crit Care Clin 2003;19:413 [PMID: 1284813].

Goldstein B et al: International pediatric sepsis consensus conference: Definitions for sepsis and organ dysfunction in pediatrics. Pediatr Crit Care Med 2005;6:2 [PMID: 15636651].

Goldstein B et al: ENHANCE: Results of a global open-label trial of drotrecogin alfa (activated) in children with severe sepsis. Pediatr Crit Care Med 2006;7:277 [PMID: 16575354].

Hollenberg SM: Vasodilators in acute heart failure. Heart Fail Rev 2007;12:143 [PMID: 17447137].

London JA, Sena MJ: Pharmacologic support of the failing heart. Surg Clin North Am 2006;86:1503 [PMID: 17116460].

Maclaren G, Butt W: ECMO and sepsis. Crit Care Resusc 2007;9:76 [PMID: 17352671].

Raghavan M, Marik PE: Management of sepsis during the early "golden hours". J Emerg Med 2006;31:185 [PMID: 17044583].

Rhodes A, Bennett ED: Early goal-directed therapy: An evidence-based review. Crit Care Med 2004;32:S448 [PMID: 15542954].

Rivers EP et al: The influence of early hemodynamic optimization on biomarker patterns of sepsis and septic shock. Crit Care Med 2007;35:2016 [PMID: 17855815].

Sharma VK, Dellinger RP: Treatment options for severe sepsis and septic shock. Expert Rev Anti Infect Ther 206;4:395 [PMID: 16771616].

Vincent JL et al and the Recombinant Human Activated Protein C Worldwide Evaluation in Severe Sepsis (PROWESS) Study Group: Effects of drotrecogin alfa (activated) on organ dysfunction in the PROWESS trial. Crit Care Med 2003;31:834 [PMID: 12626993].

Vincent JL, Gerlach H: Fluid resuscitation in severe sepsis and septic shock: An evidence-based review. Crit Care Med 2004;32:S451 [PMID: 15542955].

PAIN & ANXIETY CONTROL

Anxiety control and pain relief are important responsibilities of the critical care physician. It is well recognized that infants and children experience pain and require pain relief. Indeed, outcomes are improved in children receiving appropriate pain control. A child's anxiety in the PICU may heighten perception of pain to a level that causes deterioration of his or her condition. It is important to distinguish between anxiety and pain, because pharmacologic therapy may be directed at one or both of these symptoms (Table 13–16). Furthermore, before initiating or increasing sedative drugs, it is important to exclude or address physiologic causes of agitation, such as hypoxemia, hypercapnia, and cerebral hypoperfusion caused by low cardiac output.

Sedation

Sedative (anxiolytic) drugs are used to induce calmness without producing sleep—although at high doses, all anxiolytics will cause drowsiness and sleep. The five indications for the use of sedative drugs are (1) to allay fear and anxiety, (2) to manage acute confusional states, (3) to facilitate treatment or diagnostic procedures, (4) to facilitate mechanical ventilation, and (5) to obtund physiologic responses to stress—that is, reduce tachycardia, hypertension, or increased ICP. Parenteral administration (bolus or infusion) allows titration of response in the critically ill child. Sedatives fall into several classes, with the opioid and benzodiazepine classes serving as the mainstay of anxiety treatment in the ICU.

A. Benzodiazepines

Benzodiazepines possess anxiolytic, hypnotic, anticonvulsant, and skeletal muscle relaxant properties. Although their exact mode of action is unknown, it appears to be located within the limbic system of the CNS and to involve the neuroinhibitory transmitter γ-aminobutyric acid. Most benzodiazepines are metabolized in the liver, with their metabolites subsequently excreted in the urine; thus, patients in liver failure are likely to have long elimination times.

Benzodiazepines can cause respiratory depression if given rapidly in high doses, and they potentiate the analgesic and respiratory depressive effects of opioids and barbiturates. Therefore, it is important to monitor cardiorespiratory status and have resuscitation equipment available. Three benzodiazepines with differing half-lives are presently used in the ICU setting:

1. Midazolam—Midazolam has the shortest half-life (1.5–3.5 hours) of the benzodiazepines and is the only benzodiazepine that should be administered as a continuous IV infusion. It produces excellent retrograde amnesia lasting for 20–40 minutes after a single IV dose. Therefore, it can be used either for short-term sedation or for "awake" proce-

Table 13–16. Pain and anxiety control.

Drug	Dose and Method of Administration[a]	Advantages	Disadvantages	Usual Duration of Effect
Morphine	IV, 0.1 mg/kg; continuous infusion, 0.01–0.05 mg/kg/h	Excellent pain relief, reversible	Respiratory depression, hypotension, nausea, suppression of intestinal motility, histamine release	2–4 h
Meperidine	IV, 1 mg/kg	Good pain relief, reversible	Respiratory depression, histamine release, nausea, suppression of intestinal motility	2–4 h
Fentanyl	IV, 1–2 mcg/kg; continuous infusion, 0.5–2 mcg/kg/h	Excellent pain relief, reversible, short half-life	Respiratory depression, chest wall rigidity, severe nausea and vomiting	30 min
Diazepam	IV, 0.1 mg/kg	Sedation and seizure control	Respiratory depression, jaundice, phlebitis	1–3 h
Lorazepam	IV, 0.1 mg/kg	Longer half-life, sedation and seizure control	Nausea and vomiting, respiratory depression, phlebitis	2–4 h
Midazolam	IV, 0.1 mg/kg	Short half-life, only benzodiazepine given as continuous infusion	Respiratory depression	20–40 min

[a]Intravenous (IV) administration is most common in the ICU. The effects of morphine, meperidine, and fentanyl are reversible by administration of naloxone (opioid antagonist).

dures such as endoscopy or as a continuous infusion in the anxious, restless patient. The single IV dose is 0.05–0.1 mg/kg, whereas a continuous infusion should be started at a rate of 0.1 mg/kg/h after an initial loading dose of 0.1 mg/kg. The midazolam infusion dosage must be titrated upward to achieve the desired effect. Midazolam is not an analgesic; therefore, small doses of an analgesic such as morphine or fentanyl may be needed.

2. Diazepam—Diazepam has a longer half-life than midazolam and can be given orally (PO) as well as by the IV route. Its disadvantage in the ICU is its intermediary metabolite, nordazepam, which has a very long half-life and may accumulate, prolonging sedation. It produces excellent anxiolysis and amnesia. Additionally, it is used to treat acute status epilepticus. The IV dose is 0.1 mg/kg, which can be repeated every 15 minutes to achieve the desired effect or until undesirable side effects (somnolence and respiratory depression) occur.

3. Lorazepam—Lorazepam possesses the longest half-life of the three benzodiazepines discussed here and can be used to achieve sedation for as long as 6–8 hours. It has less effect on the cardiovascular and respiratory systems than other benzodiazepines and can be given PO, IV, or intramuscularly (IM). The IV route is most commonly used. The IV dosage is 0.1 mg/kg. Lorazepam can also be used to treat acute status epilepticus.

B. Other Drugs

1. Chloral hydrate—Chloral hydrate is an enteral sedative and hypnotic agent frequently used in children. After administration, it is rapidly metabolized by the liver to its active form trichloroethanol, which has an 8-hour half-life. A sedative dose is 6–20 mg/kg per dose, usually given every 6–8 hours, whereas the hypnotic dose is up to 50 mg/kg with a maximum dose of 1 g. The hypnotic dose is frequently used to sedate young children for outpatient radiologic procedures such as computed tomographic scanning and magnetic resonance imaging. There is little effect on respiration or blood pressure with therapeutic doses of chloral hydrate. The drug is irritating to mucous membranes, however, and may cause gastric upset if administered on an empty stomach.

2. Ketamine—Ketamine is a phencyclidine derivative that produces a trancelike state of immobility and amnesia known as dissociative anesthesia. After IM or IV administration, it causes central sympathetic nervous system stimulation with resultant increases in heart rate, blood pressure, and cardiac output. Respiration is not depressed at therapeutic doses. Because salivary and tracheobronchial mucous gland secretions are increased, atropine should be administered 20 minutes prior to the ketamine. A disadvantage of ketamine use is the occurrence of unpleasant dreams or hallucinations. This effect occurs less often in children than in adults, and can be reduced even further by the concurrent administration of a benzodiazepine. Because of its inotropic properties, ketamine is useful for the sedation of certain critically ill patients whose conditions are unstable. Additionally, its bronchodilator effects make it the induction agent of choice for patients with status asthmaticus requiring intubation. It is given as an IV injection of 1–2 mg/kg over 60 seconds, with supplementary doses of 0.5 mg/kg being required every 10–30 minutes to maintain an adequate level of anesthesia. Alternatively, it can be administered as an IM injection of 3–7 mg/kg, which usually produces the desired level of anesthesia within 3–4 minutes. If prolonged anesthesia is required, ketamine can be administered by IV infusion at doses of 3–20 mg/kg/h.

3. Antihistamines—The antihistamines diphenhydramine and hydroxyzine can be used as sedatives, but are not as effective as the benzodiazepines. Diphenhydramine produces sedation in only 50% of those patients. It can be given IV, IM, or PO at a dose of 1 mg/kg. Hydroxyzine can be given either IM or PO. It is frequently used concurrently with morphine or meperidine, adding anxiolysis and potentiating their effects. The sedative effects of both drugs can last from 4–6 hours following a single dose.

4. Propofol—Propofol is an anesthetic induction agent whose main advantages are a rapid recovery time and no cumulative effects resulting from its rapid hepatic metabolism. It has no analgesic properties and frequently causes pain on injection. Dose-related hypotension and metabolic acidosis have been reported in pediatric patients, and the FDA recommends against the use of propofol in pediatric patients outside the controlled environment of the operating room.

5. Barbiturates—Barbiturates (phenobarbital and thiopental) can cause direct myocardial and respiratory depression and are, in general, poor choices for sedation of seriously ill patients. Phenobarbital has a very long half-life (up to 4 days), and recovery from thiopental, although it is a short-acting barbiturate, can be prolonged because remobilization from tissue stores occurs.

6. Dexmedetomidine—Dexmedetomidine is an α_2-adrenoceptor agonist with sedative, analgesic, and anxiolytic effects. It produces rapid sedation while maintaining a high degree of patient rousability. Dexmedetomidine has few side effects but can produce a dose-dependent hemodynamic decline. Pediatric studies are ongoing to determine its role in the pediatric ICU.

Analgesia

A. Opioid Analgesics

Opioid analgesics (morphine, fentanyl, codeine, and meperidine) are the mainstays of therapy for most forms of acute severe pain as well as chronic cancer pain management. They possess both analgesic and dose-related sedative effects, although a range of plasma concentrations produce analgesia without sedation. In addition, opioids can cause respiratory depression, nausea, pruritus, slowed intestinal motility, miosis, urinary retention, cough suppression, biliary spasm, and vasodilation. The dose of opioid required to produce adequate analgesia varies greatly from one individual to the next. Therefore, in the intensive care setting, a continuous infusion of morphine or fentanyl allows dosages to be easily titrated to achieve the desired effect.

In general, infants younger than age 3 months are more susceptible than older children to the respiratory depressant effects of opioids. Starting dosages for these patients should be about one-third to one-half the usual pediatric dose. Most opioids (except meperidine) have minimal cardiac depressive effects, and critically ill patients generally tolerate them well. Fentanyl does not cause the histamine release that morphine does and thus produces less vasodilation and a less-pronounced drop in systemic blood pressure. Opioids are metabolized in the liver, with metabolites excreted in the urine. Thus patients with hepatic or renal impairment may have a prolonged response to their administration. Long-term (> 7 days) administration and high doses (> 1.5–2.5 mg/kg cumulative fentanyl dose) of continuous infusions of opioids or benzodiazepines can lead to tolerance and physical dependence with the development of withdrawal symptoms (agitation, tachypnea, tachycardia, sweating, and diarrhea) upon acute termination of these drugs. In these patients, gradual tapering of the opioid dosage over a 5- to 10-day period will prevent withdrawal symptoms. The mechanism of opioid tolerance is related to conformational changes in the drug-receptor interaction. The use of continuous infusions and synthetic opioids is associated with the faster development of tolerance. As with any potent sedative or analgesic used in the ICU setting, appropriate patient monitoring (pulse oximetry, cardiorespiratory monitoring, and blood pressure monitoring) should be used during the period of opioid administration, and equipment should be available to support prompt intervention if undesired side effects occur.

The ICU regimen for sedation and analgesia must be carefully modified when the patient is transferred to the ward or a lower vigilance area. Patients with baseline respiratory, hepatic, or renal insufficiencies are most predisposed to respiratory insufficiency from sedatives or opioid analgesics.

Advantages of continuous infusions of sedatives are (1) a more constant level of sedation and increased patient comfort, and (2) better tolerance of newer approaches to mechanical ventilation. Prolongation of mechanical ventilation, hospitalization, and inability to assess neurologic function and mental status are recognized as disadvantages of continuous infusions. Daily interruption of continuous sedation, allowing adult patients to "wake up," is associated with a decrease in duration of mechanical ventilation and length of stay in the ICU. Currently, similar data are not available for pediatric patients.

Frequently pediatric patients will require relatively deep levels of sedation while undergoing a procedure (eg, vascular line placement or radiographic studies). Often these patients are not intubated and are not expected to require intubation and ventilatory support—termed "moderate sedation/analgesia." A systematic approach should include the following:

1. Pertinent history to elicit underlying illnesses
2. Physical examination focusing on the anatomy and adequacy of the child's airway (ie, large tonsils or facial deformity)
3. Informed consent
4. Appropriate patient fasting from solids (6 hours) and liquids (2 hours)
5. Age- and size-appropriate equipment
6. Drug dosages calculated on a milligram per kilogram basis
7. Monitoring and documentation of vital signs (including continuous pulse oximetry, respiratory rate and pattern, and level of arousability)
8. Separate observer to monitor deeply sedated patients
9. Practitioner capable of intubating and treating patients who enter a deeper state of sedation than initially anticipated
10. Discharge criteria ensuring that the patient has recovered to his or her baseline level of consciousness

Short-acting agents are preferred. Agents typically used include an opioid (usually fentanyl or morphine) and a benzodiazepine (most often midazolam). Another option is ketamine and midazolam. It is important to select and become comfortable with a specific combination, and to learn its indications and potential complications. Using a familiar agent and following the systematic approach outlined earlier have reduced anesthetic complications in this population of patients.

Patient-controlled analgesia is a done via a computer-governed infusion pump for constant infusion or patient-regulated bolus infusion of opioid analgesics. The basal infusion mode is intended to provide a constant serum level of analgesic. The bolus mode allows the patient, by pushing a button, to self-administer additional doses for breakthrough pain. The patient is usually permitted six boluses an hour, with 10-minute lockouts. If the patient is using allotted hourly boluses, this usually means that the basal infusion rate is too low. The patient must understand the concept of patient-controlled analgesia in order to be a candidate for its use. In some circumstances in pediatrics it is more appropriate for the nurse or parent to administer the bolus dose.

Naloxone reverses the analgesic, sedative, and respiratory depressive effects of opioid agonists. Its administration should be titrated to achieve the desired effect (eg, reversal of respiratory depression) because full reversal using 1–10 mcg/kg may cause acute anxiety, dysphoria, nausea, and vomiting. Furthermore, because the duration of effect of naloxone is shorter (30 minutes) than that of most opioids, the patient must be observed carefully for reappearance of the undesired effect.

B. Nonopioid Analgesics

Nonopioid analgesics used in the treatment of mild to moderate pain include acetaminophen, aspirin, and other nonsteroidal anti-inflammatory drugs (NSAIDs) such as ibuprofen and naproxen.

1. Acetaminophen—Acetaminophen is the most commonly used analgesic in pediatrics in the United States and is the drug of choice for mild to moderate pain because of its low toxicity and lack of effect on bleeding time. It is metabolized by the liver. Suggested doses are 10–15 mg/kg PO to approximately 10–20 mg/kg per rectum every 4 hours.

2. Aspirin—Aspirin is also an effective analgesic for mild to moderate pain at doses of 10–15 mg/kg PO every 4 hours. However, its prolongation of bleeding time, association with Reye syndrome, and propensity to cause gastric irritation limit its usefulness in pediatric practice. Aspirin and other NSAIDs are still useful, especially for pain of inflammatory origin, bone pain, and pain associated with rheumatic conditions.

3. Other NSAIDs—Ibuprofen and naproxen use has been limited in pediatrics to date. Naproxen is FDA-approved for children aged 2–12 years (5–7 mg/kg PO every 8–12 hours), whereas ibuprofen requires more frequent dosing intervals (4–10 mg/kg PO every 6–8 hours).

All of the NSAIDs have a therapeutic ceiling after which no increase occurs in analgesic potency. They all can cause gastritis and should be given with antacids or with meals, and they should be used with caution in people at risk for renal compromise. In addition, the analgesic effects of acetaminophen, aspirin, and other NSAIDs are additive to those of opioids. Thus, if additional analgesia is required, their use should be continued and an appropriate oral opioid (codeine or morphine) or parenteral opioid (morphine or fentanyl) begun.

American Academy of Pediatrics; American Academy of Pediatric Dentistry, Cote CJ, Wilson S; Work Group on Sedation: Guidelines for monitoring and management of pediatric patients during and after sedation for diagnostic and therapeutic procedures. Pediatr 2006;118:2587 [PMID: 17142550].

Cray SH et al: Lactic acidemia and bradyarrhythmia in a child sedated with propofol. Crit Care Med 1998;26:2087 [PMID: 9875925].

Doyle L, Colletti JE: Pediatric procedural sedation and analgesia. Pediatr Clin North Am 2006;53:279 [PMID: 16574526].

Shankar V, Deshpande JK: Procedural sedation in the pediatric patient. Anesthesiol Clin North Am 2005;23:635 [PMID: 16310656].

Tobias JD: Dexmedetomidine: Applications in pediatric critical care and pediatric anesthesiology. Pediatr Crit Care Med 2007;8:115 [PMID: 17273114].

Skin

Joseph G. Morelli, MD

Joanna M. Burch, MD

GENERAL PRINCIPLES

DIAGNOSIS OF SKIN DISORDERS

Examination of the skin requires that the entire surface of the body be palpated and inspected in good light. The onset and duration of each symptom should be recorded, together with a description of the primary lesion and any secondary changes, using the terminology set forth in Table 14–1. In practice, the characteristics of skin lesions are described in an order opposite that shown in the table. Begin with distribution, then configuration, color, secondary changes, and primary changes. For example, guttate psoriasis could be described as generalized, discrete, red, scaly papules.

TREATMENT OF SKIN DISORDERS

Topical Therapy

Treatment should be simple and aimed at preserving normal skin physiology. Topical therapy is often preferred because medication can be delivered in optimal concentrations to the desired site.

Water is an important therapeutic agent, and optimally hydrated skin is soft and smooth. This occurs at approximately 60% environmental humidity. Because water evaporates readily from the cutaneous surface, skin hydration (stratum corneum of the epidermis) is dependent on the water concentration in the air, and sweating contributes little. However, if sweat is prevented from evaporating (eg, in the axilla, groin), local humidity and hydration of the skin are increased. As humidity falls below 15–20%, the stratum corneum shrinks and cracks; the epidermal barrier is lost and allows irritants to enter the skin and induce an inflammatory response. Replacement of water will correct this condition if evaporation is prevented. Therefore, dry and scaly skin is treated by soaking the skin in water for 5 minutes and then adding a barrier to evaporation (Table 14–2). Oils and ointments prevent evaporation for 8–12 hours, so they must be applied once or twice a day. In areas already occluded (axilla, diaper area), creams or lotions are preferred, but more frequent application may be necessary.

Overhydration (maceration) can also occur. As environmental humidity increases to 90–100%, the number of water molecules absorbed by the stratum corneum increases and the tight lipid junctions between the cells of the stratum corneum are gradually replaced by weak hydrogen bonds; the cells eventually become widely separated, and the epidermal barrier falls apart. This occurs in immersion foot, diaper areas, axillae, and the like. It is desirable to enhance evaporation of water in these areas by air drying.

Wet Dressings

By placing the skin in an environment where the humidity is 100% and allowing the moisture to evaporate to 60%, pruritus is relieved. Evaporation of water stimulates cold-dependent nerve fibers in the skin, and this may prevent the transmission of the itching sensation via pain fibers to the central nervous system. It also is vasoconstrictive, thereby helping to reduce the erythema and also decreasing the inflammatory cellular response.

The simplest form of wet dressing consists of one set of wet underwear (eg, long johns) worn under dry pajamas. The underwear should be soaked in warm (not hot) water and wrung out until no more drops come out. This should be done overnight for a few days up to 1 week. When the condition has improved, the wet dressings are discontinued.

Topical Glucocorticoids

Twice-daily application of topical corticosteroids is the mainstay of treatment for all forms of dermatitis (Table 14–3). Topical steroids can also be used under wet dressings. After wet dressings are discontinued, topical steroids should be applied only to areas of active disease. They should never be applied to normal skin to prevent recurrence. Only low-

Table 14–1. Examination of the skin.

Clinical Appearance	Description and Examples
Primary lesions (first to appear)	
Macule	Any circumscribed color change in the skin that is flat. Examples: white (vitiligo), brown (café-au-lait spot), purple (petechia).
Papule	A solid, elevated area < 1 cm in diameter whose top may be pointed, rounded, or flat. Examples: acne, warts, small lesions of psoriasis.
Plaque	A solid, circumscribed area > 1 cm in diameter, usually flat-topped. Example: psoriasis.
Vesicle	A circumscribed, elevated lesion < 1 cm in diameter and containing clear serous fluid. Example: blisters of herpes simplex.
Bulla	A circumscribed, elevated lesion > 1 cm in diameter and containing clear serous fluid. Example: bullous impetigo.
Pustule	A vesicle containing a purulent exudate. Examples: acne, folliculitis.
Nodule	A deep-seated mass with indistinct borders that elevates the overlying epidermis. Examples: tumors, granuloma annulare. If it moves with the skin on palpation, it is intradermal; if the skin moves over the nodule, it is subcutaneous.
Wheal	A circumscribed, flat-topped, firm elevation of skin resulting from tense edema of the papillary dermis. Example: urticaria.
Secondary changes	
Scales	Dry, thin plates of keratinized epidermal cells (stratum corneum). Examples: psoriasis, ichthyosis.
Lichenification	Induration of skin with exaggerated skin lines and a shiny surface resulting from chronic rubbing of the skin. Example: atopic dermatitis.
Erosion and oozing	A moist, circumscribed, slightly depressed area representing a blister base with the roof of the blister removed. Examples: burns, impetigo. Most oral blisters present as erosions.
Crusts	Dried exudate of plasma on the surface of the skin following acute dermatitis. Examples: impetigo, contact dermatitis.
Fissures	A linear split in the skin extending through the epidermis into the dermis. Example: angular cheilitis.
Scars	A flat, raised, or depressed area of fibrotic replacement of dermis or subcutaneous tissue. Examples: acne scar, burn scar.
Atrophy	Depression of the skin surface caused by thinning of one or more layers of skin. Example: lichen sclerosis.
Color	
	The lesion should be described as red, yellow, brown, tan, or blue. Particular attention should be given to the blanching of red lesions. Failure to blanch suggests bleeding into the dermis (petechiae).
Configuration of lesions	
Annular (circular)	Annular nodules represent granuloma annulare; annular scaly papules are more apt to be caused by dermatophyte infections.
Linear (straight lines)	Linear papules represent lichen striatus; linear vesicles, incontinentia pigmenti; linear papules with burrows, scabies.
Grouped	Grouped vesicles occur in herpes simplex or zoster.
Discrete	Discrete lesions are independent of each other.
Distribution	
	Note whether the eruption is generalized, acral (hands, feet, buttocks, face), or localized to a specific skin region.

potency steroids (see Table 14–3) are applied to the face or intertriginous areas.

Devillers AC, Oranje AP: Efficacy and safety of "wet wrap" dressings as an intervention treatment in children with severe and/or refractory atopic dermatitis: A critical review of the literature. Br J Dermatol 2006;154:579 [PMID: 16536797].

Isaksson M, Bruze M: Corticosteroids. Dermatitis 2005;16:3 [PMID: 15996344].

Kraft JN, Lynde CW: Moisturizers: What they are and a practical approach to product selection. Skin Therapy Lett 2005;10:1 [PMID 15986082].

DISORDERS OF THE SKIN IN NEWBORNS

TRANSIENT DISEASES IN NEWBORNS

1. Milia

Milia are tiny epidermal cysts filled with keratinous material. These 1- to 2-mm white papules occur predominantly on the face in 40% of newborns. Their intraoral counterparts are called Epstein pearls and occur in up to 60–85% of neonates. These cystic structures spontaneously rupture and exfoliate their contents.

Table 14–2. Bases used for topical preparations.

Base	Combined With	Uses
Foam		Cosmetically eloquent; increasing number of products available.
Liquids		Wet dressings: relieve pruritus, vasoconstrict
	Powder	Shake lotions, drying pastes: relieve pruritus, vasoconstrict
	Grease and emulsifier; oil in water	Cream: penetrates quickly (10–15 min) and thus allows evaporation
	Excess grease and emulsifier; water in oil	Emollient cream: penetrates more slowly and thus retains moisture on skin
Grease		Ointments: occlusive (hold material on skin for prolonged time) and prevent evaporation of water
Gel		Transparent, colorless, semisolid emulsion: nongreasy, more drying and irritating than cream
Powder		Enhances evaporation

Characteristics of bases for topical preparations:
1. Thermolabile, low-residue foam vehicle is more cosmetically acceptable and uses novel permeability pathway for delivery.
2. Most greases are triglycerides (eg, Aquaphor, petrolatum, Eucerin).
3. Oils are fluid fats (eg, Alpha Keri, olive oil, mineral oil).
4. True fats (eg, lard, animal fats) contain free fatty acids that cause irritation.
5. Ointments (eg, Aquaphor, petrolatum) should not be used in intertriginous areas such as the axillae, between the toes, and in the perineum, because they increase maceration. Lotions or creams are preferred in these areas.
6. Oils and ointments hold medication on the skin for long periods and are therefore ideal for barriers or prophylaxis and for dried areas of skin. Medication gets into the skin more slowly from ointments.
7. Creams carry medication into skin and are preferable for intertriginous dermatitis.
8. Foams, solutions, gels, or lotions should be used for scalp treatments.

2. Sebaceous Gland Hyperplasia

Prominent white to yellow papules at the opening of pilosebaceous follicles without surrounding erythema—especially over the nose—represent overgrowth of sebaceous glands in response to maternal androgens. They occur in more than half of newborns and spontaneously regress in the first few months of life.

3. Neonatal Acne

Inflammatory papules and pustules with occasional comedones predominantly on the face occur in as many as 20% of newborns. Although neonatal acne can be present at birth, it most often occurs between 2 and 4 weeks of age. Spontaneous resolution occurs over a period of 6 months to 1 year. A rare entity that is often confused with neonatal acne is **neonatal cephalic pustulosis.** This is a more monomorphic eruption with red papules and pustules on the head and neck that appears in the first month of life. There is associated neutrophilic inflammation and yeasts of the genus *Malassezia*. This eruption will resolve spontaneously, but responds to topical antiyeast preparations.

4. Harlequin Color Change

A cutaneous vascular phenomenon unique to neonates in the first week of life occurs when the infant (particularly one of low birth weight) is placed on one side. The dependent half develops an erythematous flush with a sharp demarcation at the midline, and the upper half of the body becomes pale. The color changes usually subside within a few seconds after the infant is placed supine but may persist for as long as 20 minutes.

5. Mottling

A lacelike pattern of bluish, reticular discoloration representing dilated cutaneous vessels appears over the extremities and often the trunk of neonates exposed to lowered room temperature. This feature is transient and usually disappears completely on rewarming.

6. Erythema Toxicum

Up to 50% of full-term infants develop erythema toxicum. Usually at 24–48 hours of age, blotchy erythematous macules

Table 14–3. Topical glucocorticoids.

Glucocorticoid	Concentrations
Low potency[a] = 1–9	
Hydrocortisone	0.5%, 1%, 2.5%
Desonide	0.05%
Moderate potency = 10–99	
Mometasone furoate	0.1%
Hydrocortisone valerate	0.2%
Fluocinolone acetonide	0.025%
Triamcinolone acetonide	0.01%
Amcinonide	0.1%
High potency = 100–499	
Desoximetasone	0.25%
Fluocinonide	0.05%
Halcinonide	0.1%
Super potency = 500–7500	
Betamethasone dipropionate	0.05%
Clobetasol propionate	0.05%

[a]1% hydrocortisone is defined as having a potency of 1.

2–3 cm in diameter appear, most prominently on the chest but also on the back, face, and extremities. These are occasionally present at birth. Onset after 4–5 days of life is rare. The lesions vary in number from a few up to as many as 100. Incidence is much higher in full-term versus premature infants. The macular erythema may fade within 24–48 hours or may progress to formation of urticarial wheals in the center of the macules or, in 10% of cases, pustules. Examination of a Wright-stained smear of the lesion reveals numerous eosinophils. No organisms are seen on Gram stain. These findings may be accompanied by peripheral blood eosinophilia of up to 20%. All of the lesions fade and disappear within 5–7 days. Transient neonatal pustular melanosis is a pustular eruption in newborns of African-American descent. The pustules rupture leaving a collarette of scale surrounding a macular hyperpigmentation. Unlike erythema toxicum, the pustules contain mostly neutrophils and often involve the palms and soles.

7. Sucking Blisters

Bullae, either intact or as erosions (the blister base) without inflammatory borders, may occur over the forearms, wrists, thumbs, or upper lip. These presumably result from vigorous sucking in utero. They resolve without complications.

8. Miliaria

Obstruction of the eccrine sweat ducts occurs often in neonates and produces one of two clinical pictures. Superficial obstruction in the stratum corneum causes miliaria crystallina, characterized by tiny (1- to 2-mm), superficial grouped vesicles without erythema over intertriginous areas and adjacent skin (eg, neck, upper chest). More commonly, obstruction of the eccrine duct deeper in the epidermis results in erythematous grouped papules in the same areas and is called miliaria rubra. Rarely, these may progress to pustules. Heat and high humidity predispose the patient to eccrine duct pore closure. Removal to a cooler environment is the treatment of choice.

9. Subcutaneous Fat Necrosis

This entity presents in the first 7 days of life as reddish or purple, sharply circumscribed, firm nodules occurring over the cheeks, buttocks, arms, and thighs. Cold injury is thought to play an important role. These lesions resolve spontaneously over a period of weeks, although in some instances they may calcify.

Conlon J, Drolet B: Skin lesions in the neonate. Pediatr Clin North Am 2004;51:863 [PMID: 15275979].

PIGMENT CELL BIRTHMARKS, NEVI, & MELANOMA

Birthmarks may involve an overgrowth of one or more of any of the normal components of skin (eg, pigment cells, blood vessels, lymph vessels). A nevus is a hamartoma of highly differentiated cells that retain their normal function.

1. Mongolian Spot

A blue-black macule found over the lumbosacral area in 90% of infants of Native-American, African-American, and Asian descent is called a mongolian spot. These spots are occasionally noted over the shoulders and back and may extend over the buttocks. Histologically, they consist of spindle-shaped pigment cells located deep in the dermis. The lesions fade somewhat with time as a result of darkening of the overlying skin, but some traces may persist into adult life.

2. Café-au-Lait Macule

A café-au-lait macule is a light brown, oval macule (dark brown on brown or black skin) that may be found anywhere on the body. Café-au-lait spots over 1.5 cm in greatest diameter are found in 10% of white and 22% of black children. These lesions persist throughout life and may increase in number with age. The presence of six or more such lesions over 1.5 cm in greatest diameter may be a clue to neurofibromatosis type 1 (NF-1). Patients with McCune-Albright syndrome (see Chapter 32) have a large, unilateral café-au-lait macule.

3. Spitz Nevus

A reddish-brown solitary nodule appearing on the face or upper arm of a child represents a Spitz nevus. Histologically, it consists of pigment-producing cells of bizarre shape with numerous mitoses. Although these lesions can look concerning histologically, they have a benign clinical course.

ACQUIRED MELANOCYTIC NEVI

1. Common Moles

Well-demarcated, brown to brown-black macules represent junctional nevi. They can begin to appear in the first years of life and increase with age. Histologically, these lesions are clones of melanocytes at the junction of the epidermis and dermis. Approximately 20% may progress to compound nevi—papular lesions with melanocytes both in junctional and intradermal locations. Intradermal nevi are often lighter in color and can be fleshy and pedunculated. Melanocytes in these lesions are located purely within the dermis. Nevi look dark blue (blue nevi) when they contain more deeply situated melanocytes in the dermis.

2. Melanoma

Melanoma in prepubertal children is very rare. Pigmented lesions with variegated colors (red, white, blue), notched borders, asymmetrical shape, and very irregular or ulcerated surfaces should arouse a suspicion of melanoma. Ulceration and bleeding are advanced signs of melanoma. If melanoma is suspected, wide local excision sent for pathologic examination should be done as the treatment of choice.

3. Congenital Melanocytic Nevi

One in 100 infants is born with a congenital nevus. Congenital nevi tend to be larger and darker brown than acquired nevi and may have many terminal hairs. If the pigmented plaque covers more than 5% of the body surface area, it is considered a giant or large congenital nevus; these large nevi occur in 1 in 20,000 infants. Often the lesions are so large they cover the entire trunk (bathing trunk nevi). Histologically, they are compound nevi with melanocytes often tracking around hair follicles and other adnexal structures deep in the dermis. The risk of malignant melanoma in small congenital nevi is controversial in the literature, but most likely very low. Transformation to malignant melanoma in giant congenital nevi has been estimated in the best studies to be between 1% and 5%. Two thirds of melanomas in children with giant congenital nevi develop in areas other than the skin.

Krengel S et al: Melanoma risk in congenital melanocytic naevi: A systematic review. Br J Dermatol 2006;155:1 [PMID: 16792745].

LaVigne EA et al: Clinical and dermascopic changes in common melanocytic nevi in school children: The Framingham school nevus study. Dermatology 2005;211:234 [PMID: 16205068].

Turchin I et al: Myths and misconceptions: The risk of melanoma in small congenital nevi. Skinmed 2004;3:228 [PMID: 15249787].

VASCULAR BIRTHMARKS

1. Capillary Malformations

▶ Clinical Findings

Capillary malformations are an excess of capillaries in localized areas of skin. The degree of excess is variable. The color of the lesions ranges from light red-pink to dark red. Light red macules are found over the nape of the neck, upper eyelids, and glabella of newborns. Fifty percent of infants have such lesions over their necks. Eyelid and glabellar lesions usually fade completely within the first year of life. Lesions that occupy the total central forehead area usually do not fade. Those on the neck persist into adult life.

Port-wine stains are dark red macules appearing anywhere on the body. A bilateral facial port-wine stain or one covering the entire half of the face may be a clue to Sturge-Weber syndrome, which is characterized by seizures, mental retardation, glaucoma, and hemiplegia. (See Chapter 23.) Most infants with smaller, unilateral facial port-wine stains do not have Sturge-Weber syndrome. Similarly, a port-wine stain over an extremity may be associated with hypertrophy of the soft tissue and bone of that extremity (Klippel-Trénaunay syndrome).

▶ Treatment

The pulsed dye laser is the treatment of choice for infants and children with port-wine stains.

Rallan D et al: Laser treatment of vascular lesions. Clin Dermatol 2006;24:8 [PMID: 16427501].

2. Hemangioma

▶ Clinical Findings

A red, rubbery nodule is a hemangioma. The lesion is often not present at birth but is represented by a permanent blanched area on the skin that is supplanted at age 2–4 weeks by red nodules. Histologically, these are benign tumors of capillary endothelial cells. Hemangiomas may be superficial, deep, or mixed. The terms *strawberry* and *cavernous* are misleading and should not be used. The biologic behavior of a hemangioma is the same despite its location. Fifty percent reach maximal regression by age 5 years, 70% by age 7 years, and 90% by age 9 years, leaving redundant skin, hypopigmentation, and telangiectasia. Local complications include superficial ulceration and secondary pyoderma.

▶ Treatment

Complications that require immediate treatment are (1) visual obstruction (with resulting amblyopia), (2) airway obstruction (hemangiomas of the head and neck ["beard hemangiomas"] may be associated with subglottic hemangiomas), and (3) cardiac decompensation (high-output failure). In these instances, the treatment of choice is with prednisolone, 2–3 mg/kg orally daily for 6–12 weeks. Interferon alfa-2a has been used to treat serious hemangiomas unresponsive to prednisone. Ten percent of patients with hemangiomas treated with interferon alfa-2a have developed spastic diplegia. Therefore, interferon alfa-2a therapy should be reserved for truly life-threatening hemangiomas, unresponsive to prednisolone therapy. If the lesion is ulcerated or bleeding, pulsed dye laser treatment may be helpful. The Kasabach-Merritt syndrome, characterized by platelet trapping with consumption coagulopathy, does not occur with solitary cutaneous hemangiomas. It is seen only with internal hemangiomas or the very rare vascular tumors called kaposiform hemangioendotheliomas and tufted angiomas.

Smolinski KN, Yan AC: Hemangiomas of infancy: Clinical and biological characteristics. Clin Pediatr (Phila) 2005;44:747 [PMID: 16327961].

3. Lymphatic Malformations

Lymphatic malformations may be superficial or deep. Superficial lymphatic malformations present as fluid-filled vesicles often described as looking like frog spawn. Deep lymphatic malformations are rubbery, skin-colored nodules occurring most commonly in the parotid area (cystic hygromas) or on the tongue. They often result in grotesque enlargement of soft tissues. Histologically, they can be either macrocystic or microcystic.

▶ Treatment

Therapy includes injection of picibanil, doxycycline, or surgery.

Lee BB et al: Current concepts in lymphatic malformations. Vasc Endovascular Surg 2005;39:67 [PMID: 15696250].

EPIDERMAL BIRTHMARKS

1. Epidermal Nevus

▶ **Clinical Findings**

The majority of these birthmarks present in the first year of life; however, they can first appear in adulthood. They are hamartomas of the epidermis that are warty to papillomatous plaques, often in a linear array. They range in color from skin-colored to dirty yellow to brown. Histologically they have a thickened epidermis with hyperkeratosis. The condition of widespread epidermal nevi associated with other developmental anomalies (central nervous system, eye, and skeletal), is called the epidermal nevus syndrome.

▶ **Treatment**

Treatment once or twice daily with topical calcipotriene may flatten some lesions. The only definitive cure is surgical excision.

Vujevich J, Mancini A: The epidermal nevus syndromes: Multisystem disorders. J Am Acad Dermatol 2004;50:957 [PMID: 15153903].

2. Nevus Sebaceus

▶ **Clinical Findings**

This is a hamartoma of sebaceous glands and underlying apocrine glands that is diagnosed by the appearance at birth of a yellowish, hairless plaque in the scalp or on the face. The lesions can be contiguous with an epidermal nevus on the face, and widespread lesions can constitute part of the epidermal nevus syndrome.

Histologically, nevus sebaceus represents an overabundance of sebaceous glands without hair follicles. At puberty, with androgenic stimulation, the sebaceous cells in the nevus divide, expand their cellular volume, and synthesize sebum, resulting in a warty mass.

▶ **Treatment**

Because 15% of these lesions become basal cell carcinomas after puberty, excision is recommended before puberty.

Terenzi V et al: Nevus sebaceous of Jadassohn. Craniofac Surg 2006;17:1234 [PMID: 17119437].

CONNECTIVE TISSUE BIRTHMARKS (JUVENILE ELASTOMA, COLLAGENOMA)

▶ **Clinical Findings**

Connective tissue nevi are smooth, skin-colored papules 1–10 mm in diameter that are grouped on the trunk. A solitary, larger (5–10 cm) nodule is called a shagreen patch and is histologically indistinguishable from other connective tissue nevi that show thickened, abundant collagen bundles with or without associated increases of elastic tissue. Although the shagreen patch is a cutaneous clue to tuberous sclerosis (see Chapter 23), the other connective tissue nevi occur as isolated events.

▶ **Treatment**

These nevi remain throughout life and need no treatment.

HEREDITARY SKIN DISORDERS

1. Ichthyosis

Ichthyosis is a term applied to several heritable diseases characterized by the presence of excessive scales on the skin. Major categories are listed in Table 14–4.

Table 14–4. Four major types of ichthyosis.

Name	Age at Onset	Clinical Features	Genetic Defect	Inheritance
Ichthyosis with normal epidermal turnover				
Ichthyosis vulgaris	Childhood	Fine scales, deep palmar and plantar markings	Filaggrin	Autosomal dominant
X-linked ichthyosis	Birth	Palms and soles spared; thick scales that darken with age; corneal opacities in patients and carrier mothers	Cholesterol sulfatase	X-linked
Ichthyosis with increased epidermal turnover				
Epidermolytic hyperkeratosis	Birth	Verrucous, yellow scales in flexural areas and palms and soles	Keratin 1 and 10	Autosomal dominant
Lamellar ichthyosis	Birth; collodion baby	Erythroderma, ectropion, large coarse scales; thickened palms and soles	Transglutaminase 1, ATP-binding cassette AI2	Autosomal recessive

ATP, adenosine triphosphate.

Table 14–5. Types of epidermolysis bullosa.

Name	Age at Onset	Clinical Features	Genetic Defect	Inheritance
Nonscarring types				
Epidermolysis bullosa simplex	Birth to first few years of life	Hemorrhagic blisters over lower legs; cooling prevents blisters; blisters brought out by walking	Keratins 5 and 14, plectin	Autosomal dominant
Junctional bullous dermolysis	Birth	Erosions on legs, oral mucosa; severe perioral involvement	Laminin 5, α-6- β-4 integrin, type XVII collagen	Autosomal recessive
Scarring types				
Epidermolysis bullosa dystrophica, dominant	Infancy	Numerous blisters on hands and feet; milia formation	Type VII collagen	Autosomal dominant
Epidermolysis bullosa dystrophica, recessive	Birth	Repeated episodes of blistering, secondary infection and scarring— "mitten hands and feet"	Type VII collagen	Autosomal recessive

▶ Treatment

Treatment consists of controlling scaling with lactic acid with ammonium hydroxide (Lac-Hydrin or AmLactin) 12% or urea cream 10–40% applied once daily. Daily lubrication and a good dry skin care regimen are important for these patients.

Oji V, Traupe H: Ichthyoses: Differential diagnosis and molecular genetics. Eur J Dermatol 2006;16:349 [PMID: 16935789].

2. Epidermolysis Bullosa

This is a group of heritable disorders characterized by skin fragility with blistering. Depending on the genetic defect, and therefore where the blister occurs, these disorders can be divided into scarring and nonscarring types (Table 14–5).

For the severely affected, a good deal of the surface area of the skin may have blisters and erosions, requiring daily wound care and dressings. These children are prone to frequent skin infections, have anemia, growth problems, mouth erosions and esophageal strictures, and chronic pain issues, among many others.

▶ Treatment

Treatment consists of protection of the skin with topical emollients as well as nonstick dressings. The other medical needs and potential complications of the severe forms of epidermolysis bullosa require a multidisciplinary approach. For the less severe types, protecting areas of greatest trauma with padding and dressings as well as intermittent topical or oral antibiotics for superinfection are appropriate treatments. If hands and feet are involved, reducing skin friction with 5% glutaraldehyde every 3 days is helpful.

Lucky AW: Update on epidermolysis bullosa. Yale University/Astellas Pharma Lectureship Series in Dermatology. Lecture 18, 2007.

▼ COMMON SKIN DISEASES IN INFANTS, CHILDREN, & ADOLESCENTS

ACNE

Acne affects 85% of adolescents. The onset of adolescent acne is between ages 8 and 10 years in 40% of children. The early lesions are usually limited to the face and are primarily closed comedones (whiteheads; see following discussion).

▶ Pathogenesis

The primary event in acne formation is obstruction of the sebaceous follicle and subsequent formation of the microcomedo (not evident clinically). This is the precursor to all future acne lesions. This phenomenon is androgen-dependent in adolescent acne. The keratinocytes of the sebaceous follicles contain an enzyme, 5α-reductase, which converts plasma testosterone to dihydrotestosterone (DHT). This androgen is a potent stimulus for cell proliferation. The four primary factors in the pathogenesis of acne are (1) plugging of the sebaceus follicle; (2) increased sebum production; (3) proliferation of *Propionibacterium acnes* in the obstructed follicle, and (4) inflammation. Many of these factors are influenced by androgens.

Drug-induced acne should be suspected in teenagers if all lesions are in the same stage at the same time and if involvement extends to the lower abdomen, lower back, arms, and legs. Drugs responsible for acne include corticotropin (ACTH), glucocorticoids, androgens, hydantoins, and isoniazid, each of which increases plasma testosterone.

▶ Clinical Findings

Open comedones are the predominant clinical lesion in early adolescent acne. The black color is caused not by dirt but by oxidized melanin within the stratum corneum cellular plug.

Open comedones do not often progress to inflammatory lesions. Closed comedones, or whiteheads, are caused by obstruction just beneath the follicular opening in the neck of the sebaceous follicle, which produces a cystic swelling of the follicular duct directly beneath the epidermis. Most authorities believe that closed comedones are precursors of inflammatory acne lesions (red papules, pustules, nodules and cysts). If open or closed comedones are the predominant lesions on the skin in adolescent acne, the condition is called comedonal acne.

In typical adolescent acne, several different types of lesions are present simultaneously. Severe, chronic, inflammatory lesions may rarely occur as interconnecting, draining sinus tracts. Adolescents with cystic acne require prompt medical attention, because ruptured cysts and sinus tracts result in severe scar formation. New acne scars are highly vascular and have a reddish or purplish hue. Such scars return to normal skin color after several years. Acne scars may be depressed beneath the skin level, raised, or flat to the skin. In adolescents with a tendency toward keloid formation, keloidal scars can occur following acne lesions, particularly on the chest and upper back.

▶ Differential Diagnosis

Consider rosacea, nevus comedonicus, flat warts, miliaria, molluscum contagiosum, and the angiofibromas of tuberous sclerosis.

▶ Treatment

Different treatment options are listed in Table 14–6. Recent data have indicated that combination therapy that targets multiple pathogenic factors increases the efficacy of treatment.

A. Topical Keratolytic Agents

Topical keratolytic agents address the plugging of the follicular opening with keratinocytes and include retinoids, benzoyl peroxide, and azelaic acid. The first-line treatment for both comedonal and inflammatory acne is a topical retinoid (tretinoin [retinoic acid], adapalene, and tazarotene). These are the most effective keratolytic agents. These topical agents may be used once daily, or the combination of a retinoid applied to acne-bearing areas of the skin in the evening and a benzoyl peroxide gel or azelaic acid applied in the morning may be used. This regimen will control 80–85% of cases of adolescent acne.

B. Topical Antibiotics

Topical antibiotics are less effective than systemic antibiotics and at best are equivalent in potency to 250 mg of tetracycline orally once a day. One percent clindamycin phosphate solution is the most efficacious topical antibiotic. Most *P acnes* strains are now resistant to topical erythromycin solutions. Topical antibiotic therapy alone should never be used.

Table 14–6. Acne treatment.

Type of Lesion	Treatment
Comedonal acne	One of the following: Retinoic acid, 0.025, 0.05, or 0.1% cream; 0.01 or 0.025% gel; or 0.1% microgel Adapalene, 0.1% gel or solution; 0.05% cream
Papular inflammatory acne	One from first grouping, plus one of the following: Benzoyl peroxide, 2.5, 4, 5, 8, or 10% gel or lotion; 4 or 8% wash Azaleic acid, 15% cream Clindamycin, 1% lotion, solution, or gel
Pustular inflammatory acne	One from first grouping, plus one of the following: Oral antibiotics Tetracycline, 250–500 mg, bid Minocycline or doxycycline, 50–100 mg, bid
Nodulocystic acne	Accutane, 1 mg/kg/d

Multiple studies have shown a combination of benzoyl peroxide or a retinoid and a topical antibiotic are more effective than the antibiotic alone.

C. Systemic Antibiotics

Antibiotics that are concentrated in sebum, such as tetracycline, minocycline, and doxycycline should be reserved for moderate to severe inflammatory acne. The usual dose of tetracycline is 0.5–1.0 g divided twice a day on an empty stomach; minocycline and doxycycline 50–100 mg taken once or twice daily can be taken with food. Monotherapy with oral antibiotics should never be used. Recent recommendations are that oral antibiotics should be used for a finite time period, and then discontinued as soon as possible. The tetracycline antibiotics should not be given to children younger than 8 years of age due to the effect on dentition (staining of teeth). These antibiotics have anti-inflammatory effects in addition to decreasing *P acnes* in the follicle.

D. Oral Retinoids

An oral retinoid, 13-*cis*-retinoic acid (isotretinoin; Accutane), is the most effective treatment for severe cystic acne. The precise mechanism of its action is unknown, but decreased sebum production, decreased follicular obstruction, decreased skin bacteria, and general anti-inflammatory activities have been described. The initial dosage is 40 mg once or twice daily. This therapy is reserved for severe nodulocystic acne, or acne recalcitrant to aggressive standard therapy. Side effects include dryness and scaling of the skin, dry lips, and, occasionally, dry eyes and dry nose. Fifteen percent of patients may experience some mild achiness with athletic activities. Up to 10% of patients experience mild, reversible hair loss. Elevated liver enzymes and blood lipids have rarely been described. Acute depression may occur. Isotretinoin is teratogenic in young women of childbearing age. Because of this and the other side effects, it is not recommended unless strict adherence to the Food and Drug Administration (FDA) guidelines is ensured. The FDA has implemented a strict registration program (iPLEDGE) that must be used to obtain isotretinoin.

E. Other Acne Treatments

Hormonal therapy (oral contraceptives) is often an effective option for girls who have perimenstrual flares of acne or have not responded adequately to conventional therapy. Adolescents with endocrine disorders such as polycystic ovary syndrome also see improvement of their acne with hormonal therapy. Oral contraceptives can be added to a conventional therapeutic regimen and should always be used in female patients who are prescribed oral isotretinoin unless absolute contraindications exist.

F. Avoidance of Cosmetics and Hair Spray

Acne can be aggravated by a variety of external factors that result in further obstruction of partially occluded sebaceous follicles. Discontinuing the use of oil-based cosmetics, face creams, and hair sprays may alleviate the comedonal component of acne within 4–6 weeks.

G. Patient Education and Follow-Up Visits

The multifactorial pathogenesis of acne and its role in the treatment plan must be explained to adolescent patients. Time should be set aside at the first visit to answer questions. Acne therapy is aimed at preventing the microcomedone, so therapy takes 8–12 weeks to produce improvement. This delay should be stressed to the patient. Realistic expectations should be encouraged in the adolescent patient because no therapy will prevent an adolescent from ever having another acne lesion. A written education sheet is useful.

Follow-up visits should be made every 8–12 weeks. An objective method to chart improvement should be documented by the provider, because patients' assessment of improvement tends to be inaccurate. Explain again what medications are being used and why, what the treatment is intended to achieve, and that 8–12 weeks of consistent therapy is required for improvement in most cases. Ensure on follow-up that the patient is applying the medication properly (eg, topical keratolytics are to be applied to the entire area of skin that tends to be affected, not to individual lesions already present).

Strauss JS et al: Guidelines of care for acne vulgaris management. J Am Acad Dermatol 2007;56:651 [PMID: 17276540].

BACTERIAL INFECTIONS OF THE SKIN

1. Impetigo

Erosions covered by honey-colored crusts are diagnostic of impetigo. Staphylococci and group A streptococci are important pathogens in this disease, which histologically consists of superficial invasion of bacteria into the upper epidermis, forming a subcorneal pustule.

▶ **Treatment**

Impetigo should be treated with an antimicrobial agent effective against *Staphylococcus aureus* (β-lactamase-resistant penicillins or cephalosporins, clindamycin, amoxicillin–clavulanate) for 7–10 days. Topical mupirocin and fusidic acid (three times daily) are also effective.

2. Bullous Impetigo

All impetigo is bullous, with the blister forming just beneath the stratum corneum, but in bullous impetigo there is, in addition to the usual erosion covered by a honey-colored crust, a border filled with clear fluid. Staphylococci may be isolated from these lesions, and systemic signs of circulating exfoliatin are absent. Bullous varicella is a disorder that represents bullous impetigo as a superinfection in varicella lesions.

▶ **Treatment**

Treatment with oral antistaphylococcal drugs for 7–10 days is effective. Application of cool compresses to debride crusts is a helpful symptomatic measure.

3. Ecthyma

Ecthyma is a firm, dry crust, surrounded by erythema that exudes purulent material. It represents invasion by group A β-hemolytic streptococci through the epidermis to the superficial dermis. This should not be confused with ecthyma gangrenosum. Lesions of ecthyma gangrenosum may be similar in appearance, but they are seen in a severely ill or immunocompromised patient and are due to systemic dissemination of bacteria, usually *Pseudomonas aeruginosa*, through the bloodstream.

▶ **Treatment**

Treatment is with systemic penicillin.

4. Cellulitis

Cellulitis is characterized by erythematous, hot, tender, ill-defined, edematous plaques accompanied by regional lymphadenopathy. Histologically, this disorder represents invasion of microorganisms into the lower dermis and sometimes beyond, with obstruction of local lymphatics. Group A β-hemolytic streptococci and coagulase-positive staphylococci are the most common causes; pneumococci and *Haemophilus influenzae* are rare causes. Staphylococcal infections are usually more localized and more likely to have a purulent center; streptococcal infections spread more rapidly, but these characteristics cannot be used to specify the infecting agent. An entry site of prior trauma or infection (eg, varicella) is often present. Septicemia is a potential complication.

▶ **Treatment**

Treatment is with an appropriate systemic antibiotic.

5. Folliculitis

A pustule at a follicular opening represents folliculitis. If the pustule occurs at eccrine sweat orifices, it is correctly called poritis. Staphylococci and streptococci are the most frequent pathogens.

▶ **Treatment**

Treatment consists of measures to remove follicular obstruction—either cool, wet compresses for 24 hours or keratolytics such as those used for acne.

6. Abscess

An abscess occurs deep in the skin, at the bottom of a follicle or an apocrine gland, and is diagnosed as an erythematous, firm, acutely tender nodule with ill-defined borders. Staphylococci are the most common organisms.

▶ **Treatment**

Treatment consists of incision and drainage and systemic antibiotics.

7. Scalded Skin Syndrome

This entity consists of the sudden onset of bright red, acutely painful skin, most obvious periorally, periorbitally, and in the flexural areas of the neck, the axillae, the popliteal and antecubital areas, and the groin. The slightest pressure on the skin results in severe pain and separation of the epidermis, leaving a glistening layer (the stratum granulosum of the epidermis) beneath. The disease is caused by a circulating toxin (exfoliatin) elaborated by phage group II staphylococci. Exfoliatin binds to desmoglein-1 resulting in a separation of cells in the granular layer. The causative staphylococci may be isolated not from the skin but rather from the nasopharynx, an abscess, sinus, blood culture, and so on.

▶ **Treatment**

Treatment is with systemic antistaphylococcal drugs.

Patel GK: Treatment of staphylococcal scalded skin syndrome. Expert Rev Anit Infect 2004;2:575 [PMID: 15482221].

Schachner LA: Treatment of uncomplicated skin infections in the pediatric and adolescent patient populations. J Drugs Dermatol 2005;4:s30 [PMID: 16300228].

FUNGAL INFECTIONS OF THE SKIN

1. Dermatophyte Infections

Dermatophytes become attached to the superficial layer of the epidermis, nails, and hair, where they proliferate. They grow mainly within the stratum corneum and do not invade the lower epidermis or dermis. Release of toxins from dermatophytes—especially those whose natural hosts are animals or soil, for example, *Microsporum canis* and *Trichophyton verrucosum*—results in dermatitis. Fungal infection should be suspected with any red and scaly lesion.

▶ **Classification & Clinical Findings**

A. Tinea Capitis

Thickened, broken-off hairs with erythema and scaling of underlying scalp are the distinguishing features (Table 14–7). In endemic ringworm, hairs are broken off at the surface of the scalp, leaving a "black dot" appearance. Pustule formation and a boggy, fluctuant mass on the scalp occur in *M canis* and *T tonsurans* infections. This mass, called a kerion, represents an exaggerated host response to the organism. Diffuse scaling of the scalp may also be seen. Fungal culture should be performed in all cases of suspected tinea capitis.

B. Tinea Corporis

Tinea corporis presents either as annular marginated plaques with a thin scale and clear center or as an annular confluent dermatitis. The most common organisms are *Trichophyton mentagrophytes* and *M canis*. The diagnosis is made by scraping thin scales from the border of the lesion, dissolving them in 20% KOH, and examining for hyphae.

Table 14–7. Clinical features of tinea capitis.

Most Common Organisms	Clinical Appearance	Microscopic Appearance in KOH
Trichophyton tonsurans (90%)	Hairs broken off 2-3 mm from follicle; "black dot"; diffuse pustule; seborrheic dermatitis-like; no fluorescence	Hyphae and spores within hair
Microsporum canis (10%)	Thickened broken-off hairs that fluoresce yellow-green with Wood's lamp	Small spores outside of hair; hyphae within hair

C. Tinea Cruris

Symmetrical, sharply marginated lesions in inguinal areas occur with tinea cruris. The most common organisms are *Trichophyton rubrum, T mentagrophytes,* and *Epidermophyton floccosum.*

D. Tinea Pedis

The diagnosis of tinea pedis is becoming more common in the prepubertal child, although it is still most commonly seen in postpubertal males. Presentation is with red scaly soles, blisters on the instep of the foot, or fissuring between the toes.

E. Tinea Unguium (Onychomycosis)

Loosening of the nail plate from the nail bed (onycholysis), giving a yellow discoloration, is the first sign of fungal invasion of the nails. Thickening of the distal nail plate then occurs, followed by scaling and a crumbly appearance of the entire nail plate surface. *T rubrum* and *T mentagrophytes* are the most common causes. The diagnosis is confirmed by KOH examination and fungal culture. Usually only one or two nails are involved. If every nail is involved, psoriasis, lichen planus, or idiopathic trachyonychia is a more likely diagnosis than fungal infection.

▶ Treatment

The treatment of dermatophytosis is quite simple: If hair is involved, griseofulvin is the treatment of choice. Topical antifungal agents do not enter hair or nails in sufficient concentration to clear the infection. The absorption of griseofulvin from the gastrointestinal tract is enhanced by a fatty meal; thus, whole milk or ice cream taken with the medication increases absorption. The dosage of griseofulvin is 20 mg/kg/d. With hair infections, cultures should be done every 4 weeks, and treatment should be continued for 4 weeks following a negative culture result. The side effects are few, and the drug has been used successfully in the newborn period. Itraconazole and terbinafine have been used when response to griseofulvin is unsatisfactory. For nails, daily administration of topical ciclopirox 8% (Penlac nail lacquer) can be considered, as can pulsed-dose itraconazole given in three 1-week pulses separated by 3 weeks.

Tinea corporis, tinea pedis, and tinea cruris can be treated effectively with topical medication after careful inspection to make certain that the hair and nails are not involved. Treatment with any of the imidazoles, allylamines, benzylamines, or ciclopirox applied twice daily for 3–4 weeks is recommended.

Gupta AK et al: Dermatophytosis: The management of fungal infections. Skinmed 2005;4:305 [PMID: 16282753].

2. Tinea Versicolor

Tinea versicolor is a superficial infection caused by *Pityrosporum orbiculare* (also called *Malassezia furfur*), a yeastlike fungus. It characteristically causes polycyclic connected hypopigmented macules and very fine scales in areas of sun-induced pigmentation. In winter, the polycyclic macules appear reddish brown.

▶ Treatment

Treatment consists of application of selenium sulfide (Selsun), 2.5% suspension, or topical antifungals. Selenium sulfide should be applied to the whole body and left on overnight. Treatment can be repeated again in 1 week and then monthly thereafter. It tends to be somewhat irritating, and the patient should be warned about this difficulty.

3. *Candida albicans* Infections (See also Chapter 39)

▶ Clinical Findings

In addition to being a frequent invader in diaper dermatitis, *Candida albicans* also infects the oral mucosa, where it appears as thick white patches with an erythematous base (thrush); the angles of the mouth, where it causes fissures and white exudate (perlèche); and the cuticular region of the fingers, where thickening of the cuticle, dull red erythema, and distortion of growth of the nail plate suggest the diagnosis of candidal paronychia. *Candida* dermatitis is characterized by sharply defined erythematous patches, sometimes with eroded areas. Pustules, vesicles, or papules may be present as satellite lesions. Similar infections may be found in other moist areas, such as the axillae and neck folds. This infection is more common in children who have recently received antibiotics.

▶ Treatment

A topical imidazole cream is the drug of first choice for *C albicans* infections. In diaper dermatitis, the cream form can be applied every 8–12 hours. In oral thrush, nystatin suspension should be applied directly to the mucosa with the parent's finger or a cotton-tipped applicator, because it is not absorbed and acts topically. In candidal paronychia, the antifungal agent is applied over the area, covered with occlusive plastic wrapping, and left on overnight after the application is made airtight. Refractory candidiasis will respond to a brief course of oral fluconazole.

Kyle AA, Dahl MV: Topical therapy for fungal infections. Am J Clin Dermatol 2004;5:443 [PMID: 15663341].

VIRAL INFECTIONS OF THE SKIN (SEE ALSO CHAPTER 38)

1. Herpes Simplex Infection

▶ Clinical Findings

Painful, grouped vesicles or erosions on a red base suggest herpes simplex. Rapid immunofluorescent tests for herpes simplex virus (HSV) and varicella-zoster virus (VZV) are available. A Tzanck smear is done by scraping a vesicle base with a No. 15

blade, smearing on a glass slide, and staining the epithelial cells with Wright stain. The smear is positive if epidermal multinucleated giant cells are visualized. A positive Tzanck smear indicates herpesvirus infection (HSV or VZV). In infants and children, lesions resulting from herpes simplex type 1 are seen most commonly on the gingiva, lips, and face. Involvement of a digit (herpes whitlow) will occur if the child sucks the thumb or fingers. Herpes simplex type 2 lesions are seen on the genitalia and in the mouth in adolescents. Cutaneous dissemination of herpes simplex occurs in patients with atopic dermatitis (eczema herpeticum) and appears clinically as very tender, punched out erosions among the eczematous skin changes.

► Treatment

The treatment of HSV infections is discussed in Chapter 38.

Waggoner-Fountain LA, Grossman LB: Herpes simplex virus. Pediatr Rev 2004;25:86 [PMID: 14993516].
Whitley RJ: Herpes simplex virus in children. Curr Treat Options Neurol 2004;4:231 [PMID: 11931730].

2. Varicella-Zoster Infection

► Clinical Findings

Grouped vesicles in a dermatome, usually on the trunk or face, suggest varicella-zoster reactivation. Zoster in children may not be painful and usually has a mild course. In patients with compromised host resistance, the appearance of an erythematous border around the vesicles is a good prognostic sign. Conversely, large bullae without a tendency to crusting and systemic illness imply a poor host response to the virus. Varicella-zoster and herpes simplex lesions undergo the same series of changes: papule, vesicle, pustule, crust, slightly depressed scar. Lesions of primary varicella appear in crops, and many different stages of lesions are present at the same time (eg, papules), eccentrically placed vesicles on an erythematous base ("dew drop" on a rose petal), erosions, and crusts.

► Treatment

Antihistamines may be used for pruritus; cool baths or drying lotions such as calamine lotion are usually sufficient to relieve symptoms. In immunosuppressed children, intravenous or oral acyclovir should be used.

Heininger U, Seward JF: Varicella. Lancet 2006;368:1365 [PMID: 17046469].
Leung AK et al: Herpes zoster in childhood. Pediatr Health Care 2006;20:300 [PMID: 16962434].

3. Human Immunodeficiency Virus Infection (See also Chapter 39)

► Clinical Findings

The average time of onset of skin lesions after perinatally acquired HIV infection is 4 months; after transfusion-acquired infection, it is 11 months. Persistent oral candidiasis and recalcitrant candidal diaper rash are the most frequent cutaneous features of infantile HIV infection. Severe or recurrent herpetic gingivostomatitis, varicella-zoster infection, and molluscum contagiosum infection occur. Recurrent staphylococcal pyodermas, tinea of the face, and onychomycosis are also observed. A generalized dermatitis with features of seborrhea (severe cradle cap) is extremely common. In general, persistent, recurrent, or extensive skin infections should make one suspicious of HIV infection.

► Treatment

The treatment of HIV infections is discussed in Chapter 39.

Wananukul S et al: Mucocutaneous findings in pediatric AIDS related to degree of immunosuppression. Pediatr Dermatol 2004;20:289 [PMID: 1286945].

VIRUS-INDUCED TUMORS

1. Molluscum Contagiosum

Molluscum contagiosum is a poxvirus that induces the epidermis to proliferate, forming a pale papule. Molluscum contagiosum consists of umbilicated, flesh-colored papules in groups on the genitalia or trunk. They are common in infants and preschool children, as well as sexually active adolescents.

► Treatment

Treatment for molluscum includes topical imiquimod, topical cantharidin, oral cimetidine, cryotherapy with liquid nitrogen, and curettage. Left untreated, the lesions resolve over months to years.

Dohil MA et al: The epidemiology of molluscum contagiosum in children. J Am Acad Dermatol 2006;54:47 [PMID: 16384754].

2. Warts

Warts are skin-colored papules with irregular (verrucous) surfaces. They are intraepidermal tumors caused by infection with human papillomavirus (HPV). There are over 100 types of this DNA virus, which induces the epidermal cells to proliferate, thus resulting in the warty growth. Flat warts are smoother and smaller than common warts and are often seen on the face. Certain types of HPV are associated with certain types of warts (eg, flat warts) or location of warts (eg, genital warts).

► Treatment

No therapy for warts is ideal, and 30% of warts will clear in 6 months irrespective of the therapy chosen. Liquid nitrogen is often used to treat common (vulgaris) warts. The treated lesion should stay white for 20 seconds. Aggressive treatment with prolonged freeze times and too much pressure applied with a cotton applicator can lead to blistering and scarring. The patient should be seen at treatment intervals of 2–3 weeks. Longer times between treatments result in lower efficacy. Topical salicylic acid, topical imiquimod, and oral cimetidine may also be used. Large mosaic plantar warts are treated most effectively by applying 40% salicylic acid plaster cut with a scissors to fit the lesion. The adhesive side of the plaster is placed against the lesion and taped securely in place with duct or athletic tape. The plaster and tape should be placed on Monday and removed on Friday. Over the weekend, the patient should soak the skin in warm water for 30 minutes to soften it. Then the white, macerated tissue should be pared with a pumice stone, cuticle scissors, or a nail file. This procedure is repeated every week, and the patient is seen every 4 weeks. Most plantar warts resolve in 6–8 weeks when treated in this way. Vascular pulsed dye lasers are a useful adjunct therapy for the treatment of plantar warts.

For flat warts, a good response to 0.05% tretinoin cream or topical imiquimod (Aldara) cream, applied once daily for 3–4 weeks, has been reported.

Surgical excision, electrosurgery, and nonspecific burning laser surgery should be avoided; these modalities do not have higher cure rates and result in scarring.

Venereal warts (condylomata acuminata) (see Chapter 42) may be treated with imiquimod, 25% podophyllum resin (podophyllin) in alcohol, or podofilox, a lower concentration of purified podophyllin, which is applied at home. Podophyllin should be painted on the lesions in the practitioner's office and then washed off after 4 hours. Re-treatment in 2–3 weeks may be necessary. Podofilox is applied by the patient once daily, Monday through Thursday, whereas imiquimod is used 3 times a week on alternating days. Lesions not on the vulvar mucous membrane but on the adjacent skin should be treated as a common wart and frozen.

No wart therapy is immediately and definitively successful. Realistic expectations should be set and appropriate follow-up treatments scheduled.

Keogh-Brown MR et al: To freeze or not to freeze: A cost-effectiveness analysis of wart treatment. Br J Dermatol 2007;156:687 [PMID: 17326748].

INSECT INFESTATIONS

1. Scabies

▶ **Clinical Findings**

Scabies is suggested by linear burrows about the wrists, ankles, finger webs, areolas, anterior axillary folds, genitalia, or face (in infants). Often there are excoriations, honey-colored crusts, and pustules from secondary infection. Identification of the female mite or her eggs and feces is necessary to confirm the diagnosis. Scrape an unscratched papule or burrow with a No. 15 blade and examine microscopically in immersion oil to confirm the diagnosis. In a child who is often scratching, scrape under the fingernails. Examine the parents for unscratched burrows.

▶ **Treatment**

Permethrin 5% is now the treatment of choice for scabies. It should be applied as a single overnight application. The need for re-treatment is rare.

Karthikeyan K: Scabies in children. Arch Dis Child Educ Pract Ed 2007;92:ep65 [PMID: 17517973].

2. Pediculoses (Louse Infestations)

▶ **Clinical Findings**

The presence of excoriated papules and pustules and a history of severe itching at night suggest infestation with the human body louse. This louse may be discovered in the seams of underwear but not on the body. In the scalp hair, the gelatinous nits of the head louse adhere tightly to the hair shaft. The pubic louse may be found crawling among pubic hairs, or blue-black macules may be found dispersed through the pubic region (maculae cerulea). The pubic louse is often seen on the eyelashes of newborns.

▶ **Treatment**

Initial treatment of head lice is often instituted by parents with an over-the-counter pyrethrin or permethrin product. If head lice are not eradicated after two applications 7 days apart with these products, 5% permethrin should be used. Malathion 0.5% is highly effective but is toxic if ingested, and flammable.

Lebwohl M et al: Therapy for head lice based on life cycle, resistance, and safety. Pediatrics 2007;119:965 [PMID: 17473098].

3. Papular Urticaria

▶ **Clinical Findings**

Papular urticaria is characterized by grouped erythematous papules surrounded by an urticarial flare and distributed over the shoulders, upper arms, and buttocks in infants. Although not a true infestation, these lesions represent delayed hypersensitivity reactions to stinging or biting insects and can be reproduced by patch testing with the offending insect. Fleas from dogs and cats are the usual offenders. Less commonly, mosquitoes, lice, scabies, and bird and grass mites are involved. The sensitivity is transient, lasting 4–6 months. Usually no other family members are affected. It is often difficult for the parents to understand why no one else is affected.

▶ **Treatment**

The logical therapy is to remove the offending insect, although in most cases it is very difficult to identify the exact cause. Topical corticosteroids and oral antihistamines will control symptoms.

Hernandez RG, Cohen BA: Insect bite-induced hypersensitivity and the SCRATCH principles: A new approach to papular urticaria. Pediatrics 2006;118:e189 [PMID: 16751615].

DERMATITIS (ECZEMA)

The terms *dermatitis* and *eczema* are currently used interchangeably in dermatology, although the term *eczema* truly denotes an acute weeping dermatosis. All forms of dermatitis, regardless of cause, may present with acute edema, erythema, and oozing with crusting, mild erythema alone, or lichenification. Lichenification is diagnosed by thickening of the skin with a shiny surface and exaggerated, deepened skin markings. It is the response of the skin to chronic rubbing or scratching.

Although the lesions of the various dermatoses are histologically indistinguishable, clinicians have nonetheless divided the disease group called dermatitis into several categories based on known causes in some cases and differing natural histories in others.

1. Atopic Dermatitis

▶ Pathogenesis & Clinical Findings

Atopic dermatitis is a general term for chronic superficial inflammation of the skin that can be applied to a heterogeneous group of patients. Many (not all) patients go through three clinical phases. In the first, infantile eczema, the dermatitis begins on the cheeks and scalp and frequently expresses itself as oval patches on the trunk, later involving the extensor surfaces of the extremities. The usual age at onset is 2–3 months, and this phase ends at age 18 months to 2 years. Only one third of all infants with infantile eczema progress to phase 2 childhood or flexural eczema in which the predominant involvement is in the antecubital and popliteal fossae, the neck, the wrists, and sometimes the hands or feet. This phase lasts from age 2 years to adolescence. Some children have involvement only of the soles of the feet, with cracking, redness, and pain, so-called atopic feet. Only one third of children with typical flexural eczema progress to adolescent eczema, which is usually manifested by the continuation of chronic flexural eczema alone with hand dermatitis. Atopic dermatitis is quite unusual after age 30 years.

Atopic dermatitis results from an interaction among susceptibility genes, the host environment, skin barrier defects, pharmacologic abnormalities, and immunologic response. The case for food and inhalant allergens as specific causes of atopic dermatitis is not strong. There is significant new evidence that the primary defect in atopic dermatitis is an abnormality in the skin barrier formation due to defects in the filaggrin gene.

A few patients with atopic dermatitis have immunodeficiency with recurrent pyodermas, unusual susceptibility to herpes simplex viruses, hyperimmunoglobulinemia E, defective neutrophil and monocyte chemotaxis, and impaired T-lymphocyte function. (See Chapter 31.)

A faulty epidermal barrier predisposes the patient with atopic dermatitis to dry, itchy skin. Inability to hold water within the stratum corneum results in rapid evaporation of water, shrinking of the stratum corneum, and cracks in the epidermal barrier. Such skin forms an ineffective barrier to the entry of various irritants—and, indeed, it may be clinically useful to regard atopic dermatitis as a primary-irritant contact dermatitis and simply tell the patient, "you have sensitive skin." Chronic atopic dermatitis is frequently infected secondarily with *S aureus* or *Streptococcus pyogenes*. Patients with atopic dermatitis have a deficiency of antimicrobial peptides in their skin, which may account for the susceptibility to recurrent skin infection.

▶ Treatment

A. Acute Stages

Application of wet dressings and topical corticosteroids is the treatment of choice for acute, weeping atopic eczema. A topical steroid preparation is applied two times daily and covered with wet dressings as outlined at the beginning of this chapter. Superinfection or colonization with *S aureus* is common, and appropriate systemic antibiotics may be necessary. If the expected improvement is not seen, bacterial cultures should be obtained to identify the possibility of an organism resistant to standard therapy.

B. Chronic Stages

Treatment is aimed at avoiding irritants and restoring water to the skin. No soaps or harsh shampoos should be used, and the patient should avoid woolen or any rough clothing. Bathing is minimized to every second or third day. Twice-daily lubrication of the skin is very important.

Nonperfumed lotions or creams are suitable lubricants. Plain petrolatum is an acceptable lubricant, but some people find it too greasy and during hot weather it may also cause considerable sweat retention. Liberal use of Cetaphil lotion four or five times daily as a substitute for soap is also satisfactory as a means of lubrication. A bedroom humidifier is often helpful. Topical corticosteroids should be limited to medium strength (see Table 14–3). There is never any reason to use super- or high-potency corticosteroids in atopic dermatitis. In superinfected atopic dermatitis, systemic antibiotics for 10–14 days are necessary.

Tacrolimus and pimecrolimus ointments are topical immunosuppressive agents that are effective in atopic dermatitis. Due to concerns about the development of malignancies, tacrolimus and pimecrolimus should be reserved for children older than 2 years of age with atopic dermatitis unresponsive to medium-potency topical steroids. It has been argued that an increased risk of malignancy has not been seen in immunologically normal individuals using these products. Recommendations for usage likely will change with time. Treatment failures in chronic atopic dermatitis are most often the result of patient noncompliance. This is a frustrating disease for parent and child. Return to a normal lifestyle for the parent and child is the ultimate goal of therapy.

Beck LA: The efficacy and safety of tacrolimus ointment: A clinical review. J Am Acad Dermatol 2005;53:S165 [PMID: 16021171].

Izadpanah A, Gallo RL: Antimicrobial peptides. J Am Acad Dermatol 2005;52:381 [PMID: 15761415].

Kiken DA, Silverberg NB: Atopic dermatitis in children, part 1: Clinical features and complications. Cutis 2006;78:241 [PMID: 17121059].

Kiken DA, Silverberg NB: Atopic dermatitis in children, part 2: Treatment options. Cutis 2005;78:401 [PMID: 17243427].

Sandilands A et al: Filaggrin's fuller figure: A glimpse into the genetic architecture of atopic dermatitis. J Invest Dermatol 2007;127:1282 [PMID: 17502856].

2. Nummular Eczema

Nummular eczema is characterized by numerous symmetrically distributed coin-shaped patches of dermatitis, principally on the extremities. These may be acute, oozing, and crusted or dry and scaling. The differential diagnosis should include tinea corporis, impetigo, and atopic dermatitis.

▶ Treatment

The same topical measures should be used as for atopic dermatitis, although treatment is often more difficult.

3. Primary Irritant Contact Dermatitis (Diaper Dermatitis)

Contact dermatitis is of two types: primary irritant and allergic eczematous. Primary irritant dermatitis develops within a few hours, reaches peak severity at 24 hours, and then disappears. Allergic eczematous contact dermatitis (described in the next section) has a delayed onset of 18 hours, peaks at 48–72 hours, and often lasts as long as 2–3 weeks even if exposure to the offending antigen is discontinued.

Diaper dermatitis, the most common form of primary irritant contact dermatitis seen in pediatric practice, is caused by prolonged contact of the skin with urine and feces, which contain irritating chemicals such as urea and intestinal enzymes.

▶ Clinical Findings

The diagnosis of diaper dermatitis is based on the picture of erythema and scaling of the skin in the perineal area and the history of prolonged skin contact with urine or feces. This is frequently seen in the "good baby" who sleeps many hours through the night without waking. In 80% of cases of diaper dermatitis lasting more than 3 days, the affected area is colonized with C albicans even before appearance of the classic signs of a beefy red, sharply marginated dermatitis with satel-

lite lesions. Streptococcal perianal cellulitis and infantile psoriasis should be included in the differential diagnosis.

▶ Treatment

Treatment consists of changing diapers frequently. The area should only be washed following a bowel movement. Washing should be done with a wash cloth and warm water only. Because rubber or plastic pants prevent evaporation of the contactant and enhance its penetration into the skin, they should be avoided as much as possible. Air drying is useful. Treatment of long-standing diaper dermatitis should include application of nystatin or an imidazole cream with each diaper change.

Humphrey S et al: Practical management strategies for diaper dermatitis. Skin Therapy Lett 2006;11:1 [PMID: 17021645].

4. Allergic Eczematous Contact Dermatitis (Poison Ivy Dermatitis)

▶ Clinical Findings

Plants such as poison ivy, poison sumac, and poison oak cause most cases of allergic contact dermatitis in children. Allergic contact dermatitis has all the features of delayed-type (T-lymphocyte–mediated) hypersensitivity. Many substances may cause such a reaction; nickel sulfate, potassium dichromate, and neomycin are the most common causes. Nickel is found to some degree in all metals. Nickel allergy is commonly seen on the ears secondary to the wearing of earrings, and near the umbilicus from pants snaps and belt buckles. The true incidence of allergic contact dermatitis in children is unknown. Children often present with acute dermatitis with blister formation, oozing, and crusting. Blisters are often linear and of acute onset.

▶ Treatment

Treatment of contact dermatitis in localized areas is with topical corticosteroids. In severe generalized involvement, prednisone, 1–2 mg/kg/d orally for 10–14 days, can be used.

Militello G et al: Allergic contact dermatitis in children. Curr Opin Pediatr 2006;18:385 [PMID: 16914992].

5. Seborrheic Dermatitis

▶ Clinical Findings

Seborrheic dermatitis is an erythematous scaly dermatitis accompanied by overproduction of sebum occurring in areas rich in sebaceous glands (ie, the face, scalp, and perineum). This common condition occurs predominantly in the newborn and at puberty, the ages at which hormonal stimulation of sebum production is maximal. Although it is tempting to speculate that overproduction of sebum causes the dermatitis, the exact relationship is unclear.

Seborrheic dermatitis on the scalp in infancy is clinically similar to atopic dermatitis, and the distinction may become clear only after other areas are involved. Psoriasis also occurs in seborrheic areas in older children and should be considered in the differential diagnosis.

Treatment

Seborrheic dermatitis responds well to low-potency topical corticosteroids.

Schwartz RA et al: Seborrheic dermatitis: An overview. Am Fam Physician 2006;74:125 [PMID: 16848386].

6. Dandruff

Dandruff is physiologic scaling or mild seborrhea, in the form of greasy scalp scales. The cause is unknown. Treatment is with medicated dandruff shampoos.

7. Dry Skin Dermatitis (Asteatotic Eczema, Xerosis)

Newborns and older children who live in arid climates are susceptible to dry skin, characterized by large cracked scales with erythematous borders. The stratum corneum is dependent on environmental humidity for its water, and below 30% environmental humidity the stratum corneum loses water, shrinks, and cracks. These cracks in the epidermal barrier allow irritating substances to enter the skin, predisposing the patient to dermatitis.

Treatment

Treatment consists of increasing the water content of the skin in the immediate external environment. House humidifiers are very useful. Minimize bathing to every second or third day.

Frequent soaping of the skin impairs its water-holding capacity and serves as an irritating alkali, and all soaps should therefore be avoided. Frequent use of emollients (eg, Cetaphil, Eucerin, Lubriderm) should be a major part of therapy.

8. Keratosis Pilaris

Follicular papules containing a white inspissated scale characterize keratosis pilaris. Individual lesions are discrete and may be red. They are prominent on the extensor surfaces of the upper arms and thighs and on the buttocks and cheeks. In severe cases, the lesions may be generalized. Such lesions are seen frequently in children with dry skin and have also been associated with atopic dermatitis and ichthyosis vulgaris.

Treatment

Treatment is with keratolytics such as urea cream or lactic acid, followed by skin hydration.

9. Pityriasis Alba

White, scaly macular areas with indistinct borders are seen over extensor surfaces of extremities and on the cheeks in children with pityriasis alba. Suntanning exaggerates these lesions. Histologic examination reveals a mild dermatitis. These lesions may be confused with tinea versicolor.

Treatment

Low-potency topical corticosteroids may help decrease any inflammatory component and may lead to faster return of normal pigmentation.

Lin RL, Janninger CK: Pityriasis alba. Cutis 2005;76:21 [PMID: 16144284].

COMMON SKIN TUMORS

If the skin moves with the nodule on lateral palpation, the tumor is located within the dermis; if the skin moves over the nodule, it is subcutaneous. Seventy-five percent of lumps in childhood will be either epidermoid cysts (60%) or pilomatrichomas (15%).

1. Epidermoid Cysts

Clinical Findings

Epidermoid cysts are the most common type of cutaneous cyst. Other names for epidermoid cysts are epidermal cysts, epidermal inclusion cysts, and "sebaceous" cysts. This last term is a misnomer since they contain neither sebum nor sebaceous glands. Epidermoid cysts can occur anywhere, but are most common on the face and upper trunk. They usually arise from and are lined by the stratified squamous epithelium of the follicular infundibulum. Clinically, epidermoid cysts are dermal nodules with a central punctum, representing the follicle associated with the cyst. They can reach several centimeters in diameter. **Dermoid cysts** are areas of sequestration of skin along embryonic fusion lines. They are present at birth and occur most commonly on the lateral eyebrow.

Treatment

Epidermoid cysts can rupture, causing a foreign-body inflammatory reaction, or become infected. Infectious complications should be treated with antibiotics and drainage. Definitive treatment is surgical excision. Treatment of dermoid cysts, if desired, is surgical excision.

2. Pilomatrichomas

These are benign tumors of the hair matrix. They are most commonly seen on the face and upper trunk. They are firm and may be irregular. Their color varies from flesh-colored to pink or blue. The firmness is secondary to calcification of the tumor.

Treatment

Treatment is by surgical excision.

3. Granuloma Annulare

Circles or semicircles of nontender intradermal nodules found over the lower legs and ankles, the dorsum of the hands and wrists, and the trunk, in that order of frequency, suggest granuloma annulare. Histologically, the disease appears as a central area of tissue death (necrobiosis) surrounded by macrophages and lymphocytes.

Treatment

No treatment is necessary. Lesions resolve spontaneously within 1–2 years in most children.

4. Pyogenic Granuloma

These lesions appear over 1–2 weeks following skin trauma as a dark red papule with an ulcerated and crusted surface that may bleed easily even with minor trauma. Histologically, this represents excessive new vessel formation with or without inflammation (granulation tissue). It should be regarded as an abnormal healing response.

Treatment

Pulsed dye laser for very small lesions or curettage followed by electrocautery are the treatments of choice.

5. Keloids

Keloids are scars of delayed onset that continue for up to several years to progress beyond the initial wound margins. The tendency to develop keloids is inherited. They are often found on the face, earlobes, neck, chest, and back.

Treatment

Treatment includes intralesional injection with triamcinolone acetonide, 20 mg/mL, or excision and injection with corticosteroids.

Luba MC et al: Common benign skin tumors. Am Fam Physician 2003;67:729 [PMID: 12613727].

PAPULOSQUAMOUS ERUPTIONS

Papulosquamous eruptions (Table 14–8) comprise papules or plaques with varying degrees of scale.

1. Pityriasis Rosea
Pathogenesis & Clinical Findings

Pink to red, oval plaques with fine scales that tend to align with their long axis parallel to skin tension lines (eg, "Christmas tree pattern" on the back) are characteristic lesions of

Table 14–8. Papulosquamous eruptions in children.

Psoriasis
Pityriasis rosea
Tinea corporis
Lichen planus
Pityriasis lichenoides (acute or chronic)
Dermatomyositis
Lupus erythematosus
Pityriasis rubra pilaris
Secondary syphilis

pityriasis rosea. In 20–80% of cases the generalized eruption is preceded for up to 30 days by a solitary, larger, scaling plaque with central clearing and a scaly border (the herald patch). The herald patch is clinically similar to ringworm and can be confused. In whites, the lesions are primarily on the trunk; in blacks, lesions are primarily on the extremities and may be accentuated in the axillary and inguinal areas.

This disease is common in school-aged children and adolescents and is presumed to be viral in origin. The role of human herpesvirus 7 in the pathogenesis of pityriasis rosea is debated. The condition lasts 6 weeks and may be pruritic.

Differential Diagnosis

The major differential diagnosis is secondary syphilis, and a VDRL (Venereal Disease Research Laboratories) test should be done if syphilis is suspected, especially in high-risk patients with palm or sole involvement.

Treatment

Exposure to natural sunlight may help hasten the resolution of lesions. Oral antihistamines can be used for pruritus. Often, no treatment is necessary. Pityriasis rosea that lasts more than 12 weeks should be referred to a dermatologist for evaluation.

Chuh AA et al: Interventions for pityriasis rosea. Cochrane Database Syst Rev 2007;(18):CD005068 [PMID:17443568].

2. Psoriasis
Pathogenesis & Clinical Findings

Psoriasis is characterized by erythematous papules covered by thick white scales. Guttate (droplike) psoriasis is a common form in children that often follows an episode of streptococcal pharyngitis by 2–3 weeks. The sudden onset of small papules (3–8 mm), seen predominantly over the trunk and quickly covered with thick white scales, is characteristic of guttate psoriasis. Chronic psoriasis is marked by thick, large scaly plaques (5–10 cm) over the elbows, knees, scalp, and other sites of trauma. Pinpoint pits in the nail plate are seen, as well as yellow discoloration of the nail plate resulting from onycholysis. Psoriasis occurs frequently on the scalp, elbows, knees, periumbilical area, ears, sacral area, and genitalia. It should always be included in the differential diagnosis of "dermatitis" on the scalp or genitalia of children.

The pathogenesis of psoriasis is complex and incompletely understood. It is a familial condition, and multiple psoriasis susceptibility genes have been identified. There is increased epidermal turnover; psoriatic epidermis has a turnover time of 3–4 days versus 28 days for normal skin. These rapidly proliferating epidermal cells produce excessive stratum corneum, giving rise to thick, opaque scales.

▶ Differential Diagnosis

Papulosquamous eruptions that present problems of differential diagnosis are listed in Table 14–8.

▶ Treatment

Topical corticosteroids are the initial treatment of choice. Penetration of topical steroids through the enlarged epidermal barrier in psoriasis requires that more potent preparations be used, for example, fluocinonide 0.05% (Lidex) or clobetasol 0.05% (Temovate) ointment twice daily.

The second line of therapy is topical calcipotriene (Dovonex) applied twice daily or the combination of a superpotent topical steroid twice daily on weekends and calcipotriene twice daily on weekdays for 8 weeks.

Topical retinoids such as tazarotene (0.1%, 0.5% cream, gel) can be used in combination with topical corticosteroids to help restore normal epidermal differentiation and turnover time. However, these treatments can cause skin to become dry.

Anthralin therapy is also useful. Anthralin is applied to the skin for a short contact time (eg, 20 minutes once daily) and then washed off with a neutral soap (eg, Dove). A 6-week course of treatment is recommended. This can be used in combination with topical corticosteroids.

Crude coal tar therapy is messy and stains bedclothes. The newer tar gels (Estar, PsoriGel) cause less staining and are most efficacious. They are applied twice daily for 6–8 weeks. These preparations are sold over the counter and are not usually covered by insurance plans.

Scalp care using a tar shampoo requires leaving the shampoo on for 5 minutes, washing it off, and then shampooing with commercial shampoo to remove scales. It may be necessary to shampoo daily until scaling is reduced. More severe cases of psoriasis are best treated by a dermatologist.

Liu Y et al: Psoriasis: Genetic associations and immune system changes. Genes Immunol 2007;8:1 [PMID: 17093502].

Rogers M: Childhood psoriasis. Curr Opin Pediatr 2002;14:404 [PMID: 12130902].

HAIR LOSS (ALOPECIA)

Hair loss in children (Table 14–9) imposes great emotional stress on the patient and the parent. A 60% hair loss in a

Table 14–9. Other causes of hair loss in children.

Hair loss with scalp changes
Atrophy:
Lichen planus
Lupus erythematosus
Nodules and tumors:
Epidermal nevus
Nevus sebaceus
Thickening:
Burn
Hair loss with hair shaft defects (hair fails to grow out enough to require haircuts)
Monilethrix—alternating bands of thin and thick areas
Pili annulati—alternating bands of light and dark pigmentation
Pili torti—hair twisted 180 degrees, brittle
Trichorrhexis invaginata (bamboo hair)—intussusception of one hair into another
Trichorrhexis nodosa—nodules with fragmented hair

single area is necessary before hair loss can be detected clinically. Examination should begin with the scalp to determine whether inflammation, scale, or infiltrative changes are present. Hairs should be examined microscopically for breaking and structural defects and to see whether growing or resting hairs are being shed. Placing removed hairs in mounting fluid (Permount) on a glass microscope slide makes them easy to examine. Three diseases account for most cases of hair loss in children: alopecia areata, tinea capitis (described earlier in this chapter), and hair pulling.

Silverberg NB: Helping children cope with hair loss. Cutis 2006;78:333 [PMID: 17186792].

1. Alopecia Areata

▶ Clinical Findings

Loss of every hair in a localized area is called alopecia areata. This is the most common cause of hair loss in children. An immunologic pathogenic mechanism is suspected because dense infiltration of lymphocytes precedes hair loss. Ninety-five percent of children with alopecia areata completely regrow their hair within 12 months, although as many as 40% may have a relapse in 5–6 years.

A rare and unusual form of alopecia areata begins at the occiput and proceeds along the hair margins to the frontal scalp. This variety, called ophiasis, often eventuates in total scalp hair loss (alopecia totalis). The prognosis for regrowth in ophiasis is poor.

▶ Treatment

Treatment of alopecia areata is difficult. Systemic corticosteroids given to suppress the inflammatory response will result in hair growth, but the hair may fall out again when the drug is discontinued. Systemic corticosteroids should never be used for a prolonged time period. Superpotent topical steroids, minoxidil (Rogaine), and anthralin are treatment options. In children with alopecia totalis, a wig is most helpful.

Tan E et al: A clinical study of childhood alopecia areata in Singapore. Pediatr Dermatol 2002;19:298 [PMID: 12220271].

2. Hair Pulling

▷ **Clinical Findings**

Traumatic hair pulling causes the hair shafts to be broken off at different lengths, with an ill-defined area of hair loss, petechiae around follicular openings, and a wrinkled hair shaft on microscopic examination. This behavior may be merely habit, an acute reaction to severe stress, trichotillomania, or a sign of another psychiatric disorder. Eyelashes and eyebrows rather than scalp hair may be pulled out.

▷ **Treatment**

If the behavior has a long history, psychiatric evaluation may be helpful. Oiling the hair to make it slippery is an aid to behavior modification.

Tay YK et al: Trichotillomania in childhood: Case series and review. Pediatrics 2004;113:e494 [PMID: 15121993].

REACTIVE ERYTHEMAS

1. Erythema Multiforme

▷ **Clinical Findings**

Erythema multiforme begins with papules that later develop a dark center and then evolve into lesions with central bluish discoloration or blisters and the characteristic target lesions (iris lesions) that have three concentric circles of color change. Primary injury is to endothelial cells, with later destruction of epidermal basal cells. Erythema multiforme has sometimes been diagnosed in patients with severe mucous membrane involvement, but Stevens-Johnson syndrome is the usual diagnosis when severe involvement of conjunctiva, oral cavity, and genital mucosa also occur.

Many causes are suspected, particularly concomitant herpes simplex virus; drugs, especially sulfonamides; and *Mycoplasma* infections. Recurrent erythema multiforme is usually associated with reactivation of herpes simplex virus. In the mild form, spontaneous healing occurs in 10–14 days, but Stevens-Johnson syndrome may last 6–8 weeks.

▷ **Treatment**

Treatment is symptomatic in uncomplicated erythema multiforme. Removal of offending drugs is an obvious measure. Oral antihistamines such as hydroxyzine, 2 mg/kg/d orally, are useful. Cool compresses and wet dressings will relieve pruritus. Steroids have not been demonstrated to be effective. Chronic acyclovir therapy has been successful in

Table 14–10. Common drug reactions.

Urticaria
Barbiturates
Opioids
Penicillins
Sulfonamides
Morbilliform eruption
Anticonvulsants
Cephalosporins
Penicillins
Sulfonamides
Fixed drug eruption, erythema multiforme, toxic epidermal necrolysis, Stevens-Johnson syndrome
Anticonvulsants
Nonsteroidal anti-inflammatory drugs
Sulfonamides
DRESS syndrome
Anticonvulsants
Photodermatitis
Psoralens
Sulfonamides
Tetracyclines
Thiazides

DRESS syndrome = drug eruptions with fever, eosinophilia, and systemic symptoms.

decreasing attacks in patients with herpes-associated recurrent erythema multiforme.

Lamoreaux MR et al: Erythema multiforme. Am Fam Physician 2006;74:1883 [PMID: 17168345].

2. Drug Eruptions

Drugs may produce urticarial, morbilliform, scarlatiniform, pustular, bullous, or fixed skin eruptions. Urticaria may appear within minutes after drug administration, but most reactions begin 7–14 days after the drug is first administered. These eruptions may occur in patients who have received these drugs for long periods, and eruptions continue for days after the drug has been discontinued. Drug eruptions with fever, eosinophilia, and systemic symptoms (DRESS syndrome) is most commonly seen with anticonvulsants, but may be seen with other drugs. Drugs commonly implicated in skin reactions are listed in Table 14–10.

Greenberger PA: Drug allergy. J Allergy Clin Immunol 2006;117:s464 [PMID: 16455348].

MISCELLANEOUS SKIN DISORDERS SEEN IN PEDIATRIC PRACTICE

1. Aphthous Stomatitis

Recurrent erosions on the gums, lips, tongue, palate, and buccal mucosa are often confused with herpes simplex. A smear of the base of such a lesion stained with Wright stain will aid in ruling out herpes simplex by the absence of epithelial multinucleate giant cells. A culture for herpes simplex is also useful in differential diagnostics. The cause remains unknown, but T-cell–mediated cytotoxicity to various viral antigens has been postulated.

▶ Treatment

There is no specific therapy for this condition. Rinsing the mouth with liquid antacids provides relief in most patients. Topical corticosteroids in a gel base may provide some relief. In severe cases that interfere with eating, prednisone, 1 mg/kg/d orally for 3–5 days, will suffice to abort an episode. Colchicine, 0.2–0.5 mg/d, sometimes reduces the frequency of attacks.

Scully C: Clinical practice. Aphthous ulceration. N Engl J Med 2005;355:165 [PMID: 16837680].

2. Vitiligo

Vitiligo is characterized clinically by the development of areas of depigmentation. These are often symmetrical and occur mainly on extensor surfaces. The depigmentation results from a destruction of melanocytes. The basis for this destruction is unknown, but immunologically mediated damage is likely and vitiligo sometimes occurs in individuals with autoimmune endocrinopathies, selective IgA deficiency, or graft-versus-host disease.

▶ Treatment

Treatment is not very effective. Potent topical steroids, tacrolimus, or both for 4 months are the initial treatment. Topical calcipotriene has also been used. Narrow-band ultraviolet B waves (UVB 311 nm) may be used in severe cases.

Huggins RH et al: Childhood vitiligo. Cutis 2007;79:277 [PMID: 17500374].

Eye

Rebecca Sands Braverman, MD

15

Normal vision is a sense that develops during infancy and childhood. The child must experience equally good visual inputs from well-aligned eyes during this period while the visual nervous system is still exhibiting plasticity. Thus, pediatric ophthalmology emphasizes early diagnosis and treatment of pediatric eye diseases in order to obtain the best possible visual outcome. But eye disease in children does not always originate in the ocular system. Abnormal eye findings in a child may be a sign of systemic disease.

COMMON NONSPECIFIC SIGNS & SYMPTOMS

Nonspecific signs and symptoms commonly occur as the chief complaint or as an element of the history of a child with eye disease. Five of these findings are described here, along with a sixth—leukocoria—which is less common, but often has serious implications. Do not hesitate to seek the help of a pediatric ophthalmologist when you believe the diagnosis and treatment of these signs and symptoms requires in-depth clinical experience.

REDNESS

Redness (injection) of the bulbar conjunctiva or deeper vessels is a common presenting complaint. It may be mild and localized or diffuse and bilateral. Causes include superficial or penetrating foreign bodies, infection, allergy, and conjunctivitis associated with systemic entities such as Stevens-Johnson syndrome or Kawasaki disease. Irritating noxious agents also cause injection. Subconjunctival hemorrhage may be traumatic or spontaneous or may be associated with hematopoietic disease, vascular anomalies, or inflammatory processes. Uncommonly, an injected eye can be due to an intraocular or orbital tumor.

TEARING

Tearing in infants is usually due to nasolacrimal obstruction but may also be associated with congenital glaucoma, in which case photophobia and blepharospasm may also be present. Inflammation, allergic and viral diseases, or conjunctival and corneal irritation can also cause tearing.

DISCHARGE

Purulent discharge is usually associated with bacterial conjunctivitis. In infants and toddlers with nasolacrimal obstruction, a mucopurulent discharge may be present with low-grade, chronic dacryocystitis. Watery discharge occurs with viral infection, iritis, superficial foreign bodies, and nasolacrimal obstruction. Mucoid discharge may be a sign of allergic conjunctivitis or nasolacrimal obstruction. A mucoid discharge due to allergy typically contains eosinophils; a purulent bacterial discharge contains polymorphonuclear leukocytes.

PAIN & FOREIGN BODY SENSATION

Pain in or around the eye may be due to foreign bodies, corneal abrasions, lacerations, acute infections of the globe or ocular adnexa, iritis, and angle-closure glaucoma. Large refractive errors, poor accommodative ability, and sinus disease may manifest as headaches. Trichiasis (inturned lashes) and contact lens problems also cause ocular discomfort.

PHOTOPHOBIA

Acute aversion to light may occur with corneal abrasions, foreign bodies, and iritis. Squinting of one eye in bright light is a common sign of intermittent exotropia. Photophobia is present in infants with glaucoma, albinism, aniridia, and retinal dystrophies such as achromatopsia. Photophobia is common after ocular surgery and after dilation of the pupil with mydriatic and cycloplegic agents. Photophobia in indi-

▲ **Figure 15–1.** Leukocoria of the left eye caused by retrolental membrane (persistent hyperplastic primary vitreous or persistent fetal vasculature).

viduals with no ocular pathology may be due to migraine headache, meningitis, and retrobulbar optic neuritis.

LEUKOCORIA

Although not a common sign or complaint, leukocoria (a white pupil) is associated with serious diseases and requires prompt ophthalmologic consultation. Causes of leukocoria include retinoblastoma, retinopathy of prematurity, pupillary membrane, cataract, vitreous opacities, retinal detachment, *Toxocara* infection, and retinal dysplasia (Figure 15–1).

REFRACTIVE ERRORS

Refractive error refers to the optical state of the eye (Figure 15–2). It is a physical characteristic like height or weight and can be quantitated. Not all refractive errors require correction, but severe errors can cause amblyopia (reduced vision with or without an organic lesion). Those that do can usually be corrected with glasses. Less often, contact lenses are required, usually for very high or asymmetrical refractive errors, or for adolescents who do not want to wear spectacles. Laser refractive surgery is not currently indicated for most children. There are three common refractive errors: myopia, hyperopia, and astigmatism. Inequality of the refractive state between the two eyes (anisometropia) can cause amblyopia. Children at particular risk for refractive errors requiring correction with spectacles include those who were born prematurely, those with Down syndrome, those who are offspring of parents with refractive errors, and those who have certain systemic conditions such as Stickler, Marfan, or Ehlers-Danlos syndrome.

MYOPIA (NEARSIGHTEDNESS)

For the myopic or nearsighted individual, objects nearby are in focus; those at a distance are blurred. This is because the

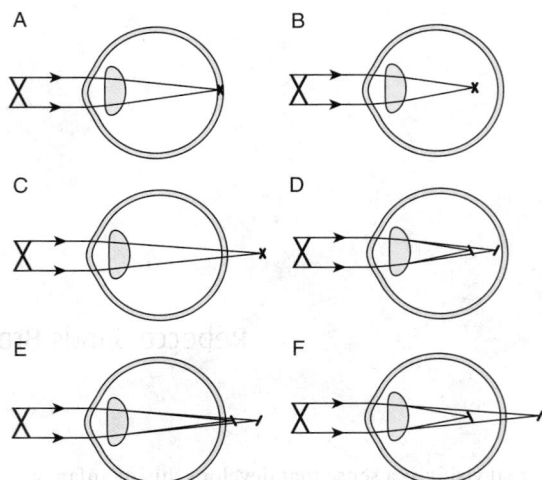

▲ **Figure 15–2.** Different refractive states of the eye. **A:** Emmetropia. Image plane from parallel rays of light falls on retina. **B:** Myopia. Image plane focuses anterior to retina. **C:** Hyperopia. Image plane focuses posterior to retina. **D:** Astigmatism, myopic type. Images in horizontal and vertical planes focus anterior to retina. **E:** Astigmatism, hyperopic type. Images in horizontal and vertical planes focus posterior to retina. **F:** Astigmatism, mixed type. Images in horizontal and vertical planes focus on either side of retina.

plane of focus is anterior to the retina. The onset is typically at about age 8 years and may progress throughout adolescence and young adulthood. A myopic person may squint to produce a pinhole effect, which improves distance vision. Divergent lenses provide clear distance vision. Many studies have been done attempting to slow or stop myopic progression. Atropine eye drops have shown some effect, but produce many side effects. A newer drug, pirenzepine, has shown promise in animal studies, and human studies are underway.

Tan DT et al, and Asian Pirenzepine Study Group: One-year multicenter, double-masked, placebo-controlled, parallel safety and efficacy study of 2% pirenzepine ophthalmic gel in children with myopia. Ophthalmology 2005;112:84 [PMID: 15629825].

HYPEROPIA (FARSIGHTEDNESS)

Saying that the hyperopic child is sighted for far (not near) vision is somewhat misleading, because the child can focus on near objects if the hyperopia is not excessive. Large amounts of uncorrected hyperopia can cause esotropia (inward deviation, or crossing, of the eyes) and amblyopia (see later section on Amblyopia & Strabismus). Most infants have a hyperopic refraction that begins to diminish during the toddler years and does not require correction.

ASTIGMATISM

When either the cornea or the crystalline lens is not perfectly spherical, an image will not be sharply focused in one plane. Schematically, there will be two planes of focus. Both of the planes can be either in front of or behind the retina, or one of the planes can be in front of the retina and the other behind it. This refractive state is described as astigmatism. Large amounts of astigmatism not corrected at an early age can cause decreased vision from amblyopia, but proper refractive correction can prevent this.

Harvey EM et al: Prescribing eyeglass correction for astigmatism in infancy and early childhood: A survey of AAPOS members. J AAPOS 2005;9:189 [PMID: 15838450].

▼ OPTHALMIC EXAMINATION

Ophthalmic examination of the pediatric patient begins with a calm demeanor and reassuring voice. Having a parent present is invaluable. The examination includes a history, assessment of visual acuity, external examination, observation of ocular alignment and motility, and ophthalmoscopic examination. Intraocular pressure is less frequently measured. Testing of binocular status and near point is desirable when age and cooperation permit.

Circumstances will dictate the use of ancillary procedures such as instilling fluorescein dye and radiologic tests (magnetic resonance imaging [MRI] and computed tomography [CT] scan). Electroretinography and electrooculography test retinal function. Visual evoked response testing assesses the function of the cortical visual pathways. Visual field testing demonstrates the presence or absence of scotomas and visual field defects occurring anywhere along the visual pathway. In the office setting, visual field testing may be done in a gross manner (confrontation) by bringing an object from the periphery of the child's field of vision into each of four quadrants or by having an older child count the examiner's fingers as they are presented in two quadrants simultaneously, but accurate results can be difficult to achieve in young children.

HISTORY

Evaluation begins by ascertaining the chief complaint and taking a history of the present illness. Elements of the history include onset of the complaint, its duration, whether it is monocular or binocular, treatment received thus far, and associated systemic symptoms. If an infectious disease is suspected, ask about possible contact with others having similar findings. The ocular history is obtained, as is the perinatal and developmental history and any history of allergy. The family history should be explored for ocular disorders that may be familial.

VISUAL ACUITY

Visual acuity testing is the single most important test of visual function and should be part of every general physical examination. This is the nonophthalmologist's most definitive test for amblyopia, refractive errors, and lesions along the optic pathways. Acuity should be tested in each eye individually, using an adhesive eye patch to prevent peeking. Glasses should be worn during vision screening if they have been prescribed in the past. In older children who can cooperate, use of a pinhole will improve vision in children not wearing the appropriate spectacle prescription.

Vision Screening

Vision screening in the pediatric age group is a challenge, especially in younger and developmentally delayed children. Accuracy of the screening test being administered to a particular population and expense in terms of time, equipment, and personnel are some factors that must be considered. Vision screening is consistent with the recommendations of the American Academy of Pediatrics (http://www.aap.org). Risk factors that should be screened for because they interfere with normal visual development and are amblyogenic include media opacities, strabismus, and refractive errors that are different in the two eyes (anisometropia) or of large magnitude in both eyes.

The type of test used to determine visual acuity is dictated by the child's age. In the sleeping newborn, the presence of a blepharospastic response to bright light is an adequate response. At age 6 weeks, eye-to-eye contact with slow following movements is becoming established and can be detected. By age 3 months, the infant should demonstrate fixing and following ocular movements for objects at a distance of 2–3 feet. At age 6 months, interest in movement across the room is the norm. Vision can be recorded for the presence or absence of fixing and following behavior and whether vision is steady (unsteady when nystagmus is present) and maintained. Vision should be tested and recorded for each eye. Visual acuity can be quantified in infants using other techniques, such as the 15-diopter prism test, preferential looking technique, or the pattern visual evoked response.

In the verbal child, the use of familiar icons will allow for a quantitative test. Allen or Lea symbols with familiar pictures can be used to test children younger than 2–3 years of age. When it is not possible to measure visual acuity or assess alignment in the preschool-aged group, random dot stereopsis testing (for depth perception) is effective in screening for manifest strabismus and amblyopia, but this test may miss some cases of anisometropic (unequal refractive error) amblyopia and small-angle strabismus. This test is not designed to detect refractive errors.

Four-year-old children are often ready to play the tumbling E game (in which the child identifies the orientation of the letter E, which is turned in one of four directions) or the

HOTV letters game (in which these four letters are shown individually at a distance and matched on a board that the child is holding). Literate children are tested with letters. Typical acuity levels in developmentally appropriate children are approximately 20/60 or better in children younger than 2–3 years, 20/40–20/30 in 3-year-old children, 20/30–20/25 in 4-year-old children, and 20/20 in literate children 5–6 years old. Perhaps more important than the absolute visual acuity is the presence of a difference of acuity between the two eyes, which might be a sign of amblyopia, uncorrected refractive error, or disease. As little as one line difference in acuity should be considered significant.

The practitioner should be aware of two situations in which vision screening is complicated by nystagmus. Children who require a face turn or torticollis (in which the head is tilted to the right or left) to quiet the nystagmus will have poor visual acuity results when tested in the absence of the compensatory head posture. When latent nystagmus is present, acuity testing is particularly challenging (see later section on Nystagmus). Nystagmus appears or worsens when an eye is occluded, degrading central vision. To minimize the nystagmus, the occluder should be held about 12 inches in front of the eye not being tested. Testing both eyes simultaneously without occlusion often gives a better visual acuity measurement than when either eye is tested individually.

Photoscreening

Traditional vision screening methods using eye charts in children aged 3–5 years require the child's cooperation as well as proficiency in testing by the examiner. Photoscreening has been developed to address the difficulties in screening young children. It requires a special camera that takes two photographs of each eye, a trained examiner to take the photographs, and a site for interpretation of the photographs. Photoscreening does not screen directly for amblyopia but for amblyogenic factors, which include strabismus, media opacities, and refractive errors. If the photographs suggest an amblyogenic factor, children are referred to an eye care professional for a complete eye examination. Problems exist with sensitivity and specificity of the instruments and poor follow-up for referrals made to eye care professionals. The cost-effectiveness of photoscreening remains an area of continued research.

Arnold RW et al: The cost and yield of photoscreening: Impact of photoscreening on overall pediatric ophthalmic costs. J Pediatr Ophthalmol Strabismus 2005;42:103 [PMID: 15825747].

Salcido AA et al: Predictive value of photoscreening and traditional screening of preschool children. J AAPOS 2005;9:114 [PMID: 15838437].

EXTERNAL EXAMINATION

Inspection of the anterior segment of the globe and its adnexa requires adequate illumination and often magnifica-

▲ **Figure 15–3.** Eversion of the upper lid. **A:** The patient looks downward. **B:** The fingers pull the lid down, and an index finger or cotton tip is placed on the upper tarsal border. **C:** The lid is pulled up over the finger. **D:** The lid is everted.

tion. A penlight provides good illumination and should be used in both straight-ahead and oblique illumination. A Wood's lamp or a blue filter cap placed over a penlight is needed for evaluation after applying a fluorescent stain. Immobilization of the child may be necessary. A drop of topical anesthetic may facilitate the examination.

In cases of suspected foreign body, pulling down on the lower lid provides excellent visualization of the inferior cul-de-sac (palpebral conjunctiva). Visualizing the upper cul-de-sac and superior bulbar conjunctiva is possible by having the patient look inferiorly while the upper lid is pulled away from the globe and the examiner peers into the upper recess. Illumination with a penlight is necessary. The upper lid should be everted to evaluate the superior tarsal conjunctiva (Figure 15–3).

When indicated for further evaluation of the cornea, a small amount of fluorescein solution should be instilled into the lower cul-de-sac. Blue light will stain defects yellow-green. Disease-specific staining patterns may be observed. For example, herpes simplex lesions of the corneal epithelium produce a dendrite or branchlike pattern. A foreign body lodged beneath the upper lid shows one or more vertical lines of stain on the cornea due to the constant movement of the foreign body over the cornea. Contact lens overwear produces a central staining pattern. A fine, scattered punctate pattern may be a sign of viral keratitis or medication toxicity. Punctate erosions of the inferior third of the cornea can be seen with staphylococcal blepharitis or exposure keratitis secondary to incomplete lid closure.

PUPILS

The child's pupils should be evaluated for reaction to light, regularity of shape, and equality of size as well as for the presence of afferent pupillary defect. This defect, occurring in optic nerve disease, is evaluated by the swinging flashlight test (see later section on Diseases of the Optic Nerve). Irregular pupils are associated with iritis, trauma, pupillary membranes, and structural defects such as iris coloboma (see later section on Iris Coloboma).

Pupils vary in size due to lighting conditions and also age. In general, infants have miotic (constricted) pupils. Children have larger pupils than either infants or adults, whereas the elderly have miotic pupils.

Anisocoria, a size difference between the two pupils, may be physiologic if the size difference is within 1 mm and is the same in light and dark. Anisocoria occurs with Horner syndrome, third nerve palsy, Adie tonic pupil, iritis, and trauma. Medication could also cause abnormal pupil size or reactivity. For example, contact with atropine-like substances (belladonna alkaloids) will cause pupillary dilation with little or no pupillary reaction. Systemic antihistamines and scopolamine patches, among other medicines, can dilate the pupils and interfere with accommodation (focusing).

ALIGNMENT & MOTILITY EVALUATION

Alignment and motility should be tested because amblyopia is associated with strabismus, a misalignment of the visual axes of the eyes. Besides alignment, ocular rotations should be evaluated in the six cardinal positions of gaze (Table 15–1; Figure 15–4). A small toy is an interesting target for testing ocular rotations in infants; a penlight works well in older children.

Alignment can be assessed in several ways. In order of increasing accuracy, these methods are observation, the corneal light reflex test, and cover testing. Observation includes an educated guess about whether the eyes are properly aligned. Corneal light reflex evaluation (Hirschberg test) is performed by shining a light beam at the patient's eyes, observing the reflections off each cornea, and estimating whether these "reflexes" appear to be positioned properly. If the reflection of light is noted temporally on the cornea, esotropia is suspected (Figure 15–5). Nasal reflection of the light suggests exotropia (outward deviation). Accuracy of these tests increases with increasing angles of misalignment.

MR = medial rectus   LR = lateral rectus
SR = superior rectus   IR = inferior rectus
SO = superior oblique   IO = inferior oblique

▲ **Figure 15–4.** Cardinal positions of gaze and muscles primarily tested in those fields of gaze. Arrow indicates position in which each muscle is tested.

Another way of evaluating alignment is with the cover test, in which the patient fixes on a target while one eye is covered. If an esotropia or an exotropia is present, the deviated eye will make a corrective movement to fixate on the target when the previously fixating eye is occluded. The other eye is tested similarly. When the occluder is removed from the eye just uncovered, a refixation movement of that eye indicates a phoria, or latent deviation, if alignment is reestablished. If the uncovered eye picks up fixation and strabismus is still present, then that eye can be presumed to be dominant and the nonpreferred eye possibly amblyopic. If the eye remains deviated after the occluder is removed, a tropia is noted to be present (Figure 15–6). A deviated eye that is blind or has very poor vision will not fixate on a target. Consequently, spurious results to cover testing may occur, as can happen with disinterest on the part of the patient, small-angle strabismus, and inexperience in administering cover tests.

OPHTHALMOSCOPIC EXAMINATION

A handheld direct ophthalmoscope allows visualization of the ocular fundus. As the patient's pupil becomes more constricted, viewing the fundus becomes more difficult. Although it is taught that pupillary dilation can precipitate

Table 15–1. Function and innervation of each of the extraocular muscles.

Muscle	Function	Innervation
Medial rectus	Adductor	Oculomotor (third)
Lateral rectus	Abductor	Abducens (sixth)
Inferior rectus	Depressor, adductor, extorter	Oculomotor
Superior rectus	Elevator, adductor, intorter	Oculomotor
Inferior oblique	Elevator, abductor, extorter	Oculomotor
Superior oblique	Depressor, abductor, intorter	Trochlear (fourth)

▲ **Figure 15–5.** Temporal displacement of light reflection showing esotropia (inward deviation) of the right eye. Nasal displacement of the reflection would show exotropia (outward deviation).

Eyes straight (maintained in position by fusion).

Position of eye under cover in orthophoria (fusion-free position). The right eye under cover has not moved.

Position of eye under cover in esophoria (fusion-free position). Under cover, the right eye has deviated inward. Upon removal of cover, the right eye will immediately resume its straight-ahead position.

Position of eye under cover in exophoria (fusion-free position). Under cover, the right eye had deviated outward. Upon removal of the cover, the right eye will immediately resume its straight-ahead position.

▲ **Figure 15–6.** Cover testing. The patient is instructed to look at a target at eye level 20 feet away. Note that in the presence of constant strabismus (ie, a tropia rather than a phoria), the deviation will remain when the cover is removed. (Reprinted, with permission, from Riordan-Eva P, Whitcher J: *Vaughan & Asbury's General Ophthalmology,* 17th ed., McGraw-Hill, 2008.)

an attack of closed-angle glaucoma in the predisposed adult, children are very rarely predisposed to angle closure. Exceptions include those with a dislocated lens, past surgery, or an eye previously compromised by a retrolental membrane, such as in retinopathy of prematurity. Therefore, if an adequate view of the fundus is precluded by a miotic pupil, use of a dilating agent (eg, 1 drop in each eye of 2.5% phenylephrine or 0.5% or 1% tropicamide) should provide adequate mydriasis (dilation). In infants, 1 drop of a combination of 1% phenylephrine with 0.2% cyclopentolate (Cyclomydril) is safer. Structures to be observed during ophthalmoscopy include the optic disk, blood vessels, the macular reflex, and retina, as well as the clarity of the vitreous media. By increasing the amount of plus lens dialed into the instrument, the point of focus moves anteriorly from the retina to the lens and finally to the cornea.

Ophthalmoscopy should include assessment of the clarity of the ocular media, that is, the quality of the red reflex. The practitioner should take the time to become familiar with this reflex. The red reflex test (Brückner test) is useful for identifying disorders such as media opacities (eg, cataracts), large refractive errors, tumors such as retinoblastoma, and strabismus. A difference in quality of the red reflexes between the two eyes constitutes a positive Brückner test and requires referral to an ophthalmologist.

The red reflex of each eye can be compared simultaneously when the observer is approximately 4 feet away from the patient. The largest diameter of light is shown through the ophthalmoscope, and no correction (zero setting) is dialed in the ophthalmoscope unless it is to compensate for the exam-iner's uncorrected refractive error. A red reflex chart is available through the American Academy of Pediatrics.

OCULAR TRAUMA

A foreign body of the globe or adnexa may be difficult to visualize due to its small size or location. The clinician should always maintain a high index of suspicion for an occult or intraocular foreign body if the history suggests this. In cases such as these, ophthalmologic referral needs to be considered.

OCULAR FOREIGN BODIES

▶ Clinical Findings

Foreign bodies on the globe and palpebral conjunctiva usually cause discomfort and red eye. The history may suggest the origin of the foreign body, such as being around a metal grinder or being outside on a windy day when a sudden foreign body sensation was encountered associated with tearing, redness, and pain. Pain with blinking suggests that the foreign body may be trapped between the eyelid and the eye.

Magnification with a slit lamp may be needed for inspection. Foreign bodies that lodge on the upper palpebral conjunctiva are best viewed by everting the lid on itself and removing the foreign body with a cotton applicator. The conjunctival surface (palpebral conjunctiva) of the lower lid presents no problem with visualization. After simple removal of a foreign body that is thought not to be contaminated, no other treatment is needed if no corneal abrasion has occurred.

Treatment

When foreign bodies are noted on the bulbar conjunctiva or cornea (Figure 15–7), removal is facilitated by using a topical anesthetic. If the foreign body is not too adherent, it can be dislodged with a stream of irrigating solution (Dacriose or saline) or with a cotton applicator after instillation of a topical anesthetic. Otherwise, a foreign body spud or needle is used to undermine the foreign body. This must be done with adequate magnification and illumination. An antibiotic ointment is then instilled. Ferrous corneal bodies often have an associated rust ring, which may be removed under slit-lamp visualization in cooperative children or under anesthesia if necessary.

A

B

▲ **Figure 15–7.** **A:** Corneal foreign body at the nasal edge of the cornea. **B:** Subconjunctival foreign body of graphite.

CORNEAL ABRASION

A corneal abrasion results in loss of the most superficial layer of corneal cells and causes severe ocular pain, tearing, and blepharospasm. An inciting event is usually identifiable as the cause of a corneal abrasion. Children often suffer corneal abrasions accidentally while playing with siblings or pets as well as participating in sports. Contact lens users frequently develop abrasions due to poorly fitting lenses, overnight wear, and use of torn or damaged lenses.

Clinical Findings

Symptoms of a corneal abrasion are sudden and severe eye pain, usually after an inciting event such as an accidental finger poke to the eye. Decreased vision secondary to pain and tearing are common complaints. Eyelid edema, tearing, injection of the conjunctiva, and poor cooperation with the ocular examination due to pain are common signs of a corneal abrasion. Fluorescein dye is instilled into the eye and a cobalt blue or Wood's lamp is used to illuminate the effected eye. The area with the abrasion will stain bright yellow.

Treatment

Ophthalmic ointment, such as erythromycin ointment, lubricates the surface of the cornea and also helps prevent infections. Patching the affected eye when a large abrasion is present may provide comfort but is not advised for corneal abrasions caused by contact lens wear or other potentially contaminated sources. Large corneal abrasions result in referred pain to the ipsilateral brow. If a brow ache is present it may be treated by the use of a topical cycloplegic agent such as 1% cyclopentolate. Daily follow-up is required until healing is complete.

INTRAOCULAR FOREIGN BODIES & PERFORATING OCULAR INJURIES

Severe trauma may result in penetration of the eye by foreign bodies or retained foreign bodies, and is an ocular emergency. Intraocular foreign bodies and penetrating injuries are most often caused by being in close proximity to high-velocity projectiles such as windshield glass broken during a motor vehicle accident, metal ground without use of protective safety goggles, and improperly detonated fireworks.

Clinical Findings

Sudden ocular pain occurs; vision loss, as well as multiple organ trauma, may be present.

Intraocular foreign bodies and corneal and scleral lacerations (ruptured globe) require emergency referral to an ophthalmologist. The diagnosis may be difficult if the obvious signs of corneal perforation (shallow anterior chamber with hyphema, traumatic cataract, and irregular pupil) are

▲ **Figure 15–8.** Corneal laceration with irregular pupil and vitreous loss.

not present (Figure 15–8). Furthermore, nonradiopaque materials such as glass will not be seen on x-ray film.

CT scan may be useful in evaluating ocular trauma, including bony injury and foreign body wound. MRI will not provide bony detail and must be avoided if a magnetic foreign body is suspected.

▶ Treatment

In cases of suspected intraocular foreign body or perforation of the globe, it may be best to keep the child at rest, gently shield the eye with a metal shield or cut-down paper cup, and keep the extent of examination to a necessary minimum to prevent expulsion of intraocular contents. In this setting, the child should be given nothing by mouth in case eye examination under anesthesia or surgical repair is required.

Aldakaf A et al: Intraocular foreign bodies associated with traumatic cataract. Oftalmologia 2006;50:90 [PMID: 17345812].

BLUNT ORBITAL TRAUMA

Blunt orbital and soft tissue trauma may produce so-called black eye or ecchymosis (blue or purplish hemorrhagic areas) of the eyelids.

Trauma to the orbit from a closed fist, collision with another player during team sports, and falls are common etiologies of blunt orbital injuries. Orbital compartment syndrome, which may result from severe orbital trauma, is caused by hemorrhaging within the orbit or severe orbital edema (or both) and may lead to permanent vision loss.

▶ Clinical Findings

Blunt trauma to the orbit may result in orbit fractures. The orbital floor is a common location for a fracture (called a blowout fracture). A specific fracture that occurs mainly in children after blunt orbit trauma is called the white-eyed blowout fracture. This results from a greenstick fracture of the orbit with entrapment of extraocular muscles. It is called "white-eyed" because the external orbital soft tissue injury may appear to be minimal, but the patient will have severe pain with eye movement, nausea, vomiting, and restriction of eye movements.

A blowout fracture must be suspected in a patient with symptoms of double vision, pain with eye movements, and restriction of extraocular muscle movements after blunt orbital trauma. CT images of an orbital floor fracture often reveal herniation of orbital fat or the inferior rectus muscle into the maxillary sinus. Assessment of ocular motility, globe integrity, and intraocular pressure will determine the extent of the blunt orbital injury. Consultation with an ophthalmologist may be necessary to determine the full spectrum of the patient's injuries.

Orbital compartment syndrome is an emergency requiring immediate treatment. Patients present with severe edema or ecchymosis of the eyelids (which makes it very difficult to open the eyelids), proptosis, and possibly an acute traumatic optic neuropathy resulting in decreased vision or an afferent papillary defect. Neuroimaging may reveal a retrobulbar hemorrhage and proptosis.

Neuroimaging of a greenstick orbital floor fracture often reveals distortion of the entrapped extraocular muscle within a small orbit fracture.

▶ Treatment

Cold compresses or ice packs for brief periods (eg, 10 minutes at a time) are recommended in older children in the first 24 hours after injury to reduce hemorrhage and swelling.

Patients with clinical signs of muscle entrapment require urgent surgical repair to help prevent permanent ischemic injury to the involved extraocular muscle. Large fractures may need repair to prevent enophthalmos, a sunken appearance to the orbit. This can usually be performed on a nonemergent basis.

Orbital compartment syndrome requires emergent lateral eyelid canthotomy and cantholysis to decompress the orbit. Treatment should not be delayed in order to image the orbits. Prompt treatment can prevent permanent vision loss.

Tse R et al: The white-eyed medial blowout fracture. Plast Reconstr Surg 2007;119:277 [PMID: 17255684].

LACERATIONS

The lids and lacrimal apparatus are susceptible to laceration. Inspection of the eyelids reveals the extent and severity of the traumatic laceration. Lacerations of the nasal third of the eyelid and involving the eyelid margin are at risk for lacrimal system injury and subsequent chronic tearing.

▶ Treatment

Except for superficial lacerations away from the globe, repair in children is best performed in the operating room under

▲ **Figure 15–9.** Laceration involving right lower lid and canaliculus.

general anesthesia. Special consideration must be given to lacerations involving the lid margin, full-thickness lacerations, lacerations that may involve the levator muscle in the upper lid, and to those that may involve the canaliculus (Figure 15–9). These injuries are best repaired by an ophthalmologist and may require intubation of the nasolacrimal system with silicone tubes.

BURNS

Severe thermal or chemical burns can cause scars resulting in ectropion or entropion of the lid and scarring of the conjunctiva and cul-de-sac.

▶ Clinical Findings

Eyelid burns can occur in toddlers from contact with a lighted cigarette. The cornea is often involved as well. Curling irons can cause similar burns. These burns usually heal following application of antibiotic ointment.

Burns of the conjunctiva and cornea may be thermal, radiant, or chemical. Radiant energy causes ultraviolet keratitis. Typical examples are welder's burn and burns associated with skiing without goggles in bright sunlight.

Chemical burns with strong acidic and alkaline agents can be blinding and constitute a true ocular emergency. Examples are burns caused by exploding batteries, spilled drain cleaner, and bleach.

Superficial thermal burns cause pain, tearing, and injection. Corneal epithelial defects can be diagnosed using fluorescein dye, which will stain areas of the cornea where the epithelium is absent. The fluorescein dye pattern will show a uniformly stippled appearance of the corneal epithelium in ultraviolet keratitis.

▶ Treatment

Management is with topical antibiotics and patching. A cycloplegic agent is added if corneal involvement is present, because pain from ciliary spasm and iritis may accompany the injury.

Alkalis tend to penetrate deeper than acids into ocular tissue. This results in damage to the conjunctival vessels which give the eye a white or blanched appearance. Immediate treatment consists of copious irrigation and removal of precipitates as soon as possible after the injury. The patient should be referred to an ophthalmologist after immediate first aid has been given.

HYPHEMA

Blunt trauma to the globe may cause a hyphema, or bleeding within the anterior chamber from a ruptured vessel located near the root of the iris or in the anterior chamber angle.

▶ Clinical Findings

A hyphema may be microscopic or may fill the entire anterior chamber (Figure 15–10). Blunt trauma severe enough to cause a hyphema may be associated with additional ocular injury, including iritis, lens subluxation, retinal edema or detachment, and glaucoma. In patients with sickle cell anemia or trait, even moderate elevations of intraocular pressure may quickly lead to optic atrophy and permanent vision loss. Therefore, all African Americans whose sickle cell status is unknown should be tested if hyphema is observed. These patients require extra vigilance in diagnosing and treating hyphema. Nontraumatic causes of hyphema include juvenile xanthogranuloma and blood dyscrasias. Rarely, hyphema is noted in the newborn after a stressful birth.

▲ **Figure 15–10.** Hyphema filling approximately 20% of the anterior chamber.

Slit-lamp examination or even penlight examination may reveal a layer of blood within the anterior chamber. Other injuries to the globe and orbit are often present.

► Treatment

A shield should be placed over the eye, the head elevated, and arrangements made for ophthalmologic referral.

NONACCIDENTAL TRAUMA & SHAKEN BABY SYNDROME

Shaken baby syndrome is a form of nonaccidental trauma characterized by a constellation of examination findings, including traumatic brain injury, retinal hemorrhages, and fractures of long bones or ribs. The history leading to the diagnosis of shaken baby syndrome is often vague and poorly correlated with the extent of injury.

► Clinical Findings

Victims often have multiple organ system involvement that includes, but is not limited to, traumatic brain injury, bone fractures and retinal hemorrhages. The presentation can vary from irritability to emesis, change in mental status, or cardiopulmonary arrest.

Neuroimaging of the brain as well as a skeletal survey are tools used to diagnose shaken baby syndrome. Ophthalmic consultation and a dilated retinal examination are necessary to document retinal hemorrhages. Hemorrhages may be unilateral or bilateral and may be located in the posterior pole or periphery. Whereas retinal hemorrhages tend to resolve fairly quickly, those in the vitreous do not. If a blood clot lies over the macula, deprivation amblyopia may occur and may require intraocular surgery by a retinal specialist. Other ocular findings associated with nonaccidental trauma include lid ecchymosis, subconjunctival hemorrhage, hyphema, retinal folds, retinoschisis, and optic nerve edema. Acute-onset esotropia can also occur.

► Differential Diagnosis

The diagnosis of shaken baby syndrome has obvious legal ramifications and is a subject of debate within the literature. The differential includes but is not limited to retinal hemorrhages secondary to a fall, seizures, chest compressions during cardiopulmonary resuscitation, blood dyscrasias, and Terson syndrome, among others. A team effort between the primary treating physician, neurosurgery, orthopedics, ophthalmology, and social services is often needed to determine the true cause of a patient's injuries.

► Treatment

Management of any systemic injuries is required. Observation by an ophthalmologist of retinal hemorrhages for resolution is the usual course of treatment. Vitreous hemor-

rhages or large preretinal hemorrhages that do not resolve within several weeks may need surgical treatment by a retinal specialist.

Dias MS et al: Preventing abusive head trauma among infants and young children: A hospital-based, parent education program. Pediatrics 2005;115:e470 [PMID: 15805350].

Newton AW, Vandeven AM: Update on child maltreatment. Curr Opin Pediatr 2007;19:223 [PMID: 17496770].

Walls C: Shaken baby syndrome education: A role for nurse practitioners working with families of small children. J Pediatr Health Care 2006;20:304 [PMID: 16962435].

PREVENTION OF OCULAR INJURIES

Air rifles, paintballs, and fireworks are responsible for many serious eye injuries in children. Golf injuries can be very severe. Bungee cords have been associated with multiple types of severe ocular trauma, including corneal abrasion, iris tears, hyphema, vitreous hemorrhage, retinal detachment, and blindness. Use of these items and associated activities should be avoided or very closely supervised. Safety goggles should be used in laboratories and industrial arts classes and when operating snow blowers, power lawn mowers, and power tools, or when using hammers and nails. Sports-related eye injuries can be prevented with protective eyewear. Sports goggles and visors of polycarbonate plastic will prevent injuries in games using fast projectiles such as tennis or racquet balls, or where opponents may swing elbows or poke at the eye.

The one-eyed individual should be specifically advised to always wear polycarbonate eyeglasses and goggles for all sports. High-risk activities such as boxing and the martial arts should be avoided by one-eyed children.

American Academy of Pediatrics, Committee on Sports Medicine and Fitness; American Academy of Ophthalmology, Eye Health and Public Information Task Force: Protective eyewear for young athletes. Ophthalmology 2004;111:600 [PMID: 15019343].

Brophy M et al: Pediatric eye injury-related hospitalizations in the United States. Pediatrics 2006;117:e1263 [PMID: 16740824].

▼ DISORDERS OF THE OCULAR STRUCTURES

DISEASES OF THE EYELIDS

The eyelids can be affected by various dermatologic and infectious conditions.

1. Blepharitis

Blepharitis is inflammation of the lid margin characterized by crusty debris at the base of the lashes; varying degrees of erythema at the lid margins; and in severe cases, secondary corneal changes such as punctate erosions, vascularization, and ulcers. When conjunctival injection accompanies blepharitis, the condition is known as blepharoconjunctivitis. *Sta-*

phylococcus is the most common bacterial cause. Treatment includes lid scrubs with a nonburning baby shampoo several times a week and application of a topical antibiotic ointment such as erythromycin or bacitracin at bedtime.

2. Rosacea

Rosacea can also occur in the pediatric age group and cause chronic blepharoconjunctivitis with corneal changes that decrease vision. Systemic antibiotics and local treatment are required.

3. Pediculosis

Pediculosis of the lids (phthiriasis palpebrarum) is caused by *Phthirus pubis*. Nits and adult lice can be seen on the eyelashes when viewed with appropriate magnification. Mechanical removal and application to the lid margins of phospholine iodide or 1% mercuric oxide ointment can be effective. Other bodily areas of involvement must also be treated if involved. Family members and contacts may also be infected (see Chapter 14).

4. Papillomavirus

Papillomavirus may infect the lid and conjunctiva. Warts may be recurrent, multiple, and difficult to treat. Treatment modalities include cryotherapy, cautery, carbon dioxide laser, and surgery.

5. Staphylococcal Infection

Localized staphylococcal infections of the glands of Zeis within the lid cause a sty (hordeolum) (Figure 15–11). When the infection coalesces and points internally or externally, it may discharge itself or require incision. The lesion is tender and red. Warm compresses help to hasten the acute process. Some practitioners prescribe a topical antibiotic ointment. Any coexisting blepharitis should be treated.

▲ **Figure 15–11.** Hordeolum and blepharitis, left upper lid.

A

B

▲ **Figure 15–12.** Chalazion. **A:** Right lower lid, external view. **B:** Right lower lid conjunctival surface.

6. Chalazion

A chalazion is an inflammation of the meibomian glands, which may produce a tender nodule over the tarsus of the upper or lower lid. In addition to localized erythema of the corresponding palpebral conjunctiva, there may be a yellow lipogranuloma (Figure 15–12). Treatment includes warm compresses for 10–15 minutes four times a day for up to 6 weeks. If incision and curettage are needed because the lesion is slow to resolve, the child will require a general anesthetic.

VIRAL LID DISEASE

Viral infections of the eyelids can result in eyelid vesicles or papules.

▶ **Clinical Findings**

Herpes simplex virus may involve the lids at the time of primary herpes simplex infection. Vesicular lesions with an erythematous base occur. Herpes zoster causes vesicular disease in association with a skin eruption in the dermatome of the ophthalmic branch of the trigeminal nerve. Molluscum contagiosum lesions are typically umbilicated papules. If near the lid margin, the lesions may shed and cause conjunctivitis.

A vesicular rash is the most common sign of viral eyelid disease. Fluorescein dye should be administered topically to both eyes followed by examination with a cobalt blue light to determine if corneal or conjunctival involvement is present. Herpes simplex or herpes zoster can be diagnosed by rapid viral culture (24–48 hours) or detection of antigen in skin lesions (3 hours).

▶ Treatment

Primary herpes simplex blepharoconjunctivitis should be treated with systemic acyclovir (a liquid formulation is available), valacyclovir, or famciclovir. When either the conjunctiva or the cornea is involved, treatment should include topical 1% trifluridine or 3% vidarabine.

Treatment of ophthalmic herpes zoster with nucleoside analogues within 5 days after onset may reduce the morbidity. When vesicles are present on the tip of the nose with herpes zoster (Hutchinson sign), ocular involvement, including iritis, may develop. Impetigo is in the differential diagnosis of vesicular lid disease.

Molluscum contagiosum lesions may be treated with cautery or excision.

LID PTOSIS

Eyelid ptosis results in a droopy eyelid that may be unilateral or bilateral. If the pupil is obstructed, deprivation amblyopia may result.

▶ Clinical Findings

Ptosis—a droopy upper lid (Figure 15–13)—may be congenital or acquired but is usually congenital in children owing to a defective levator muscle. Other causes of ptosis are myasthenia gravis, lid injuries, third nerve palsy, and Horner syndrome (see next section). Ptosis may be associated with astigmatism and amblyopia.

An association sometimes seen with congenital ptosis is the Marcus Gunn jaw-winking phenomenon. Intermittent reduction of the ptosis occurs during mastication or sucking, due to a synkinesis or simultaneous firing of either the external or internal pterygoid muscle (innervated by the trigeminal nerve) and the levator muscle (innervated by the oculomotor nerve).

▶ Treatment

Surgical correction is indicated for moderate to severe ptosis. Mild cases less often require operative management. Cosmesis may be better if surgery is delayed until most of the facial growth has occurred, usually around age 5 years.

HORNER SYNDROME

Horner syndrome, which may be congenital or acquired, presents with signs of unequal pupils (anisocoria), eyelid ptosis, iris heterochromia, and anhidrosis.

▶ Clinical Findings

Parents may notice unequal pupils or different colored eyes. Penlight examination of the eyes may reveal unequal pupils (anisocoria), iris heterochromia, and eyelid ptosis of the affected eye.

The ptosis is usually mild with a well-defined upper lid crease. This differentiates it from congenital ptosis, which typically has a poorly defined lid crease. Another key finding of congenital Horner syndrome is heterochromia of the two irides, with the lighter colored iris occurring on the same side as the lesion (Figure 15–14). Anhidrosis can occur in congenital and acquired cases. Of note, not all of the three signs must be present to make the diagnosis. The syndrome is caused by an abnormality or lesion to the sympathetic chain. The congenital variety is most commonly the result of birth trauma. Acquired cases may occur in children who have had cardiothoracic surgery, trauma, or brainstem vascular malformation. Most worrisome is a Horner syndrome caused by neuroblastoma of the sympathetic chain in the apical lung region. An excellent screening test for this is the spot urine vanillylmandelic acid/creatinine ratio.

Pharmacologic assessment of the pupils with topical cocaine and hydroxyamphetamine or epinephrine will help determine whether the Horner syndrome is due to a preganglionic or postganglionic lesion of the sympathetic chain. There are preliminary studies that suggest that topical apraclonidine may also be useful in the diagnosis of Horner syndrome. Physical examination, including palpation of the

▲ **Figure 15–13.** Congenital ptosis of severe degree, left upper lid.

▲ **Figure 15–14.** Congenital Horner syndrome. Ptosis, miosis, and heterochromia. Lighter colored iris is on the affected left side.

neck and abdomen for masses, and MRI of structures in the head, neck, chest, and abdomen should be considered.

Treatment

Management of any underlying disease is required. The ptosis and vision should be monitored by an ophthalmologist.

Mahoney NR et al: Pediatric Horner syndrome: Etiologies and roles of imaging and urine studies to detect neuroblastoma and other responsible mass lesions. Am J Ophthalmol 2006;142:651 [PMID: 17011859].

EYELID TICS

Eyelid tics may occur as a transient phenomenon lasting several days to months. Although a tic may be an isolated finding in an otherwise healthy child, it may also occur in children with multiple tics, attention-deficit/hyperactivity disorder, or Tourette syndrome. Caffeine consumption may cause or exacerbate eyelid tics. If the disorder is a short-lived annoyance, no treatment is needed.

▼ DISORDERS OF THE NASOLACRIMAL SYSTEM

NASOLACRIMAL DUCT OBSTRUCTION

Nasolacrimal obstruction occurs in up to 6% of infants. Most cases clear spontaneously during the first year. Obstruction in any part of the drainage system may result from incomplete canalization of the duct or membranous obstructions. Nasolacrimal obstruction may also occur in individuals with craniofacial abnormalities or amniotic band syndrome.

Clinical Findings

Nasolacrimal duct obstruction presents with tearing and mucoid discharge from the affected eye. Signs and symptoms include tearing (epiphora), mucoid discharge especially in the morning, erythema of one or both lids, and conjunctivitis (Figure 15–15). Light sensitivity and blepharospasm suggest possible congenital glaucoma and warrant an urgent ophthalmic referral.

Differential Diagnosis

The differential diagnosis of tearing includes nasolacrimal duct obstruction, congenital glaucoma, foreign bodies, nasal disorders, and in older children, allergies.

Treatment

Massage over the nasolacrimal sac may empty debris from the nasolacrimal sac and may clear the obstruction, although the efficacy of massage in clearing nasolacrimal obstruction is debated. Cleansing the lids and medial can-

▲ Figure 15–15. Nasolacrimal obstruction, right eye. Mattering on upper and lower lids.

thal area decreases the likelihood of infection and irritation. Superinfection may occur, and treatment with topical antibiotics may help decrease the discharge. The mainstay of surgical treatment is probing, which is successful 80% or more of the time, but the success rate may decrease after the infant reaches 1 year of age. Other surgical procedures, including infraction of the inferior nasal turbinate, balloon dilation, and silicone tube intubation, may be necessary if probing fails. Much less often, dacryocystorhinostomy is required.

Casady DR et al: Stepwise treatment paradigm for congenital nasolacrimal duct obstruction. Ophthal Plast Reconstr Surg 2006;22:243 [PMID: 16855492].
Lee DH et al: Success of simple probing and irrigation in patients with nasolacrimal duct obstruction and otitis media. J AAPOS 2005;9:192 [PMID: 15838451].

CONGENITAL DACRYOCYSTOCELE

Congenital dacryocystocele is thought to result from obstructions proximal and distal to the nasolacrimal sac. An intranasal duct cyst may be present beneath the inferior turbinate at the valve of Hasner. These cysts may be associated with respiratory distress. At birth, the nasolacrimal sac is distended and has a bluish hue that often leads to an erroneous diagnosis of hemangioma. The tense and swollen sac displaces the medial canthus superiorly (Figure 15–16). Massage and warm compresses are rarely effective. Repeated probing and endoscopic marsupialization of the intranasal cyst under general anesthesia may be required. Dacryocystitis and sepsis can result from dacryocystocele.

Becker BB: The treatment of congenital dacryocystocele. Am J Ophthalmol 2006;142:835 [PMID: 16989760].

▲ **Figure 15–16.** Congenital dacryocystocele on the left side. Raised, bluish discolored mass of enlarged nasolacrimal sac. Note superiorly displaced medial canthus.

DACRYOCYSTITIS

Dacryocystitis is an infection of the nasolacrimal sac and results in erythema and edema over the nasolacrimal sac.

Acute and chronic dacryocystitis are typically caused by bacteria that colonize the upper respiratory tract, such as *Staphylococcus aureus, Streptococcus pneumoniae, Streptococcus pyogenes, Streptococcus viridans, Moraxella catarrhalis,* and *Haemophilus* species.

▶ Clinical Findings

Acute dacryocystitis presents with inflammation, swelling, tenderness, and pain over the lacrimal sac (located inferior to the medial canthal tendon). Fever may be present. The infection may point externally (Figure 15–17). A purulent discharge and tearing can be expected, because the cause of infection is almost always nasolacrimal obstruction.

Signs of chronic dacryocystitis are mucopurulent debris on the lids and lashes, tearing, injection of the palpebral conjunctiva, and reflux of pus at the puncta when pressure is applied over the sac. Chronic dacryocystitis and recurrent episodes of low-grade dacryocystitis are caused by nasolacrimal obstruction.

▶ Treatment

Treatment of severe acute dacryocystitis is with intravenous antibiotics after attempts at identifying the offending organism by culture and staining. Oral antibiotics can be tried in milder cases. Topical antibiotic administration is adjunctive and is also used with recurrent chronic infections. Warm compresses are beneficial. After the acute episode subsides—and in chronic cases—the nasolacrimal obstruction must be relieved surgically. If it cannot be drained via the intranasal portion of the nasolacrimal duct, external drainage may be necessary. This should be done as a last resort since a fistula may develop.

▲ **Figure 15–17.** Acute dacryocystitis in an 11-week-old infant.

▼ DISEASES OF THE CONJUNCTIVA

Conjunctivitis may be infectious, allergic, or associated with systemic disease. Trauma, irritation of the conjunctiva, and intraocular inflammation also can cause injection of conjunctival vessels that can be confused with conjunctivitis (Table 15–2).

OPHTHALMIA NEONATORUM

Ophthalmia neonatorum (conjunctivitis in the newborn) occurs during the first month of life. It may be due to inflammation resulting from silver nitrate prophylaxis given at birth, bacterial infection (gonococcal, staphylococcal, pneumococcal, or chlamydial), or viral infection. In developed countries, *Chlamydia* is the most common cause. Neonatal conjunctivitis may threaten vision if caused by *Neisseria gonorrhoeae.* Herpes simplex is a rare but serious cause of neonatal conjunctivitis, since it may indicate systemic herpes simplex infection.

▶ Clinical Findings

Ophthalmia neonatorum is characterized by redness and swelling of the lids and conjunctiva and by discharge (Figure 15–18). Gram staining, Giemsa staining for elementary bodies, polymerase chain reaction amplification for *Chlamydia* and herpes simplex virus, and bacterial and viral cultures aid in making an etiologic diagnosis.

▶ Prevention & Treatment

Although no single prophylactic medication can eliminate all cases of neonatal conjunctivitis, povidone-iodine may provide broader coverage against the organisms causing this disease than silver nitrate or erythromycin ointment. Silver nitrate is not effective against *Chlamydia.* The choice of prophylactic agent is often dictated by local epidemiology and cost considerations.

Treatment of these infections requires specific systemic antibiotics because they can cause serious infections in other organs. Specifically, *Chlamydia* can cause a delayed-onset pneumonitis. Parents should be examined and receive treatment when a sexually associated pathogen is present.

Darville T: Chlamydia trachomatis infections in neonates and young children. Semin Pediatr Infect Dis 2005;16:235 [PMID: 16210104].

Woods CR: Gonococcal infections in neonates and young children. Semin Pediatr Infect Dis 2005;16:258 [PMID: 16210106].

Table 15–2. Clinical and laboratory features of conjunctivitis.

	Viral	Bacterial	Chlamydial	Allergic
Itching	Minimal	Minimal	Minimal	Severe
Hyperemia	Generalized	Generalized	Generalized	Generalized
Tearing	Profuse	Moderate	Moderate	Moderate
Exudation	Minimal, mucoid	Profuse, purulent	Profuse; mucoid or mucopurulent	Minimal, slight mucus
Preauricular adenopathy	Common	Uncommon	Common in inclusion conjunctivitis	None
Stained conjunctival smears and scrapings	Lymphocytes, plasma cells, multinucleated giant cells, eosinophilic intranuclear inclusions	Neutrophils, bacteria	Neutrophils, plasma cells, basophilic intracytoplasmic inclusions	Eosinophils
Associated systemic signs and symptoms	Rash, sore throat, fever in some patients	Occasional fever, sore throat	Pneumonia in neonates	Variable—may or may not be present

Reprinted, with permission, from Riordan-Eva P, Whitcher J: *Vaughan & Asbury's General Ophthalmology,* 17th ed., McGraw-Hill, 2008.

BACTERIAL CONJUNCTIVITIS

▶ Clinical Findings & Differential Diagnosis

In general, bacterial conjunctivitis is accompanied by a purulent discharge, whereas viral infection produces a watery discharge. One or both eyes may be involved. Regional lymphadenopathy is not a common finding in bacterial conjunctivitis except in cases of oculoglandular syndrome due to *S aureus*, group A β-hemolytic streptococci, *Mycobacterium tuberculosis* or atypical mycobacteria, *Francisella tularensis* (the agent of tularemia), and *Bartonella henselae* (the agent of cat-scratch disease).

Children with bacterial conjunctivitis usually present with mucopurulent discharge and injection of the conjunctiva of one or both eyes, which may be associated with an upper respiratory infection. The differential diagnosis includes viral or chlamydial infection, and allergic, chemical, or toxic reactions to agents accidentally instilled into the eyes. Table 15–2 outlines signs and symptoms that may help delineate the cause of conjunctivitis.

Common bacterial causes of conjunctivitis in older children include nontypable *Haemophilus* species, *S pneumoniae*, *M catarrhalis*, and *S aureus*.

▶ Treatment

If conjunctivitis is not associated with systemic illness, topical antibiotics such as erythromycin, polymyxin-bacitracin, sulfacetamide, tobramycin, and fluoroquinolones are adequate. Systemic therapy is recommended for conjunctivitis associated with *Chlamydia trachomatis, N gonorrhoeae,* and *N meningitidis*.

Silver LH et al: Clinical safety of moxifloxacin ophthalmic solution 0.5% (VIGAMOX) in pediatric and nonpediatric patients with bacterial conjunctivitis. Surv Ophthalmol 2005;50(Suppl 1):S55 [PMID: 16257311].

VIRAL CONJUNCTIVITIS

Adenovirus infection is often associated with pharyngitis, a follicular reaction and injection of the palpebral conjunctiva, and preauricular adenopathy (pharyngoconjunctival fever). Epidemics of adenoviral keratoconjunctivitis occur. Conjunctivitis can occur as part of an acute measles illness. Herpes simplex virus may cause conjunctivitis or blepharoconjunctivitis.

▶ Clinical Findings

Children with viral conjunctivitis usually present with injection of the conjunctiva of one or both eyes and watery ocular discharge; an upper respiratory infection is sometimes present. A vesicular rash involving the eyelids suggests herpes simplex virus.

▲ **Figure 15–18.** Ophthalmia neonatorum due to *Chlamydia trachomatis* infection in a 2-week-old infant. Note marked lid and conjunctival inflammation.

▶ Treatment

Treatment of adenovirus conjunctivitis is supportive. Children with presumed adenoviral keratoconjunctivitis are considered contagious 10–14 days from the day of onset. They should stay out of school and group activities as long as their eyes are red and tearing. Strict hand-washing precautions are recommended.

Herpes conjunctivitis can be treated with topical trifluridine 1% drops or 3% vidarabine ointment. Oral acyclovir may be used prophylactically in children to reduce recurrence of herpes simplex ocular disease or during the primary infection to decrease the duration and severity of the infection.

ALLERGIC CONJUNCTIVITIS

▶ Clinical Findings

In allergic conjunctivitis, the child has red and itchy eyes, may have a mucoid discharge, and often has other allergic symptoms such as sneezing and rhinitis. Vernal conjunctivitis is a seasonal form of allergic conjunctivitis occurring mostly in the spring and summer and is associated with tearing, itching, and a stringy discharge. Vernal allergic conjunctivitis is more common in males. Contact lens wear may induce a conjunctivitis that appears similar to the palpebral form of vernal conjunctivitis.

The diagnosis of allergic and vernal conjunctivitis is based predominantly on the history. Ocular itching is the major symptom of both conditions. Redness of the conjunctiva, tearing and discharge may be part of the history but need not be present on examination to make the diagnosis. Vernal conjunctivitis may present with giant cobblestone papillae (Figure 15–19) on the eyelid conjunctiva, nodules around the corneal limbus, and even sterile corneal ulcers.

▲ **Figure 15–19.** Vernal conjunctivitis. Cobblestone papillae in superior tarsal conjunctiva.

▶ Treatment

Topical ophthalmic solutions that combine both an antihistamine and mast cell stabilizers, including olopatadine 0.1%, epinastine HCl 0.05%, and ketotifen fumarate 0.025%, are very effective at treating allergic conjunctivitis. Other agents available include a combination topical vasoconstrictor plus an antihistamine (naphazoline antazoline), a nonsteroidal anti-inflammatory drug such as ketorolac tromethamine 0.5%, a mast cell stabilizer such as lodoxamide tromethamine 0.1%, or a corticosteroid such as prednisolone 0.125% (Table 15–3). Corticosteroids should be used with caution because their extended use causes glaucoma or cataracts in some patients.

Treatment of vernal conjunctivitis includes a mast cell stabilizer such as 4% cromolyn sodium or 0.1% lodoxamide tromethamine and limited use of a topical corticosteroid.

Abelson MB, Granet D: Ocular allergy in pediatric practice. Curr Allergy Asthma Rep 2006;6:306 [PMID: 16822383].

MUCOCUTANEOUS DISEASES

Systemic conditions affecting the skin or the oral and genitourinary mucosa often result in ocular involvement. Severe inflammation involving the conjunctiva may result in permanent scarring, eyelid malposition, and dry eye syndrome.

Conjunctivitis and conjunctival changes are associated with systemic syndromes, such as erythema multiforme (Stevens-Johnson syndrome; see Chapter 14), Reiter syndrome, and Kawasaki disease (see Chapter 19). The latter is also associated with iritis.

▶ Clinical Findings

With Stevens-Johnson syndrome, conjunctival changes include erythema, vesicular lesions that frequently rupture, and symblepharon (adhesions) between the raw edges of the bulbar (eye) and palpebral (lid) conjunctivae.

▶ Treatment

Management of conjunctivitis associated with mucocutaneous disease depends on its severity. Artificial tears and ointment provide comfort and a topical corticosteroid may help prevent adhesions and dry eye in severe cases. Lysis of adhesions or use of a scleral ring by an ophthalmologist may be required. Surgical treatment of severe cases of symblepharon with amniotic membrane grafts are under investigation. Topical cyclosporine may help decrease the inflammatory reaction that leads to the destruction of tear-producing glands and subsequent dry eye syndrome. Cycloplegic agents and topical corticosteroids are prescribed for iritis in Kawasaki disease.

Chang YS et al: Erythema multiforme, Stevens-Johnson syndrome, and toxic epidermal necrolysis: Acute ocular manifestations, causes, and management. Cornea 2007;26:123 [PMID: 17251797].

Table 15-3. Common ocular allergy medications.

Generic Name	Brand Name	Mechanism of Action	Side Effects	Dosage	Indications
Lodoxamide tromethamine 0.1%	Alomide	Mast cell stabilizer	Transient burning or stinging	1 drop 4 times daily—taper	Vernal keratoconjunctivitis
Cromolyn Na 4%	Crolom, Opticrom	Mast cell stabilizer	Transient burning or stinging	1 drop 4-6 times daily	Vernal keratoconjunctivitis
Olopatadine	Patanol	Mast cell stabilizer, H_1-receptor antagonist	Headache, burning or stinging	Twice daily (interval 6-8 h)	Itching due to allergic conjunctivitis
Ketorolac tromethamine 0.5%	Acular	Nonsteroidal anti-inflammatory drug	Transient burning or stinging	1 drop 4 times daily	Itching due to seasonal allergic conjunctivitis
Levocabastine HCl 0.05%	Livostin	H_1-receptor antagonist	Transient burning or stinging, headache	1 drop 4 times daily	Relief of symptoms of seasonal allergic conjunctivitis
Naphazoline HCl 0.1%	AK-Con, Naphcon, Opcon, Vasocon	Ocular decongestant, vasoconstrictor	Mydriasis, increased redness, irritation, discomfort, punctate keratitis, increased intraocular pressure, dizziness, headache, nausea, nervousness, hypertension, weakness, cardiac effects, hyperglycemia	Varies by preparation	Temporary relief of redness due to minor eye irritants
Pheniramine maleate	Component in AKCon A, Opcon-A, Naphcon-A	Antihistamine		1 drop every 3-4 h, as needed	Relief of symptoms of seasonal allergic conjunctivitis

DISORDERS OF THE IRIS

IRIS COLOBOMA

Iris coloboma is a developmental defect due to incomplete closure of the anterior embryonal fissure. The child's pupil has an elongated shape reminiscent of a keyhole or cat's eye (Figure 15-20). The effect on visual acuity is variable. Iris coloboma may occur as an isolated defect or in association with various chromosomal abnormalities and syndromes. Variable genetic expression of colobomas can include a broad spectrum, from iris coloboma, to microphthalmia-with-cyst, and clinical anophthalmia.

▶ Clinical Findings

Penlight examination of the pupils reveals a keyhole shape to the pupil rather than the normal round configuration. A dilated examination by an ophthalmologist is necessary to determine if the coloboma involves additional structures of the eye including the retina. If the retina is involved, vision may be poor. A genetic evaluation is usually recommended due to the high rate of associated genetic syndromes.

▶ Treatment

Patients with coloboma should be monitored by an ophthalmologist for signs of amblyopia, significant refractive errors, and strabismus. Rarely, if the retina is involved, detachment may occur requiring surgical intervention by a retinal specialist.

ANIRIDIA

Aniridia is a bilateral disorder that results in the absence of almost all of the iris (Figure 15-21). Cataract, corneal changes, macular hypoplasia, and glaucoma are often seen. Aniridia

▲ **Figure 15-20.** Iris coloboma located inferiorly.

▲ **Figure 15–21.** Bilateral aniridia. Iris remnants present temporally in each eye.

may occur as an autosomal dominant disease or in a sporadic form associated with Wilms tumor. The aniridia gene is located within the 11p13 chromosome region. Aniridia, genitourinary abnormalities, and mental retardation have been linked to an 11p deletion.

▶ Clinical Findings

Photophobia, nystagmus, and poor vision are present in aniridia. Abdominal ultrasonography is indicated in the sporadic form of aniridia to diagnose Wilms tumor. Genetic evaluation is indicated, as well.

▶ Treatment

An ophthalmologist should determine if cataracts or glaucoma are present in patients with aniridia. Surgical treatment is often indicated. If Wilms tumor is present, treatment by an oncologist is necessary.

ALBINISM

Albinism is caused by defective melanogenesis, usually as an autosomal recessive disease, but an X-linked form does occur. Tyrosinase is an essential enzyme in the production of melanin. Many cases of complete albinism are caused by mutations of the tyrosinase gene. Albinism with some pigment production, especially in people of African descent, is more commonly caused by mutations of the *p* gene.

▶ Clinical Findings

Affected individuals are usually legally blind and have nystagmus (see later section on Nystagmus). Iris, skin, and hair color vary with the type and severity of albinism as well as the individual's race. Iris transillumination is abnormal transmission of light through an iris with decreased pigment. This may be obvious or may require slit-lamp examination with retroillumination to detect focal areas of trans-illumination. Other ocular abnormalities include foveal hypoplasia, abnormal optic pathway projections, strabismus, and poor stereoacuity.

Albinism may be associated with other systemic manifestations. Bleeding problems occur in individuals with Her-

mansky-Pudlak syndrome (chromosome 10q23 or 5q13), in which oculocutaneous albinism is associated with a platelet abnormality. Chédiak-Higashi syndrome (chromosome 1q42–44) is characterized by neutrophil defects, recurrent infections, and oculocutaneous albinism. Other conditions associated with albinism are Waardenburg, Prader-Willi, and Angelman syndromes.

▶ Treatment

Children with albinism should be evaluated by a pediatric ophthalmologist in order to optimize their visual function. Low-vision aids such as telescopes, stand magnifiers, and large-print books are often required. Vision teachers in schools as well as ophthalmic specialists trained in treating low-vision patients can help increase the patient's ability to perform activities of daily living and function within society. Parents and patients must be advised to use sunscreen and wear protective clothing to help prevent skin cancer.

OTHER IRIS CONDITIONS

Heterochromia, or a difference in iris color, can occur in congenital Horner syndrome, after iritis, or with tumors and nevi of the iris and use of topical prostaglandins. Malignant melanoma of the iris may also cause iris heterochromia. Acquired iris nodules (Lisch nodules), which occur in type 1 neurofibromatosis, usually become apparent by age 8 years. When seen on slit-lamp examination, Lisch nodules are 1–2 mm in diameter and often beige in color, although their appearance can vary. Iris xanthogranuloma occurring with juvenile xanthogranuloma can cause hyphema and glaucoma. Patients with juvenile xanthogranuloma should be evaluated by an ophthalmologist for ocular involvement.

Ward et al: Neurofibromatosis 1: From lab bench to clinic. Pediatr Neurol 2005;32:221 [PMID: 15797177].

▼ GLAUCOMA

▶ General Considerations

Glaucoma is caused by increased intraocular pressure and results in vision loss due to optic nerve injury, corneal scarring, and amblyopia. Pediatric glaucoma can be congenital or acquired, pupillary block or angle closure, and unilateral or bilateral. Glaucoma can be classified on an anatomic basis into two types: open-angle and closed-angle. In children, precipitation of angle-closure glaucoma by dilating the pupil of an otherwise healthy eye is a very rare occurrence.

Glaucoma also occurs with ocular and systemic syndromes. Aniridia and anterior segment dysgenesis are examples. Systemic syndromes associated with glaucoma include Sturge-Weber syndrome, the oculocerebrorenal syndrome of Lowe, and the Pierre Robin syndrome. Glaucoma can also occur with hyphema, iritis, lens dislocation, intraocular tumor, and retinopathy of prematurity.

▶ Clinical Findings

Signs of glaucoma presenting within the first year of life include buphthalmos (enlargement of the globe due to low scleral rigidity in the infant eye) as well as tearing, photophobia, blepharospasm, corneal clouding due to edema, and optic nerve cupping. After age 3 years, usually only optic nerve changes occur. Findings may be unilateral or bilateral. In general, a red, inflamed eye is not typical of congenital or infantile glaucoma.

Sudden eye pain, redness, corneal clouding, and vision loss suggests possible pupillary block or angle-closure glaucoma. Urgent referral to an ophthalmologist is indicated. Genetic evaluation should be completed if other systemic abnormalities are noted.

▶ Treatment

Treatment depends on the cause, but surgery is often indicated. Topical medications, which are available to help decrease the intraocular pressure, have limited success in pediatric glaucoma.

Ishida K et al: Glaucoma drainage implants in pediatric patients. Ophthalmol Clin North Am 2005;18:431 [PMID: 16055000].
Moore W, Nischal KK: Pharmacologic management of glaucoma in childhood. Paediatr Drugs 2007;9:71 [PMID: 17407363].
Tanimoto SA, Brandt JD: Options in pediatric glaucoma after angle surgery has failed. Curr Opin Ophthalmol 2006;17:132 [PMID: 16552247].

▼ UVEITIS

Inflammation of the uveal tract can be subdivided according to the uveal tissue primarily involved (iris, choroid, or retina) or by location (anterior, intermediate, or posterior uveitis). Perhaps the most commonly diagnosed form of uveitis in childhood is traumatic iridocyclitis or iritis.

ANTERIOR UVEITIS

Iridocyclitis associated with juvenile rheumatoid arthritis occurs most often in girls with pauciarticular arthritis and a positive antinuclear antibody test. Inflammatory bowel disease is also associated with iritis—perhaps more commonly with Crohn disease than with ulcerative colitis. Other causes of anterior uveitis in children include syphilis, tuberculosis, sarcoidosis, relapsing fever (borreliosis), and Lyme disease, all but the last also causing posterior uveitis. Juvenile spondyloarthropathies, including ankylosing spondylitis, Reiter syndrome, and psoriatic arthritis, are also associated with anterior uveitis. A substantial percentage of cases are of unknown origin.

▶ Clinical Findings

Injection, photophobia, pain, and blurred vision usually accompany iritis (anterior uveitis or iridocyclitis). An exception to this is iritis associated with juvenile rheumatoid arthritis (see Chapter 27). The eye in such cases is quiet and asymptomatic, but slit-lamp examination reveals anterior chamber inflammation with inflammatory cells and protein flare. Children with juvenile rheumatoid arthritis should be screened according to a schedule recommended by the American Academy of Pediatrics (http://www.aap.org). Children with Crohn disease or ulcerative colitis should have routine periodic ophthalmologic examinations to detect ocular inflammation, which may be asymptomatic, and cataracts associated with use of systemic corticosteroids.

Other ocular findings of the anterior segment include conjunctivitis, episcleritis, and sterile corneal infiltrates. Posterior segment findings may include central serous retinochoroidopathy, panuveitis (inflammation of all uveal tissue), choroiditis, ischemic optic neuropathy, retinal vasculitis, neuroretinitis, and intermediate uveitis (see later section on Intermediate Uveitis).

Posterior subcapsular cataracts can develop in patients with or without ocular inflammation. Most, if not all, of these patients have been taking corticosteroids as part of the long-term treatment of their autoimmune disease.

▶ Treatment

Treatment with a topical corticosteroid and a cycloplegic agent is aimed at quieting the inflammation and preventing or delaying the onset of cataract and glaucoma. Methotrexate and other immunosuppressive agents can be used in refractory cases.

Levy-Clarke GA et al: Management of chronic pediatric uveitis. Curr Opin Ophthalmol 2005;16:281 [PMID: 16175040].
Reiff A: Ocular complications of childhood rheumatic diseases: Uveitis. Curr Rheumatol Rep 2006;8:459 [PMID: 17152145].

POSTERIOR UVEITIS

The terms *choroiditis, retinitis,* and *retinochoroiditis* denote the tissue layers primarily involved in posterior uveitis. Infectious agents are the most common cause of posterior uveitis in the pediatric population.

▶ Clinical Findings

Children with posterior uveitis often present with systemic manifestations of a congenital infection. Examples include deafness, developmental delay, cataracts, "salt and pepper" retinopathy, and cardiac disorders seen in congenital rubella.

Serologic analysis and retinal examination by an ophthalmologist are used to identify the cause of posterior uveitis. Active toxoplasmosis (see Chapter 41) produces a white lesion appearing as a "headlight in the fog" owing to the overlying vitreitis. Inactive lesions have a hyperpigmented border. Contiguous white satellite lesions suggest reactivation of disease.

A granular "salt and pepper" retinopathy is characteristic of congenital rubella. In infants, the TORCH complex (toxoplasmosis, other infections, rubella, cytomegalovirus [CMV], and herpes simplex virus) and syphilis must be suspected in congenital infections that cause chorioretinitis.

Congenital lymphocytic choriomeningitis is diagnosed by immunofluorescent antibody or enzyme-linked immunosorbent assay serologic testing. Congenital lymphocytic choriomeningitis virus may also present with chorioretinitis. The virus is transmitted to humans by consumption of food contaminated with rodent urine or feces. It most closely resembles congenital toxoplasmosis in presentation. If possible, pregnant women should avoid exposure to rodents.

Ocular candidiasis occurs typically in an immunocompromised host or an infant in the intensive care nursery receiving hyperalimentation. Candidal chorioretinitis appears as multifocal, whitish yellow, fluffy retinal lesions that may spread into the vitreous and produce a so-called cotton or fungus ball vitreitis.

Acute retinal necrosis syndrome is caused most often by varicella-zoster virus and occasionally by herpes simplex virus. Patients may present with vision loss and a red and painful eye. Ophthalmoscopy may show unilateral or bilateral patchy white areas of retina, arterial sheathing, vitreous haze, atrophic retinal scars, retinal detachment, and optic nerve involvement.

CMV infection must be considered as a cause of retinitis in immunocompromised and HIV-infected children. CMV retinitis appears as a white retinal lesion, typically but not always associated with hemorrhage, or as a granular, indolent-appearing lesion with hemorrhage and a white periphery. Cotton-wool spots (nerve fiber layer infarcts) also commonly occur in HIV-positive patients.

In toddlers and older youngsters, *Toxocara canis* or *T cati* infections (ocular larva migrans; see Chapter 41) occur from ingesting soil contaminated with parasite eggs. The disease is usually unilateral. Common signs and symptoms include a red injected eye, leukocoria, and decreased vision. Funduscopic examination may show endophthalmitis (vitreous abscess) or localized granuloma. Diagnosis is based on the appearance of the lesion and serologic testing using enzyme-linked immunosorbent assay for *T canis* and *T cati*.

▶ Treatment

Congenital toxoplasmosis infections must be treated with a triple drug regimen (see Chapter 41). Studies have shown improved ophthalmic and neurologic outcomes with prolonged treatment. Other infectious agents such as *Candida*, varicella, and CMV may require systemic and intraocular injections of antimicrobial agents as well as retinal surgery. Treatment of toxocariasis includes periocular corticosteroid

injections and vitrectomy. The prognosis for vision depends on the severity of retinal and systemic involvement.

Chung H et al: Retinal complications in patients with solid organ or bone marrow transplantations. Transplantation 2007;83:694 [PMID: 17414700].

INTERMEDIATE UVEITIS

Pars planitis, often of uncertain cause, can be associated with vitreous floaters. The inflammation is described as snow-banking because a heaped-up white precipitate is located in the far anterior periphery of the retina and vitreous base.

▶ Clinical Findings

Patients with pars planitis often complain of decreased vision and floaters. They may also have a history of a red eye and ocular discomfort. Patients with intermediate uveitis often have decreased vision. A prolonged duration of the disease can lead to deprivation amblyopia and strabismus.

A dilated examination is required for observation of inflammation and snowbanking of the pars plana and vitreitis. Slit-lamp and dilated funduscopic examination by an ophthalmologist often reveal chronic signs of inflammation associated with intermediate uveitis, including macular edema, cataracts, increased intraocular pressure, irregular pupil, iris adhesion to the lens, and band keratopathy.

Intermediate uveitis is often idiopathic although there are several other etiologies worth investigating. *Toxocara* infections with peripheral granuloma can be associated with intermediate uveitis, as can inflammatory bowel disease, multiple sclerosis, and sarcoidosis. Retinoblastoma and other neoplasms can imitate uveitis, causing a so-called masquerade syndrome.

▶ Treatment

The most common treatment regimen for intermediate uveitis includes subtenon steroid injections, vitrectomy by a retinal surgeon, and systemic immunosuppression. Secondary glaucoma often requires tube shunt surgery. The prognosis depends on the severity of the disease and associated secondary complications such as glaucoma and cataracts.

▼ OCULAR MANIFESTATIONS OF ACQUIRED IMMUNODEFICIENCY SYNDROME

Ocular infections are important manifestations of AIDS (see Chapter 39). As CD4 T-lymphocyte counts fall below 200/μL, opportunistic infections increase in these patients. Pathogens commonly causing eye infection include CMV and varicella-zoster virus. Acute retinal necrosis syndrome (see earlier section on Posterior Uveitis) is a severe necrotizing retinitis that often results in blindness in patients with AIDS. Most cases are thought to be caused by varicella-zoster virus. Other implicated agents are herpes simplex types 1 and 2.

Patients with CD4 counts below 50/μL are at high risk for CMV retinitis and should have a complete ocular evaluation by an ophthalmologist. Various retinal abnormalities include cotton-wool spots, retinal hemorrhages, microaneurysms, perivasculitis, and decreased visual acuity from ischemic maculopathy.

▶ Treatment

Therapy with antiviral agents is required, but the prognosis is poor. Active CMV retinitis must be treated with intravenous antiviral therapy. Ganciclovir is the usual initial therapy; foscarnet may be required if resistance develops. Intravitreal ganciclovir or ganciclovir implants in conjunction with oral valganciclovir may be required in severe cases or in individuals intolerant to intravenous therapy. The incidence of CMV retinitis has fallen dramatically with the use of multidrug antiretroviral therapy.

Esposito S et al: Effect of highly active antiretroviral therapy (HAART) on the natural history of ocular manifestations in HIV-infected children. Eye 2006;20:595 [PMID: 16410815].
Thorne JE et al: Studies of Ocular Complications of AIDS Research Group. Effect of cytomegalovirus retinitis on the risk of visual acuity loss among patients with AIDS. Ophthalmology 2007;114:591 [PMID: 17123624].

▼ DISORDERS OF THE CORNEA

CONDITIONS CAUSING CORNEAL CLOUDING

Corneal clouding can be caused by developmental abnormalities, metabolic disorders, trauma and infection.

▶ Clinical Findings

Corneal clouding, tearing, blepharospasm, and photophobia in a newborn are signs of congenital glaucoma until proven otherwise. Direct trauma to the cornea during a forceps delivery can result in corneal haze and significant amblyopia. Systemic abnormalities such as developmental delay and liver or kidney failure suggest metabolic disorders such as mucopolysaccharidoses, Wilson disease, and cystinosis. Corneal infiltrates occur with viral infections, staphylococcal lid disease, corneal dystrophies, and interstitial keratitis due to congenital syphilis.

A complete ocular evaluation by an ophthalmologist is required and should be completed urgently when congenital glaucoma is suspected.

▶ Treatment

Treatment depends on the underlying condition. Surgical treatment of glaucoma and possible corneal transplantation may be required.

MICROCORNEA & MEGALOCORNEA

Microcornea—a corneal diameter less than 10 mm in a full-term infant or older child—may be associated with other anterior segment malformations or a microphthalmic globe. Megalocornea—diameter of 12.5 mm or greater—should be regarded as due to congenital glaucoma until proved otherwise.

VIRAL KERATITIS

Herpes simplex, herpes zoster, and adenovirus can all infect the cornea. When the epithelium breaks down, a dendritic or amoeboid pattern can be seen with fluorescein staining. Corneal involvement with herpes simplex can be recurrent and lead to blindness.

▶ Clinical Findings

Patients commonly present with a painful, red eye. Photophobia and decreased vision are also common complaints. Fever, malaise, and symptoms of upper respiratory tract infection may be present.

Fluorescein administration to the involved cornea will reveal areas of staining when viewed with a blue light. Decreased visual acuity, photophobia, and conjunctivitis may also be noted. Slit-lamp examination may reveal white infiltrates beneath the corneal epithelium.

▶ Treatment

Topical antivirals such as trifluridine and vidarabine are indicated when herpes simplex infection is limited to the corneal epithelium, although additional systemic therapy is required in newborns. Topical corticosteroids may be a useful addition to antiviral therapy when stromal disease is present. The use of corticosteroids in the presence of herpetic disease should be undertaken only by an ophthalmologist because of the danger of worsening the disease. Oral acyclovir started in the early phase (first 5 days) may be helpful in treating herpes zoster eye disease. Acyclovir prophylaxis is helpful in preventing recurrent herpetic epithelial keratitis (see earlier section on Viral Conjunctivitis) and stromal keratitis caused by herpes simplex.

Adenovirus conjunctivitis may progress to keratitis 1–2 weeks after onset. Vision may be decreased. In most cases no treatment is necessary because adenovirus keratitis is most often self-limiting. However, adenovirus is highly contagious and easily spread (see section on Viral Conjunctivitis).

CORNEAL ULCERS

Bacterial corneal ulcers in healthy children who are not contact lens wearers are usually secondary to corneal trauma from corneal abrasion or a penetrating foreign body. Decreased vision, pain, injection, a white corneal infiltrate or ulcer (Figure 15–22), and hypopyon (pus in the anterior

▲ **Figure 15–22.** Corneal ulcer. Note white infiltrate located on inferior cornea.

chamber) may all be present. Prompt referral to an ophthalmologist is necessary for culture and antibiotic treatment.

▼ DISORDERS OF THE LENS

Lens disorders involve abnormality of clarity or position. Lens opacification (cataract) can affect vision depending on its density, size, and position. Visual potential is also influenced by age at onset and the success of amblyopia treatment.

CATARACTS

Cataracts in children may be unilateral or bilateral, may exist as isolated defects, or may be accompanied by other ocular disorders or systemic disease (Figure 15–23).

▶ Clinical Findings

A. Symptoms and Signs

Leukocoria, poor fixation, and strabismus or nystagmus (or both) may be the presenting complaints. Absence of a red

▲ **Figure 15–23.** Cataract causing leukocoria.

reflex in the newborn should suggest the possibility of cataract, especially if the pupil has been dilated for the examination. This requires an urgent referral to an ophthalmologist.

B. Laboratory Findings

Laboratory investigation for infectious and metabolic causes of congenital cataracts is often indicated. Such investigation would include cultures or serologic tests for toxoplasmosis, rubella, CMV, herpes simplex virus, and syphilis, as well as evaluation for metabolic errors, such as occur with galactosemia or Lowe syndrome.

▶ Treatment

Early diagnosis and treatment are necessary to prevent deprivation amblyopia in children younger than age 9 years, because they are visually immature. Cataracts that are visually significant require removal. Visually significant cataracts in infants are usually removed prior to 6 weeks of age to prevent deprivation amblyopia. Rehabilitation with an intraocular lens is commonplace, especially with cataracts removed after the age of 2 years. But contact lenses and glasses still play a role, as does occlusion of the better-seeing eye to treat the amblyopia.

Forbes BJ, Guo S: Update on the surgical management of pediatric cataracts. J Pediatr Ophthalmol Strabismus 2006;43:143 [PMID: 16761634].

Vasavada AR, Nihalani BR: Pediatric cataract surgery. Curr Opin Ophthalmol 2006;17:54 [PMID: 16436925].

DISLOCATED LENSES

Nontraumatic lens dislocation is usually bilateral. Subluxation causes refractive errors of large magnitude that are difficult to correct. Another ophthalmologic concern is pupillary block glaucoma, in which a malpositioned unstable lens interferes with the normal flow of aqueous humor from the ciliary body (posterior to the pupil), where it is produced, into the trabecular meshwork (anterior to the pupillary plane).

▶ Clinical Findings

Slit-lamp examination reveals malposition of the intraocular lens. Refraction often reveals significant astigmatism. Systemic diseases including Marfan syndrome, homocystinuria, Weill-Marchesani syndrome, sulfite oxidase deficiency, hyperlysinemia, syphilis, and Ehlers-Danlos syndrome are often associated with dislocated lenses. A complete ophthalmic evaluation, as well as genetic and metabolic evaluation, may be necessary.

▶ Treatment

Surgical lensectomy may be required if the visual acuity is not improved significantly with glasses or contact lenses.

Underlying metabolic and or genetic disorders require a multidisciplinary approach.

DISORDERS OF THE RETINA

RETINAL HEMORRHAGES IN THE NEWBORN

Retinal hemorrhages are commonly seen in the otherwise healthy newborn. Retinal hemorrhages occur most often after vaginal delivery but can also be present after suction delivery or cesarean section.

Clinical Findings

A dilated retinal examination reveals unilateral or bilateral hemorrhages that can be located anywhere in the retina. They may appear as dot, blot, subretinal, or preretinal hemorrhages. They may also break into the vitreous.

Treatment

In general, retinal hemorrhages of the newborn disappear quickly, usually within the first month of life, which may help differentiate this condition from retinal hemorrhages that occur in the shaken baby syndrome. Retinal hemorrhages also occur in association with coagulopathy.

RETINOPATHY OF PREMATURITY

Retinopathy of prematurity (ROP) continues to be an important cause of blindness, especially for infants born before 28 weeks' gestation and weighing less than 1250 g. Premature infants with incomplete retinal vascularization are at risk for developing abnormal peripheral retinal vascularization, which may lead to retinal detachment. However, most cases of ROP do not progress to retinal detachment and require no treatment.

Pathogenesis

The risk of developing visually threatening ROP is inversely proportional to birth weight and gestational age. Infants weighing less than 1500 g at birth or born at less than 33 weeks' gestation may develop visually threatening ROP. The cause of this disorder—including the role of supplemental oxygen in the neonatal period—is still not fully understood. Other risk factors for severe ROP are bronchopulmonary dysplasia, intraventricular hemorrhage, sepsis, apnea and bradycardia, and mutations of the Norrie disease gene. White males, infants with zone 1 disease, and infants with very low birth weight and gestational age have a higher risk of reaching threshold.

Recent studies suggest that vascular endothelial growth factor may play a key role in ROP development, and methods of modulating it are being investigated.

Table 15–4. Stages of retinopathy of prematurity.

Stage I	Demarcation line or border dividing the vascular from the avascular retina.
Stage II	Ridge. Line of stage I acquires volume and rises above the surface retina to become a ridge.
Stage III	Ridge with extraretinal fibrovascular proliferation.
Stage IV	Subtotal retinal detachment.
Stage V	Total retinal detachment.

Clinical Findings

The Cryotherapy for Retinopathy of Prematurity (CRYO-ROP) study outlined a standard nomenclature to describe the progression and severity of ROP (Table 15–4). Since retinal blood vessels emanate from the optic nerve and do not fully cover the developing retina until term, the optic nerve is used as the central landmark. The most immature zone of retina, zone 1, is the most posterior concentric imaginary circle around the optic nerve. Further out is zone 2, and beyond that is zone 3. Zone 1 disease is by definition more high-risk than disease in more anterior zones. Similarly, the stages of the abnormal vessels are numbered from zero, or simply incomplete vascularization, through stages I–V. When five contiguous or eight noncontiguous clock hours of stage III disease occur, "threshold" has been reached. At this stage in the CRYO-ROP study, 50% of eyes had a bad outcome without treatment, progressing to stage IV or V. This was therefore chosen as the stage for mandatory treatment. "Plus disease" (+) refers to dilation and tortuosity of the vessels around the optic nerve and is an ominous sign of active, worsening ROP. "Rush disease" refers to cases in which the disease skips intervening stages and goes rapidly to retinal detachment.

Screening guidelines recommend the first retinal examination by an ophthalmologist be done at age 4–6 weeks after birth, or 31 weeks' postconception, whichever is earlier. The frequency of follow-up examinations depends on the findings and the risk factors for developing the disease. Most infants are evaluated every 1–2 weeks. ROP often resolves when the infant reaches 40 weeks' estimated gestational age. Examinations can be discontinued when the retinas are fully vascularized, or when the infant is 45 weeks' gestational age and has never had prethreshold disease or worse, or is vascularized out to zone 3 and never had zone 1 or 2 disease.

Treatment

The treatment of threshold ROP within 72 hours of diagnosis can reduce the occurrence of bad visual outcomes by 50%. Diode laser treatment has largely replaced cryotherapy because it provides better access for treating zone 1 disease and causes less inflammation. However, some patients still progress to a retinal detachment, which can have a very poor prognosis for vision. Surgical treatment for a retinal detachment involves scleral buckling or a lens-sparing vitrectomy by an ophthalmologist specializing in vitreoretinal surgery.

With smaller, sicker infants surviving, treatment guidelines have been amended to treat earlier than threshold in some infants. The Early Treatment for Retinopathy of Prematurity (ETROP) studies showed that early treatment of high-risk prethreshold ROP significantly reduced unfavorable outcomes. Infants with zone 1 ROP are at the highest risk for complications from ROP. Studies investigating oxygen management and its influence on the progression of ROP are underway.

Children with a history of ROP require lifelong management by an ophthalmologist. They are at a much higher risk of developing strabismus, amblyopia, myopia, and glaucoma than the average child.

Drack A: Retinopathy of prematurity. Adv Pediatr 2006;53:211 [PMID: 17089868].

RETINOBLASTOMA

Retinoblastoma is the most common primary intraocular malignancy of childhood, with an incidence estimated between 1:17,000 and 1:34,000 live births (see Chapter 29). Most patients present before age 3 years; children with hereditary or bilateral retinoblastoma usually present earlier than those with unilateral, sporadic disease.

▶ Pathogenesis

Inherited forms of retinoblastoma are autosomal dominant with high penetrance. The disease may consist of a solitary mass or multiple tumors in one or both eyes. All bilateral cases and some unilateral cases are caused by germinal mutations; however, most unilateral cases are caused by a somatic retinal mutation. In both situations, the mutation occurs in the retinoblastoma gene (*Rb*) at chromosome 13q14. This is a tumor suppressor gene. One mutated copy may be inherited in an autosomal dominant fashion (germline mutation). If a second mutation spontaneously occurs in any cell, tumorigenesis is likely. Individuals with a germinal mutation are at risk for the development of tumors other than retinoblastoma (pineal tumors, osteosarcoma, and other soft tissue sarcomas). All children with unilateral or bilateral retinoblastoma must be presumed to have the germline form, and followed expectantly for other tumors in the remaining eye and at extraocular sites. Approximately 15% of patients with unilateral disease have germline mutations.

▶ Clinical Findings

A. Symptoms and Signs

The most common presenting sign in a child with previously undiagnosed retinoblastoma is leukocoria (see Figure 15–1).

Evaluation of the pupillary red reflex is important, although a normal red reflex does not rule out retinoblastoma. Examination requires indirect ophthalmoscopy with scleral depression and pupillary dilation, performed by an ophthalmologist. Other presentations include strabismus, red eye, glaucoma, or pseudo-hypopyon (appearance of puslike material in the anterior chamber).

B. Special Tests

Genetic testing is available for patients with retinoblastoma. Once the causative mutation is found in an affected individual, unaffected members of the family should be tested to determine their personal and reproductive risk. This will avoid many unnecessary examinations under anesthesia for young relatives of patients with retinoblastoma.

▶ Treatment

Treatment of unilateral cases, especially of large tumors, often requires enucleation, because at the time of presentation the eye is filled with tumor. Vision and eyes can be salvaged in some cases. Chemoreduction of intraocular tumors is a newer treatment technique used to reduce initial tumor volume. In conjunction with local treatment such as laser photocoagulation, cryotherapy, plaque radiotherapy, and thermotherapy, combined therapy can often preserve vision and spare the patient enucleation and radiation that may lead to disfigurement and the induction of secondary tumors, especially in eyes classified with less extensive disease. Agents used in chemoreduction include carboplatin, etoposide, and vincristine. Eradication of tumor before infiltration into the optic nerve or choroid carries a good prognosis for survival.

Chan HS et al: Chemotherapy for retinoblastoma. Ophthalmol Clin North Am 2005;18:55 [PMID: 15763191].
Linn Murphree A: Intraocular retinoblastoma: The case for a new group classification. Ophthalmol Clin North Am 2005;18:41 [PMID: 15763190].
Wilson WG: Retinoblastoma. Pediatr Rev 2007;28:37 [PMID: 17197460].

RETINAL DETACHMENT

Retinal detachment occurs infrequently in children. Common causes are trauma and high myopia. Other causes are ROP, Marfan syndrome, and Stickler syndrome.

▶ Clinical Findings

Symptoms of detachment are floaters, flashing lights, and loss of visual field; however, children often cannot appreciate or verbalize their symptoms. A detachment may not be discovered until the child is referred after failing a vision screening examination, strabismus supervenes, or leukocoria is noted.

Treatment

Treatment of retinal detachment is surgical. For children with conditions predisposing to retinal detachment, or a strong family history, examinations under anesthesia by an ophthalmologist, with prophylactic laser treatment, are often recommended.

DIABETIC RETINOPATHY

Diabetic retinopathy is a specific vascular complication of diabetes mellitus. Patients with type 1, or insulin-dependent, diabetes are at higher risk of developing severe proliferative retinopathy leading to visual loss than are those with type 2, or non–insulin-dependent, diabetes.

Clinical Findings

Acute onset of diabetes may be accompanied by sudden myopia and by cataracts. Sudden decreased vision in a diabetic patient may suggest the presence of severe ocular complications such as vitreous hemorrhage, macular edema, or retinal detachment.

In children older than age 9 years, referral to an ophthalmologist for screening of retinopathy should occur within 3–5 years after the onset of diabetes. Both conditions may be reversible with good glucose control. Young children with type 1 diabetes should be followed for the Wolfram, or DIDMOD, syndrome, in which diabetes mellitus occurs in conjunction with diabetes insipidus, optic atrophy, and deafness.

Treatment

Severe proliferative diabetic retinopathy requires panretinal laser photocoagulation or vitreoretinal surgery (or both). Cataracts often require surgical removal and intraocular lens placement. Intraocular steroid injections have been used to treat macular edema in adults, but their role in children is not well established.

Huo B et al: Clinical outcomes and cost-effectiveness of retinopathy screening in youth with type 1 diabetes. Diabetes Care 2007;30:362 [PMID: 17259509].

▼ DISEASES OF THE OPTIC NERVE

OPTIC NEUROPATHY

Optic nerve function is evaluated by checking visual acuity, color vision, pupillary response, and visual fields.

Clinical Findings

Poor optic nerve function results in decreased central or peripheral vision, decreased color vision, strabismus, and nystagmus. Optic nerve disorders can be due to congenital malformation, malignancy, inflammation, infection, metabolic disorders, and trauma.

▲ **Figure 15–24.** Myelinization extending from optic nerve superiorly onto the retina.

The swinging flashlight test is used to assess function of each optic nerve. It is performed by shining a light alternately in front of each pupil to check for an afferent pupillary defect or Marcus Gunn pupillary defect. An abnormal response in the affected eye is pupillary dilation when the light is directed into that eye after having been shown in the other eye with its healthy optic nerve. This results from poorer conduction along the optic nerve of the affected eye, which in turn results in less pupillary constriction of both eyes than occurs when the light is shined into the noninvolved eye. Hippus—rhythmic dilating and constricting movements of the pupil—can be confused with an afferent pupillary defect.

The optic nerve is evaluated as to size, shape, color, and vascularity. Occasionally, myelinization past the entrance of the optic nerve head occurs. It appears white, with a feathered edge (Figure 15–24). Myelinization onto the retina can be associated with myopia and amblyopia. Anatomic defects of the optic nerve include colobomatous defects and pits.

Treatment

Management of the underlying condition resulting in the optic neuropathy is necessary.

OPTIC NERVE HYPOPLASIA

Optic nerve hypoplasia may be associated with absence of the septum pellucidum and hypothalamic-pituitary dysfunction, which is known as septo-optic dysplasia, or de Morsier syndrome. Children with septo-optic dysplasia and hypocortisolism are at risk for sudden death during febrile illness from thermoregulatory disturbance and dehydration from diabetes insipidus.

Optic nerve hypoplasia may occur in infants of diabetic mothers and has also been associated with alcohol use or ingestion of quinine or phenytoin during pregnancy. Anatomically, the optic nerve may range from absent (aplasia) to almost full size, with a segmental defect. However, the nerve often appears larger than it is because it is surrounded by a depigmented halo.

▶ Clinical Findings

Visual function with optic nerve hypoplasia ranges from mildly decreased to absent light perception. If only one eye is involved, the child usually presents with strabismus. If both eyes are affected, nystagmus is usually the presenting sign. Ophthalmoscopy is performed to directly visualize the optic nerves and to determine the severity of the hypoplasia. Neuroimaging of the brain and endocrine consultation should be performed in all patients with bilateral optic nerve hypoplasia.

▶ Treatment

Sensory amblyopia and significant refractive errors should be treated by an ophthalmologist. Strabismus surgery may be necessary in certain patients. Endocrine abnormalities should be managed as necessary.

PAPILLEDEMA

Papilledema (optic disk edema or choked disk) is associated with increased intracranial pressure due to any cause, such as tumor or intracranial infection.

▶ Pathogenesis

Hydrocephalus and intracranial tumors are common causes of papilledema. In pseudotumor cerebri (idiopathic intracranial hypertension), neuroimaging is normal but papilledema, headaches, and pulsating tinnitus may be present. Papilledema occurs almost equally in boys and girls and sometimes is associated with obesity or upper respiratory tract infection. Other associated causes are viral infections, corticosteroid use and withdrawal, sinus infection, trauma, tetracycline use, growth hormone, and venous sinus thrombosis. Early in the course of the disorder, the patient may not notice a change in vision, although the blind spot may be enlarged. Transient obscuration of vision (amaurosis fugax) may occur as the process becomes more long-standing. Further effects on vision will occur as the papilledema becomes chronic and ultimately leads to optic atrophy. Workup and treatment are directed toward finding the underlying systemic or central nervous system (CNS) cause.

▶ Clinical Findings

Direct visualization of the optic nerve by ophthalmoscopy reveals an elevated disk with indistinct margins, increased vessel diameter, and hyperemia. Hemorrhages and exudates are present in more severe cases. Observed changes may be subtle to striking. Optic nerve head changes are bilateral and generally symmetrical.

▶ Treatment

Treatment of idiopathic intracranial hypertension may be pharmacologic—for example, using acetazolamide, a carbonic anhydrase inhibitor, or a corticosteroid. Diagnostic lumbar puncture may also be curative. Optic nerve sheath fenestration and ventriculoperitoneal shunt are surgical interventions used when conservative measures fail.

Thuente DD et al: Pediatric optic nerve sheath decompression. Ophthalmology 2005;112:724 [PMID: 15808268].

PAPILLITIS

Papillitis is a form of optic neuritis seen on ophthalmoscopic examination as an inflamed optic nerve head. Optic neuritis in the pediatric age group may be idiopathic or associated with multiple sclerosis, acute disseminated encephalomyelitis, Devic disease, or cat-scratch disease.

▶ Clinical Findings

Papillitis may have the same appearance as papilledema. However, papillitis may be unilateral, whereas papilledema is almost always bilateral. Papillitis can be differentiated from papilledema by an afferent pupillary defect (Marcus Gunn pupil), by its greater effect in decreasing visual acuity and color vision, and by the presence of a central scotoma. Papilledema that is not yet chronic will not have as dramatic an effect on vision. Because increased intracranial pressure can cause both papilledema and a sixth (abducens) nerve palsy, papilledema can be differentiated from papillitis if esotropia and loss of abduction are also present. However, esotropia may also develop secondarily in an eye that has lost vision from papillitis. In pseudopapilledema (a normal variant of the optic disk), the disk appears elevated, with indistinct margins and a normal vascular pattern. Pseudopapilledema sometimes occurs in hyperopic individuals. Retrobulbar neuritis, an inflamed optic nerve, but with a normal-appearing nerve head, is associated with pain and the other findings of papillitis.

Workup of the patient with papillitis includes lumbar puncture and cerebrospinal fluid analysis. *B henselae* infection can be detected by serology. MRI is the preferred imaging study. An abnormal MRI is associated with a worse visual outcome.

▶ Treatment

Treatment of the underlying disease and use of systemic corticosteroids is necessary.

OPTIC ATROPHY

Optic atrophy is pallor of the optic nerve noted on ophthalmoscopy. Optic atrophy is found in children most frequently after neurologic compromise during the perinatal period. An example would be a premature infant who develops an intraventricular hemorrhage. Hydrocephalus, glioma of the optic nerve, craniosynostosis, certain neurologic diseases, and toxins such as methyl alcohol can cause optic atrophy, as can certain inborn errors of metabolism, long-standing papilledema, or papillitis.

▶ Clinical Findings

Direct examination of the optic nerve by ophthalmoscopy reveals an optic nerve head with a cream or white color and possibly cupping. Neuroimaging may be necessary to delineate CNS abnormalities.

▶ Treatment

Treatment of the underlying condition is indicated.

▼ DISEASES OF THE ORBIT

PERIORBITAL & ORBITAL CELLULITIS

The fascia of the eyelids joins with the fibrous orbital septum to isolate the orbit from the lids. This septum serves as a barrier to the posterior spread of infection from preseptal infection. Infections arising anterior to the orbital septum are termed preseptal. Orbital cellulitis denotes infection posterior to the orbital septum and may cause serious complications, such as an acute ischemic optic neuropathy or cerebral abscess.

▶ Pathogenesis

Preseptal (periorbital) cellulitis, which indicates infection of the structures of the eyelid, is characterized by lid edema, erythema, swelling, pain, and mild fever. It usually arises from a local exogenous source such as an abrasion of the eyelid, from other infections (hordeolum, dacryocystitis, or chalazion), or from infected varicella or insect bite lesions. *Staphylococcus aureus* and *Streptococcus pyogenes* are the most common pathogens cultured from these sources. Preseptal infections in children younger than age 3 years also occur from bacteremia, although this is much less common since *Haemophilus influenzae* immunization became available. *Streptococcus pneumoniae* bacteremia is still an occasional cause of this infection. Children with periorbital cellulitis from presumed bacteremia must be examined for additional foci of infection.

Orbital cellulitis almost always arises from contiguous sinus infection, because the walls of three sinuses make up portions of the orbital walls and infection can breach these walls or extend by way of a richly anastomosing venous system. The orbital contents can develop a phlegmon (orbital cellulitis), or frank pus can develop in the orbit (orbital abscess).

▶ Clinical Findings

Children with preseptal cellulitis often present with erythematous and edematous eyelids. The vision, eye movements and eye itself are normal. Decreased vision, restricted eye movements, and an afferent papillary defect suggest orbital cellulitis.

Orbital cellulitis presents with signs of periorbital disease as well as proptosis (a protruding eye), restricted eye movement, and pain with eye movement. Fever is usually high. CT scanning or MRI is required to establish the extent of the infection within the orbit and sinuses. The pathogenic agents are those of acute or chronic sinusitis—respiratory flora and anaerobes. *S aureus* is also frequently implicated.

▶ Treatment

Therapy for preseptal and orbital cellulitis infection is with systemic antibiotics. Treatment of orbital infections may require surgical drainage for subperiosteal abscess in conjunction with intravenous antibiotics. Drainage of infected sinuses is often part of the therapy.

Hennemann S et al: Clinical inquiries. What is the best initial treatment for orbital cellulitis in children? J Fam Pract 2007;56:662 [PMID: 17669292].

CRANIOFACIAL ANOMALIES

Craniofacial anomalies can affect the orbit and visual system. Craniofacial anomalies occur with craniosynostoses and midface syndromes such as Treacher Collins and Pierre Robin syndromes. Fetal alcohol syndrome is associated with similar changes of the ocular adnexa.

▶ Clinical Finding

Ocular abnormalities associated with craniofacial disease involving the orbits include visual impairment, proptosis, corneal exposure, hypertelorism (widely spaced orbits), strabismus, amblyopia, lid coloboma, papilledema, and optic atrophy.

▶ Treatment

Orbital and ocular abnormalities associated with craniofacial anomalies often require a multispecialty approach. Management may require orbital and strabismus surgery. Ophthalmologists also treat amblyopia and corneal exposure if present.

Liasis A et al: Monitoring visual function in children with syndromic craniosynostosis: A comparison of 3 methods. Arch Ophthalmol 2006;124:1119 [PMID: 16908814].

Tay T et al: Prevalence and causes of visual impairment in craniosynostotic syndromes. Clin Experiment Ophthalmol 2006;34:434 [PMID: 16872339].

▲ **Figure 15–25.** Right upper lid hemangioma causing ptosis.

ORBITAL TUMORS

Both benign and malignant orbital lesions occur in children. The most common benign tumor is capillary hemangioma (Figure 15–25). The most common primary malignant tumor of the orbit is rhabdomyosarcoma.

▶ Clinical Findings

Capillary hemangiomas may be located superficially in the lid or deep in the orbit and can cause ptosis, refractive errors, and amblyopia. Deeper lesions may cause proptosis. Capillary hemangiomas in infants initially increase in size before involuting at about age 2–4 years.

Orbital dermoid cysts vary in size and are usually found temporally at the brow and orbital rim or supranasally. These lesions are firm, well encapsulated, and mobile. Rupture of the cyst causes a severe inflammatory reaction.

Lymphangioma occurring in the orbit is typically poorly encapsulated, increases in size with upper respiratory infection, and is susceptible to hemorrhage. Other benign tumors of the orbit are orbital pseudotumor, neurofibroma, teratoma, and tumors arising from bone, connective tissue, and neural tissue.

Orbital rhabdomyosarcoma (see Chapter 29) grows rapidly and displaces the globe. The average age at onset is 6–7 years. The tumor is often initially mistaken for orbital swelling due to insignificant trauma.

Tumors metastatic to the orbit also occur; neuroblastoma is the most common. The patient may exhibit proptosis, orbital ecchymosis (raccoon eyes), Horner syndrome, or opsoclonus (dancing eyes). Ewing sarcoma, leukemia, Burkitt lymphoma, and the histiocytosis X group of diseases may involve the orbit.

Examination of vision, eye movements, eyelids, and orbits often reveals amblyopia, eyelid malposition, strabismus, and proptosis. Neuroimaging with CT or MRI is required to delineate the location and size of orbital tumors.

▶ Treatment

Therapy for capillary hemangiomas includes observation and intralesional or systemic corticosteroids. Treatment is indicated if the lesion is large enough to cause amblyopia.

Induced astigmatism or amblyopia (or both) are treated with glasses and patching respectively. Treatment of orbital dermoids is by excision.

Rhabdomyosarcoma is treated with radiation and chemotherapy after biopsy confirms the diagnosis. With expeditious diagnosis and proper treatment, the survival rate of patients with orbital rhabdomyosarcoma confined to the orbit approaches 90%.

Treatment of metastatic disease requires management by an oncologist and may require chemotherapy and radiation therapy.

Ahuja R, Azar NF: Orbital dermoids in children. Semin Ophthalmol 2006;21:207 [PMID: 16912019].

Chung EM et al: From the archives of the AFIP: Pediatric orbit tumors and tumor like lesions: Neuroepithelial lesions of the ocular globe and optic nerve. Radiographics 2007;27:1159 [PMID: 17620473].

Gillespie MB et al: Pediatric rhabdomyosarcoma of the head and neck. Curr Treat Options Oncol 2006;7:13 [PMID: 16343365].

Schwartz SR et al: Risk factors for amblyopia in children with capillary hemangiomas of the eyelids and orbit. J AAPOS 2006;10:262 [PMID: 16814181].

NYSTAGMUS

Nystagmus is a rhythmic oscillation or jiggling of the eyes. It may be unilateral or bilateral, more pronounced in one eye, or gaze-dependent.

Nystagmus may be associated with esotropia or may occur with ocular lesions that cause deprivation amblyopia (eg, cataract and eyelid ptosis) or conditions in which the visual pathways are hypoplastic, sometimes referred to as "sensory nystagmus." Nystagmus is seen with optic nerve hypoplasia, macular hypoplasia, aniridia, and albinism. Nystagmus can also occur with normal ocular structures and seemingly normal CNS development, sometimes referred to as "motor nystagmus." In the latter instance, the nystagmus may be blocked in certain positions of gaze, in which case a face turn or torticollis may develop. Latent nystagmus occurs when one eye is occluded. This type of nystagmus occurs in patients with congenital esotropia. An associated amblyopia may be present.

Most nystagmus occurring in childhood is of ocular origin, but CNS disease and, less frequently, inner ear disease are other causes. A CNS cause is likely when the nystagmus is acquired. Patients should be referred to an ophthalmologist when nystagmus is observed.

▶ Clinical Findings

Evaluation of nystagmus begins with the pediatric ophthalmologist. Careful evaluation for iris transillumination defects caused by albinism should be performed.

An electroretinogram is usually required to rule out retinal pathology as the cause. Some types of nystagmus, usually motor nystagmus, can be treated, generally with surgery; less frequently, prisms are useful. Spasmus nutans, in which a rapid, shimmering, dysconjugate nystagmus occurs with head bobbing and torticollis, usually improves with time. Glioma of the hypothalamus can mimic spasmus nutans. Neuroimaging may be necessary to determine if the cause of the nystagmus is due to a CNS disease.

▶ Treatment

Therapy is directed at managing the underlying ocular or CNS disease. An ophthalmologist can optimize vision by correcting significant refractive errors and strabismus. The range of vision varies depending on the cause of the nystagmus.

▼ AMBLYOPIA & STRABISMUS

Visual development is a learned function. For it to proceed normally, a child must experience a normal visual environment with well-aligned eyes that are free of vision-threatening disease and significant refractive errors. The consequences of not meeting these requirements during the sensitive period of visual development in the first decade of life are strabismus and decreased vision, or amblyopia.

AMBLYOPIA

Amblyopia is a unilateral or bilateral reduction in central visual acuity due to the sensory deprivation of a well-formed retinal image that occurs with or without a visible organic lesion commensurate with the degree of visual loss. Amblyopia can occur only during the critical period of visual development in the first decade of life when the visual nervous system is plastic. Approximately 3% of the population is amblyopic.

Amblyopia is classified according to its cause. Strabismic amblyopia can occur in the nondominant eye of a strabismic child. Refractive amblyopia can occur in both eyes if significant refractive errors are untreated (ametropic or refractive amblyopia). Another type of refractive amblyopia can occur in the eye with the worse refractive error when imbalance is present between the eyes (anisometropic amblyopia). Deprivation amblyopia occurs when dense cataracts or complete ptosis prevents formation of a formed retinal image. Of the three types of amblyopia, the deprivation form of amblyopia results in the worst vision.

▶ Clinical Findings

Screening for amblyopia should be a component of periodic well-child examinations. The single best screening technique to discover amblyopia is obtaining visual acuity in each eye. In preverbal children unable to respond to visual acuity assessment, amblyogenic factors are sought, including strabismus, media opacities, unequal Brückner reflexes (pupillary red reflexes), and a family history suggestive of strabismus, amblyopia, or ocular disease occurring in childhood (see earlier section on Ophthalmic Examination).

▶ Treatment

The earlier treatment is begun, the better will be the chance of improving visual acuity. Treatment is usually discontinued after age 9 years. Amblyogenic factors such as refractive errors are addressed. Because of the extreme sensitivity of the visual nervous system in infants, congenital cataracts and media opacities must be diagnosed and treated within the first few weeks of life. Visual rehabilitation and amblyopia treatment must then be started to foster visual development.

After eradicating amblyogenic factors, the mainstay of treatment is patching the sound eye, which causes the visual nervous system to process input from the amblyopic eye and in that way permits the development of useful vision. Other treatment modalities include "fogging" the sound eye with cycloplegic drops (atropine), lenses, and filters.

Doshi NR, Rodriguez ML: Amblyopia. Am Fam Physician 2007;75:361 [PMID: 17304867].
Wu C, Hunter DG: Amblyopia: Diagnostic and therapeutic options. Am J Ophthalmol 2006;141:175 [PMID: 16386994].

STRABISMUS

▶ General Considerations

Strabismus is misalignment of the visual axes of the two eyes. Its prevalence in childhood is about 2–3%. Strabismus is categorized by the direction of the deviation and its frequency. Early diagnosis of strabismus and amblyopia, which often coexist, provides the best chance of reaching full visual potential. Strabismus may cause or be due to amblyopia.

An infant whose eyes are destined to be well aligned may appear intermittently esotropic, but this should occur less frequently over the first few months of life. By age 5 or 6 months, the eyes should be constantly well aligned.

Besides its effect on visual development, strabismus may be a marker of other ocular or systemic disease. Twenty percent of patients with retinoblastoma exhibit strabismus. Patients with CNS disorders such as hydrocephalus, space-occupying lesions, and an amaurotic (blind) eye can also exhibit strabismus. In children younger than age 3 or 4 years, blind eyes tend to assume a position of esodeviation, but after about age 4 years an amaurotic eye tends to show an exotropic shift.

Misdiagnosis of strabismus when the eyes are well-aligned—pseudostrabismus—can occur when relying on the gross observation of the appearance of the two eyes. If the child has prominent epicanthal folds, pseudoesotropia may be diagnosed erroneously. Observation of the reflection of a penlight on the cornea, the corneal light reflex, is a more accurate means of determining if the eyes are straight. If strabismus is present, the corneal light reflex will not be centered in both eyes. Observation of eye movements may reveal restriction of eye movements in certain positions of gaze.

1. Esotropia

▶ Pathogenesis & Clinical Findings

In esotropia the eyes cross. Congenital esotropia (infantile esotropia) has its onset in the first year of life in healthy infants. The deviation is large and obvious. Esotropia beginning in the first year also occurs in premature infants or in children with a complicated perinatal history associated with CNS problems such as intracranial hemorrhage and periventricular leukomalacia. The most frequent type of acquired esotropia is the accommodative type (Figure 15–26). Onset is usually between ages 2 and 5 years. The deviation is variable in magnitude and constancy and is often accompanied by amblyopia. One type of accommodative esotropia is associated with a high hyperopic refraction. In another type,

▲ **Figure 15–26.** Accommodative esotropia. Without glasses, esotropic (**A**). With glasses, well-aligned at distance (**B**), and at near with bifocal correction (**C**).

the deviation is worse with near than with distant vision. This type of esodeviation is usually associated with lower refractive errors.

Esotropia is associated with certain syndromes. In Möbius syndrome (congenital facial diplegia), a sixth nerve palsy causing esotropia is associated with palsies of the seventh and 12th cranial nerves and limb deformities. Duane syndrome can affect the medial or lateral rectus muscles (or both). It may be an isolated defect or may be associated with a multitude of systemic defects (eg, Goldenhar syndrome). Duane syndrome is often misdiagnosed as a sixth (abducens) nerve palsy. The left eye is involved more commonly than the right, but both eyes can be involved. Girls are affected more frequently than boys. Children with unilateral paretic or restrictive causes of esotropia may develop face turns toward the affected eye to maintain binocularity.

After age 5 years, any esotropia of recent onset should arouse suspicion of CNS disease. Infratentorial masses, hydrocephalus, demyelinating diseases, and idiopathic intracranial hypertension are causes of abducens palsy, which appears as an esotropia, lateral rectus paralysis or paresis, and face turn. The face turn is an attempt to maintain binocularity away from the field of action of the paretic muscle. Papilledema is often, but not invariably, present with increased intracranial pressure. Besides the vulnerability of the abducens nerve to increased intracranial pressure, it is susceptible to infection and inflammation. Otitis media and Gradenigo syndrome (inflammatory disease of the petrous bone) can cause sixth nerve palsy. Less commonly, migraine and diabetes mellitus are considerations in children with sixth nerve palsy.

Evaluation of esotropia requires examination by an ophthalmologist. Motility, cycloplegic refraction and a dilated funduscopic examination are necessary to determine the etiology of esotropia. Some children require imaging studies and neurologic consultation.

▶ Treatment

Surgery is the mainstay of treatment for congenital esotropia. Controversy exists as to how young the child should be when surgery is performed so that the child can obtain an optimal binocular result. The age range is from younger than 6 months to 2 years.

Management of accommodative esotropia includes glasses with or without bifocals, amblyopia treatment, and in some cases surgery.

Underlying neurologic disease should be referred to the appropriate specialists for further management.

2. Exotropia

▶ Pathogenesis & Clinical Findings

Exotropia is a type of strabismus in which the eyes are divergent. The patient appears wall-eyed with the visual axes of the eyes deviated in a divergent position (Figure 15–27).

▲ **Figure 15–27.** Exotropia. **A:** Fixation with left eye. **B:** Fixation with right eye.

The deviation most often begins intermittently and occurs after age 2 years. Congenital (infantile) exotropia is extremely rare in an otherwise healthy infant. Early-onset exotropia may occur in infants and children with severe neurologic problems.

Evaluation of the corneal light reflex reveals nasal decentration of the penlight's reflection in the deviated eye. All children with constant, congenital exotropia require CNS neuroimaging. Referral to an ophthalmologist is indicated.

▶ Treatment

Treatment of exotropia is with surgery, orthoptic exercises, patching, and occasionally glasses.

Archer SM et al: Social and emotional impact of strabismus surgery on quality of life in children. J AAPOS 2005;9:148 [PMID: 15838442].
Donahue SP: Clinical practice. Pediatric strabismus. N Engl J Med 2007;356:1040 [PMID: 17347457].

UNEXPLAINED DECREASED VISION IN INFANTS & CHILDREN

Some infants with delayed visual development during the first few months of life who are otherwise normal neurologically will reach an appropriate level of visual maturation.

Occult causes of poor vision and blindness in children are those for which there are no obvious ocular defects: they include Leber congenital amaurosis, a childhood form of retinitis pigmentosa; achromatopsia, the absence of functioning cones in the retina; and optic nerve abnormalities, including optic nerve hypoplasia and atrophy.

Cerebral visual impairment, also known as cortical blindness, is manifested as decreased visual attentiveness of varying degree. Cerebral visual impairment can be congenital or acquired. Insults to the optic pathways and higher cortical visual centers are responsible. Asphyxia, trauma, intracranial hemorrhage, and periventricular leukomalacia are some of the causes of cortical visual impairment.

Besides an ophthalmologic workup, electroretinogram and visual evoked response testing may be required in children with decreased vision of unexplained etiology. Imaging studies of the brain and a pediatric neurologic evaluation may be useful.

▶ Treatment

A low-vision assessment may be indicated. Low-vision aids enhance remaining vision. Devices used include magnifiers for both distance and near vision, closed-circuit television, and large-print reading materials.

▼ THE BLIND CHILD

A child's development is affected profoundly by blindness or low vision. There are psychological consequences for the child blind from birth, as well as for the family. It can be devastating to a young family to find out that their newborn is blind. Although acquired blindness may give an individual time to grow as a sighted person and make preparations for life as a nonsighted person if loss of vision is slow and predicted, psychological consequences for the child and family must be addressed.

The child who is blind from birth or from very early childhood has had little or no opportunity to form visual impressions of the physical world. Blind infants reach developmental landmarks on a different schedule from that of sighted children. In addition, some blind children are multiply handicapped. For example, the premature child who is blind from retinopathy of prematurity may also have cerebral palsy. Children with Usher syndrome become both deaf and blind.

Leading causes of blindness in the pediatric age group differ among regions of the world and between industrialized nations and developing countries. The most common causes of blindness in the pediatric age group are thought to be cerebral visual impairment, retinopathy of prematurity, and optic nerve hypoplasia. Albinism, optic atrophy, cataract, retinitis pigmentosa, microphthalmia or anophthalmia, aniridia, and glaucoma are other diseases causing blindness.

▶ Clinical Findings

Children with low vision will not fixate on visual targets and often have roving eye movements. Ophthalmic referral is necessary to determine if the etiology of the low vision is due to an ocular or neurologic disorder. Neuroimaging or specific ocular tests such as an electroretinogram may be necessary.

▶ Treatment

Blind children and their families should receive the benefit of knowledgeable therapists and support groups.

Edmond JC, Foroozan R: Cortical visual impairment in children. Curr Opin Ophthalmol 2006;17:509 [PMID: 17065917].

▼ LEARNING DISABILITIES & DYSLEXIA

Visits to the physician because of educational difficulties are common. Children often have vague complaints of ocular fatigue, headaches, and difficulty reading. Learning disabilities and dyslexia result in poor reading comprehension and writing.

Evaluation of the child with learning disabilities and dyslexia should include ophthalmologic examination to identify any ocular disorders that could cause or contribute to poor school performance. Most children with learning difficulties have no demonstrable problems on ophthalmic examination.

▶ Treatment

A multidisciplinary approach as suggested by the American Academy of Pediatrics, the American Association for Pediatric Ophthalmology and Strabismus, and the American Academy of Ophthalmology is recommended in evaluating children with learning disabilities. Although many therapies directed at "training the eyes" exist, scientific support for such approaches is weak.

Hamilton SS, Glascoe FP: Evaluation of children with reading difficulties. Am Fam Physician 2006;74:2079 [PMID: 17186715].
Smith LA et al: Developmental differences in understanding the causes, controllability and chronicity of disabilities. Child Care Health Dev 2005;31:479 [PMID: 15948885].

Web Resources

American Academy of Ophthalmology: http://www.aao.org
American Association of Pediatric Ophthalmology and Strabismus: http://www.aapos.org

Oral Medicine & Dentistry

Ulrich Klein, DMD, DDS, MS

ISSUES IN PEDIATRIC ORAL HEALTH

Concept of the Dental Home

Analogous to the American Academy of Pediatrics' (AAP) concept of a "medical home," the American Academy of Pediatric Dentistry (AAPD) supports the concept of a "dental home." This refers to a specialized primary dental care provider within the philosophical complex of the medical home and includes all aspects of oral health, involving interaction among the patient, parents, and dental and nondental professionals. A dental home is established by referring a child for an oral health examination to a dentist who provides care for infants and young children (ie, pediatric dentist) 6 months after the first tooth erupts or by 12 months of age. The intent is to implement preventive dental health habits with the goal of keeping the child free from dental and oral disease. Expectations include development of an individualized preventive health program derived from an accurate risk assessment for dental disease, anticipatory guidance about growth and development, education about proper nutrition, provision of comprehensive dental care, and referral to other dental specialists as needed.

Infant Oral Health Care

Infant oral health care is the foundation on which preventive education and dental care is built. Ideally, it begins before caries develop when preventive measures can be implemented to give the child an opportunity to grow up free from preventable oral disease. Oral evaluation of a child consists of risk assessment, anticipatory guidance, and health supervision. This approach advances dental care beyond tooth monitoring toward true health promotion. Risk assessment determines a child's risk of developing oral disease. Anticipatory guidance is proactive counseling of the parents directed toward enlisting them as allies in preventing oral health problems. Because pediatricians are far more likely to encounter new mothers and infants than are dentists, it is

essential that they be aware of the infectious pathophysiology and risk factors for early childhood caries in order to guide and intervene effectively. The most important risk factor for childhood oral disease is poverty.

The primary goals for an infant oral health program are (1) to establish with parents the goals of oral health, (2) to inform parents of their role in reaching these goals, (3) to motivate parents to learn and practice good preventive dental care, and (4) to initiate a long-term dental care relationship with parents. Such an alliance is necessary to prevent early childhood caries by preventing acquisition of harmful oral bacteria, modifying "nonnutritive sucking habits" before they become deleterious, and implementing optimal fluoride protection. Pediatricians should incorporate oral health into anticipatory guidance by providing information in their offices or by referring the child to a pediatric dental colleague.

Oral Health Risk Assessment

By 6 months of age, every child should have an oral health risk assessment by a pediatric health care provider. The Caries Risk Assessment Tool developed by the AAPD is an important component of later clinical decision making. Because the etiology of caries is multifactorial, risk assessment evaluates several contributing factors such as diet, host susceptibility, presence of aciduric oral microflora, and cultural and behavioral factors. Although the best predictor of future caries is previous caries incidence, this finding is not a practical preventative tool. Other risk factors include parental education, socioeconomic status, and age of colonization with *Streptococcus mutans* and *Lactobacillus* spp (the earlier colonization occurs, the greater the risk of severe decay). Indicators that place a patient automatically into the high-risk group are special health care needs, high maternal caries rate, nighttime breast or bottle feeding, and low socioeconomic status. High-risk individuals should be referred to a dentist as early as 6 months of age and no later than 6 months after the first tooth erupts or 12 months of age (whichever comes first) for establishment of a dental home.

Early Childhood Caries

Formerly termed "baby bottle tooth decay" or "nursing bottle caries," early childhood caries (ECC) is a particularly aggressive and rapidly progressing form of caries that begins on the smooth surfaces soon after tooth eruption. The main cause is the frequent consumption of liquids containing fermentable carbohydrates through a nursing bottle or frequent sipping from a no-spill sippy cup. Children who take a bottle to bed and those who nurse at will and fall asleep nursing are at high risk for ECC. ECC typically involves the maxillary incisors but any other teeth may be affected. When a child sucks a bottle while supine, milk pools between the backs of the front teeth and the tongue. Acid produced in this stagnant area by oral bacteria cannot dissipate, and damage to the teeth occurs.

ECC is defined as one or more decayed (d), missing (m), or filled (f) tooth surfaces (s) in any primary tooth in a child younger than 71 months of age. Any sign of smooth-surface caries in a child younger than 3 years is termed *severe ECC* (S-ECC). From 3–5 years, one or more decayed, missing, or filled smooth surfaces in maxillary front teeth or a total dmfs score of 4 or higher must be present to make a diagnosis of S-ECC. By age 5 years, a dmfs score of 6 of higher must be present to constitute S-ECC. Children with S-ECC are at higher risk for new carious lesions, more frequent hospitalizations, and emergency department visits. They are absent more often from school, may have below-normal height and weight gain, and have a diminished oral health-related quality of life. Although S-ECC can affect all children, it is 32 times more likely in children who consume sugary foods and whose mothers are of low socioeconomic status and education level.

Parents should be counseled not to put infants to sleep with a bottle containing fermentable carbohydrates. After eruption of the first tooth, ad libitum breast feeding should be discontinued and regular oral hygiene measures implemented. Infants should be weaned from the bottle at about 1 year and encouraged to drink from a cup. Frequent consumption of cariogenic liquids from a bottle or no-spill training cup should be avoided.

ORAL EXAMINATION OF THE NEWBORN & INFANT

The mouth of the normal newborn is lined with an intact, smooth, moist, shiny mucosa (Figure 16–1). The alveolar ridges are continuous and relatively smooth. Within the alveolar bone are numerous tooth buds, which at birth are mostly primary teeth.

Teeth

Hard tissue formation of primary teeth begins at approximately 4 months' gestation. At birth, all 20 primary teeth are

▲ **Figure 16–1.** Normal anatomy of the newborn mouth.

calcified. The central maxillary incisors are almost completely calcified while only the cusp tips of the maxillary and mandibular second molars are calcified. There is a trace of enamel on the first four permanent molars at birth.

The primary teeth usually begin to erupt at 6–7 months of age. On rare occasions (1:3000), natal teeth are present at birth or neonatal teeth erupt within the first month. These are most commonly (85%) mandibular primary incisors. They can be "real" primary teeth (90%) or supernumerary teeth (10%) and should be differentiated radiographically. Although the preferred approach is to leave the tooth in place, supernumerary and hypermobile immature primary teeth should be extracted. On occasion, such teeth must be smoothed or removed if their sharp incisal edge causes laceration of the tongue (Riga-Fede disease). If such teeth cause difficulties with breast feeding, pumping and bottling the milk is initially recommended while the infant is conditioned not to "bite" during suckling.

Frena

Noticeable but small maxillary and mandibular labial frena should be present (Figure 16–2). Several small accessory frena may also be present farther posteriorly. In rare cases, as in oro-facial-digital syndrome, there are multiple thick tightly bound frena. Decisions about surgical correction should be based on the ability to maintain the child's gingival health and are best left until the late preteen years. Many thick frena do not require correction.

The tongue is connected to the floor of the mouth by the lingual frenum (Figures 16–1 and 16–3). This connection should not impede the free movement of the tongue. If the

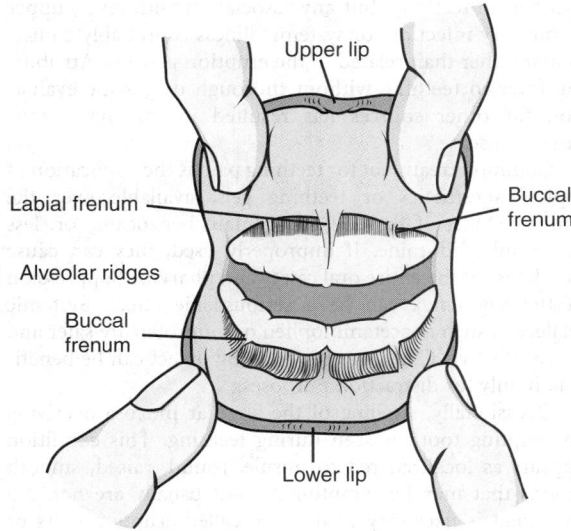

▲ **Figure 16–2.** The frena.

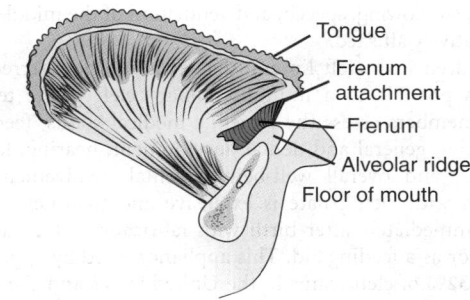

▲ **Figure 16–4.** Ankyloglossia (tongue-tie).

attachment is tight and high up on the alveolar ridge (Figure 16–4), it may restrict movement and interfere with the child's ability to produce "t," "d," and "l" sounds. This condition is called ankyloglossia (tongue-tie). Surgical correction may be indicated if the tongue cannot touch the maxillary incisors or the roof of the mouth. Earlier intervention (at age 3–4 years) is better than later, but there is usually no urgency for surgery in the neonatal period.

Cleft Lip & Palate

The palate of the newborn should be intact and continuous from the alveolar ridge anteriorly to the uvula (see Figure 16–1). Cleft lip and palate are common defects with an incidence of 0.28–3.74 in 1000 live births globally. Incidence varies widely among races and ranges from 1 in 500 among Navaho Native Americans and Japanese to more than 1 in 800 in whites and 1 in 2000 in blacks. The cleft of the palate can be

unilateral or bilateral (Figure 16–5). It can involve only the alveolar ridge, or the ridge and entire palate. Cleft palate may also present as an isolated submucous cleft, which may be detected by passing a finger posteriorly along the midline of the palate. Normally the posterior nasal spine is detectable, but if a submucous cleft is present, a bony notch will be found. Affected children sometimes have a bifid uvula. Although clefts present superficially as a cosmetic problem, they cause complex functional problems such as oro-antral communication and disruption of the maxillary alveolar ridge with a large number of associated dental problems. They disturb the muscle arrangement of the perioral and the soft palate muscles by interrupting their continuity across the midline. As a result,

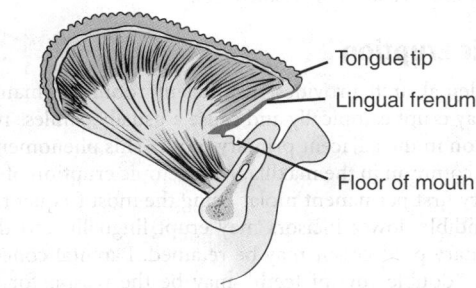

▲ **Figure 16–3.** Normal position of lingual frenum.

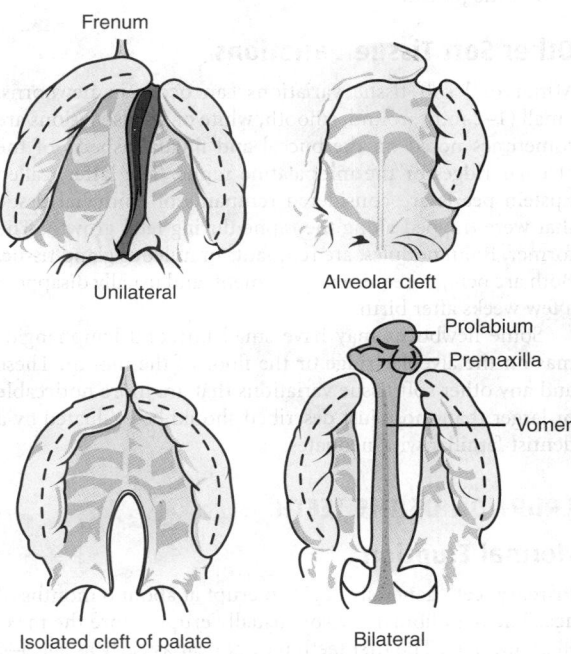

▲ **Figure 16–5.** Types of clefts.

feeding, swallowing, speech, and ventilation of the middle ear are negatively affected.

Children with cleft lip and palate should be referred as soon as possible to a multidisciplinary cleft palate team. Team members assess the patient's medical status, feeding difficulties, general and dental development, hearing, facial esthetics, and overall well-being. Dental involvement in children with cleft palate is extensive and treatment may begin immediately after birth with fabrication of a palatal obturator as a feeding aid. This appliance, used by approximately 32% of cleft teams in the United States and Canada, may also provide cross-arch stability after surgical closure of the lip and maxillary orthopedic molding before primary alveolar cleft bone grafting. Nasoalveolar molding can be used to guide the protruding premaxilla back into the oral cavity, thus making surgical lip closure easier when it is performed (usually by 10 weeks of age). However, opinions on its effectiveness, potential growth disturbances, and additional costs differ among surgeons. Palate closure to facilitate the acquisition of normal speech without nasality follows at 12–18 months of age. The associated scar formation causes significant dentofacial growth disturbance. Orthodontic treatment addresses the sagittal and transverse maxillary growth deficits as well as irregularities in tooth eruption and position. Between 7 and 10 years of age, an alveolar bone graft is often necessary to promote proper eruption of the permanent teeth adjacent to the cleft. In some patients, a combined orthodontic-surgical repositioning of the permanent dentition is needed to complete a successful rehabilitation of the patient.

Other Soft Tissue Variations

Minor oral soft tissue variations can occur in newborns. Small (1–2 mm), round, smooth, white or grayish lesions are sometimes noted on the buccal and lingual aspects of the alveolar ridges or the midpalatine raphe. The latter, called Epstein pearls are considered remnants of epithelial tissue that were trapped along the raphe during fetal growth. The former, Bohn nodules, are remnants of mucous gland tissue. Both are benign, require no treatment, and usually disappear a few weeks after birth.

Some newborns may have small intraoral lymphangiomas on the alveolar ridge or the floor of the mouth. These and any other soft tissue variations that are more noticeable or larger than those just described should be evaluated by a dentist familiar with neonates.

ERUPTION OF THE TEETH

Normal Eruption

Primary teeth generally begin to erupt at about 6 months of age. The mandibular incisors usually erupt before the maxillary incisors. The first teeth may appear as early as age 3–4 months or as late as age 12–16 months. Many symptoms are ascribed to teething, but any association with fever, upper respiratory infection, or systemic illness is probably coincidental rather than related to the eruption process. Attributing fever to teething without thorough diagnostic evaluation for other sources has resulted in missing serious organic disease.

Common treatment for teething pain is the application of topical anesthetics or teething gels, available over the counter. Most of these agents contain benzocaine or, less commonly, lidocaine. If improperly used, they can cause numbness of the entire oral cavity and pharynx. Suppression of the gag reflex can be a serious side effect. Systemic analgesics such as acetaminophen or ibuprofen are safer and more effective. Chewing on a teething object can be beneficial, if only for distraction purposes.

Occasionally, swelling of the alveolar mucosa overlying an erupting tooth is seen during teething. This condition appears as localized red to purple, round, raised, smooth lesions that may be symptomatic but usually are not. No treatment is necessary as these so-called eruption cysts or eruption hematomas resolve with tooth eruption.

Delayed Eruption

Premature loss of a primary tooth can either accelerate or delay eruption of the underlying secondary tooth. Early eruption occurs when the permanent tooth is beginning its active eruption and the overlying primary tooth is removed. This generally occurs when the primary tooth is lost within 1 year of its normal exfoliation. If loss of the primary tooth occurs more than 1 year before expected exfoliation, the permanent tooth will probably be delayed in eruption owing to healing that results in filling in of bone and gingiva over the permanent tooth. The loss of a primary tooth may cause adjacent teeth to tip into the space and lead to impaction of the underlying permanent tooth. A space maintainer should be placed by a dentist to avoid impaction.

Other local factors delaying or preventing eruption include supernumerary teeth, cysts, tumors, overretained primary teeth, ankylosed primary teeth, and impaction. A generalized delay in eruption may be associated with global developmental delays, endocrinopathies (hypothyroidism or hypopituitarism), or other systemic conditions (cleidocranial dysplasia, rickets, or trisomy 21).

Ectopic Eruption

If the dental arch provides insufficient room, permanent teeth may erupt ectopically and cause a usually painless root resorption in the adjacent primary tooth. This phenomenon is more common in the maxilla, with ectopic eruption of the maxillary first permanent molar being the most frequent. In the mandible, lower incisors may erupt lingually and thus the primary predecessor may be retained. Parental concern about a "double row of teeth" may be the reason for the child's first dental visit. If the primary teeth are not loose, they should be removed by the dentist to allow their successors to drift into proper position.

Impaction

Impaction occurs when a permanent tooth is prevented from erupting. Although crowding is the most frequent reason, overretained primary or supernumerary teeth are other causes. The teeth most often affected in the developing dentition are the maxillary canines. Generally, they are brought into correct alignment through surgical exposure and orthodontic treatment.

Variations in Tooth Number

Failure of teeth to develop—a condition called hypodontia—is rare in the primary dentition. However, it occurs about 5% of the time in the permanent dentition. The most frequently missing teeth are the third molars followed by the lateral maxillary incisors and mandibular second premolars. Oligodontia, a condition in which only a few teeth develop, occurs in patients with ectodermal dysplasias. Partial dentures should be considered as early as 3 years of age to improve the patient's ability to chew.

Occasionally, supernumerary teeth are present, most typically in the maxillary incisor area, distal to the maxillary molars, or in the mandibular bicuspid region. Mesiodentes are peg-shaped supernumerary teeth situated at the maxillary midline that occur in about 5% of individuals. If they hinder eruption of adjacent permanent incisors, their timely removal is recommended.

DENTAL CARIES

▶ General Considerations

Dental caries is biofilm-mediated acid demineralization of dental enamel or dentin. It is the most common chronic childhood disease and the most prevalent unmet health need of U.S. children. Caries is largely a disease of poverty; the 29 million children and adolescents in low-income families account for 80% of patients with tooth decay.

▶ Pathogenesis

Development of caries requires the interaction of four factors: (1) a host (tooth in the oral environment), (2) a suitable dietary substrate (fermentable carbohydrates), (3) cariogenic microorganisms that can adhere to the tooth, and (4) time, measured as the frequency of exposure to fermentable carbohydrates and the duration of the acid attack. Demineralization of the dental enamel occurs below a pH of 5.5, therefore flow and buffering capacity of saliva is an important modifier.

The main bacteria implicated in the initiation of caries are *Streptococcus mutans* and *S sobrinus*; *Lactobacillus acidophilus* and *L casei* are linked to progression of caries. *S mutans* is most commonly transmitted from mother to child. A "window of infectivity" between 19 and 33 months of age has been described, but colonization can occur as early as 3 months of age. Earlier colonization increases the risk of caries. The greatest impact physicians can have on this disease is through early referral of high-risk children to dental practitioners.

Dental plaque is an adherent film on the tooth surface that harbors bacteria in close proximity to the tooth enamel. As the bacteria metabolize sucrose, they produce lactic acid. The acidic environment causes the enamel of the teeth to decalcify. This is the first step in production of caries. After the carious process has penetrated the enamel, it advances through the dentin towards the pulp of the tooth. In response, blood vessels in the pulp dilate and inflammatory cells begin to infiltrate (pulpitis). If the carious lesion is left untreated, a frank pulp exposure will occur, triggering invasion of more inflammatory cells and the eventual formation of a small abscess in the pulp. If the abscess can drain into the oral cavity, the apical tooth tissue may remain vital. However, if the radical pulp becomes necrotic, a periapical abscess develops (Figure 16–6). Although this process is not always symptomatic, it often leads to severe pain, fever, and swelling.

▶ Clinical Findings & Treatment

The diagnosis of caries is usually made by a visual-tactile oral examination using a dental explorer supplemented by radiographs. Radiographs are used to visualize caries on the surfaces between teeth that cannot be reached with the dental explorer. The earliest sign of caries is a white spot lesion—a white, chalky, decalcified area along the gingival margin or on approximated tooth surfaces. Frank carious lesions are light to dark brown spots or cavities of varying size on a tooth. A lighter shade of brown indicates more rampant decay, whereas arrested caries are almost black in

▲ **Figure 16–6.** Tooth anatomy and progression of caries.

color. In the early stages of decay, the tooth may be sensitive to temperature changes or sweets. At this point, the tooth can be repaired by removing the carious tooth structure and filling the defect with a restorative material. As decay progresses deeper into the pulp pain increases as more of the still-vital pulp becomes necrotic. Once the entire pulp is necrotic and nonvital, a choice must be made between root canal therapy (pulpectomy) or removal of the tooth. In the presence of cellulitis or facial space abscess, extraction with antibiotic therapy is the treatment of choice.

Because cavitation is a late stage of the disease, filling cavities does nothing to address the underlying pathologic process. Unlike other infections, dental caries cannot be treated by a simple course of antibiotics. The disease can only be cured through treatment of the pervasive oral infection, a sustained reduction in the number of cariogenic bacteria, and the creation of a favorable oral environment. To achieve this, a patient's (and ideally a family's) diet must be changed to avoid the frequent intake of fermentable carbohydrates in solid and liquid form. All active cavities must be restored to eliminate sources of reinfection and meticulous oral hygiene practices embraced to prevent plaque buildup and reduce the number of bacteria. Regular dental visits must be maintained to monitor and reinforce good oral health practices. The concept of prevention through timely parent education, early diagnosis, and prompt intervention offers greater efficiency, better health outcomes, and lower costs than repeated restoration of diseased teeth.

▶ Caries Prevention

To prevent dental caries, it is necessary to remove plaque and its resident cariogenic bacteria on a regular basis.

A. Oral Hygiene

Oral hygiene should start at birth. The gums can be cleaned gently with a moist, soft cloth. Once the teeth begin to erupt, oral hygiene must be practiced in earnest. A small, soft toothbrush designed for infants should be used. Toothpaste is not necessary but should be added by age 2 years. Prior to age 8 years parents need to be involved daily in brushing and flossing. Brushing with fluoride-containing toothpaste at least twice daily and regular flossing will help to reduce the count of cariogenic bacteria in the oral flora. A second step is to decrease the amount of substrate available to the bacteria. Limiting the frequent ingestion of refined carbohydrates is most effective because each exposure produces an acidic environment for up to 30 minutes. This explains the particularly deleterious effects of frequent consumption of sugar-containing juices, sodas, and infant formulas through a nursing bottle. The primary care physician plays an invaluable role in disseminating this information and reinforcing these ideas.

Children with special health care needs require dental advice and care more frequently. Children with serious medi-cal problems or disabilities should be referred to a pediatric dentist as early as possible, usually before 1 year of age.

B. Fluoride

Fluorides are safe and effective for caries control and prevention. Fluoride can be applied professionally or by the patient under supervision. Although more than half the U.S. population has access to fluoridated community water, an increasing number of families consume processed water with unknown fluoride content. The cariostatic mechanisms of fluoride include increased resistance to demineralization, enhanced remineralization, and inhibition of bacterial colonization of dental plaque. Fluoride affects the dentin and enamel of both erupted and unerupted teeth. Systemic effects are achieved by oral ingestion from sources such as fluoridated drinking water or fluoride supplements. Fluoridated toothpaste and mouth rinses deliver topical benefits. Table 16–1 shows the current AAP and AAPD recommendations for dietary fluoride supplementation in children drinking fluoride deficient water. The patient's true exposure to fluoride must be judiciously evaluated before supplements are prescribed to avoid dental fluorosis. Because children younger than 6 years of age cannot expectorate reliably, the use of fluoridated toothpaste must be monitored by their parents and the recommendation to use only a "pea-sized" amount of toothpaste should be followed. Higher risk individuals with orthodontic appliances, reduced salivary function, or gastroesophageal reflux disease, or those who are unable to clean their teeth properly, are at dietary risk, have mothers or siblings with caries, or have active caries should be considered for additional topical fluoride therapy to supplement oral hygiene measures.

PERIODONTAL DISEASE

Periodontal disease involves a tooth's supporting structures: bone, gingiva, and periodontal ligaments (Figure 16–7). It begins as inflammation of the gingival tissue adjacent to a tooth. Bacterial accumulation in the gingival sulcus causes irritation and inflammation. This beginning phase is called dental plaque–induced gingivitis, and it is found almost universally in children and adolescents. Alterations in hormone

Table 16–1. Dietary fluoride supplementation schedule.

Age	Concentration of Fluoride in Water		
	< 0.3 ppm F	0.3–0.6 ppm F	> 0.6 ppm F
Birth–6 mo	0	0	0
6 mo–3 y	0.25 mg	0	0
3–6 y	0.50 mg	0.25 mg	0
6–at least 16 y	1.00 mg	0.50 mg	0

▲ **Figure 16–7.** Periodontal disease.

Plaque accumulation (gingivitis)

Loss of attachment

Destruction of bone (periodontitis)

levels (insulin, gonadotropin) can intensify the inflammatory response to plaque. Generally, this condition responds well to removal of bacterial deposits and improved oral hygiene.

Periodontitis is characterized by loss of attachment and destruction of bone. Patients with localized aggressive periodontitis typically have severe alveolar bone loss around permanent first molars and incisors, whereas the generalized form involves other teeth as well. The prevalence is 0.2% in Caucasians, but much higher (2.5%) in African Americans. Familial aggregation and functional defects such as anomalies of neutrophil chemotaxis, phagocytosis, and bacterial activity increase the risk of periodontitis. *Actinobacillus actinomycetemcomitans* in combination with *Bacteroides*-like species are implicated in this disease. An association between maternal periodontal disease and preterm birth has been established. It is currently unclear whether this association involves causation or it is a marker for another etiology.

Treatment consists of combined surgical and nonsurgical root debridement plus antibiotic therapy. Isolated chronic periodontitis is rare in children and adolescents but may complicate conditions such as Papillon-Lefèvre and Down syndromes, cyclic neutropenia, hypophosphatasia, agranulocytosis, and leukocyte adherence defects.

The incidence of necrotizing periodontal disease is lower (1%) in North America than in developing countries (2–5%). Necrotizing periodontal disease is characterized by interproximal ulceration and necrosis of the dental papillae, rapid onset of dental pain, and often fever. Predisposing factors include viral infections (including HIV), malnutrition, emotional stress, and systemic disease. The condition usually responds rapidly to treatment consisting of mechanical debridement with ultrasonic scalers, improved oral hygiene, and metronidazole and penicillin for febrile patients.

OROFACIAL TRAUMA

Orofacial trauma often consists only of abrasions or lacerations of the lips, gingiva, tongue, or oral mucosa (including the frena), without damage to the teeth. Lacerations should be cleansed, inspected for foreign bodies, and sutured if necessary. Occasionally, radiographs of the tongue, lips, or cheeks are needed to detect tooth fragments or other foreign bodies. All patients with facial trauma should to be evaluated for jaw fractures. Blows to the chin are among the most

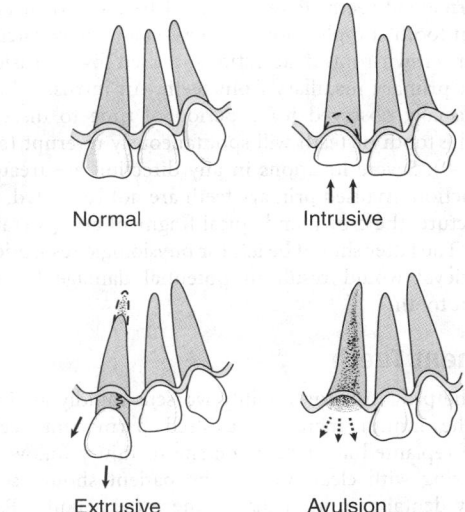

Normal   Intrusive

Extrusive   Avulsion

▲ **Figure 16–8.** Patterns of luxation injuries.

common childhood orofacial traumas. They are also a leading cause of condylar fracture in the pediatric population. Condylar fracture should be suspected if pain or deviation occurs when the jaw is opened.

Tooth-related trauma affects any or all of the dental hard tissues and the pulp, the alveolar process, and the periodontal tissues. The range of luxation injuries includes concussion; subluxation; intrusive, extrusive, and lateral luxation; and avulsion. Figure 16–8 demonstrates the different luxation injuries, and Figure 16–9 shows the different degrees of tooth fracture.

The least problematic luxation injuries are concussion (no mobility) and subluxation (mobility without displacement). Unless mobility is extensive, this condition can be followed without active intervention. Pulp vitality should be periodically assessed.

Primary Teeth

The peak age for injuries to primary teeth is toddlerhood. Any treatment must include measures to ensure the integrity

Enamel only (uncomplicated)

Exposed pulp (complicated)

Enamel and dentin (uncomplicated)

▲ **Figure 16–9.** Patterns of crown fractures.

of the permanent teeth. Parents should be advised of any permanent tooth complications such as enamel hypocalcifications or crown-root dilacerations caused by intrusion injuries of primary maxillary front teeth. An intrusive luxation is usually observed for a period of time to discern whether the tooth or teeth will spontaneously re-erupt (see Figure 16–8). Severe luxations in any direction are treated with extraction. Avulsed primary teeth are not replanted. In a root fracture, the crown and apical fragment are generally extracted. The latter should be left for physiologic resorption if its retrieval would result in potential damage to the permanent tooth.

Permanent Teeth

Because the prognosis for viability worsens rapidly as time outside the mouth increases, avulsed permanent teeth should be replanted at or near the site of injury following gentle rinsing with clean water. The patient should seek emergency dental care immediately thereafter. Hank's Balanced Salt Solution is the best storage and transport medium for avulsed teeth that are to be replanted. The next best storage media in decreasing order are milk, saline, saliva (buccal vestibule), or water. The commercially available Food and Drug Administration–approved Save-a-Tooth kit should be part of first-aid kits in schools and sports facilities (see references).

Intrusions of permanent teeth are corrected with surgical or orthodontic repositioning. Lateral and extrusive luxations are generally repositioned and splinted for a minimum of 3–4 weeks. Root canal treatment is necessary in the majority of injuries. Factors to consider during treatment planning are root development (open or closed apex) and the extent of the luxation. Pulp necrosis; surface, inflammatory, and replacement resorption; or ankylosis may occur at any time during the healing process and determine the long-term outcome. All luxated and replanted teeth need to be followed regularly by a dentist.

DENTAL EMERGENCIES

Dental emergencies other than trauma are usually associated with pain or swelling due to advanced caries. Odontogenic pain usually responds to acetaminophen or ibuprofen. Topical medications are of limited value.

A localized small swelling confined to the gingival tissue associated with a tooth is usually not an urgent situation. This "gumboil" or parulis represents infection that has spread outward from the root of the tooth through the bone and periosteum. Usually it will drain and leave a fistulous tract. Facial cellulitis results if the infection invades the facial spaces. Elevated temperature (> 38.8°C), difficulty swallowing, and difficulty breathing are signs of more serious infection. Swelling of the midface—especially the bridge of the nose and the lower eyelid—should be urgently evaluated as a potential dental infection. Extraction of teeth or root canal therapy

combined with antibiotics is the usual treatment. Hospitalization is a prudent choice for younger children with severe facial cellulitis especially if other risk factors are present—dehydration, airway compromise, or possible noncompliance. Inpatient treatment consists of intravenous antibiotics such as clindamycin or ampicillin-sulbactam (Unasyn) with incision, drainage, and removal of the source of infection.

ANTIBIOTICS IN PEDIATRIC DENTISTRY

The antibiotics of choice for odontogenic infection are clindamycin and penicillin. Several patient groups require prophylactic antibiotic coverage prior to invasive dental manipulation. These include children with artificial heart valves, previous infectious endocarditis, certain congenital heart conditions, immunodeficiency, or central venous catheters. Revised guidelines for infective endocarditis prophylaxis were published by the American Heart Association in April 2007.

SPECIAL PATIENT POPULATIONS

Children with Cancer

The most common source of systemic sepsis in the immunosuppressed patient with cancer is the oral cavity. Therefore, children with cancer should be evaluated by a dentist knowledgeable about pediatric oncology soon after diagnosis. The aim is to educate the patient and caregivers about the importance of good oral hygiene and to eliminate all existing and potential sources of infection before the child becomes neutropenic as a consequence of chemotherapy. Younger patients have more oral problems than adults. Sources of infection include abscessed teeth, extensive caries, teeth that will soon exfoliate, ragged or broken teeth, uneven fillings, and orthodontic appliances. After an initial evaluation and before the initiation of cancer therapy, a dental treatment plan should be developed in discussion with the medical team. Preventive strategies include reduction of refined sugars, fluoride therapy, lip care, and patient education. Chemotherapeutic drugs and local irradiation are cytotoxic to the oral mucosa, which becomes atrophic and develops mucositis. Oral pain may be severe and often leads to inadequate food and fluid intake, infections in the oral cavity, and an increased risk of septicemia. Meticulous oral hygiene reduces the risk of severe mucositis.

The pediatric oncology patient should be monitored throughout therapy to screen for infection, manage oral bleeding, and control oral pain. These patients can experience spontaneous oral hemorrhage, especially when the platelet count is less than 20,000/mL. Poor oral hygiene or areas of irritation can increase the chances of bleeding.

Children receiving radiation therapy to the head and neck may develop salivary dysfunction (xerostomia) if salivary glands are in the path of the beam of radiation. Xerostomia should be managed aggressively to avoid rapid and extensive destruction of the teeth. Customized fluoride applicators are used in this situation in combination with close follow-up.

Children receiving hematopoietic cell transplantation may require long periods of immunosuppression. During the neutropenic phase of pretransplant conditioning, mucositis, xerostomia, oral pain, oral bleeding, and opportunistic infections may occur. Oral graft-versus-host disease as well as oral fungal and herpes simplex virus infections can be seen during the subsequent initial engraftment and hematopoietic reconstitution period. Long-term dental follow-up includes management of salivary dysfunction and craniofacial growth abnormalities from total body radiation and treatment of oral graft-versus-host disease.

Pediatric oncology patients need regular care by a dentist familiar with young children and their growth and development. Oral and maxillofacial growth disturbances can occur after therapy. Late effects of therapy include such morphologic changes as microdontia, hypocalcification, short and blunted roots, delayed eruption, and alterations in facial bone growth.

Children with Hematologic Disorders

The child with hemophilia requires appropriate clotting factors before and after any invasive dental procedures, including local block anesthesia. Patients with factor VIII inhibitors who require oral surgical procedures should be admitted to a hospital. Some patients with very mild factor VIII deficiency or von Willebrand disease type 1 may respond to DDAVP (1-deamino-8-D-arginine vasopressin). Antifibrinolytic medications such as ε-aminocaproic and tranexamic acid are used successfully after dental treatment. Topical medications such as Gelfoam and thrombin can be used to control postoperative bleeding. Patients receiving anticoagulant therapy should generally not undergo dosage adjustment before surgical dental treatment because the risk of embolic complications is much higher than bleeding complications in those whose anticoagulant therapy is continued. However, the dentist is advised to consult with the hematologist to obtain the most recent INR (international normalized ratio) results and to discuss the most appropriate level of anticoagulation.

Children with Diabetes

Children who are insulin-dependent have significantly higher incidence of plaque, gingival inflammation, and attachment loss. They are, therefore, at high risk for periodontal disease. However, only those who are in poor metabolic control have an increased rate of caries. Care must be taken not to disturb the regular cycle of eating and insulin dosage. Anxiety associated with dental appointments can cause a major upset in the diabetic child's glycemic control. Postoperative pain or pain from dental abscess can prevent routine oral intake, necessitating adjustment of insulin doses.

MATERNAL-FETAL RELATIONSHIP

Childhood caries is an infectious disease transmitted by bacteria from the mother to the child. Infants whose mothers have high levels of S mutans are at greater risk for acquiring the organism. Dental treatment of their mothers or primary caregivers can delay or prevent the inoculation of the infant. A significant association between maternal periodontitis at 21–24 weeks' gestation and preterm birth has been reported. However, according to a more recent study, periodontal treatment of expectant mothers does not improve the incidence of preterm delivery or significantly improve birth weight. The risk of preterm birth is elevated if a mother smokes and is of low socioeconomic status, both of which also increase the risk for periodontitis. Secondhand or passive smoke increases the risk of caries in children. This association is independent of age, family income, geographic region, and frequency of dental visits. It is important to advise expectant mothers about these risk factors.

There is a higher risk of oral developmental anomalies in preterm and low birth weight infants than in full-term infants. These developmental anomalies include enamel hypoplasia of the primary dentition, crown dilaceration of the permanent maxillary incisors, and a narrow palate caused by laryngoscopy or prolonged endotracheal intubation. The role of palatal protection plates to prevent "grooving" remains unclear. It is difficult to distinguish delayed dental development of preterm infants from that associated with global developmental delays.

DENTAL & ORTHODONTIC REFERRAL

Orthodontic referral is usually made by the dentist. Early referral is indicated for any child with a craniofacial growth disorder. Other children may be referred at any time between ages 6 and 12 years, depending on their growth and oral development. Orthodontists differ about when to begin treatment. Many pediatric dentists provide early orthodontic management as a part of their practices.

REFERENCES

Print Resources

Andreasen JO et al: *Traumatic Dental Injuries,* 2nd ed. Blackwell Munksgaard, 2003.

Hale KJ; American Academy of Pediatrics Section on Pediatric Dentistry: Oral health risk assessment timing and establishment of the dental home. Pediatrics 2003;111:1113 [PMID: 1272810].

McDonald RE et al: *Dentistry for the Child and Adolescent,* 8th ed. Mosby, 2004.

Pinkham JR et al: *Pediatric Dentistry: Infancy Through Adolescence,* 4th ed. Elsevier Saunders, 2005.

Wilson W et al: Prevention of infective endocarditis: Guidelines from the American Heart Association: A guideline from the American Heart Association Rheumatic Fever, Endocarditis and Kawasaki Disease Committee, Council on Cardiovascular

Disease in the Young, and the Council on Clinical Cardiology, Council on Cardiovascular Surgery and Anesthesia, and the Quality of Care and Outcomes Research Interdisciplinary Working Group. J Am Dent Assoc 2007;138:739, 747 [PMID: 17545263].

Web Resources

American Academy of Pediatric Dentistry: http://www.aapd.org/
Save-a-Tooth emergency tooth preserving system: http://www.save-a-tooth.com/

Ear, Nose, & Throat

Peggy E. Kelley, MD

Norman R. Friedman, MD

Patricia J. Yoon, MD

▼ THE EAR

INFECTIONS OF THE EAR

The spectrum of infectious ear diseases includes the structures of the outer ear (otitis externa), the middle ear (acute otitis media), the mastoid bone (mastoiditis), and the inner ear (labyrinthitis).

1. Otitis Externa

Otitis externa is inflammation of the skin lining the ear canal and surrounding soft tissue. The most common cause is loss of the protective function of cerumen, leading to maceration of the underlying skin such as occurs with swimming. Other causes are trauma to the ear canal from using cotton-tipped applicators for cleaning or from using poorly fitted ear plugs while swimming; contact dermatitis due to hair sprays, perfumes, or self-administered ear drops; secondary infection of the canal from otitis media with a patent tympanostomy tube; and chronic drainage from a perforated tympanic membrane (TM). Infections due to *Staphylococcus aureus* or *Pseudomonas aeruginosa* are the most common.

Symptoms include pain and itching in the ear, especially with chewing or pressure on the tragus. Movement of the pinna or tragus causes considerable pain. Drainage may be minimal unless the otitis externa is from a draining pressure equalization tube or TM perforation. The ear canal is typically grossly swollen, and the patient may resist any attempt to insert an ear speculum. Debris is noticeable in the canal. It is often impossible to visualize the TM. Hearing is normal unless complete occlusion has occurred.

▶ Treatment

Topical treatment usually suffices. Fluoroquinolone drops may be more effective than traditional combination drops and are safer to use. If the TM cannot be seen, then a perforation should be presumed to exist. Children with otitis externa secondary to draining tubes or perforations should be treated with topical therapy only in the absence of systemic symptoms. The topical therapy chosen must be safe for the inner ear because the perforation or the patent tube allows the drops access to the middle and inner ear. If the ear canal is open, ototopical antibiotics are placed and prescribed for 5–7 days as indicated. If the canal is too edematous to allow the ear drop to get in, a Pope ear wick (expandable sponge) is needed for the first few days to assure antibiotic delivery. Oral antibiotics are indicated if any signs of invasive infection, such as fever, cellulitis of the auricles, or tender postauricular lymph nodes, are present. In such cases, prescribe an antistaphylococcal antibiotic while awaiting the results of the cultured ear canal discharge. Systemic antibiotics alone without topical treatment will not successfully treat otitis externa. Narcotic analgesics may be required until the infection begins to resolve in 2–3 days.

During the acute phase, the patient should avoid swimming. A cotton ear plug is not helpful and may prolong the infection. Schedule a follow-up visit in 1 week to document an intact TM (Figure 17–1). Children who have intact TMs and are predisposed to external otitis should receive 2 or 3 drops of a 1:1 solution of white vinegar and 70% ethyl alcohol into the ears before and after swimming.

Manolidis S et al: Comparative efficacy of aminoglycoside versus fluoroquinolone topical antibiotic drops. Otolaryngol Head Neck Surg 2004;130:S83 [PMID: 15054366].

Roland PS et al: Consensus panel on role of potentially ototoxic antibiotics for topical middle ear use: introduction, methodology and recommendations. Otolaryngol Head Neck Surg 2004;130:S51 [PMID: 15543836].

2. Acute Otitis Media

▶ Classification & Clinical Findings

Otitis media is an infection associated with middle ear effusion (a collection of fluid in the middle ear space) or with otorrhea (a discharge from the ear through a perforation in the TM or

Right Tympanic Membrane

Otoscopic View
(Nose is to right)

Lateral View

Attic

Pars flaccida

Short process of malleus

Chorda tympani

Incus

Umbo

Pars tensa

▲ **Figure 17–1.** Tympanic membrane.

a ventilating tube). Otitis media can be further classified by its associated clinical symptoms, otoscopic findings, duration, frequency, and complications. These more specific classifications are acute otitis media (AOM), otitis media with effusion (OME), and chronic suppurative otitis media.

AOM is commonly defined as inflammation of the middle ear resulting in an effusion and associated with rapid onset of symptoms such as otalgia, fever, irritability, anorexia, or vomiting. The 2004 Guidelines from the American Academy of Pediatrics and of the American Academy of Family Physicians specified three criteria which must be present (Table 17–1). The presence of an ear effusion is best determined by either pneumatic otoscopy or tympanometry. To distinguish

Table 17–1. Definition of acute otitis media (AOM).

A diagnosis of AOM requires (1) a history of acute onset of signs and symptoms, (2) the presence of MEE, and (3) signs and symptoms of middle-ear inflammation.
Elements of the definition of AOM are all of the following:
1. Recent, usually abrupt, onset of signs and symptoms of middle-ear inflammation and MEE
2. The presence of MEE that is indicated by any of the following:
   a. Bulging of the tympanic membrane
   b. Limited or absent mobility of the tympanic membrane
   c. Air-fluid level behind the tympanic membrane
   d. Otorrhea
3. Signs or symptoms of middle ear inflammation as indicated by either
   a. Distinct erythema of the tympanic membrane or
   b. Distinct otalgia (discomfort clearly referable to the ear[s]) that results in interference with or precludes normal activity or sleep

MEE, middle ear effusion.

AOM from OME, signs of inflammation of the TM and symptoms of acute infection must be present. Otoscopic findings specific for AOM are a bulging TM, impaired visibility of the ossicular landmarks, a yellow or white color, opacification of the eardrum, and squamous exudate or bullae on the eardrum. OME is associated with a nonbulging TM, which may be retracted or neutral, but always has decreased mobility, may have opacification, and may have white or amber discoloration. Children with OME may develop superimposed acute infection, but they will then exhibit inflammation of the eardrum as described for AOM.

A. Predisposing Factors

Factors that make otitis media more common in children than in adults include bacterial nasopharyngeal colonization in the absence of antibody, frequent upper respiratory infections, exposure to parental cigarette smoke, unfavorable eustachian tube function, and allergies.

1. Bacterial colonization—Nasopharyngeal colonization with *Streptococcus pneumoniae, Haemophilus influenzae,* or *Moraxella catarrhalis* increases the risk of otitis media, whereas colonization with normal flora such as viridans streptococci may prevent otitis episodes by inhibiting the growth of these pathogens. Colonization usually occurs sequentially with different pathogen serotypes present for about 2 months, and there is a risk of AOM with each new serotype acquired. Infants in day care acquire these serotypes at a younger age than those in home care. Since younger children are at higher risk of AOM, the increased number of children in day care over the past three decades has undoubtedly played a major role in the increase in AOM in the United States.

2. Viral upper respiratory infections—These infections increase the colonization of the nasopharynx with otitis pathogens. Viral infection also impairs eustachian tube function by causing both adenoidal swelling and edema of the tube. Therefore, factors that increase the frequency of viral respiratory infections, such as child care attendance, smoke exposure, later birth order, and absence of breast feeding, promote colonization with otitis pathogens and predispose to otitis media.

3. Smoke exposure—Passive smoking increases the risk of persistent middle ear effusion by enhancing colonization, prolonging the inflammatory response, and impeding drainage through the eustachian tube. For infants aged 12–18 months, exposure to each additional pack of cigarettes smoked at home is associated with an 11% increase in the duration of a middle ear effusion.

4. Eustachian tube dysfunction—Infants born with craniofacial disorders, such as Down syndrome or a cleft palate, are often affected by AOM and OME. The patency of the tube allows aeration of the middle ear. When the tube is obstructed, a vacuum develops in the middle ear, which can pull nasopharyngeal secretions and pathogens into the middle ear or can pull serous fluid from the middle ear lining cells. Either way, the fluid is then prone to infection.

5. Impaired host immune defenses—Immunocompromised children such as those with selective IgA deficiency usually experience recurrent AOM, rhinosinusitis, and pneumonia. However, most children who experience recurrent or persistent otitis only have selective impairments of immune defenses against specific otitis pathogens. For example, a recent study showed some children have low-to-absent IgG_2 or IgA pneumococcal polysaccharide antibody responses (or both) after vaccination, despite normal serum levels of total IgG_2 and IgA.

6. Bottle feeding—Breast feeding reduces the incidence of acute respiratory infections, provides IgA antibodies that reduce colonization with otitis pathogens, and decreases the aspiration of contaminated secretions into the middle ear space when a bottle is propped in the crib.

7. Genetic susceptibility—Although AOM is known to be multifactorial, and no gene for susceptibility has yet been identified, recent studies of twins and triplets suggest that as much as 70% of the risk is genetically determined. This has implications for the subsequent offspring of parents with a child experiencing recurrent AOM. These families might wish to consider breast feeding and home child care for later children.

B. Microbiology of Acute Otitis Media

The role of respiratory viral infection in precipitating otitis media is unquestionable, yet fewer than 12% of ear effusions culture positive for viruses. Recent studies with sensitive viral antigen or nucleic acid tests have detected virus in over 40% of infected ears. The viral infection usually precedes the

bacterial otitis media by 3–14 days and presumably causes adenoid hypertrophy and eustachian tube dysfunction. The two viruses most clearly shown to precipitate otitis media are respiratory syncytial virus and influenza, accounting for the annual surge in otitis media cases from January to May in temperate climates.

Historically, over 50% of AOM cases in the midwestern and northeastern United States were due to *S pneumoniae,* while the hotter, drier climates of southern Israel and Denver, Colorado, reported a preponderance of nontypeable *H influenzae* (Table 17–2). However, since widespread use of the pneumococcal conjugate vaccine (Prevnar; PCV7) in children younger than 2 years of age, the incidence of *H influenzae* may be on the rise and that of *S pneumoniae* may be declining. The pattern of infection in Kentucky now resembles that seen before PCV7 in Colorado. (No data are available for Denver in the post-Prevnar era.) More importantly, Prevnar has increased the percentage of cases due to non-PCV serotypes nationally from 12% in 1999 to 32% in 2002. The clinical significance of this change is to decrease the overall percentage of drug-resistant pneumococci, since the serotypes included in the vaccine are the most multiply resistant.

The third most common pathogen in some studies is *M catarrhalis,* which causes up to 25% of AOM cases in the United States. The fourth organism found is *Streptococcus pyogenes,* which is more common in school-aged children than in infants. This organism and *S pneumoniae* are the predominant causes of mastoiditis. Contrary to earlier teaching, the etiology of AOM in early infancy differs little from that in adult life. The only difference is that the risk of gram-negative enteric infection is slightly increased in infants younger than age 4 weeks who are or have been hospitalized in a neonatal intensive care nursery.

Table 17–2. Bacteriology of acute otitis media.

	Denver (Author)	Kentucky[a] Pre-PCV7 (Prevnar)	Kentucky[a] Post-PCV7
Streptococcus pneumoniae	32	48	31
Haemophilus influenzae	50	41	56
Moraxella catarrhalis	8	9	11
Streptococcus pyogenes	4	2	2
S pneumoniae + *H influenzae*	5	Not reported	Not reported

PVC7, seven-valent pneumococcal vaccine.
[a]Data used, with permission, from Block SL et al: Community-wide vaccination with the heptavalent pneumococcal conjugate significantly alters the microbiology of acute otitis media. Pediatr Infect Dis J 2004;23:829.

Drug-resistant *S pneumoniae* is a common pathogen in AOM and strains may be resistant to only one drug (ie, penicillin or macrolides) or to multiple classes. Children with resistant strains tend to be younger and to have had more unresponsive infections. Antibiotic treatment in the preceding 3 months also increases the risk of harboring resistant pathogens. Penicillin resistance develops through stepwise mutations in the structure of the three penicillin-binding proteins. Strains for which minimum inhibitory concentrations of penicillin range between 0.12 and 1.0 mcg/mL are said to exhibit "intermediate" resistance. Strains for which minimum inhibitory concentrations are equal to or higher than 2 mcg/mL are said to have "high-level resistance." The prevalence of resistant strains no longer varies significantly among geographic areas within the United States, but it does vary worldwide. Lower incidences are found in countries using fewer courses of antibiotic per person. These strains are also resistant to many other drug classes. Nationwide resistance rates include 63% for trimethoprim–sulfamethoxazole, 32% for macrolides, and 2% for amoxicillin (dosed at 90 mg/kg/d). Oral cephalosporins vary widely in efficacy, with the highest resistance rates for cefixime and cefaclor and lowest rates (about 35%) for cefuroxime, cefprozil, cefpodoxime, and cefdinir. Over 90% of highly penicillin-resistant strains are still susceptible to clindamycin, rifampin, and fluoroquinolones. Fluoroquinolones are not yet approved for children younger than 16 years; however, studies are under way to assess their safety and efficacy in this age group.

C. Examination Techniques and Procedures

1. Pneumatic otoscopy—AOM is overdiagnosed. Contributing to errors in diagnosis are the temptation to accept the diagnosis without removing enough cerumen to adequately visualize the eardrum, and the mistaken belief that a red eardrum establishes the diagnosis. In fact, redness of the eardrum is often a vascular flush caused by fever, crying, or even efforts to remove cerumen. Failure to achieve an adequate seal with the otoscope, poor visualization due to low light intensity, and mistaking the ear canal wall for the membrane can make it impossible to assess eardrum mobility.

A pneumatic otoscope with a rubber suction bulb and tube is used to assess mobility of the TM. The speculum inserted into the patient's ear canal must be large enough to provide an airtight seal. Placing a piece of rubber tubing 0.25–0.5 cm wide near the end of the ear speculum helps to create an adequate pneumatic seal. The tubing should fit snugly on the speculum at a distance about 0.5 cm from its end. The largest possible speculum (usually 3 or 4 mm) should be used to maximize the field of view. When the rubber bulb is squeezed, the TM will move freely to and fro if no fluid is present with a snapping motion; if fluid is present in the middle ear space, the mobility of the TM will be absent or resemble a fluid wave. The ability to assess mobility is compromised by low light intensity; a halogen

source is necessary. These bulbs dim but rarely ever burn out, so they must be replaced on a schedule.

Disposable ear specula have become popular but are not needed for infection control, because reusable specula can be easily disinfected. The disposable specula are sharp at the tip and often cause pain when pushed to get an airtight seal. It is advisable to consider using a smaller speculum to assess the entire TM and then place a larger speculum to stay within the outer cartilaginous ear canal when assessing mobility.

2. Cerumen removal—Cerumen removal is an essential skill for anyone who cares for children. Impacted cerumen pushed against the TM can cause itching, otalgia, or hearing loss. Parents should be advised that ear wax protects the ear (cerumen contains lysozymes and immunoglobulins that inhibit infection) and usually comes out by itself; therefore, parents should never put anything solid into the ear canal to remove the ear wax.

The physician may safely remove cerumen under direct visualization through the operating head of an otoscope, provided two adults are present to hold the child. A plastic disposable ear size 0 curette may be used. Any curette used should not be pointed or sharp.

Irrigation can also be used to remove hard or flaky cerumen. Asian children may have an ear wax variant that is flaky, called "rice bran wax." This type of wax can be softened with 1% sodium docusate solution, carbamyl peroxide solutions, mineral oil, or a few drops of detergent before irrigation is attempted. After 20 minutes, irrigation with a soft bulb syringe can be started with water warmed to 35–38°C to prevent vertigo. A commercial jet tooth cleanser (eg, Water Pik) is also an excellent device for removing cerumen, but it is important to set it at low power (2 or less) to prevent damage to the TM. A perforated TM or patent tympanostomy tube is a contraindication to any form of irrigation.

A good home remedy for recurrent cerumen impaction is a few drops of oil such as mineral or olive oil a couple of times a week warmed to body temperature to prevent dizziness.

3. Tympanometry—Tympanometry can rapidly identify an effusion in infants over about 6 months, and it requires little training. It should be preceded by pneumatic otoscopy to assure that 50% or more of the canal is wax-free. Because it does not identify inflammation, it cannot differentiate AOM and OME. Tympanometry measures TM compliance and displays it in graphic form (along the *y* axis, expressed in mm H_2O). Compliance is determined as air pressures are varied from +200 to –400 mm H_2O in the sealed external ear canal.

Tympanograms can be classified into four major patterns, as shown in Figure 17–2. The pattern shown in Figure 17–2A, characterized by maximum compliance at normal atmospheric pressure, indicates a normal TM, good eustachian tube function, and absence of effusion. The height and sharpness of the peak is not important when using the Welch-Allyn tympanometer. The pattern shown in Figure 17–2B identifies a nonmobile TM, which indicates middle

▲ **Figure 17–2.** Four types of tympanograms obtained with Welch-Allyn MicroTymp 2. **A:** Normal middle ear. **B:** Otitis media with effusion or acute otitis media. **C:** Negative middle ear pressure due to eustachian tube dysfunction. **D:** Patent tympanostomy tube or perforation in the tympanic membrane. Same as B except for a very large middle ear volume.

ear effusion. The pattern shown in Figure 17–2C indicates an intact mobile TM with poor eustachian tube function and excessive negative pressure (worse than –300 mm H₂O air pressure) in the middle ear. Figure 17–2D shows a flat tracing, which would have a very large middle ear volume on the printout, due to a patent tube or large perforation.

4. Acoustic reflectometry—Acoustic reflectometry measures the spectral gradient of the TM using a handheld instrument, without requiring an airtight seal. However, recent data suggest that this method cannot reliably distinguish negative middle ear pressure from effusion. The instrument is not commercially available at present.

▶ Treatment

A. Pain Management

Children with pain related to AOM may obtain relief from acetaminophen or ibuprofen, accompanied by a topical anesthetic drop. In a randomized controlled trial, Auralgan (benzocaine and antipyrine) ear drops were superior to olive oil in reducing pain. When severe pain is present, tympanocentesis should be considered for pain relief and to diagnose the causative pathogen.

B. The Observation Option (Watchful Waiting)

Few issues are as controversial as the necessity of immediate antibiotic treatment of otitis media. Doctors must balance the desire of the parents for symptom relief against the risk of selecting for drug resistance by overuse of antibiotics. In two recent editorials, Dr. Ellen Wald has pointed out that the major overuse of antibiotics is for the treatment of viral colds and viral pharyngitis, not otitis media. The second reason for antibiotic overuse is overdiagnosis of AOM by providers. The natural history of untreated AOM is to improve through host defenses or by perforation of the TM; but mastoiditis was not an infrequent complication before the use of antibiotics.

In Dr. Howie's classic studies in the 1970s, in which he randomized children to placebo or various antibiotics, bacteriologic cure rates determined by a second tympanocentesis while on therapy were only 32% in the placebo group. The spontaneous cure rate varied greatly by organism: 16% for *S pneumoniae*, 50% for nontypeable *H influenzae*, and about 84% for *M catarrhalis*, which he considered a contaminant. Several authors have correlated clinical cure rates at the end of therapy with bacteriologic cure on days 4–6, and clinical cure rates are always higher than bacteriologic cure rates. However, the children who are bacteriologic failures at the end of treatment have an extremely high likelihood of also experiencing clinical failure. This has important implications for study design, which has led the Food and Drug Administration (FDA) to start requiring new antibiotics to be studied for proof of bacteriologic cure in a subset of patients.

In 2004 the two academies (Family Physicians and Pediatrics) issued a clinical practice guideline that suggested nontreatment of limited groups of children with AOM (Table 17–3). Key points are that children older than age 2 years with nonsevere disease were recommended for nontreatment for the first 48–72 hours after onset of symptoms. Those younger than age 2 years and older children with severe pain or fever were always recommended to receive immediate antibiotics. Children failing observation were to begin antibiotics after 48–72 hours. Although, not mentioned, a prescription can be given at the first visit, with instructions to fill if no improvement is seen after the specified observation period.

The guidelines offer different recommendations for "certain" versus "uncertain" diagnosis, but clinicians should be able to see the eardrum and make a correct diagnosis if they master cerumen removal and pneumatic otoscopy. An "uncertain" diagnosis should only occur when pus, blood, or cerumen obscures the eardrum. For infants younger than age 6 months, antibiotics are always recommended on the first visit, regardless of the certainty of diagnosis. The guidelines also emphasize the importance of using pneumatic otoscopy or tympanometry to establish the presence of effusion, and the importance of differentiating OME from AOM by the absence of acute signs and symptoms of inflammation (see Table 17–3).

Everyone agrees that overtreatment of OME by well-meaning providers has led to overuse of antibiotics for no discernible benefit. AOM requires the recent onset of otalgia, which may be harder to diagnose in infants, but often manifests as night awakening, ear tugging, anorexia due to pain on swallowing, and unexplained crying. Although most clinicians routinely treat acute otitis with antibiotics, it is also reasonable to involve parents in the decision. There is a trade-off for the individual child between the risks of antibiotic treatment (cost, allergic reactions, side effects, and colonization with an antibiotic-resistant pathogen) and the benefit of a possibly more rapid clinical response and avoidance of potential complications. More rapid pain relief alone may justify treatment in older children. Children younger

Table 17–3. Criteria for initial antibiotic treatment in children with acute otitis media.

Age	Certain Diagnosis	Uncertain Diagnosis
< 6 mo	Antibacterial therapy	Antibacterial therapy
6 mo–2 y	Antibacterial therapy	Antibacterial therapy if severe illness; observation option[a] if nonsevere illness
≥ 2 y	Antibacterial therapy if severe illness; observation option[a] if nonsevere illness	Observation option[a]

[a]Nonsevere illness is mild otalgia and fever < 39°C in the past 24 h.

than age 2 years should be immediately treated with antibiotics because studies show an advantage over placebo, and they are more likely to develop complications.

C. Antibiotic Therapy

Amoxicillin remains the first-line antibiotic for treating otitis media, even with a high prevalence of drug-resistant *S pneumoniae*, because resistance to β-lactam antibiotics, such as amoxicillin, develops as a stepwise process over many years. A bacterial strain resistant to low levels of amoxicillin usually is eradicated by a higher dosage. Amoxicillin dosage may be raised considerably without toxicity; for example, a dosage of 200 mg/kg/d has been used to treat meningitis in children, and a maximum daily dose of 4 g has been used in adults. Studies have shown that increasing the dosage from 40 mg/kg to 90 mg/kg yields a drug concentration in middle ear fluid that surpasses the minimal level needed to inhibit 98% of all pneumococcal otitis media. A second advantage is that dosing amoxicillin at these higher levels may help delay stepwise emergence of resistance. In recognition of this new pharmacodynamic data, the federal government in June 1999 doubled the minimum inhibitory concentration used to define resistance to amoxicillin to 8 mcg/mL or greater. Because otitis media is not a life-threatening disease, it is not necessary for a first-line antibiotic to achieve 100% cure. High-dose amoxicillin will usually eradicate the most invasive pathogen, *S pneumoniae*, and if no improvement occurs, a second-line antibiotic may be chosen to cover *M catarrhalis* and β-lactamase–producing *H influenzae*.

Amoxicillin–clavulanate enhanced-strength, with 90 mg/kg/d of amoxicillin dosing (14:1 ratio of amoxicillin to clavulanate), is an appropriate choice when a child is clinically failing after 48–72 hours on amoxicillin (Table 17–4). In this situation, the most likely pathogen is *H influenzae*, and the addition of clavulanate to amoxicillin will broaden the coverage while retaining efficacy against *S pneumoniae*. The older 200- and 400-mg-per-teaspoon formulations of amoxicillin–clavulanate (7:1 ratio) should never be doubled in dosage, because the amount of clavulanate will be so high as to cause diarrhea.

Table 17–4. Treatment of acute otitis media in an era of drug resistance.

First-line therapy
1. Amoxicillin, 90 mg/kg/d, up to 4 g/d. For children over age 2 y, give for 5 d; under age 2 y, for 10 d.
2. If amoxicillin has caused a rash, give cefuroxime (Ceftin), cefdinir (Omnicef), or cefpodoxime (Vantin).
3. If urticaria or other IgE-mediated events have occurred, give trimethoprim-sulfamethoxazole or azithromycin (Zithromax).
4. If child is unable to take oral medication, give single IM dose of ceftriaxone (Rocephin).

Second-line therapy[a]
1. Amoxicillin-clavulanate (Augmentin ES-600), given so that patient receives amoxicillin at 90 mg/kg/d.
2. If amoxicillin has caused allergic symptoms, see recommendations above.

Third-line therapy
1. Tympanocentesis is recommended to determine the cause.
2. Ceftriaxone (Rocephin), two doses given IM, 48 h apart, with option of a third dose.

Recurrences > 4 wk after first episode
1. A new pathogen is likely, so restart first-line therapy.
2. Be sure diagnosis is not OME, which may be observed for 3–6 mos without treatment.

---

[a]For clinical failure after 48–72 h of treatment, or for recurrences within 4 wk. IM, intramuscular; OME, otitis media with effusion.

Three oral cephalosporins (cefuroxime, cefpodoxime, and cefdinir) are more β-lactamase-stable and these are alternative choices for antibiotic therapy in children who develop papular rashes with amoxicillin (see Table 17–4). Unfortunately, the coverage of highly penicillin-resistant pneumococci with these agents is poor and only the intermediate-resistance classes are covered. Of these three drugs, cefdinir is quite palatable in the liquid form while the other two drugs have a bitter aftertaste which is difficult, but not impossible, to conceal. Newer flavoring agents may be helpful here. A second-line antibiotic is indicated when a child experiences symptomatic infection within 1 month of stopping amoxicillin; however, repeat use of high-dose amoxicillin is indicated if more than 4 weeks have passed without symptoms, because a new pathogen is usually present. Macrolides such as azithromycin and clarithromycin are not recommended as second-line agents for two reasons. First, the national *S pneumoniae* resistance rate to macrolides is approximately 30% in respiratory isolates. Second, double tympanocentesis studies have demonstrated eradication of *H influenzae*, regardless of β-lactamase production. Virtually all strains of *H influenzae* have an intrinsic macrolide efflux pump, which pumps antibiotic out of the bacterial cell. In a recent double tympanocentesis study, the on-therapy eradication rate of all pathogens was 94.2% for high-dose amoxicillin–clavulanate and 70.3% for azithromycin ($P < .001$).

If a child remains symptomatic longer than 3 days while taking a second-line agent, a tympanocentesis is useful to identify the causative pathogen. The tap may be sterile or the organism may be sensitive. Reasons for failure to eradicate a sensitive pathogen may be nonadherence, poor drug absorption, or vomiting of drug. If a highly resistant pneumococcus is found or if tympanocentesis is not feasible, intramuscular ceftriaxone at 50 mg/kg/d for 3 consecutive days is probably the best choice based on a study performed in Israel. In addition to listing the steps of therapy, Table 17–4 also lists specific cephalosporins that may be used as alternative drugs in penicillin-allergic children. If the child has experienced anaphylaxis to amoxicillin, cephalosporins should not be substituted. However, the maculopapular rash frequently seen with amoxicillin is not IgE-mediated, and cephalosporins may be used.

With the emergence of *S pneumoniae* with minimum inhibitory concentration values of 4 mcg/mL, high-dose amoxicillin will undoubtedly fail to cure. Therefore, two new classes of antibiotics are in active clinical trials for AOM: fluoroquinolones and ketolides. Recently, however, ketolides were removed from the market. Fluoroquinolones are divided into two classes; the older class includes ciprofloxacin, ofloxacin, and levofloxacin. The newer class is the 8-methoxy-fluoroquinolones, which include gatifloxacin and moxifloxacin. The difference between the two classes is that the newer drugs have a lower tendency to select resistant *S pneumoniae*, because two mutations are required. Pneumococcal resistance has been seen in countries where fluoroquinolones were widely used in adults. Levofloxacin was evaluated in a double tympanocentesis trial and found to be highly efficacious, but the manufacturers have chosen not to apply to the FDA for use in AOM at this time. In a double tympanocentesis study of high-risk children, gatifloxacin was shown to eradicate 96% of pathogens. Cartilage toxicity has been seen only in juvenile laboratory animals, and no increased incidence of arthropathy has been seen during the compassionate use of any fluoroquinolone.

Figure 17–3 shows the recommended follow-up of AOM that resolves with a residual effusion at 3–4 weeks. Children, particularly those young enough to still be developing language skills, should be seen monthly for otoscopic examinations to determine if the effusion is persistent or occurs only with symptomatic infections. Prophylactic antibiotics and corticosteroids are no longer recommended for OME. An audiology evaluation should be performed after approximately 3 months of continuous bilateral effusion in children younger than 3 years and those at risk of language delay due to poverty or craniofacial anomalies or other risk factors. Children with hearing loss or speech delay should be referred to an otolaryngologist for possible ventilation tubes. Older children may have periodic hearing testing in the primary provider's office (see later section on Management of OME).

D. Duration of Therapy

The duration of antibiotic treatment is controversial. Only three recent trials have used stringent entry and outcome

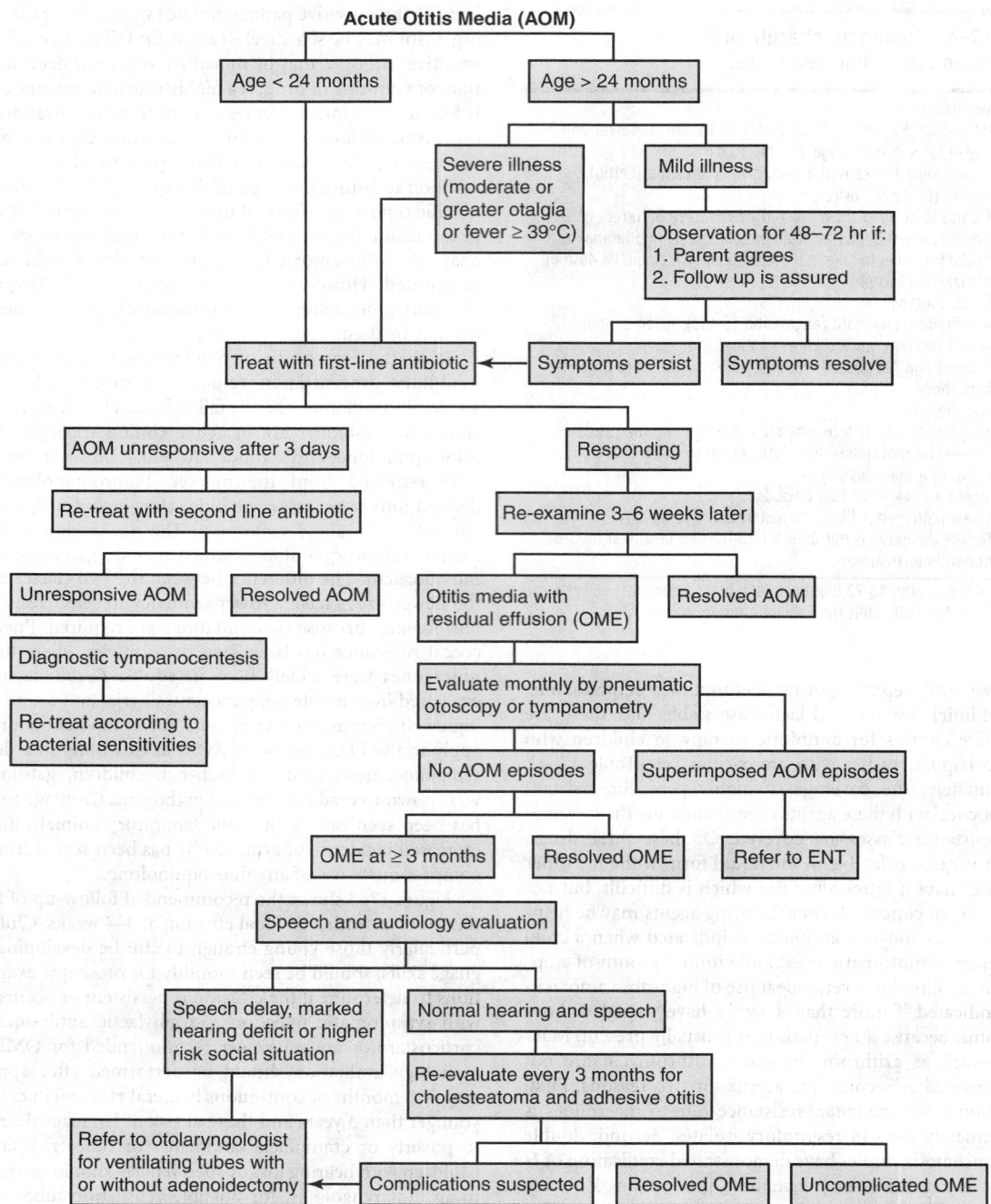

Acute Otitis Media (AOM)

▲ **Figure 17–3.** Algorithm for acute otitis media. ENT, ear, nose, and throat consult.

criteria. Success rates were higher following 10 days of therapy in all three studies, particularly for children younger than 2 years of age, and for those in day care. At this time, short-course (5-day) therapy can only be recommended for children older than 2 years and not in day care.

One side effect of using amoxicillin or penicillin is the eradication of the normal nasopharyngeal and oral flora. A recent study of preschoolers demonstrated that drug-resistant pneumococcal carriage at day 28 post-therapy was lower in a short-course high-dose amoxicillin group compared with a group given a standard course of therapy. This is an important finding, because it is now known that the nasopharyngeal flora influence the pathogen in the next episode of AOM. Normal flora resist colonization by disease-causing flora such as *S pneumoniae*.

E. Tympanocentesis

Tympanocentesis is performed by placing a needle through the TM and aspirating the middle ear fluid. Indications for tympanocentesis are (1) AOM in a patient with compromised host resistance, (2) research studies, (3) evaluation for presumed sepsis or meningitis, such as in a neonate, (4) unresponsive otitis media despite courses of two appropriate antibiotics, and (5) acute mastoiditis or other suppurative complications. The technique of tympanocentesis is as follows:

1. Premedication—In the conditions mentioned, the pain associated with tympanocentesis is only slightly greater than the pain of existing acute inflammation of the TM. Therefore, no premedication is used, but the provider should perform the procedure rapidly and return the child immediately to the parent's arms.

2. Restraint—A papoose board or a sheet can be used to immobilize the patient's body, and an extra attendant is required to hold the child's head steady. It is helpful to have the parent remain in sight of the child for reassurance.

3. Site selection—With an open-headed operating otoscope (Figure 17–4), the operator carefully selects a target. This is best done in the anteroinferior quadrant, although the posteroinferior quadrant is a safe but shallower alternative. These sites avoid damage to the ossicles, which are in the posterior superior quadrant, during the procedure.

4. Aspiration—An 8.8-cm spinal needle (No. 18 or 20) with a short bevel is attached to a 3-mL syringe. Alternatively, either an Alden-Senturia trap (Storz Instrument Co., St. Louis, MO) or the Tymp-Tap aspirator (Xomed Surgical Products, Jackson, FL) is attached to a suction pump. The operator then aspirates the middle ear effusion from the anterior inferior quadrant. Aspirate should be placed directly onto culture plates for maximum recovery, and chocolate agar is adequate to grow all common pathogens.

F. Prevention of Acute Otitis Media

1. Antibiotic prophylaxis—Prolonged use of low doses of antibiotics, for periods of 6–12 months, has been the primary method of prophylaxis. However, as the health care community tries to avoid using low doses of antibiotics (or drugs present for long time periods after therapy such as azithro-

▲ **Figure 17–4.** Operating head and Alden-Senturia trap for tympanocentesis. 18-gauge spinal needle is attached and bent.

mycin), this method should be reserved for unusual situations. Amoxicillin is the drug most studied. A situation in which prophylaxis might still be recommended is a child being considered for tympanostomy tube placement for recurrent infections who presents in late spring. A 1–2 month course of amoxicillin might prevent infection until the low-risk summer season when AOM is uncommon. Another recommendation for prophylaxis is in the child with patent tympanostomy tubes who experiences recurrent AOM and has been found to have an immune deficiency on more than one occasion. Antibiotic prophylaxis is not recommended for children with OME, despite earlier guidelines that made such a recommendation.

2. Lifestyle modifications—Parental education plays a major role in decreasing AOM, and the National Association of Daycare Providers has prepared educational materials for its centers and its parents. Here are some counseling topics to consider in children with frequent recurrences:

- Smoking is a risk factor both for upper respiratory infection and for AOM, and primary care physicians can provide literature on smoking cessation programs and on nicotine-containing gums or patches.

- Breast feeding protects children from AOM, but the mechanism is unknown. Also, propping a bottle of milk in the crib increases AOM risk.

- Removing pacifiers from infants was shown in Finland to reduce episodes of AOM by about one third compared with a control group. The mechanism is uncertain but is likely to be related to effects on the eustachian tube.

- Day care is clearly a risk factor for AOM, but working parents may have few alternatives. Suggestions include care by relatives or care of the child in a home care setting with fewer children.

- Xylitol, also known as birch sugar, is found in plums, strawberries, and raspberries. It was first studied in Europe as a chewing gum to reduce dental caries, and proved effective. Unfortunately, to prevent a single AOM episode would require a group of children to chew 4100 pieces of gum per year.

3. Surgery—Tympanostomy tubes are an effective treatment of recurrent otitis media as well as OME, which will be discussed in the next section.

4. Immunologic evaluation and allergy testing—Parents often ask if an immune deficiency may be causing their child's frequent otitis episodes. While it is known that immunoglobulin subclass deficiencies are more common in immune-deficient children, the relationship is not straightforward. Furthermore, there is no practical immune therapy. More serious immunodeficiencies such as selective IgA deficiency should be sought in children with a combination of recurrent AOM, rhinosinusitis, and pneumonia. Parents may also inquire about the role of allergy, since a generation ago many children with recurrent AOM were placed on milk elimination diets. No benefits were seen in the large group, but for certain individuals eliminating all milk and milk-containing foods can eliminate ear infections. In the school-aged child or the preschooler with an atopic background, skin testing may be beneficial in identifying allergens that predispose to AOM.

5. Vaccines—With the increasing problems of antibiotic therapy and prophylaxis, vaccines are increasingly important. The seven-valent pneumococcal vaccine (PCV7) was designed to prevent meningitis and sepsis, not AOM. However, it did produce a 55% reduction in AOM resulting from the seven serotypes found in the vaccine, and these strains include the serotypes most likely to be penicillin- and macrolide-resistant. Overall PCV7 reduced AOM by 6% in a group of children in California, compared with a control group. More impressively, it reduced pressure equalization tube placements by 20% and greatly reduced AOM incidence in children having six or more episodes per year. Furthermore, studies are showing a herd immunity effect on the older siblings of vaccinated children, which may further reduce drug-resistant serotype circulation. The vaccine should be used as a single dose for children aged 2–5 years with a history of either recurrent AOM or OME with superimposed AOM episodes.

In recent studies, intranasal influenza vaccine reduced the number of influenza-associated cases of AOM by 92%. For children older than 6 months with recurrent AOM, it seems prudent to recommend yearly influenza vaccine, although this is not yet an official recommendation.

Vaccines currently being studied in animals that hold promise for AOM prevention include a respiratory syncytial virus vaccine and a nontypeable *H influenzae* vaccine. Studies of pregnant women in the third trimester have shown that their pneumococcal antibody levels are raised by a heptavalent pneumococcal vaccine, which may also raise antibody levels in the offspring. A recent study showed that low cord blood pneumococcal antibody is a risk factor for AOM and OME, so passive transfer from the mother is a logical next step to study.

Dagan R et al: Potential role of fluoroquinolone therapy in childhood otitis media. Pediatr Infect Dis J 2004;23:390 [PMID: 15131460].

Dagan R, McCracken GH Jr: Flaws in design and conduct of clinical trials in acute otitis media. Pediatr Infect Dis J 2002;21:894 [PMID: 12394809].

Finkelstein JA et al: Watchful waiting for acute otitis media: Are parents and physicians ready? Pediatrics 2005;115:1466 [PMID: 15930205].

Hoberman A et al: Large dosage amoxicillin/clavulanate, compared with azithromycin, for the treatment of bacterial acute otitis media in children. Pediatr Infect Dis J 2005;24:525 [PMID: 15933563].

Jacobs MR, Johnson CE: Macrolide resistance: an increasing concern for treatment failure in children. Pediatr Infect Dis J 2003;22:S131 [PMID: 14566999].

McCormick DP et al: Nonsevere acute otitis media: A clinical trial comparing outcomes of watchful waiting versus immediate antibiotic treatment. Pediatrics 2005;115:1455 [PMID: 15930204].

McEllistrem MC et al: Acute otitis media due to penicillin-nonsusceptible *Streptococcus pneumoniae* before and after the introduction of the pneumococcal conjugate vaccine. Clin Infect Dis 2005;40:1738 [PMID: 15909260].

Pelton SI: Otitis media: Re-evaluation of diagnosis and treatment in the era of antimicrobial resistance, pneumococcal conjugate vaccine, and evolving morbidity. Pediatr Clin North Am 2005;52:711 [PMID: 15925659].

Ruohola A et al: Antibiotic treatment of acute otorrhea through tympanostomy tube: Randomized double-blind placebo-controlled study with daily follow-up. Pediatrics 2003;111:1061 [PMID: 12728089].

Siegel RM, Bien JP: Acute otitis media in children: A continuing story. Pediatr Rev 2004;25:187 [PMID: 15173451].

Subcommittee on Management of Acute Otitis Media: Diagnosis and management of acute otitis media. Pediatrics 2004;113:1451 [PMID: 15121972].

Wald ER: Acute otitis media: More trouble with the evidence. Pediatr Infect Dis J 2003;22:103 [PMID: 12586970].

Wald ER: To treat or not to treat. Pediatrics 2005;115:1087 [PMID: 15805394].

Web Resources

American Academy of Pediatrics (http://www.aap.org/otitismedia/www/): Information on diagnosis and treatment of AOM, written for the American Academy of Pediatrics. Features video clips of TMs being insufflated, to help clinicians learn normal landmarks and pathologic states. Requires Apple QuickTime to run.

Centers for Disease Control and Prevention: Appropriate Antibiotic Use (http://www.cdc.gov/drugresistance): Offers excellent advice for clinicians on (1) distinguishing OME from AOM, (2) careful antibiotic use for respiratory infections, and (3) patient education material on these two topics.

American Academy of Otolaryngology, Head and Neck Surgery (http://www.entnet.org): Information on diagnosis and treatment of acute and chronic ear disease, written by the Otolaryngology Academy. Information is presented for parents and treating providers.

The Ear Treatment Group at the University of Texas Medical Branch (http://www.atc.utmb.edu/aom/home.htm): An interactive site for medical students, residents, and physicians to learn about otitis media and to test their knowledge. Contains links to other otitis media–related resources as well as parent educational material.

G. Management of Otitis Media with Residual and Persistent Effusions

OME is treated to avoid the consequences of prolonged negative pressure on the TM and chronic conductive hearing loss. Available data show a causal relationship between severe sensorineural hearing loss and language delay, but not between conductive hearing loss due to OME and language delay. Studies looking at middle ear effusion (MEE) and its effects on language development in normal children of English-speaking middle- and upper-class society do not show differences at ages 5–7 years. This, however, eliminates many if not most of the children with high risk factors for otitis media. Two thirds of children with AOM have an MEE or high negative middle ear pressure 2 weeks after diagnosis and one third at 1 month after diagnosis regardless of antibiotic therapy. The management options for otitis media with residual effusion at 6 weeks to 4 months include observation. Nasal and oral corticosteroids have not been found in large studies to decrease MEE over several months but may be helpful in certain patients with nasal obstruction from adenoid hypertrophy or allergic rhinitis

If the patient clears the persistent MEE unilaterally or bilaterally, the physician should follow the patient monthly. Because of the increase in antibiotic resistance, the use of prophylaxis, even intermittently, must be restricted to carefully selected patients. The guideline recommendation developed by the Agency for Healthcare Research and Quality for the management of OME is that ventilating tubes should be placed after the effusion has persisted for 4 months and is accompanied by a bilateral hearing impairment of 20 dB or greater. Earlier placement of ventilating tubes should depend on the child's developmental and behavioral status as well as on parental preference. The value of ventilating tubes for treating unilateral effusions in otherwise healthy children is focused on preventing middle ear sequelae often seen as a retracted or atelectatic drum.

Children who have otitis media and persistent effusion have an increased incidence of cholesteatoma, adhesive otitis, retraction pockets, membrane atrophy, and persistent membrane perforation. As there is no way to identify the small proportion of candidate children for whom insertion of ventilating tubes will prevent the damage, close follow-up of children with abnormal ears may be best accomplished by an otolaryngologist. This approach is discussed further below.

Golz A et al: Reading performance in children with otitis media. Otolaryngol Head Neck Surg 2005;132:495 [PMID: 15746869].
Paradise JL et al: Effect of early or delayed insertion of tympanostomy tubes for persistent otitis media on developmental outcomes at the age of three years. N Engl J Med 2007;344:1179 [PMID: 11309632].

3. Mastoiditis

Mastoiditis is a spectrum of disease that ranges from inflammation of the mastoid periosteum to bony destruction of the mastoid air system (coalescent mastoiditis) or abscess development. Infection of the periosteum of the mastoid bone is a rare complication of AOM in the postantibiotic era. In a recent article Rosenfeld and colleagues noted a 0.01% rate of mastoiditis in a large group of children not receiving antibiotic therapy. Mastoiditis can occur in any age group, but more than 60% of the patients are younger than age 2 years. Many children do not have a prior history of recurrent AOM. The most common pathogens are *Streptococcus pneumoniae* and *S pyogenes,* with *Staphylococcus aureus* and *H influenzae* occasionally seen. Rarely gram-negative bacilli and anaerobes are isolated. Antibiotics may affect the incidence and morbidity of acute mastoiditis. However, acute mastoiditis does occur in children who are on antibiotics for an acute ear infection. In the Netherlands, where only 31% of AOM patients receive antibiotics, the incidence of acute mastoiditis is 4.2 per 100,000 person-years. In the United States, where more than 96% of patients with AOM receive antibiotics, the incidence of acute mastoiditis is 2 per 100,000 person-years. The higher antibiotic usage in the United States correlates with a higher rate of resistant organisms and more adverse drug interactions. Moreover, despite the routine use of antibiotics, the incidence of acute mastoiditis has been rising in some cities. The pattern change may be secondary to the emergence of resistant *S pneumoniae.*

Rosenfeld RM et al: Implications of the AHRQ evidence report on acute otitis media. Otolaryngol Head Neck Surg 2001;125:440 [PMID: 11700439].

▶ Clinical Findings

The principal complaints of patients with mastoiditis are usually postauricular pain, fever, and an outwardly displaced pinna. On examination, the mastoid area often appears swollen and reddened. With disease progression it may become fluctuant. The earliest finding is severe tenderness on mastoid palpation.

AOM, by otoscopy, is almost always present. Late findings are a pinna that is pushed forward by postauricular swelling and an ear canal that is narrowed in the posterosuperior wall because of pressure from the mastoid abscess. In infants younger than age 1 year, the swelling occurs superior to the ear and pushes the pinna downward rather than outward. In the acute phase, diffuse inflammatory clouding of the mastoid cells occurs, as in every case of AOM. In more severe cases, bony destruction and resorption of the mastoid air cells may occur. The best way to determine the extent of disease is by computed tomography (CT) scan.

Meningitis is a complication of acute mastoiditis and should be suspected when a child has associated high fever, stiff neck, severe headache, or other meningeal signs. Lumbar puncture should be performed for diagnosis. Brain abscess occurs in 2% of patients and may be associated with persistent headaches, recurring fever, or changes in sensorium. Facial palsy, cavernous sinus thrombosis, and thrombophlebitis may be encountered.

▶ Treatment

Treatment for mastoiditis without a posterior abscess is typically myringotomy, with or without tube placement, in order to obtain material for culture. Hospitalization for intravenous therapy follows. Reasonable initial therapy is ceftriaxone plus nafcillin or clindamycin until culture results are returned. If clinical improvement does not occur after 24–48 hours of intravenous or intramuscular therapy, or if any signs or symptoms of intracranial complications exist, immediate surgery to drain the mastoid abscess is indicated. The primary management for coalescent mastoiditis (with abscess formation and breakdown of the mastoid air cells) is a cortical mastoidectomy. A recent review from the University of Texas–Southwestern revealed that 39% of patients with mastoiditis required a mastoidectomy. After significant clinical improvement is achieved with parenteral therapy, oral antibiotics are begun and should be continued for 3 weeks. If the child has an isolated subperiosteal abscess and not coalescent mastoiditis, either needle aspiration or incision and drainage with an associated myringotomy has produced good clinical outcomes.

4. Otitis Media with Complications

Complications of otitis media may involve damage to the middle ear structures, such as tympanosclerosis, retraction pockets, adhesions, ossicular erosion, cholesteatoma, perforations, and intratemporal and intracranial injury.

A. Tympanosclerosis

A white plaquelike appearance on the TM is caused by chronic inflammation or trauma that produces granulation tissue and hyalinization. The appearance of a small defect in the posterosuperior area of the pars tensa or in the pars flaccida suggests a retraction pocket. Retraction pockets occur when chronic inflammation and negative pressure in the middle ear space produce atrophy and atelectasis of the TM.

Continued inflammation can cause adhesions between the retraction pocket and the ossicles. This condition, referred to as adhesive otitis, predisposes to formation of a cholesteatoma or fixation and erosion of the ossicles (Figure 17–5). Erosion of the ossicles results from osteitis and compromise of the blood supply to the ossicles. Ossicular discontinuity may produce a maximal hearing loss with a 50-dB threshold. A tympanogram with very high compliance suggests ossicular discontinuity.

B. Cholesteatoma

A greasy-looking mass or pearly white mass seen in a retraction pocket or perforation suggests a cholesteatoma, whether or not there is discharge (see Figure 17–5). A perforation is usually painless. If infection is absent, the middle ear cavity generally contains normal mucosa. If infection is superimposed, serous or purulent drainage will be seen, and the middle ear cavity may contain granulation tissue or even polyps. Persistent or recurrent otorrhea following appropriate medical management should make one suspect a cholesteatoma. Foul smelling otorrhea at any time should raise suspicion of potential cholesteatoma.

C. Tympanic Membrane Perforation

Occasionally, an episode of AOM is associated with otorrhea. An aural discharge indicates that the TM has perforated. Most likely the perforation will heal spontaneously. If the perforation has not healed within 3 months, surgical intervention will be necessary. A conductive hearing loss is usually

▲ Figure 17–5. Attic cholesteatoma, formed from an indrawing of an attic retraction pocket.

present, depending on the size and location of the perforation. The site of perforation is important for both cholesteatoma formation and amount of hearing loss expected. Central perforations surrounded by intact TM are usually relatively safe from cholesteatoma formation. With a peripheral perforation, especially in the pars flaccida, the perforation extends to the canal wall without any intervening TM. Peripheral perforations create a risk for cholesteatoma because the ear canal epithelium may invade the perforation. Perforations over the round window membrane in the posterior part of the TM result in more hearing loss than a perforation in either the inferior or anterior TM.

Most perforations secondary to AOM heal within 2 weeks. When perforations fail to heal after 3–6 months, surgical repair may be needed. Repair of the defect in the TM is generally delayed until the child is older and eustachian tube function has improved. Procedures include paper patch, fat myringoplasty, and tympanoplasty. Tympanoplasty is generally deferred until age 7–9 years. In otherwise healthy children without any craniofacial anomalies, some surgeons repair the perforated TM earlier if the contralateral nonperforated drum remains free of infection and effusion for 1 year. This policy does not guarantee success. The age of the child when repair is performed is the more probable indicator of success. Occasionally, a perforation is closed in a child of younger age if recurrent otorrhea is thought to be secondary to water contamination or nasopharyngeal reflux. Earlier closure of the perforation will seal the middle ear space and reestablish the air cushion provided by the mastoid air system. An older child is more likely to have a successful outcome from closure of the perforation. Water activities should be limited to surface swimming, preferably with the use of an ear mold. Diving, jumping into the water, and underwater swimming should be prohibited for 6 weeks following the reparative surgery.

D. Facial Nerve Paralysis

The facial nerve crosses the middle ear as it courses through the temporal bone to its exit at the stylomastoid foramen. Occasionally, the nerve is incompletely encased in bone, which makes it susceptible to inflammation during an episode of AOM. The acute onset of a facial nerve paralysis should not be deemed idiopathic Bell palsy until all other causes have been excluded. If middle ear fluid is present, a prompt myringotomy is indicated. Placement of a ventilation tube will allow for prolonged ventilation. CT is indicated if a cholesteatoma is suspected or acute coalescent mastoiditis is present.

E. Chronic Suppurative Otitis Media

Chronic suppurative otitis media is present when persistent otorrhea occurs in a child with tympanostomy tubes or TM perforations. Occasionally, it is an accompanying sign of cholesteatoma. Visualization of the TM, meticulous cleaning

with culture of the drainage, and appropriate antimicrobial therapy are keys to management of cases not related to cholesteatoma. The successful treatment of chronic suppurative otitis usually requires therapy with an antibiotic that covers *Pseudomonas* and anaerobes. Oral quinolone antibiotics effective against *Pseudomonas* infection are not yet approved for use in growing children. Recent studies suggest that topical quinolones for 14 days may be effective. It is very important to clean the ear canal by suction to allow penetration of drops, and it is often useful to culture the secretions. A Pope ear wick should be inserted and drops placed on the wick several times daily. The child should be seen in 7 days, the wick removed, and suction repeated if necessary. When a cholesteatoma (see Figure 17–5) is associated with chronic suppurative otitis media, medical therapy is not effective. If the discharge does not respond to 2 weeks of aggressive therapy, mastoiditis, cholesteatoma, tuberculosis, or fungal infection should be suspected. Serious central nervous system (CNS) complications such as extradural abscess, subdural abscess, brain abscess, meningitis, labyrinthitis, or lateral sinus thrombophlebitis can occur with extension of this process. Therefore, patients with facial palsy, vertigo, or other CNS signs should be referred immediately to an otolaryngologist.

Lahav J et al: Postauricular needle aspiration of subperiosteal abscess in acute mastoiditis. Ann Otol Rhinol Laryngol 2005;114:323 [PMID: 15895789].

Leskinen K: Complications of acute otitis media in children. Curr Allergy Asthma Rep 2005;5:308 [PMID: 15967073].

Leskinen K, Jero J: Complications of acute otitis media in children in southern Finland. Int J Pediatr Otorhinolaryngol 2004;68:317 [PMID: 15129942].

Oestreicher-Kedem Y et al: Complications of mastoiditis in children at the onset of a new millennium. Ann Otol Rhinol Laryngol 2005;114:147 [PMID: 15757196].

Zapalac JS et al: Suppurative complications of acute otitis media in the era of antibiotic resistance. Arch Otolaryngol Head Neck Surg 2002;128:660 [PMID: 12049560].

Web Resources

http://www.entnet.org: The official web site of the American Academy of Otolaryngology and Head and Neck Surgery. Contains patient information, clinical indications for common surgical procedures, and links to other ear, nose and throat sites.

ACUTE TRAUMA TO THE MIDDLE EAR

Head injuries, a blow to the ear canal, sudden impact with water, blast injuries, or the insertion of pointed instruments into the ear canal can lead to perforation of the TM or hematoma of the middle ear. One study reported that 50% of serious penetrating wounds of the TM were due to parental use of a cotton-tipped swab.

Treatment of middle ear hematomas consists mainly of watchful waiting. Antibiotics are not necessary unless signs of infection appear. The prognosis for unimpaired hearing depends on whether the ossicles are dislocated or fractured in the process. The patient needs to be followed with audiometry or by an otolaryngologist until hearing has returned to normal, which is expected within 6–8 weeks.

Traumatic perforations of the TM often do not heal spontaneously, in which case the patient should be referred to an otolaryngologist. Perforations caused by a foreign body should be attended to urgently, especially if accompanied by vertigo.

EAR CANAL FOREIGN BODY

Numerous objects can be inserted into the ear canal by a child. If the object is large, wedged into place, or difficult to remove with available instruments, the patient should be referred to an otolaryngologist early rather than risk traumatizing the child or the ear canal or causing edema that will require removal under anesthesia. An emergency condition exists if the foreign body is a disk-type battery used in clocks, watches, and hearing aids. An electric current is generated in the moist canal, and a severe burn with resulting scarring can occur in less than 4 hours.

Lin VY et al: Button batteries in the ear, nose and upper aerodigestive tract. Int J Pediatr Otorhinolaryngol 2004;68:473 [PMID: 15013616].

HEMATOMA OF THE PINNA

Trauma to the ear can result in a hematoma between the perichondrium and cartilage. The hematoma appears as a boggy purple swelling of the upper half of the ear. If this is not treated, it can cause pressure necrosis of the underlying cartilage and result in "cauliflower ear." To prevent this cosmetic deformity, physicians should urgently refer patients to an otolaryngologist for aspiration and application of a carefully molded pressure dressing. Recurrent or persistent hematoma of the ear may require surgical drainage.

CONGENITAL EAR MALFORMATIONS

Agenesis, known as atresia, of the external ear canal results in conductive hearing loss that requires evaluation in the first month of life by hearing specialists and an otolaryngologist.

"Lop ears," folded down or protruding ears (so-called "Dumbo" ears), are a source of much teasing and ridicule. In the past, surgical correction at age 5 or 6 years was offered. Taping the ears into a correct anatomic position is very effective if performed in the first 72–96 hours of life. Tape is applied over a molding of wax and continued for 2 weeks. Another alternative for the ear that can be molded solely by finger pressure into a normal configuration is an incisionless otoplasty, which can be performed at a much earlier age than 5–6 years and is associated with little postoperative morbidity. Because no cartilage destruction is associated with this technique, future growth is unaffected.

An ear is low-set if the upper pole is below eyebrow level. This condition is often associated with renal malformations (eg, Potter syndrome), and renal ultrasound examination is suggested.

Preauricular tags, ectopic cartilage, fistulas, sinuses, and cysts require surgical correction, mainly for cosmetic reasons. Children exhibiting any of these findings should have their hearing tested. Most preauricular pits cause no symptoms. If one should become infected, the patient should receive antibiotic therapy and be referred to an otolaryngologist for eventual excision.

Fritsch MH: Incisionless otoplasty. Facial Plast Surg 2004;20:267 [PMID: 15778913].
Yotsuyanagi T et al: Nonsurgical treatment of various auricular deformities. Clin Plast Surg 2002;29:327 [PMID: 12120687].

IDENTIFICATION & MANAGEMENT OF HEARING LOSS

Hearing loss is classified as being conductive, sensorineural, or mixed in nature. Conductive hearing loss occurs when there is a blockage of sound transmission between the opening of the external ear and the cochlear receptor cells. The most common cause of conductive hearing loss in children is fluid in the middle ear. Sensorineural hearing loss is due to a defect in the neural transmission of sound, arising from a defect in the cochlear hair cells or the auditory nerve. Mixed hearing loss is characterized by elements of both conductive and sensorineural loss.

Hearing is measured in decibels (dB). The threshold, or 0 dB, refers to the level at which a sound is perceived in normal subjects 50% of the time. Hearing is considered normal if an individual's thresholds are within 15 dB of normal. In children, severity of hearing loss is commonly graded as follows: 5–30 dB mild, 31–60 dB moderate, 61–90 dB severe, and 91+ dB profound.

Hearing loss can significantly impair a child's ability to communicate, and hinder academic, social, and emotional development. Studies suggest that periods of auditory deprivation may have enduring effects on auditory processing, even after normal hearing is restored. In the past, the effects of unilateral hearing loss were thought to be of little consequence, but studies have shown that even a unilateral loss may be associated with difficulties in school and behavioral issues. Early identification and management of any hearing impairment is therefore critical.

Conductive Hearing Loss

The most common cause of childhood conductive hearing loss is otitis media and related conditions such as middle ear effusion (MEE) and eustachian tube dysfunction. Other causes of conductive hearing loss may include external auditory canal atresia or stenosis, TM perforation, cerumen impaction, cholesteatoma, and middle ear abnormalities, such as ossicular fixation or discontinuity. Often, a conductive loss may be corrected with surgery.

MEE may be serous, mucoid, or purulent, as in AOM. Effusions are generally associated with a mild conductive hearing loss that normalizes once the effusion is gone. The American Academy of Pediatrics recommends that hearing and language skills be assessed in children who have recurrent AOM or MEE lasting longer than 3 months.

Sensorineural Hearing Loss

Sensorineural hearing loss (SNHL) arises due to a defect in the cochlear receptor cells or the auditory nerve (cranial nerve VIII). The loss may be congenital (present at birth) or acquired. In both the congenital and acquired categories, the hearing loss may be either hereditary (due to a genetic mutation) or nonhereditary. It is estimated that SNHL affects 2–3 out of every 1000 live births, making this the most common congenital sensory impairment. The incidence is thought to be considerably higher among the neonatal intensive care unit population. Well-recognized risk factors for SNHL in neonates include positive family history of childhood SNHL, birthweight less than 1500 g, low Apgar scores (0–4 at 1 minute or 0–6 at 5 minutes), craniofacial anomalies, hypoxia, in utero infections (eg, TORCH syndrome), hyperbilirubinemia requiring exchange transfusion, and mechanical ventilation for more than 5 days.

A. Congenital Hearing Loss

Nonhereditary causes account for approximately 50% of congenital hearing loss. These include prenatal infections, teratogenic drugs, and perinatal injuries. The other 50% is attributed to genetic factors. Among children with hereditary hearing loss, approximately one third of cases are thought to be due to a known syndrome, while the other two thirds are considered nonsyndromic.

Syndromic hearing impairment is associated with malformations of the external ear or other organs, or with medical problems involving other organ systems. Over 400 genetic syndromes that include hearing loss have been described. All patients being evaluated for hearing loss should also be evaluated for features commonly associated with these syndromes. These include branchial cleft cysts or sinuses, preauricular pits, ocular abnormalities, white forelock, café-au-lait spots, and craniofacial anomalies. Some of the more frequently mentioned syndromes associated with congenital hearing loss include the following: Waardenberg, branchio-oto-renal, Usher, Pendred, Jervell and Lange-Nielsen, and Alport.

Over 70% of hereditary hearing loss is nonsyndromic (ie, there are no associated visible abnormalities or related medical problems). The most common mutation associated with nonsyndromic hearing loss is in the *GJB2* gene, which encodes the protein connexin 26. The *GJB2* mutation has a carrier rate of about 3% in the general population. Most nonsyndromic hearing loss, including that due to the *GJB2* mutation, is autosomal recessive, but gene loci for autosomal dominant and X-linked hearing loss have also been identified.

B. Acquired Hearing Loss

Hereditary hearing loss may be delayed in onset, as in Alport syndrome and most types of autosomal dominant nonsyndromic hearing loss. Vulnerability to aminoglycoside-induced hearing loss has also been linked to a mitochondrial gene defect.

Nongenetic etiologies for delayed-onset SNHL include exposure to ototoxic medications, meningitis, autoimmune or neoplastic conditions, noise exposure, and trauma. Infections such as syphilis or Lyme disease have been associated with hearing impairment. Hearing loss associated with congenital cytomegalovirus infection may be present at birth, or may have a delayed onset. The loss is progressive in approximately half of all patients with congenital cytomegalovirus-associated hearing loss. Other risk factors for delayed-onset, progressive loss include a history of persistent pulmonary hypertension and extracorporeal membrane oxygenation therapy.

Identification of Hearing Loss

A. Office Clinical Assessment

In the past, the parents' report of their infant's behavior was considered an adequate assessment of hearing. However, a deaf infant's behavior can appear normal and mislead parents as well as professionals, especially if the infant has autosomal recessive deafness and is the first-born child of carrier parents. The following office screening techniques may identify only gross hearing losses, and may not detect less severe hearing loss, such as due to otitis media.

1. Birth to 4 months—In response to a sudden loud sound (70 dB or more) produced by a horn, clacker, or special electronic device, the infant should show a startle reflex or blink the eyes.

2. Four months to 2 years—While the infant is distracted with a toy or bright object, a noisemaker is sounded softly outside the field of vision at the child's waist level. Normal responses are as follows: at 4 months, there is widening of the eyes, interruption of other activity, and perhaps a slight turning of the head in the direction of the sound; at 6 months, the head turns toward the sound; at 9 months or older, the child is usually able to locate a sound originating from below as well as turn to the appropriate side; after 1 year, the child is able to locate sound whether it comes from below or above.

After responses to soft sounds are noted, a loud horn or clacker should be used to produce an eye blink or startle reflex. This latter maneuver is necessary because deaf children are often visually alert and able to scan the environment so actively that their scanning can be mistaken for an appropriate response to the softer noise test. A deaf child will not blink in response to the loud sound. Consonant sounds such as "mama," "dada," and "baba" should be present in speech by age 11 months. Children who fail to respond appropriately should be referred for audiologic assessment.

B. Newborn Hearing Screening

Prior to the institution of universal screening programs, the average age at identification of hearing loss was 30 months. Recognizing the importance of early detection, in 1993, a National Institutes of Health Consensus Panel recommended that all newborns be screened for hearing impairment prior to hospital discharge. Today, universal newborn hearing screening is mandated in a majority of states, with a goal of hearing loss identification by 3 months of age, and appropriate intervention by the age of 6 months. Subjective testing is not reliable in infants, and therefore objective, physiologic methods are used for screening. Auditory brainstem response and otoacoustic emission testing are the two commonly employed screening modalities.

C. Audiologic Evaluation of Infants and Children

Audiometry subjectively evaluates hearing. There are several different methods used, based on patient age:

- Behavioral observational audiometry: Birth to 6 months. Sounds are presented at various intensity levels, and the audiologist watches closely for a reaction, such as change in respiratory rate, starting or stopping of activity, startle, head turn, or muscle tensing. This method is highly tester-dependent and error-prone.
- Visual reinforcement audiometry: 6 months to 2.5 years. Auditory stimulus is paired with positive reinforcement. For example, when a child reacts appropriately by turning toward a sound source, the behavior is rewarded by activation of a toy that lights up. After a brief conditioning period, the child localizes toward the tone, if audible, in anticipation of the lighted toy.
- Conditioned play audiometry: 2.5 to 5 years. The child responds to sound stimulus by performing an activity, such as putting a peg into a board.
- Conventional audiometry: Age 5 and up. The child indicates when he or she hears a sound.

Objective methods such as auditory brainstem response and otoacoustic emission testing may be used if a child cannot be reliably tested using the above methods.

Referral

A child who fails newborn hearing screening or has a suspected hearing loss should be referred for further audiologic evaluation, and any child with hearing loss should be referred to an otolaryngologist for further workup and treatment. In addition to the infants who fall into the high-risk categories for SNHL as outlined above, hearing should be tested in children with a history of developmental delay,

bacterial meningitis, ototoxic medication exposure, neurodegenerative disorders, or a history of infection such as mumps or measles. Even if a newborn screening was passed, all infants who fall into a high-risk category for progressive or delayed-onset hearing loss should receive ongoing audiologic monitoring for 3 years and at appropriate intervals thereafter to avoid a missed diagnosis.

Prevention

Appropriate care may treat or prevent conditions causing hearing deficits. Aminoglycosides and diuretics, particularly in combination, are potentially ototoxic and should be used judiciously and monitored carefully. Given the association of a mitochondrial gene defect and aminoglycoside ototoxicity, use should be avoided, if possible, in patients with a known family history of aminoglycoside-related hearing loss. Reduction of repeated exposure to loud noises may help prevent high-frequency hearing loss associated with acoustic trauma. Any patient with sudden-onset sensorineural hearing loss should be seen by an otolaryngologist immediately, as in some cases, steroid therapy may reverse the loss if initiated right away.

Management of Hearing Loss

If hearing impairment is suspected, the child should be referred to an audiologist for testing, and to an otolaryngologist for further evaluation and treatment. The management of hearing loss depends on the type and severity of impairment. Conductive hearing loss is typically correctable by addressing the point in sound transmission at which efficiency is compromised. For example, hearing loss due to chronic effusions usually normalizes once the fluid has cleared, whether by natural means or by the placement of tympanostomy tubes. Conductive loss due to TM perforation may be corrected by performing a tympanoplasty. As of yet, SNHL is not reversible, although cochlear hair cell regeneration is an area of very active research. Most sensorineural loss is managed with amplification. Cochlear implantation is an option for some children with severe-profound loss, and at the time of this writing, is FDA approved down to the age of 12 months. Unlike hearing aids, the cochlear implant does not amplify sound, but works by directly stimulating the cochlea with electrical impulses. Children with hearing loss should receive ongoing audiologic monitoring.

Grundfast KM, Siparsky NF: Hearing loss. In Bluestone CD et al (editors): *Pediatric Otolaryngology*, Vol. 1. Saunders; 2003:306.

Joint Committee on Infant Hearing: Year 2000 position statement: Principles and guidelines for early hearing detection and intervention programs. Pediatrics 2000;106:798 [PMID: 11015525].

Lieu JE: Speech-language and educational consequences of unilateral hearing loss in children. Arch Otolaryngol Head Neck Surg 2004;130:524 [PMID: 15148171].

Smith RJH, Van Camp G: Deafness and hereditary hearing loss overview. Revised January 30, 2007. Available at: http://www.geneclinics.org/profiles/deafness-overview/details.html.

Yoshinaga-Itano C: Benefits of early intervention for children with hearing loss. Otolaryngol Clin North Am 1999;32:1089 [PMID: 10523454].

THE NOSE & PARANASAL SINUSES

ACUTE VIRAL RHINITIS (COMMON COLD; SEE ALSO CHAPTER 38)

The common cold (viral upper respiratory infection) is the most common pediatric infectious disease, and the incidence is higher in early childhood than in any other period of life. Children younger than age 5 years typically have 6–12 colds per year. Approximately 30–40% of these are caused by rhinoviruses. Other culprits include adenoviruses, coronaviruses, enteroviruses, influenza and parainfluenza viruses, and respiratory syncytial virus.

▶ Clinical Findings

The patient usually experiences a sudden onset of clear or mucoid rhinorrhea, nasal congestion, sneezing, and sore throat. Cough or fever may develop. Although fever is usually not a prominent feature in older children and adults, in the first 5 or 6 years of life it can be as high as 40.6°C without superinfection. The nose, throat, and tympanic membranes may appear red and inflamed. Figure 17–6 shows the duration of cough, sore throat, and rhinorrhea in adults with rhinovirus-proven infections. The average duration of symptoms is about 1 week. Nasal secretions tend to become thicker and more purulent after day 2 of infection due to shedding of epithelial cells and influx of neutrophils. This discoloration should not be assumed to be a sign of bacterial rhinosinusitis, unless it persists beyond 10–14 days, by which time the patient should be experiencing significant symptomatic improvement.

▶ Treatment

Treatment for the common cold should be symptomatic (Figure 17–7). Acetaminophen or ibuprofen is helpful for fever and pain. Nasal congestion can be treated with nasal saline drops and bulb suctioning for an infant or child unable to blow his or her nose. A topical decongestant such as oxymetazoline may provide some relief, but should be discontinued within 3 days to prevent severe rebound nasal congestion or chemical rhinitis. A cool mist vaporizer or humidifier may help the cough, but antimicrobial solution should be added to the water or the device should be cleaned at least every 3 days.

Available scientific data suggest that cold and cough medications are generally not effective in children, and may be associated with serious adverse effects. Antihistamines have not proven effective in relieving cold symptoms. In rhinoviral colds, increased levels of histamine are not observed. There is

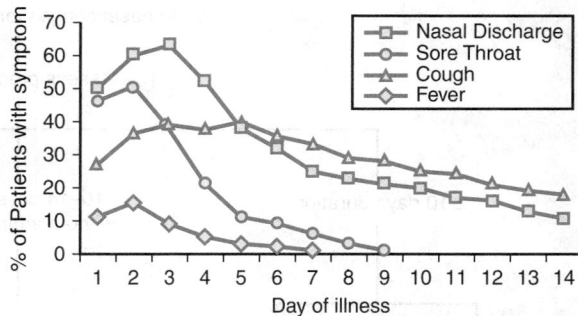

▲ **Figure 17–6.** Duration of symptoms in the common cold in adults. (Reproduced, with permission, from Gwaltney JM: Rhinovirus infections in an industrial population. II. Characteristics of illness and antibody response. JAMA 1967;202:494.)

insufficient evidence of benefit to warrant the use of antibiotics for common cold symptoms. Oral decongestants have been found to provide some symptomatic relief in adults but have not been well-studied in children. Cough suppression at night is the number one goal of many parents; however, the effectiveness of dextromethorphan is unclear. It is believed by most experts to be effective in adults and adolescents, but benefit has not been proven in younger children. Use of narcotic antitussives is discouraged, as these have been associated with severe respiratory depression.

Education and reassurance may be the most important "therapy" for the common cold. Parents should be informed about the expected nature and duration of symptoms, efficacy and potential side effects of medications, and the signs and symptoms of complications of the common cold, such as bacterial rhinosinusitis, bronchiolitis or pneumonia.

Arroll B, Kenealy T: Antibiotics for the common cold and acute purulent rhinitis. Cochrane Database Syst Rev 2005;(3):CD000247 [PMID: 16034850].

Kelly LF: Pediatric cough and cold preparations. Pediatr Rev 2004;25:115 [PMID: 15060179].

Sutter AI, et al: Antihistamines for the common cold. Cochrane Database Syst Rev 2003;(3):CD001267 [PMID: 12917904].

Taverner D, Latte J: Nasal decongestants for the common cold. Cochrane Database Syst Rev 2007;(1):CD001953 [PMID: 17253470].

RHINOSINUSITIS

The use of the term *rhinosinusitis* has replaced sinusitis. Rhinosinusitis acknowledges that the nasal *and* sinus mucosa are involved in similar and concurrent inflammatory processes.

1. Acute Bacterial Rhinosinusitis

Acute bacterial rhinosinusitis (ABRS) is a bacterial infection of the paranasal sinuses which lasts less than 30 days and in

Acute nasal congestion and rhinosinusitis

▲ **Figure 17-7.** Algorithm for acute nasal congestion and rhinosinusitis.

which the symptoms resolve completely. It is almost always preceded by a viral upper respiratory infection (cold). Other predisposing conditions include allergies, trauma, or other situations that lead to inflammation of sinonasal mucosa and obstruction of sinus drainage. The diagnosis of ABRS is made when a child with a cold does not improve by 10–14 days or worsens after 5–7 days. The maxillary and ethmoid sinuses are most commonly involved. These sinuses are present at birth, forming in the third to fourth gestational month. The sphenoid sinuses form by the age of 5 years, and the frontal sinuses form by about age 7–8 years. Frontal sinusitis is unusual before age 10 years.

A combination of anatomic, mucosal, microbial, and immune pathogenic processes is believed to underlie the development of rhinosinusitis in children. Both viral and bacterial infections play integral roles in the pathogenesis. Viral upper respiratory infections may cause sinus mucosal injury and swelling, resulting in osteomeatal obstruction, loss of ciliary activity, and mucus hypersecretion. The bacterial pathogens that commonly cause acute rhinosinusitis are

S pneumoniae, H influenzae (nontypeable), *M catarrhalis,* and β-hemolytic streptococci.

▶ **Clinical Findings**

The onset of symptoms in ABRS may be gradual or sudden, and may commonly include nasal drainage, nasal congestion, facial pressure or pain, postnasal drainage, hyposmia or anosmia, fever, cough, fatigue, maxillary dental pain, and ear pressure or fullness. The physical examination is rarely helpful in making the diagnosis, as the findings are essentially the same as those in a child with an uncomplicated cold. Occasionally, sinuses may be tender to percussion, but this is typically seen only in older children and is of questionable reliability. Transillumination of the sinuses is difficult to perform and not very helpful unless the sinuses are grossly asymmetrical.

In complicated or immunocompromised patients, sinus aspiration and culture by an otolaryngologist should be considered for diagnostic purposes and to facilitate culture-directed antibiotic therapy. Gram stain or culture of nasal discharge does not necessarily correlate with cultures of sinus aspirates. If the patient is hospitalized because of rhinosinusitis-related complications, blood cultures should also be obtained.

Imaging of the sinuses during acute illness is not indicated except when evaluating for possible complications, or for patients with persistent symptoms which do not respond to medical therapy. As with the physical examination, the radiographic findings of ABRS, such as sinus opacification, fluid, and mucosal thickening, are also seen in viral upper respiratory infections.

► Complications

Complications of ABRS occur when infection spreads to adjacent structures—the overlying tissues, the eye, or the brain. Orbital complications are the most common, arising from the ethmoid sinuses. These complications usually begin as a preseptal cellulitis, but can progress to postseptal cellulitis, subperiosteal abscess, orbital abscess, and cavernous sinus thrombosis. Associated signs and symptoms include eyelid edema, restricted extraocular movements, proptosis, chemosis, and altered visual acuity (see Chapter 15).

The most common complication of frontal sinusitis is osteitis of the frontal bone, also known as Pott's puffy tumor. Intracranial extension can lead to meningitis and to epidural, subdural, and brain abscesses. The most common maxillary complication is overlying cheek cellulites. Rarely, osteomyelitis of the maxilla can develop. For reasons that are unclear, male adolescents seem to be at higher risk for intracranial spread. Frequently, children with complicated rhinosinusitis have no prior history of sinus infection. No information is available on the rate of complications in ambulatory patients with rhinosinusitis, but the severity of the complications suggests that patients should be carefully followed while receiving treatment.

► Treatment

For children who are not improving by 10 days, or who have more severe symptoms, with fever of at least 39°C and purulent nasal drainage for at least 3–4 consecutive days, antibiotic therapy is recommended. Although some discrepancy exists, antibiotics are generally thought to decrease duration and severity of symptoms.

To minimize the number of children who receive antimicrobial therapy for uncomplicated viral upper respiratory infections, and to help combat antibiotic resistance, the American Academy of Pediatrics in 2001 issued guidelines for treatment. This algorithm is presented in Figure 17–8. Key decision points include severity of disease and risk factors for resistant organisms

For patients with mild-moderate symptoms, who are not in day care, and have not been on recent antibiotic therapy, amoxicillin is considered first-line therapy. For those with severe symptoms, in day care, or who were on antibiotics within the past 1–3 months, high-dose amoxicillin–clavulanate is recommended as first-line therapy. Cefuroxime, cefpodoxime, and cefdinir are recommended for patients with a non–type I hypersensitivity to penicillin. Macrolides should be reserved for patients with an anaphylactic reaction to penicillin. Other options for these patients include clindamycin or trimethoprim–sulfamethoxazole. However, it should be remembered that clindamycin is not effective against gram-negative organisms such as *H influenzae*.

Failure to improve after 48–72 hours suggests a resistant organism or potential complication. Second-line therapies should be initiated at this point, or, if the patient is already on amoxicillin–clavulanate or cephalosporin, intravenous antibiotic therapy should be considered. Imaging and referral for sinus aspiration should be strongly considered as well.

Patients who are toxic, or who have evidence of invasive infection or CNS complications, should be hospitalized immediately. Intravenous therapy with nafcillin or clindamycin plus a third-generation cephalosporin such as cefotaxime should be initiated until culture results become available.

Topical decongestants and oral combinations are frequently used in acute rhinosinusitis to promote drainage. Their effectiveness has not been proven, and concern has been raised about potential adverse effects related to impaired ciliary function, decreased blood flow to the mucosa, and reduced diffusion of antibiotic into the sinuses. Patients with underlying allergic rhinitis may benefit from intranasal cromolyn or corticosteroid nasal spray. Topical nasal decongestants should not be used for more than 3 days due to risk of rebound edema.

American Academy of Pediatrics: Clinical practice guidelines: Management of sinusitis. Pediatrics 2001;108:798 [PMID: 11533355].

McAlister WH et al: Sinusitis in the pediatric population: American College of Radiology. ACR appropriateness criteria. Radiology 2000;215(Suppl):811 [PMID: 11037504].

Sinus and Allergy Health Partnership: Antimicrobial treatment guidelines for acute bacterial rhinosinusitis. Otolaryngol Head Neck Surg 2004;13:1 [PMID: 14726904].

2. Recurrent or Chronic Rhinosinusitis

Recurrent rhinosinusitis occurs when episodes of ABRS clear with antibiotic therapy but recur with each or most upper respiratory infections. Chronic rhinosinusitis is diagnosed when the child has not cleared the infection in the expected time but has not developed acute complications. Both symptoms and physical findings are required to support the diagnosis, and CT scan may be a useful adjuvant in making the diagnosis. Although recent meta-analysis evaluations have resulted in recommendations for ABRS, there is a paucity of data for the treatment of recurrent or chronic rhinosinusitis. Important factors to consider include allergies, anatomic variations, and disorders in host immunity. Mucosal inflammation leading to obstruction is most com-

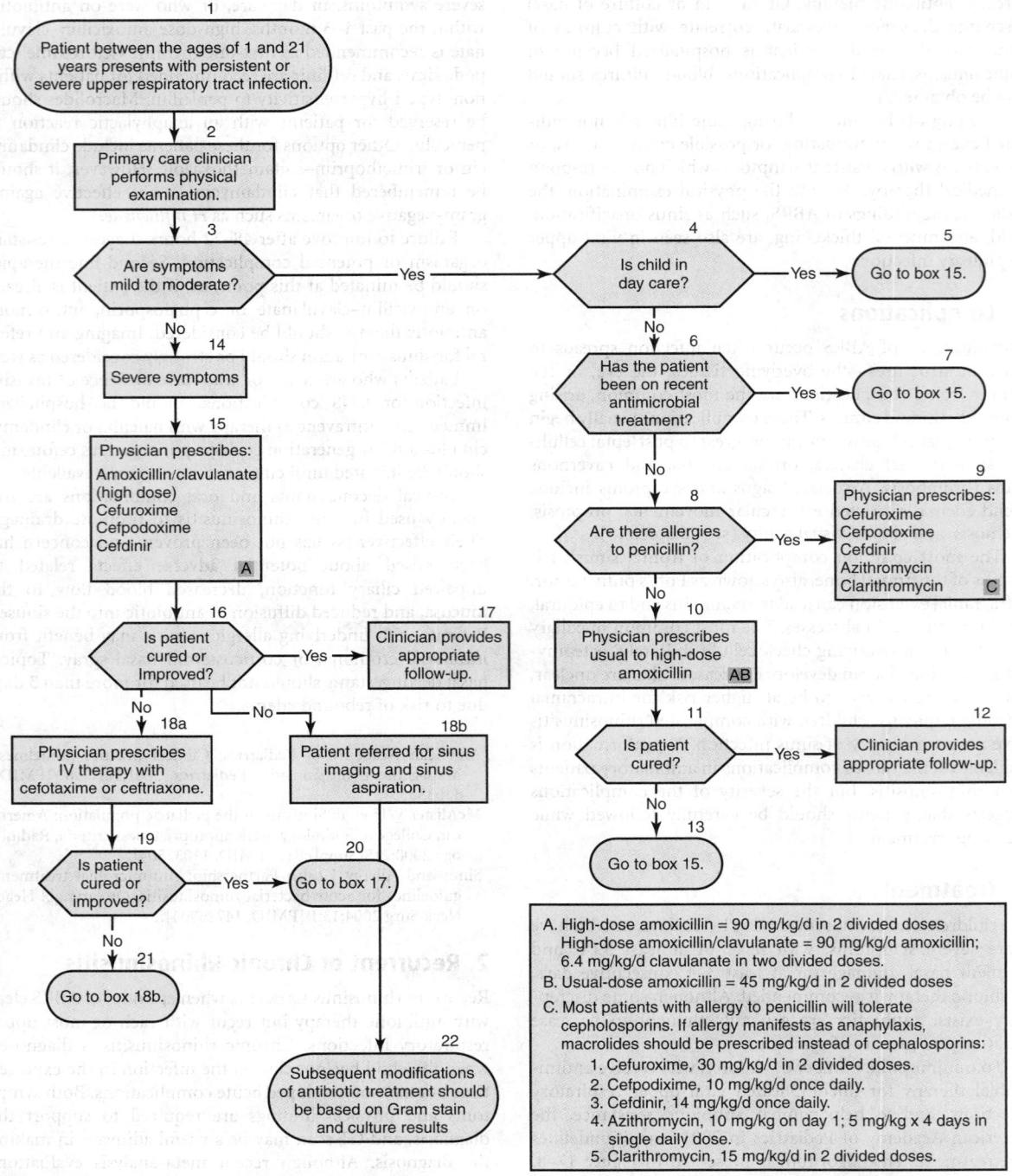

1
Patient between the ages of 1 and 21 years presents with persistent or severe upper respiratory tract infection.

2
Primary care clinician performs physical examination.

3
Are symptoms mild to moderate? — No

4
Is child in day care? — Yes → **5** Go to box 15.

No

6
Has the patient been on recent antimicrobial treatment? — Yes → **7** Go to box 15.

No

8
Are there allergies to penicillin? — Yes → **9** Physician prescribes: Cefuroxime Cefpodoxime Cefdinir Azithromycin Clarithromycin **C**

No

3 Are symptoms mild to moderate? — Yes → **4** Is child in day care?

14
Severe symptoms

15
Physician prescribes:
Amoxicillin/clavulanate (high dose)
Cefuroxime
Cefpodoxime
Cefdinir **A**

10
Physician prescribes usual to high-dose amoxicillin **AB**

11
Is patient cured? — Yes → **12** Clinician provides appropriate follow-up.

No

13
Go to box 15.

16
Is patient cured or Improved? — Yes → **17** Clinician provides appropriate follow-up.

No — No

18a
Physician prescribes IV therapy with cefotaxime or ceftriaxone.

18b
Patient referred for sinus imaging and sinus aspiration.

19
Is patient cured or improved? — Yes → **20** Go to box 17.

No

21
Go to box 18b.

22
Subsequent modifications of antibiotic treatment should be based on Gram stain and culture results

A. High-dose amoxicillin = 90 mg/kg/d in 2 divided doses
   High-dose amoxicillin/clavulanate = 90 mg/kg/d amoxicillin;
   6.4 mg/kg/d clavulanate in two divided doses.
B. Usual-dose amoxicillin = 45 mg/kg/d in 2 divided doses
C. Most patients with allergy to penicillin will tolerate cepholosporins. If allergy manifests as anaphylaxis, macrolides should be prescribed instead of cephalosporins:

   1. Cefuroxime, 30 mg/kg/d in 2 divided doses.
   2. Cefpodixime, 10 mg/kg/d once daily.
   3. Cefdinir, 14 mg/kg/d once daily.
   4. Azithromycin, 10 mg/kg on day 1; 5 mg/kg x 4 days in single daily dose.
   5. Clarithromycin, 15 mg/kg/d in 2 divided doses.

▲ **Figure 17-8.** Management of children with uncomplicated acute bacterial rhinosinusitis (ABRS). (Reproduced, with permission, from the American Academy of Pediatrics: Clinical practice guidelines: Management of sinusitis. Pediatrics 2001;108:798.)

monly caused by allergic rhinitis and occasionally by nonallergic rhinitis. Gastroesophageal reflux has also been found to be associated with chronic rhinosinusitis. Less commonly, chronic rhinosinusitis is caused by anatomic variations, such as septal deviation, polyp, or foreign body. Allergic polyps are unusual in children younger than age 10 years and should prompt a workup for cystic fibrosis. In cases of chronic or recurrent pyogenic pansinusitis, poor host resistance (eg, an immune defect, Kartagener syndrome, or cystic fibrosis)—though rare—must be ruled out by immunoglobulin studies, microscopic studies of respiratory cilia, and a sweat chloride test. Anaerobic and staphylococcal organisms are often responsible for chronic rhinosinusitis. Evaluation by an allergist and an otolaryngologist may be useful in determining the underlying causes.

▶ **Treatment**

A. Medical Therapy

Antibiotic therapy is similar to that used for ABRS, but the duration is longer, typically 3–4 weeks. Antimicrobial choice should include drugs effective against staphylococcal organisms. Adjuvant therapies such as saline nasal irrigation, decongestants, antihistamines, or topical intranasal steroids may be helpful depending on the underlying cause. A small percentage of children do not respond to medical therapy and will require surgery.

B. Surgical Therapy

1. Antral lavage—Antral lavage, generally regarded as a diagnostic procedure, may have some therapeutic value. An aspirate or a sample irrigated from the maxillary sinus is retrieved under anesthesia, either with a spinal needle or a curved-tip instrument. In the very young child, this may be the only procedure that should be performed.

2. Adenoidectomy—Adenoidectomy has been shown to be effective in 50–75% of children with chronic rhinosinusitis. The role of the adenoids in this disease is not completely understood, but it is thought that the adenoids serve as a reservoir of pathogenic bacteria, and that the adenoids may also interfere with mucociliary clearance and drainage. Biofilms have been reported in the adenoids of children with chronic rhinosinusitis, and may explain the resistance of these infections to standard antibiotic therapy.

3. Endoscopic sinus surgery—Endoscopic sinus surgery in children was controversial because of concern about alteration of developing sinuses and impairment of midface growth. However, recent studies have not supported this concern. Endoscopic sinus surgery has been shown to be effective in children, and may be indicated in addition to adenoidectomy.

4. External drainage—External drainage procedures are reserved for complications arising from ethmoid and frontal sinusitis.

Chan KH et al: Chronic rhinosinusitis in young children differs from adults: A histopathology study. J Pediatr 2004;144:206 [PMID: 14760263].

Coticchia J et al: Biofilm surface area in the pediatric nasopharynx. Arch Otolaryngol Head Neck Surg 2007;133:110 [PMID: 17309976].

Phipps CD et al: Gastroesophageal reflux contributing to chronic sinus disease in children: A prospective analysis. Arch Otolaryngol Head Neck Surg 2000;126:831 [PMID: 10888994].

Ramadan HH: Surgical management of chronic sinusitis in children. Laryngoscope 2004;114:2103 [PMID: 15564828].

CHOANAL ATRESIA

Choanal atresia occurs in approximately 1 in 7000 live births. The female-to-male ratio is 2:1, as is the unilateral-to-bilateral ratio. Bilateral atresia results in severe respiratory distress at birth and requires immediate placement of an oral airway, and otolaryngology consultation for a more permanent surgical solution. Unilateral atresia usually appears later as a unilateral chronic nasal discharge that may be mistaken for chronic rhinosinusitis. Diagnosis may be suspected if a 6F catheter cannot be passed through the nose and is confirmed by axial CT scan. Approximately 50% of patients with bilateral choanal atresia have CHARGE association (**C**oloboma, **H**eart disease, **A**tresia of the choanae, **R**etarded growth and retarded development or CNS anomalies, **G**enital hypoplasia, and **E**ar anomalies or deafness) (see Chapter 35) or other congenital anomalies.

Keller JL, Kacker A: Choanal atresia, CHARGE association, and congenital nasal stenosis. Otolaryngol Clin North Am 2000; 33:1343 [PMID: 11449791].

RECURRENT RHINITIS

Recurrent rhinitis is frequently seen in the office practice of pediatrics. The child is brought in with the chief complaint of having "one cold after another," "constant colds," or "always being sick." Approximately two thirds of these children have recurrent colds; the rest have either allergic rhinitis or recurrent rhinosinusitis.

1. Allergic Rhinitis

Allergic rhinitis has significant morbidity and may contribute to the development of rhinosinusitis and asthma exacerbations. Symptoms include nasal congestion, frequent sneezing, rubbing of the nose, and clear rhinorrhea. On physical examination the nasal turbinates are swollen and may be red or pale pink. Treatment with nasal corticosteroids is effective in decreasing the airway obstruction and rhinorrhea. Sneezing and clear drainage are controlled with nonsedating antihistamines. Montelukast, a leukotriene antagonist, has been shown to be effective in reducing nasal congestion, but it is less likely to improve the symptoms of itching, sneezing, and rhinorrhea, which are related to histamine release. Ipratropium can be used as an adjunctive therapy.

Pullerits T et al: Comparison of a nasal glucocorticoid, antileuko-triene, and a combination of antileukotriene and antihistamine in the treatment of seasonal allergic rhinitis. J Allergy Clin Immunol 2002;109:949 [PMID: 12063523].

Weinstein SF et al: Onset of efficacy of montelukast in seasonal allergic rhinitis. Allergy Asthma Proc 2005;26:41 [PMID: 15813287].

American Academy of Allergy, Asthma, and Immunology: http://www.aaaai.org/patients/allergic_conditions/rhinitis.stm

2. Vasomotor Rhinitis

Some children react to sudden changes in environmental temperature with prolonged congestion and rhinorrhea. Air pollution (especially tobacco smoke) may be a factor. Oral decongestants or nasal corticosteroids can be used to give symptomatic relief.

EPISTAXIS

The nose is an extremely vascular structure. In most cases, epistaxis (nosebleed) arises from the anterior portion of the nasal septum (Kiesselbach area), and is often due to dryness, or vigorous nose rubbing, nose blowing, or nose picking. If a patient has been using a nasal corticosteroid spray, check the patient's technique to make sure he or she is directing the nozzle laterally, away from the septum. If this does not reduce the nosebleeds, then the steroid spray should be discontinued. Examination of the anterior septum usually reveals a red, raw surface with fresh clots or old crusts. Also look for telangiectasias, hemangiomas, or varicosities.

In fewer than 5% of cases epistaxis is caused by a bleeding disorder such as von Willebrand disease. Patients need a hematologic workup if any of the following is present: a family history of a bleeding disorder; a medical history of easy bleeding, particularly with circumcision or dental extraction; spontaneous bleeding at any site; bleeding that lasts for more than 30 minutes or blood that will not clot with direct pressure by the physician; onset before age 2 years; or a drop in hematocrit due to epistaxis. High blood pressure may rarely predispose to prolonged nosebleeds in children.

A nasopharyngeal angiofibroma may be manifested by recurrent epistaxis. Adolescent boys are affected almost exclusively. CT scan of the nasal cavity and nasopharynx is diagnostic.

▶ Treatment

The following approach can be carried out in the office or offered as phone advice: The patient should sit up and lean forward so as not to swallow the blood. Swallowed blood may cause nausea and hematemesis. The nasal cavity should be cleared of clots by gentle blowing. The soft part of the nose below the nasal bones is pinched firmly enough to prevent arterial blood flow, with pressure over the bleeding site (anterior septum) being maintained for 5 minutes by the clock. For persistent bleeding, a one time only application of oxymetazoline (Afrin) into the nasal cavity may be helpful. If bleeding

continues, the bleeding site needs to be visualized. A small piece of gelatin sponge (Gelfoam) or collagen sponge (Surgicel) can be inserted over the bleeding site and held in place.

Friability of the nasal vessels can be decreased by increasing nasal moisture. This can be accomplished by daily application of a water-based ointment to the nose. A pea-sized amount of ointment is placed just inside the nose and the lubricant is spread by gently squeezing the nostrils. Twice-daily nasal saline irrigation and humidification of the patient's bedroom may also be helpful. Aspirin and ibuprofen should be avoided, as should nose picking and vigorous nose blowing. Cautery of the nasal vessels is reserved for treatment failures.

NASAL INFECTION

A nasal furuncle is an infection of a hair follicle in the anterior nares. Hair plucking or nose picking can provide a route of entry. The most common organism is S aureus. The diagnosis is made by finding an exquisitely tender, firm, red lump in the anterior nares. Treatment includes dicloxacillin or cephalexin orally for 5 days to prevent spread. The lesion should be gently incised and drained as soon as it points, usually with a needle. Topical bacitracin ointment may be of additional value. Because this lesion is in the drainage area of the cavernous sinus, the patient should be followed closely until healing is complete. Parents should be advised never to pick or squeeze a furuncle in this location—and neither should the physician. Associated cellulitis or spread requires hospitalization for administration of intravenous antibiotics.

A nasal septal abscess usually follows nasal trauma or a nasal furuncle. Examination reveals a fluctuant gray septal swelling, which is usually bilateral. The possible complications are the same as for nasal septum hematoma (see following discussion). In addition, spread of the infection to the CNS is possible. Treatment consists of immediate hospitalization and incision and drainage by an otolaryngologist.

NASAL TRAUMA

Newborn infants rarely present with subluxation of the quadrangular cartilage of the septum. In this disorder, the top of the nose deviates to one side, the inferior septal border deviates to the other side, the columella leans, and the nasal tip is unstable. This disorder must be distinguished from the more common transient flattening of the nose caused by the birth process. In the past, physicians were encouraged to reduce all subluxations in the nursery. Otolaryngologists are more likely to perform the reduction under anesthesia for more difficult cases.

Most blows to the nose result in swallowing of blood and hematoma formation without fracture. A persistent nosebleed after trauma, crepitus, instability of the bones in the nasal bridge, and deviation of the nose to one side indicate fracture. However, septal injury cannot be ruled out by radiography, and can only be ruled out by careful intranasal examination. Patients with suspected nasal fractures should be referred to an otolaryngologist for definitive therapy. Since the nasal bones begin healing within 7 days, the child must be seen by an otolaryngologist within 48–72 hours of the injury.

After nasal trauma, it is essential to examine the inside of the nose with a nasal speculum. Hematoma of the nasal septum imposes a considerable risk of pressure necrosis and resorption of the cartilage, leading to permanent nasal deformity that is very difficult to correct. This diagnosis is confirmed by the abrupt onset of nasal obstruction following trauma and the presence of a boggy, widened nasal septum. The normal nasal septum is only 2–4 mm thick. A cotton swab can be used to palpate the septum. Treatment consists of immediate referral to an otolaryngologist for evacuation of the hematoma and packing of the nose.

FOREIGN BODIES IN THE NOSE

The most common foreign bodies in the nose are seeds or beads. If the diagnosis is delayed, unilateral rhinorrhea, foul smell, halitosis, bleeding, or nasal obstruction may occur. The leading cause of halitosis in children is a nasal foreign body, and not dental disease as in adults.

There are many ways to remove nasal foreign bodies. The obvious first maneuver is vigorous nose blowing if the child is old enough. The next step in removal requires topical anesthesia, nasal decongestion, good lighting, correct instrumentation, and physical restraint. Topical tetracaine or lidocaine can be used in young children. Nasal decongestion can be achieved by topical pseudoephedrine or oxymetazoline. When the child is properly restrained, most nasal foreign bodies can be removed using a pair of alligator forceps through an operating head otoscope. If the object seems unlikely to be removed on the first attempt, is wedged in, or is quite large, the patient should be referred to an otolaryngologist rather than worsening the situation through futile attempts at removal.

Because the nose is a moist cavity, the electrical current generated by disk-type batteries—such as those used in clocks, watches, and hearing aids—can cause necrosis of mucosa and cartilage destruction in less than 4 hours. This constitutes a true foreign body emergency.

Kelley PE: Foreign bodies in the nose and pharynx. In: Burg FD et al (editors): *Gellis and Kagan's Current Pediatric Therapy*, 16th ed. WB Saunders, 1999.

THE THROAT & ORAL CAVITY

ACUTE STOMATITIS

1. Recurrent Aphthous Stomatitis

Also referred to as canker sores, these small ulcers (3–10 mm) are usually found on the inner aspect of the lips or on the tongue; rarely they may appear on the tonsils or palate. There is usually no associated fever and no cervical adenopathy. The ulcers may be painful and last 1–2 weeks. They may recur numerous times throughout life. The cause is unknown, although an allergic or autoimmune basis is suspected.

Treatment consists of coating the lesions with betamethasone valerate ointment twice daily, because unlike other topical corticosteroids, it adheres to the mucosa. Pain can also be reduced by eating a bland diet, avoiding salty or acidic foods and juices, and giving acetaminophen or ibuprofen.

Other less common causes of recurrent oral ulcers include Behçet disease, familial Mediterranean fever, and the FAPA syndrome (**F**ever, **A**phthous stomatitis, **P**haryngitis, and cervical **A**denopathy). FAPA syndrome was first described in 1987, and its cause is unknown. It usually begins before a child is 5 years of age and continues through adolescence, then resolves. It recurs at 4- to 6-week intervals, and an episode may be dramatically improved with prednisone bursts, but recurrences continue. In one case report it resolved totally with a 6-month course of cimetidine, suggesting an immune etiology. FAPA may also resolve with tonsillectomy (see later section on tonsillectomy), and an otolaryngology referral is appropriate. The ulcers in all of these syndromes respond to betamethasone valerate application. A diagnosis of Behçet disease requires two of the following: genital ulcers, uveitis, and erythema nodosum–like lesions. Patients with Mediterranean fever usually have a positive family history, serosal involvement, and recurrent fever.

Dahn KA et al: Periodic fever and pharyngitis in young children: A new disease for the otolaryngologist? Arch Otolaryngol Head Neck Surg 2000;126:1146 [PMID: 10979131].

2. Herpes Simplex Gingivostomatitis (See also Chapter 38)

Children having their first infection with the herpes simplex virus develop 10 or more small ulcers (1–3 mm) of the buccal mucosa, anterior pillars, inner lips, tongue, and especially the gingiva. The ulcers do not affect the posterior pharynx. The lesions are often associated with fever, tender cervical nodes, and generalized inflammation of the mouth, which precedes the development of the ulcers. Typically, exposure to the virus occurs 3–50 days prior to the onset of symptoms. Affected children are commonly younger than 3 years of age. Gingivostomatitis lasts 7–10 days. Treatment is symptomatic, as described earlier for recurrent aphthous stomatitis, with the exception that corticosteroids are contraindicated because they may cause spread of the infection. If the patient is seen early in the course, the physician should prescribe oral acyclovir suspension (200 mg/5 mL), 20 mg/kg per dose, four times daily for 5 days. The patient must be followed closely because dehydration occasionally develops, requiring hospitalization. Herpetic laryngotracheitis is a rare complication.

3. Thrush (See also Chapter 41)

Oral candidiasis mainly affects infants and occasionally older children in a debilitated state. *Candida albicans* is a saprophyte that normally is not invasive unless the mouth is abraded or the patient is immunocompromised. The use of broad-spectrum antibiotics and systemic or inhaled corticosteroids may be contributing factors. The symptoms include soreness of the mouth and refusal of feedings. Lesions consist of white curdlike plaques, predominantly on the buccal mucosa, which cannot be washed away after a feeding. Another less common variation of oral candidal infection is erythematous candidiasis, which produces erythematous patches on the palate and dorsum of the tongue. This condition is associated primarily with patients who are taking broad-spectrum antibiotics or corticosteroids, or are HIV-positive.

Specific treatment consists of nystatin oral suspension. Treatment may begin by removing large plaques with a moistened cotton-tipped applicator, and half the nystatin may be rubbed on the lesions with an applicator. Gentian violet is probably also effective, but it can severely stain clothing and skin. Patients who do not respond to oral therapy or who are immunocompromised may require systemic antifungal agents. The parents should be advised to replace any items, such as a pacifier, that may have become contaminated with *Candida*.

4. Traumatic Oral Ulcers

Mechanical trauma most commonly occurs on the buccal mucosa secondary to accidentally biting with the molars. Thermal trauma, from very hot foods, can also cause ulcerative lesions. Chemical ulcers can be produced by mucosal contact with aspirin, caustics, and the like. Oral ulcers can also occur with leukemia or on a recurrent basis with cyclic neutropenia.

PHARYNGITIS

Figure 17–9 is an algorithm for the management of a sore throat.

1. Acute Viral Pharyngitis & Tonsillitis

Over 90% of cases of sore throat and fever in children are due to viral infections. The findings seldom give any clue to the particular viral agent, but four types of viral pharyngitis are sufficiently distinctive to support an educated guess about the specific cause and are listed below.

▶ Clinical Findings

A. Infectious Mononucleosis

The findings are exudative tonsillitis, generalized cervical adenitis, and fever, usually in a patient older than 5 years of age. A palpable spleen or axillary adenopathy increases the likelihood of the diagnosis. The presence of more than 10% atypical lymphocytes on a peripheral blood smear or a positive mononucleosis spot test supports the diagnosis, although these tests are often falsely negative in children younger than age 5 years. Epstein-Barr virus serology showing an elevated IgM-capsid antibody is definitive. Clinicians should not prescribe amoxicillin for patients suspected of having mononucleosis because the drug often precipitates a rash and, in those with a viral infection, would be ineffective.

B. Herpangina

Herpangina ulcers are classically 3 mm in size and surrounded by a halo, and are found on the anterior pillars, the soft palate, and the uvula, but not the anterior mouth or tonsils. Herpangina is caused by several members of the coxsackie A group of viruses, and a patient may have several bouts of the ulcers. Enteroviral polymerase chain reaction testing, although now widely available, is not necessary as herpangina is a self-limiting illness.

C. Hand, Foot, and Mouth Disease

This entity is caused by several enteroviruses, only one of which (enterovirus 71) can rarely cause encephalitis. Ulcers occur anywhere in the mouth. Vesicles, pustules, or papules may be found on the palms, soles, interdigital areas, and buttocks. In younger children lesions may be seen on the distal extremities and even the face.

D. Pharyngoconjunctival Fever

This disorder is caused by an adenovirus and often is epidemic. Exudative tonsillitis, conjunctivitis, lymphadenopathy, and fever are the main findings, and treatment is symptomatic.

2. Acute Bacterial Pharyngitis

Approximately 10% of children with sore throat and fever have a group A streptococcal infection. Less common causes of bacterial pharyngitis are *Mycoplasma pneumoniae, Chlamydia pneumoniae,* groups C and G streptococci, and *Arcanobacterium hemolyticum.* Of the five, *M pneumoniae* is by far the most common and may cause over one third of all pharyngitis cases in adolescents and adults.

▶ Clinical Findings

Untreated streptococcal pharyngitis can result in acute rheumatic fever, glomerulonephritis, and suppurative complications (eg, cervical adenitis, peritonsillar abscess, otitis media, cellulitis, and septicemia). Anterior cervical nodes, palatal petechiae, a beefy-red uvula, and a tonsillar exudate suggest streptococcal infection; however, the only way to make a definitive diagnosis is by throat culture or rapid antigen test. Rapid antigen tests are very specific, but have a sensitivity of

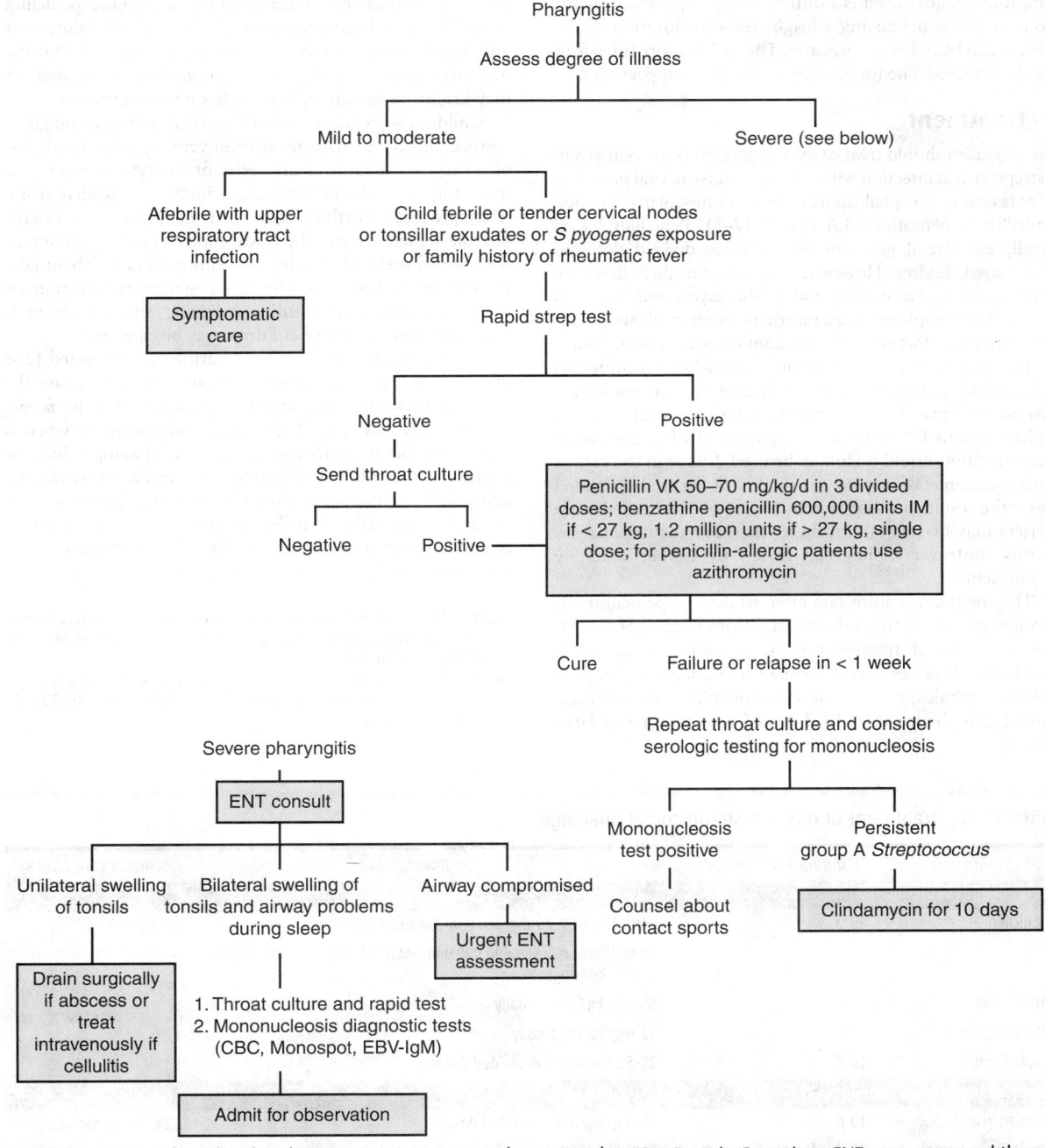

▲ **Figure 17–9.** Algorithm for pharyngitis. CBC, computed tomography; EBV, Epstein-Barr virus; ENT, ear, nose, and throat.

only 85–95%. Therefore, a positive test indicates *S pyogenes* infection, but a negative result requires confirmation by performing a culture. The presence of conjunctivitis, cough, hoarseness, symptoms of upper respiratory infection, ante-rior stomatitis, discrete ulcerative lesions, viral rash, and diarrhea should raise suspicion of a viral cause.

Occasionally, a child with group A streptococcal infection develops scarlet fever within 24–48 hours after the onset of symptoms. Scarlet fever is a diffuse, finely papular, erythematous eruption producing a bright red discoloration of the skin, which blanches on pressure. The rash is more intense in the skin creases. The tongue has a strawberry appearance.

▶ Treatment

The physician should treat cases of suspected or proven group A streptococcal infection with a 10-day course of oral penicillin V potassium, a cephalosporin, or intramuscularly injected penicillin G benzathine LA (Table 17–5). Penicillin VK is equally effective if given in two or three divided doses in school-aged children. However, in adolescents, three doses are recommended. Amoxicillin and azithromycin may be used once daily if compliance is a concern; however, both are broad-spectrum drugs that select for resistant nasopharyngeal flora.

The American Heart Association guidelines continue to recommend penicillin, with erythromycin for penicillin-allergic patients. A recent meta-analysis of trials of oral cephalosporins for streptococcal pharyngitis has concluded that penicillin should no longer be used. Just as in the case of otitis media meta-analyses, the quality of the trials included biases the results. In this case, inclusion of children who are carriers may bias certain of these trials. For further analysis of this controversy, the 2005 review by Gerber is highly recommended.

The treatment failure rate after 10 days of penicillin VK administered three times daily varies from 6–23%. However, over 50 years of treatment with penicillin, no group A streptococcal species have developed resistance to either penicillin or cephalosporins, so the cause of failure lies elsewhere. Patient compliance with 20 doses of medication is a large factor in failures, and intramuscular benzathine penicillin should be considered strongly in children who fail during or immediately after treatment. It has been suggested that the presence of β-lactamase–producing organisms in the pharynx may inactivate penicillin, but this has not been proven.

Children who fail to respond to treatment may be given amoxicillin–clavulanate or azithromycin. Approximately 5% of *S pyogenes* organisms are resistant to erythromycin, and trimethoprim–sulfamethoxazole is ineffective against group A streptococci. Further, because trimethoprim–sulfamethoxazole is ineffective in the eradication of pharyngeal organisms and is ineffective in the prevention of acute rheumatic fever when used as therapy for acute pharyngeal infections, it is not recommended. Routine culturing after treatment is not recommended, since children may be carriers.

In general, the carrier state is harmless, self-limited (2–6 months), and not contagious. An attempt to eradicate the carrier state is warranted only if the patient or another family member has frequent streptococcal infections or when a family member or patient has a history of rheumatic fever or glomerulonephritis. If eradication is chosen, a course of clindamycin for 10 days or of rifampin for 5 days should be used.

In the past, daily penicillin prophylaxis was occasionally recommended; however, to prevent development of drug resistance, tonsillectomy is now preferred.

Bisno AL: Are cephalosporins superior to penicillin for treatment of acute streptococcal pharyngitis? Clin Infect Dis 2004;38:1535 [PMID: 15156438].

Bisno AL et al: Practice guidelines for the diagnosis and management of group A streptococcal pharyngitis. Clin Infect Dis 2002;35:113 [PMID: 12087516].

Table 17–5. Treatment of group A streptococcal pharyngitis.

Drug	Duration of Therapy	Dose	Clinical Cure Rate
Treatment of acute pharyngitis			
Penicillin	10 d	Penicillin V 50-75 mg/kg/d in 3 divided doses	63–64%
		Benzathine penicillin 600,000 units IM if < 27 kg, 1.2 million units if > 27 kg, single dose	
Amoxicillin	10 d	50 mg/kg/d once daily	86%
Azithromycin	5 d	12 mg/kg once daily	82%
Cephalexin	10 d	25-50 mg/kg/d in divided doses	94%
Eradication of carrier state			
Clindamycin	10 d	20 mg/kg/d in 3 divided doses	92% for carrier state
Penicillin + rifampin	10 d (rifampin final 4 d)	Penicillin V 50-75 mg/kg/d in 3 divided doses	55%
		Benzathine penicillin 600,000 units IM if < 27 kg, 1.2 million units if > 27 kg, single dose	
		Rifampin 20 mg/kg/d twice daily for 4 d	

Reproduced, and adapted, courtesy of Children's Hospital, Denver, from Suchitra R, Todd J: Commonly asked questions about group A streptococcal pharyngitis. Contagious Comments 2007;XXII(4).

Casey JR, Pichichero ME: Meta-analysis of cephalosporin versus penicillin treatment of group A streptococcal tonsillopharyngitis in children. Pediatrics 2004;113:866 [PMID: 15156437].

Gerber MA: Diagnosis and treatment of pharyngitis in children. Pediatr Clin North Am 2005;52:729 [PMID: 15925660].

Shulman ST, Gerber MA: So what's wrong with penicillin for strep throat? Pediatrics 2004;113:1816 [PMID: 15173515].

PERITONSILLAR CELLULITIS OR ABSCESS (QUINSY)

Tonsillar infection occasionally penetrates the tonsillar capsule, spreads to the surrounding tissues, and causes peritonsillar cellulitis. If untreated, necrosis occurs and a tonsillar abscess forms. This can occur at any age. The most common cause is β-hemolytic streptococcal infection. Other pathogens are group D streptococci, β-hemolytic streptococci, S pneumoniae, and anaerobes.

The patient complains of a severe sore throat even before the physical findings become marked. A high fever is usually present, and the process is almost always unilateral. The tonsil bulges medially, and the anterior tonsillar pillar is prominent. The soft palate and uvula on the involved side are edematous and displaced toward the uninvolved side. In cases of abscess formation, trismus, ear pain, dysphagia, and eventually drooling occur. The most serious complication of inadequately treated peritonsillar abscess is a lateral pharyngeal abscess. This causes fullness and tenderness of the lateral neck as well as torticollis. Without intervention, the lateral pharyngeal abscess threatens life by airway obstruction or carotid artery erosion. If airway symptoms are present, an immediate otolaryngology consultation is indicated.

It is often difficult to differentiate peritonsillar cellulitis from abscess. In some children, it is possible to aspirate the peritonsillar space to diagnose and treat an abscess. However, it is reasonable to admit a child for 12–24 hours of intravenous antimicrobial therapy, because aggressive treatment in early cases of peritonsillar cellulitis usually prevents suppuration. Therapy with penicillin or clindamycin is appropriate. Failure to respond to therapy during the first 12–24 hours indicates a high probability of abscess formation. An otolaryngologist should be consulted for incision and drainage or for aspiration under local or general anesthesia. Prompt referral is indicated if the child is having respiratory difficulty.

Recurrent peritonsillar abscesses are so uncommon (7%) that routine tonsillectomy for a single bout is not indicated unless other tonsillectomy indications exist. Hospitalized patients can be discharged on oral antibiotics when fever has resolved for 24 hours and dysphagia has improved.

Schraff S et al: Peritonsillar abscess in children: a 10-year review of diagnosis and management. Int J Pediatr Otorhinolaryngol 2001;57:213 [PMID: 11223453].

RETROPHARYNGEAL ABSCESS

Retropharyngeal nodes drain the adenoids, nasopharynx, and paranasal sinuses and can become infected. The most common causes are β-hemolytic streptococci and S aureus. If this pyogenic adenitis goes untreated, a retropharyngeal abscess forms. The process occurs most commonly during the first 2 years of life. Beyond this age, retropharyngeal abscess usually results from superinfection of a penetrating injury of the posterior wall of the oropharynx.

The diagnosis of retropharyngeal abscess should be strongly suspected in an infant with fever, respiratory symptoms, and neck hyperextension. Dysphagia, drooling, dyspnea, and gurgling respirations are also found and are due to impingement by the abscess. Prominent swelling on one side of the posterior pharyngeal wall confirms the diagnosis. Swelling usually stops at the midline because a medial raphe divides the prevertebral space. Lateral neck soft tissue films show the retropharyngeal space to be wider than the C4 vertebral body.

Although retropharyngeal abscess is a surgical emergency, frequently it cannot be distinguished from retropharyngeal adenitis. Immediate hospitalization and intravenous antimicrobial therapy with a semisynthetic penicillin or clindamycin is the first step for most cases. Immediate surgical drainage is required when a definite abscess is seen radiographically or when the airway is compromised markedly. In most instances, a period of 12–24 hours of antimicrobial therapy will help to differentiate the two entities. In the child with adenitis, fever will decrease and oral intake will increase. A child with retropharyngeal abscess will continue to deteriorate. A surgeon should incise and drain the abscess under general anesthesia to prevent its extension.

LUDWIG ANGINA

Ludwig angina is a rapidly progressive cellulitis of the submandibular space that can cause airway obstruction and death. The submandibular space extends from the mucous membrane of the floor of the mouth to the muscular and fascial attachments of the hyoid bone. This infection is encountered infrequently in infants and children. The initiating factor in over 50% of cases is dental disease, including abscesses and extraction. Some patients have a history of lacerations and injuries to the floor of the mouth. Group A streptococci are the most common organism identified, but other pathogens cause the infection.

The manifestations are fever and tender swelling of the floor of the mouth. The tongue can become enlarged as well as tender and erythematous. Upward displacement of the tongue may cause dysphagia, drooling, and airway obstruction.

Treatment consists of giving high doses of intravenous clindamycin or ampicillin plus nafcillin until the results of cultures and sensitivity tests are available. Because the most common cause of death in Ludwig angina is sudden airway obstruction, the patient must be monitored closely in the intensive care unit and intubation provided for progressive respiratory distress. An otolaryngologist should be consulted to identify and perform a drainage procedure.

Britt JC et al: Ludwig's angina in the pediatric population: Report of a case and review of the literature. Int J Pediatr Otorhinolaryngol 2000;52:79 [PMID: 10699244].

ACUTE CERVICAL ADENITIS

Local infections of the ear, nose, and throat can involve a regional node and form an abscess. The typical case involves a unilateral, solitary, anterior cervical node. About 70% of these cases are due to β-hemolytic streptococcal infection, 20% to staphylococci, and the remainder to viruses, atypical mycobacteria, and *Bartonella henselae*. Methicillin-resistant *S aureus* (MRSA) must also be considered.

The initial evaluation of cervical adenitis should generally include a rapid group A streptococcal test, a complete blood count with differential looking for atypical lymphocytes, and a purified protein derivative skin test, looking for nontuberculous mycobacteria. If multiple enlarged nodes are found in addition to the sentinel node, a rapid mononucleosis test is useful. Early treatment with antibiotics prevents many cases of adenitis from progressing to suppuration. However, once fluctuation occurs, antibiotic therapy alone is often insufficient and needle aspiration may promote resolution. Depending on abscess size, an incision and drainage procedure may be necessary. Because of the increase in community acquired MRSA, it is a prudent to send a specimen for culture and sensitivity.

Cat-scratch disease is caused by *B henselae* and is the most frequent cause of indolent ("cold") adenopathy. The diagnosis is aided by the finding of a primary papule at the scratch site on the face. In over 90% of patients, there is a history of contact with kittens. The node is usually only mildly tender but may, over a month or more, suppurate and drain. About one third of children have fever and malaise, and rarely neurologic sequelae and prolonged fever occur. Cat-scratch disease can be diagnosed by serologic testing available at commercial laboratories, but testing is not always confirmatory. Blood should be drawn 2–8 weeks after onset of symptoms. Because most nodes caused by this pathogen spontaneously resorb within 1–3 months, the benefit of antibiotics is controversial. In a placebo-controlled trial, azithromycin for 5 days caused a more rapid decrease in node size. Other drugs likely to be effective include rifampin, trimethoprim–sulfamethoxazole, erythromycin, clarithromycin, doxycycline, ciprofloxacin, and gentamicin.

Cervical lymphadenitis can be caused by nontuberculous mycobacterial species or *Mycobacterium avium* complex. Mycobacterial disease is unilateral and may involve several matted nodes, and poor dentition may provide an entry portal. A characteristic violaceous appearance may develop over a prolonged period of time without systemic signs or much local pain. Atypical mycobacterial infections are often associated with positive purified protein derivative skin test

reactions less than 10 mm in diameter, and a second-strength (250-test-unit) purified protein derivative skin test is virtually always positive.

▶ Differential Diagnosis

A. Neoplasms and Cervical Nodes

Malignant tumors usually are not suspected until the adenopathy persists despite antibiotic treatment. Classically, the nodes are painless, nontender, and firm to hard in consistency. They may be fixed to underlying tissues. These nodes may occur as a single node, as unilateral nodes in a chain, bilateral cervical nodes, or generalized adenopathy. Common malignancies that may manifest in the neck include Hodgkin disease, non-Hodgkin lymphoma, rhabdomyosarcoma, and thyroid carcinoma.

B. Imitators of Adenitis

Several structures in the neck can become infected and resemble a node. The first three masses are of congenital origin and are listed in order of frequency.

1. Thyroglossal duct cyst—When superinfected, this congenital malformation can become acutely swollen. Helpful findings are the fact that it is in the midline, located between the hyoid bone and suprasternal notch, and moves upward when the tongue is stuck out or during swallowing. Occasionally, the cyst develops a sinus tract and opening just lateral to the midline.

2. Branchial cleft cyst—When superinfected, this malformation can become a tender mass 3–5 cm in diameter. Aids to diagnosis are the fact that the mass is located along the anterior border of the sternocleidomastoid muscle and is smooth and fluctuant. Occasionally it is attached to the overlying skin by a small dimple or a draining sinus tract.

3. Lymphatic malformation—Most of these lymphatic cysts are located in the posterior triangle just above the clavicle. The mass is soft and compressible and can be transilluminated. Over 60% of lymphatic malformations are noted at birth; the remaining malformations are usually seen by the time the child is age 2 years. If cysts become large enough, they can compromise the patient's ability to swallow and breathe.

4. Parotitis—The most common pitfall is mistaking parotitis for cervical adenitis. However, a swollen parotid crosses the angle of the jaw, is associated with preauricular percussion tenderness, and is bilateral in 70% of cases. There may be a history of exposure to mumps, but in the United States viruses such as parainfluenza are now the main cause. An amylase level will be elevated in parotitis.

5. Ranula—A ranula is a cyst in the floor of the mouth caused by obstruction of the ducts of the sublingual gland. A plunging ranula extends below the mylohyoid muscle and can appear as a neck mass.

6. Sternocleidomastoid muscle hematoma—This cervical mass is noted at age 2–4 weeks. On close examination, it is found to be part of the muscle body and not movable. An associated torticollis usually confirms the diagnosis.

Fennelly GJ: *Mycobacterium bovis* versus *Mycobacterium tuberculosis* as a cause of acute cervical lymphadenitis without pulmonary disease. Pediatr Infect Dis J 2004;23:590 [PMID: 15194851].
Peters TR, Edwards KM: Cervical lymphadenopathy and adenitis. Pediatr Rev 2000;21:399 [PMID: 11121496].

SNORING, MOUTH BREATHING, & UPPER AIRWAY OBSTRUCTION

In April 2002, the American Academy of Pediatrics published a clinical practice guideline for the diagnosis and management of uncomplicated childhood obstructive sleep apnea syndrome. Currently, OSA is considered just one component of a broader spectrum of disease known as sleep-disordered breathing (SDB) that ranges from primary snoring (isolated snoring without apnea, arousals, or gas-exchange abnormalities) to upper airway resistance syndrome (UARS) to OSA. Historically, primary snoring (PS) had not been considered to be pathologic so surgery was felt to be unnecessary. The guideline emphasizes that pediatricians should screen all children for snoring and that complex high-risk patients should be referred to a specialist.

Clinical Evaluation & Management

When parents report that their child has nightly snoring and is a mouth breather even during the day, one should be suspicious of OSA. In a healthy child, evaluation of three symptoms and signs can help determine the need for polysomnography or surgery.

1. Nighttime symptoms: habitual snoring along with gasping, pauses, or struggling to breathe.
2. Daytime symptoms: unrefreshed sleep, attention deficit, hyperactivity, emotional lability, temperamental behavior, poor weight gain, and daytime fatigue.
3. Enlarged tonsils.

If all three findings are present, some clinicians would consider proceeding with surgery without polysomnography. If the three findings cannot be confirmed but the child has other indications for an adenotonsillectomy—ie, recurrent tonsillitis, markedly enlarged (4+) tonsils with dysphagia—surgery is also scheduled.

Figure 17–10 is an algorithm for management of these complaints. The pathway relies on clinical symptoms and tonsil size. Low muscle tone also contributes to an individual's propensity to experience SDB. However, measurement of muscle tone is not straightforward. Although the pathway states that an asymptomatic child with markedly enlarged tonsils (4+) should undergo an overnight poly-

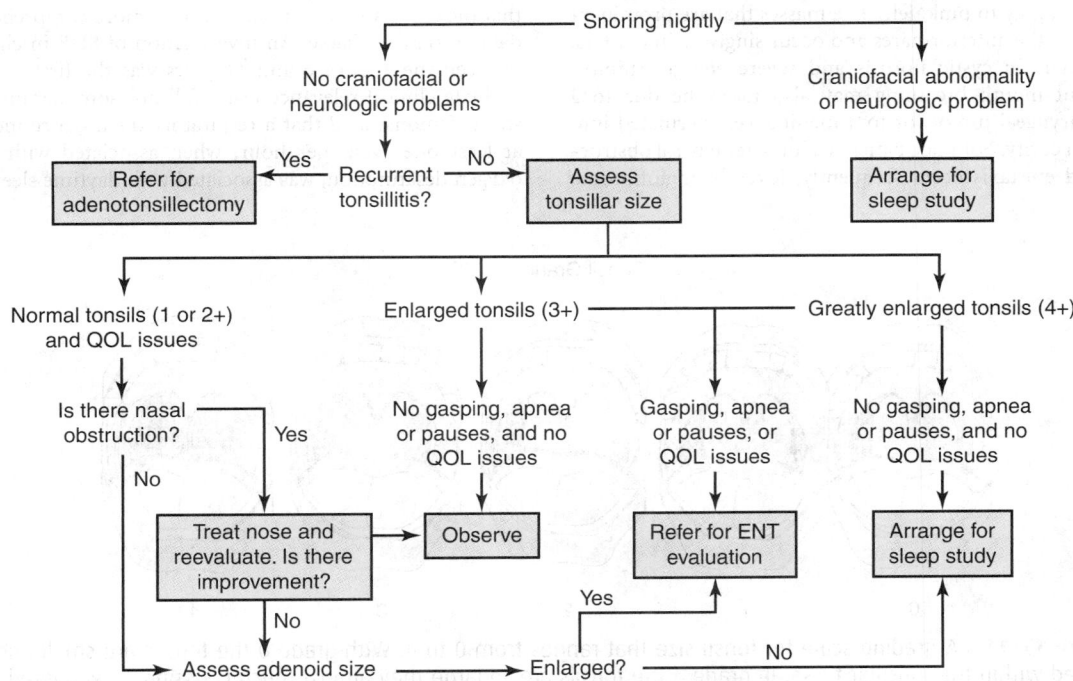

▲ **Figure 17–10.** Algorithm for snoring. ENT, ear, nose and throat; QOL, quality of life.

somnographic study, a period of observation is reasonable. One's clinical suspicion of SDB should be heightened in the presence of enlarged tonsils, especially if the parents cannot provide a reliable history. If the child has no clinical symptoms and the tonsils are only moderately enlarged (3+), observation is appropriate. Educating the parents about the risks of SDB and what to look for is paramount.

A polysomnographic study is recommended for a child who has no adenotonsillar hypertrophy with a patent nose but significant daytime symptoms of SDB. Other conditions, especially a periodic limb movement disorder, may mimic SDB. If the polysomnogram does detect SDB in a child with no adenotonsillar hypertrophy, a complete evaluation of the upper airway by flexible laryngoscopy should be performed to look for other possible sites of obstruction: base of tongue, lingual tonsils, hypopharynx or larynx.

The adenoids can also be assessed by radiographic studies. Either adenoid hypertrophy or nasal obstruction can be assumed when a child has hyponasal speech. The consonants "m," "n," and "ng" rely on the palate not touching the posterior pharyngeal wall. By having a child repeat the word "banana" or "ninety-nine" with the nose open or pinched closed, one may assess the nasal and nasopharyngeal airways. If the voice does not change with occlusion of the nostrils, then either adenoid or nasal obstruction is present.

Although nasal obstruction is usually due to allergic rhinitis and can be diagnosed by a careful allergy history, there are other less common causes. Nasal polyps appear as glistening, gray to pink, jelly-like masses that are prominent just inside the anterior nares and occur singly or in clusters. They occur in cystic fibrosis and severe allergic rhinitis. Persistent mouth breathing may also rarely be due to a nasopharyngeal tumor, or to a meningocele herniated into the nasal cavity. For male patients, if unilateral nasal obstruction and epistaxis occur frequently, juvenile angiofibroma

should be suspected. If allergic rhinitis is the suspected cause of snoring, a trial of intranasal corticosteroid spray is indicated. If enlarged tonsils (Figure 17–11) or adenoids are present, a referral to an otolaryngologist or a pediatric sleep laboratory is in order.

Polysomnography

The gold standard for diagnosis of OSA is a polysomnogram. A patient's history and clinical examination cannot predict the presence or severity of OSA. Similarly, an overnight oximetry study is a poor screening test for OSA; it may detect patients with severe disease but miss those with milder forms, such as upper airway resistance syndrome. Patients with this syndrome have an otherwise normal polysomnogram with the only evidence of obstruction being increased respiratory effort.

The criteria for diagnosing OSA differ between children and adults. An obstructive event occurs when airflow stops despite persistence of respiratory effort. A hypopnea episode is counted when airflow and respiratory effort decrease with an associated oxygen desaturation or arousal. Normative values are just being established. The revised edition of the *International Classification of Sleep Disorders,* published by the American Academy of Sleep Medicine (AASM), states that for children, the occurrence of more than one apneic or hypopneic event per hour with duration of at least two respiratory cycles is abnormal. However, the diagnostic committee of the AASM qualified its recommendation, stating that the criteria may be modified once more comprehensive data become available. An investigation of SDB in children between the ages of 6 and 11 years was the first study to evaluate clinical relevance using full polysomnograms. The study demonstrated that a respiratory disturbance index of at least one event per hour, when associated with a 3% oxygen desaturation, was associated with daytime sleepiness

Tonsil Grade

0   1   2   3   4

▲ **Figure 17–11.** A grading scale for tonsil size that ranges from 0 to 4. With grade 0 the tonsils are small and contained within the tonsillar fossa; in grade 4 the tonsils are so large they almost touch ("kissing"). (Reprinted, with permission, from Brodksy L: Modern assessment of tonsils and adenoids. Pediatr Clin North Am 1989;36:1551.)

and learning problems. If oxygen desaturations were absent, a respiratory disturbance index of five events per hour was associated with clinical symptoms.

Although an obstructive apnea index of greater than one event may be statistically significant, whether it is clinically relevant remains unclear. Any child with an apnea-plus-hypopnea index of greater than five events per hour appears to have clinically significant SDB. The dilemma is how to manage children with an apnea-plus-hypopnea index of more than one but fewer than five events per hour as some of these children do experience neurocognitive symptoms.

Complications & Sequelae

The importance of diagnosing OSA and SDB in children cannot be underestimated. Recent studies have shown that teenagers who are loud snorers exhibit impaired school performance, and that behavioral problems are associated with OSA. Likewise, a recent comprehensive review of the literature by Beebe provides a strong argument that SDB affects neurocognition and behavior.

Beebe DW: Neurobehavioral morbidity associated with disordered breathing during sleep in children: A comprehensive review. Sleep 2006;29:1115 [PMID: 17040000].

Clinical Practice Guideline: Diagnosis and management of childhood obstructive sleep apnea syndrome. Pediatrics 2002;109:704 [PMID: 11927718].

Goodwin JL et al: Clinical outcomes associated with sleep-disordered breathing in Caucasian and Hispanic children—the Tucson Children's Assessment of Sleep Apnea study (Tu-CASA). Sleep 2003;26:587 [PMID: 12853523].

Montgomery-Downs HE, et al: Snoring and sleep-disordered breathing in young children: Subjective and objective correlates. Sleep 2004;27:87 [PMID: 14998242].

O'Brien LM et al: Neurobehavioral implications of habitual snoring in children. Pediatrics 2004;114:44 [PMID: 15231906].

Ossowski K et al: Increased isolation of methicillin-resistant Staphylococcus aureus in pediatric head and neck abscesses. Arch Otolaryngol Head Neck Surg 2006;132:1176 [PMID: 17116811].

Schechter MS: Technical report: Diagnosis and management of childhood obstructive sleep apnea syndrome. Pediatrics 2002;109:e69 [PMID: 11927742].

Web Resources

American Academy of Sleep Medicine educational site: http://www.sleepeducation.com

Child-friendly web site: http://www.sleepforkids.org/

Children's Hospital web site: http://www.thechildrenshospital.org/public/cs/detail.cfm?RecordID=407

National Sleep Foundation: http://www.sleepfoundation.org/

TONSILLECTOMY & ADENOIDECTOMY

Tonsillectomy

A tonsillectomy with or without adenoidectomy is typically performed for either hypertrophy or recurrent infections. Nowadays, the most common indication for an adenotonsillectomy is adenotonsillar hypertrophy that is associated with an obstructed breathing pattern at night (see earlier discussion of OSA and SDB). Besides producing airway obstruction, adenotonsillar hypertrophy may produce dysphagia or dental malocclusion. Rarely, hypertrophied tonsils may produce pulmonary hypertension or cor pulmonale. Recurrent infections are present when a child has seven or more documented *S pyogenes* infections in 1 year, five per year for 2 years, or three per year for 3 years. A tonsillectomy is reasonable if fewer infections are present but the child has missed multiple school days or has a complicated course. Recurrent peritonsillar abscesses and persistent streptococcal carrier state are other indications, as well as unilateral tonsillar hypertrophy that appears neoplastic.

A possible new indication is FAPA syndrome (see section on Recurrent Aphthous Stomatitis, earlier), in which the fever is predictable and commonly occurs every 4–8 weeks. Removal of the tonsils was shown to relieve the symptoms in five children in one recent study.

Recently, a proliferation of new surgical techniques has occurred that can potentially reduce the morbidity associated with an adenotonsillectomy.

Dahn KA et al: Periodic fever and pharyngitis in young children. Arch Otolaryngol Head Neck Surg 2000;126:1146 [PMID: 10979131].

Darrow DH, Siemens C: Indications for tonsillectomy and adenoidectomy. Laryngoscope 2002;112(8 Pt 2 Suppl 100):6.

Derkay CS, Maddern BR: Innovative techniques for adenotonsillar surgery in children. Laryngoscope 2002;112(8 Pt 2):2 [PMID: 12172227].

Gigante J: Tonsillectomy and adenoidectomy. Pediatr Rev 2005;26:199 [PMID: 15930327].

Web Resources

American Academy of Otolaryngology/Head and Neck Surgery–sponsored site dedicated to children: http://www.entnet.org/kidsent/

Adenoidectomy

The adenoids, composed of lymphoid tissue in the nasopharynx, are a component of the Waldeyer ring of lymphoid tissue, which also includes the palatine tonsils and lingual tonsils. Enlargement of the adenoids with or without infection can obstruct the upper airway, alter normal orofacial growth, and interfere with speech, swallowing, or eustachian tube function. Most children with prolonged mouth breathing eventually develop dental malocclusion and what has been termed an adenoidal facies. The face is pinched and the maxilla narrowed because the molding pressures of the orbicularis oris and buccinator muscles are unopposed by the tongue. The role of hypertrophy and chronic infection in the pathogenesis of rhinosinusitis is unclear, but adenoidectomy has been shown to be effective in some patients with chronic rhinosinusitis.

Indications for adenoidectomy with or without tonsillectomy include pulmonary conditions such as chronic hypoxia related to upper airway obstruction; orofacial conditions such as mandibular growth abnormalities and dental malocclusion; speech abnormalities; persistent middle ear effusion; recurrent and chronic otitis media; and chronic rhinosinusitis.

Complications of Tonsillectomy & Adenoidectomy

The reported mortality rates associated with tonsillectomy and adenoidectomy now approximate that of general anesthesia alone. The rate of hemorrhage varies between 0.1% and 8.1% depending on the definition of hemorrhage; the rate of postoperative transfusion is 0.04%. Other complications include hypernasal speech (< 0.01%), and more rarely nasopharyngeal stenosis, atlantoaxial subluxation, mandible condyle fracture, and psychological trauma.

Contraindications to Tonsillectomy & Adenoidectomy

A. Short Palate

Adenoids should not be removed completely in a child with a cleft palate or submucous cleft palate because of the risk of aggravating the velopharyngeal incompetence and causing hypernasal speech and nasal regurgitation. A superior or partial adenoidectomy can be performed in a child with marked OSA who has a submucous cleft palate or ongoing conductive hearing loss from middle ear effusion.

B. Bleeding Disorder

If a chronic bleeding disorder is present, it must be diagnosed and treated before tonsillectomy and adenoidectomy.

C. Acute Tonsillitis

An elective tonsillectomy and adenoidectomy can often be postponed until acute tonsillitis is resolved. Urgent tonsillectomy may be required for tonsillitis unresponsive to medical therapy.

DISORDERS OF THE LIPS

1. Labial Sucking Tubercle

A young infant may present with a small callus in the mid-upper lip. It usually is asymptomatic and disappears after cup feeding is initiated.

2. Cheilitis

Dry, cracked, scaling lips are usually caused by sun or wind exposure. Contact dermatitis from mouthpieces or various woodwind or brass instruments has also been reported. Licking the lips accentuates the process, and the patient should be warned of this. Liberal use of lip balms gives excellent results.

3. Inclusion Cyst

Inclusion (retention) cysts are due to the obstruction of mucous glands or other mucous membrane structures. In the newborn, they occur on the hard palate or gums and are called Epstein pearls. These small cysts resolve spontaneously in 1–2 months. In older children, inclusion cysts usually occur on the palate, uvula, or tonsillar pillars. They appear as taut yellow sacs varying in size from 2–10 mm. Inclusion cysts that do not resolve spontaneously may undergo incision and drainage. Occasionally a mucous cyst on the lower lip (mucocele) requires excision for cosmetic reasons. Mucoceles pathologically are a blocked minor salivary gland.

DISORDERS OF THE TONGUE

1. Geographic Tongue (Benign Migratory Glossitis)

This condition of unknown cause occurs in 1–2% of the population with no age, sex, or racial predilection and is characterized by irregularly shaped areas on the tongue that are devoid of papillae and surrounded by parakeratotic reddish borders. The pattern changes as alternating regeneration and desquamation occurs. The lesions are generally asymptomatic and require no treatment.

2. Fissured Tongue (Scrotal Tongue)

This condition is marked by numerous irregular fissures on the dorsum of the tongue. It occurs in approximately 1% of the population and is usually a dominant trait. It is also frequently seen in children with trisomy 21 and other developmentally delayed patients who have the habit of chewing on a protruded tongue.

3. Coated Tongue (Furry Tongue)

The tongue normally becomes coated if mastication is impaired and the patient is taking a liquid or soft diet. Mouth breathing, fever, or dehydration can accentuate the process.

4. Macroglossia

Tongue hypertrophy and protrusion may be a clue to trisomy 21, Beckwith-Wiedemann syndrome, glycogen storage disease, cretinism, mucopolysaccharide storage disease, lymphangioma, or hemangioma. Tongue reduction procedures should be considered in otherwise healthy subjects when macroglossia affects airway patency.

HALITOSIS

Bad breath is usually due to acute stomatitis, pharyngitis, rhinosinusitis, a nasal foreign body, or dental hygiene problems. In older children and adolescents, halitosis can be a manifestation of chronic rhinosinusitis, gastric bezoar, bronchiectasis, or lung abscess. The presence of orthodontic devices or dentures can cause halitosis if good dental hygiene is not maintained. Halitosis can also be caused by decaying food particles embedded in cryptic tonsils. In adolescents, tobacco use is a common cause. Mouthwashes and chewable breath fresheners give limited improvement. Treatment of the underlying cause is indicated, and a dental referral may be in order.

Cicek Y et al: Effect of tongue brushing on oral malodor in adolescents. Pediatr Int 2003;45:719 [PMID: 14651548].

SALIVARY GLAND DISORDERS

1. Parotitis

A first episode of parotitis may safely be considered to be of viral origin, unless fluctuance is present. The leading cause was mumps until adoption of vaccination; now the leading viruses are parainfluenza and Epstein-Barr virus. HIV infection should be considered if the child is known to be at risk.

2. Suppurative Parotitis

Suppurative parotitis is an uncommon clinical disorder occurring chiefly in newborns and debilitated elderly patients. The parotid gland is swollen, tender, and often reddened, usually unilaterally. The diagnosis is made by expression of purulent material from the Stensen duct. The material should be smeared and cultured. Fever and leukocytosis may be present.

Treatment includes hospitalization and intravenous nafcillin because the most common causative organism is *S aureus*.

3. Recurrent Idiopathic Parotitis

Some children experience repeated episodes of parotid swelling that last 1–2 weeks and then resolve spontaneously, or can become infected and require antibiotics for resolution. There is usually pain and often no fever. The process is most often unilateral, suggesting some sort of obstructive process, but can be associated with Sjögren syndrome, another autoimmune process, HIV infection, or a calculus in the parotid duct. Serum amylase levels are normal, which speaks against a diagnosis of viral parotitis. Recently increased IgA levels have been found in these children. Many episodes occur from age 2 years on. The problem often resolves spontaneously at puberty.

Treatment includes analgesics if pain is present and an antistaphylococcal antibiotic for prophylaxis of infection and quicker resolution at the onset of symptoms. A second attack of parotid swelling without fever should result in referral to an otolaryngologist to make the diagnosis.

Fazekas T: Selective IgA deficiency in children with recurrent parotitis of childhood. Pediatr Infect Dis J 2005;24:461 [PMID: 15876950].

4. Tumors of the Parotid Gland

Mixed tumors, hemangiomas, sarcoidosis, and leukemia can be manifested in the parotid gland as a hard or persistent mass. A cystic mass or multiple cystic masses may represent an HIV infection. Workup may require consultation with oncology, infectious diseases, hematology, and otolaryngology.

5. Ranula

A ranula is a retention cyst of a sublingual salivary gland. It occurs on the floor of the mouth to one side of the lingual frenulum. Ranula has been described as resembling a frog's belly because it is thin-walled and contains a clear bluish fluid. Referral to an otolaryngologist for excision of the cyst and associated sublingual gland is the treatment of choice.

CONGENITAL ORAL MALFORMATIONS

1. Tongue-Tie (Ankyloglossia)

The tightness of the lingual frenulum varies greatly among normal people. A short frenulum prevents both protrusion and elevation of the tongue. Puckering of the midline of the tongue occurring with tongue movement is noted on physical examination.

When mild, treatment consists of reassurance. If the tongue cannot protrude past the teeth or alveolar ridge or move between the gums and cheek, referral to an otolaryngologist or dentist for evaluation is indicated. Frenulectomy may be recommended if there is a question of suckling difficulties, dental health (related to the inability to clear food from around the teeth), or articulation problems. A frenulectomy should be performed in the neonatal period if the infant is having difficulty latching onto the breast. In our practice, a neonatal frenulectomy is performed in clinic.

Messner AH, Lalakea ML: Ankyloglossia: Controversies in management. Int J Pediatr Otorhinolaryngol 2000;54:123 [PMID: 10967382].
Messner AH, Lalakea ML: The effect of ankyloglossia on speech in children. Otolaryngol Head Neck Surg 2002;127:539 [PMID: 12501105].

2. Torus Palatini

Hard midline masses on the palate are called torus palatini. They are bony protrusions that form at suture lines of bone. Usually they are asymptomatic and require no therapy. They can be surgically reduced if necessary.

3. Cleft Lip & Cleft Palate (See Chapter 35)

A. Submucous Cleft Palate

A bifid uvula is present in 3% of healthy children. However, a close association exists (as high as 75%) between bifid uvula and submucous cleft palate. A submucous cleft can be diagnosed by noting a translucent zone in the middle of the soft palate (zona pellucida). Palpation of the hard palate reveals absence of the posterior bony protrusion. Affected children have a 40% risk of developing persistent middle ear effusion. They are at risk also of incomplete closure of the palate, resulting in hypernasal speech. During feeding, some of these infants experience nasal regurgitation of food. Children with submucous cleft palate causing abnormal speech or nasal regurgitation of food require referral for surgical repair.

B. High-Arched Palate

A high-arched palate is usually a genetic trait of no consequence. It also occurs in children who are chronic mouth breathers and in premature infants who undergo prolonged oral intubation. Some rare causes of high-arched palate are congenital disorders such as Marfan syndrome, Treacher Collins syndrome, and Ehlers-Danlos syndrome.

C. Pierre Robin Sequence

This group of congenital malformations is characterized by the triad of micrognathia, cleft palate, and glossoptosis. Affected children present as emergencies in the newborn period because of infringement on the airway by the tongue. The main objective of treatment is to prevent asphyxia until the mandible becomes large enough to accommodate the tongue. In some cases, this objective can be achieved by leaving the child in a prone position while unattended. Other airway manipulations such as a nasal trumpet may be necessary. Recently distraction osteogenesis has been used to avoid tracheostomy. In severe cases, a tracheostomy is required. The child requires close observation and careful feeding until the problem is outgrown.

Denny A, Amm C: New technique for airway correction in neonates with severe Pierre Robin sequence. J Pediatr 2005;147:97 [PMID: 16027704].

Respiratory Tract & Mediastinum

Gwendolyn S. Kerby, MD

Robin R. Deterding, MD

Vivek Balasubramaniam, MD

Scott D. Sagel, MD

Keith L. Cavanaugh, MD

Monica J. Federico, MD

▼ RESPIRATORY TRACT

Pediatric pulmonary diseases account for almost 50% of deaths in children younger than age 1 year and about 20% of all hospitalizations of children younger than age 15 years. Approximately 7% of children have a chronic disorder of the lower respiratory system. Understanding the pathophysiology of many pediatric pulmonary diseases requires an appreciation of the normal growth and development of the lung.

GROWTH & DEVELOPMENT

The lung has its origins from an outpouching of the foregut during the fourth week of gestation. The development of the lung is divided into five overlapping stages.

1. *Embryonic stage* (3–7 weeks' gestation). During this stage, the primitive lung bud undergoes asymmetrical branching and then subsequent dichotomous branching, leading to the development of the conducting airways. This stage of lung development is dependent on a complex interaction of various growth factors originating in both the pulmonary epithelium and the splanchnic mesenchyme. It also sees the development of the large pulmonary arteries from the sixth aortic arch and the pulmonary veins as outgrowths of the left atrium. Abnormalities during this stage result in congenital abnormalities such as lung aplasia, tracheoesophageal fistula, and congenital pulmonary cysts.

2. *Pseudoglandular stage* (5–17 weeks' gestation). During this stage, which overlaps with the embryonic stage, the lung has a glandular appearance and witnesses the completion of the conducting airways (bronchi and bronchioles). The respiratory epithelium of these airways begins to differentiate, and the presence of cartilage, smooth muscle cells, and mucus glands are first seen. In addition, the pleuroperitoneal cavity divides into two distinct compartments. Abnormalities during this stage lead to

pulmonary sequestration, cystic adenomatoid malformation, and congenital diaphragmatic hernia.

3. *Canalicular stage* (16–26 weeks' gestation). This stage witnesses the delineation of the pulmonary acinus. The alveolar type II cells differentiate into type I cells, the pulmonary capillary network develops, and the alveolar type I cells closely approximate with the developing capillary network. Abnormalities of development during this stage include neonatal respiratory distress syndrome and lung hypoplasia.

4. *Saccular stage* (26–36 weeks' gestation). During this stage further branching of the terminal saccules takes place as well as a thinning of the interstitium and fusion of the type I cell and capillary basement membrane in preparation for the lungs' function as a gas-exchange organ.

5. *Alveolar stage* (36 weeks' gestation to 3–8 years of age). Controversy surrounds the length of this stage of lung development. This stage witnesses secondary septal formation, further sprouting of the capillary network, and the development of true alveoli. Abnormalities during this stage lead to lung hypoplasia and can result in the development of bronchopulmonary dysplasia.

At birth, the lung assumes the gas-exchanging function served by the placenta in utero, placing immediate stress on all components of the respiratory system. Abnormalities in the lung, respiratory muscles, chest wall, airway, respiratory controller, or pulmonary circulation may therefore be present at birth. Survival after delivery depends, for example, on the development of the surfactant system to maintain airspace stability and allow gas exchange. Immaturity of the surfactant system, often seen in infants born before 35 weeks' gestational age, can result in severe respiratory morbidity in the immediate neonatal period as well as subsequent chronic lung disease. A lethal form of lung disease has been recognized in infants homozygous for abnormalities in the gene for surfactant protein B. Persistent pulmonary hypertension of the newborn (failure of the normal transition to a low-resistance pulmonary circulation at birth) can complicate several neonatal respiratory diseases. There is mounting evidence that abnormalities during fetal and neonatal growth and development of the lung have long-standing effects into adulthood, such as reduced gas exchange, exercise intolerance, asthma, and an increased risk of chronic obstructive pulmonary disease.

Barker DJ: The intrauterine origins of cardiovascular and obstructive lung disease in adult life: The Marc Daniels Lecture 1990. J R Coll Physicians Lond 1991;25:129 [PMID: 2066923].

Bogue CW: Genetic and molecular basis of airway and lung development. In Haddad GG et al (editors): *Basic Mechanisms of Pediatric Respiratory Disease*. BC Decker, 2002.

Burri P: Structural aspects of prenatal and postnatal development and growth of the lung. In McDonald JA (editor): *Lung Growth and Development*. BC Dekker, 1997.

Wharburton D et al: Molecular mechanisms of early lung specification and branching morphogenesis. Pediatr Res 2005;57(5 Pt 2)26R [PMID: 15817505].

DIAGNOSTIC AIDS

PHYSICAL EXAMINATION OF THE RESPIRATORY TRACT

The four components of a complete pulmonary examination include: inspection, palpation, auscultation, and percussion. *Inspection* of respiratory rate, depth, ease, symmetry, and rhythm of respiration is critical to the detection of pulmonary disease. In young children, an elevated respiratory rate may be an initial indicator of pneumonia or hypoxemia. In a study of children with respiratory illnesses, abnormalities of attentiveness, consolability, respiratory effort, color, and movement had a good diagnostic accuracy in detecting hypoxemia. *Palpation* of tracheal position, symmetry of chest wall movement, and vibration with vocalization can help in identifying intrathoracic abnormalities. A shift in tracheal position can suggest pneumothorax or significant atelectasis. Tactile fremitus may change with the presence of consolidation or air in the pleural space. Other helpful noise transmission tests include whispered pectoriloquy, bronchophony, and egophony. Although chest radiography has replaced the utility of these tests, they can be helpful when imaging is not available. *Auscultation* should assess the quality of breath sounds and detect the presence of abnormal sounds such as fine or coarse crackles, wheezing, or rhonchi. It is important to know the lung anatomy in order to identify the location of abnormal findings (Figure 18–1). In older patients, unilateral crackles are the most valuable examination finding in pneumonia. *Percussion* may identify tympanic or dull sounds that can help define an intrathoracic process. (This component of the examination can prove challenging in young children, who may not cooperate.) Extrapulmonary manifestations of pulmonary disease include growth failure, altered mental status (from hypoxemia or hypercapnia), cyanosis, clubbing, and osteoarthropathy. Evidence of cor pulmonale (loud pulmonic

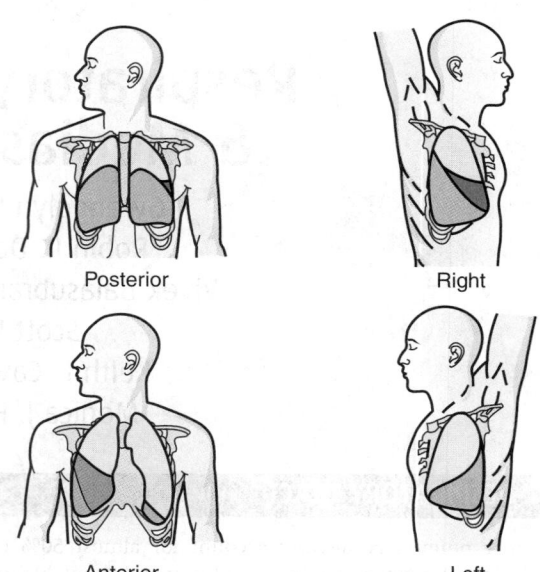

Posterior   Right

Anterior   Left

▲ **Figure 18–1.** Projections of the pulmonary lobes on the chest surface. The upper lobes are white, the right-middle lobe is the darker color, and the lower lobes are the lighter color.

component of the second heart sound, hepatomegaly, elevated neck veins, and rarely, peripheral edema) signifies advanced lung disease.

Respiratory disorders can be secondary to disease in other systems. It is therefore important to look for other conditions such as congenital heart disease (murmur or gallop), neuromuscular disease (muscle wasting or scoliosis), immunodeficiency (rash or diarrhea), and autoimmune disease or occult malignancy (arthritis or hepatosplenomegaly).

Palafox M et al: Diagnostic value of tachypnea in pneumonia defined radiologically. Arch Dis Child 2000;82:41 [PMID: 10630911].

Wipf JE et al: Diagnosing pneumonia by physical examination: Relevant or relic? Arch Intern Med 1999;159:1082 [PMID: 10335685].

PULMONARY FUNCTION TESTS

Lung function tests can help to differentiate obstructive from restrictive lung diseases, measure disease severity, define precipitants of symptoms, and evaluate response to therapy. They can help define the risks of anesthesia and surgery and assist in the planning of respiratory care in the postoperative period. However, the range of normal values for a test may be wide, and the predicted normal values change dramatically with growth. For this reason, serial determinations of lung function are often more informative than a single determination. Patient cooperation is essential for almost all physiologic assessments.

Some children are not able to perform the necessary maneuvers before age 5 years and benefit from a well-trained technician, visual incentives, and interactive computer-animated systems. Lung functions in infants and toddlers are available at specialized centers. Despite these limitations, tests of lung function are valuable in the care of children.

Spirometers are available on which forced vital capacity can be recorded either as a volume-time tracing (spirogram) or a flow-volume curve. The patient inhales maximally, holds his or her breath for a short period, and then exhales as fast as possible for at least 3 seconds. The tracing produced by the exhalation shows forced vital capacity (FVC), which is the total amount of air that is exhaled from maximum inspiration, and the forced expiratory volume in the first second of the exhalation (FEV_1). The maximum midexpiratory flow rate is the mean flow rate during the middle portion of the FVC maneuver and is also referred to as the forced expiratory flow at 25–75% of FVC (FEF_{25-75}). The FEV_1:FVC ratio is calculated from these absolute values; a ratio greater than 0.85 in children and young adults shows unlimited normal airflow.

These basic tests of lung function differentiate obstructive from restrictive processes (Table 18–1). Examples of obstructive processes include asthma, chronic bronchitis, and cystic fibrosis (CF); restrictive problems include chest wall deformities that limit lung expansion and interstitial processes due to collagen-vascular diseases, hypersensitivity pneumonitis, and interstitial fibrosis. Classically, diseases that obstruct airflow decrease the FEV_1 more than the FVC, so that the FEV_1:FVC ratio is low. In restrictive problems, however, the decreases in the FEV_1 and FVC are proportionate; thus, the ratio of FEV_1 to FVC is either normal or high. Clinical suspicion of a restrictive disease is usually an indication for referral to a specialist for evaluation.

The peak expiratory flow rate, the maximal flow recorded during an FVC maneuver, can be assessed by handheld devices. The records of the peak expiratory flow rate can be helpful in following the course of pulmonary disorders that are difficult to control and require multiple medications (eg, asthma). These devices can also be used to give patients with poor perception of their disease an awareness of a decrease in lung function, thus facilitating earlier treatment.

Beydon N et al: An official American Thoracic Society/European Respiratory Society statement: Pulmonary function testing in preschool children. Am J Respir Crit Care Med. 2007;175:1304 [PMID: 17545458].

Blonshine SB: Pediatric pulmonary function testing. Respir Care Clin North Am 2000;6:27 [PMID: 10639555].

Hammer J, Eber E (editors): *Paediatric Pulmonary Function Testing.* Karger, 2005.

Pellegrino R et al: Interpretative strategies for lung function tests. Eur Respir J 2005;26:948 [PMID: 16264058].

ASSESSMENT OF OXYGENATION & VENTILATION

Arterial blood gas determination defines the balance between respiration at the tissue level and that in the lungs.

Table 18–1. Classification of lung function abnormalities.

	Type of Lung Disease	
	Obstructive[a]	Restrictive[b]
FVC	Normal or decreased	Decreased
FEV_1	Decreased	Decreased
FEV_1:FVC ratio	Decreased	Normal or increased
FEF_{25-75}	Decreased	Normal, increased, or decreased

[a]Examples include asthma, chronic bronchitis, and cystic fibrosis.
[b]Examples include chest wall deformities, interstitial processes due to collagen-vascular disease, hypersensitivity pneumonitis, and interstitial fibrosis.
FEF_{25-75}, forced expiratory flow at 25–75% of forced vital capacity; FEV_1, forced expiratory volume in the first second of exhalation; FVC, forced vital capacity.

Assessment of blood gases is essential in critically ill children and may be used also for determining the severity of lung involvement in chronic conditions. Blood gas measurements are affected by abnormalities of respiratory control, gas exchange, respiratory mechanics, and the circulation. In pediatrics, hypoxemia (low partial pressure of arterial oxygen [PaO_2]) most commonly results from mismatching of ventilation and perfusion. Hypercapnia (elevated partial pressure of arterial carbon dioxide [$PaCO_2$]) results from inadequate alveolar ventilation (ie, inability to clear the CO_2 produced). This is termed *hypoventilation*. Causes include decreased central respiratory drive, paralysis of respiratory muscles, and low-tidal-volume breathing as seen in restrictive lung diseases, severe scoliosis, or chest wall trauma. Table 18–2 gives normal values for arterial pH, PaO_2, and $PaCO_2$ at sea level and at 5000 feet.

Exhaled or end-tidal CO_2 monitoring can be used to estimate arterial CO_2 content. It is used to monitor alveolar ventilation and is most accurate in patients without significant lung disease, particularly those with a good match of ventilation and perfusion and without airway obstruction. Monitoring of exhaled or end-tidal CO_2 is increasingly being used to confirm endotracheal tube placement and ensure endotracheal rather than esophageal intubation. This assessment is accurate in children who weigh more than 2 kg and

Table 18–2. Normal arterial blood gas values on room air.

	pH	PaO_2 (mm Hg)	$PaCO_2$ (mm Hg)
Sea level	7.38–7.42	85–95	36–42
5000 ft	7.36–7.40	65–75	35–40

$PaCO_2$, partial pressure of arterial carbon dioxide; PaO_2, partial pressure of arterial oxygen.

have a perfusing rhythm. Exhaled CO_2 can be monitored by attaching a CO_2 detector to an endotracheal tube or to a nasal cannula. Qualitative CO_2 monitors use a chemical detector in a strip of paper that changes color when CO_2 is present. Capnography devices are quantitative and measure the concentration of CO_2 by infrared absorption detectors. These display continuous exhaled CO_2 concentration as a waveform and with a digital display of end-tidal CO_2.

Transcutaneous gas monitoring is a noninvasive assessment of PaO_2 and $PaCO_2$ using electrodes that measure gas tension at the skin surface. Transcutaneous monitoring can underestimate the PaO_2 and overestimate the $PaCO_2$ unless skin perfusion is maximal. Thus heating of the skin site is required, and cardiac function should be stable.

Pulse oximetry (measuring light absorption by transilluminating the skin) is the most reliable and easiest form of noninvasive monitoring of oxygenation. Oxygenated hemoglobin absorbs red light at certain wavelengths. Measurement during a systolic pulse allows estimation of arterial oxygen saturation as the machine corrects for the light absorbed at the tissue level between pulses. No heating of the skin is necessary. Values of oxygen saturation are reliable as low as 80%. The pulse oximeter has reduced reliability during conditions causing reduced arterial pulsation such as hypothermia, hypotension, or infusion of vasoconstrictor drugs. Carbon monoxide bound by hemoglobin results in falsely high oxygen saturation readings.

Bhende MS: End-tidal carbon dioxide monitoring in pediatrics—clinical applications. J Postgrad Med 2001;47:215 [PMID: 11832630].

Hay WW Jr: Pulse oximetry: As good as it gets? J Perinatol 2000;20:181 [PMID: 10802844].

Ralston M et al (editors): *Pediatric Advanced Life Support Provider Manual*. American Heart Association and American Academy of Pediatrics, 2006.

Soubani AO: Noninvasive monitoring of oxygen and carbon dioxide. Am J Emerg Med 2001;19:141 [PMID: 11239260].

CULTURE OF MATERIAL FROM THE RESPIRATORY TRACT

Sources of respiratory tract secretions for culture include expectorated and induced sputum, oropharyngeal swabs, endolaryngeal suction, and bronchoalveolar lavage fluid. Spontaneously expectorated sputum is the easiest and most convenient sample to culture though it is rarely available from patients younger than age 6 years. Sputum induction, performed by inhaling aerosolized hypertonic saline, is a relatively safe noninvasive means of obtaining lower airway secretions and is generally successful in children older than age 10 years. Oropharyngeal swabs are widely used as a surrogate for lower airway cultures in nonexpectorating patients, particularly children with cystic fibrosis. Cultures from the lower respiratory tract can be obtained invasively by tracheal aspiration through an endotracheal tube or rigid bronchoscope, or by performing a bronchoalveolar lavage through a flexible bronchoscope. Other less commonly employed means of obtaining lung specimens include computed tomography (CT)–guided needle aspiration and lung biopsy, either open or thoracoscopic. Thoracentesis should be considered when pleural fluid is present.

Ho SA et al: Clinical value of obtaining sputum and cough swab samples following inhaled hypertonic saline in children with cystic fibrosis. Pediatr Pulmonol 2004;38:82 [PMID: 15170878].

IMAGING OF THE RESPIRATORY TRACT

The plain chest radiograph remains the foundation for investigating the pediatric thorax. Both frontal and lateral views should be obtained. The radiograph is useful for evaluating air trapping caused by airway obstruction, opacification caused by pneumonia, and interstitial problems such as pulmonary edema. Hyperinflation is best demonstrated in lateral views as flattening of the diaphragm. It is often seen because young children commonly develop small-airway obstruction and asthma. Parenchymal changes may cause increased interstitial markings, consolidation, air bronchograms, or loss of diaphragm or heart contours. When pleural fluid is suspected, lateral decubitus radiographs may be helpful in determining the extent and mobility of the fluid. When a foreign body is suspected, forced expiratory radiographs may show focal air trapping and shift of the mediastinum to the contralateral side. Lateral neck radiographs can be useful in assessing the size of adenoids and tonsils and also in differentiating croup from epiglottitis, the latter being associated with the "thumbprint" sign.

Barium swallow is indicated for patients with suspected aspiration to detect swallowing dysfunction, tracheoesophageal fistula, gastroesophageal reflux, and achalasia. This technique is also important in detecting vascular rings and slings, because most of these abnormalities compress the esophagus. Airway fluoroscopy is another important tool for assessing both fixed airway obstruction (eg, tracheal stenosis) and dynamic airway obstruction (eg, tracheomalacia). Fluoroscopy or ultrasound of the diaphragm can detect paralysis by demonstrating paradoxic movement of the involved hemidiaphragm.

High-resolution CT scanning is useful to evaluate parenchymal changes caused by interstitial lung disease and airway abnormalities including bronchiectasis. Characteristic patterns seen in interstitial lung disease (eg, ground-glass opacification) or airway disease (eg, bronchiectasis) are often missed on chest radiographs. Magnetic resonance imaging (MRI) is useful for defining subtle or complex abnormalities and vascular rings. Ventilation-perfusion scans can provide information about regional ventilation and perfusion and can help detect vascular malformations and pulmonary emboli (rare in children). Pulmonary angiography is occasionally necessary to define the pulmonary vascular bed more precisely.

Brody AS: Imaging considerations: Interstitial lung disease in children. Radiol Clin North Am 2005;43:391 [PMID: 15737375].

Long FR: Imaging evolution of airway disorders in children. Radiol Clin North Am 2005;43:371 [PMID: 15737374].

LARYNGOSCOPY & BRONCHOSCOPY

The indications for laryngoscopy include undiagnosed hoarseness, stridor, symptoms of obstructive sleep apnea, and laryngeal wheezing consistent with a diagnosis of vocal cord dysfunction; indications for bronchoscopy include wheezing, suspected foreign body, pneumonia, atelectasis, chronic cough, hemoptysis, placement of an endotracheal tube, and assessment of its patency. In general, the more specific the indication, the higher the diagnostic yield.

Pediatric bronchoscopy instruments are of either the flexible fiberoptic or the rigid open tube type. Flexible bronchoscopy has the following advantages:

1. With conscious sedation and topical anesthetics, the procedure can be done at the bedside.
2. Evaluation of the upper airway can be done with little risk in patients who are awake.
3. The distal airways of intubated patients can be examined without removing the endotracheal tube.
4. The instrument can be used as an obturator to intubate a patient with a difficult upper airway.
5. Endotracheal tube placement and patency can be checked.
6. Assessment of airway dynamics is generally better.
7. It is possible to examine more distal airways.

Improvements in digital optics have greatly enhanced the image quality. The advantages of using a rigid instrument are (1) easier removal of foreign bodies (thus rigid bronchoscopy is preferred for suspected foreign body aspiration); and (2) better airway control, allowing the patient to be ventilated through the bronchoscope. In addition, this approach to the airway allows better assessment of the subglottic space for stenosis. The choice of procedures depends largely on the expertise available.

Bronchoalveolar lavage through a flexible bronchoscope is used to detect infection. Aspiration and hemorrhage can be suspected in the presence of lipid- and hemosiderin-laden macrophages, respectively, though lipid-laden macrophages can also be found in other conditions. Analysis of lavage fluid can also be completed for cell counts, surfactant proteins, and inflammatory mediators. Transbronchial biopsy in children is limited to evaluation for infection and rejection in transplant patients due to poor diagnostic yield in most conditions. Transbronchial biopsy may have a role in diagnosing diffuse lung diseases such as sarcoidosis.

Naguib ML et al: Use of laryngeal mask airway in flexible bronchoscopy in infants and children. Pediatr Pulmonol 2005;39:56 [PMID: 15558607].

Schellhase DE: Pediatric flexible airway endoscopy. Curr Opin Pediatr 2002;14:327 [PMID: 12011674].

GENERAL THERAPY OF PEDIATRIC LUNG DISEASES

OXYGEN THERAPY

Oxygen therapy in children with respiratory disease can reduce the work of breathing, resulting in fewer respiratory symptoms; relax the pulmonary vasculature, lessening the potential for pulmonary hypertension and congestive heart failure; and improve feeding. Patients breathing spontaneously can be treated by nasal cannula, head hood, or mask (including simple, rebreathing, nonrebreathing, or Venturi masks). The general goal of oxygen therapy is to achieve an arterial oxygen tension of 65–90 mm Hg or an oxygen saturation above 92%. The actual oxygen concentration achieved by nasal cannula or mask depends on the flow rate, the type of mask used, and the patient's age. Small changes in flow rate during oxygen administration by nasal cannula can lead to substantial changes in inspired oxygen concentration in young infants. The amount of oxygen required to correct hypoxemia may vary according to the child's activity. It is not unusual, for example, for an infant with chronic lung disease to require 0.75 L/min while awake but 1 L/min while asleep or feeding.

Although the head hood is an efficient device for delivery of oxygen in young infants, the nasal cannula is used more often because it allows the infant greater mobility. The cannula has nasal prongs that are inserted in the nares. Flow through the nasal cannula should generally not exceed 3 L/min to avoid excessive drying of the mucosa. Even at high flow rates, oxygen by nasal cannula rarely delivers inspired oxygen concentrations greater than 40–45%. In contrast, partial rebreathing and nonrebreathing masks or head hoods achieve inspired oxygen concentrations as high as 90–100%.

Because the physical findings of hypoxemia are subtle, the adequacy of oxygenation should be measured as the arterial oxygen tension, or oxygen saturation can be determined by oximetry. The advantages of the latter noninvasive method include the ability to obtain continuous measurements during various normal activities and to avoid artifacts caused by crying or breath-holding during attempts at arterial puncture. For children with chronic cardiopulmonary disorders that may require supplemental oxygen therapy (eg, bronchopulmonary dysplasia or CF), frequent noninvasive assessments are essential to ensure the safety and adequacy of treatment.

Ralston M et al (editors): *Pediatric Advanced Life Support Provider Manual.* American Heart Association and American Academy of Pediatrics, 2006.

INHALATION OF MEDICATIONS

Airway obstruction that is at least partially reversed by an inhaled bronchodilator can be seen in CF, bronchiolitis, and bronchopulmonary dysplasia, as well as in acute and chronic asthma. Inhaled medications can be used to deliver anti-inflammatory medications, mucolytics, or antibiotics in patients with a variety of lung diseases.

The inhaled β-adrenergic agonists may be delivered by metered-dose inhaler, dry powder inhaler, or nebulizer. Metered-dose inhalers are convenient and best combined with valved holding chambers, especially for children who lack the ability to coordinate actuation of the metered-dose inhaler with inhalation. In contrast, the nebulizer is an effective method of delivering medication to infants and young children. Long-acting inhaled β_2-adrenergic agents that are relatively selective for the respiratory tract are described in Chapter 36. Inhaled bronchodilators are as effective as injected agents for treating acute episodes of airway obstruction and have fewer side effects. These drugs can be safely administered at home as long as both the physician and the family realize that a poor response may signify the need for corticosteroids to help restore β-adrenergic responsiveness.

Anticholinergic agents may also acutely decrease airway obstruction. Furthermore, they may yield a longer duration of bronchodilation than do many adrenergic agents. Selected patients may benefit from receiving both β-adrenergic and anticholinergic agents. In general, this class of drugs is most effective in the treatment of chronic bronchitis.

Chronic use of inhaled medications is common in children with chronic lung diseases. Inhaled corticosteroids are standard of care for persistent asthma and may be delivered by metered-dose inhaler, dry powder inhaler, or nebulizer. Dornase alfa is used as a mucolytic in CF and other disorders of mucous production. Hypertonic saline is used to induce sputum production and as a chronic medication for mucous clearance in CF. Inhaled antibiotics may be used acutely or chronically in patients with lung disease that predispose them to chronic airway infections.

Rubin BK, Fink JB: The delivery of inhaled medication to the young child. Pediatr Clin North Am 2003;50:717 [PMID: 12877243].

AIRWAY CLEARANCE THERAPY

Chest physical therapy, with postural drainage, percussion, and forced expiratory maneuvers, has been widely used to improve the clearance of lower airway secretions even though there are limited data on the efficacy of these techniques. Children with CF have been shown to benefit from routine airway clearance. Many airway clearance techniques exist, but only a few long-term studies have compared the various options. The various techniques currently available include chest physiotherapy, autogenic drainage, positive expiratory pressure (Flutter or Acapella), intrapulmonary percussive ventilation, or high-frequency chest compression. The decision about which technique to use should be based on the patient's age and preference after trying different approaches. Often bronchodilators or mucolytic medications are given prior to or during airway clearance therapy. Inhaled corticosteroids and inhaled antibiotics should be given after airway clearance therapy so that the airways are first cleared of secretions, allowing the medications to maximally penetrate into the lung.

Bradley JM et al: Evidence for physical therapies (airway clearance and physical training) in cystic fibrosis: An overview of five Cochrane systematic reviews. Respir Med 2006;100:191 [PMID: 16412951].
Marks JH: Airway clearance devices in cystic fibrosis. Paediatr Respir Rev 2007;8:17 [PMID: 17419974].

AVOIDANCE OF ENVIRONMENTAL HAZARDS

All parents or other caregivers should be counseled about environmental hazards to the lung. The list of potential hazards includes small objects that may be aspirated, allergens that can precipitate respiratory symptoms in atopic children, and tobacco smoke. The harmful effects of smoking in the home deserve special emphasis. Children from families where the parents and others smoke have decreased lung growth as well as decreased pulmonary function in comparison with children raised in smoke-free homes. Exposure of children to tobacco smoke also leads to an increased frequency of lower respiratory tract infections and an increased incidence of respiratory symptoms, including recurrent wheezing. Health care providers must increase their efforts to educate patients and their families about the hazards of smoking.

Bradley JP et al: Severity of respiratory syncytial virus bronchiolitis is affected by cigarette smoke exposure and atopy. Pediatrics 2005;115:e7 [PMID: 15629968].
DiFranza JR et al: Prenatal and postnatal environmental tobacco smoke exposure and children's health. Pediatrics 2004;113:1007 [PMID: 15060193].

DISORDERS OF THE CONDUCTING AIRWAYS

The conducting airways (the nose, mouth, pharynx, larynx, trachea, bronchi, and bronchioles) direct inspired air to the gas-exchange units of the lung; they do not participate in gas exchange themselves. Airflow obstruction in the conducting airways occurs by (1) external compression (eg, vascular ring or tumor), (2) abnormalities of the airway structure itself (eg, congenital defects or thickening of an airway wall due to inflammation), or (3) material in the airway lumen (eg, foreign body or mucus).

Airway obstruction can be fixed (airflow limited in both the inspiratory and the expiratory phases) or variable (airflow limited more in one phase of respiration than in the other). Variable obstruction is common in children because their airways are more compliant and susceptible to dynamic compression. With variable extrathoracic airway obstruction (eg, croup), airflow limitation is greater during inspiration, leading to inspiratory stridor. With variable intrathoracic obstruction (eg, bronchomalacia), limitation is greater during expiration, producing expiratory wheezing. Thus determining the phase of respiration in which obstruction is greatest may be helpful in localizing the site of obstruction.

EXTRATHORACIC AIRWAY OBSTRUCTION

Patients with abnormalities of the extrathoracic airway may present with snoring and other symptoms of obstructive apnea, hoarseness, brassy cough, or stridor. The course of the illness may be acute (eg, infectious croup), recurrent (eg, spasmodic croup), chronic (eg, subglottic stenosis), or progressive (eg, laryngeal papillomatosis). Significant risk factors are difficult delivery, ductal ligation, and intubation. Examination should determine if obstructive symptoms are present at rest or with agitation, if they are positional, or if they are related to sleep. The presence of agitation, air hunger, severe retractions, cyanosis, lethargy, or coma should alert the physician to a potentially life-threatening condition that may require immediate airway intervention. Helpful diagnostic studies in the evaluation of upper airway obstruction include chest and lateral neck radiographs, airway fluoroscopy, and barium swallow. In patients who have symptoms of severe chronic obstruction, an electrocardiogram should be obtained to evaluate for right ventricular hypertrophy and pulmonary hypertension. Patients with obstructive sleep apnea should have polysomnography (measurements during sleep of the motion of the chest wall, airflow at the nose and mouth, heart rate, oxygen saturation, and selected electroencephalographic leads to stage sleep) to determine severity and to evaluate the need for tonsillectomy and adenoidectomy, oxygen, or continuous or biphasic positive airway pressure. In older children, pulmonary function tests can differentiate fixed from variable airflow obstruction and identify the site of variable obstruction. If noninvasive studies are unable to establish the cause, direct laryngoscopy and bronchoscopy remain the procedures of choice to establish the precise diagnosis. Treatment should be directed at relieving airway obstruction and correcting the underlying condition if possible.

INTRATHORACIC AIRWAY OBSTRUCTION

Intrathoracic airway obstruction usually causes expiratory wheezing. The history should include the following:

1. Age at onset
2. Precipitating factors (eg, exercise, upper respiratory illnesses, allergens, or choking while eating)
3. Course—acute (bronchiolitis or foreign body), chronic (tracheomalacia or vascular ring), recurrent (asthma), or progressive (CF or bronchiolitis obliterans)
4. Presence and nature of cough
5. Production of sputum
6. Previous response to bronchodilators
7. Symptoms with positional changes (vascular rings)
8. Involvement of other organ systems (malabsorption in CF)

Physical examination should include growth measurements and vital signs. The examiner should look for cyanosis or pallor, barrel-shaped chest, retractions and use of accessory muscles, and clubbing. Auscultation should define the pattern and timing of respiration, detect the presence of crackles and wheezing, and determine whether findings are localized or generalized.

Routine tests include plain chest radiographs, a sweat test, and pulmonary function tests in older children. Other diagnostic studies are dictated by the history and physical findings. Treatment should be directed toward the primary cause of the obstruction, but generally includes a trial of bronchodilators.

STRIDOR & NOISY BREATHING FROM CONGENITAL DISORDERS OF THE EXTRATHORACIC AIRWAY

ESSENTIALS OF DIAGNOSIS & TYPICAL FEATURES

▶ Presentation from birth or within the first few months of life.

▶ Inspiratory sounds usually of a high-pitched ("croup") nature but can be variable depending on diagnosis.

▶ Moderate to severe symptoms require visualization of the airway.

LARYNGOMALACIA

Laryngomalacia is a benign congenital disorder in which the cartilaginous support for the supraglottic structures is underdeveloped. It is the most common cause of persistent stridor in infants and usually is seen in the first 6 weeks of life. Stridor has been reported to be worse in the supine position, with increased activity, with upper respiratory infections, and during feeding; however, the clinical presentation can be variable. Patients may have slight oxygen desaturation during sleep. Gastroesophageal reflux may also be associated with laryngomalacia requiring treatment. The condition usually improves with age and resolves by age 2 years, but in some cases symptoms persist for years. The diagnosis is established by direct laryngoscopy, which shows inspiratory collapse of an omega-shaped epiglottis (with or without long, redundant arytenoids). In mildly affected patients with a typical presentation (those without stridor at rest or retractions), this procedure may not be necessary. No treatment is usually needed. However, in patients with severe symptoms of airway obstruction associated with feeding difficulties, failure to thrive, obstructive sleep apnea, respiratory insufficiency, or severe dyspnea, surgical epiglottoplasty may be necessary.

Vicencui AG et al: Laryngomalacia and tracheomalacia: Common dynamic airway lesions. Pediatr Rev 2006;27:e33 [PMID: 16581951].

Zoumalan R et al: Etiology of stridor in infants. Ann Otol Rhinol Laryngol 2007;116:329 [PMID: 17561760].

OTHER CONGENITAL PROBLEMS

Other rare congenital lesions of the larynx (laryngeal atresia, laryngeal web, laryngocele and cyst of the larynx, subglottic hemangioma, and laryngeal cleft) are best evaluated by direct laryngoscopy. Laryngeal atresia presents immediately after birth with severe respiratory distress and is usually fatal. Laryngeal web, representing fusion of the anterior portion of the true vocal cords, is associated with hoarseness, aphonia, and stridor. Surgical correction may be necessary depending on the degree of airway obstruction.

Congenital cysts and laryngoceles are believed to have similar origin. Cysts are more superficial, whereas laryngoceles communicate with the interior of the larynx. Cysts are generally fluid-filled, whereas laryngoceles may be air- or fluid-filled. Airway obstruction is usually prominent and requires surgery or laser therapy.

Subglottic hemangiomas are seen in infancy with signs of upper airway obstruction and can be associated with similar lesions of the skin (but not always). Although these lesions tend to regress spontaneously, airway obstruction may require surgical treatment or even tracheostomy.

Laryngeal cleft is a very rare condition resulting from failure of posterior cricoid fusion. Patients with this condition may have stridor but always aspirate severely, resulting in recurrent or chronic pneumonia and failure to thrive. Barium swallow is always positive for severe aspiration, but diagnosis can be very difficult even with direct laryngoscopy. Patients often require tracheostomy and gastrostomy, because success with surgical correction can be mixed.

Vijayasekaran S et al: Open excision of subglottic hemangiomas to avoid tracheostomy. Arch Otolaryngol Head Neck Surg 2006;132:159 [PMID: 16490873].

Watson GJ et al: Acquired paediatric subglottic cysts: A series from Manchester. Int J Pediatr Otorhinolaryngol 2007;71:533 [PMID: 17239962].

STRIDOR & NOISY BREATHING FROM ACQUIRED DISORDERS OF THE EXTRATHORACIC AIRWAY

ESSENTIALS OF DIAGNOSIS & TYPICAL FEATURES

▶ Presentation with acute or subacute symptoms.

▶ Inspiratory sounds usually of a high-pitched ("croup") nature but can be variable depending on diagnosis.

▶ Life-threatening condition can occur, requiring careful patient assessment.

CROUP SYNDROME

Croup describes acute inflammatory diseases of the larynx, including viral croup (laryngotracheobronchitis), epiglottitis (supraglottitis), and bacterial tracheitis. These are the main entities in the differential diagnosis for patients presenting with acute stridor, although spasmodic croup, angioneurotic edema, laryngeal or esophageal foreign body, and retropharyngeal abscess should be considered as well.

1. Viral Croup

Viral croup generally affects younger children in the fall and early winter months and is most often caused by parainfluenza virus serotypes. Other organisms causing croup include respiratory syncytial virus (RSV), human metapneumovirus, influenza virus, rubeola virus, adenovirus, and *Mycoplasma pneumoniae*. Although inflammation of the entire airway is usually present, edema formation in the subglottic space accounts for the predominant signs of upper airway obstruction.

▶ Clinical Findings

A. Symptoms and Signs

Usually a prodrome of upper respiratory tract symptoms is followed by a barking cough and stridor. Fever is usually absent or low-grade but may on occasion be high-grade. Patients with mild disease may have stridor when agitated. As obstruction worsens, stridor occurs at rest, accompanied in severe cases by retractions, air hunger, and cyanosis. On examination, the presence of cough and the absence of drooling favor the diagnosis of viral croup over epiglottitis.

B. Imaging

Lateral neck radiographs in patients with classic presentations are not required but can be diagnostically supportive by showing subglottic narrowing without the irregularities seen in tracheitis and a normal epiglottis.

▶ Treatment

Treatment of viral croup is based on the symptoms. Mild croup, signified by a barking cough and no stridor at rest, requires supportive therapy with oral hydration and minimal handling. Mist therapy has historically been used but clinical studies do not demonstrate effectiveness. Conversely, patients with stridor at rest require active intervention. Oxygen should be administered to patients with oxygen desaturation. Nebulized racemic epinephrine (2.25% solution; 0.05 mL/kg to a maximum of 1.5 mL diluted in sterile saline) is commonly used because it has a rapid onset of action within 10–30 minutes. Both racemic epinephrine and epinephrine hydrochloride are effective in alleviating symptoms and decreasing the need for intubation.

Once controversial, the efficacy of glucocorticoids in croup is now more firmly established. Dexamethasone, 0.6 mg/kg intramuscularly as one dose, improves symptoms, reduces the duration of hospitalizations and frequency of intubations, and permits earlier discharge from the emergency department. Oral dexamethasone (0.15 mg/kg) appears equally effective.

Inhaled budesonide (2–4 mg) also improves symptoms and decreases hospital stay. Onset of action occurs within 2 hours, and this agent may be as effective as dexamethasone; however, dexamethasone is still the most cost-effective steroid of choice. Dexamethasone has also been shown to be more effective than prednisolone in equivalent doses.

If symptoms resolve within 3 hours of glucocorticoids and nebulized epinephrine, patients can safely be discharged without fear of a sudden rebound in symptoms. If, however, recurrent nebulized epinephrine treatments are required or if respiratory distress persists, patients require hospitalization for close observation, supportive care, and nebulization treatments as needed. In patients with impending respiratory failure, an airway must be established. Hospitalized patients with persistent symptoms over 3–4 days despite treatment should initiate consideration of another underlying cause.

Patients with impending respiratory failure require an artificial airway. Intubation with an endotracheal tube of slightly smaller diameter than would ordinarily be used is reasonably safe. Extubation should be accomplished within 2–3 days to minimize the risk of laryngeal injury. If the patient fails extubation, tracheostomy may be required.

▶ Prognosis

Most children with viral croup have an uneventful course and improve within a few days. Some evidence suggests that patients with a history of croup associated with wheezing may have airway hyperreactivity. It is not clear if this was present prior to the croup episode or if the croup episode itself altered airway function.

Duman M et al: Nebulised L-epinephrine and steroid combination in the treatment of moderate to severe croup. Clin Drug Investig 2005;25:183 [PMID: 17523767].

Moore M et al: Humidified air inhalation for treating croup. Cochrane Database Syst Rev 2006;(3):CD002870 [PMID: 16855994].

Sparrow A et al: Prednisolone versus dexamethasone in croup: A randomised equivalence trial. Arch Dis Child 2006;91:580 [PMID: 16624882].

2. Epiglottitis

With the introduction of the *Haemophilus influenzae* conjugate vaccine the incidence of epiglottitis has dramatically decreased and is now rare in countries with immunization programs. If disease occurs it is likely to be associated with *H influenzae* in unimmunized children or other organisms such as nontypeable *H influenzae, Neisseria meningitides,* or *Streptococcus* species in immunized populations.

▶ Clinical Findings

A. Symptoms and Signs

The classic presentation is a sudden onset of fever, dysphagia, drooling, muffled voice, inspiratory retractions, cyanosis, and soft stridor. Patients often sit in the so-called sniffing dog position, which gives them the best airway possible under the

circumstances. Progression to total airway obstruction may occur and result in respiratory arrest. The definitive diagnosis is made by direct inspection of the epiglottis, a procedure that should be done by an experienced airway specialist under controlled conditions (usually the operating room). The typical findings are cherry-red and swollen epiglottis and arytenoids.

B. Imaging

Diagnostically, lateral neck radiographs may be helpful in demonstrating a classic "thumbprint" sign. Obtaining radiographs, however, may delay important airway intervention.

▶ Treatment

Once the diagnosis of epiglottitis is made, endotracheal intubation must be performed immediately in children but not necessarily in adult populations. Most anesthesiologists prefer general anesthesia (but not muscle relaxants) to facilitate intubation. After an airway is established, cultures of the blood and epiglottis should be obtained and the patient started on appropriate intravenous antibiotics to cover *H influenzae* and *Streptococcus* species (ceftriaxone sodium or equivalent cephalosporin). Extubation can usually be accomplished in 24–48 hours, when direct inspection shows significant reduction in the size of the epiglottis. Intravenous antibiotics should be continued for 2–3 days, followed by oral antibiotics to complete a 10-day course.

▶ Prognosis

Prompt recognition and appropriate treatment usually results in rapid resolution of swelling and inflammation. Recurrence is unusual.

Faden H: The dramatic change in the epidemiology of pediatric epiglottitis. Pediatr Emerg Care 2006;22:443 [PMID: 16801849].

3. Bacterial Tracheitis

Bacterial tracheitis (pseudomembranous croup) is a severe life-threatening form of laryngotracheobronchitis. As the management of severe viral croup has been improved with the use of dexamethasone and vaccination has decreased the incidence of epiglottitis, tracheitis has now become the most common pediatric airway emergency requiring admission to the pediatric intensive care unit. This diagnosis must be high in the differential when a patient presents with severe upper airway obstruction. The organism most often isolated is *Staphylococcus aureus,* but organisms such as *H influenzae,* group A *Streptococcus pyogenes, Neisseria* species, *Moraxella catarrhalis,* and others have been reported. The disease probably represents localized mucosal invasion of bacteria in patients with primary viral croup, resulting in inflammatory edema, purulent secretions, and pseudomembranes. Although cultures of the tracheal secretions are frequently positive, blood cultures are almost always negative.

▶ Clinical Findings

A. Symptoms and Signs

The early clinical picture is similar to that of viral croup. However, instead of gradual improvement, patients develop higher fever, toxicity, and progressive or intermittent severe upper airway obstruction that is unresponsive to standard croup therapy. The incidence of sudden respiratory arrest or progressive respiratory failure is high; in such instances, airway intervention is required. Findings of toxic shock and the acute respiratory distress syndrome may also be seen. Recently, subsets of patients with tracheal membranes have been reported with a less severe clinical presentation. Aggressive medical treatment and debridement still must occur in these patients. A higher index of suspicion is required for this life-threatening condition.

B. Laboratory Findings and Imaging

The white cell count is usually elevated, with left shift. Cultures of tracheal secretions usually demonstrate one of the causative organisms. Lateral neck radiographs show a normal epiglottis but often severe subglottic and tracheal narrowing. Irregularity of the contour of the proximal tracheal mucosa can frequently be seen radiographically and should elicit concern. Bronchoscopy showing a normal epiglottis and the presence of copious purulent tracheal secretions and membranes confirm the diagnosis.

▶ Treatment

Suspected bacterial tracheitis should be managed in a fashion similar to that for epiglottitis, with visualization of the airway in a controlled environment but with the added capability to debride the airway. The incidence of respiratory arrest or progressive respiratory failure is high, necessitating intubation. Patients often have thick, purulent tracheal secretions requiring debridement, and humidification, frequent suctioning, and intensive care monitoring are required to prevent endotracheal tube obstruction. Intravenous antibiotics to cover *S aureus, H influenzae,* and the other organisms are indicated. Thick secretions persist for several days, usually resulting in longer periods of intubation for bacterial tracheitis than for epiglottitis or croup. Despite the severity of this illness, the reported mortality rate is very low if it is recognized and treated promptly.

Hopkins A et al: Changing epidemiology of life-threatening upper airway infections: The reemergence of bacterial tracheitis. Pediatrics 2006;118:1418 [PMID: 17015531].
Salamone FN et al: Bacterial tracheitis reexamined: Is there a less severe manifestation? Otolaryngol Head Neck Surg 2004;131:871 [PMID: 15577783].

VOCAL CORD PARALYSIS

Unilateral or bilateral vocal cord paralysis may be congenital, or more commonly may result from injury to the recurrent laryngeal nerves. Risk factors for acquired paralysis include difficult delivery (especially face presentation), neck and thoracic surgery (eg, ductal ligation or repair of tracheoesophageal fistula), trauma, mediastinal masses, and central nervous system disease (eg, Arnold-Chiari malformation). Patients usually present with varying degrees of hoarseness, aspiration, or high-pitched stridor. Unilateral cord paralysis is more likely to occur on the left because of the longer course of the left recurrent laryngeal nerve and its proximity to major thoracic structures. Patients with unilateral paralysis are usually hoarse but rarely have stridor. With bilateral cord paralysis, the closer to midline the cords are positioned, the greater the airway obstruction; the more lateral the cords are positioned, the greater the tendency to aspirate and experience hoarseness or aphonia. If partial function is preserved (paresis), the adductor muscles tend to operate better than the abductors, with a resultant high-pitched inspiratory stridor and normal voice.

Airway intervention (tracheostomy) is rarely indicated in unilateral paralysis but is often necessary for bilateral paralysis. Clinically, paralysis can be assessed by direct visualization of vocal cord function with laryngoscopy or more invasively by recording the electrical activity of the muscles (electromyography). Electromyogram recordings can differentiate vocal fold paralysis from arytenoid dislocation, which has prognostic value. Recovery is related to the severity of nerve injury and the potential for healing.

Miyamoto RC et al: Bilateral congenital vocal cord paralysis: A 16-year institutional review. Otolaryngol Head Neck Surg 2005;133:241 [PMID: 16087022].
Ysunza A et al: The role of laryngeal electromyography in the diagnosis of vocal fold immobility in children. Int J Pediatr Otorhinolaryngol 2007;71:949 [PMID: 17418427].

SUBGLOTTIC STENOSIS

Subglottic stenosis may be congenital, or more commonly may result from endotracheal intubation. Neonates and infants are particularly vulnerable to subglottic injury from intubation: The subglottis is the narrowest part of an infant's airway, and the cricoid cartilage, which supports the subglottis, is the only cartilage that completely encircles the airway. The clinical presentation may vary from totally asymptomatic to the typical picture of severe upper airway obstruction. Patients with signs of stridor who repeatedly fail extubation are likely to have subglottic stenosis. Subglottic stenosis should also be suspected in children with multiple, prolonged, or severe episodes of croup. Diagnosis is made by direct visualization of the subglottic space with bronchoscopy and maneuvers to size the airway. Tracheostomy is often required when airway compromise is severe. Surgical intervention is ultimately required to correct the stenosis. Depending on the type of stenosis, a cricoid split in which the cricoid cartilage is surgically opened (better for acquired than for congenital lesions) may be tried. Laryngotracheal reconstruction in which a cartilage graft from another source (eg, rib) is used to expand the airway has become the standard procedure for symptomatic subglottic stenosis in children.

Khariwala SS et al: Laryngotracheal consequences of pediatric cardiac surgery. Arch Otolaryngol Head Neck Surg 2005;131:336 [PMID: 15837903].

White DR et al: Pediatric cricotracheal resection: Surgical outcomes and risk factor analysis. Arch Otolaryngol Head Neck Surg 2005;131:896 [PMID: 16230593].

LARYNGEAL PAPILLOMATOSIS

Papillomas of the larynx are benign, warty growths that are difficult to treat and are the most common laryngeal neoplasm in children. Human papillomaviruses 6, 11, and 16 have been implicated as causative agents. A substantial percentage of mothers of patients with laryngeal papillomas have a history of genital condylomas at the time of delivery, so the virus may be acquired during passage through an infected birth canal.

The age at onset is usually 2–4 years, but juvenile-onset recurrent respiratory papillomatosis is well documented. A younger age of onset may be a worse prognostic indicator. Patients usually develop hoarseness, voice changes, croupy cough, or stridor that can lead to life-threatening airway obstruction. Diagnosis is by direct laryngoscopy. The larynx was involved at the time of diagnosis in over 95% of patients, most of whom had only one site involved.

Treatment is directed toward relieving airway obstruction, usually by surgical removal of the lesions. Tracheostomy is necessary when life-threatening obstruction or respiratory arrest occurs. Various surgical procedures (laser, cup forceps, or cryosurgery) have been used to remove papillomas, but recurrences are the rule, and frequent reoperation may be needed. The lesions occasionally spread down the trachea and bronchi, making surgical removal more difficult. The use of interferon therapy remains controversial. Fortunately, spontaneous remissions do occur, usually by puberty, so that the goal of therapy is to maintain an adequate airway until remission occurs.

Coope G et al: Juvenile laryngeal papillomatosis. Prim Care Respir J 2006;15:125 [PMID: 16701772].

Zacharisen MC et al: Recurrent respiratory papillomatosis in children: Masquerader of common respiratory diseases. Pediatrics 2006;118:1925 [PMID: 17079563].

CONGENITAL DISORDERS OF THE INTRATHORACIC AIRWAYS

MALACIA OF AIRWAYS

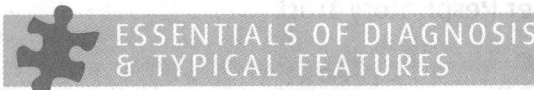

ESSENTIALS OF DIAGNOSIS & TYPICAL FEATURES

▶ Chronic monophonic wheeze with or without a barking cough.

▶ Respiratory symptoms do not respond to bronchodilators.

▶ General Considerations

Tracheomalacia or bronchomalacia exists when the cartilaginous framework of the airway is inadequate to maintain airway patency. Because cartilage of the infant airway is normally soft, all infants may have some degree of dynamic collapse of a central airway when pressure outside the airway exceeds intraluminal pressure. In tracheomalacia, whether congenital or acquired, dynamic collapse leads to airway obstruction. The congenital variety may be isolated or associated with another developmental defect. Congenital tracheomalacia and bronchomalacia may also be associated with developmental abnormalities such as tracheoesophageal fistula, vascular ring, or cardiac anomalies causing extrinsic airway compression during development. Tracheomalacia is also associated with various syndromes. Congenital tracheomalacia may be localized to part of the trachea, or more commonly may involve the entire trachea as well as the remainder of the conducting airways. In severe cases, cartilage in the involved area may be missing or underdeveloped. Acquired tracheomalacia has been associated with long-term ventilation of premature newborns that results in chronic tracheal injury, severe tracheobronchitis, and airway compression due to tumors, abscess or infection, and cysts.

▶ Clinical Findings

Coarse wheezing, cough, stridor, recurrent illnesses, recurrent wheezing that does not respond to bronchodilators, or radiographic changes are common findings. Symptoms classically present insidiously over the first few months of life and can increase with agitation, excitement, or upper respiratory tract infections. Diagnosis can be made by airway fluoroscopy or bronchoscopy. Barium swallow may be indicated to rule out coexisting conditions.

▶ Treatment

Conservative treatment is usually indicated for the isolated condition, which generally improves over time with growth. Coexisting lesions such as tracheoesophageal fistulas and vascular rings need primary repair. In severe cases of tracheomalacia, intubation or tracheostomy may be necessary. However, this alone is seldom satisfactory because airway collapse continues to exist below the tip of the artificial airway. Positive pressure ventilation may be required to stent the collapsing airway. Surgical approaches to the problem (tracheopexy or aortopexy) may be considered as alternatives prior to or in an effort to wean off of ventilatory support.

Carden KA et al: Tracheomalacia and tracheobronchomalacia in children and adults: An in-depth review. Chest 2005;127:984 [PMID: 15764786].

Masters IB, Chang AB: Interventions for primary (intrinsic) tracheomalacia in children. Cochrane Database Syst Rev 2005;(4): CD005304 [PMID: 16235399].

VASCULAR RINGS & SLINGS

The most common vascular anomaly to compress the trachea or esophagus is a vascular ring. A vascular ring can be formed by a double aortic arch, a right aortic arch with left ligamentum arteriosum, or a patent ductus arteriosus. The pulmonary sling is created when the left pulmonary artery branches off from the right pulmonary artery. Other common vascular anomalies include an anomalous innominate, a left carotid artery, and an aberrant right subclavian artery. All but the right subclavian artery can cause tracheal compression and present in infancy with symptoms of chronic airway obstruction (stridor, coarse wheezing, and croupy cough). Symptoms are often worse in the supine position. Respiratory compromise is most severe with double aortic arch and may lead to apnea, respiratory arrest, or even death. Esophageal compression, present in all but anomalous innominate or carotid artery, may result in feeding difficulties, including dysphagia and vomiting. Barium swallow showing esophageal compression is the mainstay of diagnosis. Chest radiographs and echocardiograms may miss abnormalities. Anatomy can be further defined by angiography, chest CT with contrast, MRI or magnetic resonance angiography, or bronchoscopy.

Patients with significant symptoms require surgical correction, especially those with double aortic arch. Patients usually improve following correction but may have persistent but milder symptoms of airway obstruction due to associated tracheomalacia.

Humphrey C et al: Decade of experience with vascular rings at a single institution. Pediatrics 2006;117:e903 [PMID: 16585275].

Masters IB et al: Series of laryngomalacia, tracheomalacia, and bronchomalacia disorders and their associations with other conditions in children. Pediatr Pulmonol 2002;34:189 [PMID: 12203847].

Turner A et al: Vascular rings—presentation, investigation and outcome. Eur J Pediar 2005;164:266 [PMID: 15666159].

BRONCHOGENIC CYSTS

Bronchogenic cysts generally occur in the middle mediastinum (see later section on Mediastinal Masses) near the carina and adjacent to the major bronchi but can be found elsewhere in the lung. They range in size from 2–10 cm. Cyst walls are thin and may contain pus, mucus, or blood. Cysts develop from abnormal lung budding of the primitive foregut. They can be seen in involvement with other congenital pulmonary malformations such as pulmonary sequestration or lobar emphysema.

Clinically, respiratory distress can appear acutely in early childhood due to airway compression or infection of the bronchogenic cyst or they may remain asymptomatic into adulthood. Symptoms may include chronic wheezing, chronic cough, tachypnea, recurrent pneumonia, or stridor, depending on the location and size of the cysts and the degree of airway compression. However, all asymptomatic cysts will eventually become symptomatic with chest pain being the most common presenting complaint. On examination, the trachea may deviate from the midline, breath sounds over such areas will be decreased, and percussion over involved lobes may be hyperresonant due to air trapping.

The choice of diagnostic studies for bronchogenic cysts is controversial. Chest radiographs can show air trapping and hyperinflation of the affected lobes or may show a spherical lesion with or without an air-fluid level. However, early detected or smaller lesions may not be seen on chest radiographs. CT scan is the preferred imaging study and can differentiate solid versus cystic mediastinal masses and define the cyst's relationship to the airways and the rest of the lung. A barium swallow can help determine whether the lesion communicates with the gastrointestinal tract. MRI and ultrasound are other imaging modalities used.

Treatment is surgical resection. Postoperatively, vigorous pulmonary physiotherapy is required to prevent complications (atelectasis or infection of the lung distal to the site of resection of the cyst).

McAdams HP et al: Bronchogenic cyst: Imaging features with clinical and histopathologic correlation. Radiology 2000;217:441 [PMID: 11058643].

Stewart B et al: Unusual case of stridor and wheeze in an infant: Tracheal bronchogenic cyst. Pediatric Pulmonol 2002;34:320 [PMID: 12205574].

ACQUIRED DISORDERS OF THE INTRATHORACIC AIRWAYS

FOREIGN BODY ASPIRATION

Aspiration of a foreign body into the respiratory tract is rarely observed. Onset is generally abrupt, with a history of the child running with food in the mouth or playing with seeds, small coins, or toys. Symptoms at the time of the ingestion are often abrupt and include cough, choking, or wheezing.

The foreign body can lodge itself anywhere along the respiratory tract. Often it is trapped in the supraglottic airway, triggering protective reflexes that result in laryngospasm. Small objects such as coins may pass through the glottis and obstruct the trachea. Finally, foreign bodies that lodge in the esophagus may compress the airway and cause dysphagia and respiratory distress.

The most commonly seen objects in foreign body aspiration include peanuts, hot dogs, popcorn, small coins, hard candy, and small toys. Children aged 6 months to 4 years are at highest risk, and many deaths are caused by foreign body aspiration and airway obstruction each year.

1. Foreign Bodies in the Upper Respiratory Tract

ESSENTIALS OF DIAGNOSIS & TYPICAL FEATURES

▶ Sudden onset of coughing or respiratory distress.

▶ Difficulty vocalizing.

Clinical Findings

The diagnosis is established by acute onset of choking along with *inability* to vocalize or cough and cyanosis with marked distress (complete obstruction), or with drooling, stridor, and *ability* to vocalize (partial obstruction).

Foreign bodies that lodge in the esophagus may compress the airway and cause respiratory distress. More typically, the foreign body lodges in the supraglottic airway, triggering protective reflexes that result in laryngospasm. Onset is generally abrupt, with a history of the child running with food in the mouth or playing with seeds, small coins, toys, and the like. Homes and child care centers in which an older sibling or child feeds age-inappropriate foods (eg, peanuts, hard candy, or carrot slices) to the younger child are typical. Without treatment, progressive cyanosis, loss of consciousness, seizures, bradycardia, and cardiopulmonary arrest can follow.

Treatment

The emergency treatment of upper airway obstruction due to foreign body aspiration is somewhat controversial. If *complete* obstruction is present, then one must intervene immediately. If partial obstruction is present, then the choking subject should be allowed to use his or her own cough reflex to remove the foreign body. If after a brief observation period the obstruction increases or the airway becomes completely obstructed, acute intervention is required. The American Academy of Pediatrics and the American Heart Association distinguish between children younger than and older than age 1 year. A choking infant younger than age 1 year should be placed face down over the rescuer's arm, with the head positioned below the trunk. Five measured back blows are delivered rapidly between the infant's scapulas with the heel of the rescuer's hand. If obstruction persists, the infant should be rolled over and five rapid chest compressions performed (similar to cardiopulmonary resuscitation). This sequence is repeated until the obstruction is relieved. In a choking child older than age 1 year, abdominal thrusts (Heimlich maneuver) may be performed, with special care in younger children because of concern about possible intra-abdominal organ injury.

Blind finger sweeps should *not* be performed in infants or children because the finger may actually push the foreign body further into the airway causing further obstruction. The airway may be opened by jaw thrust, and if the foreign body can be directly visualized, careful removal with the fingers or instruments (Magill forceps) can be attempted. Patients with persistent apnea and inability to achieve adequate ventilation may require emergency intubation, tracheotomy, or needle cricothyrotomy, depending on the setting and the rescuer's skills.

Ralston M et al (editors): *Pediatric Advanced Life Support Provider Manual.* American Heart Association and American Academy of Pediatrics, 2006.

2. Foreign Bodies in the Lower Respiratory Tract

ESSENTIALS OF DIAGNOSIS & TYPICAL FEATURES

► Sudden onset of coughing, wheezing, or respiratory distress.

► Asymmetrical physical findings of decreased breath sounds or localized wheezing.

► Asymmetrical radiographic findings, especially with forced expiratory view.

Clinical Findings

A. Symptoms and Signs

Respiratory symptoms and signs vary depending on the site of obstruction and the duration following the acute episode. For example, a large or central airway obstruction may cause marked distress. The acute cough or wheezing caused by a foreign body in the lower respiratory tract may diminish over time only to recur later as chronic cough or persistent wheezing, monophonic wheezing, asymmetrical breath sounds on chest examination, or recurrent pneumonia in one location. Foreign body aspiration should be suspected in children with chronic cough, persistent wheezing, or recurrent pneumonia. Long-standing foreign bodies may lead to bronchiectasis or lung abscess. Hearing asymmetrical breath sounds or localized wheezing also suggests a foreign body.

B. Imaging

Inspiratory and forced expiratory (obtained by manually compressing the abdomen during expiration) chest radiographs should be obtained if foreign body aspiration is suspected. Chest radiographs may be normal up to 25% of the time. If abnormal, the initial inspiratory view may show localized hyperinflation due to the ball-valve effect of the foreign body, causing distal air trapping or aeration within an area of atelectasis. A positive forced expiratory study shows a mediastinal shift away from the affected side. If airway obstruction is complete, atelectasis and related volume loss will be the major radiologic findings. Lateral decubitus views may be helpful if the child is too young to cooperate. Chest fluoroscopy is an alternative approach for detecting air trapping and mediastinal shift.

Treatment

When a foreign body is highly suspected, a normal chest radiograph should not rule out the possibility of an airway foreign body. If clinical suspicion persists based on two of three findings—history of possible aspiration, focal abnormal lung examination, or an abnormal chest radiograph—

then a bronchoscopy is indicated. Rigid bronchoscopy under general anesthesia is recommended. Flexible bronchoscopy may be helpful for follow-up evaluations (after the foreign object has been removed).

Children with suspected acute foreign body aspiration should be admitted to the hospital for evaluation and treatment. Chest postural drainage is no longer recommended because the foreign body may become dislodged and obstruct a major central airway. Bronchoscopy should not be delayed in children with respiratory distress but should be performed as soon as the diagnosis is made—even in children with more chronic symptoms. Following the removal of the foreign body, β-adrenergic nebulization treatments followed by chest physiotherapy are recommended to help clear related mucus or treat bronchospasm. Failure to identify a foreign body in the lower respiratory tract can result in bronchiectasis or lung abscess. This risk justifies an aggressive approach to suspected foreign bodies in suspicious cases.

Chiu CY et al: Factors predicting early diagnosis of foreign body aspiration in children. Pediatr Emerg Care 2005;21:161 [PMID: 15744193].

Dunn GR et al: Management of suspected foreign body aspiration in children. Clin Otolaryngol 2002;27:384 [PMID: 12383302].

Girardi B et al: Two new radiographic findings to improve the diagnosis of bronchial foreign body aspiration in children. Pediatr Pulmonol 2004;38:261.

Rovin JD, Rodgers BM: Pediatric foreign body aspiration. Pediatr Rev 2000;21:86 [PMID: 10702322].

BRONCHIOLITIS

ESSENTIALS OF DIAGNOSIS & TYPICAL FEATURES

▶ Clinical syndrome characterized by one or more of the following findings: coughing, tachypnea, labored breathing, and hypoxia.

▶ Irritability, poor feeding, vomiting.

▶ Wheezing and crackles on chest auscultation.

Bronchiolitis is the most common serious acute respiratory illness in infants and young children. One to 3% of infants with bronchiolitis will require hospitalization, especially during the winter months. The typical presentation is acute onset of tachypnea, cough, and expiratory wheezing after 1–2 days of rhinorrhea. RSV is by far the most common viral cause of acute bronchiolitis. Parainfluenza, human metapneumovirus, influenza, adenovirus, *Mycoplasma, Chlamydia, Ureaplasma,* and *Pneumocystis* are less common causes of bronchiolitis during early infancy. Major concerns include not only the acute effects of bronchiolitis but also the possible development of chronic airway hyperreactivity (asthma). Bronchiolitis due to RSV infection contributes substantially to morbidity and mortality in children with underlying medical disorders, including chronic lung disease of prematurity, CF, congenital heart disease, and immunodeficiency.

▶ Clinical Findings

A. Symptoms and Signs

The usual course of RSV bronchiolitis is 1–2 days of fever, rhinorrhea, and cough, followed by wheezing, tachypnea, and respiratory distress. Typically the breathing pattern is shallow, with rapid respirations. Nasal flaring, cyanosis, retractions, and rales may be present, along with prolongation of the expiratory phase and wheezing, depending on the severity of illness. Some young infants present with apnea and few findings on auscultation but may subsequently develop rales, rhonchi, and expiratory wheezing.

B. Laboratory Findings and Imaging

A viral nasal wash may be performed to identify the causative pathogen but is not necessary to make the diagnosis of bronchiolitis. The peripheral white blood cell count may be normal or may show a mild lymphocytosis. Chest radiographic findings are generally nonspecific and typically include hyperinflation, peribronchial cuffing, increased interstitial markings, and subsegmental atelectasis.

▶ Prevention & Treatment

The most effective prevention against RSV infection is to use proper handwashing techniques and to reduce exposure to potential environmental risk factors. Major challenges have impeded the development of an RSV vaccine, but a licensed product may be expected in the near future. Prophylaxis with a monoclonal antibody (palivizumab) has proven effective in reducing the rate of hospitalization and associated morbidities in high-risk premature infants and those with chronic cardiopulmonary conditions.

Although most children with RSV bronchiolitis are readily treated as outpatients, hospitalization is required in infected children with hypoxemia on room air, a history of apnea, moderate tachypnea with feeding difficulties, and marked respiratory distress with retractions. Children at high risk for hospitalization include young infants (under 6 months of age), especially with any history of prematurity, and those with underlying chronic cardiopulmonary disorders. While in the hospital, treatment should include supportive strategies such as frequent suctioning and providing adequate fluids to maintain hydration. If hypoxemia is present, supplemental oxygen should be administered. Although bronchodilators and corticosteroids may attenuate airway obstruction, their use remains controversial and empiric, and patients should be assessed individually to determine responsiveness.

In immunocompromised patients, especially bone marrow transplant recipients, a combination of RSV intravenous immune globulin and the antiviral ribavirin has been tried.

Therapy for RSV, however, remains limited, controversial, and mostly supportive.

Prognosis

The prognosis for the majority of infants with acute bronchiolitis is very good. With improved supportive care and prophylaxis with palivizumab, the mortality rate among high-risk infants has decreased substantially.

American Academy of Pediatrics Subcommittee on Diagnosis and Management of Bronchiolitis: Diagnosis and management of bronchiolitis. Pediatrics 2006;118:1774 [PMID: 17015575].

Martinez FD: Respiratory syncytial virus bronchiolitis and the pathogenesis of childhood asthma. Pediatr Infect Dis J 2003;22(Suppl):S76 [PMID: 12671456].

Simoes EA: Maternal smoking, asthma, and bronchiolitis: Clear-cut association or equivocal evidence? Pediatrics 2007;119:1210 [PMID: 17545392].

Smyth RL, Openshaw PJ: Bronchiolitis. Lancet 2006;368:312 [PMID: 16860701].

DISORDERS OF MUCOCILIARY CLEARANCE

Mucociliary clearance is the primary defense mechanism for the lung. Inhaled particles including microbial pathogens are entrapped in mucus on the airway surface, then cleared by the coordinated action of cilia. The volume and composition of airway surface liquid influence the efficiency of ciliary function and mucus clearance. The two main genetic diseases of mucociliary clearance involve disorders of ion transport (cystic fibrosis, CF) and disorders in ciliary function (primary ciliary dyskinesia, PCD).

CYSTIC FIBROSIS

ESSENTIALS OF DIAGNOSIS & TYPICAL FEATURES

▸ Greasy, bulky, malodorous stools; failure to thrive.

▸ Recurrent respiratory infections.

▸ Digital clubbing on examination.

▸ Bronchiectasis on chest imaging.

▸ Sweat chloride > 60 mmol/L.

General Considerations

CF, an autosomal recessive disease, results in a syndrome of chronic sinopulmonary infections, malabsorption, and nutritional abnormalities. It is one of the most common lethal genetic diseases in the United States, with an incidence of approximately 1:3000 among Caucasians. Although CF is characterized by abnormalities in the hepatic, gastrointestinal, and male reproductive systems, lung disease is the major cause of morbidity and mortality. Most individuals with CF develop obstructive lung disease associated with chronic infection that leads to progressive loss of pulmonary function.

The cause of CF is a defect in a single gene on chromosome 7 that encodes a cyclic adenosine monophosphate–regulated chloride channel called the cystic fibrosis transmembrane conductance regulator (CFTR) protein. CFTR functions primarily as an ion channel and controls the movement of salt and water into and out of epithelial cells lining the airways, biliary tree, intestines, vas deferens, sweat ducts, and pancreatic ducts. Approximately 1500 disease-causing mutations in the CF gene have been identified. The most common mutation, ΔF508, is a deletion of three base pairs. This and other gene mutations lead to defects or deficiencies in CFTR, causing problems in salt and water movement across cell membranes, resulting in abnormally thick secretions in various organ systems and critically altering host defense in the lung.

Clinical Findings

A. Symptoms and Signs

Approximately 15% of newborns with CF present at birth with meconium ileus, a severe intestinal obstruction resulting from inspissation of tenacious meconium in the terminal ileum. Meconium ileus is virtually diagnostic of CF, so the infant should be treated presumptively as having CF until a sweat test or genotyping can be obtained.

During infancy and beyond, a common presentation of CF is failure to thrive. These children fail to gain weight despite good appetite and typically have frequent, bulky, foul-smelling, oily stools. These symptoms are the result of severe exocrine pancreatic insufficiency, the failure of the pancreas to produce sufficient digestive enzymes to allow breakdown and absorption of fats and protein. Pancreatic insufficiency occurs in over 85% of persons with CF. (Chapter 21 describes gastrointestinal and hepatobiliary manifestations of CF; see also Table 21–9 there.) Infants with undiagnosed CF may also present with hypoproteinemia with or without edema, anemia, and deficiency of the fat-soluble vitamins A, D, E, and K, because of ongoing steatorrhea.

From a respiratory standpoint, clinical manifestations include productive cough, wheezing, chronic bronchitis and recurrent pneumonias, progressive obstructive airways disease, exercise intolerance, dyspnea, hemoptysis, anorexia, and weight loss. CF lung disease is characterized by a cycle of chronic, persistent infections with CF-related pathogens and an excessive inflammatory response that progressively damages the airways and lung parenchyma. This results in a characteristic airflow obstruction on lung function testing and bronchiectasis and other structural lung abnormalities on chest imaging (best demonstrated by high-resolution CT scans). Airway infection with bacteria, including *S aureus* and *H influenzae,* often begins in the first few months of life, even in asymptomatic infants. Eventually, *Pseudomonas aeruginosa* becomes the predominant pathogen. Acquisition of the characteristic mucoid *Pseudomonas* is associated with a more rapid decline in pulmonary function.

An acute change in respiratory signs and symptoms from the subject's baseline is generically termed a pulmonary exacerbation. Clinically, an exacerbation is typically manifested by increased cough and sputum production, decreased exercise tolerance, malaise, and anorexia. These symptoms are usually associated with decreased measures of lung function, new chest radiographic findings, or both. Treatment for pulmonary exacerbations generally consists of antibiotics and augmented airway clearance.

CF should also be considered in infants and children who present with severe dehydration and hypochloremic alkalosis. Other findings that should prompt a diagnostic evaluation for CF include unexplained bronchiectasis, rectal prolapse, nasal polyps, chronic sinusitis, and unexplained pancreatitis or cirrhosis.

B. Diagnostic Studies

The diagnosis of CF is made by a sweat chloride concentration greater than 60 mmol/L in the presence of one or more typical clinical features (chronic sinopulmonary disease, pancreatic insufficiency, salt loss syndromes) or an appropriate family history (sibling or first cousin who has CF). The most acceptable type of sweat test is performed by iontophoresis of pilocarpine into the skin to stimulate sweating. Sweat then is collected and analyzed for chloride. This test should be performed at a CF Foundation–accredited laboratory. A diagnosis can also be confirmed by genotyping that reveals two alleles that have CF-causing mutations. Many states now perform newborn screening for CF by measuring immunoreactive trypsin (IRT), a pancreatic enzyme, in blood. Most infants with CF have elevated IRT in the newborn period. In newborns with elevated IRT, the diagnosis of CF must then be confirmed by sweat testing, mutation analysis, or both.

▶ Treatment

It is strongly recommended that individuals with CF be followed at a CF Foundation–accredited CF care center (http://www.cff.org).

The cornerstone of gastrointestinal treatment is pancreatic enzyme supplementation. Persons with CF are required to take pancreatic enzyme capsules immediately prior to each meal and with snacks. Occasionally, enzyme supplementation alone does not control the malabsorption, and antacids are added to the regimen. Individuals should also take daily multivitamins that contain vitamins A, D, E, and K. Moreover, caloric supplements are often added to the patient's diet to optimize growth.

Airway clearance therapy and aggressive antibiotic use form the mainstays of treatment for CF lung disease. Antibiotic therapy appears to be one of the primary reasons for the increased life expectancy of persons with CF. Three evi-

dence-based medications that are now routinely used in many persons with CF are an inhaled mucolytic agent, recombinant human DNAse (Pulmozyme), inhaled tobramycin (TOBI), and oral azithromycin for those with chronic *Pseudomonas* infection. These therapies have been shown to maintain lung function and reduce the need for hospitalizations and intravenous antibiotics. Bronchodilators and anti-inflammatory therapies are also frequently used.

▶ Prognosis

A few decades ago, CF was fatal in early childhood. Now the median life expectancy is around 35 years of age. The rate of lung disease progression usually determines survival. Lung transplantation may be performed in those with end-stage lung disease. In addition, new treatments, including gene therapy trials and agents that modulate CFTR protein function, are being developed based on improved understanding of the disease at the cellular and molecular levels.

Ratjen F, Doring G: Cystic fibrosis. Lancet 2003;361:681 [PMID: 12606185].
Rowe SM, Clancy JP: Advances in cystic fibrosis therapies. Curr Opin Pediatr 2006;18:604 [PMID: 17099358].
Strausbaugh SD, Davis PB: Cystic fibrosis: A review of epidemiology and pathobiology. Clin Chest Med 2007;28:279 [PMID: 17467547].

PRIMARY CILIARY DYSKINESIA

ESSENTIALS OF DIAGNOSIS & TYPICAL FEATURES

- ▶ Chronic bronchitis, sinusitis, and otitis.
- ▶ Situs inversus in approximately 50% of cases.
- ▶ Unexplained respiratory distress in the newborn period.
- ▶ Consistent ultrastructural defect of cilia demonstrated by electron microscopy.

▶ General Considerations

PCD, also known as immotile cilia syndrome or Kartagener syndrome, is a human genetic disease associated with abnormal ciliary structure and function. Occurring in approximately 1 in 15,000 births, PCD is an inherited disease that causes impaired clearance of bacteria from the lung, paranasal sinuses, and middle ear. Half of the patients with PCD have their internal organs reversed (situs abnormalities), and men are usually infertile.

▶ Clinical Findings

A. Symptoms and Signs

Children with PCD have a variety of clinical features including chronic productive cough, wheezing, nasal congestion and rhinorrhea, chronic sinusitis, bronchitis, and pneumonias. Recurrent, chronic otitis media is a serious problem, and hearing loss is common. A history of transient neonatal respiratory distress and unexplained atelectasis in the newborn period is frequently elicited. Approximately 50% of PCD patients have situs inversus totalis or other organ rotation abnormalities, suggesting a role for embryonic cilia in the rotation of internal organs. The diagnosis of PCD should also be considered in any patients with unexplained bronchiectasis or in males with infertility issues.

B. Diagnostic Studies

The diagnosis of PCD currently requires a compatible clinical phenotype and specific ultrastructural defects of the cilia detected by transmission electron microscopy. Cilia samples may be obtained from either the upper airways (nasal passage) or lower airways (trachea). Semen collection from older male patients can also be obtained to analyze sperm tails, which have the same ultrastructure as cilia. Significant expertise is required to produce high-quality transmission electron micrographs of cilia, and to distinguish primary (genetic) defects from secondary (acquired) defects in ciliary ultrastructure. Functional assessments of cilia consist of crude measures of nasal mucociliary clearance (the saccharin test), or measures of lung mucociliary clearance, using radioisotopic techniques. The current limitations in diagnosis of PCD provide a compelling case to define disease-causing genetic mutations, which will allow great improvement in the identification and diagnosis of PCD through genetic testing. Although structural and functional assessments of cilia have been the diagnostic gold standard in PCD diagnosis, nasal nitric oxide has the potential to become a useful adjunctive diagnostic test for PCD. Recent studies have demonstrated extremely low levels of nasal nitric oxide in persons with PCD, suggesting that nasal nitric oxide could be used as a screening test for PCD.

Treatment

At present, no specific therapies are available to correct the ciliary dysfunction in PCD. Management includes aggressive airway clearance therapy and frequent courses of antibiotics to treat bacterial infections in the airways, sinuses, and middle ear. No randomized clinical trials have been conducted in this disease because it is so rare and most centers follow only a few PCD patients. A national consortium has been created to improve diagnostic techniques for PCD, including genetic testing to better define the pathogenesis of PCD and study treatments in this population (http://rarediseasesnetwork.epi.usf.edu/).

Prognosis

The progression of lung disease in PCD is quite variable and for most affected individuals is less severe than in CF. Importantly, though, persons with PCD are at risk for chronic lung disease with bronchiectasis. With monitoring and aggressive treatment during times of illness, most individuals with PCD should experience a normal or near-normal life span.

Bush A, O'Callaghan C: Primary ciliary dyskinesia. Arch Dis Child 2002;87:363 [PMID: 12390901].

Noone PG et al: Primary ciliary dyskinesia: Diagnostic and phenotypic features. Am J Respir Crit Care Med 2004;169:459 [PMID: 14656747].

BRONCHIECTASIS

 ESSENTIALS OF DIAGNOSIS & TYPICAL FEATURES

▶ Chronic cough with sputum production.
▶ Rhonchi or wheezes (or both) on chest auscultation.
▶ Diagnosis is confirmed by high-resolution CT scan.

General Considerations

Bronchiectasis is the permanent dilation of bronchi. The dilation may be regular, with the airway continuing to have a smooth outline (cylindric bronchiectasis); irregular, with areas of dilation and constriction (varicose bronchiectasis); or marked, with destruction of structural components of the airway wall (saccular or cystic bronchiectasis).

Bronchiectasis results from airway obstruction by retained mucus secretions or inflammation in response to chronic or repeated infection. It occurs either as a consequence of a preceding illness (severe pneumonia or foreign body aspiration) or as a manifestation of an underlying systemic disorder (CF, PCD, or immunodeficiency).

Clinical Findings

A. Symptoms and Signs

Persons with bronchiectasis will typically have chronic cough, purulent sputum, fever, and weight loss. Recurrent respiratory infections and dyspnea on exertion are also common. Hemoptysis occurs less frequently in children than in adults with bronchiectasis. On physical examination, finger clubbing may be seen. Rales, rhonchi, and decreased air entry are often noted over the bronchiectatic areas.

B. Laboratory Findings and Imaging

Cultures from the lower respiratory tract usually reveal normal oropharyngeal flora. These include *Streptococcus pneumoniae*, *Staphylococcus aureus*, and nontypeable *H influenzae*. *Pseudomonas aeruginosa* can also be found in children with bronchiectasis, even in those without CF.

Chest radiographs may be mildly abnormal with slightly increased bronchovascular markings or areas of atelectasis, or they may demonstrate cystic changes in one or more areas of the lung. The extent of bronchiectasis is best defined by high-resolution CT scan of the lung, which often reveals far wider involvement of lung than expected from the plain chest radiograph. Pulmonary function testing often reveals airflow obstruction. Evaluation of lung function after use of a bronchodilator is helpful in assessing the benefit a patient may have from bronchodilators. Serial assessments of lung function help define the progression or resolution of the disease.

Differential Diagnosis

Bronchiectasis has numerous causes. It can occur following severe respiratory tract infections by bacteria (*Bordetella pertussis*), viruses (adenovirus), or other organisms (*Mycobacterium tuberculosis*). Bronchiectasis is commonly seen in persons with CF, PCD, immunodeficiency, and collagen-vascular conditions. Other diagnostic considerations include foreign body aspiration, chronic aspiration of gastric or oropharyngeal contents, and allergic bronchopulmonary aspergillosis.

Treatment

Aggressive antibiotic therapy during pulmonary exacerbations and routine airway clearance are mainstays of treatment. Inhaled mucolytic agents and bronchodilators may also be of benefit in individual patients.

Surgical removal of an area of lung affected with severe bronchiectasis is considered when the response to medical therapy is poor. Other indications for operation include severe localized disease, repeated hemoptysis, and recurrent pneumonia in one area of lung. If bronchiectasis is widespread, surgical resection offers little advantage.

Prognosis

The prognosis depends on the underlying cause and severity of bronchiectasis, the extent of lung involvement, and the response to medical management. Good pulmonary hygiene and avoidance of infectious complications in the involved areas of lung may reverse cylindric bronchiectasis.

Barker AF: Bronchiectasis. N Engl J Med 2002;346:1383 [PMID: 11986413].

Chang AB et al: Non-CF bronchiectasis: Clinical and HRCT evaluation. Pediatr Pulmonol 2003;35:477 [PMID: 12746947].

BRONCHIOLITIS OBLITERANS

Bronchiolitis obliterans is characterized by partial or complete occlusion of the lumens of terminal and respiratory bronchioles by inflammatory and fibrous tissue. This condition follows damage to the lower respiratory tract from any of a number of insults, such as inhalation of toxic gases, infections (adenovirus, influenza virus, rubeola virus, *Bordetella,* or *Mycoplasma*), connective tissue diseases, transplan-

tation, and aspiration. Bronchiolitis obliterans may also develop in children who have Stevens-Johnson syndrome with pulmonary involvement. Many cases of bronchiolitis obliterans are idiopathic. Adenovirus-induced bronchiolitis obliterans occurs more frequently in the Native American population.

Clinical Findings

A. Symptoms and Signs

Persons with bronchiolitis obliterans usually experience dyspnea, coughing, and exercise intolerance. This diagnosis should be considered in children with persistent cough, wheezing, crackles, or hypoxemia following an episode of acute pneumonia or bronchiolitis.

B. Laboratory Findings and Imaging

Chest radiograph abnormalities include evidence of localized or generalized air trapping as well as (in some cases) nodular densities and alveolar opacification. Scattered areas of matched decreases in ventilation and perfusion are seen when the lung is scanned. Pulmonary angiograms reveal decreased vasculature in involved lung, and bronchograms show marked pruning of the bronchial tree. An assessment of lung function demonstrates an obstructive process that may be combined with evidence of restriction. Inhaled bronchodilators or corticosteroids provide little improvement in lung function.

Differential Diagnosis

Poorly treated asthma, CF, and bronchopulmonary dysplasia must be considered in children with persistent airway obstruction. A trial of medications (including bronchodilators and corticosteroids) may help to determine the reversibility of the process when the primary differential is between asthma and bronchiolitis obliterans. Although the results of imaging and pulmonary function testing are very suggestive, the most definitive way to establish a diagnosis is by lung biopsy.

Complications

Sequelae of bronchiolitis obliterans include persistent airway obstruction, recurrent wheezing, bronchiectasis, chronic atelectasis, recurrent pneumonia, and unilateral hyperlucent lung syndrome.

Treatment

Supplemental oxygen should be given to patients with oxygen desaturation during normal activities or sleep. In addition, early treatment should be directed at preventing ongoing airway damage due to problems such as aspiration, which may be either the primary insult or an acquired problem secondary to marked hyperinflation. The effectiveness of other forms of treatment may be more difficult to evaluate. Oral and inhaled bronchodilators may reverse airway obstruction if the disease has a reactive component. Many children also receive at least one course of corticosteroid treatment in an attempt to reverse the obstruction or prevent ongoing damage. Antibiotics should be used as indicated for pneumonia.

Prognosis

Prognosis may depend in part on the underlying cause as well as the age at which the insult occurred. The course varies from mild asthma-like symptoms to rapidly fatal deterioration despite therapy.

Kurland G, Michelson P: Bronchiolitis obliterans in children. Pediatr Pulmonol 2005;39:193 [PMID: 15635614].

BRONCHOPULMONARY DYSPLASIA

ESSENTIALS OF DIAGNOSIS & TYPICAL FEATURES

▶ Acute respiratory distress in the first week of life.
▶ Required oxygen therapy or mechanical ventilation, with persistent oxygen requirement at 36 weeks' gestational age.
▶ Persistent respiratory abnormalities, including physical signs and radiographic findings.

General Considerations

Bronchopulmonary dysplasia (BPD) remains one of the most significant sequelae of acute respiratory distress in the neonatal intensive care unit, with an incidence of about 30% for infants with a birth weight of less than 1000 g. This disease was first characterized in 1967 when Northway and coworkers reported the clinical, radiologic, and pathologic findings in a group of premature newborns that required prolonged mechanical ventilation and oxygen therapy to treat hyaline membrane disease. The progression from acute hyaline membrane disease to chronic lung disease was divided into four stages: acute respiratory distress shortly after birth, usually hyaline membrane disease (stage I); clinical and radiographic worsening of the acute lung disease, often due to increased pulmonary blood flow secondary to a patent ductus arteriosus (stage II); and progressive signs of chronic lung disease (stages III and IV).

The pathologic findings and clinical course of BPD in recent years have changed due to a combination of new therapies (surfactants, prenatal glucocorticoids, and different ventilation strategies) and increased survival of infants born at earlier gestational ages. Although the incidence of BPD has not changed, the severity of the lung disease has decreased. Pathologically this "new" BPD is characterized by a reduction in inflammation, decreased alveolar number, and a dysmorphic vascular structure.

Pathogenesis

The precise mechanism that results in the development of BPD is unclear. The premature lung makes insufficient functional surfactant; furthermore, the antioxidant defense mechanisms are not sufficiently mature to protect the lung from the toxic oxygen metabolites, and lungs destined to develop BPD show early inflammation and hypercellularity followed by healing with fibrosis. Thus abnormal lung mechanics due to structural immaturity, surfactant deficiency, atelectasis, and pulmonary edema—plus lung injury secondary to hyperoxia and mechanical ventilation—lead to further abnormalities of lung function, causing increases in ventilator and oxygen requirements and resulting in a vicious cycle that compounds the progression of lung injury. Excessive fluid administration, patent ductus arteriosus, pulmonary interstitial emphysema, pneumothorax, infection, pulmonary hypertension, and inflammatory stimuli secondary to lung injury or infection also play important roles in the pathogenesis of the disease. Although the exact mechanisms are not completely understood, BPD represents the consequences of lung injury caused by oxygen toxicity, barotrauma, and inflammation superimposed on a susceptible, generally immature lung.

Clinical Findings

A recent summary of a National Institutes of Health workshop on BPD proposes a definition of the disease that includes oxygen requirement for more than 28 days, a history of positive pressure ventilation or continuous positive airway pressure, and gestational age. The new definition accommodates several key observations regarding the disease, as follows: (1) although most of these children were premature and had hyaline membrane disease, full-term newborns with such disorders as meconium aspiration or persistent pulmonary hypertension can also develop bronchopulmonary dysplasia; (2) some extremely preterm newborns require minimal ventilator support yet subsequently develop a prolonged oxygen requirement despite the absence of severe acute manifestations of respiratory failure; (3) newborns dying within the first weeks of life can already have the aggressive, fibroproliferative pathologic lesions that resemble bronchopulmonary dysplasia; and (4) physiologic abnormalities (increased airway resistance) and biochemical markers of lung injury (altered protease-antiprotease ratios, and increased inflammatory cells and mediators), which may be predictive of BPD, are already present in the first week of life.

Differential Diagnosis

The radiologic appearance of BPD is changing, and severe chronic lung findings of fibrosis with infiltrate are less common. The changes in severe BPD necessitate ruling out meconium aspiration syndrome, congenital infection (eg, with cytomegalovirus or *Ureaplasma*), cystic adenomatoid malformation, recurrent aspiration, pulmonary lymphangiectasia, total anomalous pulmonary venous return, overhydration, and idiopathic pulmonary fibrosis.

▶ Treatment

A. Clinical Course

The clinical course of infants with BPD ranges from a mild increased oxygen requirement that gradually resolves over a few months to more severe disease requiring chronic tracheostomy and mechanical ventilation for the first 2 years of life. In general, patients show slow, steady improvements in oxygen or ventilator requirements but can have frequent respiratory exacerbations leading to frequent and prolonged hospitalizations. Clinical management generally includes careful attention to growth, nutrition (caloric requirements of infants with oxygen dependence and respiratory distress are quite high), metabolic status, developmental and neurologic status, and related problems, along with the various cardiopulmonary abnormalities described in a later discussion.

B. Corticosteroid Therapy

Short courses of postnatal glucocorticoid therapy have been helpful in increasing the success of weaning from the ventilator. Longer courses of postnatal glucocorticoids have been linked to an increased incidence of cerebral palsy. Inhaled glucocorticoids may help reduce the need for systemic steroids, but the overall incidence of BPD has not been affected. Early use of surfactant therapy with adequate lung recruitment increases the chance for survival without BPD and can decrease the overall mortality and reduce the need for ventilation. Thus early interventions are important prior to the development of BPD to decrease morbidity and mortality. Inhaled corticosteroids together with occasional use of β-adrenergic agonists are commonly part of the treatment plan. Part of the rationale for the use of corticosteroids is to decrease lung inflammation and enhance responsiveness to β-adrenergic drugs, as in the treatment of severe asthma. β-Adrenergic agonists followed by chest physiotherapy are often used for the thick secretions that may contribute to airway obstruction or recurrent atelectasis.

C. Airway Evaluation

Children with significant stridor, sleep apnea, chronic wheezing, or excessive respiratory distress need diagnostic bronchoscopy to evaluate for structural lesions (eg, subglottic stenosis, vocal cord paralysis, tracheal stenosis, tracheomalacia, bronchial stenosis, and granulomatous bronchial polyps). In addition, the contribution of gastroesophageal reflux and aspiration should be considered in the face of worsening chronic lung disease.

D. Diuretic Therapy

Salt and water retention secondary to chronic hypoxemia, hypercapnia, or other stimuli may be present. Chronic or intermittent diuretic therapy is commonly used if rales or signs of persistent pulmonary edema are present, and clinical studies show acute improvement in lung function with this therapy. Unfortunately, diuretics often have adverse effects, including severe volume contraction, hypokalemia, alkalosis, and hyponatremia. Potassium and arginine chloride supplements are commonly required.

E. Management of Pulmonary Hypertension

Infants with BPD are at risk of developing pulmonary hypertension, and in many of these children even mild hypoxemia can cause significant elevations of pulmonary arterial pressure. To minimize the harmful effects of hypoxemia, the arterial oxygen saturation should be kept above 93%, with care to avoid hyperoxia during retinal vascular development. Electrocardiographic and echocardiographic studies should be performed to monitor for the development of right ventricular hypertrophy. If hypertrophy persists or if it develops where it was not previously present, intermittent hypoxemia should be considered and further assessments of oxygenation pursued, especially while the infant sleeps. Infants with a history of intubation can develop obstructive sleep apnea secondary to a high-arched palate or subglottic narrowing. Barium swallow, esophageal pH probe studies, bronchoscopy, and cardiac catheterization will diagnose unsuspected cardiac or pulmonary lesions that contribute to the underlying pathophysiology, such as aspiration, tracheomalacia, obstructive sleep apnea, and anatomic cardiac lesions. Long-term care should include monitoring for systemic hypertension and the development of left ventricular hypertrophy.

F. Nutrition

Nutritional problems in infants may be due to increased oxygen consumption, feeding difficulties, gastroesophageal reflux, and chronic hypoxemia. Hypercaloric formulas and gastrostomies are often required to ensure adequate intake while avoiding overhydration. Influenza vaccination is recommended. With the onset of acute wheezing secondary to suspected viral infection, rapid diagnostic testing for RSV infection may facilitate early treatment. Immune prophylaxis of RSV reduces the morbidity of bronchiolitis in infants with BPD.

G. Ventilation

For children who remain ventilator-dependent, attempts should be made to maintain $PaCO_2$ below 60 mm Hg—even when pH is normal—because of the potential adverse effects of hypercapnia on salt and water retention, cardiac function, and perhaps pulmonary vascular tone. Changes in ventilator settings in children with severe lung disease should be slow, because the effects of many of the changes may not be apparent for days.

▶ Prognosis

Surfactant replacement therapy has had a significant effect on reducing morbidity and mortality from BPD. Infants of younger gestational age are surviving in greater numbers. Surprisingly, the effect of neonatal care has not decreased the incidence of BPD significantly, as 50% of survivors go on to develop this diagnosis. The disorder typically develops in the most immature infants, but the long-term outlook for most survivors is generally favorable. Long-term follow-up studies suggest that lung function may be altered for life. Hyperinflation and damage to small airways has been reported in children 10 years out from the first signs of BPD. In addition, these infants are at a higher risk for developing such sequelae as persistent airway hyperreactivity, exercise intolerance, pulmonary hypertension, increased risk for chronic obstructive pulmonary disease, and perhaps abnormal lung growth. As smaller, more immature infants survive, abnormal neurodevelopmental outcomes become more likely. The incidence of cerebral palsy, hearing loss, vision abnormalities, spastic diplegia, and developmental delays is increased. Feeding abnormalities, behavior difficulties, and increased irritability have all been reported. Finally, children with BPD frequently develop airway obstruction, hyperreactive airways, and decreased oxygen saturation during exercise. This should be taken into account for children residing at higher altitudes. A focus on good nutrition, prophylaxis against respiratory pathogens and airway hyperreactivity, and attention to school performance continue to provide the best outcomes. Patience, continued family support, attention to developmental issues, and speech and physical therapy help to improve the long-term outlook.

Allen J et al and the American Thoracic Society: Statement on the care of the child with chronic lung disease of infancy and childhood. Am J Respir Crit Care Med 2003;168:356 [PMID: 12888611].

Bancalari E et al: Bronchopulmonary dysplasia: Changes in pathogenesis, epidemiology and definition. Semin Neonatol 2003;8:63 [PMID: 12667831].

Chess PR et al: Pathogenesis of bronchopulmonary dysplasia. Semin Perinatol 2006;30:171 [PMID: 16860156].

Coalson JJ: Pathology of bronchopulmonary dysplasia. Semin Perinatol 2006;30:179 [PMID: 16860157].

Cole CH: Inhaled glucocorticoid therapy in infants at risk for neonatal chronic lung disease. J Asthma 2000;37:533 [PMID: 11060660].

Higgins RD et al: Executive summary of the workshop on oxygen in neonatal therapies: Controversies and opportunities for research. Pediatrics 2007;119:790 [PMID: 17403851].

Kresch MJ, Clive JM: Meta-analysis of surfactant replacement therapy of infants with birth weights less than 2000 grams. J Perinatol 1998;18:276 [PMID: 9730197].

Northway WH et al: Pulmonary disease following respiratory therapy of hyaline membrane disease: Bronchopulmonary dysplasia. N Engl J Med 1967;276:357 [PMID: 5334613].

Saugstad OD: Bronchopulmonary dysplasia—Oxidative stress and antioxidants. Semin Neonatol 2003;8:39 [PMID: 12667829].

Speer CP: Inflammation and bronchopulmonary dysplasia. Semin Neonatol 2003;8:29 [PMID: 12667828].

Stocks J, Coates A, Bush A: Lung function in infants and young children with chronic lung disease of infancy: The next steps? Pediatr Pulmonol 2007;42:3 [PMID: 17123320].

Thébaud B, Abman SH: Bronchopulmonary dysplasia: Where have all the vessels gone? Roles of angiogenic growth factors in chronic lung disease. Am J Respir Crit Care Med 2007 May 15;175:978–85 [PMID: 17272782].

Van Marter LJ: Progress in discovery and evaluation of treatments to prevent bronchopulmonary dysplasia. Biol Neonate 2006;89:303 [PMID: 16770070].

CONGENITAL MALFORMATIONS OF THE LUNG

What follows is a brief description of selected congenital pulmonary malformations.

PULMONARY AGENESIS & HYPOPLASIA

With unilateral pulmonary agenesis (complete absence of one lung), the trachea continues into a main bronchus and often has complete tracheal rings. The left lung is affected more often than the right. With compensatory postnatal growth, the remaining lung often herniates into the contralateral chest. Chest radiographs show a mediastinal shift toward the affected side, and vertebral abnormalities may be present. Absent or incomplete lung development may be associated with other congenital abnormalities, such as absence of one or both kidneys or fusion of ribs, and the outcome is primarily related to the severity of associated lesions. About 50% of patients survive; the mortality rate is higher with agenesis of the right lung than of the left lung. This difference is probably not related to the higher incidence of associated anomalies but rather to a greater shift in the mediastinum that leads to tracheal compression and distortion of vascular structures.

Pulmonary hypoplasia is incomplete development of one or both lungs, characterized by a reduction in alveolar number and a reduction in airway branches. Pulmonary hypoplasia is present in up to 10–15% of perinatal autopsies. The hypoplasia can be a result of an intrathoracic mass, resulting in lack of space for the lungs to grow; decreased size of the thorax; decreased fetal breathing movements; decreased blood flow to the lungs; or possibly a primary mesodermal defect affecting multiple organ systems. Congenital diaphragmatic hernia is the most common cause, with an incidence of 1:2200 births. Other causes include extralobar sequestration, diaphragmatic eventration or hypoplasia, thoracic neuroblastoma, fetal hydrops, and fetal hydrochylothorax. Chest cage abnormalities, diaphragmatic elevation, oligohydramnios, chromosomal abnormalities, severe musculoskeletal disorders, and cardiac lesions may also result in hypoplastic lungs. Postnatal factors may play important roles. For example, infants with advanced BPD can have pulmonary hypoplasia.

▶ Clinical Findings

A. Symptoms and Signs

The clinical presentation is highly variable and is related to the severity of hypoplasia as well as associated abnormalities. Lung hypoplasia is often associated with pneumothorax. Some newborns present with perinatal stress, severe acute respiratory distress, and persistent pulmonary hypertension of the newborn secondary to primary pulmonary hypoplasia (without associated anomalies). Children with lesser degrees of hypoplasia may present with chronic cough, tachypnea, wheezing, and recurrent pneumonia.

B. Laboratory Findings and Imaging

Chest radiographic findings include variable degrees of volume loss in a small hemithorax with mediastinal shift. Pulmonary agenesis should be suspected if tracheal deviation is evident on the chest radiograph. The chest CT scan is the optimal diagnostic imaging procedure if the chest radiograph is not definitive. Ventilation-perfusion scans, angiography, and bronchoscopy are often helpful in the evaluation, demonstrating decreased pulmonary vascularity or premature blunting of airways associated with the maldeveloped lung tissue. The degree of respiratory impairment is defined by analysis of arterial blood gases.

▶ Treatment & Prognosis

Treatment is supportive. The outcome is determined by the severity of underlying medical problems, the extent of the hypoplasia, and the degree of pulmonary hypertension.

Chinoy MR: Pulmonary hypoplasia and congenital diaphragmatic hernia: Advances in the pathogenetics and regulation of lung development. J Surg Res 2002;106:209 [PMID: 12127828].

Laudy JA, Wladimiroff JW: The fetal lung. 2: Pulmonary hypoplasia. Ultrasound Obstet Gynecol 2000;16:482 [PMID: 11169336].

Nowotny T et al: Right-sided pulmonary aplasia: Longitudinal lung function studies in two cases and comparison to results from term healthy neonates. Pediatr Pulmonol 1998;26:138 [PMID: 9727767].

Winn HN et al: Neonatal pulmonary hypoplasia and perinatal mortality in patients with midtrimester rupture of amniotic membranes—a critical analysis. Am J Obstet Gynecol 2000;182:1638 [PMID: 10871491].

PULMONARY SEQUESTRATION

Pulmonary sequestration is nonfunctional pulmonary tissue that does not communicate with the tracheobronchial tree and receives its blood supply from one or more anomalous systemic arteries. This abnormality originates during the embryonic period of lung development. It is classified as either extralobar or intralobar. Extralobar sequestration is a mass of pulmonary parenchyma anatomically separate from the normal lung, with a distinct pleural investment. Its blood supply derives from the systemic circulation (more typical), from pulmonary vessels, or from both. Rarely, it communicates with the esophagus or stomach. Pathologically, extralobar sequestration appears as a solitary thoracic lesion near the diaphragm. Abdominal sites are rare. Size varies from 0.5–12 cm. The left side is involved in over 90% of cases. In contrast to intralobar sequestrations, venous drainage is usually through the systemic or portal venous system.

Histologic findings include uniformly dilated bronchioles, alveolar ducts, and alveoli. Occasionally the bronchial structure appears normal; however, often the cartilage in the wall is deficient, or no cartilage-containing structures can be found. Lymphangiectasia is sometimes found within the lesion. Extralobar sequestration can be associated with other anomalies, including bronchogenic cysts, heart defects, and diaphragmatic hernia, the latter occurring in over half of cases.

Intralobar sequestration is an isolated segment of lung within the normal pleural investment that often receives blood from one or more arteries arising from the aorta or its branches. Intralobar sequestration is usually found within the lower lobes (98%), two thirds are found on the left side, and it is rarely associated with other congenital anomalies (< 2% versus 50% with extralobar sequestration). It rarely presents in the newborn period (unlike extralobar sequestration). Some researchers have hypothesized that intralobar sequestration is an acquired lesion secondary to chronic infection. Clinical presentation includes chronic cough, wheezing, or recurrent pneumonias. Rarely, patients with intralobar sequestration can present with hemoptysis. Diagnosis is often made by angiography, which shows large systemic arteries perfusing the lesion. Recently spiral CT scans with contrast or magnetic resonance angiography have proved useful in identifying anomalous systemic arterial supply to the lung. Treatment is usually by surgical resection.

Alton H: Pulmonary vascular imaging. Paediatr Respir Rev 2001;2:227 [PMID: 12052324].

Conran RM, Stocker JT: Extralobar sequestration with frequently associated congenital cystic adenomatoid malformation, type 2: Report of 50 cases. Pediatr Dev Pathol 1999;2:454 [PMID: 10441623].

Eber E: Antenatal diagnosis of congenital thoracic malformations: Early surgery, late surgery, or no surgery? Semin Respir Crit Care Med 2007;28:355 [PMID: 17562505].

Halkic N et al: Pulmonary sequestration: A review of 26 cases. Eur J Cardiothorac Surg 1998;14:127 [PMID: 9754996].

Salmons S: Pulmonary sequestration. Neonatal Netw 2000;19:27 [PMID: 11949021].

Zylak CJ et al: Developmental lung anomalies in the adult: Radiologic-pathologic correlation. Radiographics 2002;22(Spec No):S25 [PMID: 12376599].

CONGENITAL LOBAR EMPHYSEMA

Patients with congenital lobar emphysema—also known as infantile lobar emphysema, congenital localized emphysema, unilobar obstructive emphysema, congenital hypertrophic lobar emphysema, or congenital lobar overinflation—present most commonly with severe neonatal respiratory distress or progressive respiratory impairment during the first year of life. Rarely the mild or intermittent nature of the symptoms in older children or young adults results in delayed diagnosis. Most patients are white males. Although the cause of congenital lobar emphysema is not well understood, some lesions show bronchial cartilaginous dysplasia due to abnormal orientation or distribution of the bronchial cartilage. This leads to expiratory collapse, producing obstruction and the symptoms outlined in the following discussion.

▶ **Clinical Findings**

A. Symptoms and Signs

Clinical features include respiratory distress, tachypnea, cyanosis, wheezing, retractions, and cough. Breath sounds are reduced on the affected side, perhaps with hyperresonance to percussion, mediastinal displacement, and bulging of the chest wall on the affected side.

B. Imaging

Radiologic findings include overdistention of the affected lobe (usually an upper or middle lobe; > 99%), with wide separation of bronchovascular markings, collapse of adjacent lung, shift of the mediastinum away from the affected side, and a depressed diaphragm on the affected side. The radiographic diagnosis may be confusing in the newborn because of retention of alveolar fluid in the affected lobe causing the appearance of a homogeneous density. Other diagnostic studies include chest radiograph with fluoroscopy, ventilation-perfusion study, and chest CT scan followed by bronchoscopy, angiography, and exploratory thoracotomy.

▶ **Differential Diagnosis**

The differential diagnosis of congenital lobar emphysema includes pneumothorax, pneumatocele, atelectasis with compensatory hyperinflation, diaphragmatic hernia, and congenital cystic adenomatoid malformation. The most common site of involvement is the left upper lobe (42%) or right middle lobe (35%). Evaluation must differentiate regional obstructive emphysema from lobar hyperinflation secondary to an uncomplicated ball-valve mechanism due to extrinsic compression from a mass (ie, bronchogenic cyst, tumor, lymphadenopathy, foreign body, pseudotumor or plasma cell granuloma, or vascular compression) or intrinsic obstruction from a mucus plug due to infection and inflammation from various causes.

▶ **Treatment**

When respiratory distress is marked, a segmental or complete lobectomy is usually required. Less symptomatic older children may do equally well with or without lobectomy.

Babu R et al: Prenatal sonographic features of congenital lobar emphysema. Fetal Diagn Ther 2001;16:200 [PMID: 11399878].

Horak E et al: Congenital cystic lung disease: Diagnostic and therapeutic considerations. Clin Pediatr 2003;42:251 [PMID: 12739924].

Mandelbaum I et al: Congenital lobar obstructive emphysema: Report of eight cases and literature review. Ann Surg 1965;162:1075 [PMID: 5845589].

CONGENITAL CYSTIC ADENOMATOID MALFORMATION

Patients with congenital cystic adenomatoid malformations, which are unilateral hamartomatous lesions, generally present with marked respiratory distress within the first days of life. This disorder accounts for 95% of cases of congenital cystic lung disease.

Right and left lungs are involved with equal frequency. These lesions originate during the first 4–6 weeks of gestation during the embryonic period of lung development. They appear as glandlike space-occupying masses or have an increase in terminal respiratory structures, forming intercommunicating cysts of various sizes, lined by cuboidal or ciliated pseudostratified columnar epithelium. The lesions may have polypoid formations of mucosa, with focally increased elastic tissue in the cyst wall beneath the bronchial type of epithelium. Air passages appear malformed and tend to lack cartilage.

There are three types of such malformations. Type 1 is most common (55%) and consists of single or multiple large cysts (> 2 cm in diameter) with features of mature lung tissue. Type 1 is amenable to surgical resection. A mediastinal shift is evident on examination or chest radiograph in 80% of patients and can mimic infantile lobar emphysema. Approximately 75% of type 1 lesions are on the right side. A survival rate of 90% is generally reported.

Type 2 lesions (40% of cases) consist of multiple small cysts (< 2 cm) resembling dilated simple bronchioles and are often (60%) associated with other anomalies, especially renal agenesis or dysgenesis, cardiac malformations, and intestinal atresia. Approximately 60% of type 2 lesions are on the left side. Mediastinal shift is evident less often (10%) than in type 1, and the survival rate is worse (40%).

Type 3 lesions consist of small cysts (< 0.5 cm). They appear as bulky, firm masses. The reported survival rate is 50%.

Recently, two additional types have been described: type 0, a malformation of the proximal tracheobronchial tree (incompatible with life), and type 4, a malformation of the distal acinus. Both types are extremely uncommon.

▶ **Clinical Findings**

A. Symptoms and Signs

Clinically, respiratory distress is noted soon after birth. Expansion of the cysts occurs with the onset of breathing and produces compression of normal lung areas with mediastinal herniation. Breath sounds are decreased. With type 3 lesions, dullness to percussion may be present. Older patients can present with a spontaneous pneumothorax or with pneumonia-like symptoms.

B. Imaging

With type 1 lesions, chest radiograph shows an intrapulmonary mass of soft tissue density with scattered radiolucent areas of varying sizes and shapes, usually with a mediastinal shift and pulmonary herniation. Placement of a radiopaque feeding tube into the stomach helps in the differentiation from diaphragmatic hernia. Type 2 lesions appear similar except that the cysts are smaller. Type 3 lesions may appear as a solid homogeneous mass filling the hemithorax and causing a marked mediastinal shift. Differentiation from sequestration is not difficult because congenital cystic adenomatoid malformations have no systemic blood supply.

Treatment

Treatment of type 1 and 3 lesions involves surgical removal of the affected lobe. Resection is often indicated because of the risk of infection and air trapping, since the malformation communicates with the tracheobronchial tree but mucous clearance is compromised. Because type 2 lesions are often associated with other severe anomalies, management may be more complex. Segmental resection is not feasible because smaller cysts may expand after removal of the more obviously affected area. Cystic adenomatoid malformations have been reported to have malignant potential; therefore, expectant management with observation alone should proceed with caution. Recent development of intrauterine surgery for congenital malformations has led to promising results.

Breckenridge RL et al: Congenital cystic adenomatoid malformation of the lung. J Pediatr 1965;67:863 [PMID: 5845450].

Calvert JK et al: Outcome of antenatally suspected congenital cystic adenomatoid malformation of the lung: 10 years' experience 1991–2001. Arch Dis Child Fetal Neonatal Ed 2006;91:F26 [PMID: 16131533].

MacSweeney F et al: An assessment of the expanded classification of congenital cystic adenomatoid malformations and their relationship to malignant transformation. Am J Surg Pathol 2003;27:1139 [PMID: 12883247].

Wilson RD et al: Cystic adenomatoid malformation of the lung: Review of genetics, prenatal diagnosis, and in utero treatment. Am J Med Genet A 2006;140:151 [PMID: 16353256].

ACQUIRED DISORDERS INVOLVING ALVEOLI

BACTERIAL PNEUMONIA

ESSENTIALS OF DIAGNOSIS & TYPICAL FEATURES

- ▶ Fever, cough, dyspnea.
- ▶ Abnormal chest examination (rales or decreased breath sounds).
- ▶ Abnormal chest radiograph (infiltrates, hilar adenopathy, pleural effusion).

General Considerations

Bacterial pneumonia is inflammation of the lung classified according to the infecting organism. Patients with the following problems are particularly predisposed to this disease: aspiration, immunodeficiency or immunosuppression, congenital anomalies (intrapulmonary sequestration, tracheoesophageal fistula, or cleft palate), abnormalities in clearance of mucus (CF, ciliary dysfunction, tracheomalacia, or bronchiectasis), congestive heart failure, and perinatal contamination.

Clinical Findings

A. Symptoms and Signs

The bacterial pathogen, severity of the disease, and age of the patient may cause substantial variations in the presentation of acute bacterial pneumonia. Infants may have few or nonspecific findings on history and physical examination. Immunocompetent older patients may not be extremely ill. Some patients may present with fever only or only with signs of generalized toxicity. Others may have additional symptoms or signs of lower respiratory tract disease (respiratory distress, cough, and sputum production), pneumonia (rales, decreased breath sounds, dullness to percussion, and abnormal tactile or vocal fremitus), or pleural involvement (splinting, pain, friction rub, and dullness to percussion). Some patients may have additional extrapulmonary findings, such as meningismus or abdominal pain, due to pneumonia itself. Others may have evidence of infection at other sites due to the same organism causing their pneumonia: meningitis, otitis media, sinusitis, pericarditis, epiglottitis, or abscesses.

B. Laboratory Findings

Elevated white blood cell counts (> 15,000/μL) frequently accompany bacterial pneumonia. However, a low white blood count (< 5000/μL) can be an ominous finding in this disease.

C. Imaging

Chest radiographic findings (lateral and frontal views) define bacterial pneumonia. Patchy infiltrates, atelectasis, hilar adenopathy, or pleural effusion may be observed. Radiographs should be taken in the lateral decubitus position to identify pleural fluid. Complete lobar consolidation is not a common finding in infants and children. Severity of disease may not correlate with radiographic findings. Clinical resolution precedes resolution apparent on chest radiograph.

D. Special Tests

Invasive diagnostic procedures (bronchial brushing or washing, lung puncture, or open or thoracoscopic lung biopsy) should be undertaken in critically ill patients when other means do not adequately identify the cause (see earlier section on Culture of Material from the Respiratory Tract).

► Differential Diagnosis

The differential diagnosis of pneumonia varies with the age and immunocompetence of the host. The spectrum of potential pathogens to be considered includes aerobic, anaerobic, and acid-fast bacteria as well as *Chlamydia trachomatis, C pneumoniae, C psittaci, Coxiella burnetii* (Q fever), *Pneumocystis jiroveci, Bordetella pertussis, Mycoplasma pneumoniae, Legionella pneumophila,* and respiratory viruses. *Streptococcus pneumoniae* is the most prevalent bacterial pathogen. Vaccination with pneumococcal vaccine will aid in the prevention of pneumonia.

Noninfectious pulmonary disease (including gastric aspiration, foreign body aspiration, atelectasis, congenital malformations, congestive heart failure, malignancy, tumors such as plasma cell granuloma, chronic interstitial lung diseases, and pulmonary hemosiderosis) should be considered in the differential diagnosis of localized or diffuse infiltrates. When effusions are present, additional noninfectious disorders such as collagen diseases, neoplasm, and pulmonary infarction should also be considered.

► Complications

Empyema may occur frequently with staphylococcal, pneumococcal, and group A β-hemolytic streptococcal disease. Distal sites of infection—meningitis, otitis media, sinusitis (especially of the ethmoids), and septicemia—may be present, particularly with disease due to *S pneumoniae* or *H influenzae*. Certain immunocompromised patients, such as those who have undergone splenectomy or who have hemoglobin SS or SC disease or thalassemia, are especially prone to overwhelming sepsis with these organisms. Distal infection of the bones, joints, or other organs (eg, liver abscess) may occur in certain hosts with specific organisms.

► Treatment

Antimicrobial therapy should be guided by Gram stain of sputum, tracheobronchial secretions, or pleural fluid if available; radiographic findings; age and known or suspected immunocompetence of the host; and local epidemiologic information. Reasonable coverage for pneumonia in the sick, immunocompromised, or debilitated patient, pending the results of bronchoalveolar lavage or thoracoscopic biopsy, should include ceftazidime, clindamycin, vancomycin, a macrolide for *Legionella* and *Mycoplasma,* and possibly trimethoprim–sulfamethoxazole for *P jiroveci.* Depending on the circumstances and the level of illness, empiric antifungal or antiviral therapy may be considered. In specific circumstances such as aspiration due to neurologic impairment or in patients with tracheostomies, clindamycin is indicated, pending culture and sensitivity studies, owing to the likely presence of resistant anaerobes.

Less severe pneumonias can often be treated with oral antibiotics based on the patient's age and suspected organism. Lobar pneumonias presumed to be due to *S pneumoniae* can be treated initially with oral β-lactams, including cefuroxime axetil, amoxicillin, or amoxicillin–clavulanate. However, persistence or worsening of symptoms within 3–5 days suggests the presence of a resistant organism, and newer quinolones, clindamycin, or vancomycin may be required. When possible, therapy can be guided by the antibiotic sensitivity pattern of the organisms isolated. (For further discussion, see Chapter 37.)

Whether a child should be hospitalized depends on his or her age, the severity of illness, the suspected organism, and the anticipated reliability of adherence to the treatment regimen at home. Home treatment is adequate for most older children. With febrile pneumonias, infants generally—and toddlers often—require admission. Moderate to severe respiratory distress, apnea, hypoxemia, poor feeding, clinical deterioration on treatment, or associated complications (large effusions, empyema, or abscess) indicate the need for immediate hospitalization. Careful follow-up within 12 hours to 5 days is often indicated in those not admitted. Cefuroxime or a macrolide, depending on the clinical picture, may be appropriate initial therapy for patients in this category.

Additional therapeutic considerations include oxygen, humidification of inspired gases, hydration and electrolyte supplementation, and nutrition. Removal of pleural fluid for diagnostic purposes is indicated initially to guide antimicrobial therapy. Many experts feel that early chest tube drainage of empyema fluid is indicated. Repeat pleural taps should be considered in the patient who has persistent high fever and respiratory symptoms in association with significant pleural effusions. The persistence of organisms in this fluid or the persistence of toxicity, malaise, anorexia, and wasting in the patient suggests the potential need for pleural decortication, a procedure that can be made less morbid by thoracoscopy in skilled hands.

Endotracheal intubation or mechanical ventilation may be indicated in patients with respiratory failure or in those too debilitated or overwhelmed to handle their secretions.

► Prognosis

For the immunocompetent host in whom bacterial pneumonia is adequately recognized and treated, the survival rate is high. For example, the mortality rate from uncomplicated pneumococcal pneumonia is less than 1%. If the patient survives the initial illness, persistently abnormal pulmonary function following empyema is surprisingly uncommon, even when treatment has been delayed or inappropriate.

Kabra SK et al: Antibiotics for community acquired pneumonia in children. Cochrane Database Syst Rev 2006;(3):CD004874 [PMID: 16856067].

McIntosh K: Community-acquired pneumonia in children. N Engl J Med 2002;346:429 [PMID: 11832532].

Sinaniotis CA, Sinaniotis AC: Community-acquired pneumonia in children. Curr Opin Pulm Med 2005;11:218 [PMID: 15818183].

VIRAL PNEUMONIA

ESSENTIALS OF DIAGNOSIS & TYPICAL FEATURES

▶ Upper respiratory infection prodrome (fever, coryza, cough, hoarseness).

▶ Wheezing or rales.

▶ Myalgia, malaise, headache (older children).

General Considerations

Most pneumonias in children are caused by viruses. RSV, parainfluenza (1, 2, and 3) viruses, influenza (A and B) viruses, and human metapneumovirus are responsible for the large majority of cases. Severity of disease, severity of fever, radiographic findings, and the characteristics of cough or lung sounds do not reliably differentiate viral from bacterial pneumonias. Furthermore, such infections may coexist. However, substantial pleural effusions, pneumatoceles, abscesses, lobar consolidation with lobar volume expansion, and "round" pneumonias are generally inconsistent with viral disease.

Clinical Findings

A. Symptoms and Signs

An upper respiratory infection frequently precedes the onset of lower respiratory disease due to viruses. Although wheezing or stridor may be prominent in viral disease, cough, signs of respiratory difficulty (tachypnea, retractions, grunting, and nasal flaring), and physical findings (rales and decreased breath sounds) may not be distinguishable from those in bacterial pneumonia.

B. Laboratory Findings

The peripheral white blood cell count can be normal or slightly elevated and is not useful in distinguishing viral from bacterial disease.

Rapid viral diagnostic methods—such as fluorescent antibody tests or enzyme-linked immunosorbent assay—should be performed on nasopharyngeal secretions to confirm this diagnosis in high-risk patients and for epidemiology or infection control. Rapid diagnosis of RSV infection does not preclude the possibility of concomitant infection with other pathogens.

C. Imaging

Chest radiographs frequently show perihilar streaking, increased interstitial markings, peribronchial cuffing, or patchy bronchopneumonia. Lobar consolidation or atelectasis may occur, however, as in bacterial pneumonia. Patients with adenovirus disease may have severe necrotizing pneu-monias, resulting in the development of pneumatoceles. Hyperinflation of the lungs may occur when involvement of the small airways is prominent.

Differential Diagnosis

The differential diagnosis of viral pneumonia is the same as for bacterial pneumonia. Patients with prominent wheezing may have asthma, airway obstruction caused by foreign body aspiration, acute bacterial or viral tracheitis, or parasitic disease.

Complications

Viral pneumonia or laryngotracheobronchitis may predispose the patient to subsequent bacterial tracheitis or pneumonia as immediate sequelae. Bronchiolitis obliterans or severe chronic respiratory failure may follow adenovirus pneumonia. Bronchiolitis or viral pneumonia may contribute to persistent asthma in some patients. Bronchiectasis, chronic interstitial lung diseases, and unilateral hyperlucent lung (Sawyer-James syndrome) may follow measles, adenovirus, and influenzal pneumonias. Plasma cell granuloma may develop as a rare sequela to viral or bacterial pneumonia.

Treatment

General supportive care for viral pneumonia does not differ from that for bacterial pneumonia. Patients can be quite ill and should be hospitalized according to the level of their illness. Because bacterial disease often cannot be definitively excluded, antibiotics may be indicated.

Patients at risk for life-threatening RSV infections (eg, those with BPD or other severe pulmonary conditions, congenital heart disease, or significant immunocompromise) should be hospitalized and ribavirin should be considered. Rapid viral diagnostic tests may be a useful guide for such therapy (see Bronchiolitis section, earlier, regarding prevention). These high-risk patients and all children 6 months to 5 years of age should be immunized annually against influenza A and B viruses. Despite immunization, however, influenza infection can still occur. When available epidemiologic data indicate an active influenza A infection in the community, rimantadine, amantadine hydrochloride, or oseltamivir phosphate should be considered early for high-risk infants and children who appear to be infected. Children with suspected viral pneumonia should be placed in respiratory isolation.

Prognosis

Although most children with viral pneumonia recover uneventfully, worsening asthma, abnormal pulmonary function or chest radiographs, persistent respiratory insufficiency, and even death may occur in high-risk patients such as newborns or those with underlying lung, cardiac, or immunodeficiency disease. Patients with adenovirus infection or those concomitantly infected with RSV and second pathogens such as influenza, adenovirus, cytomegalovirus, or *P jiroveci* also have a worse prognosis.

Klig JE, Chen L: Lower respiratory infections in children. Curr Opin Pediatr 2003;15:121 [PMID: 12544283].

Klig JE: Current challenges in lower respiratory infections in children. Curr Opin Pediatr 2004;16:107 [PMID: 14758123].

CHLAMYDIAL PNEUMONIAS

ESSENTIALS OF DIAGNOSIS & TYPICAL FEATURES

▶ Cough, pharyngitis, tachypnea, rales, few wheezes, fever.

▶ Inclusion conjunctivitis, eosinophilia, and elevated immunoglobulins in some cases.

▶ General Considerations

Pulmonary disease due to *C trachomatis* usually evolves gradually as the infection descends the respiratory tract. Infants may appear quite well despite the presence of significant pulmonary illness. Infant infections are now at epidemic proportions in urban environments worldwide. *C pneumoniae* is now recognized as a common cause of respiratory infections in adults and children.

▶ Clinical Findings

A. Symptoms and Signs

About 50% of infants with *C trachomatis* pneumonia have active inclusion conjunctivitis or a history of it. Rhinopharyngitis with nasal discharge or otitis media may have occurred or may be currently present. Female patients may have vulvovaginitis. Cough is usually present. It can have a staccato character and resemble the cough of pertussis. The infant is usually tachypneic. Scattered inspiratory rales are commonly heard, wheezes rarely. Significant fever suggests a different or additional diagnosis.

In children *C pneumoniae* is a common respiratory pathogen and may cause 5–20% of all community-acquired pneumonias. Often these lower respiratory tract illnesses are mild or asymptomatic, although this can occasionally be a serious pathogen.

B. Laboratory Findings

Although patients may frequently be hypoxemic, carbon dioxide retention is not common. Peripheral blood eosinophilia (400 cells/μL) has been observed. Serum immunoglobulins are usually abnormal. IgM is virtually always elevated, IgG is high in many, and IgA is less frequently abnormal.

C trachomatis can usually be identified in nasopharyngeal washings using fluorescent antibody or culture techniques. *C pneumoniae* isolation can be difficult and the diagnosis is often made by serologic testing. These tests can be performed to confirm this diagnosis in difficult to diagnose or high-risk patients and for epidemiology or infection control.

C. Imaging

Chest radiographs may reveal diffuse interstitial and patchy alveolar infiltrates, peribronchial thickening, or focal consolidation. A small pleural reaction can be present. Despite the usual absence of wheezes, hyperexpansion is commonly present.

▶ Differential Diagnosis

Bacterial, viral, and fungal (*P jiroveci*) pneumonias should be considered. Premature infants and those with BPD may also have chlamydial pneumonia. *C pneumoniae* is often accompanied by coinfection with other pathogens, particularly *S pneumoniae* and *M pneumoniae*.

▶ Treatment

Erythromycin or sulfisoxazole therapy should be administered for 14 days. Hospitalization may be required for children with significant respiratory distress, coughing paroxysms, or posttussive apnea. Oxygen therapy may be required for prolonged periods in some patients.

▶ Prognosis

An increased incidence of obstructive airway disease and abnormal pulmonary function tests may occur for at least 7–8 years following infection.

Brunetti L et al: The role of pulmonary infection in pediatric asthma. Allergy Asthma Proc 2007;28:190 [PMID: 17479603].

Darville T: *Chlamydia trachomatis* infections in neonates and young children. Semin Pediatr Infect Dis 2005;16:235 [PMID: 16210104].

Hammerschlag MR: Pneumonia due to *Chlamydia pneumoniae* in children: Epidemiology, diagnosis, and treatment. Pediatr Pulmonol 2003;36:384 [PMID: 14520720].

Principi N, Esposito S: Emerging role of *Mycoplasma pneumoniae* and *Chlamydia pneumoniae* in paediatric respiratory tract infections. Lancet Infect Dis 2001;1:334 [PMID: 11871806].

MYCOPLASMAL PNEUMONIA

ESSENTIALS OF DIAGNOSIS & TYPICAL FEATURES

▶ Fever.

▶ Cough.

▶ Most common in children older than age 5 years.

General Considerations

M pneumoniae is a common cause of symptomatic pneumonia in older children although it may be seen in children younger than 5 years of age. Endemic and epidemic infection can occur. The incubation period is long (2–3 weeks), and the onset of symptoms is slow. Although the lung is the primary infection site, extrapulmonary complications sometimes occur.

Clinical Findings

A. Symptoms and Signs

Fever, cough, headache, and malaise are common symptoms as the illness evolves. Although cough is usually dry at the onset, sputum production may develop as the illness progresses. Sore throat, otitis media, otitis externa, and bullous myringitis may occur. Rales are frequently present on chest examination; decreased breath sounds or dullness to percussion over the involved area may be present.

B. Laboratory Findings

The total and differential white blood cell counts are usually normal. The cold hemagglutinin titer can be determined and may be elevated during the acute presentation. A titer of 1:64 or higher supports the diagnosis. Acute and convalescent titers for *M pneumoniae* demonstrating a fourfold or greater rise in specific antibodies confirm the diagnosis. Diagnosis of mycoplasmal pneumonia by polymerase chain reaction is becoming more readily available.

C. Imaging

Chest radiographs usually demonstrate interstitial or bronchopneumonic infiltrates, frequently in the middle or lower lobes. Pleural effusions are extremely uncommon.

Complications

Extrapulmonary involvement of the blood, central nervous system, skin, heart, or joints can occur. Direct Coombs-positive autoimmune hemolytic anemia, occasionally a life-threatening disorder, is the most common hematologic abnormality that can accompany *M pneumoniae* infection. Coagulation defects and thrombocytopenia can also occur. Cerebral infarction, meningoencephalitis, Guillain-Barré syndrome, cranial nerve involvement, and psychosis all have been described. A wide variety of skin rashes, including erythema multiforme and Stevens-Johnson syndrome, can occur. Myocarditis, pericarditis, and a rheumatic fever–like illness can also occur.

Treatment

Antibiotic therapy with a macrolide for 7–10 days usually shortens the course of illness. Ciprofloxacin is a possible alternative. Supportive measures, including hydration, antipyretics, and bed rest, are helpful.

Prognosis

In the absence of the less common extrapulmonary complications, the outlook for recovery is excellent. The extent to which *M pneumoniae* can initiate or exacerbate chronic lung disease is not well understood.

Brunetti L et al: The role of pulmonary infection in pediatric asthma. Allergy Asthma Proc 2007;28:190 [PMID: 17479603].
Hammerschlag MR: *Mycoplasma pneumoniae* infections. Curr Opin Infect Dis 2001;14:181 [PMID: 11979130].
Waites KB: New concepts of *Mycoplasma pneumoniae* infections in children. Pediatr Pulmonol 2003;36:267 [PMID: 12950038].

TUBERCULOSIS (SEE ALSO CHAPTER 40)

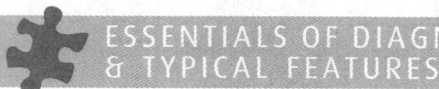

ESSENTIALS OF DIAGNOSIS & TYPICAL FEATURES

▶ Positive tuberculin skin test or anergic host.
▶ Positive culture for *Mycobacterium tuberculosis*.
▶ Symptoms of active disease (if present): chronic cough, anorexia, weight loss or poor weight gain, fever, night sweats.

General Considerations

Tuberculosis is a widespread and deadly disease resulting from infection with *M tuberculosis*. The clinical spectrum of disease includes asymptomatic primary infection, calcified nodules, pleural effusions, progressive primary cavitating lesions, contiguous spread into adjacent thoracic structures, acute miliary tuberculosis, acute respiratory distress syndrome, overwhelming reactivation infection in the immunocompromised host, occult lymphohematogenous spread, and metastatic extrapulmonary involvement at almost any site. Because transmission is usually through respiratory droplets, isolated pulmonary parenchymal tuberculosis constitutes more than 85% of presenting cases. Pulmonary tuberculosis is the focus of discussion here; additional manifestations of tuberculosis are discussed in Chapter 40.

Following a resurgence in the 1980s and early 1990s, tuberculosis has declined among all age groups in the United States, including children. This trend has continued through 2006, the most recent year for which data are available. However, the disease remains a significant cause of morbidity and mortality worldwide.

Clinical Findings

A. Symptoms and Signs

Most children with tuberculosis are asymptomatic and present with a positive tuberculin skin test. Symptoms of active disease, if present, might include chronic cough, anorexia, weight loss or poor weight gain, fever, and night sweats. Children can also present with symptoms of airway obstruction, sometimes with secondary bacterial pneumonia or airway collapse resulting from hilar adenopathy.

Because most children infected with tuberculosis are asymptomatic, a clue to infection may be contact with an individual with tuberculosis—often an elderly relative, a caregiver, or a person previously residing in a region where tuberculosis is endemic—or a history of travel to or residence in such an area. Homeless and extremely impoverished children are also at high risk, as are those in contact with high-risk adults (patients with AIDS, residents or employees of correctional institutions or nursing homes, drug users, and health care workers). Once exposed, pediatric patients at risk for developing active disease include infants and those with malnutrition, AIDS, diabetes mellitus, or immunosuppression (cancer chemotherapy or corticosteroids).

The symptoms of active disease listed previously most often occur during the first year of infection. Thereafter, infection remains quiescent until adolescence, when reactivation of pulmonary tuberculosis is common. At any stage, chronic cough, anorexia, weight loss or poor weight gain, and fever are useful clinical signs of reactivation. Of note, except in patients with complications or advanced disease, physical findings are few.

B. Tuberculin Skin Testing

A positive tuberculin skin test is defined by the size of induration as measured by a medical provider 48–72 hours after intradermal injection of 5 tuberculin units of purified protein derivative (PPD). A positive test is defined as an induration greater than or equal to 5 mm in patients who are at high risk for developing active disease (ie, immunocompromised, those with a history of a positive test or radiograph, children younger than 4 years, and those known to have close contact with someone with active disease); greater than 10 mm in patients from or exposed to high-risk populations (ie, born in countries with a high prevalence, users of injected drugs, having poor access to health care, or living in facilities such as jails, homeless shelters, or nursing homes); and greater than 15 mm in those who are at low risk. Tine tests should not be used. Appropriate control skin tests, such as those for hypersensitivity to diphtheria-tetanus, mumps, or *Candida albicans,* should be applied in patients with suspected or proven immunosuppression or in those with possible severe disseminated disease. If the patient fails to respond to PPD, the possibility of tuberculosis is not excluded.

In suspected cases, the patient, immediate family, and suspected carriers should also be tuberculin-tested. Because healing—rather than progression—is the usual course in the uncompromised host, a positive tuberculin test may be the only manifestation. The primary focus (usually single) and associated nodal involvement may not be seen radiographically. For patients born outside the United States or those who have received a previous bacillus Calmette-Guérin immunization, induration greater than 5 mm should be considered positive and further evaluated.

C. Laboratory Findings and Imaging

Anteroposterior and lateral chest radiographs should be obtained in all suspected cases. Culture for *M tuberculosis* is critical for proving the diagnosis and for defining drug susceptibility. Early morning gastric lavage following an overnight fast should be performed on three occasions in infants and children with suspected active pulmonary tuberculosis before treatment is started, when the severity of illness allows. Although stains for acid-fast bacilli on this material are of little value, this is the ideal culture site. Despite the increasing importance of isolating organisms because of multiple drug resistance, only 40% of children will yield positive cultures.

Sputum cultures from older children and adolescents can also be useful. Stains and cultures of bronchial secretions can be obtained using bronchoscopy. When pleural effusions are present, pleural biopsy for cultures and histopathologic examination for granulomas or organisms provide diagnostic information. Meningeal involvement is also possible in young children, and lumbar puncture should be considered in their initial evaluation.

▶ Differential Diagnosis

Fungal diseases that affect mainly the lungs, such as histoplasmosis, coccidioidomycosis, cryptococcosis, and North American blastomycosis, may resemble tuberculosis and in cases where the diagnosis is unclear, should be excluded by biopsy or appropriate serologic studies. Atypical tuberculous organisms may involve the lungs, especially in the immunocompromised patient. Depending on the presentation, diagnoses such as lymphoreticular and other malignancies, collagen-vascular disorders, or other pulmonary infections may be considered.

▶ Complications

In addition to those complications listed in the sections on general considerations and clinical findings, lymphadenitis, meningitis, osteomyelitis, arthritis, enteritis, peritonitis, and renal, ocular, middle ear, and cutaneous disease may occur. Infants born to parents infected with *M tuberculosis* are at great risk for developing illness. The possibility of life-threatening airway compromise must always be considered in patients with large mediastinal or hilar lesions.

▶ Treatment

Because the risk of hepatitis due to isoniazid is extremely low in children, this drug is indicated in those with a positive tuberculin skin test. This greatly reduces the risk of subsequent active disease and complications with minimal morbidity. Isoniazid plus rifampin treatment for 6 months, plus pyrazinamide during the first 2 months, is indicated when the chest radiograph is abnormal or when extrapulmonary disease is present. Without pyrazinamide, isoniazid plus rifampin must be given for 9 months. In general, the more severe tuberculous complications are treated with a larger number of drugs (see Chapter 40). Enforced, directly observed therapy (twice or three times weekly) is indicated when nonadherence is suspected. Recommendations for antituberculosis chemotherapy based on disease stage are continuously being updated. The most current edition of the American Academy of Pediatrics *Red Book* is a reliable source for these protocols.

Corticosteroids are used to control inflammation in selected patients with potentially life-threatening airway compression by lymph nodes, acute pericardial effusion, massive pleural effusion with mediastinal shift, or miliary tuberculosis with respiratory failure.

► Prognosis

In patients with an intact immune system, modern antituberculous therapy offers good potential for recovery. The outlook for patients with immunodeficiencies, organisms resistant to multiple drugs, poor drug adherence, or advanced complications is guarded. Organisms resistant to multiple drugs are increasingly common. Resistance emerges either because the physician prescribes an inadequate regimen or because the patient discontinues medications. When resistance to or intolerance of isoniazid and rifampin prevents their use, cure rates are 50% or less.

Feja K, Saiman L: Tuberculosis in children. Clin Chest Med 2005;26:295 [PMID: 15837112].

Mandalakas AM, Starke JR: Current concepts of childhood tuberculosis. Semin Pediatr Infect Dis 2005;16:93 [PMID: 15825140].

Powell DA, Hunt WG: Tuberculosis in children: An update. Adv Pediatr 2006;53:279 [PMID: 17089872].

ASPIRATION PNEUMONIA

Patients whose anatomic defense mechanisms are impaired are at risk of aspiration pneumonia (Table 18–3). Acute disease is commonly caused by bacteria present in the mouth (especially gram-negative anaerobes). Chronic aspiration often causes recurrent bouts of acute febrile pneumonia. It may also lead to chronic focal infiltrates, atelectasis, an illness resembling asthma or interstitial lung disease, bronchiectasis, or failure to thrive.

► Clinical Findings

A. Symptoms and Signs

Acute onset of fever, cough, respiratory distress, or hypoxemia in a patient at risk suggests aspiration pneumonia. Chest physical findings, such as rales, rhonchi, or decreased breath sounds, may initially be limited to the lung region into which aspiration occurred. Although any region may be affected, the right side—especially the right upper lobe in the supine patient—is commonly affected. In patients with

Table 18–3. Risk factors for aspiration pneumonia.

Seizures
Depressed sensorium
Recurrent gastroesophageal reflux, emesis, or gastrointestinal obstruction
Neuromuscular disorders with suck-swallow dysfunction
Anatomic abnormalities (laryngeal cleft, tracheoesophageal fistula, vocal cord paralysis)
Debilitating illnesses
Occult brainstem lesions
Near-drowning
Nasogastric, endotracheal, or tracheostomy tubes
Severe periodontal disease

chronic aspiration, diffuse wheezing may occur. Generalized rales may also be present. Such patients may not develop acute febrile pneumonias.

B. Laboratory Findings and Imaging

Chest radiographs may reveal lobar consolidation or atelectasis and focal or generalized alveolar or interstitial infiltrates. In some patients with chronic aspiration, perihilar infiltrates with or without bilateral air trapping may be seen.

In severely ill patients with acute febrile illnesses, and especially when the pneumonia is complicated by a pleural effusion, a bacteriologic diagnosis should be made. In addition to blood cultures and cultures of the pleural fluid, cultures of tracheobronchial secretions and bronchoalveolar lavage specimens may be considered (see earlier section on Culture of Material from the Respiratory Tract).

In patients with chronic aspiration pneumonitis, documentation of aspiration as the cause of illness may be elusive. Barium contrast studies using liquids of increasing consistency may provide evidence of suck-swallow dysfunction or laryngeal cleft. Bolus barium swallow studies with good distention of the esophagus may help to identify an occult tracheoesophageal fistula. Gastroesophageal reflux may be a risk factor for aspiration while the child is sleeping, and an overnight or 24-hour esophageal pH probe studies may also help establish the diagnosis of gastroesophageal reflux. Although radionuclide scans are commonly used, the yield from such studies is disappointingly low. Rigid bronchoscopy in infants or flexible bronchoscopy in older children can be used to identify anatomic abnormalities such as tracheal cleft and tracheoesophageal fistula. Flexible bronchoscopy and bronchoalveolar lavage specimens to search for lipid-laden macrophages can also suggest chronic aspiration.

► Differential Diagnosis

In the acutely ill patient, bacterial and viral pneumonias should be considered. In the chronically ill patient, the differential diagnosis may include disorders causing recurrent pneumonia (eg, immunodeficiencies, ciliary dysfunction, or foreign body), chronic wheezing, or interstitial lung disorders (see next section), depending on the presentation.

Complications

Empyema or lung abscess may complicate acute aspiration pneumonia. Chronic aspiration may also result in bronchiectasis.

Treatment

Antimicrobial therapy for acute aspiration pneumonia includes coverage for gram-negative anaerobic organisms. In general, clindamycin is appropriate initial coverage. However, in some hospital-acquired infections, additional coverage for multiple resistant *P aeruginosa*, streptococci, and other organisms may be required.

Treatment of recurrent and chronic aspiration pneumonia may include the following: surgical correction of anatomic abnormalities; improved oral hygiene; improved hydration; and inhaled bronchodilators, chest physical therapy, and suctioning. In patients with compromise of the central nervous system, exclusive feeding by gastrostomy and (in some) tracheostomy may be required to control airway secretions. Gastroesophageal reflux, if present in these patients, also often requires surgical correction.

Prognosis

The outlook is directly related to the disorder causing aspiration.

Brook I: Anaerobic pulmonary infections in children. Pediatr Emerg Care 2004;20:636 [PMID: 15599270].

Colombo JL, Hallberg TK: Pulmonary aspiration and lipid-laden macrophages: In search of gold (standards). Pediatr Pulmonol 1999;28:79 [PMID: 10423305].

Methany NA et al: Tracheobronchial aspiration of gastric contents in critically ill tube-fed patients: Frequency, outcomes, and risk factors. Crit Care Med 2006;34:687 [PMID: 16484901].

CHILDREN'S INTERSTITIAL LUNG DISEASE SYNDROME

ESSENTIALS OF DIAGNOSIS & TYPICAL FEATURES

▶ Occurs acutely in the neonatal period or subacutely in infancy or childhood.

▶ Infants and young children have different diagnoses than adolescents and adults.

▶ Presence of three to five of the following criteria in the absence of any identified primary etiology is suggestive of an interstitial lung disease (ILD) syndrome:

  • Symptoms of impaired respiratory function (cough, tachypnea, retractions, exercise intolerance).

  • Evidence of impaired gas exchange (resting hypoxemia or hypercarbia, desaturation with exercise).

  • Diffuse infiltrates on imaging.

  • Presence of adventitious sounds (crackles, wheezing).

  • Abnormal spirometry, lung volumes, or carbon monoxide diffusing capacity.

▶ History of exposure (eg, birds, organic dusts, drug therapy, hot tubs, molds), previous lung disease, immunosuppression, symptoms of connective tissue disease; family history of familial lung disease (especially ILD) or early infant death from lung disease.

General Considerations

Children's **I**nterstitial **L**ung **D**isease (chILD) syndrome is a constellation of signs and symptoms and not a specific diagnosis. Once recognized, chILD syndrome should elicit a search for a more specific rare ILD. Known disorders can present as chILD syndrome and must be excluded as the primary cause of symptoms. These disorders include CF, cardiac disease, asthma, acute infection, immunodeficiency, neuromuscular disease, scoliosis, thoracic cage abnormality, typical BPD or premature respiratory distress syndrome, and confirmed significant aspiration on a swallow study. However, if patients present with symptoms out of proportion to the diagnosis, consideration should be given to other ILD disorders.

Clinical Findings

A. Symptoms and Signs

chILD syndrome may present acutely in the newborn period with respiratory failure or gradually over time with a chronic dry cough or a history of dyspnea on exertion. The child with more advanced disease may have increased dyspnea, tachypnea, retractions, cyanosis, clubbing, failure to thrive, or weight loss.

B. Diagnostic Studies

Once chILD syndrome is recognized, initial evaluations should be directed at ruling out known conditions. The initial evaluations should include the following diagnostic studies: radiographs, barium swallow, pulmonary function tests, and skin tests (see earlier section on Tuberculosis); complete blood count and erythrocyte sedimentation rate; sweat chloride test for CF; electrocardiogram or echocardiogram; serum immunoglobulins and other immunologic evaluations; sputum studies (see later section on Pneumonia in the Immunocompromised Host); and possibly studies for Epstein-Barr virus, cytomegalovirus, *M pneumoniae*, *Chlamydia*, *Pneumocystis*, and *Ureaplasma urealyticum*.

Chest radiographs are normal in up to 10–15% of patients. Frequently, specific chILD disorders can be suspected by findings on controlled volume inspiratory and expiratory high-resolution CT, which should be considered early in the course of evaluation. Infants and children younger than age 5 years require sedation, which allows either infant pulmonary function testing or bronchoscopy evaluations to be completed at the same time.

On pulmonary function testing, multiple patterns can be seen depending on the specific ILD condition such as (1) a restrictive pattern of decreased lung volumes, compliance, and carbon monoxide diffusing capacity, (2) an obstructive pattern with hyperinflation, or (3) a mixed obstructive-restrictive pattern. Infant pulmonary function testing can provide insight into pulmonary mechanics and different chILD disorders. Exercise-induced or nocturnal hypoxemia is often the earliest detectable abnormality of lung function in children.

During the second evaluation phase, bronchoscopy is performed to exclude anatomic abnormalities, obtain multiple bronchial brushings to examine cilia if cilial dysfunction is considered a possibility, and obtain bronchoalveolar lavage for microbiologic and cytologic testing.

In patients with static or slowly progressing disease, one can then await results of bronchoscopic studies. In patients with acute, rapidly progressive disease, this stage should be combined with video-assisted thoracoscopic biopsy. Lung biopsy is the most reliable method for definitive diagnosis when analyzed by pathologists experienced in chILD disorders. A new chILD histology classification has been proposed to improve diagnostic yields. Tissue should be processed in a standard manner for special stains and cultures, electron microscopy, and immunofluorescence for immune complexes if indicated. Although transbronchial biopsy may be useful in diagnosing a few diffuse disorders and graft rejection in transplantation (eg, sarcoidosis), its overall usefulness in chILD is limited at this time.

C. Genetic Testing

Genomic mutational analysis of tissue or blood for surfactant proteins B and C (SP-B, SP-C) and ABCA3 is now offered in clinical laboratories and should be considered in most patients with diffuse lung disease or a strong family history of ILD.

▶ Differential Diagnosis

chILD syndrome is composed of a group of diverse conditions that can differ from adult ILD conditions. Common adult causes of ILD such as UIP (usual interstitial pneumonitis, also known as idiopathic pulmonary fibrosis), which is associated with a high mortality rate, and respiratory bronchiolitis, associated with smoking, have not been found in children. Conversely, newly identified conditions unique to infancy such as neuroendocrine cell hyperplasia of infancy (NEHI) or pulmonary interstitial glycogenosis (PIG), have not been described in adults. Other chILD conditions include the genetically recognized surfactant dysfunction mutations SP-B, SP-C, and ABCA3; developmental abnormalities; and growth disorders, especially in younger children. Older children are more likely to have SP-C or ABCA3 surfactant mutations, hypersensitivity pneumonitis, or collagen-vascular disease. Other known conditions must also be ruled out.

▶ Complications

Respiratory failure or pulmonary hypertension with cor pulmonale may occur. Mortality and morbidity can be significant in some chILD disorders.

▶ Treatment

Therapy for known causes of ILD such as infection, aspiration, or cardiac disorders should be directed toward the primary disorder. It must be recognized that treatment for chILD conditions is anecdotal and based on case reports and small case series. In noninflammatory chILD syndrome conditions such as neuroendocrine cell hyperplasia of infancy or developmental or growth abnormalities, treatment is supportive and may not require corticosteroids. For chILD conditions such as surfactant dysfunction mutations, pulmonary interstitial glycogenosis, hypersensitivity pneumonitis, and systemic collagen-vascular disease, patients are frequently treated initially with oral (2 mg/kg/d for 6 weeks) or monthly pulse glucocorticoids (IV doses of 10–30 mg/kg for 1–3 days). Many patients require even more protracted therapy with alternate-day prednisone. Chloroquine (5–10 mg/kg/d) may be useful in selected disorders such as desquamative interstitial pneumonitis, surfactant dysfunction mutations, or refractory disease. In refractory cases, azathioprine and cyclophosphamide may be tried. Newer antifibrotic agents such as interferon-γ, which are being investigated in adult patients with interstitial pulmonary fibrosis, have not been tried in children to date. Finally, some patients with severe disease may require long-term mechanical ventilation or lung transplantation for survival. chILD disorders should be evaluated and cared for by a multidisciplinary team experienced in chILD. The chILD Family Foundation can provide further supportive resources for families (http://www.childfoundation.us).

▶ Prognosis

The prognosis is guarded in children with ILD due to collagen-vascular disease, surfactant dysfunction mutations, and developmental disorders (eg, alveolar-capillary dysplasia). Other conditions such as neuroendocrine cell hyperplasia of infancy and pulmonary interstitial glycogenosis have not had deaths reported.

Deterding R: Evaluating infants and children with interstitial lung disease. Semin Respir Crit Care Med 2007;28:333 [PMID: 17562503].

Deutsch G et al: Diffuse lung disease in young children: Application of a novel classification scheme. Am J Respir Crit Care Med 2007;176:1120 [PMID: 17885266].

Hamvas A et al: Genetic disorders of surfactant proteins. Neonatology 2007;91:311 [PMID: 17575475].

HYPERSENSITIVITY PNEUMONIA

General Considerations

Hypersensitivity pneumonitis, or extrinsic allergic alveolitis, is a T-cell–mediated disease involving the peripheral airways, interstitium, and alveoli and presents as chILD. Both acute and chronic forms may occur. In children, the most common forms are brought on by exposure to domestic and occasionally wild birds or bird droppings (eg, pigeons, parakeets, parrots, or doves). However, inhalation of almost any organic dust (moldy hay, compost, logs or tree bark, sawdust, or aerosols from humidifiers or hot tubs) can cause disease. Methotrexate-induced hypersensitivity has also been described in a child with juvenile rheumatoid arthritis. Hot tub lung can be caused by exposure to aerosolized *Mycobacterium avium* complex. A high level of suspicion and a thorough history are required for diagnosis.

Clinical Findings

A. Symptoms and Signs

Episodic cough and fever can occur with acute exposures. Chronic exposure results in weight loss, fatigue, dyspnea, cyanosis, and ultimately, respiratory failure.

B. Laboratory Findings

Acute exposure may be followed by polymorphonuclear leukocytosis with eosinophilia and evidence of airway obstruction on pulmonary function testing. Chronic disease results in a restrictive picture on lung function tests. Arterial blood gases may reveal hypoxemia with a decreased $PaCO_2$ and normal pH.

The serologic key to diagnosis is the finding of precipitins (precipitating IgG antibodies) to the organic material that contain avian proteins or fungal or bacterial antigens. Ideally, to identify avian proteins, the patient's sera should be tested with antigens from droppings of the suspected species of bird. However, exposure may invoke precipitins without causing disease.

Bronchoscopy with bronchoalveolar lavage findings of lymphocytosis or *M avium* complex may be suggestive. Normal cell counts may help rule out acute hypersensitivity pneumonitis.

Differential Diagnosis

Patients with mainly acute symptoms must be differentiated from those with atopic asthma. Patients with chronic symptoms must be distinguished from those with collagen-vascular, immunologic, or primary interstitial pulmonary disorders.

Complications

Prolonged exposure to offending antigens may result in pulmonary hypertension due to chronic hypoxemia, cor pulmonale, irreversible restrictive lung disease due to pulmonary fibrosis, or respiratory failure.

Treatment & Prognosis

Complete elimination of exposure to the offending antigens is required. If drug-induced hypersensitivity pneumonitis is suspected, discontinuation is required. Corticosteroids may hasten recovery. With appropriate early diagnosis and identification and avoidance of offending antigens, the prognosis is excellent.

Fink JN et al: Needs and opportunities for research in hypersensitivity pneumonitis. Am J Respir Crit Care Med 2005;171:792 [PMID: 15657460].

Marras TK et al: Hypersensitivity pneumonitis reaction to *Mycobacterium avium* in household water. Chest 2005;127:664 [PMID: 15706013].

Stauffer EM: Bird breeder's disease: A rare diagnosis in young children. Eur J Pediatr 2006;165:55 [PMID: 16270199].

EOSINOPHILIC PNEUMONIA

General Considerations

Eosinophilic pneumonia is another rare condition that can be considered under the heading of chILD syndrome. A spectrum of diseases should be considered under this heading: (1) allergic bronchopulmonary helminthiasis (ABPH), (2) pulmonary eosinophilia with asthma (allergic bronchopulmonary aspergillosis and related disorders), (3) hypereosinophilic mucoid impaction, (4) bronchocentric granulomatosis, and (5) collagen-vascular disorders. The former term, *Löffler syndrome* (transient migratory pulmonary infiltrates and eosinophilia), is no longer used because most patients had undiagnosed ABPH, medication reactions (see http://www.pneumotox.com), or allergic bronchopulmonary aspergillosis. Many of these disorders occur in children with personal or family histories of allergies or asthma. ABPH may be related to hypersensitivity to migratory parasitic nematodes (*Ascaris, Strongyloides, Ancylostoma, Toxocara,* or *Trichuris*) and larval forms of filariae (*Wuchereria bancrofti*). Allergic bronchopulmonary aspergillosis is related to hypersensitivity to the fungus *Aspergillus*. Hypersensitivity to other fungi has also been documented. Eosinophilic pneumonias are rare but can be associated with drug hypersensitivity, sarcoidosis, Hodgkin disease or other lymphomas, and bacterial infections, including brucellosis and those caused by *M tuberculosis* and atypical mycobacteria.

Clinical Findings

A. Symptoms and Signs

Cough, wheezing, and dyspnea are common presenting complaints. In allergic bronchopulmonary helminthiasis, fever, malaise, sputum production, and rarely hemoptysis may be present. In allergic bronchopulmonary aspergillosis, patients may present with all of these findings and occasionally produce brown mucus plugs. Anorexia, weight loss, night sweats, and clubbing can also occur.

B. Laboratory Findings and Imaging

Elevated absolute peripheral blood eosinophil counts (3000/μL and often exceeding 50% of leukocytes) are present in ABPH and allergic bronchopulmonary aspergillosis. Serum IgE levels as high as 1000–10,000 IU/mL are common. In allergic bronchopulmonary aspergillosis, the serum IgE concentration appears to correlate with activity of the disease. Stools should be examined for ova and parasites—often several times—to clarify the diagnosis. Isohemagglutinin titers are often markedly elevated in ABPH.

In allergic bronchopulmonary aspergillosis and related disorders, patients may show central bronchiectasis on chest radiograph (so-called tramlines) or CT scan. Saccular proximal bronchiectasis of the upper lobes is pathognomonic. Although the chest radiograph may be normal, peribronchial haziness, focal or platelike atelectasis, or patchy to massive consolidation can occur. Positive immediate skin tests, serum IgG precipitating antibodies, or IgE specific for the offending fungus is present.

Differential Diagnosis

These disorders must be differentiated from exacerbations of asthma, CF, or other underlying lung disorders that cause infiltrates to appear on chest radiographs. Allergic bronchopulmonary aspergillosis can occur in patients with CF.

Complications

Delayed recognition and treatment of allergic bronchopulmonary aspergillosis may cause progressive lung damage and bronchiectasis. Lesions of the conducting airways in bronchocentric granulomatosis can extend into adjacent lung parenchyma and pulmonary arteries, resulting in secondary vasculitis.

Treatment

Therapy for the specific parasite causing ABPH should be given, and corticosteroids may be required when illness is severe. Treatment of disease due to microfilariae is both diagnostic and therapeutic. Allergic bronchopulmonary aspergillosis and related disorders are treated with prolonged courses of oral corticosteroids, bronchodilators, and chest physical therapy. In patients with CF, itraconazole may

decrease corticosteroid doses for those with allergic bronchopulmonary aspergillosis. Pulmonary vasculitis associated with collagen-vascular disease is usually treated with high-dose steroids or cytotoxic agents.

Jeong YJ et al: Eosinophilic lung diseases: A clinical, radiologic, and pathologic overview. Radiographics 2007;27:617 [PMID: 17495282].

Oermann CM et al: Pulmonary infiltrates with eosinophilia syndromes in children. J Pediatr 2000;136:351 [PMID: 10700692].

Wubbel C et al: Chronic eosinophilia pneumonia. Chest 2003;123:1763 [PMID: 12740299].

PNEUMONIA IN THE IMMUNOCOMPROMISED HOST

General Considerations

Immunocompromised children can present with focal pneumonia or ILD. Pneumonia in an immunocompromised host may be due to any common bacteria (streptococci, staphylococci, or *M pneumoniae*) or less common pathogens such as *Toxoplasma gondii*, *P jiroveci*, *Aspergillus* species, *Mucor*, *Candida* species, *Cryptococcus neoformans*, gram-negative enteric and anaerobic bacteria, *Nocardia*, *Legionella pneumophila*, mycobacteria, and viruses (cytomegalovirus, varicella-zoster, herpes simplex, influenza virus, RSV, human metapneumovirus, or adenovirus). Multiple organisms are commonly present.

Clinical Findings

A. Symptoms and Signs

Patients often present with subtle signs such as mild cough, tachypnea, or low-grade fever that can rapidly progress to high fever, respiratory distress, and hypoxemia or chILD syndrome. An obvious portal of infection, such as an intravascular catheter, may predispose to bacterial or fungal infection.

B. Laboratory Findings and Imaging

Fungal, parasitic, or bacterial infection, especially with antibiotic-resistant bacteria, should be suspected in the neutropenic child. Cultures of peripheral blood, sputum, tracheobronchial secretions, urine, nasopharynx or sinuses, bone marrow, pleural fluid, biopsied lymph nodes, or skin lesions or cultures through intravascular catheters should be obtained as soon as infection is suspected.

Invasive methods are commonly required to make a diagnosis. Appropriate samples should be obtained soon after a patient with pneumonia fails to respond to initial treatment. The results of these procedures usually lead to important changes in empiric preoperative therapy. Sputum is often unavailable. Bronchoalveolar lavage frequently provides the diagnosis of one or more organisms and should be done early in evaluation. The combined use of a wash, brushing, and lavage has a high yield. In patients with rapidly advancing disease, lung biopsy becomes more urgent. The morbidity and mortality of this procedure can be reduced by a surgeon skilled in video-assisted thoracoscopic surgical (VATS) techniques. Because of the multiplicity of organisms that may cause disease, a comprehensive set of studies should be done on lavage and biopsy material. These consist of rapid diagnostic studies, including fluorescent antibody studies for *Legionella;* rapid culture and antigen detection for viruses; Gram, acid-fast, and fungal stains; cytologic examination for viral inclusions; cultures for viruses, anaerobic and aerobic bacteria, fungi, mycobacteria, and *Legionella;* and rapid immunofluorescent studies for *P jiroveci.*

Chest radiographs and increasingly high-resolution CT scans may be useful in identifying the pattern and extent of disease. In *P jiroveci* pneumonia, dyspnea and hypoxemia may be marked despite minimal radiographic abnormalities.

Differential Diagnosis

The organisms causing disease vary with the type of immunocompromise present. For example, the splenectomized patient may be overwhelmed by infection with *S pneumoniae* or *H influenzae.* The infant receiving adrenocorticotropic hormone therapy may be more likely to have *P jiroveci* infection. The febrile neutropenic child who has been receiving adequate doses of intravenous broad-spectrum antibiotics may have fungal disease. The key to diagnosis is to consider all possibilities of infection.

Depending on the form of immunocompromise, perhaps only half to two thirds of new pulmonary infiltrates in such patients represents infection. The remainder are caused by pulmonary toxicity of radiation, chemotherapy, or other drugs; pulmonary disorders, including hemorrhage, embolism, atelectasis, aspiration, idiopathic pneumonia syndrome in bone marrow transplant patients, or acute respiratory distress syndrome; recurrence or extension of primary malignant growths or immunologic disorders; transfusion reactions, leukostasis, or tumor cell lysis; or interstitial lung disease, such as lymphocytic interstitial pneumonitis with HIV infection.

Complications

Progressive respiratory failure, shock, multiple organ damage, disseminated infection, and death commonly occur in the infected immunocompromised host if the primary etiology is not treated effectively.

Treatment

Broad-spectrum intravenous antibiotics are indicated early in febrile, neutropenic, or immunocompromised children. Trimethoprim–sulfamethoxazole (for *Pneumocystis*) and macrolides (for *Legionella*) are also indicated early in the treatment of immunocompromised children before an organism is identified. Further therapy should be based on studies of specimens obtained from bronchoalveolar lavage or lung biopsy. Recent data suggest that use of noninvasive ventilation strategies early in the course of pulmonary insufficiency or respiratory failure may decrease mortality.

Prognosis

Prognosis is based on the severity of the underlying immunocompromise, appropriate early diagnosis and treatment, and the infecting organisms. Intubation and mechanical ventilation have been associated with high mortality rates, especially in bone marrow transplant patients.

Efrati O et al: Fiberoptic bronchoscopy and bronchoalveolar lavage for the evaluation of pulmonary disease in children with primary immunodeficiency and cancer. Pediatr Blood Cancer 2007;48:324 [PMID: 16568442].

Gasparetto TD et al: Pulmonary infections following bone marrow transplantation: High-resolution CT findings in 35 paediatric patients. Eur J Radiol 2007 [Epub ahead of print] [PMID: 17624710].

Haung L et al: An Official ATS Workshop Summary: Recent advances and future directions in *Pneumocystis* pneumonia (PCP). Proc Am Thorac Soc 2006;3:655 [PMID: 17065370].

LUNG ABSCESS

General Considerations

Lung abscesses are most likely to occur in immunocompromised patients; in those with severe infections elsewhere (embolic spread); or in those with recurrent aspiration, malnutrition, or blunt chest trauma. Although organisms such as *S aureus, H influenzae, S pneumoniae,* and viridans streptococci more commonly affect the previously normal host, anaerobic and gram-negative organisms as well as *Nocardia, Legionella* species, and fungi (*Candida* and *Aspergillus*) should also be considered in the immunocompromised host.

Clinical Findings

A. Symptoms and Signs

High fever, malaise, and weight loss are often present. Symptoms and signs referable to the chest may or may not be present. In infants, evidence of respiratory distress can be present.

B. Laboratory Findings and Imaging

Elevated peripheral white blood cell count with a neutrophil predominance or an elevated erythrocyte sedimentation rate may be present. Blood cultures are rarely positive except in the overwhelmed host.

Chest radiographs usually reveal single or multiple thick-walled lung cavities. Air-fluid levels can be present. Local compressive atelectasis, pleural thickening, or adenopathy may also occur. Chest CT scan may provide better localization and understanding of the lesions.

In patients producing sputum, stains and cultures may provide the diagnosis. Direct percutaneous aspiration of material for stains and cultures guided by fluoroscopy or ultrasonography should be considered in the severely compromised or ill.

Differential Diagnosis

Loculated pyopneumothorax, an *Echinococcus* cyst, neoplasms, plasma cell granuloma, and infected congenital cysts and sequestrations should be considered. Pneumatoceles, non–fluid-filled cysts, are common in children with empyema and usually resolve over time.

Complications

Although complications due to abscesses are now rare, mediastinal shift, tension pneumothorax, and spontaneous rupture can occur. Diagnostic maneuvers such as lung puncture may also cause complications (pneumothorax).

Treatment

Because of the risks of lung puncture, uncomplicated abscesses are frequently conservatively treated in the uncompromised host with appropriate broad-spectrum antibiotics directed at *S aureus, H influenzae,* and streptococci. Additional coverage for anaerobic and gram-negative organisms should be provided for others. Prolonged therapy (3 weeks or more) may be required. Attempts to drain abscesses via bronchoscopy have caused life-threatening airway compromise. Surgical drainage or lobectomy is occasionally required, primarily in immunocompromised patients. However, such procedures may themselves cause life-threatening complications.

Prognosis

Although radiographic resolution may be very slow, resolution occurs in most patients without risk factors for lower respiratory tract infections or loss of pulmonary function. In the immunocompromised host, the outlook depends on the underlying disorder.

Chan PC et al: Clinical management and outcome of childhood lung abscess: A 16-year experience. J Microbiol Immunol Infect 2005;38:183 [PMID: 15986068].

DISEASES OF THE PULMONARY CIRCULATION

PULMONARY HEMORRHAGE

General Considerations

Pulmonary hemorrhage is caused by a spectrum of disorders affecting the large and small airways and alveoli. It can occur as an acute or chronic process. Hemorrhage involving the alveoli is termed diffuse alveolar hemorrhage. If pulmonary hemorrhage is subacute or chronic, hemosiderin-laden macrophages are found in the sputum and tracheal or gastric aspirate. Many cases are secondary to infection (bacterial, mycobacterial, parasitic, viral, or fungal), lung abscess, bronchiectasis (CF or other causes), foreign body, coagulopathy (often with overwhelming sepsis), or elevated pulmonary venous pressure (secondary to congestive heart failure or anatomic heart lesions). Other causes include lung contusion from trauma, arteriovenous fistula, multiple telangiectasias, pulmonary sequestration, agenesis of a single pulmonary artery, and esophageal duplication or bronchogenic cyst. Rarer causes are tumors (eg, bronchial adenoma or left atrial myxoma) and pulmonary infarction secondary to pulmonary embolus.

Diffuse alveolar hemorrhage may be idiopathic or drug-related or may occur in Goodpasture syndrome, rapidly progressive glomerulonephritis, and systemic vasculitides (often associated with such collagen-vascular diseases as systemic lupus erythematosus, rheumatoid arthritis, Wegener granulomatosis, polyarteritis nodosa, Henoch-Schönlein purpura, and Behçet's disease). Idiopathic pulmonary hemosiderosis refers to the accumulation of hemosiderin in the lung, especially the alveolar macrophage, as a result of chronic or recurrent hemorrhage (usually from pulmonary capillaries) that is not associated with the previously listed causes. Children and young adults are mainly affected, with the age at onset ranging from 6 months to 20 years. This group of disorders includes milk allergy in young infants (Heiner syndrome).

Several cases of pulmonary hemorrhage and pulmonary hemosiderosis have been reported in infants exposed to a toxigenic mold, *Stachybotrys chartarum,* and other fungi. This association was initially noted in Cleveland, Ohio. The infants were primarily African American, living in older homes, and often the homes had recent water damage. Environmental tobacco smoke was also frequently present in the environment. Other forms of hypersensitivity pneumonitis have also been reported to cause pulmonary bleeding.

Clinical Findings

A. Symptoms and Signs

Pulmonary hemorrhage has as many symptoms as it has causes. Large airway hemorrhage presents with hemoptysis and symptoms of the underlying cause, such as infection, foreign body, or bronchiectasis in CF. Hemoptysis from larger airways is often bright red or contains clots. Idiopathic pulmonary hemosiderosis usually presents with nonspecific respiratory symptoms (cough, tachypnea, and retractions) with or without hemoptysis, poor growth, and fatigue. Some children or young adults may present with massive hemoptysis, marked respiratory distress, stridor, or a pneumonia-like syndrome. Fever, abdominal pain, digital clubbing, and chest pain may be reported. Jaundice and hepatosplenomegaly may be present with chronic bleeding. Physical examination often reveals decreased breath sounds, rales, rhonchi, or wheezing.

B. Laboratory Findings and Imaging

Laboratory studies vary depending on the cause of hemorrhage. Following long-standing idiopathic pulmonary hemorrhage, iron deficiency anemia and heme-positive sputum are present. Nonspecific findings may include lymphocytosis and an elevated erythrocyte sedimentation rate. Peripheral eosinophilia is present in up to 25% of patients. Chest radiographs demonstrate a range of findings, from transient perihilar infiltrates to large, fluffy alveolar infiltrates with or without atelectasis and mediastinal adenopathy. Pulmonary function testing generally reveals restrictive impairment, with low lung volumes, poor compliance, and an increased diffusion capacity. Hemosiderin-laden macrophages are found in bronchial or gastric aspirates. The diagnostic usefulness of lung biopsy is controversial.

Diffuse alveolar hemorrhage with underlying systemic disease such as systemic lupus erythematosus, Wegener granulomatosis, and occasionally Goodpasture syndrome can occur with the histologic entity known as necrotizing pulmonary capillaritis. On lung biopsy the alveolar septa are infiltrated with neutrophils, and alveolar hemorrhage is acute or chronic. The septa can fill with edema or fibrinoid necrosis. Idiopathic pulmonary hemosiderosis may represent a mild form of capillaritis associated with alveolar hemorrhage. It might represent a process that waxes and wanes, and capillaritis may be focal or mild. Likewise, an immune-mediated process may cause idiopathic pulmonary hemosiderosis, although no serologic marker has yet been identified. Although capillaritis has been described without evidence of underlying systemic disease, the search for collagen-vascular disease, vasculitis, or pulmonary fibrosis should be exhaustive.

The investigation should include serologic studies such as circulating antineutrophilic cytoplasmic autoantibodies for Wegener granulomatosis, perinuclear antineutrophilic cytoplasmic autoantibodies for microscopic polyangiitis, antinuclear antibodies for systemic lupus erythematosus, and anti–basement membrane antibodies for Goodpasture syndrome. α_1-Antitrypsin deficiency has been associated with vasculitides and should be considered.

Suspected cases of cow's milk–induced pulmonary hemosiderosis can be confirmed by laboratory findings that include high titers of serum precipitins to multiple constituents of cow's milk and positive intradermal skin tests to various cow's milk proteins. Improvement after an empiric trial of a diet free of cow's milk also supports the diagnosis.

Differential Diagnosis

The search for the site of respiratory bleeding, underlying systemic illness, and cardiac or vascular abnormalities will help define the diagnosis. When gross hemoptysis is present, large airway bronchiectasis, epistaxis, foreign body, and arteriovenous or pulmonary malformations should be ruled out. MRI or CT-assisted angiography can localize abnormal or systemic arterial flow.

Alveolar bleeding with hemoptysis is often frothy and pink. The differential diagnosis includes the disorders causing diffuse alveolar hemorrhage listed earlier. In contrast to idiopathic pulmonary hemosiderosis, Goodpasture syndrome occurs in a slightly older age group (15–35 years), tends to have a more aggressive pulmonary course, and has renal involvement (crescentic proliferative glomerulonephritis and circulating antiglomerular basement membrane antibody). Wegener granulomatosis also has renal involvement (granulomatous glomerulitis with necrotizing vasculitis, but renal biopsy findings may be nonspecific) and other systemic manifestations, especially with upper and lower respiratory tract inflammation. Upper tract involvement includes sinusitis, rhinitis, recurrent epistaxis, otitis media, saddle-nose deformity, and subglottic stenosis. Wegener granulomatosis may occur without renal involvement early in the course of the disease. The diagnosis can be made based on biopsy findings or an elevated circulating antineutrophilic cytoplasmic autoantibody titer.

Treatment

Therapy should be aimed at direct treatment of the underlying disease. Supportive measures, including iron therapy, supplemental oxygen, and blood transfusions, may be needed. A diet free of cow's milk should be tried in infants. Systemic corticosteroids have been used for various causes of diffuse alveolar hemorrhage and have been particularly successful in those secondary to collagen-vascular disorders and vasculitis. Case reports have been published describing the variable effectiveness of steroids, chloroquine, cyclophosphamide, and azathioprine for idiopathic pulmonary hemosiderosis.

Prognosis

The outcome of idiopathic pulmonary hemosiderosis is variable, characterized by a waxing and waning course of intermittent intrapulmonary bleeds and the gradual development of pulmonary fibrosis over time. The severity of the underlying renal disease contributes to the mortality rates associated with Goodpasture syndrome and Wegener granulomatosis. Diffuse alveolar hemorrhage is considered a lethal pulmonary complication of systemic lupus erythematosus.

Ben-Abraham R et al: Diffuse alveolar hemorrhage following allogeneic bone marrow transplantation in children. Chest 2003;124:660 [PMID: 12907557].

Bull TM et al: Pulmonary vascular manifestations of mixed connective tissue disease. Rheum Dis Clin North Am 2005;31:451 [PMID: 16084318].

Etzel RA: *Stachybotrys*. Curr Opin Pediatr 2003;15:103 [PMID: 12544280].

Godfrey S: Pulmonary hemorrhage/hemoptysis in children. Pediatr Pulmonol 2004;37:476 [PMID: 15114547].

Ioachimescu OC et al: Idiopathic pulmonary haemosiderosis revisited. Eur Respir J 2004;24:162. [PMID: 15293620].

Kiper N et al: Long-term clinical course of patients with idiopathic pulmonary hemosiderosis (1979–1994): Prolonged survival with low-dose corticosteroid therapy. Pediatr Pulmonol 1999;27:180 [PMID: 10213256].

Update: Pulmonary hemorrhage/hemosiderosis among infants–Cleveland, Ohio, 1993–1996. MMWR Morb Mortal Wkly Rep 2000;49:180 (erratum in: MMWR Morb Mortal Wkly Rep 2000;49:213) [PMID: 11795499].

PULMONARY EMBOLISM

▶ General Considerations

Although pulmonary embolism is apparently rare in children, the incidence is probably underestimated because it is often not considered in the differential diagnosis of respiratory distress. It occurs most commonly in children with sickle cell anemia as part of the acute chest syndrome and with rheumatic fever, infective endocarditis, schistosomiasis, bone fracture, dehydration, polycythemia, nephrotic syndrome, atrial fibrillation, and other conditions. A recent report suggests that a majority of children with pulmonary emboli referred for hematology evaluation have coagulation regulatory protein abnormalities and antiphospholipid antibodies. Emboli may be single or multiple, large or small, with clinical signs and symptoms dependent on the severity of pulmonary vascular obstruction.

▶ Clinical Findings

A. Symptoms and Signs

Pulmonary embolism usually presents clinically as an acute onset of dyspnea and tachypnea. Heart palpitations or a sense of impending doom may be reported.

Pleuritic chest pain and hemoptysis may be present (not common), along with splinting, cyanosis, and tachycardia. Massive emboli may be present with syncope and cardiac arrhythmias. Physical examination is usually normal (except for tachycardia and tachypnea) unless the embolism is associated with an underlying disorder. Mild hypoxemia, rales, focal wheezing, or a pleural friction rub may be found.

B. Laboratory Findings and Imaging

Radiographic findings may be normal, but a peripheral infiltrate, small pleural effusion, or elevated hemidiaphragm can be present. If the emboli are massive, differential blood flow and pulmonary artery enlargement may be appreciated. The electrocardiogram is usually normal unless the pulmonary embolus is massive. Echocardiography is useful in detecting the presence of a large proximal embolus. A negative D-dimer has a more than 95% negative predictive value for an embolus. Ventilation-perfusion scans show localized areas of ventilation without perfusion.

Spiral CT with contrast may be helpful, but pulmonary angiography is the gold standard. Further evaluation may include Doppler ultrasound studies of the legs to search for deep venous thrombosis. Coagulation studies, including assessments of antithrombin III and protein C or S deficiencies or defective fibrinolysis may be indicated. Antiphospholipid antibodies and other coagulation regulatory proteins (proteins C and S, and factor V Leiden) should be checked, as abnormalities have been demonstrated in 70% of the hematology referrals in one pediatric institution.

▶ Treatment

Acute treatment includes supplemental oxygen, sedation, and anticoagulation. Current recommendations include heparin administration to maintain an activated partial thromboplastin time that is 1.5 or more times the control value for the first 24 hours. Urokinase (2000–4000 units/kg for 36 hours) can be used to help dissolve the embolus. Tissue plasminogen activator is another option via central or peripheral administration. These therapies should be followed by warfarin therapy for at least 6 weeks with an international normalized ratio (INR) greater than 2. In patients with identifiable deep venous thrombosis of the lower extremities and significant pulmonary emboli (with hemodynamic compromise despite anticoagulation), inferior vena caval interruption may be necessary. However, long-term prospective data regarding this latter therapy are lacking.

Bounameaux H: Review: ELISA D-dimer is sensitive but not specific in diagnosing pulmonary embolism in an ambulatory clinical setting. ACP J Club 2003;138:24 [PMID: 12511136].

Kearon C: Duration of therapy for acute venous thromboembolism. Clin Chest Med 2003;24:63 [PMID: 12685057].

Konstantinides S et al: Heparin plus alteplase compared with heparin alone in patients with submassive pulmonary embolism. N Engl J Med 2002;347:1143 [PMID: 12374874].

Rahimtoola A et al: Acute pulmonary embolism: An update on diagnosis and management. Curr Probl Cardiology 2005;30:61 [PMID: 15650680].

Remy-Jardin M et al: Pulmonary embolus imaging with multislice CT. Radiol Clin North Am 2003;41:507 [PMID: 12797603].

PULMONARY EDEMA

▶ General Considerations

Pulmonary edema is excessive accumulation of extravascular fluid in the lung. This occurs when fluid is filtered into the lungs faster than it can be removed, leading to changes in lung mechanics such as decreased lung compliance, worsening hypoxemia from ventilation-perfusion mismatch, bronchial compression, and if advanced, decreased surfactant function. There are two basic types of pulmonary edema: increased pressure (cardiogenic or hydrostatic) and increased permeability (noncardiogenic or primary). Hydrostatic pulmonary edema is usually due to excessive increases in pulmonary venous pressure, which is most commonly due to congestive heart failure from multiple causes. In contrast, many lung diseases, especially acute respiratory distress syndrome, are characterized by the development of pulmonary edema secondary to changes in permeability due to injury to the alveolocapillary barrier. In these settings, pulmonary edema occurs independently of the elevations of pulmonary venous pressure.

Clinical Findings

A. Symptoms and Signs

Cyanosis, tachypnea, tachycardia, and respiratory distress are commonly present. Physical findings include rales, diminished breath sounds, and (in young infants) expiratory wheezing. More severe disease is characterized by progressive respiratory distress with marked retractions, dyspnea, and severe hypoxemia.

B. Imaging

Chest radiographic findings depend on the cause of the edema. Pulmonary vessels are prominent, often with diffuse interstitial or alveolar infiltrates. Heart size is usually normal in permeability edema but enlarged in hydrostatic edema.

Treatment

Although specific therapy depends on the underlying cause, supplemental oxygen therapy is indicated and, if needed, ventilator support for respiratory failure. Diuretics, digoxin, and vasodilators may be indicated for congestive heart failure along with restriction of salt and water. Recommended interventions for permeability edema are reduction of vascular volume and maintenance of the lowest central venous or pulmonary arterial wedge pressure possible without sacrificing cardiac output or causing hypotension (see following discussion). β-Adrenergic agonists such as terbutaline have been shown to increase alveolar clearance of lung water, perhaps through the action of a sodium-potassium channel pump. Maintaining normal albumin levels and a hematocrit concentration above 30 maintains the filtration of lung liquid toward the capillaries, avoiding low oncotic pressure.

Cotter G et al: Pulmonary edema: new insight on pathogenesis and treatment. Curr Opin Cardiol 2001;16:159 [PMID: 11357010].
Redding GJ: Current concepts in adult respiratory distress syndrome in children. Curr Opin Pediatr 2001;13:261 [PMID: 11389362].
Van Kooy MA, Gargiulo RF: Postobstructive pulmonary edema. Am Fam Physician 2000;62:401 [PMID: 10929702].

CONGENITAL PULMONARY LYMPHANGIECTASIA

General Considerations

Structurally, congenital pulmonary lymphangiectasia appears as dilated subpleural and interlobular lymphatic channels and may present as part of a generalized lymphangiectasis (in association with obstructive cardiovascular lesions—especially total anomalous pulmonary venous return) or as an isolated idiopathic lesion. Pathologically, the lung appears firm, bulky, and noncompressible, with prominent cystic lymphatics visible beneath the pleura. On cut section, dilated lymphatics are present near the hilum, along interlobular septa, around bronchovascular bundles, and beneath the pleura. Histologically, dilated lymphatics have a thin endothelial cell lining overlying a delicate network of elastin and collagen.

Clinical Findings

Congenital pulmonary lymphangiectasia is a rare, usually fatal disease that generally presents as acute or persistent respiratory distress at birth. Although most patients do not survive the newborn period, some survive longer, and there are isolated case reports of its diagnosis later in childhood. It may be associated with features of Noonan syndrome, asplenia, total anomalous pulmonary venous return, septal defects, atrioventricular canal, hypoplastic left heart, aortic arch malformations, and renal malformations. Chylothorax has been reported. Chest radiographic findings include a ground-glass appearance, prominent interstitial markings suggesting lymphatic distention, diffuse hyperlucency of the pulmonary parenchyma, and hyperinflation with depression of the diaphragm.

Prognosis

Although the onset of symptoms may be delayed for as long as the first few months of life, prolonged survival is extremely rare. Most deaths occur within weeks after birth. Rapid diagnosis is essential in order to expedite the option of pulmonary transplantation.

Esther CR et al: Pulmonary lymphangiectasia: Diagnosis and clinical course. Pediatr Pulmonol 2004;38:308 [PMID: 15334508].
Huber A et al: Congenital pulmonary lymphangiectasia. Pediatr Pulmonol 1991;10:310 [PMID: 1896243].

DISORDERS OF THE CHEST WALL

EVENTRATION OF THE DIAPHRAGM

Eventration of the diaphragm occurs when striated muscle is replaced with connective tissue and is demonstrated on radiograph by elevation of part or all of the diaphragm. There are two types: congenital and acquired. The congenital type is thought to represent incomplete formation of the diaphragm in utero. The acquired type is related to atrophy of diaphragm muscles secondary to prenatal or postnatal phrenic nerve injury. The differential diagnosis of eventration includes phrenic nerve injury and partial diaphragmatic hernia. Small eventrations may be an incidental finding on a chest radiograph, commonly seen on the right side. Ultrasound provides useful information to further define a suspected eventration. When defects are small, there is no paradoxical movement of the diaphragm and little symptomatology. When defects are large, paradoxical movement of the diaphragm may be present. The degree of respiratory distress depends in large part on the amount of paradoxical motion of the diaphragm. When the diaphragm moves upward during inspiration, instability of the inferior border of the chest wall increases the work of breathing and can lead to respiratory muscle fatigue and potential failure when stressed. Symptoms include persistent increased work of breathing, particularly with feeding or failure to extubate.

Treatment is based on severity of symptoms. If symptoms persist for 2–4 weeks, the diaphragm is surgically plicated, which stabilizes it. Function returns to the diaphragm in about 50% of cases of phrenic nerve injury whether or not plication was performed. Recovery periods of up to 100 days have been reported in these cases.

Clements BS: Congenital malformations of the lungs and airways. In Taussig LM, Landau LI (editors): *Pediatric Respiratory Medicine*. Mosby, 1999.

Eren S et al: Congenital diaphragmatic eventration as a cause of anterior mediastinal mass in children: Imaging modalities and literature review. Eur J Radiol 2004;51:85 [PMID: 15186890].

SCOLIOSIS

Scoliosis is defined as lateral curvature of the spine and is commonly categorized as idiopathic, congenital, or neuromuscular. No pulmonary impairment is typically seen with a Cobb angle showing thoracic curvature of less than 35 degrees. Most cases of idiopathic scoliosis occur in adolescent girls and are corrected before significant pulmonary impairment occurs. Congenital scoliosis of severe degree or with other major abnormalities carries a more guarded prognosis. Patients with progressive neuromuscular disease, such as Duchenne muscular dystrophy, can be at risk for respiratory failure due to severe scoliosis. Severe scoliosis can also lead to impaired lung function and possible death from cor pulmonale if uncorrected. (See also Chapter 24.)

Greiner KA: Adolescent idiopathic scoliosis: Radiologic decision-making. Am Fam Physician 2002;65:1817 [PMID: 12018804].

Kearon C et al: Factors determining pulmonary function in adolescent idiopathic thoracic scoliosis. Am Rev Respir Dis 1993;148:288 [PMID: 8342890].

PECTUS EXCAVATUM

Pectus excavatum is anterior depression of the chest wall that may be symmetrical or asymmetrical with respect to the midline. Its presence can be psychologically difficult for the patient. Whether or not it is cause for cardiopulmonary limitations is controversial. While subjective exertional dyspnea can be reported and may improve with repair, objective cardiopulmonary function may not change postoperatively. Therefore, the decision to repair the deformity may be based on cosmetic or physiologic considerations.

Surgical literature is providing more information regarding long-term outcomes following repair. Timing of repair is critical in light of growth plate maturation. Pectus excavatum may be associated with congenital heart disease.

Borowitz D et al: Pulmonary function and exercise response in patients with pectus excavatum after Nuss repair. J Pediatr Surg 2003;38:544 [PMID: 12677562].

Lawson ML et al: Impact of pectus excavatum on pulmonary function before and after repair with the Nuss procedure. J Pediatr Surg 2005;40:174 [PMID: 15868581].

Malek MH et al: Ventilatory and cardiovascular responses to exercise in patients with pectus excavatum. Chest 2003;124:870 [PMID: 12970011].

PECTUS CARINATUM

Pectus carinatum is a protrusion of the upper or lower (more common) portion of the sternum, more commonly seen in males. Again, although the disorder may have a psychological impact, impedance of cardiopulmonary function is debated. The decision to repair this deformity is often based on cosmetic grounds, but research has shown that those with reduced endurance or dyspnea with mild exercise experienced marked improvement within 6 months following repair, suggesting possible physiologic indications. Pectus carinatum may be associated with systemic diseases such as the mucopolysaccharidoses and congenital heart disease.

Fonkalsrud EW, Anselmo DM: Less extensive techniques for repair of pectus carinatum: The undertreated chest deformity. J Am Coll Surg 2004;198:898 [PMID: 15194071].

Williams AM, Crabbe DC: Pectus deformities of the anterior chest wall. Paediatr Respir Rev 2003;4:237 [PMID: 12880759].

NEUROMUSCULAR DISORDERS

Neuromuscular disorders are discussed in detail in Chapter 23. Weakness of the respiratory and pharyngeal muscles leads to chronic or recurrent pneumonia secondary to aspiration and infection, atelectasis, hypoventilation, and respiratory failure in severe cases. Scoliosis, which frequently accompanies long-standing neuromuscular disorders, may further compromise respiratory function. Typical physical findings are a weak cough, decreased air exchange, crackles, wheezing, and dullness to percussion. Signs of cor pulmonale (loud pulmonary component to the second heart sound, hepatomegaly, and elevated neck veins) may be evident in advanced cases. Chest radiographs generally show small lung volumes. If chronic aspiration is present, increased interstitial infiltrates and areas of atelectasis or consolidation may be present. Arterial blood gases demonstrate hypoxemia in the early stages and compensated respiratory acidosis in the late stages. Typical pulmonary function abnormalities include low lung volumes and decreased inspiratory force generated against an occluded airway.

Treatment is supportive and includes vigorous pulmonary toilet, antibiotics with infection, and oxygen to correct hypoxemia. Consideration of bilevel positive airway pressure and mechanical airway clearance support, like mechanical in-exsufflation, should be introduced before respiratory failure is present. Unfortunately, despite aggressive medical therapy, many neuromuscular conditions progress to respiratory failure and death. The decision to intubate and ventilate is a difficult one; it should be made only when there is real hope that deterioration, though acute, is potentially reversible or when chronic ventilation is wanted. Chronic mechanical ventilation using either noninvasive or invasive techniques is being used more frequently in patients with chronic respiratory insufficiency.

Birnkrant DJ: The assessment and management of the respiratory complications of pediatric neuromuscular diseases. Clin Pediatr 2002;41:301 [PMID: 12086195].

Finder JD et al: Respiratory care of the patient with Duchenne muscular dystrophy: ATS consensus statement. Am J Respir Crit Care Med 2004;170:456 [PMID: 15302625].

Mallory GB: Pulmonary complications of neuromuscular disease. Pediatr Pulmonol 2004;(Suppl 26):138 [PMID: 15029630].

Miske LJ et al: Use of the mechanical in-exsufflator in pediatric patients with neuromuscular disease and impaired cough. Chest 2004;125:1406 [PMID: 15078753].

Simonds AK: Nocturnal ventilation in neuromuscular disease—When and how? Monaldi Arch Chest Dis 2002;57:273 [PMID: 12814040].

DISORDERS OF THE PLEURA & PLEURAL CAVITY

The *parietal* pleura covers the inner surface of the chest wall. The visceral pleura covers the outer surface of the lungs. Disease processes can lead to accumulation of air or fluid in the pleural space. Pleural effusions are classified as transudates or exudates. Transudates occur when there is imbalance between hydrostatic and oncotic pressure, so that fluid filtration exceeds reabsorption (eg, congestive heart failure). Exudates form as a result of inflammation of the pleural surface leading to increased capillary permeability (eg, parapneumonic effusions). Other pleural effusions include chylothorax and hemothorax.

Thoracentesis is helpful in characterizing the fluid and providing definitive diagnosis. Recovered fluid is considered an exudate (as opposed to a transudate) if any of the following are found: a pleural fluid–serum protein ratio greater than 0.5, a pleural fluid–serum lactate dehydrogenase ratio greater than 0.6, or a pleural fluid lactate dehydrogenase level greater than 200 units/L. Important additional studies on pleural fluid include cell count; pH and glucose; Gram, acid-fast, and fungal stains; cultures; counterimmunoelectrophoresis for specific organisms; and occasionally, amylase concentration. Cytologic examination of pleural fluid should be performed to rule out leukemia or other neoplasm.

Hilliard TN et al: Management of parapneumonic effusion and empyema. Arch Dis Child 2003;88:915 [PMID: 14500314].

PARAPNEUMONIC EFFUSION & EMPYEMA

▶ General Considerations

Bacterial pneumonia is often accompanied by pleural effusion. Some of these effusions harbor infection, and others are inflammatory reactions to pneumonia. The nomenclature in this area is somewhat confusing. Some authors use the term *empyema* for grossly purulent fluid and *parapneumonic effusion* for nonpurulent fluid. It is clear, however, that some nonpurulent effusions will also contain organisms and represent either partially treated or early empyema. It is probably best to refer to all effusions associated with pneumonia as parapneumonic effusions, some of which are infected and some not.

The most common organism associated with empyema is *S pneumoniae*. Other common organisms include *H influenzae* and *S aureus*. Less common causes are group A streptococci, gram-negative organisms, anaerobic organisms, and *M pneumoniae*. Effusions associated with tuberculosis are almost always sterile and constitute an inflammatory reaction.

▶ Clinical Findings

A. Symptoms and Signs

Patients usually present with typical signs of pneumonia, including fever, tachypnea, and cough. They may have chest pain, decreased breath sounds, and dullness to percussion on the affected side and may prefer to lie on the affected side. With large effusions, there may be tracheal deviation to the contralateral side.

B. Laboratory Findings

The white blood cell count is often elevated, with left shift. Blood cultures are sometimes positive. The tuberculin skin test is positive in most cases of tuberculosis. Thoracentesis reveals findings consistent with an exudate. Cells in the pleural fluid are usually neutrophils in bacterial disease and lymphocytes in tuberculous effusions. In bacterial disease, pleural fluid pH and glucose are often low. pH less than 7.2 suggests active bacterial infection. The pH of the specimen should be determined in a blood gas syringe sent to the laboratory on ice. Extra heparin should not be used in the syringe as it can falsely lower the pH. Although in adults the presence of low pH and glucose necessitates aggressive and thorough drainage procedures, the prognostic significance of these findings in children is unknown. Gram stain, cultures, and counterimmunoelectrophoresis are often positive for the offending organism.

C. Imaging

The presence of pleural fluid is suggested by a homogeneous density that obscures the underlying lung on chest radiograph. Large effusions may cause a shift of the mediastinum to the contralateral side. Small effusions may only blunt the costophrenic angle. Lateral decubitus radiographs may help to detect freely movable fluid by demonstrating a layering-out effect. If the fluid is loculated, no such effect is perceived. Ultrasonography can be extremely valuable in localizing the fluid and detecting loculations, especially when thoracentesis is contemplated, but availability may be limited. Chest CT scan can help determine if loculations are present and direct further care of complicated pneumonias.

▶ Treatment

After initial thoracentesis and identification of the organism, appropriate intravenous antibiotics and adequate drainage of the fluid remain the mainstay of therapy, but the approach is debated. Although there is a trend toward managing smaller pneumococcal empyemas without a chest tube, most larger effusions require chest tube drainage. Often the empyema has been present for more than 7 days, increasing the chance for loculation of fluid. Evidence of early decortication using thoracoscopic techniques such as video-assisted thoraco-scopic surgery (VATS) may reduce morbidity and has been shown to shorten length of hospital stay when done by an experienced surgeon. While there is growing use of VATS as first-line therapy, it is not standard of care. Aggressive management with drainage of pleural cavity fluid and release of adhesions with fibrinolytics is often sought in many institutions where the chest tube is placed in the operating room under anesthesia. The decision on therapeutic choice will vary depending on the resources available to the clinician.

▶ Prognosis

The prognosis is related to the severity of disease but is generally excellent, with complete or nearly complete recovery expected in most instances.

Efrati O, Barak A: Pleural effusions in the pediatric population. Pediatr Rev 2002;23:417 [PMID: 12456894].
Gates RL et al: Drainage, fibrinolytics, or surgery: A comparison of treatment options in pediatric empyema. J Pediatr Surg 2004;39:1638 [PMID: 15547825].
Quadri A, Thomson AH: Pleural fluids associated with chest infection. Paediatr Respir Rev 2002;3:349 [PMID: 12457606].
Rodgers BM: The role of thoracoscopy in pediatric surgical practice. Semin Pediatr Surg 2003;12:62 [PMID: 12520474].

HEMOTHORAX

Accumulation of blood in the pleural space can be caused by surgical or accidental trauma, coagulation defects, and pleural or pulmonary tumors. With blunt trauma, hemopneumothorax may be present. Symptoms are related to blood loss and compression of underlying lung parenchyma. There is some risk of secondary infection, resulting in empyema.

▶ Treatment

Drainage of a hemothorax is required when significant compromise of pulmonary function is present, as with hemopneumothorax. In uncomplicated cases, observation is indicated because blood is readily absorbed spontaneously from the pleural space.

VATS has been used successfully in the management of hemothorax. Chest CT scan is helpful to select patients who may require surgery, as identification of blood and the volume of blood may be more predictive by this method than by chest radiograph.

Bliss D, Silen M: Pediatric thoracic trauma. Crit Care Med 2002;30(Suppl):S409 [PMID: 12528782].

CHYLOTHORAX

The accumulation of chyle, fluid of intestinal origin containing fat digestion products, in the pleural space usually results from accidental or surgical trauma to the thoracic duct. In the newborn, chylothorax can be congenital or secondary to birth trauma. This condition also occurs as a result of superior vena caval obstruction secondary to central venous lines and following Fontan procedures for tricuspid atresia. Symptoms of chylothorax are related to the amount of fluid accumulation and the degree of compromise of underlying pulmonary parenchyma. Thoracentesis reveals typical milky fluid (unless the patient has been fasting) containing chiefly T lymphocytes.

▶ Treatment

Treatment should be conservative because many chylothoraces resolve spontaneously. Oral feedings with medium-chain triglycerides reduce lymphatic flow through the thoracic duct. Recent literature has shown somatostatin as a viable therapeutic option. Drainage of chylous effusions should be performed only for respiratory compromise because the fluid often rapidly reaccumulates. Repeated or continuous drainage may lead to protein malnutrition and T-cell depletion, rendering the patient relatively immunocompromised. If reaccumulation of fluid persists, surgical ligation of the thoracic duct or sclerosis of the pleural space can be attempted, although the results may be less than satisfactory.

Beghetti M et al: Etiology and management of pediatric chylothorax. J Pediatr 2000;136:653 [PMID: 10802499].
Romero S: Nontraumatic chylothorax. Curr Opin Pulm Med 2000;6:287 [PMID: 10912634].

PNEUMOTHORAX & RELATED AIR LEAK SYNDROMES

Pneumothorax can occur spontaneously in newborns and in older children, or more commonly, as a result of birth trauma, positive pressure ventilation, underlying obstructive or restrictive lung disease, and rupture of a congenital or acquired lung cyst. Pneumothorax can also occur as an acute complication of tracheostomy. Air usually dissects from the alveolar spaces into the interstitial spaces of the lung. Migration to the visceral pleura ultimately leads to rupture into the pleural space. Associated conditions include pneumomediastinum, pneumopericardium, pneumoperitoneum, and subcutaneous emphysema. These conditions are more commonly associated with dissection of air into the interstitial spaces of the lung with retrograde dissection along the bronchovascular bundles toward the hilum.

Clinical Findings

A. Symptoms and Signs

The clinical spectrum can vary from asymptomatic to severe respiratory distress. Associated symptoms include cyanosis, chest pain, and dyspnea. Physical examination may reveal decreased breath sounds and hyperresonance to percussion on the affected side with tracheal deviation to the opposite side. When pneumothorax is under tension, cardiac function may be compromised, resulting in hypotension or narrowing of the pulse pressure. Pneumopericardium is a life-threatening condition that presents with muffled heart tones and shock. Pneumomediastinum rarely causes symptoms by itself.

B. Imaging

Chest radiographs usually demonstrate the presence of free air in the pleural space. If the pneumothorax is large and under tension, compressive atelectasis of the underlying lung and shift of the mediastinum to the opposite side may be demonstrated. Cross-table lateral and lateral decubitus radiographs can aid in the diagnosis of free air. Pneumopericardium is identified by the presence of air completely surrounding the heart, whereas in patients with pneumomediastinum, the heart and mediastinal structures may be outlined with air, but the air does not involve the diaphragmatic cardiac border. Chest CT scan may be helpful with recurrent spontaneous pneumothoraces to look for subtle pulmonary disease not seen on chest radiograph, but this is debated.

Differential Diagnosis

Acute deterioration of a patient on a ventilator can be caused by tension pneumothorax, obstruction or dislodgment of the endotracheal tube, or ventilator failure. Radiographically, pneumothorax must be distinguished from diaphragmatic hernia, lung cysts, congenital lobar emphysema, and cystic adenomatoid malformation, but this task is usually not difficult.

Treatment

Small or asymptomatic pneumothoraces usually do not require treatment and can be managed with close observation. Larger or symptomatic ones usually require drainage, although inhalation of 100% oxygen to wash out blood nitrogen can be tried.

Needle aspiration should be used to relieve tension acutely, followed by chest tube or pigtail catheter placement.

Pneumopericardium requires immediate identification, and if clinically symptomatic, needle aspiration to prevent death, followed by pericardial tube placement.

In older patients with spontaneous pneumothorax, recurrences are common; sclerosing and surgical procedures are often required.

Baumann MH et al: Management of spontaneous pneumothorax: An American College of Chest Physicians Delphi Consensus Statement. ACCP Pneumothorax Consensus Group. Chest 2001;119:590 [PMID: 11171742].

Damore DT, Dayan PS: Medical causes of pneumomediastinum in children. Clin Pediatr 2001;40:87 [PMID: 11261455].

Panitch HB et al: Abnormalities of the pleural space. In Taussig LM, Landau LI (editors): *Pediatric Respiratory Medicine.* Mosby, 1999.

SLEEP-DISORDERED BREATHING

General Considerations

Sleep apnea is recognized as a major public health problem in adults, with the risk of excessive daytime sleepiness, driving accidents, poor work performance, and effects on mental health. Pediatric sleep disorders are less commonly recognized because of a lack of training in sleep problem recognition and the presentation, risks, and outcome all differ from those in adults. The spectrum of sleep-disordered breathing includes obstructive sleep apnea, upper airway resistance disorder, and primary snoring. Sleep apnea is defined as cessation of breathing and can be classified as obstructive (the attempt to breathe through an obstructed airway) or central (the lack of effort to breathe). Snoring, mouth breathing, and upper airway obstruction are further discussed in Chapter 17.

Clinical Findings & Differential Diagnosis

A. Obstructive Sleep Apnea

Obstructive sleep apnea occurs in normal children with an incidence of about 2%, increasing in children with craniofacial abnormalities, neuropathies, or other medical problems. The incidence also increases when children are medicated with hypnotics, sedatives, or anticonvulsants. While not all children who snore have sleep apnea, there is recent literature that raises concerns that snoring without apnea has neurobehavioral consequences. (See Chapter 17.) Obstructive sleep apnea should be suspected whenever a child presents with nightly snoring, witnessed apnea, labored breathing, frequent nighttime arousals, failure to thrive, oxygen desaturations, life-threatening events, behavior abnormalities, obesity, or craniofacial abnormalities. Upper airway resistance syndrome is characterized by the presence of daytime fatigue or sleepiness in the presence of a normal polysomnogram and oxygen saturations. Symptoms are similar to obstructive sleep apnea, including change in appetite, poor performance in school, and problems with behavior.

B. Central Sleep Apnea

Central apneas are common in infants and children. They are considered significant if longer than 20 seconds or associated with bradycardia or desaturations. Clinical significance is uncertain, but may be relevant if they occur frequently or gas exchange problems exist. Healthy children have been shown to have central apneas lasting 25 seconds without clear consequences. In comparison, central hypoventilation syndrome patients have intact voluntary control of ventilation, but lack automatic control. During sleep, they will hypoventilate to the point at which they need ventilatory support that may require treatment with positive airway pressure and a rated tidal volume via tracheostomy. Central sleep apnea may be present with this syndrome, but is not usually noted.

C. Diagnostic Studies

When sleep apnea is suspected, the polysomnogram is the diagnostic test of choice. This test measures sleep state with electroencephalogram leads and electromyography, airflow at the nose, heart rate and rhythm, gas exchange (CO_2 and oxygenation), and leg movements, along with other potential data including esophageal pH, end-tidal CO_2, body position, muscle activity, and other optional additions. Polysomnography allows diagnosis of various forms of apnea, sleep fragmentation, periodic limb movement disorder, or other sleep disorders of children. Overnight oximetry is not an ideal study to diagnose obstructive sleep apnea. While it may identify subjects with severe obstructive sleep apnea, its sensitivity is low. Literature has shown normal oximetry studies in half a population of subjects with polysomnogram-confirmed obstructive sleep apnea.

▶ Treatment

First-line therapy for obstructive sleep apnea in children is adenotonsillectomy, which improves the clinical status for most children with normal craniofacial structure. Even children with craniofacial anomalies or neuromuscular disorders may benefit, although additional treatment with continuous positive airway pressure may be indicated. Down syndrome presents unique challenges: Up to half of these children can still have obstructive sleep apnea despite adenotonsillectomy. Treatment of young or developmentally delayed children with apnea also presents several challenges. (See Chapter 17 for additional discussion.)

Because the differential diagnosis of sleepiness is quite varied among children, pediatric sleep disorder centers are the referral of choice for testing and initiation of therapy.

Carroll JL: Obstructive sleep-disordered breathing in children: New controversies, new directions. Clin Chest Med 2003;24:261 [PMID: 12800783].

Marcus CL: Sleep-disordered breathing in children. Am J Respir Crit Care Med 2001;164:16 [PMID: 11435234].

Sateia MJ (editor): *The International Classification of Sleep Disorders,* 2nd ed. American Academy of Sleep Medicine, 2005.

Schechter MS et al: Technical report: Diagnosis and management of childhood obstructive sleep apnea syndrome. Pediatrics 2002;109:e69 [PMID: 11927742].

Section on Pediatric Pulmonology, Subcommittee on Obstructive Sleep Apnea Syndrome, American Academy of Pediatrics: Clinical practice guideline: Diagnosis and management of childhood obstructive sleep apnea syndrome. Pediatrics 2002;109:704 [PMID: 11927718].

APPARENT LIFE-THREATENING EVENTS IN INFANCY

▶ General Considerations

Apparent life-threatening events (ALTEs) are characterized as being frightening to the observer and commonly include some combination of apnea, color change (usually cyanosis or pallor), a marked change in muscle tone (usually extreme limpness), choking, or gagging. The observer sometimes fears the infant has died. The most frequent problems associated with an ALTE are gastrointestinal (~50%), neurologic (30%), respiratory (20%), cardiovascular (5%), metabolic and endocrine (< 5%), or diverse other problems, including child abuse. Up to 50% of ALTEs remain unexplained and are referred to as apnea of infancy. The relationship between ALTE and future risk of sudden infant death syndrome (SIDS) is not clear. The term *apparent life-threatening event* replaced "near-miss SIDS" in order to distance the event from a direct association with SIDS. Literature has reported an increased risk when extreme cardiopulmonary events were present at the time of the ALTE. Fewer than 10% of SIDS victims have had a prior history of ALTE.

The mechanism for ALTEs is unknown, but because they do not occur after infancy, immaturity is felt to play a major role. Indeed, classic studies on the nervous system, reflexes, and responses to apnea or hypoxia during sleep show profound cardiovascular compromise in infants during stimulation of the immature autonomic nervous system; adults would not be affected.

The following section describes an approach to the patient who has undergone an ALTE, taking note of the very broad differential diagnosis and uncertainties in both evaluation and treatment.

▶ Clinical Findings & Differential Diagnosis

A. History and Physical Examination

Table 18–4 classifies disorders associated with ALTEs. A careful history is often the most helpful part of the evaluation. It is useful to determine whether the infant has been chronically ill or essentially well. A history of several days of poor feeding, temperature instability, or respiratory or gastrointestinal symptoms suggests an infectious process. Reports of "struggling to breathe" or "trying to breathe" imply airway obstruction. Association of the episodes with feeding implies discoordinated swallowing, gastroesophageal reflux, or airway obstruction. Episodes that typically follow crying may be related to breath-holding. Association of

Table 18–4. Potential causes of apparent life-threatening events.

Infectious	Viral: respiratory syncytial virus and other respiratory viruses
	Bacterial: sepsis, pertussis, chlamydia
Gastrointestinal	Gastroesophageal reflux with or without obstructive apnea
Respiratory	Airway abnormality; vascular rings, pulmonary slings, tracheomalacia
	Pneumonia
Neurologic	Seizure disorder
	Central nervous system infection: meningitis, encephalitis
	Vasovagal response
	Leigh encephalopathy
	Brain tumor
Cardiovascular	Congenital malformation
	Dysrhythmias
	Cardiomyopathy
Nonaccidental trauma	Battering
	Drug overdose
	Münchhausen syndrome by proxy
No definable cause	Apnea of infancy

episodes with sleeping may also suggest gastroesophageal reflux, apnea of infancy, or sleep-disordered breathing. Attempts should be made to determine the duration of the episode, but this is often difficult. It is helpful to role-play the episode with the family. Details regarding the measures taken to resuscitate the infant and the infant's recovery from the episode are often useful in determining severity.

The physical examination provides further direction in pursuing the diagnosis. Fever or hypothermia suggests infection. An altered state of consciousness implies a postictal state or drug overdose. Respiratory distress implies cardiac or pulmonary lesions.

Apneic episodes have been linked to child abuse in several ways. Head injury following nonaccidental trauma may be first brought to medical attention because of apnea. Other signs of abuse are usually immediately apparent in such cases. Drug overdose, either accidental or intentional, may also present with apnea. Several series document that apneic episodes may be falsely reported by parents seeking attention (ie, Münchhausen syndrome by proxy). Parents may physically interfere with a child's respiratory efforts, in which case pinch marks on the nares are sometimes found.

B. Laboratory Findings

Most patients are hospitalized for observation in order to reduce stress on the family and allow prompt completion of the evaluation. Laboratory evaluation includes a complete blood count for evidence of infection. Serum electrolytes are usually obtained. Elevations in serum bicarbonate suggest chronic hypoventilation, whereas decreases suggest acute acidosis, perhaps due to hypoxia during the episode. Chronic acidosis suggests an inherited metabolic disorder. Arterial blood gas studies provide an initial assessment of oxygenation and acid-base status, and low Pa_{O_2} or elevated Pa_{CO_2} (or both) implies cardiorespiratory disease. A significant base deficit suggests that the episode was accompanied by hypoxia or circulatory impairment. Oxygen saturation measurements in the hospital assess oxygenation status during different activities and are more comprehensive than a single blood gas sample.

Because apnea has been associated with respiratory infections, diagnostic studies for RSV and other viruses, pertussis, and *Chlamydia* may help with diagnosis. Apnea occurring with infection often precedes other physical findings.

C. Imaging

The chest radiograph is examined for infiltrates suggesting acute infection or chronic aspiration and for cardiac size as a clue to intrinsic cardiac disease. If the episode might have involved airway obstruction, the airway should be examined either directly, by fiberoptic bronchoscopy, or radiographically, by CT or barium swallow. Barium swallow is a useful tool to rule out the possibility of anatomic abnormalities such as vascular ring and tracheoesophageal fistula. This study may also demonstrate reflux and aspiration. If reflux is suspected, it should be documented by esophageal pH monitoring coupled with respiratory pattern recording. Most infants with reflux and apnea can be given medical antireflux treatment. Infants with reflux and repeated episodes of apnea may benefit from a surgical antireflux procedure.

D. Polysomnography and Other Studies

ALTEs occur in the same age group as infants who die of sudden death (2–4 months is the peak age). Sleep-disordered breathing has been implicated as a possible cause of ALTEs and perhaps sudden death. Depending on the discretion of the clinician in appropriate scenarios, polysomnograms can be useful to determine abnormalities of cardiorespiratory function, sleep state, oxygen saturation, CO_2 retention, and seizure activity. They can be used in conjunction with pH monitoring to determine the contribution of reflux to apnea. Esophageal pressure manometry can be useful to detect subtle changes in respiratory effort related to partial obstructive breathing (hypopnea). Infants may be at more risk of adverse events from sleep-disordered breathing due to their immature nervous system.

There are several neurologic causes of ALTEs. Apnea as the sole manifestation of a seizure disorder is unusual but may occur. In cases of repeated episodes, 24-hour electroencephalographic monitoring may be helpful in detecting a seizure disorder. Leigh disease, a brainstem disorder characterized pathologically by neuronal dropout, may present with apneic episodes.

Treatment

Therapy is directed at the underlying cause if one is found. After blood cultures are taken, antibiotics should be given to infants who appear toxic. Seizure disorders are treated with anticonvulsants. Gastroesophageal reflux should be treated, but may not prevent future episodes of ALTE. Vascular rings and pulmonary slings must be corrected surgically because of severe morbidity and high mortality rates when untreated.

The approach to care of infants with ALTEs where no definable cause can be ascertained is controversial. Home monitoring has been used in the past as treatment, but the efficacy of monitoring has not been demonstrated in controlled trials. The rationale for use of monitors is that infants at risk for subsequent severe episodes can be identified. With over 20 years of home monitoring, the sudden infant death rate did not change due to this intervention. Although monitors can detect apnea or bradycardia, they do not predict which children will have future ALTEs. Parents should be taught cardiopulmonary resuscitation prior to discharge. They should also be aware of the possibility of frequent false alarms. It must be noted that many parents cannot handle the stress associated with having a monitor in the home.

The decision to monitor these infants involves the participation of the family. Infants with severe initial episodes or repeated severe episodes are now thought to be at significantly increased risk and should probably be monitored in the home. Episodes in these children are so severe that the parents want to know the infant's condition at all times. The decision to discontinue monitoring is usually based on the infant's ability to go several months without triggering the alarm.

Oxygen has been used as therapy for ALTEs for several reasons. First, it reduces periodic breathing of infancy, an immature pattern of breathing that can cause some degree of oxygen desaturation. Second, infants have small chest capacities with increased chest wall compliance that reduces lung volume. Oxygen can increase the baseline saturation, reducing the severity of desaturation with short apneas. Respiratory stimulants such as caffeine and aminophylline have been used in specific cases of central apnea or periodic breathing.

Davies F, Gupta R: Apparent life threatening events in infants presenting to an emergency department. Emerg Med J 2002;19:11 [PMID: 11777863].

Farrell PA et al: SIDS, ALTE, apnea, and the use of home monitors. Pediatr Rev 2002;23:3 [PMID: 11773587].

Kahn A, European Society for the Study and Prevention of Infant Death: Recommended clinical evaluation of infants with an apparent life-threatening event. Consensus document of the European Society for the Study and Prevention of Infant Death, 2003. Eur J Pediatr 2004;163:108 [PMID: 14652748].

SUDDEN INFANT DEATH SYNDROME

► General Considerations

SIDS is defined as the sudden death of an infant younger than age 1 year that remains unexplained after a thorough case investigation, including performance of a complete autopsy, examination of the death scene, and review of the clinical history. The postmortem examination is an important feature of the definition because approximately 20% of cases of sudden death can be explained by autopsy findings. The incidence of SIDS in the United States has declined to less than 1 in 1000 live births. The part of the decline that has occurred since 1994 is likely due to alterations of risk factors (see following discussion).

► Epidemiology & Pathogenesis

Epidemiologic and pathologic data constitute most of what is known about SIDS. The number of deaths peaks between ages 2 and 4 months, and most deaths occur in infants a few weeks to 6 months of age. Most deaths occur between midnight and 8 AM, while the infant and often the caregiver are sleeping. In fact, the only unifying features of all SIDS cases are age and sleep. Previous studies showed a peak in SIDS during the respiratory virus season, but the association becomes weaker when the data are controlled for risk factors such as tobacco exposure. SIDS is more common among ethnic and racial minorities and socioeconomically disadvantaged populations. Racial disparity in the prevalence of prone positioning may also be contributing to the continued disparity in SIDS rates between black and white infants. There is a 3:2 male predominance in most series. Other risk factors include low birth weight, teenage or drug-addicted mothers, maternal smoking, and a family history of SIDS. Most of these risk factors are associated with a two- to threefold elevation of incidence but are not specific enough to be useful in predicting which infants will die unexpectedly. Recent immunization is not a risk factor.

The most consistent pathologic findings are intrathoracic petechiae and mild inflammation and congestion of the respiratory tract. Subtler pathologic findings include brainstem gliosis, extramedullary hematopoiesis, and increases in periadrenal brown fat. These latter findings suggest that infants who succumb to SIDS have had intermittent or chronic hypoxia before death.

The mechanism or mechanisms of death in SIDS are unknown. For example, it is unknown whether the initiating event at the time of death is cessation of breathing, cardiac arrhythmia, or asystole. Hypotheses have included upper airway obstruction, catecholamine excess, and increased fetal hemoglobin. However, maldevelopment or delay in maturation of the brainstem, which is responsible for arousal, remains the predominant theory. It has been recognized that some infants who presented with apneic episodes subsequently died from SIDS; however, study of these infants and prospective studies of large numbers of newborns have indicated that most infants with apnea do not die from SIDS and that most infants with SIDS have no identifiable episodes of apnea. The American Academy of Pediatrics has recommended that infant home monitoring not be used as a strategy to prevent SIDS, but may be useful in some infants who have had an ALTE (see section on Apparent Life-Threatening Events, earlier).

A history of mild symptoms of upper respiratory infection before death is not uncommon, and SIDS victims are sometimes seen by physicians a day or so before death. When infants are discovered blue, cold, and motionless by parents or caregivers, they are most commonly taken to the emergency department, where resuscitation usually fails. Families must then be supported following the death. The National SIDS Resource Center (http://www.sidscenter.org) provides information about psychosocial support groups and counseling for families of SIDS victims. The postmortem examination is essential for the diagnosis of SIDS and may help the family by excluding other possible causes of death. A death scene investigation is also important in determining the cause of sudden unexpected deaths in infancy.

▶ Prevention

Since 1990, SIDS rates have declined more than 60% worldwide. Population studies in New Zealand and Europe identified risk factors, which when changed had a major effect on the incidence of SIDS. Since 1994 the American Academy of Pediatrics' "Back-to-Sleep" campaign has promoted education about SIDS risk factors in the United States. Modifiable risk factors include sleeping position, bottle feeding, maternal smoking, and infant overheating; sleeping position and smoke exposure may have the largest influence. The prone sleep position could contribute to SIDS through decreased arousal during sleep or during hypoxia, rebreathing of exhaled gases, or effects on the immature autonomic nervous system. The side position, often used in hospitals and then mimicked at home, also shows increased risk of SIDS compared with the supine position. Maternal smoking, especially prenatal maternal smoking, increases the risk of SIDS. Investigations of tobacco effects on the autonomic nervous system of the developing fetus, pulmonary growth and function of the newborn, or its combination with viral infection all point to differences in SIDS compared with control subjects. Although the mechanism is not known, recent literature review has shown a reduced risk of SIDS associated with pacifier use. While beneficial for many reasons, breast feeding is debated regarding decreasing SIDS risk.

The health care provider is instrumental in parental education regarding the modifiable risk factors for SIDS (Table 18–5). Education includes promotion of the supine sleeping position, firm sleep surface, pacifier use at nap or bedtime, avoidance of overheating, and smoking cessation; and identification of child care settings, as many parents rely on others to watch their children, where the impor-

Table 18–5. American Academy of Pediatrics recommendations regarding sudden infant death syndrome (SIDS) risk reduction.

"Back-to-Sleep" (supine sleeping position)
Firm sleep surface
Soft objects/loose bedding out of crib
Do not smoke during pregnancy
Separate but proximate sleeping environment
Consider offering a pacifier at nap and bed time
Avoid overheating
Avoid commercial devices marketed to reduce the risk of SIDS
Do not use home monitors as a strategy to reduce the risk of SIDS
Avoid development of positional plagiocephaly

Data from American Academy of Pediatrics Task Force on Sudden Infant Death Syndrome: The changing concept of sudden infant death syndrome: Diagnostic coding shifts, controversies regarding the sleeping environment, and new variables to consider in reducing risk. Pediatrics 2005;116:1245.

tance of infant sleep position may not recognized. Hospitals should set an example by placing infants in the supine position. With education, the mortality rate may continue to decline.

American Academy of Pediatrics Task Force on Sudden Infant Death Syndrome: The changing concept of sudden infant death syndrome: Diagnostic coding shifts, controversies regarding the sleeping environment, and new variables to consider in reducing risk. Pediatrics 2005;116:1245 [PMID: 16216901].

Committee on the Fetus and Newborn, American Academy of Pediatrics: Apnea, sudden infant death syndrome, and home monitoring. Pediatrics 2003;111:914 [PMID: 12671135].

Hunt CE: Sudden infant death syndrome and other causes of infant mortality: Diagnosis, mechanisms, and risk for recurrence in siblings. Am J Respir Crit Care Med 2001;164:346 [PMID: 11500332].

Nagler J: Sudden infant death syndrome. Curr Opin Pediatr 2002;14:247 [PMID: 11981299].

Ramanathan R et al: Cardiorespiratory events recorded on home monitors: Comparison of healthy infants with those at increased risk for SIDS. JAMA 2001;285:2199 [PMID: 11325321].

Toomey S, Bernstein H: Sudden infant death syndrome. Curr Opin Pediatr 2001;13:207 [PMID: 11317067].

▼ MEDIASTINUM

MEDIASTINAL MASSES

▶ General Considerations

Children with mediastinal masses may present because of symptoms produced by pressure on the esophagus, airways, nerves, or vessels within the mediastinum, or the masses may be discovered on a routine chest radiograph. Once the mass is identified, localization to one of four mediastinal compartments aids in the differential diagnosis. The superior mediastinum is the area above the pericardium that is bordered inferiorly by an imaginary line from the manubrium to the fourth thoracic vertebra. The anterior mediastinum is bordered by the sternum anteriorly and the pericardium posteriorly, and the posterior mediastinum is defined by the pericardium and diaphragm anteriorly and the lower eight thoracic vertebrae posteriorly. The middle mediastinum is surrounded by these three compartments.

Clinical Findings

A. Symptoms and Signs

Respiratory symptoms, when present, are due to pressure on an airway (cough or wheezing) or an infection (unresolving pneumonia in one area of lung). Hemoptysis can also occur but is an unusual presenting symptom. Dysphagia may occur secondary to compression of the esophagus. Pressure on the recurrent laryngeal nerve can cause hoarseness due to paralysis of the left vocal cord. Superior vena caval obstruction can lead to dilation of neck vessels and other signs and symptoms of obstruction of venous return from the upper part of the body (superior mediastinal syndrome).

B. Laboratory Findings and Imaging

The mass is initially defined by frontal and lateral chest radiographs together with thoracic CT scans and perhaps MRI. A barium swallow may also help define the extent of a mass. Other studies that may be required include angiography (to define the blood supply to large tumors), electrocardiography, echocardiography, ultrasound of the thorax, fungal and mycobacterial skin tests, and urinary catecholamine assays. MRI or myelography may be necessary in children suspected of having a neurogenic tumor in the posterior mediastinum.

Differential Diagnosis

The differential diagnosis of mediastinal masses is determined by their location. Within the superior mediastinum, one may find cystic hygromas, vascular or neurogenic tumors, thymic masses, teratomas, intrathoracic thyroid tissue, and esophageal lesions. A mediastinal abscess may also be found in this region. Within the anterior mediastinum, thymic tissue (thymomas, hyperplasia, and cysts) and teratomas, vascular tumors, and lymphatic tissue (lymphomas or reactive lymphadenopathy) give rise to masses. An intrathoracic thyroid and a pleuropericardial cyst may also be found in this region. Within the middle mediastinum one may again find lymphomas and hypertrophic lymph nodes, granulomas, bronchogenic or enterogenous cysts, metastases, and pericardial cysts. Abnormalities of the great vessels and aortic aneurysms may also present as masses in this compartment. Within the posterior mediastinum, neurogenic tumors, enterogenous cysts, thoracic meningoceles, or aortic aneurysms may be present.

In some series, more than 50% of mediastinal tumors occur in the posterior mediastinum and are mainly neurogenic tumors or enterogenous cysts. Most neurogenic tumors in children younger than age 4 years are malignant (neuroblastoma or neuroganglioblastoma), whereas a benign ganglioneuroma is the most common histologic type in older children. In the middle and anterior mediastinum, tumors of lymphatic origin (lymphomas) are the primary concern. Bulky anterior mediastinal tumors that compress the trachea and the great vessels can lead to a superior mediastinal syndrome, which presents a diagnostic problem because of anesthesia hazards. Definitive diagnosis in most instances relies on surgery to obtain the mass or a part of the mass for histologic examination. In cases of lymphoma, the scalene nodes may also contain tumor, and a biopsy should be performed in an attempt to establish a diagnosis.

Treatment & Prognosis

The appropriate therapy and the response to therapy depend on the cause of the mediastinal mass.

Franco A et al: Imaging evaluation of pediatric mediastinal masses. Radiol Clin North Am 2005;43:325 [PMID: 15737372].

Williams HJ, Alton HM: Imaging of paediatric mediastinal abnormalities. Paediatr Respir Rev 2003;4:55 [PMID: 12615033].

Cardiovascular Diseases

Henry M. Sondheimer, MD

Jeffrey R. Darst, MD

Elizabeth M. Shaffer, MD

Shelley D. Miyamoto, MD

Eight in 1000 infants are born with a congenital heart defect. Acquired heart diseases such as Kawasaki disease, myocarditis, and rheumatic heart disease also cause significant morbidity and mortality in children. Advances in medical and surgical care now allow more than 90% of children with congenital heart defects to enter adulthood. It is therefore important that current pediatric cardiac care include not only the diagnosis and treatment of congenital heart disease but also the prevention of risk factors for adult cardiovascular disease—obesity, smoking and hyperlipidemia. Subspecialty clinics addressing the needs of adults with repaired or palliated congenital heart disease are needed to assess and advise patients regarding such adult issues as the impact of pregnancy, the risks of anticoagulation during pregnancy, and appropriate adult career choices.

▼ DIAGNOSTIC EVALUATION

The presence of a heart murmur suggests the possibility of heart disease. Murmurs, however, may be functional or innocent, and not all serious cardiovascular disorders are accompanied by an easily detectable murmur.

HISTORY

Most congenital defects lead either to decreased pulmonary blood flow or increased pulmonary blood flow with pulmonary congestion. Symptoms vary according to the alteration in pulmonary blood flow (Table 19–1). The presence of other cardiovascular symptoms such as palpitations and chest pain should also be determined by history in the older child, paying particular attention to the timing (at rest or activity-related), onset, and termination (gradual versus sudden), and precipitating and relieving factors.

PHYSICAL EXAMINATION

General

The examination should begin with a visual assessment of skin perfusion and skin color. Heart rate, respiratory rate, blood pressure (in all four extremities), and oxygen saturation are required. Many congenital cardiac defects occur as part of a genetic syndrome (Table 19–2) and the complete assessment includes an evaluation for dysmorphic features that may be clues to the associated cardiac defect.

CARDIOVASCULAR DISEASE ABBREVIATIONS	
ASD	Atrial septal defect
AVSD	Atrioventricular septal defect
ccTGA	Congenitally corrected transposition of the great arteries
DCM	Dilated cardiomyopathy
HCM	Hypertrophic cardiomyopathy
HF	Heart failure
HLHS	Hypoplastic left heart syndrome
LVH	Left ventricular hypertrophy
MVP	Mitral valve prolapse
PA/IVS	Pulmonary atresia with intact ventricular septum
PDA	Patent (persistent) ductus arteriosus
PPH	Primary pulmonary hypertension
RVH	Right ventricular hypertrophy
TAPVR	Total anomalous pulmonary venous return
TGA	Transposition of the great arteries
ToF	Tetralogy of Fallot
VSD	Ventricular septal defect
WPW	Wolff-Parkinson-White syndrome

Table 19–1. Symptoms of increased and decreased pulmonary blood flow.

Decreased Pulmonary Blood Flow	Increased Pulmonary Blood Flow
Infant/Toddler	
Cyanosis	Tachypnea with activity/feeds
Squatting	Diaphoresis
Loss of consciousness	Poor weight gain
Older Child	
Dizziness	Exercise intolerance
Syncope	Dyspnea on exertion, diaphoresis

Cardiovascular Examination

A. Inspection and Palpation

Chest conformation should be noted in the supine position. A precordial bulge indicates cardiomegaly. Palpation may reveal increased precordial activity, right ventricular lift, or left-sided heave; a diffuse point of maximal impulse; or a precordial thrill caused by a grade IV/VI murmur. The thrill of aortic stenosis is found in the suprasternal notch. In patients with severe pulmonary hypertension, a palpable pulmonary closure (P_2) is frequently noted at the upper left sternal border.

B. Auscultation

1. Heart sounds—The first heart sound (S_1) is the sound of atrioventricular (AV) valve closure. It is best heard at the lower left sternal border and is usually medium-pitched. Although S_1 has multiple components only one of these (M_1) is usually audible.

Table 19–2. Cardiac defects in common syndromes.

Genetic Syndrome	Commonly Associated Cardiac Defect
Down syndrome	AVSD
Turner syndrome	Bicuspid aortic valve, coarctation
Noonan syndrome	Dysplastic pulmonic valve, HCM
Williams-Beuren syndrome	Supravalvular aortic stenosis, PPS
Marfan syndrome	MVP, MR, dilated aortic root
Fetal alcohol syndrome	VSD, ASD
Maternal rubella	PDA, PPS

ASD, atrial septal defect; AVSD, atrioventricular septal defect; HCM, hypertrophic cardiomyopathy; MR, mitral regurgitation; MVP, mitral valve prolapse; PDA, patent ductus arteriosus; PPS, peripheral pulmonary stenosis; VSD, ventricular septal defect.

The second heart sound (S_2) is the sound of semilunar valve closure. It is best heard at the upper left sternal border. S_2 has two component sounds, A_2 and P_2 (aortic and pulmonic valve closure). Splitting of S_2 varies with respiration, widening with inspiration and narrowing with expiration. Abnormal splitting of S_2 may be an indication of cardiac disease (Table 19–3).

The third heart sound (S_3) is the sound of rapid left ventricular filling. It occurs in early diastole, after S_2, and is medium- to low-pitched. In healthy children, S_3 diminishes or disappears when going from supine to sitting or standing. A persistent S_3 is often heard in the presence of a dilated left ventricle (LV) caused by cardiomyopathy or a large left-to-right shunt. The fourth heart sound (S_4) is associated with atrial contraction and increased atrial pressure and has a low pitch similar to that of S_3. It occurs just prior to S_1 and is not normally audible. It is heard in the presence of atrial contraction into a noncompliant ventricle as in hypertrophic or restrictive cardiomyopathy or hypertrophied LV from other causes.

Ejection clicks are usually related to dilated great vessels or valve abnormalities. They can be heard throughout ventricular systole and are classified as early, mid, or late. Early ejection clicks at the mid left sternal border are from the pulmonic valve. Aortic clicks are typically best heard at the apex. In contrast to aortic clicks, pulmonic clicks vary with respiration, becoming louder during inspiration. A mid to late ejection click at the apex is most typically caused by mitral valve prolapse.

2. Murmurs—A heart murmur is the most common cardiovascular finding leading to a cardiology referral. Innocent or functional heart murmurs are common, and 40–45% of children have an innocent murmur at some time during childhood.

A. CHARACTERISTICS—All murmurs should be described based on the following characteristics:

(1) *Location and radiation*—Where the murmur is best heard and where the sound extends.

(2) *Relationship to cardiac cycle and duration*—Systolic ejection (immediately following S_1 with a crescendo/decrescendo change in intensity), pansystolic (occurring through-

Table 19–3. Abnormal splitting of S_2.

Causes of wide split S_2
RV volume overload: ASD, anomalous pulmonary venous return, PI
RV pressure overload: Pulmonary valve stenosis
Delayed RV conduction: RBBB
Causes of narrow split S_2
Pulmonary hypertension
Single semilunar valve (aortic atresia, pulmonary atresia, truncus arteriosus)

ASD, atrial septal defect; PI, pulmonic insufficiency; RBBB, right bundle branch block; RV, right ventricle.

Table 19–4. Pathologic murmurs.

Systolic Ejection	Pansystolic	Diastolic	Continuous
Semilunar valve stenosis (AS/PS/truncal stenosis)	VSD	Semilunar valve regurgitation	Runoff lesions
ASD	AVVR (MR/TR)	(AI/PI/truncal insufficiency)	(PDA/AVM/aortopulmonary collaterals)
Coarctation		AV valve stenosis (MS/TS)	

AI/PI, aortic insufficiency/pulmonic insufficiency; AS/PS, aortic stenosis/pulmonic stenosis; ASD, atrial septal defect; AV, atrioventricular; MS/TS, mitral stenosis/tricuspid stenosis; AVVR, atrioventricular valve regurgitation; MR/TR, mitral regurgitation/tricuspid regurgitation; PDA/AVM, patent ductus arteriosus/arteriovenous malformation; VSD, ventricular septal defect.

out most of systole and of constant intensity), diastolic, and continuous. The timing of the murmur provides valuable clues as to underlying pathology (Table 19–4).

(3) Intensity—Grade I describes a soft murmur heard with difficulty; grade II, soft but easily heard; grade III, loud but without a thrill; grade IV, loud and associated with a precordial thrill; grade V, loud, with thrill, and audible with the edge of the stethoscope; grade VI, very loud and audible with the stethoscope off the chest.

(4) Quality—Harsh, musical, or rough; high, medium, or low in pitch.

(5) Variation with position—Audible when the patient is supine, sitting, standing, or squatting.

B. Innocent murmurs—The six most common innocent murmurs of childhood are:

(1) Newborn murmur—Heard in the first few days of life, this murmur is at the lower left sternal border, without significant radiation. It has a soft, short, vibratory grade I–II/VI quality that often subsides when mild pressure is applied to the abdomen. It usually disappears by age 2–3 weeks.

(2) Peripheral arterial pulmonary stenosis—This murmur, often heard in newborns, is caused by the normal branching of the pulmonary artery. It is heard with equal intensity at the upper left sternal border, at the back, and in both axillae. It is a soft, short, high-pitched, grade I–II/VI systolic ejection murmur and usually disappears by age 2. This murmur must be differentiated from true peripheral pulmonary stenosis (Williams syndrome, Alagille syndrome, or rubella syndrome), coarctation of the thoracic aorta, and valvular pulmonary stenosis.

(3) Still murmur—This is the most common innocent murmur of early childhood. It is typically heard between 2 and 7 years of age. It is loudest midway between the apex and the lower left sternal border. Still murmur is a musical or vibratory, short, high-pitched, grade I–III early systolic murmur. It is loudest when the patient is supine. It diminishes or disappears with inspiration or when the patient is sitting. The Still murmur is louder in patients with fever, anemia, or sinus tachycardia from any reason.

(4) Pulmonary ejection murmur—This is the most common innocent murmur in older children and adults. It is

heard from age 3 years onward. It is usually a soft systolic ejection murmur, grade I–II in intensity at the upper left sternal border. The murmur is louder when the patient is supine or when cardiac output is increased. The pulmonary ejection murmur must be differentiated from murmurs of pulmonary stenosis, coarctation of the aorta, atrial septal defect (ASD), and peripheral pulmonary artery stenosis.

(5) Venous hum—A venous hum is usually heard after age 2 years. It is located in the infraclavicular area on the right. It is a continuous musical hum of grade I–III intensity and may be accentuated in diastole and with inspiration. It is best heard in the sitting position. Turning the child's neck, placing the child supine, and compressing the jugular vein obliterates the venous hum. Venous hum is caused by turbulence at the confluence of the subclavian and jugular veins.

(6) Innominate or carotid bruit—This murmur is more common in the older child and adolescent. It is heard in the right supraclavicular area. It is a long systolic ejection murmur, somewhat harsh and of grade II–III intensity. The bruit can be accentuated by light pressure on the carotid artery and must be differentiated from all types of aortic stenosis.

When functional murmurs are found in a child, the physician should assure the parents that these are normal heart sounds of the developing child and that they do not represent heart disease.

Extracardiac Examination

A. Arterial Pulse Rate and Rhythm

Cardiac rate and rhythm vary greatly during infancy and childhood, so multiple determinations should be made. This is particularly important for infants (Table 19–5) whose heart rate varies with activity. The rhythm may be regular or there may be a phasic variation with respiration (sinus arrhythmia), which is normal.

B. Arterial Pulse Quality and Amplitude

The pulses of the upper and lower extremities should be compared. A bounding pulse is characteristic of run-off lesions, including patent ductus arteriosus (PDA), aortic regurgitation, arteriovenous malformation, or any condition

Table 19–5. Resting heart rates.

Age	Low	High
< 1 mo	80	160
1–3 mo	80	200
2–24 mo	70	120
2–10 y	60	90
11–18 y	40	90

with a low diastolic pressure (fever, anemia, or septic shock). Narrow or thready pulses occur in patients with conditions reducing cardiac output such as cardiomyopathy, myocarditis, pericardial tamponade, or severe aortic stenosis. A reduction in pulse amplitude or blood pressure (> 10 mm Hg) with inspiration is referred to as pulsus paradoxus and is a telltale sign of pericardial tamponade. The femoral pulse should be palpable and equal in amplitude and simultaneous with the brachial pulse. A femoral pulse that is absent or weak, or that is delayed in comparison with the brachial pulse, suggests coarctation of the aorta.

C. Arterial Blood Pressure

Blood pressures should be obtained in the upper and lower extremities. Systolic pressure in the lower extremities should be greater than or equal to that in the upper extremities. The cuff must cover the same relative area of the arm and leg. Measurements should be repeated several times.

D. Cyanosis of the Extremities

Cyanosis results from an increased concentration (> 4–5 g/dL) of reduced hemoglobin in the blood. Bluish skin color is usually, but not always, a sign. Visible cyanosis accompanies low cardiac output, hypothermia, and systemic venous congestion, even in the presence of adequate oxygenation. Cyanosis should be judged only by the color of the mucous membranes (lips). Bluish discoloration around the mouth (acrocyanosis) is a feature of skin that has not been exposed to sun, and it does not correlate with cyanosis.

E. Clubbing of the Fingers and Toes

Clubbing is often associated with severe cyanotic congenital heart disease. It usually appears after age 1 year. Hypoxemia with cyanosis is the most common cause, but clubbing also occurs in patients with endocarditis, chronic liver disease, inflammatory bowel diseases, chronic pulmonary disease, and lung abscess. Digital clubbing may be a benign genetic variant.

F. Edema

Edema of dependent areas (lower extremities in the older child and the face and sacrum in the younger child) is

characteristic of elevated right heart pressure, which may be seen with tricuspid valve pathology or right ventricle (RV) dysfunction (right heart failure) from a variety of causes including LV dysfunction.

G. Abdomen

Hepatomegaly is the cardinal sign of right heart failure in the infant and child. Hepatomegaly may also be seen in the child with pulmonary edema from lesions causing left-to-right shunting or left heart failure. Splenomegaly may be present in patients with long-standing heart failure (HF), and is characteristic of infective endocarditis. Ascites is also a feature of chronic right heart failure. Examination of the abdomen may reveal shifting dullness or a fluid wave.

Finley JP et al: Assessing children's heart sounds at a distance with digital recordings. Pediatrics 2006;118:2322 [PMID: 17142514].

Murphy DJ: The patient population and requirements for optimal care: Adult congenital heart disease. Prog Pediatr Cardiol 2003;17:1.

Pierpont ME at al. Genetic basis for congenital heart defects: Current knowledge: A scientific statement from the American Heart Association Congenital Cardiac Defects Committee, Council on Cardiovascular Disease in the Young: endorsed by the American Academy of Pediatrics. Circulation 2007;115:3015 [PMID: 17519398].

Williams CL et al: Cardiovascular health in childhood: A statement for health professionals. Circulation 2002;106:143 [PMID: 12093785].

ELECTROCARDIOGRAPHY

The electrocardiogram (ECG) is essential in the evaluation of the cardiovascular system. The heart rate should first be determined, then the cardiac rhythm (Is the patient in a normal sinus rhythm or other rhythm as evidenced by a P wave with a consistent PR interval before every QRS complex?), and then the axis (Are the P and QRS axes normal for patient age?). Once this initial assessment of rate, rhythm, and axis is performed, attention can be directed toward assessment of chamber enlargement and finally to assessment of cardiac intervals and ST segments.

Age-Related Variations

The ECG evolves with age. The rate decreases and intervals increase with age. RV dominance in the newborn changes to LV dominance in the older infant, child, and adult. The normal ECG of the 1-week-old infant is abnormal for a 1-year-old child, and the ECG of a 5-year-old child is abnormal for an adult.

Electrocardiographic Interpretation

Figure 19–1 defines the events recorded by the ECG.

A. Rate

The heart rate varies markedly with age, activity, and state of emotional and physical well-being. In most infants and

▲ **Figure 19–1.** Complexes and intervals of the electrocardiogram.

younger children, the heart rate ranges from 70–200 beats per minute depending on the above.

B. Rhythm

Sinus rhythm should always be present in normal children. In contrast to adults, premature atrial and ventricular contractions are uncommon during childhood.

C. Axis

1. P wave axis—The P wave is generated from atrial contraction beginning in the high right atrium at the site of the sinus node. The impulse proceeds leftward and inferiorly, thus leading to a positive deflection in all left-sided and inferior leads (II, III, and aVF). The P wave in patients in normal sinus rhythm should be negative in lead aVR.

2. QRS axis—The net voltage should be positive in leads I and aVF in children with a normal axis. In the young child, RV dominance may persist, leading to a negative deflection in lead I. Several congenital cardiac lesions are associated with alterations in the normal QRS axis (Table 19–6).

D. P Wave

In the pediatric patient, the amplitude of the P wave is normally no greater than 3 mm and the duration no more than 0.08 second. The P wave is best seen in leads II and V_1.

E. PR Interval

The PR is measured from the beginning of the P wave to the beginning of the QRS complex. It increases with age and with slower rates. The PR interval ranges from a minimum of 0.10 second in infants to a maximum of 0.18 second in older children with slow rates. The PR interval is commonly prolonged in patients who have rheumatic heart disease and by digitalis.

F. QRS Complex

This represents ventricular depolarization, and its amplitude and direction of force (axis) reveal the relative size of the

Table 19–6. QRS axis deviation.

Right Axis Deviation	Left Axis Deviation
Tetralogy of Fallot	Atrioventricular septal defect
Dextro transposition of the great arteries	Pulmonary atresia with intact ventricular septum
Total anomalous pulmonary venous return	Tricuspid atresia
Atrial septal defect	

Table 19–7. Causes of QT prolongation.[a]

Cardiac medications
Antiarrhythmics: IA (quinidine, procainamide, disopyramide) class III (amiodarone, sotalol)
Inotropic agents: dobutamine, dopamine, epinephrine, isoproterenol
Noncardiac medications
Antibiotics/antivirals: azithromycin, clarithromycin, levofloxacin, amantadine
Antipsychotics: risperidol, thioridazine, lithium, haloperidol
Sedatives: chloral hydrate, methadone
Other: albuterol, levalbuterol, ondansetron, phenytoin, pseudoephedrine
Electrolyte disturbances: hypokalemia, hypomagnesemia, hypocalcemia

[a]Partial list only.

ventricular mass in hypertrophy, hypoplasia, and infarction. Abnormal ventricular conduction (ie, right or left bundle-branch block) is also revealed.

G. QT Interval

This interval is measured from the beginning of the QRS complex to the end of the T wave. The QT duration may be prolonged as a primary condition or secondarily due to drugs or electrolyte imbalances (Table 19–7). The normal QT duration is rate-related and must be corrected using the Bazett formula:

$$QTC = \frac{QT \ interval(s)}{\sqrt{R - R \ interval(s)}}$$

The normal QTc is less than or equal to 0.44 second.

H. ST Segment

This segment, lying between the end of the QRS complex and the beginning of the T wave, is affected by drugs, electrolyte imbalances, or myocardial injury.

I. T Wave

The T wave represents myocardial repolarization and is altered by electrolytes, myocardial hypertrophy, and ischemia.

J. Impression

The ultimate impression of the ECG is derived from a systematic analysis of the features described earlier as compared with expected normal values for the child's age.

Al-Khatib SM et al: What clinicians should know about the QT interval. JAMA 2003;289:2120 [PMID: 12709470].
Benson DW Jr: The normal electrocardiogram. In Emmanouilides GC et al (editors): *Moss and Adams Heart Disease in Infants, Children, and Adolescents*, 5th ed. Williams & Wilkins, 1995.
Viskin S et al: Long QT syndrome caused by noncardiac drugs. Prog Cardiovasc Dis 2003;45:415 [PMID: 12704598].

Table 19–8. Radiographic changes with cardiac chamber enlargement.

Chamber Enlarged	Change in Cardiac Silhouette on Anteroposterior Film
Right ventricle	Apex of the heart is tipped upward
Left ventricle	Apex of the heart is tipped downward
Left atrium	Double shadow behind cardiac silhouette
	Increase in subcarinal angle
Right atrium	Prominence of right atrial border of the heart

CHEST RADIOGRAPH

Evaluation of the chest radiograph for cardiac disease should focus on (1) position of the heart, (2) position of the abdominal viscera, (3) cardiac size, (4) cardiac configuration, and (5) character of the pulmonary vasculature.

Cardiac position is either levocardia (heart predominantly in the left chest), dextrocardia (heart predominantly in the right chest), or mesocardia (midline heart). The position of the liver and stomach bubble is either in the normal position (abdominal situs solitus), inverted with the stomach bubble on the right (abdominal situs inversus), or variable with midline liver (abdominal situs ambiguous). The heart appears relatively large in normal newborns and decreases on the chest radiograph with age. The heart size should be less than 50% of the chest diameter in children older than age 1 year. The cardiac configuration on chest radiograph may provide useful diagnostic information, as certain cardiac lesions have a characteristic radiographic appearance (Tables 19–8 and 19–9). The pulmonary vasculature should be assessed. The presence of increased or decreased pulmonary blood flow provides a clue to cardiac diagnosis, particularly in the cyanotic infant (Table 19–10).

The standard posteroanterior and left lateral chest radiographs are used (Figure 19–2).

Table 19–9. Lesion-specific chest radiographic findings.

Diagnosis	Chest Radiograph Appearance
D-transposition of the great arteries	Egg on a string
Tetralogy of Fallot	Boot-shaped heart
Unobstructed total anomalous pulmonary venous drainage	Snowman
Obstructed total anomalous pulmonary venous drainage	Small heart with congested lungs
Coarctation	Figure 3 sign + rib notching

Table 19–10. Alterations in pulmonary blood flow in cyanotic cardiac lesions.

Increased Pulmonary Blood Flow	Decreased Pulmonary Blood Flow
Total anomalous Tricuspid Atresia with pulmonary venous return	Pulmonic stenosis
Tricuspid Atresia with large ventricular septal defect	Tricuspid atresia/restrictive ventricular septal defect
Transposition of the great arteries	Tetralogy of Fallot
Truncus arteriosus	Pulmonary atresia with intact ventricular septum
	Hypoplastic left heart syndrome

Burrows PE et al: Imaging of the neonate with congenital heart disease. In Freedom RM (editor): *Neonatal Heart Disease.* Springer-Verlag, 1992.

Dextrocardia

Dextrocardia is a radiographic term used when the heart is on the right side of the chest. When dextrocardia occurs with reversal of position of the other important organs of the chest and abdomen (eg, liver, lungs, and spleen), the condition is called situs inversus totalis, and the heart is usually normal. When dextrocardia occurs with the other organs normally located (situs solitus), the heart usually has severe defects.

Rarely, the abdominal organs and lungs are in situs ambiguous. The liver is central and anterior in the upper abdomen, with the stomach pushed posteriorly. Bilateral right-sidedness (asplenia syndrome) or bilateral left-sidedness (polysplenia syndrome) may occur, but in virtually all cases of situs ambiguous, congenital heart disease is present.

ECHOCARDIOGRAPHY

Echocardiography is a fundamental tool of pediatric cardiology. Using multiple ultrasound modalities (two-dimensional imaging, Doppler, and M-mode), cardiac anatomy, blood flow, intracardiac pressures, and ventricular function can be assessed. Echocardiography is based on the physical principles of sound waves. The ultrasound frequencies utilized in cardiac imaging range from 2–10 million cycles/s.

M-mode echocardiography uses short bursts of ultrasound sent from a transducer. At acoustic interfaces, sound waves are reflected back to the transducer. The time it takes for the sound wave to return to the transducer is measured and the distance to the interface is calculated. That calculated distance is displayed against time, and a one-dimensional image is constructed that demonstrates cardiac motion. **Two-dimensional imaging** extends this technique by sending a rapid series of ultrasound bursts across a 90-degree sector, which allows construction of a two-dimensional image of the heart. **Doppler ultrasound** measures blood flow. The ultrasound transducer sends out a known frequency of sound which reflects off moving red blood cells. The transducer receives the reflected frequency and compares it with the transmitted frequency. The blood flow velocity can be calculated from the measured frequency shift. This information is used to estimate pressure gradients by the simplified Bernouli equation, in which the pressure gradient is equal to four times the calculated velocity (Pressure gradient = $4(V^2)$).

A transthoracic echocardiogram is obtained by placing the transducer on areas of the chest where there is minimal lung interference. At each transducer position, the beam is swept through the heart and a three-dimensional image of the heart is constructed in the interpreter's mind. Complex intracardiac anatomy and spatial relationships can be described, making possible the accurate diagnosis of simple and complex congenital heart disease. In addition to structural details, Doppler gives information about intracardiac blood flow and pressure gradients. Commonly used Doppler techniques include color flow imaging, pulsed wave, and continuous wave Doppler. Color flow imaging gives general information on the direction and velocity of flow. Pulsed and continuous wave Doppler imaging give more precise measurements of blood velocity. The role of M-mode in the ultrasound examination has decreased as other ultrasound modalities have been developed. M-mode is still used to measure LV end-diastolic and end-systolic dimensions and

Posteroanterior

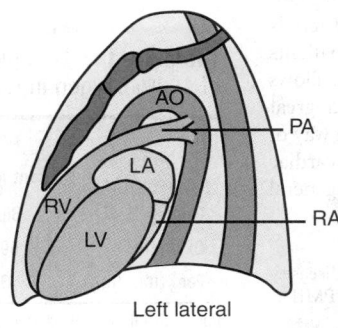

Left lateral

▲ **Figure 19–2.** Position of cardiovascular structures in principal radiograph views. AO, aorta; IVC, inferior vena cava; LA, left atrium; LA APP, left atrial appendage; LV, left ventricle; PA, pulmonary artery; RA, right atrium; RV, right ventricle; SVC, superior vena cava.

permits calculation of the LV shortening fraction, a standard estimate of LV function (SF = LV end-diastolic volume – LV systolic volume/LV end-diastolic volume).

A typical transthoracic echocardiogram performed by a skilled sonographer takes about 30 minutes, and patients must be still for the examination. Frequently infants and children cannot cooperate for the examination and sedation may be required.

Although echocardiography is an excellent tool for cardiac examination, there are drawbacks to the technique. Two-dimensional imaging can accurately diagnose intracardiac anatomy, but extracardiac structures such as pulmonary arteries and the aortic arch are more difficult to assess. Doppler imaging measures pressure gradients accurately but does not obtain exactly the same information obtained by cardiac catheterization. The indications for pediatric echocardiography are summarized in the American College of Cardiology/American Heart Association (ACC/AHA) practice guidelines published in 2003.

Snider AR et al: *Echocardiography in Congenital Heart Disease.* Mosby, 1997.

NUCLEAR CARDIOLOGY

Nuclear imaging is a useful adjunct to cardiopulmonary exercise testing in assessing both fixed and reversible areas of myocardial ischemia. It is valuable in evaluating myocardial perfusion in patients with Kawasaki disease, repaired anomalous left coronary artery or other coronary anomalies, myocardial bridging in the setting of hypertrophic cardiomyopathy, or chest pain in association with ECG changes with exercise.

MAGNETIC RESONANCE IMAGING

Magnetic resonance imaging (MRI) is valuable for evaluation and noninvasive follow-up of many congenital heart defects. It is particularly useful in imaging the thoracic vessels, which are difficult to image by transthoracic echocardiogram. Cardiac gated imaging allows dynamic evaluation of structure and blood flow of the heart and great vessels. It is invaluable to diagnose and follow aortic coarctation, to follow the progress of aortic dilation in Marfan syndrome, to quantify regurgitant lesions such as pulmonary insufficiency after repair of tetralogy of Fallot, and to measure ventricular function in patients with inadequate echocardiographic images. Because it allows computer manipulation of the images of heart and great vessels, three-dimensional MRI is an ideal noninvasive way of obtaining accurate reconstructions of the heart. If a cardiac MRI is performed in a child younger than age 8 years, general anesthesia is often required.

Boxt LM, Rozenshtein A: MR imaging of congenital heart disease. Magn Reson Imaging Clin North Am 2003;11:27 [PMID: 12797509].

CARDIOPULMONARY STRESS TESTING

Most children with heart disease are capable of normal activity. Data on cardiac function after exercise are essential to preventing unnecessary restriction of activities. The response to exercise is helpful in determining the need for and the timing of cardiovascular surgery as well as a useful objective outcome measure of the results of medical and surgical interventions.

Bicycle ergometers or treadmills can be used in children as young as age 5 years. The addition of a metabolic cart enables one to assess whether exercise impairment is secondary to cardiac limitation, pulmonary limitation, deconditioning, or lack of effort. Exercise variables include the ECG, blood pressure response to exercise, oxygen saturation, ventilation, maximal oxygen consumption, and peak work load attained. Cardiopulmonary stress testing is routine in children with congenital cardiac lesions to ascertain limitations, develop exercise prescriptions, assess the effect of therapies, and decide on the need for cardiac transplantation. Stress testing is also employed in children with structurally normal hearts to rule out cardiac or pulmonary pathology in children with symptoms during exertion. Significant stress ischemia or dysrhythmias warrant physical restrictions or appropriate therapy. Children with poor performance due to suboptimal conditioning benefit from a planned exercise program.

McManus A, Leung M: Maximizing the clinical use of exercise gaseous exchange testing in children with repaired cyanotic congenital heart defects: The development of an appropriate test strategy. Sports Med 2000;29:229 [PMID: 10783899].

ARTERIAL BLOOD GASES

Quantitating the partial oxygen pressure (Po_2) or O_2 saturation (eg, by pulse oximetry) during the administration of 100% oxygen is the most useful method of distinguishing cyanosis produced primarily by heart disease or by lung disease in sick infants. In cyanotic heart disease, the partial arterial oxygen pressure (Pao_2) increases very little when 100% oxygen is administered over the values obtained while breathing room air. However, Pao_2 usually increases very significantly when oxygen is administered to a patient who has lung disease. Table 19–11 illustrates the

Table 19–11. Examples of responses to 10 minutes of 100% oxygen in lung disease and heart disease.

	Lung Disease		Heart Disease	
	Room Air	100% O_2	Room Air	100% O_2
Color	Blue →	Pink	Blue →	Blue
Oximetry	60% →	99%	60% →	62%
Pao_2 (mm Hg)	35 →	120	35 →	38

Pao_2, partial arterial oxygen pressure.

responses seen in patients with heart or lung disease during the hyperoxic test. Routine pulse oximetry has been advocated as an adjunct to the current newborn screening evaluation, as it is a simple, cost-effective means of screening for major cardiac defects prior to hospital discharge.

Koppel RI et al. Effectiveness of pulse oximetry screening for congenital heart disease in asymptomatic newborns. Pediatrics 2003;111:451 [PMID: 12612220].

CARDIAC CATHETERIZATION & ANGIOCARDIOGRAPHY

Cardiac catheterization precisely defines the anatomic and physiologic abnormalities in simple and complex cardiac malformations. Cardiac catheterization may be performed for diagnostic purposes when further anatomic or physiologic data are needed prior to a therapeutic decision or may be performed for therapeutic purposes when the cardiac condition can be palliated or treated in the catheterization laboratory.

Therapeutic Cardiac Catheterization

Therapeutic procedures performed during cardiac catheterization include coil embolization of a PDA, balloon angioplasty with or without stent placement for aortic coarctation or branch pulmonary artery stenoses, balloon atrial septostomy, valvuloplasty of stenotic aortic or pulmonic valves, and placement of ASD and ventricular septal defect (VSD) devices. Cardiac catheterization is also performed to evaluate the effects of pharmaceutical therapy. An example of this use of catheterization is monitoring changes in pulmonary vascular resistance during the administration of nitric oxide or prostacyclin in a child with primary pulmonary hypertension. Electrophysiologic evaluation and ablation of abnormal electrical pathways in children can be performed by qualified personnel in the pediatric catheterization laboratory.

The risks of cardiac catheterization (morbidity and mortality) must be explained to the patient's family. Although the risks are very low for elective studies in older children (< 0.1%), the risk of major complications in distressed infants is about 2%. Interventional procedures such as balloon valvuloplasty increase these risks further.

Cardiac Catheterization Data

Figure 19–3 shows oxygen saturation (in percent) and pressure (in millimeters of mercury) values obtained at cardiac catheterization from the chambers and great arteries of the heart. These values are within the normal range for a child.

A. Oxygen Content and Saturation; Pulmonary (Q_p) and Systemic (Q_s) Blood Flow (Cardiac Output)

In most laboratories, left-to-right shunting is determined by changes of blood oxygen content or saturation during sam-

▲ **Figure 19–3.** Pressures (in millimeters of mercury) and oxygen saturation (in percent) obtained by cardiac catheterization in a healthy child. 3, mean pressure of 3 mm Hg in the right atrium; 5, mean pressure of 5 mm Hg in the left atrium.

pling through the right side of the heart. A significant increase in oxygen saturation between one right chamber and the other indicates the presence of a left-to-right shunt at the site of the increase. The oxygen saturation of the peripheral arterial blood should always be determined during cardiac catheterization. Normal arterial oxygen saturation is 95–97% at sea level and 92–94% at 5280 feet. Subnormal saturations suggest the presence of a right-to-left shunt, underventilation, or pulmonary disease.

The size of a left-to-right shunt is usually expressed as a ratio of pulmonary to systemic blood flow (Q_p/Q_s) or as liters per minute as determined by the Fick principle:

$$\frac{\text{Cardiac}}{\text{output (L/min)}} = \frac{\text{Oxygen consumption (mL/min)}}{\text{Arteriovenous difference (mL/L)}}$$

B. Pressures

Pressures should be determined in all chambers and major vessels entered. It is not normal for systolic pressure in the ventricles to exceed systolic pressure in the great arteries, or mean diastolic pressure in the atria to exceed end-diastolic pressure in the ventricles. If a gradient in pressure exists, an obstruction is present, and the severity of the gradient is one criterion for the necessity of operative repair or catheter intervention. An RV systolic pressure of 100 mm Hg and a pulmonary artery systolic pressure of 20 mm Hg yield a gradient of 80 mm Hg. In this case, the patient would be classified as having severe pulmonary stenosis requiring balloon dilation of the pulmonic valve or surgery if valvuloplasty fails to significantly reduce the gradient.

C. Pulmonary and Systemic Vascular Resistance

The vascular resistance is calculated from the following formula and reported in units or in dynes $\times$ cm^{-5}/m^2:

$$\text{Resistance} = \frac{\text{Pressure}}{\text{Flow}}$$

The pressure drop used to determine pulmonary vascular resistance is calculated by subtracting the mean pulmonary artery wedge or left atrial pressure from the mean pulmonary artery pressure. This pressure drop is divided by pulmonary blood flow per square meter of body surface area. (Pulmonary blood flow is determined by thermodilution or from the Fick principle, as noted earlier.) Similarly, systemic vascular resistance is determined by subtracting the mean central venous pressure from the mean systemic arterial pressure and dividing this pressure drop by systemic blood flow.

Normally, the pulmonary vascular resistance ranges from 1–3 U/m^2, or from 80–240 dynes $\times$ cm^{-5}/m^2. Systemic vascular resistance ranges from 15–20 U/m^2, or from 1200–1600 dynes $\times$ cm^{-5}/m^2. If pulmonary resistance is greater than 10 units or the ratio of pulmonary to systemic resistance is greater than 0.5, the child may have pulmonary vascular disease and therefore be inoperable.

Freedom RM et al: *Congenital Heart Disease: Textbook of Angiography.* Futura, 1997.
Simpson JM et al: Cardiac catheterization of low birth weight infants. Am J Cardiol 2001;87:1372 [PMID: 11397356].

PERINATAL & NEONATAL CIRCULATION

At birth, two events occur that affect the cardiovascular and pulmonary system (1) the umbilical cord is clamped, removing the placenta from the maternal circulation; and (2) breathing commences. As a result, marked changes in the circulation occur. During fetal life, the placenta offers low resistance to blood flow. In contrast, the pulmonary arterioles are markedly constricted and offer high resistance to the flow of blood into the lungs. Pulmonary blood flow accounts for only 7–10% of the combined in utero ventricular output. At birth, pulmonary blood flow dramatically increases with the fall in pulmonary vascular resistance and pressure. The causes of prolonged high pulmonary vascular resistance include physical factors (lack of an adequate air-liquid interface or ventilation), low oxygen tension, and vasoactive mediators such as elevated endothelin peptide levels or

leukotrienes. Clamping the cord produces an immediate increase in resistance to flow in the systemic circuit. As breathing commences, the PO$_2$ of the small pulmonary arterioles increases, causing their constriction to decrease and producing a decrease in pulmonary vascular resistance. Increased oxygen tension, rhythmic lung distention, and production of nitric oxide as well as prostacyclin play major roles in the fall in pulmonary vascular resistance at birth. The pulmonary vascular resistance falls below that of the systemic circuit, resulting in a reversal in direction of blood flow across the ductus arteriosus.

Functional closure of the ductus arteriosus begins shortly after birth. The ductus arteriosus usually remains patent for 3–5 days. During the first hour after birth, a small right-to-left shunt is present (as in the fetus). However, after 1 hour, bidirectional shunting occurs, with the left-to-right direction predominating. In most cases, right-to-left shunting disappears completely by 8 hours. In patients with severe hypoxia (eg, in the syndrome of persistent pulmonary hypertension of the newborn), pulmonary vascular resistance remains high, resulting in a continued right-to-left shunt. Increased PO$_2$ of the arterial blood causes spasm of the ductus. Although flow through the ductus arteriosus usually is gone by 5 days of life, the vessel does not close anatomically for 7–14 days.

In fetal life, the foramen ovale serves as a one-way valve shunting blood from the inferior vena cava through the right atrium into the left atrium. At birth, because of the changes in the pulmonary and systemic vascular resistance and the increase in the quantity of blood returning from the pulmonary veins to the left atrium, the left atrial pressure rises above that of the right atrium. This functionally closes the flap of the foramen ovale, preventing flow of blood across the septum. The foramen ovale remains probe patent in 10–15% of adults.

Persistent pulmonary hypertension is a clinical syndrome of full-term infants. The neonate develops tachypnea, cyanosis, and pulmonary hypertension during the first 8 hours after delivery. These infants have massive right-to-left ductal or foramen shunting (or both) for 3–7 days because of high pulmonary vascular resistance. Progressive hypoxia and acidosis will cause early death unless the pulmonary resistance can be lowered. Postmortem findings include increased thickness of the pulmonary arteriolar media. Increase alveolar PO$_2$ with hyperventilation, alkalosis, paralysis, surfactant administration, high-frequency ventilation, and cardiac pressors can usually reverse the resistance. Inhaled nitric oxide selectively dilates pulmonary vasculature, produces a sustained improvement in oxygenation, and has reduced the need for extracorporeal membrane oxygenation.

In the normal newborn, pulmonary vascular resistance and pulmonary arterial pressure continue to fall during the first weeks of life as a result of demuscularization of the pulmonary arterioles. Adult levels of pulmonary resistance and pressure are normally achieved by 4–6 weeks of age. It is at this time typically that signs of pulmonary overcirculation associated with left-to-right shunts (VSD or atrioventricular septal defect [AVSD]) appear.

Fineman JR, Soifer SJ: The fetal and neonatal circulations. In Rudolph AR (editor): *Congenital Diseases of the Heart: Clinical Physiologic Considerations,* 2nd ed. Futura, 2001.

HEART FAILURE

Heart failure (HF) is the clinical condition in which the heart fails to meet the circulatory and metabolic needs of the body. The term *congestive heart failure* is falling out of favor, as some patients with significant cardiac dysfunction have symptoms of exercise intolerance and fatigue without evidence of congestion. Almost all infants who develop HF from congenital heart lesions do so by 6 months of age. Common causes of HF in infants include VSD, PDA, coarctation of the aorta, AV septal defect, large arteriovenous malformations, and chronic atrial tachyarrhythmias. Metabolic, mitochondrial, and neuromuscular disorders with associated cardiomyopathy present at various ages depending on the diagnosis. HF due to acquired conditions such as myocarditis occur at any age. Children with HF may present with irritability, diaphoresis with feeds, fatigue, exercise intolerance, or evidence of pulmonary congestion (see Table 19–1).

Treatment of Heart Failure

The therapy of HF should be directed toward the underlying cause as well as the symptoms. Regardless of the cause, neurohormonal activation occurs early when ventricular systolic dysfunction is present. Plasma catecholamine levels (eg, norepinephrine) increase and cause tachycardia, diaphoresis, and, by activating the renin-angiotensin system, peripheral vasoconstriction and salt and water retention. There is no gold standard diagnostic or therapeutic approach to HF in children. Treatment must be individualized and

therapies should be aimed at improving cardiac performance by targeting the three determinants of cardiac performance: (1) preload, (2) afterload, and (3) contractility.

Inpatient Management of Heart Failure

Patients with cardiac decompensation may require hospitalization for initiation or augmentation of HF therapy. Table 19–12 demonstrates intravenous inotropic agents used to augment cardiac output and their relative effect on heart rate, systemic vascular resistance, and cardiac index. The drug used will depend in part on the cause of the HF.

A. Intravenous Inotropic Support

1. Afterload reduction

A. MILRINONE—This selective phosphodiesterase inhibitor increases cyclic adenosine monophosphate, thereby improving the inotropic state of the heart. In addition to a dose-dependent increase in cardiac contractility, milrinone is a systemic and pulmonary vasodilator and thus an effective agent in both right and left ventricular systolic dysfunction. Milrinone reduces the incidence of low cardiac output syndrome following open heart surgery. The usual dosage range is 0.25–0.75 mcg/kg/min.

B. NITROGLYCERIN—Nitroglycerin functions primarily as a dilator of venous capacitance vessels and causes a reduction of right and left atrial pressure. Systemic blood pressure may also fall, and reflex tachycardia may occur. Nitroglycerin is used to improve coronary blood flow and may be especially useful when cardiac output is reduced because of coronary underperfusion following congenital heart surgery. The usual intravenous dosage range is 1–3 mcg/kg/min.

2. Enhancement of contractility

A. DOPAMINE—This naturally occurring catecholamine increases myocardial contractility primarily via cardiac β-adrenergic activation. Dopamine also directly acts on renal dopamine receptors to improve renal perfusion. The usual dose range for HF is 3–10 mcg/kg/min.

Table 19–12. Intravenous inotropic agents.

Drug	Dose	Renal Perfusion	Heart Rate	Cardiac Index	SVR
Dopamine	2–5 mcg/kg/min	↑ via vasodilation	0	0	0
	5–10	↑ via ↑ cardiac index	↑	↑	0
	> 10	↓	↑	↑	↑
Dobutamine	2.5–10 mcg/kg/min	↑ via ↑ cardiac index	↑	↑	↑↓
Epinephrine	0.2–2.0 mcg/kg/min	↓	↑	↑	↑
Norepinephrine	0.05–0.1 mcg/kg/min	↓	0	↑	↑↑
Isoproterenol	0.05–2.0 mcg/kg/min	0	↑↑	↑	↓↓

SVR, systemic vascular resistance.

B. Dobutamine—This synthetic catecholamine increases myocardial contractility secondary to cardiospecific β-adrenergic activation and produces little peripheral vasoconstriction. Dobutamine does not usually cause marked tachycardia, which is a distinct advantage. However, the drug does not selectively improve renal perfusion as does dopamine. The usual dose range is essentially the same as for dopamine.

3. Mechanical circulatory support—Mechanical support is indicated in children with severe, refractory myocardial failure secondary to cardiomyopathy, myocarditis, or following cardiac surgery. Mechanical support is used for a limited time while cardiac function improves, or as a bridge to cardiac transplantation.

A. Extracorporeal membrane oxygenation (ECMO)— ECMO is a temporary means of providing oxygenation, carbon dioxide removal, and hemodynamic support to patients with cardiac or pulmonary failure refractory to conventional therapy. Flow from a catheter positioned in the venous system (eg, right atrium) passes through a membrane oxygenator and then is delivered back to the patient via a catheter in the arterial system (eg, aorta or common carotid artery). Flow rates are adjusted to maintain adequate systemic perfusion, as judged by mean arterial blood pressure, acid-base status, end-organ function, and mixed venous oxygen saturation. The patient is monitored closely for improvement in cardiac contractility. Risks are significant and include severe internal and external bleeding, infection, thrombosis, and pump failure.

B. Ventricular assist devices—Use of pulsatile assist devices is limited in children by patient size, availability, and institutional expertise. These devices allow for less invasive hemodynamic support than ECMO. A cannula positioned in the apex of the ventricle removes blood from the ventricle using a battery-operated pump. Blood is then returned to the patient through a separate cannula positioned in the aorta or pulmonary artery, depending on the ventricle being supported. Ventricular assist carries lower risk of bleeding and pump failure than ECMO, but the risk of infection and thrombosis remain.

Outpatient Management of Heart Failure

A. Medications

1. Afterload-reducing agents—Oral afterload-reducing agents improve cardiac output by decreasing systemic vascular resistance. Angiotensin-converting enzyme (ACE) inhibitors (captopril, enalapril, and lisinopril) are first-line therapy in patients with HF requiring long-term treatment. These agents block angiotensin II–mediated systemic vasoconstriction and are particularly useful in children with structurally normal hearts but reduced LV myocardial function (ie, myocarditis or dilated cardiomyopathies). They are also useful in ameliorating mitral and aortic insufficiency and

have a role in controlling refractory HF in patients with large left-to-right shunts in whom systemic vascular resistance is elevated.

2. β-Blockade—β-Blockers may be useful adjunctive therapy in children with refractory HF already taking ACE inhibitors. Excessive circulating catecholamines are present due to the activation of the sympathetic nervous system by HF. Although beneficial acutely, this compensatory response over time produces myocardial fibrosis, myocyte hypertrophy, and myocyte apoptosis that contribute to the progression of HF. β-Blockers (eg, carvedilol and metoprolol) antagonize this sympathetic activation and may offset these deleterious effects. Side effects of β-blockers are significant and include bradycardia, hypotension, and worsening HF in some patients.

3. Diuretics—Diuretic therapy may be necessary in HF to maintain the euvolemic state.

A. Furosemide—This rapid-acting loop diuretic may be given intravenously or orally. It removes large amounts of potassium and chloride from the body, producing hypochloremic metabolic alkalosis when used chronically. Electrolytes should be monitored during long-term therapy.

B. Thiazides—Thiazides are distal tubular diuretics used to complement furosemide in severe cases of HF.

C. Spironolactone—Spironolactone is a potassium-sparing aldosterone inhibitor. It is used frequently in conjunction with furosemide or thiazides for its enhanced diuretic function. Because it spares potassium, supplemental potassium may be avoided. Spironolactone may also be used as a neurohormonal antagonist with potential benefit in HF regardless of its diuretic effect.

4. Digitalis—Digitalis is a cardiac glycoside with a positive inotropic effect on the heart and an associated decrease in systemic vascular resistance. The preparation of digitalis used in clinical practice is digoxin. Large studies in adult patients with HF have not demonstrated decreased mortality of HF with digoxin use, but treatment is associated with reduced hospitalization rates for HF exacerbations.

A. Dosing—The routine schedule consists of giving one half of the total digitalizing dose initially, then one quarter of the total digitalizing dose at 6 and 12 hours of therapy (Table 19–13). Twenty-four hours after the last digitalizing dose, maintenance therapy is started. Serum digoxin levels are not routinely monitored unless there are concerns regarding compliance or toxicity.

B. Digitalis toxicity—Any dysrhythmia that occurs during digoxin therapy should be attributed to the drug until proven otherwise. Ventricular bigeminy and first-, second-, or third-degree AV block are characteristic of digoxin toxicity. A trough level should be obtained if digoxin toxicity is suspected.

Table 19–13. Digoxin dosing schedule.

Age	Parenteral	Oral
Premature	0.035 mg/kg	0.04 mg/kg
1 wk–2 y	0.05 mg/kg	0.06 mg/kg
< 1 wk or > 2 y	0.04 mg/kg	0.05 mg/kg

c. DIGITALIS POISONING—This acute emergency must be treated without delay. Digoxin poisoning most commonly occurs in toddlers who have taken their parents' or grandparents' medications. The child's stomach should be emptied immediately by gastric lavage even if several hours have passed since ingestion. Patients who have ingested massive amounts of digoxin should receive large doses of activated charcoal. In advanced heart block, atropine or temporary ventricular pacing may be needed. Digoxin immune Fab can be used to reverse potentially life-threatening intoxication. Antiarrhythmic agents may be useful.

5. Fluid restriction—Fluid restriction is rarely used in pediatric cardiology due to the effectiveness of diuretics. Ensuring adequate caloric intake to promote growth is a more important goal in children with HF.

Azeka E et al: Delisting of infants and children from the heart transplantation waiting list after carvedilol treatment. J Am Coll Cardiol 2002;40:2034 [PMID: 12475466].

Fiser WP et al: Pediatric arteriovenous ECMO as a bridge to cardiac transplantation. J Heart Lung Transplant 2003;22:770 [PMID: 12873545].

Hoffman TM et al: Efficacy and safety of milrinone in preventing low cardiac output syndrome in infants and children after corrective surgery for congenital heart disease. Circulation 2003;107:996 [PMID: 12600913].

Rosenthal D et al: International Society for Heart and Lung Transplantation: Practice guidelines for management of heart failure in children. J Heart Lung Transplant 2004;23:1313 [PMID: 15607659].

GENETIC BASIS OF CONGENITAL HEART DISEASE

Congenital heart disease often has a genetic basis. The most common genetic abnormality is a microdeletion in the long arm of chromosome 22 (22q11) associated with DiGeorge syndrome. These children often have conotruncal abnormalities such as truncus arteriosus, tetralogy of Fallot, or double-outlet RV. Intrauterine factors such as maternal diabetes, alcohol consumption, progesterone use, viral infection, and other maternal teratogen exposure are associated with an increased incidence of cardiac malformations. Genetic diagnosis may allow for more accurate prediction of recurrence risk in subsequent pregnancies.

Park IS et al: Cardiovascular anomalies in patients with chromosome 22q11.2 deletion: A Korean multicenter study. Int J Cardiol 2007;114:230 [PMID: 16824627].

ACYANOTIC CONGENITAL HEART DISEASE

DEFECTS IN SEPTATION

1. Atrial Septal Defect (Ostium Secundum Variant)

 ESSENTIALS OF DIAGNOSIS & TYPICAL FEATURES

▸ Fixed, widely split S_2, RV heave.

▸ Grade I–III/VI ejection systolic murmur at the pulmonary area.

▸ Large shunts cause a diastolic flow murmur at the lower left sternal border.

▸ ECG shows rsR' in lead V_1.

▸ Frequently asymptomatic.

▸ **General Considerations**

Atrial septal defect (ASD) is an opening in the atrial septum permitting the shunting of blood between the atria. There are three major types: ostium secundum, ostium primum, and sinus venosus. Ostium secundum is the most common type. Ostium primum defect is associated with atrioventricular septal defect. The sinus venosus defect is frequently associated with abnormal pulmonary venous return, as the location of the sinus venosus is intimately related to the right upper pulmonary vein.

Ostium secundum ASD occurs in 10% of patients with congenital heart disease and is two times more common in females than males. The defect is most often sporadic but may be familial. Pulmonary hypertension and growth failure are uncommon complications in infancy and childhood. After the third decade, atrial arrhythmias or pulmonary vascular disease may develop. In the setting of pulmonary vascular disease, left-to-right shunting decreases, and right-to-left shunting becomes the major clinical abnormality (Eisenmenger syndrome).

▸ **Clinical Findings**

A. Symptoms and Signs

Most infants and children with ASD have no cardiovascular symptoms. With age, some never develop symptoms. Others develop easy fatigability as older children or adults, or rarely, HF. The direction of flow across the ASD is determined by the compliance of the underlying ventricle. Therefore, cyanosis does not occur unless RV dysfunction occurs, usually as a result of pulmonary hypertension that causes reversal of the shunt across the defect.

Peripheral pulses are normal and equal. The heart is usually hyperactive, with an RV heave felt best at the mid to lower left sternal border. S_2 at the pulmonary area is widely split and often fixed. The pulmonary component is normal in intensity. A grade I–III/VI ejection-type systolic murmur is heard best at the left sternal border in the second intercostal space. This murmur is caused by increased flow across the pulmonic valve, not flow across the ASD. A mid-diastolic murmur is often heard in the fourth intercostal space at the left sternal border. This murmur is caused by increased flow across the tricuspid valve during diastole. The presence of this murmur suggests high flow with a pulmonary-to-systemic blood flow ratio greater than 2:1.

B. Imaging

Radiographs may show cardiac enlargement. The main pulmonary artery may be dilated and pulmonary vascular markings increased in large defects owing to the increased pulmonary blood flow.

C. Electrocardiography

The usual ECG shows right axis deviation. In the right precordial leads, an rsR′ pattern is usually present. In patients with a mutation in the cardiac homeobox gene (*NKX2-5*), AV heart block may be present.

D. Echocardiography

Echocardiography shows a dilated right atrium and RV. Direct visualization of the ASD by two-dimensional echocardiography, plus demonstration of a left-to-right shunt through the defect by color-flow Doppler, confirms the diagnosis and has eliminated the need for cardiac catheterization prior to surgical or catheter closure of the defect. Assessment of all pulmonary veins should be made to rule out associated anomalous pulmonary venous return.

E. Cardiac Catheterization

Oximetry shows significant increase in oxygen saturation at the atrial level. The pulmonary artery pressure and pulmonary vascular resistance are usually normal. The $Q_p:Q_s$ may vary from 1.5:1 to 4:1. Cardiac catheterization is rarely needed for diagnostic purposes but transcatheter closure of an ostium secundum ASD is now the preferred method of closure.

▶ Treatment

Surgical or catheterization closure is generally recommended for symptomatic children with a large atrial level defect and associated right heart dilation. In the asymptomatic child with a large hemodynamically significant defect, closure is performed electively at age 1–3 years. Many defects are amenable to nonoperative device closure during cardiac catheterization, but the defect must have adequate tissue rims on all sides on which to anchor the device. The mortality for surgical closure is less than 1%. When closure is performed by age 3 years, late complications of RV dysfunction and dysrhythmias are avoided.

▶ Course & Prognosis

Patients usually tolerate an ASD well in the first two decades of life, and the defect often goes unnoticed until middle or late adulthood. Pulmonary hypertension and reversal of the shunt are rare late complications. Infective endocarditis is uncommon. Spontaneous closure occurs, most frequently in children with a defect less than 4 mm in diameter. Exercise tolerance and oxygen consumption in surgically corrected children are generally normal, and restriction of physical activity is unnecessary.

Arrington CB et al: An assessment of the electrocardiogram as a screening test for large atrial septal defects in children. J Electrocardiol 2007;40:484 [PMID: 17673249].
Kozlik-Feldmann R et al: First experience with the 2005 modified Gore Helex ASD occluder system. Clin Res Cardiol 2006;95:468 [PMID: 16845573].
Sigler M et al: Histological confirmation of complete endothelialisation of a surgically removed Amplatzer ASD occluder. Heart 2006;92:1723 [PMID: 17105877].

2. Ventricular Septal Defect

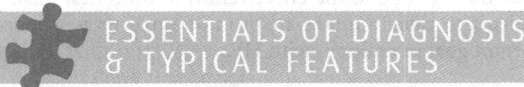
ESSENTIALS OF DIAGNOSIS & TYPICAL FEATURES

▶ Holosystolic murmur at lower left sternal border with RV heave.

▶ Presentation and course depend on size of defect and the pulmonary vascular resistance.

▶ Clinical features are HF, failure to thrive, and diaphoresis with feeds.

▶ Left-to-right shunt with normal pulmonary vascular resistance.

▶ Large defects may cause Eisenmenger syndrome if not repaired early.

▶ General Considerations

Simple ventricular septal defect (VSD) is the most common congenital heart malformation, accounting for about 30% of all congenital heart disease. Defects in the ventricular septum occur both in the membranous portion of the septum (most common) and the muscular portion. VSDs follow one of four courses:

A. Small, Hemodynamically Insignificant Ventricular Septal Defects

Between 80% and 85% of VSDs are small (< 3 mm in diameter) at birth and will close spontaneously. In general, small defects in the muscular interventricular septum will close sooner than those in the membranous septum. In most cases, a small VSD never requires surgical closure. Fifty percent of small VSDs will close by age 2 years, and 90% by age 6 years. The remaining 10% will close during the school years. Parents should be told at the time of diagnosis and echocardiographic confirmation that all small VSDs will eventually close.

B. Moderate Ventricular Septal Defects

Asymptomatic patients with moderate VSDs (3–5 mm in diameter) account for 3–5% of children with VSDs. In general these children do not have clear indicators for surgical closure. Historically, in those who had cardiac catheterization, the ratio of pulmonary to systemic blood flow is usually less than 2:1, and serial cardiac catheterizations demonstrate that the shunts get progressively smaller. If there is neither HF nor pulmonary hypertension, these defects can be followed until spontaneous closure.

C. Large Ventricular Septal Defects with Normal Pulmonary Vascular Resistance

These defects are usually 6–10 mm in diameter. Unless they become markedly smaller within a few months after birth, they will require surgery. The timing of surgery depends on the clinical situation. Many infants with large VSDs and normal pulmonary vascular resistance develop HF and failure to thrive by age 3–6 months, and require correction at that time. In all cases, surgery before age 2 years is required to decrease the risk of pulmonary vascular disease.

D. Large Ventricular Septal Defects with Pulmonary Vascular Obstructive Disease

The direction of flow across a VSD is determined by the downstream resistance, explaining why flow is usually left-to-right. In large VSDs, ventricular pressures are equal, causing increased pulmonary artery pressure. In addition, shear stress caused by increased volume in the pulmonary circuit causes increased resistance over time. The vast majority of patients with inoperable pulmonary hypertension develop the condition progressively. The combined data of the multicenter National History Study indicate that almost all cases of irreversible pulmonary hypertension can be prevented by surgical repair of a large VSD before age 2 years.

► Clinical Findings

A. Symptoms and Signs

Patients with small or moderate left-to-right shunts usually have no cardiovascular symptoms. Patients with large left-to-right shunts are usually ill early in infancy. These infants have frequent respiratory infections and gain weight slowly. Dyspnea, diaphoresis, and fatigue are common. HF can develop as early as 1 to 6 months of age. After the first year, symptoms usually improve, although easy fatigability may persist. Older children may experience exercise intolerance. Over time, in children with persistent large left-to-right shunt, the pulmonary vascular bed undergoes structural changes, leading to increased pulmonary vascular resistance and reversal of the shunt from left-to-right, to right-to-left (Eisenmenger syndrome). Cyanosis will then be present.

1. Small left-to-right shunt—No lifts, heaves, or thrills are present. The first sound at the apex is normal, and the second sound at the pulmonary area is split physiologically. A grade II–IV/VI, medium- to high-pitched, harsh pansystolic murmur is heard best at the left sternal border in the third and fourth intercostal spaces. The murmur radiates over the entire precordium. No diastolic murmurs are heard.

2. Moderate left-to-right shunt—Slight prominence of the precordium with moderate LV heave is evident. A systolic thrill may be palpable at the lower left sternal border between the third and fourth intercostal spaces. The second sound at the pulmonary area is most often split but may be single. A grade III–IV/VI, harsh pansystolic murmur is heard best at the lower left sternal border in the fourth intercostal space. A mitral diastolic flow murmur indicates that the pulmonary blood flow is significantly increased by the large shunt.

3. Large ventricular septal defects with pulmonary hypertension—The precordium is prominent, and the sternum bulges. Both LV and RV heaves are palpable. S_2 is palpable in the pulmonary area. A thrill may be present at the lower left sternal border. S_2 is usually single or narrowly split, with accentuation of the pulmonary component. The murmur ranges from grade I to grade IV/VI and is usually harsh and pansystolic. Occasionally, when the defect is large or ventricular pressures approach equivalency, a murmur is difficult to hear. A diastolic flow murmur may be heard, depending on the size of the shunt.

B. Imaging

In patients with small shunts, the chest radiograph may be normal. Patients with large shunts have significant cardiac enlargement involving both the left and right ventricles and the left atrium. The main pulmonary artery segment may be dilated. The pulmonary vascular markings are increased.

C. Electrocardiography

The ECG is normal in small left-to-right shunts. Left ventricular hypertrophy (LVH) usually occurs in patients with large left-to-right shunts and normal pulmonary vascular resistance. Combined ventricular enlargement occurs in patients with pulmonary hypertension caused by increased flow, increased resistance, or both. Pure RV hypertrophy occurs in patients with pulmonary hypertension secondary to pulmonary vascular obstruction induced by long-standing left-to-right shunt (Eisenmenger syndrome).

D. Echocardiography

Two-dimensional echocardiography can reveal the size of a VSD and pinpoint its anatomic location. Color-flow Doppler allows detection of the smallest VSDs. Multiple defects can be detected by combining two-dimensional and color-flow imaging. Doppler can further evaluate the VSD by estimating the pressure difference between the left and right ventricles. A pressure difference greater than 50 mm Hg confirms the absence of severe pulmonary hypertension.

E. Cardiac Catheterization and Angiocardiography

The ability to describe the VSD anatomy and estimate the pulmonary artery pressures on the basis of the gradient across the VSD, allows for the vast majority of isolated defects to be repaired without cardiac catheterization and angiocardiography. Catheterization is indicated in those patients with increased pulmonary vascular resistance. The pulmonary artery pressure may vary from normal to systemic level (equal to the aortic pressure). Pulmonary artery wedge pressure (a surrogate for direct left atrial pressure) may be normal to increased. Pulmonary vascular resistance varies from normal to markedly increased. Angiocardiographic examination defines the number, size, and location of the defects.

▶ Treatment

A. Medical Management

Patients who develop HF should receive anticongestive measures (see section on Heart Failure, earlier), particularly diuretics and systemic afterload reduction. If the patient does not respond to anticongestive measures, or if he or she shows progressive pulmonary hypertension, surgery is indicated without delay.

B. Surgical Treatment

Patients with cardiomegaly, poor growth, poor exercise tolerance, or other clinical abnormalities who have a significant shunt (> 2:1) without significant pulmonary hypertension typically undergo surgical repair at age 3–6 months. A synthetic or pericardial patch is used for primary closure. The age of elective surgery has decreased and most defects are now closed in infancy. Patients with pulmonary artery pressures equal to systemic pressure undergo surgical repair well before age 2 years to avoid pulmonary vascular disease. In most centers these children have surgery before age 1 year. As a result, Eisenmenger syndrome has been virtually eliminated. In all cases of VSD, the surgical mortality rate is below 2%.

Transcatheter closure of muscular VSDs is now becoming common. Perimembranous VSDs have also been closed in children during catheterization, but an alarmingly high incidence of complete heart block after placement of the occluding device has slowed the acceptance of this approach.

▶ Course & Prognosis

Significant late dysrhythmias are uncommon. Functional exercise capacity and oxygen consumption are usually nor-

mal, and physical restrictions are unnecessary. Adults with corrected defects have normal quality of life. With complete VSD closure, antibiotic prophylaxis for bacterial endocarditis can be discontinued 6 months after surgery.

Bol Raap G et al: Long-term follow-up and quality of life after closure of ventricular septal defect in adults. Eur J Cardiothorac Surg 2007;32:215 [PMID: 17566753].

Butera G et al: Transcatheter closure of perimembranous ventricular septal defects: Early and long-term results. J Am Coll Cardiol 2007;50:1189 [PMID: 17868812].

Sondheimer HM, Rahimi-Alangi K: Current management of ventricular septal defect. Cardiol Young 2006;16(Suppl 3):131 [PMID: 17378052].

3. Atrioventricular Septal Defect

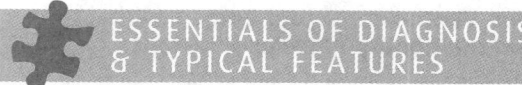

ESSENTIALS OF DIAGNOSIS & TYPICAL FEATURES

▶ Murmur often inaudible in neonates.

▶ Loud pulmonary component of S_2.

▶ Common in infants with Down syndrome.

▶ ECG with extreme left axis deviation.

▶ General Considerations

Atrioventricular septal defect (AVSD) results from incomplete fusion of the embryonic endocardial cushions. The endocardial cushions help to form the "crux" of the heart, which includes the lower portion of the atrial septum, the membranous portion of the ventricular septum, and the septal leaflets of the tricuspid and mitral valves. AVSD accounts for about 4% of all congenital heart disease. Sixty percent of children with Down syndrome have congenital heart disease, and of these, 35–40% has AVSD.

AV septal defects are defined as partial or complete. The physiology of the defect is determined by the location of the AV valves. If the valves are located in the midportion of the defect (complete AVSD), both atrial and ventricular components of the septal defect are present and the left- and right-sided AV valves share a common ring or orifice. In the partial form there is a low insertion of the AV valves resulting in primum ASD without a ventricular component. In partial AVSD, there are two separate AV valve orifices and usually a cleft in the left-sided valve

Partial AVSD behaves like an isolated ASD with variable amounts of regurgitation through the cleft in the left AV valve. The complete form causes large left-to-right shunts at both the ventricular and atrial levels with AV valve regurgitation. It there is increased pulmonary vascular resistance, the shunts may be bidirectional. Bidirectional shunting is more common in Down syndrome or in older children who have not undergone repair.

Clinical Findings

A. Symptoms and Signs

The partial form may produce symptoms similar to ostium secundum ASD. Patients with complete AVSD usually are severely affected. HF often develops in infancy, and recurrent bouts of pneumonia are common.

In the neonate with the complete form, the murmur may be inaudible due to relatively equal systemic and pulmonary vascular resistance (PVR). After 4–6 weeks, as PVR drops, a nonspecific systolic murmur develops. The murmur is usually not as harsh as that of isolated VSD. There is both right- and left-sided cardiac enlargement. S_2 is loud, and a pronounced diastolic flow murmur may be heard at the apex and the lower left sternal border.

If severe pulmonary vascular obstructive disease is present, there is usually dominant RV enlargement. S_2 is palpable at the pulmonary area and no thrill is felt. A nonspecific short systolic murmur is heard at the lower left sternal border. No diastolic flow murmurs are heard. In severe cases predominant right-to-left shunting causes cyanosis.

B. Imaging

Cardiac enlargement is always present. In the complete form, all four chambers are enlarged. Pulmonary vascular markings are increased. In patients with pulmonary vascular obstructive disease, only the main pulmonary artery segment and its branches are prominent and the peripheral pulmonary vascular markings are usually decreased.

C. Electrocardiography

In all forms of AVSD, there is extreme left axis deviation with a counterclockwise loop in the frontal plane. The ECG is an important diagnostic tool. Only 5% of isolated VSDs have this ECG abnormality. First-degree heart block occurs in over 50% of patients. Right, left, or combined ventricular hypertrophy is present depending on the particular defect and the presence or absence of pulmonary hypertension.

D. Echocardiography

Echocardiography is the diagnostic test of choice. The anatomy can be well visualized by two-dimensional echocardiography. Both AV valves are at the same level, compared with the normal heart in which the tricuspid valve is more apically positioned. The size of the atrial and ventricular components of the defect can be measured. AV valve regurgitation can be detected. The LV outflow tract is elongated (gooseneck appearance), which produces systemic outflow obstruction.

E. Cardiac Catheterization and Angiocardiography

Cardiac catheterization is not routinely used to evaluate AVSD but may be used to assess pulmonary artery pressures in the older infant with Down syndrome, as this patient group is predisposed to early-onset pulmonary hypertension. Increased oxygen saturation in the RV or the right atrium identifies the level of the shunt. Angiocardiography reveals the characteristic gooseneck deformity of the LV outflow tract in the complete form.

Treatment

Spontaneous improvement does not occur. Surgery is always required. In the partial form, surgery carries a low mortality rate (1–2%), but patients require follow-up because of late-occurring LV outflow tract obstruction and mitral valve dysfunction. The complete form carries a higher mortality rate. Complete correction in the first year of life, prior to the onset of irreversible pulmonary hypertension, is obligatory. If possible, primary correction should be performed when the child is well and weighs more than 5 kg. During surgery, transesophageal echocardiography is used to assess the adequacy of repair before discontinuing cardiopulmonary bypass.

Craig B: Atrioventricular septal defect: From fetus to adult. Heart 2006;92:1879 [PMID: 17105897].
Kobayashi M et al: Ideal timing of surgical repair of isolated complete atrioventricular septal defect. Interact Cardiovasc Thorac Surg 2007;6:24 [PMID: 17669760].

PATENT (PERSISTENT) DUCTUS ARTERIOSUS

General Considerations

PDA is the persistence of the normal fetal vessel joining the pulmonary artery to the aorta. It closes spontaneously in normal term infants at 3–5 days of age. PDA accounts for 10% of all congenital heart disease. The incidence of PDA is higher in infants born at altitudes over 10,000 ft. It is twice as common in females as in males. The frequency of PDA in preterm infants weighing less than 1500 g ranges from 20–60%. The defect may occur as an isolated abnormality or with associated lesions, commonly coarctation of the aorta and VSD. It is critical to recognize patients with a PDA, but without readily apparent findings of other associated lesions, who are being kept alive by the patent ductus (eg, a patient with PDA and unsuspected pulmonary atresia).

Clinical Findings

A. Symptoms and Signs

The clinical findings and course depend on the size of the shunt and the degree of pulmonary hypertension.

1. Typical patent ductus arteriosus—Pulses are bounding, and pulse pressure is widened due to diastolic runoff through the ductus. S_1 is normal and S_2 is usually narrowly split. In large shunts, S_2 may have a paradoxical split (ie, S_2 closes on inspiration and splits on expiration). Paradoxical splitting is caused by volume overload of the LV and pro-longed ejection of blood from this chamber.

The murmur is characteristic. It is a rough machinery murmur maximal at the second left intercostal space. It begins shortly after S_1, rises to a peak at S_2, and passes through the S_2 into diastole, where it becomes a decrescendo murmur and fades before the S_1. The murmur tends to radiate well to the anterior lung fields but relatively poorly to the posterior lung fields. A diastolic flow murmur is often heard at the apex.

2. Patent ductus arteriosus with increased pulmonary vascular resistance—Flow across the ductus is diminished. S_2 is single and accentuated, and no significant heart murmur is present. The pulses are normal rather than bounding.

B. Imaging

In simple PDA, the radiographic appearance depends on the size of the shunt. If the shunt is small, the heart is not enlarged. If the shunt is large, both left atrial and LV enlargement may be seen. The aorta and the main pulmonary artery segment may be prominent.

C. Electrocardiography

The ECG may be normal or may show LVH, depending on the size of the shunt. In patients with pulmonary hypertension caused by increased blood flow, biventricular hypertrophy usually occurs. In pulmonary vascular obstructive disease, pure right ventricular hypertrophy (RVH) occurs.

D. Echocardiography

Echocardiography provides direct visualization of the ductus and confirms the direction and degree of shunting. High-velocity left-to-right flow argues against abnormally elevated pulmonary vascular resistance, and as pulmonary vascular resistance drops during the neonatal period, higher velocity left-to-right shunting is usually seen. If suprasystemic pulmonary vascular resistance is present, flow across the ductus will be seen from right-to-left. Ductal-dependent pulmonary or systemic blood flow must be recognized by echocardiography, as closure of a PDA in this setting would obviously be contraindicated.

E. Cardiac Catheterization and Angiocardiography

Children with PDA never require a cardiac catheterization for diagnostic purposes. However, children more than 5 kg with PDA routinely undergo PDA closure in the catheterization laboratory.

▶ Treatment

Treatment is surgical when the PDA is large and the patient is small, except in patients with pulmonary vascular obstructive disease. Patients with large left-to-right shunts require repair by age 1 year to prevent the development of progressive pulmonary vascular obstructive disease. Symptomatic PDA with normal pulmonary artery pressure can be safely coil or device-occluded in the catheterization laboratory after the child has reached 5 kg.

Patients with nonreactive pulmonary vascular obstruction with resistance greater than 10 Wood units (normal, < 3) and a ratio of pulmonary to systemic resistance greater than 0.7 (normal, < 0.3) despite vasodilator therapy (eg, nitric oxide) should not undergo PDA closure. These patients are made worse by PDA closure because the flow through the ductus maintains cardiac output to the systemic circulation in the presence of high pulmonary vascular resistance.

Symptomatic PDA is common in preterm infants. Indomethacin, a prostaglandin synthesis inhibitor, is often used to close PDA in premature infants. Indomethacin does not close the PDA of full-term infants or children. The success of indomethacin therapy is as high as 80–90% in premature infants with a birth weight greater than 1200 g, but it is less successful in smaller infants. Indomethacin (0.1–0.3 mg/kg orally every 8–24 hours or 0.1–0.3 mg/kg parenterally every 12 hours) can be used if there is adequate renal, hematologic, and hepatic function. Because indomethacin may impair renal function, urine output, BUN, and creatinine should be monitored during therapy. If indomethacin is not effective and the ductus remains hemodynamically significant, surgical ligation should be performed. If the ductus closes substantially so that it is no longer hemodynamically significant, even with some residual flow from left to right, surgery is not needed, and a second course of indomethacin may be used. Recent studies from Europe indicate that ibuprofen may be as effective as indomethacin for medical closure of preterm PDA.

▶ Course & Prognosis

Patients with simple PDA and small-to-moderate shunts usually do well without surgery. However, in the third or fourth decade of life, symptoms of easy fatigability, dyspnea on exertion, and exercise intolerance appear, usually as a consequence of progressive pulmonary hypertension or HF.

Spontaneous closure of a PDA may occur up to age 1 year, especially in preterm infants. After age 1 year, spontaneous closure is rare. Because infective endocarditis is a potential complication, closure is recommended if the defect persists beyond age 1 year.

The prognosis for patients with large shunts or pulmonary hypertension is not as good. Poor growth and development, frequent pneumonias, and HF occur in these children. Patients beyond the newborn period with PDA and large shunts should have transcatheter device closure of their PDA.

Cherif A et al: Oral ibuprofen in early curative closure of patent ductus arteriosus in very premature infants. Am J Perinatol 2007;24:339 [PMID: 17564958].

Rao PS: Percutaneous closure of patent ductus arteriosus: State of the art. J Invasive Cardiol 2007;19:299 [PMID: 17620674].

RIGHT-SIDED OBSTRUCTIVE LESIONS

1. Pulmonary Valve Stenosis

ESSENTIALS OF DIAGNOSIS & TYPICAL FEATURES

▸ No symptoms in mild or moderate stenosis.

▸ Cyanosis and a high incidence of right-sided HF in ductal-dependent lesions.

▸ RV lift with systolic ejection click heard at the third left intercostal space.

▸ S_2 widely split with soft to inaudible P_2; grade I–VI/VI systolic ejection murmur, maximal at the pulmonary area.

▸ Dilated pulmonary artery on chest radiograph.

▸ General Considerations

Pulmonic valve stenosis accounts for 10% of all congenital heart disease. In the usual case, the cusps of the pulmonary valve are fused to form a membrane or diaphragm with a hole in the middle from 2–10 mm in diameter. Occasionally, only two cusps are fused, producing a bicuspid pulmonary valve. In more severe cases, secondary infundibular (sub-valve) stenosis occurs. The pulmonary valve annulus is usually small with moderate to marked poststenotic dilation of the main pulmonary arteries.

Obstruction to blood flow across the pulmonary valve causes an increase in RV pressure. Pressures greater than systemic are potentially life-threatening and are associated with critical obstruction. Because of the increased RV strain, severe RVH and eventual RV failure can occur.

When obstruction is severe and the ventricular septum is intact, a right-to-left shunt will often occur at the atrial level through a patent foramen ovale. In neonates with severe obstruction, pulmonary blood flow will shunt through the ductus, making prostaglandin a necessary intervention at the time of birth. Patients with this condition are cyanotic.

▸ Clinical Findings

A. Symptoms and Signs

Patients with mild or even moderate valvular pulmonary stenosis are acyanotic and asymptomatic. Patients with severe valvular obstruction may develop cyanosis early. Patients with mild to moderate obstruction are usually well developed and well nourished. They are not prone to pulmonary infections. The pulses are normal. The precordium may be prominent, often with palpable RV heave. A systolic thrill is often present in the pulmonary area. In patients with mild to moderate stenosis, a prominent ejection click of pulmonary origin is heard at the third left intercostal space. The click varies with respiration, being more prominent during expiration than inspiration. In severe stenosis, the click tends to merge with S_1. S_2 varies with the degree of stenosis. In mild pulmonic stenosis, S_2 is normal. In moderate pulmonic stenosis, S_2 is more widely split and the pulmonary component is softer. In severe pulmonary stenosis, S_2 is single because the pulmonary component cannot be heard. A rough systolic ejection murmur is best heard at the second left interspace. It radiates well to the back. With severe pulmonary valve obstruction, the murmur is usually short. No diastolic murmurs are audible.

B. Imaging

The heart size is normal. Post-stenotic dilation of the main pulmonary artery and the left pulmonary artery often occurs.

C. Electrocardiography

The ECG is usually normal with mild obstruction. RVH is present with moderate to severe pulmonic stenosis. In severe obstruction, RV hypertrophy with an RV strain pattern (deep inversion of the T wave) occurs in the right precordial leads (V_{3R}, V_1, V_2). Right atrial enlargement may be present. Right axis deviation occurs in moderate to severe stenosis.

D. Echocardiography

The diagnosis often is made by physical examination, but the echocardiogram supports the diagnosis when the pulmonary valve is unusually thickened with reduced valve leaflet excursion. The transvalvular pressure gradient can be estimated accurately by Doppler, which provides evidence of the RV pressure and can assist in determining the appropriate time to intervene.

E. Cardiac Catheterization and Angiocardiography

Pulmonic stenosis is easily diagnosed by physical examination, ECG, and echocardiography. Catheterization is reserved for therapeutic balloon pulmonic valvuloplasty. In severe cases with RV dysfunction, a right-to-left shunt at the atrial level is indicated by a lower left atrial saturation than pulmonary vein saturation. Pulmonary artery pressure is normal. The gradient across the pulmonary valve varies from 10–200 mm Hg. In severe cases, the right atrial pressure is elevated, with a predominant "a" wave. Angiocardiography in the RV shows a thick pulmonary valve with a narrow opening producing a jet of contrast into the pulmonary artery. Infundibular (RV outflow tract) hypertrophy may be present.

▸ Treatment

Relief of pulmonic stenosis is recommended for children with RV systolic pressure greater than two thirds of systemic pressure. Immediate correction is indicated for patients with systemic or suprasystemic RV pressure. Percutaneous balloon valvuloplasty is the procedure of choice. It is as effective as surgery in relieving obstruction and causes less valve insufficiency. Surgery is needed to treat pulmonic valve stenosis when balloon pulmonic valvuloplasty is unsuccessful.

▶ Course & Prognosis

Patients with mild pulmonary stenosis live normal lives. Even those with moderate stenosis are rarely symptomatic. Those with severe valvular obstruction may develop cyanosis in infancy.

After balloon pulmonary valvuloplasty or surgery, most patients have good maximum exercise capacity unless they have significant pulmonary insufficiency (PI). Limitation of physical activity is unwarranted. The quality of life of adults with successfully treated pulmonary stenosis and minimal PI is normal. Patients with PI, a frequent side effect of intervention, may be significantly limited in exercise performance. Severe PI leads to progressive RV dilation and dysfunction, which may precipitate ventricular arrhythmias or right heart failure in adulthood. Patients with severe PI may benefit from replacement of the pulmonic valve.

Davidson MJ et al. Percutaneous therapies for valvular heart disease. Cardiovasc Pathol 2006;15:123 [PMID: 16697924].
Davlouros PA et al. The right ventricle in congenital heart disease. Heart 2006;92(Suppl 1):i27 [PMID: 16543599].

2. Subvalvular Pulmonary Stenosis

Pure infundibular (subvalvular) pulmonary stenosis is rare. Infundibular hypertrophy, often associated with a small perimembranous VSD, may lead to a "double-chambered RV" characterized by obstruction between the inflow and outflow portion of the RV. One should suspect such an abnormality if there is a prominent precordial thrill, no audible pulmonary ejection click, and a murmur maximal in the third and fourth intercostal spaces rather than in the second intercostal space. The clinical picture is otherwise identical to that of pulmonic valve stenosis. Intervention, if indicated, is always surgical because this condition does not improve with balloon catheter dilation.

3. Supravalvular Pulmonary Stenosis

Supravalvular pulmonary stenosis is a relatively rare condition caused by narrowing of the main pulmonary artery. The clinical picture may be identical to valvular pulmonary stenosis, although the murmur is maximal in the first intercostal space at the left sternal border and in the suprasternal notch. No ejection click is audible, as the valve itself is not involved. The murmur radiates toward the neck and over the lung fields. This condition occurs most often in children with Noonan syndrome.

4. Peripheral (Branch) Pulmonary Artery Stenosis

In peripheral pulmonary stenosis, there are multiple narrowings of the branches of the pulmonary artery at the bifurcation of the main pulmonary artery or in the periphery of the lung. Systolic murmurs may be heard over both lung fields, anteriorly and posteriorly. Mild pulmonary branch stenosis produces a murmur in infancy that resolves by 6 months of age. Severe forms of peripheral pulmonary stenosis persist. The three most common causes of pulmonary artery branch stenosis are Williams syndrome, Alagille syndrome, and congenital rubella. Surgery is often unsuccessful, as stenoses near and in the hilum of the lung are not surgically correctable. Transcatheter balloon angioplasty is currently being used to treat this condition, with moderate success. In some instances, the stenoses improve spontaneously with age.

5. Ebstein Malformation of the Tricuspid Valve

In Ebstein malformation of the tricuspid valve, the septal leaflet of the tricuspid valve is displaced toward the apex of the heart and is attached to the endocardium of the RV rather than at the tricuspid annulus. As a result, the upper portion of the RV is physiologically within the right atrium. This "atrialized" portion of the RV is thin-walled and does not contribute to RV output. The portion of the ventricle below the displaced tricuspid valve is diminished in volume and represents the functioning RV.

▶ Clinical Findings

A. Symptoms and Signs

The clinical picture of Ebstein malformation varies with the degree of displacement of the tricuspid valve. In the most extreme form, the septal leaflet is markedly displaced into the RV outflow tract, causing obstruction of antegrade flow into the pulmonary artery. The degree of tricuspid insufficiency may be so severe that forward flow out the RV outflow tract is further diminished leading to cyanosis. At the opposite extreme, symptoms may not develop until adulthood when tachyarrhythmias associated with right atrial dilation or associated reentrant electrical pathway occur. These older patients typically have less displacement of the septal leaflet of the tricuspid valve.

B. Imaging

The chest radiograph usually shows cardiomegaly with prominence of the right heart border. The extent of cardiomegaly depends on the degree of tricuspid valve insufficiency and the presence and size of the atrial level shunt. Massive cardiomegaly with a "wall-to-wall heart" occurs with severe displacement and a restrictive atrial level defect.

C. Electrocardiography

ECG may be normal but usually shows right atrial enlargement and right bundle-branch block (RBBB). There is an association between Ebstein anomaly and Wolff-Parkinson-White (WPW) syndrome. In these cases a delta wave is present.

D. Echocardiography

Echocardiography is necessary to confirm the diagnosis and may aid in predicting outcome. Degree of displacement, size of the right atrium, and presence of associated atrial level shunt all affect outcome. The size of the atrialized portion of the RV is determined by echocardiography, and in severe cases, the RV can become so enlarged that it encroaches on the LV mass, impeding LV filling.

▶ Course & Prognosis

In cyanotic neonates, prostaglandin E is used to maintain pulmonary blood flow until pulmonary vascular resistance decreases, facilitating antegrade pulmonary artery flow. If the neonate remains significantly cyanotic, surgical intervention is required but the outcome is poor. Intervention in older children or adults has a better outcome.

Surgical repair consists of an annuloplasty to modify the level of the tricuspid orifice and diminish tricuspid insufficiency. The success of the procedure is highly variable. Late arrhythmias are common due to the preexisting atrial dilation. If a significant Ebstein malformation is not treated, atrial tachyarrhythmias frequently begin during adolescence. Postoperative exercise tolerance improves but remains lower than age-related norms.

6. Other Rare Right-Sided Malformations

A. Absence of a Pulmonary Artery

Absence of a pulmonary artery (left or right) may be an isolated malformation or may occur in association with other congenital heart diseases. It occurs occasionally in patients with tetralogy of Fallot.

B. Absence of the Pulmonary Valve

Absence of the pulmonary valve is rare and usually associated with VSD. In about 50% of cases, infundibular pulmonary stenosis is also present (termed tetralogy of Fallot with absent pulmonary valve).

Alsoufi B et al: Surgical outcomes in the treatment of patients with tetralogy of Fallot and absent pulmonary valve. Eur J Cardiothorac Surg 2007;31:354 [PMID: 17215132].

Knott-Craig CJ et al: Repair of neonates and young infants with Ebstein's anomaly and related disorders. Ann Thorac Surg 2007;84:587 [PMID: 17643640].

LEFT-SIDED OBSTRUCTIVE LESIONS

1. Coarctation of the Aorta

▶ Absent or diminished femoral pulses.

▶ Upper to lower extremity systolic blood pressure gradient of > 20 mm Hg.

▶ Blowing systolic murmur in the back or left axilla.

▶ General Considerations

Coarctation accounts for about 6% of all congenital heart disease. Three times as many males as females are affected. Many affected females have Turner syndrome (45,XO). Coarctation usually occurs in the proximal descending aorta near the takeoff of the left subclavian artery next to the ductus arteriosus. The abdominal aorta is rarely involved. The incidence of associated bicuspid aortic valve with coarctation is 80–85%.

▶ Clinical Findings

A. Symptoms and Signs

The cardinal physical finding is decreased or absent femoral pulses. Infants with severe coarctation have equal upper and lower extremity pulses from birth until the ductus arteriosus closes. This is either because the coarctation is so severe that the ductus supplies blood flow to the descending aorta, or because the coarctation itself is the result of ductal tissue in the aorta sufficient to cause aortic obstruction. Approximately 40% of children with coarctation will present as young infants. Coarctation alone, or in combination with VSD, ASD, or other congenital cardiac anomalies, is the leading cause of HF in the first month of life.

Coarctation presents insidiously in the 60% of children with no symptoms in infancy. Coarctation is usually diagnosed by a pulse discrepancy between the arms and legs on physical examination or by right arm hypertension on blood pressure measurement. The pulses in the legs are diminished or absent. The left subclavian artery is occasionally involved in the coarctation, in which case the left brachial pulse is also weak. The pathognomonic murmur of coarctation is heard in the left axilla and the left back. The murmur is usually systolic but may spill into diastole, as forward flow continues across the narrow coarctation site throughout the cardiac cycle. A systolic ejection murmur is often heard at the aortic area and the lower left sternal border along with an apical ejection click from a bicuspid aortic valve.

B. Imaging

In the older child, radiographs may show a normal-sized heart, or more often some degree of LV enlargement. The aorta proximal to the coarctation is prominent. The aortic outline may indent at the level of the coarctation. The post-stenotic segment is often dilated. This combination of abnormalities results in the "figure 3" sign on chest radiograph. Notching of the ribs caused by marked enlargement of the intercostal collaterals can be seen. In patients with severe coarctation and associated HF, marked cardiac enlargement and pulmonary venous congestion occur.

C. Electrocardiography

ECGs in older children may be normal or may show LVH. ECG usually shows RVH in infants with severe coarctation because the RV has been a "systemic" ventricle during fetal life.

D. Echocardiography

Two-dimensional echocardiography and color-flow Doppler are used to visualize the coarctation directly, and continuous-wave Doppler estimates the degree of obstruction. Diastolic run-off flow is detected by continuous-wave Doppler if the obstruction is severe. In neonates with a PDA, a coarctation cannot be ruled out, as one may develop as the PDA closes. Associated lesions such as a bicuspid aortic valve or mitral abnormalities may suggest the presence of a coarctation. In the face of poor LV systolic function, the gradient across the coarctation will be falsely low, as the LV is unable to generate adequate pressure proximal to the narrowing.

E. Cardiac Catheterization and Angiocardiography

Cardiac catheterization and angiocardiography are rarely performed for diagnosis in infants or children with coarctation, but are used if transcatheter intervention is planned. If completed, these studies demonstrate the anatomy and severity of the coarctation and assess the adequacy of collateral circulation.

▶ Treatment

Infants with coarctation of the aorta and HF may present in extremis secondary to LV dysfunction and low cardiac output. Resuscitative measures include prostaglandin infusion (0.05–0.1 mcg/kg/min) to reopen the ductus arteriosus. End-organ damage distal to the coarctation is not rare, and inotropic support is frequently needed. Once stabilized, the infant should undergo corrective repair. In patients with poor LV function, balloon angioplasty is sometimes performed as a palliative measure. Recent data suggest that balloon angioplasty of the aorta can be the definitive procedure in many patients with good LV function. Surgery also has a high success rate. The main complication of both surgery and balloon angioplasty is recurrent coarctation. Fortunately, this complication is treatable in the catheter-

ization laboratory. In older patients, particularly those of adult size, transcatheter stent placement is effective for recurrent coarctation.

▶ Course & Prognosis

Children who survive the neonatal period without developing HF do well through childhood and adolescence. Fatal complications (eg, hypertensive encephalopathy or intracranial bleeding) are uncommon in childhood. Infective endarteritis is rare before adolescence. Children with coarctation corrected after age 5 years are at increased risk for systemic hypertension and myocardial dysfunction even with successful surgery. Exercise testing is mandatory for these children prior to their participation in athletic activities.

Golden AB et al: Coarctation of the aorta: Stenting in children and adults. Catheter Cardiovasc Interv 2007;69:289 [PMID: 17191237].

2. Aortic Stenosis

ESSENTIALS OF DIAGNOSIS & TYPICAL FEATURES

► Harsh systolic ejection murmur at the upper right sternal border.

► Thrill in the carotid arteries.

► Systolic click at the apex.

► Dilation of the ascending aorta on chest radiograph.

▶ General Considerations

Aortic stenosis is defined as obstruction to outflow from the LV at or near the aortic valve producing a systolic pressure gradient of more than 10 mm Hg between the LV and the aorta. Aortic stenosis accounts for approximately 7% of congenital heart disease. There are three anatomic types of congenital aortic stenosis.

A. Valvular Aortic Stenosis (75%)

In critical aortic stenosis presenting in infancy, the aortic valve is usually a unicuspid diaphragm-like structure without well-defined commissures. Preschool- and school-aged children more commonly have bicuspid aortic valve. Teenagers and young adults characteristically have a tricuspid valve with partially fused leaflets. This lesion is more common in males than in females.

B. Subvalvular Aortic Stenosis (23%)

In this type, a membranous or fibrous ring occurs just below the aortic valve that causes obstruction to LV outflow. The aortic valve itself and the anterior leaflet of the mitral valve are often malformed.

C. Supravalvular Aortic Stenosis (2%)

In this type, constriction of the ascending aorta occurs just above the coronary arteries. The condition is often familial, and two different genetic patterns are found, one with abnormal facies and mental retardation (Williams syndrome) and one with normal facies and no developmental delay.

▶ **Clinical Findings**

A. Symptoms and Signs

Most patients with aortic stenosis have no cardiovascular symptoms. Except in the most severe cases, patients do well until the third to fifth decades of life. Some patients have mild exercise intolerance and fatigability. In a small percentage of patients significant symptoms (ie, dizziness and syncope) manifest in the first decade. Sudden death is uncommon but may occur in all forms of aortic stenosis with the greatest risk in patients with subvalvular obstruction (similar to hypertrophic cardiomyopathy).

Although isolated valvular aortic stenosis seldom causes symptoms in infancy, severe HF occasionally occurs when critical obstruction is present at birth. Response to medical therapy is poor; therefore, an aggressive approach using interventional catheterization or surgery is required. The physical findings vary depending on the anatomic type of lesion:

1. Valvular aortic stenosis—Patients are well developed and well nourished. Pulses are usually normal and equal throughout. If the stenosis is severe with a gradient greater than 80 mm Hg, the pulses are diminished with a slow upstroke. Cardiac examination reveals an LV thrust at the apex. A systolic thrill at the right base, the suprasternal notch, and over both carotid arteries may accompany moderate disease.

A prominent aortic ejection click is best heard at the apex. The click corresponds to the opening of the aortic valve. It is separated from S_1 by a short but appreciable interval. It does not vary with respiration. S_2 at the pulmonary area is normal. A loud, rough, medium- to high-pitched ejection-type systolic murmur is evident. It is loudest at the first and second intercostal spaces, radiating well into the suprasternal notch and along the carotids. The grade of the murmur correlates well with the severity of the stenosis.

2. Discrete membranous subvalvular aortic stenosis—The findings are the same as those of valvular aortic stenosis except for the absence of a click. The murmur and thrill are usually somewhat more intense at the left sternal border in the third and fourth intercostal spaces. A diastolic murmur of aortic insufficiency is commonly heard after age 5 years.

3. Supravalvular aortic stenosis—The thrill and murmur are best heard in the suprasternal notch and along the carotids but are well transmitted over the aortic area and near the mid left sternal border. There may be a difference in pulses and blood pressure between the right and left arms if the narrowing is just distal to the takeoff of the innominate artery, with more prominent pulse and pressure in the right arm (the Coanda effect).

B. Imaging

In most cases the heart is not enlarged. The LV, however, may be slightly prominent. In valvular aortic stenosis, dilation of the ascending aorta is frequently seen.

C. Electrocardiography

Patients with mild aortic stenosis have normal ECGs. Some patients with severe obstruction have LVH and LV strain but even in severe cases, 25% of ECGs are normal. Progressive LVH on serial ECGs indicates a significant obstruction. LV strain is an indication for surgery.

D. Echocardiography

This is a reliable noninvasive technique for the evaluation of all forms of aortic stenosis. Doppler accurately estimates the transvalvular gradient, and the level of obstruction can be confirmed by both two-dimensional echocardiographic images and by the level of flow disturbance revealed by color Doppler.

E. Cardiac Catheterization and Angiocardiography

Left heart catheterization demonstrates the pressure differential between the LV and the aorta and the anatomic level at which the gradient exists. Echocardiography is the standard method for following the severity of aortic valve stenosis, and catheterization is reserved for patients whose resting gradient has reached 60–80 mm Hg and in whom intervention is planned. For those with valvular aortic stenosis, balloon valvuloplasty is usually the first option. In subvalvular or supravalvular aortic stenosis, interventional catheterization is not effective and surgery is required.

▶ **Treatment**

Percutaneous balloon valvuloplasty is now standard initial treatment. Surgery should be considered in patients with symptoms, a high resting gradient (60–80 mm Hg) despite balloon angioplasty, or coexisting aortic insufficiency. In many cases, the gradient cannot be significantly diminished without producing aortic insufficiency. Patients who develop significant aortic insufficiency require surgical intervention to repair or replace the valve, In the Ross procedure, the patient's own pulmonic valve is moved to the aortic position, and an RV-to-pulmonary artery conduit is used to replace the pulmonic valve. Discrete subvalvular aortic stenosis is usually surgically repaired at a lesser gradient because continued trauma to the aortic valve by the subvalvular jet may damage the valve and produce aortic insufficiency. Unfortunately, simple resection is followed by recurrence in more than 25% of patients with subvalvular aortic stenosis.

Course & Prognosis

All forms of LV outflow tract obstruction tend to be progressive. Pediatric patients with LV outflow tract obstruction—with the exception of those with critical aortic stenosis of infancy—are usually asymptomatic. Symptoms accompanying severe unoperated obstruction (angina, syncope, or HF) are rare but imply serious disease. Preoperative or postoperative children whose obstruction is mild to moderate have normal oxygen consumption and maximum voluntary working capacity. Children in this category with normal heart size and normal resting and exercising ECGs may safely participate in vigorous physical activity, including nonisometric competitive sports. Children with severe aortic stenosis are predisposed to ventricular dysrhythmias.

McLean KM et al: Current treatments for congenital aortic stenosis. Curr Opin Cardiol 2006;21:200 [PMID: 16601457].

Mertens L et al: The role of imaging techniques in diagnosis and evaluation of congenital aortic stenosis. Acta Cardiol 2006;61:208 [PMID: 16716029].

3. Mitral Valve Prolapse

ESSENTIALS OF DIAGNOSIS & TYPICAL FEATURES

► Midsystolic click.

► Late systolic "whooping" or "honking" murmur.

► Typical symptoms include chest pain, palpitations, and dizziness.

► Often overdiagnosed on routine cardiac ultrasound.

General Considerations

In this condition the mitral valve prolapses, moving posteriorly or superiorly into the left atrium during ventricular systole as the mitral valve closes. A midsystolic click occurs at the time of this movement and is the hallmark of this entity. Mitral insufficiency may occur late in systole, causing a short, atypical murmur with variable radiation. Mitral valve prolapse (MVP) occurs in about 2% of thin female adolescents, a minority of whom have concomitant mitral insufficiency. Although MVP is usually an isolated lesion, it can occur in association with Marfan syndrome and Ehlers-Danlos syndrome. These coexisting conditions should be ruled out by clinical examination.

Clinical Findings

A. Symptoms and Signs

Most patients with MVP are asymptomatic. Chest pain, palpitations, and dizziness may be reported, but it is unclear whether these symptoms are more common in affected patients than in the normal population. Chest pain on exertion is rare and should be assessed with cardiopulmonary stress testing. Significant dysrhythmias have been reported, including increased ventricular ectopy and nonsustained ventricular tachycardia. If significant mitral regurgitation is present, atrial arrhythmias may also occur. Standard auscultation technique must be modified to diagnose MVP. Clicks, with or without systolic murmur, are elicited best in the standing position due to the decrease in LV volume. Conversely, maneuvers that increase LV volume, such as squatting or handgrip exercise, will cause delay or obliteration of the click-murmur complex. The systolic click usually is heard at the apex but may be audible at the left sternal border. A systolic murmur after the click implies mitral insufficiency and is much less common than isolated prolapse. The murmur is not holosystolic, in contrast to rheumatic mitral insufficiency.

B. Imaging

Most chest radiographs are normal. They are not indicated in this condition. In the rare case of significant mitral valve insufficiency, the left atrium may be enlarged.

C. Electrocardiography

The ECG may be normal. Diffuse flattening or inversion of T waves may occur in the precordial leads. U waves are sometimes prominent.

D. Echocardiography

Significant posterior systolic movement of the mitral valve leaflets to the atrial side of the mitral annulus is diagnostic. Echocardiography assesses the degree of myxomatous change of the mitral valve and the degree of mitral insufficiency.

E. Other Testing

Invasive procedures are rarely indicated. Holter monitoring or event recorders may be useful in establishing the presence of ventricular dysrhythmias in patients with palpitations.

Treatment & Prognosis

Propranolol may be effective in treatment of coexisting arrhythmias. Prophylaxis for infectious endocarditis is no longer indicated, based on 2007 AHA guidelines.

The natural course of this condition is not well defined. Twenty years of observation indicate that isolated MVP in childhood is usually a benign entity. Surgery for mitral insufficiency is rarely needed.

Knackstedt C et al: Ventricular fibrillation due to severe mitral valve prolapse. Int J Cardiol 2007;116:e101 [PMID: 17137658].

Mechleb BK et al. Mitral valve prolapse: Relationship of echocardiography characteristics to natural history. Echocardiography 2006;23:434 [PMID: 16686634].

4. Other Congenital Left Heart Valvular Lesions

A. Congenital Mitral Stenosis

Congenital mitral stenosis is a rare disorder in which the valve leaflets are thickened and fused, producing a diaphragm-like or funnel-like structure with a central opening. When mitral stenosis occurs with other left-sided obstructive lesions, such as subaortic stenosis and coarctation of the aorta, the complex is called Shone syndrome. Most patients develop symptoms early in life with tachypnea, dyspnea, and failure to thrive. Physical examination reveals an accentuated S_1 and a loud pulmonary closure sound. No opening snap can be heard. In most cases, a presystolic crescendo murmur is heard at the apex. Occasionally, only a mid-diastolic murmur can be heard. Rarely, no murmur is present. ECG shows right axis deviation, biatrial enlargement, and RVH. Chest radiograph reveals left atrial enlargement and frequently pulmonary venous congestion. Echocardiography shows abnormal mitral valve structures with reduced leaflet excursion and left atrial enlargement. Cardiac catheterization reveals an elevated pulmonary capillary wedge pressure and pulmonary hypertension, owing to the elevated left atrial pressure.

Mitral valve repair or mitral valve replacement with a prosthetic mitral valve may be performed, even in young infants, but is a technically difficult procedure. Mitral valve repair is the preferred surgical option, as valve replacement has a poor outcome in very young children.

B. Cor Triatriatum

Cor triatriatum is a rare abnormality in which the pulmonary veins join at their confluence but the confluence is not completely incorporated into the left atrium. The confluence communicates with the left atrium through an opening of variable size, and may be obstructed. The consequences are similar to those of mitral stenosis. Clinical findings depend on the size of the opening. If the opening is small, symptoms develop early in life. Echocardiography reveals a linear density in the left atrium with a gradient between the pulmonary venous chamber and the true left atrium. Cardiac catheterization may be needed if the diagnosis is in doubt. High pulmonary wedge pressure and low left atrial pressure (with the catheter passed through the foramen ovale into the true left atrium) support the diagnosis. Angiocardiography identifies both the proximal and distal left atria. Surgical repair is always required in the presence of an obstructive membrane, and long-term results are good. Coexisting mitral valve abnormalities may be noted, including a supravalvular mitral ring or a dysplastic mitral valve.

C. Congenital Mitral Regurgitation

Congenital mitral regurgitation is a rare abnormality usually associated with other congenital heart lesions, such as ccTGA, AV septal defect, and anomalous left coronary artery. Isolated congenital mitral regurgitation is very rare. It is sometimes present in patients with Marfan syndrome, usually associated with a myxomatous prolapsing mitral valve.

D. Congenital Aortic Regurgitation

Congenital aortic regurgitation is rare. The most common causes are bicuspid aortic valve, with or without coarctation of the aorta; VSD with aortic cusp prolapse and aortic insufficiency; and fenestration of the aortic valve cusp (one or more holes in the cusp).

Beierlein W et al: Long-term follow-up after mitral valve replacement in childhood: Poor event-free survival in the young child. Eur J Cardiothorac Surg 2007;31:860 [PMID: 17383889].

DISEASES OF THE AORTA

Although more common in mid to late adulthood, aortic dilation and dissection may occur in children. Although the aorta may not be dilated at birth, the structural abnormality that predisposes to dilation is presumed to be congenital. Patients at risk for progressive aortic dilation and dissection include those with isolated bicuspid aortic valve, Marfan syndrome, Turner syndrome, and type IV Ehlers-Danlos syndrome.

1. Bicuspid Aortic Valve

Patients with bicuspid aortic valves have an increased incidence of aortic dilation and dissection, regardless of the presence of aortic stenosis. Histologic examination demonstrates cystic medial degeneration of the aortic wall, similar to that seen in patients with Marfan syndrome. Patients with isolated bicuspid aortic valve require regular follow-up even in the absence of aortic insufficiency or aortic stenosis. Significant aortic root dilation requiring surgical intervention typically does not occur until adulthood.

2. Marfan Syndrome

Marfan syndrome is an autosomal dominant disorder of connective tissue caused by a mutation in the fibrillin-1 gene. Spontaneous mutations account for 25–30% of cases, and thus family history is not always helpful. Patients are diagnosed by the Ghent criteria and must have at a minimum, major involvement of two body systems plus involvement of a third body system or a positive family history. Body systems involved include cardiovascular, ocular, musculoskeletal, pulmonary, and integumentary. Cardiac manifestations include aortic root dilation and MVP, which may be present at birth. Patients are at risk for aortic dilation and dissection and are restricted from competitive athletics, contact sports, and isometric activities. β-Blockers or ACE inhibitors are used to lower blood pressure and slow the rate of aortic dilation. More recently, studies are ongoing to evaluate the effectiveness of angiotensin receptor blockers (losartan). Elective surgical intervention is performed in patients of adult size when the aortic root dimension reaches 50 mm. The ratio of actual to expected aortic root dimension is used to determine the need for surgery in the young child. Surgical options include replacement of the dilated aortic root with a composite valve graft (Bentall technique) or a David procedure in which the patient's own aortic valve is spared and a Dacron tube graft is used to replace the dilated ascending aorta. Young age at diagnosis was previously thought to confer a poor prognosis; however, early diagnosis with close follow-up and early medical therapy has been associated with more favorable outcome. Ventricular dysrhythmias may contribute to the mortality in Marfan syndrome.

3. Turner Syndrome

Cardiovascular abnormalities are common in Turner syndrome. Patients are at risk for aortic dissection, typically during adulthood. Risk factors include hypertension regardless of cause, aortic dilation, bicuspid aortic valve, and coarctation of the aorta. There are rare reports of aortic dissection in adult Turner syndrome patients in the absence of any risk factors. Patients with Turner syndrome require routine follow-up from adolescence onward to monitor this potentially lethal complication.

Beroukhim RS et al: Comparison of the pattern of aortic dilation in children the Marfan syndrome versus children with bicuspid aortic valve. Am J Cardiol 2006;98:1094 [PMID: 17027578].

Silberbach M: Aortic dissection in Turner's syndrome: A "perfect storm"? Cardiol Young 2006;16:430 [PMID: 16984695].

Yetman AT: Cardiovascular pharmacotherapy in patients with Marfan syndrome. Am J Cardiovasc Drugs 2007;7:117 [PMID: 17503882].

CORONARY ARTERY ABNORMALITIES

Several anomalies involve the origin, course, and distribution of the coronary arteries. The only abnormality seen with regularity, and which has disastrous consequences if unrecognized, is anomalous origin of the left coronary artery.

Anomalous Origin of the Left Coronary Artery from the Pulmonary Artery (ALCAPA)

In this condition, the left coronary artery arises from the pulmonary artery rather than the aorta. In neonates, whose pulmonary artery pressure is high, perfusion of the left coronary artery may be adequate and the infant may be asymptomatic. By age 2 months the pulmonary arterial pressure falls, causing a progressive decrease in myocardial perfusion by the left coronary artery. Ischemia and infarction of the LV occur. Immediate surgery is needed to reimplant the left coronary artery and restore myocardial perfusion. The surgery is relatively high-risk, especially if infarction of the papillary muscles supporting the mitral apparatus has occurred. Mitral valve replacement will then sometimes be needed.

▶ Clinical Findings

A. Symptoms and Signs

Neonates appear healthy and growth and development are relatively normal for a few months while pulmonary artery pressure is dropping. Detailed questioning may disclose a history of intermittent abdominal pain, pallor, and sweating, especially during or after feeding. Presentation may be subtle, with nonspecific complaints of "fussiness" or intermittent "colic." The colic and fussiness are probably attacks of true angina. Presentation may be fulminant at age 2–4 months with sudden, severe HF due to LV dysfunction and mitral insufficiency. On physical examination, the infants are usually well developed and well nourished. The pulses are typically weak but equal. A prominent left precordial bulge is present. A holosystolic murmur of mitral regurgitation is sometimes present, though frequently auscultation alone reveals no obvious abnormalities.

B. Imaging

Chest radiographs show cardiac enlargement and left atrial enlargement and may show pulmonary venous congestion if left ventricular function has been compromised.

C. Electrocardiography

The ECG is very helpful. There is T-wave inversion in leads I and aVL. The precordial leads also show T-wave inversion from V_4–V_7. Deep and wide Q waves are present in leads I, aVL, and sometimes in V_4–V_6. These findings of myocardial infarction are similar to those in adults.

D. Echocardiography

The diagnosis can be made with two-dimensional echo techniques by visualizing a single large right coronary artery arising from the aorta and visualization of the anomalous left coronary artery arising from the main pulmonary artery. Flow reversal in the left coronary (heading *toward* the aorta, rather than away) confirms the diagnosis. LV dysfunction, echo-bright (ischemic) papillary muscles, and mitral regurgitation may be seen.

E. Cardiac Catheterization and Angiocardiography

Angiogram of the aorta fails to show the origin of the left coronary artery. A large right coronary artery fills directly from the aorta, and contrast flows from the right coronary system via collaterals into the left coronary arteries and finally into the pulmonary artery. Angiogram of the RV or main pulmonary artery may show the origin of the anomalous vessel. Rarely, a left-to-right shunt may be detected as oxygenated blood passes through the collateral system without delivering oxygen to the myocardium, and passes into the pulmonary artery.

Treatment & Prognosis

Anomalous left coronary artery is a high-risk diagnosis. The prognosis is guarded at best. Medical management with diuretics and afterload reduction can help stabilize the ill patient, but surgical intervention should not be delayed. Most surgeons relocate the anomalous coronary button into the aorta. The mitral valve may have to be replaced, depending on the degree of mitral insufficiency.

Lange R et al: Long-term results of repair of anomalous origin on the left coronary artery from the pulmonary artery. Ann Thorac Surg 2007;83:1463 [PMID: 17383358].

CYANOTIC CONGENITAL HEART DISEASE

TETRALOGY OF FALLOT

ESSENTIALS OF DIAGNOSIS & TYPICAL FEATURES

- ▶ Hypoxemic spells during infancy.
- ▶ Right-sided aortic arch in 25% of patients.
- ▶ Systolic ejection murmur at the upper left sternal border.

General Considerations

In tetralogy of Fallot (ToF), a single embryologic abnormality causes multiple morphologic problems. Anterior deviation of the infundibular (pulmonary outflow) septum causes narrowing of the right ventricular outflow tract. This deviation also causes a VSD and the aorta overrides the crest of the ventricular septum. The RV hypertrophies, not because of pulmonary stenosis, but because it is pumping against systemic resistance across a (usually) large VSD. ToF is the most common cyanotic cardiac lesion and accounts for 10% of all congenital heart disease. A right-sided aortic arch is present in 25% of cases, and ASD occurs in 15%.

Obstruction to RV outflow with a large VSD causes a right-to-left shunt at the ventricular level with arterial desaturation. The greater the obstruction and the lower the systemic vascular resistance, the greater is the right-to-left shunt. ToF is associated with deletions in the long arm of chromosome 22 (22q11) in as many as 15% of affected children.

Clinical Findings

A. Symptoms and Signs

Clinical findings vary with the degree of RV outflow obstruction. Patients with mild obstruction are minimally cyanotic or acyanotic. Those with maximal obstruction are deeply cyanotic from birth. Few children are asymptomatic. Most have cyanosis by age 4 months, and the cyanosis usually is progressive, as subvalvular obstruction increases. Growth and development are not typically delayed, but easy fatigability and dyspnea on exertion are common. The fingers and toes show variable clubbing depending on age and severity of cyanosis. Historically, older children with ToF would frequently squat to increase systemic vascular resistance. This decreased the amount of right-to-left shunt, forcing blood through the pulmonary circuit, and would help ward off cyanotic spells. Squatting is rarely seen as the diagnosis is now made much earlier.

Hypoxemic spells, also called cyanotic or "Tet spells," are one of the hallmarks of severe ToF. They are characterized by (1) sudden onset of cyanosis or deepening of cyanosis; (2) dyspnea; (3) alterations in consciousness, from irritability to syncope; and (4) decrease or disappearance of the systolic murmur (as RV outflow tract flow becomes completely obstructed). These episodes most commonly start at age 4–6 months. Cyanotic spells are treated acutely by administration of oxygen and placing the patient in the knee-chest position. Intravenous morphine should be administered cautiously. Propranolol produces β-blockade and may reduce the obstruction across the RV outflow tract. Acidosis, if present, should be corrected with intravenous sodium bicarbonate. Chronic oral prophylaxis of cyanotic spells with propranolol may be useful to delay surgery but the onset of Tet spells usually prompts expedient intervention.

An RV lift is palpable. S_2 is predominantly aortic and single. A grade II–IV/VI, rough, systolic ejection murmur is present at the left sternal border in the third intercostal space and radiates well to the back.

B. Laboratory Findings

Hemoglobin, hematocrit, and red blood cell count are usually elevated secondary to arterial desaturation.

C. Imaging

Chest radiographs show a normal size heart. The RV is hypertrophied, often shown by an upturning of the apex (boot-shaped heart). The main pulmonary artery segment is usually concave and, if there is a right aortic arch, the aortic knob is to the right of the trachea. The pulmonary vascular markings are usually decreased.

D. Electrocardiography

The QRS axis is rightward, ranging from +90 to +180 degrees. The P waves are usually normal. RVH is always present, but RV strain patterns are rare.

E. Echocardiography

Two-dimensional imaging is diagnostic, revealing thickening of the RV wall, overriding of the aorta, and a large subaortic VSD. Obstruction at the level of the infundibulum and pulmonary valve can be identified, and the size of the proximal pulmonary arteries can be measured. The anatomy of the coronary arteries should be visualized, as abnormal branches crossing the RV outflow tract are at risk for transection during surgical enlargement of the area.

F. Cardiac Catheterization and Angiocardiography

Cardiac catheterization reveals a right-to-left shunt at the ventricular level in most cases. Arterial desaturation of varying degrees is present. The RV pressure is at systemic levels and the pressure tracing in the RV is identical to that in the LV if the VSD is large. The pulmonary artery pressure is invariably low. Pressure gradients may be noted at the valvular level, the infundibular level, or both. RV angiography reveals RV outflow obstruction and a right-to-left shunt at the ventricular level. The major indications for cardiac catheterization are to establish coronary artery and distal pulmonary artery anatomy.

▶ Treatment

A. Palliative Treatment

A few centers currently advocate complete repair of ToF during the neonatal period regardless of patient size. Many centers prefer palliative treatment for small infants in whom complete correction is deemed risky. Medical palliation with long-term oral β-blocking agents may delay surgery. Some patients may be palliated by balloon dilation of the RV outflow tract during infancy. While this may improve the pulmonary blood flow and delay surgical intervention, hypercyanotic spells are frequent when the RV outflow tract is manipulated, making this procedure somewhat risky.

The most common surgical palliation is the insertion of a GoreTex shunt from the subclavian artery to the ipsilateral pulmonary artery (modified Blalock-Taussig shunt). This improves pulmonary blood flow regardless of the level of infundibular or valvular obstruction, and some believe, allows for growth of the patient's pulmonary arteries (which are usually small) prior to complete surgical correction.

B. Total Correction

Open-heart surgery for repair of ToF is performed at ages ranging from birth to 2 years, depending on the experience of each center. The current surgical trend is toward earlier repair for symptomatic infants. The major limiting anatomic feature of total correction is the size of the pulmonary arteries. During surgery, the VSD is closed and the obstruction to RV outflow removed. Surgical mortality is low.

▶ Course & Prognosis

Infants with severe ToF are usually deeply cyanotic at birth. These children require early surgery, either a Blalock-Taussig shunt or primary correction. All children with ToF require open-heart surgery. Complete repair before age 2 years usually produces a good result, and patients are currently living well into adulthood. Depending on the extent of the repair required, patients frequently require additional surgery 10–15 years after their initial repair for replacement of the pulmonary valve. Transcatheter pulmonary valves are under investigation and may help these patients avoid additional open-heart surgery in the future. The greatest risk for death in ToF patients is ventricular dysrhythmias. A competent pulmonary valve without a dilated RV appears to diminish arrhythmias and enhance exercise performance.

Nordmeyer J et al: Current experience with percutaneous pulmonary valve implantation. Semin Thorac Cardiovasc Surg 2006;18:122 [PMID: 17157232].
Shinebourne EA et al: Tetralogy of Fallot: From fetus to adult. Heart 2006;92:1353 [PMID: 16908723].

PULMONARY ATRESIA WITH VENTRICULAR SEPTAL DEFECT

This condition, complete atresia of the pulmonary valve in association with VSD, is essentially an extreme form of ToF. Because there is no antegrade flow from the RV to the pulmonary artery, pulmonary blood flow must be derived from a PDA or from multiple aortopulmonary collateral arteries (MAPCAs). Symptoms depend on the amount of pulmonary blood flow. If flow is significant, patients may be stable. If pulmonary flow is inadequate, severe hypoxemia occurs and immediate palliation is required. Newborns are stabilized with intravenous prostaglandin E_1 (PGE$_1$) to maintain the PDA while being prepared for surgery. Rarely, if the ductus does not contribute significantly to pulmonary blood flow (ie, the MAPCAs alone are sufficient), PGE$_1$ may be discontinued. Once stabilized, palliative aortopulmonary shunt or primary correction is undertaken. In most centers, a palliative shunt is performed in the newborn to augment pulmonary blood flow, and open-heart surgical correction planned for age 9–18 months.

Echocardiography is usually diagnostic. Cardiac catheterization and angiocardiography are required to confirm the source(s) of pulmonary blood flow. With small native pulmonary arteries and inadequate blood flow, an aortopulmonary shunt is created, either by rerouting the patient's own vessels or by creating a shunt with artificial material. When the pulmonary arteries are large enough, relocation of the MAPCAs from the aorta to the pulmonary trunk (unifocalization) is performed to complete the repair.

Pulmonary vascular disease is common in pulmonary atresia with VSD, due both to intrinsic abnormalities of the pulmonary vasculature and to abnormal amounts of pulmonary blood flow. Even patients who have undergone surgical correction as infants are at risk. Pulmonary vascular disease is a common cause of death as early as the third decade of life.

Ishibashi N et al: Clinical results of staged repair with complete unifocalization for pulmonary atresia with ventricular septal defect and major aortopulmonary collateral arteries. Eur J Cardiothorac Surg 2007;32:202 [PMID: 17512210].

PULMONARY ATRESIA WITH INTACT VENTRICULAR SEPTUM

ESSENTIALS OF DIAGNOSIS & TYPICAL FEATURES

▶ Completely different from pulmonary atresia with VSD.

▶ Cyanosis at birth.

▶ Always ductal dependent with rare aortopulmonary collateral arteries.

▶ RV-dependent coronary arteries sometimes are present.

▶ General Considerations

Although pulmonary atresia with intact ventricular septum (PA/IVS) sounds as if it might be related to pulmonary atresia with VSD, it is a distinct cardiac condition. As the name suggests, the pulmonary valve is atretic. The pulmonic annulus usually has a small diaphragm consisting of the fused valve cusps. The ventricular septum is intact. The main pulmonary artery segment is usually present and closely approximated to the atretic valve, but is somewhat hypoplastic. Although the RV is always reduced in size, the degree of reduction is variable. The size of the RV is critical to the success of surgical repair. In some children with PA/IVS, the RV is adequate for ultimate two-ventricular repair. A normal RV has three component parts (inlet, trabecular or body, and outlet). The absence of any one of the components makes adequate RV function unlikely. Even with all three components, some RVs are inadequate.

After birth, the pulmonary circulation is maintained by the ductus arteriosus. Multiple aortopulmonary collateral arteries are usually not present in this disease, in contrast to pulmonary atresia with VSD. A continuous infusion of PGE_1 must be started as soon as possible after birth to maintain ductal patency.

▶ Clinical Findings

A. Symptoms and Signs

Neonates are usually cyanotic and become more so as the ductus arteriosus closes. A blowing systolic murmur resulting from the associated PDA may be heard at the pulmonary area. A holosystolic murmur is often heard at the lower left sternal border, as many children develop tricuspid insufficiency if the RV is of good size and egress from that ventricle is only through the tricuspid valve.

B. Imaging

The heart size varies from small to markedly enlarged depending on the degree of tricuspid insufficiency. With severe tricuspid insufficiency, right atrial enlargement may be massive and the cardiac silhouette may fill the chest on radiograph.

C. Electrocardiography

ECG reveals a left axis for age (45–90 degrees) in the frontal plane. Left ventricular forces dominate the ECG, and there is a paucity of RV forces, particularly with hypoplastic RV. Findings of right atrial enlargement are usually striking.

D. Echocardiography

Echocardiography shows atresia of the pulmonary valve with varying degrees of RV cavity and tricuspid annulus hypoplasia. The severity of tricuspid regurgitation correlates with RV size.

E. Cardiac Catheterization and Angiocardiography

RV pressure is almost always suprasystemic. Angiogram of the RV reveals no filling of the pulmonary artery. It also demonstrates the size of the RV chamber, relative hypoplasia of the three components of the RV, and the presence or absence of tricuspid regurgitation. Some children with pulmonary atresia and an intact ventricular septum have sinusoids between the RV and the coronary arteries. The presence of sinusoids indicates that the coronary circulation may depend on high right ventricular pressure. Any attempt to decompress the RV in patients with RV-dependent coronary circulation causes myocardial infarction and death because of the precipitous decrease in coronary perfusion.

▶ Treatment & Prognosis

As in all ductal-dependent lesions, PGE_1 is used to stabilize the patient and maintain patency of the ductus until surgery can be performed. Surgery is usually undertaken in the first week of life. Unrestricted flow through the ASD is a necessity, since the only outflow from the right atrium is via the atrial defect and into the left atrium.

A Rashkind balloon atrial septostomy may be required, depending on RV size, to open a communication across the atrial septum. If the RV is tripartite and an eventual two-chamber repair is planned, the pulmonary valve plate may be perforated and dilated during cardiac catheterization in the newborn to allow antegrade flow from the RV to the pulmonary artery and thus encourage RV cavity growth. If the RV is inadequate, if significant sinusoids are present, or if the pulmonic valve cannot be opened successfully during cardiac catheterization, a Blalock-Taussig shunt is performed to establish pulmonary blood flow. Later in infancy, a communication between the RV and pulmonary artery can be created to stimulate RV cavity growth. If either RV dimension or function is inadequate for two-ventricular repair, an approach similar to that taken for a single ventricle pathway best serves these children (see section on Hypoplastic Left Heart Syndrome, later). Children with significant sinusoids are often considered for cardiac transplantation if they are at risk for coronary insufficiency and sudden death.

The prognosis in this condition is guarded. Experience strongly favors opening the atretic valve in the catheterization laboratory in the newborn period if possible. Ultimate plans for two-ventricular repair, Fontan procedure, or cardiac transplantation depend on the anatomy.

Hirata Y et al: Pulmonary atresia with intact ventricular septum: Limitations of catheter-based intervention. Ann Thorac Surg 2007;84;574 [PMID: 17643638].

McLean KM et al: Pulmonary atresia with intact ventricular septum: Initial management. Ann Thorac Surg 2006;82:2214 [PMID: 17126137].

TRICUSPID ATRESIA

 ESSENTIALS OF DIAGNOSIS & TYPICAL FEATURES

▶ Marked cyanosis present from birth.
▶ ECG with left axis deviation, right atrial enlargement, and LVH.

▶ General Considerations

In tricuspid atresia, there is complete atresia of the tricuspid valve with no direct communication between the right atrium and the RV. There are two types of tricuspid atresia based on the relationship of the great arteries. The entire systemic venous return must flow through the atrial septum (either ASD or patent foramen ovale) to reach the left atrium. The left atrium thus receives both the systemic venous return and the pulmonary venous return. Complete mixing occurs in the left atrium, resulting in variable degrees of arterial desaturation.

Because there is no flow to the RV, development of the RV depends on the presence of a ventricular left-to-right shunt. Severe hypoplasia of the RV occurs when there is no VSD or when the VSD is small.

▶ Clinical Findings

A. Symptoms and Signs

Symptoms usually develop in early infancy with cyanosis present at birth in most infants. Growth and development are poor, and the infant usually exhibits exhaustion during feedings, tachypnea, and dyspnea. Patients with an increased pulmonary blood flow—types 1(c) and 2(b)—may develop HF with less prominent cyanosis. A murmur from the VSD is usually present and heard best at the lower left sternal border. Digital clubbing is present in older children with long standing cyanosis.

B. Imaging

The heart is slightly to markedly enlarged. The main pulmonary artery segment is usually small or absent. The size of the right atrium is moderately to massively enlarged, depending on the size of the communication at the atrial level. The pulmonary vascular markings are usually decreased. Pulmonary vascular markings may be increased if pulmonary blood flow is not restricted by the VSD or pulmonary stenosis.

C. Electrocardiography

The ECG shows marked left axis deviation. The P waves are tall and peaked, indicative of right atrial hypertrophy. LVH or LV dominance is found in almost all cases. RV forces on the ECG are usually low or absent.

D. Echocardiography

Two-dimensional methods are diagnostic and show absence of the tricuspid valve, the relationship between the great arteries, and the size of the pulmonary arteries. Color-flow Doppler imaging can help identify levels of restriction of pulmonary blood flow, either at the VSD or in the RV outflow tract.

E. Cardiac Catheterization and Angiocardiography

Catheterization reveals a right-to-left shunt at the atrial level. Because of mixing in the left atrium, oxygen saturations in the LV, RV, pulmonary artery, and aorta are identical to that in the left atrium. Right atrial pressure is increased if the ASD is restrictive. LV and systemic pressures are normal. The catheter cannot be passed through the tricuspid valve from the right atrium to the RV. A balloon atrial septostomy is performed if a restrictive foramen ovale or ASD is present.

▶ Treatment & Prognosis

In infants with unrestricted pulmonary blood flow, conventional anticongestive therapy with diuretics and afterload reduction should be given until the infant begins to outgrow the VSD. Sometimes, a pulmonary artery band is needed to protect the pulmonary bed from excessive flow.

Staged palliation of tricuspid atresia is the usual surgical approach. In infants with diminished pulmonary blood flow, PGE$_1$ is given until an aortopulmonary shunt can be performed. A Glenn procedure (superior vena cava to pulmonary artery anastomosis) is done with takedown of the aortopulmonary shunt at 4–6 months when saturations begin to fall, and completion of the Fontan procedure (redirection of inferior vena cava and superior vena cava to pulmonary artery) is performed when the child reaches around 15 kg.

The prognosis for patients with tricuspid atresia depends on achieving a pulmonary blood flow that permits adequate oxygenation of the tissues without producing HF. The long-term prognosis for children treated by the Fontan procedure is unknown, although patients now are living into their late 20s and early 30s. In the short term, the best results for the Fontan procedure occur in children with low pulmonary artery pressures prior to open-heart surgery.

Wald RM et al: Outcome after prenatal diagnosis of tricuspid atresia: A multicenter experience. Am Heart J 2007;153:772 [PMID: 17452152].

HYPOPLASTIC LEFT HEART SYNDROME

 ESSENTIALS OF DIAGNOSIS & TYPICAL FEATURES

- ▸ Mild cyanosis at birth.
- ▸ Minimal auscultatory findings.
- ▸ Rapid onset of shock with ductal closure.

▸ General Considerations

Hypoplastic left heart syndrome (HLHS) includes several conditions in which lesions of the left heart result in hypoplasia of the LV. The syndrome occurs in 1.4–3.8% of infants with congenital heart disease.

Stenosis or atresia of the mitral and aortic valves is the rule. In the neonate, survival depends on a PDA because antegrade flow into the systemic circulation is inadequate or nonexistent. The PDA provides the only flow to the aorta. Children with HLHS are usually stable at birth, but they deteriorate rapidly as the ductus closes in the first week of life. Untreated, the average age at death is the first week of life. Rarely, the ductus remains patent and infants may survive for several months without PGE1 therapy.

Currently, in settings with the expertise, the diagnosis is made prepartum by fetal echocardiography. Prepartum diagnosis aids greatly in planning for the delivery of the infant at or near a center with experience in treating HLHS.

▸ Clinical Findings

A. Symptoms and Signs

Neonates with HLHS appear stable at birth because the ductus is patent. They deteriorate rapidly as the ductus closes, with shock and acidosis secondary to inadequate systemic perfusion. Oxygen saturation may initially increase as more blood flows to the lungs with ductal closure.

B. Imaging

Chest radiograph at presentation shows cardiac enlargement with severe pulmonary venous congestion if the PDA has begun closing. Chest radiograph in the first day of life may be relatively unremarkable, with the exception of a small cardiac silhouette.

C. Electrocardiography

The ECG shows right axis deviation, right atrial enlargement, and RVH with a relative paucity of LV forces. The small Q wave in lead V_6 may be absent, and a qR pattern is often seen in lead V_1.

D. Echocardiography

Echocardiography is diagnostic. A very small aorta and LV with atretic or severely stenotic mitral and aortic valves are diagnostic. The systemic circulation is dependent on the PDA. Color-flow Doppler imaging shows retrograde flow in the ascending aorta, as the coronary arteries must be supplied by the ductus via the small native aorta.

▸ Treatment & Prognosis

PGE1 is essential initially, as systemic circulation depends on a patent ductus arteriosus. Later management depends on balancing pulmonary and systemic blood flow both of which depend on the RV. At a few days of age the pulmonary resistance falls, favoring pulmonary overcirculation and systemic underperfusion. Therapy is then directed at encouraging systemic blood flow. Nitrogen is used to decrease inspired oxygen to as low as 17%. This therapy must be carefully monitored but results in increased pulmonary arterial tone and better systemic perfusion. Systemic afterload reduction will also increase systemic perfusion. Adequate perfusion can usually be obtained by keeping systemic O_2 saturation between 65% and 80%, or more accurately a P_{O_2} of 40 mm Hg.

A choice must be made shortly after birth among several treatment options. In the Norwood procedure, the relatively normal main pulmonary artery is transected and connected to the small ascending aorta. The aortic arch must be reconstructed due to its small size. Then, either a Blalock-Taussig shunt (from the subclavian artery to the pulmonary artery) or a Sano shunt (from the RV to the pulmonary artery) must be created to restore pulmonary blood flow. Children who have a Norwood procedure will later require a Glenn anastomosis (superior vena cava to pulmonary artery with takedown of the systemic-pulmonary shunt) and then a Fontan (inferior vena cava to pulmonary artery, completing the systemic venous bypass of the heart) at ages 6 months and 2–3 years, respectively. Although this is a major improvement over nonsurgical intervention, HLHS remains one of the most challenging lesions in pediatric cardiology, as survival is still only 60% at 5 years.

Orthotopic heart transplantation is also a treatment for HLHS. Survival after transplantation is better than survival after the Norwood operation, but death while awaiting transplantation increases overall mortality to the same level as the Norwood.

Recently, many centers have moved toward a "hybrid" approach to HLHS as a result of collaboration between surgeons and interventional cardiologists. In the hybrid procedure, the chest is opened surgically and the pulmonary arteries are banded, to limit pulmonary blood flow. Then, also through the open chest, a PDA stent is placed by the interventionalist to maintain systemic output. The second stage is considered a "comprehensive Glenn," in which the pulmonary artery bands and ductal stent are taken down, and the superior vena cava is surgically connected to the pulmonary arteries. Aortic arch reconstruction is done during the second stage, in contrast to the Norwood operation. Survival after the first-stage "hybrid" is greater than 90% at the most experienced centers. Long-term follow-up is not yet available.

Artrip JH et al: Birth weight and complexity are significant factors for the management of hypoplastic left heart syndrome. Ann Thorac Surg 2006t;82:1252 [PMID: 16996917].

Pedra CA et al: New transcatheter techniques for creation or enlargement of atrial septal defects in infants with complex congenital heart disease. Catheter Cardiovasc Interv 2007;70:731 [PMID: 17621660].

TRANSPOSITION OF THE GREAT ARTERIES

ESSENTIALS OF DIAGNOSIS & TYPICAL FEATURES

▶ Cyanotic newborn without respiratory distress.
▶ More common in males.

General Considerations

Transposition of the great arteries (TGA) is the second most common cyanotic congenital heart disease, accounting for 5% of all cases of congenital heart disease. The male-to-female ratio is 3:1. It is caused by an embryologic abnormality in the spiral division of the truncus arteriosus in which the aorta arises from the RV and the pulmonary artery from the LV. This is referred to as "ventriculoarterial discordance." Patients may have a VSD, or the ventricular septum may be intact. Left unrepaired, transposition is associated with a high incidence of early pulmonary vascular obstructive disease. Because pulmonary and systemic circulations are in parallel, survival is impossible without mixing between the two circuits. The PDA and the patent foramen ovale are critically important. The majority of mixing occurs at the atrial and ductal levels. These communications are frequently inadequate at birth, and patients are therefore severely cyanotic.

Clinical Findings

A. Symptoms and Signs

Many neonates are large (up to 4 kg) and profoundly cyanotic without respiratory distress or a significant murmur. Infants with a large VSD may be less cyanotic and they usually have a prominent murmur. The findings on cardiovascular examination depend on the intracardiac defects. Obstruction to outflow from either ventricle is possible, and coarctation must be ruled out.

B. Imaging

The chest radiograph in transposition is usually nondiagnostic. Sometimes there is an "egg on a string" appearance because the aorta is directly anterior to the main pulmonary artery, giving the image of a narrow mediastinum.

C. Electrocardiography

Because the newborn ECG normally has RV predominance, the ECG in transposition is of little help, as it will frequently look normal.

D. Echocardiography

Two-dimensional imaging and Doppler evaluation demonstrate the anatomy and physiology well. The aorta arises from the RV and the pulmonary artery arises from the LV. Associated defects, such as a VSD, RV or LV outflow tract obstruction, or coarctation, must be evaluated. The atrial septum should be closely evaluated, as any restriction could prove detrimental as the child awaits repair. The coronary anatomy is variable and must be defined prior to surgery.

E. Cardiac Catheterization and Angiocardiography

A Rashkind balloon atrial septostomy is frequently performed in complete transposition to open the atrial septum no true ASD exists. The coronary anatomy can be delineated by ascending aortography if not well seen by echocardiography.

Treatment

Early corrective surgery is recommended. The arterial switch operation (ASO) has replaced the previously performed atrial switch procedures (Mustard and Senning operations). The ASO is performed at age 4–7 days. The arteries are switched in the anterior chest, and the coronaries are separately reimplanted. Small associated VSDs may be left to close on their own, but large VSDs are closed at this time. The atrial septum is also closed. The LV must be able to function against systemic vascular resistance, so the longer the LV faces only the falling pulmonary vascular resistance, the more deconditioned it becomes. For this reason, the ASO is rarely delayed beyond age 14 days in infants with an intact ventricular septum or small VSD. If a large, unrestrictive VSD is present to maintain LV pressure at systemic levels, the LV does not become deconditioned, and corrective surgery can be delayed for a few months. Surgery should still be performed by age 3–4 months because of the high risk of early pulmonary vascular disease associated with transposition.

Survival after the ASO is greater than 95% in major centers. The switch procedure greatly shortens the duration of severe cyanosis before corrective surgery. Early relief of cyanosis may improve the developmental outcome. Finally, the switch procedure leaves the LV as the systemic ventricle. The older atrial corrective procedures left the RV in this role and there was a significant late RV failure.

Bellinger DC et al: Developmental and neurological status of children at 4 years of age after heart surgery with hypothermic circulatory arrest or low flow cardiopulmonary bypass. Circulation 1999;100:526 [PMID: 10430767].

Cohen MS et al: Is the arterial switch operation as good over the long term as we thought it would be? Cardiol Young 2006;16(Suppl 3):117 [PMID: 17378050].

Warnes CA: Transposition of the great arteries. Circulation 2006;114:2699 [PMID: 17159076].

1. Congenitally Corrected Transposition of the Great Arteries

Congenitally corrected transposition of the great arteries (ccTGA) is a relatively uncommon congenital heart disease. Patients may present with cyanosis, depending on the associated lesions. In ccTGA, both atrioventricular and ventriculoarterial discordance occurs so that the right atrium connects to a morphologic LV, which supports the pulmonary artery. Conversely, the left atrium empties via a tricuspid valve into a morphologic RV, which supports the aorta. Common associated lesions are VSD and pulmonary stenosis. A dysplastic left-sided tricuspid valve is almost always present. In the absence of associated lesions, patients with ccTGA are often undiagnosed until adulthood when they present with left-sided AV valve insufficiency or arrhythmias.

Previously, surgical repair was directed at VSD closure and relief of pulmonary outflow tract obstruction—a technique that maintained the RV as the systemic ventricle supporting the aorta. It is now recognized that these patients have a reduced life span; thus other surgical techniques have been advocated. The double-switch procedure is one such technique. An atrial level switch (Mustard or Senning technique) is performed, in which pulmonary and systemic venous blood are baffled across the atrial mass in a way that prevents mixing and drains into the contralateral ventricle. An ASO then restores the morphologic LV to its position as systemic ventricle.

Patients with ccTGA have an increased incidence of complete heart block with an estimated risk of 1% per year and an overall frequency of 50%.

Bove EL et al: Anatomic correction of congenitally corrected transposition and its close cousins. Cardiol Young 2006;16(Suppl 3):85 [PMID: 17378045].

2. Double-Outlet Right Ventricle

In this uncommon malformation, both great arteries arise from the RV. There is always a VSD that allows blood to exit the LV. Presenting symptoms depend on the relationship of the VSD to the semilunar valves. The VSD can be in variable positions, and the great arteries could be normally related or malposed. In the absence of outflow obstruction, a large left-to-right shunt exists and the clinical picture resembles that of a large VSD. Pulmonary stenosis may be present, particularly if the VSD is remote from the pulmonary artery. This physiology is similar to ToF. Alternatively, if the VSD is nearer the pulmonary artery, aortic outflow may be obstructed (called the Taussig-Bing malformation). Early primary correction is the goal. LV flow is directed to the aorta across the VSD, and frequently an RV-pulmonary artery conduit is placed to maintain an unobstructed pulmonary circuit. If the aorta is far from the VSD, an arterial switch may be necessary. Echocardiography is usually sufficient to make the diagnosis and determine the orientation of the great vessels and their relationship to the VSD.

Cetta F et al: Double outlet right ventricle: Opinions regarding management. Curr Treat Options Cardiovasc Med 2005;7:385 [PMID: 16138957].

Kim N et al: Diagnosis and prognosis of fetuses with double outlet right ventricle. Prenat Diagn 2006;26:740 [PMID: 16807954].

TOTAL ANOMALOUS PULMONARY VENOUS RETURN

ESSENTIALS OF DIAGNOSIS & TYPICAL FEATURES

▶ Abnormal pulmonary venous connection *leading to* cyanosis.

▶ Occurs with or without murmur and may have accentuated P$_2$.

▶ Right atrial enlargement and RVH.

▶ General Considerations

This malformation accounts for 2% of all congenital heart lesions. The pulmonary venous blood drains into a confluence behind the left atrium, but the confluence is not connected to the left atrium. The pulmonary venous blood finds another route to rejoin the circulation via the larger systemic veins. This leads to complete mixing at the level of the right atrium. The presentation of total anomalous pulmonary venous return (TAPVR) depends on the route of return to the systemic circulation and whether or not the return is obstructed.

The malformation is classified by the site of entry of the pulmonary venous drainage into the right side of the heart. Supradiaphragmatic return is defined as a confluence that drains into the right superior vena cava, innominate vein or persistent left superior vena cava. In infradiaphragmatic return the confluence returns below the diaphragm usually into the portal venous system which empties into the inferior vena cava. Infradiaphragmatic pulmonary venous return is essentially always obstructed. It is a surgical emergency. Supradiaphragmatic veins may also be obstructed, though less commonly. Rarely, pulmonary veins can drain directly to the right atrium, or a single confluence may drain to more than one location, called mixed TAPVR.

Because the entire venous drainage from the body comes to the right atrium, a right-to-left shunt must be present at the atrial level, either as an ASD or a patent foramen ovale. Occasionally the atrial septum is restrictive and balloon septostomy is needed at birth to allow filling of the left heart.

▶ Clinical Findings

A. Unobstructed Pulmonary Venous Return

Patients with a large atrial communication tend to have high pulmonary blood flow and typically present with cardiomegaly and HF rather than cyanosis. Oxygen saturations in the high 80s or low 90s are common. Most patients in this group have mild to moderate elevation of pulmonary artery pressure owing to elevated pulmonary blood flow. In most instances, PA pressure does not reach systemic levels.

1. Symptoms and signs—Patients may have mild cyanosis in the neonatal period and early infancy. Thereafter, they do relatively well except for frequent respiratory infections. They are usually small and thin, resembling patients with other large left-to-right shunts. Examination discloses dusky nail beds and mucous membranes, but overt cyanosis and digital clubbing are usually absent. The arterial pulses are normal. An RV heave is palpable, and P_2 is increased. A systolic and diastolic murmur may be heard as a result of increased flow across the pulmonary and tricuspid valves, respectively.

2. Imaging—Chest radiography reveals cardiomegaly involving the right heart and pulmonary artery. Pulmonary vascular markings are increased. The characteristic cardiac contour called a "snowman" or "figure 8" is often seen when the anomalous veins drain via a persistent left superior vena cava to the innominate vein and then the right superior vena cava, but this is not apparent until about 3 months of age when the vertical and innominate vein have dilated.

3. Electrocardiography—ECG shows right axis deviation and varying degrees of right atrial enlargement and right ventricular hypertrophy. A qR pattern is often seen over the right precordial leads.

4. Echocardiography—Demonstration by echocardiography of a discrete chamber posterior to the left atrium is strongly suggestive of the diagnosis. The availability of two-dimensional echocardiography plus color-flow Doppler has increased diagnostic accuracy such that diagnostic cardiac catheterization is rarely required.

B. With Obstructed Pulmonary Venous Return

This group includes all patients with infradiaphragmatic TAPVR and a few of the patients in whom venous drainage is into a systemic vein above the diaphragm.

1. Symptoms and signs—Infants usually present shortly after birth with severe cyanosis and require early corrective surgery. Cardiac examination discloses a striking RV impulse. S_1 is accentuated and S_2 is markedly accentuated and single. There is no murmur in many cases. Sometimes, a systolic murmur is heard over the pulmonary area with radiation over the lung fields. Diastolic murmurs are uncommon.

2. Imaging—The heart is usually small and pulmonary venous congestion severe with associated air bronchograms. The chest radiographic appearance may lead to an erroneous diagnosis of severe lung disease. In less severe cases, the heart size may be normal or slightly enlarged with mild pulmonary venous congestion.

3. Electrocardiography—The ECG shows right axis deviation, right atrial enlargement, and RVH.

4. Echocardiography—Echocardiography shows a small left atrium and LV. For infradiaphragmatic TAPVR, appearance of a vessel lying parallel and anterior to the descending aorta and to the left of the inferior vena cava may represent the vein draining the confluence caudally toward the diaphragm. Color-flow Doppler echocardiography may reveal flow disturbance, commonly near the confluence or in the liver, where flow is obstructed.

5. Cardiac catheterization and angiocardiography— If echocardiography does not confirm the anatomy, cardiac catheterization and angiography demonstrate the site of entry of the anomalous veins. Catheterization can also assist in calculating the ratio of pulmonary to systemic blood flow and the degree of pulmonary hypertension and pulmonary vascular resistance.

▶ Treatment

Surgery is always required for TAPVR. If pulmonary venous return is obstructed, surgery must be performed immediately. In unobstructed TAPVR, surgery may be delayed for weeks to months. The timing of surgery is determined by the child's weight gain and the risk of pulmonary infection. If early surgery is not required and the atrial septum is restrictive, a balloon atrial septostomy can be performed in newborns.

▶ Course & Prognosis

Most children with TAPVR do well after surgery. Some surgical survivors develop late stenosis of the pulmonary veins. Pulmonary vein stenosis is an intractable condition that is difficult to treat either with interventional catheterization or surgery and has a poor prognosis. By avoiding direct suturing at the pulmonary venous ostia, the chance of recurrent stenosis at the anastomotic site is lessened. Unfortunately, any manipulation of the pulmonary veins increases the risk of stenosis.

Lacour-Gayet F: Surgery for pulmonary venous obstruction after repair of total anomalous pulmonary venous return. Semin Thorac Cardiovasc Surg Pediatr Card Surg Annu 2006;45 [PMID: 16638547].

TRUNCUS ARTERIOSUS

 ESSENTIALS OF DIAGNOSIS & TYPICAL FEATURES

▶ Early HF with or without cyanosis.
▶ Systolic ejection click.

▶ General Considerations

Truncus arteriosus accounts for less than 1% of congenital heart malformations. A single great artery arises from the heart, giving rise to the systemic, pulmonary, and coronary circulations. Truncus develops embryologically as a result of failure of the division of the common truncus arteriosus into the aorta and the pulmonary artery. A VSD is always present. The number of truncal valve leaflets varies from two to six, and the valve may be insufficient or stenotic.

Truncus arteriosus is divided into subtypes by the anatomy of the pulmonary circulation. A single main pulmonary artery may arise from the base of the trunk and gives rise to branch pulmonary arteries (type 1). Alternatively, the pulmonary arteries may arise separately from the common trunk, either in close association with one another (type 2) or widely separated (type 3).

In patients with truncus, blood from both ventricles leaves the heart through a single exit. Thus, oxygen saturation in the pulmonary artery is equal to that in the systemic arteries. The degree of systemic arterial oxygen saturation depends on the ratio of pulmonary to systemic blood flow. If pulmonary vascular resistance is normal, the pulmonary blood flow is greater than the systemic blood flow and the saturation is relatively high. If pulmonary vascular resistance is elevated because of pulmonary vascular obstructive disease or small pulmonary arteries, pulmonary blood flow is reduced and oxygen saturation is low. The systolic pressures are systemic in both ventricles.

▶ Clinical Findings

A. Symptoms and Signs

High pulmonary blood flow characterizes most patients with truncus arteriosus. These patients are usually acyanotic and present in HF. Examination of the heart reveals a hyperactive precordium. A systolic thrill is common at the lower left sternal border. A loud early systolic ejection click is commonly heard. S_2 is single and accentuated. A loud holosystolic murmur is audible at the left lower sternal border. A diastolic flow murmur can often be heard at the apex due to increased pulmonary venous return crossing the mitral valve. An additional diastolic murmur of truncal insufficiency may be present.

Patients with decreased pulmonary blood flow are cyanotic early. The most common manifestations are growth retardation, easy fatigability, and HF. The heart is not hyperactive. S_1 and S_2 are single and loud. A systolic murmur is heard at the lower left sternal border. No mitral flow murmur is heard, as pulmonary venous return is decreased. A loud systolic ejection click is commonly heard.

B. Imaging

The common radiographic findings are a boot-shaped heart, absence of the main pulmonary artery segment, and a large aorta that has a right arch 30% of the time. The pulmonary vascular markings vary with the degree of pulmonary blood flow.

C. Electrocardiography

The axis is usually normal. RVH or combined ventricular hypertrophy is commonly present.

D. Echocardiography

Images generally show override of a single great artery (similar to ToF, but no second great artery arises directly from the heart). The origin of the pulmonary arteries and the degree of truncal valve abnormality can be seen. Color-flow Doppler can aid in the description of pulmonary flow and the function of the truncal valve, both of which are critical to management.

E. Angiocardiography

Cardiac catheterization is not routinely performed but may be of value in older infants in whom pulmonary vascular disease must be ruled out. The single most important angiogram would be from the truncal root, as both the origin of the pulmonary arteries and the amount of truncal insufficiency would be seen from one injection.

▶ Treatment

Anticongestive measures are needed for patients with high pulmonary blood flow and congestive failure. Surgery is always required in this condition. Because of HF, surgery is usually performed in the neonatal period. The VSD is closed to allow LV egress to the truncal valve. The pulmonary artery (type 1) or arteries (types 2–3) are separated from the truncus as a block, and a valved conduit is fashioned from the RV to the pulmonary circulation.

▶ Course & Prognosis

Children with a good surgical result generally do well. Similar to patients with ToF, they almost always outgrow the RV-to-pulmonary artery conduit placed in infancy and require revision of the conduit in later childhood. The risk of early pulmonary vascular obstructive disease is high in the unrepaired patient and a decision to delay open-heart surgery beyond age 4–6 months is not wise even in stable patients.

Kalavrouziotis G et al: Truncus arteriosus communis: Early and midterm results of early primary repair. Ann Thorac Surg 2006;82;2200 [PMID: 17126135].

McElhinney DB et al: Reinterventions after repair of common arterial trunk in neonates and young infants. J Am Coll Cardiol 2000;35:1317 [PMID: 10758975].

▼ ACQUIRED HEART DISEASE

RHEUMATIC FEVER

Rheumatic fever remains a major cause of morbidity and mortality in developing countries that suffer from poverty, overcrowding, and poor access to health care. Even in developed countries, rheumatic fever has not been entirely eradicated. The overall incidence in the United States is less than 1 per 100,000. There have been regional resurgences, such as in Utah in the 1980s, with an incidence of nearly 12 per 100,000 children between the ages of 3 and 17 years.

Group A β-hemolytic streptococcal infection of the upper respiratory tract is the essential trigger in predisposed individuals. Only certain serotypes of group A *Streptococcus* cause rheumatic fever. The latest attempts to define host susceptibility implicate immune response genes that are present in approximately 15% of the population. The immune response triggered by colonization of the pharynx with group A streptococci consists of (1) sensitization of B lymphocytes by streptococcal antigens, (2) formation of antistreptococcal antibody, (3) formation of immune complexes that cross-react with cardiac sarcolemma antigens, and (4) myocardial and valvular inflammatory response.

The peak age of risk in the United States is 5–15 years. The disease is slightly more common in girls and in African Americans. The annual death rate from rheumatic heart disease in school-aged children (whites and nonwhites) recorded in the 1980s was less than 1 per 100,000.

▶ Clinical Findings

Two major or one major and two minor manifestations (plus supporting evidence of streptococcal infection) based on the modified Jones criteria are needed for the diagnosis of acute rheumatic fever (Table 19–14). Except in cases of rheumatic fever manifesting solely as Sydenham chorea or long-standing carditis, there should be clear evidence of a streptococcal infection such as scarlet fever, a positive throat

Table 19–14. Jones criteria (modified) for diagnosis of rheumatic fever.

Major manifestations
Carditis
Polyarthritis
Sydenham chorea
Erythema marginatum
Subcutaneous nodules
Minor manifestations
Clinical
Previous rheumatic fever or rheumatic heart disease
Polyarthralgia
Fever
Laboratory
Acute phase reaction: elevated erythrocyte sedimentation rate, C-reactive protein, leukocytosis
Prolonged PR interval
plus
Supporting evidence of preceding streptococcal infection, that is, increased titers of antistreptolysin O or other streptococcal antibodies, positive throat culture for group A *Streptococcus*

culture for group A β-hemolytic *Streptococcus*, and increased antistreptolysin O or other streptococcal antibody titers. The antistreptolysin O titer is significantly higher in rheumatic fever than in uncomplicated streptococcal infections.

A. Carditis

Carditis is the most serious consequence of rheumatic fever and varies from minimal to life-threatening HF. The term *carditis* implies pancardiac inflammation, but it may be limited to valves, myocardium, or pericardium. Valvulitis is frequently seen, with the mitral valve most commonly affected. Mitral insufficiency is the most common valvular residua of acute rheumatic carditis. Mitral stenosis after acute rheumatic fever is rarely encountered until 5–10 years after the first episode. Thus, mitral stenosis is much more commonly seen in adults than in children.

An early decrescendo diastolic murmur consistent with aortic insufficiency is occasionally encountered as the sole valvular manifestation of rheumatic carditis. The aortic valve is the second most common valve affected in polyvalvular as well as in single-valve disease. The aortic valve is involved more often in males and in African Americans. Dominant aortic stenosis of rheumatic origin does not occur in pediatric patients. In one large study, the shortest length of time observed for a patient to develop dominant aortic stenosis secondary to rheumatic heart disease was 20 years.

B. Polyarthritis

The large joints (knees, hips, wrists, elbows, and shoulders) are most commonly involved and the arthritis is typically migratory. Joint swelling and associated limitation of movement should be present. This is one of the more common major criteria, occurring in 80% of patients. Arthralgia alone is not a major criterion.

C. Sydenham Chorea

Sydenham chorea is characterized by involuntary and purposeless movements and is often associated with emotional lability. These symptoms become progressively worse and may be accompanied by ataxia and slurring of speech. Muscular weakness becomes apparent following the onset of the involuntary movements. Chorea is self-limiting, although it may last up to 3 months. Chorea may not be apparent for months to years after the acute episode of rheumatic fever.

D. Erythema Marginatum

A macular, serpiginous, erythematous rash with a sharply demarcated border appears primarily on the trunk and the extremities. The face is usually spared.

E. Subcutaneous Nodules

These usually occur only in severe cases, and then most commonly over the joints, scalp, and spinal column. The nodules vary from a few millimeters to 2 cm in diameter and are nontender and freely movable under the skin.

▶ Treatment & Prophylaxis

A. Treatment of the Acute Episode

1. Anti-infective therapy—Eradication of the streptococcal infection is essential. Long-acting benzathine penicillin is the drug of choice. Depending on the age and weight of the patient, give a single intramuscular injection of 0.6–1.2 million units; alternatively, give penicillin V, 125–250 mg orally four times a day for 10 days. Erythromycin, 250 mg orally four times a day, may be substituted if the patient is allergic to penicillin.

2. Anti-inflammatory agents

A. ASPIRIN—Aspirin, 30–60 mg/kg/d, is given in four divided doses. This dose is usually sufficient to effect dramatic relief of arthritis and fever. Higher dosages carry a greater risk of side effects and there are no proven short- or long-term benefits of high doses that produce salicylate blood levels of 20–30 mg/dL. The duration of therapy is tailored to meet the needs of the patient, but 2–6 weeks of therapy with reduction in dose toward the end of the course is usually sufficient. Other nonsteroidal anti-inflammatory agents used because of concerns about Reye syndrome are less effective than aspirin.

B. CORTICOSTEROIDS—Corticosteroids are seldom indicated except in the rare patient with severe carditis and HF, in whom they may be lifesaving. Steroids are given as follows: prednisone, 2 mg/kg/d orally for 2 weeks; reduce prednisone to 1 mg/kg/d during the third week, and begin aspirin, 50

mg/kg/d; stop prednisone at the end of 3 weeks, and continue aspirin for 8 weeks or until the C-reactive protein is negative and the sedimentation rate is falling.

3. Therapy in heart failure—Treatment for HF is based on symptoms and severity of valve involvement and cardiac dysfunction (see section on Heart Failure, earlier).

4. Bed rest and ambulation—Bed rest is not required in most cases. Activity level should be commensurate with symptoms and children should be allowed to self-limit their activity level while affected. Children should not return to school while there is clear evidence of rheumatic activity. Most acute episodes of rheumatic fever are managed on an outpatient basis.

B. Treatment after the Acute Episode

1. Prevention—Prevention is critical, as patients who have had rheumatic fever are at greater risk of recurrence if future group A β-hemolytic streptococcal infections are inadequately treated. Follow-up visits are essential to reinforce the necessity for prophylaxis with regular long-acting benzathine penicillin. Intramuscular rather than oral medication is associated with better adherence and is the preferred method of prophylaxis. If myocardial or valvular disease persists, antibacterial prophylaxis is a lifelong commitment. More commonly with transient or no cardiac involvement, 3–5 years of therapy or discontinuance in early adulthood (age 21) is an effective approach.

The following preventive regimens are in current use:

A. PENICILLIN G BENZATHINE—1.2 million units intramuscularly every 21–28 days is the drug of choice.

B. SULFADIAZINE—500 mg daily as a single oral dose for patients weighing more than 27 kg is the drug of second choice. Blood dyscrasias and lesser effectiveness in reducing streptococcal infections make this drug less satisfactory than penicillin benzathine G.

C. PENICILLIN V—250,000 units orally twice daily offers approximately the same protection afforded by sulfadiazine but is much less effective than intramuscular penicillin benzathine G (5.5 versus 0.4 streptococcal infections per 100 patient-years).

D. ERYTHROMYCIN—250 mg orally twice a day may be given to patients who are allergic to both penicillin and sulfonamides.

2. Residual valvular damage—As described above, the mitral and aortic valves are most commonly affected by rheumatic fever and the severity of carditis is quite variable. In the most severe cases, cardiac failure or the need for a valve replacement can occur in the acute setting. In less severe cases, valve abnormalities can persist, requiring lifelong medical management and eventual valve replacement. Other patients fully recover without residual cardiac sequelae.

Ayoub EM: Resurgence of rheumatic fever in the United States: The changing picture of a preventable illness. Postgrad Med 1992;92:139 [PMID: 1518750].

Cilliers AM: Rheumatic fever and its management. BMJ 2006;333:1153 [PMID: 17138996].

Dajani A et al: Treatment of acute streptococcal pharyngitis and prevention of rheumatic fever: A statement for health professionals. Committee on Rheumatic Fever, Endocarditis, and Kawasaki Disease of the Council on Cardiovascular Disease in the Young, the American Heart Association. Pediatrics 1996;96(4 Pt 1):758 [PMID: 7567345].

KAWASAKI DISEASE

Kawasaki disease was first described in Japan in 1967 and was initially called mucocutaneous lymph node syndrome. The cause is unclear and there is no specific diagnostic test. Kawasaki disease is the leading cause of acquired heart disease in children in the United States. Eighty percent of patients are younger than 5 years old (median age at diagnosis is 2 years), and the male-to-female ratio is 1.5:1. Diagnostic criteria are fever for more than 5 days and at least four of the following features: (1) bilateral, painless, nonexudative conjunctivitis; (2) lip or oral cavity changes (eg, lip cracking and fissuring, strawberry tongue, and inflammation of the oral mucosa); (3) cervical lymphadenopathy ≥ 1.5 cm in diameter and usually unilateral); (4) polymorphous exanthema; and (5) extremity changes (redness and swelling of the hands and feet with subsequent desquamation). Clinical features not part of the diagnostic criteria, but frequently associated with Kawasaki disease, are shown in Table 19–15.

The potential for cardiovascular complications is the most serious aspect of Kawasaki disease. Complications during the acute illness include myocarditis, pericarditis, valvular heart disease (usually mitral or aortic regurgitation), and coronary arteritis. Patients with fever for at least 5 days

Table 19–15. Noncardiac manifestations of Kawaski disease.

System	Associated Signs and Symptoms
Gastrointestinal	Vomiting, diarrhea, gallbladder hydrops, elevated transaminases
Blood	Elevated ESR or CRP, leukocytosis, hypoalbuminemia, mild anemia in acute phase and thrombocytosis in subacute phase (usually second to third week of illness)
Renal	Sterile pyuria, proteinuria
Respiratory	Cough, rhinorrhea, infiltrate on chest radiograph
Joint	Arthralgia and arthritis
Neurologic	Mononuclear pleocytosis of cerebrospinal fluid, irritability, facial palsy

CRP, C-reactive protein; ESR, erythrocyte sedimentation rate.

but fewer than four of the diagnostic features can be diagnosed with atypical Kawasaki disease if they have coronary artery abnormalities detected by echocardiography.

Coronary artery lesions range from mild transient dilation of a coronary artery to large aneurysms. Aneurysms rarely form before day 10 of illness. Untreated patients have a 15–25% risk of developing coronary aneurysms. Those at greatest risk of aneurysm are males, young children (< 6 months), and those not treated with intravenous immunoglobulin (IVIG). Most coronary artery aneurysms resolve within 5 years of diagnosis; however, as aneurysms resolve, associated obstruction or stenosis (19% of all aneurysms) may develop, which may result in coronary ischemia. Giant aneurysms (> 8 mm) are less likely to resolve, and nearly 50% eventually become stenotic. Of additional concern, acute thrombosis of an aneurysm can occur, resulting in myocardial infarction that is fatal in approximately 20% of cases.

▶ Treatment

Immediate management of Kawasaki disease is IVIG and high-dose aspirin. This therapy is effective in decreasing the incidence of coronary artery dilation and aneurysm formation. The currently recommended regimen is 2 g/kg of IVIG administered over 10–12 hours and 80–100 mg/kg/d of aspirin in four divided doses. The duration of high-dose aspirin is institution-dependent: many centers reduce the dose once the patient is afebrile for 48–72 hours; others continue through day 14 of the illness. Once high-dose aspirin is discontinued, low-dose aspirin (3–5 mg/kg/d) is given through the subacute phase of the illness (6–8 weeks) or until coronary artery abnormalities resolve. If fever recurs within 48–72 hours of the initial treatment course and no other source of the fever is detected, a second dose of IVIG is often recommended; however, the effectiveness of this approach has not been clearly demonstrated. A recent multicenter, randomized, double-blind, placebo-controlled study (Newburger et al) demonstrated no beneficial effect of pulsed corticosteroids on the development of coronary abnormalities in patients responsive to IVIG. However, corticosteroids should be considered for patients with persistent fever despite at least two infusions of IVIG.

Follow-up of patients with treated Kawasaki disease depends on the degree of coronary involvement. In those with no or minimal coronary disease at the time of diagnosis, an echocardiogram 2 weeks and again 6–8 weeks after diagnosis is sufficient. Repeat echocardiography more than 8 weeks after diagnosis in those with no coronary abnormalities is optional. In 2004, the AHA published updated guidelines for the long-term management of Kawasaki disease based on the risk level of the patient. The risk stratification and recommended follow-up can be reviewed in Table 19–16.

Burns JC et al: Intravenous gamma-globulin treatment and retreatment in Kawasaki disease. US/Canadian Kawasaki Syndrome Group. Pediatr Infect Dis J 1998;17:1144 [PMID: 9877364].

Table 19–16. Long-term management in Kawasaki disease.

Risk Level	Definition	Management Guidelines
I	No coronary artery changes at any stage of the illness	No ASA is needed beyond the sub-acute phase (6–8 wk). No follow-up beyond the first year.
II	Transient ectasia of coronary arteries during the acute phase	Same as above, or clinical follow-up ± ECG every 3–5 y.
III	Single small to medium coronary aneurysm	ASA until abnormality resolves. Annual follow-up with ECG and echo if younger than age 10 y and every-other-year stress testing if older than 10 y.
IV	Giant aneurysm or multiple small to medium aneurysms without obstruction	Long-term ASA ± warfarin. Annual follow-up with ECG, echo, and stress testing (in those older than 20 y).
V	Coronary artery obstruction	Long-term ASA ± warfarin ± calcium channel blocker to reduce myocardial oxygen consumption. Echo and ECG every 6 months. Stress testing and Holter examination annually.

ASA, acetyl salicylic acid; ECG, electrocardiogram; echo, echocardiogram.

Kavey RE et al: Cardiovascular risk reduction in high-risk pediatric patients: A scientific statement from the American Heart Association. Circulation 2006;114:2710 [PMID: 17545824].

Newburger JW et al: Diagnosis, treatment, and long-term management of Kawasaki disease: A statement for health professionals from the Committee on Rheumatic Fever, Endocarditis, and Kawasaki Disease, Council on Cardiovascular Disease in the Young, American Heart Association. Circulation 2004;110:2747 [PMID: 15574639].

Newburger JW et al: Randomized trial of pulsed corticosteroid therapy for primary treatment of Kawasaki disease. N Engl J Med 2007;356:663 [PMID: 17301297].

CARDIOMYOPATHY

The three most common forms of cardiomyopathy in children are (1) dilated, (2) hypertrophic, and (3) restrictive. Two other cardiomyopathies recently classified as distinct entities include arrhythmogenic right ventricular dysplasia (ARVD) and left ventricular noncompaction.

1. Dilated Cardiomyopathy

This most frequent of the childhood cardiomyopathies occurs with an annual incidence of 4–8 cases per 100,000 population in the United States and Europe. Although usually idiopathic, identifiable causes of dilated cardiomyopathy

(DCM) include viral myocarditis, untreated tachyarrhythmias, left heart obstructive lesions, congenital abnormalities of the coronary arteries, toxicity (eg, anthracycline), and genetic (eg, dystrophin gene defects, responsible for Duchenne and Becker muscular dystrophies) and metabolic diseases (inborn errors of fatty acid oxidation and mitochondrial oxidative phosphorylation defects). Genetic causes are being discovered at an increasing rate with commercial testing now available for some of the more common genes.

▶ **Clinical Findings**

A. Signs and Symptoms

As myocardial function fails and the heart dilates, cardiac output falls, and affected children develop decreased exercise tolerance, failure to thrive, diaphoresis, and tachypnea. As the heart continues to deteriorate, congestive signs such as hepatomegaly and rales develop, and a prominent gallop can be appreciated on examination. The initial diagnosis in a previously healthy child can be difficult, as presenting symptoms can resemble a viral respiratory infection, pneumonia, or asthma.

B. Imaging

Chest radiograph shows generalized cardiomegaly with or without pulmonary venous congestion.

C. Electrocardiography

Sinus tachycardia with ST-T segment changes is commonly seen on ECG. The criteria for right and left ventricular hypertrophy may also be met. Evaluation for the presence of supraventricular arrhythmias on ECG is critical, as this is one of the few treatable and reversible causes of DCM in children.

D. Echocardiography

The echocardiogram shows LV and left atrial enlargement with decreased LV shortening fraction and ejection fraction. The calculated end-diastolic and end-systolic dimensions are increased and mitral insufficiency is commonly seen. A careful evaluation for evidence of structural abnormalities (especially coronary artery anomalies) must be performed in infant patients.

E. Other Testing

Cardiac catheterization is useful to evaluate hemodynamic status and coronary artery anatomy. Endomyocardial biopsies can aid in diagnosis. Biopsy specimens may show inflammation consistent with acute myocarditis, abnormal myocyte architecture and myocardial fibrosis. Electron micrographs may reveal evidence of mitochondrial or other metabolic disorders. Polymerase chain reaction (PCR) testing may be performed on biopsied specimens to detect viral genome products in infectious myocarditis. Skeletal muscle biopsy may be helpful in patients with evidence of skeletal muscle involvement. Cardiopulmonary stress testing is useful for measuring response to medical therapy and as an objective assessment of the cardiac limitations on exercise.

▶ Treatment & Prognosis

Outpatient management of pediatric DCM usually entails combinations of afterload-reducing agents, digoxin, and diuretics (see section on Heart Failure, earlier). A recently completed multicenter, placebo-controlled, double-blind trial of carvedilol in children with HF will help determine the efficacy of β-blocker therapy as an adjunct in these patients. Aspirin or warfarin may be used to prevent thrombus formation in the dilated and poorly contractile cardiac chambers. Arrhythmias are more common in dilated hearts. Antiarrhythmic agents that do not suppress myocardial contractility, such as amiodarone, are used. Despite widespread use of internal defibrillators in the adult population, the technical difficulty of implanting internal defibrillators and the risk of adverse events (eg, inappropriate discharge) in children limit their use.

Therapy of the underlying cause of cardiomyopathy is always indicated if possible. Unfortunately despite complete evaluation, a diagnosis is discovered in less than 30% of patients with DCM. If medical management is unsuccessful, cardiac transplantation is considered.

2. Hypertrophic Cardiomyopathy

The most common cause of hypertrophic cardiomyopathy (HCM) is familial hypertrophic cardiomyopathy, which is found in 1 in 500 individuals. HCM is the leading cause of sudden cardiac death in young persons. The most common presentation is an older child, adolescent, or adult, although it may occur in neonates. Other causes of HCM in neonates and children are glycogen storage disease, Noonan syndrome, Friedreich ataxia, maternal gestational diabetes, mitochondrial disorders, and other metabolic disorders.

A. Familial Hypertrophic Cardiomyopathy

In the familial form, HCM is most commonly caused by a mutation in one of the several genes that encode proteins of the cardiac sarcomere (B-myosin heavy chain, cardiac troponin T or I, α-tropomyosin, and myosin-binding protein C).

1. Clinical findings—Patients may be asymptomatic despite having significant hypertrophy, or may present with symptoms of inadequate coronary perfusion such as angina, syncope, palpitations, or exercise intolerance. Patients may experience sudden cardiac death as their initial presentation, often precipitated by sporting activities. Although the cardiac examination may be normal on presentation, eventually patients develop a left precordial bulge with a diffuse point of maximal impulse. An LV heave or an S_4 gallop may be present. If outflow tract obstruction exists, a systolic ejection murmur will be audible. A murmur may not be audible at rest but may be provoked with exercise or positional maneuvers that decrease left ventricular volume (standing) thereby increasing the outflow tract obstruction.

A. ECHOCARDIOGRAPHY—The diagnosis of HCM is usually made by echocardiography and in most familial cases demonstrates asymmetrical septal hypertrophy. Young patients with metabolic or other nonfamilial causes are more likely to have concentric hypertrophy. Systolic anterior motion of the mitral valve leaflet may occur and contribute to LV outflow tract obstruction. The mitral valve leaflet may become distorted and cause mitral insufficiency over time. LV outflow tract obstruction may be present at rest or provoked with either amyl nitrate or monitored exercise. Systolic function is most often hypercontractile in young children but may deteriorate over time, resulting in poor contractility and LV dilation. Diastolic function is almost always abnormal.

B. ELECTROCARDIOGRAPHY—The ECG may be normal, but more typically demonstrates deep Q waves in the inferolateral leads (II, III, aVF, V_5, and V_6) secondary to the increased mass of the hypertrophied septum. ST segment abnormalities may be seen in the same leads. Age-dependent criteria for LVH are often present as are criteria for left atrial enlargement.

C. OTHER TESTING—Cardiopulmonary stress testing is valuable to evaluate for provocable LV outflow tract obstruction, ischemia, and arrhythmias, and to determine prognosis. A blunted blood pressure response and ventricular arrhythmias with exercise have both been associated with increased mortality in children. Nuclear stress testing allows for assessment of myocardial perfusion defects. Patients are at risk for myocardial ischemia, possibly as a result of systolic compression of the intramyocardial septal perforators, myocardial bridging of epicardial coronary arteries, or an imbalance of coronary artery supply and demand due to the presence of massive myocardial hypertrophy.

D. CARDIAC CATHETERIZATION—Cardiac catheterization should be performed in patients with HCM who have angina, syncope, resuscitated sudden death, or a worrisome stress test. Hemodynamic findings include elevated left atrial pressure secondary to impaired diastolic filling. If midcavitary LV outflow tract obstruction is present, an associated pressure gradient will be evident. Provocation of LV outflow tract obstruction with either rapid atrial pacing or isoproterenol may be sought. Angiography demonstrates a "ballerina slipper" configuration of the LV secondary to the midcavitary LV obliteration during systole. The myocardial biopsy specimen demonstrates myofiber disarray.

2. Treatment and prognosis—Treatment varies depending on symptoms and phenotype. Patients are usually restricted from competitive athletics and isometric exercise. Patients with resting or latent LV outflow tract obstruction may be treated with β-blockers, verapamil, or disopyramide with variable success in alleviating obstruction. Patients with severe symptoms despite medical therapy and an LV outflow tract gradient may require additional intervention. Surgical myectomy with resection of part of the hypertrophied septum has been used with good results. At the time of myectomy, the mitral valve may require repair or replacement in patients with a long history of systolic anterior motion of the mitral valve. Ethanol ablation is being used increasingly in adults with HCM and LV outflow tract obstruction. This procedure involves selective infiltration of ethanol in a coronary septal artery branch to induce a small myocardial infarction. This leads to a reduction in septal size and improvement of obstruction. The long-term effects of this procedure are unknown and it is not currently employed in children. Although dual-chamber pacing has been used in children with good relief of obstruction, larger series demonstrate no significant improvement in obstruction. Risk stratification with respect to sudden death is important in HCM. Internal defibrillators are placed in patients with severe hypertrophy (> 3 cm septal thickness in adults), documented ventricular arrhythmias, resuscitated sudden death, or a strong family history of HCM with associated sudden death.

B. Glycogen Storage Disease of the Heart

There are at least 10 types of glycogen storage disease. The type that primarily involves the heart is Pompe disease (GSD IIa) in which acid maltase, necessary for hydrolysis of the outer branches of glycogen, is absent. There is marked deposition of glycogen within the myocardium. Affected infants are well at birth, but symptoms of growth and developmental delay, feeding problems, and cardiac failure occur by the sixth month of life. Physical examination reveals generalized muscular weakness, a large tongue, and cardiomegaly without significant heart murmurs. Chest radiographs reveal cardiomegaly with or without pulmonary venous congestion. The ECG shows a short PR interval and LVH with ST depression and T-wave inversion over the left precordial leads. Echocardiography shows severe concentric LVH. Children with Pompe disease usually die before age 1 year. Death may be sudden or result from progressive HF.

3. Restrictive Cardiomyopathy

Restrictive cardiomyopathy is a rare entity in the pediatric population, accounting for less than 5% of all cases of cardiomyopathy. The cause is usually idiopathic but can be familial or secondary to an infiltrative process (eg, amyloidosis).

▶ Clinical Findings

Patients present with signs of HF as outlined previously. Physical examination is remarkable for a prominent S_4 and jugular venous distention.

A. Electrocardiography

ECG demonstrates marked right and left atrial enlargement with normal ventricular voltages. ST-T–wave abnormalities including a prolonged QTc interval may be present.

B. Echocardiography

The diagnosis is confirmed echocardiographically by the presence of normal sized ventricles with normal systolic function and massively dilated atria. Cardiac MRI is useful in ruling out pericardial abnormalities that can result in similar echocardiographic and clinical findings consistent with restrictive or constrictive pericarditis.

▶ Treatment & Prognosis

Anticongestive therapy is used for symptomatic relief. The high risk of sudden death in restrictive cardiomyopathy and the propensity for rapid progression of pulmonary hypertension warrant close follow-up with early consideration of cardiac transplantation in most patients.

Colan SD et al: Epidemiology and cause-specific outcome of hypertrophic cardiomyopathy in children: Findings from the Pediatric Cardiomyopathy Registry. Circulation 2007;115:773 [PMID: 17261650].

Malcíc I et al: Epidemiology of cardiomyopathies in children and adolescents: A retrospective study over the last 10 years. Cardiol Young 2002;12:253 [PMID: 12365172].

Maron BJ et al: American College of Cardiology/European Society of Cardiology clinical expert consensus document on hypertrophic cardiomyopathy. J Am Coll Cardiol 2003;42:1687 [PMID: 14607462].

Towbin JA et al: Incidence, causes, and outcomes of dilated cardiomyopathy in children. JAMA 2006;296:1867 [PMID: 17047217].

MYOCARDITIS

The most common causes of viral myocarditis are adenovirus, coxsackie A and B viruses, echovirus, cytomegalovirus, parvovirus, and influenza A virus. Human immunodeficiency virus can also cause myocarditis. The ability to identify the pathogen has been enhanced by PCR technology, which replicates identifiable segments of the viral genome from the myocardium of affected children.

▶ Clinical Findings

A. Symptoms and Signs

There are two major clinical patterns. In the first, sudden-onset HF occurs in an infant or child who was relatively healthy 12–24 hours previously. This malignant form of the disease is usually secondary to overwhelming viremia with tissue invasion in multiple organ systems including the heart. In the second pattern, the onset of cardiac symptoms is gradual and there is often a history of upper respiratory tract infection or gastroenteritis in the previous month. This more insidious form may have a late postinfectious or autoimmune component. Acute and chronic presentations occur at any age and with all types of myocarditis.

The signs of HF include pale gray skin; rapid, weak, and thready pulses; and edema of the face and extremities.

Patients are breathless and often orthopneic. The heart sounds may be muffled and distant, an S_3 or S_4 gallop (or both) are common. Murmurs are usually absent, although a murmur of tricuspid or mitral insufficiency may be heard. Moist rales are usually present at both lung bases. The liver is enlarged and frequently tender.

B. Imaging

Generalized cardiomegaly is seen on radiographs along with moderate to marked pulmonary venous congestion.

C. Electrocardiography

The ECG is variable. Classically, there is low-voltage QRS in all frontal and precordial leads with ST-segment depression and inversion of T waves in leads I, III, and aVF (and in the left precordial leads during the acute stage). Dysrhythmias are common, and AV and intraventricular conduction disturbances may be present.

D. Echocardiography

Echocardiography demonstrates four-chamber dilation with poor ventricular function and AV valve regurgitation. A pericardial effusion may be present.

E. Myocardial Biopsy

An endomyocardial biopsy may be helpful in the diagnosis of viral myocarditis. An inflammatory infiltrate with myocyte damage can be seen by hematoxylin and eosin staining. Viral PCR testing of the biopsy specimen may yield a positive result in 30–40% of patients suspected to have myocarditis.

▶ Treatment

The use of digitalis in a rapidly deteriorating child with myocarditis is dangerous and should be undertaken with great caution, as it may cause ventricular dysrhythmias. The inpatient cardiac support measures outlined previously in the section on heart failure are used in the treatment of these patients.

Administration of immunomodulating medications such as corticosteroids for myocarditis is controversial. If the patient's condition deteriorates despite anticongestive measures, corticosteroids are commonly used, although conclusive data supporting their effectiveness are lacking. Subsequent to the successful use of IVIG in children with Kawasaki disease, there have been several trials of IVIG in presumed viral myocarditis. The therapeutic value of IVIG remains unconfirmed.

▶ Prognosis

The prognosis of myocarditis is determined by the age at onset and the response to therapy. In patients younger than 6 months or older than 3 years with poor response to therapy, the prognosis is poor. Although complete recovery is possible, many patients recover clinically but have persistent LV dysfunction and a need for ongoing medical therapy for HF. It is possible that subclinical myocarditis in childhood is the pathophysiologic basis for some of the idiopathic dilated cardiomyopathies later in life. Children with myocarditis whose ventricular function fails to return to normal may be candidates for cardiac transplantation.

Baboonian C, McKenna W: Eradication of viral myocarditis: Is there hope? J Am Coll Cardiol 2003;42:473 [PMID: 12906975].

Bowles NE et al: Detection of viruses in myocardial tissues by polymerase chain reaction. Evidence of adenovirus as a common cause of myocarditis in children and adults. J Am Coll Cardiol 2003;42:466 [PMID: 12906974].

Mahrholdt H et al: Presentation, patterns of myocardial damage, and clinical course of viral myocarditis. Circulation 2006;114:1581 [PMID: 17015795].

INFECTIVE ENDOCARDITIS

 ESSENTIALS OF DIAGNOSIS & TYPICAL FEATURES

▶ Positive blood culture.

▶ Intracardiac oscillating mass, abscess, or new valve regurgitation on echocardiogram.

▶ Fever.

▶ Elevated erythrocyte sedimentation rate or C-reactive protein.

▶ General Considerations

Bacterial or fungal infection of the endocardium of the heart is rare and usually occurs in the setting of a preexisting abnormality of the heart or great arteries. It may occur in a normal heart during septicemia or as a consequence of infected indwelling central catheters.

The frequency of infective endocarditis (IE) appears to be increasing for a several reasons: (1) increased survival in children with congenital heart disease, (2) greater use of central venous catheters, and (3) increased use of prosthetic material and valves. Pediatric patients without preexisting heart disease are also at increased risk for IE because of (1) increased survival rates for children with immune deficiencies, (2) long-term use of indwelling lines in ill newborns and patients with chronic diseases, and (3) increased intravenous drug abuse.

Patients at greatest risk are children with unrepaired or palliated cyanotic heart disease (especially in the presence of an aorta to pulmonary shunt), those with implanted prosthetic material, and patients who have had a prior episode of IE. Common organisms causing IE are viridans streptococci

(30–40% of cases), *Staphylococcus aureus* (25–30%), and fungal agents (about 5%).

Clinical Findings

A. History

Almost all patients with IE have a history of heart disease. There may or may not be an antecedent infection or surgical procedure (cardiac surgery, tooth extraction, tonsillectomy). Transient bacteremia occurs frequently during normal daily activities such as flossing or brushing teeth, using a toothpick and even when chewing food. Although dental and nonsterile surgical procedures also can result in transient bacteremias these episodes are much less frequent for a given individual. This may be why a clear inciting event is often not identified in association with IE.

B. Symptoms, Signs, and Laboratory Findings

Although IE can present in a fulminant fashion with cardiovascular collapse, often it presents in an indolent manner with fever, malaise, and weight loss. Joint pain and vomiting are less common. On physical examination, there may be a new or changing murmur, splenomegaly and hepatomegaly. Classic findings of Osler nodes (tender nodules, usually on the pulp of the fingers), Janeway lesions (nontender hemorrhage macules on palms and soles), splinter hemorrhages, and Roth spots (retinal hemorrhage) are rarely noted. Laboratory findings include positive blood culture, elevated erythrocyte sedimentation rate or C-reactive protein, and hematuria. Transthoracic echocardiography can identify large vegetations in some patients, but transesophageal imaging has better sensitivity and may be necessary if the diagnosis remains in question.

Prevention

In 2007, the AHA revised criteria for patients requiring prophylaxis for IE (Table 19–17). Only these high-risk patients require antibiotics before dental work (tooth extraction or cleaning) and procedures involving the respiratory tract or infected skin or musculoskeletal structures. IE prophylaxis is *not* recommended for gastrointestinal or genitourinary procedures, body piercing, or tattooing.

Table 19-17. Conditions requiring antibiotic prophylaxis for the prevention of infective endocarditis (IE).

Prosthetic cardiac valves
Prior episode of IE
Congenital heart disease (CHD)
Palliated cyanotic CHD
For 6 months post-procedure if CHD repair involves implanted prosthetic material
Repair of CHD with residual defect bordered by prosthetic material
Cardiac transplant with valvulopathy

The following schedule is recommended: under 40 kg, 50 mg/kg of oral amoxicillin; over 40 kg, 2000 mg. This dose is to be given 1 hour prior to the above defined procedures. If the patient is allergic to amoxicillin, an alternative prophylactic antibiotic is used.

Treatment

In general appropriate antibiotic therapy should be initiated as soon as IE is suspected. Therapy can be tailored once the pathogen and sensitivities are defined. Vancomycin, with or without gentamicin, for a 6-week course is the most common regimen. If HF occurs and progresses in the face of adequate antibiotic therapy, surgical excision of the infected area and prosthetic valve replacement must be considered.

Course & Prognosis

Factors associated with a poor outcome are delayed diagnosis, presence of prosthetic material, perioperative associated IE and *S aureus* infection. Mortality for bacterial endocarditis in children ranges from 10–25% with fungal infections having a much greater mortality at 50% or more.

Ferrieri P et al: Unique features of infective endocarditis in childhood. Circulation 2002;105:2115 [PMID: 11980694].

Wilson W et al: Prevention of infective endocarditis: Guidelines from the American Heart Association: a guideline from the American Heart Association Rheumatic Fever, Endocarditis, and Kawasaki Disease Committee, Council on Cardiovascular Disease in the Young, and the Council on Clinical Cardiology, Council on Cardiovascular Surgery and Anesthesia, and the Quality of Care and Outcomes Research Interdisciplinary Working Group. Circulation. 2007;116:1736 [PMID: 17446442].

PERICARDITIS

ESSENTIALS OF DIAGNOSIS & TYPICAL FEATURES

▶ Chest pain made worse by deep inspiration and decreased by leaning forward.
▶ Fever and tachycardia.
▶ Shortness of breath.
▶ Pericardial friction rub.
▶ ECG with elevated ST segments.

General Considerations

Pericarditis is an inflammation of the pericardium and is commonly related to an infectious process. The most common cause of pericarditis in children is viral infection (eg, coxsackievirus, mumps, Epstein-Barr, adenovirus, influenza, and HIV). Purulent pericarditis results from bacterial infection (eg, pneumococci, streptococci, staphylococci, and *Haemophilus influenzae*) and is less common but potentially life-threatening.

In some cases, pericardial disease occurs in association with a generalized process. Associations include rheumatic fever, rheumatoid arthritis, uremia, systemic lupus erythematosus, malignancy, and tuberculosis. Pericarditis after cardiac surgery (postpericardiotomy syndrome) is most commonly seen after surgical closure of an ASD. Postpericardiotomy syndrome appears to be autoimmune in nature with high titers of anti-heart antibody and evidence of fresh or reactivated viral illness. The syndrome is often self-limited and responds well to short courses of aspirin or corticosteroids.

▶ Clinical Findings

A. Symptoms and Signs

Childhood pericarditis usually presents with sharp stabbing mid chest, shoulder, and neck pain made worse by deep inspiration or coughing, and decreased by sitting up and leaning forward. Shortness of breath and grunting respirations are common. Physical findings depend on the presence of fluid accumulation in the pericardial space (effusion). In the absence of significant accumulation, a characteristic scratchy, high-pitched friction rub may be heard. If the effusion is large, heart sounds are distant and muffled. A friction rub may not be present. In the absence of cardiac tamponade, the peripheral, venous, and arterial pulses are normal.

Cardiac tamponade occurs in association with a large effusion, or one that has rapidly accumulated. Tamponade is characterized by jugular venous distention, tachycardia, hepatomegaly, peripheral edema, and pulsus paradoxus, in which systolic blood pressure drops more than 10 mm Hg during inspiration. Decreased cardiac filling and subsequent decrease in cardiac output result in signs of right heart failure and the potential for cardiovascular collapse.

B. Imaging

In pericarditis with a significant pericardial effusion the cardiac silhouette is enlarged. The cardiac silhouette can appear normal if the effusion has developed over an extremely short period of time.

C. Electrocardiography

The ST segments are commonly elevated in acute pericarditis. Low voltages or electrical alternans (alteration in QRS amplitude between beats) can be seen with large pericardial effusions.

D. Echocardiography

Echocardiography is essential in diagnosis and management of pericarditis. Serial studies allow direct, noninvasive estimate of the volume of fluid and its change over time. Echocardiography also demonstrates cardiac tamponade if there is compression of the atria or respiratory alteration of ventricular inflow.

▶ Treatment

Treatment depends on the cause of pericarditis and the size of associated effusion. Viral pericarditis is usually self-limited and symptoms can be improved with nonsteroidal anti-inflammatory therapy. Purulent pericarditis requires immediate evacuation of the fluid and appropriate antibiotic therapy. Cardiac tamponade from any cause must be treated by immediate removal of the fluid, usually via pericardiocentesis. Pericardiocentesis should also be considered if the underlying cause is unclear or identification of the pathogen is necessary for targeted therapy. In the setting of recurrent or persistent effusions, a surgical pericardiectomy or pericardial window may be necessary. Diuretics should be avoided in the patient with cardiac tamponade because they reduce ventricular preload and can exacerbate the degree of cardiac decompensation.

▶ Prognosis

Prognosis depends to a great extent on the cause of pericardial disease. Constrictive pericarditis can develop following infectious pericarditis (especially if bacterial) and can be a difficult problem to manage. Cardiac tamponade will result in death unless the fluid is evacuated.

Cakir O et al: Purulent pericarditis in childhood: Ten years of experience. J Pediatr Surg 2002;37:1404 [PMID: 12378443].
Demmler GJ: Infectious pericarditis in children. Pediatr Infect Dis J 2006;25:165 [PMID: 16462296].
Roodpeyma S, Sadeghian N: Acute pericarditis in childhood: A 10-year experience. Pediatr Cardiol 2000;21:363 [PMID: 10865014].

HYPERTENSION

Blood pressure should be determined at every pediatric visit beginning at 3 years. Because blood pressure is being more carefully monitored, systemic hypertension has become more widely recognized as a pediatric problem. Pediatric standards for blood pressure have been published. Blood pressures in children must be obtained when the child is relaxed and an appropriate-size cuff must always be used. The widest cuff that fits between the axilla and the antecubital fossa should be used (covers 60–75% of the upper arm). Most children aged 10–11 years need a standard adult cuff (bladder width of 12 cm), and many high school students need a large adult cuff (width of 16 cm) or leg cuff (width of 18 cm). The pressure coinciding with the onset (K_1) and the loss (K_5) of the Korotkoff sounds determine the systolic and diastolic blood pressure respectively. The 95th percentile value for blood pressure (Table 19–18) is similar for both sexes and all three major ethnic groups. If a properly measured blood pressure exceeds the 95th percentile, the measurement should be repeated several times over a 2- to 4-week interval. If it is elevated persistently, a search for the

Table 19–18. The 95th percentile value for blood pressure (mm Hg) taken in the sitting position.[a]

Age (y)	Sea Level			10,000 ft		
	S	Dm	Dd	S	Dm	Dd
5				92	72	62
6	106	64	60	96	74	66
7	108	72	66	98	76	70
8	110	76	70	104	80	70
9	114	80	76	106	80	70
10	118	82	76	108	80	70
11	124	82	78	108	80	72
12	128	84	78	108	80	72
13	132	84	80	116	84	76
14	136	86	80	120	84	76
15	140	88	80	120	84	80
16	140	90	80	120	84	80
17	140	92	80	122	84	80
18	140	92	80	130	84	80

[a]Blood pressures: S, systolic (Korotkoff sound 1; onset of tapping); Dm, diastolic muffling (Korotkoff sound 4); Dd, diastolic disappearance (Korotkoff sound 5).

cause should be undertaken. Although most hypertension in children is essential, the incidence of treatable causes is higher in children than in adults; these include conditions such as coarctation of the aorta, renal artery stenosis, chronic renal disease, and pheochromocytoma, as well as medication side effects (eg, steroids). If no cause is identified, and hypertension is deemed essential, antihypertensive therapy should be initiated and nutritional and exercise counseling given. β-Blockers or ACE inhibitors are the usual first-line medical therapies for essential hypertension in children.

Falkner B, Daniels SR: Summary of the Fourth Report on the Diagnosis, Evaluation, and Treatment of High Blood Pressure in Children and Adolescents. Hypertension 2004;44:387 [PMID: 15353515].

Gidding SS et al. Higher self-reported physical activity is associated with lower systolic blood pressure: The Dietary Intervention Study in Childhood (DISC). Pediatrics 2006;118:2388 [PMID: 17142523].

ATHEROSCLEROSIS & DYSLIPIDEMIAS

Awareness of coronary artery risk factors in general—and atherosclerosis in particular—has risen dramatically in the general population since the mid-1970s. Although coronary artery disease is still the leading cause of death in the United States, the age-adjusted incidence of death from ischemic heart disease has been decreasing as a result of improved diet, decreased smoking, awareness and treatment of hypertension, and an increase in physical activity. The level of serum lipids in childhood usually remains constant through adolescence. Biochemical abnormalities in the lipid profile appearing early in childhood correlate with higher risk for coronary artery disease in adulthood. Low-density lipoprotein (LDL) is atherogenic, while its counterpart, high-density lipoprotein (HDL) has been identified as an anti-atherogenic factor.

Routine lipid screening of children at age 3 years remains controversial. The National Cholesterol Education Program recommends selective screening in children with high-risk family members, defined as a parent with total cholesterol greater than 240 mg/dL or a parent or grandparent with early-onset cardiovascular disease. When children have LDL levels greater than 130 mg/dL on two successive tests, dietary lifestyle counseling is appropriate. Dietary modification may decrease cholesterol levels by 5–20%. If the patient is unresponsive to diet change and at extreme risk (ie, LDL > 160 mg/dL, HDL less than 35 mg/dL, and a history of cardiovascular disease in a first-degree relative at an age younger than 40 years), drug therapy may be indicated. Cholestyramine, a bile acid binding resin, is rarely used today due to poor adherence. The 3-hydroxy-3-methylglutaryl coenzyme A (HMG-CoA) reductase inhibitors (statins) are more commonly used in the pediatric population. Niacin is useful for treatment of hypertriglyceridemia.

De Jongh S et al: Efficacy and safety of statin therapy in children with familial hypercholesterolemia: A randomized double-blind placebo-controlled trial with simvastatin. Circulation 2002;106:2231 [PMID: 12390953].

Gidding SS: Dietary recommendations for children and adolescents: a guide for practitioners: consensus statement from the American Heart Association. Circulation 2005;112:2061 [PMID: 16186441].

CHEST PAIN

Overview

Chest pain is a common pediatric complaint, accounting for 6 in 1000 visits to urban emergency departments and urgent care clinics. Although children with chest pain are commonly referred for cardiac evaluation, chest pain in children is rarely cardiac in origin. Other more likely causes of chest pain in children include reactive airways disease, musculoskeletal pain, esophagitis, gastritis, and functional pain.

Detailed history and physical examination should guide the pediatrician to the appropriate workup of chest pain. Rarely is there a need for laboratory tests or evaluation by a specialist. The duration, location, intensity, frequency, and radiation of the pain should be documented, and possible triggering events preceding the pain should be explored. For instance, chest pain following exertion may lead to a more elaborate evaluation for a cardiac disorder. The timing of the pain in relation to meals may suggest a gastrointestinal cause.

The patient should also be asked about how pain relief is achieved. A social history to reveal psychosocial stressors and cigarette smoke exposure may be revealing. On physical examination, attention must be placed on the vital signs; general appearance of the child; the chest wall musculature; cardiac, pulmonary, and abdominal examination findings; and quality of peripheral pulses. If the pain can be reproduced through direct palpation of the chest wall, it is almost always musculoskeletal in origin.

Etiology

Cardiac disease is a rare cause of chest pain, but if misdiagnosed it may be life-threatening. Although myocardial infarction rarely occurs in healthy children, patients with diabetes mellitus, chronic anemia, anomalous left coronary artery, or hypertrophic cardiomyopathy may be at increased risk for ischemia. It is also important to ask the family about a history of Kawasaki disease, as these children are at risk for myocardial infarction secondary to thrombosis of coronary aneurysms. More than 50% of children and adolescents who exhibit sequelae from Kawasaki disease arrive at the emergency department with chest pain.

Young children may mistake palpitations for chest pain. Supraventricular tachycardia (SVT), atrial flutter, premature ventricular contractions (PVCs), or ventricular tachycardia may be associated with chest pain in children. Structural lesions that can cause chest pain include aortic stenosis, pulmonary stenosis, and mitral valve prolapse. Structural cardiac lesions are usually accompanied by significant findings on cardiac examination. Of children with mitral valve prolapse, 30% will complain of chest pain presumably caused by papillary muscle ischemia. Other cardiac lesions causing chest pain include dilated cardiomyopathy, myocarditis, pericarditis, rheumatic carditis, and aortic dissection.

Noncardiac chest pain may be due to a respiratory illness, reactive airway disease, pneumonia, pneumothorax, or pulmonary embolism. Gastrointestinal causes of chest pain include reflux, esophagitis, and foreign body ingestion. The most common cause of chest pain (30% of children) is inflammation of musculoskeletal structures of the chest wall. Costochondritis is caused by inflammation of the costochondral joints and is usually unilateral.

In most cases sophisticated testing is not required. However, if a cardiac origin is suspected, a pediatric cardiologist should be consulted. Evaluation in these instances may include an ECG, chest radiograph, echocardiogram, Holter monitor, or serum troponin levels.

Cava JR, Sayger PL: Chest pain in children and adolescents. Pediatr Clin North Am 2004;51:1553 [PMID: 15561173].

Cardiac Transplantation

Cardiac transplantation has become an effective therapeutic modality for infants and children with end-stage cardiac disease. Indications for transplantation include (1) progressive HF despite maximal medical therapy, (2) complex congenital heart diseases that are not amenable to surgical repair or palliation or in instances in which the surgical palliative approach has an equal or higher risk of mortality compared with transplantation, and (3) malignant arrhythmias unresponsive to medical therapy, catheter ablation, or automatic implantable cardiodefibrillator. Approximately 300–400 pediatric cardiac transplant procedures are performed annually in the United States. Infant (< 1 year of age) transplants account for 30% of pediatric cardiac transplants. The current estimated half-life for children undergoing cardiac transplantation is approximately 13 years. This is a rapidly evolving field, and the most recent data indicate an optimistic future for the transplant recipient.

Careful evaluation of the recipient and the donor is performed prior to cardiac transplantation. Assessment of the recipient's pulmonary vascular resistance is critical, as irreversible and severe pulmonary hypertension is a risk factor for post-transplant right heart failure and early death. End-organ function of the recipient may also influence post-transplant outcome and should be evaluated closely. Donor-related factors that can have an impact on outcome include cardiac function, amount of inotropic support needed, active infection (HIV and hepatitis B and C are contraindications to donation), donor size, and ischemic time to transplantation.

Immunosuppression

The ideal post-transplant immunosuppressive regimen allows the immune system to continue to recognize and respond to foreign antigens in a productive manner while avoiding graft rejection. Although there are many different regimens, calcineurin inhibitors (eg, cyclosporine and tacrolimus) are the mainstay of maintenance immunosuppression in pediatric heart transplantation. Calcineurin inhibitors may be used in isolation. Double-drug therapy includes the addition of antimetabolite or antiproliferative medications such as azathioprine, mycophenolate mofetil, or sirolimus. Due to the significant adverse side effects of corticosteroids in children, attempts have been made in some centers to discontinue triple-drug therapy that would include steroid use. Growth retardation, susceptibility to infection, impaired wound healing, hypertension, and a cushingoid appearance are some of the consequences of long-term steroid use.

Graft Rejection

Despite advances in immunosuppression, graft rejection remains the leading cause of death in the first 3 years after transplantation. The pathophysiologic mechanisms of rejection are not entirely known. T cells are required for rejection, but multiple cell lines and mechanisms are likely involved. Because graft rejection can present in the absence of clinical symptomatology, monitoring for and diagnosing rejection in a timely fashion can be difficult. Screening regimens include serial physical examinations, electrocardiography, echocardiography, and cardiac catheterization with endomyocardial biopsy.

Rejection Surveillance

A. Symptoms and Signs

Acute graft rejection may not cause symptoms in the early stages. With progression patients may develop tachycardia, tachypnea, rales, a gallop rhythm, or hepatosplenomegaly. Infants and young children may present with irritability, poor feeding, vomiting, or lethargy. The goal is to detect rejection prior to the development of hemodynamic compromise, as there is 50% mortality in the year following an episode of rejection resulting in cardiovascular compromise.

B. Imaging

Chest radiographs may show cardiomegaly, pulmonary edema, or pleural effusions.

C. Electrocardiography

Abnormalities in conduction can be present, although the most typical finding is reduced QRS voltages. Both atrial and ventricular arrhythmias can occur in rejection.

D. Echocardiography

Echocardiography is a noninvasive rejection surveillance tool that is especially useful in infant recipients, but helpful in all ages. Changes in ventricular compliance and function may initially be subtle, but are progressive with increasing duration of the rejection episode. A new pericardial effusion or worsening valvular insufficiency may also indicate rejection.

E. Cardiac Catheterization and Endomyocardial Biopsy

Hemodynamic assessment including ventricular filling pressures, cardiac output, and oxygen consumption can be obtained via cardiac catheterization. The endomyocardial biopsy has been considered the gold standard for diagnosing acute graft rejection. However, because not all episodes of symptomatic rejection result in a positive biopsy result, this tool is not universally reliable. The appearance of infiltrating lymphocytes with myocellular damage is the hallmark of graft rejection and is helpful if present.

▶ Treatment of Graft Rejection

The goal of graft rejection treatment is to reverse the immunologic inflammatory cascade. High-dose corticosteroids are the first line of treatment. Occasionally additional therapy with antithymocyte biologic preparations such as antithymocyte globulin or OKT-3 (a murine monoclonal antibody to the CD3 T-lymphocyte epitope) is needed to reverse rejection. Most rejection episodes can be treated effectively if diagnosed promptly. Usually graft function returns to its baseline state, although severe rejection episodes can result in graft loss and patient death even with optimal therapy.

▶ Course & Prognosis

The course of cardiac transplantation in pediatric patients is usually quite good. The risk of infection is low after the immediate post-transplant period in spite of chronic immunosuppression. Cytomegalovirus is the most common pathogen responsible for infection-related morbidity and mortality in heart transplant recipients. Most children tolerate environmental pathogens well. Nonadherence with lifetime immunosuppression is of great concern especially in adolescent patients. Several recent studies have identified nonadherence as the leading cause of late death. Post-transplant lymphoproliferative disorder, a syndrome related to Epstein-Barr virus infection, can result in a Burkitt-like lymphoma that usually responds to a reduction in immunosuppression, but occasionally must be treated with chemotherapy. The overwhelming majority of children are not physically limited and do not require restrictions related to the cardiovascular system.

The greatest long-term concern after heart transplantation is related to cardiac allograft vasculopathy. Cardiac allograft vasculopathy results from concentric intimal proliferation of the coronary arteries that can ultimately result in complete luminal occlusion. These lesions are diffuse and often involve distal vessels and thus are usually not amenable to bypass grafting, angioplasty, or stent placement. Overall, despite the concerns of immunosuppression, the risk of late rejection, and coronary disease, the majority of pediatric patients enjoy a good quality of life with survival rates that are improving. Currently, 10-year survival is 80% for infant recipients and 70% overall for all pediatric recipients. Newer, more specific, and more effective immunosuppressive agents are currently being tried in clinical studies or are being evaluated in preclinical studies, making the future almost certainly better for children after cardiac transplantation. Donor availability remains a major limitation to the expansion of indications for cardiac transplantation.

Boucek MM et al: Prospective evaluation of echocardiography for primary rejection surveillance after heart transplantation: Comparison with endomyocardial biopsy. J Heart Lung Transplant 1994;13(1 Pt 1):66 [PMID: 8167130].

Boucek MM et al: Registry of the International Society for Heart and Lung Transplantation: Tenth official pediatric heart transplantation report—2007. J Heart Lung Transplant 2007;26:1223 [PMID: 18096472].

Canter CE et al: Indications for heart transplantation in pediatric heart disease: A scientific statement from the American Heart Association. Circulation 2007;115:658 [PMID: 17261651].

Pietra BA: Transplantation immunology 2003: A simplified approach. Pediatr Clin North Am 2003;50:1233 [PMID: 14710779].

PRIMARY PULMONARY HYPERTENSION

ESSENTIALS OF DIAGNOSIS & TYPICAL FEATURES

► Often subtle with symptoms of dyspnea, fatigue, chest pain, and syncope.

► Loud pulmonary component of S_2; ECG with RVH.

► Implies exclusion of secondary causes of pulmonary hypertension.

► Rare, progressive, and often fatal disease without treatment.

► General Considerations

Unexplained or primary pulmonary hypertension (PPH) in children is a rare disease with an estimated overall incidence of 1–2 persons per million worldwide. Pulmonary hypertension is defined as a mean pulmonary pressure greater than 25 mm Hg at rest or greater than 30 mm Hg during exercise. PPH is a diagnosis made after exclusion of all other causes of pulmonary hypertension. Secondary pulmonary hypertension is most commonly associated with congenital heart disease, pulmonary parenchymal disease, causes of chronic hypoxia (upper airway obstruction), thrombosis, liver disease, hemoglobinopathies and collagen vascular disease. PPH is difficult to diagnose in the early stages because of its subtle manifestations. Most patients with PPH are young adult women, although the sex incidence is equal in children. As recently as 1991, the diagnosis of PPH in individuals younger than 16 years of age carried a medial survival of only 10 months. Fortunately, survival is improving with the advent of new therapies. Familial PPH occurs in 6–12% of affected individuals. When a clear familial association is known, the disease shows evidence of genetic anticipation, presenting at younger ages in subsequent generations.

► Clinical Findings

A. Symptoms and Signs

The clinical picture varies with the severity of pulmonary hypertension, and usually early symptoms are subtle, delaying the diagnosis. Initial symptoms may be dyspnea, palpitations, or chest pain, often brought on by strenuous exercise or competitive sports. Syncope may be the first symptom, which usually implies severe disease. As the disease progresses, patients have signs of low cardiac output and right heart failure. Right heart failure may be manifested by increasing

hepatomegaly, peripheral edema, and an S_3 gallop on examination. Murmurs of pulmonary regurgitation and tricuspid regurgitation may be present, and the pulmonary component of S_2 is usually pronounced.

B. Imaging

The chest radiograph most often reveals a prominent main pulmonary artery, and the RV may be enlarged. The peripheral pulmonary vascular markings may be normal or diminished. However, in 6% of patients with confirmed PPH, the chest radiograph is normal.

C. Electrocardiography

The ECG usually shows right ventricular hypertrophy with an upright T wave in V_1 (from age 7 days to 7 years) or a qR complex in lead V_1 or V_3. Also present may be evidence of right axis deviation and right atrial enlargement.

D. Echocardiography

The echocardiogram is an essential tool for excluding other congenital heart diseases. It frequently shows RVH and dilation. In the absence of other structural disease, any tricuspid and pulmonary insufficiency jets can be used to estimate pulmonary artery systolic and diastolic pressures, respectively. Other echocardiographic modalities such as myocardial performance index and input vascular impedance are in the early stages of use in evaluation of pulmonary hypertension.

E. Cardiac Catheterization and Angiocardiography

Cardiac catheterization is the best method of diagnosing PPH. As an invasive test, it carries with it associated risks and should be performed with caution. The procedure is performed to rule out cardiac causes of pulmonary hypertension, determine the severity of disease, and define treatment strategies. The reactivity of the pulmonary vascular bed to short-acting vasodilator agents (oxygen, nitric oxide, or prostacyclin) can be assessed and used to determine treatment options. Angiography may show a decrease in the number of small pulmonary arteries with tortuous vessels.

F. Other Evaluation Modalities

Cardiac MRI is used in some patients to measure heart function and blood flow. Cardiopulmonary exercise testing using cycle ergometry correlates with disease severity. More simply, a 6-minute walk test, in which distance walked and perceived level of exertion are measured, has a strong independent association with mortality in late disease.

► Treatment

The goal of therapy is to reduce pulmonary artery pressure and increase cardiac output. Cardiac catheterization data are used to determine treatment. Patients responsive to pulmonary vasodilators are given calcium channel blockers such as nifedipine or diltiazem. Patients unresponsive to vasodilators initially receive one of three classes of drugs: prostanoids (such as epoprostenol), endothelin receptor antagonists (such as bosentan), or phosphodiesterase inhibitors (such as sildenafil). All of these agents have distinct mechanisms of action that can reduce pulmonary vascular resistance. Warfarin is commonly used for anticoagulation to prevent thromboembolic events, usually with a goal to maintain the INR between 1.5 and 2.0.

Atrial septostomy is indicated in some patients with refractory pulmonary hypertension. Cardiac output falls as pulmonary vascular resistance rises, so an interatrial shunt can preserve left heart output, albeit with deoxygenated blood. Lung transplantation should be considered in patients with intractable pulmonary hypertension and in those with associated anatomic lesions that contribute to high pulmonary arterial pressure, like pulmonary vein stenosis. Heart-lung transplant procedures appear to have survival benefits over isolated lung transplantation in patients with pulmonary hypertension.

Although survival is less than 10 months in children with untreated pulmonary hypertension, recent studies have showed improved survival rates of more than 95% at 5 years with calcium channel blockade, and more than 80% at 5 years in children requiring epoprostenol.

Ivy DD: Chronic pulmonary hypertension. In Munoz R et al (editors): Handbook of Pediatric Cardiac Intensive Care. Springer-Verlag, 2008.

DISORDERS OF RATE & RHYTHM

As more children are surviving cardiac surgery and living with chronically altered hemodynamics there has been an increase in the incidence of arrhythmias in the pediatric population.

The introduction of invasive electrophysiology with recordings from the endocardium has greatly improved understanding of the conduction system. Cardiac ablation techniques offer some children with arrhythmias a cure rather than lifelong antiarrhythmia treatment.

Sinus Arrhythmia

Phasic variation in the heart rate (sinus arrhythmia) is normal. Typically, the sinus rate varies with the respiratory cycle, whereas P-QRS-T intervals remain stable. Marked sinus arrhythmia is defined as more than 100% variation in heart rate. It may occur in association with respiratory distress or increased intracranial pressure, or it may be present in normal children. In isolation, it never requires treatment; however, it may be associated with sinus node dysfunction or autonomic nervous system dysfunction.

Sinus Bradycardia

Depending on age, sinus bradycardia is defined as either (1) a heart rate below the normal limit for age (neonates to 6 years, 60 beats/min; 7–11 years, 45 beats/min; older than 12 years, 40 beats/min) or (2) a heart rate inappropriately slow for the functional status of the patient (chronotropic incompetence). In critically ill patients, common causes of sinus bradycardia include hypoxia, central nervous system damage, eating disorders, and medication side effects. Only symptomatic bradycardia (syncope, low cardiac output, or exercise intolerance) requires treatment (atropine, isoproterenol, or cardiac pacing).

Sinus Tachycardia

The heart rate normally accelerates in response to stress (eg, fever, hypovolemia, anemia, or HF). Although sinus tachycardia in the normal heart is well tolerated, symptomatic tachycardia with decreased cardiac output warrants evaluation for structural heart disease or true tachyarrhythmias. Treatment may be indicated for correction of the underlying cause of sinus tachycardia (eg, transfusion for anemia or correction of hypovolemia or fever).

PREMATURE ATRIAL CONTRACTIONS

Premature atrial contractions are triggered by an ectopic focus in the atrium. They are one of the most common premature beats occurring in pediatric patients, particularly during the fetal and newborn periods. They may be conducted (followed by a QRS) or nonconducted (not followed by a QRS, as the beat has occurred so early that the AV node is still refractory) (Figure 19–4). A less-than-compensatory pause usually occurs until the next normal sinus beat. Depending on the location of the ectopic focus of the premature contraction, the P-wave morphology may be normal or abnormal. As an isolated finding, premature atrial contractions are benign and require no treatment. They need to be treated with antiarrhythmic agents only when they trigger tachyarrhythmias or produce bradycardia secondary to nonconduction.

PREMATURE JUNCTIONAL CONTRACTIONS

Premature junctional contractions arise in the AV node or the bundle of His. They usually induce a normal QRS complex with no preceding P wave. When conducted aberrantly to the ventricles, they cannot be distinguished from PVCs except by invasive electrophysiologic study. Premature junctional contractions are usually benign and require no specific therapy.

PREMATURE VENTRICULAR CONTRACTIONS

PVCs may originate in either ventricle and are characterized by an abnormal QRS of more than 80 ms duration in

▲ **Figure 19–4.** Lead II rhythm strip with premature atrial contractions. Beats 1, 3, 7, and 8 are conducted to the ventricles, whereas beats 2, 4, 5, and 6 are not.

newborns and more than 120 ms in adolescents and adults (Figure 19–5). PVCs originating from a single ectopic focus all have the same configuration; those of multifocal origin show varying configurations. The consecutive occurrence of two PVCs is referred to as a ventricular couplet and of three or more as ventricular tachycardia.

Most unifocal PVCs in otherwise normal patients are benign. The significance of PVCs can be confirmed by having the patient exercise. As the heart rate increases, benign PVCs usually disappear. If exercise results in an increase or coupling of contractions, underlying disease may be present. Multifocal PVCs are always abnormal and may be more dangerous. They may be associated with drug overdose (tricyclic antidepressants or digoxin toxicity), electrolyte imbalance, myocarditis, or hypoxia. Treatment is directed at correcting the underlying disorder.

SINUS NODE DYSFUNCTION

Sinus node dysfunction, or sick sinus syndrome, is a clinical syndrome of inappropriate sinus nodal function and rate. The abnormality may be a true anatomic defect of the sinus node or its surrounding tissue, or it may be an abnormality of autonomic input. It is defined as one or more of the following:

1. Sinus bradycardia
2. Marked sinus arrhythmia
3. Chronotropic incompetence
4. Sinus pause or arrest
5. Sinoatrial exit block
6. Combined bradyarrhythmias and tachyarrhythmias
7. Sinus node reentry
8. Atrial muscle reentry tachycardia

It is usually associated with postoperative repair of congenital heart disease (most commonly the Mustard or Senning repair for complete transposition of the great arteries or the Fontan procedure), but it is also seen in unoperated congenital heart disease, in acquired heart diseases, and in normal hearts. In some cases the disorder is inherited. Symptoms usually manifest between ages 2 and 17 years and consist of episodes of syncope, presyncope, or disorientation. Some patients may experience palpitations, pallor, or exercise intolerance.

Lead V₅

▲ **Figure 19–5.** Lead V$_5$ rhythm strip with unifocal premature ventricular contractions in a bigeminy pattern. The arrow shows a ventricular couplet.

The evaluation of sinus node dysfunction involves both surface ECG and invasive electrophysiologic testing. Exercise testing and ambulatory monitoring help define any arrhythmias and correlate rhythm changes with symptoms.

Treatment for sinus node dysfunction is indicated only in symptomatic patients. Asymptomatic patients can be observed for the onset of exercise intolerance or syncope because there is little chance of sudden death prior to the onset of such symptoms. Bradyarrhythmias are treated with vagolytic (atropine) or adrenergic (aminophylline) agents or permanent cardiac pacemakers. Antiarrhythmic treatment of tachyarrhythmias often produces or enhances bradycardia, thus requiring permanent cardiac pacing. A pacemaker is inserted prophylactically prior to the initiation of antiarrhythmic medications.

The prognosis is excellent when appropriate treatment is provided, with morbidity and mortality rates nearly equal to those of the underlying heart disease. In severe untreated cases, sinus node dysfunction may become chronic and may lead to sudden death.

Miller MS et al: Neonatal bradycardia. Prog Pediatr Cardiol 2000;11:19 [PMID: 10822186].

SUPRAVENTRICULAR TACHYCARDIA

SVT, also known as paroxysmal SVT or paroxysmal atrial tachycardia, is defined as an abnormal arrhythmia mechanism arising above or within the bundle of His. The mode of presentation depends on the heart rate, the presence of underlying cardiac structural or functional abnormalities, coexisting illness, and patient age. Tachycardia may be poorly tolerated in a child with preexisting HF or an under-

lying systemic disease such as anemia or sepsis. It may go unnoticed in an otherwise healthy child. Incessant tachycardia in an otherwise healthy individual, even if fairly slow (120–150 beats/min), may cause myocardial dysfunction and HF if left untreated. The mechanisms of tachycardia are divided into three groups: reentry, enhanced automaticity, and triggered dysrhythmias.

Reentry is conduction through two or more pathways, creating a sustained repetitive circular loop. The circuit can be confined to the atrium (intra-atrial reentry, a form of atrial flutter) (Figure 19–6). It may be confined within the AV node (AV nodal reentrant tachycardia), or it may encompass an accessory connection between atria and ventricle (atrioventricular tachycardia). The arrhythmia circuit includes conduction through the normal pathway (the AV node) as well as the accessory AV connection. If during tachycardia the electrical impulse travels antegrade (from atria to ventricles) through the AV node and retrograde (from ventricle to atria) back up the accessory pathway, orthodromic reciprocating tachycardia is present. If instead the impulse travels antegrade through the accessory pathway and retrograde up through the AV node, antidromic reciprocating tachycardia is present.

Wolff-Parkinson-White (WPW) syndrome is a subclass of reentrant tachycardia in which, during sinus rhythm, the impulse travels antegrade down the accessory connection, bypassing the AV node and creating ventricular preexcitation (early eccentric activation of the ventricle with a short PR interval and slurred upstroke of the QRS, a delta wave) (Figure 19–7). Reentrant tachycardia represents approximately 80% of pediatric arrhythmias, has a wide range of rates, and may or may not demonstrate P waves. Reentrant tachycardia initiates and terminates abruptly. Most patients

▲ **Figure 19–6.** Leads aVF (F) and V_1, showing atrial flutter with "sawtooth" atrial flutter waves.

with WPW have otherwise structurally normal hearts. However, WPW has been noted to occur with increased frequency in association with the following congenital cardiac lesions: tricuspid atresia, Ebstein anomaly of the tricuspid valve, hypertrophic cardiomyopathy, and congenitally corrected transposition of the great arteries (ccTGA).

Enhanced automaticity (also known as automatic or ectopic tachycardia) is created when a focus of cardiac tissue develops an abnormally fast spontaneous rate of depolarization. These arrhythmias represent approximately 20% of childhood arrhythmias and are usually under autonomic influence. ECG demonstrates a normal QRS complex preceded by an abnormal P wave (Figure 19–8). Junctional ectopic tachycardia does not have a P wave preceding the QRS waves and may be associated with AV dissociation or 1:1 retrograde conduction. Ectopic tachycardias demonstrate a gradual onset and offset and may be paroxysmal or incessant. When they are incessant, they are usually associated with HF and a clinical picture of dilated cardiomyopathy.

Triggered dysrhythmia is extremely rare. It is caused by afterdepolarizations. These tachycardias are usually associated with diseased atrial myocardium, are triggered by premature atrial contractions or sinus tachycardia, initiate and terminate abruptly, and mimic intra-atrial reentry (atrial flutter). However, they can be distinguished from atrial flutter: they terminate with the administration of adenosine, whereas atrial flutter does not (see later section on Atrial Flutter and Fibrillation).

► **Clinical Findings**

A. Symptoms and Signs

Presentation varies with age. Infants tend to turn pale and mottled with onset of tachycardia and may become irritable. With long duration of tachycardia, symptoms of HF develop. Heart rates range from 240–300 beats/min. Older children complain of dizziness, palpitations, fatigue, and chest pain. Heart rates range from 240 beats/min in the younger child to 150–180 beats/min in the teenager. HF is less common in children than in infants. Tachycardia may be associated with either congenital heart defects or acquired conditions such as cardiomyopathies and myocarditis.

B. Imaging

Chest radiographs are normal during the early course of tachycardia. If HF is present, the heart is enlarged and pulmonary venous congestion is evident.

C. Electrocardiography

ECG is the most important tool in the diagnosis of SVT.

1. The heart rate is rapid and out of proportion to the patient's physical status (ie, a rate of 140 beats/min with an abnormal P wave while quiet and asleep).
2. The rhythm is extremely regular. There is little variation in the rate throughout the entire tracing.

Spontaneous Intermittent Preexcitation

Delta   Delta   No delta   Delta   Delta   Delta   No delta

▲ **Figure 19–7.** Leads I and II with spontaneous intermittent ventricular preexcitation (Wolff-Parkinson-White syndrome).

▲ **Figure 19–8.** Lead II rhythm strip of ectopic atrial tachycardia. The tracing demonstrates a variable rate with a maximum of 260 beats/min, an abnormal P wave, and a gradual termination.

3. P waves may or may not be present. If they are present, the PR interval and appearance do not vary. P waves may be difficult to find because they are superimposed on the preceding T wave. Furthermore, if the abnormal focus is located within the AV node, the P waves will not be seen.

4. The QRS complex is usually the same as during normal sinus rhythm. However, the QRS complex is occasionally widened (SVT with aberrant ventricular conduction), in which case the condition may be difficult to differentiate from ventricular tachycardia.

▶ **Treatment**

A. Acute Treatment

During the initial episodes of SVT, patients require close monitoring. Correction of acidosis and electrolyte abnormalities is also indicated.

1. Vagal maneuvers—The "diving reflex" produced by placing an ice bag on the nasal bridge for 20 seconds (for infants) or by immersing the face in ice water (for children or adolescents) will increase parasympathetic tone and terminate some tachycardias. The Valsalva maneuver, which can be performed by older compliant children, may also terminate SVT.

2. Adenosine—Adenosine transiently blocks AV conduction and terminates tachycardias that incorporate the AV node.

Adenosine does not convert tachycardias whose mechanism is confined to the atria (atrial ectopic tachycardia or

intra-atrial reentry). However, it serves as a diagnostic tool in these arrhythmias by demonstrating continuation of the atrial tachycardia during AV block, implying that AV node conduction is not a crucial element of the tachycardia circuit. The dose is 50–250 mcg/kg by rapid intravenous bolus. It is antagonized by aminophylline and should be used with caution in patients with sinus node dysfunction or asthma.

3. Transesophageal atrial pacing—Atrial overdrive pacing and termination can be performed from a bipolar electrode-tipped catheter positioned in the esophagus adjacent to the left atrium. Overdrive pacing at rates approximately 30% faster than the tachycardia rate will interrupt the tachycardia circuit and restore sinus rhythm.

4. Direct current cardioversion—Direct current cardioversion (0.5–2 synchronized J/kg) should be used immediately when a patient presents in cardiovascular collapse.

B. Chronic Treatment

1. Digitalis—Digoxin is still used for long-term treatment and maintenance of sinus rhythm. The doses used are the same as those for HF. Conversion should be accomplished within 8–12 hours. In some patients, digoxin accelerates conduction over an accessory pathway. In such children, digitalis products are contraindicated. Patients with an accessory pathway (eg, those with WPW syndrome) often have primary atrial tachycardias (atrial flutter or fibrillation or atrial ectopic tachycardias), and with enhanced conduction in the accessory pathway these primary atrial tachycardias can transmit to the ventricles, causing ventricular fibrillation. Therefore, an evaluation of the effect of digoxin on the accessory pathway should be performed in the electrophysiology lab before chronic digoxin use in patients with WPW syndrome.

2. β-Adrenergic blocking agents—Propranolol decreases sinus heart rate and AV nodal conduction. It is effective in the treatment of both reentrant and ectopic arrhythmias in doses ranging from 1–4 mg/kg/d. Long-acting β-blockers, such as atenolol and nadolol, are used because they have fewer central nervous system side effects than propranolol and may be given only once or twice a day.

3. Calcium channel antagonists—Verapamil and other calcium channel blockers markedly prolong conduction through the AV node and are effective in interrupting and preventing reentrant tachycardias that incorporate the AV node. They are ineffective in terminating atrial tachycardias but may be useful in controlling the ventricular response by producing AV blockade. Verapamil comes in short- and long-acting preparations; the dose is 3–5 mg/kg/d. It may cause myocardial dysfunction and is contraindicated in infants.

4. Other drugs—Recently introduced antiarrhythmic medications (eg, flecainide, propafenone, sotalol, and amiodarone) have increased pharmacologic actions and are extremely effective. However, these drugs also have serious side effects, including proarrhythmia (production of arrhythmias) and sudden death, and should be used only under the direction of a pediatric cardiologist.

5. Radiofrequency ablation—This is a nonsurgical transvascular catheter technique that desiccates an arrhythmia focus or accessory pathway and permanently cures an arrhythmia. The success rate is approximately 90%, with a recurrence risk of 10%. The risk of developing complete heart block is approximately 2–5% when applying burns in the vicinity of the AV node/His bundle. The procedure can be performed in infants or adults. In children younger than age 4 years, the risks are higher, and the procedure should be reserved for those whose arrhythmias are refractory to medical management. In well-tolerated SVTs that respond to vagal maneuvers, no further treatment is necessary. However, the high success rate, low complication and recurrence rates, and the elimination of the need for chronic antiarrhythmic medications have made radiofrequency ablation the primary treatment option in most pediatric cardiovascular centers.

▶ Prognosis

SVT has an excellent prognosis. When it occurs in early infancy, 90% will respond to initial treatment. Approximately 30% will recur at an average age of 8 years.

Basson CT: A molecular basis for Wolff-Parkinson-White syndrome. N Engl J Med 2001;344:1861 [PMID: 11407351].

Dubin AM et al: Radiofrequency catheter ablation: Indications and complications. Pediatr Cardiol 2000;21:551 [PMID: 11050279].

Moak JP: Supraventricular tachycardia in the neonate and infant. Prog Pediatr Cardiol 2000;11:25 [PMID: 10822187].

ATRIAL FLUTTER & FIBRILLATION

Atrial flutter and fibrillation are rare in children and are most often associated with organic heart disease—particularly postoperative congenital heart disease and sinus node dysfunction. Atrial flutter can occur in infancy and can mimic SVT. The atrial rate is usually more than 240 beats/min and often more than 300 beats/min. The ventricular rate depends on the rate of AV conduction and is usually slower than the atrial rate.

▶ Treatment & Prognosis

Transesophageal atrial pacing is the treatment of choice to terminate atrial flutter. When it is not successful, antiarrhythmic medications (eg, digoxin, sotalol, and amiodarone) may succeed; however, direct current cardioversion is frequently necessary.

The prognosis in neonates without structural heart disease is excellent, and after conversion these patients may need no further treatment.

POSTOPERATIVE INCISIONAL INTRA-ATRIAL REENTRY

Improved surgical survival for patients with congenital heart disease has created a new, increasingly prevalent, chronic arrhythmia: incisional intra-atrial reentry, or postoperative atrial flutter. In these tachycardias, electrically isolated corridors of atrial myocardium (eg, the tricuspid valve–inferior vena cava isthmus, or the region between an atrial incision and the crista terminalis) act as pathways for sustained reentrant circuits of electrical activity. These tachycardias are chronic, medically refractory, and clinically incapacitating. Electromagnetic mapping permits precise localization of these corridors. Long linear radiofrequency or surgical lesions are then used to interrupt the reentrant circuits.

Delacretaz E et al: Multiple atrial macro-reentry circuits in adults with repaired congenital heart disease: Entrainment mapping combined with three-dimensional electroanatomic mapping. J Am Coll Cardiol 2001;37:1665 [PMID: 11345382].

Van Hare GF: Intra-atrial reentry tachycardia in pediatric patients. Prog Pediatr Cardiol 2001;13:41 [PMID: 11413057].

VENTRICULAR TACHYCARDIA

Ventricular tachycardia is uncommon in childhood (Figure 19–9). It is usually associated with underlying abnormalities of the myocardium (myocarditis, cardiomyopathy, myocardial tumors, or postoperative congenital heart disease) or toxicity (hypoxia, electrolyte imbalance, or drug toxicity). Sustained tachycardia is generally an unstable

▲ **Figure 19–9.** Twelve-lead ECG from a child with imipramine toxicity and ventricular tachycardia.

situation, and if left untreated will usually degenerate into ventricular fibrillation.

Accelerated idioventricular rhythm is a sustained ventricular tachycardia occurring in neonates with normal hearts. The rate is within 10% of the preceding sinus rate, and it is a self-limiting arrhythmia that requires no treatment.

Acute termination of ventricular tachycardia involves restoration of the normal myocardium when possible (correction of electrolyte imbalance, drug toxicity, and so on) and direct current cardioversion (1–4 J/kg), cardioversion with lidocaine (1 mg/kg), or both. Chronic suppression of ventricular arrhythmias with antiarrhythmic drugs has many side effects (including proarrhythmia and death), and it must be initiated in the hospital under the direction of a pediatric cardiologist.

Alexander ME et al: Ventricular arrhythmias: When to worry. Pediatr Cardiol 2000;21:532 [PMID: 11050277].
Batra A et al: Ventricular arrhythmias. Prog Pediatr Cardiol 2000;11:39 [PMID: 10822188].

LONG QT SYNDROME

The congenital long QT syndromes (types 1–6) in children are arrhythmic disorders in which ventricular repolarization is irregular and prolonged (QTc > 0.44 second, or 0.46 second in postpubertal females). Some myocardial ion channelopathies predispose patients to torsade de pointes (multifocal ventricular tachycardia) and manifest as syncope, seizures, or sudden death, often in response to exercise. If untreated, they account for a very high mortality rate (5% per year). They are inherited genetically in an autosomal dominant or recessive pattern (the latter being associated with congenital deafness, the Jervell and Lange-Nielsen syndrome) or they may arise spontaneously. Treatment with β-blockade and exercise limitation is only partially successful.

In recurrent, medically refractory cases, implantable cardioverter defibrillators are necessary to prevent sudden death. Congenital long QT syndrome has now been demonstrated to be one of the causes of sudden infant death syndrome.

Acquired long QT syndrome—resulting from altered ventricular repolarization secondary to myocardial toxins, ischemia, or inflammation—also predisposes a patient to ventricular arrhythmias. Numerous medications as outlined previously can also cause QT prolongation. ECGs are recommended before therapy (for a baseline measurement) and after steady state is achieved.

Gutgesell H et al: Cardiovascular monitoring of children and adolescents receiving psychotropic drugs. A statement for healthcare professionals from the Committee on Congenital Cardiac Defects, Counsel on Cardiovascular Diseases in the Young–American Heart Association. Circulation 1999;99:979 [PMID: 10027824].
Kimbrough J et al: Clinical implications for affected parents and siblings of probands with long QT syndrome. Circulation 2001;104:557 [PMID: 11479253].
Li H et al: Current concepts in long QT syndrome. Pediatr Cardiol 2000;21:542 [PMID: 11050278].
Moss AJ et al: Effectiveness and limitations of β-blocker therapy in congenital long QT syndrome. Circulation 2000;101:616 [PMID: 10673253].
Wedekind H et al: De novo mutation in the SCN5A gene associated with early onset of sudden infant death. Circulation 2001;104:1158 [PMID: 11535573].
Zhang L et al: Spectrum of ST-T wave patterns and repolarization parameters in congenital long QT syndrome: ECG findings identify genotypes. Circulation 2000;102:2849 [PMID: 11104743].

SUDDEN DEATH

Hypertrophic cardiomyopathy (the most common cause of sudden death in young athletes) and other cardiomyopathies (dilated cardiomyopathies, restrictive cardiomyopathy, or arrhythmogenic RV dysplasia) may be hereditary

Lead I

▲ **Figure 19–10.** Lead I rhythm strip with Mobitz type I (Wenckebach) second-degree heart block. There is progressive lengthening of the PR interval prior to the nonconducted P wave (*arrows*).

and should be looked for in patients with resuscitated cardiac arrest or family members of those who have died suddenly. Congenital structural anomalies of the coronary arteries are the second most common cause of sudden death in young athletes. These anomalies are not hereditary. The coronary arteries need to be evaluated in survivors of sudden death events. Arrhythmias in patients with postoperative congenital heart disease are important causes of morbidity and mortality and may present as sudden death events. All survivors of cardiac arrest require thorough evaluation for arrhythmias, including invasive electrophysiology. Episodes of seizures, syncope, and presyncope in patients with congenital heart disease should be evaluated for the possibilities of arrhythmias, and they may also require thorough electrophysiologic evaluation and treatment.

When a child dies suddenly and unexpectedly, or is resuscitated from cardiac arrest that had no apparent cause, it is necessary to conduct a detailed family history looking for seizures, syncope, or early sudden death. Family members should be examined with an arrhythmia screen, physical examination, ECG, and echocardiography to detect arrhythmias or cardiomyopathies.

Corrado D et al: Right bundle branch block, right precordial ST-segment elevation, and sudden death in young people. Circulation 2001;103:710 [PMID: 11156883].

Gatzoulis MA et al: Risk factors for arrhythmia and sudden cardiac death later after repair of tetralogy of Fallot: A Multicentre Study. Lancet 2000;356:975 [PMID: 11041398].

HEART BLOCK

1. First-Degree Heart Block

First-degree heart block is an ECG diagnosis of prolongation of the PR interval. The block does not in itself cause problems. It may be associated with structural congenital heart defects, namely AV septal defects and ccTGA, and with diseases such as rheumatic carditis. The PR interval is prolonged in patients receiving digoxin therapy.

2. Second-Degree Heart Block

Mobitz type I (Wenckebach) heart block is recognized by progressive prolongation of the PR interval until there is no QRS following a P wave (Figure 19–10). Mobitz type I heart block occurs in normal hearts at rest and is usually benign. In Mobitz type II heart block, there is no progressive lengthening of the PR interval before the dropped beat (Figure 19–11). Mobitz type II heart block is frequently associated with organic heart disease, and a complete evaluation is necessary.

3. Complete Heart Block

In complete heart block, the atria and ventricles beat independently. Ventricular rates can range from 40–80 beats/min, whereas atrial rates are faster (Figure 19–12).

Congenital complete heart block, the most common form of complete heart block, has a very high association with maternal systemic lupus erythematosus antibodies. Serologic screening should be performed in the mother of an infant with complete heart block, even if she has no symptoms of collagen vascular disease. Congenital complete heart block is also associated with congenitally corrected transposition of the great vessels and AV septal defect. Acquired complete heart block may be secondary to acute myocarditis, drug toxicity, electrolyte imbalance, hypoxia, and cardiac surgery.

▶ Clinical Findings

Prenatal bradycardia is frequently noted in infants with congenital complete heart block, and emergent delivery is required if hydrops fetalis develops. Postnatal adaptation largely depends on the heart rate; infants with heart rates less than 55 beats/min are at significantly greater risk for low

Lead III

▲ **Figure 19–11.** Lead III rhythm strip with Mobitz type II second-degree heart block. There is a consistent PR interval with occasional loss of AV conduction (*arrow*).

cardiac output, HF, and death. Wide QRS complexes and a rapid atrial rate are also poor prognostic signs. Most patients have an innocent flow murmur from increased stroke volume. In symptomatic patients, the heart can be quite enlarged, and pulmonary edema may be present. In older patients, syncope can be the presenting symptom, or heart block may be found unexpectedly on routine physical examination. Complete cardiac evaluation, including echocardiography and Holter monitoring, is necessary to assess the patient for ventricular dysfunction and to relate any symptoms to concurrent arrhythmias.

▷ **Treatment**

In patients thought to be at risk for syncope, HF, or sudden death, the treatment of choice for complete heart block is insertion of a permanent pacemaker. Until permanent pacing can be instituted, patients can be assisted temporarily by infusions of isoproterenol or by temporary transcutaneous pacemakers.

Eronen M et al: Short- and long-term outcome of children with congenital complete heart block diagnosed in utero or as a newborn. Pediatrics 2000;106(1 Pt 1):86 [PMID: 10878154].

▲ **Figure 19–12.** Twelve-lead ECG and lead II rhythm strip of complete heart block. The atrial rate is 150 beats/min, and the ventricular rate is 60 beats/min.

Moak JP et al: Congenital heart block: Development of late-onset cardiomyopathy, a previously underappreciated sequela. J Am Coll Cardiol 2001;37:238 [PMID: 11153745].

SYNCOPE (FAINTING)

Syncope is a sudden transient loss of consciousness that resolves spontaneously. The common form of syncope (simple fainting) occurs in 15% of children and is a disorder of control of heart rate and blood pressure by the autonomic nervous system that causes hypotension or bradycardia. It is often associated with rapid rising and postural hypotension, prolonged standing, or hypovolemia. Patients exhibit vagal symptoms such as pallor, nausea, or diaphoresis. Syncope, also known as autonomic dysfunction, can be evaluated with head-up tilt table testing. The patient is placed supine on a tilt table, and then—under constant heart rate and blood pressure monitoring—is tilted to the upright position. If symptoms develop, they can be classified as vasodepressor (hypotension), cardioinhibitory (bradycardia), or mixed.

Syncope is usually self-limited (lasting approximately 6 months to 2 years) and can be controlled with dietary salt and volume loading to prevent hypovolemia. In refractory cases, medications to manipulate the autonomic nervous system have been useful. Fludrocortisone (0.1 mg/kg/d) is a mineralocorticoid that causes renal salt resorption and thus increases intravascular volume. β-Blockade (atenolol, 0.5–2.0 mg/kg/d) can inhibit the catecholamine surge and help prevent the rebound bradycardia and hypotension. Vagolytic agents (disopyramide, 2.5 mg/kg four times daily) help control hypervagotonia, and the selective serotonin reuptake inhibitors have also been effective in alleviating symptoms. Syncope that occurs during exercise or stress or is associated with a positive family history is a warning sign that a serious underlying dysrhythmia may be present, calling for further investigation.

Johnsrude CL: Current approach to pediatric syncope. Pediatr Cardiol 2000;21:522 [PMID: 11050276].

Gastrointestinal Tract

Judith M. Sondheimer, MD
Shikha Sundaram, MD, MSCI

DISORDERS OF THE ESOPHAGUS

GASTROESOPHAGEAL REFLUX

ESSENTIALS OF DIAGNOSIS & TYPICAL FEATURES

▶ Recurrent post-prandial spitting and vomiting in healthy infants that resolves spontaneously.

▶ Heartburn and regurgitation in older children.

▶ Chronic complications—esophagitis, stricture, anemia, and Barrett esophagus.

▶ Diagnosis is clinical in infancy with upper gastrointestinal (GI) radiograph and upper endoscopy to rule out other GI disease.

▶ Clinical Findings

A. Infants with Reflux

Gastroesophageal (GE) reflux is common in young infants. Frequent post-prandial regurgitation, ranging from effortless to forceful, is the most common infant symptom. Infant reflux is usually benign but in rare cases causes failure to thrive, food refusal, colic, rumination, and neck contortions (Sandifer syndrome). Apneic spells in young infants, especially occurring with position change after feeding, may be caused by reflux. GE reflux is common in neurologically impaired infants.

Reflux of gastric contents into the esophagus occurs during spontaneous relaxations of the lower esophageal sphincter that are unaccompanied by swallowing. Low pressures in the lower esophageal sphincter or developmental immaturity of the sphincter are not causes of GE reflux in infants. Normal factors promoting reflux in infants are their small stomach capacity, frequent large-volume feedings, short esophageal length, supine positioning, and slow swallowing response to

the flow of refluxed material up the esophagus. Infants' individual responses to the stimulus of reflux, particularly the maturity of their self-settling skills, are important factors determining the severity of reflux-related symptoms.

An important differential point in evaluating infants with GE reflux is whether the vomited material contains bile. Bile-stained emesis in an infant requires immediate evaluation as it may be a symptom of intestinal obstruction (malrotation with volvulus, intussusception).

B. Older Children with Reflux

GE reflux disease (GERD) is diagnosed clinically in older children when reflux causes persistent symptoms with or without inflammation of the esophagus. Older children with GERD have less frequent vomiting than infants, and more often complain of adult-type symptoms of regurgitation into the mouth, heartburn, and dysphagia. Esophagitis occurs in children with GERD and requires endoscopic evaluation. Children with asthma, cystic fibrosis, developmental handicaps, hiatal hernia, and repaired tracheoesophageal fistula are at increased risk of GERD.

C. Diagnostic Studies

In thriving infants, GE reflux is a clinical diagnosis. An upper GI series rules out anatomic causes of vomiting but is not an accurate test for GE reflux because of a 30% false-positive rate. In older children with heartburn, a trial of acid-suppressing medication may be both diagnostic and therapeutic. Persistent symptoms should be investigated by upper GI radiographs and endoscopy to rule out other organic causes. pH probe or esophageal impedance studies may be helpful in recognizing an association between episodic or unusual symptoms and reflux events. pH studies quantify the number and duration of acid reflux events. Esophageal intraluminal impedance monitoring is a pH-independent method of detecting fluid movements in the esophagus. These studies have shown that episodes of nonacid reflux occur as frequently as acid reflux episodes and that treatment with acid-suppressing medications changes the proportions of acid versus nonacid events, not the total number of events. Esophagoscopy is not diagnostic of reflux, but esophagitis can be identified.

Treatment & Prognosis

Reflux resolves spontaneously in 85% of affected infants by 12 months of age, coincident with assumption of erect posture and initiation of solid feedings. Until then, regurgitation volume may be reduced by offering small feedings at frequent intervals and by thickening feedings with rice cereal (2–3 tsp/oz of formula). Prethickened "anti-reflux" formulas are available. Histamine-2 (H2)–receptor antagonists (ranitidine, 5 mg/kg/d in two doses) or proton pump inhibitors (omeprazole, 0.5–1.0 mg/kg/d in one dose) do not reduce the frequency of reflux but may reduce pain behavior. Prokinetic agents such as metoclopramide hasten gastric emptying and improve esophageal motor function, but studies have not shown efficacy in controlling symptoms. A short trial of protein hydrolysate formula (hypoallergenic) sometimes controls emesis and pain behavior in infants with protein sensitivity. Special formulas and acid suppression agents are costly and should be discontinued if there is no improvement of symptoms in 1 week.

Spontaneous resolution is less likely in older children with GERD. Episodic heartburn pain may be controlled with intermittent use of acid blockers. Patients with more severe heartburn or esophagitis require regular acid suppression. Untreated esophagitis may cause esophageal stricture and anemia from blood loss. Barrett esophagus, a precancerous condition, is rare in childhood but can occur in patients with very long-standing esophagitis.

Antireflux surgery (fundoplication) is indicated when GERD causes severe symptoms unresponsive to medications: (1) persistent vomiting with failure to thrive, (2) esophagitis or esophageal stricture, (3) life-threatening apneic spells, or (4) chronic pulmonary disease unresponsive to 2–3 months of medical therapy. Fundoplication also may be considered early in patients whose response to medication is likely to be poor—those with large hiatal hernia, neurologic handicap, previous tracheoesophageal (TE) fistula surgery, or severe esophagitis.

Rudolph CD et al: Guidelines for evaluation and treatment of gastroesophageal reflux in infants and children: Recommendations of the North American Society for Pediatric Gastroenterology and Nutrition. J Pediatr Gastroenterol Nutr 2001;23(Suppl):1 [PMID: 11525610].

EOSINOPHILIC ESOPHAGITIS

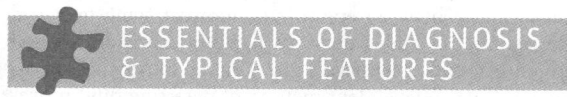

ESSENTIALS OF DIAGNOSIS & TYPICAL FEATURES

▶ Dysphagia, esophageal food impaction, and heartburn.

▶ Most common in adolescent boys.

▶ Grossly, esophagoscopy shows white eosinophilic exudates, ringlike esophageal folds, and esophageal stricture. Esophageal mucosal biopsy shows dense eosinophilic infiltrate and hyperplasia of the basal layer of the epithelium.

Clinical Findings

A. Symptoms and Signs

This recently recognized entity occurs most often in teenage boys but is reported in both sexes and all ages. A common initial presentation is an acute food impaction. The patient may have a long history of recurrent impactions and dysphagia. Heartburn is sometimes reported and suggests the diagnosis of GERD. There often is a family or personal history of atopy, asthma, and dysphagia in male relatives.

B. Laboratory Findings

The esophageal mucosa is thick and inflamed with long, shallow, linear mucosal fissures and visible circumferential mucosal rings that look a bit like the trachea (so-called trachealization). The esophagus is often sprinkled with innumerable pinpoint white exudates that superficially resemble *Candida*. On microscopic examination the white spots are composed of eosinophils. The basal cell layer of the esophageal mucosa is hypertrophied and infiltrated by eosinophils (usually more than 40 per 40 × light microscopic field). A lengthy stricture is often seen which tends to split during endoscopy. Serum IgE often is elevated but this is not a diagnostic finding. Specific allergens are rarely identified by skin testing even though the patient can sometimes identify foods that precipitate pain and dysphagia.

Differential Diagnosis

The most common differential conditions are peptic esophagitis and candidal esophagitis. Eosinophilic esophagitis may be part of a generalized eosinophilic gastroenteropathy, a very rare, steroid-responsive entity. Patients with eosinophilic gastroenteropathy often present with intestinal obstruction or gastric outlet obstruction caused by large local infiltrates of eosinophils in the antrum, duodenum, and cecum.

Treatment

An extremely hypoallergenic diet is effective in controlling symptoms. Such diets are useful in infants, but adherence to the diet in older children usually is poor. Beclomethasone, puffed or swallowed from a metered dose pulmonary inhaler, improves symptoms. Two puffs of beclomethasone from an inhaler twice daily using an age-appropriate metered dose is a common recommendation. Systemic corticosteroids, oral sodium cromolyn, and montelukast sodium also have been used with benefit in some patients. Esophageal dilation may be required to treat strictures. Repeat endoscopy after therapy often shows persistent inflammation despite good control of symptoms. The relationship between eosinophilic esophagitis and later esophageal malignancy has not been determined.

Furuta GT, Straumann A: Review article: The pathogenesis and management of eosinophilic oesophagitis. Aliment Pharmacol Ther 2006;24:173 [PMID: 1682447].

ACHALASIA OF THE ESOPHAGUS

ESSENTIALS OF DIAGNOSIS & TYPICAL FEATURES

► Gradual onset of distal esophageal obstruction.

► Dysphagia, esophageal food impaction, chronic pulmonary aspiration.

► Failure of lower esophageal relaxation during swallowing with abnormalities of esophageal peristalsis.

► High or low resting pressure of the lower esophageal sphincter.

► Clinical Findings

A. Symptoms and Signs

Achalasia is uncommon in children younger than 5 years, but cases in those younger than 12 months have been reported. Symptoms include retrosternal pain and fullness, vomiting, and solid food impaction. Patients eat slowly and may drink large amounts of fluid with solid food. Dysphagia is relieved by repeated forceful swallowing or by vomiting. Familial cases occur in Allgrove syndrome (alacrima, adrenal insufficiency, and achalasia) and familial dysautonomia. Chronic cough, wheezing, recurrent aspiration pneumonitis, anemia, and poor weight gain are common.

B. Imaging and Manometry

Barium esophagram shows a dilated esophagus with a tapered "beak" at the GE junction. Esophageal dilation may not be present in infants because of the short duration of distal obstruction. Fluoroscopy shows disordered esophageal peristalsis. Esophageal manometry may show high resting pressure of the lower esophageal sphincter, failure of sphincter relaxation after swallowing, and abnormal esophageal peristalsis. The cause is unknown. There is a decrease in neuronal nitric oxide synthetase (nNOS) in the tissues of the lower esophageal sphincter and, possibly, local nitric oxide deficiency prevents sphincter relaxation. It is unclear whether the lack of nNOS is a secondary or primary phenomenon.

► Differential Diagnosis

Congenital or peptic esophageal stricture, esophageal webs, and esophageal masses may mimic achalasia. Intestinal pseudo-obstruction, multiple endocrine neoplasia type 2b, systemic amyloidosis, and postvagotomy syndrome cause esophageal dysmotility and symptoms similar to achalasia. Teenage girls may be suspected of having an eating disorder. In Chagas disease, caused by the parasite *Trypanosoma cruzi*, nNOS and ganglion cells are diminished or absent in the muscular layers of the lower esophageal sphincter causing an acquired achalasia.

► Treatment & Prognosis

Pneumatic dilation of the lower esophageal sphincter produces temporary relief of obstruction that may last weeks to years. Local injection of botulinum toxin paralyzes the lower esophageal sphincter and temporarily relieves obstruction. More long-lasting relief of obstruction is achieved by surgically dividing the lower esophageal sphincter (Heller myotomy). The procedure can be performed laparoscopically or thoracoscopically. Because of the shorter duration of esophageal obstruction in children, there is less secondary dilation of the esophagus. Thus, the prognosis for return or retention of some normal esophageal motor function after surgery is better than in adults.

Hussain SZ et al: A review of achalasia in 33 children. Dig Dis Sci 2002;47:2538 [PMID: 12452392].

CAUSTIC BURNS OF THE ESOPHAGUS

Ingestion of caustic solids or liquids (pH > 12) produces esophageal lesions ranging from superficial inflammation to coagulative necrosis with ulceration, perforation, mediastinitis, or peritonitis. The severity of immediate oral or laryngeal injury after ingestion does not correlate with the degree of esophageal injury. Esophageal or laryngeal obstruction from edema and exudate may occur within 24 hours. Pain may be severe. Esophageal strictures develop in areas of anatomic narrowing (thoracic inlet, GE junction, or point of compression where the left bronchus crosses the esophagus), where contact with the caustic agent is more prolonged. Strictures may develop quickly or gradually over several months. Strictures occur only with full-thickness esophageal necrosis. Shortening of the esophagus is a late complication that may cause hiatal hernia.

The lips, mouth, and airway should be examined in suspected alkali ingestion. Vomiting should not be induced. Drooling is common and is not an accurate reflection of severity of esophageal burns. Oral injury is common with solid caustic agents. Intravenous corticosteroids (eg, methylprednisolone, 1–2 mg/kg/d) are given immediately to reduce oral swelling and laryngeal edema. Intravenous fluids are necessary if dysphagia prevents oral intake. Esophagoscopy, if needed, should be done within 24–48 hours after ingestion before liquefaction of tissues is complete. Treatment may be stopped if there are only first-degree burns at endoscopy. Corticosteroids may be beneficial in first- and second-degree burns but do not prevent stricture formation from circumferential third-degree burns. Repeated esophageal dilations may be necessary as a stricture develops but are not performed acutely. When radiographs show erosion into the mediastinum or peritoneum, antibiotics are mandatory. Intraluminal esophageal stenting may be beneficial during early management. Surgical replacement of the esophagus by colonic interposition or gastric tube may be needed for long strictures resistant to dilation.

Although agents such as bleach, detergents, and acids may cause esophageal irritation, it is rare for any but the strongest acids and detergents to produce full-thickness necrosis and stricture.

Turner A, Robinson P: Respiratory and gastrointestinal complications of caustic ingestion in children. Emerg Med J 2005;22:359 [PMID: 1584706].

FOREIGN BODIES IN THE ALIMENTARY TRACT

The most common foreign bodies ingested by children are coins. Most foreign bodies pass through the GI tract without difficulty, although objects longer than 5 cm may be unable to pass the ligament of Treitz. Ingested foreign bodies tend to lodge in areas of natural constriction—valleculae, thoracic inlet, GE junction, pylorus, ligament of Treitz, and ileocecal junction. Foreign bodies lodged in the esophagus for more than 24 hours, or those causing pain or respiratory distress, should be removed. Disk-shaped batteries lodged in the esophagus should be removed immediately.

Smooth foreign bodies in the stomach, such as buttons or coins, may be monitored without attempting removal for up to several months if the child is free of symptoms. Disk-shaped batteries in the stomach will generally pass uneventfully. Straight pins, screws, and nails generally pass without incident. Large, open safety pins should be removed from the stomach because they may not pass the pyloric sphincter and may cause perforation. Wooden toothpicks should be removed. They have usually been chewed prior to accidental swallowing and carry mouth flora which may cause abscess formation if the toothpick becomes imbedded in the bowel wall. The use of balanced electrolyte lavage solutions containing polyethylene glycol may help the passage of small, smooth foreign bodies lodged in the stomach or intestine. Lavage is especially useful in hastening the passage of disk-shaped batteries or ingested tablets that may be toxic. Failure of a smooth foreign body to exit the stomach after several days suggests the possibility of gastric outlet obstruction.

Most foreign bodies can be removed from the esophagus or stomach by a skilled endoscopist. Under fluoroscopy, a Foley catheter with balloon inflated below the foreign body can be used to extract smooth, round esophageal foreign bodies if the foreign body has been present for less than a few days and if the child has not had previous esophageal surgery. Only an experienced radiologist should attempt this maneuver.

TRACHEOESOPHAGEAL FISTULA

See Chapter 1.

DISORDERS OF THE STOMACH & DUODENUM

HIATAL HERNIA

In *paraesophageal hiatal hernias*, the esophagus and GE junction are in their normal anatomic position, but the gastric cardia is herniated through the diaphragmatic hiatus along side the GE junction. In *sliding hiatal hernias*, the GE junction and a portion of the proximal stomach are displaced above the diaphragmatic hiatus. Paraesophageal hernias are rare in childhood; patients present with pain, esophageal obstruction, or respiratory compromise. The most common cause of paraesophageal hernia is previous fundoplication surgery. *Sliding hiatal hernias* are common. GE reflux may accompany sliding hiatal hernias, although most produce no symptoms. Surgery is indicated if paraesophageal or sliding hiatal hernias produce persistent symptoms.

PYLORIC STENOSIS

ESSENTIALS OF DIAGNOSIS & TYPICAL FEATURES

▶ Postnatal muscular hypertrophy of the pylorus.
▶ Progressive gastric outlet obstruction, nonbilious vomiting, dehydration, and alkalosis in infants younger than 12 weeks.
▶ Upper GI contrast radiographs or abdominal ultrasound are diagnostic.

The cause of postnatal pyloric muscular hypertrophy with gastric outlet obstruction is unknown. The incidence is 1–8 per 1000 births, with a 4:1 male predominance. A positive family history is present in 13% of patients. Recent studies suggest that erythromycin in the neonatal period is associated with a higher incidence of pyloric stenosis in infants younger than 30 days.

▶ Clinical Findings

A. Symptoms and Signs

Vomiting usually begins between 2 and 4 weeks of age but may start as late as 12 weeks. Vomiting rapidly becomes projectile after every feeding. Vomiting starts at birth in about 10% of cases. Onset of symptoms may be delayed in preterm infants. The vomitus is rarely bilious but may be blood-streaked. Infants are usually hungry and nurse avidly. Constipation, weight loss, fretfulness, dehydration, and finally apathy occur. The upper abdomen may be distended after feeding, and prominent gastric peristaltic waves from left to right may be seen. An oval mass, 5–15 mm in longest dimension can be felt on deep palpation in the right upper abdomen, especially after vomiting.

B. Laboratory Findings

Hypochloremic alkalosis with potassium depletion occurs. Dehydration causes elevated hemoglobin and hematocrit. Mild unconjugated bilirubinemia occurs in 2–5% of cases.

C. Imaging

A barium upper GI series reveals retention of contrast in the stomach and a long narrow pyloric channel with a double track of barium. The hypertrophied muscle mass produces typical semilunar filling defects in the antrum. Isolated pylorospasm is common in young infants, and by itself is insufficient to make a diagnosis of pyloric stenosis. Ultrasonography shows a hypoechoic muscle ring greater than 4-mm thick with a hyperdense center.

▶ Treatment & Prognosis

Pyloromyotomy is the treatment of choice and consists of incision down to the mucosa along the pyloric length. The procedure can be performed laparoscopically. Treatment of dehydration and electrolyte imbalance is mandatory before surgical treatment, even if it takes 24–48 hours. The outlook after surgery is excellent. Patients often vomit postoperatively as a consequence of gastritis, esophagitis, or associated GE reflux. The postoperative barium radiograph remains abnormal for many months despite relief of symptoms.

Aspelund G, Langer JC: Current management of hypertrophic pyloric stenosis. Semin Pediatr Surg 2007;16:27 [PMID: 17210480].

Mahon BE et al: Maternal and infant use of erythromycin and other macrolide antibiotics as risk factors for infantile hypertrophic pyloric stenosis. J Pediatr 2001;139:380 [PMID: 11562617].

GASTRIC & DUODENAL ULCER

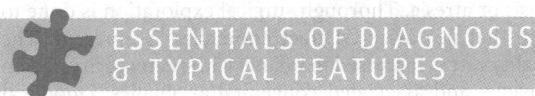

ESSENTIALS OF DIAGNOSIS & TYPICAL FEATURES

- ▶ Localized erosions of gastric or duodenal mucosa.
- ▶ Pain and bleeding are the most common symptoms.
- ▶ Underlying severe illness, *Helicobacter pylori* infection, and nonsteroidal anti-inflammatory drugs (NSAIDs) are the most common causes.
- ▶ Diagnosis by endoscopy.

▶ General Considerations

Gastric and duodenal ulcers occur at any age. Boys are affected more frequently than girls. In the United States, most childhood gastric and duodenal ulcers are associated with underlying illness, toxins, or drugs that cause breakdown in mucosal defenses.

Worldwide, the most common cause of gastric and duodenal ulcer is infection of the gastric mucosa with *H pylori*. Infection causes nodular gastritis and duodenal or gastric ulcer. Long-standing infection is associated with gastric lymphoid tumors and adenocarcinoma. Between 10% and 20% of North American children have antibodies against *H pylori*. Antibody prevalence increases with age, poor sanitation, crowded living conditions, and family exposure. In some developing countries, over 90% of schoolchildren have serologic evidence of past or present infection.

Illnesses predisposing to secondary ulcers include central nervous system disease, burns, sepsis, multi-organ system failure, chronic lung disease, Crohn disease, cirrhosis, and rheumatoid arthritis. The most common drugs causing secondary ulcers are aspirin, alcohol, and NSAIDs. NSAID use causes ulcers throughout the upper GI tract but most often in the stomach and duodenum.

▶ Clinical Findings

A. Symptoms and Signs

In children younger than 6 years, vomiting and upper GI bleeding are the most common symptoms of gastric and duodenal ulcer. Older children are more likely to complain of abdominal pain. The first attack of acute *H pylori* gastritis may be accompanied by vomiting and hematemesis. Ulcers in the pyloric channel may cause gastric outlet obstruction. Chronic blood loss may cause iron-deficiency anemia. Deep penetration of the ulcer may erode into a mucosal arteriole and cause acute hemorrhage. Penetrating duodenal ulcers (especially common during cancer chemotherapy, immunosuppression and in the intensive care setting) may perforate the duodenal wall causing peritonitis or abscess.

B. Diagnostic Studies

Upper GI endoscopy is the most accurate diagnostic examination. It also allows for identification of other causes of peptic symptoms such as esophagitis, eosinophilic enteropathy, and celiac disease. Upper GI barium radiographs may show an ulcer crater. Soft signs suggestive of peptic disease in adults (duodenal spasticity and thick irregular folds) are not reliable indicators in children. Urease activity is assessed on gastric biopsies, or by evaluation of breath after administration of radiolabeled urea by mouth. *H pylori* antigens can be measured in stool and may be an effective, noninvasive test for infection. Serum antibodies against *H pylori* do not prove that there is active infection or that treatment is needed.

Treatment

Acid suppression or neutralization is the mainstay of ulcer therapy. Liquid antacids in the volumes needed to neutralize gastric acid are usually unacceptable to children. H2-receptor antagonists and proton pump inhibitors are more effective and usually produce endoscopic healing in 4–8 weeks. Bland "ulcer diets" do not speed healing, but foods causing pain should be avoided. Caffeine should be avoided because it increases gastric acid secretion. Aspirin, alcohol, NSAIDs, and other gastric irritants should be avoided.

Treatment of *H pylori* infection requires eradication of the organism. Spontaneous clearance of infection may occur. The optimal medical regimen is still undetermined. Combinations of amoxicillin, metronidazole, and bismuth subsalicylate for 10–14 days, or amoxicillin for 14 days with omeprazole for 6 weeks are both effective. Clarithromycin for 7 days with a proton pump inhibitor for 6 weeks also is also effective. Resistance to antibiotics is common. An unresolved clinical question is whether recurrent courses of antibiotics should be used to eradicate resistant *H pylori* infection. Some epidemiologic data suggest that the incidence of GERD and Barrett esophagus is increasing in white males as a consequence of aggressive eradication of *H pylori*.

Bourke B et al: Canadian Helicobacter Study Group Consensus Conference: Update on the approach to *Helicobacter pylori* infection in children and adolescents—an evidence-based evaluation. Can J Gastroenterol 2005;19:478 [PMID: 16010300].

Crone J et al: *Helicobacter pylori* in children and adolescents: Increasing primary clarithromycin resistance 1997–2000. J Pediatr Gastroenterol Nutr 2003;36:368 [PMID: 12604976].

Vakil N: Primary and secondary treatment of *Helicobacter pylori* in the United States. Rev Gastroenterol Disord 2005;5:67 [PMID: 15976737].

CONGENITAL DIAPHRAGMATIC HERNIA

Herniation of abdominal contents through the diaphragm usually occurs through a posteriolateral defect in the diaphragm (foramen of Bochdalek). In about 5% of cases, the diaphragmatic defect is retrosternal (foramen of Morgagni). Hernias result from failure of the diaphragmatic anlagen to fuse and divide the thoracic and abdominal cavities at 8–10 weeks' gestation. All degrees of protrusion of the abdominal viscera through the diaphragmatic opening may occur. Eighty percent of posteriolateral defects involve the left diaphragm. In eventration of the diaphragm, a leaf of the diaphragm with hypoplastic muscular elements balloons into the chest and leads to similar but milder symptoms. Occasionally, diaphragmatic hernia is first identified in an older infant or child during incidental radiograph or routine physical examination. These children usually have a much more favorable prognosis than neonates (see Chapter 1).

CONGENITAL DUODENAL OBSTRUCTION

General Considerations

Extrinsic duodenal obstruction is usually due to congenital peritoneal bands associated with intestinal malrotation, annular pancreas, or duodenal duplication. Intrinsic obstruction is caused by stenosis, mucosal diaphragm (so-called wind sock deformity), or duodenal atresia. The duodenal lumen may be obliterated by a membrane or completely interrupted with a fibrous cord between the two segments. Atresia is more often distal to the ampulla of Vater than proximal.

Clinical Findings

A. Duodenal Atresia

Maternal polyhydramnios is common and often leads to prenatal diagnosis by ultrasonography. Vomiting (usually bile-stained) and epigastric distention begin within a few hours of birth. Meconium may be passed normally. Duodenal atresia is often associated with other congenital anomalies (30%), including esophageal atresia, intestinal atresias, and cardiac and renal anomalies. Prematurity (25–50%) and Down syndrome (20–30%) are also associated. Abdominal plain radiographs show gaseous distention of the stomach and proximal duodenum (the "double-bubble" radiologic sign). With protracted vomiting, there is less air in the stomach and less abdominal distention. Absence of distal intestinal gas suggests atresia or severe extrinsic obstruction, whereas a pattern of intestinal air scattered over the lower abdomen may indicate partial duodenal obstruction. Barium enema may be helpful in determining the presence of malrotation or atresia in the lower GI tract.

B. Duodenal Stenosis

In this condition, duodenal obstruction is not complete. Onset of obvious obstructive symptoms may be delayed for weeks or years. Although the stenotic area is usually distal to the ampulla of Vater, the vomitus does not always contain bile. Children with Down syndrome have an increased risk of duodenal stenosis.

Treatment & Prognosis

Duodenoduodenostomy is performed to bypass the area of stenosis or atresia. Thorough surgical exploration is done to ensure that no lower GI tract anomalies are present. The mortality rate is increased in infants with prematurity, Down syndrome, and associated congenital anomalies. Duodenal dilation and hypomotility from antenatal obstruction may cause duodenal dysmotility with obstructive symptoms even after surgical treatment.

ANNULAR PANCREAS

Annular pancreas is a rotational defect in which normal fusion of the dorsal and ventral pancreatic anlagen does

Table 20–1. Localization and relative frequency of congenital gastrointestinal atresias and stenoses.

	Area Involved	Type of Lesion	Relative Frequency
Pylorus		Atresia; web or diaphragm	1%
Duodenum	80% are distal to the ampulla of Vater	Atresia, stenosis; web or diaphragm	45%
Jejunoileal	Proximal jejunum and distal ileum	Atresia (multiple in 6–29%); stenosis	50%
Colon	Left colon and rectum	Atresia (usually associated with atresias of the small bowel)	5–9%

not occur, and a ring of pancreatic tissue encircles the duodenum. The presenting symptom is duodenal obstruction. Down syndrome and congenital anomalies of the GI tract occur frequently. Polyhydramnios is common. Symptoms may develop late in childhood or even in adulthood if the obstruction is not complete in infancy. Treatment consists of duodenoduodenostomy or duodenojejunostomy without operative dissection or division of the pancreatic annulus.

DISORDERS OF THE SMALL INTESTINE

INTESTINAL ATRESIA & STENOSIS

Excluding anal anomalies, intestinal atresia or stenosis accounts for one third of all cases of neonatal intestinal obstruction (see Chapter 1). Antenatal ultrasound can identify intestinal atresia in utero; polyhydramnios occurs in most affected pregnancies. Prematurity and other congenital anomalies may be present. The localization and relative incidence of atresias and stenoses are listed in Table 20–1.

Bile-stained vomiting and abdominal distention begin in the first 48 hours of life. Multiple sites in the intestine may be affected. The overall length of the small intestine may be significantly shortened. Radiographic features include dilated loops of small bowel and absence of colonic gas. Barium enema reveals narrow-caliber microcolon because of lack of intestinal flow distal to the atresia. In over 10% of patients with intestinal atresia the mesentery is absent, and the superior mesenteric artery cannot be identified beyond the origin of the right colic and ileocolic arteries. The ileum coils around one of these two arteries, giving rise to the so-called Christmas tree deformity on contrast radiographs. The tenuous blood supply often compromises surgical anastomoses. The differential diagnosis of intestinal atresia includes Hirschsprung disease, paralytic ileus secondary to sepsis, midgut volvulus, and meconium ileus. Surgery is mandatory. Postoperative complications include short bowel syndrome and small bowel hypomotility secondary to antenatal obstruction.

INTESTINAL MALROTATION

▶ General Considerations

The midgut extends from the duodenojejunal junction to the mid transverse colon. It is supplied by the superior mesenteric artery, which runs in the root of the mesentery. During gestation, the midgut elongates into the umbilical sac, returning to an intra-abdominal position during the 10th week of gestation. The root of the mesentery rotates in a counterclockwise direction during retraction causing the colon to cross the abdominal cavity ventrally. The cecum moves from the left to the right lower quadrant, and the duodenum crosses dorsally becoming partly retroperitoneal. When rotation is incomplete, the dorsal fixation of the mesentery is defective and shortened, so that the bowel from the ligament of Treitz to the mid transverse colon may rotate around its narrow mesenteric root and occlude the superior mesenteric artery (volvulus).

▶ Clinical Findings

A. Symptoms and Signs

Malrotation with volvulus accounts for 10% of neonatal intestinal obstructions. Most infants present in the first 3 weeks of life with bile-stained vomiting or with overt small bowel obstruction. Intrauterine volvulus may cause intestinal obstruction or perforation at birth. The neonate may present with ascites or meconium peritonitis. Later presenting signs include intermittent intestinal obstruction, malabsorption, protein-losing enteropathy, or diarrhea. Associated congenital anomalies, especially cardiac, occur in over 25% of symptomatic patients.

B. Imaging

An upper GI series shows the duodenojejunal junction and the jejunum on the right side of the spine. The diagnosis of malrotation can be further confirmed by barium enema, which may demonstrate a mobile cecum located in the midline, right upper quadrant, or left abdomen.

▶ Treatment & Prognosis

Surgical treatment of malrotation is the Ladd procedure. In young infants the Ladd procedure should be performed even if volvulus has not occurred. The duodenum is mobilized and the short mesenteric root is extended. The bowel is then fixed in a more normal distribution. Treatment of malrotation discovered in children older than age 12 months is uncertain. Because volvulus can occur at any age, surgical repair is usually recommended, even in asymptomatic children. Laparoscopic repair of malrotation is possible but is technically difficult and is never performed in the presence of volvulus.

Midgut volvulus is a surgical emergency. Bowel necrosis results from occlusion of the superior mesenteric artery. When necrosis is extensive, it is recommended that a first operation include only reduction of the volvulus with lysis of mesenteric bands. Resection of necrotic bowel should be delayed if possible until a second-look operation 24–48 hours later can be undertaken in the hope that more bowel can be salvaged. The prognosis is guarded if perforation, peritonitis, or extensive intestinal necrosis is present.

SHORT BOWEL SYNDROME

The most common cause of short bowel syndrome is neonatal intestinal resection. Necrotizing enterocolitis is the most common reason for resection (45%). Other causes include intestinal atresias (23%), gastroschisis (15%), volvulus (15%), and, less commonly, congenital short bowel, long-segment Hirschsprung disease, and bowel ischemic events. If bowel resection is extensive, the infant may be left with an intestine of insufficient length to support normal absorption and growth. Estimates of the small bowel length of a newborn range from 150–300 cm. Neonatal short bowel syndrome is defined as removal of more than 50% of the small intestinal length. In patients with 50% resection, it is almost certain that intravenous nutrition will be required for months to years to support growth.

The intestine remaining after resection does not undergo compensatory increase in length. However, if nutrition can be maintained, enterocytes will proliferate, villi will lengthen, and the intestine will elongate in proportion to the child's increasing height. These adaptations may eventually be sufficient for the patient's nutritional needs. Achieving independence from intravenous nutrition is less likely when less than 30 cm of small intestine remain after surgery. An intact colon and intact ileocecal sphincter are factors improving prognosis in short bowel syndrome. Liver failure (a consequence of intravenous nutrition, recurrent infection, and other injuries) is the most common cause of death in patients with short bowel syndrome. Mortality among all infants with short bowel syndrome is about 10–15%. Intestinal transplantation is an option for children with very short residual intestinal segments.

Goulet O, Ruemmele F: Causes and management of intestinal failure in children. Gastroenterology 2006;130:S16 [PMID: 16473066].

INTUSSUSCEPTION

Intussusception is the most frequent cause of intestinal obstruction in the first 2 years of life. It is three times more common in males than in females. In 85% of cases the cause is not apparent. Small bowel polyp, Meckel diverticulum, omphalomesenteric remnant, duplication, Henoch-Schönlein purpura, lymphoma, lipoma, parasites, foreign bodies, and viral enteritis with hypertrophy of Peyer patches all have been implicated as causes. Intussusception of the small intestine occurs in patients with celiac disease and cystic fibrosis related to the bulk of stool in the terminal ileum. In children older than 6 years, lymphoma is the most common cause. Intermittent small bowel intussusception is a rare cause of recurrent abdominal pain.

In its usual form, the intussusception starts just proximal to the ileocecal valve and extends for varying distances into the colon. The terminal ileum telescopes into the colon. Swelling, hemorrhage, incarceration, arterial and venous compromise, and necrosis of the intussuscepted ileum may occur, as well as intestinal perforation and peritonitis.

▶ Clinical Findings

Characteristically, a thriving infant 3–12 months of age develops recurring paroxysms of abdominal pain with screaming and drawing up of the knees. Vomiting and diarrhea occur soon afterward (90% of cases), and bloody bowel movements with mucus appear within the next 12 hours (50%). The child is characteristically lethargic between paroxysms and may be febrile. The abdomen is tender and often distended. A sausage-shaped mass may be palpated, usually in the upper mid abdomen. An intussusception can persist for several days if obstruction is not complete, and patients may present with intermittent attacks of enterocolitis. In older children, sudden attacks of abdominal pain may be related to chronic recurrent intussusception with spontaneous reduction.

▶ Treatment

Barium enema and air enema are both diagnostic and therapeutic. Reduction of the intussusception by barium enema should not be attempted if signs of strangulated bowel, perforation, or toxicity are present. Air insufflation of the colon under fluoroscopic guidance is a safe alternative to barium enema that has excellent diagnostic sensitivity and specificity without the risk of contaminating the abdominal cavity with barium. Care is required in performing either air or barium enema because ischemic damage to the colon secondary to vascular compromise increases the risk of perforation.

Surgery is required in extremely ill patients, in patients with evidence of bowel perforation, or in those in whom hydrostatic or pneumatic reduction has been unsuccessful (25%). Surgery has the advantage of identifying a lead point such as a Meckel diverticulum. Surgical reduction of intussusception is associated with a lower recurrence rate than pneumatic reduction.

Prognosis

The prognosis relates directly to the duration of the intussusception before reduction. The mortality rate with treatment is 1–2%. The patient should be observed carefully after hydrostatic or pneumatic reduction because intussusception recurs within 24 hours in 3–4% of patients.

INGUINAL HERNIA

A peritoneal sac precedes the testicle as it descends from the genital ridge to the scrotum. The lower portion of this sac envelops the testis as the tunica vaginalis, and the remainder normally atrophies by the time of birth forming a cord (processus vaginalis). In some cases, peritoneal fluid may become trapped in the tunica vaginalis (noncommunicating hydrocele). If the processus vaginalis remains open, peritoneal fluid or an abdominal structure may be forced into it (indirect inguinal hernia).

Inguinal hernias are most often indirect and occur more frequently (9:1) in boys than in girls. Hernias may be present at birth or may appear at any age. The incidence in preterm male infants is close to 5%. Inguinal hernia is reported in 30% of male infants weighing 1000 g or less.

Clinical Findings

No symptoms are associated with an empty processus vaginalis. In most cases, a hernia is a painless inguinal swelling. The mother of the infant may be the only person to see the mass, as it may retract when the infant is active, cold, frightened, or agitated during the physical examination. There may be a history of inguinal fullness associated with coughing or long periods of standing, or there may be a firm, globular, and tender swelling, sometimes associated with vomiting and abdominal distention. In some instances, a herniated loop of intestine may become partially obstructed, leading to pain and partial intestinal obstruction. Rarely, bowel becomes trapped in the hernia sac, and complete intestinal obstruction occurs. Gangrene of the hernia contents or testis may occur. In girls, the ovary may prolapse into the hernia sac presenting as a mass below the inguinal ligament. A suggestive history is often the only criterion for diagnosis, along with the "silk glove" feel of the rubbing together of the two walls of the empty hernia sac.

Differential Diagnosis

Inguinal lymph nodes may be mistaken for a hernia. Nodes are usually multiple with more discrete borders. A hydrocele of the cord should transilluminate. An undescended testis is usually mobile in the canal and is associated with absence of the gonad in the scrotum.

Treatment

Incarceration of an inguinal hernia is more likely to occur in boys and in children younger than 10 months of age. Manual reduction of incarcerated inguinal hernias can be attempted after the sedated infant is placed in the Trendelenburg position with an ice bag on the affected side. Manual reduction is contraindicated if incarceration has been present for more than 12 hours or if bloody stools are noted. Surgery is usually indicated if a hernia has ever incarcerated. Hydroceles frequently resolve by age 2 years. Controversy remains about whether the side opposite a unilateral hernia should be surgically explored. Exploration of the unaffected groin can document an open processus vaginalis, but patency does not always guarantee that herniation will occur, especially in patients older than age 1 year, in whom the risk of contralateral hernia is about 10%.

Nicholls E: Inguino-scrotal problems in children. Practitioner 2003;247:226 [PMID: 12640831].

UMBILICAL HERNIA

Umbilical hernias are more common in preterm than in fullterm infants and more common in black than in white infants. Small bowel may incarcerate in small-diameter umbilical hernias. Most umbilical hernias regress spontaneously if the fascial defect has a diameter of less than 1 cm. Large defects and hernias persisting after age 4 years should be treated surgically. Reducing the hernia and strapping the skin over the abdominal wall defect does not accelerate the healing process.

PATENT OMPHALOMESENTERIC DUCT

The omphalomesenteric duct is an embryonic remnant connecting the ileum to the undersurface of the umbilicus. It may be patent, completely occluded as a fibrous cord, or may have blind cystic areas. Fecal discharge from the umbilicus suggests a patent omphalomesenteric duct. A fibrous cord may become the focal point of an intestinal volvulus. Mucoid umbilical discharge may indicate a mucocele in the omphalomesenteric remnant with an opening at the umbilicus. A closed mucocele may protrude through the umbilicus and be mistaken for an umbilical granuloma because it is firm and bright red. Cauterization of a mucocele is not recommended. Surgical excision of omphalomesenteric remnants is indicated. Ultrasound examination or abdominal computed tomography (CT) can help confirm the diagnosis of omphalomesenteric duct remnant.

MECKEL DIVERTICULUM

Meckel diverticulum is the most common form of omphalomesenteric duct remnant. It is usually located on the antimesenteric border of the mid to distal ileum. It occurs in 1.5% of the population and in the majority of cases causes no symptoms. Diverticula may be lined by ileal, gastric, pancreatic, jejunal, or colonic mucosa. Familial cases have been reported. If complications occur, they are three times more common in males than in females. More than 50% of complications occur in the first 2 years of life.

► Clinical Findings

A. Symptoms and Signs

Forty to 60% of symptomatic patients have painless episodes of maroon or melanotic rectal bleeding. The bleeding is due to deep ileal ulcers adjacent to the diverticulum caused by acid secreted by heterotopic gastric tissue. Bleeding may be voluminous enough to cause shock and anemia. Occult bleeding is less common. Intestinal obstruction occurs in 25% of symptomatic patients as a result of ileocolonic intussusception. Intestinal volvulus may occur around a fibrous remnant of the vitelline duct extending from the tip of the diverticulum to the abdominal wall. In some patients, entrapment of bowel under a band running between the diverticulum and the base of the mesentery occurs. Meckel diverticula may be trapped in an inguinal hernia (Littre hernia). Diverticulitis occurs in 10–20% of symptomatic patients and is clinically indistinguishable from acute appendicitis. Perforation and peritonitis may occur. Chronic recurrent abdominal pain is rarely the only symptom.

B. Imaging

Diagnosis of Meckel diverticulum is seldom made on barium radiograph. Technetium-99 (^{99m}Tc)-pertechnetate is taken up by the heterotopic gastric mucosa in the diverticulum and outlines the diverticulum on a nuclear scan. Giving pentagastrin or cimetidine before administering the radionuclide increases ^{99m}Tc-pertechnetate uptake and retention by the heterotopic gastric mucosa and can increase the sensitivity of the test. Angiography or tagged red cell scan may be useful when bleeding is brisk.

► Treatment & Prognosis

Treatment is surgical. At laparoscopy or laparotomy, the ileum proximal and distal to the diverticulum may reveal ulcerations and heterotopic gastric tissue adjacent to the neck of the diverticulum. The prognosis for Meckel diverticulum is good.

ACUTE APPENDICITIS

► General Considerations

Acute appendicitis is the most common indication for emergency abdominal surgery in childhood. The frequency increases with age and peaks between 15 and 30 years. Obstruction of the appendix by fecalith (25%) is a common predisposing factor. Parasites may rarely cause obstruction (especially ascarids) and most of the remaining cases are idiopathic.

The incidence of perforation is high in childhood (40%), especially in children younger than age 2 years, in whom pain is often poorly localized and symptoms nonspecific. To avoid delay in diagnosis, it is important to maintain close communication with parents and perform a thorough initial physical examination with sequential examinations at frequent intervals over several hours to correctly interpret the evolving symptoms and signs.

► Clinical Findings

A. Symptoms and Signs

The typical patient has fever and periumbilical abdominal pain, which then localizes to the right lower quadrant with signs of peritoneal irritation. Anorexia, vomiting, constipation, and diarrhea also occur. Contrary to the vomiting of acute gastroenteritis which usually precedes abdominal pain, vomiting in appendicitis usually follows the onset of pain and is often bilious. The clinical picture is frequently atypical, especially in young children and infants. A rectal examination may clarify the site of tenderness or reveal a localized appendiceal mass. Serial examinations are critical in differentiating appendicitis from the many other conditions that transiently mimic its symptoms.

B. Laboratory Findings

The white blood cell count is seldom higher than 15,000/μL. Pyuria, fecal leukocytes, and guaiac-positive stool are sometimes present.

C. Imaging

A radio-opaque fecalith reportedly is present in two thirds of cases of ruptured appendix. In experienced hands, ultrasonography of the appendix shows a noncompressible, thickened appendix in 93% of cases. A localized fluid collection adjacent to or surrounding the appendix may also be seen. Abdominal CT after rectal instillation of contrast with thin cuts in the area of the appendix may be diagnostic. Indium-labeled white blood cell scan may localize to an inflamed appendix. Enlarged mesenteric lymph nodes are a nondiagnostic finding.

► Differential Diagnosis

The presence of pneumonia, pleural effusion, urinary tract infection, right-sided kidney stone, cholecystitis, perihepatitis, and pelvic inflammatory disease may mimic appendicitis. Other medical and surgical conditions causing acute abdomen should also be considered (see Table 20–8).

► Treatment & Prognosis

Exploratory laparotomy or laparoscopy is indicated when the diagnosis of appendicitis cannot be ruled out after a period of close observation. Postoperative antibiotic therapy is reserved for patients with gangrenous or perforated appendix. A single intraoperative dose of cefoxitin or cefotetan is recommended for all patients to prevent postoperative infection. The mortality rate is less than 1% during childhood, despite the high incidence of perforation. In uncomplicated nonruptured appendicitis, a laparoscopic approach is associated with a shortened hospital stay.

Bundy DG et al: Does this child have appendicitis? JAMA 2007;298:438 [PMID: 17652298].

DUPLICATIONS OF THE GASTROINTESTINAL TRACT

Duplications are congenital spherical or tubular structures found most commonly in the ileum. The other common locations of duplication are the duodenum, rectum, and esophagus. Duplications usually contain fluid and sometimes blood if necrosis has taken place. Most duplications are attached to the mesenteric side of the gut. They generally do not communicate with the intestinal lumen but share a common muscular coat. The epithelial lining of the duplication is usually of the same type as the bowel from which it originates. Some duplications (neuroenteric cysts) are attached to the spinal cord and are associated with hemivertebrae and anterior or posterior spina bifida.

Symptoms of vomiting, abdominal distention, colicky pain, rectal bleeding, partial or total intestinal obstruction, or an abdominal mass may start in infancy. Diarrhea and malabsorption may result from bacterial overgrowth in communicating duplications. Physical examination may reveal a rounded, smooth, movable mass, and barium radiograph or CT of the abdomen may show a noncalcified cystic mass displacing other organs. ^{99m}Tc-pertechnetate scan may help identify duplications containing gastric mucosa. Duplications of the ileum can give rise to an intussusception. Prompt surgical treatment is indicated.

DISORDERS OF THE COLON

CONGENITAL AGANGLIONIC MEGACOLON (HIRSCHSPRUNG DISEASE)

General Considerations

Hirschsprung disease results from an absence of ganglion cells in the mucosal and muscular layers of the colon. Neural crest cells fail to migrate into the mesodermal layers of the gut during gestation, possibly secondary to abnormal end-organ cell surface receptors or local deficiency of nitric oxide synthesis. The absence of ganglion cells results in failure of the colonic muscles to relax in front of an advancing bolus. The rectum (30%) or rectosigmoid (44%) is usually affected. The entire colon may be aganglionic (8%). Segmental aganglionosis is rare and is probably an acquired ischemic lesion.

The aganglionic segment has normal or slightly narrowed caliber with dilation of the normal colon proximal to the obstructing aganglionic segment. The mucosa of the dilated colonic segment may become thin and inflamed, causing diarrhea, bleeding, and protein loss (enterocolitis).

A familial pattern has been described, particularly in total colonic aganglionosis. The disease is four times more common in boys than girls, and 10–15% of patients have Down syndrome. Mutations in the *ret* proto-oncogene have been identified in about 15% of cases.

Clinical Findings

A. Symptoms and Signs

Failure of the newborn to pass meconium, followed by vomiting, abdominal distention, and reluctance to feed, suggest the diagnosis of Hirschsprung disease. Enterocolitis manifested by fever, explosive diarrhea, and prostration, is reported in approximately 50% of affected newborns. Enterocolitis may lead to inflammatory and ischemic changes in the colon, with perforation and sepsis. In some patients, especially those with short segments involved, symptoms are not obvious at birth. In later infancy, alternating obstipation and diarrhea predominate. The older child is more likely to have constipation alone. The stools are foul-smelling and ribbon-like. The abdomen is distended with prominent veins. Peristaltic waves are visible and fecal masses palpable. Intermittent bouts of intestinal obstruction, hypochromic anemia, hypoproteinemia, and failure to thrive are common. Encopresis is rare.

On digital rectal examination, the anal canal and rectum are devoid of fecal material despite obvious retained stool on abdominal examination or radiographs. If the aganglionic segment is short, there may be a gush of flatus and stool as the finger is withdrawn.

Infants of diabetic mothers may have similar symptoms and, in this setting, small left colon syndrome should be suspected. Meglumine diatrizoate (Gastrografin) enema is both diagnostic and therapeutic in small left colon syndrome as it reveals a meconium plug in the left colon, which is often passed during the diagnostic radiograph. The left colon is narrow but usually functional. In a small proportion of patients with small left colon, Hirschsprung disease may later be found.

B. Laboratory Findings

Ganglion cells are absent in both the submucosal and muscular layers of involved bowel. Special stains may show nerve trunk hypertrophy and increased acetylcholinesterase activity. Ganglionated bowel above the aganglionic segment is sometimes found to contain more than normal numbers of ganglion cells in abnormal locations (neuronal dysplasia). This finding is sometimes associated with persistent motor dysfunction of the remnant colon.

C. Imaging

Plain abdominal radiographs may reveal dilated proximal colon and absence of gas in the pelvic colon. Barium enema using a catheter without a balloon and with the tip inserted barely beyond the anal sphincter usually demonstrates a narrow distal segment with a sharp transition to the proximal dilated (normal) colon. The transition zone may not be seen in neonates since the normal proximal bowel has not had time to become dilated. Retention of barium for 24–48 hours is not diagnostic of Hirschsprung disease in older children as it typically occurs in retentive constipation as well. Barium retention is a more reliable sign in neonates.

D. Special Examinations

Rectal manometric testing reveals failure of reflex relaxation of the internal anal sphincter after distention of the rectum in all patients with Hirschsprung disease, regardless of the length of the aganglionic segment. In occasional patients, a nonrelaxing internal anal sphincter is the only abnormality. This condition is often called "ultrashort segment Hirschsprung disease."

Differential Diagnosis

Hirschsprung disease accounts for 15–20% of cases of neonatal intestinal obstruction. It must be differentiated from the small left colon syndrome by biopsy. In childhood, Hirschsprung disease must be differentiated from retentive constipation. In older infants and children it can also be confused with celiac disease because of the striking abdominal distention and failure to thrive.

Treatment & Prognosis

Treatment is surgical. Diverting colostomy (or ileostomy) is performed proximal to the aganglionic segment. In unstable infants, resection of the aganglionic segment may be postponed. At the time of definitive surgery, the transition zone between ganglionated and nonganglionated bowel is identified. Aganglionic bowel is resected, and a pull-through of ganglionated bowel to the preanal rectal remnant is made. Several surgical techniques, including laparoscopic pull-through, are in use. In children with ultrashort segment disease, an internal anal sphincter myotomy or botulinum toxin injection of the internal anal sphincter may control symptoms.

Complications after surgery include fecal retention, fecal incontinence, anastomotic breakdown, or anastomotic stricture. Postoperative obstruction may result from inadvertent retention of a distal aganglionic colon segment or postoperative destruction of ganglion cells secondary to vascular impairment. Neuronal dysplasia of the remaining bowel may produce a pseudo-obstruction syndrome. Enterocolitis occurs postoperatively in 15% of patients.

Gariepy CE: Developmental disorders of the enteric nervous system: Genetic and molecular bases. J Pediatr Gastroenterol Nutr 2004;39:5 [PMID: 15187773].

CONSTIPATION

Chronic constipation in childhood is defined as two or more of the following characteristics for 2 months: (1) less than 3 bowel movements per week; (2) more than 1 episode of encopresis per week; (3) impaction of the rectum with stool; (4) passage of stool so large it obstructs the toilet; (5) retentive posturing and fecal withholding; and (6) pain with defecation. Retention of feces in the rectum results in encopresis (involuntary fecal leakage) in 60% of children with constipation. Most constipation in childhood is a result of voluntary or involuntary retentive behavior (chronic retentive constipation). About 2% of healthy primary school children have chronic retentive constipation. The ratio of males to females may be as high as 4:1. Constipation due to organic causes is much rarer.

Clinical Findings

Infants younger than age 3 months often grunt, strain, and turn red in the face while passing normal stools. This pattern may be viewed erroneously as constipation. Failure to appreciate this normal developmental pattern may lead to the unwise use of laxatives or enemas. Infants and children may, however, develop the ability to ignore the sensation of rectal fullness and retain stool. Many factors reinforce this behavior, which results in impaction of the rectum and overflow incontinence or encopresis. Among these are painful defecation; skeletal muscle weakness; psychological issues, especially those relating to control and authority; modesty and distaste for school bathrooms; medications; and other factors listed in Table 20–2. The dilated rectum gradually becomes less sensitive to fullness, thus perpetuating the problem.

Differential Diagnosis

It is important to distinguish chronic retentive constipation from Hirschsprung disease. Features distinguishing these two entities are summarized in Table 20–3.

Treatment

Increased intake of high-residue foods such as bran, whole wheat, fruits, and vegetables may be sufficient therapy in mild constipation. Although extremes of dehydration may result in constipation, the most likely response to increased fluid intake in normal children is increased urination with little effect on defecation.

If diet change alone is ineffective, medications may be required. Barley malt extract (Maltsupex), 1–2 tsp added to feedings two or three times daily, or polyethylene glycol solution (MiraLax), 0.8–1 g/kg/d, are safe stool softeners in infants and children. Stool softeners such as dioctyl sodium sulfosuccinate, 5–10 mg/kg/d, may be less effective in children with voluntary stool retention. Stimulant laxatives such as standardized extract of senna fruit (Senokot syrup, Ex-Lax) can be used for short periods to relieve fecal impaction.

Table 20–2. Causes of constipation.

Functional or retentive causes	**Abnormalities of myenteric ganglion cells**
Dietary causes	Hirschsprung disease
Undernutrition, dehydration	Waardenburg syndrome
Excessive milk intake	Multiple endocrine neoplasia 2a
Lack of bulk	**Hypo- and hyperganglionosis**
Cathartic abuse	von Recklinghausen disease
Drugs	Multiple endocrine neoplasia 2b
Narcotics	Intestinal neuronal dysplasia
Antihistamines	Chronic intestinal pseudo-obstruction
Some antidepressants	**Spinal cord defects**
Vincristine	**Metabolic and endocrine disorders**
Structural defects of gastrointestinal tract	Hypothyroidism
Anus and rectum	Hyperparathyroidism
Fissure, hemorrhoids, abscess	Renal tubular acidosis
Anterior ectopic anus	Diabetes insipidus (dehydration)
Anal and rectal stenosis	Vitamin D intoxication (hypercalcemia)
Presacral teratoma	Idiopathic hypercalcemia
Small bowel and colon	**Skeletal muscle weakness or incoordination**
Tumor, stricture	Cerebral palsy
Chronic volvulus	Muscular dystrophy/myotonia
Intussusception	
Smooth muscle diseases	
Scleroderma and dermatomyositis	
Systemic lupus erythematosus	
Chronic intestinal pseudo-obstruction	

Modified and reproduced, with permission, from Silverman A, Roy CC: *Pediatric Clinical Gastroenterology*, 3rd ed. Mosby, 1983.

If encopresis is present, treatment should start with relieving fecal impaction. Disimpaction can be achieved in several ways, including medications such as hypertonic phosphate or saline enemas, mineral oil (2–3 mL/kg/d), and nonabsorbable

Table 20–3. Differentiation of retentive constipation and Hirschsprung disease.

	Retentive Constipation	Hirschsprung Disease
Onset	2–3 years	At birth
Abdominal distention	Rare	Present
Nutrition and growth	Normal	Poor
Soiling and retentive behavior	Intermittent or constant	Rare
Rectal examination	Ampulla full	Ampulla may be empty
Rectal biopsy	Ganglion cells present	Ganglion cells absent
Rectal manometry	Normal rectoanal reflex	Nonrelaxation of internal anal sphincter after rectal distention
Barium enema	Distended rectum	Narrow distal segment with proximal megacolon

osmotic agents such as polyethylene glycol (MiraLax, 1 g/kg/d) and milk of magnesia (1–2 mL/kg/d). Effective stool softeners should thereafter be given regularly in doses sufficient to induce two or three loose bowel movements per day. After several weeks to months of regular loose stools, stool softeners can be tapered and stopped. Mineral oil should not be given to nonambulatory infants, physically handicapped or bed-bound children, or any child with GE reflux. Aspiration of mineral oil may cause lipid pneumonia. A multiple vitamin supplement is recommended while mineral oil is given. Recurrence of encopresis is common and should be treated promptly with a short course of stimulant laxatives or an enema. Psychiatric consultation may be indicated for patients with resistant symptoms or severe emotional disturbances.

Benninga M et al: The Paris Consensus on Childhood Constipation Terminology (PACCT) Group. J Pediatr Gastroenterol Nutr 2005;40:273 [PMID: 15735478].

Constipation Guidelines Committee of the North American Society for Pediatric Gastroenterology, Hepatology and Nutrition: Evaluation and treatment of constipation in infants and children: Recommendations of the North American Society for Pediatric Gastroenterology, Hepatology and Nutrition. J Pediatr Gastroenterol Nutr 2006;43:e1 [PMID: 16954945].

ANAL FISSURE

Anal fissure is a slitlike tear in the squamous epithelium of the anus, usually secondary to the passage of large, hard fecal masses. Anal stenosis, anal crypt abscess, and trauma can be contributory factors. Sexual abuse must be considered in children with large, irregular, or multiple anal fissures. Anal fissures may be the presenting sign of Crohn disease in older children.

The infant or child with anal fissure typically cries with defecation and will try to hold back stools. Sparse, bright red bleeding is seen on the outside of the stool or on the toilet tissue following defecation. The fissure can often be seen if the patient is examined in a knee-chest position with the buttocks spread apart. When a fissure cannot be identified, it is essential to rule out other causes of rectal bleeding such as juvenile polyp, perianal inflammation due to group A β-hemolytic streptococcus, or inflammatory bowel disease. Anal fissures should be treated promptly to break the constipation → fissure → pain → retention → constipation cycle. A stool softener should be given. Anal dilation relieves sphincter spasm. Warm sitz baths after defecation may be helpful. Rarely, silver nitrate cauterization or surgery is indicated. Anal surgery should be avoided in patients with Crohn disease because of the high risk of recurrence and progression after surgery.

CONGENITAL ANORECTAL ANOMALIES

1. Anterior Displacement of the Anus

Anterior displacement of the anus is a common anomaly of infant girls. Its usual presentation in infants is constipation and straining with stool. On physical examination, the anus looks normal but is ventrally displaced, located close to the vaginal fourchette (in females) or to the base of the scrotum (in males). The diagnosis is made in girls if the distance from the vaginal fourchette to the center of the anal opening is less than 25% of the total distance from fourchette to coccyx. In boys the diagnosis is made if the distance from the base of the scrotum to the anal aperture is less than 33% of the total distance from scrotum to coccyx. In severe anterior displacement, when the anal opening is located less than 10% of the distance from the vaginal fourchette to the coccyx, the anal sphincter muscle may not completely encircle the anal opening and severe obstipation similar to that seen in imperforate anus may occur. Indeed, extreme anterior displacement of the anus may be a form of imperforate anus. Surgery is not needed in most cases. Stool softeners or occasional glycerin suppositories usually relieve straining. This problem improves significantly by age 3–4 years as normal toddler lordosis disappears. A thorough investigation for imperforate anus should be performed in children with severe persistent symptoms, and an anal cutback operation may be needed.

2. Anal Stenosis

Anal stenosis usually presents in the newborn period. The anal aperture may be very small and filled with a dot of meconium. Defecation is difficult, with ribbon-like stools, blood and mucus per rectum, fecal impaction, and abdominal distention. This malformation accounts for about 10% of anorectal anomalies. Anal stenosis may not be apparent at birth because the anus looks normal. Rectal bleeding in a straining infant often leads to a rectal examination which reveals a tight ring in the anal canal. Dilation of the anal ring is usually curative but may have to be repeated daily for several weeks.

3. Imperforate Anus

Imperforate anus in its numerous forms accounts for 75% of all anorectal anomalies. These anomalies are often complicated by associated anomalies of the urinary and genital tract. They are more common in males than in females and require careful diagnostic evaluation immediately to assess the extent of bowel, urinary, genital, and other organ system anomalies, including spinal cord and heart.

Infants with low imperforate anus fail to pass meconium. There may be a greenish bulging membrane obstructing the anal aperture. Perforation of the anal membrane is a relatively simple surgical procedure. A skin tag shaped like a "bucket handle" is seen on the perineum of some males below which a stenotic aperture can be seen. The aperture is sometimes surrounded by normal anal musculature, but in many cases the aperture is a rectoperineal fistula and the anal musculature is displaced posteriorly or is absent. Eighty to 90% of patients with low imperforate anus are continent after surgery.

In high imperforate anus, physical examination usually shows no anal musculature. There may be a rectoperineal, rectovesicular, rectourethral, or rectovaginal fistula; hypoplastic buttocks; cloacal anomalies; and sometimes, evidence of distal neurologic deficit. It is critical in these cases to fully evaluate the complex anatomy and neurologic function before attempting corrective surgery. A diverting colostomy is usually performed to protect the urinary tract and relieve obstruction. After reparative surgery, only 30% of patients with high imperforate anus achieve fecal continence.

Levitt MA, Pena A: Outcomes from the correction of anorectal malformations. Curr Opin Pediatr 2005;17:394 [PMID: 15891433].

PSEUDOMEMBRANOUS ENTEROCOLITIS

Pseudomembranous enterocolitis occurs when previous antibiotic use allows overgrowth of *Clostridium difficile* in the colon and toxin production. The onset of colitis occurs from 1–14 days after initiation of antibiotic therapy and can occur up to 30 days after antibiotics have been discontinued. Clindamycin was one of the first antibiotics associated with pseudomembranous colitis. Almost all antibiotics are now recognized to be potential causes, although erythromycin seems less likely than most. In pediatric patients, amoxicillin and cephalosporins are commonly associated with pseudomembranous enterocolitis, probably because of their widespread use. Although antibiotic use is the most common antecedent of pseudomembranous colitis, previous GI surgery and antimetabolite therapy in cancer patients are also associated with its development.

C difficile secretes enterotoxins that cause necrotizing inflammation of the colon mucosa. The patient characteristically has fever, abdominal distention, tenesmus, diarrhea, and generalized abdominal tenderness. Chronic presentations with low-grade fever, diarrhea, and abdominal pain have been described. Diarrheal stools contain sheets of neutrophils and sometimes gross blood. Plain abdominal radiographs show a thickened colon wall and ileus. On colonoscopy, the colon is covered by small, raised white plaques (pseudomembranes) with areas of apparently normal bowel in between. Biopsy specimens show "exploding crypts"—an eruption of white cells that appears to be shooting out of affected crypts. Stool cultures often show overgrowth of *Staphylococcus aureus,* which is probably an opportunistic organism growing in the necrotic tissue. *C difficile* can be cultured in specialized laboratories. Identification of stool toxins is the usual method of diagnosis. Infants up to 18–24 months of age may have toxins in the stool but do not develop disease or require therapy. Infants do not have sufficient receptors for the toxins to produce disease.

The treatment of pseudomembranous colitis consists of stopping antibiotics and instituting therapy with oral vancomycin (30–50 mg/kg/d) or metronidazole (30 mg/kg/d). Vancomycin is many times more expensive than metronidazole and no more efficacious. Metronidazole can be given intravenously in patients with vomiting or ileus. Relapse occurs after treatment in 10–50% of patients because of exsporulation of residual spores in the colon. Retreatment with the same antibiotic regimen is usually effective, but multiple relapses are possible and may be a significant management problem. Ulcerative colitis may be an underlying problem in cases of apparent recurrent *C difficile.*

▼ DISORDERS OF THE PERITONEAL CAVITY

PERITONITIS

Primary bacterial peritonitis accounts for less than 2% of childhood peritonitis. The most common causative organisms are *Escherichia coli,* other enteric organisms, hemolytic streptococci, and pneumococci. Primary peritonitis occurs in patients with splenectomy, splenic dysfunction, or ascites (nephrotic syndrome, advanced liver disease, kwashiorkor). It also occurs in infants with pyelonephritis or pneumonia.

Secondary peritonitis is much more common. It is associated with peritoneal dialysis, penetrating abdominal trauma, or ruptured viscus. The organisms associated with secondary peritonitis vary with the cause. Organisms not commonly pathogenic such as *Staphylococcus epidermidis* and *Candida* may cause secondary peritonitis in patients

receiving peritoneal dialysis. Multiple enteric organisms may be isolated after penetrating abdominal injury, bowel perforation, or ruptured appendicitis. Intra-abdominal abscesses may form in pelvic, subhepatic, or subphrenic areas, but discrete localization of infection is less common in young infants than in adults.

Symptoms of peritonitis include abdominal pain, fever, nausea, vomiting, acidosis, and shock. Respirations are shallow. The abdomen is tender, rigid, and distended, with involuntary guarding. Bowel sounds may be absent. Diarrhea is fairly common in primary peritonitis and less so in secondary peritonitis. Most peritonitis is an acute medical emergency. In patients receiving peritoneal dialysis, peritonitis can be a chronic infection causing milder symptoms.

Leukocyte count is high initially (> 20,000/μL) with a predominance of immature forms, and later may fall to neutropenic levels, especially in primary peritonitis. Plain abdominal radiographs and CT scan will confirm the presence of ascites. Bacterial peritonitis should be suspected if paracentesis fluid contains more than 500 leukocytes/μL or more than 32 mg/dL of lactate; if it has a pH less than 7.34; or if the pH is over 0.1 pH unit less than arterial blood pH. Diagnosis is made by Gram stain and culture, preferably of 5–10 mL of fluid for optimal yield. The blood culture is often positive in primary peritonitis.

Antibiotic treatment and supportive therapy for dehydration, shock, and acidosis are indicated. Surgical treatment of the underlying cause of secondary peritonitis is critical. Removal of infected peritoneal dialysis catheters in patients with secondary peritonitis is sometimes necessary and almost always required if *Candida* infection is present.

CHYLOUS ASCITES

Neonatal chylous ascites may be due to congenital infection or developmental abnormality of the lymphatic system (intestinal lymphangiectasia). If the thoracic duct is involved, chylothorax may be present. Later in life, chylous ascites may result from congenital lymphangiectasia, retroperitoneal or lymphatic tumors, peritoneal bands, abdominal trauma, or infection, or it may occur after cardiac or abdominal surgery. It may be associated with intestinal malrotation.

▶ Clinical Findings

A. Symptoms and Signs

Both congenital and acquired lymphatic obstruction cause chylous ascites, diarrhea, and failure to thrive. The abdomen is distended, with a fluid wave and shifting dullness. Unilateral or generalized peripheral edema may be present.

B. Laboratory Findings

Laboratory findings include hypoalbuminemia, hypogammaglobulinemia, and lymphopenia. Ascitic fluid contains lymphocytes and has the biochemical composition of chyle if the patient has just been fed; otherwise, it is indistinguishable from ascites secondary to cirrhosis.

▶ Differential Diagnosis

Chylous ascites must be differentiated from ascites due to liver disease and in the older child, from constrictive pericarditis, chronic elevated right heart pressure, malignancy, infection, or inflammatory diseases causing lymphatic obstruction. In the newborn, urinary ascites from anatomic abnormalities of the kidney or collecting system must be considered. A simple test to diagnose urinary ascites is urea nitrogen or creatinine concentration of abdominal fluid. Neither of these is present in chylous or hepatic ascites

▶ Complications & Sequelae

Chylous ascites caused by intestinal lymphatic obstruction is associated with fat malabsorption and protein loss. Intestinal loss of albumin and γ-globulin may lead to edema and increase the risk of infection. Rapidly accumulating chylous ascites may cause respiratory complications. The primary infections and malignancies causing chylous ascites may be life-threatening.

▶ Treatment & Prognosis

Little can be done to correct congenital abnormalities due to hypoplasia, aplasia, or ectasia of the lymphatics unless they are surgically resectable. Treatment is supportive, consisting mainly of a very high-protein diet and careful attention to infections. Shunting of peritoneal fluid into the venous system is sometimes effective. A fat-free diet supplemented with medium-chain triglycerides decreases the formation of chylous ascites. Total parenteral nutrition may rarely be necessary. Infusions of albumin generally provide only temporary relief and are rarely used for chronic management. In the neonate, congenital chylous ascites may spontaneously disappear following one or more paracenteses and a medium-chain triglyceride diet.

Chye JK et al: Neonatal chylous ascites: Report of 3 cases and review of the literature. Pediatr Surg Int 1997;12:296 [PMID: 9099650].

GASTROINTESTINAL TUMORS & MALIGNANCIES

JUVENILE POLYPS

Juvenile polyps are usually pedunculated and solitary. The head of the polyp is composed of hyperplastic glandular and vascular elements, often with cystic transformation. Juvenile polyps are benign, and 80% occur in the rectosigmoid. Their incidence is highest between ages 3 and 5 years, and they are rare before age 1 year and usually autoamputate by age 15 years. They are more frequent in boys. The painless passage of small amounts of bright red blood on a normal or constipated stool is the most frequent manifestation. Abdominal pain is rare, but a juvenile polyp can be the lead point for an intussusception. Low-lying polyps may prolapse during defecation.

Rarely, many juvenile polyps may be present in the colon, causing anemia, diarrhea, and protein loss. A few cases of generalized juvenile polyposis involving the stomach, small bowel, and colon have been reported. These cases are associated with a slightly increased risk of cancer.

Colonoscopy is diagnostic and therapeutic when polyps are suspected. After removal of the polyp by electrocautery, nothing further should be done if histologic findings confirm the diagnosis. There is a slight risk of developing further juvenile polyps. Other polyposis syndromes are summarized in Table 20–4.

CANCERS OF THE ESOPHAGUS, SMALL BOWEL, & COLON

Esophageal cancer is rare in childhood. Cysts, leiomyomas, and hamartomas predominate. Caustic injury of the esophagus increases the very long-term risk of squamous cell carcinoma. Chronic peptic esophagitis is associated with Barrett esophagus, a precancerous lesion. Simple GE reflux in infancy without esophagitis is not a risk for cancer of the esophagus.

The most common **gastric or small bowel cancer** in children is lymphoma or lymphosarcoma. Intermittent abdominal pain, abdominal mass, intussusception, or a celiac-like picture may be present. Carcinoid tumors are usually benign and most often an incidental finding in the appendix. Metastasis is rare. The carcinoid syndrome (flushing, sweating, hypertension, diarrhea, and vomiting), associated with serotonin secretion, only occurs with metastatic carcinoid tumors.

Adenocarcinoma of the colon is rare in childhood. The transverse colon and rectosigmoid are the two most commonly affected sites. The low 5-year survival rate relates to the nonspecificity of presenting complaints and the large percentage of undifferentiated types. Children with a family history of colon cancer, chronic ulcerative colitis, or familial polyposis syndromes are at greater risk.

MESENTERIC CYSTS

These rare tumors may be small or large, single or multiloculated. They are thin-walled and contain serous, chylous, or hemorrhagic fluid. They are commonly located in the small bowel mesentery but are also found in the mesocolon. Most mesenteric cysts cause no symptoms. Traction on the mesentery may lead to colicky abdominal pain, which can be mild and recurrent but may appear acutely with vomiting. Volvu-

Table 20-4. Gastrointestinal polyposis syndromes.

	Location	Number	Histology	Extraintestinal Findings	Malignant Potential	Recommended Therapy
Juvenile polyps	Colon	Single (70%) Several (30%)	Hyperplastic, hamartomatous	None	None	Remove polyp for continuous bleeding or prolapse.
Familial juvenile polyposis coli[a]	Colon	> 10	Hyperplastic with focal adenomatous change	None	10–25%; higher if familial	Remove all polyps. Consider colectomy if very numerous or adenomatous.
Generalized juvenile polyposis[a]	Stomach, small bowel, colon	Multiple	Hyperplastic with focal adenomatous change	Hydrocephaly, cardiac lesions, mesenteric lymphangioma, malrotation	10–25%	Colectomy and close surveillance.
Familial adenomatous polyposis[a]	Colon; less commonly, stomach and small bowel	Multiple	Adenomatous	None	95–100%	Colectomy by age 18 years.
Peutz-Jeghers syndrome[a]	Small bowel, stomach, colon	Multiple	Hamartomatous	Pigmented cutaneous and oral macules; ovarian cysts and tumors; bony exostoses	2–3%	Remove accessible polyps or those causing obstruction or bleeding.
Gardner syndrome	Colon; less commonly, stomach and small bowel	Multiple	Adenomatous	Cysts, tumors, and desmoids of skin and bone; ampullary tumors; other tumors, retinal pigmentations can be a screening tool in families	95–100%	Colectomy by age 18 y. Upper tract surveillance.
Cronkhite-Canada syndrome	Stomach, colon; less commonly, esophagus and small bowel	Multiple	Hamartomatous	Alopecia; onychodystrophy; hyper-pigmentation	Rare	None.
Turcot syndrome[b]	Colon	Multiple	Adenomatous	Thyroid and brain tumors are the usual presentation	Possible	Central nervous system screening most important.

[a]Autosomal dominant.
[b]Autosomal recessive.

lus may occur around a cyst, and hemorrhage into a cyst may be mild or hemodynamically significant. A rounded mass can occasionally be palpated or seen on radiograph displacing adjacent intestine. Abdominal ultrasonography is usually diagnostic. Surgical removal is indicated.

INTESTINAL HEMANGIOMA

Hemangiomas of the bowel may cause acute or chronic blood loss. They may also cause intussusception, local stricture, or intramural hematoma. Thrombocytopenia and consumptive coagulopathy are occasional complications. Some lesions are telangiectasias (Rendu-Osler-Weber syndrome), and others are capillary hemangiomas. The largest group is cavernous hemangiomas, which are composed of large, thin-walled vessels arising from the submucosal vascular plexus.

They may protrude into the lumen as polypoid lesions or may invade the intestine from mucosa to serosa.

MAJOR GASTROINTESTINAL SYMPTOMS & SIGNS

ACUTE DIARRHEA

Viruses are the most common cause of acute gastroenteritis in developing and developed countries. Bacterial and parasitic enteric infections are discussed in Chapters 40 and 41. Of the viral agents causing enteric infection, rotavirus, a 67-nm double-stranded RNA virus with at least eight serotypes, is the most common. As with most viral pathogens, rotavirus affects the small intestine, causing voluminous watery diarrhea without leukocytes or blood. In the United States, rotavirus mainly affects infants between 3 and 15 months. Peak incidence in the United States is in the winter with sporadic cases occurring at other times. The virus is transmitted via the fecal-oral route and survives for hours on hands and for days on environmental surfaces.

1. Rotavirus Infection

The incubation period for rotavirus is 24–48 hours. Vomiting is the first symptom in 80–90% of patients, followed within 24 hours by low-grade fever and watery diarrhea. Diarrhea usually lasts 4–8 days but may last longer in young infants or immunocompromised patients. The white blood cell count is rarely elevated. The stool sodium level is usually less than 40 mEq/L. As patients become dehydrated from unreplaced fecal water loss, they may become hypernatremic. The stool does not contain blood or white cells. Metabolic acidosis results from bicarbonate loss in the stool, ketosis from poor intake, and lactic acidemia from hypotension and hypoperfusion

Replacement of fluid and electrolyte deficits and ongoing losses is critical, especially in small infants. (Oral and intravenous therapy are discussed in Chapter 43.) The use of oral rehydration fluid is appropriate in most cases. The use of clear liquids or hypocaloric (dilute formula) diets for more than 48 hours is not advisable in uncomplicated viral gastroenteritis because starvation depresses digestive function and prolongs diarrhea.

Intestinal lactase levels are reduced during rotavirus infection. Brief use of a lactose-free diet is associated with a shorter period of diarrhea but is not critical to successful recovery in healthy infants. Reduced fat intake during recovery may decrease nausea and vomiting.

Antidiarrheal medications are ineffective (kaolin-pectin combinations) or even dangerous (loperamide, tincture of opium, diphenoxylate with atropine). Bismuth subsalicylate preparations may reduce stool volume but are not critical to recovery. Oral immunoglobulin or specific antiviral agents have occasionally been useful in limiting duration of disease in immunocompromised patients.

Specific identification of rotavirus is not required in every case, especially in outbreaks. Rotavirus antigens can be identified in stool or virus can be seen by scanning electron microscopy. False-positive results (which may actually be nonpathogenic rotavirus) are seen in neonates. Most children are infected with rotavirus more than once, with the first infection being the most severe. Some protective immunity is imparted by the first infection. Prevention of infection occurs primarily by good hygiene and prevention of fecal-oral contamination. The American Academy of Pediatrics issued guidelines in January 2007 recommending the routine use of bovine-based pentavalent rotavirus vaccine to be given orally to infants at 2, 4, and 6 months of age.

2. Other Viral Infections Causing Acute Diarrhea

Other viral pathogens causing diarrhea in children can be identified in stool by electron microscopy, viral culture, or enzyme-linked immunoassay. Depending on the geographic location, enteric adenoviruses (serotypes 40 and 41) or caliciviruses are the next most common viral pathogens in infants. The symptoms of enteric adenovirus infection are similar to those of rotavirus, but infection is not seasonal and duration of illness may be longer. The Norwalk agent (now called norovirus) is a calicivirus, a small RNA virus that mainly causes vomiting but can also cause diarrhea in older children and adults, usually in common source outbreaks. The duration of symptoms is short, usually 24–48 hours. Other potentially pathogenic viruses include astroviruses, corona-like viruses, and other small round viruses.

Cytomegalovirus rarely causes diarrhea in immunocompetent children but may cause erosive colitis or enteritis in immunocompromised hosts. Cytomegalovirus enteritis is particularly common after bone marrow transplantation and in late stages of HIV infection.

American Academy of Pediatrics Committee on Infectious Diseases: Prevention of rotavirus disease: Guidelines for the use of rotavirus vaccine. Pediatrics 2007;119:171 [PMID: 17200286].

Caeiro JP et al: Etiology of outpatient pediatric nondysenteric diarrhea: A multicenter study in the United States. Pediatr Infect Dis J 1999;18:94 [PMID: 10048678].

CHRONIC DIARRHEA

Bowel habits are variable, making specific diagnosis of chronic diarrhea difficult. Some infants normally have 5–8 stools daily. A gradual or sudden increase in the number and volume of stools to more than 15 g/kg/d combined with an increase in fluidity should raise a suspicion that an organic cause of chronic diarrhea is present. Diarrhea may result from (1) interruption of normal cell transport processes for water, electrolytes, or nutrients; (2) decrease in the surface area available for absorption secondary to shortened bowel or mucosal disease; (3) increase in intestinal motility; (4) increase in unabsorbable osmotically active molecules in the intestinal lumen; (5) increase in intestinal permeability, leading to increased loss of water and electrolytes; and (6) stimulation of enterocyte secretion by toxins or cytokines. The most common entities causing chronic diarrhea are listed below. Malabsorption syndromes, which also cause chronic or recurrent diarrhea, are considered separately.

1. Noninfectious Causes of Chronic Diarrhea

A. Antibiotic Therapy

Diarrhea is reported in up to 60% of children receiving antibiotics. Only a tiny fraction of these patients have *C difficile*–related pseudomembranous enterocolitis. Eradication of normal gut flora and overgrowth of other organisms may cause diarrhea. Most antibiotic-associated diarrhea is watery, is not associated with systemic symptoms, and decreases when antibiotic therapy is stopped.

B. Extraintestinal Infections

Infections of the urinary tract and upper respiratory tract (especially otitis media) are at times associated with diarrhea. The mechanism is obscure. Antibiotic treatment of the primary infection, toxins released by infecting organisms, and local irritation of the rectum (in patients with bladder infection) may play a role.

C. Malnutrition

Malnutrition is associated with an increased frequency of enteral infections. Decreased bile acid synthesis, decreased pancreatic enzyme output, decreased disaccharidase activity, altered motility, and changes in the intestinal flora all may cause diarrhea. Severely malnourished children are at higher risk of enteric infections because of depressed immune functions, both cellular and humoral.

D. Diet and Medications

Overfeeding may cause diarrhea, especially in young infants. Relative deficiency of pancreatic amylase in young infants causes osmotic diarrhea after starchy foods. Fruit juices, especially those high in fructose or sorbitol, produce diarrhea because these osmotically active sugars are poorly absorbed. Intestinal irritants (spices and foods high in fiber) and histamine-containing or histamine-releasing foods (eg, citrus fruits, tomatoes, fermented cheeses, red wines, and scombroid fish) also cause diarrhea.

Laxative abuse in association with eating disorders or Münchausen syndrome by proxy can cause unpredictable diarrhea. A high concentration of magnesium in the stool may indicate overuse of milk of magnesia or other magnesium-containing laxatives. Detection of other laxative preparations in the stool or circulation requires sophisticated analysis not available in most laboratories. A high index of suspicion and careful observation may be required to make this diagnosis.

E. Allergic Diarrhea

Diarrhea resulting from allergy to dietary proteins is a frequently entertained but rarely proven diagnosis. Gastrointestinal symptoms from protein allergy are more common in infants younger than age 12 months, who may experience mild to severe colitis with diarrhea and rectal bleeding in response to cow's milk protein—either ingested directly or in minute quantities in maternal breast milk. A personal or family history of atopy is common in these infants. Skin testing is not reliable. Double-blind oral challenge with the suspected food under careful observation is necessary to confirm intestinal protein allergy. In the breast-fed infant, maternal avoidance of milk protein may be effective in reducing the signs of colitis. Substituting a protein hydrolysate formula for cow's milk–based formula may reduce symptoms. Allergic colitis in young infants is self-limited, usually disappearing by 8–12 months of age. The condition does not require treatment if the infant is thriving and the colitic symptoms are mild. Colonoscopy is not required for diagnosis, but rectal biopsies, if performed, show mild lymphonodular hyperplasia, mucosal edema, and slight eosinophilia. Allergies to fish, peanuts, and eggs are more likely to be lifelong and more likely to be IgE mediated. Multiple food allergy (more than three) is rare.

Older children may develop a celiac-like syndrome secondary to milk protein with flattening of small bowel villi, steatorrhea, hypoproteinemia, occult blood loss, and chronic diarrhea. Skin testing is not reliable since it detects circulating antibodies, not the T-cell–mediated responses that are probably responsible for food sensitivity reactions. Double-blind oral challenge with the suspected food under careful observation is necessary to confirm intestinal protein allergy. Small bowel biopsy findings are obvious but nonspecific. The diagnosis is often confirmed by dietary trial followed by disappearance of occult blood in the stool and improvement in other symptoms.

Anaphylactic, IgE-mediated reactions to foods can occur. After ingestion, the patient quickly develops vomiting, then diarrhea, pallor, and hypotension. In these cases, skin testing is positive. Food challenges should be undertaken in a setting in which resuscitation can be performed as there is often a progressively more severe reaction with subsequent ingestions. The close association between ingestion and symptoms usually leaves little doubt about the diagnosis.

F. Chronic Nonspecific Diarrhea

Chronic nonspecific diarrhea is the most common cause of loose stools in thriving children. The typical patient is a healthy child aged 6–20 months who has three to six loose mucoid stools per day during the waking hours. The diarrhea worsens with a low-residue, low-fat, or high-carbohydrate diet and during periods of stress and infection. It clears spontaneously at about age 3½ years (usually coincident with toilet training). No organic disease is discoverable. Possible causes include abnormalities of bile acid absorption in the terminal ileum, incomplete carbohydrate absorption (excessive fruit juice ingestion seems to worsen the condition or in some cases is the primary cause), and abnormal motor function. Family history of functional bowel disease is common. Stool tests for blood, white cells, fat, parasites, and bacterial pathogens are negative.

The following measures are helpful: use of a slightly high-fat (about 40% of total calories), low-carbohydrate, high-fiber diet; avoidance of between-meal snacks; avoidance of chilled fluids, especially fruit juices. Loperamide (0.1–0.2 mg/kg/d in two or three divided doses) is often helpful. Cholestyramine (2–4 g in divided doses) or psyllium agents (1–2 tsp twice daily) are sometimes used.

G. Secretory Diarrhea

Certain malignancies of childhood (neuroblastoma, ganglioneuroma, metastatic carcinoid, pancreatic VIPoma, or gastrinoma) may secrete substances such as gastrin and vasoactive intestinal polypeptide (VIP) that promote small intestinal secretion of water and electrolytes. Children may present with large-volume, chronic and intermittent watery diarrhea that does not cease when they discontinue oral feedings. Fat malabsorption is not characteristic. The serum potassium level is often low because of stool losses. The hallmark of the diarrhea is that, unlike osmotic and infectious viral diarrheas, the sodium content of stool water is high, usually between 90 and 140 mEq/L of stool. Other signs and symptoms are associated with specific tumors. Neuroblastoma and ganglioneuroma produce elevations in urinary homovanillic acid and vanillylmandelic acid. Metastatic carcinoid produces characteristic flushing and sweating. Gastrinoma may produce multiple duodenal ulcers (Zollinger-Ellison syndrome).

In all secretory diarrheas, a careful radiologic search for a tumor is indicated. Intraendoscopic ultrasound examination may reveal small tumors in the bowel wall or pancreatic head. Bacterial overgrowth of the small bowel in patients with short bowel, cancer chemotherapy, or anatomic abnormalities may be associated with enterotoxins that promote secretory diarrhea. Cholera is the best known bacterial secretory diarrhea. Its enterotoxin stimulates cyclic adenosine monophosphate in the enterocyte, which promotes salt and water secretion.

2. Infectious Causes of Chronic Diarrhea

Most infections of the GI tract are acute and resolve spontaneously or with specific antibiotic therapy. Organisms most prone to cause chronic or recurrent diarrhea in immunocompetent children are *Giardia lamblia*, *Entameba histolytica*, *Salmonella* spp, and *Yersinia*.

Chronic diarrhea is common in immune deficiency states, especially IgA deficiency and T-cell abnormalities. The cause of is often common bacterial, viral, fungal, or parasitic organisms usually considered nonpathogenic (rotavirus, *Blastocystis hominis*, *Candida*), or unusual organisms (cytomegalovirus, *Cryptosporidium*, *Isospora belli*, *Mycobacterium* spp, microsporidia, and algal organisms such as cyanobacteria).

Between 50% and 60% of patients with idiopathic acquired hypogammaglobulinemia have steatorrhea and intestinal villous atrophy. Lymphonodular hyperplasia of the small intestine is prominent. Patients with congenital or Bruton-type agammaglobulinemia usually have diarrhea and abnormal intestinal morphology. Patients with isolated IgA deficiency have chronic diarrhea, a celiac-like picture, lymphoid nodular hyperplasia, and are prone to giardiasis. Patients with isolated cellular immunity defects, combined cellular and humoral immune incompetence, and HIV infec-

tion may have severe chronic diarrhea leading to malnutrition. Often the cause is not found. The incidence of disaccharidase deficiency is high. Chronic granulomatous disease may be associated with intestinal symptoms suggestive of chronic inflammatory bowel disease. A rectal biopsy may reveal the presence of typical macrophages.

Treatment must be directed toward correcting the immunologic defect. Specific treatments are available or are being developed for many of the unusual pathogens causing diarrhea in the immunocompromised host. Thus, a vigorous diagnostic search for specific pathogens is warranted in these individuals.

GASTROINTESTINAL BLEEDING

Vomiting blood and passing blood per rectum are alarming symptoms. The history is the key to identifying the bleeding source. The following questions should be answered:

1. Is it really blood, and is it coming from the GI tract? A number of substances simulate hematochezia or melena (Table 20–5). The presence of blood should be confirmed chemically. Coughing, tonsillitis, lost teeth, or epistaxis may cause what appears to be occult or overt GI bleeding. An adolescent female may be experiencing menarche.

Table 20–5. Pitfalls in the diagnosis of gastrointestinal bleeding in children.

Exogenous blood
Maternal blood[a]
Epistaxis
Uncooked meat
Pseudoblood
Medications in red syrup
Red Kool-Aid, fruit punch, red gelatin
Tomato skin
Tomato juice
Cranberry juice
Beets
Peach skin
Red diaper syndrome[b]
Red cherries
Black stools
Iron preparations[c,d]
Pepto-Bismol
Grape juice
Purple grapes
Spinach
Chocolate

[a]From cracked nipples in a breast-fed infant.
[b]Red pigmentation of soiled diapers due to *Serratia marcescens* in stool.
[c]Ferrous sulfate and ferrous gluconate with guaiac and orthotoluidine-based tests.
[d]High false-positive rate with orthotoluidine-based tests.
Modified and reproduced, with permission, from Treem WR: Gastrointestinal bleeding in children. Gastrointest Endosc Clin North Am 1994;4:75.

2. How much blood is there and what is its color and character? Table 20–6 lists the sites of GI bleeding predicted by the appearance of the blood in the stools. Table 20–7 lists causes of rectal bleeding.

3. Is the child acutely or chronically ill? The physical examination should be thorough. Physical signs of portal hypertension, intestinal obstruction, or coagulopathy are particularly important. The nasal passages should be inspected for signs of recent epistaxis, the vagina for menstrual blood, and the anus for fissures and hemorrhoids. A systolic blood pressure below 100 mm Hg and a pulse rate above 100 beats/min in an older child suggest at least a 20% reduction of blood volume. A pulse rate increase of 20 beats/min or a drop in systolic blood pressure greater than 10 mm Hg when the patient sits up is also a sensitive index of volume depletion.

4. Is the child still bleeding? Serial determination of vital signs and hematocrit are essential to assess ongoing bleeding. Detection of blood in the gastric aspirate confirms a bleeding site proximal to the ligament of Treitz. However, its absence does not rule out the duodenum as the source. Testing the stool for occult blood will help in monitoring ongoing loss of blood.

▶ **Treatment**

If a hemorrhagic diathesis is detected, vitamin K should be given intravenously. In severe bleeding, the need for volume replacement is monitored by measurement of central venous pressure. In less severe cases, vital signs, serial hematocrits, and gastric aspirates are sufficient.

Table 20–6. Identification of sites of gastrointestinal bleeding.

Symptom or Sign	Location of Bleeding Lesion
Effortless bright red blood from the mouth	Nasopharyngeal or oral lesions; tonsillitis; esophageal varices; lacerations of esophageal or gastric mucosa (Mallory-Weiss syndrome)
Vomiting of bright red blood or of "coffee grounds"	Lesion proximal to ligament of Treitz
Melanotic stool	Lesion proximal to ligament of Treitz, upper small bowel. Blood loss in excess of 50–100 mL/24 h
Bright red or dark red blood in stools	Lesion in the ileum or colon. (Massive upper gastrointestinal bleeding may also be associated with bright red blood in stool.)
Streak of blood on outside of a stool	Lesion in the rectal ampulla or anal canal

If blood is recovered from the gastric aspirate, gastric lavage with saline should be performed until only a blood-tinged return is obtained. Upper intestinal endoscopy is then done to identify the bleeding site. Endoscopy is superior to barium contrast study for lesions such as esophageal varices, stress ulcers, and gastritis. Colonoscopy may identify the source of bright red rectal bleeding but should be performed as an emergency procedure only if the extent of bleeding warrants immediate investigation and if plain abdominal radiographs show no signs of intestinal obstruction. Colonoscopy on an unprepped colon is often inadequate for making a diagnosis. Capsule endoscopy may help identify the site of bleeding if colonoscopy and upper endoscopy findings are negative. Small or large bowel lesions that bleed briskly (> 0.5 mL/min) may be localized by angiography or radionuclide scanning following injection of labeled red cells.

Persistent vascular bleeding (varices, vascular anomalies) may be relieved temporarily using intravenous octreotide, 25–30 µg/m²/h. Sustained infusion of octreotide may be used for up to 48 hours if needed. Bleeding from esophageal varices may be stopped by compression with a Sengstaken-Blakemore tube. Endoscopic sclerosis or banding of bleeding varices is effective treatment.

If gastric decompression, acid suppressive therapy, and transfusion are ineffective in stopping ulcer bleeding, laser therapy, local injection of epinephrine, electrocautery, or emergency surgery may be necessary.

Fox VL: Gastrointestinal bleeding in infancy and childhood. Gastroenterol Clin North Am 2000;29:37 [PMID: 10752017].

VOMITING

Vomiting is an extremely complex, poorly understood activity. The centers controlling and coordinating vomiting are in the paraventricular nuclei of the brain. These nuclei receive afferent input from many sources: drugs and neurotransmitters in cerebrospinal fluid, the chemoreceptor trigger zone (CTZ) near the distal fourth ventricle, the vestibular apparatus of the ear, the GI tract and other abdominal organs, and even from higher cortical areas. Vagal afferents from gut to brain are stimulated by ingested drugs and toxins, mechanical stretch, inflammation, and local neurotransmitters. Additionally, local feedback loops in the gut also appear capable of initiating vomiting.

Vomiting is the presenting symptom of many pediatric conditions. It is the pediatrician's difficult job to find the underlying cause. The most common cause of vomiting in childhood is probably acute viral gastroenteritis. However, obstruction and acute or chronic inflammation of the GI tract and associated structures are also major causes. Central nervous system inflammation, pressure, or tumor may cause vomiting. Metabolic derangements associated with inborn errors of metabolism, sepsis, and drug intoxication can stimulate either the CTZ or the brain directly to promote vomiting.

Table 20–7. Differential diagnosis of gastrointestinal bleeding in children by symptoms and age at presentation.

	Infant	Child (2–12 y)	Adolescent (> 12 y)
Hematemesis	Swallowed maternal blood Peptic esophagitis Mallory-Weiss tear Gastritis Gastric ulcer Duodenal ulcer	Epistaxis Peptic esophagitis Caustic ingestion Mallory-Weiss tear Esophageal varices Gastritis Gastric ulcer Duodenal ulcer Hereditary hemorrhagic telangiectasia Hemobilia Henoch-Schönlein purpura	Esophageal ulcer Peptic esophagitis Mallory-Weiss tear Esophageal varices Gastric ulcer Gastritis Duodenal ulcer Hereditary hemorrhagic telangiectasia Hemobilia Henoch-Schönlein purpura
Painless melena	Duodenal ulcer Duodenal duplication Ileal duplication Meckel diverticulum Gastric heterotopia[a]	Duodenal ulcer Duodenal duplication Ileal duplication Meckel diverticulum Gastric heterotopia[a]	Duodenal ulcer Leiomyoma (sarcoma)
Melena with pain, obstruction, peritonitis, perforation	Necrotizing enterocolitis Intussusception[b] Volvulus	Duodenal ulcer Hemobilia[c] Intussusception[b] Volvulus Ileal ulcer (isolated)	Duodenal ulcer Hemobilia[c] Crohn disease (ileal ulcer)
Hematochezia with diarrhea, crampy abdominal pain	Infectious colitis Pseudomembranous colitis Eosinophilic colitis Hirschsprung enterocolitis	Infectious colitis Pseudomembranous colitis Granulomatous (Crohn) colitis Hemolytic-uremic syndrome Henoch-Schönlein purpura Lymphonodular hyperplasia	Infectious colitis Pseudomembranous colitis Granulomatous (Crohn) colitis Hemolytic-uremic syndrome Henoch-Schönlein purpura
Hematochezia without diarrhea or abdominal pain	Anal fissure Eosinophilic colitis Rectal gastric mucosa heterotopia Colonic hemangiomas	Anal fissure Solitary rectal ulcer Juvenile polyp Lymphonodular hyperplasia	Anal fissure Hemorrhoid Solitary rectal ulcer Colonic arteriovenous malformation

[a]Ectopic gastric tissue in jejunum or ileum without Meckel diverticulum.
[b]Classically, "currant jelly" stool.
[c]Often accompanied by vomiting and right upper quadrant pain.
Reproduced, with permission, from Treem WR: Gastrointestinal bleeding in children. Gastrointest Endosc Clin North Am 1994;4:75.

Regurgitation associated with GE reflux of infants should be distinguished from vomiting. In this instance, spontaneous relaxation of the lower esophageal sphincter creates a common cavity between the stomach and esophagus. Because the resting pressure of the thorax is negative, the mildly positive pressure of the abdominal cavity (~ 6 mm Hg) pushes gastric contents into the esophagus, causing an effortless flow into the mouth. Occasionally, regurgitated fluid stimulates the pharyngeal afferents and provokes gagging or even a complete vomiting complex.

Control of vomiting with medication is rarely needed in acute gastroenteritis and should not be attempted in other patients until the source is clear. Antihistamines and anticholinergics are appropriate for motion sickness because of their labyrinthine effects. 5-HT$_3$ receptor antagonists (ondansetron, granisetron) are useful for vomiting associated with surgery and chemotherapy. Benzodiazepines, corticosteroids, and substituted benzamides are also used in chemotherapy-induced vomiting. Butyrophenones (droperidol, haloperidone) are powerful drugs that block the D2 receptor in the CTZ and are used for intractable vomiting in acute gastritis, chemotherapy, and after surgery. Phenothiazines are helpful in chemotherapy, cyclic vomiting, and acute GI infection but are not recommended for outpatient use because of extrapyramidal side effects.

1. Cyclic Vomiting Syndrome

▷ Clinical Findings

Cyclic vomiting syndrome (CVS) is characterized by recurrent episodes of stereotypical vomiting in children usually older than 1 year of age. The emesis is forceful and frequent, occurring up to six times per hour for up to 72 hours or more. Episode frequency ranges from two to three per month to less than one per year. Nausea, retching, and small-volume bilious emesis continue even after the stomach is emptied. Hematemesis secondary to forceful vomiting may occur. Patients experience abdominal pain, anorexia, and rarely, diarrhea. Autonomic symptoms, such as pallor, sweating, temperature instability, and lethargy are common and give the patient a very ill appearance. The episodes end suddenly, often after a period of sleep. In some children, dehydration, electrolyte imbalance, and shock may occur. Between episodes, the child is completely healthy.

The cause of CVS is unknown; however, a similarity to migraine has long been recognized. Family history is positive for migraine in 50–70% of cases and many patients develop migraine headaches as adults. Research suggests that abnormalities of neurotransmitters and hormones provoke CVS. About one quarter of patients have typical migraine symptoms during episodes: premonitory sensation, headache, photophobia, and phonophobia. Identifiable triggers include infection, positive or negative emotional stress, diet (chocolate, cheese, monosodium glutamate), menses, or motion sickness.

▷ Differential Diagnosis

Conditions that mimic CVS include drug toxicity, increased intracranial pressure, seizures, brain tumor, Chiari malformation, recurrent sinusitis, choledochal cyst, gallstones, recurrent small bowel obstruction, inflammatory bowel disease, familial pancreatitis, obstructive uropathy, recurrent urinary infection, diabetes, mitochondrial diseases, disorders of fatty and organic acid metabolism, adrenal insufficiency, and Münchausen syndrome by proxy. Although tests for GE reflux are often positive in these patients, it is unlikely that GE reflux and CVS are related.

▷ Treatment

Avoidance of triggers prevents spells in some patients. Sleep can also end a spell although some children awaken and resume vomiting. Diphenhydramine or lorazepam are used at the onset of spells in some children to reduce nausea and induce sleep. Early use of antimigraine medications (sumatriptan), antiemetics (ondansetron), or antihistamines can abort spells in some patients. Once a spell is well established, intravenous fluids are often required to end it. With careful supervision, some children with predictable spells can receive intravenous fluids at home. Several approaches usually are tried before an effective therapy is found. Preventing spells with prophylactic propranolol, amitriptyline, or antihistamines is effective in some patients with frequent or disabling spells. Some patients have been successfully treated with anticonvulsants.

Sudel B, Li BU: Treatment options for cyclic vomiting syndrome. Curr Treat Options Gastroenterol 2005;8:387 [PMID: 16162304].

RECURRENT ABDOMINAL PAIN

About 10% of healthy schoolchildren between 5 and 15 years of age will at some time have recurrent episodes of unexplained abdominal pain severe enough to interfere with normal activities. An organic cause is found in fewer than 10% of patients.

▷ Clinical Findings

A. Symptoms and Signs

Attacks of pain are characteristically of variable duration and intensity. It is not rare for the parent or patient to report that the pain is constant, all day, every day. Although the pain is usually located in the periumbilical area, a location far from the umbilicus does not rule out recurrent abdominal pain. Pain occurs both day and night. Weight loss is rare. Pain may be associated with dramatic reactions—frantic crying, clutching the abdomen, doubling over. Parents may be alarmed, and children are often taken to emergency departments, where the evaluation is negative for an abdominal crisis. School attendance may suffer, and enjoyable family events may be disrupted. The pain may be associated with pallor, nausea, vomiting, and slight temperature elevation.

The pain usually bears little relationship to bowel habits and physical activity. However, some patients have a symptom constellation suggestive of irritable bowel syndrome—bloating, postprandial pain, lower abdominal discomfort, and erratic stool habits with a sensation of obstipation or incomplete evacuation of stool. A precipitating or stressful situation in the child's life at the time the pains began can sometimes be elicited. School phobia may be a precipitant. A history of functional GI complaints is often found in family members.

A thorough physical examination is essential and usually normal. Complaints of abdominal tenderness elicited during palpation sometimes seem out of proportion to visible signs of distress.

B. Laboratory Findings

Complete blood count, sedimentation rate, urinalysis, and stool test for occult blood usually suffice. In the adolescent female patient, ultrasound of the abdomen may be helpful to detect gallbladder or ovarian pathology. If the pain is atypi-

Table 20–8. Causes of acute abdomen.

Infection and Inflammation	Other Causes
Appendicitis	Midgut volvulus
Severe infectious enteritis and colitis	Intussusception
	Ovarian torsion
Pseudomembranous enterocolitis	Incarcerated hernia
Toxic megacolon associated with Hirschsprung disease or ulcerative colitis	Abdominal trauma
	Diabetic ketoacidosis
	Peritonitis
Mesenteric adenitis	Intussusception with obstruction
Pelvic inflammatory disease	Distal intestinal obstruction syndrome
Pancreatitis	
Cholecystitis	Testicular torsion
Abdominal vasculitis (Henoch-Schönlein purpura, polyarteritis nodosa)	Intestinal pseudo-obstruction
	Sickle cell abdominal crisis
	Metabolic conditions (eg, porphyria, lead poisoning)
Peritonitis	

cal, further testing suggested by symptoms and family history should be done.

▶ Differential Diagnosis

Abdominal pain secondary to disorders causing acute abdomen are listed in Table 20–8. Pinworms, mesenteric lymphadenitis, and chronic appendicitis are improbable causes of recurrent abdominal pain. *H pylori* infection is rarely the cause of recurrent abdominal pain. Lactose intolerance usually causes abdominal distention, gas, and diarrhea with milk ingestion. At times, however, abdominal discomfort may be the only symptom. Abdominal migraine and abdominal epilepsy are rare conditions with an episodic character often associated with vomiting. The incidence of peptic gastritis, esophagitis, duodenitis, and ulcer disease is probably underappreciated. Upper intestinal endoscopy may be useful.

▶ Treatment & Prognosis

Treatment consists of reassurance based on a thorough physical appraisal and a sympathetic, age-appropriate explanation of the nature of functional pain. The concept of "visceral hyperalgesia" or increased pain signaling from physiologic stimuli such as gas, acid secretion, or stool is one that parents can understand and helps them to respond appropriately to the child's complaints. Reassurance without education is rarely helpful. Regular activity should be resumed, especially school attendance. Therapy for emotional problems is sometimes required, but drugs should be avoided. In older patients, and in those with what appears to be visceral hyperalgesia, amitriptyline in low doses may occasionally be helpful. Antispasmodic medications are rarely helpful and should be reserved for patients with more typical irritable bowel complaints.

Rasquin A et al: Childhood functional gastrointestinal disorders: Child/adolescent. Gastroenterology 2006;130:1527 [PMID: 16678566].

ACUTE ABDOMEN

An acute abdomen is a constellation of findings indicating an intra-abdominal process that may require surgery. A degree of urgency is implied when this diagnosis is suspected. The pain of an acute abdomen intensifies over time and is rarely relieved without definitive treatment. Pain is often accompanied by nausea, vomiting, diarrhea, fever, and anorexia. Pain may be localized or generalized. The abdomen may be distended and tense and bowel sounds reduced or obstructive. Patients appear ill and are reluctant to be examined or moved. The acute abdomen is usually a result of infection of the intra-abdominal or pelvic organs but also occurs with intestinal obstruction, intestinal perforation, inflammatory conditions, trauma, and some metabolic disorders. Some conditions causing acute abdomen are listed in Table 20–8. Reaching a speedy and accurate diagnosis is critical and requires skill in physical diagnosis, recognition of the symptoms of a large number of conditions, and a judicious selection of laboratory and radiologic tests. (Acute appendicitis is discussed earlier in the section on Disorders of the Small Intestine.)

▼ MALABSORPTION SYNDROMES

Malabsorption of ingested food has many causes (Table 20–9). Shortening of the small bowel (usually via surgical resection) and mucosal damage (celiac disease) both reduce surface area. Impaired motility of the small intestine may interfere with normal propulsive movements and mixing of food with pancreatic and biliary secretions. Anaerobic bacteria proliferate under these conditions and impair fat absorption by deconjugation of bile acids (intestinal pseudo-obstruction, postoperative blind loop syndrome). Impaired intestinal lymphatic (congenital lymphangiectasia) or venous drainage also causes malabsorption. Diseases reducing pancreatic exocrine function (cystic fibrosis, Shwachman syndrome) or the production and flow of biliary secretions cause nutrient malabsorption. Malabsorption of specific nutrients may be genetically determined (disaccharidase deficiency, glucose-galactose malabsorption, and abetalipoproteinemia).

▶ Clinical Findings

Diarrhea, vomiting, anorexia, abdominal pain, failure to thrive, and abdominal distention are common. Stool may be bulky, foul, and pale with fat malabsorption or loose when diarrhea is osmotically induced. Microscopic examination of stools for neutral fat and fatty acids is a useful screen because most malabsorption syndromes involve some fat malabsorption. Pancreatic insufficiency is associated with neutral fat (triglycerides) in the stool. Fatty acids are the major fatty material found in the stool of patients with mucosal and liver disease.

Quantitation of fat malabsorption requires measuring fat excreted in the feces as a proportion of fat intake for a defined

Table 20–9. Malabsorption syndromes.

Intraluminal phase abnormalities
  Acid hypersecretion (eg, Zollinger-Ellison syndrome)
  Exocrine pancreatic insufficiency
    Cystic fibrosis
    Shwachman syndrome
    Malnutrition
    Specific enzyme defects
  Decreased intraluminal bile acids
    Chronic parenchymal liver disease
    Biliary obstruction
    Bile acid loss (short gut, ileal disease)
    Bile acid deconjugation by bacterial overgrowth
Intestinal phase abnormalities
  Mucosal infection (*Giardia, Cryptosporidium*)
  Celiac disease
  Mucosal enzyme deficiency (primary or secondary)
  Allergic enteropathy
  Radiation enteritis
  Dumping syndrome
  Short bowel syndrome
Vascular phase abnormalities
  Whipple disease
  Intestinal lymphangiectasia
  Congestive heart failure
Metabolic genetic disease
  Abetalipoproteinemia
  Glucose-galactose malabsorption
  Acrodermatitis enteropathica
  Congenital chloride diarrhea

---

period. Excretion of 5% of ingested fat is normal for a child older than age 1 year; 10–15% is normal in a younger infant. Prothrombin time and serum carotene, vitamin E, and vitamin D levels may be depressed by long-standing fat malabsorption. Accurate assessment of protein absorption is difficult and requires isotopic labeling of amino acids. Loss of serum proteins across the intestinal mucosa can be estimated by measurement of fecal α_1-antitrypsin. Malabsorption of complex carbohydrate is rarely measured. Disaccharide or monosaccharide malabsorption is estimated by reduction in stool pH, increased breath hydrogen after ingestion of carbohydrate, or decreased intestinal mucosal disaccharidase activity.

Other screening tests suggesting a specific diagnosis include sweat chloride concentration (cystic fibrosis), intestinal mucosal biopsy (celiac disease, intestinal lymphangiectasia, giardiasis, inflammatory bowel disease), liver and gallbladder function tests, and pancreatic secretion after stimulation with secretin and cholecystokinin. Some of the most common disorders associated with malabsorption in pediatric patients are detailed below.

1. Protein-Losing Enteropathy

Loss of plasma proteins into the GI tract occurs in association with intestinal inflammation, intestinal graft-versus-host disease, acute and chronic intestinal infections, venous and lym-

phatic obstruction or malformations, and infiltration of the intestine or its lymphatics and vasculature by malignant cells. Chronic elevation of venous pressure in children with the Fontan procedure may produce protein-losing enteropathy.

► Clinical Findings

Signs and symptoms are mainly those caused by hypoproteinemia, and in some instances by fat malabsorption: edema, ascites, poor weight gain, and specific vitamin and mineral deficiencies. Serum albumin and globulins may be decreased. Fecal α_1-antitrypsin is elevated (> 3 mg/g dry weight stool; slightly higher in breast-fed infants). Disorders associated with protein-losing enteropathy are listed in Table 20–10. In the presence of intestinal bleeding, fecal α_1-antitrypsin measurements are falsely high.

► Differential Diagnosis

Hypoalbuminemia may be due to increased catabolism, poor protein intake, impaired hepatic protein synthesis, or congenital malformations of lymphatics outside the GI tract. Protein losses in the urine from nephritis and nephrotic syndrome may also cause hypoalbuminemia.

Table 20–10. Disorders associated with protein-losing enteropathy.

Vascular obstruction
  Congestive heart failure
  Constrictive pericarditis
  Atrial septal defect
  Primary myocardial disease
  Increased right atrial pressure[a]
Stomach
  Giant hypertrophic gastritis (Ménétrier disease), often secondary to cytomegalovirus infection
  Polyps
  Gastritis secondary to *Helicobacter pylori* infection
Small intestine
  Celiac disease
  Intestinal lymphangiectasia
  Blind loop syndrome
  Abetalipoproteinemia
  Chronic mucosal ischemia (eg, from chronic volvulus or radiation enteritis)
  Allergic enteropathy
  Malrotation
  Inflammatory bowel disease
Colon
  Ulcerative colitis
  Hirschsprung disease
  Pseudomembranous colitis
  Polyposis syndromes
  Villous adenoma
  Solitary rectal ulcer

---

[a]Children who undergo Fontan procedure for tricuspid atresia are especially prone.

▶ Treatment

Albumin infusion, diuretics, and a high-protein, low-fat diet may control symptoms. Treatment must be directed toward identifying and treating the underlying cause.

2. Celiac Disease (Gluten Enteropathy)

ESSENTIALS OF DIAGNOSIS
& TYPICAL FEATURES

- ▶ Diarrhea, fatty stools, failure to thrive, irritability, hypoproteinemia, edema.
- ▶ Mean age of onset is 18 months.
- ▶ Tissue transglutaminase antibody testing is positive.
- ▶ Intestinal biopsy confirms the diagnosis.

Celiac disease results from intestinal sensitivity to the gliadin fraction of glutens from wheat, rye, barley, and (possibly) oats. Most children present during the second year of life, but the age at onset and the severity are variable. Up-to-date estimates of disease frequency are being revised with the widespread use of sensitive screening tests such as the tissue transglutaminase. Screening with antigliadin antibodies is not recommended because of the high frequency of false-positive tests. The frequency of celiac disease in the United States is around 1:300. It is thought that intestinal damage and villous atrophy result from a cell-mediated immune response initiated by exposure to a polypeptide fragment of gliadin. Ten percent of first-degree relatives may be affected. The inheritance is probably polygenic but may result from a single gene in combination with an environmental precipitant such as intestinal viral infection. The increased incidence of celiac disease in children with type 1 diabetes mellitus, IgA deficiency, and Down syndrome is consistent with possible immunologic factors in the development of celiac disease. Individuals with HLA DR4 and perhaps DR3 tissue types are at higher risk.

▶ Clinical Findings

A. Symptoms and Signs

1. Diarrhea—Affected children usually have diarrhea starting 6–12 months after the introduction of grains. Initially, the diarrhea may be intermittent; subsequently it is continuous, with bulky, pale, frothy, greasy, foul-smelling stools. During celiac crises, dehydration, shock, and acidosis occur. If anorexia is severe (about 10% of cases), diarrhea may be absent.

2. Constipation, vomiting, and abdominal pain—This triad of symptoms may occasionally dominate the clinical picture and suggest a diagnosis of intestinal obstruction. Constipation generally results from a combination of anorexia, dehydration, muscle weakness, and bulky stools.

3. Failure to thrive—Active celiac disease is often accompanied by loss of appetite, failure to gain weight, and irritability. Weight loss is most marked in the limbs and buttocks. The abdomen becomes distended secondary to intestinal gas and fluid accumulation. Short stature and delayed puberty may be the only sign in some older children.

4. Anemia and vitamin deficiencies—Anemia usually responds to iron supplementation and is rarely megaloblastic. Anemia is a more common presenting problem in adults than in children. Fat-soluble vitamin deficiency is common. Rickets can be seen in growing children but osteomalacia even with pathologic fractures is more common. Hypoprothrombinemia secondary to vitamin K malabsorption can cause easy bleeding.

5. Silent celiac disease—Serologic screening in children with nonspecific GI complaints, growth failure, type 1 diabetes, thyroid disease, vitiligo, IgA deficiency, and Down syndrome, and in family members of celiac patients is widespread. The therapy for a symptom-free child with positive serology is unclear. Intestinal biopsy specimens from children with positive serology are usually abnormal and the prudent response is to recommend a gluten-free diet. In patients with positive serology but normal intestinal biopsies, careful follow-up without diet therapy is the most appropriate current recommendation.

B. Laboratory Findings

1. Fat content of stools—A 3-day collection of stools usually reveals excessive fecal fat excretion. A normal child excretes 5–10% of ingested fat. In untreated celiac disease fat excretion is more than 15% of daily fat intake. Anorexia may be so severe that steatorrhea may not be present in 10–25% of patients until normal intake is established.

2. Carbohydrate absorption—A low oral glucose tolerance curve is seen. Absorption of D-xylose is impaired, with blood levels lower than 20 mg/dL 60 minutes after ingestion.

3. Hypoproteinemia—Hypoalbuminemia can be severe enough to lead to edema. There is evidence of increased protein loss in the gut lumen and poor hepatic synthesis secondary to malnutrition.

4. Serologic and genetic testing—The most sensitive and specific screening test for celiac disease in IgA-sufficient patients is a tissue transglutaminase antibody test. In the presence of IgA deficiency, this test may be falsely negative. IgG tissue transglutaminase antibody testing is available. The tissue transglutaminase antibody results can be used to roughly gauge dietary compliance. Antigliadin antibodies are not reliable for screening. Genetic screening for typical tissue type may be an indication of risk but it is not diagnostic.

C. Imaging

A small bowel series shows a malabsorptive pattern characterized by segmentation, clumping of the barium column, and hypersecretion. These changes are nonspecific and can be found in patients with other malabsorption states.

D. Biopsy Findings

Intestinal biopsy is the most reliable test for celiac disease. By light microscopy, the celiac mucosa has shortened or absent villi, lengthened crypts of Lieberkühn, intense plasma cell infiltration of the lamina propria, and numerous intraepithelial lymphocytes. Extent of change is quantitated from 0 (normal) to 4 (complete villous atrophy) using the Marsh scoring system.

▶ Differential Diagnosis

The differential diagnosis includes disorders causing malabsorption. Strict adherence to two diagnostic criteria is essential—the characteristic small bowel microscopic changes and clinical improvement on a gluten-free diet. Repeat mucosal biopsies to prove histologic recovery on gluten-free diet and relapse on gluten challenge are not indicated in typical patients.

▶ Treatment

A. Diet

Treatment is dietary gluten restriction for life. All sources of wheat, rye, and barley are eliminated. Some patients can tolerate oats, but this should be tested only after recovery has occurred. Lactose is poorly tolerated in the acute stage because mucosal atrophy causes secondary disaccharidase deficiency. Normal amounts of fat are advisable. Supplemental calories, vitamins, and minerals are indicated only in the acute phase. Clinical improvement usually starts within a week, but complete clinical recovery and histologic normality may require 3–12 months. Tissue transglutaminase titers may decrease on a gluten-free diet, but usually do not disappear.

B. Corticosteroids

Corticosteroids can hasten clinical improvement but are indicated only in very ill patients with profound anorexia, malnutrition, diarrhea, edema, abdominal distention, and hypokalemia.

▶ Prognosis

Clinical and histologic recovery is the rule but may be slow. Malignant lymphoma of the small bowel occurs with increased frequency in adults with long-standing disease. Dietary treatment seems to decrease the risk of this complication.

Fasano A et al: The prevalence of celiac disease in at-risk and not-at-risk groups in the United States: A multicenter study. Arch Intern Med 2003;163:286 [PMID: 12578508].

Hill I et al: Guidelines for the diagnosis and treatment of celiac disease in children: Recommendations of the North American Society for Pediatric Gastroenterology, Hepatology and Nutrition. J Pediatr Gastroenterol Nutr 2005;40:1 [PMID: 15625418].

3. Disaccharidase Deficiency

Starches and the disaccharides sucrose and lactose are the most important dietary carbohydrates. Dietary disaccharides and oligosaccharide products of pancreatic amylase action on starch require hydrolysis by intestinal brush border disaccharidases before absorption takes place. Disaccharidase levels are higher in the jejunum and proximal ileum than in the distal ileum and duodenum. In primary disaccharidase deficiency, a single enzyme is affected; disaccharide intolerance is permanent; intestinal histologic findings are normal; and a positive family history is common. Because disaccharidases are located on the luminal surface of intestinal enterocytes, they are susceptible to mucosal damage. Many conditions cause secondary disaccharidase deficiency and lactase is usually the most severely depressed.

A. Lactase Deficiency

Congenital lactase deficiency is rare. All human ethnic groups are lactase-sufficient at birth. Genetic or familial lactase deficiency begins to appear in children as young as 3–5 years. In Asians, Alaskan natives, and Native Americans, genetic lactase deficiency develops in virtually 100%. In Africans, the incidence in most tribes is over 80%. In African Americans, the incidence is about 70%, and among Caucasian Americans, the incidence is between 30% and 60%. Acquired or secondary lactase deficiency caused by intestinal injury due to viral infection, inflammatory disease, radiation, and drugs is very common. Lactase deficiency secondary to viral gastroenteritis is usually self-limited, lasting days or, at most, weeks after recovery from infection.

Lactose ingestion in deficient individuals causes variable degrees of diarrhea, gassy distention, and abdominal pain depending on the residual enzyme activity and the dose of lactose. Stools are liquid or frothy, with a pH below 4.5 owing to the presence of organic acids. Vomiting is common. Severe malnutrition may occur in a milk-fed infant with lactase deficiency. Reducing substances are present in fresh stools. The blood glucose fails to rise more than 10 mg/dL after ingestion of 1 g/kg of lactose. A rise in breath hydrogen after oral administration of lactose (from hydrogen produced by normal colon flora during fermentation of unabsorbed carbohydrate) is also diagnostic.

Symptoms disappear when dietary lactose is restricted. Lactase extracted from *Aspergillus* and *Kluyvera* species can be added to milk products or taken with meals to enhance lactose hydrolysis.

B. Sucrase-Isomaltase Deficiency

This is a combined defect inherited as an autosomal recessive trait. Ten percent of Alaskan natives are affected. The condition is rare in other groups. Abdominal distention, failure to thrive, and chronic diarrhea may be the presenting symptoms. Intestinal mucosal damage from viral infection reduces the activity of all disaccharidases including sucrase, but symptoms of sucrose intolerance are usually masked by the more striking symptoms of lactose intolerance. Distaste for and avoidance of sucrose occurs even in young infants with genetic sucrase-isomaltase deficiency.

Because sucrose is not a reducing sugar, the results of tests for reducing substances in the stool are negative unless the sucrose in the stool is hydrolyzed by colon bacteria. Oral sucrose tolerance testing (1 g/kg) is abnormal. Breath hydrogen will be elevated after ingestion of sucrose. Treatment of primary sucrase-isomaltase deficiency requires elimination of most sucrose. A preparation of yeast sucrase taken with meals is also effective.

Treem WR et al: Saccharosidase therapy for congenital sucrase-isomaltase deficiency. J Pediatr Gastroenterol Nutr 1999;28:137 [PMID: 9932843].

4. Glucose-Galactose Malabsorption

Glucose-galactose malabsorption is a rare disorder in which the sodium-glucose transport protein is defective. The gene has been localized to the long arm of chromosome 22. Transport of glucose in the intestinal epithelium and renal tubule is impaired. Diarrhea begins with the first feedings, accompanied by reducing sugar in the stool and acidosis. Small bowel histologic findings are normal. Glycosuria and aminoaciduria may occur. The glucose tolerance test is flat. Fructose is well tolerated. Diarrhea subsides promptly on withdrawal of glucose and galactose from the diet. The acquired form of glucose-galactose malabsorption occurs mainly in infants younger than age 6 months, usually following acute viral or bacterial enteritis.

In the congenital disease, exclusion of glucose and galactose from the diet is mandatory. A satisfactory formula is one with a carbohydrate-free base plus added fructose. The prognosis is good if the disease is diagnosed early, because tolerance for glucose and galactose improves with age. In secondary monosaccharide intolerance, prolonged parenteral nutrition may be required until intestinal transport mechanisms for monosaccharides return.

El-Naggar W et al: Nephrocalcinosis in glucose-galactose malabsorption: Association with renal tubular acidosis. Pediatr Nephrol 2005;20:1336 [PMID: 16010597].

Wright EM et al: Molecular basis for glucose-galactose malabsorption. Cell Biochem Biophys 2002;36:115 [PMID: 12139397].

5. Intestinal Lymphangiectasia

This form of protein-losing enteropathy results from a congenital ectasia of the bowel lymphatic system, often associated with abnormalities of the lymphatics in the extremities. Obstruction of lymphatic drainage of the intestine leads to rupture of the intestinal lacteals with leakage of lymph into the lumen of the bowel. Fat loss in the stool may be significant. Chronic loss of lymphocytes and immunoglobulins increases the susceptibility to infections.

▶ Clinical Findings

Peripheral edema, diarrhea, abdominal distention, chylous effusions, and repeated infections are common. Laboratory findings are reduced serum albumin, decreased immunoglobulin levels, lymphocytopenia, and anemia. Serum calcium and magnesium are frequently depressed as these cations are lost in complex with unabsorbed fatty acids. Lymphocytes may be seen on a stool smear. Fecal α_1-antitrypsin is elevated. Radiographic studies reveal an edematous small bowel mucosal pattern, and biopsy findings reveal dilated lacteals in the villi and lamina propria. If only the lymphatics of the deeper layers of bowel or intestinal mesenteries are involved, laparotomy may be necessary to establish the diagnosis. Capsule (camera) endoscopy shows diagnostic brightness secondary to the fat-filled lacteals.

▶ Differential Diagnosis

Other causes of protein-losing enteropathy must be considered, although an associated lymphedematous extremity strongly favors this diagnosis.

▶ Treatment & Prognosis

A high-protein diet (6–7 g/kg/d may be needed) enriched with medium-chain triglycerides as a fat source usually allows for adequate nutrition and growth in patients with intestinal mucosal lymphangiectasia. The serum albumin may not normalize. Vitamin and calcium supplements should be given. Parenteral nutritional supplementation may be needed temporarily. Surgery may be curative if the lesion is localized to a small area of the bowel or in cases of constrictive pericarditis or obstructing tumors. Intravenous albumin and immune globulin may also be used to control symptoms but are usually not needed chronically. The prognosis is not favorable, although remission may occur with age. Malignant degeneration of the abnormal lymphatics may occur, and intestinal lymphoma of the B-cell type may be a long-term complication.

6. Cow's Milk Protein Intolerance

Milk protein intolerance is more common in males than females and in young infants with a family history of atopy. The estimated prevalence is 0.5–1.0%. Colic, vomiting, and diarrhea are the major symptoms in young infants whose stools often contain small flecks of blood and mucus. Children with these symptoms are generally healthy and gain weight normally. The diagnosis is usually made clinically. Elimination of whole milk from the maternal diet sometimes relieves symptoms. A switch to a protein hydrolysate formula almost always results in improvement. Because the blood loss and diarrhea are rarely severe, it is not essential that breast feeding be stopped. If symptoms are severe or prolonged, a trial of semielemental formula is recommended. Allergic colitis in infants usually clears spontaneously by age 6–12 months. When there is uncertainty or when symptoms are severe, sigmoidoscopic examination reveals a superficial colitis, often with edema, a mild eosinophilic infiltrate, and lymphonodular hyperplasia. Pneumatosis intestinalis rarely is found on radiographs. Viral gastroenteritis sometimes precedes the onset of symptoms. Early reports that patients with milk protein allergy have a 30% incidence of sensitivity to soy protein, with similar symptoms, have not been uniformly confirmed.

In older children, milk protein sensitivity may induce eosinophilic gastroenteritis with protein-losing enteropathy, iron deficiency, hypoalbuminemia, and hypogammaglobulinemia. A celiac-like syndrome with villous atrophy, malabsorption, hypoalbuminemia, occult blood in the stool, and anemia can occur.

IgE-mediated anaphylactic shock is a rare but potentially life-threatening manifestation of milk protein sensitivity in infancy. If the symptoms suggest an anaphylactic response to milk or other protein, food challenge should be performed only in a setting in which resuscitation can be carried out.

7. Pancreatic Insufficiency

The most common cause of pancreatic exocrine insufficiency in childhood is cystic fibrosis. Decreased secretion of pancreatic digestive enzymes is caused by obstruction of the exocrine ducts by thick secretions, which destroys pancreatic acinar cells. Destruction of acinar cells may occur antenatally. Some genotypes of cystic fibrosis have partially or completely preserved pancreatic exocrine function. Other conditions associated with exocrine pancreatic insufficiency are discussed in Chapter 21.

8. Other Genetic Disorders Causing Malabsorption

A. Abetalipoproteinemia

Abetalipoproteinemia is an autosomal recessive condition in which the secretion of triglyceride-rich lipoproteins from the small intestine (chylomicrons) and liver (very low-density lipoproteins) is abnormal. Profound steatosis of the intestinal enterocytes (and hepatocytes) and severe fat malabsorption occur. Deficiencies of fat-soluble vitamins develop with neurologic complications of vitamin E deficiency and atypical retinitis pigmentosa. Serum cholesterol level is very low, and red cell membrane lipids are abnormal, causing acanthosis of red blood cells, which may be the key to diagnosis.

B. Acrodermatitis Enteropathica

Acrodermatitis enteropathica is an autosomal recessive condition in which the intestine has a selective inability to absorb zinc. The condition usually becomes obvious at the time of weaning and is characterized by rash on the extremities, rashes around the body orifices, eczema, profound failure to thrive, steatorrhea, diarrhea, and immune deficiency. Zinc supplementation by mouth results in rapid improvement.

▼ INFLAMMATORY BOWEL DISEASE

▶ General Considerations

Inflammatory bowel disease is most commonly differentiated into Crohn disease (CD) and ulcerative colitis (UC). The etiology is most likely multifactorial, involving a complex interaction of immune, environmental (eg, smoking, breast feeding, diet), and genetic factors. The genetic association is clear, with frequency as high as 40% in first-degree relatives. Monozygotic twins have a 37% concordance for CD and 10% concordance for UC. Mutations in the *NOD2/CARD15* gene on chromosome 16 have been implicated in CD. This gene has an important role in activating nuclear factor-κ, which mediates the inflammatory response and the production of proinflammatory cytokines.

▶ Clinical Findings

A. Symptoms and Signs

The clinical presentation of inflammatory bowel disease depends on the site of inflammation. Most (50–70%) children with CD have terminal ileal disease, and more than half have colonic involvement, typically of the ascending colon. Ten to 20% have isolated colonic disease, and 10–15% have small bowel disease. Gastroduodenal inflammation is common, although isolated gastric disease is rare. CD patients may have nonspecific symptoms at presentation, leading to delays in diagnosis. The most common presentation is abdominal pain, sometimes with diarrhea and weight loss. Some patients may have anal skin tags or fistulas on examination. Rectal bleeding and nonspecific symptoms such as fever, anorexia, fatigue, nausea and vomiting, aphthous ulcerations, short stature, and delayed puberty may also occur.

The most common symptoms in UC are rectal bleeding, diarrhea, and abdominal pain. In contrast to CD, the colon is the major site of inflammation with 44–49% of patients having rectosigmoid disease; 36–41%, left-sided colonic disease; and 14–37%, pancolitis. The younger the child, the more likely it is that he or she will have pancolitis and the more aggressive the inflammatory process is likely to be.

Extraintestinal symptoms and signs are common in both CD and UC and may precede the onset of GI symptoms. Arthritis is the most common extraintestinal manifestation of inflammatory bowel disease. Nephrolithiasis, erythema nodosum, and pyoderma gangrenosum can also occur. Uveitis, conjunctivitis, and primary sclerosing cholangitis may also be seen.

B. Diagnostic Testing

Patients with inflammatory bowel disease often have low hemoglobin and serum albumin levels and increased platelet count, erythrocyte sedimentation rate, and C-reactive protein. These findings are not always present. Serum antibodies to *Saccharomyces cerevisiae* (ASCA) are detected in 40–60% of patients with CD. Serum perinuclear antineutrophil cytoplasmic antibodies (pANCA) are present in approximately 70% of UC patients. Both of these antibodies, if positive, may be helpful screens, but they are neither sensitive nor specific enough to be diagnostic. In patients with diarrhea, it is important to evaluate for infectious and malabsorptive problems.

Barium upper GI study with small bowel follow-through shows small bowel disease. CT scan and magnetic resonance imaging may show mucosal and mural edema but are not specific. Intestinal wall thickening is often reported on CT scans performed as part of an urgent evaluation to rule out appendicitis. This finding is probably an acute reaction to infection and should not prompt an extensive evaluation for CD without other supporting symptoms or signs.

Upper endoscopy and colonoscopy including the terminal ileum are essential in diagnosing inflammatory bowel disease. Mucosal involvement in CD is typically patchy with disease-free skip areas. It can be found in any part of the GI tract (including esophagus and stomach) with transmural inflammation manifested by ulcers, fistulas, strictures, and granulomas. UC is usually localized to the colon, and generally the inflammation is mucosal or submucosal. Although inflammation seems to spread proximally from the rectum, rectal sparing sometimes occurs.

▶ Differential Diagnosis

When extraintestinal symptoms predominate, CD can be mistaken for rheumatoid arthritis, systemic lupus erythematosus, or hypopituitarism. The acute onset of ileocolitis may be mistaken for appendicitis. Symptoms sometimes suggest celiac disease, peptic ulcer, intestinal obstruction, intestinal lymphoma, anorexia nervosa, or growth failure from endocrine causes. In the acute stage, bacterial pathogens and toxins causing colitis must be ruled out. These include *Shigella, Salmonella, Yersinia, Campylobacter, Entamoeba histolytica,* enteroinvasive *Escherichia coli* (*E coli* O157), *Aeromonas hydrophila, Giardia,* and *Clostridium difficile.* Mild UC sometimes mimics irritable bowel syndrome. Eosinophilic gastroenteropathy and vasculitic lesions should also be considered. Finally, Behçet disease should be considered. It is characterized by oral aphthous ulcerations along with at least two of the following: genital ulcers, synovitis, posterior uveitis, meningoencephalitis, and pustular vasculitis. Patients with Behçet disease also may have anorexia, vomiting, diarrhea, abdominal pain, distention, and dyspepsia.

▶ Complications

A. Crohn Disease

Malnutrition is caused by anorexia and compounded by malabsorption, protein-losing enteropathy, iron-deficiency anemia, disaccharidase deficiency, and bile salt malabsorption in poorly controlled disease. Growth failure, delayed bone age, and delayed puberty are common results of malnutrition and steroid use. Controlling active disease to the point of remission usually allows for improved nutrition and resumption of normal growth velocity. Most patients today achieve reasonable final adult height. Intestinal obstruction, fistulae, abdominal abscess, perianal disease, pyoderma gangrenosum, arthritis, and amyloidosis occur. The risk of colon cancer is increased in patients with CD colitis although not to the extent seen in UC.

B. Ulcerative Colitis

Arthritis, uveitis, pyoderma gangrenosum, and malnutrition all occur. Growth failure and delayed puberty are less common than in CD. Liver disease (chronic active hepatitis, sclerosing cholangitis) is more common. In patients with pancolitis, carcinoma of the colon occurs with an incidence of 1–2% per year after the first 10 years of disease. Cancer risk is a function of disease duration, not age at onset. The mortality rate from colon cancer is high because the usual signs (occult blood in stool, pain, and abnormal radiologic findings) are not specific and may be ignored in a patient with colitis. Routine cancer screening (colonoscopy with multiple biopsies and evaluation of specimens for metaplasia and aneuploidy) is recommended in pediatric patients after 10 years of pancolitis. Dysplasia that persists in the absence of inflammation is an indication for colectomy, as is aneuploidy in multiple biopsy specimens.

▶ Treatment

A. Medical Treatment

Medical treatment of CD and UC is similar and includes anti-inflammatory, antidiarrheal, and antibiotic medication. No medical therapy is uniformly effective in all patients.

1. Diet—The main priority in patients with inflammatory bowel disease is ensuring adequate caloric intake. Restrictive or bland diets are counterproductive because they usually result in poor intake. A high-protein, high-carbohydrate diet with normal amounts of fat is recommended. A diet with decreased fiber may prevent symptoms during active colitis or partial intestinal obstruction; however, increased fiber may benefit mucosal health via bacterial production of fatty acids when disease is inactive. Lactose is poorly tolerated when disease is active. Supplemental calories in the form of liquid diets are well tolerated and promote catch-up growth. Enteral administration of low-residue or elemental liquid diets is widely used outside of the United States to induce remission in patients with CD. It is less effective in UC. Total parenteral nutrition for periods of 4–6 weeks may induce remission and promote linear growth and sexual development.

2. Nonabsorbable 5-aminosalicylates (5-ASA)—Multiple preparations of 5-ASA derivatives are available and are used to induce remission in mild CD and UC. 5-ASA derivatives are also used for maintenance therapy in patients in remission. Sulfasalazine, a common form of 5-ASA, is not absorbed systemically. Intact drug is hydrolyzed by colon flora into sulfapyridine and 5-aminosalicylate. The sulfonamide moiety is probably inactive but is responsible for the allergic side effects of the drug. The salicylate moiety has local anti-inflammatory activity. Side effects include skin rash, nausea, headache, and abdominal pain. Rarely, serum sickness, hemolytic anemia, aplastic anemia, and pancreatitis occur. Response to therapy may be slow. Sulfasalazine inhibits folic acid absorption, and supplemental folic acid is required. The recommended dosage is 2–3 g/d in three divided doses for children older than 10 years or 50 mg/kg/d for younger children. Half of this dosage is used as a maintenance medication for well-controlled UC. Salicylate polymers for oral and rectal use (olsalazine, mesalamine) are available. A variety of pH-sensitive tablet coatings and microencapsulation allow release of these products at specific locations in the GI tract, thereby improving efficacy. These drugs are no more effective than sulfasalazine but are used in sulfonamide-sensitive patients and have fewer side effects.

3. Corticosteroids—Patients with moderate to severe CD and UC require corticosteroids. Methylprednisolone (2 mg/kg/d, maximum 60 mg/d) may be given intravenously when disease is severe. For moderate disease, prednisone (1–2 mg/kg/d orally in one to two divided doses) is given for 6–8 weeks followed by gradual tapering. Alternate-day steroids produce fewer side effects as the dosage of drug is tapered. Chronic use of corticosteroids does not prevent relapse. Prednisone is usually given with a 5-ASA derivative. The patient's varicella immunity should be confirmed by history or antibody screen and parents counseled as to risks and therapy after varicella exposure. Hydrocortisone enemas or rectal foam can be used to treat tenesmus or ulcerative proctitis. Budesonide, which has "one pass metabolism" in the liver, is available in oral and rectal preparations. These preparations are most useful in rectal disease (enemas and suppositories) and right-sided colon disease (oral), and in appropriate doses have fewer corticoid side effects. Calcium and vitamin D supplementation should be considered while patients are being treated with corticosteroids.

4. Azathioprine and 6-mercaptopurine—Azathioprine (Imuran), 2–3 mg/kg/d orally, or 6-mercaptopurine (1–2 mg/kg) provides effective maintenance therapy for moderate to severe CD. These medications are used for frequently relapsing disease or when high-dose corticosteroids are necessary to control disease. The optimal dose depends on the patient's ability to metabolize the compound. Metabolites of azathioprine should be monitored to avoid over- and under-dosing in patients with variable metabolizing capacity and to assess compliance. Testing prior to initiating therapy is indicated to identify patients at risk for serious side effects such as bone marrow failure. Maximum therapeutic efficacy

may not be seen for 12–16 weeks after beginning treatment. Side effects include pancreatitis, hepatotoxicity, and bone marrow suppression.

5. Antibiotics—Metronidazole has been used to treat perianal CD. It may also be effective in treating CD of the colon. The dosage of metronidazole is 15–30 mg/kg/d in three divided doses. Peripheral neuropathy may occur with prolonged use. Ciprofloxacin has similar therapeutic effect and is occasionally used in combination with metronidazole.

6. Biologic therapies—Infliximab, a chimeric monoclonal antibody against tumor necrosis factor-β (TNFβ), is used for moderate to severe CD, especially in patients with resistant perianal and fistulizing disease unresponsive to milder therapy. Most patients require repeated intravenous infusion at 4–12-week intervals to remain in remission. Anaphylactic reactions have been reported. The concomitant use of azathioprine decreases the incidence of severe allergic reactions and may help maintain responsiveness to therapy. Side effects include flushing, rash, dyspnea, delayed hypersensitivity reactions, opportunistic infections, and lymphoproliferative disorders. Infliximab is also effective in severe colitis and in steroid-dependent colitis.

7. Other Agents—Cyclosporine can be used in severe, steroid-resistant UC. Because it has significant side effects and is followed by rapid relapse after discontinuation, cyclosporine is usually used to "buy time" and improve symptoms of severe colitis in patients prior to surgery. Oral or subcutaneous methotrexate has been used to treat severe, refractory CD. Liver toxicity is a risk with prolonged use. Thalidomide has been used, especially in patients with oral and vaginal ulcers secondary to CD. Its mechanism of action may include prevention of TNF secretion or antiangiogenic activity. This medication must be used under strict supervision in postpubescent female patients because of the risk of teratogenesis.

B. Surgical Treatment

1. Crohn disease—CD is not cured by surgery. Surgery is typically recommended for complications such as obstruction, perforation, abscess, stricture, fistula, and sometimes for intractable symptoms, growth retardation, and pubertal delay. Up to 50% of patients with CD eventually require a surgical procedure. There is a high relapse rate after surgery, typically at the site of anastomosis within 2 years. Recurrence rate may be less in patients with disease limited to the colon. Surgery to correct growth retardation must be performed before the completion of puberty.

2. Ulcerative colitis—Surgery is curative and is recommended for patients with uncontrolled hemorrhage, toxic megacolon, unrelenting pain and diarrhea, growth failure, high-grade mucosal dysplasia, or malignant tumors. Several surgical approaches (ileoanal anastomosis, Koch-type continent ileostomy) are available that allow a near-normal lifestyle after colectomy. Liver disease associated with UC (sclerosing cholangitis) is not improved by colectomy.

Bariol C et al: Early studies on the safety and effectiveness of thalidomide for symptomatic inflammatory bowel disease. J Gastroenterol Hepatol 2002;17:135 [PMID: 11966942].

deRidder L et al: Infliximab use in children and adolescents with inflammatory bowel disease. J Pediatr Gastroenterol Nutr 2007;45:3 [PMID: 17592358].

Differentiating ulcerative colitis from Crohn disease in children and young adults: Report of the working group of the North American Society for Pediatric Gastroenterology, Hepatology and Nutrition and the Crohn and Colitis Foundation of America. J Pediatr Gastroenterol Nutr 2007;44:53 [PMID: 17460505].

Newman B, Siinovich KA: Recent advances in the genetics of inflammatory bowel disease. Curr Opin Gastroenterol 2005;21:401 [PMID: 15930978].

Rufo RA, Bousvaros A. Challenges and progress in pediatric inflammatory bowel disease. Cur Opin Gastroenterol 2007; 23:406-12 [PMID: 17545777].

REFERENCES

Web Resources

http://www.naspghn.org/: The web site of the North American Society for Pediatric Gastroenterology, Hepatology and Nutrition (NASPGHAN) has an excellent selection of educational materials on many pediatric gastroenterologic conditions with information for parents and recommendations for evaluation and therapy.

General References

Silverman A, Roy CC: *Pediatric Clinical Gastroenterology*, 4th ed. Mosby, 1995.

Suchy FJ, Sokol RJ, Balistreri WF (editors): *Liver Disease in Children*, 3rd ed. Mosby, 2007.

Walker WA et al (editors): *Pediatric Gastrointestinal Disease*, 4th ed. BC Decker, 2004.

Wyllie R et al: (editors): *Pediatric Gastrointestinal and Liver Disease*, 3rd ed. WB Saunders, 2006.

Liver & Pancreas

21

Ronald J. Sokol, MD

Michael R. Narkewicz, MD

PROLONGED NEONATAL CHOLESTATIC JAUNDICE

The main clinical features of disorders causing prolonged neonatal cholestasis are (1) jaundice with elevated serum conjugated (or direct) bilirubin fraction (> 2 mg/dL or > 20% of total bilirubin), (2) variably acholic stools, (3) dark urine, and (4) hepatomegaly.

Prolonged neonatal cholestasis (conditions with decreased bile flow) has intrahepatic and extrahepatic causes. Specific clinical clues (Table 21–1) distinguish these two major categories of jaundice in 85% of cases. Histologic examination of tissue obtained by percutaneous liver biopsy increases the accuracy of differentiation to 95% (Table 21–2).

INTRAHEPATIC CHOLESTASIS

 ESSENTIALS OF DIAGNOSIS & TYPICAL FEATURES

- ► Elevated total and conjugated bilirubin.
- ► Hepatomegaly and dark urine.
- ► Patency of extrahepatic biliary tree.

► General Considerations

Intrahepatic cholestasis is characterized by hepatocyte dysfunction and patency of the extrahepatic biliary system. A specific cause can be identified in about 50% of cases. Patency of the extrahepatic biliary tract is suggested by pigmented stools and lack of bile duct proliferation on liver biopsy. It can be confirmed least invasively by hepatobiliary scintigraphy using technetium-99m (^{99m}Tc)-diethyliminodi-

acetic acid (diethyl-IDA [DIDA]). Radioactivity in the bowel within 4–24 hours is evidence of bile duct patency. Finding bilirubin in duodenal aspirates also confirms patency. Patency can also be determined by cholangiography carried out intraoperatively, percutaneously by transhepatic cholecystography, or endoscopic retrograde cholangiopancreatography (ERCP) using a pediatric-size side-viewing endoscope. Magnetic resonance cholangiopancreatography in infants is of limited use and highly dependent on the operator and equipment.

1. Perinatal or Neonatal Hepatitis Resulting from Infection

This diagnosis is considered in infants with jaundice, hepatomegaly, vomiting, lethargy, fever, and petechiae. It is important to identify perinatally acquired viral, bacterial, or protozoal infections (Table 21–3). Infection may occur transplacentally, by ascent through the cervix into amniotic fluid, from swallowed contaminated fluids (maternal blood, urine) during delivery, from blood transfusions administered in the early neonatal period, or from breast milk or environmental exposure. Infectious agents associated with neonatal intrahepatic cholestasis include herpes simplex virus, varicella virus, enteroviruses (coxsackievirus and echovirus), cytomegalovirus (CMV), rubella virus, adenovirus, parvovirus, human herpesvirus type 6 (HHV-6), hepatitis B virus (HBV), human immunodeficiency virus (HIV), *Treponema pallidum,* and *Toxoplasma gondii.* Although hepatitis C may be transmitted vertically, it rarely causes neonatal cholestasis. The degree of liver cell injury caused by these agents is variable, ranging from massive hepatic necrosis (herpes simplex, enteroviruses) to focal necrosis and mild inflammation (CMV, HBV). Serum bilirubin, bile acids, alanine aminotransferase (ALT), aspartate aminotransferase (AST), and alkaline phosphatase are elevated. The infant is jaundiced, may have petechiae or rash, and generally appears ill.

Table 21–1. Characteristic clinical features of intrahepatic and extrahepatic neonatal cholestasis.

Intrahepatic	Extrahepatic
Preterm infant, small for gestational age, appears ill	Full-term infant, seems well
Hepatosplenomegaly, other organ or system involvement	Hepatomegaly (firm to hard)
Incomplete cholestasis (stools with some pigment)	Complete cholestasis (acholic stools)
Associated cause identified (infections, metabolic, familial, etc)	Polysplenia syndrome, equal right and left hepatic lobes

Table 21–2. Characteristic histologic features of intrahepatic and extrahepatic neonatal cholestasis.

	Intrahepatic	Extrahepatic
Giant cells	+++	+
Lobules	Disarray	Normal
Portal reaction	Inflammation, minimal fibrosis	Fibrosis, lymphocytic infiltrate
Neoductular proliferation	Rare	Marked
Other	Steatosis, extramedullary hematopoiesis	Portal bile duct plugging, bile lakes

▶ Clinical Findings

A. Symptoms and Signs

Clinical symptoms usually appear in the first 2 weeks of life, but may appear as late as age 2–3 months. Jaundice may be noted as early as the first 24 hours of life. Poor oral intake, poor sucking reflex, lethargy, and vomiting are frequent. Stools may be normal to pale in color but are seldom acholic. Dark urine stains the diaper. Hepatomegaly is present, and the liver has a uniform firm consistency. Splenomegaly is variably present. Macular, papular, vesicular, or petechial rashes may occur. In less severe cases, failure to thrive may be the major complaint. Unusual presentations include neonatal liver failure, hypoproteinemia, anasarca (nonhemolytic hydrops), and hemorrhagic disease of the newborn.

Table 21–3. Infectious causes of neonatal hepatitis.

Infectious Agent	Diagnostic Tests	Specimens	Treatment
Cytomegalovirus	Culture and PCR, liver histology, IgM/[a]IgG	Urine, blood, liver	Ganciclovir (Foscarnet)[b]
Herpes simplex	PCR and culture, liver histology, Ag (skin)	Liver, blood, eye, throat, rectal, CSF, skin	Acyclovir
Rubella	Culture, IgM/[a]IgG	Liver, blood, urine	Supportive
Varicella	Culture, PCR, Ag (skin)	Skin, blood, CSF, liver	Acyclovir (Foscarnet)[b]
Parvovirus	Serum IgM/[a]IgG, PCR	Blood	Supportive, IVIG
Enteroviruses	Culture and PCR	Blood, urine, CSF, throat, rectal, liver	Pleconaril (investigative), IVIG
Adenovirus	Culture and PCR	Nasal/throat, rectal, blood, liver, urine	Cidofovir, ?IVIG
Hepatitis B virus (HBV)	HBsAg, HBcAg IgM	Serum	Supportive for acute infection
Hepatitis C virus (HCV)	HCV PCR, HCV-IgG	Serum	Supportive for acute infection
Treponema pallidum	Serology; darkfield exam	Serum, CSF	Penicillin
Toxoplasma gondii	IgM/[a]IgG, PCR, culture	Serum, liver	Pyrimethamine and sulfadiazine with folinic acid for 6 mo; followed by this therapy alternating with spiramycin for 6 mo
Mycobacterium tuberculosis	PPD, chest radiograph, liver tissue histologic stains and culture, gastric aspirate stain and culture	Serum, liver, gastric aspirate	INH, pyrazinamide, rifampin (add streptomycin for severe disease[c])

[a]IgG = positive indicates maternal infection and transfer of antibody transplacentally; negative indicates unlikelihood of infection in mother and infant.
[b]Use foscarnet for resistant viruses. Treat only if symptomatic.
[c]Discontinue streptomycin as soon as possible.
Ag, viral antigen testing; CSF, cerebrospinal fluid; HBcAg, hepatitis B core antigen; HBsAg, hepatitis B surface antigen; INH, isoniazid; IVIG, intravenous gamma globulin; PCR, polymerase chain reaction test for viral DNA or RNA; PPD, purified protein derivative.

B. Diagnostic Studies

Neutropenia, thrombocytopenia, and signs of mild hemolysis are common. Mixed hyperbilirubinemia, elevated aminotransferases with near-normal alkaline phosphatase, prolongation of clotting studies, mild acidosis, and elevated cord serum IgM suggest congenital infection. Nasopharyngeal washings, urine, stool, serum, and cerebrospinal fluid (CSF) should be cultured for virus and tested for pathogen-specific nucleic acid. Specific IgM antibody may be useful, as are long-bone radiographs to determine the presence of "celery stalking" in the metaphyseal regions of the humeri, femurs, and tibias. When indicated, computed tomography (CT) and magnetic resonance imaging (MRI) scans can identify intracranial calcifications (especially with CMV and toxoplasmosis). Hepatobiliary scintigraphy shows decreased hepatic clearance of the circulating isotope with excretion into the gut. Careful ophthalmologic examination may be useful for diagnosis of herpes simplex virus, CMV, toxoplasmosis, and rubella.

A percutaneous liver biopsy is useful in distinguishing intrahepatic from extrahepatic cholestasis, but may not identify a specific infectious agent (see Table 21–2). However, typical inclusions of CMV in hepatocytes or bile duct epithelial cells, the presence of intranuclear acidophilic inclusions of herpes simplex, or positive immunohistochemical stains for several viruses can be diagnostic. Variable degrees of lobular disarray characterized by focal necrosis, multinucleated giant-cell transformation, and ballooned pale hepatocytes with loss of cordlike arrangement of liver cells are usual. Intrahepatocytic and canalicular cholestasis may be prominent. Portal changes are not striking, but modest neoductular proliferation and mild fibrosis may occur. Viral cultures or polymerase chain reaction (PCR) testing of biopsy material may be helpful.

▶ Differential Diagnosis

Great care must be taken to distinguish infectious causes of intrahepatic cholestasis from genetic or metabolic disorders because the clinical presentations are similar. Galactosemia, congenital fructose intolerance, and tyrosinemia must be investigated promptly, because specific dietary therapy is available. These infants may also have concomitant bacteremia. α_1-Antitrypsin deficiency, cystic fibrosis, bile acid synthesis defects, mitochondrial respiratory chain disorders, and neonatal iron storage disease must also be considered. Specific physical features may be helpful when considering Alagille or Zellweger syndrome. Idiopathic neonatal hepatitis may be indistinguishable from infectious causes.

Patients with intrahepatic cholestasis frequently appear ill, whereas infants with extrahepatic cholestasis do not appear ill, have stools that are usually completely acholic, and have an enlarged, firm liver. Histologic findings are described in Table 21–2.

▶ Treatment

Most forms of viral neonatal hepatitis are treated symptomatically. However, infections with herpes simplex virus, varicella, CMV, parvovirus, adenovirus, and toxoplasmosis have specific treatments. Fluids and adequate calories are encouraged. Intravenous dextrose is needed if feedings are not well tolerated. The consequences of cholestasis are treated as indicated (Table 21–4). Vitamin K orally or by injection and vitamins D and E orally should be provided. Choleretics (ursodeoxycholic acid [UDCA] or cholestyramine) are used if cholestasis persists. Corticosteroids are contraindicated. Penicillin for suspected syphilis, specific antiviral therapy, or antibiotics for bacterial hepatitis, need to be administered promptly.

▶ Prognosis

Multiple organ involvement is commonly associated with neonatal infectious hepatitis and has a poor outcome. Death from hepatic or cardiac failure, intractable acidosis, or intracranial hemorrhage may occur, especially in herpesvirus or enterovirus infection, and occasionally in CMV or rubella infection. HBV rarely causes fulminant neonatal hepatitis; most infected infants become asymptomatic carriers of hepatitis B. Persistent liver disease results in mild chronic hepatitis, portal fibrosis, or cirrhosis. The liver in most infants who recover from congenital viral infection is left without fibrosis. Chronic cholestasis, although rare following infections, may lead to dental enamel hypoplasia, failure to thrive, biliary rickets, severe pruritus, and xanthoma.

2. Specific Infectious Agents

A. Neonatal Hepatitis B Virus Disease

Infection with HBV may occur at any time during perinatal life, but the risk is higher when acute maternal disease occurs during the last trimester of pregnancy. However, most cases of neonatal disease are acquired from mothers who are asymptomatic carriers of HBV. Although HBV has been found in most body fluids, including breast milk, neonatal transmission occurs occasionally transplacentally and primarily from exposure to maternal blood at delivery. In chronic hepatitis B surface antigen (HBsAg)–carrier mothers, fetal and infant acquisition risk is greatest if the mother (1) is also hepatitis B "e" antigen (HBeAg)–positive and hepatitis B "e" antibody (HBeAb)–negative, (2) has detectable levels of serum-specific hepatitis B DNA polymerase, (3) has high serum levels of hepatitis B core antibody (HBcAb), or (4) has high blood levels of HBV DNA. These findings are markers for circulating infectious virus; however, hepatitis B can be transmitted even if HBsAg is the only marker present.

Neonatal liver disease resulting from HBV is extremely variable. The infant has a 70–90% chance of acquiring HBV at birth from an HBsAg-positive mother if the infant does not receive prophylaxis. Most infected infants become prolonged asymptomatic "carriers" of HBV. Fulminant hepatic necrosis

Table 21–4. Treatment of complications of chronic cholestatic liver disease.

Indication	Treatment	Dose	Toxicity
Intrahepatic cholestasis	Phenobarbital	3–10 mg/kg/d	Drowsiness, irritability, interference with vitamin D metabolism
	Cholestyramine or colestipol hydrochloride	250–500 mg/kg/d	Constipation, acidosis, binding of drugs, increased steatorrhea
	Ursodeoxycholic acid	15–20 mg/kg/d	Transient increase in pruritus
Pruritus	Phenobarbital	3–10 mg/kg/d	Drowsiness, irritability, interference with vitamin D metabolism
	Cholestyramine or colestipol	250–500 mg/kg/d	Constipation, acidosis, binding of drugs, increased steatorrhea
	Antihistamines: diphenhydramine hydrochloride	5–10 mg/kg/d	Drowsiness
	Hydroxyzine	2–5 mg/kg/d	
	Ultraviolet light B	Exposure as needed	Skin burn
	Carbamazepine	20–40 mg/kg/d	Hepatotoxicity, marrow suppression, fluid retention
	Rifampin	10 mg/kg/d	Hepatotoxicity, marrow suppression
	Ursodeoxycholic acid	15–20 mg/kg/d	Transient increase in pruritus
Steatorrhea	Formula containing medium-chain triglycerides (eg, Pregestimil or Alimentum)	120–150 kcal/kg/d for infants	Expensive
	Oil supplement containing medium-chain triglycerides	1–2 mL/kg/d	Diarrhea, aspiration
Malabsorption of fat-soluble vitamins	Vitamin A	10,000–25,000 U/d	Hepatitis, pseudotumor cerebri, bone lesions
	Vitamin D	800–5000 U/d	Hypercalcemia, hypercalciuria
	25-Hydroxycholecalciferol (25-OH vitamin D)	3–5 mcg/kg/d	Hypercalcemia, hypercalciuria
	1,25-Dihydroxycholecalciferol (1,25 OH$_2$ vitamin D)	0.05–0.2 mcg/kg/d	Hypercalcemia, hypercalciuria
	Vitamin E (oral)	25–200 IU/kg/d	Potentiation of vitamin K deficiency
	Vitamin E (oral, TPGS[a])	15–25 IU/kg/d	Potentiation of vitamin K deficiency
	Vitamin E (intramuscular)	1–2 mg/kg/d	Muscle calcifications
	Vitamin K (oral)	2.5 mg twice per week to 5 mg/d	
	Vitamin K (intramuscular)	2–5 mg each 4 wk	
Malabsorption of other nutrients	Multiple vitamin	1–2 times the standard dose	
	Calcium	25–100 mg/kg/d	Hypercalcemia, hypercalciuria
	Phosphorus	25–50 mg/kg/d	Gastrointestinal intolerance
	Zinc	1 mg/kg/d	Interference with copper and iron absorption

[a]D-α-Tocopheryl polyethylene glycol-1000 succinate.

has rarely been reported. In such cases, progressive jaundice, stupor, shrinking liver size, and coagulation abnormalities dominate the clinical picture. Respiratory, circulatory, and renal failure usually follow. Histologically, the liver shows massive hepatocyte necrosis, collapse of the reticulum framework, minimal inflammation, and occasional pseudoacinar structures. Survival without liver transplantation is rare, but is associated with reasonable repair of liver architecture.

In less severe cases, focal hepatocyte necrosis occurs with a mild portal inflammatory response. Cholestasis is intracellular and canalicular. Chronic hepatitis may be present for many years, with serologic evidence of persisting antigenemia (HBsAg) and mildly elevated serum aminotransferases. Chronic hepatitis may rarely progress to cirrhosis within 1–2 years. Most infected infants have only mild evidence, if any, of liver injury.

To prevent perinatal transmission, all infants of mothers who are HBsAg-positive (regardless of HBeAg status) should receive hepatitis B immunoglobulin (HBIG) and hepatitis B vaccine within the first 24 hours after birth and vaccine again at ages 1 and 6 months. (See Chapter 9.) This prevents HBV infection in 85–95% of infants. HBIG can provide some protection when given as late as 72 hours after birth. If not given at birth it can be administered as late as 7 days postpartum as long as the infant has received the vaccine. Universal HBV immunization at birth, with two follow-up doses, is recommended for all infants.

B. Neonatal Bacterial Hepatitis

Most bacterial liver infections in newborns are acquired by transplacental invasion from amnionitis with ascending spread from maternal vaginal or cervical infection. Onset is abrupt, usually within 48–72 hours after delivery, with signs of sepsis and often shock. Jaundice appears early and is of the mixed type. The liver enlarges rapidly, and the histologic picture is that of diffuse hepatitis with or without microabscess. The most common organisms involved are *Escherichia coli, Listeria monocytogenes,* and group B streptococci. Isolated neonatal liver abscess caused by *E coli* or *Staphylococcus aureus* is associated with omphalitis or umbilical vein catheterization. Bacterial hepatitis and neonatal liver abscesses require specific antibiotics in large doses and, rarely, surgical or radiologic interventional drainage. Deaths are common, but survivors show no long-term consequences of liver disease.

C. Neonatal Jaundice with Urinary Tract Infection

Jaundice in affected infants—usually males—typically appears between the second and fourth weeks of life. This disorder causes lethargy, fever, poor appetite, jaundice, and hepatomegaly. Except for mixed hyperbilirubinemia, other liver function tests (LFTs) are mildly abnormal. Leukocytosis is present, and infection is confirmed by urine culture. The mechanism for the liver impairment is the inhibitory action on bile secretion produced by bacterial products (endotoxins) and inflammatory cytokines.

Treatment of the infection leads to prompt resolution of the cholestasis without hepatic sequelae. Metabolic liver diseases, such as galactosemia and tyrosinemia, may present with gram-negative bacterial urinary tract infection and should be excluded.

Chang MH: Hepatitis B virus infection. Semin Fetal Neonatal Med. 2007;12:160 [PMID: 17336170].

Kane MA: Hepatitis viruses and the neonate. Clin Perinatol 1997;24:181 [PMID: 9099509].

Kimberlin DW: Herpes simplex virus infections in neonates and early childhood. Semin Pediatr Infect Dis. 2005;16:271 [PMID: 16210107].

Rosenthal P: Neonatal hepatitis and congenital infections. In: Suchy FJ, Sokol RJ, Balistreri WF (editors): *Liver Disease in Children*, 3rd ed. Cambridge University Press, 2007:232–246.

3. Intrahepatic Cholestasis Resulting from Inborn Errors of Metabolism, Familial, & "Toxic" Causes

These cholestatic syndromes caused by specific enzyme deficiencies, other genetic disorders, or certain precipitants associated with neonatal liver disease feature intrahepatic cholestasis (ie, jaundice, hepatomegaly, and normal to completely acholic stools). Some of the specific clinical conditions have characteristic clinical signs.

A. Enzyme Deficiencies and Other Inherited Disorders

Early specific diagnosis is important because dietary or pharmacologic treatment may be available (Table 21–5). Reversal of liver disease and clinical symptoms is prompt and permanent in several disorders as long as the diet is maintained. As with other genetic disorders, parents of the affected infant should be offered genetic counseling. For some disorders, prenatal genetic diagnosis is available.

Cholestasis caused by metabolic diseases such as galactosemia, fructose intolerance, and tyrosinemia may be accompanied by vomiting, lethargy, poor feeding, hypoglycemia, and irritability. Hepatomegaly is a constant finding. The infants often appear septic; gram-negative bacteria can be cultured from blood in 25–50% of cases, especially in patients with galactosemia. Neonatal screening programs for galactosemia usually detect the disorder before cholestasis develops. Other inherited conditions associated with neonatal intrahepatic cholestasis are outlined in Table 21–5. Treatment of these disorders is discussed in Chapter 34.

B. "Toxic" Causes of Neonatal Cholestasis

1. Neonatal ischemic-hypoxic conditions—Perinatal events that result in hypoperfusion of the gastrointestinal system are sometimes followed within 1–2 weeks by cholestasis. This occurs in premature infants with respiratory distress, severe hypoxia, hypoglycemia, shock, and acidosis. When these perinatal conditions develop in association with gastrointestinal lesions, such as ruptured omphalocele, gastroschisis, or necrotizing enterocolitis, a subsequent cholestatic picture is common (25–50% of cases). Liver function studies reveal mixed hyperbilirubinemia, elevated alkaline phosphatase and γ-glutamyl transpeptidase (GGT) values, and variable elevation of the aminotransferases. Stools are seldom persistently acholic.

Table 21–5. Metabolic and genetic causes of neonatal cholestasis.

Disease	Inborn Error	Hepatic Pathology	Diagnostic Studies
Galactosemia	Galactose-1-phosphate uridylyltransferase	Cholestasis, steatosis, necrosis, pseudoacini, fibrosis	Galactose-1-phosphate uridylyl-transferase assay of red blood cells
Fructose intolerance	Fructose-1-phosphate aldolase	Steatosis, necrosis, pseudoacini, fibrosis	Liver fructose-1-phosphate aldolase assay or genotyping of leukocyte DNA
Tyrosinemia	Fumarylacetoacetase	Necrosis, steatosis, pseudoacini, portal fibrosis	Urinary succinylacetone, fumarylacetoacetase assay of red blood cells
Cystic fibrosis	Cystic fibrosis transmembrane conductance regulator gene	Cholestasis, neoductular proliferation, excess bile duct mucus, portal fibrosis	Sweat test and genotyping of leukocyte DNA
Hypopituitarism	Deficient production of pituitary hormones	Cholestasis, giant cells	Thyroxine, TSH, cortisol levels
α_1-Antitrypsin deficiency	Abnormal α_1-antitrypsin molecule (Pi ZZ phenotype)	Giant cells, cholestasis, steatosis, neoductular proliferation, fibrosis, PAS-diastase–resistant cytoplasmic globules	Serum α_1-antitrypsin phenotype or genotype
Gaucher disease	β-Glucosidase	Cholestasis, cytoplasmic inclusions in Kupffer cells (foam cells)	β-Glucosidase assay in leukocytes
Niemann-Pick disease	Lysosomal sphingomyelinase	Cholestasis, cytoplasmic inclusions in Kupffer cells	Sphingomyelinase assay of leukocytes or liver or fibroblasts (type C); genotyping of leukocyte DNA
Glycogen storage disease type IV	Branching enzyme	Fibrosis, cirrhosis, PAS-diastase–resistant cytoplasmic inclusions	Branching enzyme analysis of leukocytes or liver, genotyping of leukocyte DNA
Neonatal hemochromatosis	Transplacental alloimmunization	Giant cells, portal fibrosis, hemosiderosis, cirrhosis	Histology, iron stains, lip biopsy, abdominal MRI
Peroxisomal disorders (eg, Zellweger syndrome)	Deficient peroxisomal enzymes or assembly	Cholestasis, necrosis, fibrosis, cirrhosis, hemosiderosis	Plasma very long chain fatty acids, qualitative bile acids, plasmalogen, pipecolic acid, liver electron microscopy
Abnormalities in bile acid metabolism	Several enzyme deficiencies defined	Cholestasis, necrosis, giant cells	Urine, serum, duodenal fluid analyzed for bile acids by fast atom bombardment–mass spectroscopy
Byler disease (familial progressive intrahepatic cholestasis)	*FIC-1* and *BSEP* genes	Cholestasis, necrosis, giant cells, fibrosis	Histology, family history, normal cholesterol, low or normal γ-glutamyl transpeptidase, genotyping of leukocyte DNA
MDR3 deficiency	*MDR3* gene	Cholestasis, bile duct proliferation, portal fibrosis	Bile phospholipid level, genotyping of leukocyte DNA
Alagille syndrome (syndromic paucity of interlobular bile ducts)	*JAGGED1* gene and *NOTCH2* mutations	Cholestasis, paucity of interlobular bile ducts, increased copper levels	Three or more clinical features, liver histology, genotyping of leukocyte DNA
Mitochondrial hepatopathies (respiratory chain disease)	*POLG, BCS1l, SCO1, DGUOK,* and *MPV17* gene mutations	Cholestasis, steatosis, portal fibrosis, abnormal mitochondria on electron microscopy	mtDNA depletion studies, respiratory chain studies on liver or muscle, genotyping

MDR3, multiple drug resistance protein type 3; MRI, magnetic resonance imaging; mtDNA, mitochondrial DNA; PAS, periodic acid–Schiff; TSH, thyroid-stimulating hormone.

Choleretics (UDCA), introduction of enteral feedings as soon as possible, and nutritional support are the mainstays of treatment until the cholestasis resolves (see Table 21–4). In some cases, this resolution may take 3–6 months. As long as no severe intestinal problem is present (eg, short gut syndrome), complete resolution of the hepatic abnormalities is the rule. But portal fibrosis with periportal scarring is occasionally found on follow-up biopsy.

2. Prolonged parenteral nutrition—Cholestasis may develop after 1–2 weeks in premature newborns receiving parenteral nutrition. Even full-term infants with significant intestinal disease, resections, or dysmotility may develop parenteral nutrition–related cholestasis. Contributing factors may include toxicity of intravenous amino acids, diminished stimulation of bile flow from prolonged absence of feedings, small intestinal bacterial overgrowth with translocation of intestinal bacteria and their cell wall products, missing nutrients or antioxidants, photooxidation of amino acids, infusion of lipid hydroperoxides or lipid sterols, and the "physiologic cholestatic" propensity of the premature infant. Histology of the liver may resemble that of extrahepatic biliary obstruction. Early introduction of feedings has reduced the frequency of this disorder. The prognosis is generally good. Occasional cases of cirrhosis, liver failure, and hepatoma may develop, particularly in infants with intestinal resections or malformations that require prolonged parenteral nutrition. A recent study suggests that oral erythromycin as a prokinetic agent may reduce the incidence of cholestasis in very low birth infants.

3. Inspissated bile syndrome—This syndrome is the result of accumulation of bile in canaliculi and in the small- and medium-sized bile ducts in hemolytic disease of the newborn (Rh, ABO) and in some infants receiving parenteral nutrition. The same mechanisms may cause intrinsic obstruction of the common bile duct. An ischemia-reperfusion injury may also contribute to cholestasis in Rh incompatibility. In extreme hemolysis, the cholestasis may be seemingly complete, with acholic stools. Levels of bilirubin, primarily conjugated, may reach 40 mg/dL. If inspissation of bile occurs within the extrahepatic biliary tree, differentiation from biliary atresia may be difficult. A trial of choleretics is indicated. Once stools show a return to normal color or ^{99m}Tc-DIDA scanning shows biliary excretion into the duodenum, patency of the extrahepatic biliary tree is assured. Although most cases improve slowly over 2–6 months, persistence of complete cholestasis for more than 1–2 weeks requires further studies (ultrasonography, DIDA scanning, liver biopsy) with possible cholangiographic or MRI of the extrahepatic biliary tree. Irrigation of the common bile duct is sometimes necessary to dislodge the obstructing inspissated biliary material.

Balistreri WF et al: Intrahepatic cholestasis: Summary of an American Association for the Study of Liver Diseases single-topic conference. Hepatology 2005;42:222 [PMID: 15898074].

Ng PC et al: High-dose oral erythromycin decreased the incidence of parenteral nutrition-associated cholestasis in preterm infants. Gastroenterology 2007;132:1726 [PMID: 17484870].
Teitelbaum DH et al: Use of cholecystokinin-octapeptide for the prevention of parenteral nutrition-associated cholestasis. Pediatrics 2005;115:1332 [PMID: 15867044].

4. Idiopathic Neonatal Hepatitis (Giant-Cell Hepatitis)

This type of cholestatic jaundice of unknown cause presents with features of cholestasis and a typical liver biopsy appearance; it accounts for 25–40% of cases of neonatal intrahepatic cholestasis. The degree of cholestasis is variable, and the disorder may be indistinguishable from extrahepatic causes in 10% of cases. Viral infections, α_1-antitrypsin deficiency, Alagille syndrome, Niemann-Pick type C disease (NPC), progressive familial intrahepatic cholestasis (PFIC), and bile acid synthesis defects may present in a similar clinical and histologic manner. In idiopathic neonatal hepatitis, PFIC types 1 and 2, and disease due to bile acid synthesis defects the GGT levels are normal or low. Electron microscopy of the liver biopsy (and genotyping) may help distinguish NPC and PFIC.

Intrauterine growth retardation, prematurity, poor feeding, emesis, poor growth, and partially or intermittently acholic stools are characteristic of intrahepatic cholestasis. Patients with neonatal lupus erythematosus may present with giant-cell hepatitis; however, thrombocytopenia, skin rash, or congenital heart block is usually also present.

In cases of suspected idiopathic neonatal hepatitis (diagnosed in the absence of infectious, metabolic, and toxic causes), patency of the biliary tree should be verified to exclude extrahepatic surgical disorders. DIDA scanning and ultrasonography may be helpful in this regard if stools are acholic. Some clinicians have used the enteral string test during DIDA scanning to confirm bile duct patency. Liver biopsy findings are usually diagnostic after age 6–8 weeks (see Table 21–2), but may be misleading before age 6 weeks. Failure to detect patency of the biliary tree, nondiagnostic liver biopsy findings, or persisting complete cholestasis (acholic stools) are indications for minilaparotomy and intraoperative cholangiography performed by an experienced surgeon, ERCP, percutaneous cholecystography, or magnetic resonance cholangiopancreatography (MRCP). Occasionally, a small but patent (hypoplastic) extrahepatic biliary tree is demonstrated (as in Alagille syndrome); it is probably the result, rather than the cause, of diminished bile flow. Surgical reconstruction of hypoplastic biliary trees should not be attempted.

Once a patent extrahepatic tree is confirmed, therapy should include choleretics, a special formula with medium-chain triglycerides (eg, Pregestimil, Alimentum), and supplemental fat-soluble vitamins in water-soluble form (see Table 21–4). This therapy is continued as long as significant cholestasis remains (conjugated bilirubin > 1 mg/dL). Fat-soluble vitamin serum levels should be monitored while supplements are given and at least once after their discontinuation.

Eighty percent of patients recover without significant hepatic fibrosis. However, in 20% of cases the patient has PFIC and is likely to progress to cirrhosis. In general, failure to resolve the cholestatic picture by age 6–12 months is associated with progressive liver disease and evolving cirrhosis. This may occur with either normal or diminished numbers of interlobular bile ducts (paucity of interlobular ducts). Liver transplantation has been successful when signs of hepatic decompensation are noted (rising bilirubin, coagulopathy, intractable ascites).

Balistreri WF, Bezerra JA: Whatever happened to "neonatal hepatitis"? Clin Liver Dis 2006;10:27 [PMID: 16376793].

Roberts EA: Neonatal hepatitis syndrome. Semin Neonatol 2003;8:357 [PMID: 15001124].

Yerushalmi B et al: Niemann-Pick disease type C in neonatal cholestasis at a North American Center. J Pediatr Gastroenterol Nutr 2002;35:44 [PMID: 12142809].

5. Paucity of Interlobular Bile Ducts

Forms of intrahepatic cholestasis caused by decreased numbers of interlobular bile ducts (< 0.5 bile ducts per portal tract) may be classified according to whether they are associated with other malformations. Alagille syndrome (syndromic paucity or arteriohepatic dysplasia) is caused by mutations in the gene *JAGGED1*, located on chromosome 20p, which codes for a ligand of the notch receptor, or more rarely in the gene *NOTCH2*. Alagille syndrome is sometimes recognized by identification of the characteristic facies, which becomes more obvious with age. The forehead is prominent, as is the nasal bridge. The eyes are set deep and sometimes widely apart (hypertelorism). The chin is small and slightly pointed and projects forward. The ears are prominent. The stool color varies with the severity of cholestasis. Pruritus begins by age 3–6 months. Firm, smooth hepatomegaly may be present. Cardiac murmurs are present in 95% of patients, and butterfly vertebrae (incomplete fusion of the vertebral body or anterior arch) are present in 50%. Xanthomas develop later in the disease as hypercholesterolemia becomes a problem. Occasionally, early cholestasis is mild and not recognized or the patient presents with complex congenital heart disease (eg, tetralogy of Fallot).

Conjugated hyperbilirubinemia may be mild to severe (2–15 mg/dL). Serum alkaline phosphatase, GGT, and cholesterol are markedly elevated, especially early in life. Serum bile acids are always elevated. Aminotransferases are mildly increased, but clotting factors and other liver proteins are usually normal.

The cardiovascular abnormalities include peripheral pulmonary artery, branch pulmonary artery, or pulmonary valvular stenoses (most common), atrial septal defect, coarctation of the aorta, and tetralogy of Fallot. Up to 10–15% of patients have intracranial vascular abnormalities and may develop intracranial hemorrhage early in childhood.

Eye abnormalities (posterior embryotoxon in 90%) and renal abnormalities (dysplastic kidneys, renal tubular ectasia, single kidney, hematuria) can also be present. Growth retardation with normal to increased levels of growth hormone (growth hormone resistance) is common. A variable proportion of patients may have pancreatic insufficiency that may contribute to the fat malabsorption. Although variable, the intelligence quotient is frequently low. Hypogonadism with micropenis may be present. A weak, high-pitched voice may develop. Neurologic disorders resulting from vitamin E deficiency (areflexia, ataxia, ophthalmoplegia) eventually develop in many unsupplemented children and may be profound.

In the nonsyndromic form, paucity of interlobular bile ducts occurs in the absence of the extrahepatic malformations. Paucity of interlobular bile ducts may also occur in α_1-antitrypsin deficiency, Zellweger syndrome, in association with lymphedema (Aagenaes syndrome), PFIC, cystic fibrosis, CMV or rubella infection, and inborn errors of bile acid metabolism.

High doses (250 mg/kg/d) of cholestyramine may control pruritus, lower cholesterol, and clear xanthomas. UDCA (15–25 mg/kg/d) appears to be more effective and causes fewer side effects than cholestyramine. Nutritional therapy to prevent wasting and deficiencies of fat-soluble vitamins is of particular importance because of the severity of cholestasis (see Table 21–4).

Prognosis is more favorable in the syndromic than in the nonsyndromic varieties. In the former, only 30–40% of patients have severe complications of disease, whereas over 70% of patients with nonsyndromic varieties progress to cirrhosis. Many of this latter group may have PFIC. In Alagille syndrome, cholestasis may improve by age 2–4 years, with minimal residual hepatic fibrosis. Survival into adulthood despite raised serum bile acids, aminotransferases, and alkaline phosphatase occurs in about 50% of cases. Several patients have developed hepatocellular carcinoma. Hypogonadism has been noted; however, fertility is not obviously affected in most cases. Cardiovascular anomalies may shorten life expectancy. Some patients have persistent, severe cholestasis, rendering their quality of life poor. Recurrent bone fractures may result from metabolic bone disease. Liver transplantation has been successfully performed under these circumstances. Intracranial hemorrhage may occur in up to 10–12% of affected children.

Emerick KM et al: Intracranial vascular abnormalities in patients with Alagille syndrome. J Pediatr Gastroenterol Nutr 2005; 41:99 [PMID: 15990638].

Kamath BM et al: Alagille syndrome. In Suchy FJ, Sokol RJ, Balistreri WF (editors): *Liver Disease in Children*, 3rd ed. Cambridge University Press, 2007:326–345.

Mattei P et al: Relief of intractable pruritus in Alagille syndrome by partial external biliary diversion. J Pediatr Surg 2006;41:104 [PMID: 16410117].

PROGRESSIVE FAMILIAL INTRAHEPATIC CHOLESTASIS (BYLER DISEASE)

PFIC is a group of disorders presenting as pruritus, diarrhea, jaundice, and failure to thrive in the first 6–12 months of life. PFIC type I (Byler disease), caused by mutations in the *FIC1* gene, is associated with low to normal serum levels of GGT and cholesterol and elevated levels of bilirubin, aminotransferases, and bile acids. Diarrhea and pruritus are common. Liver biopsy demonstrates cellular cholestasis, sometimes with a paucity of interlobular bile ducts and centrolobular fibrosis that progresses to cirrhosis. Electron microscopy shows diagnostic granular "Byler bile" in canaliculi.

Treatment includes administration of UDCA, partial biliary diversion if the condition is unresponsive to UDCA, and liver transplantation. With partial biliary diversion or ileal exclusion surgery, many patients show improved growth and liver histology, reduction in symptoms and, thus, avoidance of liver transplantation. PFIC type II is caused by mutations in the bile salt export pump (*BSEP*) gene, which codes for an adenosine triphosphate–dependent canalicular bile salt transport protein. These patients are clinically and biochemically similar to PFIC type I patients and have similar liver histology except for more "giant cells" and treatment options. There is an increased incidence of hepatocellular carcinoma in these patients. PFIC type III is caused by mutations in the multiple drug resistance protein type 3 (*MDR3)* gene, which encodes a canalicular protein that pumps phospholipid into bile. Serum GGT and bile acid levels are elevated, bile duct proliferation and portal tract fibrosis are seen in liver biopsies, and bile phospholipid levels are low. Treatment is similar to that for other forms of PFIC except for partial biliary diversion. Bile acid synthesis defects are clinically similar to PFIC I and PFIC II, with low serum levels of GGT and cholesterol; however, the serum level of total bile acids is inappropriately normal or low and urine bile acid analysis may identify a synthesis defect. Treatment is with oral cholic acid and UDCA.

Knisely AS et al: Hepatocellular carcinoma in ten children under five years of age with bile salt export pump deficiency. Hepatology 2006;44:478 [PMID: 16871584].

Kurbegov AC et al: Biliary diversion for progressive familial intrahepatic cholestasis: Improved liver morphology and bile acid profile. Gastroenterology 2003;125:1227 [PMID: 14517804].

Trauner M, Boyer JL: Cholestatic syndromes. Curr Opin Gastroenterol 2004;20:220 [PMID: 15703646].

Wanty C et al: Fifteen years single center experience in the management of progressive familial intrahepatic cholestasis of infancy. Acta Gastroenterol Belg 2004;67:313 [PMID: 15727074].

EXTRAHEPATIC NEONATAL CHOLESTASIS

Extrahepatic neonatal cholestasis is characterized by complete and persistent cholestasis (acholic stools) in the first 3 months of life; lack of patency of the extrahepatic biliary tree proved by intraoperative, percutaneous, or endoscopic cholangiography; firm to hard hepatomegaly; and typical features on histologic examination of liver biopsy tissue (see Table 21–2). Causes include biliary atresia, choledochal cyst, spontaneous perforation of the extrahepatic ducts, and intrinsic or extrinsic obstruction of the common duct.

1. Biliary Atresia

▶ General Considerations

Biliary atresia is the progressive fibroinflammatory obliteration of the lumen of all, or part of, the extrahepatic biliary tree presenting within the first 3 months of life. In Americans of European origin, biliary atresia occurs in 1:10,000–1:18,000 births, and the incidence in both sexes is equal. In Asian Americans the incidence is higher and the disorder is more common in girls. The abnormality found most commonly is complete atresia of all extrahepatic biliary structures. There appear to be at least two types of biliary atresia: the perinatal form (80% of cases), in which a perinatal insult is believed to initiate inflammatory obstruction and fibrosis of the biliary tree, and the fetal-embryonic form (20% of cases), in which the extrahepatic biliary system did not develop normally. In the perinatal form, meconium and first-passed stools are usually normal in color, suggesting early patency of the ducts. Evidence obtained from surgically removed remnants of the extrahepatic biliary tree suggests an inflammatory or sclerosing cholangiopathy. Although an infectious cause seems reasonable, no agent has been consistently found in such cases. A role for reovirus type 3 and rotavirus group C has been suggested. In the fetal-embryonic type, the bile duct presumably developed abnormally and is associated with other nonhepatic congenital anomalies. The association of biliary atresia with the polysplenia syndrome (heterotaxia, preduodenal portal vein, interruption of the inferior vena cava, polysplenia, and midline liver) and asplenia syndrome supports an embryonic origin of biliary atresia in these cases.

▶ Clinical Findings

A. Symptoms and Signs

Jaundice may be noted in the newborn period and persists beyond age 2–3 weeks. The urine stains the diaper; and the stools are often pale yellow, buff-colored, gray, or acholic. Seepage of bilirubin products across the intestinal mucosa may give some yellow coloration to the stools. Hepatomegaly is common, and the liver may feel firm to hard; splenomegaly develops later. Pruritus, digital clubbing, xanthomas, and a rachitic rosary may be noted in older patients. By age 2–6 months, the growth curves reveal poor weight gain. Late in the course, ascites, failure to thrive, bone fractures and bleeding complications occur.

B. Laboratory Findings and Imaging

No single laboratory test will consistently differentiate biliary atresia from other causes of complete obstructive jaundice. A study of hepatic 2,6-dimethyliminodiacetic acid (HIDA) excretion performed early in the course of disease may help to distinguish intrahepatic from extrahepatic causes of cholestasis, although there is considerable overlap. A HIDA scan showing lack of intestinal excretion is always present in biliary atresia also but may be seen with intrahepatic cholestasis. MRCP may be of value as an imaging study to define biliary atresia. Although biliary atresia is suggested by persistent elevation of serum GGT or alkaline phosphatase levels, high cholesterol levels, and prolonged prothrombin times, these findings have also been reported in severe neonatal hepatitis, α_1-antitrypsin deficiency, and bile duct paucity. Furthermore, these tests will not differentiate the location of the obstruction within the extrahepatic system. Generally, the aminotransferases are elevated only modestly in biliary atresia. Serum proteins and blood clotting factors are not affected early in the disease. Routine chest radiograph may reveal abnormalities suggestive of polysplenia syndrome. Ultrasonography of the biliary system should be performed to exclude the presence of choledochal cyst and intra-abdominal anomalies. Liver biopsy specimens can differentiate intrahepatic causes of cholestasis from biliary atresia in over 90% of cases (see Table 21–2).

▶ Differential Diagnosis

The major diagnostic dilemma is distinguishing between this entity and neonatal hepatitis, bile duct paucity, metabolic liver disease (particularly α_1-antitrypsin deficiency), choledochal cyst, or intrinsic bile duct obstruction (stones, bile plugs). Although spontaneous perforation of extrahepatic bile ducts leads to jaundice and acholic stools, the infants are usually quite ill with chemical peritonitis from biliary ascites, and hepatomegaly is not found.

If the diagnosis of biliary atresia cannot be excluded by the diagnostic evaluation, surgical exploration should be performed as soon as possible. Laparotomy or laparoscopy must include liver biopsy and an operative cholangiogram if a gallbladder is present. The presence of yellow bile in the gallbladder implies patency of the proximal extrahepatic duct system. Radiographic visualization of cholangiographic contrast in the duodenum excludes obstruction to the distal extrahepatic ducts.

▶ Treatment

In the absence of surgical correction or transplantation, biliary cirrhosis, hepatic failure, and death occur, almost always by age 18–24 months.

Except for the occasional example of correctable biliary atresia, in which choledochojejunostomy is feasible, the standard procedure is hepatoportoenterostomy (Kasai procedure). Occasionally, portocholecystostomy (gallbladder Kasai procedure) may be performed if the gallbladder is present and the passage from it to the duodenum is patent. These procedures are best done in specialized centers where experienced surgical, pediatric, and nursing personnel are available. Surgery should be performed as early as possible (ideally before 45–60 days of life); the Kasai procedure should generally not be undertaken in infants older than age 4 months, because the likelihood of bile drainage at this age is very low. Orthotopic liver transplantation is now indicated for patients who do not undergo the Kasai procedure, who fail to drain bile after the Kasai procedure, or who progress to end-stage biliary cirrhosis despite surgical treatment. The 3–5-year survival rate following liver transplantation for biliary atresia is 80–90%.

Whether or not the Kasai procedure is performed, supportive medical treatment measures consist of vitamin and caloric support (vitamins A, D, K, and E and formulas containing medium-chain triglycerides [Pregestimil or Alimentum]) (see Table 21–4). Suspected bacterial infections (eg, ascending cholangitis) should be treated promptly with broad-spectrum antibiotics, and any bleeding tendency should be corrected with intramuscular vitamin K. Ascites can be managed initially with reduced sodium intake and spironolactone. Choleretics and bile acid–binding products (cholestyramine, aluminum hydroxide gel) are of little use. The value of UDCA remains to be determined. The role of postoperative corticosteroids is controversial.

▶ Prognosis

When bile flow is sustained following portoenterostomy, the 10-year survival rate without liver transplantation is 25–35%. Death is usually caused by liver failure, sepsis, acidosis, or respiratory failure secondary to intractable ascites. Esophageal variceal hemorrhage develops in 40% of patients. Surprisingly, terminal hemorrhage is unusual. Occasional long-term survivors develop hepatopulmonary syndrome (intrapulmonary right to left shunting of blood resulting in hypoxia) or portopulmonary hypertension (pulmonary arterial hypertension in patients with portal hypertension). Liver transplantation has dramatically changed the outlook for these patients.

Escobar MA et al: Effect of corticosteroid therapy on outcomes in biliary atresia after Kasai portoenterostomy. J Pediatr Surg 2006;41:99 [PMID: 16410116].

Nio M et al: Japanese Biliary Atresia Registry: Five- and 10-year survival rates after surgery for biliary atresia: A report from the Japanese Biliary Atresia Registry. J Pediatr Surg 2003;38:997 [PMID: 12861525].

Shneider BL et al: A multicenter study of the outcome of biliary atresia in the United States, 1997 to 2000. J Pediatr 2006;148:467 [PMID: 16647406].

Sokol RJ et al: Screening and outcomes in biliary atresia: Summary of a National Institutes of Health workshop. Hepatology 2007;46:566 [PMID: 17661405].

2. Choledochal Cyst

Choledochal cysts cause 2–5% of cases of extrahepatic neonatal cholestasis; the incidence is fourfold higher in girls and higher in patients of Asian descent. In most cases, the clinical manifestations, basic laboratory findings, and histopathologic features on liver biopsy are indistinguishable from those associated with biliary atresia. Neonatal symptomatic cysts are usually associated with atresia of the distal common duct—accounting for the diagnostic dilemma—and may simply be part of the spectrum of biliary atresia. Ultrasonography or MRI reveals the presence of a cyst. Immediate surgery is indicated once abnormalities in clotting factors have been corrected and bacterial cholangitis, if present, has been treated with intravenous antibiotics. In older children, choledochal cyst presents as recurrent episodes of right upper quadrant abdominal pain, vomiting, obstructive jaundice, or pancreatitis, or as a right abdominal mass.

Excision of the cyst and choledocho–Roux-en-Y jejunal anastomosis are recommended. In some cases, because of technical problems, only the mucosa of the cyst can be removed with jejunal anastomosis to the proximal bile duct. Anastomosis of cyst to jejunum or duodenum is not recommended.

The prognosis depends on the presence or absence of associated evidence of atresia and the appearance of the intrahepatic ducts. If atresia is found, the prognosis is similar to that described in the preceding section. If an isolated extrahepatic cyst is encountered, the outcome is generally excellent, with resolution of the jaundice and return to normal liver architecture. However, bouts of ascending cholangitis may occur, particularly if intrahepatic cysts are present or obstruction of the anastomotic site develops. The risk of biliary carcinoma developing within the cyst is about 5–15% at adulthood; therefore, cystectomy or excision of cyst mucosa should be undertaken whenever possible.

Bismuth H, Krissat J: Choledochal cyst malignancies. Ann Oncol 1999;10:94 [PMID: 10436795].

He X et al: Congenital choledochal cyst—Report of 56 cases. Chin Med Sci J 2000;15:52 [PMID: 12899402].

Miyano G et al: Cholecystectomy alone is inadequate for treating forme fruste choledochal cyst: Evidence from a rare but important case report. Pediatr Surg Int 2005;21:61 [PMID: 15316725].

Wong AM et al: Prenatal diagnosis of choledochal cyst using magnetic resonance imaging: A case report. World J Gastroenterol 2005;11:5082 [PMID: 16124073].

3. Spontaneous Perforation of the Extrahepatic Bile Ducts

The sudden appearance of obstructive jaundice, acholic stools, and abdominal enlargement with ascites in a sick newborn is suggestive of this condition. The liver is usually normal in size, and a yellow-green discoloration can often be discerned under the umbilicus or in the scrotum. In 24% of cases, stones or sludge obstructs the common bile duct. DIDA scan or ERCP shows leakage from the biliary tree, and ultrasonography confirms ascites or fluid around the bile duct.

Treatment is surgical. Simple drainage, without attempts at oversewing the perforation, is sufficient in primary perforations. A diversion anastomosis is constructed in cases associated with choledochal cyst or stenosis. The prognosis is generally good.

Barnes BH et al: Spontaneous perforation of the bile duct in a toddler: The role of endoscopic retrograde cholangiopancreatography in diagnosis and therapy. J Pediatr Gastroenterol Nutr 2006;43:695 [PMID: 17503309].

Sahnoun L et al: Spontaneous perforation of the extrahepatic bile duct in infancy: Report of two cases and literature review. Eur J Pediatr Surg 2007;17:132 [PMID: 17503309].

OTHER NEONATAL HYPERBILIRUBINEMIC CONDITIONS (NONCHOLESTATIC NONHEMOLYTIC)

This group of disorders is associated with hyperbilirubinemia of two types: (1) unconjugated hyperbilirubinemia, present in breast milk jaundice, Lucey-Driscoll syndrome, congenital hypothyroidism, upper intestinal obstruction, Gilbert disease, Crigler-Najjar syndrome, and drug-induced hyperbilirubinemia; and (2) conjugated noncholestatic hyperbilirubinemia, present in the Dubin-Johnson syndrome and Rotor syndrome.

1. Unconjugated Hyperbilirubinemia

A. Breast Milk Jaundice

Persistent elevation of the indirect bilirubin fraction may occur in up to 36% of breast-fed infants. Enhanced β-glucuronidase activity in breast milk is one factor that increases absorption of unconjugated bilirubin. Substances (eg, L-aspartic acid) in casein hydrolysate formulas inhibit this enzyme. The increased enterohepatic shunting of unconjugated bilirubin exceeds the normal conjugating capacity in the liver of these infants. The mutation for Gilbert syndrome predisposes to breast milk jaundice and to more prolonged jaundice. Low volumes of ingested breast milk may also contribute to jaundice in the first week of life.

Hyperbilirubinemia does not usually exceed 20 mg/dL, with most cases in the range of 10–15 mg/dL. In patients whose bilirubin levels are above 4–5 mg/dL, the jaundice is noticeable by the fifth to seventh day of breast feeding. It may accentuate the underlying physiologic jaundice—especially early, when total fluid intake may be less than optimal. Except for jaundice, the physical examination is usually normal; urine does not stain the diaper, and the stools are golden yellow.

The jaundice peaks before the third week of life and clears before age 3 months in almost all infants, even when breast feeding is continued. All infants who remain jaundiced past age 2–3 weeks should have measurements of conjugated bilirubin to exclude hepatobiliary disease.

Kernicterus has rarely been reported in association with this condition. In special situations, breast feeding may be discontinued temporarily and replaced by formula feedings for 2–3 days until serum bilirubin decreases by 2–8 mg/ dL. Cow's milk formulas inhibit the intestinal reabsorption of unconjugated bilirubin. When breast feeding is reinstituted, the serum bilirubin may increase slightly, but not to the previous level. Phototherapy is not indicated in the healthy full-term infant with this condition unless bilirubin levels meet high-risk levels as defined by the American Academy of Pediatrics.

American Academy of Pediatrics, Subcommittee on Hyperbilirubinemia: Management of hyperbilirubinemia in the newborn infant 35 or more weeks of gestation. Pediatrics 2004;114:297 [PMID: 15231951].

Gourley GR: A controlled, randomized, double-blind trial of prophylaxis against jaundice among breastfed newborns. Pediatrics 2005;116:385 [PMID: 16061593].

Mauro Y et al: Prolonged unconjugated hyperbilirubinemia associated with breast milk and mutations of the bilirubin uridine diphosphate-glucuronosyl transferase gene. Pediatrics 2000;106:E59 [PMID: 11061796].

Moyer V et al: Guideline for the evaluation of cholestatic jaundice in infants: Recommendations of the North American Society for Pediatric Gastroenterology, Hepatology and Nutrition. J Pediatr Gastroenterol Nutr 2004;39:115 [PMID: 15269615].

B. Congenital Hypothyroidism

Although the differential diagnosis of indirect hyperbilirubinemia should always include congenital hypothyroidism, the diagnosis may be obvious from other clinical and physical clues or from the newborn screening results. The jaundice clears quickly with replacement thyroid hormone therapy, although the mechanism is unclear.

Tiker F: Congenital hypothyroidism and early severe hyperbilirubinemia. Clin Pediatr (Phila) 2003;42:365 [PMID: 12800733].

C. Upper Intestinal Obstruction

The association of indirect hyperbilirubinemia with high intestinal obstruction (eg, duodenal atresia, annular pancreas, pyloric stenosis) in the newborn has been observed repeatedly; the mechanism is unknown. Diminished levels of hepatic glucuronyl transferase have been found on liver biopsy in pyloric stenosis, and genetic studies suggest that this indirect hyperbilirubinemia is an early sign of Gilbert syndrome.

Treatment is that of the underlying obstructive condition (usually surgical). Jaundice disappears once adequate nutrition is achieved.

Trioche P et al: Jaundice with hypertrophic pyloric stenosis is an early manifestation of Gilbert's syndrome. Arch Dis Child 1999;81:301 [PMID: 10490432].

D. Gilbert Syndrome

Gilbert syndrome is a common form (3–7% of the population) of familial hyperbilirubinemia associated with a partial reduction of hepatic bilirubin uridine diphosphate-glucuronyl transferase activity and perhaps an abnormality in the function or amount of one or more hepatocyte membrane protein carriers. Accelerated jaundice of the newborn, breast milk jaundice, and jaundice with intestinal obstruction may be present in affected infants. During puberty and beyond, mild fluctuating jaundice, especially with illness, and vague constitutional symptoms are common. Shortened red blood cell survival time in some patients is thought to be caused by reduced activity of enzymes involved in heme biosynthesis (protoporphyrinogen oxidase). Subsidence of hyperbilirubinemia has been achieved in patients by administration of phenobarbital (5–8 mg/kg/d), although this therapy is not justified.

The disease is inherited as an abnormality of the promoter region of uridine diphosphate-glucuronyl transferase-1; however, another factor is necessary for disease expression. The homozygous (16%) and heterozygous states (40%) are common. Males are affected more often than females (4:1). Serum unconjugated bilirubin is generally less than 3–6 mg/dL, although unusual cases may exceed 8 mg/dL. The findings on liver biopsy and most other LFTs are normal except for prolonged indocyanine green and bromosulfophthalein retention. An increase of 1.4 mg/dL or more in the level of unconjugated bilirubin after a 2-day fast (300 kcal/d) is consistent with the diagnosis of Gilbert syndrome. Genetic testing is available but rarely needed. No treatment is necessary.

Laforgia N et al: Neonatal hyperbilirubinemia and Gilbert's syndrome. J Perinat Med 2002;30:166 [PMID: 12012638].

Ulgenalp A et al: Analyses of polymorphism for UGT1*1 exon 1 promoter in neonates with pathologic and prolonged jaundice. Biol Neonate 2003;83:258 [PMID: 12743455].

E. Crigler-Najjar Syndrome

Infants with type 1 Crigler-Najjar syndrome usually develop rapid severe elevation of unconjugated bilirubin (> 30–40 mg/dL) with neurologic consequences (kernicterus). Consanguinity is often present. Prompt recognition of this entity and treatment with exchange transfusions are required, followed by phototherapy. Some patients have no neurologic signs until adolescence or early adulthood, at which time deterioration may occur suddenly. For diagnosis of this condition it is useful to obtain a duodenal bile specimen, which characteristically will be colorless and contain a predominance of unconjugated bilirubin, small amounts of monoconjugates, and only traces of diconjugated bilirubin. Phenobarbital administration does not significantly alter these findings, nor does it lower serum bilirubin levels. The deficiency in uridine diphosphate-glucuronyl transferase-1 is inherited in an autosomal recessive pattern. A combination of phototherapy and cholestyramine may keep bilirubin levels below 25 mg/dL. The use of tin protoporphyrin or tin mesoporphyrin remains experimental. Orlistat therapy may decrease bilirubin in a subset of patients. Liver transplantation is curative and may prevent kernicterus if performed early. An auxiliary orthotopic transplantation also relieves the jaundice while the patient retains native liver. Hepatocyte transplantation is experimental.

A milder form (type 2) with both autosomal dominant and recessive inheritance is rarely associated with neurologic complications. Hyperbilirubinemia is less severe, and the bile is pigmented and contains bilirubin monoglucuronide and diglucuronide. Patients with this form respond to phenobarbital with lowering of serum bilirubin levels. An increased proportion of monoconjugated and diconjugated bilirubin in the bile follows phenobarbital treatment. Liver biopsy findings and LFTs are consistently normal in both types.

Ambrosino G et al: Isolated hepatocyte transplantation for Crigler-Najjar syndrome type 1. Cell Transplant 2005;14:151 [PMID: 15881424].
Hafkamp AM et al: Orlistat treatment of unconjugated hyperbilirubinemia in Crigler-Najjar disease: A randomized controlled trial. Pediatr Res 2007;62:725 [PMID: 17957158].
Strauss KA et al: Management of hyperbilirubinemia and prevention of kernicterus in 20 patients with Crigler-Najjar disease. Eur J Pediatr 2006;165:306 [PMID: 16456422].

F. Drug-Induced Hyperbilirubinemia

Vitamin K_3 (menadiol) may elevate indirect bilirubin levels by causing hemolysis. Vitamin K_1 (phytonadione) can be used safely in neonates. Carbamazepine can cause conjugated hyperbilirubinemia in infancy. Rifampin and antiretroviral protease inhibitors may cause unconjugated hyperbilirubinemia. Other drugs (eg, ceftriaxone, sulfonamides) may displace bilirubin from albumin, potentially increasing the risk of kernicterus—especially in the sick premature infant.

2. Conjugated Noncholestatic Hyperbilirubinemia (Dubin-Johnson Syndrome & Rotor Syndrome)

These diagnoses are suspected when persistent or recurrent conjugated hyperbilirubinemia and jaundice occur and liver function tests are normal. The basic defect in Dubin-Johnson syndrome is in the multiple organic anion transport protein (MRP2) of the bile canaliculus, causing impaired hepatocyte excretion of conjugated bilirubin into bile. A variable degree of impairment in uptake and conjugation complicates the clinical picture. Transmission is autosomal recessive, so a positive family history is occasionally obtained. In Rotor syndrome, the defect lies in hepatic uptake and storage of bilirubin. Bile acids are metabolized normally, so that cholestasis does not occur. Bilirubin values range from 2–5 mg/dL, and other LFTs are normal.

In Rotor syndrome, the liver is normal; in Dubin-Johnson syndrome, it is darkly pigmented on gross inspection and may be enlarged. Microscopic examination reveals numerous dark-brown pigment granules consisting of polymers of epinephrine metabolites, especially in the centrilobular regions. However, the amount of pigment varies within

families, and some jaundiced family members may have no demonstrable pigmentation in the liver. Otherwise, the liver is histologically normal. Oral cholecystography fails to visualize the gallbladder in Dubin-Johnson syndrome, but is normal in Rotor syndrome. Differences in the excretion patterns of bromosulfophthalein, in results of DIDA cholescintigraphy, in urinary coproporphyrin I and III levels, and in the serum pattern of monoglucuronide and diglucuronide conjugates of bilirubin can help distinguish between these two conditions. Genotyping of *MRP2* is available.

Choleretic agents (eg, UDCA) may help reduce the cholestasis in infants with Dubin-Johnson syndrome.

Kaplan M et al: Bilirubin genetics for the nongeneticist: Hereditary defects of neonatal bilirubin conjugation. Pediatrics 2003;111(4 Pt 1):886 [PMID: 12671128].
Lee JH et al: Neonatal Dubin-Johnson syndrome: Long-term follow-up and MRP2 mutations study. Pediatr Res 2006;59:584 [PMID: 16549534].
Regev RH et al: Treatment of severe cholestasis in neonatal Dubin-Johnson syndrome with ursodeoxycholic acid. J Perinat Med 2002;30:185 [PMID: 12012642].

HEPATITIS A

ESSENTIALS OF DIAGNOSIS & TYPICAL FEATURES

▶ Gastrointestinal upset (anorexia, vomiting, diarrhea).

▶ Jaundice.

▶ Liver tenderness and enlargement.

▶ Abnormal LFTs.

▶ Local epidemic of hepatitis A infection.

▶ Positive anti–hepatitis A virus (HAV) IgM antibody.

▶ General Considerations

Hepatitis A virus (HAV) infection occurs in both epidemic and sporadic fashion (Table 21–6). Transmission by the fecal-oral route explains epidemic outbreaks from contaminated food or water supplies, including by food handlers. Viral particles are found in stools during the acute phase of hepatitis A infection and are similar in appearance to the enteroviruses. Sporadic cases usually result from contact with an infected individual. Transmission through blood products obtained during the viremic phase is a rare event, although it has occurred in a newborn nursery. The overt form of the disease is easily recognized by the clinical manifestations. However, two thirds of children are asymptomatic, and two thirds of symptomatic children are anicteric. Therefore, most symptomatic children with HAV are believed to have gastroenteritis. Lifelong immunity to HAV follows infection. In developing countries, most children are

Table 21–6. Hepatitis viruses.

	HAV	HBV	HCV	HDV	HEV
Type of virus	Enterovirus (RNA)	Hepadnavirus (DNA)	Flavivirus (RNA)	Deltavirus (RNA)	Calicivirus (RNA)
Transmission routes	Fecal-oral	Parenteral, sexual, vertical	Parenteral, sexual, vertical	Parenteral, sexual	Fecal-oral
Incubation period (days)	15–40	45–160	30–150	20–90	14–65
Diagnostic test	Anti-HAV IgM	HBsAg, anti-HBc IgM	Anti-HCV, PCR-RNA test	Anti-HDV antibody	Anti-HEV IgM
Mortality rate (acute)	0.1–0.2%	0.5–2%	1–2%	2–20%	1–2% (10–20% in pregnant women)
Carrier state	No	Yes	Yes	Yes	No
Vaccine available	Yes	Yes	No	Yes (HBV)	No
Treatment	None	Interferon-α (pegylated interferon in adults), nucleoside analogues (lamivudine, tenofovir, adefovir, entecavir)	Interferon-α or pegylated interferon plus ribavirin	Treatment for HBV	None

HAV, hepatitis A virus; HBc, hepatitis B core; HBsAg, hepatitis B surface antigen; HBV, hepatitis B virus; HDV, hepatitis D (delta) virus; HEV, hepatitis E virus; PCR, polymerase chain reaction.

exposed to HAV by age 10 years, while only 20% are exposed by age 20 years in developed countries.

Antibody to HAV appears within 1–4 weeks of clinical symptoms. Although the great majority of children with infectious hepatitis are asymptomatic or have mild disease and recover completely, some will develop fulminant hepatitis leading to death or requiring liver transplantation.

HEPATITIS VIRUS ABBREVIATIONS

HAV	Hepatitis A virus
Anti-HAV IgM	IgM antibody to HAV
HBV	Hepatitis B virus
HBsAg	HBV surface antigen
HBcAg	HBV core antigen
HBeAg	HBVe antigen
Anti-HBs	Antibody to HBsAg
Anti-HBc	Antibody to HBcAg
Anti-HBc IgM	IgM antibody to HBcAg
Anti-HBe	Antibody to HBeAg
HCV	Hepatitis C virus
Anti-HCV	Antibody to HCV
HDV	Hepatitis D (delta) virus
Anti-HDV	Antibody to HDV
HEV	Hepatitis E virus
Anti-HEV	Antibody to HEV

▶ Clinical Findings

A. History

Features of the patient's history may include direct exposure to a previously jaundiced individual, consumption of seafood, contaminated water or imported fruits or vegetables, attendance in a day care center, or recent travel to an area of endemic infection. Following an incubation period of 15–40 days, the initial nonspecific symptoms usually precede the development of jaundice by 5–10 days.

B. Symptoms and Signs

Fever, anorexia, vomiting, headache, and abdominal pain are typical symptoms. Dark urine precedes jaundice, which peaks in 1–2 weeks and then begins to subside. The stools may become light or clay-colored during this time. Clinical improvement can occur as jaundice develops. Tender hepatomegaly and jaundice are typically present; splenomegaly is variable.

C. Laboratory Findings

Aminotransferases and conjugated and unconjugated bilirubin levels are elevated. The leukocyte count is normal to low; the sedimentation rate is elevated. Serum proteins are generally normal, but an elevation of the γ-globulin fraction (> 2.5 g/dL) can occur and indicates a worse prognosis. Hypoalbuminemia, hypoglycemia, and marked prolongation of prothrombin time (international normalized ratio [INR] > 2.0) are serious prognostic findings. Diagnosis is made by serology. A positive anti-HAV IgM indicates acute disease, whereas IgG anti-HAV persists after recovery.

Percutaneous liver biopsy is rarely indicated. "Balloon cells" and acidophilic bodies are characteristic histologic findings. Liver cell necrosis may be diffuse or focal, with accompanying infiltration of inflammatory cells containing polymorphonuclear leukocytes, lymphocytes, macrophages, and plasma cells, particularly in portal areas. Some bile duct proliferation may be seen in the perilobular portal areas alongside areas of bile stasis. Regenerative liver cells and proliferation of reticuloendothelial cells are present. Occasionally massive hepatocyte necrosis occurs, portending a bad prognosis.

▶ Differential Diagnosis

Before jaundice appears, the symptoms are those of nonspecific viral enteritis. Other diseases with somewhat similar onset include pancreatitis, infectious mononucleosis, leptospirosis, drug-induced hepatitis, Wilson disease, autoimmune hepatitis, and other hepatitis viruses. Acquired CMV disease may also mimic HAV, although lymphadenopathy is usually present in the former.

▶ Prevention

Isolation of the patient during initial phases of illness is indicated, although most patients with hepatitis A are noninfectious by the time the disease becomes overt. Stool, diapers, and other fecally stained clothing should be handled with care for 1 week after the appearance of jaundice.

Passive-active immunization of exposed susceptible persons can be achieved by giving standard immune globulin, 0.02–0.04 mL/kg intramuscularly. Illness is prevented in 80–90% of individuals if immune globulin is given within 1–2 weeks of exposure. Alternatively, HAV vaccine can be given following exposure, with equal efficacy at preventing symptomatic HAV infection. Individuals traveling to endemic disease areas should receive HAV vaccine or 0.02–0.06 mL/kg of immune globulin as prophylaxis if there is insufficient time (< 2 weeks) for the initial dose of vaccine. All children older than 12 months with chronic liver disease should receive two doses of HAV vaccine 6 months apart. It is currently recommended that all children 12–23 months of age receive HAV vaccination in the United States.

▶ Treatment

No specific treatment measures are required. Sedatives and corticosteroids should be avoided. At the start of the illness, a light diet is preferable. During the icteric phase, lower-fat foods may diminish gastrointestinal symptoms but do not affect overall outcome. Drugs and elective surgery should be avoided.

▶ Prognosis

Ninety-nine percent of children recover without sequelae. In rare cases of fulminant hepatitis, the patient may die in 5 days or may survive as long as 1–2 months without liver transplantation. The prognosis is poor if hepatic coma or ascites develop; orthotopic liver transplantation is indicated under these circumstances. Incomplete resolution can cause a prolonged hepatitis; however, resolution invariably occurs without long-term hepatic sequelae. Rare cases of aplastic anemia following acute infectious hepatitis have been reported. A benign relapse of symptoms may occur in 10–15% of cases after 6–10 weeks of apparent resolution.

American Academy of Pediatrics Committee on Infectious Diseases: Hepatitis A vaccine recommendations. Pediatrics 2007;120:189 [PMID: 17606579].

Armstrong GL et al: The economics of routine childhood hepatitis A immunization in the United States: The impact of herd immunity. Pediatrics 2007;119:e22 [PMID: 17200247].

Belmaker I et al: Elimination of hepatitis A infection outbreaks in day care and school settings in southern Israel after introduction of the national universal toddler hepatitis a immunization program. Pediatr Infect Dis J 2007;26:36 [PMID: 17195703].

Victor JC et al: Hepatitis A vaccine versus immune globulin for postexposure prophylaxis. N Engl J Med 2007;357:1685 [PMID: 17947390].

HEPATITIS B

ESSENTIALS OF DIAGNOSIS & TYPICAL FEATURES

▶ Gastrointestinal upset, anorexia, vomiting, diarrhea.

▶ Jaundice, tender hepatomegaly, abnormal LFTs.

▶ Serologic evidence of hepatitis B disease: HBsAg, HBeAg, anti-HBc IgM.

▶ History of parenteral, sexual, or household exposure or maternal HBsAg carriage.

▶ General Considerations

In contrast to hepatitis A, hepatitis B virus (HBV) infection has a longer incubation period of 45–160 days (see Table 21–6). The disease is caused by a DNA virus that is usually acquired perinatally from a carrier mother, or later in life from exposure to contaminated blood through shared needles, needle sticks, skin piercing, or tattoos. It is also sexually transmitted. Transmission via blood products has been almost eliminated by anti-HBc antibody donor-screening protocols. The complete HBV particle is composed of a core (28-nm particle) that is found in the nucleus of infected liver cells and a double outer shell (surface antigen). The surface antigen in blood is termed HBsAg. The antibody to it is anti-HBs. The core antigen is termed HBcAg and its antibody is anti-HBc. A specific anti-HBc IgM antibody occurs during primary viral replication.

Another important antigen-antibody system associated with HBV disease is the "e" antigen system. HBeAg, a truncated soluble form of HBcAg, appears in the serum of infected patients early and correlates with active virus replication. Persistence of HBeAg is a marker of infectivity, whereas the appearance of anti-HBe generally implies termination of viral replication. However, HBV mutant viruses (precore mutant) may replicate with negative HBeAg tests and positive tests for anti-HBe antibody. Other serologic markers indicating viral replication include the presence of HBV DNA polymerase and circulating HBV DNA.

▶ Clinical Findings

A. Symptoms and Signs

Symptoms of acute hepatitis B infection include slight fever (which may be absent) and mild gastrointestinal upset. Visible jaundice is usually the first significant finding. It is accompanied by darkening of the urine and pale or clay-colored stools. Many patients, particularly infants, are asymptomatic. Hepatomegaly is frequently present. Occasionally a symptom complex (caused by antigen-antibody complexes) of macular rash, urticarial lesions, and arthritis antedates the appearance of icterus. Occasionally, HBV infection presents as a glomerulonephritis or nephrotic syndrome from immune complexes. When acquired vertically at birth, the disease is usually asymptomatic despite ongoing liver injury.

B. Laboratory Findings

To diagnose acute HBV infection, the HBsAg and anti-HBc IgM are the only tests needed. To document recovery, immunity, or response to the HBV vaccine, the anti-HBs is useful. To document previous HBV infection, the anti-HBc is most useful. If HBsAg persists after 8 weeks in acute infections, it may signify a chronic infection, although chronic infection is defined as lasting 6 months or more. Vertical transmission to newborns is documented by positive HBsAg. LFT results are similar to those discussed earlier for hepatitis A. Liver histology is similar for HAV and HBV disease, although specific stains may detect HBcAg or HBsAg in the liver, and ground-glass appearance to hepatocytes may be present. Renal involvement may be suspected on the basis of urinary findings suggesting glomerulonephritis or nephrotic syndrome.

▶ Differential Diagnosis

The differentiation between HAV and HBV disease is made easier by a history of parenteral exposure, an HBsAg-positive parent, or an unusually long period of incubation. HBV and hepatitis C virus (HCV) infection or Epstein-Barr virus (EBV) infection are differentiated serologically. The history may suggest a drug-induced hepatitis, especially if a serum sickness prodrome is reported. Autoimmune hepatitis, Wilson disease, hemochromatosis, nonalcoholic fatty liver disease, and α_1-antitrypsin deficiency should also be considered. Drug-induced hepatitis is diagnosed if there is a history of specific drug exposure; autoimmune hepatitis is diag-

nosed if autoimmune markers are present; Wilson disease is diagnosed if ceruloplasmin levels are abnormal; hemochromatosis is diagnosed if transferrin saturation is high; α_1-antitrypsin deficiency is diagnosed if serum α_1-antitrypsin concentration is decreased; and steatohepatitis is diagnosed if liver biopsy findings are suggestive.

▶ Prevention

Control of hepatitis B in the population is based on screening of blood donors and pregnant women, use of properly sterilized needles and surgical equipment, avoidance of sexual contact with carriers, and vaccination of all infants and adolescents, as well as household contacts, sexual partners, medical personnel, and those at high risk. Universal immunization of all infants born in the United States and of adolescents is now recommended, as it is in most other countries. The vaccine is highly effective for preexposure prophylaxis. (See Chapter 9.) For postexposure prophylaxis, administration of HBIG (0.06 mL/kg intramuscularly, given as soon as possible after exposure, up to 7 days) and initiation of vaccination are recommended. The risk of vertical transmission is dramatically reduced with the combination of postpartum vaccination and immunoprophylaxis.

▶ Treatment

Supportive measures such as bed rest and a nutritious diet are used during the active symptomatic stage of disease. Corticosteroids are contraindicated. No other treatment is needed for acute HBV infection. For patients with progressive disease (chronic hepatitis with fibrosis), there are currently two treatment options. Treatment with α-interferon (5–6 million U/m^2 body surface area injected subcutaneously three times a week for 4–6 months) inhibits viral replication in 30–40% of patients, normalizes the ALT level, and leads to the disappearance of HBeAg and the appearance of anti-HBe. Side effects are common. Younger children may respond better than older children. Orally administered lamivudine therapy (3 mg/kg/d up to 100 mg/d for 12 months) leads to a successful response in 25% of treated children, with minimal side effects. However, resistant organisms can emerge. Pegylated interferon, several oral antiviral agents, and combination therapy are promising options being tested in children. Asymptomatic HBsAg carriers (normal serum ALT, no hepatomegaly) do not respond to either therapy. Liver transplantation is successful in acute fulminant hepatitis B; however, reinfection is common following liver transplantation for chronic hepatitis B. Chronic HBIG therapy or lamivudine therapy reduces recurrence after transplantation.

▶ Prognosis

The prognosis is good, although fulminant hepatitis or chronic hepatitis and cirrhosis may supervene in up to 10% of patients. The course of the acute disease is variable, but jaundice seldom persists for more than 2 weeks. HBsAg disappears in 95% of cases at the time of clinical recovery. Persistent asymptomatic infection may occur, particularly in children with vertical transmission, Down syndrome, or leukemia, and in those undergoing chronic hemodialysis. Persistence of neonatally acquired HBsAg occurs in 70–90% of infants without immunoprophylaxis or vaccination, and the presence of HBeAg in the HBsAg carrier indicates ongoing viral replication. However, 1–2% of children infected at birth will show spontaneous seroconversion of HBeAg each year. If HBV infection is acquired later in childhood, HBV is cleared and recovery occurs in 90–95% of patients. Chronic hepatitis B disease predisposes the patient to development of hepatocellular carcinoma. Once chronic HBV infection is established, surveillance for development of hepatocellular carcinoma with serum α-fetoprotein is performed biannually and ultrasonography yearly. Routine HBV vaccination of newborns in endemic countries has reduced the incidence of fulminant hepatic failure, chronic hepatitis, and hepatocellular carcinoma in children.

Dentinger CM et al: Persistence of antibody to hepatitis B and protection from disease among Alaska natives immunized at birth. Pediatr Infect Dis J 2005;24:786 [PMID: 16148845].

Jonas MM: Treatment of hepatitis B in children. J Pediatr Gastroenterol Nutr 2006;43:S56 [PMID: 16819403].

Kansu A et al: Comparison of two different regimens of combined interferon-alpha2a and lamivudine therapy in children with chronic hepatitis B infection. Antivir Ther 2006;11:255 [PMID: 16640106].

Ni YH et al: Lamivudine treatment in maternally transmitted chronic hepatitis B virus infection patients. Pediatr Int 2005;47:372 [PMID: 16091071].

Shepard CW et al: Epidemiology of hepatitis B and hepatitis B virus infection in United States children. Pediatr Infect Dis J 2005;24:755 [PMID: 16148839].

HEPATITIS C

General Considerations

Hepatitis C virus (HCV) virus is the most common cause of non-B chronic hepatitis (90% of post-transfusion hepatitis cases) (see Table 21–6). Risk factors in adults and older children include illicit use of intravenous drugs (40%), occupational or sexual exposure (10%), and transfusions (10%); 30% of cases have no known risk factors. In children, most cases are now associated with transmission from an infected mother or other household transmission. In the past, children with hemophilia or on chronic hemodialysis were at significant risk. The risk from transfused blood products has diminished greatly (from 1–2:100 to 1:100,000 units of blood) since the advent of blood testing for ALT and anti-HCV. HCV infection has also been caused by contaminated immune serum globulin preparations. Vertical transmission from HCV-infected mothers occurs more commonly with mothers who are HIV-positive (15–20%) compared with those who are HIV-negative (5–6%). About 0.4% of adolescents and 1.5% of adults in the United States have serologic evidence of infection. Vertically infected infants often have elevated ALT levels, but do not appear ill; long-term outcome is unknown, however 20–30% of infants recover completely. Transmission of the virus from breast milk is probably rare. HCV rarely causes fulminant hepatitis in children or adults in Western countries, but different serotypes do so in Asia.

HCV is a single-stranded RNA virus in the flavivirus family. At least seven genotypes of HCV exist. Several well-defined HCV antigens are the basis for serologic antibody tests. The third-generation enzyme-linked immunosorbent assay (ELISA) test for anti-HCV is highly accurate. Anti-HCV is generally present when symptoms occur; however, test results may be negative in the first few months of infection. The presence of HCV RNA in serum indicates active infection.

Clinical Findings

A. Symptoms and Signs

The incubation period is 1–5 months, with insidious onset of symptoms. Many childhood cases, especially those acquired vertically, are asymptomatic despite development of chronic hepatitis. Flulike prodromal symptoms and jaundice occur in less than 25% of cases. Hepatosplenomegaly may or may not be evident in chronic hepatitis. Ascites, clubbing, palmar erythema, or spider angiomas are rare and indicate progression to cirrhosis.

B. Laboratory Findings

Fluctuating mild to moderate elevations of aminotransferases over long periods are characteristic of chronic HCV infection. Diagnosis is established by the presence of anti-HCV (third-generation ELISA) confirmed by the radioimmunoblot assay or HCV RNA by PCR. Anti-HCV is acquired passively at birth from infected mothers and cannot be used to confirm disease in the neonate for the first 15 months. HCV RNA testing should be performed in suspected cases. Results of this test may be negative in the first month of life, but become positive by 4 months.

Percutaneous liver biopsy should be considered in chronic cases. Histologic examination shows portal triaditis with chronic inflammatory cells, occasional lymphocyte nodules in portal tracts, mild macrovesicular steatosis, and variable bridging necrosis, fibrosis, and cirrhosis; most children have only mild to moderate fibrosis on liver biopsy. Cirrhosis in adults generally requires 20–30 years of chronic HCV infection, but it has occasionally developed sooner in children.

Differential Diagnosis

HCV disease should be distinguished from HAV and HBV disease by serologic testing. Other causes of cirrhosis in children should be considered in cases of chronic illness, such as Wilson disease or α_1-antitrypsin deficiency. Chronic hepatitis may also be caused by drug reactions, autoimmune disease, or steatohepatitis.

Treatment

Treatment of acute HCV hepatitis is supportive. Indications for treatment of chronic infection will be determined by current clinical trials. Chronic hepatitis caused by HCV responds to combined interferon-α (3 million U/m^2 three times a week for 6–12 months) and ribavirin (15 mg/kg/d), with sustained response rates of 30–50%. The response is poorer in those who have infections with genotype 1a or 1b and very good for genotypes 2 and 3. Long-acting (pegylated) interferon (with or without ribavirin), which has been studied in adults, is more effective, with sustained response rates up to 60–70%. This therapy is being tested in children. End-stage liver disease secondary to HCV responds well to liver transplantation, although reinfection is common and is occasionally rapidly progressive. Pre- and post-transplant antiviral therapy may reduce the risk of reinfection. There is no vaccine, and no benefit from using immune globulin in infants born to infected mothers. Elective cesarean delivery of HCV-infected pregnant women with a high titer of circulating virus may lessen the likelihood for vertical transmission.

Prognosis

In adults, 70–80% of HCV patients develop chronic hepatitis, and cirrhosis develops in 20% of those with chronic infection for 10–30 years. Alcohol intake, and concomitant obesity and fatty liver, increase this risk. HCV is now the leading indication for liver transplantation in adults. A strong association exists between chronic HCV disease and the development of hepatocellular carcinoma after as little as 15 years. The outcome in children is less well defined, although cirrhosis may develop rapidly in rare cases or after decades. About 50% of children infected by transfusion in the first few years of life develop chronic infection. The prognosis for infants infected at birth with concomitant HIV infection is unknown, but the course appears benign for the first 10 years of life. In adults, chronic HCV infection has been associated with mixed cryoglobulinemia, polyarteritis nodosa, a sicca-like syndrome, and membranoproliferative glomerulonephritis.

Elisofon SA, Jonas M: Hepatitis B and C in children: Current treatment and future strategies. Clin Liver Dis 2006;10:133 [PMID: 16376798].

Gonzalez-Peralta RP et al: Interferon alfa-2b in combination with ribavirin for the treatment of chronic hepatitis C in children: Efficacy, safety, and pharmacokinetics. Hepatology 2005;42:1010 [PMID: 16250032].

Narkewicz MR et al: The "C" of viral hepatitis in children. Semin Liv Dis 2007;27:295 [PMID: 17682976].

Schwarz KB et al: Safety, efficacy and pharmacokinetics of peginterferon alpha2a (40 kd) in children with chronic hepatitis C. J Pediatr Gastroenterol Nutr 2006;43:499 [PMID: 17033526].

Syriopoulou V et al: Mother to child transmission of hepatitis C virus: Rate of infection and risk factors. Scand J Infect Dis 2005;37:350 [PMID: 16051571].

HEPATITIS D (DELTA AGENT)

The hepatitis D virus (HDV) is a 35-nm defective virus that requires a coat of HBsAg to be infectious (see Table 21–6). Thus, HDV infection can occur only in the presence of HBV infection. In developing countries, transmission is by intimate contact; in western countries, by parenteral exposure. HDV is rare in North America. HDV can infect simultaneously with HBV, causing acute hepatitis, or can superinfect a patient with chronic HBV infection, predisposing the individual to chronic hepatitis or fulminant hepatitis. In children, the association between chronic HDV coinfection with HBV and chronic hepatitis and cirrhosis is strong. Vertical HDV transmission is rare. The diagnosis of HDV is made by anti-HDV IgM or detection of HDV by PCR. Treatment is directed at therapy for HBV infection or for fulminant hepatic failure.

Niro GA et al: Treatment of hepatitis D. J Viral Hepat 2005;12:2 [PMID: 15655042].

HEPATITIS E

Hepatitis E virus (HEV) infection is a cause of enterically transmitted, epidemic non-A, non-B hepatitis (see Table 21–6). It is rare in the United States. HEV is a calicivirus-like agent that is transmitted via the fecal-oral route. It occurs predominantly in developing countries in association with waterborne epidemics, and has only a 3% secondary attack rate in household contacts. Areas reporting epidemics include Southeast Asia, China, the Indian subcontinent, the Middle East, northern and western Africa, Mexico, and Central America. Its clinical manifestations resemble HAV infection except that symptomatic disease is rare in children, more common in adolescents and adults, and is associated with a high mortality (10–20%) in pregnant women, particularly in the third trimester. Diagnosis is established by detecting anti-HEV antibody. The outcome in nonpregnant individuals is benign, with no chronic hepatitis or chronic carrier state reported. A recombinant vaccine is being tested. There is no effective treatment.

Panda SK et al: Hepatitis E virus. Rev Med Virol 2007;17:151 [PMID: 17051624].

Shrestha MP et al: Safety and efficacy of a recombinant hepatitis E vaccine. N Engl J Med 2007;356:895 [PMID: 17329696].

OTHER HEPATITIS VIRUSES

Other undiscovered viruses may be the cause of cases of fulminant hepatitis in children that can be associated with the development of aplastic anemia in a small proportion of patients recovering from hepatitis and in 10–20% of those undergoing liver transplantation for indeterminate fulminant hepatitis. Parvovirus has been associated with fulminant hepatitis; the prognosis is relatively good in children. Infectious mononucleosis (EBV) is commonly associated with acute hepatitis. CMV, adenovirus, herpes simplex virus, HHV-6, HIV, brucella, and leptospirosis are other infectious causes of acute hepatitis.

Aydim M et al: Detection of human parvovirus B19 in children with acute hepatitis. Ann Trop Paediatr 2006;26:25 [PMID: 16494701].
Cacheux W et al: HHV-6-related acute liver failure in two immunocompetent adults: Favourable outcome after liver transplantation and/or ganciclovir therapy. J Intern Med. 2005;258:573 [PMID: 16313481].

ACUTE LIVER FAILURE (FULMINANT HEPATIC FAILURE)

 ESSENTIALS OF DIAGNOSIS & TYPICAL FEATURES

▶ Acute hepatitis with deepening jaundice.
▶ Extreme elevation of AST and ALT.
▶ Prolonged prothrombin time and INR.
▶ Encephalopathy and cerebral edema.
▶ Asterixis and fetor hepaticus.

General Considerations

Acute liver failure (ALF) is defined as acute liver dysfunction resulting in hepatic coma and coagulopathy (INR > 2.0) within 6 weeks after onset. In young children, encephalopathy may be difficult to detect or absent. Mortality is approximately 50% in children (without liver transplantation). An unusually virulent infectious agent or aggressive host immune response is postulated in many cases. In the first few weeks of life, ALF can be caused by herpes simplex, enteroviruses, adenovirus, galactosemia, fructose intolerance, tyrosinemia, neonatal iron storage disease, respiratory chain and fatty acid oxidation defects, familial erythrophagocytic histiocytosis, bile acid synthesis defects, and peroxisomal diseases. In older infants and children, the most common identified diagnoses are idiopathic, acetaminophen toxicity, autoimmune hepatitis, and infections. HBV, parvovirus, and HEV are sometimes causative. HAV rarely is responsible in the United States. Patients with immunologic deficiency diseases and those receiving immunosuppressive drugs are vulnerable to herpesviruses. In children with HIV infection, nucleoside reverse transcriptase inhibitors have triggered lactic acidosis and liver failure. In patients with underlying respiratory chain defects, valproic acid may trigger ALF. In older children, Wilson disease, acute fatty liver of pregnancy, Reye syndrome, drugs (eg, acetaminophen, anesthetic agents, valproic acid) or toxins (eg, poisonous mushrooms, herbs, "ecstasy"), leukemia, and cardiac dysfunction must also be considered. Some 30–40% of cases in children are without identifiable cause and labeled indeterminate.

Clinical Findings

In some patients, the disease proceeds in a rapidly fulminant course with deepening jaundice, coagulopathy, hyperammonemia, ascites, a rapidly shrinking liver, and progressive coma. Terminally, AST and ALT, which were greatly elevated (2000–10,000 U/L), may improve at the time when the liver is getting smaller and undergoing massive necrosis and collapse. Some patients start with a course typical of benign hepatitis and then suddenly become severely ill during the second week of the disease. Fever, anorexia, vomiting, and abdominal pain may be noted, and worsening of LFTs parallels changes in sensorium or impending coma. Hyperreflexia and a positive extensor plantar response are seen. A characteristic breath odor (fetor hepaticus) is present. A severe coagulopathy precedes impairment of renal function, manifested by either oliguria or anuria, which is an ominous sign. Characteristic laboratory findings include elevated serum bilirubin levels (usually > 15–20 mg/dL), sustained very high AST and ALT (> 3000 U/L) that may decrease terminally, low serum albumin, hypoglycemia, and prolonged prothrombin time and INR. Blood ammonia levels become elevated, whereas blood urea nitrogen is often very low. Hyperpnea is frequent, and mixed respiratory alkalosis and metabolic acidosis are present.

Differential Diagnosis

Infectious, autoimmune, metabolic, and drug or toxin causes are most common. Patients with Reye syndrome or urea cycle defects are typically anicteric. Wilson disease, autoimmune hepatitis, acute leukemia, cardiomyopathy, and Budd-Chiari syndrome should be considered. Acetaminophen overdose, herbal remedies, and other toxins (eg, "ecstasy") need to be considered even if the history is negative.

Complications

The development of renal failure and depth of hepatic coma determine the prognosis. Patients in grade 4 coma (unresponsiveness to verbal stimuli, decorticate or decerebrate posturing) rarely survive without transplantation and may have residual central nervous system deficits. Cerebral edema, which usually accompanies coma, is frequently the cause of death. Extreme prolongation of prothrombin time or INR greater than 4 predicts poor recovery except with acetaminophen overdose. Sepsis, hemorrhage, renal failure, or cardiorespiratory arrest is a common terminal event. The rare survivor of advanced disease without transplantation may have residual fibrosis or even cirrhosis.

Treatment

The most effective therapy is excellent critical care. Several therapies have failed to affect outcome, including exchange transfusion, plasmapheresis with plasma exchange, total body washout, charcoal hemoperfusion, and hemodialysis using a special high-permeability membrane. Hyperammonemia and bleeding should be controlled. Extracorporeal hepatic support devices are being developed to help bridge patients to liver transplantation or allow for liver regeneration. Orthotopic liver transplantation is successful in 60–85% of cases; however, patients in grade 4 coma may not always recover cerebral function. Therefore, patients in ALF should be transferred prior to the development of hepatic coma to centers where liver transplantation can be performed. Criteria for deciding when to perform transplantation are not firmly established; however, serum bilirubin over 20 mg/dL, INR greater than 4, and factor V levels less than 20% indicate a poor prognosis. Living related donors may be required for transplantation in a timely fashion. The prognosis is better for acetaminophen ingestion, particularly when N-acetylcysteine treatment is given.

Corticosteroids may be harmful, except in autoimmune hepatitis for which steroids may reverse the ALF. Acyclovir is essential in herpes simplex infection. Sterilization of the colon with oral antibiotics such as metronidazole, neomycin, or gentamicin is recommended. An alternative is acidification of the colon with lactulose, 1–2 mL/kg three or four times daily, which reduces blood ammonia levels and traps ammonia in the colon. Some centers use N-acetylcysteine in all patients, although it is only of proven benefit in acetaminophen toxicity.

Close monitoring of fluid and electrolytes is mandatory and requires a central venous line. Ten percent dextrose solutions should be infused (6–8 mg/kg/min) to maintain normal blood glucose. Diuretics, sedatives, and tranquilizers should be used sparingly. Early signs of cerebral edema are treated with infusions of mannitol (0.5–1.0 g/kg). Comatose patients are intubated, given mechanical ventilatory support, and monitored for signs of infection. Coagulopathy is treated with fresh-frozen plasma, recombinant factor VIIa, other clotting factor concentrates, platelet infusions, or exchange transfusion. Plasmapheresis and hemodialysis may help stabilize a patient while awaiting liver transplantation. Epidural monitoring for increased intracranial pressure (hepatic coma stages 3 and 4) in patients awaiting liver transplantation is advocated by some. Artificial hepatic support devices are being developed. Continuous venous–venous dialysis may be helpful to maintain fluid balance. Prophylactic immune globulin, 0.02 mL/kg intramuscularly, should be given to close contacts of patients with HAV infection.

Prognosis

The prognosis is primarily dependent on etiology and depth of coma. Children with acute acetaminophen toxicity have a high rate of spontaneous survival. Only 20–30% of children with stage 3 or 4 hepatic encephalopathy will have a spontaneous recovery. In children with indeterminate ALF, 40% will have a spontaneous recovery. Data from a recent large study suggest that the spontaneous recovery rate is about 40–50% when all causes of ALF are combined; 30% of patients will receive a liver transplant; and 20% will die without a transplant. Exchange transfusions or other modes of heroic therapy do not improve survival figures. The presence of nests of liver cells amounting to more than 25% of the total cells seen on liver biopsy examination and rising levels of clotting factors V and VII, coupled with rising levels of serum α-fetoprotein, may signify a more favorable prognosis. The survival rate in patients who undergo liver transplantation is 60–85%.

Dhawan A et al: Approaches to acute liver failure in children. Pediatr Transplant 2004;8:584 [PMID: 15598330].

Lee WS et al: Etiology, outcome and prognostic indicators of childhood fulminant hepatic failure in the United Kingdom. J Pediatr Gastroenterol Nutr 2005;40:575 [PMID: 15861019].

Liu E et al: Characterization of acute liver failure and development of a continuous risk of death staging system in children. J Hepatol 2006;44:134 [PMID: 16169116].

Squires RH et al: Acute liver failure in children: The first 348 patients in the pediatric acute liver failure study group. J Pediatr 2006;148:652 [PMID: 16737880].

AUTOIMMUNE HEPATITIS

ESSENTIALS OF DIAGNOSIS & TYPICAL FEATURES

► Acute or chronic hepatitis.

► Hypergammaglobulinemia.

► Positive antinuclear antibodies (ANA), anti–smooth muscle antibodies (ASMA), anti–liver-kidney microsomal (LKM) antibodies, or anti–soluble liver antibodies (SLA).

General Considerations

Autoimmune hepatitis (AIH) is most common in adolescent girls, although it occurs at all ages and in either sex. Rarely, AIH evolves from drug-induced hepatitis (eg, minocycline) or may develop in conjunction with such diseases as ulcerative colitis, Sjögren syndrome, or autoimmune hemolytic anemia. Wilson disease, α_1-antitrypsin deficiency, cystic fibrosis, and bile acid synthesis defects may present similarly as chronic hepatitis. A positive HBsAg test implicates HBV, and a positive HCV PCR suggests HCV infection. Positive autoantibodies, elevated serum IgG, and systemic manifestations (eg, arthralgia, weight loss, acne, and amenorrhea) are characteristic of AIH.

A genetic susceptibility to development of this entity is suggested by the increased incidence of the histocompatibility antigens HLA-A1 and HLA-B8. Increased autoimmune disease in families of patients and a high prevalence of seroimmunologic abnormalities have been noted in relatives. Occasionally patients have an "overlap syndrome" of AIH and primary sclerosing cholangitis.

Clinical Findings

Fever, malaise, recurrent or persistent jaundice, skin rash, arthritis, amenorrhea, gynecomastia, acne, pleurisy, pericarditis, or ulcerative colitis may be found in the history of these patients, or asymptomatic hepatomegaly or splenomegaly may be found on examination. Occasionally patients present in acute liver failure. Cutaneous signs of chronic liver disease may be noted (eg, spider angiomas, palmar erythema, and digital clubbing). Hepatosplenomegaly is frequently present.

LFTs reveal moderate elevations of serum bilirubin, AST, ALT, and serum alkaline phosphatase. Serum albumin may be low. Serum IgG levels are strikingly elevated (in the range of 2–6 g/dL). Low levels of C3 complement have been reported. Three subtypes of disease have been described based on autoantibodies present: type 1—anti–smooth muscle (antiactin); type 2—anti-LKM (anti–cytochrome P-450); and type 3—anti-SLA.

Histologic examination of liver biopsy specimens shows loss of the lobular limiting plate, and interface hepatitis ("piecemeal" necrosis). Portal fibrosis, an inflammatory reaction of lymphocytes and plasma cells in the portal areas and perivascularly, and some bile duct and Kupffer cell proliferation and pseudolobule formation may be present. Cirrhosis may exist at diagnosis in up to 50% of patients.

Differential Diagnosis

Laboratory and histologic findings differentiate other types of chronic hepatitis (eg, HBV, HCV, and HDV infection; steatohepatitis; Wilson disease; α_1-antitrypsin deficiency; primary sclerosing cholangitis). Primary sclerosing cholangitis occasionally presents in a manner similar to AIH, including the presence of autoantibodies. Wilson disease and α_1-antitrypsin deficiency must be excluded if HBV and HCV studies are negative. Anti-HCV antibodies can be falsely positive and should be confirmed by HCV PCR. Drug-induced (minocycline, isoniazid, methyldopa, pemoline) chronic hepatitis should be ruled out.

Complications

Untreated disease that continues for months to years eventually results in postnecrotic cirrhosis, with complications of portal hypertension. Persistent malaise, fatigue, amenorrhea, and anorexia parallel disease activity. Bleeding from esophageal varices and development of ascites usually usher in hepatic failure.

Treatment

Corticosteroids (prednisone, 2 mg/kg/d) decrease the mortality rate during the early active phase of the disease. Azathioprine or 6-mercaptopurine (6MP), 1–2 mg/kg/d, is of value in decreasing the side effects of long-term corticosteroid therapy but should not be used alone during the induction phase of treatment. Steroids are reduced over a 3- to 12-month period, and azathioprine is continued for 1–2 years if AST and ALT remain consistently normal. Liver biopsy is performed before stopping azathioprine therapy; if inflammation persists, then azathioprine is continued. Thiopurine methyltransferase activity should be assessed prior to starting azathioprine, to prevent extremely high blood levels and severe bone marrow toxicity. Relapses are treated similarly. Many patients require chronic azathioprine or 6MP therapy. UCDA, cyclosporine, tacrolimus, or methotrexate may be helpful in poorly responsive cases. Mycophenolate mofetil can be substituted for azathioprine, but it is more expensive. Liver transplantation is indicated when disease progresses to decompensated cirrhosis despite therapy or in unresponsive cases presenting in acute liver failure. Steroid therapy may be lifesaving in those presenting in acute liver failure.

Prognosis

The overall prognosis for AIH is improved significantly with early therapy. Some studies report cures (normal histologic findings) in 15–20% of patients. Relapses (seen clinically and histologically) occur in 40–50% of patients after cessation of therapy; remissions follow repeat treatment. Survival for 10 years is common despite residual cirrhosis. Of children with AIH, 20–50% eventually require liver transplantation. Complications of portal hypertension (bleeding varices, ascites, spontaneous bacterial peritonitis, and hepatopulmonary syndrome) require specific therapy. Liver transplantation is successful 70–90% of the time. Disease recurs after transplantation 10–50% of the time and is treated similarly to pretransplant disease.

Alvarez F: Autoimmune hepatitis and primary sclerosing cholangitis. Clin Liver Dis 2006;10:89 [PMID: 16376796].

Ishibashi H et al: Guidelines for therapy of autoimmune liver disease. Semin Liver Dis 2007;27:214 [PMID: 17520519].

Krawitt EL: Autoimmune hepatitis. N Engl J Med. 2006;354:54 [PMID: 16394302].

NONALCOHOLIC FATTY LIVER DISEASE

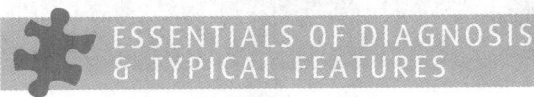

ESSENTIALS OF DIAGNOSIS & TYPICAL FEATURES

▶ Hepatomegaly in patient with BMI > 95th percentile.

▶ Elevated ALT > AST.

▶ Detection of fatty infiltration of the liver on ultrasound.

▶ Histologic evidence of fat in the liver.

▶ Insulin resistance.

Nonalcoholic fatty liver disease (NAFLD) is increasingly diagnosed in children. Patients with NAFLD present with asymptomatic soft hepatomegaly. If nonalcoholic steatohepatitis (NASH) is present, mild to moderately elevated aminotransferases (2–10 times the upper limit of normal) are also present. ALT is frequently higher than AST. Alkaline phosphatase and GGT may be mildly elevated, but bilirubin is normal. Ultrasonography or CT scanning indicates fat density in the liver. Liver biopsy shows micro- or macrovesicular steatosis in simple NAFLD, with the addition of portal tract inflammation, Mallory bodies, and variable degrees of portal fibrosis to cirrhosis in NASH. Most cases are associated with overweight state or type 2 diabetes mellitus. The prevalence of NAFLD is related to the prevalence of obesity in the population. The prevalence is estimated at 10% for children and adolescents with significant racial and ethic variability. One to 3% of adolescents in the United States may have NASH, based on the observation that 15–25% of American adolescents are overweight or obese and that roughly 40% will have NAFLD and 10% will have NASH. Steatohepatitis is also associated with Wilson disease, hereditary fructose intolerance, tyrosinemia, HCV hepatitis, cystic fibrosis, fatty acid oxidation defects, kwashiorkor, Reye syndrome, respiratory chain defects, and toxic hepatopathy (ethanol and others). Treatment is weight reduction and exercise for obesity or treatment for the other causes. A pilot trial suggests that vitamin E may be helpful and is currently under study. In addition, improved control of insulin resistance with metformin or pioglitazone is also under study in NASH. Cirrhosis and liver failure have been described in adults with this disease.

Patton HM et al: Pediatric nonalcoholic fatty liver disease: A critical appraisal of current data and implications for future research. J Pediatr Gastroenterol Nutr 2006;43:413 [PMID: 17033514].

Schwimmer JB et al: Obesity, insulin resistance, and other clinico-pathological correlates of pediatric nonalcoholic fatty liver disease. J Pediatr 2003;143:500 [PMID: 14571229].

Schwimmer JB et al: Prevalence of fatty liver in children and adolescents. Pediatrics 2006;118:1388 [PMID: 17015527].

Wieckowska A, Feldstein AE: Nonalcoholic fatty liver disease in the pediatric population: A review. Curr Opin Pediatr 2005; 17:636 [PMID: 16160540].

α_1-ANTITRYPSIN DEFICIENCY LIVER DISEASE

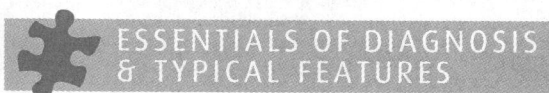

ESSENTIALS OF DIAGNOSIS & TYPICAL FEATURES

▶ Serum α_1-antitrypsin level < 50–80 mg/dL.

▶ Identification of a specific protease inhibitor (Pi) phenotype (PiZZ, PiSZ) or genotype.

▶ Detection of diastase-resistant glycoprotein deposits in periportal hepatocytes.

▶ Histologic evidence of liver disease.

▶ Family history of early-onset pulmonary disease or liver disease.

▶ General Considerations

The disease is caused by a deficiency in α_1-antitrypsin, a protease inhibitor (Pi) system, predisposing patients to chronic liver disease and an early onset of pulmonary emphysema. It is most often associated with the Pi phenotypes ZZ and SZ. Heterozygotes may have a slightly higher incidence of liver disease. The exact relationship between low levels of serum α_1-antitrypsin and the development of liver disease is unclear. Emphysema develops because of a lack of inhibition of neutrophil elastase, which destroys pulmonary connective tissue. The accumulation of misfolded aggregates of α_1-antitrypsin protein in the liver causes the liver injury by unclear mechanisms. Although all patients with the ZZ genotype eventually have antitrypsin inclusions in hepatocytes, only about 15–20% develop significant liver disease. Thus another genetic or environmental modifier must be involved. An associated abnormality in the microsomal disposal of accumulated aggregates may contribute to the liver disease phenotype.

About 10–20% of affected individuals present with neonatal cholestasis. About 10% of individuals with α_1-antitrypsin deficiency have clinically significant liver injury by age 18 years. Very few children have significant pulmonary involvement. Most affected children are completely asymptomatic, with no laboratory or clinical evidence of liver or lung disease.

▶ Clinical Findings

A. Symptoms and Signs

α_1-Antitrypsin deficiency should be considered in all infants with neonatal cholestasis. Serum GGT is usually, but not always, elevated. Jaundice, acholic stools, and malabsorption may also be present. Infants are often small for gestational age, and hepatosplenomegaly may be present. The family history may be positive for emphysema or cirrhosis.

In older children, hepatomegaly or physical findings suggestive of cirrhosis and portal hypertension, especially in the face of a negative history of liver disease, should always lead one to consider α_1-antitrypsin deficiency. Recurrent pulmonary disease (bronchitis, pneumonia) may be present in a few older children.

B. Laboratory Findings

Levels of the α_1-globulin fraction may be less than 0.2 mg/dL on serum protein electrophoresis. α_1-Antitrypsin level is low (< 50–80 mg/dL) in homozygotes (ZZ). Specific Pi phenotyping should be done to confirm the diagnosis. Genotyping is also available. LFTs often reflect underlying hepatic pathologic changes. Hyperbilirubinemia (mixed) and elevated aminotransferases, alkaline phosphatase, and GGT are present early. Hyperbilirubinemia generally resolves, while aminotransferase and GGT elevation may persist. Signs of cirrhosis and hypersplenism may develop even when LFTs are normal.

Liver biopsy findings after age 6 months show diastase-resistant, periodic acid–Schiff staining intracellular globules, particularly in periportal zones. These may be absent prior to age 6 months, but when present are characteristic of α_1-antitrypsin deficiency.

Differential Diagnosis

In newborns, other specific causes of neonatal cholestasis need to be considered, including biliary atresia. In older children, other causes of insidious cirrhosis (eg, HBV or HCV infection, autoimmune hepatitis, Wilson disease, cystic fibrosis, hemochromatosis, and glycogen storage disease) should be considered.

Complications

Of all infants with PiZZ α_1-antitrypsin deficiency, only 15–20% develop liver disease in childhood, and many have clinical recovery. The complications of portal hypertension, cirrhosis, and chronic cholestasis predominate in affected children. Occasionally, children develop paucity of interlobular bile ducts.

Early-onset pulmonary emphysema occurs in young adults (age 30–40 years), particularly in smokers. An increased susceptibility to hepatocellular carcinoma has been noted in cirrhosis associated with α_1-antitrypsin deficiency.

Treatment

There is no specific treatment for the liver disease of this disorder. Replacement of the protein by transfusion therapy is used to prevent or treat pulmonary disease in affected adults. The neonatal cholestatic condition is treated with choleretics, medium-chain triglyceride-containing formula, and water-soluble preparations of fat-soluble vitamins (see Table 21–4). UCDA may reduce AST, ALT, and GGT, but its effect on outcome is unknown. Portal hypertension, esophageal bleeding, ascites, and other complications are treated as described elsewhere. Hepatitis A and B vaccines should be given to children with α_1-antitrypsin deficiency. Genetic counseling is indicated when the diagnosis is made. Diagnosis by prenatal screening is possible. Liver transplantation, performed for development of end-stage liver disease, cures the deficiency. Passive and active cigarette smoke exposure should be eliminated to help prevent pulmonary manifestations, and obesity should be avoided.

Prognosis

Of those patients presenting with neonatal cholestasis, approximately 10–25% will need liver transplantation in the first 5 years of life, 15–25% during childhood or adolescence, and 50–75% will survive into adulthood with variable degrees of liver fibrosis. A correlation between histologic patterns and clinical course has been documented in the infantile form of the disease. Liver failure

can be expected 5–15 years after development of cirrhosis. Recurrence or persistence of hyperbilirubinemia along with worsening coagulation studies indicates the need for evaluation for possible liver transplantation. Decompensated cirrhosis caused by this disease is an excellent indication for liver transplantation; the survival rate should reach 80–90%. Pulmonary involvement is prevented by liver transplantation.

Rudnick DA, Perlmutter DH: Alpha-1-antitrypsin deficiency: A new paradigm for hepatocellular carcinoma in genetic liver disease. Hepatology 2005;42:514 [PMID: 16044402].
Stoller JK, Aboussouan LS: Alpha 1-antitrypsin deficiency. Lancet 2005;365:2225-36 [PMID: 15978931].
Sveger T, Eriksson S: The liver in adolescents with α_1-antitrypsin deficiency. Hepatology 1995;22:514 [PMID: 7635419].
Teckman JH: Alpha 1-antitrypsin deficiency in childhood. Semin Liv Dis 2007;27:274 [PMID: 17682974].

WILSON DISEASE (HEPATOLENTICULAR DEGENERATION)

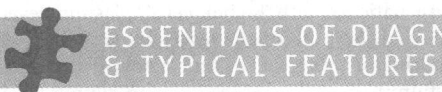

ESSENTIALS OF DIAGNOSIS & TYPICAL FEATURES

▶ Acute or chronic liver disease.

▶ Deteriorating neurologic status.

▶ Kayser-Fleischer rings.

▶ Elevated liver copper.

▶ Abnormalities in levels of ceruloplasmin and serum and urine copper.

General Considerations

Wilson disease is caused by mutations in the gene *ATP7B* on chromosome 13 coding for a specific P-type adenosine triphosphatase involved in copper transport. This results in impaired bile excretion of copper and incorporation of copper into ceruloplasmin by the liver. The accumulated hepatic copper causes oxidant (free-radical) damage to the liver. Subsequently, copper accumulates in the basal ganglia and other tissues. The disease should be considered in all children older than age 3 years with evidence of liver disease (especially with hemolysis) or with suggestive neurologic signs. A family history is often present, and 25% of patients are identified by screening asymptomatic homozygous family members. The disease is autosomal recessive and occurs in 1:30,000 live births in all populations.

Clinical Findings

A. Symptoms and Signs

Hepatic involvement may be fulminant; may present as an acute hepatitis; may masquerade as chronic liver disease; or may progress insidiously to postnecrotic cirrhosis. Findings include jaundice; hepatomegaly early in childhood; splenomegaly; Kayser-Fleischer rings; and later onset of neurologic manifestations, such as tremor, dysarthria, and drooling beginning after age 10 years. Deterioration in school performance is often the earliest neurologic expression of disease. Psychiatric symptoms may also occur. The Kayser-Fleischer rings can sometimes be detected by unaided visual inspection as a brown band at the junction of the iris and cornea, but slit-lamp examination is always necessary. Absence of Kayser-Fleischer rings does not exclude this diagnosis.

B. Laboratory Findings

The laboratory diagnosis is sometimes difficult. Serum ceruloplasmin levels (measured by the oxidase method) are usually less than 20 mg/dL. (Normal values are 23–43 mg/dL.) Low values, however, occur normally in infants younger than 3 months, and in at least 10% of homozygotes the levels may be within the lower end of the normal range (20–30 mg/dL), particularly if immunoassays are used to measure ceruloplasmin. Rare patients with higher ceruloplasmin levels have been reported. Serum copper levels are low, but the overlap with normal is too great for satisfactory discrimination. In acute fulminant Wilson disease serum copper levels are elevated markedly, owing to hepatic necrosis and release of copper. The presence of anemia, hemolysis, very high serum bilirubin levels (> 20–30 mg/dL), low alkaline phosphatase, and low uric acid are characteristic of acute Wilson disease. Urine copper excretion in children older than 3 years is normally less than 30 mcg/d; in Wilson disease, it is generally greater than 150 mcg/d. Finally, the tissue content of copper from a liver biopsy, normally less than 50 mcg/g dry tissue, is greater than 250 mcg/g in Wilson disease.

Glycosuria and aminoaciduria have been reported. Hemolysis and gallstones may be present; bone lesions simulating those of osteochondritis dissecans have also been found.

The coarse nodular cirrhosis, steatosis, and glycogenated nuclei seen on liver biopsy may distinguish Wilson disease from other types of cirrhosis. Early in the disease, vacuolation of liver cells, steatosis, and lipofuscin granules can be seen, as well as Mallory bodies. The presence of Mallory bodies in a child is strongly suggestive of Wilson disease. Stains for copper may sometimes be negative despite high copper content in the liver. Therefore, liver copper levels must be determined biochemically on biopsy specimens. Electron microscopy findings of abnormal mitochondria may be helpful.

▶ Differential Diagnosis

During the icteric phase, acute viral hepatitis, α_1-antitrypsin deficiency, autoimmune hepatitis, Indian childhood cirrhosis, and drug-induced hepatitis are the usual diagnostic possibilities. Nonalcoholic steatohepatitis may have similar histology and be confused with Wilson disease in overweight patients. Later, other causes of cirrhosis and portal hypertension require consideration. Laboratory testing for serum ceruloplasmin, 24-hour urine copper excretion, liver copper concentration, and a slit-lamp examination of the cornea will differentiate Wilson disease from the others. Urinary copper excretion during penicillamine challenge (500 mg twice a day in the older child or adult) may help differentiate Wilson disease from other causes. Genetic testing may be necessary in confusing cases. Other copper storage diseases that occur in early childhood include Indian childhood cirrhosis, Tyrolean childhood cirrhosis, and idiopathic copper toxicosis. However, ceruloplasmin concentrations are normal in these conditions.

▶ Complications

Progressive liver disease, postnecrotic cirrhosis, hepatic coma, progressive neurologic degeneration, and death are the rule in the untreated patient. The complications of portal hypertension (variceal hemorrhage, ascites) are poorly tolerated by these patients. Progressive degenerating central nervous system disease and terminal aspiration pneumonia are common in untreated older people. Acute hemolytic disease may result in acute renal failure and profound jaundice as part of the presentation of fulminant hepatitis.

▶ Treatment

Copper chelation with D-penicillamine or trientine hydrochloride, 1000–2000 mg/d orally, is the treatment of choice, whether or not the patient is symptomatic. The target dose for children is 20 mg/kg/d; begin with 250 mg/d and increase the dose weekly by 250 mg increments. Strict dietary restriction of copper intake is not practical. Supplementation with zinc acetate (25–50 mg orally, three times daily) may reduce copper absorption. Copper chelation is continued for life, although doses may be reduced transiently at the time of surgery or early in pregnancy. Vitamin B_6 (25 mg) is given daily during therapy with penicillamine to prevent optic neuritis. In some countries, after a clinical response to penicillamine or trientine, zinc therapy is substituted and continued for life. Tetrathiomolybdate is being tested as an alternative therapy. Noncompliance with the drug regimen can lead to sudden fulminant liver failure and death.

Liver transplantation is indicated for all cases of acute fulminant disease with hemolysis and renal failure, progressive hepatic decompensation despite several months of penicillamine, and severe progressive hepatic insufficiency in patients who unadvisedly discontinue penicillamine, triene, or zinc therapy.

▶ Prognosis

The prognosis of untreated Wilson disease is poor. Without liver transplantation, all patients with the fulminant presentation succumb. Copper chelation reduces hepatic copper content, reverses many of the liver lesions, and can stabilize the clinical course of established cirrhosis. Neurologic symptoms generally respond to therapy. All siblings should be immediately screened and homozygotes given treatment with copper chelation or zinc acetate therapy, even if asymptomatic. Genetic testing (haplotype analysis or genotyping) is available clinically if there is any doubt about the diagnosis and for family members.

Arnon R et al: Wilson disease in children: Serum aminotransferases and urinary copper on triethylene tetramine dihydrochloride (trientine) treatment. J Pediatr Gastroenterol Nutr 2007;44:596 [PMID: 17460493].

Dhawan A et al: Wilson's disease in children: 37-year experience and revised King's score for liver transplantation. Liver Transpl 2005;11:441 [PMID: 15776453].

Marcellini M et al: Treatment of Wilson's disease with zinc from the time of diagnosis in pediatric patients: A single-hospital, 10-year follow-up study. J Lab Clin Med 2005;145:139 [PMID: 15871305].

Roberts EA, Schilsky ML: A practice guideline on Wilson disease. Hepatology 2003;37:1475 [PMID: 12774027].

Wang XH et al: Living-related liver transplantation for Wilson's disease. Transpl Int 2005;18:651 [PMID: 15910288].

CIRRHOSIS

ESSENTIALS OF DIAGNOSIS & TYPICAL FEATURES

▶ Underlying liver disease.

▶ Nodular hard liver.

▶ Nodular liver on abdominal imaging.

▶ Liver biopsy demonstrating cirrhosis.

General Considerations

Cirrhosis is a histologically defined condition of the liver characterized by diffuse hepatocyte injury and regeneration, an increase in connective tissue (bridging fibrosis), and disorganization of the lobular and vascular architecture (regenerative nodules). It may be micronodular or macronodular in appearance. It is the vasculature distortion that leads to increased resistance to blood flow, producing portal hypertension and its consequences.

Many liver diseases may progress to cirrhosis. In children, the two most common forms of cirrhosis are postnecrotic and biliary, with different causes, symptomatology, and treatment requirements. Both forms can eventually lead to liver failure and death.

In the pediatric population, postnecrotic cirrhosis is often a result of acute or chronic liver disease (eg, idiopathic neonatal giant-cell hepatitis, viral hepatitis [HBV, HCV], autoimmune or drug-induced hepatitis); more recently, NAFLD; or certain inborn errors of metabolism (see Table 21–5). Cirrhosis is an exceptional outcome of HAV infection and only follows massive hepatic necrosis. The evolution to

cirrhosis may be insidious, with no recognized icteric phase, as in some cases of HBV or HCV infection, Wilson disease, hemochromatosis, or α_1-antitrypsin deficiency. At the time of diagnosis of cirrhosis, the underlying liver disease may be active, with abnormal LFTs; or it may be quiescent, with normal LFTs. Most cases of biliary cirrhosis result from congenital abnormalities of the bile ducts (biliary atresia, choledochal cyst), tumors of the bile duct, Caroli disease, PFIC, primary sclerosing cholangitis, paucity of the intrahepatic bile ducts, and cystic fibrosis.

Occasionally, cirrhosis may follow a hypersensitivity reaction to certain drugs such as phenytoin. Parasites (*Opisthorchis sinensis, Fasciola,* and *Ascaris*) may be causative in children living in endemic areas.

▶ Clinical Findings

A. Symptoms and Signs

Malaise, loss of appetite, failure to thrive, and nausea are frequent complaints, especially in anicteric varieties. Easy bruising may be reported. Jaundice may or may not be present. The first indication of underlying liver disease may be ascites, gastrointestinal hemorrhage, or hepatic encephalopathy. Variable hepatosplenomegaly, spider angiomas, warm skin, palmar erythema, or digital clubbing may be present. A small, shrunken liver may present. Most often, the liver is enlarged slightly, especially in the subxiphoid region, where it has a firm to hard quality and an irregular edge. Ascites may be detected as shifting dullness or a fluid wave. Gynecomastia may be noted in males. Digital clubbing occurs in 10–15% of cases. Pretibial edema often occurs, reflecting underlying hypoproteinemia. In adolescent girls, irregularities of menstruation and amenorrhea may be early complaints.

In biliary cirrhosis, patients often have jaundice, dark urine, pruritus, hepatomegaly, and sometimes xanthomas in addition to the previously mentioned clinical findings. Malnutrition and failure to thrive due to steatorrhea may be more apparent in this form of cirrhosis.

B. Laboratory Findings

Mild abnormalities of aminotransferases (AST, ALT) are often present, with a decreased level of albumin and a variable increase in the level of γ-globulins. Prothrombin time is prolonged and may be unresponsive to vitamin K administration. Burr and target red cells may be noted on the peripheral blood smear. Anemia, thrombocytopenia, and leukopenia are present if hypersplenism exists. However, cirrhosis may be present despite normal blood tests.

In biliary cirrhosis, elevated conjugated bilirubin, bile acids, GGT, alkaline phosphatase, and cholesterol are common.

C. Imaging

Hepatic ultrasound or CT examination may demonstrate abnormal hepatic texture and nodules. In biliary cirrhosis, abnormalities of the biliary tree may be apparent by ultrasonography, CT, hepatobiliary scintigraphy, or cholangiography.

D. Pathologic Findings

Liver biopsy findings of regenerating nodules and surrounding fibrosis are hallmarks of cirrhosis. Pathologic features of biliary cirrhosis also include canalicular and hepatocyte cholestasis, as well as plugging of bile ducts. The interlobular bile ducts may be increased or decreased, depending on the cause and the stage of the disease process.

▶ Complications & Treatment

Major complications of cirrhosis in childhood include progressive nutritional disturbances, hormonal disturbances, and the evolution of portal hypertension and its complications. Hepatocellular carcinoma occurs with increased frequency in the cirrhotic liver, especially in patients with the chronic form of hereditary tyrosinemia or after long-standing HBV or HCV disease. At present, there is no proven medical treatment for cirrhosis, but whenever a treatable condition is identified (eg, Wilson disease, galactosemia, congenital fructose intolerance, autoimmune hepatitis) or an offending agent eliminated (HBV, HCV, drugs, toxins), disease progression can be altered; occasionally regression of fibrosis has been noted. Children with cirrhosis should receive the hepatitis A and B vaccines, and they should be monitored for the development of hepatocellular carcinoma with serial serum α-fetoprotein determinations and abdominal ultrasound for hepatic nodules. Liver transplantation may be appropriate in patients with cirrhosis whose disease is continuing to progress, with evidence of worsening hepatic synthetic function, or in whom the complications of cirrhosis are no longer manageable.

▶ Prognosis

Postnecrotic cirrhosis has an unpredictable course. Without transplantation, affected patients may die from liver failure within 10–15 years. Patients with a rising bilirubin, a vitamin K–resistant coagulopathy, or diuretic refractory ascites usually survive less than 1–2 years. The terminal event in some patients may be generalized hemorrhage, sepsis, or cardiorespiratory arrest. For patients with biliary cirrhosis, the prognosis is similar, except for those with surgically corrected lesions that result in regression or stabilization of the underlying liver condition. With liver transplantation, the long-term survival rate is 70–90%.

Hardy SC, Kleinman RE: Cirrhosis and chronic liver failure. In Suchy FJ, Sokol RJ, Balistreri WF (editors): *Liver Disease in Children,* 3rd ed. Cambridge University Press, 2007:97–137.

Okuda H: Hepatocellular carcinoma development in cirrhosis. Best Pract Res Clin Gastroenterol 2007;21:161 [PMID: 17223503].

PORTAL HYPERTENSION

ESSENTIALS OF DIAGNOSIS & TYPICAL FEATURES

▶ Splenomegaly.
▶ Recurrent ascites.
▶ Variceal hemorrhage.
▶ Hypersplenism.

▶ General Considerations

Portal hypertension is defined as an increase in the portal venous pressure to more than 5 mm Hg greater than the inferior vena caval pressure. Portal hypertension is most commonly a result of cirrhosis. Portal hypertension without cirrhosis may be divided into prehepatic, suprahepatic, and intrahepatic causes. Although the specific lesions vary somewhat in their clinical signs and symptoms, the consequences of portal hypertension are common to all.

A. Prehepatic Portal Hypertension

Prehepatic portal hypertension from acquired abnormalities of the portal and splenic veins accounts for 30–50% of cases of variceal hemorrhage in children. A history of neonatal omphalitis, sepsis, dehydration, or umbilical vein catheterization may be present. Causes in older children include local trauma, peritonitis (pyelophlebitis), hypercoagulable states, and pancreatitis. Symptoms may occur before age 1 year, but in most cases the diagnosis is not made until age 3–5 years. Patients with a positive neonatal history tend to be symptomatic earlier.

A variety of portal or splenic vein malformations, some of which may be congenital, have been described, including defects in valves and atretic segments. Cavernous transformation is probably the result of attempted collateralization around the thrombosed portal vein rather than a congenital malformation. The site of the venous obstruction may be anywhere from the hilum of the liver to the hilum of the spleen.

B. Suprahepatic Vein Occlusion or Thrombosis (Budd-Chiari Syndrome)

No cause can be demonstrated in most instances. One suggested cause is endothelial injury to hepatic veins by bacterial endotoxin, which has been demonstrated experimentally. The occasional association of hepatic vein thrombosis in inflammatory bowel disease favors the presence of endogenous toxins traversing the liver. Vasculitis leading to endophlebitis of the hepatic veins has been described. In addition, hepatic vein obstruction may be secondary to tumor, abdominal trauma, hyperthermia, or sepsis, or it may occur following the repair of an omphalocele or gastroschisis. Congenital vena caval bands, webs, a membrane, or stricture above the hepatic veins are sometimes causative. Hepatic vein thrombosis may be a complication of oral contraceptive medications. Underlying thrombotic conditions (deficiency of antithrombin III, protein C or S, or factor V Leiden; antiphospholipid antibodies; or mutations of the prothrombin gene) should be evaluated.

C. Intrahepatic Portal Hypertension

1. Cirrhosis—See previous section.

2. Veno-occlusive disease (acute stage)—This entity now occurs most frequently in bone marrow transplant recipients. It may also develop after chemotherapy for acute leukemia, particularly with thioguanine. Additional causes include the ingestion of pyrrolizidine alkaloids ("bush tea") or other herbal teas, and a familial form of the disease occurring in congenital immunodeficiency states. The acute form of the disease generally occurs in the first month after bone marrow transplantation and is heralded by the triad of weight gain (ascites), tender hepatomegaly, and jaundice.

3. Congenital hepatic fibrosis—This is a rare autosomal recessive cause of intrahepatic presinusoidal portal hypertension (see Table 21–8). Liver biopsy is generally diagnostic, demonstrating Meyenburg complexes. On angiography, the intrahepatic branches of the portal vein may be duplicated. Autosomal recessive polycystic kidney disease is often associated with the hepatic lesion; therefore, renal ultrasonography and urography should be routinely performed.

4. Other rare causes—Hepatoportal sclerosis (idiopathic portal hypertension, noncirrhotic portal fibrosis), noncirrhotic nodular transformation of the liver, and schistosomal hepatic fibrosis are also rare causes of intrahepatic presinusoidal portal hypertension.

▶ Clinical Findings

A. Symptoms and Signs

For prehepatic portal hypertension, splenomegaly in an otherwise well child is the most constant physical sign. Recurrent episodes of abdominal distention resulting from ascites may be noted. The usual presenting symptoms are hematemesis and melena.

The presence of prehepatic portal hypertension is suggested by the following: (1) an episode of severe infection in the newborn period or early infancy—especially omphalitis, sepsis, gastroenteritis, severe dehydration, or prolonged or difficult umbilical vein catheterizations; (2) no previous evidence of liver disease; (3) a history of well-being prior to onset or recognition of symptoms; and (4) normal liver size and tests with splenomegaly.

Most patients with suprahepatic portal hypertension present with abdominal pain, tender hepatomegaly of acute onset, and abdominal enlargement caused by ascites. Jaundice is present in only 25% of patients. Vomiting, hematemesis, and diarrhea are less common. Cutaneous signs of chronic liver disease are often absent, as the obstruction is usually acute. Distended superficial veins on the back and the anterior abdomen, along with dependent edema, are seen when inferior vena cava obstruction affects hepatic vein outflow. Absence of hepatojugular reflux (jugular distention when pressure is applied to the liver) is a helpful clinical sign.

The symptoms and signs of intrahepatic portal hypertension are generally those of cirrhosis (see earlier section on Cirrhosis).

B. Laboratory Findings and Imaging

Most other common causes of splenomegaly or hepatosplenomegaly may be excluded by appropriate laboratory tests. Cultures, EBV titers, hepatitis serologies, blood smear examination, bone marrow studies, and LFTs may be necessary. In prehepatic portal hypertension, LFTs are generally normal. In Budd-Chiari syndrome and veno-occlusive disease, mild to moderate hyperbilirubinemia with modest elevations of aminotransferases and prothrombin time are often present. Significant early increases in fibrinolytic parameters (especially plasminogen activator inhibitor 1) have been reported in veno-occlusive disease. Hypersplenism with mild leucopenia and thrombocytopenia is often present. Upper endoscopy may reveal varices in symptomatic patients.

Doppler-assisted ultrasound scanning of the liver, portal vein, splenic vein, inferior vena cava, and hepatic veins may assist in defining the vascular anatomy. In prehepatic portal hypertension, abnormalities of the portal or splenic vein may be apparent, whereas the hepatic veins are normal. When noncirrhotic portal hypertension is suspected, angiography often is diagnostic. Selective arteriography of the superior mesenteric artery or MRI is recommended prior to surgical shunting to determine the patency of the superior mesenteric vein.

For suprahepatic portal hypertension, an inferior venacavogram using catheters from above or below the suspected obstruction may reveal an intrinsic filling defect, an infiltrating tumor, or extrinsic compression of the inferior vena cava by an adjacent lesion. A large caudate lobe of the liver suggests Budd-Chiari syndrome. Care must be taken in interpreting extrinsic pressure defects of the subdiaphragmatic inferior vena cava if ascites is significant.

Simultaneous wedged hepatic vein pressure and hepatic venography are useful to demonstrate obstruction to major hepatic vein ostia and smaller vessels. In the absence of obstruction, reflux across the sinusoids into the portal vein branches can be accomplished. Pressures should also be taken from the right heart and supradiaphragmatic portion of the inferior vena cava to eliminate constrictive pericarditis and pulmonary hypertension from the differential diagnosis.

Differential Diagnosis

All causes of splenomegaly must be included in the differential diagnosis. The most common ones are infections, immune thrombocytopenic purpura, blood dyscrasias, lipidosis, reticuloendotheliosis, cirrhosis of the liver, and cysts or hemangiomas of the spleen. When hematemesis or melena occurs, other causes of gastrointestinal bleeding are possible, such as gastric or duodenal ulcers, tumors, duplications, and inflammatory bowel disease.

Because ascites is almost always present in suprahepatic portal hypertension, cirrhosis resulting from any cause must be excluded. Other suprahepatic (cardiac, pulmonary) causes of portal hypertension must also be ruled out. Although ascites may occur in prehepatic portal hypertension, it is uncommon.

Complications

The major manifestation and complication of portal hypertension is bleeding from esophageal varices. Fatal exsanguination is uncommon, but hypovolemic shock or resulting anemia may require prompt treatment. Hypersplenism with leukopenia and thrombocytopenia occurs, but seldom causes major symptoms. Rupture of the enlarged spleen secondary to trauma is always a threat. Retroperitoneal edema has been reported (Clatworthy sign).

Without treatment, complete and persistent hepatic vein obstruction leads to liver failure, coma, and death. A nonportal type of cirrhosis may develop in the chronic form of hepatic veno-occlusive disease in which small- and medium-sized hepatic veins are affected. Death from renal failure may occur in rare cases of congenital hepatic fibrosis.

Treatment

Definitive treatment of noncirrhotic portal hypertension is generally lacking. Aggressive medical treatment of the complications of prehepatic portal hypertension is generally quite effective. The early experience with surgical portosystemic shunts was unfavorable. Recently, several centers have reported excellent results with either portosystemic shunt or the mesorex (mesenterico–left portal bypass) shunt. When possible, the mesorex shunt is the preferred technique. Veno-occlusive disease may be prevented somewhat by the prophylactic use of UCDA or defibrotide prior to conditioning for bone marrow transplantation. Treatment with defibrotide and withdrawal of the suspected offending agent, if possible, may increase the chance of recovery. Transjugular intrahepatic portosystemic shunts have been successful bridging to recovery in veno-occlusive disease. For suprahepatic portal hypertension, efforts should be directed at correcting the underlying cause, if possible. Either surgical or angiographic relief of obstruction should be attempted if a defined obstruction of the vessels is apparent. Liver transplantation, if not contraindicated, should be considered early if direct correction is not possible. In most cases, management of portal hypertension is directed at management of the complications (Table 21–7).

Prognosis

For prehepatic portal hypertension, the prognosis depends on the site of the block, the effectiveness of variceal eradication, the availability of suitable vessels for shunting procedures, and the experience of the surgeon. In patients treated by medical means, bleeding episodes seem to diminish with adolescence.

Table 21–7. Treatment of complications of portal hypertension.

Complication	Diagnosis	Treatment
Bleeding esophageal varices	Endoscopic verification of variceal bleeding.	Endosclerosis or variceal band ligation. Octreotide, 30 mcg/m^2/h intravenous. Pediatric Sengstaken-Blakemore tube. Surgical variceal ligation, selective venous embolization, surgical portosystemic shunt, TIPS, OLT. Propranolol may be useful to prevent recurrent bleeding.
Ascites	Clinical examination (fluid wave, shifting dullness), abdominal ultrasonography.	Sodium restriction (1-2 mEq/kg/d), spironolactone (3–5 mg/kg/d), furosemide (1-2 mg/kg/d), intravenous albumin (0.5–1 g/kg per dose), paracentesis, peritoneovenous (LeVeen) shunt, TIPS, surgical portosystemic shunt, OLT.[a]
Hepatic encephalopathy	Abnormal neurologic examination, elevated plasma ammonia.	Protein restriction (0.5–1 g/kg/d), intravenous glucose (6–8 mg/kg/min), neomycin (2–4 g/m^2 BSA PO in 4 doses), rifaximin (200 mg 3 times a day in children > 12 y), lactulose (1 mL/kg per dose [up to 30 mL] every 4-6 h PO), plasmapheresis, hemodialysis, OLT.[a]
Hypersplenism	Low WBC count, platelets, and/or hemoglobin. Splenomegaly.	No intervention, partial splenic embolization, TIPS, surgical portosystemic shunt, OLT. Splenectomy may worsen variceal bleeding.

[a]In order of sequential management.

BSA, body surface area; OLT, orthotopic liver transplantation; TIPS, transjugular intrahepatic portosystemic shunt; WBC, white blood cell.

The prognosis in patients treated by medical and supportive therapy may be better than in the surgically treated group, especially when surgery is performed at an early age, although no comparative study has been done. Portacaval encephalopathy is unusual after shunting except when protein intake is excessive, but neurologic outcome may be better in patients who receive a mesorex shunt when compared with medical management alone.

The mortality rate of hepatic vein obstruction is very high (95%). In veno-occlusive disease, the prognosis is better, with complete recovery possible in 50% of acute forms and 5–10% of subacute forms.

Botha JF et al: Portosystemic shunts in children: A 15-year experience. J Am Coll Surg 2004;199:179 [PMID: 15275870].

Chalandon Y et al: Prevention of veno-occlusive disease with defibrotide after allogeneic stem cell transplantation. Biol Blood Marrow Transplant 2004;10:347 [PMID: 15111934].

Fuchs J et al: Mesenterico-left portal vein bypass in children with congenital extrahepatic portal vein thrombosis: A unique curative approach. J Pediatr Gastroenterol Nutr 2003;36:213 [PMID: 12548056].

McKiernan PJ: Treatment of variceal bleeding. Gastrointest Endosc Clin North Am 2001;11:789 [PMID: 11689366].

Menon P et al: Extrahepatic portal hypertension: Quality of life and somatic growth after surgery. Eur J Pediatr Surg 2005;15:82 [PMID: 15877255].

Price MR et al: Management of esophageal varices in children by endoscopic variceal ligation. J Pediatr Surg 1996;31:1056 [PMID: 8863233].

Sarin SK, Kumar A: Noncirrhotic portal hypertension. Clin Liver Dis 2006;10:627 [PMID: 17162232].

Sartori MT et al: Role of fibrinolytic and clotting parameters in the diagnosis of liver veno-occlusive disease after hematopoietic stem cell transplantation in a pediatric population. Thromb Haemost 2005;93:682 [PMID: 15142875].

Vora A et al: Toxicity and efficacy of 6-thioguanine versus 6-mercaptopurine in childhood lymphoblastic leukaemia: A randomised trial. Lancet 2006;368:1339 [PMID: 17046466].

Zimmerman MA et al: Budd-Chiari syndrome. Clin Liver Dis 2006;10:259 [PMID: 16971261].

BILIARY TRACT DISEASE

1. Cholelithiasis

ESSENTIALS OF DIAGNOSIS & TYPICAL FEATURES

▶ Episodic right upper quadrant abdominal pain.

▶ Elevated bilirubin, alkaline phosphatase, and GGT.

▶ Stones or sludge seen on abdominal ultrasound.

▶ General Considerations

Gallstones may develop at all ages in the pediatric population and in utero. Gallstones may be divided into cholesterol stones (which contain more than 50% cholesterol) and pig-

ment (black [sterile bile] and brown [infected bile]) stones. Pigment stones predominate in the first decade of life, while cholesterol stones account for up to 90% of gallstones in adolescence. For some patients, gallbladder dysfunction is associated with biliary sludge formation, which may evolve into "sludge balls" or tumefaction bile and then into gallstones. The process is reversible in many patients.

▶ Clinical Findings

A. History

Most symptomatic gallstones are associated with acute or recurrent episodes of moderate to severe, sharp right upper quadrant or epigastric pain. The pain may radiate substernally or to the right shoulder. On rare occasions, the presentation may include a history of jaundice, back pain, or generalized abdominal discomfort, when it is associated with pancreatitis, suggesting stone impaction in the common duct or ampulla hepatopancreatica. Nausea and vomiting may occur during attacks. Pain episodes often occur postprandially, especially after ingestion of fatty foods. The groups at risk for gallstones include patients with known or suspected hemolytic disease; females; teenagers with prior pregnancy; obese individuals; individuals with rapid weight loss; children with portal vein thrombosis; certain racial or ethnic groups, particularly Native Americans (Pima Indians) and Hispanics; infants and children with ileal disease (Crohn disease) or prior ileal resection; patients with cystic fibrosis or Wilson disease; and infants on prolonged parenteral hyperalimentation. Other, less certain risk factors include a positive family history, use of birth control pills, and diabetes mellitus.

B. Symptoms and Signs

During acute episodes of pain, tenderness is present in the right upper quadrant or epigastrium, with a positive inspiratory arrest (Murphy sign), usually without peritoneal signs. While rarely present, scleral icterus is helpful. Evidence of underlying hemolytic disease in addition to icterus may include pallor (anemia), splenomegaly, tachycardia, and high-output cardiac murmur. Fever is unusual in uncomplicated cases.

C. Laboratory Findings

Laboratory tests are usually normal unless calculi have lodged in the extrahepatic biliary system, in which case the serum bilirubin and GGT (or alkaline phosphatase) may be elevated. Amylase and lipase levels may be increased if stone obstruction occurs at the ampulla hepatopancreatica.

D. Imaging

Ultrasound evaluation is the best imaging technique, showing abnormal intraluminal contents (stones, sludge) as well as anatomic alterations of the gallbladder or dilation of the biliary ductal system. The presence of an anechoic acoustic shadow differentiates calculi from intraluminal sludge or sludge balls.

Ceftriaxone may cause similar findings. Plain abdominal radiographs will show calculi with a high calcium content in the region of the gallbladder in up to 15% of patients. Lack of visualization of the gallbladder with hepatobiliary scintigraphy suggests chronic cholecystitis. In selected cases, ERCP, MRCP, or endoscopic ultrasound may be helpful in defining subtle abnormalities of the bile ducts and locating intraductal stones.

Differential Diagnosis

Other abnormal conditions of the biliary system with similar presentation are summarized in Table 21–8. Liver disease (hepatitis, abscess, or tumor) can cause similar symptoms or signs. Peptic disease, reflux esophagitis, paraesophageal hiatal hernia, cardiac disease, and pneumomediastinum must be considered when the pain is epigastric or substernal in location. Renal or pancreatic disease is a possible explanation if the pain is localized to the right flank or mid back. Subcapsular or supracapsular lesions of the liver (abscess, tumor, or hematoma) or right lower lobe infiltrate may also be a cause of nontraumatic right shoulder pain.

Complications

Major problems are related to stone impaction in either the cystic or common duct and may lead to stricture formation or perforation. Acute distention and subsequent perforation of the gallbladder may occur when gallstones cause obstruction of the cystic duct. Stones impacted at the level of the ampulla hepatopancreatica often cause gallstone pancreatitis.

Treatment

Symptomatic cholelithiasis is treated by laparoscopic cholecystectomy or open cholecystectomy in selected cases. Intraoperative cholangiography via the cystic duct is recommended so that the physician can be certain the biliary system is free of retained stones. Calculi in the extrahepatic bile ducts may be removed at ERCP.

Gallstones developing in premature infants on parenteral nutrition can be followed by ultrasound examination. Most of the infants are asymptomatic, and the stones will resolve in 3–36 months. Gallstone dissolution using cholelitholytics (UCDA) or mechanical means (lithotripsy) has not been approved for use in children. Asymptomatic gallstones do not usually require treatment, as less than 20% will eventually cause problems.

Prognosis

The prognosis is excellent in uncomplicated cases that come to standard cholecystectomy.

Bruch SW et al: The management of nonpigmented gallstones in children. J Pediatr Surg 2000;35:729 [PMID: 10813336].

Jaffray B: Minimally invasive surgery. Arch Dis Child 2005;90:537 [PMID: 15851444].

Lobe, TE: Cholelithiasis and cholecystitis in children. Semin Pediatr Surg 2000;9:170 [PMID: 11112834].

Mah D et al: Management of suspected common bile duct stones in children: Role of selective intraoperative cholangiogram and endoscopic retrograde cholangiopancreatography. J Pediatr Surg 2004;39:808 [PMID: 15185201].

Sanders G, Kingsnorth AN: Gallstones. BMJ 2007;335:295 [PMID: 17690370].

2. Primary Sclerosing Cholangitis

ESSENTIALS OF DIAGNOSIS & TYPICAL FEATURES

▶ Pruritus and jaundice.

▶ Elevated GGT.

▶ Associated with inflammatory bowel disease.

▶ Abnormal ERCP or MRCP.

General Considerations

Primary sclerosing cholangitis (PSC) is a progressive liver disease of unknown cause, characterized by chronic inflammation and fibrosis of the intrahepatic or extrahepatic bile ducts (or both), with eventual obliteration of peripheral bile ducts, cholangiographic evidence of strictures, and dilation of all or parts of the biliary tree. PSC is more common in males with inflammatory bowel disease, particularly ulcerative colitis. It can also be seen with histiocytosis X, sicca syndromes, congenital and acquired immunodeficiency syndromes, and cystic fibrosis.

Clinical Findings

A. Symptoms and Signs

PSC often has an insidious onset. Clinical symptoms may include abdominal pain, fatigue, pruritus, and jaundice. Acholic stools and steatorrhea can occur. Physical findings include hepatomegaly, splenomegaly, and jaundice.

B. Laboratory Findings

The earliest finding may be asymptomatic elevation of the GGT. Subsequent laboratory abnormalities include elevated levels of alkaline phosphatase and bile acids. Later, cholestatic jaundice and elevated AST and ALT may occur. Patients with associated inflammatory bowel disease often test positive for perinuclear antineutrophil cytoplasmic antibodies. Other markers of autoimmune liver disease (ANA and anti–smooth muscle antibodies [ASMA]) are often found but are not specific for PSC. Sclerosing cholangitis due to cryptosporidia is common in immunodeficiency syndromes.

C. Imaging

Ultrasound may show dilated intrahepatic bile ducts behind strictures. MRCP is now the diagnostic study of choice, demonstrating irregularities of the biliary tree. ERCP may be more sensitive for the diagnosis of irregularities of the intrahepatic biliary tree.

Table 21–8. Biliary tract diseases of childhood.

	Acute Hydrops Transient Dilation of Gallbladder[a,b]	Choledochal Cyst[c] (see Figure 21-1)	Acalculous Cholecystitis[d]	Caroli Disease[e] (Idiopathic Intrahepatic Bile Duct Dilation)	Congenital Hepatic Fibrosis[f]	Biliary Dyskinesia[g]
Predisposing or associated conditions	Premature infants with prolonged fasting or systemic illness. Hepatitis. Abnormalities of cystic duct. Kawasaki disease. Bacterial sepsis, EBV.	Congenital lesion. Female sex. Asians. Rarely with Caroli disease or congenital hepatic fibrosis.	Systemic illness, sepsis (Streptococcus, Salmonella, Klebsiella, etc), HIV infection. Gallbladder stasis, obstruction of cystic duct (stones, nodes, tumor).	Congenital lesion. Also found in congenital hepatic fibrosis or with choledochal cyst. Female sex. Autosomal recessive polycystic kidney disease.	Familial (autosomal recessive) 25% with autosomal recessive polycystic kidney disease. Choledochal cyst. Caroli disease. Meckel-Gruber, Ivemark, or Jeune syndrome.	Adolescents.
Symptoms	Absent in premature infants. Vomiting, abdominal pain in older children.	Abdominal pain, vomiting, jaundice.	Acute severe abdominal pain, vomiting, fever.	Recurrent abdominal pain, vomiting. Fever, jaundice when cholangitis occurs.	Hematemesis, melena from bleeding esophageal varices.	Intermittent RUQ pain.
Signs	RUQ abdominal mass. Tenderness in some.	Icterus, acholic stools, dark urine in neonatal period. RUQ abdominal mass or tenderness in older children.	Tenderness in mid and right upper abdomen. Occasional palpable mass in RUQ.	Icterus, hepatomegaly.	Hepatosplenomegaly.	Usually normal exam.
Laboratory abnormalities	Most are normal. Increased WBC count in sepsis (may be decreased in premature infants). Abnormal LFTs in hepatitis.	Conjugated hyperbilirubinemia, elevated GGT, slightly increased AST. Elevated pancreatic serum amylase common.	Elevated WBC count, normal or slight abnormality of LFTs.	Abnormal LFTs. Increased WBC count with cholangitis. Urine abnormalities if associated with congenital hepatic fibrosis.	Low platelet and WBC count (hypersplenism), slight elevation of AST, GGT. Inability to concentrate urine.	Usually normal.
Diagnostic studies most useful	Gallbladder ultrasonography.	Gallbladder ultrasonography hepatobiliary scintigraphy, MRCP, or ERCP.	Scintigraphy to confirm nonfunction of gallbladder. Ultrasonography or abdominal CT scan to rule out other neighboring disease.	Transhepatic cholangiography, MRCP, ERCP, scintigraphy, ultrasonography, intravenous pyelography.	Liver biopsy. Ultrasonography of liver and kidneys. Upper endoscopy.	CCK stimulated scintigraphy demonstrating reduced ejection fraction.
Treatment	Treatment of associated condition. Needle or tube cystostomy rarely required. Cholecystectomy seldom indicated.	Surgical resection and choledocho-jejunostomy.	Broad-spectrum antibiotic coverage, then cholecystectomy.	Antibiotics and surgical or endoscopic drainage for cholangitis. Liver transplantation for some. Lobectomy for localized disease.	Treatment of portal hypertension. Liver and kidney transplantation for some.	Cholecystectomy in well selected cases.

(continued)

Table 21-8. Biliary tract diseases of childhood. (*Continued*)

	Acute Hydrops Transient Dilation of Gallbladder[a,b]	Choledochal Cyst[c] (see Figure 21-1)	Acalculous Cholecystitis[d]	Caroli Disease[e] (Idiopathic Intrahepatic Bile Duct Dilation)	Congenital Hepatic Fibrosis[f]	Biliary Dyskinesia[g]
Complications	Perforation with bile peritonitis rare.	Progressive biliary cirrhosis. Increased incidence of cholangiocarcinoma. Cholangitis in some.	Perforation and bile peritonitis, sepsis, abscess or fistula formation. Pancreatitis.	Sepsis with episodes of cholangitis, biliary cirrhosis, portal hypertension. Intraductal stones. Cholangiocarcinoma.	Bleeding from varices. Splenic rupture, severe thrombocytopenia. Progressive renal failure.	Continued pain after surgery.
Prognosis	Excellent with resolution of underlying condition. Consider cystic duct obstruction if disorder fails to resolve.	Depends on anatomic type of cyst, associated condition, and success of surgery. Liver transplantation required in some.	Good with early diagnosis and treatment.	Poor, with gradual deterioration of liver function. Multiple surgical procedures expected. Liver transplantation should improve long-term prognosis.	Good in absence of serious renal involvement and with control of portal hypertension. Slightly increased risk of cholangiocarcinoma.	Good short-term outcome in well-selected patients.

[a]Crankson S et al: Acute hydrops of the gallbladder in childhood. Eur J Pediatr 1992;151:318 [PMID: 9788647].

[b]Zulian F et al: Acute surgical abdomen as presenting manifestation of Kawasaki disease. J Pediatr 2003;142:731 [PMID: 12838207].

[c]deVries JS et al: Choledochal cysts: Age of presentation, symptoms and late complications related to Todani's classification. J Pediatr Surg 2002;37:1568 [PMID: 12407541].

[d]Imamoglu M et al: Acute acalculous cholecystitis in children: Diagnosis and treatment. J Pediatr Surg 2002;37:36 [PMID: 11781983].

[e]Yonem O, Bayraktar Y: Clinical characteristics of Caroli's syndrome. World J Gastroenterol 2007;13:1934 [PMID: 17461493].

[f]Perisic VN: Long term studies on congenital hepatic fibrosis in children. Acta Paediatr 1995;85:695 [PMID: 7670259].

[g]Telega G: Biliary dyskinesia in pediatrics. Curr Gastroenterol Rep 2006;8:172 [PMID: 16533482].

AST, aspartate aminotransferase; CCK, cholecystokinin; CT, computed tomography; ERCP, endoscopic retrograde cholangiopancreatography; GGT, glutamyl transpeptidase; LFT, liver function tests; MRCP, magnetic resonance cholangiopancreatography; RUQ, right upper quadrant; WBC, white blood count.

Differential Diagnosis

The differential diagnosis includes infectious hepatitis, secondary cholangitis, autoimmune hepatitis, metabolic liver disease, cystic fibrosis, choledochal cyst, or other anomalies of the biliary tree, including Caroli disease and congenital hepatic fibrosis (see Table 21–8).

Complications

Complications include secondary bacterial cholangitis, pancreatitis, biliary fibrosis, and cirrhosis. Progression to liver failure is common, and the risk of cholangiocarcinoma is higher in PSC.

Treatment

No completely effective treatment is available. Patients with early disease may benefit from high-dose UCDA (25–30 mg/kg/d). Patients with autoimmune markers may benefit from treatment with corticosteroids and azathioprine. Antibiotic treatment of cholangitis and dilation and stenting of dominant bile duct strictures can reduce symptoms.

Prognosis

The majority of patients will eventually require liver transplantation, and PSC is the fifth leading indication for liver transplantation in the United States. The median duration from the time of diagnosis to end-stage liver disease is 12–15 years.

Alvarez F: Autoimmune hepatitis and primary sclerosing cholangitis. Clin Liver Dis 2006;10:89 [PMID: 16376796].

Charatcharoenwitthava P, Lindor KD: Primary sclerosing cholangitis: Diagnosis and management. Curr Gastroenterol Rep 2006;8:75 [PMID: 16510038].

Mieli-Vergani G, Vergani D: Sclerosing cholangitis in the paediatric patient. Best Pract Res Clin Gastroenterol 2001;15:681 [PMID: 11492976].

3. Other Biliary Tract Disorders

For a schematic representation of the various types of choledochal cysts, see Figure 21–1. For summary information on acute hydrops, choledochal cyst, acalculous cholecystitis, Caroli disease, biliary dyskinesia, and congenital hepatic fibrosis, see Table 21–8.

PYOGENIC & AMEBIC LIVER ABSCESS

ESSENTIALS OF DIAGNOSIS & TYPICAL FEATURES

▶ Fever and painful enlarged liver.

▶ Ultrasound of liver demonstrating an abscess.

▶ Positive serum ameba antibody or positive bacterial culture of abscess fluid.

TYPE		FINDINGS
I	GB — CBD	Spherical dilation of the common duct
II		Congenital diverticulum of the common bile duct
III		Intraduodenal diverticulum of the common bile duct (choledochocele)
IVa		Multiple intrahepatic communicating cysts (Caroli disease)
IVb		Mixed extrahepatic and intrahepatic fusiform or cystic dilation (possibly variants of Caroli disease, congenital hepatic fibrosis)

▲ **Figure 21–1.** Classification of cystic dilation of the bile ducts. Types I, II, and III are extrahepatic choledochal cysts. Type IVa is solely intrahepatic, and type IVb is both intrahepatic and extrahepatic. GB, gallbladder; CBD, common bile duct.

General Considerations

Pyogenic liver abscesses are often caused by intestinal bacteria seeded via the portal vein from infected viscera and occasionally from ascending cholangitis or gangrenous cholecystitis. Blood cultures are positive in up to 60% of patients. The resulting lesion tends to be solitary and located in the right hepatic lobe. Bacterial seeding may also occur from infected burns, pyodermas, and osteomyelitis. Unusual causes include omphalitis, subacute infective endocarditis, pyelonephritis, Crohn disease, and perinephric abscess. In immunocompromised patients, *S aureus,* gram-negative organisms, and fungi may seed the liver from the arterial system. Multiple pyogenic liver abscesses are associated with severe sepsis. Children receiving anti-inflammatory and immunosuppressive agents and children with defects in white blood cell function (chronic granulomatous disease) are prone to pyogenic hepatic abscesses, especially those caused by *S aureus.*

Amoebic liver abscess is rare in children. An increased risk is associated with travel in areas of endemic infection (Mexico, Southeast Asia) within 5 months of presentation. *Entamoeba histolytica* invasion occurs via the large bowel, although a history of diarrhea (colitis-like picture) is not always obtained.

Clinical Findings

With pyogenic liver abscess, nonspecific complaints of fever, chills, malaise, and abdominal pain are frequent. Weight loss is very common, especially in delayed diagnosis. A few patients have shaking chills and jaundice. The dominant complaint is a constant dull pain over an enlarged liver that is tender to palpation. An elevated hemidiaphragm with reduced or absent respiratory excursion may be demonstrated on physical examination and confirmed by fluoroscopy. Laboratory studies show leukocytosis and, at times, anemia. LFTs may be normal or reveal mild elevation of transaminases and alkaline phosphatase. Fever and abdominal pain are the two most common symptoms of amebic liver abscess. Abdominal tenderness and hepatomegaly are present in over 50%. Early in the course, LFTs may suggest mild hepatitis. An occasional prodrome may include cough, dyspnea, and shoulder pain when rupture of the abscess into the right chest occurs. Consolidation of the right lower lobe is common (10–30% of patients).

Ultrasound liver scan is the most useful diagnostic aid in evaluating pyogenic and amebic abscesses, detecting lesions as small as 1–2 cm. MRI, CT, or nuclear scanning with gallium or technetium sulfur colloid may be useful in differentiating tumor or hydatid cyst.

The distinction between pyogenic and amebic abscesses is best made by indirect hemagglutination test for specific antibody (which is positive in more than 95% of patients with amebic liver disease) and the prompt clinical response of the latter to antiamebic therapy (metronidazole). Examination of material obtained by needle aspiration of the abscess using ultrasound guidance is often diagnostic.

▶ Differential Diagnosis

Hepatitis, hepatoma, hydatid cyst, gallbladder disease, or biliary tract infections can mimic liver abscess. Subphrenic abscesses, empyema, and pneumonia may give a similar picture. Inflammatory disease of the intestines or of the biliary system may be complicated by liver abscess.

▶ Complications

Spontaneous rupture of the abscess may occur with extension of infection into the subphrenic space, thorax, peritoneal cavity, and, occasionally, the pericardium. Bronchopleural fistula with large sputum production and hemoptysis can develop in severe cases. Simultaneously, the amebic liver abscess may be secondarily infected with bacteria (in 10–20% of patients). Metastatic hematogenous spread to the lungs and the brain has been reported.

▶ Treatment

Ultrasound- or CT-guided percutaneous needle aspiration for aerobic and anaerobic culture with simultaneous placement of a catheter for drainage, combined with appropriate antibiotic therapy, is the treatment of choice for solitary pyogenic liver abscess. Multiple liver abscesses may also be treated successfully by this method. Surgical intervention

may be indicated if rupture occurs outside the capsule of the liver or if enterohepatic fistulae are suspected.

Amebic abscesses in uncomplicated cases should be treated promptly with oral metronidazole, 35–50 mg/kg/d, in three divided doses for 10 days. Intravenous metronidazole can be used for patients unable to take oral medication. Failure to improve after 72 hours of drug therapy suggests superimposed bacterial infection or an incorrect diagnosis. At this point, needle aspiration or surgical drainage is indicated. Once oral feedings can be tolerated, a luminal amebicide such as iodoquinol should be initiated. Resolution of the abscess cavity occurs over 3–6 months.

▶ Prognosis

An unrecognized and untreated pyogenic liver abscess is universally fatal. With drainage and antibiotics, the cure rate is about 90%. Most amebic abscesses are cured with conservative medical management; the mortality rate is less than 3%. If extrahepatic complications occur (empyema, bronchopleural fistula, or pericardial complications), 10–15% of patients will succumb.

Kurland JE, Brann OS: Pyogenic and amebic liver abscesses. Curr Gastroenterol Rep 2004;6:273 [PMID: 15245694].

Rajak CL et al: Percutaneous drainage of liver abscesses: Needle aspiration versus catheter drainage. AJR Am J Roentgenol 1998;170:1035 [PMID: 9530055].

Sharma MP, Kumar A: Liver abscess in children. Indian J Pediatr 2006;73:813 [PMID: 17006041].

HEPATOMA

ESSENTIALS OF DIAGNOSIS & TYPICAL FEATURES

- ▶ Abdominal enlargement and pain, weight loss, anemia.
- ▶ Hepatomegaly with or without a definable mass.
- ▶ Mass lesion on imaging studies.
- ▶ Laparotomy and tissue biopsy.

▶ General Considerations

Primary epithelial neoplasms of the liver represent 0.2–5.8% of all malignant conditions in children. After Wilms tumor and neuroblastoma, hepatomas are the third most common intra-abdominal cancer. The incidence is higher in Southeast Asia, where childhood cirrhosis is more common. There are two basic morphologic types with certain clinical and prognostic differences. Hepatoblastoma predominates in male infants and children and accounts for 79% of liver cancer in children, with most cases appearing before age 5 years. There is an increased risk of hepatoblastoma in Beckwith-Wiedemann syndrome, hemihypertrophy, familial adenomatosis polyposis coli, and in premature or low-birth-weight infants. Most lesions are found in the right lobe of the liver. Pathologic differentiation from hepatocellular carcinoma, the other major malignant tumor of the liver, may be difficult. Hepatocellular carcinoma occurs more frequently after age 3 years, carries a worse prognosis than hepatoblastoma, and causes more abdominal discomfort.

Patients with chronic HBV or HCV infection, cirrhosis, glycogen storage disease type I, tyrosinemia, or α_1-antitrypsin deficiency have an increased risk for hepatocellular carcinoma. The late development of hepatocellular carcinoma in patients receiving androgens for treatment of Fanconi syndrome and aplastic anemia must also be kept in mind. The use of anabolic steroids by body-conscious adolescents poses a risk of hepatic neoplasia.

An interesting aspect of primary epithelial neoplasms of the liver has been the increased incidence of associated anomalies and endocrine abnormalities. Virilization has been reported as a consequence of gonadotropin activity of the tumor. Feminization with bilateral gynecomastia may occur in association with high estradiol levels in the blood, the latter a consequence of increased aromatization of circulating androgens by the liver. Leydig cell hyperplasia without spermatogenesis is found on testicular biopsy. Hemihypertrophy, congenital absence of the kidney, macroglossia, and Meckel diverticulum have been found in association with hepatocellular carcinoma.

Clinical Findings

A noticeable increase in abdominal girth with or without pain is the most constant feature of the history. A parent may note a bulge in the upper abdomen or report feeling a hard mass. Constitutional symptoms (eg, anorexia, fatigue, fever, and chills) may be present. Teenage boys may complain of gynecomastia.

A. Symptoms and Signs

Weight loss, pallor, and abdominal pain associated with a large abdomen are common. Physical examination reveals hepatomegaly with or without a definite tumor mass, usually to the right of the midline. In the absence of cirrhosis, signs of chronic liver disease are usually absent. However, evidence of virilization or feminization in prepubertal children may be noted.

B. Laboratory Findings

Normal LFTs are the rule. Anemia frequently occurs, especially in cases of hepatoblastoma. Cystathioninuria has been reported. α-Fetoprotein levels are often elevated, especially in hepatoblastoma. Estradiol levels are sometimes elevated. Tissue diagnosis is best obtained at laparotomy, although ultrasound- or CT-guided needle biopsy of the liver mass can be used.

C. Imaging

Ultrasonography, CT, and MRI are useful for diagnosis, staging, and to follow tumor response to therapy. A scintigraphic study of bone and lung and selective angiography are generally part of the preoperative workup to evaluate metastatic disease.

Differential Diagnosis

In the absence of a palpable mass, the differential diagnosis is that of hepatomegaly with or without anemia or jaundice. Hematologic and nutritional conditions should be ruled out, as well as HBV and HCV infection, α_1-antitrypsin deficiency disease, lipid storage diseases, histiocytosis X, glycogen storage disease, tyrosinemia, congenital hepatic fibrosis, cysts, adenoma, focal nodular hyperplasia, inflammatory pseudotumor, and hemangiomas. If fever is present, hepatic abscess (pyogenic or amebic) must be considered. Veno-occlusive disease and hepatic vein thrombosis are rare possibilities. Tumors in the left lobe may be mistaken for pancreatic pseudocysts.

Complications

Progressive enlargement of the tumor, abdominal discomfort, ascites, respiratory difficulty, and widespread metastases (especially to the lungs and the abdominal lymph nodes) are the rule. Rupture of the neoplastic liver and intraperitoneal hemorrhage have been reported. Progressive anemia and emaciation predispose the patient to an early septic death.

Treatment

An aggressive surgical approach has resulted in the only reports of long-term survival. Complete resection of the lesion offers the only chance for cure. It appears that every isolated lung metastasis should also be surgically resected. Radiotherapy and chemotherapy have been disappointing in the treatment of primary liver neoplasms, although they may be used for initial cytoreduction of tumors found to be unresectable at the time of primary surgery (see Chapter 29 for additional discussion). Second-look celiotomy has, in some cases, allowed resection of the tumor, resulting in a reduced mortality rate. Liver transplantation can be an option in hepatoblastoma with 85% 10-year survival in patients with unresectable disease limited to the liver. For hepatocellular carcinoma, the survival rate is poor due to the typically advanced stage at diagnosis. The survival rate may be better for those patients in whom the tumor is incidental to another disorder (tyrosinemia, biliary atresia, cirrhosis). In HBV-endemic areas, childhood HBV vaccination has reduced the incidence of hepatocellular carcinoma.

Prognosis

If the tumor is completely removed the survival rate is 90% for hepatoblastoma and 33% for hepatocellular carcinoma. If metastases are present, survival is reduced to 40% for hepatoblastoma.

Chien YC et al: Nationwide hepatitis B vaccination program in Taiwan: Effectiveness in the 20 years after it was launched. Epidemiol Rev 2006;28:126 [PMID: 16782778].

Otte JB, de Ville de Goyet J: The contribution of transplantation to the treatment of liver tumors in children. Semin Pediatr Surg 2005;14:233 [PMID: 16226698].

Tiao GM et al: The current management of hepatoblastoma: A combination of chemotherapy, conventional resection, and liver transplantation. J Pediatr 2005;146:204 [PMID: 15689909].

von Schweinitz D: Management of liver tumors in childhood. Semin Pediatr Surg 2006;15:17 [PMID: 16458842].

LIVER TRANSPLANTATION

Orthotopic liver transplantation is indicated in children with end-stage liver disease, acute fulminant hepatic failure, or complications from metabolic liver disorders. Recent advances in immunosuppression (eg, cyclosporine and tacrolimus, use of monoclonal antibodies against T cells, introduction of mycophenolate mofetil and sirolimus), better candidate selection, improvements in surgical techniques, antiviral medications, and experience in postoperative management have contributed to improved results.

The major indications for childhood transplantation are:

1. A failed Kasai operation or decompensated cirrhosis caused by biliary atresia.
2. α_1-Antitrypsin deficiency causing end-stage liver disease.
3. Posthepatitic (autoimmune chronic hepatitis, hepatitis B or C disease) cirrhosis.
4. Tyrosinemia.
5. Crigler-Najjar syndrome type 1.
6. Wilson disease.
7. Acute liver failure when recovery is unlikely.
8. Primary sclerosing cholangitis.
9. Hepatic-based malignancies.
10. Cases in which the consequences of chronic cholestasis severely impair the patient's quality of life (eg, Alagille syndrome).

Children should be referred early for evaluation because the limiting factor for success is the small donor pool. Pared-down adult livers, organs from living related donors, and split adult donor livers have expanded the donor pool, in addition to whole pediatric donor organs. Ten percent of recipients require retransplantation. In general, 80–90% of children survive at least 2–5 years after transplantation, with long-term survival expected to be comparable. Lifetime immunosuppression therapy, using combinations of tacrolimus, cyclosporine, prednisone, azathioprine, mycophenolate mofetil, or sirolimus, with its incumbent risks, is generally necessary to prevent rejection. Several studies have examined immunosuppression withdrawal, which can occasionally be performed successfully; however, criteria for which patients can survive off of immunosuppression have not been determined. The minimal amount of immunosuppression that will prevent allograft rejection should be chosen. The overall quality of life for children with a transplanted liver appears to be excellent. There is an increased risk (up to 25%) of renal dysfunction. The lifelong risk of EBV-induced lymphoproliferative disease is approximately 5% and is related to age, EBV exposure status at time of transplantation, and intensity of immunosuppression. Various protocols are being tested for prevention and treatment of lymphoproliferative disease.

Alonso EM et al: Functional outcomes of pediatric liver transplantation. J Pediatr Gastroenterol Nutr 2003;37:155 [PMID: 12883302].

Buell JF et al: Malignancy in pediatric transplant recipients. Semin Pediatr Surg 2006;15:179 [PMID: 16818139].

Campbell KM et al: High prevalence of renal dysfunction in long-term survivors after pediatric liver transplantation. J Pediatr 2006;148:475 [PMID: 16647407].

Taylor RM et al: Liver transplantation in children: Part 2—long-term issues. J Child Health Care 2005;9:274 [PMID: 16275665].

Tiao G, Ryckman FC: Pediatric liver transplantation. Clin Liver Dis 2006;10:169 [PMID: 16376800].

Utterson EC et al; The Split Research Group: Biliary atresia: Clinical profiles, risk factors, and outcomes of 755 patients listed for liver transplantation. J Pediatr 2005;147:180 [PMID: 16126046].

PANCREATIC DISORDERS

ACUTE PANCREATITIS

ESSENTIALS OF DIAGNOSIS & TYPICAL FEATURES

▶ Epigastric abdominal pain radiating to the back.
▶ Nausea and vomiting.
▶ Elevated serum amylase and lipase.
▶ Evidence of pancreatic inflammation by CT or ultrasound.

▶ General Considerations

Most cases of acute pancreatitis are the result of drugs, viral infections, systemic diseases, abdominal trauma, or obstruction of pancreatic flow. More than 20% are idiopathic. Causes of pancreatic obstruction include stones, choledochal cyst, tumors of the duodenum, pancreas divisum, and ascariasis. Acute pancreatitis has been seen following treatment with sulfasalazine, thiazides, valproic acid, azathioprine, mercaptopurine, asparaginase, antiretroviral drugs (especially didanosine), high-dose corticosteroids, and other drugs. It may also occur in cystic fibrosis, systemic lupus erythematosus, α_1-antitrypsin deficiency, diabetes mellitus, Crohn disease, glycogen storage disease type I, hyperlipidemia types I and V, hyperparathyroidism, Henoch-Schönlein purpura, Reye syndrome, organic acidopathies, Kawasaki disease, or chronic renal failure; during rapid refeeding in cases of malnutrition; following spinal fusion surgery; and in familial cases. Alcohol-induced pancreatitis should be considered in the teenage patient.

Clinical Findings

A. Symptoms and Signs

An acute onset of persistent (hours to days), moderate to severe upper abdominal and midabdominal pain occasionally referred to the back, and vomiting, is the common presenting picture. The abdomen is tender, but not rigid, and bowel sounds are diminished, suggesting peritoneal irritation. Abdominal distention is common in infants and younger children. Jaundice is unusual. Ascites may be noted, and a left-sided pleural effusion is present in some patients. Periumbilical and flank bruising indicate hemorrhagic pancreatitis.

B. Laboratory Findings

Leukocytosis and an elevated serum amylase (more than three times normal) should be expected early, except in infants younger than 6 months who may have hypoamylasemia. Serum lipase is elevated and persists longer than serum amylase. The immunoreactive trypsinogen may also be elevated. Pancreatic amylase isoenzyme determination can help differentiate nonpancreatic causes (eg, salivary, intestinal, or tubo-ovarian) of serum amylase elevation. Hyperglycemia (serum glucose > 300 mg/dL), hypocalcemia, falling hematocrit, rising blood urea nitrogen, hypoxemia, and acidosis may all occur in severe cases and imply a poor prognosis.

C. Imaging

Plain radiographic films of the abdomen may show a localized ileus (sentinel loop). Ultrasonography shows decreased echodensity of the gland in comparison with the left lobe of the liver. Pseudocyst formation can occasionally be seen early in the course. CT scanning is better for detecting pancreatic phlegmon, or abscess formation. ERCP or MRCP may be useful in confirming patency of the main pancreatic duct in cases of abdominal trauma; in recurrent acute pancreatitis; or in revealing stones, ductal strictures, and pancreas divisum.

Differential Diagnosis

Other causes of acute upper abdominal pain include lesions of the stomach, duodenum, liver, and biliary system; acute gastroenteritis or atypical appendicitis; pneumonia; volvulus; intussusception; and nonaccidental trauma.

Complications

Complications early in the disease include shock, fluid and electrolyte disturbances, ileus, acute respiratory distress syndrome, and hypocalcemia. Hypervolemia is seen between the

third and fifth day, at which time renal tubular necrosis may occur. The gastrointestinal, neurologic, musculoskeletal, hepatobiliary, dermatologic, and hematologic systems may also be involved.

Later, 5–20% of patients develop a pseudocyst heralded by recurrence of abdominal pain and rise in the serum amylase. Up to 60–70% of pseudocysts resolve spontaneously. Infection, hemorrhage, rupture, or fistulization may occur. Phlegmon formation is common and may extend from the gland into the retroperitoneum or into the lesser sac. Most regress, but some require drainage. Infection in this inflammatory mass may occur. Pancreatic abscess formation, which is rare (3–5%), develops 2–3 weeks after the initial insult. Fever, leukocytosis, and pain suggest this complication; diagnosis is made by ultrasound or CT scanning. Chronic pancreatitis, exocrine or endocrine pancreatic insufficiency, and pancreatic lithiasis are rare sequelae of acute pancreatitis.

Treatment

Medical management includes careful attention to fluids, electrolytes, and respiratory status. Gastric decompression may be helpful if there is significant vomiting. Pain should be controlled with opioids. Acid suppression may be helpful. Nutrition is provided by the parenteral or enteral (jejunal) route. Broad-spectrum antibiotic coverage is useful only in necrotizing pancreatitis. Drugs known to produce acute pancreatitis should be discontinued. Surgical treatment is reserved for traumatic disruption of the gland, intraductal stone, other anatomic obstructive lesions, and unresolved or infected pseudocysts or abscesses. Early endoscopic decompression of the biliary system reduces the morbidity associated with pancreatitis caused by obstruction of the common bile duct.

Prognosis

In the pediatric age group, the prognosis is surprisingly good with conservative management. The mortality rate is 5–10% in patients treated surgically and 1% in those treated only with medication. The morbidity rate is high with surgery as a result of fistula formation.

Lowe ME: Pancreatitis in childhood. Curr Gastroenterol Rep 2004;6:240 [PMID: 15128492].
Nydegger A et al: Childhood pancreatitis. J Gastroenterol Hepatol 2006;21:499 [PMID: 16638090].

CHRONIC PANCREATITIS

Chronic pancreatitis is differentiated from acute pancreatitis in that the pancreas remains structurally or functionally abnormal after an attack.

The causes are multiple and can be divided into toxic-metabolic (eg, alcohol, chronic renal failure, hypercalcemia), idiopathic, genetic, autoimmune, recurrent and severe acute pancreatitis, and obstructive pancreatitis (eg, pancreas divisum, choledochal cyst).

Clinical Findings

The diagnosis often is delayed by the nonspecificity of symptoms and the lack of persistent laboratory abnormalities.

A. Symptoms and Signs

There is usually a prolonged history of recurrent upper abdominal pain of variable severity. Radiation of the pain into the back is a frequent complaint. Fever and vomiting are not common. Steatorrhea and symptoms of diabetes may develop later in the course, and malnutrition secondary to failure of pancreatic exocrine secretions may also occur.

B. Laboratory Findings

Serum amylase and lipase levels are usually elevated during early acute attacks but are often normal later. Pancreatic insufficiency and reduced volume and bicarbonate response may be found during pancreatic stimulation testing or by determination of fecal pancreatic elastase 1. Mutations of the cationic trypsinogen gene, the pancreatic secretory trypsin inhibitor, and the cystic fibrosis transmembrane conductance regulator gene (*CFTR*) are associated with recurrent acute and chronic pancreatitis. Elevated blood glucose and glycohemoglobin levels and glycosuria frequently occur in protracted disease. Sweat chloride should be checked for cystic fibrosis and serum calcium for hyperparathyroidism.

C. Imaging

Radiographs of the abdomen may show pancreatic calcifications in up to 30% of patients. Ultrasound or CT examination demonstrates pancreatic enlargement, ductal dilation, and calculi in up to 80%. CT is the initial imaging procedure of choice. MRCP or ERCP can show ductal dilation, stones, strictures, or stenotic segments. Endoscopic ultrasound in the diagnosis and staging of chronic pancreatitis is being evaluated.

Differential Diagnosis

Other causes of recurrent abdominal pain must be considered. Specific causes of pancreatitis such as hyperparathyroidism; systemic lupus erythematosus; infectious disease; and ductal obstruction by tumors, stones, or helminths must be excluded by appropriate tests.

Complications

Disabling abdominal pain, steatorrhea, malnutrition, pancreatic pseudocysts, and diabetes are the most frequent long-term complications. Pancreatic carcinoma occurs more frequently in chronic pancreatitis, and in up to 40% of patients with hereditary pancreatitis by age 70.

Treatment

Medical management of acute attacks is indicated (see Acute Pancreatitis section). If ductal obstruction is strongly suspected, endoscopic therapy (balloon dilation, stenting, stone removal, or sphincterotomy) should be pursued. Relapses occur in most patients. Orally ingested nonenteric-coated pancreatic enzymes at mealtime may reduce pain episodes in some patients. Antioxidant therapy is being investigated. Pseudocysts may be marsupialized to the surface or drained into the stomach or into a loop of jejunum if they fail to regress spontaneously. Experience in pediatric patients indicates that lateral pancreaticojejunostomy or the Frey procedure can reduce pain in patients with a dilated pancreatic duct and may prevent or delay progression of functional pancreatic impairment. Pancreatectomy and islet cell autotransplantation have been used in selected cases of chronic pancreatitis.

Prognosis

In the absence of a correctable lesion, the prognosis is not good. Disabling episodes of pain, pancreatic insufficiency, diabetes, and pancreatic cancer may ensue. Narcotic addiction and suicide are risks in teenagers with disabling disease.

Kandula L et al.: Genetic issues in pediatric pancreatitis. Curr Gastroenterol Rep 2006;8:248 [PMID: 16764792].

Witt H: Gene mutations in children with chronic pancreatitis. Pancreatology 2001;1:432 [PMID: 12120220].

GASTROINTESTINAL & HEPATOBILIARY MANIFESTATIONS OF CYSTIC FIBROSIS

Cystic fibrosis is a disease with protean manifestations. Although pulmonary and pancreatic involvement dominate the clinical picture for most patients (see Chapter 18), various other organs can be involved. Table 21–9 lists the important gastrointestinal, pancreatic, and hepatobiliary conditions that may affect patients with cystic fibrosis along with their clinical findings, incidence, most useful diagnostic studies, and preferred treatment.

Baker SS et al: Pancreatic enzyme therapy and clinical outcomes in patients with cystic fibrosis. J Pediatr 2005;146:189 [PMID: 15689904].

Borwitz D et al: Gastrointestinal outcomes and confounders in cystic fibrosis. J Pediatr Gastroenterol Nutr 2005;41:273 [PMID: 16131979].

Borowitz D et al: Use of fecal elastase-1 to classify pancreatic status in patients with cystic fibrosis. J Pediatr 2004;145:322 [PMID: 15343184].

Corbett K et al: Cystic fibrosis-associated liver disease: A population-based study. J Pediatr 2004;145:327 [PMID: 15343185].

Littlewood JM et al: Diagnosis and treatment of intestinal malabsorption in cystic fibrosis. Pediatr Pulmonol 2006;41:35 [PMID: 16288483].

Table 21-9. Gastrointestinal and hepatobiliary manifestations of cystic fibrosis.

Organ	Condition	Symptoms	Age at Presentation	Incidence (%)	Diagnostic Evaluation	Management
Esophagus	Gastroesophageal reflux, esophagitis	Pyrosis, dysphagia, epigastric pain, hematemesis.	All ages	10–20	Endoscopy and biopsy, overnight pH study	H₂ blockers, antacids, sucralfate, PPIs, surgical antireflux procedure.
	Varices	Hematemesis, melena.	Childhood and adolescents	3–10	Endoscopy	Endosclerosis, band ligation, drugs (see text), TIPS, liver transplantation (see Table 21–7).
Stomach	Gastritis	Upper abdominal pain, vomiting, hematemesis.	School age and older	10–25	Endoscopy and biopsy	H₂ blockers, antacids, sucralfate, PPIs.
	Hiatal hernia	Reflux symptoms (see above), epigastric pain.	School age and older	3–5	Endoscopy; UGI	As above. Surgery in some.
Intestine	Meconium ileus	Abdominal distention, bilious emesis.	Neonate	10–15	Radiologic studies, plain abdominal films; contrast enema shows microcolon	Dislodgement of obstruction with Gastrografin enema. Surgery if unsuccessful or if case complicated by atresia, perforation, or volvulus.
	Distal intestinal obstruction syndrome	Abdominal pain, acute and recurrent; distention; occasional vomiting.	Any age, usually school age through adolescence	10–15	Palpable mass in right lower quadrant, radiologic studies	Gastrografin enema, intestinal lavage solution, diet, bulk laxatives, adjustment of pancreatic enzyme intake.
	Fibrosing colonopathy	As above. History of high enzyme dosage.	≥ 3 y	< 1	Barium enema or UGI/SBFT, abdominal ultrasound, or CT	Reduce pancreatic enzyme dose to < 2000 U/kg of lipase per dose if indicated. Surgical resection may be necessary.
	Intussusception	Acute, intermittent abdominal pain; distention; emesis.	Infants through adolescence	1–3	Radiographic studies, barium enema	Reduction by barium or air enema or surgery if needed. Diet. Bulk laxatives. Adjustment of pancreatic enzyme intake.
	Rectal prolapse	Anal discomfort, rectal bleeding.	Infants and children to age 4–5 y	15–25	Visual mass protruding from anus	Manual reduction, adjustment of pancreatic enzyme dosage, reassurance as problem resolves by age 3–5 y.
	Carbohydrate intolerance	Abdominal pain, flatulence, continued diarrhea with adequate replacement therapy.	Any age	10–25	Intestinal mucosal biopsy and disaccharidase analysis. Breath hydrogen after lactose load.	Reduce lactose intake; lactase; reduction of gastric hyperacidity if mucosa shows partial villous atrophy. Beware concurrent celiac disease or *Giardia* infection.
Pancreas	Total exocrine insufficiency	Diarrhea, steatorrhea, malnutrition, failure to thrive. Specific fat-soluble vitamin deficiency states.	Neonate through infancy	85–90	72-h fecal fat evaluation, fecal pancreatic elastase, direct pancreatic function tests	Pancreatic enzyme replacement, may need elemental formula, fat-soluble vitamin and vitamin E supplements.

(continued)

Table 21-9. Gastrointestinal and hepatobiliary manifestations of cystic fibrosis. *(Continued)*

Organ	Condition	Symptoms	Age at Presentation	Incidence (%)	Diagnostic Evaluation	Management
	Pancreatic sufficiency (partial exocrine insufficiency)	Occasional diarrhea, mild growth delay.	Any age	10–15	72-h fecal fat evaluation, direct pancreatic function tests, fecal pancreatic elastase	Pancreatic enzyme replacement in selected patients. Fat-soluble vitamin supplements as indicated by biochemical evaluation.
	Pancreatitis	Recurrent abdominal pain, vomiting.	Older children through adolescence. Primarily in patients with partial pancreatic sufficiency.	0.1	Increased serum lipase and amylase, pancreatic provocative test, MRCP, ERCP	Addition of pancreatic enzymes to feeds, endoscopic removal of sludge or stones if present, endoscopic papillotomy.
	Diabetes	Weight loss, polyuria, polydipsia.	Older children through adolescence	5–7	Glucose tolerance test and insulin levels	Diet, insulin, oral hypoglycemics.
Liver	Steatosis	Hepatomegaly.	Neonates and infants, but can be seen at all ages	20–60	Liver biopsy	Improved nutrition, replacement of pancreatic enzymes, vitamins, and essential fatty acids.
	Focal biliary cirrhosis	Hepatomegaly.	Infants and older patients. Prevalence increases with age.	10–70	Liver biopsy	As above. Ursodeoxycholic acid.
	Multilobular biliary cirrhosis	Hepatosplenomegaly, hematemesis from esophageal varices; hypersplenism, jaundice, ascites late in course.	School age through adolescence	5–15	Liver biopsy, endoscopy	Improved nutrition, ursodeoxycholic acid, endosclerosis or band ligation of varices, or partial splenic embolization, liver transplantation.
	Neonatal jaundice	Cholestatic jaundice hepatomegaly; often seen with meconium ileus.	Neonates	0.1–1	Sweat chloride test, liver biopsy	Nutritional support, special formula with medium-chain triglyceride-containing oil, pancreatic enzyme replacement, vitamin supplements.
Gallbladder	Microgallbladder	None.	Congenital—present at any age	30	Ultrasound or hepatobiliary scintigraphy	None needed.
	Cholelithiasis	Recurrent abdominal pain, rarely jaundice.	School age through adolescence	1–10	Ultrasound	Surgery if symptomatic and low risk, trial of cholelitholytics in others.
Extrahepatic bile ducts	Intraluminal obstruction (sludge, stones, tumor)	Jaundice, hepatomegaly, abdominal pain.	Neonates, then older children through adolescence	Rare in neonates (< 0.1)	Ultrasound and hepatobiliary scintigraphy, MRCP	Surgery in neonates; ERCP in older patients or surgery.
	Extraluminal obstruction (intrapancreatic compression, tumor)	As above.	Older children to adults	Rare (< 1)	As above	Surgical biliary drainage procedure or ERCP.

CT, computed tomography; ERCP, endoscopic retrograde cholangiopancreatography; MRCP, magnetic resonance cholangiopancreatography; PPI, proton pump inhibitor; TIPS, transjugular intrahepatic portosystemic shunt; UGI/SBFT, upper gastrointestinal/small bowel follow-through radiologic series.

SYNDROMES WITH PANCREATIC EXOCRINE INSUFFICIENCY

Several syndromes are associated with exocrine pancreatic insufficiency. Clinically, patients present with a history of failure to thrive, diarrhea, fatty stools, and an absence of respiratory symptoms. Laboratory findings include a normal sweat chloride; low fecal pancreatic elastase 1; and low to absent pancreatic lipase, amylase, and trypsin levels on duodenal intubation. Each disorder has several associated clinical features that aid in the differential diagnosis. In Shwachman syndrome, pancreatic exocrine hypoplasia with widespread fatty replacement of the glandular acinar tissue is associated with neutropenia because of maturational arrest of the granulocyte series. Metaphyseal dysostosis and an elevated fetal hemoglobin level are common; immunoglobulin deficiency and hepatic dysfunction are also reported. CT examination of the pancreas demonstrates the widespread fatty replacement. Serum immunoreactive trypsinogen levels are extremely low.

Other associations of exocrine pancreatic insufficiency include (1) aplastic alae, aplasia cutis, deafness (Johanson-Blizzard syndrome); (2) sideroblastic anemia, developmental delay, seizures, and liver dysfunction (Pearson bone marrow pancreas syndrome); (3) duodenal atresia or stenosis; (4) malnutrition; and (5) pancreatic hypoplasia or agenesis.

The complications and sequelae of deficient pancreatic enzyme secretion are malnutrition, diarrhea, and growth failure. The degree of steatorrhea may lessen with age. Intragastric lipolysis primarily caused by lingual lipase may compensate in patients with low or absent pancreatic function. In Shwachman syndrome, the major sequela is short stature. Increased numbers of infections may result from chronic neutropenia. Neutrophil mobility is also impaired in many patients. In addition, an increased incidence of leukemia has been noted in these patients.

Pancreatic enzyme and fat-soluble vitamin replacement are required therapy in most patients. The prognosis appears to be good for those able to survive the increased number of bacterial infections early in life and those patients without severe associated defects.

Boocock GR et al: Mutations in SBDS are associated with Shwachman-Diamond syndrome. Nat Genet 2003;33:97 [PMID: 12496757].

Durie PR: Pancreatic aspects of cystic fibrosis and other inherited causes of pancreatic dysfunction. Med Clin North Am 2000;84:609 [PMID: 10872418].

Dror Y: Shwachman-Diamond syndrome. Pediatr Blood Cancer 2005;45:892 [PMID: 16047374].

Sarles J et al: Pancreatic function and congenital duodenal abnormalities. J Pediatr Gastroenterol Nutr 1993;16:284 [PMID: 8492257].

Seneca S et al: Pearson marrow pancreas syndrome: A molecular study and clinical management. Clin Genet 1997;51:338 [PMID: 9212183].

Wright NM et al: Permanent neonatal diabetes mellitus and pancreatic exocrine insufficiency resulting from congenital pancreatic agenesis. Am J Dis Child 1993;147:607 [PMID: 8506821].

ISOLATED EXOCRINE PANCREATIC ENZYME DEFECT

Normal premature infants and most newborns produce little, if any, pancreatic amylase following meals or exogenous hormonal stimulation. This temporary physiologic insufficiency may persist for the first 3–6 months of life and be responsible for diarrhea when complex carbohydrates (cereals) are introduced into the diet.

Congenital pancreatic lipase deficiency and congenital colipase deficiency are extremely rare disorders, causing diarrhea and variable malnutrition with malabsorption of dietary fat and fat-soluble vitamins. The sweat chloride level is normal, and neutropenia is absent. Treatment is oral replacement of pancreatic enzymes and a low-fat diet or formula containing medium-chain triglycerides.

Exocrine pancreatic insufficiency of proteolytic enzymes (eg, trypsinogen, trypsin, chymotrypsin) is caused by enterokinase deficiency, a duodenal mucosal enzyme required for activation of the pancreatic proenzymes. These patients present with malnutrition associated with hypoproteinemia and edema but are free of respiratory symptoms and have a normal sweat test. They respond to pancreatic enzyme replacement therapy and feeding formulas that contain a casein hydrolysate (eg, Nutramigen, Pregestimil).

Durie PR: Pancreatic aspects of cystic fibrosis and other inherited causes of pancreatic dysfunction. Med Clin North Am 2000;84:609 [PMID: 10872418].

Mann NS, Mann SK: Enterokinase. Proc Soc Exp Biol Med 1994;206:114 [PMID: 8208733].

McKenna LL: Pancreatic disorders in the newborn. Neonatal Netw 2000;19:13 [PMID: 11949098].

Stormon MO, Durie PR: Pathophysiologic basis of exocrine pancreatic dysfunction in childhood. J Pediatr Gastroenterol Nutr 2002;35:8 [PMID: 12142803].

PANCREATIC TUMORS

Pancreatic tumors, whether benign or malignant, are rare. They most often arise from ductal or acinar epithelium (malignant adenocarcinoma) or from islet (endocrine) components within the gland, such as the benign insulinoma (adenoma) derived from β cells. Other pancreatic tumors also originate from these pluripotential endocrine cells (gastrinoma, VIPoma, glucagonoma). These malignant lesions produce diverse symptoms, because they release biologically active polypeptides from this ectopic location. The clinical features of these tumors are summarized in Table 21–10. The differential diagnosis of pancreatic tumors includes Wilms tumor, neuroblastoma, and malignant lymphoma. In older children, endoscopic ultrasonography can aid in localizing these tumors.

Table 21–10. Pancreatic tumors.

	Age	Major Findings	Diagnosis	Treatment	Associated Conditions
Insulinoma	Any age	Hypoglycemia, seizures; high serum insulin; weight gain; abdominal pain and mass infrequent	CT scan, MRI, EUS, SRS	Surgery, diazoxide, SSTA	
Adenocarcinoma	Any age	Epigastric pain, mass weight loss, anemia, biliary obstruction	Ultrasound, CT scan, MRI, EUS	Surgery	Chronic pancreatitis
Gastrinoma	Older than age 5-8 y	Male sex, gastric hypersecretion, peptic symptoms, multiple ulcers, gastrointestinal bleeding, anemia, diarrhea	Elevated fasting gastrin and postsecretin suppression test (> 300 pg/mL), CT scan, MRI, EUS, SRS, laparotomy	PPI, surgical resection, total gastrectomy, SSTA	Zollinger-Ellison syndrome, multiple endocrine neoplasia syndrome type I, neurofibromatosis
VIPoma	Any age	Secretory diarrhea, hypokalemia, hypochlorhydria, weight loss, flushing	Elevated VIP levels; sometimes, elevated serum gastrin and pancreatic polypeptide; SRS	Surgery, SSTA, IV fluids	
Glucagonoma	Older patients	Diabetes, necrolytic rash, diarrhea, anemia, thrombotic events, depression	Elevated glucagon, gastrin, VIP, MRI, SRS	Surgery, SSTA	

CT, computed tomography; EUS, endoscopic ultrasound; MRI, magnetic resonance imaging; PPI, proton pump inhibitor; SRS, somatostatin-receptor scintigraphy; SSTA, somatostatin analogue; VIP, vasoactive intestinal polypeptide.

Doherty GM: Rare endocrine tumours of the GI tract. Best Pract Res Clin Gastroenterol 2005;19:807 [PMID: 16253902].

Jaksic T et al: A 20-year review of pediatric pancreatic tumors. J Pediatr Surg 1992;27:1315 [PMID: 1328584].

Johnson PRV, Spitz L: Cysts and tumors of the pancreas. Semin Pediatr Surg 2000;9:209 [PMID: 11112838].

Vossen S et al: Therapeutic management of rare malignant pancreatic tumors in children. World J Surg 1998;22:879 [PMID: 9673563].

REFERENCES

Suchy FJ, Sokol RJ, Balistreri WF (editors): *Liver Disease in Children*, 3rd ed. Cambridge University Press, 2007.

Walker WA et al (editors): *Pediatric Gastrointestinal Disease: Pathophysiology, Diagnosis, Management*, 4th ed. BC Decker, 2004.

Wyllie R, Hyams JS (editors): *Pediatric Gastrointestinal and Liver Disease*, 3rd ed. Elsevier, 2006.

Kidney & Urinary Tract

Gary M. Lum, MD

▼ EVALUATION OF THE KIDNEY & URINARY TRACT

HISTORY

When renal disease is suspected, the history should include:

1. Family history of cystic disease, hereditary nephritis, deafness, dialysis, or renal transplantation.
2. Preceding acute or chronic illnesses (eg, urinary tract infection, pharyngitis, impetigo, or endocarditis).
3. Rashes or joint pains.
4. Growth delay or failure to thrive.
5. Polyuria, polydipsia, enuresis, urinary frequency, or dysuria.
6. Documentation of hematuria, proteinuria, or discolored urine.
7. Pain (abdominal, costovertebral angle, or flank) or trauma.
8. Sudden weight gain or edema.
9. Drug or toxin exposure.
10. Data pertaining to the newborn with suspected urinary tract disease: prenatal ultrasonographic studies, birth asphyxia, Apgar scores, oligohydramnios, dysmorphic features, abdominal masses, voiding patterns, anomalous development, and umbilical artery catheterization.

PHYSICAL EXAMINATION

Important aspects of the physical examination include the height, weight, skin lesions (café-au-lait or ash leaf spots), pallor, edema, or skeletal deformities. Anomalies of the ears, eyes, or external genitalia may be associated with renal anomalies or disease. The blood pressure should be measured in a quiet setting. The cuff should cover two thirds of the child's upper arm, and peripheral pulses should be noted. The abdomen should be palpated, with attention to the kidneys, abdominal masses, musculature, and the presence of ascites. An ultrasonic device is useful for measurements in infants.

LABORATORY EVALUATION OF RENAL FUNCTION

Serum Analysis

The standard indicators of renal function are serum levels of urea nitrogen and creatinine; their ratio is normally about 10:1. This ratio may increase when renal perfusion or urine flow is decreased, as in urinary tract obstruction or dehydration. Because serum urea nitrogen levels are more affected by these and other factors (eg, nitrogen intake, catabolism, use of corticosteroids) than are creatinine levels, the most reliable single indicator of glomerular function is the serum level of creatinine. For example, an increase in serum creatinine from 0.5 mg/dL to 1.0 mg/dL represents a 50% decrease in glomerular filtration rate. The serum creatinine level of small children should be well under 0.8 mg/dL. Only larger adolescents should have levels exceeding 1 mg/dL. Less precise but nonetheless important indicators of possible renal disease are abnormalities of serum electrolytes, pH, calcium, phosphorus, magnesium, albumin, or complement.

Glomerular Filtration Rate

The endogenous creatinine clearance (C_{cr}) in milliliters per minute estimates the glomerular filtration rate (GFR). A 24-hour urine collection is usually obtained; however, in small children from whom collection is difficult, a 12-hour daytime specimen, collected when urine flow rate is greatest, is acceptable. The procedure for collecting a timed urine specimen should be explained carefully so that the parent or patient understands fully the rationale of (1) first emptying the bladder (discarding that urine) and noting the time; and (2) putting all urine subsequently voided into the collection receptacle, including the last void, 12 or 24 hours later. Reliability of the 24-hour collection can be checked by measuring the total 24-hour creatinine excretion in the specimen. Total daily creatinine excretion (creatinine index) should be 14–20 mg/kg. Creatinine indices on either side of this range suggest collections that were either inadequate or excessive. Calculation by the following formula requires measurements of plasma creatinine (P_{cr}) in mg/mL, urine creatinine (U_{cr}) in mg/mL, and urine volume (V) expressed as mL/min:

$$C_{cr} = \frac{U_{cr}V}{P_{cr}}$$

Creatinine is a reflection of body muscle mass. Because accepted ranges of normal C_{cr} are based on adult parameters, correction for size is needed to determine normal ranges in children. Clearance is corrected to a standard body surface area of 1.73 m^2 in the formula:

$$\text{"Corrected" } C = \frac{\text{Patient's } C_{cr} \times 1.73 \text{ m}^2}{\text{Patient's body surface area}}$$

Although 80–125 mL/min/1.73 m^2 is the normal range for C_{cr}, estimates at the lower end of this range may indicate problems.

A reliable formula for quick approximation of C_{cr} is based on plasma creatinine level and length in centimeters:

$$C_{cr}(\text{mL/min/1.73 m}^2) = \frac{0.55 \times \text{Height in cm}}{P_{cr} \text{ in mg/dL}}$$

Note: Because this formula takes into account the body surface area, further correction is not necessary. Use 0.45 × length in centimeters for newborns and for infants younger than age 1 year. This method of calculation does not replace creatinine clearance determinations, but is useful when a suspicious plasma creatinine needs to be checked.

Urine Concentrating Ability

Inability to concentrate urine causes polyuria, polydipsia, or enuresis and is often the first sign of chronic renal failure. The first morning void should be concentrated. Evaluation of other abnormalities of urinary concentration or dilution is discussed later in the sections on specific disease entities, such as diabetes insipidus.

Urinalysis

Commercially available dipsticks can be used to check the urine for red blood cells (RBCs), hemoglobin, leukocytes, nitrites, and protein and to approximate its pH. Positive results for blood should always be confirmed by microscopy, as should any suspicion of crystalluria. Significant proteinuria (> 150 mg/dL) detected by dipstick should be confirmed by quantitation, either with a 24-hour collection or by the protein/creatinine ratio (see following section) of a random specimen.

In children with asymptomatic hematuria or proteinuria, the search for renal origins will yield the most results.

Isolated proteinuria may reflect urologic abnormalities, benign excretion, or glomerular alterations. RBC casts suggest glomerulonephritis (GN), but the absence of casts does not rule out this disease. Anatomic abnormalities such as cystic disease may also cause hematuria.

Benign hematuria, including benign familial hematuria, is diagnosed by exclusion. In this group are children whose hematuria is caused by asymptomatic hypercalciuria. Figure 22–1 suggests an approach to the renal workup of hematuria. GN is discussed in more detail later in this chapter.

Combined proteinuria and hematuria is characteristic of more significant glomerular disease. Quantitation of proteinuria is customarily accomplished by a timed collection (eg, over a 24-hour period). However, the degree of proteinuria may be estimated by the ratio of protein/creatinine in a random urine sample. A protein-to-creatinine ratio above 0.2 is abnormal.

In the evaluation of asymptomatic proteinuria, orthostatic or postural proteinuria should be ruled out. The protein present in urine voided on arising in the morning is compared with that in urine formed in the upright position during the rest of the day. This can be accomplished simply by comparing the protein/creatinine ratios of the two urine samples. When quantitation is accomplished by evaluating the "upright" and "supine" portions of a 24-hour collection, a diagnosis of benign postural proteinuria is indicated if the upright collection contains 80–100% of the entire 24-hour protein excretion, and if there are no other markers of renal disease.

An approach to the workup of isolated proteinuria is shown in Figure 22–2. Note that corticosteroid therapy is indicated in the algorithm because this may be initiated prior to referral. Other renal lesions with proteinuric manifestations are discussed later in this chapter.

Special Tests of Renal Function

Measurements of urinary sodium, creatinine, and osmolality are useful in differentiating prerenal from renal causes of renal insufficiency, such as acute tubular necrosis. The physiologic response to decreased renal perfusion is decreased urinary output, increased urine osmolality, increased urinary solutes (eg, creatinine), and decreased urinary sodium (usually < 20 mEq/L). Prolonged underperfusion causes varying increases in serum creatinine and blood urea nitrogen (BUN) concentrations, prompting the need to differentiate between this state and acute tubular necrosis (see section on Acute Renal Failure, later).

The presence of certain substances in urine may suggest tubular dysfunction. For example, urine glucose should be less than 5 mg/dL. Hyperphosphaturia occurs with significant tubular abnormalities (eg, Fanconi syndrome). Measurement of the phosphate concentration of a 24-hour urine specimen and evaluation of tubular reabsorption of phosphorus (TRP) will help document renal tubular diseases as

▲ **Figure 22–1.** Approach to the renal workup of hematuria. (Exclude UTI, lithiasis, trauma, bleeding disorders, sickle cell disease.) Complement is depressed in acute poststreptococcal type of glomerulonephritis (about 30 days), chronic glomerulonephritis (persistent), and lupus. ANA, antinuclear antibody; ASO, antistreptolysin antibody; BP, blood pressure; BUN, blood urea nitrogen; C3, complement; Ca, calcium; CBC, complete blood count; Cr, creatinine; IgA, immunoglobulin A; RBC, red blood cell; SLE, systemic lupus erythematosus; U/A, urinalysis.

well as hyperparathyroid states. TRP (expressed as percentage of reabsorption) is calculated as follows:

$$TRP = 100\left[1 - \frac{S_{cr} \times U_{PO_4}}{S_{PO_4} \times U_{cr}}\right]$$

where S_{cr} = serum creatinine; U_{cr} = urine creatinine; S_{PO_4} = serum phosphate; and U_{PO_4} = urine phosphate. All values for creatinine and phosphate are expressed in milligrams per deciliter for purposes of calculation. A TRP value of 80% or more is considered normal, although it depends somewhat on the value of SPO_4.

The urinary excretion of amino acids in generalized tubular disease reflects a quantitative increase rather than a qualitative change. Diseases affecting proximal tubular reabsorption of bicarbonate—including isolated renal tubular acidosis (RTA), Fanconi syndrome (which occurs in diseases

such as cystinosis), and chronic renal failure—are discussed later in the chapter.

LABORATORY EVALUATION OF IMMUNOLOGIC FUNCTION

Many parenchymal renal diseases are thought to have immune causation, although the mechanisms are largely unknown. Examples include (1) deposition of circulating antigen-antibody complexes that are directly injurious or incite injurious responses and (2) formation of antibody directed against the glomerular basement membrane (rare in children).

Total serum complement and the C3 and C4 complement components should be measured when immune-mediated renal injury or chronic GN is suspected. Where clinically indicated, antinuclear antibodies, hepatitis B surface antigen, and rheumatoid factor should be obtained. In rare cases cold-

▲ **Figure 22–2.** Approach to the workup of isolated proteinuria. BP, blood pressure; Cr, creatinine; hpf, high-power field; RBC, red blood cell; U/A, urinalysis; VCUG, voiding cystourethrogram. Rules out benign postural proteinuria with urine protein/creatine ratio of first morning void (recumbent urine) vs day void (upright). Will normalize within a month in post-streptococcal glomerulonephritis.

precipitable proteins (cryoglobulins), C3 "nephritic" factor, or antiglomerular basement membrane (anti-GBM) antibody measurements may help confirm a specific diagnosis. At some point in the workup, the diagnosis may be supported or confirmed by histologic examination of renal tissue.

RADIOGRAPHIC EVALUATION

Renal ultrasonography is a useful noninvasive tool for evaluating renal parenchymal disease, urinary tract abnormalities,

or renal blood flow. Excretory urography is used to assess the anatomy and function of the kidney, collecting system, and bladder. Radioisotope studies provide information about renal anatomy, blood flow, and integrity and function of the glomerular, tubular, and collecting systems. Renal stones are best seen by computed tomography.

Voiding cystourethrography or cystoscopy is indicated when vesicoureteral reflux or bladder outlet obstruction is suspected. Cystoscopy is rarely useful in the evaluation of asymptomatic hematuria or proteinuria in children.

Renal arteriography or venography is indicated to define vascular abnormalities (eg, renal artery stenosis) prior to surgical intervention or transluminal angiography. Less invasive measures such as ultrasonography and Doppler studies can demonstrate renal blood flow or thromboses. More specific identification of stenoses of the renal artery is accomplished by magnetic resonance arteriography.

RENAL BIOPSY

Histologic information is valuable for diagnosis, treatment, and prognosis. Satisfactory evaluation of renal tissue requires examination by light, immunofluorescence, and electron microscopy.

When a biopsy is anticipated, a pediatric nephrologist should be consulted. In children, percutaneous renal biopsy with a biopsy needle is an acceptable low-risk procedure—avoiding the risks of general anesthesia—when performed by an experienced physician. A surgeon should perform the biopsy procedure if operative exposure of the kidney is necessary, if a risk factor (eg, bleeding disorder) is present, or if a "wedge" biopsy is preferred.

CONGENITAL ANOMALIES OF THE URINARY TRACT

RENAL PARENCHYMAL ANOMALIES

About 10% of children have congenital anomalies of the genitourinary tract, which range in severity from asymptomatic to lethal. Some asymptomatic abnormalities may have significant complications. For example, patients with "horseshoe" kidney (kidneys fused in their lower poles) have a higher incidence of renal calculi. Unilateral agenesis is usually accompanied by compensatory hypertrophy of the contralateral kidney and thus should be compatible with normal renal function. Supernumerary and ectopic kidneys are usually of no significance. Abnormal genitourinary development is associated with varying degrees of renal dysgenesis and dysfunction ranging from mild forms to complete renal agenesis. In neonates, bilateral renal agenesis is associated with severe oligohydramnios, pulmonary hypoplasia, abnormal (Potter) facies, and early death.

1. Renal Dysgenesis

Renal dysgenesis is a spectrum of anomalies. In simple hypoplasia, which may be unilateral or bilateral, the affected kidneys are smaller than normal. In some forms of dysplasia, immature, undifferentiated renal tissue persists. In some dysplasias, the number of normal nephrons is insufficient to sustain life once the child reaches a critical body size. The lack of renal tissue may not be readily discernible in the newborn period because the infant's urine production, though poor in concentration, may be adequate in volume.

Often, the search for renal insufficiency is initiated only when growth fails or chronic renal failure develops.

Other forms of renal dysplasia include oligomeganephronia (characterized by the presence of only a few large glomeruli) and the cystic dysplasias (characterized by the presence of renal cysts). This group includes microcystic disease (congenital nephrosis). A simple cyst within a kidney may be clinically unimportant because it does not predispose to progressive polycystic development. An entire kidney lost to multicystic development with concomitant hypertrophy and normal function of the contralateral side may also be of little clinical consequence. Nonetheless, even a simple cyst could pose problems if it becomes a site for stone formation, infection, or bleeding.

2. Polycystic Kidney Disease

Autosomal recessive polycystic kidney disease is increasingly diagnosed by prenatal ultrasound. In its most severe form the cystic kidneys are nonfunctional in utero, and, therefore, newborns can have Potter facies and other complications of oligohydramnios. In infancy and childhood, kidney enlargement by cysts may initially be recognized by abdominal palpation of renal masses. Hypertension is an early problem. The rate of the progression of renal insufficiency varies, as does growth failure and other complications of chronic renal failure. Two genes (*ADPKD1* and *ADPKD2*) account for 80% and 10% of cases of autosomal dominant polycystic kidney disease, respectively. Susceptibility of family members is detected by gene linkage studies. Renal ultrasound identifies cysts in about 80% of affected children by age 5 years. Children with this diagnosis need close monitoring for the development and treatment of hypertension, and their families should be offered genetic counseling. Management of end-stage renal failure is by dialysis or renal transplantation.

3. Medullary Cystic Disease (Juvenile Nephronophthisis)

Medullary cystic disease is characterized by cysts of varying sizes in the renal medulla with tubular and interstitial nephritis. Children present with renal failure and signs of tubular dysfunction (decreased concentrating ability, Fanconi syndrome). This lesion should not be confused with medullary sponge kidney (renal tubular ectasia), a frequently asymptomatic disease occurring in adults.

DISTAL URINARY TRACT ANOMALIES

1. Obstructive Uropathy

Obstruction at the ureteropelvic junction may be the result of intrinsic muscle abnormalities, aberrant vessels, or fibrous bands. The lesion can cause hydronephrosis and usually presents as an abdominal mass in the newborn. Obstruction can occur in other parts of the ureter, especially at its entrance into the bladder, causing proximal hydroureter and hydronephrosis. Renal radionuclide scan with furosemide "wash-out" will reveal or rule out obstruction as the cause of the hydronephrosis. Whether intrinsic or extrinsic, urinary tract obstruction should be relieved surgically as soon as possible to minimize damage to the kidneys.

Severe bladder malformations such as exstrophy are clinically obvious and a surgical challenge. More subtle—but urgent in terms of diagnosis—is obstruction of urine flow from vestigial posterior urethral valves. This anomaly, which occurs almost exclusively in males, usually presents in newborns with anuria or a poor voiding stream secondary to severe obstruction of urine flow. The kidneys and bladder may be easily palpable. Leakage proximal to the obstruction may produce urinary ascites. Surgical drainage of urine is urgently required to prevent irreversible damage.

Prune belly syndrome is an association of urinary tract anomalies with cryptorchidism and absent abdominal musculature. Although complex anomalies, especially renal dysplasia, usually cause early death or the need for dialysis or transplantation, some patients have lived into the third decade with varying degrees of renal insufficiency. Timely urinary diversion is essential to sustain renal function.

Other complex malformations and external genital anomalies such as hypospadias are beyond the scope of this text. The challenge presented by urologic abnormalities resulting in severe compromise and destruction of renal tissue is to preserve all remaining renal function and treat the complications of progressive chronic renal failure. Involvement of a specialist in pediatric urology in early management is essential.

2. Reflux Nephropathy

The retrograde flow of urine from the bladder into the ureter (vesicoureteral reflux), may cause renal scarring and subsequent renal insufficiency or hypertension, or both, especially in the presence of urinary tract infection. A finding of hydronephrosis on renal ultrasound is suggestive of vesicoureteral reflux. Its presence can be confirmed or eliminated by a voiding cystourethrogram, which would also be obtained to rule out reflux in the evaluation of urinary tract infection. Low-grade reflux may resolve in the absence of infection, in which case antibiotic prophylaxis is undertaken while awaiting signs of resolution. Surgery may be required for chronic severe reflux.

Chevalier RL: Pathogenesis of renal injury in obstructive uropathy. Curr Opin Pediatr 2006;18:153 [PMID: 16601495].

Greenbaum LA. Mesrobian HG: Vesicoureteral reflux. Pediatr Clin North Am 2006;53:413 [PMID: 16716788].

Jodal U et al: Ten-year results of randomized treatment of children with severe vesicoureteral reflux. Final report of the International Reflux Study in children. Pediatr Nephrol 2006;21:757 [PMID: 16565873].

HEMATURIA & GLOMERULAR DISEASE

MICROHEMATURIA

Children with painful hematuria should be investigated for urinary tract infection or direct injury to the urinary tract. Dysuria is common in cystitis or urethritis; associated back pain suggests the possibility of pyelonephritis; colicky flank pain may indicate the passage of a stone. Bright red blood or clots in the urine are associated with bleeding disorders, trauma, and arteriovenous malformations. Abdominal masses suggest the presence of urinary tract obstruction, cystic disease, or tumors of the renal or perirenal structures.

Asymptomatic hematuria is a challenge because clinical and diagnostic data are required to decide whether to refer the child to a nephrologist. The diagnosis of hematuria should not rely solely on a urine "dipstick" evaluation, but should be verified by a microscopic RBC count. Ruling out hypercalciuria as a cause of hematuria by a random urine calcium/creatinine ratio is one of the initial steps in the evaluation of hematuria. A value above 0.2 requires verification with a 24-hour collection. Hypercalciuria is excretion of calcium in excess of 4 mg/kg/d. Figure 22–1 delineates the outpatient approach to renal hematuria. The concern regarding the differential diagnosis is the possible presence of glomerular disease.

GLOMERULONEPHRITIS

The various types of GN have similar manifestations. Table 22–1 lists the most commonly encountered disorders in the differential diagnosis of childhood GN, including their clinical and histopathologic abnormalities. Severe glomerular histopathologic and clinical entities, such as anti-GBM antibody disease (Goodpasture syndrome), Wegener granulomatosis, and idiopathic, rapidly progressive GN, may be considered in the differential diagnosis of acute GN, but these disorders are exceedingly rare in children.

1. Poststreptococcal Glomerulonephritis

The diagnosis of poststreptococcal disease is supported by a recent history (7–14 days previously) of group A β-hemolytic streptococcal infection. If a positive culture is not available, recent infection may be supported by an elevated antistreptolysin O titer or by high titers of other antistreptococcal antibodies. Other infections can cause similar glomerular injury; thus, "postinfection" glomerulonephritis (GN) may be a better term for this type of acute GN. In most cases, recovery is expected and usually complete within weeks. If the diagnosis is in question, or if the renal function of a patient with postinfection GN progressively deteriorates, a renal biopsy should be performed.

The clinical presentation of GN is usually gross hematuria. Urine may be coffee-colored or tea-colored. Microscopic examination of urine reveals RBCs too numerous to

Table 22–1. Glomerular diseases encountered in childhood.

Entity	Clinical Course	Prognosis
Postinfection glomerulonephritis (GN). Onset occurs 10–14 d after acute illness, commonly streptococcal. Characteristics include acute onset, tea-colored urine, mild to severe renal insufficiency, and edema.	Acute phase is usually over in 2 wk. Complete resolution occurs in 95% of cases. Severity of renal failure and hypertension varies. Microhematuria may persist to 18 mo. Hypocomplementemia resolves in 1–30 d.	Excellent. Chronic disease is rare. Severe proteinuria, atypical presentation or course, or persistent hypocomplementemia suggest another entity.
Membranoproliferative GN. Presentation ranges from mild microhematuria to acute GN syndrome. Diagnosis is made by renal biopsy. Etiology is unknown. Types I and II are most common. Lesion is chronic.	Course can be mild to severe (rapid deterioration in renal function); may mimic postinfection GN. Proteinuria can be severe. Complement depression is intermittent to persistent. Hypertension is usually significant.	Type I may respond to corticosteroids. Type II (dense deposit disease) is less treatable; function decrease varies from immediate to as long as 15 y in 30–50% of untreated cases.
IgA nephropathy. Classic presentation is asymptomatic gross hematuria during acute unrelated illness, with microhematuria between episodes. Occasional instances of acute GN syndrome occur. Etiology is unknown. Diagnosis is made by biopsy.	90% of cases resolve in 1–5 y. Gross hematuric episodes resolve with recovery from acute illness. Severity of renal insufficiency and hypertension varies. Proteinuria occurs in more severe, atypical cases.	Generally good; a small percentage develops chronic renal failure. Proteinuria in the nephrotic range is a poor sign. There is no universally accepted medication. (Corticosteroids may be useful in severe cases.)
Henoch–Schönlein purpura GN. Degree of renal involvement varies. Asymptomatic microhematuria is most common, but GN syndrome can occur. Renal biopsy is recommended in severe cases; it can provide prognostic information.	Presentation varies with severity of renal lesion. In rare cases, may progress rapidly to serious renal failure. Hypertension varies. Proteinuria in the nephrotic range and severe decline in function can occur.	Overall, prognosis is good. Patients presenting with > 50% reduction in function or proteinuria exceeding 1 g/24 h may develop chronic renal failure. Severity of renal biopsy picture can best guide approach in such cases. There is no universally accepted medication.
GN of systemic lupus erythematosus (SLE). Microhematuria and proteinuria are rarely first signs of this systemic disease. Renal involvement varies, but severe GN may ensue with remissions and exacerbations throughout the course.	Renal involvement is mild to severe. Clinical complexity depends on degree of renal insufficiency and other systems involved. Hypertension is significant. Manifestations of the severity of the renal lesion guide therapeutic intervention.	Renal involvement accounts for most significant morbidity in SLE. Control of hypertension affects renal prognosis. Medication is guided by symptoms, serology, and renal lesion. End-stage renal failure can occur.
Hereditary GN (eg, Alport syndrome). Transmission is autosomal-dominant/X-linked, with family history marked by end-stage renal failure, especially in young males. Deafness and eye abnormalities are associated.	There is no acute syndrome. Females are generally less affected but are carriers. Hypertension and increasing proteinuria occur with advancing renal failure. There is no known treatment.	Progressive proteinuria and hypertension occur early, with gradual decline in renal function in those most severely affected. Disease progresses to end-stage renal failure in most males.

count. Microscopy may reveal RBC casts. If present, these are diagnostic of GN, but their absence does not exclude the diagnosis. Edema is often seen (periorbital, facial, extremities), caused by sodium and water retention resulting from alteration in glomerular function. Symptoms are usually nonspecific. In cases accompanied by hypertension (a common finding), headache may be present. Fever is uncommon. Severe glomerular injury (which usually occurs in severe, acute presentations of the more chronic or destructive forms of GN) may be accompanied by massive proteinuria (nephrotic syndrome), anasarca, ascites, and severe compromise of renal function.

Typical poststreptococcal GN has no specific treatment. Antibiotic therapy is indicated if an infection is still present. Disturbances in renal function and resulting hypertension may require close monitoring, reduction in salt intake, diuretics or other antihypertensive drugs. In severe cases of renal failure, hemodialysis or peritoneal dialysis may be

necessary. Corticosteroids may also be administered in an attempt to influence the course of the GN.

The acute abnormalities generally resolve in 2–3 weeks. Serum complement (C3) may be normal as early as 3 days or as late as 30 days after onset. Complement-consuming glomerulonephritides also include membranoproliferative GN (chronic GN with persistent complement depression) and lupus GN. (See Chapter 27.) Although microscopic hematuria may persist for as long as a year, 85% of children recover completely. Persistent deterioration in renal function, urinary abnormalities beyond 18 months, persistent hypocomplementemia, and nephrotic syndrome are ominous signs. If any of these is present, a renal biopsy is indicated.

2. IgA Nephropathy

When asymptomatic gross hematuria appears to accompany a minor acute febrile illness or other stressful occurrence, the diagnosis of IgA nephropathy may be entertained. In contrast to postinfection GN, IgA nephropathy is not associated with prior streptococcal infection, complement is not depressed, and in 50% of cases, serum immunoglobin A is elevated. Often there are no associated symptoms or signs. Gross hematuria resolves within days, and there are no serious sequelae in 85% of cases. Treatment is not indicated, and the prognosis is good in most cases. Prognosis is guarded, however, if severe proteinuria, hypertension, or renal insufficiency is present or develops. In such instances, although no treatment is universally accepted, corticosteroids and other immunosuppressive drugs are used. Omega-3 fatty acids from fish oils are thought to be helpful.

3. Henoch-Schönlein Purpura

The diagnosis of Henoch-Schönlein purpura rests on the presence of a typical maculopapular rash found primarily, but not exclusively, on the dorsal surfaces of the lower extremities and buttocks. Most children have abdominal pain and bloody diarrhea. Joint pain is common, and, depending on the extent of renal involvement, hypertension may be present. Joint and abdominal pain responds to treatment with corticosteroids. Renal involvement ranges from mild GN with microhematuria to severe GN and varying degrees of renal insufficiency. GN with massive proteinuria and renal insufficiency carries a poor prognosis. Twenty percent of such cases result in end-stage renal failure. There is no universally accepted treatment, but corticosteroids are often administered (see Chapter 28).

4. Membranoproliferative Glomerulonephritis

The most common "chronic" form of GN in childhood is membranoproliferative GN. The diagnosis is established from the histologic appearance of the glomeruli on biopsy tissue. There are two major histologic types of membranoproliferative GN. Clinically, type II carries the worse prognosis, as end-stage renal failure develops in most cases. Type I more often responds to treatment with corticosteroids. C3 is depressed (in both types) and may be useful as a marker of response to treatment.

5. Lupus Glomerulonephritis

The diagnosis of systemic lupus erythematosus is based on its numerous clinical features and abnormal laboratory findings that include a positive antinuclear antibody test, depressed serum complement, and increased serum double-stranded DNA. Renal involvement is indicated by varying degrees of hematuria and proteinuria. More severe cases are accompanied by renal insufficiency and hypertension. Significant renal involvement requires treatment with immunosuppressive drugs and close monitoring. End-stage renal failure develops in 10–15% of patients with childhood SLE.

6. Hereditary Glomerulonephritis

The most commonly encountered hereditary glomerulonephritis is Alport syndrome, characterized by hearing loss and GN, occurring predominantly in males. It is a chronic form of GN and thus does not present with the clinical features typically seen in patients with acute processes. A family history is generally present, but there is a spontaneous mutation rate of about 18%. In individuals with the progressive form of GN, end-stage renal failure occurs, usually in the second to third decade of life. Although currently there is no treatment for this disorder, careful management of associated hypertension may slow the process.

ACUTE INTERSTITIAL NEPHRITIS

Acute interstitial nephritis is characterized by diffuse or focal inflammation and edema of the renal interstitium and secondary involvement of the tubules. The condition is most commonly drug related (eg, β-lactam–containing antibiotics, such as methicillin).

Fever, rigor, abdominal or flank pain, and rashes may occur in drug-associated cases. Urinalysis usually reveals leukocyturia and hematuria. Hansel staining of the urinary sediment often demonstrates eosinophils. The inflammation can cause significant deterioration of renal function. If the diagnosis is unclear because of the absence of a history of drug or toxin exposure or the absence of eosinophils in the urine, a renal biopsy may be performed to demonstrate the characteristic tubular and interstitial inflammation. Immediate identification and removal of the causative agent is imperative and may be all that is necessary. Treatment with corticosteroids is helpful in patients with progressive renal insufficiency or nephrotic syndrome. Severe renal failure requires supportive dialysis.

Bergstein J et al: The clinical significance of asymptomatic gross and microscopic hematuria in children. Arch Pediatr Adolesc Med 2005;159:398 [PMID: 15809388].

Youn T et al: Clinical spectrum of gross hematuria in pediatric patients. Clin Pediatr (Phila) 2006;45:135 [PMID: 16528433].

PROTEINURIA & RENAL DISEASE

Urine is rarely completely protein-free, but the average excretion is well below 150 mg/24 h. Small increases in urinary protein can accompany febrile illnesses or exertion and in some cases occur while in the upright posture.

An algorithm for investigation of isolated proteinuria is presented in Figure 22–2. In idiopathic nephrotic syndrome without associated features of GN, treatment with corticosteroids may be initiated. Nephrologic advice or follow-up should be sought, especially in patients with difficult or frequently relapsing unexplained proteinuria.

CONGENITAL NEPHROSIS

Congenital nephrosis is a rare autosomal recessive disorder. The kidneys are pale and large and may show microcystic dilations (microcystic disease) of the proximal tubules and glomerular abnormalities, including proliferation, crescent formation, and thickening of capillary walls. The pathogenesis is not well understood.

Infants with congenital nephrosis commonly have low birth weight, a large placenta, wide cranial sutures, and delayed ossification. Mild edema may be seen after the first few weeks of life. Anasarca follows, and the abdomen can become greatly distended by ascites. Massive proteinuria associated with typical-appearing nephrotic syndrome and hyperlipidemia is the rule. Hematuria is common. If the patient lives long enough, progressive renal failure occurs. Most affected infants succumb to infections at the age of a few months.

Treatment prior to dialysis and transplantation has little to offer other than nutritional support and management of the chronic renal failure.

IDIOPATHIC NEPHROTIC SYNDROME OF CHILDHOOD (NIL DISEASE, LIPOID NEPHROSIS, MINIMAL CHANGE DISEASE)

Nephrotic syndrome is characterized by proteinuria, hypoproteinemia, edema, and hyperlipidemia. It may occur as a result of any form of glomerular disease and may rarely be associated with a several extrarenal conditions. In young children, the disease usually takes the form of idiopathic nephrotic syndrome of childhood (nil disease, lipoid nephrosis, minimal change disease), which has characteristic clinical and laboratory findings, but no well-understood cause.

▶ Clinical Findings

Affected patients are generally younger than age 6 years at onset. Typically, periorbital swelling and oliguria are noted, often following an influenza-like syndrome. Within a few days, increasing edema—even anasarca—becomes evident. Most children have few complaints other than vague malaise or abdominal pain. With significant "third spacing" of plasma volume, however, some children may present with hypotension. With marked edema, dyspnea due to pleural effusions may also occur.

Despite heavy proteinuria, the urine sediment is usually normal, although microscopic hematuria may be present. Plasma albumin concentration is low, and lipid levels increased. When azotemia occurs, it is usually secondary to intravascular volume depletion.

Glomerular morphology is unremarkable except for fusion of foot processes of the glomerular basement membrane. This nonspecific finding is associated with many proteinuric states.

▶ Complications

Infections (eg, peritonitis) sometimes occur, and pneumococci are frequently the cause. Hypercoagulability may be present, and thromboembolic phenomena are commonly reported. In patients with minimal change disease, hypertension can still be noted, and renal insufficiency can result from decreased renal perfusion.

▶ Treatment & Prognosis

As soon as the diagnosis of idiopathic nephrotic syndrome is made, corticosteroid treatment should be started. Prednisone, 2 mg/kg/d (maximum, 60 mg/d), is given for 6 weeks as a single daily dose. The same dose is then administered on an alternate-day schedule for 6 weeks; thereafter, the dose is tapered gradually and discontinued over the ensuing 2 months. The goal of this regimen is the disappearance of proteinuria. If remission is not achieved during the initial phase of corticosteroid treatment, additional nephrologic consultation should be obtained. If remission is achieved, only to be followed by relapse, the treatment course may be repeated. A renal biopsy is often considered when there is little or no response to treatment. One should take into account that the histologic findings may not alter the treatment plan, which is designed to eliminate the nephrotic syndrome regardless of underlying renal histology.

Unless the edema causes symptoms such as respiratory compromise due to ascites, diuretics should be used with extreme care. Patients may have decreased circulating volume and are also at risk for intravenous thrombosis. Careful restoration of compromised circulating volume with intravenous albumin infusion and administration of diuretics is helpful in mobilizing edema. Infections such as peritonitis should be treated promptly to reduce morbidity. Immunization with pneumococcal vaccine is advised.

A favorable response of proteinuria to corticosteroids and subsequent favorable response during relapse suggests a good prognosis. Failure to respond or early relapse usually heralds a prolonged series of relapses. This not only may indicate the presence of more serious nephropathy, but presents a challenge in choosing future therapy. Chlorambucil or cyclophosphamide drug therapy is usually effective only in children who respond to corticosteroids. Patients who do not respond to corticosteroids or who relapse frequently should be referred to a pediatric nephrologist. Intravenous Solu-Medrol may be helpful in more refractory cases. When the protracted use of corticosteroids raises concerns of toxicity, concomitant treatment with either cyclosporin A or tacrolimus appears to be helpful.

FOCAL GLOMERULAR SCLEROSIS

Focal glomerular sclerosis is one cause of corticosteroid-resistant or frequent relapsing nephrotic syndrome. The cause is unknown. The diagnosis is made by renal biopsy, which shows normal-appearing glomeruli as well as some partially or completely sclerosed glomeruli. The lesion has serious prognostic implications because as many as 15–20% of cases can progress to end-stage renal failure. The response to corticosteroid treatment is variable. In difficult cases, cyclosporin A or tacrolimus have been used in addition to corticosteroids. There are increasing reports that poorly responsive cases may respond to rituximab, a monoclonal antibody against the B-cell surface antigen CD20. Recurrence of focal glomerular sclerosis may occur after renal transplantation. The recurrence is usually treated with plasmapheresis or rituximab (this drug is finding encouraging utility in membranous or mesangial nephropathy as well as minimal change disease).

MESANGIAL NEPHROPATHY (MESANGIAL GLOMERULONEPHRITIS)

Mesangial nephropathy is another form of corticosteroid-resistant nephrotic syndrome. The renal biopsy shows a distinct increase in the mesangial matrix of the glomeruli. Very often the expanded mesangium contains deposits of IgM demonstrable on immunofluorescent staining. The cause is unknown. Corticosteroid therapy may induce remission, but relapses are common. Choices for treating this type of nephrotic syndrome are the same as noted earlier.

MEMBRANOUS NEPHROPATHY (MEMBRANOUS GLOMERULONEPHRITIS)

Although largely idiopathic in nature, membranous nephropathy can be found in association with hepatitis B antigenemia, systemic lupus erythematosus, congenital and secondary syphilis, renal vein thrombosis; with immunologic disorders such as autoimmune thyroiditis; and with administration of drugs such as penicillamine. The pathogenesis is unknown, but the glomerular lesion is thought to be the result of prolonged deposition of circulating antigen–antibody complexes.

The onset of membranous nephropathy may be insidious or may resemble that of idiopathic nephrotic syndrome of childhood (see earlier section). It occurs more often in older children and adults. The proteinuria of membranous nephropathy responds poorly to corticosteroid therapy, although low-dose corticosteroid therapy may reduce or delay development of chronic renal insufficiency. The diagnosis is made by renal biopsy.

Fine RN: Recurrence of nephrotic syndrome/focal segmental glomerulosclerosis following renal transplantation in children. Pediatr Nephrol 2007;22:496 [PMID: 17186280].

Gipson DS et al: Differential risk of remission and ESRD in childhood FSGS. Pediatr Nephrol 2006;21:344 [PMID: 16395603].

Kim JS et al: High incidence of initial and late steroid resistance in childhood nephrotic syndrome. Kidney Int 2005;68:1275 [PMID: 16105061].

▼ DISEASES OF THE RENAL VESSELS

RENAL VEIN THROMBOSIS

In newborns, renal vein thrombosis may complicate sepsis or dehydration. It may be observed in infants of diabetic mothers; may be associated with umbilical vein catheterization; or may result from any condition that produces a hypercoagulable state (eg, clotting factor deficiency, systemic lupus erythematosus, or thrombocytosis). Renal vein thrombosis is less common in older children and adolescents. It may develop following trauma or without any apparent predisposing factors. Spontaneous renal vein thrombosis has been associated with membranous glomerulonephropathy. Nephrotic syndrome may either cause or result from renal vein thrombosis.

▶ Clinical Findings

Renal vein thrombosis in newborns is generally characterized by the sudden development of an abdominal mass. If the thrombosis is bilateral, oliguria may be present; urine output may be normal with a unilateral thrombus. In older children, flank pain, sometimes with a palpable mass, is a common presentation.

No single laboratory test is diagnostic of renal vein thrombosis. Hematuria usually is present; proteinuria is less constant. In the newborn, thrombocytopenia may be found, but it is rare in older children. The diagnosis is made by ultrasonography and Doppler flow studies.

▶ Treatment

Anticoagulation with heparin is the treatment of choice in newborns and older children. In the newborn, a course of heparin combined with treatment of the underlying problem is usually all that is required. Management in other cases is less straightforward. The tendency for recurrence and embolization has led some to recommend long-term anticoagulation. If an underlying membranous GN is suspected, biopsy should be performed.

▶ Course & Prognosis

The mortality rate in newborns from renal vein thrombosis depends on the underlying cause. With unilateral thromboses, the prognosis for adequate renal function is good. Renal vein thrombosis may rarely recur in the same kidney or occur in the other kidney years after the original episode of thrombus formation. Extension into the vena cava with pulmonary emboli is possible.

RENAL ARTERIAL DISEASE

Arterial disease (eg, fibromuscular hyperplasia, congenital stenosis) is a rare cause of hypertension in children. Although few clinical clues are specific to underlying arterial lesions, they should be suspected in children with severe hypertension, with onset at or before age 10 years, or with delayed visualization on nuclear scan of the kidneys. The diagnosis is established by renal arteriography with selective renal vein renin measurements. Some of these lesions may be approached by transluminal angioplasty or surgery (see section on Hypertension, later), but repair may be technically impossible in small children. Although thrombosis of renal arteries is rare, it should be considered in a patient with acute onset of hypertension and hematuria in an appropriate setting (eg, in association with hyperviscosity or umbilical artery catheterization). Early diagnosis and treatment provides the best chance of reestablishing renal blood flow.

HEMOLYTIC-UREMIC SYNDROME

Hemolytic-uremic syndrome is the most common glomerular vascular cause of acute renal failure in childhood. It is usually the result of infection with Shigatoxin-producing (also called verotoxin-producing) strains of *Shigella* or *Escherichia coli*. Ingestion of undercooked ground beef or unpasteurized foods is a common source. There are many serotypes, but the most common pathogen in the United States is *E coli* O157:H7. Bloody diarrhea is the usual presenting complaint, followed by hemolysis and renal failure. Circulating verotoxin causes endothelial damage, which leads to platelet deposition, microvascular occlusion with subsequent hemolysis, and thrombocytopenia. Similar microvascular endothelial activation may also be triggered by drugs (eg, cyclosporin A); by viruses (HIV); and by pneumococcal infections, in which bacterial neuraminidase exposes the Thomsen-Friedenreich antigen on RBCs, platelets, and endothelial cells, thereby causing platelet aggregation, endothelial damage, and hemolysis. Rare cases are caused by genetic factors (eg, congenitally depressed C3 complement and factor H deficiency).

▶ Clinical Findings

The epidemic form begins with a prodrome of abdominal pain, diarrhea, and vomiting. Oliguria, pallor, and bleeding manifestations, principally gastrointestinal, occur next. Hypertension and seizures develop in some children—especially those who develop severe renal failure and fluid overload. There may also be significant endothelial involvement in the central nervous system (CNS).

Anemia is profound, and RBC fragments are seen on blood smears. A high reticulocyte count confirms the hemolytic nature of the anemia, but may not be noted in the presence of renal failure. Thrombocytopenia is profound, but other coagulation abnormalities are less consistent. Serum fibrin split products are often present, but fulminant disseminated intravascular coagulation is rare. Hematuria and proteinuria are often present. The serum complement level is normal except in those cases related to congenital predisposition.

▶ Complications

These usually result from renal failure. Neurologic problems, particularly seizures, may result from hyponatremia, hyper-

tension, or CNS vascular disease. Severe bleeding, transfusion requirements, and hospital-acquired infections must be anticipated.

▶ Treatment

Meticulous attention to fluid and electrolyte status is crucial. The use of antimotility agents and antibiotics is believed to worsen the disease. Antibiotics may up-regulate and cause the release of large amounts of bacterial Shiga toxin. Timely dialysis improves the prognosis. Since prostacyclin-stimulating factor, a potent inhibitor of platelet aggregation, may be absent in some cases, plasma infusion or plasmapheresis has been advocated in severe cases (generally in those cases with severe CNS involvement). Platelet inhibitors have also been tried, but the results have not been impressive, especially late in the disease. Nonetheless, using a platelet inhibitor early in the disease in an attempt to halt platelet consumption and microvascular occlusion may obviate the need for platelet transfusions and reduce the progression of renal failure. RBC and platelet transfusions may be necessary. Although the risk of volume overload is significant, this can be minimized by dialysis. Erythropoietin (epoetin alfa) treatment may reduce RBC transfusion needs. Although no therapy is universally accepted, strict control of hypertension, adequate nutrition support, and the timely use of dialysis reduce morbidity and mortality. If renal failure is "nonoliguric," and if urine output is sufficient to ensure against fluid overload and electrolyte abnormalities, management of renal failure without dialysis is possible.

▶ Course & Prognosis

Most commonly, children recover from the acute episode within 2–3 weeks. Some residual renal disease (including hypertension) occurs in about 30%, and end-stage renal failure occurs in about 15%. Thus follow-up of children recovering from hemolytic-uremic syndrome should include serial determinations of renal function for 1–2 years and monitoring of blood pressure for 5 years. Mortality (about 3–5%) is most likely in the early phase, primarily resulting from CNS or cardiac complications.

Repetto HA: Long-term course and mechanisms of progression of renal disease in hemolytic uremic syndrome. Kidney Int Suppl 2005;97:S102 [PMID: 16014085].

Siegler R, Oakes R: Hemolytic uremic syndrome; pathogenesis, treatment and outcome. Curr. Opin Pediatr 2005;17:200 [PMID: 15800412].

RENAL FAILURE

ACUTE RENAL FAILURE

Acute renal failure is the sudden inability to excrete urine of sufficient quantity or composition to maintain body fluid homeostasis. The most common cause in children is dehy-

Table 22–2. Classification of renal failure.

Prerenal
   Dehydration due to gastroenteritis, malnutrition, or diarrhea
   Hemorrhage, aortic or renal vessel injury, trauma, cardiac disease
     or surgery, renal arterial thrombosis
   Diabetic acidosis
   Hypovolemia associated with capillary leak or nephrotic syndrome
   Shock
   Heart failure
Renal
   Hemolytic-uremic syndrome
   Acute glomerulonephritis
   Prolonged renal hypoperfusion
   Nephrotoxins
   Acute tubular necrosis or vascular nephropathy
   Renal (cortical) necrosis
   Intravascular coagulation: septic shock, hemorrhage
   Diseases of renal vessels
   Iatrogenic disorders
   Severe infections
   Drowning, especially fresh water
   Crystalluria: sulfonamide or uric acid
   Hypercalcemia from cancer treatment
   Hepatic failure
Postrenal
   Obstruction due to tumor, hematoma, posterior urethral valves,
     ureteropelvic junction stricture, ureterovesical junction stricture,
     ureterocele
   Stones
   Trauma to a solitary kidney or collecting system
   Renal vein thrombosis

dration. However, encountering signs of acute renal insufficiency in a hospitalized patient raises many other possibilities: impaired renal perfusion or renal ischemia, acute renal disease, renal vascular compromise, acute tubular necrosis, or obstructive uropathy. Table 22–2 lists such prerenal, renal, and postrenal causes.

▶ Clinical Findings

The hallmark of early renal failure is oliguria. Although an exact etiologic diagnosis may be unclear at the onset, classifying oliguria as outlined in Table 22–2 is helpful in determining if an immediately reversible cause is present.

If the cause of elevation in serum BUN and creatinine or oliguria is unclear, entities that can be quickly addressed and corrected (eg, volume depletion) should be considered first. Once normal renal perfusion is ensured and no clinical evidence for de novo renal disease is present, a diagnosis of acute tubular necrosis (vasomotor nephropathy, ischemic injury) may be entertained.

A. Prerenal Causes

The most common cause of decreased renal function in children is compromised renal perfusion. It is usually sec-

Table 22–3. Urine studies.

	Prerenal Failure	Acute Tubular Necrosis
Urine osmolality	50 mOsm/kg > plasma osmolality	≤ plasma osmolality
Urine sodium	< 10 mEq/L	> 20 mEq/L
Ratio of urine creatinine to plasma creatinine	> 40:1	< 40:1
Specific gravity	> 1.020	1.012–1.018

ondary to dehydration, although abnormalities of renal vasculature and poor cardiac performance may also be considered. Table 22–3 lists the urinary indices helpful in distinguishing these "prerenal" conditions from true renal parenchymal insult, such as in acute tubular necrosis.

B. Renal Causes

Causes of renal failure intrinsic to the kidney include acute glomerulonephritides, hemolytic-uremic syndrome, acute interstitial nephritis, and nephrotoxic injury. The diagnosis of acute tubular necrosis (vasomotor nephropathy)—which is reserved for those cases in which renal ischemic insult is believed to be the likely cause—should be considered when correction of prerenal or postrenal problems does not improve renal function and there is no evidence of de novo renal disease.

C. Postrenal Causes

Postrenal failure, usually found in newborns with urologic anatomic abnormalities, is accompanied by varying degrees of renal insufficiency. The approach to the problem in the very young is addressed earlier in the chapter, but one should always keep in mind the possibility of acute urinary tract obstruction in acute renal failure, especially in the setting of anuria of acute onset.

▶ Complications

The clinical severity of the complications depends on the degree of renal functional impairment and oliguria. Common complications include (1) fluid overload (hypertension, congestive heart failure, pulmonary edema), (2) electrolyte disturbances (hyperkalemia), (3) metabolic acidosis, (4) hyperphosphatemia, and (5) uremia.

▶ Treatment

An indwelling bladder catheter is inserted to ascertain urine output. If urine volume is insignificant and renal failure is established, the catheter should be removed to minimize infection risk. Prerenal or postrenal factors should be excluded or rectified, and normal circulating volume maintained with appropriate fluids. Strict measurement of input and output must be maintained, and input adjusted as reduction in output dictates. The patient's response is assessed by physical examination and urinary output. Measurement of central venous pressure may be indicated. Increasing urine output with diuretics, such as furosemide (1–5 mg/kg, per dose, intravenously, maximum of 200 mg), can be attempted. The effective dose will depend on the amount of functional compromise (if < 50% function, initiate attempt at diuresis with maximum dose). If a response does not occur within 1 hour and the urine output remains low (< 0.5 mL/kg/h), the furosemide dose, if not already maximized, should be increased up to 5 mg/kg. In some cases the addition of a long-acting thiazide diuretic, such as metolazone, may improve the response. If no diuresis occurs with maximum dosing, further administration of diuretics should cease.

If these maneuvers stimulate some urine flow but biochemical evidence of acute renal failure persists, the resulting non-oliguric acute renal failure should be more manageable. Fluid overload and dialysis may be averted. However, if the medications and nutrients required exceed the urinary output, dialysis is indicated. Institution of dialysis before the early complications of acute renal failure develop is likely to improve clinical management and outcome. It is important to adjust medication dosage according to the degree of renal function.

A. Acute Dialysis: Indications

Immediate indications for dialysis are (1) severe hyperkalemia; (2) unrelenting metabolic acidosis (usually in a situation where fluid overload prevents sodium bicarbonate administration); (3) fluid overload with or without severe hypertension or congestive heart failure (a situation that would seriously compromise nutrition or drug administration); and (4) symptoms of uremia, usually manifested in children by CNS depression.

B. Methods of Dialysis

Peritoneal dialysis is generally preferred in children because of the ease of performance and patient tolerance. Although peritoneal dialysis is technically less efficient than hemodialysis, hemodynamic stability and metabolic control can be better sustained because this technique can be applied on a relatively continuous basis. Hemodialysis should be considered (1) if rapid removal of toxins is desired, (2) if the size of the patient makes hemodialysis less technically cumbersome and hemodynamically well tolerated, or (3) if impediments to efficient peritoneal dialysis are present (eg, ileus, adhesions). Furthermore, if vascular access and usage of anticoagulation are not impediments, a slow, continuous hemodialytic process (continuous renal replacement treatment) may be applied.

C. Complications of Dialysis

Complications of peritoneal dialysis include peritonitis, volume depletion, and technical complications such as dialysate leakage and respiratory compromise from intra-abdominal dialysate fluid. Peritonitis can be avoided by strict aseptic technique. Peritoneal fluid cultures are obtained as clinically indicated. Leakage is reduced by good catheter placement technique and appropriate intra-abdominal dialysate volumes. Dialysis is useful in maintaining electrolyte balance. Potassium (absent from standard dialysate solutions) can be added to the dialysate as required. Phosphate is also absent because hyperphosphatemia is an expected problem in renal failure. Nonetheless, if phosphate intake is inadequate, hypophosphatemia must be addressed. Correction of fluid overload is accomplished by using high osmolar dialysis fluids. Higher dextrose concentrations (maximum 4.25%) can correct fluid overload rapidly at the risk of causing hyperglycemia. Fluid removal may also be increased with more frequent exchanges of the dialysate, but rapid osmotic transfer of water may result in hypernatremia.

Even in small infants, hemodialysis can rapidly correct major metabolic and electrolyte disturbances, as well as volume overload. The process is highly efficient, but the speed of the changes can cause problems such as hemodynamic instability. Anticoagulation is usually required. Careful monitoring of the appropriate biochemical parameters is important. Note that during or immediately following the procedure, blood sampling will produce misleading results because equilibration between extravascular compartments and the blood will not have been achieved. Vascular access must be obtained and carefully monitored.

▶ Course & Prognosis

If severe oliguria occurs, it usually lasts about 10 days. Anuria or oliguria lasting longer than 3 weeks makes the diagnosis of acute tubular necrosis unlikely and favors alternative diagnoses such as vascular injury, severe ischemia (cortical necrosis), GN, or obstruction. The diuretic phase begins with an increase in urinary output to large volumes of isosthenuric urine containing sodium levels of 80–150 mEq/L. During the recovery phase, signs and symptoms subside rapidly, although polyuria may persist for several days or weeks. Urinary abnormalities usually disappear completely within a few months. If renal recovery does not ensue, arrangements are made for chronic dialysis and eventual renal transplantation.

Boydstun II: Acute renal failure. Adolesc Med Clin 2005;16:1 [PMID: 15844380].

Hui-Stickle S et al: Pediatric ARF epidemiology at a tertiary care center from 1999 to 2001. Am. J. Kidney Dis 2005;45:96 [PMID: 15696448].

CHRONIC RENAL FAILURE

Chronic renal failure in children most commonly results from developmental abnormalities of the kidneys or urinary tract. Infants with renal agenesis are not expected to survive. Depending on the degree of dysgenesis (including multicystic development) the resulting renal function will determine outcome. Abnormal development of the urinary tract may not permit normal renal development. Obstructive uropathy or severe vesicoureteral reflux nephropathy, without (or despite) surgical intervention, continues to cause a significant amount of progressive renal insufficiency in children. In older children, the chronic glomerulonephritides and nephropathies, irreversible nephrotoxic injury, or hemolytic-uremic syndrome may also cause chronic renal failure.

When chronic renal failure is congenital, the inability to concentrate urine results in polyuria. Affected patients often fail to thrive. Without medical care, children with long-standing chronic renal failure may present with complications such as rickets or anemia.

Chronic renal failure may follow acute GN or develop with chronic GN in the absence of an obvious acute episode. Growth failure depends on age at presentation and the rapidity of functional decline. Some of the chronic glomerulonephritides (eg, membranoproliferative GN) can progress unnoticed if subtle abnormalities of the urinary sediment are undetected or ignored. Any child with a history of chronic GN or significant renal injury needs close follow-up and monitoring of renal function and blood pressure.

Complications

Any remaining unaffected renal tissue can compensate for gradual loss of functioning nephrons in progressive chronic renal failure, but complications of renal insufficiency appear when compensatory ability is overwhelmed. In children who have developmentally reduced function and are unable to concentrate the urine, polyuria and dehydration are more likely to be problems than fluid overload. Output may be expected to gradually diminish as renal failure progresses to end stage; however, some children can continue to produce generous quantities of urine (but not of good quality) even though they require dialysis. A salt-wasting state can also occur. In contrast, children who develop chronic renal failure due to glomerular disease or renal injury will characteristically retain sodium and water and develop hypertension.

Metabolic acidosis and growth retardation occur early in chronic renal failure. Disturbances in calcium, phosphorus, and vitamin D metabolism leading to renal osteodystrophy require prompt attention. Although renal compensation and increased parathyroid hormone can maintain a normal serum phosphate level early in the course, this pathophysiologic response to hyperphosphatemia will be reflected by an increase in parathyroid hormone and alkaline phosphatase.

Uremic symptoms occur late in chronic renal failure, and include anorexia, nausea, and malaise. CNS features range from confusion, apathy, and lethargy to stupor and coma. Associated electrolyte abnormalities may precipitate seizures. More commonly, seizures are a result of untreated hypertension or hypocalcemia (especially with rapid correction of acidosis). Anemia (normochromic and normocytic from decreased renal erythropoietin synthesis) is common. Platelet dysfunction and other abnormalities of the coagula-

tion system may be present. Bleeding—especially gastrointestinal bleeding—may be a problem. Uremic pericarditis, congestive heart failure, pulmonary edema, and hypertension may occur.

▶ Treatment

A. Management of Complications

Treatment of chronic renal failure is primarily aimed at controlling the associated complications. Hypertension, hyperkalemia, hyperphosphatemia, acidosis, and anemia are among the early problems. Acidosis may be treated with sodium citrate solutions, as long as the added sodium will not aggravate hypertension. Sodium restriction is advisable when hypertension is present. Hyperphosphatemia is controlled by dietary restriction and dietary phosphate binders (eg, calcium carbonate). Vitamin D should be given to maintain normal serum calcium. When the BUN level exceeds approximately 50 mg/dL, or if the child is lethargic or anorexic, dietary protein should be restricted. Potassium restriction will be necessary as the GFR falls to a level where urinary output decreases sharply. Diet must be maintained to provide the child's daily requirements.

Renal function must be monitored regularly (creatinine and BUN), and serum electrolytes, calcium, phosphorus, alkaline phosphatase, and hemoglobin and hematocrit levels monitored to guide changes in fluid and dietary management as well as dosages of phosphate binder, citrate buffer, vitamin D, blood pressure medications, and epoetin alfa. Growth failure may be treated with human recombinant growth hormone. These treatment areas require careful monitoring to minimize symptoms while the need for chronic dialysis and transplantation continues to be assessed.

Care must be taken to avoid medications that aggravate hypertension; increase the body burden of sodium, potassium, or phosphate; or increase production of BUN. Successful management relies greatly on education of the patient and family.

Attention must also be directed toward the psychosocial needs of the patient and family as they adjust to chronic illness and the eventual need for dialysis and kidney transplantation.

B. Dialysis and Transplantation

At present the graft survival rate for living-related kidney transplants is 90% at 1 year, 85% at 2 years, and 75% at 5 years. With cadaveric transplantation, graft survivals are 76%, 71%, and 62%, respectively. Overall, the mortality rate is 4% for recipients of living-related donors and 6.8% for recipients of cadaver organs. These percentages are affected by the increased mortality, reported to be as high as 75% in infants younger than age 1 year, primarily due to technical issues and complications of immunosuppression. A body weight of at least 15 kg is associated with a significantly improved survival rate. Adequate growth and well-being are directly related to acceptance of the graft, the degree of normal function, and the side effects of medications.

Chronic peritoneal dialysis (home-based) and hemodialysis provide life-saving treatment for children awaiting renal transplantation. The best measure of the success of chronic dialysis in children is the level of physical and psychosocial rehabilitation achieved, such as continued participation in day-to-day activities and school attendance. Although catch-up growth rarely occurs, patients can grow at an acceptable rate even though they may remain in the lower percentiles. Use of epoetin alfa, growth hormone, and better control of renal osteodystrophy contribute to improved outcome.

Carey WA et al: Outcomes of dialysis initiated during the neonatal period for treatment of end-stage renal disease: A North American Pediatric Renal Trials and Collaborative Studies special analysis. Pediatrics 2007;119:468 [PMID: 17224455].

Chadha V, Warady BA: Epidemiology of pediatric chronic kidney disease. Adv Chronic Kidney Dis. 2005;12:343 [PMID: 16198273].

Gonzáles Celedón C et al: Progression of chronic renal failure in children with dysplastic kidneys. Pediatr Nephrol 2007;22:1014 [PMID: 17380351].

Seikaly MG et al: Stature in children with chronic kidney disease: analysis of NAPRTCS database. Pediatr Nephrol 2006;21:793 [PMID: 16583244].

HYPERTENSION

Hypertension in children is commonly of renal origin. It is anticipated as a complication of known renal parenchymal disease, but it may be found on routine physical examination in an otherwise normal child. Increased understanding of the roles of water and salt retention and overactivity of the renin-angiotensin system has done much to guide therapy; nevertheless, not all forms of hypertension can be explained by these two mechanisms.

The causes of renal hypertension in the newborn period include (1) congenital anomalies of the kidneys or renal vasculature, (2) obstruction of the urinary tract, (3) thrombosis of renal vasculature or kidneys, and (4) volume overload. Some instances of apparent paradoxic elevations of blood pressure have been reported in clinical situations in which chronic diuretic therapy is used, such as in bronchopulmonary dysplasia. Hypertensive infants should be examined for renal, vascular, or aortic abnormalities (eg, thrombosis, neurofibromatosis, coarctation) as well as some endocrine disorders, including pheochromocytoma and glucocorticoid-remedial aldosteronism.

Clinical Findings

A child is normotensive if the average recorded systolic and diastolic blood pressures are lower than the 90th percentile for age and sex. The 90th percentile in the newborn period is approximately 85–90/55–65 mm Hg for both sexes. In the first year of life, the acceptable levels are 90–100/60–67 mm Hg. Incremental increases with growth occur, gradually approaching young adult ranges of 100–120/65–75 mm Hg in the late teens. Careful measurement of blood pressure requires correct cuff size and reliable equipment. The cuff should be wide enough to cover two thirds of the upper arm and should encircle the arm completely without an overlap in the inflatable bladder. Although an anxious child may have an elevation in blood pressure, abnormal readings must not be too hastily attributed to this cause. Repeat measurement is helpful, especially after the child has been consoled.

Routine laboratory studies include a complete blood count, urinalysis, and urine culture. Radiography and ultrasonography are used to study the anatomy of the urinary tract, the blood flow to the kidneys, and their function. A renal biopsy (which rarely reveals the cause of hypertension unless clinical evidence of renal disease is present) should always be undertaken with special care in the hypertensive patient and preferably after pressures have been controlled by therapy. Figure 22–3 presents a suggested approach to the outpatient workup of hypertension.

Treatment

A. Acute Hypertensive Emergencies

A hypertensive emergency exists when CNS signs of hypertension appear, such as papilledema or encephalopathy. Retinal hemorrhages or exudates indicate a need for prompt and effective control. In children, end-organ abnormalities secondary to hypertension commonly are not present. Treatment varies with the clinical presentation. The primary classes of useful antihypertensive drugs are (1) diuretics, (2) α- and β-adrenergic blockers, (3) angiotensin-converting enzyme inhibitors, (4) calcium channel blockers, and (5) vasodilators.

Whatever method is used to control emergent hypertension, medications for sustained control should also be initiated so that normal blood pressure will be maintained when the emergent measures are discontinued (Table 22–4). Acute elevations of blood pressure not exceeding the 95th percentile for age may be treated with oral antihypertensives, aiming for progressive improvement and control within 48 hours.

1. Sublingual nifedipine—This calcium channel blocker is rapid acting, and, in appropriate doses, should not result in hypotensive blood pressure levels. The liquid from a 10-mg capsule can be drawn into a syringe and the dosage approximated. The exact dosage for children who weigh less than 10–30 kg is difficult to ascertain by this method, but 5 mg is a safe starting point. Because the treatment is given for rising blood pressure, it is unlikely that the effects will be greater than desired. Larger children with malignant hypertension require 10 mg. In such cases, the capsule may simply be pierced and the medication squeezed under the patient's tongue.

2. Intravenous hydralazine—This vasodilator is sometimes effective. Dosage varies according to the severity of the hypertension and should begin at about 0.15 mg/kg.

Initial data: Physical examination, including BP (for extremity history), UA, BUN, Cr, electrolytes, peripheral renin (electrocardiogram, chest x-ray, urine metanephrines, catechols). Obtain cardiac ECHO when suspecting coarctation of aorta. If present refer for surgical correction.

Normal initial data → Mild ↑BP, older age child, and family history → Treat and follow → Difficult Treatment; Severe or difficult to control BP (suspected renovascular hypertension)

Renal ultrasound with Doppler study — — — — Captopril enhanced scan or mRA

Abnormal initial data → Renal → C3, ANA, renal ultrasound → Nephrology referral; Nonrenal → Appropriate diagnostic steps and referral

Normal anatomy Treat BP and follow → Repeat initial workup, renal vein renin, or arteriography (digital subtraction angiography)

Abnormal renal anatomy (eg. scarring, atrophy, cysts) → Surgical → Resolved / Persistent ↑BP; Nonsurgical

Vascular flow discrepancy → Digital subtraction angiography or arteriography, ± renal vein renins → Normal / Abnormal → Transluminal angioplasty or vascular surgery

Abnormal; Normal

Continue treatment and follow ← Continued ↑BP ← Transluminal angioplasty or vascular surgery

Reevaluate? ← ; Follow-up ← Resolution ←

▲ **Figure 22–3.** Approach to the outpatient workup of hypertension. ANA, antinuclear antibody; BP, blood pressure; BUN, blood urea nitrogen; C3, complement; Cr, creatinine; mRA, magnetic resonance angiography; UA, urinalysis.

3. Sodium nitroprusside—In an intensive care setting, this powerful vasodilator is very effective for reducing severely elevated blood pressure. Intravenous administration of 0.5–10 mg/kg/min will reduce blood pressure in seconds; the dose must be monitored carefully. Metabolism of the drug results in thiocyanate; thus, with prolonged usage, levels of thiocyanate must be monitored, especially in renal insufficiency.

4. Furosemide—Administered at 1–5 mg/kg intravenously, this diuretic reduces blood volume and enhances the effectiveness of antihypertensive drugs.

B. Sustained Hypertension

Several choices are available (Table 22–5). A single drug such as a β-blocker (unless contraindicated, eg, in reactive airway disease) may be adequate to treat mild hypertension. Diuretics are useful to treat renal insufficiency, but the disadvantages of possible electrolyte imbalance must be considered. Single-drug therapy with an angiotensin-converting enzyme inhibitor is useful, especially because most hypertension in children is renal in origin. Calcium channel blockers are increasingly useful, and appear well tolerated in children. The use of the vasodilator type of antihypertensive drug requires concomitant

Table 22–4. Antihypertensive drugs for emergent treatment.

Drug	Oral Dose	Major Side Effects[a]
Nifedipine	0.25–0.5 mg/kg SL	Flushing, tachycardia
Labetalol	1–3 mg/kg/h IV	Secondary to β-blocking activity
Sodium nitroprusside	0.5–10 mg/kg/min IV drip	Cyanide toxicity, sodium and water retention
Furosemide	1–5 mg/kg IV	Secondary to severe volume contraction, hypokalemia
Diazoxide	2–10 mg/kg IV bolus	Hyperglycemia, hyperuricemia, sodium and water retention
Hydralazine	0.1–0.2 mg/kg IV	Sodium and water retention, tachycardia, flushing

[a]Many more side effects than those listed have been reported.
IV, intravenous; SL, sublingual.

Table 22–5. Antihypertensive drugs for ambulatory treatment.

Drug	Oral Dose	Major Side Effects[a]
Hydrochlorothiazide	2–4 mg/kg/24 h as single dose or in 2 individual doses	Potassium depletion, hyperuricemia
Furosemide	1–5 mg/kg per dose, 2–3 doses per day	Potassium and volume depletion
Hydralazine	0.75 mg/kg/24 h in 4–6 divided doses	Lupus erythematosus, tachycardia, headache
Amlodipine	0.2–0.5 mg/kg/d in 2 divided doses	Fatigue, headache, facial flushing
Propranolol	0.2–5 mg/kg per dose, 2–3 doses per day	Syncope, cardiac failure, hypoglycemia
Minoxidil	0.15 mg/kg per dose, 2–3 doses per day	Tachycardia, angina, fluid retention, hirsutism
Captopril	0.3–2 mg/kg per dose, 2–3 doses per day	Rash, hyperkalemia, glomerulopathy
Enalapril	0.2–0.5 mg/kg/d in 2 divided doses	Proteinuria, cough, hyperkalemia
Nifedipine	0.5–1 mg/kg/d, 3 doses per day	Flushing, tachycardia
Verapamil	3–7 mg/kg/d in 2 or 3 divided doses	AV conduction disturbance

[a]Many more side effects than those listed have been reported.
AV, atrioventricular.

administration of a diuretic to counter the effect of vasodilation on increasing renal sodium and water retention and a β-blocker to counter reflex tachycardia. Minoxidil, considered the most powerful of the orally administered vasodilators, can be extremely efficacious in the treatment of severe, sustained hypertension, but its effect is greatly offset by the other effects described. Hirsutism is a significant side effect. Hydralazine hydrochloride may still be the most common vasodilator in pediatric use—but, again, the necessity of using two additional drugs for maximum benefit relegates to severe situations calling for management with three or four drugs. The advice of a pediatric nephrologist should be sought.

Falkner B: Hypertension in children. Pediatr Ann. 2006;35:795 [PMID: 17153125].

Hogg RJ et al: A multicenter study of the pharmacokinetics of lisinopril in pediatric patients with hypertension. Pediatr Nephrol 2007;22:695 [PMID: 17216247].

INHERITED OR DEVELOPMENTAL DEFECTS OF THE KIDNEY

There are many developmental, hereditary, or metabolic defects of the kidneys and collecting system. The clinical consequences include metabolic abnormalities, failure to thrive, nephrolithiasis, renal glomerular or tubular dysfunction, and chronic renal failure. Table 22–6 lists some of the major entities; discussion of the rarer conditions is beyond the scope of this book.

DISORDERS OF THE RENAL TUBULES

Three subtypes of renal tubular acidosis (RTA) are recognized: (1) the classic form, called type I or distal RTA; (2) the bicarbonate-wasting form, called type II or proximal RTA; and (3) type IV, or hyperkalemic RTA (rare in children), which is associated with hyporeninemic hypoaldosteronism. Type I and type II and their variants are encountered most frequently in children. Type III is a combination of types I and II.

Primary tubular disorders in childhood, such as glycinuria, hypouricemia, or renal glycosuria, may result from a defect in a single tubular transport pathway (see Table 22–6).

1. Distal Renal Tubular Acidosis (Type I)

The most common form of distal RTA in childhood is the hereditary form. The clinical presentation is one of failure to thrive, anorexia, vomiting, and dehydration. Hyperchloremic metabolic acidosis, hypokalemia, and a urinary pH exceeding 6.5 is found. Acidosis is more severe in the presence of a bicarbonate "leak." This variant of distal RTA with bicarbonate wasting has been called type III but for clinical purposes need not be considered as a distinct entity. Concomitant hypercalciuria may lead to rickets, nephrocalcinosis, nephrolithiasis, and renal failure.

Other situations that may be responsible for distal RTA are found in some of the entities listed in Table 22–6.

Table 22–6. Inherited or developmental defects of the urinary tract.

Cystic diseases of genetic origin	**Hereditary renal diseases associated with tubular transport defects**
Polycystic disease	Hartnup disease
Autosomal recessive form (infantile)	Fanconi anemia
Autosomal dominant form (adult)	Oculocerebrorenal syndrome of Lowe
Other syndromes that include either form	Cystinosis (infantile, adolescent, adult types)
Cortical cysts	Wilson disease
Several syndromes are known to have various renal cystic manifesta-	Galactosemia
tions, including "simple" cysts; may not have significant effect on	Hereditary fructose intolerance
renal functional status or be associated with progressive disease	Renal tubular acidosis (many types)
Medullary cysts	Hereditary tyrosinemia
Medullary sponge kidney	Renal glycosuria
Medullary cystic disease (nephronophthisis)	Vitamin D-resistant rickets
Hereditary and familial cystic dysplasia	Pseudohypoparathyroidism
Congenital nephrosis	Vasopressin-resistant diabetes insipidus
"Finnish" disease	Hypouricemia
Dysplastic renal diseases	**Hereditary diseases associated with lithiasis**
Renal aplasia (unilateral, bilateral)	Hyperoxaluria
Renal hypoplasia (unilateral, bilateral, total, segmental)	L-Glyceric aciduria
Multicystic renal dysplasia (unilateral, bilateral, multilocular, postobstructive)	Xanthinuria
Familial and hereditary renal dysplasias	Lesch-Nyhan syndrome and variants, gout
Oligomeganephronia	Nephropathy due to familial hyperparathyroidism
Hereditary diseases associated with nephritis	Cystinuria (types I, II, III)
Hereditary nephritis with deafness and ocular defects (Alport syndrome)	Glycinuria
Nail-patella syndrome	**Miscellaneous**
Familial hyperprolinemia	Hereditary intestinal vitamin B_{12} malabsorption
Hereditary nephrotic syndrome	Total and partial lipodystrophy
Hereditary osteolysis with nephropathy	Sickle cell anemia
Hereditary nephritis with thoracic asphyxiant dystrophy syndrome	Bartter syndrome
Hereditary diseases associated with intrarenal deposition of metabolites	
Angiokeratoma corporis diffusum (Fabry disease)	
Heredopathia atactica polyneuritiformis (Refsum disease)	
Various storage diseases (eg, G_{M1} monosialogangliosidosis, Hurler syndrome,	
Niemann-Pick disease, familial metachromatic leukodystrophy, glycogeno-	
sis type I [von Gierke disease], glycogenosis type II [Pompe disease])	
Hereditary amyloidosis (familial Mediterranean fever, heredofamilial urti-	
caria with deafness and neuropathy, primary familial amyloidosis with	
polyneuropathy)	

Distal RTA results from a defect in the distal nephron, in the tubular transport of hydrogen ion, or in the maintenance of a steep enough gradient for proper excretion of hydrogen ion. This defect can be accompanied by degrees of bicarbonate wasting.

The classic test for distal RTA is an acid load from NH_4Cl. The test is cumbersome and can produce severe acidosis. A clinical trial of alkali administration should be used to rule out proximal (type II) RTA. The dose of alkali required to achieve a normal plasma bicarbonate concentration in patients with distal RTA is low (seldom exceeding 2–3 mEq/kg/24 h)—in contrast to that required in proximal RTA (> 10 mEq/kg/24 h). Higher doses are needed, however, if distal RTA is accompanied by bicarbonate wasting. Correction of acidosis can result in reduced complications and improved growth.

Distal RTA is usually permanent, although it sometimes occurs as a secondary complication. If the defect is not caused by a significant tubular disorder and renal damage is prevented, the prognosis is good.

2. Proximal Renal Tubular Acidosis (Type II)

Proximal RTA, the most common form of RTA in childhood, is characterized by an alkaline urine pH, loss of bicarbonate in the urine, and mildly reduced serum bicarbonate concentration. This occurs as a result of a lower than normal bicarbonate threshold, above which bicarbonate appears in the urine. Thus, urinary acidification can occur when the concentration of serum bicarbonate drops below that threshold, and bicarbonate disappears from the urine; this ability to eventually acidify the urine thus reflects normal distal tubular function.

Proximal RTA is often an isolated defect, and in the newborn can be considered an aspect of renal immaturity. Onset in infants is accompanied by failure to thrive, hyperchloremic acidosis, hypokalemia, and, rarely, nephrocalcinosis. Secondary forms result from reflux or obstructive uropathy or occur in association with other tubular disorders (see Table 22–6). Proximal RTA requires more than 3 mEq/kg of alkali per day to correct the acidosis. Serum bicarbonate should be monitored weekly until a level of at least 20 mEq/L is attained.

Citrate solutions (eg, Bicitra, Polycitra) are somewhat more easily tolerated than sodium bicarbonate. Bicitra contains 1 mEq/mL of Na^+ and citrate. Polycitra contains 2 mEq/mL of citrate and 1 mEq each of Na^+ and K^+. The required daily dosage is divided into three doses. Potassium supplementation may be required, because the added sodium load presented to the distal tubule may exaggerate potassium losses.

The prognosis is excellent in cases of isolated defects, especially when the problem is related to renal immaturity. Alkali therapy can usually be discontinued after several months to 2 years. Growth should be normal, and the gradual increase in the serum bicarbonate level to greater than 22 mEq/L heralds the presence of a raised bicarbonate threshold in the tubules. If the defect is part of a more complex tubular abnormality (Fanconi syndrome with attendant phosphaturia, glycosuria, and amino aciduria), the prognosis depends on the underlying disorder or syndrome.

OCULOCEREBRORENAL SYNDROME (LOWE SYNDROME)

Lowe syndrome results from various mutations in the *ORCL1* gene, which codes for a Golgi apparatus phosphatase. Affected males have anomalies involving the eyes, brain, and kidneys. The physical stigmata and degree of mental retardation vary with the location of the mutation. In addition to congenital cataracts and buphthalmos, the typical facies includes prominent epicanthal folds, frontal prominence, and a tendency to scaphocephaly. Muscle hypotonia is a prominent finding. The renal abnormalities are of tubule function and include hypophosphatemic rickets with low serum phosphorus levels, low to normal serum calcium levels, elevated serum alkaline phosphatase levels, RTA, and aminoaciduria. Treatment includes alkali therapy, phosphate replacement, and vitamin D. Antenatal diagnosis is possible.

CONGENITAL HYPOKALEMIC ALKALOSIS (BARTTER SYNDROME & GITELMAN SYNDROME)

Bartter syndrome is characterized by severe hypokalemic, hypochloremic metabolic alkalosis, extremely high levels of circulating renin and aldosterone, and a paradoxic absence of hypertension. On renal biopsy, a striking juxtaglomerular hyperplasia is seen.

A neonatal form of Bartter syndrome is thought to result from mutations in two genes affecting either $Na^+–K^+$ or K^+ transport. These patients have life-threatening episodes of fever and dehydration with hypercalciuria and early-onset nephrocalcinosis. Classic Bartter syndrome presenting in infancy with polyuria and growth retardation (but not nephrocalcinosis) is thought to result from mutations in a chloride channel gene. Gitelman syndrome occurs in older children and features episodes of muscle weakness, tetany, hypokalemia, and hypomagnesemia. These children have hypocalciuria.

Treatment with prostaglandin inhibitors and potassium-conserving diuretics (eg, amiloride combined with magnesium supplements) and potassium may be beneficial. Although the prognosis is guarded, a few patients seem to have less severe forms of the disease that are compatible with long survival times.

CYSTINOSIS

There are three types of cystinosis: adult, adolescent, and infantile. The adolescent type is characterized by cystine deposition, which if not treated with phosphocysteamine (Cystagon), is accompanied by the development of the renal Fanconi syndrome and varying degrees of renal failure. Growth is usually normal. The infantile type is the most common and the most severe. Characteristically, children present in the first or second year of life with Fanconi syndrome and, without the metabolic benefit of Cystagon treatment, progress to end-stage renal failure.

Cystinosis results from mutations in the *CTNS* gene, which codes for a cystine transporter. About 50% of patients share an identical deletion. Inheritance is autosomal recessive. Cystine is stored in cellular lysosomes in virtually all tissues. Eventually, cystine accumulation results in cell damage and cell death, particularly in the renal tubules. Renal failure between ages 6 and 12 years is common.

Whenever the diagnosis of cystinosis is suspected, slit-lamp examination of the corneas should be performed. Cystine crystal deposition causes an almost pathognomonic ground-glass "dazzle" appearance. Increased white cell cystine levels are diagnostic. Hypothyroidism is common.

Cystagon therapy is helpful in the treatment of cystinosis. Depending on the progression of chronic renal failure, management is directed toward all side effects of renal failure, with particular attention paid to the control of renal osteodystrophy. Dialysis and transplantation may be needed.

NEPHROGENIC DIABETES INSIPIDUS

The congenital X-linked recessive form of nephrogenic diabetes insipidus results from mutations in the vasopressin receptor, *AVPR2*. Autosomal (recessive and dominant) forms of nephrogenic diabetes insipidus are caused by mutations of the *AQP2* gene that codes for a water channel protein, aquaporin-2. Genetic counseling and mutation testing are available.

The symptoms are polyuria, polydipsia, and failure to thrive. In some children, particularly if the solute intake is unrestricted, adjustment to an elevated serum osmolality may develop. These children are particularly susceptible to episodes of dehydration, fever, vomiting, and convulsions.

The diagnosis can be suspected on the basis of a history of polydipsia and polyuria insensitive to the administration of vasopressin, desmopressin acetate, or lypressin. The diagnosis is confirmed by performing a vasopressin test. Carefully monitored water restriction does not increase the tubular reabsorption of water (TcH_2O) to above 3 mL/min/m^2. Urine osmolality remains lower than 450 mOsm/kg, whereas serum osmolality rises and total body weight falls. Before weight reduction of more than 5% occurs or before serum osmolality exceeds 320 mOsm/kg, vasopressin should be administered. Urine concentrating ability is impaired in a number of conditions—sickle cell anemia, pyelonephritis, potassium depletion, hypercalcemia, cystinosis and other renal tubular disorders, and obstructive uropathy—and as a result of nephrotoxic drugs. Children receiving lithium treatment should be monitored for the development of nephrogenic diabetes insipidus.

In infants, it is usually best to allow water as demanded and to restrict salt. Serum sodium levels should be evaluated at intervals to avoid hyperosmolality from inadvertent water restriction. In later childhood, sodium intake should continue to be restricted to 2.0–2.5 mEq/kg/24 h.

Treatment with hydrochlorothiazide is helpful, and many patients show improvement with administration of prostaglandin inhibitors such as indomethacin or tolmetin.

NEPHROLITHIASIS

Renal calculi in children may result from inborn errors of metabolism, such as cystine in cystinosis, glycine in hyperglycinuria, urates in Lesch-Nyhan syndrome, and oxalates in oxalosis. Stones may occur secondary to hypercalciuria in distal tubular acidosis, and large stones are quite often seen in children with spina bifida who have paralyzed lower limbs. Treatment is limited to that of the primary condition, if possible. Surgical removal of stones should be considered only for obstruction, intractable severe pain, and chronic infection.

1. Cystinuria

Cystinuria, like Hartnup disease and several other disorders, is primarily an abnormality of amino acid transport across both the enteric and proximal renal tubular epithelium. There are at least three biochemical types. In the first type, the bowel transport of basic amino acids and cystine is impaired, but transport of cysteine is not impaired. In the renal tubule, basic amino acids are again rejected by the tubule, but cystine absorption appears to be normal. The reason for cystinuria remains obscure. Heterozygous individuals have no aminoaciduria. The second type is similar to the first except that heterozygous individuals excrete excess cystine and lysine in the urine, and cystine transport in the bowel is normal. In the

third type, only the nephron is involved. The only clinical manifestations are related to stone formation: ureteral colic, dysuria, hematuria, proteinuria, and secondary urinary tract infection (UTI). Urinary excretion of cystine, lysine, arginine, and ornithine is increased.

The most reliable way to prevent stone formation is to maintain a constantly high free-water clearance. This involves generous fluid intake. Alkalinization of the urine is helpful. If these measures do not prevent significant renal lithiasis, the use of tiopronin (Thiola) is recommended.

2. Primary Hyperoxaluria

Oxalate in humans is derived from the oxidative deamination of glycine to glyoxylate, from the serine-glycolate pathway, and from ascorbic acid. At least two enzymatic blocks have been described. Type I is a deficiency of liver-specific peroxisomal alanine–glyoxylate aminotransferase. Type II is glyoxylate reductase deficiency.

Excess oxalate combines with calcium to form insoluble deposits in the kidneys, lungs, and other tissues, beginning during childhood. The joints are occasionally involved, but the main effect is on the kidneys, where progressive oxalate deposition leads to fibrosis and eventual renal failure.

Pyridoxine supplementation and a low-oxalate diet have been tried as therapy, but the overall prognosis is poor, and most patients succumb to uremia by early adulthood. Renal transplantation is not very successful because of destruction of the transplant kidney. However, encouraging results have been obtained with concomitant liver transplantation, correcting the metabolic defect.

Hyperoxaluria may also be a consequence of severe ileal disease or ileal resection.

URINARY TRACT INFECTIONS

It is estimated that 8% of girls and 2% of boys will acquire UTIs in childhood. Girls older than age 6 months have UTIs far more commonly than boys, whereas uncircumcised boys younger than 3 months of age have more UTIs than girls. Circumcision reduces the risk of UTI in boys. The density of distal urethral and periurethral bacterial colonization with uropathogenic bacteria correlates with the risk of UTI in children. Most UTIs are ascending infections. Specific adhesins present on the fimbria of uropathogenic bacteria allow colonization of the uroepithelium in the urethra and bladder and increase the likelihood of UTI.

▶ Pathogenesis

Dysfunctional voiding, which is uncoordinated relaxation of the urethral sphincter during voiding, leads to incomplete emptying of the bladder, increasing the risk of bacterial colonization. Similarly, any condition that interferes with complete emptying of the bladder, such as constipation or neurogenic bladder, increases the risk of UTI. Poor perineal hygiene, structural abnormalities of the urinary tract, catheterization, instrumentation of the urinary tract, and sexual activity increase the risk as well.

The inflammatory response to pyelonephritis may produce renal parenchymal scars. Such scars in infancy and childhood may contribute to hypertension, renal disease, and renal failure later in life. The organisms most commonly responsible for UTI are fecal flora, most commonly *E coli* (> 85%), *Klebsiella, Proteus,* other gram-negative bacteria, and, less frequently, *Enterococcus* or coagulase-negative staphylococci.

► Clinical Findings

A. Symptoms and Signs

Newborns and infants with UTI have nonspecific signs, including fever, hypothermia, jaundice, poor feeding, irritability, vomiting, failure to thrive, and sepsis. Strong, foul-smelling or cloudy urine may be noted. Preschool children may have abdominal or flank pain, vomiting, fever, urinary frequency, dysuria, urgency, or enuresis. School-aged children commonly have classic signs of cystitis (frequency, dysuria, and urgency) or pyelonephritis (fever, vomiting, and flank pain). Costovertebral tenderness is unusual in young children, but may be demonstrated by school-aged children. Physical examination should include attention to blood pressure determination, abdominal examination, and a genitourinary examination. Urethritis, poor perineal hygiene, herpes simplex virus, or other genitourinary infections may be apparent on examination.

B. Laboratory Findings

Collection of urine for urinalysis and culture is difficult in children due to frequent contamination of the sample. In toilet-trained, cooperative, older children, a midstream, clean-catch method is satisfactory. Although cleaning of the perineum does not improve specimen quality, straddling of the toilet to separate the labia in girls, retraction of the foreskin in boys, and collecting midstream urine significantly reduce contamination. In infants and young children, bladder catheterization or suprapubic collection is necessary in most cases to avoid contaminated samples. Bagged urine specimens are helpful only if negative.

Screening urinalysis indicates pyuria (> 5 WBCs/high-power field) in most children with UTI, but many children with pyuria do not have UTI. White cells from the urethra or vagina may be present in urine or may be in the urine because of a systemic infection. The leukocyte esterase test correlates well with pyuria, but has a similar false-positive rate. The detection of urinary nitrite by dipstick is highly correlated with enteric organisms being cultured from urine. Most young children (70%) with UTI have negative nitrite tests. They empty their bladders frequently, and it requires several hours for bacteria to convert ingested nitrates to nitrite in the bladder. The sensitivity of nitrite detection is highest on a first morning void. Gram stain of unspun urine correlates well with culture recovery of 10^5 colony-forming units (cfu)/mL or more, but this test is frequently unavailable outside the hospital.

The gold standard for diagnosis remains the culture of a properly collected urine specimen. Specimens that are not immediately cultured should be refrigerated and kept cold during transport. Any growth is considered significant from a suprapubic culture. Quantitative recovery of 10^5 cfu/mL or more is considered significant on clean-catch specimens, and 10^4–10^5 is considered significant on catheterized specimens. Usually the recovery of multiple organisms indicates contamination, but some contaminated specimens yield only a single species.

Asymptomatic bacteriuria is detected in 0.5–1.0% of children who are screened with urine culture. Asymptomatic bacteriuria is believed to represent colonization of the urinary tract with nonuropathogenic bacteria. Treatment may increase the risk of symptomatic UTI by eliminating non-pathogenic colonization. Screening urine cultures in non-symptomatic children are, therefore, generally discouraged. Repeated urine cultures are often helpful in differentiating asymptomatic bacteriuria from contamination of the culture versus true UTI.

Urinary function during UTI should be assessed by measurement of BUN and serum creatinine concentration.

C. Imaging

Because congenital urologic abnormalities increase the risk of UTI, radiologic evaluation of first UTI has been routinely recommended. These recommendations usually include routine ultrasound of the kidneys and voiding cystourethrogram (VCUG). Vesicoureteral reflux (VUR) is a congenital abnormality present in about 1% of the population. VUR is graded using the international scale (I—reflux into ureter; II—reflux to the kidney; III—reflux to kidney with dilation of ureter only; IV—reflux with dilation of ureter and mild blunting of renal calyces; V—reflux with dilation of ureter and blunting of renal calyces). Reflux is detected in 30–50% of children 1 year of age and younger. The natural history of reflux is to improve, and 80% of reflux of grades I, II, or III will resolve or significantly improve within 3 years following detection.

VCUG should be done selectively on children with a first UTI. Children with a suspected urologic abnormality due to weak stream, dribbling, or perineal abnormalities should be studied with VCUG. Boys with a first UTI should be studied to detect posterior urethral valves, an important congenital abnormality that requires surgery. Children older than 3 years of age who are otherwise healthy and growing well usually can be followed clinically and do not need VCUG for a first UTI. The yield in sexually active teenagers is also very low.

Ultrasonographic examination of kidneys should be done in children with acute pyelonephritis who have not improved after 3–5 days of antimicrobial treatment adjusted for the susceptibility of the organism. The examination is done to detect renal or perirenal abscesses or obstruction of the kidney.

Treatment

A. Antibiotic Therapy

Management of UTI is influenced by clinical assessment. Very young children (younger than 3 months) and children with dehydration, toxicity, or sepsis should be admitted to the hospital and treated with parenteral antimicrobials. Older infants and children who are not seriously ill can be treated as outpatients. Initial antimicrobial therapy is based on prior history of infection and antimicrobial use, as well as location of the infection in the urinary tract.

Uncomplicated cystitis can be treated with amoxicillin, trimethoprim–sulfamethoxazole, or a first-generation cephalosporin. These antimicrobials are concentrated in the lower urinary tract, and high cure rates are common. There are significant differences in the rates of antimicrobial resistance, so knowledge of the rates in the local community is important. More seriously ill children are initially treated parenterally with a third-generation cephalosporin or aminoglycoside. The initial antimicrobial choice is adjusted after culture and susceptibility are known. The recommended duration of antimicrobial therapy for uncomplicated cystitis is 7–10 days. For sexually mature teenagers with cystitis, fluoroquinolones such as ciprofloxacin and levofloxacin for 3 days are effective and cost-effective. Short-course therapy of cystitis is not recommended in children, because differentiating upper and lower tract disease may be difficult, and higher failure rates are reported in most studies of short-course therapy.

Acute pyelonephritis is usually treated for 10 days. The duration of parenteral therapy in uncomplicated pyelonephritis is not well defined, but most children can complete therapy orally once symptomatic improvement has occurred.

A repeat urine culture 24–48 hours after beginning therapy is not needed if the child is improving and doing well.

B. Follow-Up

Children with UTI should be followed with screening urinalysis 1 and 2 months after resolution of UTI. Dipstick nitrate determination can be used at home by parents on first morning voided urine in children with frequently recurring UTI.

C. Prophylactic Antimicrobials

Selected children with frequently recurring UTI may benefit from prophylactic antimicrobials. In children with high-grade VUR, prophylactic antimicrobials may be beneficial in reducing UTI, as an alternative to surgical correction, or in the interval prior to surgical therapy. Many experts recommend surgical correction of higher-grade reflux, particularly grade V. Trimethoprim–sulfamethoxazole and nitrofurantoin are approved for prophylaxis. The use of broader-spectrum antimicrobials leads to colonization and infection with resistant strains.

Children with dysfunctional voiding generally do not benefit from prophylactic antimicrobials; rather, addressing the underlying dysfunctional voiding is most important.

Conway PH et al: Recurrent urinary tract infections in children: Risk factors and association with prophylactic antimicrobials. JAMA 2007;298:179 [PMID: 17622599].

Feldman AS, Bauer SB: Diagnosis and management of dysfunctional voiding. Curr Opin Pediatr 2006;18:139 [PMID: 16601493].

Mak RH, Kuo HJ: Pathogenesis of urinary tract infection: An update. Curr Opin Pediatr 2006;18:148 [PMID: 16601494].

REFERENCES

Barratt TM et al: *Pediatric Nephrology,* 5th ed. Lippincott Williams & Wilkins, 2003.

Webb N, Postlethwaite R: *Clinical Paediatric Nephrology,* 3rd ed. Oxford University Press, 2003.

Neurologic & Muscular Disorders

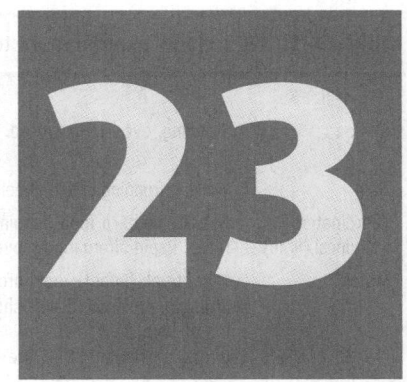

23

Paul G. Moe, MD

Timothy A. Benke, MD, PhD

Timothy J. Bernard, MD

Paul Levisohn, MD

NEUROLOGIC ASSESSMENT & NEURODIAGNOSTIC PROCEDURES

HISTORY & EXAMINATION

A general physical examination (albeit sometimes truncated) and an age-appropriate developmental assessment are part of every neurologic visit. Information provided in several earlier chapters is relevant in this context. Chapter 2 delineates age-appropriate developmental landmarks (see Tables 2–1 and 2–2); the Denver II schedule (see Figure 2–12) is helpful, especially in infancy. Growth and head circumference charts (*you* should measure the head) are also included in Chapter 2. Details of the standard pediatric history and physical examination are presented in Chapter 8. Expected newborn-infant reflexes and automations and other examination suggestions pertinent to that age group are included in Chapter 1.

Table 23–1 outlines components of the neurologic examination. Examination of a frightened or wary infant can begin on the mother's lap. Playing games will engage a toddler or preschooler: retrieving, casting a ball, stacking blocks, hopping, jogging, counting, and drawing (circles, lines) can reduce anxiety and exhibit fine and gross motor coordination, balance, and handedness. On occasion beyond preschool age, describing a picture, drawing, writing, calculating, and spelling will aid in assessing speech and intelligence.

Emphasis (or fine tuning) of both history and physical examination strongly depends on the chief complaint. Insidious developmental delay or weakness might demand detailed exploration of pregnancy, family, and social history; developmental landmarks; and general physical, motor, and speech achievements. Headaches or seizures in an older child warrant more emphasis on precise details preceding and during these events.

LUMBAR PUNCTURE

Spinal fluid is usually obtained by inserting a small-gauge needle (eg, No. 22) through the L3–L4 intervertebral space into the thecal sac while the patient is lying on his or her side. After an opening pressure is measured, a small amount of fluid is removed most frequently to examine for evidence of infection or inflammation (Table 23–2). Fluid is sent for red and white cell counts, for determination of the concentrations of protein and glucose, and for viral and bacterial cultures. In some cases, additional information is obtained with special staining techniques for mycobacteria and fungus. Additional fluid may be sent for polymerase chain reaction (PCR) testing for specific viral agents, antibody titer determinations, cytopathologic study, lactate and pyruvate concentrations, and amino acid and neurotransmitter analysis. Lumbar puncture is imperative when bacterial meningitis is suspected. Caution must be exercised, however, when signs of increased intracranial pressure (eg, papilledema) or focal neurologic signs are present that might indicate a substantial risk of precipitating tentorial or tonsillar herniation.

ELECTROENCEPHALOGRAPHY

Electroencephalography (EEG), a widely used noninvasive electrophysiologic method for recording cerebral activity, has its greatest clinical applicability in the study of seizure disorders. EEG is particularly helpful in showing epileptiform activity. Sometimes the findings are diagnostic, as in the hypsarrhythmia EEG of infantile spasms or the prolonged generalized 3/s spike-wave of absence seizures.

EEG is also used in the evaluation of tumors, cerebrovascular accidents, neurodegenerative diseases, and other neurologic disorders causing brain dysfunction. Recordings over a 24-hour period or all-night recordings are invaluable in the diagnosis of sleep disturbances and narcolepsy. EEG with telemetry or simultaneous monitoring of behavior on videotape has great usefulness in selected cases. The EEG can be helpful in determining a possible cause or mechanism of coma and whether subclinical seizures are contributing to the coma, and can help determine whether coma is irreversible and brain death has occurred.

Table 23–1. Neurologic examination: toddler age and up.

Category	Operation	Assesses
Station	Standing, eyes open, closed, hands out (Romberg test): truncal balance.	Cerebellum (vermis) Posterior columns
Gait	Walking (running in hall); heel-toe (tandem gait) forward, backward. Balance on each foot.	Cerebellum (vermis)
Coordination (truncal, limb)	Balance on each foot; hopping; finger-nose-finger pursuit. Stack blocks. Reach for a rattle. Rapid alternating movements.	Cerebellum: lateral lobes
Motor	Tone: trunk (infant)—hold prone, supine; manipulate relaxed limbs; hold under arms. Strength: proximal/distal—shoulder abduction/grasp; get up from floor (hips); dorsiflexion of foot. 0 = no movement; 1 = trace; 3 = against gravity; 5 = normal (0–5 grading strength)	Brain: "suprasegmental" influence Cord: lower motor neuron-"segmental" component
Reflexes	Tendon reflexes: biceps, triceps, brachioradialis, knee, ankle. Cutaneous: abdominal (cremasteric).	Pyramidal tract Spinal cord: sensory/motor nerve arc
Sensory	Light touch, sharp (pain), vibration (tuning fork-toe, finger, on bone), position (same). Cortical: 2 point, finger writing, object identification, position limb in space, barognosis (weight).	Peripheral nerve Posterior column Anterior/lateral column Parietal lobe
Cranial nerves	CN I: omit most of the time (smell). CN II: pupils (light reflex), vision (acuity), fields, fundi. CN III, IV, VI: extraocular movements, pupils, convergence, (strabismus?). CN V: facial sensation (upper, middle, lower; V_1, V_2, V_3); motor—move jaw laterally, open, close against resistance. CN VII: upper—eye closure, brow; lower—grimace, show teeth. CN VIII: whispered voice from 10–20 ft each ear. Tuning fork tests. CN IX, X: sensation? Movement of palate to "ahh" or tongue blade ("gagging"—often omit). CN XI: turning head right, left; flexing against resistance. CN XII: protrude tongue, push it out cheek. Push left, right against resistance (examiner's thumb).	

The limitations of EEG are considerable. In most cases, the duration of the actual tracing is about 45 minutes and reflects only surface cortical function. Many drugs, especially barbiturates and benzodiazepines, may cause artifact on the tracing and may confuse interpretation. Moreover, about 15% of nonepileptic individuals, especially children, may have an abnormal EEG. EEG findings such as those occasionally seen in migraine, learning disabilities, or behavior disorders are often nonspecific and do not reflect structural brain damage.

Computed tomography (CT) scans, evoked potentials, positron emission tomography (PET), regional cerebral blood flow studies, single-photon emission computed tomography (SPECT), and magnetic resonance imaging (MRI) supplement the EEG as a diagnostic and prognostic tool.

EVOKED POTENTIALS

Cortical visual, auditory, or somatosensory evoked potentials (evoked responses) may be recorded from the scalp surface over the temporal, occipital, or frontoparietal cortex after repetitive stimulation of the retina by light flashes, the cochlea by sounds, or a nerve by galvanic stimuli of varying frequency and intensity, respectively. Computer averaging is used to recognize and enhance these responses while subtracting or suppressing the asynchronous background EEG activity. The presence or absence of evoked potential waves and their latencies (time from stimulus to wave peak or time between peaks) figures in the clinical interpretation.

The reproducible and quantifiable results obtained from brainstem auditory, pattern-shift visual, and short-latency somatosensory evoked potentials (see section on short-latency somatosensory evoked potentials) indicate the level of function of the relevant sensory pathway or system and identify the site of anatomic disruption. Although results of these tests alone are usually not diagnostic, the tests are noninvasive, sensitive, objective, and relatively inexpensive extensions of the clinical neurologic examination. Because the auditory and somatosensory tests and one type of visual test are completely passive, requiring only that the patient remain still, they are particularly useful in the evaluation of neonates, young children, and patients unable to cooperate. Knowledge of normal values and experience in testing are mandatory.

Brainstem Auditory Evoked Potentials

A brief auditory stimulus (click) of varying intensity and frequency is delivered to the ear to activate the auditory

Table 23–2. Characteristics of cerebrospinal fluid in the normal child and in central nervous system infections and inflammatory conditions.

Condition	Initial Pressure (mm H$_2$O)	Appearance	Cells/μL	Protein (mg/dL)	Glucose (mg/dl)	Other Tests	Comments
Normal	< 160	Clear	0–5 lymphocytes; first 3 months, 1–3 PMNs; neonates, up to 30 lymphocytes, rare RBCs	15–35 (lumbar), 5–15 (ventricular); up to 150 (lumbar) for short time after birth; to 6 months up to 65	50–80 (two thirds of blood glucose); may be increased after seizure	CSF-IgG index[a] < 0.7[a]; LDH 2–27 U/L	CSF protein in first month may be up to 170 mg/dL in small-for-date or premature infants; no increase in WBCs due to seizure
Bloody tap	Normal or low	Bloody (sometimes with clot)	One additional WBC/700 RBCs[b]; RBCs not crenated	One additional milli-gram per 800 RBCs[b]	Normal	RBC number should fall between first and third tubes; wait 5 min between tubes	Spin down fluid, supernatant will be clear and colorless[c]
Bacterial meningitis, acute	200–750+	Opalescent to puru-lent	Up to thousands, mostly PMNs; early, few cells	Up to hundreds	Decreased; may be none	Smear and culture mandatory; LDH > 24 U/L; lactate, IL-8, TNF elevated, correlate with prognosis	Very early, glucose may be normal; PCR meningococci and pneumococci in plasma, CSF may aid diagnosis
Bacterial meningitis, partially treated	Usually increased	Clear or opalescent	Usually increased; PMNs usually pre-dominate	Elevated	Normal or decreased	LDH usually > 24 U/L; PCR may still be pos-itive	Smear and culture may be negative if antibiotics have been in use
Tuberculous meningitis	150–750+	Opalescent; fibrin web or pellicle	250–500, mostly lymphocytes; early, more PMNs	45–500; parallels cell count; increases over time	Decreased; may be none	Smear for acid-fast organism: CSF culture and inoculation; PCR	Consider AIDS, a com-mon comorbidity of tuberculosis
Fungal meningitis	Increased	Variable; often clear	10–500; early, more PMNs; then mostly lymphocytes	Elevated and increasing	Decreased	India ink prepara-tions, cryptococcal antigen, PCR, culture, inoculations, immu-nofluorescence tests	Often superimposed in patients who are debilitated or on immuno-suppressive therapy
Aseptic meningo-encephalitis (viral meningitis, or parameningeal disease); enceph-alitis is similar	Normal or slightly increased	Clear unless cell count > 300/μL	None to a few hun-dred, mostly lym-phocytes; PMNs predominate early	20–125	Normal; may be low in mumps, herpes, or other viral infec-tions	CSF, stool, blood, throat washings for viral cultures; LDH < 28 U/L; PCR for HSV, CMV, EBV, enterovirus, etc	Acute and convales-cent antibody titers for some viruses; in mumps, up to 1000 lymphocytes; serum amylase often ele-vated; up to 1000 cells present in enteroviral infection

(continued)

Table 23–2. Characteristics of cerebrospinal fluid in the normal child and in central nervous system infections and inflammatory conditions. *(Continued)*

Condition	Initial Pressure (mm H₂0)	Appearance	Cells/μL	Protein (mg/dL)	Glucose (mg/dL)	Other Tests	Comments
Parainfectious encephalomyelitis (ADEM)	80–450, usually increased	Usually clear	0–50+, mostly lymphocytes; lower numbers, even 0, in MS	15–75	Normal	CSF-IgG index, oligoclonal bands variable; in MS, moderate increase	No organisms; fulminant cases resemble bacterial meningitis
Polyneuritis	Normal and occasionally increased	Early: normal; late: xanthochromic if protein high	Normal; occasionally slight increase	Early: normal; late: 45–1500	Normal	CSF-IgG index may be increased; oligoclonal bands variable	Try to find cause (viral infections, toxins, lupus, diabetes, etc)
Meningeal carcinomatosis	Often elevated	Clear to opalescent	Cytologic identification of tumor cells	Often mildly to moderately elevated	Often depressed	Cytology	Seen with leukemia, medulloblastoma, meningeal melanosis, histiocytosis X
Brain abscess	Normal or increased	Usually clear	5–500 in 80%; mostly PMNs	Usually slightly increased	Normal; occasionally decreased	Imaging study of brain (MRI)	Cell count related to proximity to meninges; findings as in purulent meningitis if abscess ruptures

ᵃCSF-IgG index = CSF IgG/serum IgG ÷ CSF albumin/serum albumin.

ᵇMany studies document pitfalls in using these ratios due to WBC lysis. Clinical judgment and repeat lumbar punctures may be necessary to rule out meningitis in this situation.

ᶜCSF WBC (predicted) = CSF RBC × (blood WBC/blood RBC). O:P ratio = observed CSF WBC + predicted CSF WBC. Also, do WBC:RBC ratio. If O:P ratio ≤0.01, and WBC:RBC ratio ≤1:100, meningitis is absent. ADEM, acute disseminated encephalomyelitis; AIDS, acquired immunodeficiency syndrome; CMV, cytomegalovirus; CSF, cerebrospinal fluid; EBV, Epstein-Barr virus; HSV, herpes simplex virus; IL-8, interleukin 8; LDH, lactate dehydrogenase; MRI, magnetic resonance imaging; MS, multiple sclerosis; PCR, polymerase chain reaction; PMN, polymorphonuclear neutrophil; RBC, red blood cell; TNF, tumor necrosis factor; WBC, white blood cell.

nerve (nerve VIII) and sequentially activate the cochlear nucleus, tracts and nuclei of the lateral lemniscus, and inferior colliculus. Thus this technique assesses hearing and function of the brainstem auditory tracts.

Hearing in the neonate or uncooperative patient can be assessed objectively, making the technique particularly useful in high-risk infants and in mentally retarded or autistic patients. Because high doses of anesthetic agents or barbiturates do not seriously affect results, the test is used to assess and monitor brainstem function of surgical patients (in the operating room) and those in hypoxic-ischemic coma or coma following head injury. Absence of evoked potential waves beyond the first wave from the auditory nerve usually signifies brain death. Brainstem auditory evoked potentials are also useful in the early evaluation of diseases affecting myelin such as the leukodystrophies and multiple sclerosis, although auditory evoked potentials are less valuable than visual evoked potentials in the evaluation of multiple sclerosis. Intrinsic brainstem gliomas and brainstem encephalitis (eg, enterovirus 71) can also be evaluated with auditory evoked potentials. They are sometimes useful in evaluation of hereditary ataxias, Wilson disease, and other degenerative disorders of the brainstem.

Pattern-Shift Visual Evoked Potentials

The preferred stimulus is a shift (reversal) of a checkerboard pattern, and the response is a single wave (called P-100) generated in the striate and parastriate visual cortex. The absolute latency of P-100 (time from stimulus to wave peak) and the difference in latency between the two eyes are sensitive indicators of disease. The amplitude of response is affected by any process resulting in poor fixation on the stimulus screen or affecting visual acuity. Ability to focus on a checkerboard pattern is necessary. An LED (light-emitting diode) in goggles, or bright flash stimulus can be used in younger and uncooperative children, but the norms are less standardized. This is a less sensitive whole retina (rather than only macula) stimulation that may give normal results in a child who is legally blind.

Clinical applications of the test include detection and monitoring of strabismus (eg, in amblyopia ex anopsia), optic neuritis, and lesions near the optic nerve and chiasm such as optic gliomas and craniopharyngiomas. Degenerative and immunologic diseases that affect visual transmission may be detected early and followed by serial evaluations. Examples of such diseases include adrenoleukodystrophy, Pelizaeus-Merzbacher disease, some spinocerebellar degenerations, sarcoidosis, and even multiple sclerosis. Flash visual evoked potentials are used to monitor function during surgery on the eyes or optic nerve, to assess cortical or hysterical blindness, and to evaluate patients with photosensitive epilepsy, who may have exaggerated responses.

Short-Latency Somatosensory Evoked Potentials

Responses are commonly produced by electrical stimulation of peripheral sensory nerves, because this evokes potentials of greatest amplitude and clarity. Finger tapping and muscle stretching may also be used to stimulate somatosensory potentials. The function of this test is similar to that of the auditory test in closely correlating waveforms with function of the sensory pathways and permitting localization of conduction defects.

Short-latency somatosensory evoked potentials are used in the assessment of a wide variety of lesions of the peripheral nerve, root, spinal cord, and central nervous system (CNS) following trauma, neuropathies (eg, in diabetes mellitus or Guillain-Barré syndrome), myelodysplasias, Arnold-Chiari malformation, and achondroplasia.. The procedure is often performed on an outpatient basis. One method is stimulation of the median nerve at the wrist with small (nonpainful) electrical shocks and recording of responses from the brachial plexus above the clavicle, the neck (cervical cord), and the opposite scalp area overlying the sensorimotor cortex. After stimulation from the knee (peroneal nerve) or ankle (tibial nerve), impulses are recorded from the lower lumbar spinal cord, cervical cord, and sensorimotor cortex. Such potentials are used to monitor spinal cord sensory functioning during surgery for scoliosis, myelodysplasias, tumors, and other lesions of the spinal cord or its blood vessels. The technique is also used in leukodystrophies involving peripheral nerves, in multiple sclerosis, and in the evaluation of hysteria and malingering (anesthetic limbs). In the diagnosis of coma and brain death, somatosensory evoked potentials supplement the results of auditory evoked potentials.

PEDIATRIC NEURORADIOLOGIC PROCEDURES

Sedation for Procedures

Oral chloral hydrate, 30–60 mg/kg per dose, is safest. Many radiology departments, however, use intravenously administered agents because of the risks of vomiting and aspiration. One favorite is pentobarbital, 6 mg/kg for children weighing less than 15 kg and 5 mg/kg for larger children (up to a maximum of 200 mg) given intramuscularly or rectally (at least 20 minutes before a procedure), or 2–4 mg/kg given intravenously. Equipment to support blood pressure and respiration must be available. This dosage usually achieves sedation for up to 2 hours. If, however, sedation is inadequate 30 minutes after injection, and if the child's condition permits a second dose of pentobarbital, 2 mg/kg is given. Midazolam, 0.1 mg/kg IV or 0.2 mg/kg intranasally, is gaining popularity for brief procedures (eg, Botox injection).

Computed Tomography

CT scanning consists of a series of cross-sectional (axial) roentgenograms. Radiation exposure is approximately the same as that from a skull radiographic series. CT images record variations in tissue density and can be viewed on a television screen as the scan is being done, and later examined on films. CT scanning is of high sensitivity (88–96% of lesions larger than 1–2 cm can be seen) but low specificity (tumor, infection, or infarct may look the same). Sedation is usually not needed. CT scan is occasionally repeated after intravenous injection of iodized contrast for enhancement, which reflects the vascularity of a lesion or its surrounding tissues. Most CT scans do not require enhancement. Lastly, CT angiography (CTA; no injection is needed) is often "more available" in an acute stroke evaluation, gives excellent cross-sectional views of major arteries, and may identify the site of an acute thrombosis. Radiation dose is a disadvantage of all CT scanning.

Magnetic Resonance Imaging

MRI is a noninvasive technique that uses the magnetic properties of certain nuclei to produce diagnostically useful signals. Currently the technique is based on detecting the response (resonance) of hydrogen proton nuclei to applied radiofrequency electromagnetic radiation. These nuclei are abundant in the body and more sensitive to MRI than other nuclei. The strength of MRI signals varies with the relationship of water to protein and the amount of lipid in the tissue. The MRI image displayed provides high-resolution contrast of soft tissues. MRI can provide information about the histologic, physiologic, and biochemical status of tissues in addition to gross anatomic data. Sedation is necessary in children younger than age 6 years to avoid any movement artefact.

MRI has been used to delineate brain tumors, edema, ischemic and hemorrhagic lesions, hydrocephalus, vascular disorders, inflammatory and infectious lesions, and degenerative processes. MRI can be used to study myelination and demyelination, and through the demonstration of changes in relaxation time, metabolic disorders of the brain, muscles, and glands. Because bone causes no artifact in the images, the posterior fossa and its contents can be studied far better using MRI than with CT scans. Even blood vessels and the cranial nerves can be imaged. In contrast, the lesser ability of MRI to detect calcification limits its usefulness in the investigation of calcified lesions such as craniopharyngioma and leptomeningeal angiomatosis.

Magnetic resonance angiography (MRA) or venography (MRV) is a noninvasive (no arterial or venous puncture or dye injection) technique to show large extra- and intracranial blood vessels. It often replaces the more hazardous intraarterial injection angiogram. An advantage over CTA (see previous section) is the lack of radiation exposure.

Perfusion imaging involving a paramagnetic contrast agent is used in stroke patients to evaluate brain ischemic penumbra. Similarly, diffusion imaging (measuring random motion of water molecules) may show reduced diffusion in areas of cytotoxic edema, and is useful in acute strokes and toxic or metabolic brain injuries. The area of involvement often exceeds the T1 hypodense or T2 hyperdense stroke area, and this penumbra possibly reflects recoverable tissue injury as compared with totally infarcted tissue, cell death, or apoptosis (programmed cell death) in the center of the stroke.

Another new MRI technique, proton MR spectroscopy, measures signals of increased cellular activity and oxidative metabolism; neuronal acetyl aspartate, phosphocreatinine, and phosphomonoester are increased. Ratios are often calculated to choline and P_i (inorganic phosphate). Increased lactate (anaerobic metabolism), choline, and creatinine, reflecting increased cell surface area—as in gliosis or scarring—can be assessed in a chosen voxel or tiny area of interest. An epileptic focus in the medial temporal lobe is an example; an active seizure site might show increased metabolism. Sclerosis and gliosis ("scar") would show the converse.

Functional MRI can be performed at the same time as an ongoing regular MRI. Blood oxygenation changes in an area of interest (eg, an area of language acquisition) during rest and then during a verbal work paradigm can identify and lateralize the language cortex. A change in the ratio of oxyhemoglobin to deoxyhemoglobin results in a detectable MRI signal.

Positron Emission Tomography

PET is an imaging technique that measures the metabolic rate at a given site by CT scanning. For measurement of local cerebral metabolism, the radiolabeled substrate most frequently used has been intravenously administered fluorodeoxyglucose. Gray matter and white matter are clearly distinguishable; the skull and air- or fluid-filled cavities are least active metabolically.

PET has been used to study the cerebral metabolism of neonates and brain activation by visual or auditory stimuli. Pathologic states that have been studied include epilepsy, brain infarcts, brain tumors, and dementias. This functional test of brain metabolism is useful in preoperative evaluation for epilepsy surgery. The epileptogenic zone will often be hypermetabolic during seizures and hypoactive during the time between seizures. The information from PET scan complements EEG and MRI findings to aid in the decision about tissue removal. In infants with infantile spasms, PET scan has occasionally detected focal lesions, thereby leading to successful surgical removal. Clinical application is limited by the cost of the procedure and the clinician's need for access to a nearby cyclotron for preparation of the radiopharmaceuticals.

Ultrasonography

Ultrasonography offers a pictorial display of the varying densities of tissues in a given anatomic region by recording the echoes of ultrasonic waves reflected from it. These waves, modulated by pulsations, are introduced into the tissue by means of a piezoelectric transducer. The many advantages of ultrasonography include the ability to assess a structure and its positioning quickly with easily portable equipment, without ionizing radiation, and at about one fourth the cost of CT scanning. Sedation is usually not necessary, and the procedure can be repeated as often as needed without risk to the patient. In brain imaging, B-mode and real-time sector scanners are usually used, permitting excellent detail in the coronal and sagittal planes. Contiguous structures can be studied by a continuous sweep and reviewed on videotape.

Ultrasonography has been used for in-utero diagnosis of hydrocephalus and other anomalies. In neonates, the thin skull and the open anterior fontanelle have facilitated imaging of the brain, and ultrasonography is used to screen and follow infants of less than 32 weeks' gestation or weighing less than 1500 g for intracranial hemorrhage. Other uses in neonates include detection of hydrocephalus, major brain and spine malformations, and calcifications from intrauterine infection with cytomegalovirus (CMV) or *Toxoplasma*. In skilled hands, sonography of the neonatal spine can be used as a screening test for anomalies at the lumbosacral level.

Cerebral Angiography

Arteriography remains a useful procedure in the diagnosis of many cerebrovascular disorders, particularly in cerebrovascular accidents or in potentially operable vascular malformations. In some brain tumors, arteriography may be necessary to define the precise location or vascular bed, to differentiate among tumors, or to distinguish tumor from abscess or infarction. Noninvasive CT, MRI, and MRA scans can diagnose many cases of static or flowing blood disorders (eg, sinus thromboses). If necessary, the more risky invasive arteriography is usually done via femoral artery-aorta catheterization.

Myelography

Radiographic examination of the spine may be indicated in cases of spinal cord tumors, myelitis, or various forms of spinal dysraphism and in the rare instance of herniated disks in children. MRI has largely replaced sonography, CT, and myelography for examination of the spinal cord.

Aydin K et al: Utility of electroencephalography in the evaluation of common neurologic conditions in children. J Child Neurol 2003;18:394 [PMID: 128896973].

Baxter AL et al: Local anesthetic and stylet styles: Factors associated with resident lumbar puncture success. Pediatrics 2006;117;876 [PMID: 16510670].

Baxter AL et al: Pain, position, and stylet styles: Infant lumbar puncture practices of pediatric emergency attending physicians. Pediatr Emerg Care 2004;20:816 [PMID: 15572969].

Bonsu BK, Harper MB: Accuracy and test characteristics of ancillary tests of cerebrospinal fluid for predicting acute bacterial meningitis in children with low white blood cell counts in cerebrospinal fluid. Acad Emerg Med 2005;12:303 [PMID: 15805320].

Cecil KM, Kos RS: Magnetic resonance spectroscopy and metabolic imaging in white matter diseases and pediatric disorders. Top Magn Reson Imaging 2006;17:275 [PMID: 17415001].

Dooley JM et al: The utility of the physical examination and investigations in the pediatric neurology consultation. Pediatr Neurol 2003;28:96 [PMID: 12699858].

Ellenby MS et al: Videos in clinical medicine. Lumbar puncture. N Engl J Med 2006;355:e12 [PMID: 17005943].

Lowe LH et al: Sonography of the neonatal spine: Part 2, Spinal disorders. AJR Am J Roentgenol 2007;188:739 [PMID: 17312062].

Mazor SS et al: Interpretation of traumatic lumbar punctures: Who can go home? Pediatrics 2003;111:525 [PMID: 12612231].

Sood S, Chugani HT: Functional neuroimaging in the preoperative evaluation of children with drug-resistant epilepsy. Childs Nerv Syst 2006;22:810 [PMID: 16799821].

Straussberg R et al: Absolute neutrophil count in aseptic and bacterial meningitis related to time of lumbar puncture. Pediatr Neurol 2003;28:365 [PMID: 12878298].

DISORDERS AFFECTING THE NERVOUS SYSTEM IN INFANTS & CHILDREN

ALTERED STATES OF CONSCIOUSNESS

ESSENTIALS OF DIAGNOSIS & TYPICAL FEATURES

▶ Reduction or alteration in cognitive and affective mental functioning and in arousability or attentiveness.

▶ Acute onset.

▶ General Considerations

Many terms are used to describe the continuum from full alertness to complete unresponsiveness and deep coma, including clouding, obtundation, somnolence or stupor, semicoma or light coma, and deep coma. Several scales have been used to grade the depth of unconsciousness (Table 23–3). The commonly used Glasgow Coma Scale is summarized in Table 11–5. Physicians should use one of these tables and provide further descriptions in case narratives. These descriptions help subsequent observers quantify unconsciousness and evaluate changes in the patient's condition.

The neurologic substrate for consciousness is the reticular activating system in the brainstem, up to and including the thalamus and paraventricular hypothalamus. Large lesions of the cortex, especially of the left hemisphere, can also cause coma. The term *locked-in syndrome* describes patients who are conscious but have no access to motor or verbal expression because of massive loss of motor function of the brainstem. *Coma vigil* refers to patients who seem comatose but have some spontaneous motor behavior, such as eye opening or eye tracking, almost always at a reflex level. *Persistent vegetative state* denotes a chronic condition in which there is preservation of the sleep-wake cycle but no awareness and no recovery of mental function.

▶ Treatment

A. Emergency Measures

The clinician's first response is to ensure that the patient will survive. The ABCs of resuscitation are pertinent. The airway must be kept open with positioning or even endotracheal

Table 23–3. Gradation of coma.

	Deep Coma		Light Coma		
	Grade 4	Grade 3	Grade 2	Grade 1	Stupor
Response to pain	0	+	Avoidance	Avoidance	Arousal unsustained
Tone/posture	Flaccid	Decerebrate	Variable	Variable	Normal
Tendon reflexes	0	+/−	+	+	+
Pupil response	0	+	+	+	+
Response to verbal stimuli	0	0	0	0	+
Other corneal reflex	0	+	+	+	+
Gag reflex	0	+	+	+	+

intubation. Breathing and adequate air exchange can be assessed by auscultation; hand bag respiratory assistance with oxygen may be needed. Circulation must be ensured by assessing pulse and blood pressure. An intravenous line is always necessary. Fluids, plasma, blood, or even a dopamine drip (1–20 mcg/kg/min) may be required in cases of hypotension. An extremely hypothermic or febrile child may require vigorous cooling or warming to save life. The assessment of vital signs may signal the diagnosis. Slow, insufficient respirations suggest poisoning by hypnotic drugs; apnea may indicate diphenoxylate hydrochloride poisoning. Rapid, deep respirations suggest acidosis, possibly metabolic, as with diabetic coma; toxic, such as that due to aspirin; or neurogenic, as in Reye syndrome. Hyperthermia may indicate infection or heat stroke; hypothermia may indicate cold exposure, ethanol poisoning, or hypoglycemia (especially in infancy).

The signs of impending brain herniation are another priority of the initial assessment. Bradycardia, high blood pressure, irregular breathing, increased extensor tone, and third nerve palsy with the eye deviated outward and the pupil dilated are possible signs of impending temporal lobe or brainstem herniation. These signs suggest a need for slight hyperventilation, reducing cerebral edema, prompt neurosurgical consultation, and possibly, in an infant with a bulging fontanelle, subdural or ventricular tap (or both). Initial intravenous fluids should contain glucose until further assessment disproves hypoglycemia as a cause.

A history obtained from parents or witnesses is desirable. Sometimes the only history will be obtained from ambulance attendants. An important point is whether the child is known to have a chronic illness, such as diabetes, hemophilia, epilepsy, or cystic fibrosis. Recent acute illness raises the possibility of coma caused by viral or bacterial meningitis. Trauma is a common cause of coma. Lack of a history of trauma, especially in infants, does not rule it out. Nonaccidental trauma or a fall not witnessed by caregivers may have occurred. In coma of unknown cause, poisoning is always a possibility. Absence of a history of ingestion of a toxic substance or of medication in the home does not rule out poisoning as a cause.

Often the history is obtained concurrently with a brief pediatric and neurologic screening examination. After the assessment of vital signs, the general examination proceeds with a trauma assessment. Palpation of the head and fontanelle, inspection of the ears for infection or hemorrhage, and a careful examination for neck stiffness are indicated. If circumstances suggest head or neck trauma, the head and neck must be immobilized so that any fracture or dislocation will not be aggravated. The skin must be inspected for petechiae or purpura that might suggest bacteremia, infection, bleeding disorder, or traumatic bruising. Examination of the chest, abdomen, and limbs is important to exclude enclosed hemorrhage or traumatic fractures.

Neurologic examination quantifies the stimulus response and depth of coma, such as responsiveness to verbal or painful stimuli. Examination of the pupils, optic fundi, and eye movements is important. Are the eye movements spontaneous, or is it necessary to do the doll's-eye maneuver (rotating the head rapidly to see whether the eyes follow)? Motor and sensory examinations assess reflex asymmetries, Babinski sign, and evidence of spontaneous posturing or posturing induced by noxious stimuli (eg, decorticate or decerebrate posturing).

If the cause of the coma is not obvious, emergency laboratory tests must be obtained. Table 23–4 lists some of the causes of coma in children. Most comas (90%) in children have a medical (versus structural) cause. Infection is a common cause (30%). An immediate blood glucose (or Dextrostix), complete blood count, urine obtained by catheterization if necessary, pH and electrolytes (including bicarbonate), serum urea nitrogen, and aspartate aminotransferase are initial screens. Urine, blood, and even gastric contents must be saved for toxin screen if the underlying cause is not obvious. Blood culture and lumbar puncture often are necessary to rule out CNS infection. Papilledema is a relative contraindication to lumbar puncture. Occasionally, blood culture is obtained, antibiotics started, and imaging study of the brain done prior to a diagnostic lumbar puncture. If meningitis is suspected and a lumbar puncture is delayed or believed to be hazardous, antibiotics should be started and the diagnostic lumbar punc-

Table 23–4. Some causes of coma in childhood.

Mechanism of Coma	Likely Cause	
	Newborn Infant	Older Child
Anoxia		
Asphyxia	Birth asphyxia, HIE	Carbon monoxide (CO) poisoning
Respiratory obstruction	Meconium aspiration, infection (especially respiratory syncytial virus)	Croup, tracheitis, epiglottitis
Severe anemia	Hydrops fetalis	Hemolysis, blood loss
Ischemia		
Cardiac	Shunting lesions, hypoplastic left heart	Shunting lesions, aortic stenosis, myocarditis
Shock	Asphyxia, sepsis	Blood loss, infection
Head trauma (structural cause)	Birth contusion, hemorrhage, nonaccidental trauma (NAT)	Falls, auto accidents, athletic injuries
Infection (most common cause in childhood)	Gram-negative meningitis, enterovirus, herpes encephalitis, sepsis	Bacterial meningitis, viral encephalitis, postinfectious encephalitis, sepsis, typhoid, malaria
Vascular (CVA or stroke, often of unknown cause)	Intraventricular hemorrhage, sinus thrombosis	Arterial or venous occlusion with congenital heart disease, head or neck trauma
Neoplasm (structural cause)	Rare this age. Choroid plexus papilloma with severe hydrocephalus.	Brainstem glioma, increased pressure with posterior fossa tumors
Drugs (toxidrome)	Maternal sedatives; injected pudendal and paracervical analgesics	Overdose, salicylates, lithium, sedatives, psychotropic agents
Epilepsy	Constant minor motor seizures; electrical seizure without motor manifestations	Nonconvulsive or, absence status, postictal state; drugs given to stop seizures
Toxins (toxidrome)	Maternal sedatives or injections	Arsenic, alcohol, CO, pesticides, mushroom, lead
Hypoglycemia	Birth injury, diabetic progeny, toxemic progeny	Diabetes, "prediabetes," hypoglycemic agents
Increased intracranial pressure (metabolic or structural cause)	Anoxic brain damage, hydrocephalus, metabolic disorders (urea cycle; amino-, organic acidurias)	Toxic encephalopathy, Reye syndrome, head trauma, tumor of posterior fossa
Hepatic causes	Hepatic failure, inborn metabolic errors in bilirubin conjugation	Hepatic failure
Renal causes, hypertensive encephalopathy	Hypoplastic kidneys	Nephritis, acute (AGN) and chronic, uremia, uremic syndrome
Hypothermia, hyperthermia	Iatrogenic (head cooling)	Cold weather exposure, drowning; heat stroke
Hypercapnia	Congenital lung anomalies, bronchopulmonary dysplasia	Cystic fibrosis (hypercapnia, anoxia)
Electrolyte changes		
Hyper- or hyponatremia	Iatrogenic (NaHCO₃ use), salt poisoning (formula errors)	Diarrhea, dehydration
Hyper- or hypocalcemia	SIADH, adrenogenital syndrome, dialysis (iatrogenic)	Lactic acidosis
Severe acidosis, lactic acidosis	septicemia, metabolic errors, adrenogenital syndrome	Infection, diabetic coma, poisoning (eg, aspirin) hyperglycemic nonketotic coma
Purpuric	Disseminated intravascular coagulation (DIC)	DIC, leukemia, thrombotic thrombocytopenic purpura

AGN, acute glomerulonephritis; SIADH, syndrome of inappropriate antidiuretic hormone.
Modified and reproduced, with permission, from Lewis J, Moe PG: The unconscious child. In Conn H, Conn R (editors): *Current Diagnosis,* 5th ed. WB Saunders, 1977.

ture done later. Tests that are helpful in obscure cases of coma include oxygen and carbon dioxide partial pressures, ammonia levels, serum and urine osmolality, porphyrins, lead levels, and urine and serum amino acids and urine organic acids.

If head trauma or increased pressure is suspected, an emergency CT scan or MRI is necessary. Bone windows on the former study or skull radiographs can be done at the same sitting. The absence of skull fracture does not rule out coma caused by closed head trauma. Injury that results from shaking a child is one example. In a child with an open fontanelle, a real-time ultrasound may be transiently substituted for the other, more definitive imaging studies if there is good local expertise. Treatment of head injury associated with coma is discussed in detail in Chapter 11.

Rarely, an emergency EEG aids in diagnosing the cause of coma. Nonconvulsive status epilepticus or a focal finding seen with herpes encephalitis (periodic lateralized epileptiform discharges) and focal slowing as seen with stroke or cerebritis are cases in which the EEG might be helpful. The EEG also may correlate with the stage of coma and add prognostic information.

B. General Measures

Vital signs must be monitored and maintained. Most emergency departments and intensive care units have flow sheets that provide space for repeated monitoring of the coma; a coma scale can be a useful tool for this purpose. The patient's response to vocal or painful stimuli and orientation to time, place, and situation are monitored. Posture and movements of the limbs, either spontaneously or in response to pain, are serially noted. Pupillary size, equality, and reaction to light, and movement of the eyes to the doll's-eye maneuver or ice-water caloric tests should be recorded. Intravenous fluids can be tailored to the situation, as for treatment of acidosis, shock, or hypovolemia. Nasogastric suction is initially important. The bladder should be catheterized for monitoring urine output and for urinalysis.

C. Seizure Management

An EEG should be ordered if seizures are suspected. If obvious motor seizures have occurred, treatment for status epilepticus is given with intravenous drugs (see later section on Seizure Disorders). If brainstem herniation or increased pressure is possible, intracranial monitoring may be necessary. This procedure is described in more detail in Chapter 13. Initial treatment of impending herniation includes keeping the patient's head up (15–30 degrees) and providing slight hyperventilation. The use of mannitol, diuretics, corticosteroids, and drainage of cerebrospinal fluid (CSF) are more heroic measures covered in detail in Chapter 13.

▶ Prognosis

About 50% of children with nontraumatic causes of coma have a good outcome. In studies of adults assessed on admission or within the first days after the onset of coma, an analysis of multiple variables was most helpful in assessing prognosis. Abnormal neuro-ophthalmologic signs (eg, the absence of pupillary reaction or of eye movement in response to the doll's-eye maneuver or ice water caloric testing and the absence of corneal responses) were unfavorable. Delay in the return of motor responses, tone, or eye opening was also unfavorable. In children, the assessment done on admission is about as predictive as one done in the succeeding days. Approximately two thirds of outcomes can be successfully predicted at an early stage on the basis of coma severity, extraocular movements, pupillary reactions, motor patterns, blood pressure, temperature, and seizure type. Other characteristics, such as the need for assisted respiration, the presence of increased intracranial pressure, and the duration of coma, are not significantly predictive. Published reports suggest that an anoxic (in contrast to traumatic, metabolic, or toxic) coma, such as that caused by near drowning, has a much grimmer outlook.

BRAIN DEATH

Many medical and law associations have endorsed the following definition of death: An individual who has sustained either (1) irreversible cessation of circulatory and respiratory functions or (2) irreversible cessation of all functions of the entire brain, including the brainstem, is dead. A determination of death must be made in accordance with accepted medical standards. Representatives from several pediatric and neurologic associations have endorsed the Guidelines for the Determination of Brain Death in Children. The criteria in full-term infants (ie, those born at greater than 38 weeks' gestation) were applicable 1 week after the neurologic insult. Difficulties in assessing premature infants and full-term infants shortly after birth were acknowledged.

Prerequisites

In assessment of brain death, the history is important. The physician must determine proximate causes to make sure no remediable or reversible conditions are present. Examples of such causes are metabolic conditions, toxic agents, sedative-hypnotic drugs, surgically remediable conditions, hypothermia, and paralytic agents.

Physical Examination Criteria

(See also Chapter 13.) The following criteria are those established by the Task Force on Brain Death in Children:

1. **Coexistence of coma and apnea:** The patient must exhibit complete loss of consciousness, vocalization, and volitional activity.
2. **Absence of brainstem function:** As defined by the following: (a) Midposition or fully dilated pupils that do not respond to light; drugs may influence and invalidate pupillary assessment. (b) Absence of spontaneous eye movements and those induced by side-to-side passive head movements (oculocephalic reflex) and ice water instillation in the external auditory canal (ice water caloric test; intact tympanic membranes must be documented). (c) Absence of movement of bulbar musculature, including facial and oropharyngeal muscles; the corneal, gag, cough, sucking, and rooting reflexes are absent. (d) Absence of respiratory movements when the patient is off the respirator; apnea testing using standardized methods can be performed but is done after other criteria are met.
3. **Temperature and blood pressure:** The patient must not be significantly hypothermic or hypotensive for age.
4. **Tone:** Tone is flaccid, and spontaneous or induced movements are absent, excluding spinal cord events such as reflex withdrawal or spinal myoclonus.
5. **General examination findings:** The examination should remain consistent with brain death throughout the observation and testing period.

Confirmation

Apnea testing should be carried out at a partial carbon dioxide pressure level greater than 60 mm Hg, and with normal oxygenation maintained throughout the test period. This level may be reached 3–15 minutes after taking the patient off the respirator. The recommended observation period to confirm brain death (repeated examinations) is 12–24 hours (longer in infants); reversible causes must be ruled out. If an irreversible cause is documented, laboratory testing is not essential. Helpful tests to support the clinical assertion of brain death include EEG and angiography. Electrocerebral silence on EEG should persist for 30 minutes, and drug concentrations must be insufficient to suppress EEG activity. Absence of intracerebral arterial blood flow can be confirmed by carotid angiography and cerebral radionuclide angiography. Persistence of dural sinus flow does not invalidate the diagnosis of brain death.

Cerebral evoked potentials, intracranial blood pulsations on ultrasound, and xenon-enhanced CT have not been sufficiently studied to be considered definitive in the diagnosis of brain death. In rare cases, preserved intracranial perfusion in the presence of EEG silence has been documented, and the converse has also been reported.

Ashwal S et al: Use of advanced neuroimaging techniques in the evaluation of pediatric traumatic brain injury. Dev Neurosci 2006;28:309 [PMID: 16943654].

Ashwal S, Serna-Fonseca T: Brain death in infants and children. Crit Care Nurse 2006;26:117, 126 [PMID: 16565286].

Atabaki SM: Pediatric head injury. Pediatr Rev 2007;28:215 [PMID: 17545333].

Avner JR: Altered states of consciousness. Pediatr Rev 2006;27:331 [PMID: 16950938].

Claassen J et al: Detection of electrographic seizures with continuous EEG monitoring in critically ill patients. Neurology 2004;62:1743 [PMID: 15159471].

Hosain SA et al: Electroencephalographic patterns in unresponsive pediatric patients. Pediatr Neurol 2005;32:162 [PMID: 15730895].

Oropello JM: Determination of brain death: Theme, variations, and preventable errors. Crit Care Med 2004;32:1417 [PMID: 15187532].

Posner JB et al: *Diagnosis of Stupor and Coma.* Oxford University Press, 2007.

Shemie SD et al: Diagnosis of brain death in children. Lancet Neurol 2007;6:87 [PMID: 17166805].

Shewmon DA: Coma prognosis in children. Part II: Clinical application. J Clin Neurophysiol 2000;17:467 [PMID: 11085550].

Worrall K: Use of the Glasgow coma scale in infants. Paediatr Nurs 2004;16:45 [PMID: 15160621].

SEIZURE DISORDERS (EPILEPSIES)

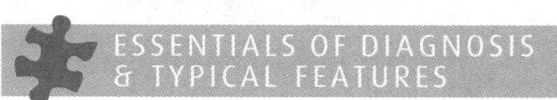

ESSENTIALS OF DIAGNOSIS
& TYPICAL FEATURES

▶ Recurrent unprovoked seizures.
▶ Often, interictal electroencephalographic changes.

▶ General Considerations

A seizure is a sudden, transient disturbance of brain function, manifested by involuntary motor, sensory, autonomic, or psychic phenomena, alone or in any combination, often accompanied by alteration or loss of consciousness. Seizures can be caused by any factor that disturbs brain function. They may occur after a metabolic, traumatic, anoxic, or infectious insult to the brain (classified as remote symptomatic seizures), or spontaneously without prior known CNS insult.

Repeated seizures without evident acute symptomatic cause (eg, fever) are defined as epilepsy. Epilepsy occurs most often in individuals at the extremes of the life span. The incidence is highest in the newborn period, and higher in childhood than in later life, with another peak in the elderly. Prevalence flattens out after age 10–15 years. The chance of having a second seizure after an initial unprovoked episode in a child is about 50%. The risk of recurrence after a second unprovoked seizure is 85%. Sixty-five to 70% of children with epilepsy will achieve seizure remission with appropriate medication. Epilepsy with childhood onset remits in about 50% of children.

▶ Classification

The International League Against Epilepsy (ILAE) has established classifications of seizures and epilepsy syndromes. Seizures are classified as either as partial (with localized onset) or generalized, involving the whole brain. Seizures and epilepsy syndromes may be partial at onset and then secondarily generalize (partial seizures with secondary generalization), or generalized from the onset.

Epilepsy syndromes are defined by the nature of the seizures (ie, localized vs generalized), age of onset, EEG findings, and other clinical factors. Epilepsy is classified as symptomatic (the cause is identified or presumed and may be due to a remote CNS injury), cryptogenic (undetermined etiology, presumably symptomatic and often due to congenital CNS abnormalities), or idiopathic (often genetic). In general, symptomatic and cryptogenic epilepsy have their onset early in life. Idiopathic (genetic) epilepsy syndromes are usually age specific, occurring at any age from early infancy to adolescence, depending on the specific syndrome. The specific epilepsy syndrome is helpful in defining prognosis, with idiopathic epilepsy more likely to be controlled and eventually remit than symptomatic epilepsy.

1. Seizures & Epilepsy in Childhood

Classifying the seizure is necessary for accurate diagnosis, which will determine the nature of further evaluation and treatment and help in prognostication (Tables 23–5 and 23–6).

Table 23-5. Seizures by age at onset, pattern, and preferred treatment.

Seizure Type	Age at Onset	Clinical Manifestations	Causative Factors	EEG Pattern	Other Diagnostic Studies	Treatment and Comments
Neonatal seizures	Birth–2 wk	Often subtle; sudden limpness or tonic posturing, brief apnea, and cyanosis; odd cry; eyes rolling up; blinking or mouthing or chewing movements; nystagmus, twitchiness or clonic movements (focal, multifocal, or generalized). Some seizures are nonepileptic: decerebrate, or other posturings, release from forebrain inhibition. Poor response to drugs.	Neurologic insults (hypoxia/ischemia; intracranial hemorrhage) present more in first 3 or after 8th day; metabolic disturbances alone between 3rd and 8th days; hypoglycemia, hypocalcemia, hyper- and hyponatremia. Pyridoxine dependency, CNS infections. Structural abnormalities.	May correlate poorly with clinical seizures. Focal spikes or slow rhythms; multifocal discharges. Electroclinical dissociation may occur: EEG-electrical seizure without clinical manifestations and vice versa.	Lumbar puncture; CSF PCR for herpes, enterovirus; serum Ca^{2+}, PO_4^{3-}, glucose, Mg^{2+}; BUN, amino acid screen, blood ammonia, organic acid screen, TORCHS IgM. Ultrasound or CT/MRI for suspected intracranial hemorrhage and structural abnormalities.	Phenobarbital, IV or IM; if seizures not controlled, add phenytoin IV (loading dose 20 mg/kg each). Diazepam, 0.3 mg/kg. Recent experience with levetiracetam and topiramate. Treat underlying disorder. Seizures due to brain damage often resistant to anticonvulsants. When cause in doubt, stop protein feedings until enzyme deficiencies of urea cycle or amino acid metabolism ruled out.
West syndrome (infantile spasms)	3–18 mo	Sudden, usually but not always symmetrical adduction or flexion of limbs with flexion of head and trunk; or abduction and extensor movements (similar to Moro reflex). Occur in clusters. Associated irritability and regression in development.	Symptomatic in approximately two thirds. Acquired CNS injury in approximately one third; biochemical, infectious, degenerative in approximately one third; cryptogenic in approximately one third. With early onset, pyridoxine dependency, inherited metabolic disorders. Tuberous sclerosis in 5–10%. TORCHS, homeobox gene mutations.	Hypsarrhythmia; chaotic high-voltage slow waves or random spikes (90%); other abnormalities in 10%. Rarely normal at onset. EEG normalization early in course usually correlates with reduction of seizures; not helpful prognostically regarding mental development.	Funduscopic and skin examination, trial of pyridoxine. Amino and organic acid screen. Chronic inflammatory disease. TORCHS screen, CT, or MRI scan should be done to (1) establish definite diagnosis, (2) aid in genetic counseling. Occasionally, surgical resection of cortical malformation useful.	ACTH gel (40 U/d to 150 U/m^2) IM once daily. Vigabatrin, especially if tuberous sclerosis. B_6 (pyridoxine) trial. In resistant cases, zonisamide, valproic acid, topiramate, lamotrigine, ketogenic diet. Mental retardation of varying degree in 90% of cases.
Febrile convulsions	3 mo–5 y (maximum 6–18 mo); most common childhood seizure (incidence 2%)	Usually generalized seizures, < 15 min; rarely focal in onset. May lead to status epilepticus. Recurrence risk of second febrile seizure 30% (50% if under 1 y of age); recurrence risk is same after status epilepticus.	Non-neurologic febrile illness (temperature rises to 39°C or higher); Risk factors: positive family history, day care, slow development, prolonged neonatal hospitalization.	Normal interictal EEG, especially when obtained 8–10 d after seizure.	Lumbar puncture in infants or whenever suspicion of meningitis exists.	Treat underlying illness, fever. Diazepam orally, 0.3–0.5 mg/kg, divided 3 times daily during illness may be considered. Diastat rectally for prolonged (> 5 min) seizure. Prophylaxis with phenobarbital or valproic acid rarely needed.

	Age	Clinical Features	Etiology	EEG	Workup	Treatment
Cryptogenic generalized epilepsies of early childhood, including Lennox-Gastaut syndrome and myoclonic-astatic epilepsy (Doose syndrome)	Any time in childhood (usually 2–7 y)	Mixed seizures dependent on particular syndrome, including tonic, myoclonic (shocklike violent contractions of one or more muscle groups, singly or irregularly repetitive); atonic ("drop attacks") and atypical absence with episodes of absence status epilepticus.	Multiple causes, usually resulting in diffuse neuronal damage. History of West syndrome; prenatal or perinatal brain damage; viral meningoencephalitis; CNS degenerative disorders; structural cerebral abnormalities (eg, migrational abnormalities). Doose syndrome may be genetic.	Atypical slow (1–2.5 Hz) spike-wave complexes and bursts of high-voltage generalized spikes, often with diffusely slow background frequencies. Electro-decremental and fast spikes during sleep.	As dictated by index of suspicion. Consider inherited metabolic disorders, neuronal ceroid lipofuscinosis, others. Skin or conjunctival biopsy for electron microscopy, MRI scan, WBC lysosomal enzymes, nerve conduction studies if degenerative disease suspected.	Difficult to treat. Topiramate, ethosuximide, felbamate, levetiracetam, zonisamide, valproate, clonazepam, ketogenic diet, vagus nerve stimulation. Avoid phenytoin, carbamazepine, oxcarbazepine, gabapentin.
Childhood absence epilepsy	3–12 y	Lapses of consciousness or vacant stares, lasting about 3–10 s, often in clusters. Automatisms of face and hands; clonic activity in 30–45%. Often confused with complex partial seizures but no aura or postictal confusion.	Unknown. Genetic component. Abnormal thalamocortical circuitry.	3/s bilaterally synchronous, symmetrical, high-voltage spikes and waves. EEG normalization correlates closely with control of seizures.	Hyperventilation often provokes attacks. Imaging studies rarely of value.	Valproic acid, lamotrigine, or ethosuximide. In resistant cases, zonisamide, topiramate, levetiracetam, acetazolamide, ketogenic diet.
Juvenile absence epilepsy	10–15 y	Absence seizures less frequent than in childhood absence epilepsy. May have greater risk of convulsive seizures.	Unknown (idiopathic); possibly genetic.	3-Hz spike wave and atypical generalized discharges.	Not always triggered by hyperventilation.	Same as childhood absence epilepsy but may be more difficult to treat successfully.
Simple partial or focal seizures (motor/sensory/jacksonian).	Any age	Seizure may involve any part of body; may spread in fixed pattern (jacksonian march), becoming generalized. In children, epileptogenic focus often "shifts," and epileptic manifestations may change concomitantly.	Often unknown; birth trauma, inflammatory process, vascular accidents, meningo-encephalitis, etc. If seizures are coupled with new or progressive neurologic deficits, a structural lesion (eg, brain tumor) is likely. If epilepsia partialis continua (simple partial status epilepticus), Rasmussen syndrome is likely.	EEG may be normal; focal spikes or slow waves in appropriate cortical region; sometimes diffusely abnormal or even normal. "Rolandic spikes" (centrotemporal spikes) are typical. Possibly genetic.	If seizures are difficult to control or progressive deficits occur, neuroradio-diagnostic studies, particularly MRI brain scan, are imperative.	Carbamazepine; oxcarbazepine; phenytoin, lamotrigine, gabapentin, topiramate, levetiracetam, and zonisamide. Valproic acid useful adjunct.

(continued)

Table 23–5. Seizures by age at onset, pattern, and preferred treatment. (*Continued*)

Seizure Type	Age at Onset	Clinical Manifestations	Causative Factors	EEG Pattern	Other Diagnostic Studies	Treatment and Comments
Complex partial seizures (psychomotor, temporal lobe, or limbic seizures are older terms).	Any age	Aura may be a sensation of fear, epigastric discomfort, odd smell or taste (usually unpleasant), visual or auditory hallucination. Aura and seizure stereotyped for each patient. Seizure may consist of vague stare; facial, tongue, or swallowing movements and throaty sounds; or various complex automatisms. Usually brief, 15–90 s, followed by confusion. History of aura and of automatisms involving more than face and hands establish diagnosis.	As above. Temporal lobes especially sensitive to hypoxia; seizure may be a sequela of birth trauma, febrile convulsions, viral encephalitis, especially herpes. Remediable other causes are small cryptic tumors or vascular malformations. May be genetic.	As above, but occurring in temporal lobe and its connections (eg, frontotemporal, temporoparietal, temporo-occipital regions).	MRI when structural lesions suspected. PCR of CSF in acute febrile situation for herpes or enteroviral encephalitis. SPECT, PET scan, video EEG monitoring when epilepsy surgery considered.	Carbamazepine, phenytoin. More than one drug may be necessary. Valproic acid may be useful. In cases uncontrolled by drugs and where a primary epileptogenic focus is identifiable, excision of anterior third of temporal lobe. Oxcarbazepine, topiramate, lamotrigine, levetiracetam, and zonisamide.
Benign epilepsy of childhood with centrotemporal spikes (BECTS/rolandic epilepsy)	5–16 y	Partial motor or generalized seizures. Similar seizure patterns may be observed in patients with focal cortical lesions. Usually nocturnal simple partial seizures of face, tongue, hand.	Seizure history or abnormal EEG findings in relatives of 40% of affected probands and 18–20% of parents and siblings, suggesting transmission by a single autosomal dominant gene, possibly with age-dependent penetrance.	Centrotemporal spikes or sharp waves ("rolandic discharges") appearing paroxysmally against a normal EEG background.	Seldom need CT or MRI scan.	Carbamazepine or other agent. (See complex partial seizures.) Often no medication is necessary, especially if seizure is exclusively nocturnal and infrequent. Lamotrigine, topiramate, levetiracetam, zonisamide.
Juvenile myoclonic epilepsy (of Janz)	Late childhood and adolescence, peaking at 13 y	Mild myoclonic jerks of neck and shoulder flexor muscles after awakening. Intelligence usually normal. Often absence seizures, and generalized tonic-clonic seizures as well.	40% of relatives have myoclonias, especially in females; 15% have the abnormal EEG pattern with clinical attacks.	Interictal EEG shows variety of spike-and-wave sequences or 4–6-Hz multi-spike-and-wave complexes ("fast spikes").	If course is unfavorable, differentiate from progressive myoclonic syndromes by appropriate biopsies (muscles, liver, etc).	Valproic acid, lamotrigine, topiramate, ?levetiracetam, zonisamide.
Generalized tonic-clonic seizures (grand mal) (GTCS)	Any age	Loss of consciousness; tonic-clonic movements; often preceded by vague aura or cry. Postictal confusion; sleep. Often mixed with or masking other seizure patterns. Incontinence in 15%.	Often unknown. Genetic component. May be seen with metabolic disturbances, trauma, infection, intoxication, degenerative disorders, brain tumors.	Bilaterally synchronous, symmetrical multiple high-voltage spikes, spikes-waves (eg, 3/s). EEG often normal in those younger than age 4 y. Focal spikes may become "secondarily generalized."	As above.	Phenobarbital in infants; carbamazepine or valproic acid; phenytoin; topiramate, lamotrigine. Combinations may be necessary.

ACTH, adrenocorticotropic hormone; BUN, blood urea nitrogen; CNS, central nervous system; CSF, cerebrospinal fluid; CT, computed tomography; EEG, electroencephalogram; IM, intramuscularly; IV, intravenously; MRI, magnetic resonance imaging; PCR, polymerase chain reaction; PET, positron emission tomography; SPECT, single photon emission tomography; TORCHS, toxoplasmosis, other infections, rubella, cytomegalovirus, herpes simplex, and syphilis; WBC, white blood cell.

Table 23–6. Benign childhood epileptic syndromes.

Syndrome	Characteristics
Benign idiopathic neonatal convulsions (BINC)	So-called "5th day fits" (97% have onset on 3rd to 7th day of life); 6% of neonatal convulsions; clonic, multifocal, usually brief; occasional status epilepticus
Benign familial neonatal convulsions (BFNC)	Autosomal dominant; onset in 2–90 d; genes, *KCNQ2* or *KCNQ3*; clonic; 86% recover
Generalized tonic-clonic seizures (GTCS)	Age at onset, 3–11 y; may have family or personal history of febrile convulsions; 50% have 3/s spike-wave EEG; may have concurrent absence seizures
Childhood absence seizures	Incidence higher in girls than in boys; age at onset, 3–12 y (peak 6–7 y); 10–200 seizures per day; 3/s spike-wave EEG; up to 40% have GTCS
Juvenile absence seizures	Incidence higher in boys than in girls; age at onset, 10–12 y; uncommon; less frequent seizures; 3–4/s general spike-wave EEG; most have GTCS; some remit
Juvenile myoclonic epilepsy (Janz syndrome)	Age at onset, 12–18 y (average, 15 y); myoclonic jerks upper limbs, seldom fall; 4–6/s general spike-wave EEG; untreated, 90% have GTCS, mostly on waking; 20–30% have absence seizures; 25–40% are photosensitive; 10% remission rate (90% do not remit)
Benign epilepsy with centrotemporal spikes (BECTS); "rolandic epilepsy"	Age at onset 3–13 y (most at 4–10 y); 80% have brief, 2–5 min sleep seizures only; usually simple partial seizures (face, tongue, cheek, hand) sensory or motor; occasionally have GTCS; bilateral independent spikes on EEG; may not need medication if seizures infrequent; remits at puberty
Benign epilepsy of childhood with occipital paroxysms (Panayiotopoulos syndrome)	6% of children with epilepsy; age at onset 3–6 y in 80% of patients (mean age, 5 y; range, 1–12 y); autonomic symptoms and visual aura may suggest migraine

EEG, electroencephalogram.

▶ Clinical Findings

A. History, Symptoms, and Signs

Seizures are clinical events; the key to diagnosis is the clinical history. Not all paroxysmal events are epileptic. A description of seizure onset is important in determining if there is localized onset (partial or focal seizure). Events prior to, during, and after the seizure need to be described (although observers often recall little except generalized convulsive activity because of its dramatic appearance). An aura (actu-ally a simple partial seizure) may precede the clinically apparent seizure and indicates focal onset. The patient may describe a feeling of fear, numbness or tingling in the fingers, or bright lights in one visual field. The specific symptoms may help define the location of seizure onset (eg, déjà vu suggests temporal lobe onset). Often, the child does not recall or cannot define the aura though the family may note alterations in behavior at the onset.

Details of the seizure's semiology can help determine the seizure type and, if partial, the site of onset. Did the patient become extremely pale before falling? Was the patient able to respond to queries during the episode? Was the patient unconscious or was there just impaired awareness? Did the patient fall stiffly or gradually slump to the floor? Was there an injury? How long did the tonic stiffening or clonic jerking last? Where in the body did the clonic activity take place? Postictal states can be helpful in diagnosis. After complex partial and generalized convulsive seizures, postictal sleep typically occurs, but postictal changes are not seen after generalized absence seizures. Was there loss of speech after the seizure (suggesting left temporal lobe seizure) or was the patient able to respond and speak in short order? The parent may report lateralized motor activity (eg, the child's eyes may deviate to one side or the child may experience dystonic posturing of a limb). Motor activity without impaired awareness supports the diagnosis of simple partial seizures. Impaired awareness and automatisms define the event as a complex partial seizure.

In contrast, primary generalized seizures manifest with acute loss of consciousness, usually with generalized motor activity. Tonic posturing, tonic-clonic activity or myoclonus (spasms) may occur. In children with generalized absence seizures, behavioral arrest may be associated with automatisms such as blinking, chewing, or hand movements, making it difficult to differentiate between absence seizures and partial seizures.

Description of the semiology of the event may help determine if the child experienced an epileptic seizure or a nonepileptic event mimicking or misinterpreted as an epileptic seizure. Frequently the child presenting with a presumed first seizure has experienced unrecognized seizures before the event that brings the child to medical attention. In particular, partial and absence seizures may not be recognized except in retrospect. Thus careful questioning regarding prior events is important in the child being evaluated for new onset of seizures.

B. Diagnostic Evaluation

The extent and urgency of the diagnostic evaluation is determined, in general, by the child's age, the severity and type of seizure, whether the child is ill or injured, and the clinician's suspicion about the underlying cause. Seizures in early infancy are often symptomatic. Therefore, the younger the child, the more extensive must be the diagnostic assessment (Table 23–7).

Table 23–7. Diagnostic evaluation in seizures.

After a first seizure	
Well infant (not neonatal)	Emergent imaging if persistent abnormal neurologic examination (especially Todd paresis), or concern about trauma (rule out nonaccidental trauma). EEG (may be deferred unless concern about nonconvulsive status epilepticus). If clinical suspicion, calcium, BUN, or others.
Well older child	Same as above.
Ill infant	Depending on presentation consider CT, Ca^{2+}, Mg^{2+}, CBC, BUN, glucose, electrolytes, blood culture, lumbar puncture performed acutely. Nonemergent EEG (emergent if concern about nonconvulsive status epilepticus). Possibly MRI.
Ill older child	Depending on presentation consider CT, CBC, BUN, lumbar puncture. Nonemergent EEG. Possibly MRI.
Generalized tonic-clonic seizure	Practice parameter: EEG only. Circumstances may suggest need for toxicology screen, calcium, glucose, CBC, BUN, electrolytes, lumbar puncture, and others if concern about infection (especially HSV).
For new-onset epilepsy	
Infant (< 1 y)	Imaging (MRI is preferred study); EEG. Evaluation for inherited metabolic disorder: lumbar puncture including CSF (and serum) glucose, lactate, glycine; serum and urine amino and organic acids; high-resolution chromosome analysis; other genetic testing including Rett syndrome; FISH for Angelman syndrome.
Older child	EEG; imaging (MRI). Other evaluation dependant on epilepsy syndrome. Consider CBC and AST before initiation of treatment.
Childhood absence seizure	EEG only.
Symptomatic/cryptogenic generalized epilepsy (Lennox-Gastaut and variants; myoclonic epilepsy)	EEG. Evaluation for causes of mental retardation: MRI; serum and urine amino and organic acids; high-resolution chromosome analysis; other genetic testing including Rett syndrome; FISH for Angelman syndrome, progressive myoclonic epilepsy (neuronal ceroid lipofuscinosis [NCL]. Consider lysosomal enzymes, lumbar puncture including glucose (CSF and serum) lactate, glycine, neurotransmitters, long-chain fatty acids, skin or conjunctival biopsies.
Infantile spasms (West syndrome)	Consider tuberous sclerosis complex (including Wood's lamp, renal and cardiac scans). Evaluation as for symptomatic generalized epilepsy.
Cryptogenic focal epilepsy	EEG including video-EEG monitoring if necessary for clarification of diagnosis. MRI with attention to possible focal cortical dysplasia.
Idiopathic focal epilepsy (BECTS)	EEG.

AST, aspartate aminotransferase; BECTS, benign epilepsy with centrotemporal spikes; BUN, blood urea nitrogen; CBC, complete blood count; CSF, cerebrospinal fluid; CT, computed tomography; EEG, electroencephalogram; FISH, florescent in-situ hybridization; HSV, herpes simples virus.

It is generally accepted that every child with new onset of unprovoked seizures should be evaluated with an EEG, although this need not be done emergently. An EEG is very unlikely to yield clinically useful information in the child with a febrile seizure. Other diagnostic studies should be used selectively.

Metabolic abnormalities are seldom found in the well child with seizures. Unless there is a high clinical suspicion of serious medical conditions (eg, uremia, hyponatremia, hypocalcemia, etc), "routine" laboratory tests rarely yield clinically significant information. Special studies may be necessary in circumstances that suggest an acute systemic etiology for a seizure, for example, in the presence of apparent renal failure, sepsis, or substance abuse.

Emergent imaging of the brain is usually not necessary in the absence evidence of trauma or of acute abnormalities on examination. Nonurgent MRI should be performed in any child with a significant cognitive or motor impairment, or abnormalities on neurologic examination of unknown etiology, a seizure of partial (focal) onset, or an EEG that does not

represent benign partial epilepsy of childhood or primary generalized epilepsy, and should be seriously considered in infants younger than 1 year of age.

The child with a simple febrile seizure or an unprovoked generalized seizure with normal examination and normal EEG often will not require imaging. Clinically significant abnormalities rarely are found on imaging of children with new onset of idiopathic epilepsy syndromes such as benign focal epilepsy of childhood (BECTS or rolandic epilepsy) and absence epilepsy with a normal neurologic examination and diagnostic EEG. Conversely, in children with symptomatic epileptic syndromes such as infantile spasms and Lennox-Gastaut syndrome, MRI (the preferred study) will be abnormal in as many as 60–80% of patients. Evidence of localization related epilepsy is an indication for MRI of the brain. Imaging is not necessary in children with BECTS, but the yield with other focal seizures is 15–30%, with findings supportive of the diagnosis (eg, focal cortical dysplasia) and useful in defining the prognosis. Other indications for MRI scan include difficulty in controlling seizures, progressive neurologic findings on serial examinations, worsening focal findings on the EEG, or other evidence of progressive neurologic dysfunction, even in the instance where a prior imaging scan was normal.

C. Electroencephalography

Appropriate use of EEG requires awareness of its limitations as well as its utility. The limitations of EEG even with epilepsy, for which it is most useful, are considerable. A routine EEG captures electrical activity during a very short period of time, usually 30–40 minutes. Thus it is useful primarily for defining interictal activity (except for the fortuitous recording of a clinical seizure or in the case of childhood absence epilepsy). A seizure is a clinical phenomenon; an EEG showing epileptiform activity may confirm and even extend the clinical diagnosis, but it is only occasionally diagnostic.

1. Diagnostic value—The greatest value of the EEG in convulsive disorders is to help classify seizure types and epilepsy syndromes. This can aid in prognostication and in selecting appropriate therapy (see Table 23–5). Hypomotor seizures (absence and complex partial seizures) are sometimes difficult to distinguish. The differing EEG patterns of these seizures will then prove most helpful. The presence of a mixed seizure EEG pattern in a child with clinically generalized convulsive seizures or only focal seizures may lead to identification of specific epilepsy syndromes and help the clinician select anticonvulsants effective for the seizure types identified by the EEG. Similarly, the EEG may help in diagnosing seizures in a young infant with minimal or atypical clinical manifestations; it may show hypsarrhythmia (high-amplitude spikes and slow waves with a chaotic background) in West syndrome (infantile spasms) or the 1–4/s slow spike-wave pattern of the Lennox-Gastaut syndrome. The EEG may show focal slowing that, if constant, particularly when corresponding focal seizure manifestations and abnormal neurologic findings are present, will alert the physician to the presence of a structural lesion. In this case, brain imaging may establish the cause and help determine further investigation and treatment.

The EEG need not be abnormal in a child with epilepsy. Normal EEGs are seen following a first generalized seizure in one third of children younger than age 4 years. The initial EEG is normal in about 20% of older epileptic children and in about 10% of epileptic adults. These percentages are reduced when serial tracings are obtained. Focal spikes and generalized spike-wave discharges are seen in 30% of close nonepileptic relatives of patients with epilepsy.

2. Prognostic value—A normal EEG following a first convulsion suggests (but does not guarantee) a favorable prognosis. Hypsarrhythmia or slow spike and wave patterns support the diagnosis of West syndrome and Lennox-Gastaut syndrome respectively. Both are expressions of diffuse brain dysfunction (epileptic encephalopathy) and are generally of grave significance. Central-temporal (rolandic spikes) and occipital spike wave activity (occipital paroxysms) are the EEG correlates of idiopathic focal epilepsies of childhood.

Following successful treatment, abnormal EEGs may become normal and may aid in the decision to discontinue medications. The normalization of the EEG in childhood absence epilepsy confirms the efficacy of treatment. Normalization can also be seen in infants with West syndrome who have been successfully treated and, less commonly, in children with epileptic encephalopathies.

Electroencephalography should be repeated when the severity and frequency of seizures increase despite adequate anticonvulsant therapy, when the clinical seizure pattern changes significantly, or when progressive neurologic deficits develop. Emergence of new focal or diffuse slowing may indicate a progressive lesion or neurodegenerative disorder.

The EEG may be helpful in determining when to discontinue anticonvulsant therapy. The presence or absence of epileptiform activity on the EEG prior to withdrawal of anticonvulsants after a seizure-free period of 2 years on medications has been shown to correlate with the degree of risk of seizure recurrence.

▶ Differential Diagnosis

It is extremely important to be accurate in the diagnosis of epilepsy and not to make the diagnosis without ample proof. To the layperson, epilepsy often has connotations of brain damage and limitation of activity. A person so diagnosed may be excluded from certain occupations in later life. It is often very difficult to change an inaccurate diagnosis of many years' standing.

Misinterpretation of behaviors in children is the most common reason for misdiagnosis. Psychogenic seizures are much less common in children than in adults but must be considered even in the young or cognitively impaired child. The most commonly misinterpreted behaviors are inattention in school-aged children with attention disorders, stereotypes in children with autistic spectrum disorder, sleep-related movements, habit movements such as head-banging and so-called infantile masturbation (sometimes referred to as gratification movements), and gastroesophageal reflux in very young (often impaired) infants.

Some of the common nonepileptic events that mimic seizure disorder are listed in Table 23–8.

▶ Complications & Sequelae

A. Psychosocial Impact

Emotional disturbances, especially depression but also including anxiety, anger, and feelings of guilt and inadequacy, often occur in the patient as well as the parents of a child with epilepsy. Actual or perceived stigma as well as issues regarding "disclosure" are common. There may be an increased risk of suicide in people with epilepsy. Schools often limit activities of children with epilepsy inappropriately and stigmatize children by these limitations.

Table 23–8. Nonepileptic paroxysmal events.

Breath-holding attacks (cyanotic and pallid)

Cyanotic: Age 6 mo–3 y. Always precipitated by trauma and fright. Cyanosis; sometimes stiffening, tonic (or jerking-clonic) convulsion (anoxic seizure). Patient may sleep following attack. Family history positive in 30%. Electroencephalogram (EEG) normal. Treatment is interpretation and reassurance.

Pallid: No external precipitant (perhaps internal pain, cramp, or fear?). Pallor may be followed by seizure (anoxic-ischemic). Vagally (heart-slowing) mediated, like adult syncope. EEG normal; may see cardiac slowing with vagal stimulation (cold cloth on face) during EEG. May be seen in children with cyanotic spells as well.

Tics (Tourette syndrome)

Simple or complex stereotyped jerks or movements, coughs, grunts, sniffs. Worse at repose or with stress. May be suppressed during physician visit. Family history often positive for tics or for obsessive compulsive disorder. Diagnosis is clinical. MRI and EEG are negative. Medications may benefit.

Parasomnias (Night terrors, sleep talking, walking, "sit-ups")

Ages 3–10 y. Usually occur in first sleep cycle (30–90 min after going to sleep), with crying, screaming, and autonomic discharge (pupils dilated, perspiring, etc). May last only a few minutes or be more prolonged. Child goes back to sleep and has no recall of event next day. Sleep studies (polysomnogram and EEG) are normal. Sleep talking and walking and short "sit-ups" in bed are fragmentary arousals. If a spell is recorded, EEG shows arousal from deep sleep, but behavior seems wakeful. Child needs to be protected from injury and gradually settled down and taken back to bed. Medications may be considered in rare instances.

Nightmares

Nightmares or vivid dreams occur in subsequent cycles of sleep, often in early morning hours, and generally are partially recalled the next day. The bizarre and frightening behavior may sometimes be confused with complex partial seizures but occurs during REM (rapid eye movement) sleep, whereas epilepsy usually does not. In extreme or difficult cases, an all-night sleep EEG may help differentiate seizures from nightmares.

Migraine

One migraine variant can be associated with an acute confusional state. Usual migraine prodrome of spots before the eyes, dizziness, visual field defects, and then agitated confusion may be present. History of other, more typical migraine with severe headache and vomiting but without confusion may aid in diagnosis. Severe headache with vomiting as child comes out of spell may aid in distinguishing the attack from epilepsy. Other seizure manifestations are practically never seen (eg, tonic-clonic movements, falling, complete loss of consciousness). EEG in migraine is usually normal and seldom has epileptiform abnormalities often seen in patients with epilepsy. Migraine and epilepsy are sometimes linked: migraine-caused ischemia on the surface sometimes leads to later epilepsy. Are both channelopathies?

Benign nocturnal myoclonus

Common in infants and may last even up to school age. Focal or generalized jerks (the latter also called hypnic or sleep jerks) may persist from onset of sleep on and off all night. A video record for physician review can aid in diagnosis. EEG taken during jerks is normal, proving that these jerks are not epilepsy. Treatment is reassurance.

Shuddering

Shuddering or shivering attacks can occur in infancy and be a forerunner of essential tremor in later life. Often, family history is positive for tremor. Shivering may be very frequent. EEG is normal. There is no clouding or loss of consciousness.

Gastroesophageal reflux (Sandifer syndrome)

Seen more commonly in children with cerebral palsy or brain damage; reflux of acid gastric contents may cause pain that cannot be described by child. Unusual posturing (dystonic or other) of head and neck or trunk may occur, an apparent attempt to stretch the esophagus or close the opening. There is no loss of consciousness, but eye rolling, apnea, and occasional vomiting may simulate a seizure. An upper gastrointestinal series, cine of swallowing, sometimes even an EEG (normal during episode) may be necessary to distinguish from seizures.

Infantile masturbation

Rarely in infants, repetitive rocking or rubbing motions may simulate seizures. Infant may look out of contact, be poorly responsive to environment, and have autonomic expressions (eg, perspiration, dilated pupils) that may be confused with seizures. Observation by a skilled individual, sometimes even in a hospital setting, may be necessary to distinguish from seizures. EEG is normal between or during attacks. Interpretation and reassurance are the only necessary treatment.

Conversion reaction/pseudoseizures

Up to 50% of patients with pseudoseizures have epilepsy. Episodes may involve writhing, intercourse-like movements, tonic movements, bizarre jerking and thrashing, or even apparently sudden unresponsiveness. Often, there is ongoing psychological trauma. Often, but not invariably, children are developmentally delayed. Spells must often be seen or recorded on videotape in a controlled situation to distinguish from epilepsy but are sometimes so bizarre they are easily differentiated. A normal EEG during a spell is a key diagnostic feature. Sometimes, pseudoseizures can be precipitated by suggestion with injection of normal saline in a controlled situation. Combativeness is common; self-injury and incontinence, rare.

Temper tantrums and rage attacks

Sometimes confused with epilepsy. Child is often amnesic or at least claims amnesia for events during spell. Attacks are usually precipitated by frustration or anger, often directed either verbally or physically, and subside with behavior modification and isolation. EEGs are generally normal but unfortunately seldom obtained during an attack. Anterior temporal leads may help rule out temporal or lateral frontal abnormalities, the latter sometimes seen in partial complex seizures. Improvement of attacks with psychotherapy, milieu therapy, or behavioral modification helps rule out epilepsy.

Benign paroxysmal vertigo

Brief attacks of vertigo in which child often appears frightened and pale and clutches parent. Attacks last 5–30 s. Sometimes, nystagmus is identified. There is no loss of consciousness. Usually, child is well and returns to play immediately afterward. Attacks may occur in clusters, then disappear for months. Attacks are usually seen in infants and preschoolers aged 2–5 y. EEG is normal. If caloric tests can be obtained (often very difficult in this age group), abnormalities with hypofunction of one side are sometimes seen. Medications are usually not desirable or necessary.

Staring spells

Teachers often make referral for absence or petit mal seizures in children who stare or seem preoccupied at school. Helpful in the history is the lack of these spells at home (eg, before breakfast, a common time for absence seizures). Lack of other epilepsy in child or family history often is helpful. These children sometimes have difficulties with school and cognitive or learning disabilities. Child can generally be brought out of spell by a firm command. EEG is sometimes necessary to confirm that absence seizures are not occurring. A 24-hour ambulatory EEG to record attacks during child's everyday school activities is occasionally necessary.

Epilepsy with onset in childhood has an impact on adult function. Adults with early onset of epilepsy are less likely to complete high school, have less adequate employment, and are less likely to marry. Persistent epilepsy results in significant dependence; even when epilepsy is successfully treated, patients with long-standing epilepsy often do not become independent.

Rarely, psychosis may be seen in patients with epilepsy; usually in older children and adults.

B. Cognitive Delay

There remains considerable debate about the impact of seizures and epilepsy on cognition. Clearly, epileptic encephalopathy (ie, regression in cognitive ability and development associated with uncontrolled seizures) does occur, particularly in young children with catastrophic epilepsies such as West syndrome and Lennox-Gastaut syndrome. It is less clear whether persistent partial seizures have an impact on development. It is even less likely that interictal epileptiform activity contributes to cognitive impairment. However, continuous epileptiform activity in sleep is associated with Landau-Kleffner syndrome (acquired epileptic aphasia).

Pseudodementia may occur in children with poorly controlled epilepsy because their seizures interfere with their learning. Depression is a common cause of impaired cognitive function in children with epilepsy. Anticonvulsants are less likely to cause such interference at usual therapeutic doses. However, all antiepileptic drugs carry some risk for adverse impact on cognition. Phenobarbital in particular, but also topiramate, valproate, and others, may be implicated.

Mental retardation and autistic spectrum disorders may be part of the same pathologic process that causes the seizures but may occasionally be worsened when seizures are frequent, prolonged, and accompanied by hypoxia.

C. Injury and Death

Physical injuries, especially lacerations of the forehead and chin, are frequent in astatic or akinetic seizures (so-called drop attacks), necessitating protective headgear. In all other seizure disorders in childhood, injuries as a direct result of an attack are not as common although drowning, injuries related to working in kitchens, and falls from heights remain a potential risk for all children with active epilepsy. It is therefore extremely important to stress "seizure precautions," in particular, water safety.

Sudden unexpected death with epilepsy (SUDEP) is a very rare event. The greatest fear of a parent of a child with new-onset of epilepsy is the possibility of death or brain injury. Although children with epilepsy have an increased risk of death, SUDEP is very rare (1–2:10,000 patient-years). Nearly all of the mortality in children with epilepsy is related to the underlying neurologic disorder, not the seizures. The greatest risk for SUDEP is in children with medically uncontrolled epilepsy, especially with symptomatic epilepsy (associated with identifiable CNS etiology). Normal children with epilepsy do not have an increased risk of death compared with the general population. There is no current proven strategy to prevent SUDEP. The mechanism for SUDEP is unclear but is probably most commonly related to postictal respiratory insufficiency. Occasionally the cause is a cardiac arrhythmia induced by a seizure. Vigorous attempts to control intractable seizure disorders remain the most important approach. Identifying life-threatening disorders (eg, identifying patients with cardiac arrhythmias, especially prolonged QT syndrome) as the cause of misdiagnosed epilepsy is clearly of utmost importance.

▶ Treatment

The ideal treatment of seizures is the correction of specific causes. However, even when a biochemical disorder, a tumor, meningitis, or another specific cause is being treated, anticonvulsant drugs are often still required.

A. First Aid

Caregivers should be instructed to protect the patient against self-injury. Turning the child to the side is useful for preventing aspiration. Thrusting a spoon handle, tongue depressor or finger into the clenched mouth of a convulsing patient or trying to restrain tonic-clonic movements may cause worse injuries than a bitten tongue or bruised limb. Parents are often concerned that cyanosis will occur during generalized convulsive seizures but it is rare for clinically significant hypoxia to occur. Mouth-to-mouth resuscitation is rarely necessary and is unlikely to be effective.

For prolonged seizures (those lasting over 5 minutes), rectal diazepam gel (Diastat) may be administered to prevent the development of status epilepticus. Diastat has proven to be safe even when administered by nonmedical professionals, including teachers and day-care providers, when appropriately instructed.

B. Antiepileptic Drug (AED) Therapy

1. Drug selection—Treat with the drug appropriate to the clinical situation, as outlined in Table 23–5.

2. Treatment strategy—The child with a single seizure has a 50% chance of recurrence. Thus, it is usually not necessary to initiate AED therapy until the diagnosis of epilepsy is established, that is, there is a second seizure. The seizure type and epilepsy syndrome as well as potential side-effects will determine which drug to initiate (see Table 23–5). Start with one drug in moderate dosage and increase the dosage until seizures are controlled. If seizures are not controlled on the maximal tolerated dosage of one major AED, gradually switch to another before using two-drug therapy. Polytherapy (ie, the use of more than two medications concurrently) is rarely sufficiently effective to warrant the considerable risk of adverse side effects from the synergistic impact of multiple medications.

Dosages and usually target serum levels of commonly prescribed AEDs are listed in Table 23–9. Individual variations

Table 23–9. Guide to pediatric antiepileptic drug (AED) therapy.[a]

Drug/Target Dose	Target Serum Levels	Idiosyncratic Reactions	Dose-Related Toxicity	Other Effects
Carbamazepine Adult: 1000–2000 mg/d Pediatric: 10–30 mg/kg/d	4–12 mcg/mL	Dermatologic (rash, including Stevens-Johnson syndrome), rare hematologic, hepatic	Vertigo, visual disturbance (diplopia), leukopenia	Hyponatremia in adults; leukopenia; liver induction; myoclonus in patients with general spike-wave discharges, increased bone metabolism
Ethosuximide Adult: 1000 mg/d Pediatric: 15–40 mg/kg/d	40–100 mcg/mL	Leukopenia, SLE, nephrotic syndrome, rash	Sedation, GI upset	Behavioral changes
Felbamate Adult: 2400–3600 mg/d Pediatric: 45–60 mg/kg/d; has been used up to 200 mg/kg/d	30–100 mcg/mL	Aplastic anemia (adults only?), hepatic failure, rash (rare)	Anorexia, insomnia, headache, irritability	Aplastic anemia (postpubertal?); drug interactions
Gabapentin Adult: 1800–3600 mg/d Pediatric: 30–100 mg/kg/d	4–20 mcg/mL	Rash (rare)	Somnolence, irritability, weight gain	Renal excretion, no drug interactions
Lamotrigine Adult: 300–500 mg/d Pediatric: 1–15 mg/kg/d; dose depends on concomitant medication	3–20 mcg/mL	Rash, hypersensitivity reaction	Ataxia, diplopia, GI upset, headache	Rash (probably 5%, especially in children), Stevens-Johnson syndrome
Levetiracetam Adult: 1200–2400 mg/d Pediatric: 40–100 mg/kg/d	5–50 mcg/mL	None reported to date	Somnolence, ataxia	Agitation, aggression, depression (5–10%?)
Oxcarbazepine Adult: 1200–2400 mg/d Pediatric: 15–45 mg/kg/d	MHD: 10–45 mcg/mL	Rash (25% cross-reactivity with carbamazepine)	CNS effects, diplopia	Hyponatremia (3% of adults) behavior, ?weight gain
Phenobarbital Adult: 60–120 mg/d Pediatric: 2–6 mg/kg/d	15–40 mcg/mL	Rash, Stevens-Johnson syndrome, SLE	Somnolence, irritability	Possible irreversible cognitive effects, liver induction, increased bone metabolism
Phenytoin Adult: 200–600 mg/d Pediatric: 4–8 mg/kg/d; may need higher does in infants	10–20 mcg/mL	Rash (5–10%), hematologic, hepatic, lymphadenopathy others	Cosmetic, CNS, ataxia, nystagmus	Elevated LFTs, induction; reduced vitamin D levels; ?cerebellar degeneration; increased bone metabolism
Primidone Adult: 750–2000 mg/d Pediatric: 5–20 mg/kg/d	4–12 mcg/mL	Rash	Sedation, irritability, GI upset	Similar to phenobarbital
Tiagabine Adult: 32–56 mg/d Pediatric: 0.25–1.25 mg/kg/d	5–70 mcg/mL	Psychiatric effects	CNS, tremor, weakness, gastroesophageal reflux, gait difficulty	
Topiramate Adult: 100–400 mg/d Pediatric: 5–25 mg/kg/d; can increase if side effects are tolerated	3–25 mcg/mL	Rash (rare), acute glaucoma (rare)	Somnolence, language disturbance, renal stones anorexia, paresthesias	Language disturbance (especially with polytherapy); avoid ketogenic diet; oligohidrosis

(continued)

Table 23–9. Guide to pediatric antiepileptic drug (AED) therapy.[a] *(Continued)*

Drug/Target Dose	Target Serum Levels	Idiosyncratic Reactions	Dose-Related Toxicity	Other Effects
Valproic acid Adult: 750–1500 mg/d Pediatric: 20–60 mg/kg/d	50–150 mcg/mL	Hepatic failure; pancreatitis	Tremor, weight gain, alopecia, sedation and cognitive changes, thrombocytopenia, prolonged bleeding time	Hepatic failure (in 1:500 children < age 2 y receiving polytherapy), elevated LFTs; GI upset with syrup; incidence of PCOS unknown, liver enzyme inhibition
Vigabatrin Adult: maximum 3000 mg/d Pediatric: 40–150 mg/kg/d	—	Visual field constriction, sedation, CNS effects	Psychiatric symptoms (rare), visual field constriction	Especially effective for infantile spasms and tuberous sclerosis
Zonisamide Adult: 200–600 mg/d Pediatric: 4–10 mg/kg/d	10–30 mcg/mL	Rash, hematologic, hepatic	Renal stones, anorexia, somnolence	Oligohidrosis in children; cross-sensitivity with sulfa drugs

[a]For newer drugs, doses, levels, and adverse effects are based on reported clinical experience and not on adequate scientific information from clinical trials in most cases. Some medications do not have FDA approval for children. The package insert for each medication lists indications, potential adverse effects, warnings, etc. Practitioners should with familiar with current published information as regards specific dosing, as well as potential adverse effects.
CNS, central nervous system; GI, gastrointestinal; LFT, liver function test; MHD, monohydroxy derivative; PCOS, polycystic ovary syndrome; SLE, systemic lupus erythematosus.

must be expected, both in tolerance and efficacy. The therapeutic range may also vary somewhat with the method used to determine levels, and published levels are not always reflective of clinical efficacy and tolerability.

3. Counseling—Advise the parents and the patient that the prolonged use of AEDs will not produce significant or permanent mental slowing (although the underlying cause of the seizures might) and that prevention of seizures for 1–2 years substantially reduces the chances of recurrence. Advise them also that AEDs are given to prevent further seizures and that they should be taken as prescribed. Changes in medications or dosages should not be made without the physician's knowledge. Unsupervised sudden withdrawal of AEDs may precipitate severe seizures or even status epilepticus. Medications must be kept where they cannot be ingested by small children or suicidal patients.

Older children should be encouraged to manage their medications on their own, but some degree of supervision by parents is often necessary to guarantee adherence to treatment regimens. Medications are invariably missed on occasions. Making up a single dose is reasonable, but making up multiple doses should be discouraged.

4. Follow-up—Regular follow-up evaluations of the patient are appropriate at intervals that depend on the degree of control, underlying cause of the seizures, and toxic properties of the AEDs used. Blood counts and liver function tests (aspartate aminotransferase; AST) are often obtained periodically in patients taking the older AEDs, such as valproate, phenytoin, and carbamazepine. Periodic neurologic reevaluation is important. Repeat EEGs are useful for confirming

seizure-freedom in children with absence epilepsy and West syndrome but otherwise are usually not useful as measures of medication efficacy.

5. Long-term management and discontinuation of treatment—AEDS should be continued until the patient is free of seizures for at least 1–2 years. In about 75% of patients, seizures may not recur. Variables such as younger age at onset, normal EEG, idiopathic etiology and ease of controlling seizures carry a favorable prognosis, whereas symptomatic etiology, later onset, continued epileptiform EEG, difficulty in establishing initial control of the seizures, polytherapy, generalized tonic-clonic or myoclonic seizures, as well as an abnormal neurologic examination are associated with a higher risk of recurrence. Most AEDs (with the exception of barbiturates and clonazepam) can be withdrawn over 6–8 weeks. There does not appear to be an advantage to slower withdrawal.

Recurrent seizures affect up to 25% of children who attempt withdrawal from medications. Recurrence of seizures is most likely within 6–12 months of discontinuing medications. Therefore, seizure safety precautions will need to be reinstituted, including driving restriction. If seizures recur during or after withdrawal, AED therapy should be reinstituted and maintained for at least another 1–2 years. The vast majority of children will again achieve remission of their seizures.

6. Blood levels of AEDs

A. GENERAL COMMENTS—Most AEDs take two or three times their half-life to reach the target serum levels indicated in Table 23–9. This must be considered when blood levels are assessed after AEDs are started or dosages are changed. Individuals vary in their metabolism and their particular pharmacokinetic characteristics. These and external factors, including, for example, food intake or illness, also affect the blood level. Thus the level reached on a milligram per kilogram basis varies among patients. Experience and clinical research in the determination of AED blood levels have shown that there is some correlation between (1) drug dose and blood level, (2) blood level and therapeutic effect, and (3) blood level and some toxic effects.

B. EFFECTIVE LEVELS—The target serum levels listed in Table 23–9 are those within which seizure control without toxicity will be achieved in most patients. The level for any given individual will vary not only with metabolic makeup (including biochemical defects) but also with the nature and severity of the seizures and their underlying cause, and with other medications being taken, among other factors. Seizure control may be achieved at lower levels in some patients, and higher levels may be reached without toxicity in others. When control is achieved at a lower level, the dosage should not be increased merely to move the level into the therapeutic range. Likewise, toxic side effects will be experienced at different levels even within the therapeutic range. Lowering the dosage may relieve the problem, but sometimes the drug must be withdrawn or another added (or both). Some serious toxic effects, including allergic reactions and bone marrow or liver toxicity, are independent of dosage.

C. INTERACTION OF AEDs—Blood levels of older AEDs may be affected by other drugs but this is less often the case with the newer medications. In addition to pharmacokinetic interaction, pharmacodynamic interactions may be observed, with increased side-effects despite "therapeutic" levels. Likewise, adverse effects noted with introduction of a second medication may be due to drug interactions and not to toxicity of the newly introduced medication per se.

D. INDICATIONS FOR DETERMINATION OF BLOOD LEVELS— There is rarely an indication for obtaining "routine" blood levels of AEDs. Thus levels should be determined for specific reasons. After a drug is introduced and seizure control is achieved, it may be useful to determine the effective level for that patient. Blood level monitoring is also useful when expected control on a usual dosage has not been achieved, when seizures recur in a patient with previously well-controlled seizures, or when there is a question of adherence to recommended treatment ("noncompliance"). A low level may indicate inadequate dosage, drug interaction, or nonadherence with the prescribed regimen. A high level may indicate slowed metabolism or excretion or drug interaction.

Blood levels are most commonly obtained when signs and symptoms of toxicity are present, especially when more than one drug is being used or when the dosage of a single drug has been changed. Blood levels may be the only means of detecting intoxication in a comatose patient, very young child, or child with severe cognitive impairment. Toxic levels also occur with drug abuse and in the presence of liver or renal disease. Blood levels are unnecessary when the patient's seizure control is satisfactory and he or she is free of toxic signs or symptoms.

7. Side effects of AEDs—(See also Table 23–9.)

A. IDIOSYNCRATIC REACTIONS—Serious **allergic rash** usually necessitates discontinuance of a drug. The risk of significant allergic rash is probably about 5–10% with carbamazepine, lamotrigine, oxcarbazepine, and phenobarbital, phenytoin. Stevens-Johnson syndrome is a risk in any child with a cutaneous eruption due to AEDs, although the degree of this risk is unclear. Not every rash in a child receiving an AED is drug-related. If a useful AED is discontinued and the rash disappears, restarting the drug in a smaller dosage may be warranted to see if the rash recurs.

Hepatic toxicity, pancreatitis, blood dyscrasias, renal stones, and other adverse **systemic effects** have been reported with various medications. It is not clear that routine surveillance is effective in preventing these complications of treatment. Nevertheless, routine laboratory testing is often undertaken by clinicians managing patients with epilepsy.

B. TREATMENT-EMERGENT TOXICITY—Signs of **dose-related drug toxicity** such as ataxia often disappear with relatively small decreases in medication dose. The exception is phenytoin, where protein binding and so called "zero-order kinetics" can make dose adjustments difficult.

Sedation is the most common treatment-emergent side effect of AED treatment. The sedative effect of many of these drugs may be avoided by slowly titrating mediation to a moderate dose over several weeks.

Familiarity with potential side effects can allow **anticipatory counseling.** Gingival hyperplasia secondary to phenytoin is best minimized through good dental hygiene but occasionally requires gingivectomy. The hypertrichosis associated with phenytoin does not regress when the drug is discontinued. The risk of weight gain with valproate and gabapentin and weight loss with topiramate, zonisamide, and felbamate should be discussed on initiation of treatment. Adequate hydration and avoiding overheating on hot days can prevent the hypothermia associated with hypohidrosis in some patients treated with topiramate and zonisamide.

C. Alternative Treatments

1. Adrenocorticotropic hormone (ACTH) and corticosteroids

A. INDICATIONS—ACTH is indicated for treatment of West syndrome. The utility of other immunotherapy is less clear. Duration of ACTH therapy is guided by cessation of clinical seizures and normalization of the EEG. No specific recommendations can be made regarding dosing and duration of therapy, and multiple protocols have been advocated with initial dosing ranging from 20 U/d to 150 U/m^2. ACTH is often continued in full doses for 2 or more weeks and then, if seizures have ceased, tapered over a variable length of time, usually several weeks. If seizures recur, the dosage is increased to the last effective level. Alternatively, vigabatrin may be tried. Some neurologists use longer durations of treatment, keeping the patient at the effective dosage of ACTH for up to 6 months before attempting withdrawal. There is no strong evidence, however, that longer courses of treatment are more beneficial.

Oral corticosteroids and intravenous immune globulin (IVIG) are occasionally used for pharmacoresistant epilepsy. However, dosing regimens and indications are not well established. Landau-Kleffner syndrome (acquired epileptic aphasia) is reported to respond to oral steroid treatment.

B. Dosages—For ACTH (Acthar Gel), start with 40–80 U/d or up to 150 U/m^2 intramuscularly in a single morning dose. Parents can be taught to give injections. For prednisone, start with 2–4 mg/kg/d orally in two or three divided doses.

C. Precautions—Give additional potassium, guard against infections, follow for possible hypertension, and discuss the cushingoid appearance and its disappearance. Do not withdraw oral corticosteroids suddenly. Side effects in some series occur in up to 40% of patients, especially with higher dosages than those listed here (used by some authorities). With long-term use, prophylaxis against *Pneumocystis* infection may be required. Careful and frequent follow-up is necessary. Visiting nurse services can be very helpful in surveillance such as monitoring blood pressure, weight, and potential adverse effects.

2. Ketogenic diet—A diet high in fats and low in protein and carbohydrates will result in ketosis as fatty acids replace glucose as a source of energy for cellular metabolism. Such a diet has been observed to decrease and even control seizures in some children. A ketogenic diet should be recommended in children with pharmacoresistant epilepsy, particularly those with symptomatic generalized epilepsies (astatic and myoclonic seizures and absence seizures) not responsive to drug therapy. Other seizure types may also respond. Ketosis is induced by a diet high in fats and very limited in carbohydrates with sufficient protein for body maintenance and growth. The ratio of fat-derived calories to carbohydrate and protein-derived calories is usually 4:1 in young children and somewhat lower in older children. Adding medium-chain triglycerides to the diet induces ketosis more readily than does a high level of dietary fats and thus requires less carbohydrate restriction. However, medium chain triglycerides are often not well tolerated.

Recent reports suggest efficacy with the Atkins diet or a low-glycemic index diet in older and higher functioning children who will not accept the ketogenic diet. A prepared commercially available formula is available for children receiving tube feedings. The mechanism for the anticonvulsant action of the ketogenic diet is not understood. It is, however, the ketosis, not the acidosis, that raises the seizure threshold.

The ketogenic diet requires close adherence and is often difficult for families as well as the children who cannot participate in family meals or special occasions (eg, birthday parties where cake is served). Full cooperation of all family members is required, including the patient if old enough. However, when seizure control is achieved by this method, acceptance of the diet is usually excellent.

As with all therapies, potential adverse effects can occur with the ketogenic diet. These include acidosis and hypoglycemia, particularly on initiation of the diet. Thus it is prudent to admit the child for initiation of the diet after screening laboratory studies are performed to rule out underlying metabolic disorders. Renal stones can occur, and acidosis and carnitine deficiency are often seen.

3. Vagus nerve stimulator—The vagus nerve stimulator (VNS) is a recently developed treatment for medically intractable epilepsy. A pacemaker-like device is implanted below the clavicle on the left and attached to the left vagus nerve. A cycle of stimulation of the nerve is established (typically 30 seconds of stimulation every 5 minutes), which has an antiepileptic effect, reducing seizures by at least 50% in over half the children so treated. In addition, turning on the stimulator by the use of a magnet may interrupt a seizure (ie, an anticonvulsant effect). With current technology, the battery in the stimulator will last 7 or more years in many patients.

D. Surgery

An evaluation for epilepsy surgery is indicated for all children with medically intractable partial epilepsy. The evaluation and surgery should be performed at a center with expertise in epilepsy surgery and which has a dedicated neurosurgeon as well as a team of physicians and other providers.

The first surgery for treatment of epilepsy took place over 100 years ago, and surgery is now established as the appropriate treatment for adults and children with epilepsy refractory to medical treatment. Evaluation for possible surgical treatment should begin as soon as it is clear that the child is not responding to standard therapy and there is evidence of focal onset of seizures. Advances in technology allow for definition and removal of the epileptogenic focus even in young infants. Many centers now have access to video-EEG monitoring, PET, and similar noninvasive techniques that can be used to identify lesions such as cortical dysplasias that are amenable to resection. Freedom from seizures is reported in 80% or more of children who have been treated surgically. Some patients such as those with Rasmussen encephalitis or extensive perinatal strokes may be candidates for hemispherectomy. Increasingly, surgery is being performed on children with tuberous sclerosis after identification of the epileptogenic tuber.

Corpus callostomy remains an option for children who are experiencing uncontrolled drop attacks. A marked reduction in injuries due seizure-related falls is usually seen.

E. General Management of the Child with Epilepsy

1. Education—The initial diagnosis is often devastating for families. Some have been told that their child has a seizure disorder but the term *epilepsy* has been avoided. The patient and parents must be helped to understand the nature of epilepsy and its management, including etiology, prognosis, safety issues, and treatment options. Many children—some even as young as age 3 years—are capable of cooperating with the physician in problems of seizure control.

Excellent educational materials are available for families of a child with epilepsy, both in print and online. Two excellent web sites are http://www.epilepsyfoundation.org and http://www.epilepsy.com. Materials on epilepsy—including pamphlets, monographs, films, and videotapes suitable for children and teenagers, parents, teachers, and medical professionals—may be purchased through the Epilepsy Foundation: 8301 Professional Place, Landover, MD 20785; (800) 332-1000. The Foundation's local chapter and other community organizations are able to provide guidance and other services. Support groups exist in many cities for older children and adolescents and for their parents and others concerned.

2. Privileges and precautions in daily life—*"No seizures and no side effects"* is a motto established by the Epilepsy Foundation. The child should be encouraged to live as normal a life as possible. Children should engage in physical activities appropriate to their age and social group. After seizure control is established, swimming is generally permissible with a buddy system or adequate lifeguard coverage. Scuba diving, gymnastic activities involving heights, and high climbing should not be permitted. There are no absolute contraindications to any other sports, although some physicians recommend against contact sports. Physical training and sports are usually to be welcomed rather than restricted. Driving is discussed in the next section.

Loss of sleep should be avoided. Emotional disturbances may need to be treated. Alcohol intake should be avoided because it may precipitate seizures. Prompt attention should be given to infections. Further neurologic disturbances should be brought to the physician's attention promptly.

Although every effort should be made to control seizures, this must not interfere with a child's ability to function. Sometimes a child is better off having an occasional mild seizure than being so heavily sedated that function at home, in school, or at play is impaired. Therapy and medication adjustment often require much art and fortitude on the physician's part. Some patients with infrequent seizures, especially if only nocturnal partial seizures (eg, rolandic seizures) may not need AEDs.

3. Driving—Driving becomes important to most young people at age 15 or 16 years. Restrictions vary from state to state. In most states, a learner's permit or driver's license will be issued to an individual with epilepsy if he or she has been under a physician's care and free of seizures for at least 1 year (although restrictions vary from state to state in the United States and in other countries), provided that the treatment or basic neurologic problems do not interfere with the ability to drive. A guide to this and other legal matters pertaining to persons with epilepsy is published by the Epilepsy Foundation, and the Foundation's legal department may be able to provide additional information.

4. Pregnancy—Contraception (especially interaction of oral contraceptive with some AEDs) childbearing, potential teratogenicity of AEDs, and the management of pregnancy should be discussed as soon as appropriate with the adolescent young woman with epilepsy. Daily use of vitamin preparations containing folic acid is recommended. For the pregnant teenager with epilepsy, management by an obstetrician conversant with the use of AEDs in pregnancy is appropriate. The patient should be cautioned against discontinuing her medications during pregnancy. The possibility of teratogenic effects of AEDs, such as facial clefts (two to three times increased risk), must be weighed against the risks from seizures All AEDs appear to have some risk for teratogenicity, although valproate carries a particularly high risk for spinal dysraphism.

5. School intervention and seizure response plans—Most schools will work with parents to establish a seizure action plan for their child with epilepsy. A template for such a plan is available on the Epilepsy Foundation web site at http://www.epilepsyfoundation.org/programs/upload/snactionplan.pdf. These plans usually require the approval of the child's physician. Schools are sometimes hesitant to administer Diastat or to activate the vagal nerve stimulator. Often, information from the physician, especially that obtained from the Epilepsy Foundation web site, will relieve anxieties. School authorities should be encouraged to avoid needless restrictions and to address the emotional and educational needs of all children with disabilities, including epilepsy. The local affiliates of the Epilepsy Foundation can often provide support for families in their interactions with the school.

2. Status Epilepticus

Status epilepticus is a clinical or electrical seizure lasting at least 30 minutes, or a series of seizures without complete recovery over the same period of time. After 30 minutes of seizure activity, hypoxia and acidosis occur, with depletion of energy stores, cerebral edema, and structural damage. Eventually, high fever, hypotension, respiratory depression, and even death may occur. Status epilepticus is a medical emergency.

Status epilepticus is classified as (1) convulsive (the common tonic-clonic, or grand mal, status epilepticus) or (2) nonconvulsive (characterized by altered mental status or behavior with subtle or absent motor components). Absence status, or spike-wave stupor, and complex partial status epilepticus are examples of the nonconvulsive type (Table 23–10). An EEG may be necessary to aid in diagnosing nonconvulsive status

Table 23–10. Status epilepticus: clinical types.

Generalized seizure (common)
  Convulsive (tonic, clonic, myoclonic): 90%
  Nonconvulsive (absence, atypical absence, atonic): 10%
Focal (partial) seizures (rare)
  Simple partial
  Complex partial
Neonatal
  Many clinical varieties
  May show electroclinical dissociation (on EEG with no visible clinical correlate)
Other (very rare)
  Continuous epileptiform activity in sleep (Landau-Kleffner syndrome and syndrome of continuous spike-wave in slow wave sleep)

because patients sometimes appear merely stuporous and lack typical convulsive movements.

▶ **Clinical Findings**

A child with status epilepticus may have a high fever with or without intracranial infection. Studies show that 25–75% of children with status epilepticus experience it as their initial seizure. Often it is a reflection of a acute or remote insult. Tumor and stroke, which are common causes of status epilepticus in adults, are uncommon causes in childhood. Fifty percent of pediatric status epilepticus is due to acute (25%) or chronic (25%) CNS disorders. Infection and metabolic disorders are common causes of status epilepticus in children. The cause is unknown in 50% of patients, but many of these patients will be febrile. In the child with known epilepsy, medication nonadherence should be considered. Status epilepticus occurs most commonly in children aged 5 years and younger (85%). The most common age is 1 year or younger (37%); the distribution is even for each year thereafter (approximately 12% per year).

▶ **Treatment**

For treatment options, see Table 23–11.

3. Febrile Seizures

Criteria for febrile seizures are (1) age 3 months to 5 years (most occur between ages 6 and 18 months), (2) fever of greater than 38.8°C, and (3) non-CNS infection. More than 90% of febrile seizures are generalized, last less than 5 minutes, and occur early in the illness causing the fever. Febrile seizures occur in 2–3% of children. Acute respiratory illnesses are most commonly associated with febrile seizures. Gastroenteritis, especially when caused by *Shigella* or *Campylobacter*, and urinary tract infections are less common causes. Roseola infantum is a rare but classic cause. One study implicated viral causes in 86% of cases. Immunizations may be a cause.

Table 23–11. Status epilepticus treatment.

1. ABCs
   a. Airway: maintain oral airway; intubation may be necessary.
   b. Breathing: oxygen.
   c. Circulation: assess pulse, blood pressure; support with IV fluids, drugs. Monitor vital signs.
2. Start glucose-containing IV; evaluate serum glucose; electrolytes, HCO_3^-, CBC, BUN, anticonvulsant levels.
3. May need arterial blood gases, pH.
4. Give 50% glucose if serum glucose low (1–2 mL/kg).
5. Begin IV drug therapy; goal is to control status epilepticus in 20–60 min.
   a. Diazepam, 0.3–0.5 mg/kg over 1–5 min (20 mg maximum); may repeat in 5–20 min; or, lorazepam, 0.05–0.2 mg/kg (less effective with repeated doses, longer-acting than diazepam). [a]Midazolam: IV, 0.1–0.2 mg/kg; intranasally, 0.2 mg/kg.
   b. Phenytoin, 10–20 mg/kg IV (not IM) over 5–20 min; 1000 mg maximum); monitor with blood pressure and ECG. Fosphenytoin may be given more rapidly in the same dosage; order 10–20 mg/kg of "phenytoin equivalent."
   c. Phenobarbital, 5–20 mg/kg (sometimes higher in newborns or refractory status in intubated patients).
6. Correct metabolic perturbations (eg, low-sodium, acidosis).
7. Other drug approaches in refractory status:
   a. Repeat phenytoin, phenobarbital (10 mg/kg). Monitor blood levels. Support respiration, blood pressure as necessary.
   b. [a]Midazolam drip: 1–5 mcg/kg/min (even to 20 kg/min). Valproate sodium, available as 100 mg/mL for IV use; give 15–30 mg/kg over 5–20 min.
   c. Pentobarb coma. Propofol. General anesthetic.
8. Consider underlying causes:
   a. Structural disorders or trauma: MRI or CT scan.
   b. Infection: lumbar puncture, blood culture, antibiotics.
   c. Metabolic disorders: consider lactic acidosis, toxins, uremia. May need to evaluate medication levels. Toxin screen. Judicious fluid administration.
9. Give maintenance drug (if diazepam only was sufficient to halt status epilepticus): phenytoin (10 mg/kg); phenobarbital (5 mg/kg); daily dose IV (or by mouth) divided every 12 h.

[a]Much supportive data.
BUN, blood urea nitrogen; CBC, complete blood count; CT, computed tomography; ECG, electrocardiogram; IM, intramuscularly; IV, intravenously; MRI, magnetic resonance imaging.

Rarely status epilepticus may occur during a febrile seizure. Febrile seizures rarely (1–3%) lead to recurrent unprovoked seizures (epilepsy) in later childhood and adult life (risk is increased two- to fivefold compared with children who do not have febrile seizures). The chance of later epilepsy is higher if the febrile seizures have complex features, such as duration longer than 15 minutes, more than one seizure in the same day, or focal features. Other adverse factors are an abnormal neurologic status preceding the seizures (eg, cerebral palsy or mental retardation), early onset of febrile seizure (before age 1 year), and a family history of epilepsy. Even with adverse factors, the risk of epilepsy after febrile seizures is still only in the range of 15–20%, although it is increased if more than one risk factor is present. Recurrent febrile seizures occur in 30–50% of cases but in general do not worsen the long-term outlook.

Generalized epilepsy with febrile seizures plus (GEFS+) is an autosomal dominant form of epilepsy first described in 1997. The most frequently observed GEFS+ phenotype includes childhood onset of multiple febrile seizures persisting beyond the age of 6 years, and unprovoked (afebrile) seizures, including absence, myoclonic, or atonic seizures, and rarely, myoclonic-astatic epilepsy. Originally associated with a point mutation in *SCN1B*, GEFS+ is now known to have other channelopathies.

▶ Clinical Findings

A. Diagnostic Evaluation

The child with a febrile seizure must be evaluated for the source of the fever, in particular to exclude CNS infection. Routine studies such as serum electrolytes, glucose, calcium, skull radiographs, or brain imaging studies are seldom helpful. A white count above 20,000/μL or an extreme left shift may correlate with bacteremia. Complete blood count and blood cultures may be appropriate. Serum sodium is often slightly low but not low enough to require treatment or to cause the seizure. Meningitis and encephalitis must be considered. Signs of meningitis (eg, bulging fontanelle, stiff neck, stupor, and irritability) may all be absent, especially in a child younger than age 18 months.

B. Lumbar Puncture

After controlling the fever and stopping an ongoing seizure, the physician must decide whether to do a lumbar puncture. The fact that the child has had a previous febrile seizure does not rule out meningitis as the cause of the current episode. The younger the child, the more important is the procedure, because physical findings are less reliable in diagnosing meningitis. Although the yield is low, a lumbar puncture should probably be done if the child is younger than age 18 months, if recovery is slow, if no other cause for the fever is found, or if close follow-up will not be possible. Occasionally observation in the emergency department for several hours obviates the need for a lumbar puncture. A negative finding does not exclude the possibility of emergence of CNS infection during the same febrile illness. Sometimes a second procedure must be done.

▶ Treatment & Prognosis

Prophylactic anticonvulsants are not recommended after an uncomplicated febrile seizure.

If febrile seizures are complicated or prolonged, or if medical reassurance fails to relieve family anxiety, anticonvulsant prophylaxis may be indicated and can reduce the incidence of recurrent febrile seizures. Only phenobarbital and valproic acid have demonstrated efficacy in preventing febrile seizures; phenytoin and carbamazepine have been

show to be ineffective. Newer antiepileptic drugs have not been studied. Diazepam started at the first onset of fever for the duration of the febrile illness (0.5 mg/kg two or three times per day orally or rectally) may be effective but will sedate a child. Prophylactic diazepam is also limited by the fact that a seizure is often the first evidence of fever associated with an acute illness. Diastat (rectal diazepam gel) can be used to prevent febrile status epilepticus in the child with a prolonged febrile seizure (one lasting over 5 minutes), often the greatest concern.

Phenobarbital, 3–5 mg/kg/d as a single bedtime dose, is an inexpensive long-term prophylaxis. However, significant behavioral disturbance is seen in about one third of toddlers treated with phenobarbital. Often, increasing the dosage gradually (eg, starting with 2 mg/kg/d the first week, increasing to 3 mg/kg/d the second week, and so on) decreases side effects and nonadherence. A plasma phenobarbital level in the range of 15–40 mg/mL is desirable.

Valproate sodium is potentially more hazardous. In infants, the commonly used liquid suspension has a short half-life and causes more gastrointestinal upset than do the sprinkle capsules. The dosage is 15–60 mg/kg/d in divided doses. Precautionary laboratory studies are necessary. In the infant younger than age 2 years, there is an increased risk of hepatic toxicity. Thrombocytopenia may occur, particularly in the face of an acute illness.

Measures to control fever such as sponging or tepid baths, antipyretics, and the administration of antibiotics for proven bacterial illness are reasonable but unproven to prevent recurrent febrile seizures.

Simple febrile seizures do not have any long-term adverse consequences. An EEG may be considered if the febrile seizure is complicated, focal, or otherwise unusual. In uncomplicated febrile seizures, the EEG is usually normal. Ideally the EEG should be done at least a week after the illness to avoid transient changes due to fever or the seizure itself. In older children, 3/s spike-wave discharges, suggestive of a genetic propensity to epilepsy, may occur. In the young infant, EEG findings seldom aid in assessing the chance of recurrence of febrile seizures or in long-term prognosis.

Aldenkamp AP et al: Optimizing therapy of seizures in children and adolescents with ADHD. Neurology 2006;67(Suppl 4):S49 [PMID: 17190923].

Barkovich AJ et al: A developmental and genetic classification for malformations of cortical development. Neurology 2005;65:1873 [PMID: 16192428].

Bartha AI et al: Neonatal seizures: Multicenter variability in current treatment practices. Pediatr Neurol 2007;37:85 [PMID: 17675022].

Berg AT et al: How long does it take for epilepsy to become intractable? A prospective investigation. Ann Neurol 2006;60:73 [PMID: 16685695].

Berg AT et al. Longitudinal assessment of adaptive behavior in infants and young children with newly diagnosed epilepsy: Influences of etiology, syndrome, and seizure control. Pediatrics 2004;114:645 [PMID: 15342834].

Berg AT et al: Status epilepticus after the initial diagnosis of epilepsy in children. Neurology 2004;63:1027 [PMID: 15452294].

Berkovic SF et al: De-novo mutations of the sodium channel gene SCN1A in alleged vaccine encephalopathy: A retrospective study. Lancet Neurol 2006;5:488 [PMID: 16713920].

Bough KJ, Rho JM: Anticonvulsant mechanisms of the ketogenic diet. Epilepsia 2007;48:43 [PMID: 17241207].

Bruhn K et al: Screen sensitivity in photosensitive children and adolescents: Patient-dependant and stimulus-dependant factors. Epileptic Disord 2007;9:57 [PMID: 17307713].

Buchhalter JR, Jarrar RG: Therapeutics in pediatric epilepsy, Part 2: Epilepsy surgery and vagus nerve stimulation. Mayo Clin Proc 2003;78:371 [PMID: 12630591].

Camfield P, Camfield C: Childhood epilepsy: What is the evidence for what we think and what we do? J Child Neurol 2003;18:272 [PMID: 12760431].

Camfield P, Camfield C: Sudden unexpected death in people with epilepsy: A pediatric perspective. Semin Pediatr Neurol 2005;12:10 [PMID: 15929460].

Caplan R et al: Depression and anxiety disorders in pediatric epilepsy. Epilepsia 2005;46:720 [PMID: 15857439].

Caraballo RH et al: Ketogenic diet in patients with myoclonic-astatic epilepsy. Epileptic Disord 2006;8:151 [PMID: 16793577].

Ceulemans BP et al: Clinical correlations of mutations in the SCN1A gene: From febrile seizures to severe myoclonic epilepsy in infancy. Pediatr Neurol 2004;30:236 [PMID: 15087100].

Chahine LM, Mikati MA: Benign pediatric localization-related epilepsies. Epileptic Disord 2006;8:243 [PMID: 17150437].

Chin RF et al: Meningitis is a common cause of convulsive status epilepticus with fever. Arch Dis Child 2005;90:66 [PMID: 15613516].

Deltour L et al: Children with benign epilepsy with centrotemporal spikes (BECTS) show impaired attentional control: evidence from an attentional capture paradigm. Epileptic Disord 2007;9:32 [PMID: 17307709].

Dion MH et al: Lamotrigine therapy of epilepsy with Angelman's syndrome. Epilepsia 2007;48:593 [PMID: 17326790].

Donati F et al; Oxcarbazepine Cognitive Study Group: Effects of oxcarbazepine on cognitive function in children and adolescents with partial seizures. Neurology 2006;67:679 [PMID: 16924022].

Evans D et al: Anticonvulsants for preventing mortality and morbidity in full term newborns with perinatal asphyxia. Cochrane Database Syst Rev 2007:CD001240 [PMID: 17636659].

Ferrie C et al: Panayiotopoulos syndrome: A consensus view. Dev Med Child Neurol 2006;48:236 [PMID: 16483404].

Gardiner M: Genetics of idiopathic generalized epilepsies. Epilepsia 2005;46(Suppl 9):15 [PMID: 16302872].

Gerstner T et al: Valproic acid induced encephalopathy–19 new cases in Germany from 1994 to 2003–a side effect associated to VPA-therapy not only in young children. Seizure 2006;15:443 [PMID: 16787750].

Glauser TA et al: Pharmacokinetics of levetiracetam in infants and young children with epilepsy. Epilepsia 2007;48:1117 [PMID: 17442002].

Glauser TA et al: Topiramate monotherapy in newly diagnosed epilepsy in children and adolescents. J Child Neurol 2007;22:693 [PMID: 17641254].

Goh S et al: Infantile spasms and intellectual outcomes in children with tuberous sclerosis complex. Neurology 2005;65:235 [PMID: 16043792].

Grosso S et al: Efficacy and safety of levetiracetam in infants and young children with refractory epilepsy. Seizure 2007;16:345 [PMID: 17368928].

Guillet R, Kwon J: Seizure recurrence and developmental disabilities after neonatal seizures: Outcomes are unrelated to use of phenobarbital prophylaxis. J Child Neurol 2007;22:389 [PMID: 17621516].

Hedera P et al: Identification of a novel locus for febrile seizures and epilepsy on chromosome 21q22. Epilepsia 2006;47:1622 [PMID: 17054683].

Hirtz D et al: Practice parameter: Evaluating a first nonfebrile seizure in children: Report of the Quality Standards Subcommittee of the American Academy of Neurology, the Child Neurology Society, and the American Epilepsy Society. Neurology 2000;55:616 [PMID: 10980722].

Hirtz D et al: Practice parameter: Treatment of the child with a first unprovoked seizure: Report of the Quality Standards Subcommittee of the American Academy of Neurology and the Practice Committee of the Child Neurology Society. Neurology 2003;60:166 [PMID: 12552027].

Holmes GL, Stafstrom CE, Tuberous Sclerosis Study Group: Tuberous sclerosis complex and epilepsy: Recent developments and future challenges. Epilepsia 2007;48:617 [PMID: 17386056].

Jansen FE et al: Epilepsy surgery in tuberous sclerosis: A systematic review. Epilepsia 2007;48:1477 [PMID: 17484753].

Kang HC et al: Early- and late-onset complications of the ketogenic diet for intractable epilepsy. Epilepsia 2004;45:1116 [PMID: 15329077].

Kivity S et al: Long-term cognitive outcomes of a cohort of children with cryptogenic infantile spasms treated with high-dose adrenocorticotropic hormone. Epilepsia 2004;45:255 [PMID: 15009227].

Knudsen JF et al: Oligohydrosis and fever in pediatric patients treated with zonisamide. Pediatr Neurol 2003;28:184 [PMID: 12770670].

Koenig SA et al: Valproic acid-induced hepatopathy: Nine new fatalities in Germany from 1994 to 2003. Epilepsia 2006;47:2027 [PMID: 17201699].

Korinthenberg R, Schreiner A: Topiramate in children with West syndrome: A retrospective multicenter evaluation of 100 patients. J Child Neurol 2007;22:302 [PMID: 17621500].

Kossoff EH et al: A modified Atkins diet is effective for the treatment of intractable pediatric epilepsy. Epilepsia 2006;47:421 [PMID: 16499770].

Mackay MT et al; American Academy of Neurology, Child Neurology Society: Practice parameter: Medical treatment of infantile spasms: Report of the American Academy of Neurology and the Child Neurology Society. Neurology 2004;62:1668 [PMID: 15159460].

Majorie JF et al: Vagus nerve stimulation in patients with catastrophic childhood epilepsy, a 2-year follow-up study. Seizure 2005;14:10 [PMID: 15642494].

Mancardi MM et al: Familial occurrence of febrile seizures and epilepsy in severe myoclonic epilepsy of infancy (SMEI) patients with SCN1A mutations. Epilepsia 2006;47:1629 [PMID: 17054684].

Ozdemir D et al: Efficacy of continuous midazolam infusion and mortality in childhood refractory generalized convulsive status epilepticus. Seizure 2005;14:129 [PMID: 15694567].

Pfeifer HH, Thiele EA: Low-glycemic-index treatment: a liberalized ketogenic diet for treatment of intractable epilepsy. Neurology 2005;65:1810[PMID: 16344529].

Posner EB et al: A systematic review of treatment of typical absence seizures in children and adolescents with ethosuximide, sodium valproate or lamotrigine. Seizure 2005;14:117 [PMID: 15694565].

Rankin PM et al: Pyridoxine-dependent seizures: A family phenotype that leads to severe cognitive deficits, regardless of treatment regime. Dev Med Child Neurol 2007;49:300 [PMID: 17376142].

Rennie J, Boylan G: Treatment of neonatal seizures. Arch Dis Child Fetal Neonatal Ed 2007;92:F148 [PMID: 17337664].

Rho JM, Rogawski MA: The ketogenic diet: stoking the powerhouse of the cell. Epilepsy Curr 2007;7:58 [PMID: 17505556].

Riikonen R: The latest on infantile spasms. Curr Opin Neurol 2005;18:91 [PMID: 15791136].

Sabaz M et al: The impact of epilepsy surgery on quality of life in children. Neurology 2006;66:557 [PMID: 16505311].

Sadleir LG, Scheffer IE: Febrile seizures. BMJ 2007;334:307 [PMID: 17289734].

Sahin M et al: Prolonged treatment for acute symptomatic refractory status epilepticus. Neurology 2003;61:398 [PMID: 12913208].

Sazgar M, Bourgeois BF: Aggravation of epilepsy by antiepileptic drugs. Pediatr Neurol 2005;33:227 [PMID: 16194719].

Shoemaker MT, Rotenberg JS: Levetiracetam for the treatment of neonatal seizures. J Child Neurol 2007;22:95 [PMID: 17608315].

Shostak S, Ottman R: Ethical, legal, and social dimensions of epilepsy genetics. Epilepsia 2006;47:1595 [PMID: 17054679].

Sillanpaa M, Schmidt D: Natural history of treated childhood-onset epilepsy: Prospective, long-term population-based study. Brain 2006;129:617 [PMID: 16401617].

Silverstein FS, Jensen FE: Neonatal seizures. Ann Neurol 2007;62:112 [PMID: 17683087].

Sinclair DB: Prednisone therapy in pediatric epilepsy. Pediatr Neurol 2003;28:194 [PMID: 12770672].

Sullivan JE, Dlugos DJ: Idiopathic generalized epilepsy. Curr Treat Options Neurol 2004;6:231 [PMID: 15043806].

Than KD et al: Can you predict an immediate, complete, and sustained response to the ketogenic diet? Epilepsia 2005;46:580 [PMID: 15816955].

Tromp SC et al: Relative influence of epileptic seizures and of epilepsy syndrome on cognitive function. J Child Neurol 2003;18:407 [PMID: 12886976].

Tuchman R: Autism and epilepsy: What has regression got to do with it? Epilepsy Curr 2006;6:107 [PMID: 17260027].

van Gestel JP et al: Propofol and thiopental for refractory status epilepticus in children. Neurology 2005;65:591 [PMID: 16116121].

Verrotti A et al: Intermittent oral diazepam prophylaxis in febrile convulsions: Its effectiveness for febrile seizure recurrence. Eur J Paediatr Neurol 2004;8:131 [PMID: 15120684].

Vining EP: Struggling with Rasmussen's syndrome. Epilepsy Curr 2006;6:20 [PMID: 16477319].

Waruiru C, Appleton R: Febrile seizures: An update. Arch Dis Child 2004;89:751 [PMID: 15269077].

Wheless JW et al: Treatment of pediatric epilepsy: Expert opinion, 2005. J Child Neurol 2005;(Suppl 1):S1 [PMID: 16615562].

Zaccara G et al: Idiosyncratic adverse reactions to antiepileptic drugs. Epilepsia 2007;48:1223 [PMID: 17386054].

Zupanc ML: Neonatal seizures. Pediatr Clin North Am 2004;51:961 [PMID: 15275983].

SYNCOPE & FAINTING

Fainting is transient loss of consciousness and postural tone due to cerebral ischemia or anoxia. Up to 20–50% of children (birth–20 years) will faint at some time. There may be a prodrome of dizziness, lightheadedness, nausea, so-called gray-out, sweating, and pallor. After falling, many children stiffen or have jerking motions when unconscious, a tonic-clonic, anoxic-ischemic seizure mimicking epilepsy. Watching or undergoing a venipuncture is a common precipitant of fainting, as is prolonged standing, fatigue, illness, over-heating and sweating, dehydration, hunger, and athleticism with slow baseline pulse. The family history is positive for similar episodes in 90% of patients.

▶ Classification

Ninety-five percent of cases of syncope are of the vasovagal-vasodepressive or neurocardiogenic type (Table 23–12). Vasodilation, cardiac slowing, and hypotension cause transient (1–2 minutes) cerebral ischemia and result in the patient passing out. The patient arouses in 1–2 minutes, but full recovery may take an hour or more. Besides those already listed, rare precipitants include hair grooming, cough, micturition, neck stretching, and emotional stress. More ominous is cardiac syncope, which often occurs during exercise. Angina or palpitations may occur. An obstructive lesion such as aortic stenosis, cardiomyopathy, coronary disease, or dysrhythmia may be the cause. Other spells that may mimic syncope are listed in Table 23–12.

▶ Clinical Findings

A. Symptoms and Signs

The workup of fainting includes a personal and a detailed family history, and a physical examination with emphasis on blood pressure and cardiac and neurologic features. In the adolescent, a blood pressure drop of more than 30 mm Hg after standing for 5–10 minutes or a baseline systolic pressure of less than 80 mm Hg suggests orthostasis.

B. Laboratory Findings and Imaging

Hemoglobin should be checked if anemia is suggested by the history. Electrocardiography should be done. Consider cardiology referral, Holter monitoring, and echocardiography if cardiac causes seem likely (eg, fainting during exercise). Tilt

Table 23–12. Classification of syncope in childhood.

Vasovagal, neurocardiogenic (neurally mediated)
Orthostatic
Athleticism
Pallid breath-holding
Situational (stress, blood drawing)
Cardiac
Obstructive
Arrhythmia
Prolonged QTc
Hypercyanotic (eg, in tetralogy of Fallot)
Nonsyncope mimicker
Migraine with confusion or stupor
Seizure
Hypoglycemia
Hysteria
Hyperventilation
Vertigo

testing (though norms are vague) may have a role in frequent recurrent syncope to confirm a vasodepressive cause and avoid more expensive diagnostic investigations.

▶ Treatment

Treatment consists mostly of giving advice about the benign nature of fainting and about avoiding precipitating situations. The patient should be cautioned to lie down if prodromal symptoms occur. Good hydration and reasonable salt intake are advisable. In some cases β-blockers and, rarely, fludrocortisone may have a role.

Allan WC, Gospe SM Jr: Seizures, syncope, or breath-holding presenting to the pediatric neurologist—when is the etiology a life-threatening arrhythmia? Semin Pediatr Neurol 2005;12:2 [PMID: 15929459].

Britton JW: Syncope and seizures—differential diagnosis and evaluation. Clin Auton Res 2004;14:148 [PMID: 15241643].

DiVasta AD, Alexander ME: Fainting freshmen and sinking sophomores: cardiovascular issues of the adolescent. Curr Opin Pediatr 2004;16:350 [PMID: 15273492].

Grubb BP: Clinical practice. Neurocardiogenic syncope. N Engl J Med 2005;352:1004 [PMID: 15758011].

Singh A, Silberbach M: Consultation with the specialist: Cardiovascular preparticipation sports screening. Pediatr Rev 2006;27:418 [PMID: 17079507].

Verma S et al: Syncope in athletes: A guide to getting them back on their feet. J Fam Pract 2007;56:545 [PMID: 17605946].

Vlahos AP et al: Provocation of neurocardiogenic syncope during head-up tilt testing in children: Comparison between isoproterenol and nitroglycerin. Pediatrics 2007;119:e419 [PMID: 17224456].

HEADACHES

Headache is one of the most common complaints in pediatric neurology clinics, accounting for 25–30% of all referrals. Epidemiologic studies indicate that headache occurs in 37% of children by age 7 years and in 69% of children by age 14 years. Migraine headache occurs in 5% and 15%, respectively, of children at these ages. Successful treatment requires an accurate diagnosis and proper classification of headache. Based on the patient's history, a simplified initial categorization as summarized in Table 23–13 can be made. A more exhaustive classification scheme has been developed by the International Headache Society and modified for use in children. Muscle contraction tension headaches are common in older children and adolescents. They are frequently generalized over the head with a "hat band" pressure or squeezing quality. Although appetite may be diminished, nausea and vomiting are usually not present. Symptoms specifically referable to the CNS are absent. If this type of headache becomes very frequent (three or more days per week) consideration should be given to drug (analgesic) overuse or misuse, depression, or sleep disorder. The neurologic examination is normal, neuroimaging tests are generally not needed, and treatment is judicious use of ibuprofen with or without a prophylactic (daily, at bedtime) trial of amitriptyline. If simple measures are not satisfactory, biofeedback, hypnosis, other relaxation methods, psychotherapy, or a combination of these methods may be useful.

Between 65% and 75% of children referred to neurology clinics for consultation regarding headaches have migraine. Many of these children are referred after they have seen ophthalmologists for "eye strain" or otolaryngologists to rule out sinusitis. Approximately 30% of children are referred after already undergoing one or more neuroimaging tests, the vast majority of which show normal results.

▶ Clinical Findings

The diagnosis and proper classification of migraine depends primarily on a thorough and detailed history (Table 23–14). Migraine headaches are paroxysmal, recurrent events separated by symptom-free intervals in a child with normal growth

Table 23–13. Differential features of headaches in children.

	Muscle Contraction (Tension/Psychogenic)	Vascular (Migraine)	Traction and Inflammatory (Increased Intracranial Pressure)
Time course	Chronic, recurrent; if headache persists > 2 h and occurs > 15 days per month, diagnose "chronic daily headache"	Acute, paroxysmal, recurrent	Chronic or intermittent but increasingly frequent; progressive severity
Prodromes	No	Yes (sometimes in children)	No
Description	Diffuse, bandlike, tight; usually mild severity, 1–5 on a 1–10 scale	Intense, pulsatile, unilateral in older child (70%); usually forehead in or behind one or both eyes; 6–10 severity	Diffuse; more occipital with infratentorial mass, more frontal with supratentorial mass
Characteristic findings	Feelings of inadequacy, depression, or anxiety	Neurologic symptoms and signs usually transient	Positive neurologic signs, especially papilledema
Predisposing factors	Problems at home or school or socially (sexually)	Positive family history (75%); trivial head trauma may precipitate	None

Table 23–14. Proposed revised IHS classification of migraine.

Pediatric Migraine without Aura (Common)	Pediatric Migraine with Aura[a] (Rare)

Diagnostic criteria
 A. At least five attacks fulfilling B–D
 B. Headache attack lasting 1–48 h
 C. Headache has at least two of the following:
   1. Bilateral location (frontal/temporal) or unilateral location
   2. Pulsating quality
   3. Moderate to severe intensity
   4. Aggravation by routine physical activity
 D. During headache, at least one of the following
   1. Nausea or vomiting (or both)
   2. Photophobia and/or phonophobia
	Diagnostic criteria
	 A. At least two attacks fulfilling B
	 B. At least three of the following:
	   1. One or more fully reversible aura symptoms indicating focal cortical and/or brainstem dysfunction
	   2. At least one aura developing gradually over more than 4 min or 2 or more symptoms occurring in succession
	   3. No auras lasting more than 60 min
	   4. Headache follows in less than 60 min

[a]Idiopathic recurring disorder; headache usually lasts 1–48 h.
IHS, International Headache Society.
Adapted, with permission, from: Winner P et al: Classification of pediatric migraine: Proposed revisions of the IHS criteria. Headache 1995;35:407.

and development and whose neurologic examination is normal. Migraine affects children of all ages but is difficult to diagnose before age 4 years. The family history is positive for vascular, migrainous headaches in 75% of patients. The headaches have a pulsatile quality and are located unilaterally or bilaterally in the frontal or temporal regions, or commonly in the retro-orbital and cheek regions. The headaches last from 2 to more than 24 hours. A nonspecific prodrome of decreased or increased appetite and change in mood and temperament may precede the headache by hours or days. Headaches may be triggered by specific foods, minor head injuries, sleep deprivation, or irregular eating patterns, but more often no precipitant can be identified. An aura such as visual scotomata is uncommon in children. The headache is frequently accompanied by nausea, vomiting, photophobia, sensitivity to sound, vertigo, lightheadedness, fatigue, and mood alterations. Occasionally children may have loss of speech, hemiparesis, ataxia, confusional states, and bizarre visual distortions (so-called Alice in Wonderland syndrome). Very young children may experience recurrent or cyclical vomiting, abdominal pain, or recurrent self-limited bouts of ataxia or vertigo as the early manifestations of migraine.

Occasionally the frequency of migraine may spontaneously increase and become an almost daily occurrence, a condition referred to as transformed migraine. When this change in frequency happens, it should at least raise suspicion of medication overuse with development of rebound headache; successful treatment requires medication withdrawal for 6–12 weeks or longer.

In contrast to tension and migraine headaches, headaches caused by intracranial disorders or increased intracranial pressure rarely occur in children who are otherwise healthy and well and who have completely normal examinations.

Laboratory studies and neuroimaging tests are rarely needed if a thorough history has been taken and the neurologic examination is normal. If the progression of headache is atypical for migraine or tension-type headaches or if the neurologic examination is abnormal, an MRI scan should be considered. When papilledema is present but the MRI is normal, a lumbar puncture may be needed to diagnose pseudotumor cerebri.

▶ Treatment

Successful treatment of migraine is usually achieved with the systematic use of simple analgesics such as ibuprofen. The key to successful results is to take enough early enough to do the job. As soon as possible after the headache starts, the child is given ibuprofen, 10 mg/kg, followed in 45 minutes by 5 mg/kg if needed. Additional doses of analgesics rarely provide additional benefit. The addition of 40–65 mg of caffeine, caffeine-ergotamine combinations, or 65 mg of isometheptene (Midrin) to ibuprofen may provide more reliable relief for some patients. Nausea and vomiting can be treated with metoclopramide, taken 10–20 minutes before other medications. For frequently recurring migraine, prophylaxis (twice daily or single dose at bedtime) with propranolol, amitriptyline, cyproheptadine, valproate, or topiramate should be considered; however, none of these agents has had carefully double-blinded, controlled trials in children or teens. At this time experience with using triptan and dihydroergotamine (nasal spray) in young children is limited; in teens, studies show sumatriptan and zolmitriptan nasal sprays to be effective (although after-taste can be sometimes daunting). Oral triptans and dihydroergotamine have been shown to be effective compared with placebo and are safe and inexpensive; most studies have been done in adolescents. Biofeedback, relaxation therapy, and other nonpharmacologic approaches to managing headache may be useful in children, and they provide an alternative method of treatment that avoids medication-related side effects.

Allen KD: Using biofeedback to make childhood headaches less of a pain. Pediatr Ann 2004;33:241 [PMID: 15101230].

Anttila P: Tension-type headache in childhood and adolescence. Lancet Neurol 2006;5:268 [PMID: 16488382].

Curran MP et al: Intranasal sumatriptan in adolescents with migraine. CNS Drugs 2005;19:335 [PMID: 15813647].

Damen L et al: Prophylactic treatment of migraine in children. Part 1. A systematic review of non-pharmacological trials. Cephalalgia 2006;26:373 [PMID: 16556238].

Eiland LS et al: Pediatric migraine: Pharmacologic agents for prophylaxis. Ann Pharmacother 2007;41:1181 [PMID: 17550953].

Hershey AD et al: Chronic daily headaches in children. Curr Pain Headache Rep 2006;10:370 [PMID: 16945254].

Lewis DW: Pediatric migraine. Pediatr Rev 2007;28:43 [PMID: 17272520].

Lewis DW et al: Efficacy of zolmitriptan nasal spray in adolescent migraine. Pediatrics 2007;120:390 [PMID: 17671066].

Lewis DW et al: Practice parameter: Pharmacological treatment of migraine headache in children and adolescents. Neurology 2004;28:2215 [PMID: 15623677].

Saadat H, Kain ZN: Hypnosis as a therapeutic tool in pediatrics. Pediatrics 2007;120:179 [PMID: 17606576].

Schreiber CP et al: Prevalence of migraine in patients with a history of self-reported or physician-diagnosed "sinus" headache. Arch Intern Med 2004;164:1769 [PMID: 15364670].

Termine C et al: Alternative therapies in the treatment of headache in childhood, adolescence and adulthood. Funct Neurol 2005;20:9 [PMID: 15948561].

Wang SJ et al: Chronic daily headache in adolescents: Prevalence, impact and medication overuse. Neurol 2006;66:193 [PMID: 16434652].

SLEEP DISORDERS

This discussion focuses on neurologic features of several sleep disorders affecting children. Chapter 2 discusses behavioral considerations in the treatment of sleep disorders. Obstructive sleep apnea and sleep-disordered breathing are described in detail in Chapters 17 and 18.

1. Sleep Apnea Syndrome in Older Children (See also Chapters 17 & 18)

Children with sleep apnea frequently have hypertrophied tonsils or adenoids, causing partial airway obstruction. Sleep apnea may also be associated with facial dysmorphism, neuromuscular disorders with poor pharyngeal muscle control, and conditions causing enlargement of soft tissue in the pharynx and neck such as obesity (pickwickian syndrome). Discovery and correction of sleep apnea may have a favorable effect on persistent parasomnias.

2. Narcolepsy

Narcolepsy, a primary disorder of sleep, is characterized by chronic, excessive daytime sleeping that occurs regardless of activity or surroundings and is not relieved by increased sleep at night. Onset occurs as early as age 3 years. Of children with narcolepsy, 18% are younger than age 10, and 60% are between puberty and their late teens. Narcolepsy usually interferes severely with normal living. Months to years after onset, there may also be cataplexy (transient partial or total loss of muscle tone, often triggered by laughter, anger, or other emotional upsurge), hypnagogic hallucinations (visual or auditory), and sensations of paralysis on falling asleep. Studies have shown that rapid eye movement (REM) sleep, with loss of muscle tone and an EEG low-amplitude mixed frequency pattern, occurs soon after sleep onset in patients with cataplexy, whereas normal subjects experience 80–100 minutes or longer of non-REM (NREM) sleep before the initial REM period.

Recent research suggests absence of a hypothalamic neuropeptide, hypocretin, causes narcolepsy and cataplexy. Spinal fluid (but not plasma) levels of hypocretin-1 (also called orexin) are diagnostic (level will be zero). The condition persists throughout life.

Modafinil is a new effective treatment for narcolepsy or excessive daytime sleepiness. Other CNS stimulants may have a role. Amphetamine mixtures (Adderall) or long-acting methylphenidate are examples. Cataplexy responds to venlafaxine, fluoxetine, or clomipramine. Rarely, acute narcolepsy/cataplexy (autoimmune) responds to IVIG.

3. Somnambulism (Sleepwalking) (See also Chapter 2)

Somnambulism and somniloquy (sleep talking) are among a group of sleep disturbances known as disorders of arousal. The onset is abrupt, usually early in the night. It is characterized by coordinated activity (eg, walking and sometimes moving objects seemingly without purpose) in a state of veiled consciousness. The episode is relatively brief and ceases spontaneously. There is poor recall of the event on waking in the morning. Somnambulism may be related to mental activities occurring in stages 3 and 4 of NREM sleep. Incidence has been estimated at only 2–3%, but up to 15% of cases are reported in children aged 6–16 years. Boys are affected more often than girls, and many have recurrent episodes. Psychopathologic features are rarely demonstrated, but a strong association (30%) between childhood migraine and somnambulism has been noted. Episodes of somnambulism may be triggered in predisposed children by stresses, including febrile illnesses. No treatment of somnambulism is required, and it is not necessary to seek psychiatric consultation.

4. Night Terrors (See also Chapter 2)

Night terrors (pavor nocturnus) are a disorder of arousal from NREM sleep. Most cases occur in children aged 3–8 years, and the disorder rarely occurs after adolescence. It is characterized by sudden (but only partial) waking, with the severely frightened child unable to be fully roused or comforted. Concomitant autonomic symptoms include rapid breathing, tachycardia, and perspiring. The child has no recall of any nightmare. Psychopathologic mechanisms are unclear, but falling asleep after watching scenes of violence on television or hearing frightening stories may play a role. Elimination of such causes and consideration of a sleep study (polysomnogram) to rule out obstructive apnea and partial complex seizures may have a role. Most of the time, watchful waiting and reassurance of the family are sufficient.

5. Restless Legs Syndrome (See also Chapter 2)

Restless legs syndrome refers to continuous, bothersome leg movements occurring at rest and producing unpleasant paresthesias (sensory symptoms) that often interfere with restful sleep. Occasionally, anemia (low ferritin) has been noted in adults with the disorder; in these cases improvement has occurred with ferrous sulfate treatment. Avoidance of caffeine, nicotine, alcohol, and some drugs (antidepressants, neuroleptics) has helped in adult series. No pediatric medication studies exist; anecdotally, clonazepam, possibly clonidine, and gabapentin are safe options. Dopa agonists, ropinirole, and pramipexole, used in adults, are unproven in children but also likely safe. (See also Chapter 2.)

Arii J et al: DSF hypocretin-1 (orexin-A) levels in childhood narcolepsy and neurologic disorders. Neurology 2004;63:2440 [PMID: 15623725].

Blum NJ, Mason TB: Restless legs syndrome: What is a pediatrician to do? Pediatrics 2007;120:253 [PMID: 17671070].

Dauvillirs Y et al: Narcolepsy with cataplexy. Lancet 2007;369:499 [PMID: 17292770].

Dauvilliers Y et al: Successful management of cataplexy with intravenous immunoglobulins at narcolepsy onset. Ann Neurol 2004;56:905 [PMID: 15562415].

Fauroux B: What's new in pediatric sleep. Paediatr Respir Rev 2007;8:85 [PMID: 17419982].

Kass LJ: Sleep problems. Pediatr Rev 2006;27:455 [PMID: 17142467].

Kotagal S, Pianosi P: Sleep disorders in children and adolescents. BMJ 2006;332:828 [PMID: 16601043].

Meltzer LJ, Mindell JA: Sleep and sleep disorders in children and adolescents. Psychatr Clin North Am 2006;29:1059 [PMID: 17118282].

Moore M et al: A review of pediatric nonrespiratory sleep disorders. Chest 2006;130;1252 [PMID: 17035465].

Petit D et al: Dyssomnias and parasomnias in early childhood. Pediatrics 2007;119:e1016 [PMID: 17438080].

Picchietti D et al: Restless legs syndrome: Prevalence and impact in children and adolescents—the Peds REST study. Pediatrics 2007;120:253 [PMID: 17671050].

Turner K et al: Index of suspicion. Pediatr Rev 2006;27:231 [PMID: 16740807].

PSEUDOTUMOR CEREBRI

Pseudotumor cerebri is characterized by increased intracranial pressure in the absence of an identifiable intracranial mass or hydrocephalus. An obese teenage girl (or adult) is the typical phenotype. Symptoms are headache, tinnitus, and visual loss; signs are those of increased intracranial pressure as outlined in Table 23–15. The cause is usually unknown, but pseudotumor cerebri has been described in association with a variety of

Table 23–15. Signs of increased intracranial pressure.

Acute, Subacute
Headache, vomiting
Excessive rate of head growth
Altered behavior
Decreased level of consciousness
Blurred or double vision
Optic disk swelling
Abducens nerve paresis
Chronic
Macrocephaly
Growth impairment
Developmental delay
Optic atrophy
Visual field loss

inflammatory, metabolic, toxic, and connective tissue disorders (Table 23–16). The diagnosis of pseudotumor cerebri is one of exclusion. MRI scan of the head is needed to exclude hydrocephalus and intracranial masses. This study demonstrates ventricles of small or normal size but no other structural abnormalities. Venous thrombosis, an underrecognized cause, must be ruled out by magnetic resonance venogram or even injected venograms of cerebral sinuses. Lumbar puncture should be performed to document elevated CSF pressure. Examination of CSF reveals normal findings except for elevated pressure. In some inflammatory and connective tissue diseases, however, the CSF protein concentration may be increased.

Treatment of pseudotumor cerebri is aimed at correcting the identifiable predisposing condition. In addition, some

Table 23–16. Conditions associated with pseudotumor cerebri.

Metabolic-toxic disorders
Hypervitaminosis A
Obesity
Prolonged steroid therapy
Steroid withdrawal
Tetracycline, minocycline toxicity
Nalidixic acid toxicity
Iron deficiency
Clotting disorders
Hypocalcemia
Hyperparathyroidism
Adrenal insufficiency
Systemic lupus erythematosus
Chronic CO_2 retention
Infectious and parainfectious disorders
Chronic otitis media (Lateral sinus thrombosis)
Guillain-Barré syndrome
Lyme disease
Dural sinus thrombosis
Minor head injury

patients may benefit from the use of furosemide or acetazolamide to decrease the volume and pressure of CSF within the CNS. These drugs may be used in combination with repeated lumbar punctures to remove CSF. If a program of repeated CSF removal and medical management is not successful or if central vision or visual field loss is detected despite these measures, lumboperitoneal or ventriculoperitoneal shunt or optic nerve fenestration may be necessary to prevent irreparable visual loss and damage to the optic nerves.

Ball AK, Clarke CE: Idiopathic intracranial hypertension. Lancet Neurol 2006;5:433 [PMID: 16632314].

De Lucia D et al: Benign intracranial hypertension associated to blood coagulation derangements. Thromb J 2006;4:21 [PMID: 17187688].

Kesler A, Bassan H: Pseudotumor cerebri—idiopathic intracranial hypertension in the pediatric population. Pediatr Endocrinol Rev 2006;3,387 [PMID: 16816807].

Lim M et al: Visual failure without headache in idiopathic intracranial hypertension. Arch Dis Child 2005;90:206 [PMID: 15665183].

Rajpal S et al: Transverse venous sinus stent placement as treatment for benign intracranial hypertension in a young male: Case report and review of the literature. J Neurosurg 2005;102:342 [PMID: 15881764].

Stiebel-Kalish H et al: Puberty as a risk factor for less favorable visual outcome in idiopathic intracranial hypertension. Am J Ophthalmol 2006;142:279 [PMID: 16876509].

Thambisetty M et al: Fulminant idiopathic intracranial hypertension. Neurol 2007;68:229 [PMID: 17224579].

CEREBROVASCULAR DISEASE

Pediatric arterial ischemic stroke is subdivided into two categories: neonatal arterial ischemic stroke (neonatal stroke) and childhood arterial ischemic stroke (childhood stroke). Generally, neonatal stroke is defined as arterial ischemia occurring in a patient younger than age 28 days and older than 28 weeks' gestation. Childhood stroke is any stroke occurring in a patient between 28 days and 18 years old.

1. Childhood Stroke

Childhood stroke is emerging as a serious and increasingly recognized disorder, affecting 2–8:100,000 children. There are numerous adverse outcomes, which include death in 10%, neurologic deficits or seizures in 60–85%, and recurrent strokes in 20–35%. The initial approach to the patient should recognize that childhood stroke represents a neurologic emergency, for which promptness in diagnosis can affect treatment considerations and outcome. Unfortunately, most pediatric stroke is not recognized until 24–36 hours after onset; treatment considerations matter most in the first hours after stroke onset. When possible, all children who present with stroke should be transferred to a tertiary care center that specializes in pediatric stroke management. The evaluation should include a thorough history of prior illnesses, especially those associated with varicella (even in the prior 1–2 years) influenza, parvovirus B19, HIV, minor trauma to the head and neck, and familial clotting tendencies. A systematic search for evidence of cardiac, vascular,

Table 23-17. Etiologic risk factors for stroke.

Cardiac disorders
  Cyanotic heart disease
  Valvular disease
    Rheumatic
    Endocarditis
  Cardiomyopathy
  Cardiac dysrhythmia
Vascular occlusive disorders
  Arterial trauma (carotid dissections)
  Homocystinuria/homocystinemia
  Vasculitis
    Meningitis
    Polyarteritis nodosa
    Systemic lupus erythematosus
    Drug abuse (amphetamines)
    Varicella
    Mycoplasma
  Human immunodeficiency virus
  Fibromuscular dysplasia
  Moyamoya disease
  Diabetes
  Nephrotic syndrome
  Systemic hypertension
  Dural sinus and cerebral venous thrombosis
  Cortical venous thrombosis
Hematologic disorders
  Iron deficiency anemia
  Polycythemia
  Thrombotic thrombocytopenia
  Thrombocytopenic purpura
  Hemoglobinopathies
    Sickle cell disease
  Coagulation defects
    Hemophilia
    Vitamin K deficiency
  Hypercoagulable states
    Prothrombin gene mutation
    Methylenetetrahydrofolate reductase mutation
    Lipoprotein (a)
    Factor V Leiden deficiency
    Antiphospholipid antibodies
    Hypercholesterolemia
    Hypertriglyceridemia
    Factor VIII elevation
    Pregnancy
    Systemic lupus erythematosus
    Use of oral contraceptives
    Antithrombin III deficiency
    Protein C and S deficiencies
  Leukemia
Intracranial vascular anomalies
  Arteriovenous malformation
  Arterial aneurysm
  Carotid-cavernous fistula
  Transient cerebral arteriopathy

hematologic, or intracranial disorders should be undertaken (Table 23–17). Although many strokes are not associated with a single underlying systemic disorder, previously diagnosed congenital heart disease is the most common predisposing illness, followed by hematologic and neoplastic disorders. In many instances the origin is multifactorial, necessitating a thorough investigation even when the cause may seem obvious. As a result, the cause of childhood stroke is increasingly determined, whereas in past studies up to 30% remained idiopathic. This is particularly important when considering that recurrence risk may be as high as 35%.

▶ Clinical Findings

A. Symptoms and Signs

Manifestations of stroke in childhood vary according to the vascular distribution to the brain structure that is involved. Because many conditions leading to childhood stroke result in emboli, multifocal neurologic involvement is common. Children may present with acute hemiplegia similarly to stroke in adults. Symptoms of unilateral weakness, sensory disturbance, dysarthria, and dysphagia may develop over a period of minutes, but at times progressive worsening of symptoms may evolve over several hours. Bilateral hemispheric involvement may lead to a depressed level of consciousness. The patient may also demonstrate disturbances of mood and behavior and experience focal or multifocal seizures. Physical examination of the patient is aimed not only at identifying the specific deficits related to impaired cerebral blood flow, but also at seeking evidence for any predisposing disorder. Retinal hemorrhages, splinter hemorrhages in the nail beds, cardiac murmurs, rash, neurocutaneous stigmata, and signs of trauma are especially important findings.

B. Laboratory Findings and Ancillary Testing

In the acute phase, certain investigations should be carried out emergently with consideration of treatment options. This should include complete blood count, erythrocyte sedimentation rate, basic chemistries, blood urea nitrogen, creatinine, prothrombin time/partial thromboplastin time, chest radiography, electrocardiography, urine toxicology, and imaging (see following section). Subsequent studies can be carried out systemically, with particular attention paid to disorders involving the heart, blood vessels, platelets, red cells, hemoglobin, and coagulation proteins. Twenty to 50% of all pediatric stroke patients will have a prothrombotic state. Additional laboratory tests for systemic disorders such as vasculitis, mitochondrial disorders, and metabolic disorders are sometimes indicated.

Examination of CSF is indicated in patients with fever, nuchal rigidity, or obtundation when the diagnosis of intracranial infection requires exclusion. Lumbar puncture may be deferred until a neuroimaging scan (excluding brain abscess or a space-occupying lesion that might contraindicate lumbar puncture) has been obtained. In the absence of infection and frank intracranial subarachnoid hemorrhage, CSF examination is rarely helpful in defining the cause of the cerebrovascular disorder.

When seizures are prominent, an EEG may be used as an adjunct in the patient's evaluation. An EEG and sequential EEG monitoring may help in patients with severely depressed consciousness.

Electrocardiography and echocardiography are useful both in the diagnostic approach to the patient and in ongoing monitoring and management, particularly when hypotension or cardiac arrhythmias complicate the clinical course.

C. Imaging

CT and MRI scans of the brain are helpful in defining the extent of cerebral involvement with ischemia or hemorrhage. CT scans may be normal within the first 12–24 hours of an ischemic stroke and may need to be repeated. CT scan early after the onset of neurologic deficits is valuable in excluding intracranial hemorrhage. This information may be helpful in the early stages of management and in the decision to treat with anticoagulants. State-of-the-art management of stroke in the adult population omits CT scanning but proceeds directly to urgent MRI, MRA, and diffusion-weighted imaging since these modalities are sensitive to acute stroke in the initial 3 hours, when intravenous thrombolytics might be considered. Increasingly, MRI with diffusion-weighed imaging is becoming the standard of care in diagnosing pediatric stroke.

Vascular imaging is an important part of pediatric stroke management and may include CTA, MRA, or conventional angiography. In studies in which both MRA and cerebral angiography have been used, up to 80% of patients with ischemic stroke have demonstrated a vascular abnormality. Vascular imaging is helpful in diagnosing disorders such as transient cerebral arteriopathy, arteriopathy associated with sickle cell disease, moyamoya disease, arterial dissection, aneurysm, fibromuscular dysplasia, and chronic inflammatory vasculitis. Recent studies have demonstrated that patients with vascular abnormalities on MRA or conventional angiography have a much greater recurrence risk than patients with normal vessels. When vessel imaging is performed, all major vessels should be studied from the aortic arch. If evidence of fibromuscular dysplasia is present in the intracranial or extracranial vessels, renal arteriography is indicated.

▶ Differential Diagnosis

Patients with an acute onset of neurologic deficits must be evaluated for other disorders that can cause focal neurologic deficits. Hypoglycemia, prolonged focal seizures, a prolonged postictal paresis (Todd paralysis), acute disseminated encephalomyelitis, meningitis, encephalitis, and brain abscess should all be considered. Migraine with focal neurologic deficits may be difficult to differentiate initially from ischemic stroke. Occasionally the onset of a neurodegenerative disorder (eg, adrenoleukodystrophy or mitochondrial disorder) may begin with the abrupt onset of seizures and focal neurologic deficits. The possibility of drug abuse (particularly cocaine) and other toxic exposures must be investigated diligently in any patient with acute mental status changes.

▶ Treatment

The initial management of stroke in a child is aimed at providing support for pulmonary, cardiovascular, and renal function. Patients should be administered oxygen. Typically, maintenance fluids without added glucose are indicated to augment vascular volume. Specific treatment of stroke, including blood pressure management, fluid management, and anticoagulation measures, depends partly on the underlying pathogenesis. Meningitis or varicella infections should be treated. Sickle cell patients require specialists in hematology to perform urgent exchange transfusion and most patients will require chronic transfusions after hospital discharge. Moyamoya is usually treated with surgical revascularization. In most idiopathic cases of childhood stroke without hemorrhage, anticoagulation or aspirin therapy is indicated. The Royal College of Physicians Pediatric Stroke Working Group recommends aspirin, 5 mg/kg daily, as soon as the diagnosis is made. Aspirin use appears safe and has not been associated with Reye syndrome in pediatric stroke patients. Other groups, such as the American College of Chest Physicians, recommend initial treatment with anticoagulants, such as low-molecular-weight heparin or unfractionated heparin, for 5–7 days (while excluding cardiac sources and dissection) and then switching to aspirin (3–5 mg/d). In some situations, such as arterial dissection, stuttering stroke, emboli, and consumptive coagulopathies, emergent heparinization is usually indicated. In adults with cerebrovascular thrombosis, thrombolytic agents (tissue plasminogen activator) used systemically or delivered directly to a vascular thrombotic lesion using interventional radiologic techniques has been shown to improve outcome. Although case reports exist, studies in children have not been completed. Given the time-lag to diagnosis and the lack of evidence in children, tissue plasminogen activator is currently used in less than 2% of U.S. children with stroke.

Long-term management requires intensive rehabilitation efforts and therapy aimed at improving the child's language, educational, and psychological performance. Length of treatment with various agents, such as low-molecular-weight heparin and aspirin, is still being studied and depends on the etiology. Constraint therapy may be particularly helpful in cases of hemiparesis. Multidisciplinary stroke teams are the best resource for making these decisions.

▶ Prognosis

The outcome of stroke in infants and children is variable. Roughly 40% may have minimal or no deficits, 30% are moderately affected, and 30% are severely affected. Underlying predisposing conditions and the vascular territory involved all play a role in dictating the outcome for an individual patient. When the stroke involves extremely large portions of one hemisphere or large portions of both hemispheres and cerebral edema develops, the patient's level of consciousness may deteriorate rapidly, and death may occur within the first few days. Some patients may achieve almost complete recovery of neurologic function within several days if the cerebral territory is small. Seizures, either focal or generalized, may occur in 30–50% of patients at some point in the course of their cerebrovascular disorder. Recurrence is 20–35%, and is more prominent in some conditions, such as protein C deficiency, lipoprotein (a) abnormalities and arteriopathies. Chronic problems with learning, behavior, and activity are common. Long-term follow-up with a multidisciplinary stroke team is indicated.

2. Neonatal Stroke

Neonatal stroke is more common than childhood stroke, affecting 1:4000 children. Neonatal stroke has two distinct presentations: acute and delayed. Most patients with an acute presentation develop neonatal seizures during the first week of life, usually in association with a perinatal event. The seizures in acute neonatal stroke are often focal motor seizures of the contralateral arm and leg. The presentation is stereotypical because of the predilection of the stroke to occur in the middle cerebral artery. The presence of diffusion-weighted abnormalities on an MRI scan confirms an acute perinatal stroke during the first week of life. Others patients present with delayed symptoms, typically with an evolving hemiparesis at an average of 4–8 months.

Acute treatment of a neonatal stroke is usually limited to neonates with seizures. Unless an embolic source is identified, aspirin and anticoagulation are usually deferred. Management is based on supportive care, identification of comorbid conditions, and treatment of seizures. In acute neonatal stroke, treatable causes of the stroke such as infection, cardiac embolus, metabolic derangement, and dissection must be ruled out. In appropriate cases, echocardiography, MRA, and lumbar puncture are indicated. Supportive management focuses on general measures, such as normalizing glucose levels, monitoring blood pressure, and optimizing oxygenation.

Long-term management of neonatal stroke usually starts with identifying risk factors, which might include prothrombotic states, cardiac disease, drugs, and dehydration. Although prothrombotic abnormalities with the best evidence of association are factor V Leiden, protein C deficiency, and lipoprotein (a), many neurologists perform an extensive hematologic workup. Maternal risk factors such as infertility, antiphospholipid antibodies, placental infection, premature rupture of membranes, and cocaine exposure are all independently associated with neonatal stroke.

The prognosis for children who sustain neonatal strokes is generally better than for children or adults with strokes, presumably because of the plasticity of the neonatal brain. Twenty to 40% of patients who experience neonatal strokes are neurologically normal. Motor impairment affects about

40% of patient and is predominantly hemiplegic cerebral palsy. In acute presentations, MRI can be predictive of motor impairment, as descending corticospinal tract diffusion-weighted MRI signal is associated with a higher incidence of hemiplegia. Language delays, behavioral abnormalities, and cognitive deficits are seen in 20–30% of infants who experience neonatal strokes. Patients are also at an increased risk for seizures. Stroke recurs in 3% of neonates and is usually associated with a prothrombotic abnormality or an underlying illness, such as cardiac malformation or infection. Given the low incidence of recurrence, long-term management is largely rehabilitative, including constraint therapies.

Barnes C et al: Prothrombotic abnormalities in childhood ischaemic stroke. Thromb Res 2005;1 [PMID: 16039697].

deVeber G: In pursuit of evidence-based treatments for paediatric stroke: The UK and Chest guidelines. Lancet Neurol 2005;7:432 [PMID: 15963446].

Duran R et al: Factor V Leiden mutation and other thrombophilia markers in childhood ischemic stroke. Clinical and applied thrombosis/hemostasis. Clin Appl Thromb Hemost 2005;11:83 [PMID: 15678277].

Friefeld S et al: Health-related quality of life and its relationship to neurological outcome in child survivors of stroke. CNS Spectr 2004;6:465 [PMID: 15162094].

Fullerton H et al: Risk of recurrent childhood arterial ischemic stroke in a population-based cohort: The importance of cerebrovascular imaging. Pediatrics 2007;119:3 [PMID: 17332202].

Gabis L et al: Time lag to diagnosis of stroke in children. Pediatrics 2002;110:924 [PMID: 12415031].

Ganesan V et al: Clinical guidelines for the management of childhood stroke. Hosp Med 2005;1:4 [PMID: 15686158].

Ganesan V et al: Investigation of risk factors in children with arterial ischemic stroke. Ann Neurol 2003;53:167 [PMID: 12557282].

Janjua N et al: Thrombolysis for ischemic stroke in children data from the nationwide inpatient sample. Stroke 2007;38 [PMID: 17431210].

Kirton A et al: Cerebral palsy secondary to perinatal ischemic stroke. Clin Perinatol 2006;367 [PMID: 16765730]

Kirton A et al: Quantified corticospinal tract diffusion restriction predicts neonatal stroke outcome. Stroke 2007;38:3 [PMID: 17272775].

Kurnik K et al: Recurrent thromboembolism in infants and children suffering from symptomatic neonatal arterial stroke. Stroke 2003;34:2887 [PMID: 14631084].

Lee J et al: Maternal and infant characteristics associated with perinatal arterial stroke in the infant. JAMA 2005;293:723 [PMID: 15701914].

Lee J et al: Predictors of outcome in perinatal arterial stroke: A population-based study. Ann Neurology 2005;58:303 [PMID: 16010659].

Lee M et al: Stroke prevention trial in sickle cell anemia (STOP): Extended follow-up and final results for the STOP Study Investigators. Blood 2006;108:847 [PMID: 16861341].

Lynch J et al: Pediatric stroke: What do we know and what do we need to know? Semin Neurol 2005;4:410 [PMID: 16341997].

Monagle et al: Antithrombotic therapy in children: The seventh ACCP conference on antithrombotic and thrombolytic therapy. Chest 2004;126:645 [PMID: 15383489].

Nelson K et al: Stroke in newborn infants. Lancet Neurol 2004;3:150 [PMID: 14980530].

Sebire G et al: Toward the definition of cerebral arteriopathies of childhood. Curr Opin Pediatr 2004;16:617 [PMID: 15548922].

Shellhaas R et al: Mimics of childhood stroke: Characteristics of a prospective cohort. Pediatrics 2006;118:704 [PMID: 16882826].

Sofronas M et al: Pediatric stroke initiatives and preliminary studies: What is known and what is needed? Pediatr Neurol 2006;34:439 [PMID: 16765821].

Taub E et al: Pediatric CI therapy for stroke-induced hemiparesis in young children. Dev Neurorehabil 2007;10:3 [PMID: 17608322].

Zahuranec DB et al: Is it time for a large, collaborative study of pediatric stroke? Stroke 2005;36:1825 [PMID: 16100029].

CONGENITAL MALFORMATIONS OF THE NERVOUS SYSTEM

Malformations of the nervous system occur in 1–3% of living neonates and are present in 40% of infants who die. Developmental anomalies of the CNS may result from a variety of causes, including infectious, toxic, metabolic, and vascular insults that affect the fetus. The specific type of malformation that results from such insults, however, may depend more on the gestational period during which the insult occurs than on the specific cause. The period of induction, days 0–28 of gestation, is the period during which the neural plate appears and the neural tube forms and closes. Insults during this phase can result in a major absence of neural structures, such as anencephaly, or in a defect of neural tube closure, such as spina bifida, meningomyelocele, or encephalocele. Cellular proliferation and migration characterize neural development that occurs after 28 days' gestation. Lissencephaly, pachygyria, agyria, and agenesis of the corpus callosum may be the result of disruptions (genetic, toxic, infectious, or metabolic) that can occur during the period of cellular proliferation and migration.

1. Abnormalities of Neural Tube Closure

Defects of neural tube closure constitute some of the most common congenital malformations affecting the nervous system, occurring in 1:1000 live births. Spina bifida with associated meningomyelocele or meningocele is commonly found in the lumbar region. Depending on the extent and severity of the involvement of the spinal cord and peripheral nerves, lower extremity weakness, bowel and bladder dysfunction, and hip dislocation may be present. Delivery via cesarean section followed by early surgical closure of meningoceles and meningomyeloceles is usually indicated. Additional treatment is necessary to manage chronic abnormalities of the urinary tract, orthopedic abnormalities such as kyphosis and scoliosis, and paresis of the lower extremities. Hydrocephalus associated with meningomyelocele usually requires ventriculoperitoneal shunting.

A. Arnold-Chiari Malformations

Arnold-Chiari malformation type I consists of elongation and displacement of the caudal end of the brainstem into the spinal canal with protrusion of the cerebellar tonsils through the foramen magnum. In association with this hindbrain malformation, minor to moderate abnormalities of the base of the skull often occur, including basilar impression (platybasia) and small foramen magnum. Arnold-Chiari malformation type I may remain asymptomatic for years, but in older children and young adults it may cause progressive ataxia, paresis of the lower cranial nerves, and progressive vertigo; rarely it may present with apnea or disordered breathing. Posterior cervical laminectomy may be necessary to provide relief from cervical cord compression. Ventriculoperitoneal shunting is required for hydrocephalus.

Arnold-Chiari malformation type II consists of the malformations found in Arnold-Chiari type I plus an associated lumbar meningomyelocele. Hydrocephalus develops in approximately 90% of children with Arnold-Chiari malformation type II. These patients may also have aqueductal stenosis, hydromyelia or syringomyelia, and cortical dysplasias. The clinical manifestations of Arnold-Chiari malformation type II are most commonly caused by the associated hydrocephalus and meningomyelocele. In addition, dysfunction of the lower cranial nerves may be present. Up to 25% of patients may have epilepsy, likely secondary to the cortical dysplasias. Higher lesions of the thoracic or upper lumbar cord are associated with mild mental retardation in about half of patients, while over 85% of patients with lower level lesions have normal intelligence quotients (IQs). Many patients will develop a latex sensitivity or allergy.

Arnold-Chiari malformation type III is characterized by occipital encephalocele, a closure defect of the rostral end of the neural tube. Hydrocephalus is extremely common with this malformation.

B. Diagnosis and Prevention

In general, the diagnosis of neural tube defects is obvious at the time of birth. The diagnosis may be strongly suspected prenatally on the basis of ultrasonographic findings and the presence of elevated α-fetoprotein in the amniotic fluid. All women of childbearing age should take prophylactic folate, which can prevent these defects and decrease the risk of recurrence by 70%.

2. Disorders of Cortical Development

Malformations of cortical development are increasingly recognized with the advent of MRI techniques and the explosion of newly identified genetic syndromes. They are subdivided into disorders based on their etiology: neuronal migration, cortical organization, abnormal proliferation or apoptosis, and unclassified. In this section we provide some common examples of these subtypes. Lissencephaly is the most common disorder of neuronal migration. Polymicrogyria and schizencephaly are examples of organizational abnormalities. Agenesis of the corpus callosum, described below, is an example of abnormal apoptosis. Finally, some abnormalities such as Dandy-Walker syndrome remained unclassified.

A. Lissencephaly

Lissencephaly is a severe malformation of the brain characterized by an extremely smooth cortical surface with minimal sulcal and gyral development. Such a smooth surface is characteristic of fetal brain at the end of the first trimester. In addition, lissencephalic brains have a primitive cytoarchitectural construction with a four-layered cerebral mantle instead of the mature six-layered mantle. Pachygyria (thick gyri) and agyria (absence of gyri) may vary in an anterior to posterior gradient, which can be suggestive of the underlying genetic defect. Patients with lissencephaly usually have severe neurodevelopmental delay, microcephaly, and seizures (including infantile spasms); however, there is significant phenotypic heterogeneity, which can depend on the specific mutation. These disorders are autosomal recessive, except for the X-linked disorders. LIS1 mutations on chromosome 17 are associated with dysmorphic features (Miller-Dieker syndrome). Another autosomal recessive mutation, involving the RELN gene, results in a lissencephaly with severe hippocampal and cerebellar hypoplasia. X-linked syndromes involving mutations in DCX (double cortin) and ARX (associated with ambiguous genitalia) affect males with lissencephaly and females with band heterotopias or agenesis of the corpus callosum. Lissencephaly in association with hydrocephalus, cerebellar malformations, and muscular dystrophy may occur in Walker-Warburg syndrome (POMT1 mutation), Fukuyama muscular dystrophy (fukutin mutation), and muscle-eye-brain disease (POMGnT1 mutation). It is particularly important to identify these syndromes not only because clinical tests are available, but also because of their genetic implications. Lissencephaly may also be a component of Zellweger syndrome, a metabolic peroxisomal abnormality associated with the presence of elevated concentrations of very-long-chain fatty acids in plasma. No specific treatment for lissencephaly is available, and seizures are often difficult to control with standard medications.

MRI scans have helped to define several presumed migrational defects that are similar to but anatomically more restricted than lissencephaly. A distinctive example is bilateral perisylvian cortical dysplasia. Patients with this disorder have pseudobulbar palsy, variable cognitive deficits, facial diplegia, dysarthria, developmental delay, and epilepsy. Seizures are often difficult to control with antiepileptic drugs; some patients have benefited from corpus callosotomy. The cause of this syndrome is as yet unknown, although intrauterine cerebral ischemic injury has been postulated. Therapy is aimed at improving speech and oromotor functions and controlling seizures.

B. Agenesis of the Corpus Callosum

Agenesis of the corpus callosum, once thought to be a rare cerebral malformation, is more frequently diagnosed with modern neuroimaging techniques; occurring in 1:4000 births. The cause of this malformation is unknown. Occasionally it appears to be inherited in either an autosomal dominant or recessive pattern. X-linked recessive patterns have also been described (*ARX* as mentioned earlier). Agenesis of the corpus callosum has been found in some patients with pyruvate dehydrogenase deficiency and in others with nonketotic hyperglycinemia. Most cases are sporadic. Maldevelopment of the corpus callosum may be partial or complete. No specific syndrome is typical of agenesis of the corpus callosum, although many patients have seizures, developmental delay, microcephaly, or mental retardation. Neurologic abnormalities may be related to microscopic cytoarchitectural abnormalities of the brain that occur in association with agenesis of the corpus callosum. The malformation may be found coincidentally by neuroimaging studies in otherwise normal patients and has been described as a coincidental finding at autopsy in neurologically normal individuals. A special form of agenesis of the corpus callosum occurs in Aicardi syndrome. In this X-linked disorder, agenesis of the corpus callosum is associated with other cystic intracerebral abnormalities, infantile spasms, mental retardation, lacunar chorioretinopathy, and vertebral body abnormalities.

C. Dandy-Walker Syndrome

Despite being described nearly a century ago, the exact definition of the Dandy-Walker syndrome is still debated. Classically, it is characterized by aplasia of the vermis, cystic enlargement of the fourth ventricle, rostral displacement of the tentorium, and absence or atresia of the foramina of Magendie and Luschka. Although hydrocephalus is usually not present congenitally, it develops within the first few months of life. Ninety percent of patients who develop hydrocephalus do so by age 1 year. On physical examination, a rounded protuberance or exaggeration of the cranial occiput often exists. In the absence of hydrocephalus and increased intracranial pressure, few physical findings may be present to suggest neurologic dysfunction. An ataxic syndrome occurs in fewer than 20% of patients and is usually late in appearing. Many long-term neurologic deficits result directly from hydrocephalus. Diagnosis of Dandy-Walker syndrome is confirmed by CT or MRI scanning of the head. Treatment is directed at the management of hydrocephalus.

3. Craniosynostosis

Craniosynostosis, or premature closure of cranial sutures, is usually sporadic and idiopathic. However, some patients have hereditary disorders, such as Apert syndrome and Crouzon disease, that are associated with abnormalities of the digits, extremities, and heart. Occasionally craniosynostosis may be associated with an underlying metabolic disturbance such as hyperthyroidism and hypophosphatasia. The most common form of craniosynostosis involves the sagittal suture and results in scaphocephaly, an elongation of the head in the anterior to posterior direction. Premature clo-

sure of the coronal sutures causes brachycephaly, an increase in cranial growth from left to right. Unless many or all cranial sutures close prematurely, intracranial volume will not be compromised, and the brain's growth will not be impaired. Closure of only one or a few sutures will not cause impaired brain growth or neurologic dysfunction. Management of craniosynostosis is directed at preserving normal skull shape and consists of excising the fused suture and applying material to the edge of the craniectomy to prevent reossification of the bone edges. The best cosmetic effect on the skull is achieved when surgery is performed during the first 6 months of life.

4. Hydrocephalus

Hydrocephalus is characterized by an increased volume of CSF in association with progressive ventricular dilation. In communicating hydrocephalus, CSF circulates through the ventricular system and into the subarachnoid space without obstruction. In noncommunicating hydrocephalus, an obstruction blocks the flow of CSF within the ventricular system or blocks the egress of CSF from the ventricular system into the subarachnoid space. A wide variety of disorders, such as hemorrhage, infection, tumors, and congenital malformations, may play a causal role in the development of hydrocephalus. Attention to an X-linked inheritance pattern, the presence of radialized thumbs and aqueductal stenosis, is suggestive of X-linked hydrocephalus due to the clinically testable neural cell adhesion molecule-L1 deficiency.

Clinical features of hydrocephalus include macrocephaly, an excessive rate of head growth, irritability, vomiting, loss of appetite, impaired upgaze, impaired extraocular movements, hypertonia of the lower extremities, and generalized hyperreflexia. Without treatment, optic atrophy may occur. In infants, papilledema may not be present, whereas older children with closed cranial sutures can eventually develop swelling of the optic disk. Hydrocephalus can be diagnosed on the basis of the clinical course, findings on physical examination, and CT or MRI scan.

Treatment of hydrocephalus is directed at providing an alternative outlet for CSF from the intracranial compartment. The most common method is ventriculoperitoneal shunting. Other treatment should be directed, if possible, at the underlying cause of the hydrocephalus.

For genetic testing, see http://www.genetests.org

Barkovich R et al: A developmental and genetic classification for malformations of cortical development. Neurology 2005;65:1873 [PMID: 16192428].

Doherty D et al: Pediatric perspective on prenatal counseling for myelomeningocele. Birth Defects Res A Clin Mol Teratol 2006;76:645 [PMID: 17001678].

Forman M et al: Genotypically defined lissencephalies show distinct pathologies. J Neuropathol Exp Neurol 2005;64:847 [PMID: 16215456].

Kotrikova B et al: Diagnostic imaging in the management of craniosynostoses. Eur Radiol 2007;17:1968 [PMID: 17151858].

Paul L et al: Agenesis of the corpus callosum: genetic, developmental and functional aspects of connectivity. Nat Rev Neurosci 2007;8:287 [PMID: 17375041].

Vertinsky A et al: Macrocephaly, increased intracranial pressure, and hydrocephalus in the infant and young child. Top Magn Reson Imaging 2007;18:31 [PMID: 17607142].

ABNORMAL HEAD SIZE

Bone plates of the skull have almost no intrinsic capacity to enlarge or grow. Unlike long bones, they depend on extrinsic forces to stimulate new bone formation at the suture lines. Although gravity and traction on bone by muscle and scalp probably stimulate some growth, the single most important stimulus for head growth during infancy and childhood is brain growth. Therefore, accurate assessment of head growth is one of the most important aspects of the neurologic examination of young children. A head circumference that is two standard deviations above or below the mean for age requires investigation and explanation.

1. Plagiocephaly

An abnormal skull shape is plagiocephaly ("oblique head"). Flatness of the head (brachycephaly) is a common complaint, and nowadays is usually secondary to supine sleep position ("back to sleep"), not from occipital lambdoid suture craniosynostosis.

Repositioning the head during naps (eg, with a rolled towel under one shoulder), and "tummy time" when awake are remedies. Rarely is a skull film or consultation necessary to rule out craniosynostosis. Most positional nonsynostotic plagiocephaly resolves by age 2 years.

2. Microcephaly

A head circumference more than two standard deviations below the mean for age and sex is by definition microcephaly. More important, however, than a single head circumference measurement is the rate or pattern of head growth over time. Head circumference measurements that progressively drop to lower percentiles with increasing age are indicative of a process or condition that has impaired the brain's capacity to grow. The causes of microcephaly are numerous. Some examples are listed in Table 23–18.

▶ Clinical Findings

A. Symptoms and Signs

Microcephaly may be suspected in the full-term newborn and in infants up to age 6 months whose chest circumference exceeds the head circumference (unless the child is very obese). Microcephaly may be discovered when the child is examined because of delayed developmental milestones or neurologic problems, such as seizures or spasticity. There may be a marked backward slope of the forehead (as in familial microcephaly) with narrowing of the bitemporal

Table 23–18. Causes of microcephaly.

Causes	Examples
Chromosomal	Trisomies 13, 18, 21
Malformation	Lissencephaly, schizencephaly
Syndromes	Rubenstein-Taybi, Cornelia de Lange, Angelman
Toxins	Alcohol, anticonvulsants (?), maternal phenylketonuria (PKU)
Infections (intrauterine)	TORCHS[a]
Radiation	Maternal pelvis, first and second trimester
Placental insufficiency	Toxemia, infection, small for gestational age
Familial	Autosomal dominant, autosomal recessive
Perinatal hypoxia, trauma	Birth asphyxia, injury
Infections (perinatal)	Bacterial meningitis (especially group B streptococci)
	Viral encephalitis (enterovirus, herpes simplex)
Metabolic	Glut-1 deficiency, PKU, maple syrup urine disease
Degenerative disease	Tay-Sachs, Krabbe

[a]TORCHS is a mnemonic for toxoplasmosis, other infections, rubella, cytomegalovirus, herpes simplex, and syphilis.

diameter. The fontanelle may close earlier than expected, and sutures may be prominent.

B. Laboratory Findings

Laboratory findings vary with the cause. Abnormal dermatoglyphics may be present when the injury occurred before 19 weeks' gestation. In the newborn, IgM antibody titers for toxoplasmosis, rubella, cytomegalovirus (CMV), herpes simplex virus, and syphilis may be assessed. Elevated specific IgM titer is indicative of congenital infection. The urine culture for CMV will be positive at birth when this virus is the cause of microcephaly. Eye, cardiac, and bone abnormalities may also be clues to congenital infection. The child's serum and urine amino and organic acid determinations are occasionally diagnostic. The mother may require screening for phenylketonuria. Karyotyping should be considered.

C. Imaging

CT or MRI scans may aid in diagnosis and prognosis. These studies may demonstrate calcifications, malformations, or atrophic patterns that suggest specific congenital infections or genetic syndromes. Plain skull radiographs are of limited value. Genetic counseling should be offered to the family of any infant with significant microcephaly.

Differential Diagnosis

Congenital craniosynostosis involving multiple sutures is easily differentiated by inspection of the head, history, identification of syndromes, hereditary pattern, and sometimes signs and symptoms of increased intracranial pressure. Common forms of craniosynostosis involving sagittal, coronal, and lambdoidal sutures are associated with abnormally shaped heads but do not cause microcephaly. Recognizing treatable causes of undergrowth of the brain such as hypopituitarism or hypothyroidism and severe protein-calorie undernutrition is critical so that therapy can be initiated as early as possible.

Treatment & Prognosis

Except for the treatable disorders already noted, treatment is usually supportive and directed at the multiple neurologic and sensory deficits, endocrine disturbances (eg, diabetes insipidus), and seizures. Many, but not all, children with microcephaly are developmentally delayed. The notable exceptions are found in cases of hypopituitarism (rare) or familial autosomal dominant microcephaly.

Bishop FS et al: Glutaric aciduria type 1 presenting as bilateral subdural hematomas mimicking nonaccidental trauma. Case report and review of the literature. J Neurosurg 2007;106(Suppl):222 [PMID: 17465389].

Chiu S et al: Early acceleration of head circumference in children with fragile X syndrome and autism. J Dev Behav Pediatr 2007;28:31 [PMID: 17353729].

Freeman JM, Carson BS: Management of infants with potentially misshapen heads. Pediatrics 2003;111:918.

Glass RB et al: The infant skull: A vault of information. Radiographics 2004;507:22 [PMID: 15026597].

Gnamey DK et al: Primary autosomal recessive microcephaly: A novel clinical phenotype. Genet Couns 2005;16:107 [PMID: 15844788].

Hutchison BL et al: Plagiocephaly and brachycephaly in the first two years of life: A prospective cohort study. Pediatrics 2004;114:970 [PMID: 15466093].

Losee JE et al: Nonsynostotic occipital plagiocephaly: Factors impacting onset, treatment, and outcomes. Plast Reconstr Surg 2007;119:1866 [PMID: 17440367].

Purugganan OH: Abnormalities in head size. Pediatr Rev 2006;27:473 [PMID: 17142470].

Sztriha L et al: Microcephaly associated with abnormal gyral pattern. Neuropediatrics 2004;35:346 [PMID: 15627942].

Wang D et al: Glut-1 deficiency syndrome: Clinical, genetic, and therapeutic aspects. Ann Neurol 2005;57:111 [PMID: 15622525].

3. Macrocephaly

A head circumference more than two standard deviations above the mean for age and sex denotes macrocephaly. Rapid head growth rate suggests increased intracranial pressure, most likely caused by hydrocephalus, extra-axial fluid collections, or neoplasms. Macrocephaly with normal head growth

Table 23–19. Causes of macrocephaly.

Causes	Examples
Pseudomacrocephaly, pseudohydrocephalus, catch-up growth crossing percentiles	Growing premature infant; recovery from malnutrition, congenital heart disease, postsurgical correction
Increased intracranial pressure	
With dilated ventricles	Progressive hydrocephalus, subdural effusion
With other mass	Arachnoid cyst, porencephalic cyst, brain tumor
Benign familial macrocephaly (idiopathic external hydrocephalus)	External hydrocephalus, benign enlargement of the subarachnoid spaces (synonyms)
Megalencephaly (large brain)	
With neurocutaneous disorder	Neurofibromatosis, tuberous sclerosis, etc
With gigantism	Sotos syndrome
With dwarfism	Achondroplasia
Metabolic	Mucopolysaccharidoses
Lysosomal	Metachromatic leukodystrophy (late)
Other leukodystrophy	Canavan spongy degeneration
Thickened skull	Fibrous dysplasia (bone), hemolytic anemia (marrow), sicklemia, thalassemia

rate suggests familial macrocephaly or true megalencephaly, as might occur in neurofibromatosis. Other causes and examples of macrocephaly are listed in Table 23–19.

Clinical Findings

Clinical and laboratory findings vary with the underlying process. In infants, transillumination of the skull with an intensely bright light in a completely darkened room may disclose subdural effusions, hydrocephalus, hydranencephaly, and cystic defects. A surgically or medically treatable condition must be ruled out. Thus the first decision is whether and when to perform an imaging study.

A. Imaging Study Deferred

1. Catch-up growth—Catch-up growth may be evident, as it is in the thriving, neurologically intact premature infant whose rapid head enlargement is most marked in the first weeks of life, or the infant in the early phase of recovery from deprivation dwarfism. As the expected normal size is reached, head growth slows and then resumes a normal growth pattern. If the fontanelle is open, cranial ultrasonography can assess ventricular size and diagnose or exclude hydrocephalus.

2. Familial macrocephaly—This condition may exist when another family member has an unusually large head with no signs or symptoms referable to such disorders as neurocutaneous dysplasias (especially neurofibromatosis) or cerebral gigantism (Sotos syndrome), or when there are no significant mental or neurologic abnormalities in the child.

B. Imaging Study

CT or MRI scans (or ultrasonography, if the anterior fontanelle is open) are used to define any structural cause of macrocephaly and to identify an operable disorder. Even when the condition is untreatable (or does not require treatment), the information gained may permit more accurate diagnosis and prognosis, guide management and genetic counseling, and serve as a basis for comparison should future abnormal cranial growth or neurologic changes necessitate a repeat study. An imaging study is necessary if signs or symptoms of increased intracranial pressure are present (see Table 23–15).

Cutting LE et al: Megalencephaly in NF1. Neurology 2002;59:1388 [PMID: 12427889].

Dementieva YA et al: Accelerated head growth in early development of individuals with autism. Pediatr Neurol 2005;32:102 [PMID: 15664769].

Riel-Romero RM et al: Megalencephalic leukoencephalopathy with subcortical cysts in two siblings owing to two novel mutations: Case reports and review of the literature. J Child Neurol 2005;20:230 [PMID: 1583614].

NEUROCUTANEOUS DYSPLASIAS

Neurocutaneous dysplasias are diseases of the neuroectoderm and sometimes involve endoderm and mesoderm. Birthmarks—and skin growths appearing later—often suggest a need to look for brain, spinal cord, and eye disease. Hamartomas (histologically normal tissue growing abnormally rapidly or in aberrant sites) are common. The most common dysplasias are dominantly inherited. Benign and even malignant tumors may develop.

Johnson KJ et al: Childhood cancer and birthmarks in the Collaborative Perinatal Project. Pediatrics 2007;119:e1088 [PMID: 17473081].

Kandt RS: Tuberous sclerosis complex and neurofibromatosis type 1: The two most common neurocutaneous diseases. Neurol Clin 2003;21:983 [PMID: 14743661].

Korf BR: The phakomatoses. Clin Dermatol 2005;23:78 [PMID: 15708292].

1. Neurofibromatosis (von Recklinghausen Disease)

ESSENTIALS OF DIAGNOSIS & TYPICAL FEATURES

▶ More than six café-au-lait spots 5 mm in greatest diameter in prepubertal individuals and over 15 mm in greatest diameter in postpubertal individuals.

▶ Two or more neurofibromas of any type or one plexiform neurofibroma.

▶ Freckling in the axillary or inguinal regions.

▶ Optic glioma.

▶ Two or more Lisch nodules (iris hamartomas).

▶ Distinctive bony lesions, such as sphenoid dysplasia or thinning of long bone with or without pseudarthroses.

▶ First-degree relative (parent, sibling, offspring) with neurofibromatosis type 1 by above criteria.

▶ General Considerations

Neurofibromatosis is a multisystem disorder with a prevalence of 1:3000–4000. Fifty percent of cases are due to new mutations in the *NF1* gene. Forty percent of patients will develop medical complications of the disorder in their lifetime.

▶ Clinical Findings

A. Symptoms and Signs

The most common presenting symptoms are cognitive or psychomotor problems; 40% of patients have learning disabilities, and mental retardation occurs in 8%. The family history is important in identifying dominant gene manifestations in parents. Parents should be examined in detail. The history should focus on lumps or masses causing disfigurement, functional problems, or pain. Café-au-lait spots are seen in most affected children by age 1 year. The typical skin lesion is 10–30 mm, ovoid, and smooth-bordered. Discrete tumors are more common, are well demarcated, and can occur at any age. Plexiform neurofibromas are more diffuse and can invade normal tissue. They are congenital and are frequently detected during periods of rapid growth. If the face or a limb is involved, there may be associated hypertrophy or overgrowth.

The clinician should ask about visual problems. Strabismus or amblyopia dictates a search for optic glioma, a common tumor in neurofibromatosis. Any progressive neurologic deficit calls for studies to rule out tumor of the spinal cord or CNS. Tumors of cranial nerve VIII virtually never occur in neurofibromatosis type 1 but are the rule in neurofibromatosis type 2, a rare autosomal dominant disease.

The physician should check blood pressure and examine the spine for scoliosis and the limbs for pseudarthroses. Head measurement often shows macrocephaly. Hearing and vision need to be assessed. The eye examination should include a check for proptosis and iris Lisch nodules. The optic disk should be examined for atrophy or papilledema. Short stature and precocious puberty are occasional findings. An examination for neurologic manifestations of tumors (eg, asymmetrical reflexes or spasticity) is important.

B. Laboratory Findings

Laboratory tests are not likely to be of value in asymptomatic patients. Selected patients require brain MRI with special cuts through the optic nerves to rule out optic glioma. Hypertension necessitates evaluation of renal arteries for dysplasia and stenosis. Cognitive and school achievement testing may be indicated. Scoliosis or limb abnormalities should be studied by appropriate roentgenograms such as an MRI scan of the spinal cord and roots.

▶ Differential Diagnosis

Patients with McCune-Albright syndrome often have larger café-au-lait spots with precocious puberty, polyostotic fibrous dysplasia, and hyperfunctioning endocrinopathies. One or two café-au-lait spots are often seen in normal children. A large solitary café-au-lait spot is usually innocent, not neurofibromatosis type 1.

▶ Complications

Seizures, deafness, short stature, early puberty, and hypertension occur in less than 25% of patients with neurofibromatosis. Optic glioma occurs in about 15%. Although the tumor may be apparent at an early age, it rarely causes functional problems and is usually nonprogressive. Patients have a slightly increased risk (5% life risk) for various malignancies. Other tumors may be benign but may cause significant morbidity and mortality because of their size and location in a vital or enclosed space.

▶ Treatment

Genetic counseling is important. The risk to siblings is up to 50%. The disease may be progressive, with serious complications occasionally seen. Patients sometimes worsen during puberty or pregnancy. Genetic screening of family members is required. Annual or semiannual visits are important in the early detection of school problems or bony or neurologic abnormalities. The following parameters should be recorded at each annual visit:

1. Child's development and progress at school
2. Visual symptoms, visual acuity, and funduscopy until age 7 years (to detect optic pathway glioma, glaucoma)
3. Head circumference (rapid increase might indicate tumor or hydrocephalus)
4. Height (to detect abnormal pubertal development)
5. Weight (to detect abnormal pubertal development)
6. Pubertal development (to detect delayed or precocious puberty due to pituitary or hypothalamic lesion)
7. Blood pressure (to detect renal artery stenosis or pheochromocytoma)
8. Cardiovascular examination (for congenital heart disease, especially pulmonary stenosis)
9. Evaluation of spine (for scoliosis and underlying plexiform neurofibromas)
10. Evaluation of the skin (for cutaneous, subcutaneous, and plexiform neurofibromas)
11. Examination of other systems, depending on specific symptoms

Multidisciplinary clinics at medical centers around the United States are excellent resources. Prenatal diagnosis is probably on the horizon, but the variability of manifestations (trivial to severe) will make therapeutic abortion an unlikely option. Chromosomal linkage studies are under way (chromosome 17q11.2). Information for lay people and physicians is available from the National Neurofibromatosis Foundation (http://www.nf.org).

Acosta MT et al: Neurofibromatosis type 1: New insights in to neurocognitive issues. Curr Neurol Neurosci Rep 2006;6:136 [PMID: 16522267].

Al-Otibi M, Rutka JT: Neurosurgical implications of neurofibromatosis type 1 in children. Neurosurg Focus 2006;20:E2 [PMID: 16459992].

Arun D, Gutmann DH: Recent advances in neurofibromatosis type 1. Curr Opin Neurol 2005;17:101 [PMID: 15021234].

Ferner RE et al: Guidelines for the diagnosis and management of individuals with neurofibromatosis 1. J Med Genet 2007;44:81 [PMID: 17105749].

Gonzalez G et al: Bilateral segmental neurofibromatosis: A case report and review. Pediatr Neurol 2007;36:51.

Han M, Criado E: Renal artery stenosis and aneurysms associated with neurofibromatosis. J Vasc Surg 2005;41:539 [PMID: 15838492].

Kanowitz SJ et al: Auditory brainstem implantation in patients with neurofibromatosis type 2. Laryngoscope 2004;114:3135 [PMID: 15564834].

Listrnick R et al: Optic pathway gliomas in neruofibromatosis-1: Controversies and recommendations. Ann Neurol 2007;61:189 [PMID: 17387725].

Rosser TL et al: Cerebrovascular abnormalities in a population of children with neurofibromatosis type 1. Neurology 2005;64:553 [PMID: 15699396].

Ruggieri M et al: Earliest clinical manifestations and natural history of neurofibromatosis type 2 (NF2) in childhood: A study of 24 patients. Neuropediatrics 2005;36:21 [PMID: 15776319].

2. Tuberous Sclerosis (Bourneville Disease)

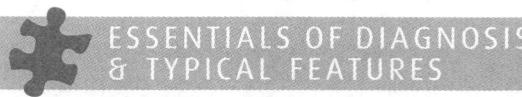

ESSENTIALS OF DIAGNOSIS & TYPICAL FEATURES

▶ Facial angiofibromas or subungual fibromas.

▶ Often hypomelanotic macules, gingival fibromas.

▶ Retinal hamartomas.

▶ Cortical tubers or subependymal glial nodules, often calcified.

▶ Renal angiomyolipomas.

General Considerations

Tuberous sclerosis is a dominantly inherited disease. Almost all patients have deletions on chromosome 9 (*TSC1* gene) or 16 (*TSC2* gene). The gene products hamartin and tuberin have tumor-suppressing effects. A triad of seizures, mental retardation, and adenoma sebaceum occurs in only 33% of patients. The disease was earlier thought to have a high rate of mutation. As a result of more sophisticated techniques such as MRI, parents formerly thought not to harbor the gene are now being diagnosed as asymptomatic carriers.

Like neurofibromatosis, tuberous sclerosis is associated with a wide variety of symptoms. The patient may be asymptomatic except for skin findings or may be devastated by severe infantile spasms in early infancy, by continuing epilepsy, and by mental retardation. Seizures in early infancy correlate with later mental retardation.

Clinical Findings

A. Symptoms and Signs

1. Dermatologic features—Skin findings bring most patients to the physician's attention. Ninety-six percent of patients have one or more hypomelanotic macules, facial angiofibromas, ungual fibromas, or shagreen patches. Adenoma sebaceum, the facial skin hamartomas, may first appear in early childhood, often on the cheek, chin, and dry sites of the skin where acne is not usually seen. They often have a reddish hue. The off-white hypomelanotic macules are seen more easily in tanned or dark-skinned individuals than in those with lighter skin. The macules often are oval or "ash leaf" in shape and follow dermatomes. A Wood's lamp (ultraviolet light) shows the macules more clearly, a great help in the light-skinned patient. In the scalp, poliosis (whitened hair) is the equivalent. In infancy, the presence of these macules accompanied by seizures is virtually diagnostic of the disease. Subungual or periungual fibromas are more common in the toes. Leathery, orange peel–like shagreen patches support the diagnosis. Café-au-lait spots are occasionally seen. Fibrous or raised plaques may resemble coalescent angiofibromas.

2. Neurologic features—Seizures are the most common presenting symptom. Five percent of patients with infantile spasms (a serious epileptic syndrome) have tuberous sclerosis. Thus any patient presenting with infantile spasms (and the parents as well) should be evaluated for this disorder. An imaging study of the CNS, such as a CT scan, may show calcified subependymal nodules; MRI may show dysmyelinating white matter lesions or cortical tubers. Virtually any kind of symptomatic seizure (eg, atypical absence, partial complex, and generalized tonic-clonic seizures) may occur.

3. Mental retardation—Mental retardation occurs in up to 50% of patients referred to tertiary care centers; the incidence is probably much lower in randomly selected patients. Patients with seizures are more prone to mental retardation or learning disabilities.

4. Renal lesions—Renal cysts or angiomyolipomas may be asymptomatic. Hematuria or obstruction of urine flow sometimes occurs; the latter requires operation. Ultrasonography of the kidneys should be done in any patient suspected of tuberous sclerosis, both to aid in diagnosis if lesions are found and to rule out renal obstructive disease.

5. Cardiopulmonary involvement—Rarely cystic lung disease may occur. Rhabdomyomas of the heart may be asymptomatic but can lead to outflow obstruction, conduction difficulties, and death. Chest radiographs and echocardiograms can detect these rare manifestations. Cardiac rhabdomyoma may be detected on prenatal ultra-sound examination.

6. Eye involvement—Retinal hamartomas are often near the disk.

7. Skeletal involvement—Findings sometimes helpful in diagnosis are cystic rarefactions of the bones of the fingers or toes.

B. Diagnostic Studies

Plain radiographs may detect areas of thickening within the skull, spine, and pelvis, and cystic lesions in the hands and feet. Chest radiographs may show lung honeycombing. More helpful is CT scanning, which can show the virtually pathognomonic subependymal nodular calcifications and sometimes widened gyri or tubers and brain tumors. Contrast material may show the often classically located tumors near the interventricular foramen. Hypomyelinated lesions may be seen with MRI. Electroencephalography is helpful in delineating the presence of seizure discharges.

Treatment

Therapy is as indicated by underlying disease (eg, seizures and tumors of the brain, kidney, and heart). Skin lesions on the face may need dermabrasion or laser treatment. Genetic counseling emphasizes identification of the carrier. The risk of appearance in offspring if either parent is a carrier is 50%. The patient should be seen annually for counseling and reexamination in childhood. Identification of the chromosomes (9,16; *TSC1* and *TSC2* genes) may in the future make intrauterine diagnosis possible.

Au KS et al: Molecular genetic basis of tuberous sclerosis complex: From bench to bedside. J Child Neurol 2004;19:699 [PMID: 15563017].

Devlin La et al: Tuberous sclerosis complex: Clinical features, diagnosis, and prevalence within Northern Ireland. Dev Med Child Neurol 2006;48:495 [PMID: 16700943].

Leung AK, Robson WL: Tuberous sclerosis complex: A review. J Pediatr Health Care 2007;21:108 [PMID: 17321910].

Roach ES, Sparagana SP: Diagnosis of tuberous sclerosis complex. J Child Neurol 2004;19:643 [PMID: 15563009].

Rosser T et al: The diverse clinical manifestations of tuberous sclerosis complex: A review. Semin Pediatr Neurol 2006;13:27 [PMID: 16818173].

Thiele EA: Managing epilepsy in tuberous sclerosis complex. J Child Neurol 2004;19:680 [PMID: 15563014].

3. Encephalofacial Angiomatosis (Sturge-Weber Disease)

Sturge-Weber disease consists of a facial port wine nevus involving the upper part of the face (in the first division of cranial nerve V), a venous angioma of the meninges in the occipitoparietal regions, and choroidal angioma. The syndrome has been described without the facial nevus (rare, type III, exclusive leptomeningeal angioma).

▶ Clinical Findings

In infancy, the eye may show congenital glaucoma, or buphthalmos, with a cloudy, enlarged cornea. In early stages, the facial nevus may be the only indication, with no findings in the brain even on radiologic studies. The characteristic cortical atrophy, calcifications of the cortex, and meningeal angiomatosis may appear with time, solidifying the diagnosis.

Physical examination may show focal seizures or hemiparesis on the side opposite the cerebral lesion. The facial nevus may be much more extensive than the first division of cranial nerve V; it can involve the lower face, mouth, lip, neck, and even torso. Hemiatrophy of the opposite limbs may occur. Mental handicap may result from poorly controlled seizures. Late-appearing glaucoma and rarely CNS hemorrhage occur.

Radiologic studies may show calcification of the cortex; CT scanning may show this much earlier than plain radiographic studies. MRI often shows underlying brain involvement.

The EEG often shows depression of voltage over the involved area in early stages; later, epileptiform abnormalities may be present focally.

▶ Treatment

Sturge-Weber disease is sporadic. Early control of seizures is important to avoid consequent developmental setback. If seizures do not occur, normal development can be anticipated. Careful examination of the newborn, with ophthalmologic assessment to detect early glaucoma, is indicated.

Rarely, surgical removal of the involved meninges and the involved portion of the brain may be indicated, even hemispherectomy.

Comi AM et al: Encephalofacial angiomatosis sparing the occipital lobe and without facial nevus: On the spectrum of Sturge-Weber syndrome variants? J Child Neurol 2003;18:35 [PMID: 12661936].

Feller L, Lemmer J: Encephalotrigeminal angiomatosis. SADJ 2003;58:370 [PMID: 14964051].

Heyer GL et al: The neurologic aspect os PHACE: Case report and review of the literature. Pediatr Neurol 2006;35:419 [PMID: 17138012].

Janner D et al: Index of suspicion: Sturge-Weber. Pediatr Rev 2007;28:27 [PMID: 17197457].

Kossoff EH et al: Outcomes of 32 hemispherectomies for Sturge-Weber syndrome worldwide. Neurology 2002;59:1735 [PMID: 12473761].

Miyama S, Goto T: Leptomeningeal angiomatosis with infantile spasms. Pediatr Neurol 2004;31:353 [PMID: 15519118].

Slasky SE et al: Sturge-Weber syndrome: Deep venous occlusion and the radiologic spectrum. Pediatr Neurol 2006;35:343 [PMID: 17074605].

Taddeucci G et al: Migraine-like attacks in a child with Sturge-Weber syndrome without facial nevus. Pediatr Neurol 2005;32:131 [PMID: 15664776].

Welty LD: Sturge-Weber syndrome: A case study. Neonatal Netw 2006;25:89 [PMID: 16610482].

4. von Hippel-Lindau Disease (Retinocerebellar Angiomatosis)

von Hippel-Lindau disease is a rare, dominantly inherited condition with retinal and cerebellar hemangioblastomas; cysts of the kidneys, pancreas, and epididymis; and sometimes renal cancers. The patient may present with ataxia, slurred speech, and nystagmus due to a hemangioblastoma of the cerebellum or with a medullary spinal cord cystic hemangioblastoma. Retinal detachment may occur from hemorrhage or exudate in the retinal vascular malformation. Rarely a pancreatic cyst or renal tumor may be the presenting symptom.

The diagnostic criteria for the disease are a retinal or cerebellar hemangioblastoma with or without a positive family history, intra-abdominal cyst, or renal cancer.

Fitz EW, Newman SA: Neuro-ophthalmology of von Hippel-Lindau. Curr Neurol Neurosci Rep 2004;4:384 [PMID: 15324605].

Maher ER: von Hippel-Lindau disease. Curr Mol Med 2004;4:833 [PMID: 15579030].

Richard S et al: von Hippel-Lindau disease. Lancet 2004;363:1231 [PMID: 15081659].

CENTRAL NERVOUS SYSTEM DEGENERATIVE DISORDERS OF INFANCY & CHILDHOOD

The CNS degenerative disorders of infancy and childhood are characterized by arrest of psychomotor development and loss, usually progressive but at variable rates, of mental and motor functioning and often of vision as well (Tables 23–20 and 23–21). Seizures are common in some disorders. Symptoms and signs vary with age at onset and primary sites of involvement of specific types.

These disorders are fortunately rare. An early clinical pattern of decline often follows normal early development. Referral for sophisticated biochemical testing is usually necessary before a definitive diagnosis can be made. Recently, many physicians have been involved in experimental bone marrow transplantation and enzyme replacement therapy for some of these disorders, with variable results. Patients with metachromatic leukodystrophy, Krabbe disease, and adrenoleukodystrophy are candidates for experimental bone marrow transplantation, but results are uncertain. Treatment of some lysosomal storage diseases, such as Gaucher disease, with experimental enzyme replacement therapy has shown promising results.

Augestad L et al: Occurrence of and mortality from childhood neuronal ceroid lipofuscinoses in Norway. J Child Neurol 2006;21:917 [PMID: 17092455].

Auvin S, Valee L: Neuronal lipofuscinosis. Lancet 2004;364:786 [PMID: 15337405].

Aydin A et al: Nonconvulsive status epilepticus on electroencephalography in a case with subacute sclerosing panencephalitis. J Child Neurol 2006;21:256 [PMID: 1690143].

Bindu P et al: Clinical heterogeneity in Hallervorden-Spatz syndrome: A clinicoradiological study in 13 patients from South India. Brain Dev 2006;28:343 [PMID: 16504438].

de Bie P et al: Molecular pathogenesis of Wilson and Menkes disease: Correlation of mutations with molecular defects and disease phenotypes. J Med Genet 2007;23 [PMID: 17717039].

Deusterhus P: Huntington disease: A case study of early onset presenting as depression. J Am Acad Child Adolesc Psychiatry 2004;43:1293 [PMID: 15381897].

Dubey P et al: Adrenal insufficiency in asymptomatic adrenoleukodystrophy patients identified by very long-chain fatty acid screening. J Pediatr 2005;146:528 [PMID: 15812458].

Fogel B et al: Clinical features and molecular genetics of autosomal recessive cerebellar ataxias. Lancet Neurol 2007;6:245 [PMID: 17303531].

Garbern J: Pelizaeus-Merzbacher disease: Genetic and cellular pathogenesis. Cell Mol Life Sci 2007;64:50 [PMID: 17115121].

Gordon N: Alpers syndrome: Progressive neuronal degeneration of children with liver disease. Dev Med Child Neurol 2006;48:1001 [PMID: 17109792].

Gordon N: Infantile neuroaxonal dystrophy (Seitelberger's disease). Dev Med Child Neurol 2002;44:849 [PMID: 12455862].

Huntsman RJ et al: A typical presentation of Leigh syndrome: A case series and review. Pediatr Neurol 2005;32:335 [PMID: 15866434].

Kolter T et al: Sphingolipid metabolism diseases. Biochim Biophys Acta 2006;1758:2057 [PMID: 16854371].

Krupp L et al: Consensus definitions proposed for pediatric multiple sclerosis and related disorders. Neurology 2007;68:S7 [PMID: 17438241].

Lyon G et al: Leukodystrophies: Clinical and genetic aspects. Top Magn Reson Imaging 2006;17:219 [PMID: 17414998].

Moser HW et al: Follow-up of 89 asymptomatic patients with adrenoleukodystrophy treated with Lorenzo's oil. Arch Neurol 2005;62:1073 [PMID: 16009761].

Riel-Romero RM et al: Megalencephalic leukoencephalopathy with subcortical cysts in two siblings owing to two novel mutations: Case reports and review of the literature. J Child Neurol 2005;20:230 [PMID: 15832614].

Roze E et al: Dystonia and parkinsonism in GM1 type 3 gangliosidosis. Mov Disord 2005;20:1366 [PMID: 15986423].

Sauer M et al: Hematopoietic stem cell transplantation for mucopolysaccharidoses and leukodystrophies. Klin Padiatr 2004;216:163 [PMID: 15175961].

Schiffmann R, van der Knaap MS: The latest on leukodystrophies. Curr Opin Neurol 2004;17:187 [PMID: 15021247].

Sparks S: Inherited disorders of glycosylation. Mol Genet Metab 2006;87:1 [PMID: 16511948].

Vermeulen G et al: Fright is a provoking factor in vanishing white matter disease. Ann Neurol 2005;57:560 [PMID: 15786451].

Walker F: Huntington's disease. Lancet 2007;369:218 [PMID: 17240289].

Wilson CG et al: Vanishing white matter disease in a child presenting with ataxia. J Paediatr Child Health 2005;41:65 [PMID: 15670229].

Worgall S: Neurological deterioration in late infantile neuronal ceroid lipofuscinosis. Neurology 2007;69:521 [PMID: 17679671].

ATAXIAS OF CHILDHOOD

1. Acute Cerebellar Ataxia

Acute cerebellar ataxia occurs most commonly in children aged 2–6 years. The onset is abrupt, and the evolution of symptoms is rapid. In about 50% of patients, a prodromal illness occurs with fever, respiratory or gastrointestinal symptoms, or an exanthem within 3 weeks of onset. Associated viral infections include varicella, rubeola, mumps, rubella, echovirus infections, poliomyelitis, infectious mononucleosis, and influenza. Bacterial infections such as scarlet fever and salmonellosis have also been incriminated.

▶ Clinical Findings

A. Symptoms and Signs

Ataxia of the trunk and extremities may be so severe that the child exhibits a staggering, reeling gait and inability to sit without support or to reach for objects; or he or she may show only mild unsteadiness. Hypotonia, tremor of the extremities, and horizontal nystagmus may be present. Speech may be slurred. The child is frequently irritable, and vomiting may occur.

There are no clinical signs of increased intracranial pressure. Sensory and reflex testing usually shows no abnormalities.

B. Laboratory Findings and Imaging

CSF pressure and protein and glucose levels are normal; slight lymphocytosis (≤ 30 cells/mL) may be present. Attempts should be made to identify the etiologic viral agent. CT scans are normal; MRI may show cerebellar postinfectious demyelinating lesions. The EEG may be normal or may show nonspecific slowing.

Table 23–20. Central nervous system degenerative disorders of infancy.

Disease	Enzyme Defect and Genetics	Onset	Early Manifestations	Vision and Hearing	Somatic Findings
WHITE MATTER					
Globoid (Krabbe) leukodystrophy	Recessive galactocerebroside β-galactosidase deficiency. Chromosome 14q21–14q31.	Infantile form first 6 mo. Late-onset form 2–6 y. Adolescent and adult forms are rare.	Feeding difficulties. Shrill cry. Irritability. Arching of back.	Optic atrophy, midcourse to late. Hyperacusis occasionally.	Head often small. Often underweight.
Metachromatic leukodystrophy	Recessive. Arylsulfatase A deficiency. 22q13.	Most common is late-infantile form, presenting at 18–24 mo. Juvenile and adult forms present later.	Incoordination, especially gait disturbance; then general regression. Reverse in juveniles.	Optic atrophy, usually late. Hearing normal.	Head enlarged late. No change in juvenile form.
Pantothenate kinase–associated neurodegeneration (previously Hallervorden-Spatz syndrome)	Autosomal recessive; most common mutation is in *PANK2* gene on chromosome 20.	Early onset is by age 10 y.	Rigidity, dystonia, gait disturbance, tremor.	Abnormal ERG. Retinal degeneration.	Dystonia, gait disturbance.
Pelizaeus-Merzbacher disease	X-linked recessive; rare female. Proteolipid protein (myelin) decreased. Xq22.	Birth (connatal) to 2 y.	Eye rolling often shortly after birth. Head bobbing. Slow loss of intellect.	Slowly developing optic atrophy. Hearing normal. Nystagmus.	Head and body normal.
DIFFUSE, BUT PRIMARILY GRAY MATTER					
Poliodystrophy (Alpers disease or syndrome)	Occasionally familial, recessive. Metabolic forms.	Infancy to adolescence.	Variable: loss of intellect, seizures, incoordination. Vomiting, hepatic failure.	Cortical blindness and deafness.	Head normal initially; may fail to grow.
Tay-Sachs disease and G_{M2} gangliosidosis variants: Sandhoff disease; juvenile; chronic-adult	Recessive. Hexosaminidase deficiencies caused by *HEXA* gene on chromosome 15q23–24.62,63. Tay-Sachs (93% East European Jewish), hexosaminidase A deficiency. Sandhoff hexosaminidase A and B deficiency. Juvenile partial hexosaminidase A.	Tay-Sachs, and Sandhoff 3–6 mo; others 2–6 y or later.	Variable: shrill cry, loss of vision, infantile spasms, arrest of development. In juvenile and chronic forms: motor difficulties; later, mental difficulties.	Cherry-red macula, early blindness. Hyperacusis early. Strabismus in juvenile form, blindness late.	Head enlarged late. Liver occasionally enlarged. None in juvenile chronic forms.
Niemann-Pick disease and variants	50% Jewish. Recessive. Sphingomyelinase deficiency in types A and C involving the CNS.	First 6 mo. In variants, later onset: often non-Jewish.	Slow development. Protruding belly.	Cherry-red macula in 35–50%. Blindness late. Deafness occasionally.	Head usually normal. Spleen enlarged more than liver. Occasional xanthomas of skin. Vertical gaze palsy.
Infantile Gaucher disease (glucosylceramide lipidosis)	Recessive. Glucocerebrosidase deficiency.	First 6 mo; rarely, late infancy.	Stridor or hoarse cry; retraction; feeding difficulties.	Occasional cherry-red macula. Convergent squint. Deafness occasionally.	Head usually normal. Liver and spleen equally enlarged.

Motor System	Seizures	Laboratory and Tissue Studies	Course
Early spasticity, occasionally preceded by hypotonia. Prolonged nerve conduction.	Early. Myoclonic and generalized, decerebrate posturing.	CSF protein elevated; usually normal in late-onset forms. Sural nerve; nonspecific myelin breakdown. Enzyme deficiency in leukocytes, cultured skin fibroblasts. Demyelination, gliosis with low-signal CT scan, high-signal T_2-weighted MRI.	Rapid. Death usually by 1.5–2 y. Late-onset cases may live 5–10 y. Hematopoietic stem cell transplantation is an experimental treatment with variable results.
Combined upper and lower motor neuron signs. Ataxia. Prolonged nerve conduction.	Infrequent, usually late and generalized.	Metachromatic cells in urine: negative sulfatase A test. CSF protein elevated. Urine sulfatide increased. Sural nerve biopsy; metachromasia. Enzyme deficiency in leukocytes, cultured skin fibroblasts. Imaging: Same as globoid leukodystrophy.	Moderately slow. Death in infantile form by 3–8 y, in juvenile form by 10–15 y. Hematopoietic stem cell transplantation is an experimental treatment with variable results.
Extrapyramidal signs, dysarthria, increased deep tendon reflexes.	Variable, EEG may be abnormal.	Axonal degeneration (spheroids). Iron deposits in basal ganglia on MRI: eye-of-the-tiger appearance.	Progressive mental/motor deterioration.
Cerebellar signs early, hyperactive deep reflexes. Spasticity.	Usually only late.	None specific. Brain biopsy: extensive demyelination with small perivascular islands of intact myelin. Point mutations or duplications of *PLP* gene account for 65–90% of cases.	Very slow, often seemingly stationary.
Variable: incoordination, spasticity.	Often initial manifestation: myoclonic, akinetic, and generalized.	*POLG1* mutation: multiple deletions, depletions of mitochondrial DNA. Neuronal loss in cortex: may occur very late. Variably increased serum pyruvate, lactate; liver steatosis, cirrhosis late. Muscle and liver biopsy show evidence of mitochondrial dysfunction.	Usually rapid, with death within 1–3 y after onset. Variants in older children, adults.
Initially floppy. Eventual decerebrate rigidity. In juvenile and chronic forms: dysarthria, ataxia, spasticity.	Frequent, in mid-course and late. Infantile spasms and generalized.	Blood smears: vacuolated lymphocytes; basophilic hypergranulation. Enzyme deficiencies in serum, leukocytes, culture, skin fibroblasts. High-density thalami on CT scan, low-density white matter.	Moderately rapid. Death usually by 2–5 y. In juvenile form, 5–15 y.
Initially floppy. Eventually spastic. Occasionally extrapyramidal signs. Ataxia, dystonia.	Rare and late.	Blood: vacuolated lymphocytes; increased lipids. X-rays: "mottled" lungs, decalcified bones. "Foam cells" in bone marrow, spleen, lymph nodes. WBC, fibroblast enzyme studies are diagnostic.	Moderately slow. Death usually by 3–5 y.
Opisthotonos early, followed rapidly by decerebrate rigidity.	Rare and late.	Anemia. Increased acid phosphatase. X-rays: thinned cortex, trabeculation of bones. "Gaucher cells" in bone marrow, spleen. Enzyme deficiency in leukocytes or cultured skin fibroblasts.	Very rapid. Experimental enzyme replacement therapy is underway.

(continued)

Table 23–20. Central nervous system degenerative disorders of infancy. *(Continued)*

Disease	Enzyme Defect and Genetics	Onset	Early Manifestations	Vision and Hearing	Somatic Findings
Generalized gangliosidosis and juvenile type (G_{M1} gangliosidoses)	Recessive; β-galactosidase deficiency.	1–2 y in infantile form.	Arrest of development. Protruding belly. Coarse facies in infantile (generalized) form. In juvenile form, ataxia and dysarthria.	50% "cherry-red spot." Hearing usually normal. In juvenile type. Occasionally retinitis pigmentosa.	Head enlarged early; liver enlarged more than spleen.
Subacute necrotizing encephalomyelopathy (Leigh disease)	Recessive or variable. May have deficiency of pyruvate carboxylase, pyruvate dehydrogenase, cytochrome enzymes.	Infancy to late childhood.	Difficulties in feeding; feeble or absent cry; floppiness; apnea; developmental regression; ataxia. Presentation can be highly variable.	Optic atrophy, often early. Roving eye movements. Ophthalmoplegia.	Head usually normal, occasionally small; cardiac and renal tubular dysfunction occasionally.
Menkes disease (kinky hair disease)	X-linked recessive; defect in copper absorption.	Infancy.	Peculiar facies; secondary hair white, twisted, split; hypothermia.	May show optic disk pallor and microcysts of pigment epithelium.	Growth retardation.
Carbohydrate-deficient glycoprotein syndrome	Recessive glycoprotein abnormality; glycosylation faulty.	Infancy.	Failure to thrive, retardation, protein-losing enteropathy.	Strabismus, retinopathy.	Dysmorphic facies. Prominent fat pads. Inverted nipples.
Abetalipoproteinemia (Bassen-Kornzweig disease)	Recessive; primary defect is microsomal triglyceride transfer protein (MTP) on chromosome 4q22–24.	Early childhood.	Diarrhea in infancy.	Retinitis pigmentosa; late ophthalmoplegia.	None.

▶ Differential Diagnosis

Acute cerebellar ataxia must be differentiated from acute cerebellar syndromes due to phenytoin, phenobarbital, primidone, or lead intoxication. For phenytoin, the toxic level in serum is usually above 25 mcg/mL; for phenobarbital, above 50 mcg/mL; for primidone, above 14 mcg/mL. (See section on Seizure Disorders, earlier.) Papilledema, anemia, basophilic stippling of erythrocytes, proteinuria, typical radiographs, and elevated CSF protein are clinical clues to lead intoxication, which is confirmed by serum, urine, or hair lead levels. Polymyoclonus-opsoclonus syndrome with an occult neuroblastoma (see following section) occasionally begins as acute cerebellar ataxia.

In rare cases, acute cerebellar ataxia may be the presenting sign of acute bacterial meningitis or may be mimicked by corticosteroid withdrawal, vasculitides such as in polyarteritis nodosa, trauma, the first attack of ataxia in a metabolic disorder such as Hartnup disease, or the onset of acute disseminated encephalomyelitis or of multiple sclerosis. The history and physical findings may differentiate these disturbances, but appropriate laboratory studies are often necessary. For ataxias with more chronic onset and course, see the sections on spinocerebellar degeneration and the other degenerative disorders.

▶ Treatment & Prognosis

Treatment is supportive. Corticosteroids have not been shown to be of benefit; IVIG has been used. Between 80% and 90% of children with acute cerebellar ataxia not secondary to drug toxicity recover without sequelae within 6–8 weeks. In the remainder, neurologic disturbances, including disorders of behavior and of learning, ataxia, abnormal eye movements, and speech impairment, may persist for months or years, and recovery may remain incomplete.

Blokker RS et al: A boy with acute cerebellar ataxia without opsoclonus caused by neuroblastoma. Ned Tijdschr Geneeskd 2006;150:799. [PMID: 16649400].

Bodensteiner JB, Johnsen SD: Cerebellar injury in the extremely premature infant: Newly recognized but relatively common outcome. J Child Neurol 2005;20:139 [PMID: 15794181].

De Bruecker Y et al: MRI findings in acute cerebellitis. Eur Radiol 2004;14:1478 [PMID: 14968261].

Motor System	Seizures	Laboratory and Tissue Studies	Course
Initially floppy, eventually spastic.	Usually late.	Blood: vacuolated lymphocytes. X-rays: dorsolumbar kyphosis, "beaking" of vertebrae. "Foam cells" similar to those in Niemann-Pick disease.	Very rapid. Death within a few years. Slower in juvenile type (to 10 y).
Flaccid and immobile; may become spastic. Spinocerebellar forms; ataxia, myelopathy.	Rare and late tonic seizures.	Increased CSF and blood lactate and pyruvate. High-signal MRI T$_2$ foci in thalami; globus pallidus, putamen, subthalamic nuclei. May be considered a mitochondrial disorder. DNA, enzyme tests on muscle.	Usually rapid in infants, but may be slow with death after several years. Central hypoventilation a frequent cause of death.
Variable: floppy to spastic.	Myoclonic infantile spasms, status epilepticus.	Defective absorption of copper. Cerebral angiography shows elongated arteries. Hair shows pili torti, split shafts. Copper and ceruloplasmin low.	Moderately rapid. Death usually by 3–4 y.
Variable hypotonia, neuropathy.	Rare.	Normal transferrin decreased. Carbohydrate-deficient transferrin increased. Liver steatosis. Cerebellar hypoplasia.	Cardiomyopathy, thrombosis. Hepatic fibrosis.
Ataxia, late extrapyramidal movement disorder.	None.	Abetalipoproteinemia: acanthocytosis, low serum vitamin E; cerebellar atrophy on imaging.	Progression arrested with vitamin E.

CNS, central nervous system; CSF, cerebrospinal fluid; CT, computed tomography; EEG, electroencephalogram; EMG, electromyelogram; MRI, magnetic resonance imaging; WBC, white blood cell.

Go T: Intravenous immunoglobulin therapy for acute cerebellar ataxia. Acta Paediatr 2003;92:504 [PMID: 12801122].

Ryan MM, Engle EC: Acute ataxia I childhood. J Child Neurol 2003;18:309 [PMID: 12822814].

Shiihara T et al: Acute cerebellar ataxia and consecutive cerebellitis produced by glutamate receptor delta2 autoantibody. Brain Dev 2007;29:254 [PMID: 17049194].

Uchibori A et al: Autoantibodies in postinfectious acute cerebellar ataxia. Neurology 2005;65:1114 [PMID: 16217070].

2. Polymyoclonus-Opsoclonus Syndrome of Childhood (Infantile Myoclonic Encephalopathy, "Dancing Eyes-Dancing Feet" Syndrome)

The symptoms and signs of this syndrome are at first similar to those of acute cerebellar ataxia. Often of sudden onset, polymyoclonus-opsoclonus syndrome is characterized by severe incoordination of the trunk and extremities with lightning-like jerking or flinging movements of a group of muscles, causing the child to be in constant motion while awake. Extraocular muscle involvement results in sudden irregular eye movements (opsoclonus). Irritability and vomiting are often present, but there is no depression of level of consciousness. This syndrome occurs in association with viral infections and tumors of neural crest origin among other disorders. Immunologic mechanisms have been postulated. Usually no signs of increased intracranial pressure are present. CSF may show normal or mildly increased protein levels. Special techniques show increased CSF levels of plasmacytes and abnormal immunoglobulins. The EEG may be slightly slow, but when performed together with EMG, it shows no evidence of association between cortical discharges and the muscle movements. An assiduous search must be made to rule out tumor of neural crest origin by chest radiographs and CT, MRI, or ultrasound of the adrenal area as well as by assays of urinary catecholamine metabolites (vanillylmandelic acid and others) and cystathionine.

The symptoms respond variably to ACTH or to IVIG. Plasmapheresis has been successful. Usually the underlying neural crest tumor is benign (ganglioneuroblastoma); surgical excision may be the only oncologic therapy needed. Life span is determined by the biologic behavior of the tumor. The syndrome is usually self-limited but may be characterized by exacerbations and remissions, even after the removal of the neural crest tumor and without other evidence of its

Table 23–21. Central nervous system degenerative disorders of childhood.[a]

Disease	Enzyme Defect and Genetics	Onset	Early Manifestations	Vision and Hearing	Motor System	Seizures	Laboratory and Tissue Studies	Course
Adrenoleukodystrophy and variants (peroxisomal disease)	X-linked recessive. Neonatal form recessive Xq28. Acyl-CoA synthetase deficiency.	5–10 y. May also present as newborn, adolescent or adult.	Impaired intellect; behavioral problems.	Cortical blindness and deafness.	Ataxia, spasticity; motor deficits may be asymmetrical or one-sided initially; adrenomyeloneuropathy in adults.	Occasionally.	Hyperpigmentation and adrenocortical insufficiency. ACTH elevated. Accumulation of very-long-chain fatty acids in plasma. ?Stem cell, marrow transplantation early.	Variable course, many mildly involved. Severe variant with death in 2–5 y.
Neuronal ceroid lipofuscinosis (NCL; cerebromacular degeneration); infantile NCL (INCL); late infantile (LINCL); juvenile NCL (JNCL; Batten disease)	Recessive; multiple gene mutations, polymorphisms.	INCL: 6–24 mo; LINCL: 2–4 y; JNCL: 4–8 y.	Ataxia; visual difficulties; arrested intellectual development. Seizures.	Pigmentary degeneration of macula; optic atrophy; ERG, VER abnormal	Ataxia; spasticity progressing to decerebrate rigidity.	Often early: myoclonus and later generalized; refractory.	Blood: vacuolated lymphocytes. Biopsy, EM of skin, conjunctiva; WBC: "curvilinear bodies, fingerprint profiles." Molecular testing of *CLN1*, *CLN2*, *CLN3* genes. Protein gene product testing for CLN1 and CLN2.	Moderately slow. Death in 3–8 y.
Subacute sclerosing panencephalitis (Dawson disease)	None. Measles "slow virus" infection. Also reported as result of rubella.	3–22 y; rarely earlier or later.	Impaired intellect; emotional lability; incoordination.	Occasionally chorioretinitis or optic atrophy; hearing normal.	Ataxia; slurred speech; occasionally involuntary movements; spasticity progressing to decerebrate rigidity.	Myoclonic and akinetic seizures relatively early; later, focal and generalized.	CSF protein normal to moderately elevated. High CSF IgG,[b] oligoclonal bands. Elevated CSF (and serum) measles (or rubella) antibody titers. Characteristic EEG. Brain biopsy: inclusion (acidophilic) body encephalitis; culturing of measles virus, perhaps rubella virus.	Variable, death in months to years. Remissions occasional. Treatment: INF-α intrathecal?
Megalencephalic leukodystrophy with subcortical cysts (MLC)	*MLC1* gene defect usually 22q.	Infancy.	Macrocephaly.		Ataxia; spasticity; ?dystonia.	Varied; epilepsy.	Characteristic MRI dysmyelination.	Slowly progressive to adulthood.
Vanishing white matter/childhood ataxia with CNS hypomyelination (VWM/CACH)	eIF2B 3q27 autosomal recessive.	Fatal infancy variant; other (slower) variants.	Episodic deterioration with fever, head trauma, fear.		Ataxia, spasticity.		MRI: dramatic disappearance of white matter.	Fatal infantile form. Slowly progressive form. Adult variant (autosomal dominant) with ovarian dysgenesis.

Disease	Genetics	Onset				Seizures	Laboratory/Pathology	Comments
Alexander disease	*GFAP* gene mutation autosomal dominant.	Infancy.	Macrocephaly key finding.		As above.	Rare: focal or generalized.	Demyelination; Rosenthal fibers characteristic of biopsy.	Fatal infantile. Juvenile: bulbar signs, less retardation.
Multiple sclerosis	None. Diagnosis difficult in childhood.	Adolescent; rare in childhood.	Highly variable: may strike one or more sites of CNS; paresthesias common.	Optic neuritis; diplopia, nystagmus at some time; vestibulocochlear nerves occasionally affected.	Motor weakness; spasticity; ataxia; sphincter disturbances; slurred speech; mental difficulties.		CSF may show slight pleocytosis, elevation of protein and γ-globulin,[b] oligoclonal bands present. CT scan may show areas of demyelination. Auditory, visual, and somatosensory evoked responses often show lesions in respective pathways. Changes in T-cell subsets.	Variable: complete remission possible. Recurrent attacks and involvement of multiple sites are prerequisites for diagnosis.
Cerebrotendinous xanthomatosis	?Recessive. Abnormal accumulation of cholesterol.	Late childhood to adolescence.	Xanthomas in tendons; mental deterioration.	Cataracts; xanthelasma.	Cerebellar defects; bulbar paralysis late.	Myoclonus.	Xanthomas may appear in lungs. Xanthomas in tendons (especially Achilles).	Very slowly progressive into middle life. Replace deficient bile acid.
Huntington disease	Dominant. Chromosome 4p CAG repeat.	10% childhood onset.	Rigidity; dementia.	Ophthalmoplegia late.	Rigidity; chorea frequently absent in children.	50% with major motor seizures.	CT scan may show "butterfly" atrophy of caudate and putamen.	Moderately rapid with death in 15 y.
Refsum disease (peroxisomal disease)	Recessive. Phytanic acid oxidase deficiency.	5–10 y.	Ataxia; ichthyosis; cardiomyopathy.	Retinitis pigmentosa; nystagmus.	Ataxia; neuropathy; tendon reflexes absent.	None.	Serum phytanic acid elevated. Slow nerve conduction velocity. Elevated CSF protein. Peroxisomal disease.	Treat with low phytanic acid diet.

[a] For late infantile metachromatic leukodystrophy, Pelizaeus-Merzbacher disease, poliodystrophy, Gaucher disease of later onset, and subacute necrotizing encephalomyelopathy, see Table 23-20.

[b] CSF γ-globulin (IgG) is considered elevated in children when IgG is > 9% of total protein (possibly even > 8.3%); definitively elevated when > 14%.

ACTH, adrenocorticotropic hormone; CLN, ceroid lipofuscinosis; CNS, central nervous system; CSF, cerebrospinal fluid; CT, computed tomography; EEG, electroencephalogram; EM, electron microscopy ERG, electroretinogram; IFN-α, interferon-α; MRI, magnetic resonance imaging; VER, visual evoked response; WBC, white blood cell.

recurrence, symptoms may reappear. Mild mental retardation may be a sequela.

Burke MJ, Cohn SL: Rituximab for treatment of opsoclonus-myoclonus syndrome in neuroblastoma. Pediatr Blood Cancer 2008;50:679 [PMID: 16900484].

Gesundheit B et al: Ataxia and secretory diarrhea: Two unusual paraneoplastic syndromes occurring concurrently in the same patient with ganglioneuroblastoma. J Pediatr Hematol Oncol 2004;26:549 [PMID: 15342979].

Glatz K et al: Parainfectious opsoclonus-myoclonus syndrome: High dose intravenous immunoglobulins are effective. J Neurol Neurosurg Psychiatry 2003;74:279 [PMID: 12531974].

Kincaid CR et al: Index of suspicion: Opsoclonus. Pediatr Rev 2006;27:307 [PMID: 16882760].

Pranzatelli MR et al: Evidence of cellular immune activation in children with opsoclonus-myoclonus: Cerebrospinal fluid neopterin. J Child Neurol 2004;19:919 [PMID: 15704863].

Pranzatelli MR et al: Immunologic and clinical responses to rituximab in a child with opsoclonus-myoclonus syndrome. Pediatrics 2005;115:115 [PMID: 15601813].

Rostasy K et al: High dose pulsatile dexamethasone therapy in children with opsoclonus-myoclonus syndrome. Neuropediatrics 2006;37:291 [PMID: 17236108].

Tate ED et al: Neuroepidemiologic trends in 105 US cases of pediatric opsoclonus-myoclonus syndrome. J Pediatr Oncol Nurs 2005;22:8 [PMID: 15574722].

Wilken B et al: Chronic relapsing opsoclonus-myoclonus syndrome: Combination of cyclophosphamide and dexamethasone pulses. Eur J Paediatr Neurol 2008;12:51 [PMID: 17625938].

Wilson J: Neuroimmunology of dancing eye syndrome in children. Dev Med Child Neurol 2006;48:693 [PMID: 16836785].

3. Spinocerebellar Degeneration Disorders

Spinocerebellar degeneration disorders may be hereditary or may occur in sporadic fashion. Hereditary disorders include Friedreich ataxia, dominant hereditary ataxia, and a group of miscellaneous diseases.

A. Friedreich Ataxia

This is a recessive disorder characterized by onset of gait ataxia or scoliosis before puberty that becomes progressively worse. Reflexes, light touch, and position sensation are reduced. Dysarthria becomes progressively more severe. Cardiomyopathy usually develops, and diabetes mellitus occurs in 40% of patients, half of whom require insulin. Pes cavus typically is found. The GAA trinucleotide repeats on chromosome 9 can be used for laboratory diagnosis.

Treatment includes surgery for scoliosis and intervention as needed for cardiac disease and diabetes. Antioxidants may slow cardiac deterioration. Patients are usually confined to a wheelchair after age 20 years. Death occurs, usually from heart failure or dysrhythmias, in the third or fourth decade; some patients survive longer.

B. Dominant Ataxia

These diseases (in the past known as olivopontocerebellar atrophy, Holmes ataxia, Marie ataxia, and the like) occur with varying manifestations, even among members of the same family. Ataxia occurs at onset, and progression continues with ophthalmoplegias (in some patients), extrapyramidal syndromes, polyneuropathy, and dementia. Several types have been found to be caused by CAG trinucleotide repeats. Levodopa may ameliorate rigidity and bradykinesia, but no other therapy is available. Only 10% of patients experience onset in childhood, and the course in these patients is often more rapid.

C. Miscellaneous Hereditary Ataxias

Associated findings permit identification of these recessive disorders. These include ataxia-telangiectasia (telangiectasia and immune defects; see below); Wilson disease (Kayser-Fleischer rings); Refsum disease (ichthyosis, cardiomyopathy, retinitis pigmentosa, and large nerves); Rett syndrome (regression to autism at age 7–18 months in girls, loss of use of hands, and progressive failure of brain growth); and abetalipoproteinemia (infantile diarrhea, acanthocytosis, and retinitis pigmentosa). Gluten sensitivity may cause ataxia. Patients with juvenile and chronic gangliosidoses and some hemolytic anemias and long-term survivors of Chédiak-Higashi disease may develop spinocerebellar degeneration. Idiopathic familial ataxia is called Behr syndrome. Neuropathies such as Charcot-Marie-Tooth disease produce ataxia.

Berry-Kravis E et al: Fragile X-associated tremor/ataxia syndrome: Clinical features, genetics, and testing guidelines. Mov Disord 2007;22:2018 [PMID: 17618523].

Di Prospero NA et al: Safety, tolerability and pharmacokinetics of high-dose idebenone in patients with Friedreich ataxia. Arch Neurol 2007;64:803 [PMID: 17562928].

Herrmann A et al: Episodic ataxias. Tidsskr Nor Laegeforen 2005;125:2005 [PMID: 16100538].

Jacquemont S et al: Fragile-X syndrome and fragile X-associated tremor/ataxia syndrome: Two faces of FMR1. Lancet Neurol 2007;6:45 [PMID: 17166801].

LeBer I et al: Muscle coenzyme Q10 deficiencies in ataxia with oculomotor apraxia 1. Neurology 2007;68:295 [PMID: 17242337].

Mahajnah M et al: Familial cognitive impairment with ataxia with oculomotor apraxia. J Child Neurol 2005;20:523 [PMID: 15996403].

Morrison PJ: Hereditary ataxias and paediatric neurology: New movers and shakers enter the field. Eur J Paediatr Neurol 2003;7:217 [PMID: 14511625].

Shahwan A et al: Atypical presentation of ataxia-oculomotor apraxia type 1. Dev Med Child Neurol 2006;48:529 [PMID: 16700949].

Van der Knaap MS et al: Vanishing white matter disease. Lancet Neurol 2006;5:413 [PMID: 16632312].

Vedanarayanan VV: Mitochondrial disorders and ataxia. Semin Pediatr Neurol 2003;10:200 [PMID: 14653408].

Yapici Z, Eraksoy M: Non-progressive congenital ataxia with cerebellar hypoplasia in three families. Acta Paediatr 2005;94:248 [PMID: 15981765].

ATAXIA-TELANGIECTASIA (LOUIS-BAR SYNDROME)

Ataxia-telangiectasia is a multisystem disorder inherited as an autosomal recessive trait. It is characterized by progressive ataxia; telangiectasia of the bulbar conjunctivae, external ears, nares, and (later) other body surfaces, appearing in the third to sixth year; and recurrent respiratory, sinus, and ear infections. Ocular dyspraxia, slurred speech, choreoathetosis, hypotonia and areflexia, and psychomotor and growth retardation may be present. Endocrinopathies are common. Nerve conduction velocities may be reduced. The entire nervous system may be affected in late stages of the disease. A spectrum of involvement may be seen in the same family. Immunodeficiencies of IgA and IgE are common (see Chapter 31), and the incidence of certain cancers is high. Elevated serum α-fetoprotein is a screen for this disease.

Bott L et al: Lung disease in ataxia-telangiectasia. Acta Paediatr 2007;96:1021 [PMID: 17524020].

Buoni S et al: Betamethasone and improvement of neurological symptoms in ataxia-telangiectasia. Arch Neurol 2006;63:1479 [PMID: 17030666].

Moin M et al: Ataxia-telangiectasia in Iran: Clinical and laboratory features of 104 patients. Pediatr Neurol 2007;37:21 [PMID: 17628218].

Nowak-Wegrzyn A et al: Immunodeficiency and infections in ataxia telangiectasia. J Pediatr 2004;144:505 [PMID: 15069401].

Sandoval C, Swift M: Hodgkin disease in ataxia-telangiectasia patients with poor outcomes. Med Pediatr Oncol 2003;40:162 [PMID: 12518345].

Tavani F et al: Ataxia-telangiectasia: The pattern of cerebellar atrophy on MRI. Neuroradiology 2003;45:315 [PMID: 12740724].

EXTRAPYRAMIDAL DISORDERS

Extrapyramidal disorders are characterized by the presence in the waking state of one or more of the following features: dyskinesias, athetosis, ballismus, tremors, rigidity, and dystonias.

For the most part, the precise pathologic and anatomic localization of these disorders is not understood. Motor pathways synapsing in the striatum (putamen and caudate nucleus), globus pallidus, red nucleus, substantia nigra, and the body of Luys are involved; this system is modulated by pathways originating in the thalamus, cerebellum, and reticular formation.

1. Sydenham Post-Rheumatic Chorea

Sydenham chorea is characterized by an acute onset of choreiform movements and variable degrees of psychological disturbance. It is frequently associated with rheumatic endocarditis and arthritis. Although the disorder follows infections with group A β-hemolytic streptococci, the interval between infection and chorea may be greatly prolonged; throat cultures and antistreptolysin O titers may therefore be negative. Chorea has also been associated with hypocalcemia; with vascular lupus erythematosus; and with toxic, viral, infectious, parainfectious, and degenerative encephalopathies. Paraneoplastic chorea is not seen in children.

▶ Clinical Findings

A. Symptoms and Signs

Chorea, or rapid involuntary movements of the limbs and face, is the hallmark physical finding. In addition to the jerky incoordinate movements, the following are noted: emotional lability, waxing and waning ("milkmaid's") grip, darting tongue, "spooning" of the extended hands and their tendency to pronate, and knee jerks slow to return from the extended to their prestimulus position ("hung up"). Seizures, while uncommon, may be masked by choreic jerks.

B. Laboratory Findings

Anemia, leukocytosis, and an increased erythrocyte sedimentation rate and C-reactive protein may be present. The antistreptolysin O or anti-DNase titer (or both) may be elevated, and C-reactive protein present. Throat culture is sometimes positive for group A β-hemolytic streptococci.

ECG and echocardiography are often essential to detect cardiac involvement. Antineuronal antibodies are present in most patients but are not specific for this disease. Specialized radiologic procedures (MRI and SPECT) may show basal ganglia abnormalities.

▶ Differential Diagnosis

The diagnosis of Sydenham chorea is usually not difficult. Tics, drug-induced extrapyramidal syndromes, Huntington chorea, and hepatolenticular degeneration (Wilson disease), as well as other rare movement disorders, can usually be ruled out on historical and clinical grounds. Immunologic linkages among chorea, tics, and obsessive-compulsive disorder are being studied in pediatric patients. Stroke is a rare cause for unilateral chorea. Other causes of chorea can be ruled out by laboratory tests, such as antinuclear antibody for lupus, thyroid screening tests, serum calcium for hypocalcemia, and immunologic and virologic tests for (rare) HIV, parvovirus B19, and Epstein-Barr virus infection.

▶ Treatment

There is no specific treatment. Dopaminergic blockers such as haloperidol (0.5 mg to 3–6 mg/d) and pimozide (2–10 mg/d) have been used. Parkinsonian side effects such as rigidity and masked facies, and with high doses tardive dyskinesia, rarely occur in childhood. Other drugs have been used with success in individual cases; these include the anticonvulsant sodium valproate (50–60 mg/kg/d in divided doses) and prednisone (0.5–2 mg/kg/d in divided doses). IVIG has been successful in severe cases. Emotional lability and depression sometimes warrant administration of antidepressants. All patients should be given antistreptococcal rheumatic fever prophylaxis, possibly through childbearing age.

Prognosis

Sydenham chorea is a self-limited disease that may last from a few weeks to months. Relapse of chorea may occur with nonspecific stress or illness—or with breakthrough streptococcal infections (if penicillin prophylaxis is not done). Two thirds of patients relapse one or more times, but the ultimate outcome does not appear to be worse in those with recurrences. In older studies, eventual valvular heart disease occurs in about one third of patients, particularly if other rheumatic manifestations appear. Psychoneurotic disturbances occur in a significant percentage of patients.

Barash J et al: Corticosteroid treatment in patients with Sydenham's chorea. Pediatr Neurol 2005;32:205 [PMID: 15730904].

Cardoso F: Chorea: Non-genetic causes. Curr Opin Neurol 2004;17:433 [PMID: 15247538].

Citak EC et al: Functional brain imaging in Sydenham's chorea and streptococcal tic disorders. J Child Neurol 2004;19:387 [PMID: 15224712].

Fong CY, de Sousa C: Childhood chorea-encephalopathy associated with human parvovirus B19 infection. Dev Med Child Neurol 2006;48:526 [PMID: 16700948].

Garvey MA et al: Treatment of Sydenham's chorea with intravenous immunoglobulin, plasma exchange, or prednisone. J Child Neurol 2005;20:424 [PMID: 15968928].

Korn-Lubetzki I et al: Recurrence of Sydenham chorea: Implications for pathogenesis. Arch Neurol 2004;61:1261 [PMID: 15313844].

Pavone P et al: Autoimmune neuropsychiatric disorders associated with streptococcal infection: Sydenham chorea, PANDAS, and PANDAS variants. J Child Neurol 2006;21:727 [PMID: 16970875].

Singer HS, Williams PN: Autoimmunity and pediatric movement disorders. Adv Neurol 2006;99:166 [PMID: 16536363].

van Toorn R et al: Distinguishing PANDAS from Sydenham's chorea: Case report and review of the literature. Eur J Paediatr Neurol 2004;8:211 [PMID: 15261885].

Zomorrodi A, Wald ER: Sydenham's chorea in western Pennsylvania. Pediatrics 2006;117:e675 [PMID: 16533893].

2. Tics (Habit Spasms)

Clinical Findings

Tics, or habit spasms, are quick repetitive but irregular movements, often stereotyped, and briefly suppressible. Coordination and muscle tone are not affected. A psychogenic basis is seldom discernible. Transient tics of childhood (12–24% incidence in school-aged children) last from 1 month to 1 year and seldom need treatment. Many children with tics have a history of encephalopathic past events, neurologic soft signs, and school problems. Facial tics such as grimaces, twitches, and blinking predominate, but the trunk and extremities are often involved and twisting or flinging movements may be present. Vocal tics are less common.

Tourette syndrome is characterized by multiple fluctuating motor and vocal tics with no obvious cause lasting more than 1 year. Tics evolve slowly, new ones being added to or replacing old ones. Coprolalia and echolalia are relatively infrequent. Partial forms are common. The usual age at onset is 2–15 years, and the familial incidence is 35–50%.

The disorder occurs in all ethnic groups. Tourette syndrome may be triggered by stimulants such as methylphenidate and dextroamphetamine. An imbalance of or hypersensitivity to neurotransmitters, especially dopaminergic and adrenergic, has been hypothesized.

In mild cases, tics are self-limited, and when disregarded disappear. When attention is paid to one tic, it may disappear only to be replaced by another that is often worse. If the tic and its underlying anxiety or compulsive neuroses are severe, psychiatric evaluation and treatment are needed.

Important comorbidities are attention-deficit/hyperactivity disorder and obsessive-compulsive disorder. Learning disabilities, sleep difficulties, anxiety states, and mood swings are also common. Medications such as methylphenidate and dextroamphetamine should be carefully titrated to treat attention-deficit/hyperactivity disorder and avoid worsening tics. Fluoxetine and clomipramine may be useful for obsessive-compulsive disorder and rage episodes in patients with tics.

Treatment

The most effective medications for treating Tourette syndrome are dopamine blockers; however, many pediatric patients can manage without drug treatment. Medications are generally reserved for patients with disabling symptoms; treatment may be relaxed or discontinued when the symptoms abate (Table 23–22). Nonpharmacologic treatment of Tourette syndrome includes education of patients, family members, and school personnel. In some cases, restructuring the school environment to prevent tension and teasing may be necessary. Supportive counseling, either at or outside school, should be provided. Medications usually do not eradicate the tics. The goal of treatment should be to reduce

Table 23–22. Medications for Tourette syndrome and tics.

Dopamine blockers (many are antipsychotics)[c]
Haloperidol (Haldol)
Pimozide (Orap)
Aripiprazole (Abilify)[c]
Olanzapine (Zyprexa)[c]
Risperidone (Risperdal)
Serotonergic drugs[a]
Fluoxetine (Prozac)
Anafranil (Clomipramine)
Noradrenergic drugs[b]
Clonidine (Catapres)
Guanfacine (Tenex)
Other
Selegiline (Eldepryl)[d]
Baclofen (Lioresal)
Pergolide (Permax)[d]

[a]Useful for obsessive-compulsive disorder.
[b]Useful for attention-deficit/hyperactivity disorder.
[c]Some off-label use.
[d]Dopamine-modulating.

the tics to tolerable levels without inducing undesirable side effects. Medication dosage should be increased at weekly intervals until a satisfactory response is obtained. Often a single dose at bedtime is sufficient. The two neuroleptic agents used most often are pimozide and risperidone. Sleepiness and weight gain are the most common side effects; rare are prolonged QT interval (ECG), akathisia, and tardive dyskinesia. Clonidine, guanfacine, and dopamine modulators have been used in individual patients with some success. Sometimes these agents are used in combination (eg, clonidine with pimozide). IVIG has been unsuccessful.

Sydenham chorea is a well-documented pediatric autoimmune disorder associated with streptococcal infections (pediatric autoimmune neuropsychiatric disorder associated with streptococcal infection; PANDAS). Patients with tic disorders occasionally have obsessive-compulsive disorder precipitated or exacerbated by streptococcal infections. Less definite (much less frequent) are tic flare-ups with streptococcal infection. Active prospective antibody (antineuronal and antistreptococcal) and clinical studies are in progress. Research centers have used experimental treatments (IVIG, plasmapheresis, and corticosteroids) in severe cases. At present, most patients with a tic do not worsen with group A streptococcal infections; with rare exceptions, penicillin prophylaxis is not generally necessary for the majority of patients with tic disorders.

Bubl E et al: Aripiprazole in patients with Tourette syndrome. World J Biol Psychiatry 2006;7:123 [PMID: 16684686].

Goodman WK et al: Obsessive-compulsive disorder in Tourette syndrome. J Child Neurol 2006;21:704 [PMID: 16970872].

Himle MB et al: Brief review of habit reversal training for Tourette syndrome. J Child Neurol 2006;21:719 [PMID: 16970874].

Hoekstra J et al: Lack of effect of intravenous immunoglobulins on tics: A double-blind placebo-controlled study. J Clin Psychiatry 2004;65:537 [PMID: 14119917].

March JS: Pediatric autoimmune neuropsychiatric disorders associated with streptococcal infection (PANDAS): Implications for clinical practice. Arch Pediatr Adolesc Med 2004;158:926 [PMID: 15351762].

Mell LK et al: Association between streptococcal infection and obsessive-compulsive disorder, Tourette syndrome and tic disorder. Pediatrics 2005;116:56 [PMID: 15995031].

Qasaymeh MM, Mink JW: New treatments for tic disorders. Curr Treat Options Neurol 2006;8:465 [PMID: 17032567].

Swedo SE, Grant PJ: Annotation: PANDAS: A model for human autoimmune disease. J Child Psychol Psychiatry 2005;46:227 [PMID: 15755299].

3. Paroxysmal Dyskinesias/Chronic Dystonia

Sudden-onset, short-duration choreoathetosis or dystonia episodes occur in childhood. Most often these episodes are of familial or genetic origin. Episodes may occur spontaneously or be set off by actions ("kinesigenic," or movement-induced) such as rising from a chair, reaching for a glass, or walking. Sometimes only hard sustained exercise will induce the dyskinesia. (Nocturnal dyskinesia/dystonic episodes are currently thought to be frontal lobe seizures.)

The diagnosis is clinical. Onset is usually in childhood (1.5–14 years). The patient is alert and often disconcerted during an episode.

Episodes may last seconds to 5–20 minutes and occur several times daily or monthly. Laboratory work is normal. EEG is normal between or during an attack; brain imaging is normal. Inheritance is usually autosomal dominant. Anticonvulsants (eg, carbamazepine) usually prevent further attacks. Patients often grow out of this disease in one or two decades.

Nonkinesigenic dyskinesia is often secondary to an identifiable brain lesion, less or not responsive to medications, and nongenetic.

Disorders of ion channels underlie many of the genetic cases; some cases are linked to epilepsy and hemiplegic migraine. Chromosome loci are known.

The diagnosis of chronic persistent dystonia (sometimes L-dopa–responsive; DYT5) may be aided by spinal fluid neurotransmitter (DYT5) and genetic chromosome studies: DYT1 is the most common. Rarely, dyskinesia (eg, dystonia) may be precipitated by fever. Persistent chorea (rarely) may be a benign lifelong genetic disease.

Bruno MK et al: Clinical evaluation of idiopathic paroxysmal kinesigenic dyskinesia: New diagnostic criteria. Neurology 2004;63:2280 [PMID: 15623687].

Bruno MK et al: Genotype-phenotype correlations of paroxysmal nonkinesigenic dyskinesia. Neurology 2007;68:1782 [PMID: 17515540].

Chaila EC et al: Broadening the phenotype of childhood-onset dopa-responsive dystonia. Arch Neurol 2006;63:1185 [PMID: 16908750].

Dressler D, Benedke R: Diagnosis and management of acute movement disorders. J Neurol 2005;252:1299 [PMID: 16208529].

Jankovic J: Treatment of dystonia. Lancet Neurol 2006;5:864 [PMID: 16987733].

Kleiner-Fisman G et al: Benign hereditary chorea: Clinical, genetic and pathological findings. Ann Neurol 2003:54:244 [PMID: 12891678].

Li Z et al: Childhood paroxysmal kinesigenic dyskinesia: Report of seven cases with onset at an early age. Epilepsy Behav 2005;6:435 [PMID: 15820356].

Tarsy D, Simon DK: Dystonia. N Engl J Med 2006;355:818 [PMID: 16928997].

4. Tremor

The most common cause of persisting tremors in childhood is essential tremor. Of those with this lifelong malady, 4.6% have onset in childhood (2–16 years). A genetic dominant inheritance is probable; 20–80% afflicted report a relative with tremors. Tremor, a mild fine motor and cosmetic handicap, is worsened by anxiety, fatigue, stress, physical activity, and caffeine, and transiently improved by alcohol. Comorbidities include attention-deficit/hyperactivity disorder, dystonia, and possibly Tourette syndrome. Hand/arm tremor is the major manifestation; voice and head tremors are rare. Sometimes, "shuddering attacks" in infancy are a forerunner.

Laboratory studies are normal. Progression is usually minimal. Some patients develop other movement disorders over a lifetime. Helpful medications (rarely needed long-term) include propranolol or primidone.

Differential diagnosis includes birth asphyxia, Wilson disease, hyperthyroidism, and hypocalcemia; history and laboratory tests rule out these rare possibilities.

Recent research studies in adults utilizing proton MRS (magnetic resonance spectroscopy) suggest decreased nerve cells in the cerebellar cortex and increased harmane, a neurotoxin, at the same site. The latter suggests a possible environmental contribution to essential tremor.

Deng H et al: Genetics of essential tremor. Brain 2007;130:1456 [PMID: 17353225].

Jankovic J et al: Essential tremor among children. Pediatrics 2004;114:1203 [PMID: 15520096].

Louis ED, Zheng W: Blood harmane is correlated with cerebellar metabolism in essential tremor. Neurology 2007;69:515 [PMID: 17679670].

Schlaggar BL, Mink JW: Movement disorders in children. Pediatr Rev 2003;24:39 [PMID: 15972843].

Zesiewicz TA et al: Practice parameter: Therapies for essential tremor. Neurology 2005;64:2008 [PMID: 15972843].

INFECTIONS & INFLAMMATORY DISORDERS OF THE CENTRAL NERVOUS SYSTEM

Infections of the CNS are among the most common neurologic disorders encountered by pediatricians. Although infections are among the CNS disorders most amenable to treatment, they also have a very high potential for causing catastrophic destruction of the nervous system. It is imperative for the clinician to recognize infections early in order to treat and prevent massive tissue destruction.

▶ Clinical Findings

A. Symptoms and Signs

Patients with CNS infections, whether caused by bacteria, viruses, or other microorganisms, present with similar manifestations. Systemic signs of infection include fever; malaise; and impaired heart, lung, liver, or kidney function. General features suggesting CNS infection include headache, stiff neck, fever or hypothermia, changes in mental status (including hyperirritability evolving into lethargy and coma), seizures, and focal sensory and motor deficits. Meningeal irritation is manifested by the presence of Kernig and Brudzinski signs. In very young infants, signs of meningeal irritation may be absent, and temperature instability and hypothermia are often more prominent than fever. In young infants, a bulging fontanelle and an increased head circumference are common. Papilledema may eventually develop, particularly in older children and adolescents. Cranial nerve palsies may develop acutely or gradually during the course of neurologic infections. No specific clinical sign or symptom is reliable in distinguishing bacterial infections from infections caused by other microbes.

During the initial clinical assessment, conditions that predispose the patient to infection of the CNS should be sought. Infections involving the sinuses or other structures in the head and neck region can result in direct extension of infection into the intracranial compartment. Open head injuries, recent neurosurgical procedures, immunodeficiency, and the presence of a mechanical shunt may predispose to intracranial infection.

B. Laboratory Findings

When CNS infections are suspected, blood should be obtained for a complete blood count, general chemistry panel, and culture. Most important, however, is obtaining CSF. In the absence of focal neurologic deficits or signs of brainstem herniation, CSF should be obtained immediately from any patient in whom serious CNS infection is suspected. When papilledema or focal motor signs are present, a lumbar puncture may be delayed until a neuroimaging procedure has been done to exclude space-occupying lesions. Treatment must be started even if lumbar puncture is delayed. It is generally safe to obtain spinal fluid from infants with nonfocal neurologic examination even if the fontanelle is bulging. Spinal fluid should be examined for the presence of red and white blood cells, protein concentration, glucose concentration, bacteria, and other microorganisms; a sample should be cultured. In addition, serologic, immunologic, and nucleic acid detection (PCR) tests may be performed on the spinal fluid in an attempt to identify the specific organism. Spinal fluid that contains a high proportion of polymorphonuclear leukocytes, a high protein concentration, and a low glucose concentration strongly suggests bacterial infection (see Chapter 40). CSF containing predominantly lymphocytes, a high protein concentration, and a low glucose concentration suggests infection with mycobacteria, fungi, uncommon bacteria, and some viruses such as lymphocytic choriomeningitis virus, herpes simplex virus, mumps virus, and arboviruses (see Chapters 38 and 41). CSF that contains a high proportion of lymphocytes, normal or only slightly elevated protein concentration, and a normal glucose concentration is most suggestive of viral infections, although partially treated bacterial meningitis and parameningeal infections may also result in this type of CSF formula. Typical CSF findings in a variety of infectious and inflammatory disorders are shown in Table 23–2.

In some cases, brain biopsy may be needed to identify the presence of specific organisms and clarify the diagnosis. Herpes simplex virus infections can be confirmed using the PCR test to assay for herpes DNA in spinal fluid. This test has 95% sensitivity and 99% specificity. Brain biopsy may be needed to detect the rare PCR-negative case of herpes simplex and various parasitic infections, or in a suspected noninfectious cause with ambiguous spinal fluid findings (eg, vasculitis).

C. Imaging

Neuroimaging with CT and MRI scans may be helpful in demonstrating the presence of brain abscess, meningeal inflammation, or secondary problems such as venous and arterial infarctions, hemorrhages, and subdural effusions when these are suspected. In addition, these procedures may identify sinus or other focal infections in the head or neck region that are related to the CNS infection. CT bone windows may demonstrate bony abnormalities such as basilar fractures.

EEGs may be helpful in the assessment of patients who have had seizures at the time of presentation. The changes are often nonspecific and characterized by generalized slowing. In some instances, such as herpes simplex virus or focal enterovirus infection, lateralized epileptiform discharges may be seen early in the course and may be one of the earliest laboratory abnormalities to suggest the diagnosis. EEGs may also show focal slowing over regions of infarcts or (rare) abscesses.

BACTERIAL MENINGITIS

Bacterial infections of the CNS may present acutely (symptoms evolving rapidly over 1–24 hours), subacutely (symptoms evolving over 1–7 days), or chronically (symptoms evolving over more than 1 week). Diffuse bacterial infections involve the leptomeninges, superficial cortical structures, and blood vessels. Although the term *meningitis* is used to describe these infections, it should not be forgotten that the brain parenchyma is also inflamed and that blood vessel walls may be infiltrated by inflammatory cells that result in endothelial cell injury, vessel stenosis, and secondary ischemia and infarction. Overall clinical characteristics of bacterial meningitis (and viral meningoencephalitis) are outlined in Table 23–23.

Pathologically, the inflammatory process involves all intracranial structures to some degree. Acutely, this inflammatory process may result in cerebral edema or impaired CSF flow through and out of the ventricular system, resulting in hydrocephalus.

▶ Treatment

A. Specific Measures

(See also Chapters 37, 38, and the section on bacterial infections in Chapter 40.)

While awaiting the results of diagnostic tests, the physician should start broad-spectrum antibiotic coverage as noted in the following discussion. After specific organisms are identified, antibiotic therapy can be tailored based on antibiotic sensitivity patterns. Bacterial meningitis in children younger than age 3 months is treated initially with cefotaxime (or ceftriaxone if the child is older than age 1 month) and ampicillin; the latter agent is used to treat *Listeria* and enterococci infections, which rarely affect older children. Children older than age 3 months are given ceftriaxone, cefotaxime, or ampicillin plus gentamicin. If *Streptococcus pneumoniae* cannot be ruled out by the initial Gram stain, vancomycin or rifampin is added until cultures are reported, because penicillin-resistant pneumococci are common in the United States. Therapy may be narrowed when organism sensitivity allows. Duration of therapy is 7 days for meningococcal infections, 10 days for *Haemophilus influenzae* or pneumococcal infection, and 14–21 days for other organisms. Slow clinical response or the occurrence of complications may prolong the need for therapy.

B. General and Supportive Measures

Children with bacterial meningitis are often systemically ill. The following complications should be looked for and treated aggressively: hypovolemia, hypoglycemia, hyponatremia, acidosis, septic shock, increased intracranial pressure, seizures, disseminated intravascular coagulation, and metastatic infection (eg, pericarditis, arthritis, or pneumonia). Children should initially be monitored closely (cardiorespiratory monitor, strict fluid balance and frequent urine specific gravity assessment, daily weights, and neurologic assessment every few hours), not fed until neurologically very stable, isolated until the organism is known, rehydrated with isotonic solutions until euvolemic, and then given intravenous fluids containing dextrose and sodium at no more than maintenance rate (assuming no unusual losses occur).

▶ Complications

Abnormalities of water and electrolyte balance result from either excessive or insufficient production of antidiuretic hormone and require careful monitoring and appropriate adjustments in fluid administration. Monitoring serum sodium every 8–12 hours during the first 1–2 days, and urine sodium if the inappropriate secretion of antidiuretic hormone is suspected, usually uncovers significant problems.

Table 23–23. Encephalitis.

Definition: brain inflammation (usually acute)
  Clinical: (fever, headache) seizures, motor paralysis, impaired consciousness
  Laboratory: CSF cells, protein increased; culture/PCR; serology CSF/blood
  Radiographic: swelling (?focal), dysmyelination, ?infarcts
  Pathologic: perivascular cells, gray matter, even neuronophagia; edema, dysmyelination, gliosis
Infectious: (95%) enteroviruses, *Mycoplasma,* herpes, EBV, other viral
  Unusual: bacteria, fungi, protozoa
  Some causes are mosquito- or tick-borne; seasonal.
Para-/Postinfectious (ADEM): (25%) during or after banal respiratory infection, exanthem; most often no etiologic agent is identified
Treatment: supportive
  Herpes: acyclovir
  ADEM: steroids, ?IVIG

ADEM, acute disseminated encephalomyelitis; EBV, Epstein-Barr virus; IVIG, intravenous immune globulin; PCR, polymerase chain reaction.
Data from Lewis P, Glaser CA: Encephalitis. Pediatr Rev 2005;26:347.

Seizures occur in up to 30% of children with bacterial meningitis. Seizures tend to be most common in neonates and less common in older children. Persistent focal seizures or focal seizures associated with focal neurologic deficits strongly suggest subdural effusion, abscess, or vascular lesions such as arterial infarct, cortical venous infarcts, or dural sinus thrombosis. Because generalized seizures in a metabolically compromised child may have severe sequelae, early recognition and therapy are critical; some practitioners prefer phenytoin for acute management because it is less sedating than phenobarbital.

Subdural effusions occur in as many as 50% of young children with *S pneumoniae* meningitis. Subdural effusions are often seen on CT scans of the head during the course of meningitis. They do not require treatment unless they are producing increased intracranial pressure or progressive mass effect. Although subdural effusions may be detected in children who have persistent fever, such effusions do not usually have to be sampled or drained if the infecting organism is *H influenzae*, meningococcus, or pneumococcus. These are usually sterilized with the standard treatment duration, and slowly waning fever during an otherwise uncomplicated recovery may be followed clinically. Under any other circumstance, however, aspiration of the fluid for documentation of sterilization or for relief of pressure should be considered. Interestingly, prognosis is not worsened by subdural effusions.

Cerebral edema can participate in the production of increased intracranial pressure, requiring treatment with dexamethasone, osmotic agents, diuretics, or hyperventilation; continuous pressure monitoring may be needed.

Long-term sequelae of meningitis result from direct inflammatory destruction of brain cells, vascular injuries, or secondary gliosis. Focal motor and sensory deficits, visual impairment, hearing loss, seizures, hydrocephalus, and a variety of cranial nerve deficits can result from meningitis. Sensorineural hearing loss in *H influenzae* meningitis occurs in approximately 5–10% of patients during long-term follow-up. Recent studies have suggested that early addition of dexamethasone to the antibiotic regimen may modestly decrease the risk of hearing loss in some children with *bacterial* meningitis (see Chapter 40).

In addition to the variety of disorders mentioned earlier in this section, some patients with meningitis have mental retardation and severe behavioral disorders that limit their function at school and later performance in life.

BRAIN ABSCESS

▶ Clinical Findings

Patients with brain abscess often appear to have systemic illness similar to patients with bacterial meningitis, but in addition they show signs of focal neurologic deficits, papilledema, and other evidence of increased intracranial pressure or a mass lesion. Symptoms may be present for a week or more; children with bacterial meningitis usually present within a few days. Conditions predisposing to development of brain abscess include penetrating head trauma; chronic infection of the middle ear, mastoid, or sinuses (especially the frontal sinus); chronic dental or pulmonary infection; cardiovascular lesions allowing right-to-left shunting of blood (including arteriovenous malformations); and endocarditis. Sinus infections more characteristically cause subdural-epidural, orbital and forehead abscesses or empyemas, or cellulitis rather than intrabrain abscesses. Recent reports have identified a predisposition to brain abscess in patients with congenital heart disease and acute immunosuppression, with a fungal cause in the latter, and *Citrobacter* infection in infants.

When brain abscess is strongly suspected, a neuroimaging procedure such as CT or MRI scans with contrast enhancement should be done prior to lumbar puncture. (CT scan can miss an epidural collection.) If a brain abscess is identified, lumbar puncture may be dangerous and rarely alters the choice of antibiotic or clinical management since the CSF abnormalities usually reflect only parameningeal inflammation or are often normal. With spread from contiguous septic foci, streptococci and anaerobic bacteria are most common. Staphylococci most often enter from trauma or spread from distant or occult infections. Enteric organisms may form an abscess from chronic otitis. Unfortunately, cultures from a large number of brain abscesses remain negative.

The diagnosis of brain abscess is based primarily on a strong clinical suspicion and confirmed by a neuroimaging procedure. Strongly positive inflammatory markers (erythrocyte sedimentation rate, C-reactive protein) are useful in screening. Normal results would be unlikely in patients with brain abscess. EEG changes are nonspecific but frequently demonstrate focal slowing in the region of brain abscess.

▶ Differential Diagnosis

Differential diagnosis of brain abscess includes any condition that produces focal neurologic deficits and increased intracranial pressure, such as neoplasms, subdural effusions, cerebral infarctions, and certain infections (herpes simplex, cysticercosis, and toxocariasis).

▶ Treatment

Initial therapy for infection from presumed contiguous foci uses penicillin and metronidazole. Cefotaxime is a good alternative to penicillin, especially if enteric organisms are suspected. Enteric organisms are also often susceptible to trimethoprim–sulfamethoxazole. Suspicion of infection by staphylococci, or their recovery from an aspirate, should be treated with nafcillin or vancomycin (for discussion of methicillin-resistant *Staphylococcus aureus* [MRSA], see Chapter 37). Treatment may include neurologic consultation and anticonvulsant and edema therapy if necessary. In their early stages, brain abscesses are areas of focal cerebritis and can be "cured" with antibiotic treatment alone. Encapsulated abscesses require surgical drainage.

▶ Prognosis

The surgical mortality rate in the treatment of brain abscess is lower than 5%. Untreated cerebral abscesses lead to irreversible tissue destruction and may rupture into the ventricle, producing catastrophic deterioration in neurologic function and death. Because brain abscesses are often associated with systemic illness and systemic infections, the death rate is frequently high in these patients.

VIRAL INFECTIONS

Viral infections of the CNS can involve primarily meninges (meningitis) (see Chapter 38) or cerebral parenchyma (encephalitis) (see Table 23–23). All patients, however, have some degree of involvement of both the meninges and cerebral parenchyma (meningoencephalitis). Many viral infections are generalized and diffuse, but some viruses, notably herpes simplex and some enteroviruses, characteristically cause prominent focal disease. Focal cerebral involvement is clearly evident on neuroimaging procedures. Some viruses have an affinity for specific CNS cell populations. Poliovirus and other enteroviruses can selectively infect anterior horn cells (poliomyelitis) and some intracranial motor neurons.

Although most viral infections of the nervous system have an acute or subacute course in childhood, chronic infections can occur. Subacute sclerosing panencephalitis, for example, represents a chronic indolent infection caused by altered measles virus and is characterized clinically by progressive neurodegeneration and seizures.

Inflammatory reactions within the nervous system may occur during the convalescent stage of systemic viral infections. Parainfectious or postinfectious inflammation of the CNS results in several well-recognized disorders: acute disseminated encephalomyelitis (ADEM; 25% of encephalitis), transverse myelitis, optic neuritis, polyneuritis, and Guillain-Barré syndrome. MRI findings in ADEM are distinctive: demyelinating lesions, seen on T_2 and FLAIR images, are key to the diagnosis. Small and large white matter lesions can mimic findings in multiple sclerosis (MS) but, unusually for MS, may involve gray matter such as cortex, basal ganglia, especially thalamus. Radiologic changes are usually florid when the patient is first seen but occasionally emerge only days to weeks later. Thus serial or repeat scans may be necessary.

Corticosteroids are beneficial. Current practice is to administer massive doses over 5 days, followed by tapering of the dosage over 2–4 weeks. (Older studies used 2–4 mg/kg/d; no comparative dose studies are available.) In refractory patients, IVIG or plasmapheresis (or both) may be effective.

Rarely, ADEM relapses (biphasic acute disseminated encephalomyelitis; biDEM or BDEM). Recurrence more than 3 months after treatment should raise strong suspicion of MS. Congenital viral infections can also affect the CNS. CMV, herpes simplex virus, varicella and (rare now, because of immunization) rubella virus are the most notable causes of viral brain injury in utero.

Treatment of CNS viral infections is usually limited to symptomatic and supportive measures, except for herpes simplex virus: Acyclovir is utilized in some patients with varicella-zoster virus infections of the CNS. West Nile virus, new in the United States, is an arthropod-borne flavivirus. It is found in mosquitoes, birds, and horses, and in 1991 accounted for 27% of hospitalized patients with encephalitis and muscle weakness in New York. Fourteen percent had encephalitis alone, and 6% had aseptic meningitis. CSF antibody studies and PCR (57% positive for viral RNA) were diagnostic aids. The infection is now endemic as far as the western United States, particularly in California.

This disease is often asymptomatic or mild in pediatric patients; paralysis and death occur mostly in the elderly.

▼ ENCEPHALOPATHY OF HUMAN IMMUNODEFICIENCY VIRUS INFECTION

Neurologic syndromes associated directly with HIV infection include subacute encephalitis, meningitis, myelopathy, polyneuropathy, and myositis. In addition, secondary opportunistic infections of the CNS occur in patients with HIV-induced immunosuppression. *Pneumocystis, Toxoplasma,* and CMV infections are particularly common. Progressive multifocal leukoencephalopathy, a secondary papillomavirus infection, and herpes simplex and varicella-zoster infections also occur frequently in patients with HIV infection. Various fungal (especially cryptococcal), mycobacterial, and bacterial infections have been described.

Neurologic abnormalities in these patients can also be the result of noninfectious neoplastic disorders. Primary CNS lymphoma and metastatic lymphoma to the nervous system are the most frequent neoplasms of the nervous system in these patients. See Chapters 31, 37, and 39 for diagnosis and management of HIV infection.

OTHER INFECTIONS

A wide variety of other microorganisms, including *Toxoplasma,* mycobacteria, spirochetes, rickettsiae, amoebae, and mycoplasmas, can cause CNS infections. CNS involvement in these infections is usually secondary to systemic infection or other predisposing factors. Appropriate cultures and serologic testing are required to confirm infections by these organisms. Parenteral antimicrobial treatment for these infections is discussed in Chapter 37.

NONINFECTIOUS INFLAMMATORY DISORDERS OF THE CENTRAL NERVOUS SYSTEM

The differential diagnosis of bacterial, viral, and other microbial infections of the CNS includes disorders that cause inflammation but for which no specific causal organism has been identified. Sarcoidosis, Behçet disease, systemic lupus erythematosus, other collagen-vascular disorders, and Kawasaki disease are examples. In these disorders, CNS inflammation usually occurs in association with characteristic systemic manifestations that allow proper diagnosis. Management of CNS involvement in these disorders is the same as the treatment of the systemic illness.

OTHER PARAINFECTIOUS ENCEPHALOPATHIES

In association with systemic infections or other illnesses, CNS dysfunction may occur in the absence of direct CNS inflammation or infection. Reye syndrome is a prominent example of this type of encephalopathy that often occurs in association with varicella virus or other respiratory or systemic viral infections. In Reye syndrome, cerebral edema and cerebral dysfunction occur, but there is no evidence of any direct involvement of the nervous system by the associated microorganism or inflammation. Cerebral edema in Reye syndrome is accompanied by liver dysfunction and fatty infiltration of the liver. As a result of efforts to discourage use of aspirin in childhood febrile illnesses, the number of patients with Reye syndrome has markedly decreased. The precise relationship, however, between aspirin and Reye syndrome is unclear.

MULTIPLE SCLEROSIS

Multiple sclerosis (MS) can begin in childhood; 2–5% of individuals with MS have symptom onset before age 16 years. Formation of a Pediatric MS Study Group led to a supplementary issue of *Neurology*, summarizing pediatric MS and related disorders. (See Krupp and Hertz citation, included in the references below.) Essential points follow:

- Multiple sclerosis starts with clinical isolated symptoms (CSI) of CNS demyelination. Examples include optic neuritis; transverse myelitis; or brainstem, cerebellar, or hemispheric dysfunction, without fever or encephalopathy (whereas ADEM usually has both).

- Atypical clinical features (think of *other* diagnoses) include fever and involvement of the peripheral nervous system or other organ systems. Aberrant (for MS) laboratory results might include elevated erythrocyte sedimentation rate or marked CSF pleocytosis.

- A diagnosis of MS demands multiple episodes of CNS demyelination, separated in time and space. MRI (many fine-tuned criteria) and spinal fluid changes (oligoclonal bands, IgG index) are key laboratory tests.

- Differential diagnosis includes especially ADEM. Excellent tables, examples, and criteria abound in the supplementary issue of *Neurology*. Many other infections, metabolic disorders, and degenerative diseases can mimic MS.

- Acute treatment (mainly corticosteroids) and prevention or modulation of relapses is extrapolated from adult studies; pediatric trials are in their infancy.

Adame N et al: Sinogenic intracranial empyema in children. Pediatrics 2005;116:e461 [PMID: 16190693].

Alshekhlee A et al: Opsoclonus persisting during sleep in West Nile encephalitis. Arch Neurol 2006;63:1324 [PMID: 16966514].

Avery RA et al: Prediction of Lyme meningitis in children from a Lyme disease-endemic region. Pediatrics 2006;117:e1 [PMID: 16396843].

Chang LY et al: Neurodevelopment and cognition in children after enterovirus 71 infection. N Engl J Med 2007;356:1226 [PMID: 17377160].

Chavez-Bueno S, McCracken GH Jr: Bacterial meningitis in children. Pediatr Clin North Am 2005;52:795 [PMID: 15925663].

Christie LJ et al: Pediatric encephalitis: What is the role of Mycoplasma pneumoniae? Pediatrics 2007;120:305 [PMID: 17671056].

Davis LE et al: West Nile virus neuroinvasive disease. Ann Neurol 2006;60:286 [PMID: 16983682].

Feigin RD: Use of corticosteroids in bacterial meningitis. Pediatr Infect Dis J 2004;23:355 [PMID: 15071293].

Goodkin HP et al: Intracerebral abscess in children: Historical tends at Children's Hospital Boston. Pediatrics 2004;113:1765 [PMID: 15173504].

Grose C: The puzzling picture of acute necrotizing encephalopathy after influenza A and B virus infection in young children. Pediatr Infect Dis J 2004;23:253 [PMID: 15014302].

Hayes EB: West Nile virus disease in children. Pediatr Infect Dis J 2006;25:1065 [PMID: 17072131].

Helperin JJ et al: Practice parameter: Treatment of nervous system Lyme disease (and evidence-based review). Neurology 2007;69:91 [PMID: 17522387].

Huang MC et al: Long-term cognitive and motor deficits after enterovirus 71 brainstem encephalitis in children. Pediatrics 2006;118:e1785 [PMID: 17116698].

Kennedy PG: Neurological infection. Lancet Neurol 2004;3:13 [PMID: 14693102].

Khurana DS et al: Acute disseminated encephalomyelitis in children: Discordant neurologic and neuroimaging abnormalities and response to plasmapheresis. Pediatrics 2004;116:431 [PMID: 16061599].

Krupp LB, Hertz DP (editors): Pediatric multiple sclerosis and related disorders. Neurology 2007;68(Suppl 2) [PMID: 17438241].

Lewis P, Glaser CA: Encephalitis. Pediatr Rev 2005;26:353 [PMID: 16199589].

Pasquinelli L: Enterovirus infections. Pediatr Rev 2006;27:e14 [PMID: 16473836].

Sejvar JJ et al: Neurologic manifestations and outcome of West Nile virus infection. JAMA 2003;290:511 [PMID: 12876094].

Silvia MT, Licht DJ: Pediatric central nervous system infections and inflammatory white matter disease. Pediatr Clin North Am 2005;52:1107 [PMID: 16009259].

Torok M: Neurological infections: Clinical advances and emerging threats. Lancet Neurol 2007;6:16 [PMID: 17166795].

Vam de Beek D et al: Corticosteroids for acute bacterial meningitis. Cochrane Database Syst Rev 2003;24:CD004405 [PMID: 17253505].

Tyler KL: West Nile virus infection in the United States. Arch Neurol 2004;61:1190 [PMID: 15313835].

Whitley RJ, Kimberlin DW: Herpes simplex encephalitis: Children and adolescents. Semin Pediatr Infect Dis 2005;16:17 [PMID: 15685145].

SYNDROMES PRESENTING AS ACUTE FLACCID PARALYSIS

Flaccid paralysis evolving over hours or a few days suggests involvement of the lower motor neuron complex (see section on Floppy Infant Syndrome, later). Anterior horn cells (spinal cord) may be involved by viral infection (paralytic poliomyelitis) or by paraviral or postviral immunologically mediated disease (acute transverse myelitis). The nerve trunks (polyneuritis) may be diseased as in Guillain-Barré syndrome or affected by toxins (diphtheria or porphyria). The neuromuscular junction may be blocked by tick toxin or botulinum toxin. The paralysis rarely will be due to metabolic (periodic paralysis) or inflammatory muscle disease (myositis). A lesion compressing the spinal cord must be ruled out. The back often is tender to percussion at that site. Plain films may show disk or bone erosion; MRI, a displaced or compressed spinal cord. Several examples with pertinent discussions are included in a recent issue of *Pediatrics in Review* (2007, volume 28; see references at the end of this section).

▶ Clinical Findings

A. Symptoms and Signs

Features assisting diagnosis are age, a history of preceding or waning illness, the presence (at time of paralysis) of fever, rapidity of progression, cranial nerve findings, and sensory findings (Table 23–24). The examination may show long tract findings (pyramidal tract), causing increased reflexes and a positive Babinski sign. The spinothalamic tract may be interrupted, causing loss of pain and temperature. Back pain, even tenderness to percussion, may occur, as well as bowel and bladder incontinence. Often the paralysis is ascending, symmetrical, and painful (muscle tenderness or myalgia). Laboratory findings occasionally are diagnostic.

B. Laboratory Findings (See Table 23–24)

Examination of CSF is helpful. Imaging studies of the spinal column (plain radiographs) and spinal cord (MRI) are occasionally essential. Viral cultures (CSF, throat, and stool) and titers aid in diagnosing poliomyelitis. A high sedimentation rate may suggest tumor or abscess; the presence of antinuclear antibody may suggest lupus arteritis.

EMG and nerve conduction velocity can be helpful in diagnosing polyneuropathy. Nerve conduction is usually slowed after 7–10 days. Findings in botulism and tick-bite paralysis can be specific and diagnostic. Rarely, elevation of muscle enzymes or even myoglobinuria may aid in diagnosis of myopathic paralysis. Porphyrin urine studies and heavy-metal assays (arsenic, thallium, and lead) can reveal those rare toxic causes of polyneuropathic paralysis.

▶ Differential Diagnosis

The child who has been well and becomes paralyzed often has polyneuritis. Acute transverse myelitis sometimes occurs in an afebrile child. The child who is ill and febrile at the time of paralysis often has acute transverse myelitis or poliomyelitis. Acute epidural spinal cord abscess (or other compressive lesion) must be ruled out. Poliomyelitis is very rare among the immunized population in the United States. Enterovirus 71 and West Nile disease are two new causes. Paralysis due to tick bites occurs seasonally (spring and summer). The tick is usually found in the occipital hair. Removal is curative.

Paralysis due to botulinum toxin occurs most commonly in those younger than age 6 months (see Chapter 40). Intravenous drug abuse can lead to myelitis and paralysis. Furthermore, chronic myelopathy occurs with two human immunodeficiency virus infections: HTLVI and HTLV-III (now called HIV-1).

▶ Complications

A. Respiratory Paralysis

Early and careful attention to oxygenation is essential. Administration of oxygen, intubation, mechanical respiratory assistance, and careful suctioning of secretions may be required. Increasing anxiety and a rise in diastolic and systolic blood pressures are early signs of hypoxia. Cyanosis is a late sign. Deteriorating spirometric findings (forced expiratory volume in 1 second and total vital capacity) may indicate the need for controlled intubation and respiratory support. Blood gases (usually late changes with increased CO_2 and decreased O_2) can aid decisions.

B. Infections

Pneumonia is common, especially in patients with respiratory paralysis. Antibiotic therapy is best guided by results of cultures. Bladder infections occur when an indwelling catheter is required because of bladder paralysis. Recovery from myelitis may be delayed by urinary tract infection.

C. Autonomic Crisis

This may be a cause of death in Guillain-Barré syndrome. Strict attention to vital signs to detect and treat hypotension or hypertension and cardiac arrhythmias in an intensive care setting is advisable, at least early in the course and in severely ill patients.

▶ Treatment

Most of these syndromes have no specific treatment. Ticks causing paralysis must be removed. Other therapies include the use of erythromycin in *Mycoplasma* infections and botulism immune globulin in infant botulism. Recognized associated disorders (eg, endocrine, neoplastic, or toxic) should

Table 23–24. Acute flaccid paralysis in children.

	Poliomyelitis (Paralytic, Spinal, and Bulbar), with or without Encephalitis	Guillain-Barré Syndrome (AIDP)	Botulism	Tick-Bite Paralysis	Transverse Myelitis and Neuromyelitis Optica
Etiology	Poliovirus types I, II, and III; other enteroviruses, eg, EV-71; vaccine strain poliovirus (rare); West Nile virus: epidemic in birds; mosquitoes infect horses, humans. EV-71 is hand-foot-mouth disease, rarely paralytic.	Likely delayed hypersensitivity—with T-cell-mediated antiganglioside antibodies. Mycoplasmal and viral infections (EBV, CMV), *Campylobacter jejuni,* hepatitis B.	*Clostridium botulinum* toxin. Block at neuromuscular junction. Under age 1, toxin synthesized in bowel by organisms in ingested dust or honey. At older ages toxin ingested in food. Rarely from wound infection.	Probable interference with transmission of nerve impulse caused by toxin in tick saliva.	Usually unknown; multiple viruses (herpes, EBV, varicella, hepatitis A) often postviral (see Guillain-Barré syndrome).
History	None, or inadequate polio immunization. Upper respiratory or GI symptoms followed by brief respite. Bulbar paralysis more frequent after tonsillectomy. Often in epidemics, in summer and early fall.	Nonspecific respiratory or GI symptoms in preceding 5–14 d common. Any season, though slightly lower incidence in summer.	Infancy: dusty environment (eg, construction area), honey. Older: food poisoning. Multiple cases hours to days after ingesting contaminated food.	Exposure to ticks (dog tick in eastern United States; wood ticks). Irritability 12–24 h before onset of a rapidly progressive ascending paralysis.	Rarely symptoms compatible with multiple sclerosis or optic neuritis. Progression from onset to paraplegia often rapid, usually without a history of bacterial infection.
Presenting complaints	Febrile at time of paralysis. Meningeal signs, muscle tenderness, and spasm. Asymmetrical weakness widespread or segmental (cervical, thoracic, lumbar). Bulbar symptoms early or before extremity weakness; anxiety; delirium.	Symmetrical weakness of lower extremities, which may ascend rapidly to arms, trunk, and face. Verbal child may complain of paresthesias. Fever uncommon. Facial weakness early. Miller-Fisher variant presents as ataxia and ophthalmoplegia (rare).	Infancy: constipation, poor suck and cry. "Floppy." Apnea. Lethargy. Choking (cause of SIDS?). Bulbar palsy. Older: blurred vision, diplopia, ptosis, choking, weakness.	Rapid onset and progression of ascending flaccid paralysis; often accompanied by pain and paresthesias. Paralysis of upper extremities 2nd day after onset. Sometimes acute ataxia presentation.	Root and back pain in about 30–50% of cases. Sensory loss below level of lesion accompanying rapidly developing paralysis. Sphincter difficulties common. Fever (58%).
Findings	Flaccid weakness, usually asymmetrical. Cord level: Lumbar: legs, lower abdomen. Cervical: shoulder, arm, neck, diaphragm. Bulbar: respiratory, lower cranial nerves. Encephalopathy accompanies paralysis in West Nile.	Flaccid weakness, symmetrical, usually greater proximally, but may be more distal or equal in distribution. Rarely cranial nerves IX-XI, III-VI. Miller-Fisher variant: ophthalmoplegia, ataxia. Bulbar involvement may occur. Slight distal impairment of position, vibration, touch; difficult to assess in young children.	Infants: Flaccid weakness. Alert. Eye, pupil, facial weakness. Deep tendon reflexes decreased. Absent suck, gag. Constipation. Older: paralysis accommodation, eye movements. Weak swallow. Respiratory paralysis.	Flaccid, symmetrical paralysis. Cranial nerve and bulbar (respiratory) paralysis, ataxia, sphincter disturbances, and sensory deficits may occur. Some fever. Diagnosis rests on finding tick, which is especially likely to be on occipital scalp.	Paraplegia with areflexia below level of lesion early; later, may have hyperreflexia. Sensory loss below and hyperesthesia or normal sensation above level of lesion. Paralysis of bladder and rectum. Optic neuritis rarely may be present.
CSF	Pleocytosis (20–500+ cells) with PMN predominance in first few days, later monocytic preponderance. Protein frequently elevated (50–150 mg/dL). CSF IgM-positive in West Nile.	Cytoalbuminologic dissociation; ten or fewer mononuclear cells with high protein after first week. Normal glucose. IgG may be elevated. West Nile will have cells; nerves can be involved in a myeloradiculitis.	Normal.	Normal.	Usually no manometric block; CSF may show increased protein, pleocytosis with predominantly mononuclear cells, increased IgG.

(continued)

Table 23–24. Acute flaccid paralysis in children. *(Continued)*

	Poliomyelitis (Paralytic, Spinal, and Bulbar), with or without Encephalitis	Guillain-Barré Syndrome (AIDP)	Botulism	Tick-Bite Paralysis	Transverse Myelitis and Neuromyelitis Optica
EMG	Denervation after 10–21 d. Nerve conduction normal. Amplitude reduced in West Nile.	Nerve conduction velocities markedly decreased; may be normal early, or if axon only damage (AMAN[a]).	EMG distinctive: BSAP (brief small abundant potentials). Helpful if present; not diagnostic.	Nerve conduction slowed; returns rapidly to normal after removal of tick.	Normal early. Denervation at level of lesion after 10–21 d.
Other studies	Virus in stool and throat. Serial serologic titers IgG, IgM in West Nile. Hyponatremia 30% in West Nile.	Search for specific cause such as infection, intoxication, autoimmune disease. Antiganglioside antibodies to GM_1 (GQ1b in Miller-Fisher).	Infancy: stool culture, toxin. Rare serum toxin positive. Older: serum (or wound) toxin.	Leukocytosis, often with moderate eosinophilia.	Normal spine x-rays do not exclude spinal epidural abscess. MRI to rule out cord-compressive lesions. Cord may be swollen in myelitis.
Course and prognosis	Paralysis usually maximal 3–5 d after onset. Transient bladder paralysis may occur. Outlook varies with extent and severity of involvement. *Note:* Mortality greatest from respiratory failure and superinfection. West Nile paralysis may be permanent.	Course progressive over a few days to about 2 wk. *Note:* Threat greatest from respiratory failure (10%), autonomic crises (eg, widely variable blood pressure, arrhythmia), and superinfection. Majority recover completely. Plasmapheresis may have a role. IVIG. Relapses occasionally occur.	Infancy: supportive. Penicillin. Botulism immune globulin intravenous (BIGIV). Respiratory support, gavage feeding. Avoid aminoglycosides. Older: penicillin, antitoxin, prolonged respiratory support. Prognosis: excellent. Fatality 3%.	Total removal of tick is followed by rapid improvement and recovery. Otherwise, mortality rate due to respiratory paralysis is very high.	Large degree of functional recovery possible. Corticosteroids are of controversial benefit in shortening duration of acute attack or altering the overall course. Plasmapheresis, IVIG: anecdotal benefit.

[a]AMAN is acute motor axonal neuropathy (uncommon variant in the United States).
AIDP, acute inflammatory demyelinating neuropathy; CMV, cytomegalovirus; CSF, cerebrospinal fluid; EBV, Ebstein–Barr virus; EMG, electromyogram; EV-71, enterovirus 71; GI, gastrointestinal; IVIG, intravenous immune globulin; MRI, magnetic resonance imaging; PMN, polymorphonuclear neutrophil; SIDS, sudden infant death syndrome.

be treated by appropriate means. Supportive care also involves pulmonary toilet, adequate fluids and nutrition, bladder and bowel care, prevention of decubitus ulcers, and in many cases, psychiatric support.

A. Corticosteroids

These agents are believed by most to be of no benefit in Guillain-Barré syndrome. Autonomic symptoms (eg, hypertension) in polyneuritis may require treatment.

B. Plasmapheresis, Intravenous Immunoglobulin

Plasma exchange or IVIG has been beneficial in moderate or severe cases of Guillain-Barré syndrome. Some clinicians use inability to ambulate as a criterion to use IVIG.

C. Physical Therapy

Rehabilitative measures are best instituted when acute symptoms have subsided and the patient is stable.

D. Antibiotics

Appropriate antibiotics and drainage are required for epidural abscess.

Baldovsky M et al: Index of suspicion, case 1. Pediatr Rev 2006;27:147 [PMID: 16581956].

Banwell BL: The long (-itudinally extensive) and the short of it: transverse myelitis in children. Neurology 2007;68:1447 [PMID: 17470744].

Dalakas MC: Intravenous immunoglobulin in autoimmune neuromuscular diseases. JAMA 2004;291:2367 [PMID: 15150209].

Defresne P et al: Acute transverse myelitis in children: Clinical course and prognostic factors. J Child Neurol 2003;18:401 [PMID: 12886975].

Dimario FJ Jr: Intravenous immunoglobulin in the treatment of childhood Guillain-Barré syndrome: A randomized trial. Pediatrics 2005;116:226 [PMID: 15995056].

Fox CK et al: Recent advances in infant botulism. Pediatr Neurol 2005;32:149 [PMID: 15730893].

Francisco AM, Arnon SS: Clinical mimics of infant botulism. Pediatrics 2007;119:826 [PMID: 17403857].

Greenberg BM et al: Idiopathic transverse myelitis. Neurology 2007;68:1614 [PMID: 17485649].

Hughes RA, Cornblath DR: Guillain-Barré syndrome. Lancet 2005;366:1653 [PMID: 16271648].

Janner D, Barron SA: Index of suspicion, case 1 (Back pain). Pediatr Rev 2007;28:27 [PMID: 17197457].

Kincaid O, Lipton HL: Viral myelitis: An update. Curr Neurol Neurosci Rep 2006;6:469 [PMID: 17074281].

Li Z, Turner RP: Pediatric tick paralysis: Discussion of two cases and literature review. Pediatr Neurol 2004;31:304 [PMID: 15464647].

Qualia CM et al: Index of suspicion, case 3 (Fever and leg weakness). Pediatr Rev 2007;28:193 [PMID: 17473124].

Risko W: Infant botulism. Pediatr Rev 2006;27:36 [PMID: 16473839].

Sejvar JJ et al: West Nile virus-associated flaccid paralysis. Emerg Infect Dis 2005;11:1021 [PMID: 16022775].

Shafqat S et al: Guillain-Barré syndrome in Pakistan: Similarity of demyelinating and axonal variants. Eur J Neurol 2006;13:662 [PMID: 16796593].

Shahar E: Current therapeutic options in severe Guillain-Barré syndrome. Clin Neuropharmacol 2006;29:45 [PMID: 16518134].

Taylor Z et al: Index of suspicion. Pediatr Rev 2006;27:463 [PMID: 17671863].

Thompson JA et al: Infant botulism in the age of botulism immune globulin. Neurology 2005;64:2029 [PMID: 15917401].

Tsiodras S et al: *Mycoplasma pneumoniae*-associated myelitis: A comprehensive review. Eur J Neurol 2006;13:112 [PMID: 16490040].

Wingerchuk DM: Diagnosis and treatment of neuromyelitis optica. Neurologist 2007;13:2 [PMID: 17215722].

DISORDERS OF CHILDHOOD AFFECTING MUSCLES (TABLE 23–25)

DIAGNOSTIC STUDIES

Serum Enzymes

Creatine kinase reflects muscle damage or "leaks" from muscle into plasma. Blood should be drawn before EMG or muscle biopsy, which may lead to release of the enzyme. Corticosteroids may suppress levels despite very active muscle disease, for example, as in polymyositis.

Electromyography

Electromyography is often helpful in grossly differentiating myopathic from neurogenic processes. Fibrillations occur in both. In the myopathies, very low spikes are more typical, and the motor unit action potentials seen during contraction characteristically are of short duration, are polyphasic, and are increased in number for the strength of the contraction (increased interference pattern). Neurogenic findings include decreased numbers of motor units, which may be polyphasic, larger than normal, or both. The interference pattern is decreased. In myotonic dystrophy, the EMG is characterized by prolonged discharge of electrical activity on movement of the probing needle (so-called "dive-bomber" sound).

Muscle Biopsy

Properly executed (by open biopsy or by using the Bergstrom muscle biopsy needle), this procedure is usually helpful. Histochemical techniques, histogram analysis of muscle fiber types and sizes, and electron microscopy are offering new classifications of the myopathies. Findings common to the muscular dystrophies include variation in the size and shape of muscle fibers, increase in connective tissue, interstitial infiltration of fatty tissue, degenerative changes in muscle fibers, and central location of nuclei.

Dystrophin is a normal intracellular plasma membrane protein in muscle, the gene product missing in Duchenne and Becker muscular dystrophies. Staining the muscle for dystrophin aids in differentiating Duchenne and Becker muscular dystrophies; dystrophin is absent in Duchenne muscular dystrophy and reduced in Becker muscular dystrophy. Electrophoresis can confirm whether the dystrophin is absent or present in small amounts and whether there is a qualitative difference from normal dystrophin, the latter two patterns being characteristic of Becker muscular dystrophy.

Genetic Testing & Carrier Detection

Previously, detection of carriers for Duchenne muscular dystrophy (mothers and sisters of affected boys) rested on creatine kinase elevations (two thirds of patients will have this finding); physical findings of mild dystrophy (large calves and muscle weakness); abnormal muscle EMGs; or biopsy results. All are unreliable for diagnostic purposes.

DNA probes are now available for carrier detection and prenatal diagnosis of Duchenne and Becker muscular dystrophies. Deletions are often (60%) found on the short arm of the X chromosome; it is postulated that all patients and most mothers will show deletions when sufficient probes are developed to search the whole Duchenne genome (perhaps 4000 kb in length).

Amplification of DNA by the PCR test can detect the deletion. Moreover, this technique plus Southern blot analysis can detect abnormal DNA base repeats. For example, in myotonic dystrophy, a GCT triplet excess is currently the most sensitive test for that disease. The tests can be used for intrauterine diagnosis and prediction of whether the triplet is within the normal or mutant range. Thus, in many cases, the greater the number of repeats, the more severely involved the fetus or patient.

Mutations (especially deletions) of survivor motor neuron and neuronal apoptosis inhibitory protein genes on chromosome 5q13 are present in 95% of patients with spinal muscular atrophy (SMA). SMA is the most common cause of inherited neonatal death, occurring in 1 in 10,000 live births.

Finally, Kearns-Sayre progressive external ophthalmoplegia with retinopathy is inherited via maternal cytoplasmic mitochondria. Assay of mutations and deletions from blood or muscle samples are now commercially available.

Genetic testing is increasingly available for common disorders, such as Duchenne and spinal muscle atrophy, as well as less common disorders found in Table 23–25.

Therapy for Duchenne muscular dystrophy continues to be frustrating. Prednisone in low doses has increased muscle strength and prolonged ambulation. Research emphasis is on gene therapy, but there is great difficulty in finding viral vectors able to carry the very large dystrophin gene into muscle cells.

Dubowitz V: Prednisone for Duchenne muscular dystrophy. Lancet Neurol 2005;4:264 [PMID: 15847833].

Escolar D et al: CINRG randomized controlled trial of creatine and glutamine in Duchenne muscular dystrophy. Ann Neurol 2005;58:151 [PMID: 15984021].

Goebel H: Congenital myopathies in the new millennium. J Child Neurol 2005;20:94 [PMID: 15794172].

Grewal PK, Hewitt JE: Glycosylation defects: A new mechanism for muscular dystrophy? Hum Mol Genet 2003;12(Spec No 2):R259 [PMID: 12925572].

Heatwole C et al: The nondystrophic myotonias. Neurotherapeutics 2007;4:238 [PMID: 17395134].

Kesari A et al: SMNI dosage analysis in spinal muscular atrophy from India. BMC Med Genet 2005;6:22 [PMID: 15910686].

Komura K et al: Effectiveness of creatine monohydrate in mitochondrial encephalomyopathies. Pediatr Neurol 2003;28:53 [PMID: 12657421].

Lisi M et al: Congenital muscular dystrophies: New aspects of an expanding group of disorders. Biochim Biophys Acta 2007;1772:159 [PMID: 17097859].

Lois M et al: Beneficial effects of creatine supplementation in dystrophic patients. Muscle Nerve 2003;27:604 [PMID: 12707981].

Mathrew KD, Moore SA: Limb-girdle muscular dystrophy. Curr Neurol Neurosci Rep 2003;3:78 [PMID: 12507416].

Mendell JR: Congenital muscular dystrophy (editorial). Neurology 2001;56:993 [PMID: 11320168].

Meola G et al: Cerebral involvement in myotonic dystrophies. Muscle Nerve 2007;36:294 [PMID: 17486579].

Moxley RT 3rd et al: Practice parameter: Corticosteroid treatment of Duchenne dystrophy. Neurology 2005;64:13 [PMID: 15642897].

Muntoni F et al: Defective glycosylation in muscular dystrophy. Lancet 2002;360:1419 [PMID: 12424008].

Ryan M et al: Spinal muscular atrophy type 1: Is long-term mechanical ventilation ethical? J Paediatr Child Health 2007;43:237 [PMID: 17444824].

Schara U et al: Myotonic dystrophies type 1 and 2: A summary on current aspects. Semin Pediatr Neurol 2006;13:71 [PMID: 17027856].

Stanley C: Carnitine deficiency disorders in children. Ann N Y Acad Sci 2004;1033:42 [PMID: 15591002].

Straub V et al: The childhood limb-girdle muscular dystrophies. Semin Pediatr Neurol 2006;13:104 [PMID: 17027860].

Strober J: Therapeutics in Duchenne muscular dystrophy. NeuroRx 2006;3:225 [PMID: 16554260].

Sumner C: Therapeutics development for spinal muscular atrophy. NeuroRx 2006;3:235 [PMID: 16554261].

Tawil R et al: Facioscapulohumeral muscular dystrophy. Muscle Nerve 2006;34:1 [PMID: 16508966].

Young T et al: Kearns-Sayre syndrome: A case report and review of cardiovascular complications. Pacing Clin Electrophysiol 2005;28:454 [PMID: 15869681].

BENIGN ACUTE CHILDHOOD MYOSITIS

Benign acute childhood myositis (myalgia cruris epidemica) is characterized by transient severe muscle pain and weakness affecting mainly the calves and occurring 1–2 days following an upper respiratory tract infection. Although symptoms involve mainly the gastrocnemius muscles, all skeletal muscles appear to be invaded directly by virus; recurrent episodes are due to different viral types. By seroconversion or isolation of the virus, acute myositis has been shown to be largely due to influenza types B and A and occasionally due to parainfluenza and adenovirus.

Agyeman P et al: Influenza-associated myositis in children. Infection 2004;32:199 [PMID: 15293074].

MYASTHENIA GRAVIS

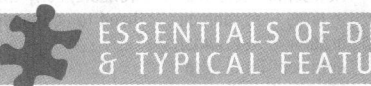

ESSENTIALS OF DIAGNOSIS & TYPICAL FEATURES

▶ Weakness, chiefly of muscles innervated by the brainstem, usually coming on or increasing with use (fatigue).

▶ Positive response to neostigmine and edrophonium.

▶ Acetylcholine receptor antibodies in serum (except in congenital form).

▶ General Considerations

Myasthenia gravis is characterized by easy fatigability of muscles, particularly the extraocular muscles and those of mastication, swallowing, and respiration. In the neonatal period, however, or in early infancy, the weakness may be so constant and general that an affected infant may present nonspecifically as a "floppy infant." Girls are affected more frequently than boys. The age at onset is older than 10 years in 75% of patients, often shortly after menarche. If diagnosed before age 10 years, congenital myasthenia should be considered in retrospect. Thyrotoxicosis is found in almost 10% of affected female patients. The essential abnormality is a circulating antibody that binds to the acetylcholine receptor protein and thus reduces the number of motor end plates for binding by acetylcholine.

▶ Clinical Findings

A. Symptoms and Signs

1. Neonatal (transient) myasthenia gravis—This disorder occurs in 12–19% of infants born to myasthenic mothers. The condition is due to maternal acetylcholine receptor antibody transferred across the placenta; a thymic factor in the infant may also be involved. Maternal thymectomy may reduce the transference rate.

Table 23–25. Muscular dystrophies, myopathies, myotonias and anterior horn diseases of childhood.

Disease	Genetic Pattern	Age at Onset	Early Manifestation	Involved Muscles	Reflexes
Muscular dystrophies					
Duchenne muscular dystrophy (pseudo-hypertrophic infantile)	X-linked recessive; autosomal-recessive unusual. 30–50% have no family history.	2–6 y; rarely in infancy.	Clumsiness, easy fatigability on walking, running, and climbing stairs. Walking on toes; waddling gait. Lordosis. (Climbing up on legs rising from supine position—Gower maneuver.)	Axial and proximal before distal. Pelvic girdle; pseudohypertrophy of gastrocnemius (90%), triceps brachii, and vastus lateralis. Shoulder girdle usually later, also articulation difficulties. Eventually cardiomyopathy (50%).	Knee jerks +/− or 0; ankle jerks + to ++.
Becker muscular dystrophy (late onset)	X-linked recessive. (Allele at Xp21.)	Childhood (usually later than in Duchenne).	Similar to Duchenne.	Similar to Duchenne.	Similar to Duchenne.
Limb-girdle muscular dystrophy	Autosomal-recessive in 60%; high sporadic incidence. Autosomal dominant forms also identified. 17 known genetic mutations.	Variable; early childhood to adulthood.	Weakness, with distribution according to type. Waddling gait, difficulty climbing stairs. Lordosis.	Characteristic pattern involves the shoulder and pelvic girdle muscles. Truncal and distal muscles affected later.	Usually present.
Facioscapulohumeral muscular dystrophy (Landouzy-Déjérine) Scapuloperoneal variant (rare)	Autosomal dominant; sporadic cases not uncommon. Linkage to 4q35; variable number of (decreased) D4Z4 repeats.	Usually late in childhood and adolescence; rare in infancy, not uncommon in 20s.	Diminished facial movements with inability to close eyes, smile, or whistle. Face may be flat; unlined. Difficulty in raising arms over heard. Lordosis. Tripping in scapuloperoneal type.	Facial muscles followed by shoulder girdle, with occasional spread to hips or distal legs (scapuloperoneal variant). (Face may be uninvolved.)	Present
Spinal muscular atrophy (SMA)					
Infantile SMA (Werdnig-Hoffman disease)	Autosomal-recessive. Survival motor neuron on chromosome 5q.	0–2 y.	Floppy infant.	Pelvic and shoulder girdle. Tongue. Intercostal. Fingers and toes spared.	0 or nearly so.
Juvenile SMA (Kugelburg-Welander disease)	Autosomal-recessive. Survival motor neuron on chromosome 5q.	Onset usually after age 2 y (ages 5–15 typical).	Weakness. "Fasciculations" 50%. Rarely a cause of floppy infant.	Same.	Same.
Metabolic myopathies					
Carnitine deficiency (lipid storage myopathy) Primary (rare) Secondary: multiple forms	Genetics variable, often autosomal recessive. Most common variant *OCTN2* on chromosome 5q.	Infancy to adolescence.	Fasting hypoglycemia and coma; less ketosis than expected. Myopathy. Cardiomyopathy. Fatty liver. Do not confuse with Reye, SIDS.	Weakness variable; may be precipitated by exercise (with resultant myoglobulinuria) or fasting.	Normal to decreased.
Kearns-Sayre syndrome					
"Oculocraniosomatic syndrome" (ophthalmoplegia and ragged red fibers; progressive external ophthalmoplegia)	Mitochondrial DNA deletion; other hereditary neurologic disorders may be found in patient or family.	Variable; from infancy to second decade; most at about age 10 y.	Ptosis and limitation of eye movements; hearing and visual loss (retinitis pigmentosa); intellectual loss; cerebellar disturbance (ataxia).	Extraocular muscles, often asymmetrical. Variable involvement of axial muscles; cardiac muscles, with conduction defect.	Depressed to +/− or 0.

Muscle Biopsy Findings	Other Diagnostic Tests	Treatment	Prognosis
Degeneration and variation in fiber size; proliferation of connective tissue. Basophilia, phagocytosis. Poor differentiation of fiber types on ATPase reaction; deficiency of type IIB fibers. Dystrophin absent.	EMG myopathic. CK (4000–5000 IU) very high with decrease towards normal over the years. 60% have C-terminal Xp21 deletion on blood, amniotic fluid or chorionic villi. Positive test obviates need for muscle biopsy.	Physical therapy, braces, wheelchair eventually, weight control. Prednisone, deflazacort improve motor function temporarily. Creatine shows some benefit. Stem cell therapies and gene therapies benefit mouse models and may eventually provide new therapeutic options for patients.	10% show nonprogressive mental retardation. Osteoporosis, scoliosis common. Death from cardiac or respiratory failure 10–15 y after diagnosis with 75% of patients dead by age 20.
Similar to above, except type IIB fibers present. Reduced or abnormal size dystrophin.	Similar to above, although muscle enzymes may not be as elevated.	As above. Wheelchair in late childhood or early adult life.	Slower progression than Duchenne, with death usually in adulthood.
Dystrophic muscle changes (see Duchenne). Dystrophin normal. Special stains for sarcoglycan (dystrophin associated glycoprotein [DAG] deficiency).	EMG myopathic. CK variable; many severe cases have sarcoglycan deficiency (severe autosomal recessive type). Must exclude dystrophinopathy and SMA.	Physical therapy, weight control and regular echocardiograms.	Mildly progressive: spread from lower to upper limbs may take 15–20 y. Life expectancy mid to late adulthood.
Predominantly large fibers with scattered tiny atrophic fibers, "moth-eaten" and whorled fibers. Inflammatory response. Little or no fiber splitting, fibrosis, or type 1 fiber predominance.	EMG myopathic. Muscle enzymes usually normal to mildly elevated. 4q35ter deletion. If blood test positive, biopsy unnecessary.	Physical therapy where indicated. Wheelchair in 20%. Inflammation seen in 40% of biopsies; however, corticosteroids are ineffective.	Very slowly progressive, often with plateaus, except in infantile form where there may be difficulties in walking by adolescences. Usually normal life span. Hearing loss in 60%.
Small, group atrophy. Twin peak fiber size. Fiber type grouping. Minimal fibrosis. Group atrophy and fiber type grouping. Small angular fibers.	EMG neuropathic. Nerve conduction, CSF, muscle enzymes normal. 90–95% have deletions or abnormalities in SMN (survival motor neuron) or other genes at band 5q13. Carrier detection available.	Supportive respiratory care, positioning, secretion management. Genetic and ethical counseling. Physical therapy, wheelchair positioning to avoid scoliosis. May walk, usually later lose this ability.	80–95% of patients 4 y or younger die of pneumonia and respiratory failure. Fairly normal life expectancy. 4–40+ y.
Lipid droplets [+/-] ragged red fibers may be present.	Muscle biochemistry (carnitine, CPT enzyme). Urine organic acids (at time of illness). Plasma carnitine: deficiency may be in blood alone or blood and muscle.	Avoid fasting and mitochondrial toxins, eg, ASA, valproic acid. Carbohydrate. Treat acidosis. Carnitine orally.	Variable: occasionally fatal in infants. Progressive weakness, developmental delay, cardiomyopathy may occur.
Mitochondrial abnormalities. Ragged red fibers. Changes in fiber size, usually due to type 2 fiber atrophy.	CK usually normal. ECG with conduction block. CSF protein elevated. Nerve conduction slowed. MRI of brain and brainstem auditory evoked response may be abnormal. Mitochondrial deletions.	Plastic retraction of eyelids. Cardiac support and surveillance. Anticipate diabetes mellitus. Many clinicians treat with mitochondrial cocktail.	Dysphagia may develop (50%) as well as generalized muscle weakness, cardiac conduction block, endocrinopathies and hearing loss. Prognosis poor. In severe cases, spongy vacuolization of brain and brainstem causing dementia.

(continued)

Table 23–25. Muscular dystrophies, myopathies, myotonias and anterior horn diseases of childhood. *(Continued)*

Disease	Genetic Pattern	Age at Onset	Early Manifestation	Involved Muscles	Reflexes
Congenital myopathies					
Myotonic dystrophy (neonatal onset)	Autosomal dominant triple repeat. Most common form is DM1 on chromosome 19.	At birth.	Decreased fetal movement, respiratory insufficiency, facial weakness, and difficulties in feeding, sucking, and swallowing.	Diffuse hypotonia. Facial and pharyngeal involvement prominent.	Decreased to 0.
"Other" myopathies Central core Nemaline (rod body) Nuclear (including myotubular and Emery-Dreifuss)	Dominant or rarely autosomal recessive. Myotubular and Emery-Dreifuss are both X-linked.	Severe variants present at birth; milder variants (more common) infancy, childhood.	Severe variant, newborns with severe hypotonia and respiratory failure is rare. Later presentation: facial weakness, mild to moderate weakness, even "toe walking" only.	Similar to myotonic dystrophy.	Decreased to 0.
Congenital muscular dystrophy: dystro-glycanopathies Fukayama (FCMD) Walker-Warburg (WW) Muscle-eye-brain (MEB)	Recessive; 6 genes identified (including *POMT*). Associated with abnormalities of glycosylation of dystroglycan.	Birth to 9 mo.	Hypotonia, joint contractures, moderate to severe mental retardation and eye abnormalities (cataracts, microphthalmia, optic nerve hypoplasia).	Heterogenous. Facial (cranial) and somatic. Contracture common.	Variable.
Congenital muscular dystrophy: nondys-troglycanopathies	Most common is MDC1A autosomal recessive form. Some forms demonstrate merosin deficiency.	Birth (or early infancy).	Normal IQ in most patients. Hypotonia, hypoventilation and occasional spine stiffness.	Same (merosin negative may involve heart, nerves, and brain).	Same.
Benign congenital hypotonia (Oppenheim)	Variable	Variable	Hypotonia only. Deep tendon reflexes positive. Laboratory tests, biopsy normal.	Somatic muscles (respiratory muscles spared).	Normal to decreased.
Myotonias					
Myotonia congenita (Thomsen)	Autosomal dominant on chromosome 7q. (autosomal recessive cases reported).	Early infancy to late childhood.	Difficulty in relaxing muscles after contracting them, especially after sleep; aggravated by cold, excitement.	Hands especially; muscles may be diffusely enlarged, giving patient herculean appearance.	Normal
Myotonic dystrophy I (Steinert) (childhood and adult form) Myotonic dystrophy II [Proximal myotonic myopathy (PROMM)]	Autosomal dominant triple repeat. Most common form is DM1 on chromosome 19. DM2 is a CCTG repeat in zinc finger protein gene.	Late childhood to adolescence; neonatal and infantile forms increasingly recognized (see above).	Myotonia of grasp, tongue; worsened by cold, emotions. "Hatchet-face." Nasal voice. Weakness and easy fatigability. Mild to moderate mental retardation noted.	Wasting, weakness of facial muscles, (mastication); sternocleidomastoids, hands. Myotonic phenomena: "bunching up" of muscles of tongue, thenar eminence, finger extensors after tapping with percussion hammer.	In infantile form, marked hyporeflexia.

2. Congenital (persistent) myasthenia gravis—In this form of the disease, the mothers of the affected infants rarely have myasthenia gravis, but other relatives may. Sex distribution is equal. Symptoms are often subtle and not recognized initially. Differential diagnosis includes many other causes of the "floppy infant" syndrome, such as infant botulism, ocular myopathy, congenital ptosis, and Möbius syndrome (facial nuclear aplasia and other anomalies). Congenital myasthenia

Muscle Biopsy Findings	Other Diagnostic Tests	Treatment	Prognosis
Generalized fiber hypertrophy, delay in maturation. Type I atrophy. Internal nuclei.	EMG myotonic in some (waning amplitude and pitch). Test mother. CK often normal. DNA testing (chromosome 19) for CTG repeat.	Supportive, even respiratory support. Genetic counseling. Cardiac referral for all affected family members to evaluate for heart block.	Severely involved infant may improve dramatically over months; expect mental retardation in this same variant. Life expectancy is shortened.
Distinctive diagnostic histochemistry, eg, "central cores," "nemaline rods," myotubes type II–I fibers of unequal size. Type I fiber predominance and atrophy.	Myopathic EMG.	Supportive. Genetic counseling.	Variable. May shorten life. Death in infancy or severe handicap in severe neonatal form. Scoliosis prominent.
"Dystrophic" changes. Fibrosis. Necrotic fibers. Internal nuclei. ?Regenerative fibers.	Myopathic EMG. CK increased. MRI scans often demonstrate neuronal migration abnormalities in WW and MEB.	Supportive.	Physical and mental handicap lifelong. Virtually all FCMD are of Japanese ancestry. WW has life expectancy of < 3 y. Mental retardation is common in FCMD and MEB, but clinical outcome is variable.
Same. Evaluate for merosin (alaminen-2 deficiency).	Brain imaging normal in pure form. Merosin-deficient form may have white matter abnormalities.	Supportive.	May improve, walk. Scoliosis.
Normal with sophisticated studies (histochemistry, electron microscopy, even metabolic studies).	Use of this diagnosis is shrinking with increasingly sophisticated biochemical (eg, cytochrome oxidase) studies.	Supportive.	Good (by definition). Few documented long-term studies.
Nonspecific and minor changes; type IIB fibers may be absent.	EMG myotonic.	Usually none. Phenytoin, especially in cold weather, may improve muscle functioning.	Normal life expectancy, with only mild disability.
Type I fiber atrophy, type II hypertrophy, sarcoplasmic masses, internal nuclei, phagocytosis, fibrosis, and cellular reaction.	EMG markedly myotonic. Glucose tolerance test, thyroid tests. ECG. Chest x-ray and pulmonary function tests. Immunoglobulins. PCR amplification of CTG repeat on chromosome 19q13 to distinguish DM1 from DM2 form.	Monitor developmental progress. May be candidate for speech and occupational therapy. Ongoing cardiac monitoring.	Frontal baldness, cataracts (85%), gonadal atrophy (85% of males), thyroid dysfunction, diabetes mellitus (20%). Cardiac conduction defects; impaired pulmonary function. Low IgG. Life expectancy decreased. Type II: slowly progressive weakening; good outlook.

ASA, acetylsalicylic acid; CK, creatine kinase; CPT, carnitine palmityl transferase; CSF, cerebrospinal fluid; CT, computed tomography; ECG, electrocardiogram; EMG, electromyogram; MRI, magnetic resonance imaging; PCR, polymerase chain reaction; SIDS, sudden infant death syndrome.

gravis is not caused by receptor antibodies and often responds poorly to therapy. It may result from a genetic abnormality of the acetylcholine receptor protein, postsynaptic membrane structure, or other myoneural transmission defects.

3. Juvenile myasthenia gravis—In this autoimmune form, the symptoms and signs are similar to those in adults. Receptor antibodies are usually present. The patient may be first seen by an ophthalmologist or psychiatrist. The more prominent signs are difficulty in chewing, dysphagia, a nasal voice, ptosis, and ophthalmoplegia. Pathologic fatigability of limbs, chiefly involving the proximal limb and neck muscles, may be more prominent than the bulbar signs and may lead to an initial diagnosis of conversion hysteria, muscular dystrophy, or polymyositis. Weakness may be limited to ocular muscles only. Associated disorders include autoimmune conditions, especially thyroid disease.

An acute fulminant form of myasthenia gravis has been reported in children aged 2–10 years, who present with rapidly progressive respiratory difficulties. Bulbar paralysis may evolve within 24 hours. The differential diagnosis includes Guillain-Barré syndrome and bulbar poliomyelitis. Administration of anticholinesterase agents establishes the diagnosis and is lifesaving. Rarely, myasthenia can be postinfectious, and slowly resolve to normal.

B. Laboratory Findings

1. Neostigmine test—In newborns and very young infants, the neostigmine test may be preferable to the edrophonium (Tensilon) test because the longer duration of its response permits better observation, especially of sucking and swallowing movements. There is a delay of about 10 minutes before the effect may be manifest. The physician should be prepared to suction secretions, and adminster atropine if necessary.

2. Edrophonium test—Testing with edrophonium is used in older children who are capable of cooperating in certain tasks, such as raising and lowering their eyelids and squeezing a sphygmomanometer bulb or the examiner's hands. Ophthalmologic tests of ocular motility with edrophonium are often positive in patients able to cooperate. Maximum improvement occurs within 2 minutes.

3. Other laboratory tests—Serum acetylcholine receptor antibodies or muscle-specific receptor tyrosine kinase (MuSK) are often found in the neonatal and juvenile forms. In juveniles, thyroid studies are appropriate.

C. Electrical Studies of Muscle

Repetitive stimulation of a motor nerve at slow rates (3/s) with recording over the appropriate muscle reveals a progressive fall in amplitude of the muscle potential in myasthenic patients. A maximal stimulus must be given. At higher rates of stimulation (50/s), there may be a transient repair of this defect before the progressive decline is seen. If this study is negative, single-fiber EMG may be helpful diagnostically.

D. Imaging

Chest radiograph and CT scanning in older children may disclose benign thymus enlargement. Thymus tumors are rare in children.

▶ Treatment

A. General and Supportive Measures

In the newborn or in a child in myasthenic or cholinergic crisis (see item 5 in the following section), suctioning of secretions is essential. Respiratory assistance may be required. Treatment should be conducted by physicians with experience in this disorder.

B. Anticholinesterase Drug Therapy

1. Pyridostigmine bromide—The dosage must be adjusted for each patient. A frequent starting oral dosage is 15–30 mg orally every 6 hours, or 1 mg/kg per dose every 6 hours in pediatric patients.

2. Neostigmine—Fifteen milligrams of neostigmine are roughly equivalent to 60 mg of pyridostigmine bromide. Neostigmine often causes gastric hypermotility with diarrhea, but it is the drug of choice in newborns, in whom prompt treatment may be lifesaving. It may be given parenterally.

3. Atropine—Atropine may be added on a maintenance basis to control mild cholinergic side effects such as hypersecretion, abdominal cramps, and nausea and vomiting.

4. Immunologic intervention—Such intervention is achieved primarily with prednisone and recently with mycophenolate mofetil. Plasmapheresis is effective in removing acetylcholine receptor antibody in severely affected patients. More potent immunomodulators, such as azathioprine, are occasionally necessary.

5. Myasthenic crisis—Relatively sudden difficulties in swallowing and respiration may be observed in myasthenic patients. Edrophonium results in dramatic but brief improvement; this may make evaluation of the condition of the small child difficult. Suctioning, tracheostomy, respiratory assistance, and fluid and electrolyte maintenance may be required.

6. Cholinergic crisis—Cholinergic crisis may result from overdosage of anticholinesterase drugs. The resulting weakness may be similar to that of myasthenia, and the muscarinic effects (diarrhea, sweating, lacrimation, miosis, bradycardia, and hypotension) are often absent or difficult to evaluate. The edrophonium test may help to determine whether the patient is receiving too little of the drug or is manifesting toxic symptoms due to overdosage. Improvement after the drugs are withdrawn suggests cholinergic crisis. A respirator should be available. The patient may require atropine and tracheostomy.

C. Surgical Measures

Early video thoracoscopic thymectomy is beneficial in many patients whose disease is not confined to ocular symptoms; the effects may be delayed. Experienced surgical and postsurgical care are prerequisites. Thymectomy demonstrates a cure rate of 10–75% and improves symptoms in over half of patients.

▶ Prognosis

Neonatal (transient) myasthenia presents a great threat to life, primarily because of secretion aspiration. With proper treatment, the symptoms usually begin to disappear within a few days to 2–3 weeks, after which the child usually requires no further treatment. In the congenital (persistent) form, the symptoms may initially be as acute as in the transient variety. More commonly, however, they are relatively benign and constant, with gradual worsening as the child grows older. Fatal cases occur. In the juvenile form, patients may become resistant or unresponsive to anticholinesterase compounds and require corticosteroids or treatment in a hospital where respiratory assistance can be given. The overall prognosis for survival, for remission, and for improvement after therapy with prednisone and thymectomy is favorable. Death in myasthenic or cholinergic crisis may occur unless prompt treatment is given.

Andrews PI: Autoimmune myasthenia gravis in childhood. Semin Neurol 2004;24:101 [PMID: 15229797].

Felice KJ et al: Postinfectious myasthenia gravis: Report of two children. J Child Neurol 2005;20:441 [PMID: 15968930].

Hetherington K et al: Myasthenia gravis: Myasthenia vs. cholinergic crisis. Pediatr Emerg Care 2005;21:546 [PMID: 16096606].

Hoff J et al: Myasthenia gravis in pregnancy and birth: Identifying risk factors, optimising care. Eur J Neurol 2007;14:43 [PMID: 17222111].

Juel VC, Massey JM: Autoimmune myasthenia gravis: Recommendations for treatment and immunologic modulation. Curr Treat Opt Neurol 2005;7:3 [PMID: 15610702].

PERIPHERAL NERVE PALSIES

1. Facial Weakness

Facial asymmetry may be present at birth or may develop later, either suddenly or gradually, unilaterally or bilaterally. Nuclear or peripheral involvement of the facial nerves results in sagging or drooping of the mouth and inability to close one or both eyes, particularly when newborns and infants cry. Inability to wrinkle the forehead may be demonstrated in infants and young children by getting them to follow a light moved vertically above the forehead. Loss of taste of the anterior two thirds of the tongue on the involved side may be demonstrated in cooperative children by age 4 or 5 years. Playing with a younger child and the judicious use of a tongue blade may enable the physician to note whether the child's face puckers up when something sour (eg, lemon juice) is applied with a swab to the anterior tongue. Ability to wrinkle the forehead is preserved, owing to bilateral innervation, in supranuclear facial paralysis.

Injuries to the facial nerve at birth occur in 0.25–6.5% of consecutive live births. Forceps delivery is the cause in some cases; in others, the side of the face affected may have abutted in utero against the sacral prominence. Often, no cause can be established.

Acquired peripheral facial weakness (Bell palsy) of sudden onset and unknown cause is common in children. It often follows a viral illness (postinfectious) or physical trauma (eg, cold). It may be a presenting sign of Lyme disease, infectious mononucleosis, herpes simplex, or Guillain-Barré syndrome and is usually diagnosable by the history, physical examination, and appropriate laboratory tests. Chronic cranial nerve VII palsy may be a sign of brainstem tumor.

Bilateral facial weakness in early life may be due to agenesis of the facial nerve nuclei or muscles (part of Möbius syndrome) or may even be familial. Myasthenia gravis, polyneuritis (Miller-Fisher syndrome), and myotonic dystrophy or other congenital myopathies must be considered.

Asymmetrical crying facies, in which one side of the lower lip depresses with crying (this is the normal side) and the other does not, is usually an innocent form of autosomal dominant inherited congenital malformation. The defect in the parent (the asymmetry often improves with age) may be almost inapparent. EMG suggests congenital absence of the depressor anguli oris muscle of the lower lip. Forceps pressure is often erroneously incriminated as a cause of this innocent congenital anomaly. Occasionally other major (eg, cardiac septal defects) congenital defects accompany the palsy. Authorities vary in the incidence of major anomalies (10%?) and extent of investigations; testing for chromosome 22q11 deletion, careful cardiac evaluation, and assessment of serum calcium level may be pertinent.

In the vast majority of cases of isolated peripheral facial palsy—both those due to birth trauma and those acquired later—improvement begins within 1–2 weeks, and near or total recovery of function is observed within 2 months. In severe palsy with inefficient blinking, methylcellulose drops, 1%, should be instilled into the eyes to protect the cornea during the day; at night the lid should be taped down with cellophane tape. Upward massage of the face for 5–10 minutes three or four times a day may help maintain muscle tone. Prednisone therapy (2–4 mg/kg orally for 5–7 days) likely does not aid recovery. In the older child, acyclovir or valacyclovir (herpes antiviral agent) therapy or antibiotics (Lyme disease) may have a role in Bell palsy.

In the few children with permanent and cosmetically disfiguring facial weakness, plastic surgical intervention at age 6 years or older may be of benefit. New procedures, such as attachment of facial muscles to the temporal muscle and transplantation of cranial nerve XI, are being developed.

Akcakus M et al: Asymmetric crying facies associated with congenital hypoparathyroidism and 22q11 deletion. Turk J Pediatr 2004;46:191 [PMID: 15214756].

Ashtekar CS et al: Best evidence topic report. Do we need to give steroids in children with Bell's palsy? Emerg Med J 2005;22:505 [PMID: 15983089].

Gilden DH: Clinical practice. Bell's palsy: N Engl J Med 2004;351:1323 [PMID: 15385659].

Hato N et al: Valcyclovir and prednisolone treatment for Bell's palsy: A multicenter, randomized, placebo-controlled study. Otol Neurotology 2007;28:408 [PMID: 17414047].

Kawaguchi K et al: Reactivation of herpes simplex virus type 1 and varicella-zoster virus and therapeutic effects of combination therapy with prednisolone and valacyclovir in patients with Bell's palsy. Laryngoscope 2007;117:147 [PMID: 17202945].

Salinas RA et al: Corticosteroids for Bell's palsy (idiopathic facial paralysis). Cochrane Database Syst Rev 2004;(4):CD001942 [PMID: 15495021].

Sapin SO et al: Neonatal asymmetric crying facies: A new look at an old problem. Clin Pediatr (Phila) 2005;44:109 [PMID: 15735828].

Terada K et al: Bilateral facial nerve palsy associated with Epstein-Barr virus infection with a review of the literature. Scand J Infect Dis 2004;36:75 [PMID: 15000569].

Vorstman JA, Kuiper H: Peripheral facial palsy in children: Test for Lyme borreliosis only in the presence of other clinical signs. Ned Tijdschr Geneeskd 2004;148:655 [PMID: 15106315].

CHRONIC POLYNEUROPATHY

ESSENTIALS OF DIAGNOSIS & TYPICAL FEATURES

▶ Insidious onset of weakness and fatigability of the limbs, sometimes with pain or numbness; decreased strength and reflexes.

General Considerations

Polyneuropathy is usually insidious in onset and slowly progressive. Children present with disturbances of gait and easy fatigability in walking or running, and slightly less often, weakness or clumsiness of the hands. Pain, tenderness, or paresthesias are mentioned less frequently. Neurologic examination discloses muscular weakness, greatest in the distal portions of the extremities, with steppage gait and depressed or absent deep tendon reflexes. Cranial nerves are sometimes affected. Sensory deficits occur in a stocking-and-glove distribution. The muscles may be tender, and trophic changes such as glassy or parchment skin and absent sweating may occur. Rarely, thickening of the ulnar and peroneal nerves may be felt. In sensory neuropathy the patient may not feel minor trauma or burns, and thus allows trauma to occur.

Known causes include (1) toxins (lead, arsenic, mercurials, vincristine, and benzene); (2) systemic disorders (diabetes mellitus, chronic uremia, recurrent hypoglycemia, porphyria, polyarteritis nodosa, and lupus erythematosus); (3) inflammatory states (chronic or recurrent Guillain-Barré syndrome and neuritis associated with mumps or diphtheria); (4) hereditary, often degenerative conditions, which in some classifications include certain storage diseases, leukodystrophies, spinocerebellar degenerations with neurogenic components, and Bassen-Kornzweig syndrome; and (5) hereditary sensory or combined motor and sensory neuropathies. Polyneuropathies associated with malignancies, vitamin deficiencies, or excessive vitamin B_6 intake are not reported or are exceedingly rare in children.

The most common chronic motor neuropathy of insidious onset often has no identifiable cause. This chronic inflammatory demyelinating neuropathy (CIDP) is assumed to be immunologically mediated and may have a relapsing course. Sometimes facial weakness occurs. CSF protein levels are elevated. Nerve conduction is slowed, and findings on nerve biopsy are abnormal. Immunologic abnormalities are seldom demonstrated, although nerve biopsy findings may show round cell infiltration. Corticosteroids, repeated IVIG, and, occasionally, immunosuppressants may give long-term benefit.

Clinical Findings

Hereditary neuropathy is the most common documented cause of chronic neuropathy in childhood. A careful genetic history (pedigree) and examination and electrical testing (motor and sensory nerve conduction and EMG) of patient and relatives are keys to diagnosis. Genetic tests are available for many of the variants. Nerve biopsy is rarely necessary.

Other hereditary neuropathies may have ataxia as a prominent finding, often overshadowing the neuropathy. Examples are Friedreich ataxia, dominant cerebellar ataxia, and Marinesco-Sjögren syndrome. Finally, some hereditary neuropathies are associated with identifiable and occasionally treatable metabolic errors (see Tables 23–20 and 23–21). These disorders are described in more detail in Chapter 34.

Laboratory diagnosis of chronic polyneuropathy is made by measurement of motor and sensory nerve conduction velocities. EMG may show a neurogenic polyphasic pattern. CSF protein levels are often elevated, sometimes with an increased IgG index. Nerve biopsy, with teasing of the fibers and staining for metachromasia, may demonstrate loss of myelin, and to a lesser degree, loss of axons and increased connective tissue or concentric lamellas (so-called onion-skin appearance) around the nerve fiber. Muscle biopsy may show the pattern associated with denervation. Other laboratory studies directed toward specific causes mentioned above include screening for heavy metals and for metabolic, renal, or vascular disorders.

Treatment & Prognosis

Therapy is directed at specific disorders whenever possible. Corticosteroid therapy is used first when the cause is unknown or neuropathy is considered to be due to chronic inflammation (this is not the case in acute Guillain-Barré syndrome (AIDP; acute inflammatory demyelinating neuropathy). Prednisone is initiated at 2–4 mg/kg/d orally, with tapering to the lowest effective dose; it may need be reinstituted when symptoms recur. (Prednisone should probably not be used for treatment of hereditary neuropathy.) Immunomodulating therapy may be safer or "steroid-sparing";

IVIG, plasmapheresis, mycophenolate mofetil, and ritux-imab are choices.

The long-term prognosis varies with the cause and the ability to offer specific therapy. In the corticosteroid-dependent group, residual deficits are more frequent.

Finsterer J: Treatment of immune-mediated, dysimmune neuropathies. Acta Neurol Scand 2005;112:115 [PMID: 16008538].

Fudge E et al: Chronic inflammatory demyelinating polyradiculoneuropathy in two children with type 1 diabetes mellitus. Pediatr Diabetes 2005;6:244 [PMID: 16390395].

Gorson KC et al: Efficacy of mycophenolate mofetil in patients with chronic immune demyelinating polyneuropathy. Neurology 2004;63:715 [PMID: 15326250].

Kararizou E et al: Polyneuropathies in teenagers: A clinicopathological study of 45 cases. Neuromuscul Disord 2006;16:304 [PMID: 16616844].

Pareyson D: Differential diagnosis of Charcot-Marie-Tooth disease and related neuropathies. Neurol Sci 2004;25:72. [PMID: 15221625].

Ropper AH: Current treatments for CIDP. Neurology 2003;60(Suppl 3):S16 [PMID: 12707418].

Rossignol E et al: Evolution and treatment of childhood chronic inflammatory polyneuropathy. Pediatr Neurol 2007;36:88 [PMID: 17275659].

Ruts L et al: Distinguishing acute-onset CIDP from Guillain-Barré syndrome with treatment related fluctuations: Neurology 2005;65:138 [PMID: 16009902].

van Doorn PA: Treatment of Guillain-Barré syndrome and CIDP. J Peripher Nerv Syst 2005;10:113 [PMID: 15958124].

Visudtibhan A: Cyclosporine in chronic inflammatory demyelinating polyradiculoneuropathy. Pediatr Neurol 2005;33:368 [PMID: 16243226].

MISCELLANEOUS NEUROMUSCULAR DISORDERS

FLOPPY INFANT SYNDROME

ESSENTIALS OF DIAGNOSIS & TYPICAL FEATURES

▶ In early infancy, decreased muscular activity, both spontaneous and in response to postural reflex testing and to passive motion.

▶ In young infants, "frog posture" or other unusual positions at rest.

▶ In older infants, delay in motor milestones.

▶ General Considerations

In the young infant, ventral suspension (ie, supporting the infant with a hand under the chest) normally results in the infant's holding its head slightly up (45 degrees or less), the back straight or nearly so, the arms flexed at the elbows and slightly abducted, and the knees partly flexed. The "floppy" infant droops over the hand like an inverted U. The normal newborn attempts to keep the head in the same plane as the body when pulled up from supine to sitting by the hands (traction response). Marked head lag is characteristic of the floppy infant. Hyperextensibility of the joints is not a dependable criterion.

The usual reasons for seeking medical evaluation in older infants are delays in walking, running, or climbing stairs or motor difficulties and lack of endurance. Hypotonia or decreased motor activity is a frequent presenting complaint in neuromuscular disorders but may also accompany a variety of systemic (non-neuromuscular) conditions or, rarely, may be due to certain disorders of connective tissue.

1. Paralytic Group

The hypotonic infant who is weak (appearing paralyzed) usually has a lesion of the lower motor neuron complex (Table 23–26). The child has significant lack of movement against gravity (eg, fails to kick the legs, hold up the arms, or attempt to stand when held) or in response to stimuli such as tickling or slight pain. Infantile progressive spinal muscular atrophy (Werdnig-Hoffman disease) is the most common cause. Neuropathy is rare. Botulism and myasthenia gravis (rare) are neuromuscular junction causes. Myotonic dystrophy and rare myopathies (eg, central core myopathy) are muscle disease entities.

In anterior horn cell or muscle disease, weakness is proximal (ie, in shoulders and hips); finger movement is preserved. Tendon reflexes are absent or depressed; strength (to noxious stimuli) is decreased (paralytic). Intelligence is preserved. Fine motor, language, and personal and social milestones are normal, as measured, for example, on a Denver Developmental Screening Test (DDST, or Denver II) (see Chapter 2).

A. Myopathies

The congenital, relatively nonprogressive myopathies, muscular dystrophy, myotonic dystrophy, polymyositis, and periodic paralysis were discussed earlier in this chapter. Most cases of congenital or early infantile muscular dystrophy reported in the past probably represented congenital myopathies (see Table 23–25). Congenital muscular dystrophy, diagnosed by muscle biopsy, occurs in two forms: (1) a benign form, with gradual improvement in strength; and (2) a severe form, in which either weakness progresses rapidly and death occurs in the first months or year of life or severe disability is present with little or no progression but lifelong marked limitation of activity.

B. Glycogenosis with Muscle Involvement

Glycogen storage diseases are described in Chapter 34. Patients with type II disease (Pompe disease, due to a deficiency of acid maltase) are most likely to present as floppy infants. Muscle cramps on exertion or easy fatigabil-

Table 23–26. Floppy infant: paralytic causes.

Disease	Genetic	Early Manifestations
Infantile progressive spinal muscular atrophy (IPSMA) "Malignant" form (often fatal in infancy-respiratory failure)	Autosomal recessive; diagnose by SMN deletion exon 7,8 (98% of cases). Rarely, X-linked SMA, a new (also fatal) variant.	In-utero movements decreased in one third. Gradual weakness, delay in gross motor milestones. Weak cry. Abdominal breathing. Poor limb motion ("no kicking"). No deep tendon reflexes. Fasciculations of tongue. Normal personal-social behavior.
"Intermediate" form	Autosomal recessive; same as above. EMG helpful.	Onset before age 1 y usual. *Progression slower:* may be impossible to predict early course of IPSMA. Hand tremors common.
Infantile botulism	Acquired younger than age 1 y (mostly before age 6 mo); botulism spore in stool makes toxin.	Poor feeding. Constipation. Weak cry. Failure to thrive. Lethargy. Facial weakness, ptosis, ocular muscle palsy. Inability to suck, swallow. Apnea. Source: soil dust (outdoor construction workers or family gardeners may bring it home on clothes), honey. EMG helpful, RMNS.
Myasthenia gravis Neonatal transient	12% of infants born from a myasthenic mother.	Floppiness. Poor sucking and feeding; choking. Respiratory distress. Weak cry. Autoimmune antibodies from mother.
Congenital persistent	Mother normal. Rare autosomal recessive (autosomal dominant).	As above; may improve and later exacerbate. Multiple syndromes (rare).
Myotonic dystrophy	Autosomal dominant: in 99% mother transmits gene. DNA testing 98% accurate.	Polyhydramnios; failure of suck, respirations. Facial diplegia. Ptosis. Arthrogryposis. Thin ribs. Later, developmental delay. Examine mother for myotonia, physiognomy. EMG variable in infant.
Neonatal "rare myopathy," severe variant Nemaline, central core, "minimal change," etc	Autosomal recessive or dominant.	Virtually all of the rare myopathies may have a severe (even fatal) neonatal or early infant form. Clinical features similar in infancy to infantile myotonic dystrophy. Muscle biopsy for definitive diagnosis.
Congenital muscular dystrophy Fukayama (FCMD)	Genetic.	Early onset. Facial weakness. Joint contractures. Severe mental retardation. Seizures. Brain structural abnormalities; MRI helpful.
Other		Severe or benign. No mental retardation (see text).
Infantile neuropathy Hypomyelinating (rare)	HSMN most common cause.	Demyelinating or axonal; a rare cause. Rule out mimicking IPSMA (deletion study). EMG, NCV are key studies. Nerve biopsy.
Benign congenital hypotonia	Unknown cause.	Diagnosis of exclusion. Family history variable. Mild to moderate hypotonia with weakness. (This term being used less with increasing genetic, microscopy advances.) Improves with time.

AD, autosomal dominant; AR, autosomal recessive; EMG, electromyogram; HSMN, hereditary sensory motor neuropathy; MRI, magnetic resonance imaging; NCV, nerve conduction velocity; RMNS, repetitive motor nerve stimulation; SMN, survival motor neuron.

ity, rather than floppiness in infancy, is the presenting complaint in type V disease (McArdle phosphorylase deficiency) or in the glycogenosis due to phosphofructokinase deficiency or phosphohexose isomerase inhibition.

C. Myasthenia Gravis

Neonatal transient and congenital persistent myasthenia gravis, with patients presenting as paralytic floppy infants, is described earlier in this chapter.

D. Arthrogryposis Multiplex (Congenital Deformities About Multiple Joints)

This symptom complex, sometimes associated with hypotonia, may be of neurogenic or myopathic origin (or both) and may be associated with a variety of other anomalies. Orthopedic aspects are discussed in Chapter 24.

E. Spinal Cord Lesions

Severe limpness in newborns following breech extraction with stretching or actual tearing of the lower cervical to upper thoracic spinal cord is rarely seen today, owing to improved obstetric delivery. Klumpke lower brachial plexus paralysis may be present; the abdomen is usually exceedingly soft, and the lower extremities are flaccid. Urinary retention is present initially; later, the bladder may function autonomously. MRI of the cervical cord should define the lesion. After a few weeks, spasticity of the lower limbs becomes obvious. Treatment is symptomatic and consists of bladder and skin care and eventual mobilization on crutches or in a wheelchair.

2. Nonparalytic Group

The nonparalytic hypotonic infant often has a damaged brain (Table 23–27). Rarely, tendon reflexes may be depressed or

Table 23–27. Floppy infant: nonparalytic causes.

	Causes	Manifestations
Central nervous system disorders		
Atonic diplegia (prespastic diplegia)	Intrauterine, perinatal asphyxia, cord injury.	Limpness, stupor; poor suck, cry, Moro reflex, and grasp; later, irritability, increased tone and reflexes.
Choreoathetosis	As above; kernicterus.	Hypotonic early; movement disorder emerges later (6–18 mo).
Ataxic cerebral palsy	Same as choreoathetosis.	Same as choreoathetosis.
Syndromes with hypotonia (CNS origin)		
Trisomy 21	Genetic.	All have hypotonia early.
Prader-Willi syndrome	Genetic deletion 15q11.	Hypotonia, hypomentia, hypogonadism, obesity ("H$_3$O").
Marfan syndrome	Autosomal dominant.	Arachnodactyly.
Dysautonomia	Autosomal recessive.	Respiratory infections, corneal anesthesia.
Turner syndrome	45X, or mosaic.	Somatic stigmata (see Chapter 34).
Degenerative disorders		
Tay-Sachs disease	Autosomal recessive.	Cherry-red spot on macula.
Metachromatic leukodystrophy	Autosomal recessive.	Deep tendon reflexes increased early, polyneuropathy late; mental retardation.
Systemic diseases[a]		
Malnutrition	Deprivation, cystic fibrosis, celiac disease.	
Chronic illness	Congenital heart disease; chronic pulmonary disease (eg, bronchopulmonary dysplasia); uremia, renal acidosis.	
Metabolic disease	Mitochondrial; Lowe, Pompe, Leigh disease; hypercalcemia.	
Endocrinopathy	Hypothyroid.	

[a]See elsewhere in text for manifestations.
CNS, central nervous system.

absent; usually, brisk reflexes (with hypotonia) point to "supra-segmental" or cerebral dysfunction. Intrauterine or perinatal insults to brain or upper cord, while sometimes difficult to document, are major causes. (Occasionally, severe congenital myopathies presenting in the newborn period simulate nonparalytic hypotonia.) Persisting severe hypotonia is ominous. Tone will often vary. Spasticity and other forms of cerebral palsy may emerge; hypertonia and hypotonia may occur at varying times or sites in the same infant. Associated choreoathetoid or ataxic movements and developmental delay can clarify the diagnosis. Tendon reflexes are usually increased; pathologic infant reflexes (Babinski and tonic neck) may persist or worsen.

The creatine kinase level and the EMG are usually normal. Prolonged nerve conduction velocities (rare in this situation) point to polyneuritis or leukodystrophy. Muscle biopsy evaluation, using special stains and histographic analysis, often shows a reduction in size of type II fibers associated with decreased voluntary motor activity.

Limpness in the neonatal period and early infancy and subsequent delay in achieving motor milestones are the presenting features in a large number of children with a variety of CNS disorders, including mental retardation, as in trisomy 21. In many such cases, no specific diagnosis can be made. Close observation and scoring of motor patterns and adaptive behavior, as by the DDST, are helpful.

Anagnostou E et al: Type I spinal muscular atrophy can mimic sensory-motor axonal neuropathy. J Child Neurol 2005;20:147 [PMID: 15794183].

Birdi K et al: The floppy infant: Retrospective analysis of clinical experience (1990–2000) in a tertiary care facility. J Child Neurol 2005;20:803 [PMID: 16417874].

Clemmens MR, Bell L: Infant botulism presenting with poor feeding and lethargy: A review of 4 cases. Pediatr Emerg Care 2007;23:492 [PMID: 17666936].

Darras BT, Jones HR Jr: Neuromuscular problems of the critically ill neonate and child. Semin Pediatr Neurol 2004;11:147 [PMID: 15259868].

Howell RR et al: Diagnostic challenges for Pompe disease: An underrecognized cause of floppy baby syndrome. Genet Med 2006;8:289 [PMID: 16702878].

Kim CT et al: Neuromuscular rehabilitation and electrodiagnosis. 4. Pediatric issues. Arch Phys Med Rehabil 2005:86(3 Suppl 1):S28 [PMID: 15761797].

Kroksmark AK et al: Myotonic dystrophy: Muscle involvement in relation to disease type and size of expanded CTG-repeat sequence. Dev Med Child Neurol 2005;47:478 [PMID: 15991869].

Lee JS et al: Mitochondrial respiratory complex 1 deficiency simulating spinal muscular atrophy. Pediatr Neurol 2007;36:45 [PMID: 17162196].

Paro-Panjan D, Neubauer D: Congenital hypotonia: Is there an algorithm? J Child Neurol 2005;19:439 [PMID: 15446393].

Premasiri MK, Lee YS: The myopathology of floppy and hypotonic infants in Singapore. Pathology 2003;35:409 [PMID: 14555385].

Richer LP et al: Diagnostic profile of neonatal hypotonia: An 11-year study. Pediatr Neurol 2001;25:32 [PMID: 11483393].

Thompson JA et al: Infant botulism in the age of botulism immune globulin. Neurology 2005;64:2029 [PMID: 15917401].

Vasta I et al: Can clinical signs identify newborns with neuromuscular disorders? J Pediatr 2005;146:73 [PMID: 1564482].

CEREBRAL PALSY

The term *cerebral palsy* is a nonspecific term used to describe a chronic, static impairment of muscle tone, strength, coordination, or movements. The term implies that the condition is nonprogressive and originated from some type of cerebral insult or injury before birth, during delivery, or in the perinatal period. Other neurologic deficits or disorders (eg, blindness, deafness, or epilepsy) often coexist. Some form of cerebral palsy occurs in about 0.2% of neonatal survivors. The fundamental course, severity, precise manifestations, and prognosis vary widely.

The most common forms of cerebral palsy (75% of cases) involve spasticity of the limbs. A variety of terms denote the specific limb or combination of limbs affected: monoplegia (one limb); hemiplegia (arm and leg on same side of body, but arm more affected than leg); paraplegia (both legs affected with arms unaffected); quadriplegia (all four limbs affected equally).

Ataxia is the second most common form of cerebral palsy, accounting for about 15% of cases. The ataxia frequently affects fine coordinated movements of the upper extremities, but may also involve lower extremities and trunk. An involuntary movement disorder usually in the form of choreoathetosis accounts for 5% of cases and persistent hypotonia without spasticity for 1%.

Depending on the type and severity of the motor deficits, associated neurologic deficits or disorders may occur: seizures in up to 50%, mild mental retardation in 26%, and severe retardation in up to 27%. Disorders of language, speech, vision, hearing, and sensory perception are found in varying degrees and combinations.

The findings on physical examination are variable and are predominantly those of spasticity, hyperreflexia, ataxia, and involuntary movements. Microcephaly is frequently present. In patients with hemiplegia, the affected arm and leg may be smaller and shorter than the unaffected limbs. Cataracts, retinopathy, and congenital heart defects may be indicative of congenital infections such as CMV and rubella.

Appropriate laboratory studies depend on the history and physical findings. MRI scans may be helpful in understanding the full extent of cerebral injury, and occasionally neuroimaging results suggest specific etiologies (eg, periventricular calcifications in congenital CMV infections). Other diagnostic tests that may be considered include genetic studies based on history or MRI findings; urine amino acids and organic acids; and blood amino acids, lactate, pyruvate, and ammonia concentrations.

The determination that a child has cerebral palsy is based in part on excluding other neurologic disorders and following the child for a sufficient amount of time to ascertain the usually static, nonprogressive nature of the disorder.

Treatment and management are directed at assisting the child to attain maximal physical functioning and potential physical, occupational, and speech therapy; orthopedic monitoring and intervention and special educational assistance may all contribute to an improved outcome. Medications and injections (eg, botulinum toxin) for spasticity and seizures are needed in many children. A new treatment, constraint-induced (CI) movement therapy is being studied in controlled trials. Also important is the general support of the parents and family with counseling, educational programs, and support groups.

The prognosis for patients with cerebral palsy depends greatly on the child's IQ, severity of the motor deficits, and degree of incapacity. Aspiration, pneumonia, or other intercurrent infections are the most common causes of death.

In contrast, patients with mild cerebral palsy may improve with age. Some patients experience resolution of their motor deficits by age 7 years. Many children with normal intellect have normal life spans and are able to lead productive, satisfying lives.

The cause is often obscure or multifactorial. No definite etiologic diagnosis is possible in 25% of cases. The incidence is high among infants small for gestational age. Intrauterine hypoxia is a frequent cause. Other known causes are intrauterine bleeding, infections, toxins, congenital malformations, obstetric complications (including birth hypoxia), neonatal infections, kernicterus, neonatal hypoglycemia, metabolic disorders, and a small number of genetic syndromes.

Cooley WD: Providing a primary care medical home for children and youth with cerebral palsy. Pediatrics 2004;114:1106 [PMID: 15466117].

Garvey MA et al: Cerebral palsy: New approaches to therapy. Curr Neurol Neurosci Rep 2007;7:147 [PMID: 17324366].

Hoare BJ et al: Constraint-induced movement therapy in the treatment of the upper limb in children with hemiplegic cerebral palsy. Cochrane Database Syst Rev. 2007;2:CD004149 [PMID: 17443542].

Oskoui M, Shevell MI: Profile of pediatric hemiparesis. J Child Neurol 2005;20:471 [PMID: 15996394].

Pidcock FS: The emerging role of therapeutic botulinum toxin in the treatment of cerebral palsy. J Pediatr 2004;145(Suppl):S33 [PMID: 15292885].

Russman BS, Ashwal S: Evaluation of the child with cerebral palsy. Semin Pediatr Neurol 2004;11:47 [PMID: 15132253].

Taub E et al: Pediatric CI therapy for stroke-induced hemiparesis in young children. Dev Neurorehabil 2007;10:3 [PMID: 17608322].

Wood E. The child with cerebral palsy: diagnosis and beyond. Semin Pediatr Neurol 2006;13:286 [PMID: 17178359].

Wu YW et al: Prognosis for ambulation in cerebral palsy: A population-based study. Pediatrics 2004;14:1264 [PMID: 15520106].

REFERENCES

Web Resources

American Association of Child and Adolescent Psychiatry: http://www.aacp.org
Contains practice parameters and other information.
American Epilepsy Society: http://www.aesnet.org
Gives information about the society and general information about epilepsy; includes a good section on drugs.

Child Neurology Foundation: http://www.childneurologyfoundation.org/index.html
Describes sites, resources, and tests related to child neurology.
Child Neurology Society: http://www.childneurologysociety.org
Contains information about new developments and research and has practice parameters.
Epilepsy Foundation of America: http://www.epilepsyfoundation.org
Describes epilepsy research and some basics about epilepsy.
Gene tests: http://www.genetests.org
Lengthy descriptions of many genetic disorders.
National Institute of Neurological Disorders and Stroke: http://www.ninds.nih.gov
Brief descriptions of neurologic disorders.
Neurofibromatosis Foundation: http://www.nf.org
Tuberous Sclerosis Association: http://www.tsalliance.org

Orthopedics

John D. Polousky, MD
Robert E. Eilert, MD

Orthopedics is the medical discipline that deals with disorders of the neuromuscular and skeletal systems. The most common complaints in orthopedics are pain, loss of function, and deformity. Although the medical history reveals the patient's expectations, the physical examination and radiographic imaging are the most important tools of orthopedic diagnosis.

DISTURBANCES OF PRENATAL ORIGIN

CONGENITAL AMPUTATIONS & LIMB DEFICIENCIES

▶ General Considerations

Congenital amputations are caused by teratogens (eg, drugs or viruses), amniotic bands, or metabolic diseases (eg, diabetes in the mother). Children with congenital limb deficiencies, such as absence of the femur, tibia, or fibula, also have a high incidence of associated congenital anomalies, including genitourinary and cardiac defects and cleft palate. A limb deficiency usually consists of partial absence of structures in the extremity along one side or the other. The effect on structures distal to the amputation varies. For example, in radial club hand, the entire radius is absent, while the thumb may be hypoplastic or absent. Longitudinal bone deficiency is almost always associated with complex tissue defects in the extremity because of abnormalities of the associated nerves and muscles.

▶ Treatment

Mild limb deficiencies can be treated with limb lengthening or contralateral limb shortening, or both. More severe deficiencies are treated with prostheses to compensate for the length discrepancy. For some severe anomalies, surgery to remove a portion of the malformed extremity (eg, foot) is indicated so that a prosthesis can be fitted early.

Lower extremity prostheses are best fitted between ages 12 and 15 months, when walking starts. They are consistently well accepted, because they are necessary for balance and walking. In unilateral upper extremity amputation, fitting the child with a dummy-type prosthesis as early as age 6 months is advantageous because the child becomes accustomed to an extremity of the proper length and to the habit of bimanual manipulation. Children quickly learn how to function with a prosthesis and can lead active lives, even participating in sports. Although myoelectric prostheses have a technologic appeal, most patients find that simpler constructs are more useful in the long run.

Fixsen JA: Major lower limb shortening: A mini review. J Pediatr Orthop B 2003;12:1 [PMID: 12488764].

Kant P et al: Treatment of longitudinal deficiency affecting the femur: Comparing patient mobility and satisfaction outcomes of Syme amputation against extension prosthesis. J Pediatr Orthop 2003;23:236 [PMID: 12604957].

DEFORMITIES OF THE EXTREMITIES

1. Metatarsus Varus

Metatarsus varus is a common congenital foot deformity characterized by inward deviation of the forefoot. A vertical crease in the arch is present in rigid deformities. The angulation is located at the base of the fifth metatarsal, and this bone is prominent. Most flexible deformities are secondary to intrauterine positioning pressure and usually resolve spontaneously. Ten to 15% of children with metatarsus varus also have hip dysplasia. A careful hip examination is mandatory. If the deformity is rigid and cannot be manipulated past the midline, it is worthwhile to use a cast changed at intervals of 2 weeks to correct the deformity. So-called corrective shoes do not live up to their name, although they can be used to maintain correction obtained by casting.

Lincoln TL, Suen PW: Common rotational variations in children. J Am Acad Orthop Surg 2003;11:312 [PMID: 14565753].

2. Clubfoot (Talipes Equinovarus)

The diagnosis of classic talipes equinovarus, or clubfoot, requires three features: (1) plantarflexion of the foot at the ankle joint (equinus), (2) inversion deformity of the heel (varus), and (3) medial deviation of the forefoot (varus). The incidence of clubfoot is approximately 1:1000 live births. There are three major categories of clubfoot: (1) idiopathic, (2) neurogenic, and (3) those associated with syndromes such as arthrogryposis and Larsen syndrome. Any infant with a clubfoot should be examined carefully for associated anomalies, especially of the spine. Idiopathic clubfeet may be hereditary.

▶ Treatment

Treatment consists of manipulation of the foot to stretch the contracted tissues on the medial and posterior aspects, followed by splinting to hold the correction. When treatment is instituted shortly after birth, correction is rapid. When treatment is delayed, the foot tends to become more rigid within a matter of days. After full correction is obtained, a night brace is necessary for long-term maintenance of correction. Treatment by casting requires patience and experience, but fewer patients require surgery when attention is paid to details of the Ponsetti technique. If the foot is rigid and resistant to casting, surgical correction by tendon release is appropriate. Fifteen to 50% of patients require surgical correction.

Colburn M, Williams M: Evaluation of the treatment of idiopathic clubfoot by using the Ponsetti method. J Foot Ankle Surg 2003;42:259 [PMID: 14566717].
Clubfoot: http://www.marchofdimes.com/professionals/681_1211.asp.

3. Developmental Dysplasia of the Hip Joint

The definition of dysplasia is abnormal growth or development. Dysplasia of the hip encompasses a spectrum of conditions in which there is an abnormal relationship between the proximal femur and the acetabulum. In the most severe condition, the femoral head is not in contact with the acetabulum and is classified as a *dislocated hip*. A *dislocatable hip* is one in which the femoral head lies within the acetabulum at rest but can be dislocated with a provocative maneuver. A *subluxatable hip* is one in which the femoral head comes partially out of the joint with a provocative maneuver. *Acetabular dysplasia* is a term describing insufficient acetabular development on radiograph.

Congenital dislocation of the hip occurs in approximately 1 in 1000 live births. At birth, both the acetabulum and femur are underdeveloped. Dysplasia becomes worse with growth unless the dislocation is corrected. If the dislocation is corrected in the first few days or weeks of life, the dysplasia is completely reversible and a normal hip will develop. In older children with persistent dislocation or subluxation, especially those who have begun walking, dysplasia will worsen to the point that it is irreversible. For this reason, it is important to recognize the deformity early.

▶ Clinical Findings

A. Newborn Infant

The diagnosis of hip dislocation in the newborn depends on demonstrating instability of the joint. The infant is placed supine and complete relaxation is obtained by feeding with a bottle if necessary. The examiner's long finger is then placed over the greater trochanter and the thumb over the inner side of the thigh. Both hips are flexed 90 degrees and then slowly abducted from the midline, one hip at a time. With gentle pressure, an attempt is made to lift the greater trochanter forward. A feeling of slipping as the head relocates is a sign of instability (Ortolani sign). When the joint is more stable, the deformity must be provoked by applying slight pressure with the thumb on the medial side of the thigh as the thigh is adducted, thus slipping the hip posteriorly and eliciting a jerk as the hip dislocates (Barlow sign). The signs of instability are more reliable than a radiograph for diagnosing developmental dislocation of the hip in the newborn. Ultrasonography can be used but tends to result in overdiagnosis in the newborn. Asymmetrical skinfolds are present in about 40% of newborns and therefore are not particularly helpful.

B. Infants Aged 1–12 Months

After the first month of life, the signs of instability become less evident. Contractures begin to develop about the hip joint, limiting abduction to less than 90 degrees. It is important to hold the pelvis level to detect asymmetry of abduction. If the knees are at unequal heights when the hips and knees are flexed, the dislocated hip is on the side with the lower knee. If abduction is incomplete on examination, radiographs of the hips are indicated. After 6 weeks of age, radiologic examination is more accurate. Lateral displacement of the femoral head is the most reliable sign. In mild cases, the only radiologic abnormality may be an increased steepness of acetabular alignment and an acetabular angle greater than 35 degrees.

C. Children Older Than 1 Year

If dysplasia of the hip has not been diagnosed during the first year of life and the child begins to walk, there will be a painless limp and a lurch to the affected side. When the child stands on the affected leg, a dip of the pelvis will be evident on the opposite side, owing to weakness of the gluteus medius muscle. This is the Trendelenburg sign and accounts for the unusual swaying gait of children with unilateral hip dislocation. In children with bilateral dislocation, the loss of abduction is almost symmetrical and the findings may not be obvious. As a child with bilateral dislocation of the hips begins to walk, the gait is waddling. The perineum is widened as a result of lateral displacement of the hips, and there is flexion contracture as a result of posterior displacement of the femoral head. Flexion contracture contributes to a marked lumbar lordosis, and the greater trochanters are easily palpable in their elevated position. Treatment is still possible in the first 2 years of life, but the results are not nearly as good as in children receiving treatment early.

Treatment

Dislocation or dysplasia diagnosed in the first few weeks or months of life can be treated by Pavlik harness, which maintains reduction by placing the hip in a flexed and abducted position. Forced abduction is contraindicated, because this can lead to avascular necrosis of the femoral head. The use of double or triple diapers is ineffective. An experienced pediatric orthopedic surgeon should supervise treatment of children requiring splints.

In the first 4 months of life, reduction can be obtained by flexing and abducting the hip; no other manipulation is usually necessary. In late cases, preoperative traction for 2–3 weeks relaxes the soft tissues about the hip and draws the femoral head down so it is opposite the acetabulum. Reduction can be then be achieved without force under general anesthesia. After reduction, a hip spica cast is used for 6 months. After closed reduction, if the hip is not stable with a reasonable range of motion, open reduction is indicated. If reduction is done at an older age, operations to correct the deformities of the acetabulum and femur may be necessary in addition to the open reduction.

Weinstein SL et al: Developmental hip dysplasia and dislocation: Part I. Instr Course Lect 2004;53:523 [PMID: 15116641].

Weinstein SL et al: Developmental hip dysplasia and dislocation: Part II. Instr Course Lect 2004;53:531 [PMID: 15116642].

4. Torticollis

Wryneck deformities in infants may be due either to injury to the sternocleidomastoid muscle during delivery or to disease affecting the cervical spine. When contracture of the sternocleidomastoid muscle causes torticollis, the chin is rotated to the side opposite the affected muscle, and the head is tilted toward the side of the contracture. A mass palpable in the midportion of the sternocleidomastoid muscle is not a true tumor but rather fibrous transformation within the muscle. Torticollis is occasionally associated with congenital deformities of the cervical spine, and radiographs of the spine are indicated in all cases. In addition, there is a 20% incidence of hip dysplasia.

In most cases, passive stretching is effective. If the deformity has not been corrected by passive stretching within the first year of life, surgical release of the muscle origin and insertion will correct it. Excising the "tumor" of the sternocleidomastoid muscle creates an unsightly scar and is unnecessary. If the deformity is left untreated, a striking facial asymmetry will persist.

Acute torticollis may follow upper respiratory infection or mild trauma. Rotatory subluxation of the upper cervical spine requires computed tomography for accurate imaging. Traction or a cervical collar usually results in resolution of the symptoms within 1–2 days. Other causes of torticollis include spinal cord or cerebellar tumors, syringomyelia, and rheumatoid arthritis.

Fernandez Cornejo VJ et al: Inflammatory atlantoaxial subluxation (Grisel's syndrome) in children: Clinical diagnosis and management. Childs Nerv Syst 2003;19:342 [PMID: 12783261].

GENERALIZED DISORDERS OF SKELETAL OR MESODERMAL TISSUES

1. Arthrogryposis Multiplex Congenita (Amyoplasia Congenita)

Clinical Findings

Arthrogryposis multiplex congenita is characterized by incomplete fibrous ankylosis (usually bilateral) of many or all joints of the body. Upper extremity contractures usually produce adduction of the shoulders; extension of the elbows; flexion of the wrists; and stiff, straight fingers with poor muscle control of the thumbs. In the lower extremities, common deformities are dislocation of the hips, extension contractures of the knees, and severe clubfeet. The joints are fusiform and the joint capsules decreased in volume due to lack of movement during fetal development. Various investigations have attributed the basic defect to an abnormality of muscle or the lower motor neurons. Muscle development is poor, and muscles may be represented only by fibrous bands.

Treatment

Passive mobilization of joints is the early treatment. Prolonged casting to correct deformities is contraindicated because it causes further stiffness. Removable splints combined with vigorous physical therapy are the most effective conservative treatments. Surgical release of the affected joints is often necessary. The clubfoot associated with arthrogryposis is very stiff and nearly always requires surgery. Surgery, including capsulotomy, osteotomy, and tendon lengthening, is used to correct deformities of the knees. In the young child, a dislocated hip may be reduced operatively by the medial approach. Multiple operative procedures on the hip joint are contraindicated because worsening stiffness and impaired of range of motion may be produced. Affected children are often able to walk if the dislocations and contractures are reduced surgically. The long-term prognosis for physical and vocational independence is guarded. These patients have normal intelligence.

Bernstein RM: Arthrogryposis and amyoplasia. J Am Acad Orthop Surg 2002;10:417 [PMID: 12470044].

2. Marfan Syndrome

Marfan syndrome is a connective tissue disorder characterized by unusually long fingers and toes (arachnodactyly); hypermobility of the joints; flatfeet; subluxation of the ocular lenses; other eye abnormalities, including cataract, coloboma, megalocornea, strabismus, and nystagmus; a high-arched palate; a strong tendency to scoliosis; pectus carinatum; and thoracic aortic aneurysms due to weakness of the media of the vessels (see Chapter 35). Serum mucoproteins may be decreased, and urinary excretion of hydroxyproline increased. The condition is easily confused with homocystinuria, because the phenotypic presentation is identical. The two diseases are differentiated by detecting homocystine in the urine of patients with homocystinuria.

Treatment of flatfeet is usually supportive. Scoliosis may require more vigorous treatment by bracing or spine fusion. The long-term prognosis has improved for patients because better treatment for their aortic aneurysms has been devised.

ter Heide H et al: Neonatal Marfan syndrome: Clinical report and review of the literature. Clin Dysmorphol 2005;14:81 [PMID: 15770129].

3. Klippel-Feil Syndrome

In Klippel-Feil syndrome some or all of the cervical vertebrae fail to separate. Multiple congenital spinal anomalies may be present, with hemivertebrae and scoliosis. The neck is short and stiff, the hairline is low, and the ears are low-set. Common associated defects include congenital scoliosis, cervical rib, spina bifida, torticollis, web neck, high scapula, renal anomalies, and deafness. If there is evidence of abnormal renal function, renal ultrasound is indicated as well as a hearing test. Scoliotic deformities, if progressive, are an indication for spinal arthrodesis.

Tracy MR et al: Klippel-Feil syndrome: Clinical features and current understanding of etiology. Clin Orthop Relat Res 2004;424:183 [PMID: 15241163].

4. Sprengel Deformity

Sprengel deformity is a congenital condition in which one or both scapulas are elevated and small. The child cannot raise the arm completely on the affected side, and torticollis may be present. The deformity occurs alone or in association with Klippel-Feil syndrome. If the deformity is functionally limiting, the scapula may be surgically relocated lower in the thorax. Excision of the upper portion of the scapula improves cosmetic appearance but has little effect on function.

Williams MS: Developmental anomalies of the scapula—the "omo"st forgotten bone. Am J Med Genet 2003;120A:583 [PMID: 12884444].

5. Osteogenesis Imperfecta

Osteogenesis imperfecta is a rare genetic connective tissue disease characterized by multiple and recurrent fractures.

The severe fetal type (osteogenesis imperfecta congenita) is characterized by multiple intrauterine or perinatal fractures. Moderately affected children have numerous fractures and are dwarfed as a result of bony deformities and growth retardation. Intelligence is not affected. The shafts of the long bones are reduced in cortical thickness, and wormian bones are present in the skull. Other features include blue scleras, thin skin, hyperextensibility of ligaments, otosclerosis with hearing loss, and hypoplastic and deformed teeth. In the tarda type, fractures begin to occur at variable times after the perinatal period. There are relatively fewer fractures and deformities in these children. Affected patients are sometimes suspected of having suffered abuse. Osteogenesis imperfecta tarda should be ruled out in any case of nonaccidental trauma with multiple fractures.

Molecular genetic studies have identified more than 150 mutations of the COL1A1 and COL1A2 genes, which encode for type I procollagen. Parents without this mutation can be counseled that the likelihood of a second affected child is negligible.

Bisphosphonates show promise for decreasing the incidence of fractures. Surgical treatment involves correction of deformity of the long bones. Multiple intramedullary rods have been used to prevent deformity from fracture malunion. Patients are often confined to wheelchairs during adulthood.

Millington-Ward S et al: Emerging therapeutic approaches for osteogenesis imperfecta. Trends Mol Med 2005;11:299 [PMID: 15949772].

6. Osteopetrosis (Osteitis Condensans Generalisata, Marble Bone Disease, Albers-Schönberg Disease)

Osteopetrosis is a rare disorder of osteoclastic resorption of bone, resulting in abnormally dense bones. The marrow spaces are reduced, resulting in anemia. There are two types: a milder autosomal dominant type and a more malignant autosomal recessive type. The findings may appear at any age. On radiologic examination, the bones show increased density, transverse bands in the shafts, clubbing of ends, and vertical striations of long bones. Thickening about the cranial foramina is present, and heterotopic calcification of soft tissues is possible.

The autosomal recessive form of osteopetrosis can be treated successfully by allogeneic bone marrow transplantation.

Tolar J et al: Osteopetrosis. N Engl J Med 2004;351:2839 [PMID: 15625335].

7. Achondroplasia (Classic Chondrodystrophy)

Achondroplasia is the most common form of short-limbed dwarfism. The upper arms and thighs are proportionately shorter than the forearms and legs. Findings include bowing of the extremities, a waddling gait, limitation of motion of major joints, relaxation of the ligaments, short stubby fingers of almost equal length, frontal bossing, moderate hydrocephalus, depressed nasal bridge, and lumbar lordosis. Intelligence and sexual function are normal. The disorder is transmitted in an autosomal dominant manner, but 80% of cases result from new mutations of the fibroblast growth factor receptor-3 (*FGFR3*) gene. Radiographs demonstrate short, thick tubular bones and irregular epiphysial plates. The ends of the bones are thick, with broadening and cupping. Epiphysial ossification may be delayed. Because the spinal canal is narrowed, a herniated disk in adulthood may lead to acute paraplegia. Growth hormone is given to some children with bone dysplasia. Limb lengthening surgery remains controversial.

Carter EM et al: Advances in understanding etiology of achondroplasia and review of management. Curr Opin Pediatr 2007;19:32 [PMID: 17224659].
Achondroplasia: http://www.achondroplasia.co.uk/.

8. Osteochondrodystrophy (Morquio Disease)

Morquio disease is an autosomal recessive disorder of mucopolysaccharide storage. Skeletal abnormalities include shortening of the spine, kyphosis, scoliosis, shortened extremities, pectus carinatum, genu valgum, and a hypoplastic odontoid with atlantoaxial instability. The child generally appears normal at birth and begins to develop deformities between ages 1 and 4 years as a result of abnormal deposition of mucopolysaccharides.

Radiographs demonstrate wedge-shaped flattened vertebrae and irregular, malformed epiphyses. The ribs are broad and have been likened to canoe paddles. The lower extremities are more severely involved than the upper ones.

The major treatment issue revolves around the prevention of cervical myelopathy. Bone marrow transplantation has been successful in alleviating some of the symptoms.

Krivit W: Allogeneic stem cell transplantation for the treatment of lysosomal and peroxisomal metabolic diseases. Springer Semin Immunopathol 2004;26:119 [PMID: 15452666].

GROWTH DISTURBANCES OF THE MUSCULOSKELETAL SYSTEM

SCOLIOSIS

▷ General Considerations

Scoliosis is characterized by lateral curvature of the spine associated with rotation of the involved vertebrae. Scoliosis is classified by its anatomic location—thoracic, lumbar, and rarely, cervical. The convexity of the curve is designated right or left. Thus a right thoracic scoliosis would denote a thoracic curve in which the convexity is to the right, which is the most common type of idiopathic curve. A mild degree of posterior curvature of the spine (kyphosis) is normal in the thoracic area. Excessive curvature is pathologic. Mild anterior curvature of the spine (lordosis) is normal in the lumbar and cervical spines. Idiopathic scoliosis generally begins at age 8 or 10 years and usually progresses during growth. In rare instances, infantile scoliosis may be seen in children aged 2 years or younger.

Idiopathic scoliosis is four to five times more common in girls than boys. Eighty percent of cases of scoliosis are idiopathic. Because 30% of family members are also affected, siblings of an affected child should be examined. The disorder is usually asymptomatic in adolescence, but severe curvature can cause pain or loss of pulmonary function in later years. The screening examination for scoliosis is performed by having the patient bend forward 90 degrees with the hands joined in the midline. Asymmetry of the height of the ribs or paravertebral muscles on one side indicates the rotation of the trunk associated with lateral curvature.

Diseases associated with scoliosis include neurofibromatosis, Marfan syndrome, cerebral palsy, muscular dystrophy, poliomyelitis, and myelodysplasia. Between 5% and 7% of cases of scoliosis are due to congenital vertebral anomalies such as a hemivertebra or unilateral vertebral bridge. These curves are more rigid than the common idiopathic curve (see later discussion) and often increase with growth, especially during adolescence.

Idiopathic infantile scoliosis, occurring in children age 2–4 years, is uncommon in the United States but more common in Great Britain. If the rib-vertebral angle of Mehta is less than 20 degrees, the curve will resolve spontaneously. If the angle is greater, the curve will progress. Sciatic scoliosis may result from pressure on the spinal cord or roots by infectious processes or herniation of the nucleus pulposus; the underlying cause must be sought. Secondary curvature will resolve as the primary problem is treated.

▷ Clinical Findings

A. Symptoms and Signs

Scoliosis in adolescents does not cause significant pain. If a patient has significant pain, seek the underlying cause because the scoliosis is usually secondary to another disorder such as bone or spinal cord tumor. Deformity of the rib cage and asymmetry of the waistline are evident with curvatures of 30 degrees or more. Less severe curvature may be detected by the forward bending test described earlier. This test is designed to detect early abnormalities of rotation that may not be apparent when the patient is standing erect.

B. Imaging

The most valuable radiographs are those taken of the entire spine in the standing position in both the anteroposterior and lateral planes. Usually one primary curvature is evident with a compensatory curvature that develops to balance the body. At times two primary curvatures may be seen, usually in the right thoracic and left lumbar regions. Any left thoracic curvature should be suspected of being secondary to neurologic disease and should prompt a more meticulous neurologic examination. If the curvatures of the spine are balanced (compensated), the head is centered over the center of the pelvis and the patient is "in balance." If the spinal alignment is uncompensated, the head will be displaced to one side, which produces an unsightly deformity. Rotation of the spine may be measured by scoliometer. Rotation is associated with a marked rib hump as the lateral curvature increases in severity. Deformity of the rib cage causes long-term problems when lung volumes are reduced.

▶ Treatment

Treatment of scoliosis depends on curve magnitude, skeletal maturity, and risk of progression. Curvatures less than 20 degrees usually do not require treatment unless they show progression. Bracing is controversial but often used for curvatures of 20–40 degrees in a skeletally immature child. Treatment is indicated for any curvature that demonstrates progression on serial radiologic examination. Curvatures greater than 40 degrees are resistant to treatment by bracing. Thoracic curvatures greater than 60 degrees have been correlated with poor pulmonary function in adult life. Curvatures of such severity are an indication for surgical correction and posterior spinal fusion to maintain the correction. Curvatures of 40–60 degrees may also require spinal fusion if they are progressive, are causing decompensation of the spine, or cause unacceptable deformity.

Surgical fusion involves decortication of the bone over the laminas and spinous processes, with the addition of bone graft. Rods, hooks, or pedicle screws maintain postoperative correction, with activity restriction for several months until the bone fusion is solid. Treatment requires a team approach and is best done in centers with full support facilities.

▶ Prognosis

Compensated small curves that do not progress may be well tolerated throughout life, with minor deformity. Counsel the parents regarding the genetic transmission of scoliosis and caution that their children's backs should be examined as part of routine physical examinations. Early detection allows for simple brace treatment. Severe scoliosis may require correction by spinal arthrodesis, although fusionless techniques are being developed.

Braun JT et al: The use of animal models in fusionless scoliosis investigations. Spine 2005;30(Suppl):S35 [PMID: 16138065].
Lonstien JE: Scoliosis: Surgical versus nonsurgical treatment. Clin Orthop 2006;443:248 [PMID: 16462448].

SLIPPED CAPITAL FEMORAL EPIPHYSIS

Slipped capital femoral epiphysis (SCFE) is caused by displacement of the proximal femoral epiphysis due to disruption of the growth plate. The head of the femur is usually displaced medially and posteriorly relative to the femoral neck. The condition occurs in adolescence and is most common in obese males. The cause is unclear, although some authorities have shown experimentally that the strength of the perichondrial ring stabilizing the epiphysial area is sufficiently weakened by hormonal changes during adolescence that excessive body weight can cause a fracture through the growth plate. Hormonal studies in these children are usually normal, although SCFE is associated with hypothyroidism.

Clinically, SCFE is classified as stable or unstable. The condition is stable if the child is able to bear weight on the affected extremity. In unstable SCFE, the child is unable to bear weight. Inability to bear weight in SCFE correlates with increasing rate of avascular necrosis.

The condition occasionally occurs acutely following a fall or direct trauma to the hip. More commonly, vague symptoms occur over a protracted period in an otherwise healthy child who presents with pain and limp. The pain can be referred into the thigh or the medial side of the knee. The hip joint should be examined in any obese child complaining of knee pain. The consistent finding on physical examination is limitation of internal rotation of the hip. The diagnosis may be clearly apparent only in the lateral radiographic view.

Treatment is based on the same principles that govern treatment of any fracture of the femoral neck. The head of the femur is internally fixed to the neck of the femur and the fracture line allowed to heal. The long-term prognosis is guarded because most of these patients continue to be overweight, placing chronic stress on the hip joints. Follow-up studies have shown a high incidence of premature degenerative arthritis in this disease, even in those who do not develop avascular necrosis. The development of avascular necrosis almost guarantees a poor prognosis, because new bone does not readily replace the dead bone at this late stage of skeletal development. About 30% of patients have bilateral involvement, which may occur as late as 1–2 years after the primary episode.

GENU VARUM & GENU VALGUM

Genu varum (bowleg) is normal from infancy through age 2 years. The alignment then changes to genu valgum (knock-knee) until about age 8 years, at which time adult alignment is attained. Criteria for referral to an orthopedist include persistent bowing beyond age 2 years, bowing that is increasing rather than decreasing, bowing of one leg only, and knock-knee associated with short stature.

Bracing may be appropriate. Rarely, an osteotomy is necessary for a severe problem such as Blount disease (proximal tibial epiphysial dysplasia).

Sass P, Hassan G: Lower extremity abnormalities in children. Am Fam Physician 2003;68:461 [PMID: 12924829].

TIBIAL TORSION

"Toeing in" in small children is a common parental concern. Tibial torsion is rotation of the leg between the knee and the ankle. Internal rotation amounts to about 20 degrees at birth but decreases to neutral rotation by age 16 months. The deformity is sometimes accentuated by laxity of the knee ligaments, allowing excessive internal rotation of the leg in small children. In children who have a persistent internal rotation of the tibia beyond age 16–18 months, the condition is often due to sleeping with feet turned in and can be reversed with an external rotation splint worn only at night.

FEMORAL ANTEVERSION

Toeing in beyond age 2 or 3 years is usually secondary to femoral anteversion, which is characterized by more internal rotation of the hip compared with external rotation. This femoral alignment follows a natural history of progressive decrease toward neutral during growth. Studies comparing the results of treatment with shoes or braces to the natural history have shown that little is gained by active treatment. Active external rotation exercises, such as skating or bicycle riding, can be encouraged. Osteotomy for rotational correction is rarely required. Children who have no external rotation of hip in extension are candidates for orthopedic consultation.

Lincoln TL, Suen PW: Common rotational variations in children. J Am Acad Orthop Surg 2003;11:312 [PMID: 14565753].

COMMON FOOT PROBLEMS

When a child begins to stand and walk, the long arch of the foot is flat with a medial bulge over the inner border of the foot. The forefeet are mildly pronated or rotated inward, with a slight valgus alignment of the knees. As the child grows and joint laxity decreases, the long arch is better supported and more normal relationships occur in the lower extremities. (See also sections on Metatarsus Varus and Clubfoot, earlier.)

1. Flatfoot

Flatfoot is a normal condition in infants. If the heel cord is of normal length, full dorsiflexion is possible with the heel in the neutral position. As long as the heel cord is of normal length and a longitudinal arch is noted when the child is sitting in a non–weight-bearing position, the parents can be assured that a normal arch will probably develop. There is usually a familial incidence of relaxed flatfeet in children who have no apparent arch. In any child with a shortened heel cord or stiffness of the foot, other causes of flatfoot such as tarsal coalition or vertical talus should be ruled out by a complete orthopedic examination and radiograph.

In the child with an ordinary relaxed flatfoot, no active treatment is indicated unless calf or leg pain is present. In children who have leg pains attributable to flatfoot, a supportive shoe with scaphoid pad, such as a good-quality sports shoe, is useful. An orthotic that holds the heel in neutral and supports the arch may relieve discomfort if more support is needed. An arch insert should not be prescribed unless passive correction of the arch is easily accomplished; otherwise, the skin over the medial side of the foot will be irritated.

2. Talipes Calcaneovalgus

Talipes calcaneovalgus is characterized by excessive dorsiflexion at the ankle and eversion of the foot. It is often present at birth and is due to intrauterine position. Treatment consists of passive exercises, stretching the foot into plantarflexion. In rare instances, it may be necessary to use plaster casts to help with manipulation and positioning. Complete correction is the rule.

Gore AI, Spencer JP: The newborn foot. Am Fam Physician 2004;69:865 [PMID: 14989573].

3. Cavus Foot

This deformity consists of an unusually high longitudinal arch of the foot. It may be hereditary or associated with neurologic conditions such as poliomyelitis, Charcot-Marie-Tooth disease, Friedreich ataxia, and diastematomyelia. There is usually an associated contracture of the toe extensor, producing a claw toe deformity in which the metatarsophalangeal joints are hyperextended and the interphalangeal joints acutely flexed. Any child presenting with cavus feet should receive a careful neurologic examination and radiographs of the spine.

Conservative therapy is ineffective. In symptomatic cases, surgery may be necessary to lengthen the contracted extensor and flexor tendons and to release the plantar fascia and other tight plantar structures. The associated varus heel deformity causes more problems than the high arch.

Statler TK, Tullis BL: Pes cavus. J Am Podiatr Med Assoc 2005; 95:42 [PMID: 15659413].

4. Bunions (Hallux Valgus)

Adolescents may present with lateral deviation of the great toe associated with a prominence over the head of the first metatarsal. This deformity is painful only with shoe wear and almost always can be relieved by fitting shoes that are wide enough in the toe. Surgery should be avoided in the adolescent, because further growth tends to cause recurrence of the deformity.

Talab YA: Hallux valgus in children: A 5–14-year follow-up study of 30 feet treated with a modified Mitchell osteotomy. Acta Orthop Scand 2002;73:195 [PMID: 12079019].

DEGENERATIVE PROBLEMS (ARTHRITIS, BURSITIS, & TENOSYNOVITIS)

ESSENTIALS OF DIAGNOSIS & TYPICAL FEATURES

▶ Chronic condition.

▶ May result from overuse in adolescent athletes.

▶ Rule out more serious conditions first.

Degenerative arthritis may follow childhood skeletal problems, such as infection, slipped capital femoral epiphysis, avascular necrosis, or trauma, or it may occur in association with hemophilia. Early effective treatment of these disorders can prevent arthritis. Degenerative changes in the soft tissues around joints may occur as a result of overuse syndrome in adolescent athletes. Young boys throwing excessive numbers of pitches, especially curve balls, may develop "Little League" elbow, consisting of degenerative changes around the humeral condyles associated with pain, swelling, and limitation of motion (see Chapter 25). Limitation of the number of pitches thrown by Little League pitchers is the key to prevention.

Acute bursitis is uncommon in childhood, and other causes should be ruled out before this diagnosis is accepted.

Tenosynovitis is most common in the region of the knees and feet. Children taking dancing lessons, particularly toe dancing, may have pain around the flexor tendon sheaths in the toes or ankles. Rest is effective treatment. At the knee level, the patellar ligament may be irritated, with associated swelling in the infrapatellar fat pad. Synovitis in this area is usually due to overuse and is treated by rest and nonsteroidal anti-inflammatory drugs. Corticosteroid injections are contraindicated.

TRAUMA

ESSENTIALS OF DIAGNOSIS & TYPICAL FEATURES

▶ Directed physical examination shows swelling, tenderness, deformity, or instability.

▶ Radiographic findings are consistent with forceful injury.

▶ Rule out physeal fracture.

SOFT TISSUE TRAUMA (SPRAINS, STRAINS, & CONTUSIONS)

A *sprain* is the stretching of a ligament. A *strain* is a stretch of a muscle or tendon. *Contusions* are generally due to tissue compression, with damage to blood vessels within the tissue and the formation of hematoma. A severe sprain is one in which the ligament is completely disrupted, resulting in instability of the joint. In a mild or moderate sprain, tearing of the ligament is incomplete, but local pain and swelling results. Mild or moderate sprain is not associated with instability of the joint.

The initial treatment of mild or moderate sprain consists of ice, compression, and elevation. Brief splinting followed by early range of motion of the affected joint protects against further injury and relieves swelling and pain. Ibuprofen and other nonsteroidal anti-inflammatory drugs are useful for pain.

In more severe trauma with tearing of a ligament, instability of the joint may be demonstrated by gross examination or by stress testing with radiographic documentation. Such deformity of the joint may cause persistent instability resulting from inaccurate apposition of the ligament ends during healing. If instability is evident, surgical repair of the torn ligament may be indicated. If a muscle is torn at its tendinous insertion, it should be repaired.

1. Ankle Sprains

The history will indicate that the injury was by either forceful inversion or eversion. The more common inversion injury results in tearing or injury to the lateral ligaments, whereas an eversion injury will injure the medial ligaments of the ankle. The injured ligaments may be identified by means of careful palpation for point tenderness around the ankle. The joint should be supported or immobilized at a right angle, which is the functional position. Use of an air splint produces joint rest, and the extremity can be protected by using crutches. Functional rehabilitation, including edema control, range-of-motion exercises, strengthening, and restitution of proprioceptive sensation, can prevent long-term disability.

Ivins D: Acute ankle sprain: An update. Am Fam Physician 2006;74:1714 [PMID: 17137000].

2. Knee Sprains

Sprains of the collateral and cruciate ligaments are uncommon in children. These ligaments are so strong that it is more common to injure the growth plates, which are the weakest structures in the knees of children. In adolescence, however, the physes have started to close, and the knee joint is more like that of an adult. Rupture of the anterior cruciate ligament can result from a rotational injury (see Chapter 25). If the injury produces avulsion of the tibial spine, anatomic reduction and fixation is often required.

Effusion of the knee after trauma should be referred to an orthopedic specialist. The differential diagnosis includes torn ligament, torn meniscus, and osteochondral fracture. Nontraumatic effusion should be evaluated for inflammatory conditions (eg, juvenile rheumatoid arthritis) or patellar malalignment.

Vaquero J et al: Intra-articular traumatic disorders of the knee in children and adolescents. Clin Orthop Relat Res 2005;432:97 [PMID: 15738809].

3. Internal Derangements of the Knee

Meniscal injuries are uncommon in children younger than age 12 years. Clicking or locking of the knee may occur in young children as a result of a discoid lateral meniscus, a rare congenital anomaly. As the child approaches adolescence, internal damage to the knee from a torsion weight-bearing injury may cause tearing and displacement of a meniscus and result in locking of the knee. Osteochondral fractures secondary to osteochondritis dissecans may also present as internal derangements of the knee in adolescence. Post-traumatic synovitis may mimic a meniscal lesion. In any severe injury to the knee, epiphysial injury should be suspected. Stress films will sometimes demonstrate separation of the distal femoral epiphysis in such cases. Epiphysial injury should be suspected whenever tenderness is present on both sides of the metaphysis of the femur after injury.

Smith AD: The skeletally immature knee: What's new in overuse injuries. Instr Course Lect 2003;52:691 [PMID: 12690894].

4. Back Sprains

Sprains of the ligaments and muscles of the back are unusual in children but may occur as a result of violent trauma from automobile accidents or athletic injuries. Back pain in a child may be the only symptom of significant disease and warrants clinical investigation. Inflammation, infection, renal disease, or tumors can cause back pain in children, and sprain should not be accepted as a routine diagnosis.

Balagué F et al: Low-back pain in children. Lancet 2003;361:1403 [PMID: 12727390].

Wall EJ et al: Backpacks and back pain: Where's the epidemic? J Pediatr Orthop 2003;23:437 [PMID: 12826938].

5. Contusions

Contusion of muscle with hematoma formation produces the familiar "charley horse" injury. Treatment of such injuries is by application of ice, compression, and rest. Exercise should be avoided for 5–7 days. Local heat may hasten healing once the acute phase of tenderness and swelling is past.

6. Myositis Ossificans

Ossification within muscle occurs when there is sufficient trauma to cause a hematoma that later heals in the manner of a fracture. The injury is usually a contusion and occurs most commonly in the quadriceps of the thigh or the triceps of the arm. When a severe injury with hematoma is recognized, it is important to splint the extremity and avoid activity. If further trauma causes recurrent injury, ossification may reach spectacular proportions and resemble an osteosarcoma.

Disability is great, with local swelling and heat and extreme pain on the slightest motion of the adjacent joint. The limb should be rested until the local reaction has subsided (5–7 days). After local heat and tenderness have decreased, gentle active exercises may be initiated. Passive stretching exercises are not indicated, because they may stimulate the ossification reaction. If surgery is necessary, it should not be attempted before 9 months to 1 year after injury, because it may restart the process and lead to an even more severe reaction.

TRAUMATIC SUBLUXATIONS & DISLOCATIONS

Dislocation of a joint is always associated with severe damage to the ligaments and joint capsule. In contrast to fracture reduction, which may be safely postponed, dislocations must be reduced immediately. Dislocations can usually be reduced by gentle sustained traction. It often happens that no anesthetic is necessary for several hours after the injury, because of the protective anesthesia produced by the injury. Following reduction, the joint should be splinted for transportation of the patient. A thorough neurovascular examination should be performed and documented before and after reduction.

The dislocated joint should be treated initially by immobilization followed by graduated active exercises through a full range of motion. Vigorous passive manipulation of the joint by a therapist may be harmful.

1. Subluxation of the Radial Head (Nursemaid Elbow)

Infants may sustain subluxation of the radial head as a result of being lifted or pulled by the hand. The child presents with a painful, fully pronated elbow. The usual complaint is that the child's elbow will not bend. Radiographic findings are normal, but there is point tenderness over the radial head. When the elbow is placed in full supination and slowly moved from full extension to full flexion, a click may be palpated at the level of the radial head. The relief of pain is remarkable, as the child usually stops crying immediately. The elbow may be immobilized briefly in a sling for comfort. Occasionally, symptoms last for several days, requiring more prolonged immobilization.

Pulled elbow may be a clue to child abuse. This should be considered during examination, especially if the problem is recurrent.

2. Recurrent Dislocation of the Patella

Recurrent dislocation of the patella is more common in loose-jointed individuals, especially adolescent girls. If the patella completely dislocates, it nearly always goes laterally. Pain is severe, and the patient is brought to the physician with the knee slightly flexed and an obvious bony mass lateral to the knee joint associated with a flat area over the anterior knee. Radiologic examination confirms the diagnosis. The patella may be reduced by extending the knee and placing slight pressure on the patella while gentle traction is exerted on the leg. In subluxation of the patella, the symptoms may be more subtle, and the patient will complain that the knee "gives out" or "jumps out of place."

In patients with first-time dislocation, the initial treatment should be nonoperative, consisting of physical therapy to strengthen the quadriceps, hips, and core stabilizers. Surgery is reserved for individuals with reparable osteochondral injuries, loose bodies, and recurrent dislocation following appropriate nonoperative therapy.

Stefancin JJ, Parker RD: First-time traumatic patellar dislocation: A systematic review. Clin Orthop 2007;455:93 [PMID: 17279039].

FRACTURES

1. Epiphysial Separations

In children, epiphysial separations and fractures are more common than ligamentous injuries. This finding is based on the fact that the ligaments of the joints are generally stronger than the associated growth plates. In instances in which dislocation is suspected, a radiograph should be taken to rule out epiphysial fracture. Radiographs of the opposite extremity, especially for injuries around the elbow, may be valuable for comparison. Reduction of a fractured epiphysis should be done under anesthesia to align the growth plate with the least amount of force. Fractures across the growth plate may produce bony bridges that will cause premature cessation of growth or angular deformities of the extremity. Epiphysial fractures around the shoulder, wrist, and fingers can usually be treated by closed reduction, but fractures of the epiphyses around the elbow often require open reduction. In the lower extremity, accurate reduction of the epiphysial plate is necessary to prevent joint deformity if a joint surface is involved. If angular deformities result, corrective osteotomy may be necessary.

Mehlman CT: Growth plate fractures. Available at: http://www.emedicine.com/orthoped/topic627.htm.

2. Torus Fractures

Torus fractures consist of "buckling" of the cortex due to compression of the bone. They usually occur in the distal radius or ulna. Alignment is usually satisfactory, and simple immobilization for 3 weeks is sufficient.

3. Greenstick Fractures

Greenstick fractures involve frank disruption of the cortex on one side of the bone but no discernible cleavage plane on the opposite side. These fractures are angulated but not displaced, because the bone ends are not separated. Reduction is achieved by straightening the arm into normal alignment, and reduction is maintained by a snugly fitting plaster cast. Follow-up radiographs should be obtained after 7–10 days to ensure that the reduction has been maintained in the cast. A slight angular deformity can be corrected by remodeling of the bone. The farther the fracture is from the growing end of the bone, the longer the time required for remodeling. The fracture can be considered healed when no tenderness or local heat is present and when adequate bony callus is seen on radiograph.

4. Fracture of the Clavicle

Clavicular fractures are very common injuries in infants and children. The arm can be immobilized in a sling for comfort. The healing callus will be apparent when the fracture has consolidated, but this unsightly lump will generally resolve over a period of months to a year. (See also Chapter 25.)

5. Supracondylar Fractures of the Humerus

Supracondylar fractures tend to occur in children aged 3–6 years and are potentially dangerous because of the proximity to the brachial artery in the distal arm. As they are usually associated with significant trauma, swelling may be severe. Most often, these fractures are treated by closed reduction and percutaneous pinning. Complications associated with supracondylar fractures include Volkmann ischemic contracture of the forearm due to vascular compromise and cubitus varus (decreased carrying angle) secondary to poor reduction. The so-called gunstock deformity of the elbow may be somewhat unsightly but does not usually interfere with joint function.

Gosens T, Bongers KJ: Neurovascular complications and functional outcome in displaced supracondylar fractures of the humerus in children. Injury 2003;34:267 [PMID: 12667778].

6. General Comments on Other Fractures in Children

Reduction of fractures in children is usually accomplished by simple traction and manipulation; open reduction is indicated if a satisfactory alignment is not obtained. Remodeling of the fracture callus usually produces an almost normal appearance of the bone over a matter of months. The younger the child, the more remodeling is possible. Angular deformities remodel reliably. Rotatory malalignment does not remodel.

The physician should be suspicious of child abuse whenever the age of a fracture does not match the history given or when the severity of the injury is more than the alleged accident would have produced. In suspected cases of battering in which no fracture is present on the initial radiograph, a repeat radiograph 10 days later is in order. Bleeding beneath the periosteum will be calcified by 7–10 days, and the radiographic appearance is almost diagnostic of severe closed trauma characteristic of a battered child.

INFECTIONS OF THE BONES & JOINTS

OSTEOMYELITIS

Osteomyelitis is an infectious process that usually starts in the spongy or medullary bone and then extends to involve compact or cortical bone. The lower extremities are most often affected, and there is commonly a history of trauma. Osteomyelitis may occur as a result of direct bacterial invasion through a penetrating wound or open fracture, but hematogenous spread of infection (eg, pyoderma or upper respiratory tract infection) from other infected areas is much more common. The most common infecting organism is *Staphylococcus aureus,* which has a tendency to infect the metaphyses of growing bones. Anatomically, circulation in the long bones is such that the blood supply to the metaphysis just below the growth plate is provided by end arteries, which turn sharply to end in venous sinusoids, causing a relative stasis. In the infant younger than age 1 year, there is direct vascular communication with the epiphysis across the growth plate, so that direct spread may occur from the metaphysis to the epiphysis and subsequently into the joint. In the older child, the growth plate provides an effective barrier, the epiphysis is usually not involved. In the older child, infection spreads retrograde from the metaphysis into the diaphysis, and by rupture through the cortical bone and along the diaphysis beneath the periosteum.

1. Exogenous Osteomyelitis

To avoid osteomyelitis by direct extension, all wounds must be carefully cleansed. Osteomyelitis is a common occurrence from pressure sores in anesthetic areas, as in patients with spina bifida. Cultures of the wound at the time of exploration and debridement may be useful if signs of infection develop subsequently. Copious irrigation is necessary, and all nonviable skin, subcutaneous tissue, fascia, and muscle must be excised. In extensive or contaminated wounds, antibiotic coverage is indicated. Contaminated lacerations should be left open and secondary closure performed 3–5 days later. At the time of delayed closure, any remaining necrotic tissue should be excised. Leaving the wound open allows the infection to stay at the surface rather than extend inward to the bone. Puncture wounds are especially liable to cause osteomyelitis and should be carefully debrided.

Initially, broad-spectrum antibiotics should be administered, but the final choice of antibiotics is directed by culture results. A tetanus toxoid booster may be indicated. Gas gangrene is best prevented by adequate debridement. After exogenous osteomyelitis has become established, treatment becomes more complicated, requiring extensive surgical debridement and intravenous antibiotics.

2. Hematogenous Osteomyelitis

Hematogenous osteomyelitis is usually caused by pyogenic bacteria; 85% of cases are due to staphylococci. Streptococci are a less common cause of osteomyelitis. *Pseudomonas* organisms are common in cases of nail puncture wounds. Children with sickle cell anemia are especially prone to osteomyelitis caused by *Salmonella* spp.

▶ Clinical Findings

A. Symptoms and Signs

In infants, the manifestations of osteomyelitis may be subtle, presenting as irritability, diarrhea, or failure to feed properly; the temperature may be normal or slightly low; and the white blood cell count may be normal or only slightly elevated. There may be pseudoparalysis of the involved limb. In older children, the manifestations are more striking, with local tenderness and pain, high fever, rapid pulse, and elevated white blood cell count, erythrocyte sedimentation rate (ESR), and C-reactive protein. Osteomyelitis of a lower extremity often occurs around the knee joint in children aged 7–10 years. Tenderness is most marked over the metaphysis of the bone where the process originates. Lower extremity osteomyelitis should be ruled out in any child who refuses to bear weight.

B. Laboratory Findings

Blood cultures are often positive early. The most significant test in infancy is the aspiration of pus. It is useful to needle the bone in the area of suspected infection and aspirate any fluid present. This fluid should be stained for organisms and cultured. Even edema fluid may be useful for determining the causative organism. Elevation of the ESR above 50 mm/h is typical for osteomyelitis. C-reactive protein is elevated earlier than the ESR.

C. Imaging

Nonspecific local swelling is the first radiographic finding, followed by elevation of the periosteum. Formation of new bone from the cambium layer of the periosteum occurs after 3–6 days. As the infection becomes chronic, areas of cortical bone are isolated by pus spreading down the medullary canal, causing rarefaction and demineralization of the bone. Such isolated pieces of cortex become ischemic and form sequestra (dead bone fragments). These radiographic findings are late but specific. Osteomyelitis should be diagnosed clinically before significant radiographic findings are present. Bone scan is sensitive but nonspecific and should be interpreted in the clinical context before radiographic findings become positive. Magnetic resonance imaging can demonstrate edema early or soft-tissue thickening later.

▶ Treatment

A. Specific Measures

Antibiotics should be started intravenously as soon as the diagnosis of osteomyelitis is made. Oral antibiotics are begun when tenderness, fever, the white cell count, and the C-reactive protein are all decreasing and the culture is positive. Agents that cover *S aureus* and *Streptococcus pyogenes* (eg, oxacillin, nafcillin, cefazolin, and clindamycin) are appropriate for most cases. For specific recommendations and for possible *Pseudomonas* infection, see Chapter 40. Chronic infections are treated for months. Following surgical debridement, *Pseudomonas* foot infections usually respond to 1–2 weeks of antibiotic treatment.

B. General Measures

Splinting of the limb minimizes pain and decreases spread of the infection by lymphatic channels through the soft tissue. The splint should be removed periodically to allow active use of adjacent joints and prevent stiffening and muscle atrophy. In chronic osteomyelitis, splinting may be necessary to guard against fracture of the weakened bone.

C. Surgical Measures

Aspiration of the metaphysis for culture and Gram stain is the most useful diagnostic measure in any case of suspected osteomyelitis. In the first 24–72 hours, it may be possible to treat osteomyelitis with antibiotics alone. If frank pus is aspirated from the bone, however, surgical drainage is indicated. If the infection has not shown a dramatic response within 24 hours, surgical drainage is also indicated. It is important that all devitalized soft tissue be removed and adequate exposure of the bone obtained to permit free drainage. Excessive amounts of bone should not be removed when draining acute osteomyelitis, because it will not be completely replaced by the normal healing process. Bone damage is limited by surgical drainage, whereas failure to evacuate pus in acute cases may lead to widespread damage.

▶ Prognosis

When osteomyelitis is diagnosed in the early clinical stages and prompt antibiotic therapy is begun, the prognosis is excellent. If the process has been unattended for 7–10 days, there is almost always some permanent loss of bone structure, as well as the possibility of growth abnormality.

Moumile K et al: Bacterial aetiology of acute osteoarticular infections in children. Acta Paediatr 2005;94:419 [PMID: 16092454].

PYOGENIC ARTHRITIS

The source of pyogenic arthritis varies with age. In the infant, pyogenic arthritis often develops by spread from adjacent osteomyelitis. In the older child, it presents as an isolated infection, usually without bony involvement. In teenagers with pyogenic arthritis, an underlying systemic disease or infection with an organism (eg, gonococcus) that has an affinity for joints is usually the cause.

The infecting organism also varies with age: group B streptococcus and *S aureus* in those younger than age 4 months; *Haemophilus influenzae* and *S aureus* in those aged 4 months to 4 years; and *S aureus* and *S pyogenes* in older children and adolescents. *H influenzae* is now uncommon because of effective immunization. *Kingella kingae* is a gram-negative bacterium that occasionally causes pyarthrosis.

▶ Clinical Findings

A. Symptoms and Signs

In older children, the signs may be striking, with fever, malaise, vomiting, and restriction of motion. In infants, paralysis of the limb due to inflammatory neuritis may be evident. Infection of the hip joint in infants should be suspected if decreased abduction of the hip is present in an infant who is irritable or feeding poorly. A history of umbilical catheter treatment in the newborn nursery should alert the physician to the possibility of pyogenic arthritis of the hip.

B. Laboratory Findings

The initial effusion of the joint rapidly becomes purulent. An effusion of the joint may accompany osteomyelitis in the adjacent bone. A white cell count exceeding 50,000/μL in the joint fluid indicates a definite purulent infection. Generally, spread of infection is from the bone into the joint, but unattended pyogenic arthritis may also affect adjacent bone. The ESR is often above 50 mm/h.

C. Imaging

Early distention of the joint capsule is nonspecific and difficult to measure on radiograph. In the infant with unrecognized pyogenic arthritis, dislocation of the joint may follow within a few days as a result of distention of the capsule by pus. Later changes include destruction of the joint space, resorption of epiphysial cartilage, and erosion of the adjacent bone of the metaphysis. The bone scan shows increased flow and increased uptake about the joint.

▶ Treatment

Aspiration of the joint is the key to diagnosis. In the hip joint, pyogenic arthritis is most easily treated by surgical drainage because the joint is deep, difficult to aspirate, and inaccessible to thorough cleaning by needle aspiration. Arthroscopic irrigation and debridement have been successful in treating pyogenic arthritis of the knee. If fever and clinical symptoms do not subside within 24 hours after initial treatment, open surgical drainage is indicated. Antibiotics can be selected based on the child's age, results of the Gram stain, and culture of the aspirated pus. Reasonable empiric therapy for infants is nafcillin or oxacillin plus a third-generation cephalosporin. An antistaphylococcal agent alone is usually adequate for children older than age 5 years.

For staphylococcal infections, 3 weeks of therapy is recommended; for other organisms, 2 weeks is usually sufficient. Oral therapy may be begun when clinical signs have improved markedly. It is not necessary to give intra-articular antibiotics, because good levels are achieved in the synovial fluid with parenteral administration.

▶ Prognosis

The prognosis for the patient with pyogenic arthritis is excellent if the joint is drained early, before damage to the articular cartilage has occurred. If infection is present for more than 24 hours, dissolution of the proteoglycans in the articular cartilage takes place, with subsequent arthrosis and fibrosis of the joint. Damage to the growth plate may also occur, especially within the hip joint, where the epiphyseal plate is intracapsular.

Frank G et al: Musculoskeletal infections in children. Pediatr Clin North Am 2005;52:1083 [PMID: 16009258].

TUBERCULOUS ARTHRITIS

Tuberculous arthritis is now a rare disease in the United States, but children in poor social circumstances are at risk for the infection. Generally tuberculous arthritis may be ruled out by negative skin testing. The joints most commonly affected in children are the intervertebral disks, resulting in gibbus or dorsal angular deformity at the site of involvement. Treatment is by local drainage of the abscess, followed by antituberculous therapy. Prolonged immobilization in a plaster cast or prolonged bed rest is necessary to promote healing. Spinal fusion may be required to preserve stability of the vertebral column.

Mkandawire NC, Kaunda E: Bone and joint TB at Queen Elizabeth Central Hospital 1986 to 2002. Trop Doct 2005;35:14 [PMID: 15712533].

DISKITIS

Diskitis is pyogenic infectious spondylitis in children; supportive treatment and intravenous antibiotics are likely to lead to rapid relief of symptoms and signs without recurrence.

McCarthy JJ et al: Musculoskeletal infections in children: Basic treatment principles and recent advancements. Instr Course Lect 2005;54:515 [PMID: 15948476].

TRANSIENT SYNOVITIS OF THE HIP

The most common cause of limping and pain in the hip in children in the United States is transitory synovitis, an acute inflammatory reaction that often follows an upper respiratory infection. It is generally self-limited. In questionable cases, aspiration of the hip joint yields only yellowish fluid with low protein and few if any neutrophils. Toxic synovitis of the hip

is rarely associated with elevation of the ESR, white blood cell count, or temperature above 38.3°C. It usually affects children aged 3–10 years and is more common in boys than girls. Motion of the hip joint is limited, particularly internal rotation, and radiographic changes are nonspecific, with some swelling apparent in the soft tissues around the joint.

Treatment consists of bed rest and mild traction with slight flexion of the hip. Nonsteroidal anti-inflammatory drugs shorten the course of the disease, although even with no treatment, the disease usually runs its course in days. Follow-up radiographs of the hip are important because toxic synovitis may be the precursor of avascular necrosis of the femoral head in a small percentage of patients. Radiographs can be obtained at 6 weeks, or earlier if either a persistent limp or pain is present.

Yagupsky P: Differentiation between septic arthritis and transient synovitis of the hip in children. J Bone Joint Surg Am 2005;87:459; author reply 459 [PMID: 15687174].

▼ VASCULAR LESIONS & AVASCULAR NECROSIS (OSTEOCHONDROSES)

ESSENTIALS OF DIAGNOSIS & TYPICAL FEATURES

▶ Diagnosis is made by characteristic radiographic findings.

▶ Radiographic resolution lags behind symptomatic resolution.

Osteochondrosis due to vascular lesions may affect several growth centers. Table 24–1 indicates the common sites and the typical ages at presentation. Although the pathologic and radiographic features of avascular necrosis of the epiphyses are well known, the cause is not generally agreed upon. Necrosis may follow trauma or infection, but idiopathic lesions are common and often occur during periods of rapid growth of the epiphyses.

In contrast to other body tissues that undergo infarction, infarcted bone heals by removal of necrotic tissue replacement with living bone in a process called creeping substitution. Replacement of necrotic bone may be so perfect that a completely normal bone results. Adequacy of replacement depends on the patient's age, the presence or absence of associated infection, the congruity of the involved joint, and other physiologic and mechanical factors.

Because of their rapid growth in relation to their blood supply, the secondary ossification centers in the epiphyses are very susceptible to avascular necrosis. Despite the number of different names referring to avascular necrosis of the epiphyses, the process is identical: necrosis of bone followed by replacement (see Table 24–1).

Table 24–1. The osteochondroses.

Ossification Center	Eponym	Typical Age (y)
Capital femoral	Legg-Calvé-Perthes disease	4–8
Tarsal navicular	Köhler bone disease	6
Second metatarsal head	Freiberg disease	12–14
Vertebral ring	Scheuermann disease	13–16
Capitellum	Panner disease	9–11
Tibial tubercle	Osgood-Schlatter disease	11–13
Calcaneus	Sever disease	8–9

AVASCULAR NECROSIS OF THE PROXIMAL FEMUR (LEGG-CALVÉ-PERTHES DISEASE)

The vascular supply of the proximal femur is precarious, and when it is interrupted, necrosis results.

▶ Clinical Findings

A. Symptoms and Signs

The highest incidence of Legg-Calvé-Perthes disease is between ages 4 and 8 years. Persistent pain is the most common symptom, and the patient may present with limp or limitation of motion.

B. Laboratory Findings

Laboratory findings, including studies of joint aspirates, are normal.

C. Imaging

Radiographic findings correlate with the progression of the process and the extent of necrosis. The early finding is effusion of the joint associated with slight widening of the joint space and periarticular swelling. Decreased bone density in and around the joint is apparent after a few weeks. The necrotic ossification center appears denser than the surrounding viable structures, and the femoral head is collapsed or narrowed.

As replacement of the necrotic ossification center occurs, rarefaction of the bone occurs in a patchwork fashion, producing alternating areas of rarefaction and relative density, referred to as "fragmentation" of the epiphysis.

In the hip, widening of the femoral head may occur associated with flattening, or coxa plana. If infarction has extended across the growth plate, a radiolucent lesion will be evident within the metaphysis. If the growth center of the femoral head has been damaged so that normal growth is arrested, shortening of the femoral neck results.

Eventually, complete replacement of the epiphysis develops as living bone replaces necrotic bone by creeping substitution. The final shape of the head depends on the extent of the necrosis and collapse of weakened bone.

▶ Differential Diagnosis

Differential diagnosis includes inflammation, infection, and dysplasia. Transient synovitis of the hip may be distinguished from Legg-Calvé-Perthes disease by serial radiographs.

▶ Treatment

The principle of treatment is protection of the joint. If the joint is deeply seated within the acetabulum and normal joint motion is maintained, a reasonably functional hip can result. Little benefit has been shown from bracing.

▶ Prognosis

The prognosis for complete replacement of the necrotic femoral head in a child is excellent, but the functional result depends on the amount of deformity that develops during the time the softened structure exists. In Legg-Calvé-Perthes disease, the prognosis depends on the extent of involvement of the epiphysial center. In general, patients with metaphysial defects, those in whom the disease develops late in childhood, and those who have more complete involvement of the femoral head have a worse prognosis.

Hesse B, Kohler G: Does it always have to be Perthes' disease? What is epiphyseal dysplasia? Clin Orthop 2003;414:219 [PMID: 12966296].

Joseph B et al: Natural evolution of Perthes disease: A study of 610 children under 12 years of age at disease onset. J Pediatr Orthop 2003;23:590 [PMID: 12960621].

OSTEOCHONDRITIS DISSECANS

In osteochondritis dissecans, a wedge-shaped necrotic area of bone and cartilage develops adjacent to the articular surface. The fragment of bone may be broken off from the host bone and displaced into the joint as a loose body. If it remains attached, the necrotic fragment may be completely replaced by creeping substitution.

The pathologic process is the same as that described previously for avascular necrosing lesions of ossification centers. Because these lesions are adjacent to articular cartilage, however, joint damage may occur. The most common sites of these lesions are the knee (medial femoral condyle), the elbow joint (capitellum), and the talus (superior lateral dome). Joint pain is the usual presenting complaint. However, local swelling or locking may be present, particularly if a fragment is free in the joint. Laboratory studies are normal.

Treatment consists of protecting the involved area from mechanical damage. If a fragment is free-floating within the joint, it must be removed. For some marginal lesions, it may be worthwhile to drill the necrotic fragment to encourage more rapid vascular ingrowth and replacement. If large areas of a weight-bearing joint are involved, secondary degenerative arthritis may result. Adolescents have less favorable outcomes with nonoperative therapy.

Wall E, Von Stein D: Juvenile osteochondritis dissecans. Orthop Clin North Am 2003;34:341 [PMID: 12974484].

NEUROLOGIC DISORDERS INVOLVING THE MUSCULOSKELETAL SYSTEM

ORTHOPEDIC ASPECTS OF CEREBRAL PALSY

Early physical therapy to encourage completion of the normal developmental patterns may benefit patients with cerebral palsy. The greatest gains from this therapy are obtained during the first few years of life, and therapy should not be continued when no improvement is apparent.

Bracing and splinting are of questionable benefit, although night splints may be useful in preventing equinus deformity of the feet or adduction contractures of the hips. Orthopedic surgery is useful for treating joint contractures that interfere with function. In general, muscle transfers are unpredictable in cerebral palsy, and most orthopedic procedures are directed at tendon lengthening or bony stabilization by osteotomy or arthrodesis.

Flexion and adduction of the hip due to hyperactivity of the adductors and flexors may produce a progressive paralytic dislocation of the hip, which can lead to pain and dysfunction. Treatment of this dislocation is difficult and unsatisfactory. The principal preventive measure is abduction bracing, but this must often be supplemented by release of the adductors and hip flexors in order to prevent dislocation. In severe cases, osteotomy of the femur may also be necessary to correct the bony deformities of femoral anteversion and coxa valga that are invariably present. Patients with a predominantly athetotic pattern are poor candidates for any surgical procedure or bracing.

Because it is difficult to predict the outcome of surgical procedures in cerebral palsy, the surgeon must examine patients on several occasions before any operative procedure is undertaken. Follow-up care by a physical therapist to maximize the anticipated long-term gains should be arranged before the operation.

Aiona MD, Sussman MD: Treatment of spastic diplegia in patients with cerebral palsy: Part II. J Pediatr Orthop B 2004;13:S13 [PMID: 15083127].
Sussman MD, Aiona MD: Treatment of spastic diplegia in patients with cerebral palsy. J Pediatr Orthop B 2004;13:S1 [PMID: 15076595].

ORTHOPEDIC ASPECTS OF MYELODYSPLASIA

Patients born with spina bifida cystica (aperta) should be examined early by an orthopedic surgeon. The level of neurologic involvement determines the muscle imbalance that will be present and apt to produce deformity with growth. The involvement is often asymmetrical and tends to change during the first 12–18 months of life. Early closure of the sac is the rule, although there has been some hesitancy to provide treatment to all of these patients because of the extremely poor prognosis associated with congenital hydrocephalus, high levels of paralysis, and associated congenital anomalies. A high percentage of these children have hydrocephalus, which may be evident at birth or shortly thereafter, requiring shunting. Associated musculoskeletal problems may include clubfoot, congenital dislocation of the hip, arthrogryposis-type changes of the lower extremities, and congenital scoliosis. The most common lesions are at the level of L3–4 and tend to affect the hip joint, with progressive dislocation occurring during growth. Foot deformities may be in any direction and are complicated by the fact that sensation is generally absent. Spinal deformities develop in a high percentage of these children, with scoliosis present in approximately 40%. Ambulation may require long leg braces. Careful urologic follow-up must be obtained to prevent complications from bladder dysfunction.

In children who have a reasonable likelihood of walking, operative treatment consists of reduction of the hip and alignment of the feet in the weight-bearing position as well as stabilization of the scoliosis. In children who lack active quadriceps function and extensor power of the knee, the likelihood of ambulation is greatly decreased. In such patients, aggressive surgery in the hip region may result in stiffening of the joints, thus preventing sitting. Multiple foot operations are also contraindicated in these children.

The overall treatment of the child with spina bifida should be coordinated in a multidisciplinary clinic where various medical specialists work with therapists, social workers, and teachers to provide the best possible care.

Mazur JM, Kyle S: Efficacy of bracing the lower limbs and ambulation training in children with myelomeningocele. Dev Med Child Neurol 2004;46:352 [PMID: 15132267].

NEOPLASIA OF THE MUSCULOSKELETAL SYSTEM

Neoplastic diseases of the musculoskeletal system are a serious problem because of the poor prognosis of malignant tumors arising in bone or other tissues derived from mesoderm. Fortunately, few of the benign lesions undergo malignant transformation. Accurate diagnosis depends on correlation of the clinical, radiographic, and microscopic findings. Complaints about the knee should be investigated for tumor, although the usual causes of knee pain are traumatic, infectious, or developmental in origin.

Lewis VO: Limb salvage in the skeletally immature patient. Curr Oncol Rep 2005;7:285 [PMID: 15946588].

OSTEOCHONDROMA

Osteochondroma is the most common bone tumor in children. It usually presents as a pain-free mass. When present, pain is caused by adventitious bursitis or tendinitis due to irritation by the tumor. The lesion may be single or multiple. Pathologically, the lesion is a bone mass capped with cartilage. These masses tend to grow during childhood and adolescence in proportion to the child's growth.

On radiograph, the tumors tend to be in the metaphysial region of long bones and may be pedunculated or sessile. The cortex of the underlying bone "flows" into the base of the tumor.

An osteochondroma should be excised if it interferes with function, is frequently traumatized, or is large enough to be deforming. The prognosis is excellent. Malignant transformation is very rare.

Bottner F et al: Surgical treatment of symptomatic osteochondroma: A three- to eight-year follow-up study. J Bone Joint Surg Br 2003;85:1161 [PMID: 14653600].

OSTEOID OSTEOMA

Osteoid osteoma classically produces night pain that can be relieved by nonsteroidal anti-inflammatory drugs. On physical examination there usually is tenderness over the lesion. An osteoid osteoma in the upper femur may cause pain referred to the knee.

On radiograph, the lesion is a radiolucent nidus surrounded by dense osteosclerosis that may obscure the nidus. Bone scan shows intense uptake in the lesion.

Surgical incision or radiofrequency ablation of the nidus is curative and may be done using computed tomography imaging and minimally invasive technique. The prognosis is excellent, with no known cases of malignant transformation, although the lesion has a tendency to recur.

ENCHONDROMA

Enchondroma is usually a silent lesion unless it produces a pathologic fracture. On radiograph it is radiolucent, usually in a long bone. A speckled calcification may be present. The classic lesion looks as though someone dragged his or her fingernails through clay, making streaks in the bones. Enchondroma is treated by surgical curettage and bone grafting. The prognosis is excellent. Malignant transformation may occur but is very rare in childhood.

CHONDROBLASTOMA

In chondroblastoma, the presenting complaint is pain around a joint. This neoplasm may produce a pathologic fracture. On radiograph, the lesion is radiolucent and usually located in the epiphysis. Calcification is unusual, with little or no reactive bone. The lesion is treated by surgical curettage and bone grafting. The prognosis is excellent if complete curettage is performed. There is no known malignant transformation.

Masui F et al: Chondroblastoma: A study of 11 cases. Eur J Surg Oncol 2002;28:869 [PMID: 12477480].

NONOSSIFYING FIBROMA

Nonossifying fibroma is also called benign cortical defect and is nearly always an incidental finding on radiograph. The most frequent sites are the distal femur and proximal tibia. Nonossifying fibroma is a radiolucent lesion eccentrically located in the bone. Usually a thin sclerotic border is evident. Multiple lesions may be present. No treatment is needed because these lesions heal as they ossify with maturation of the bone and growth.

OSTEOSARCOMA

In osteosarcoma, the presenting complaint is usually pain in a long bone, although functional loss, the mass of the tumor, or limp may be the complaint. Pathologic fracture is common. The malignant osseous tumor produces a destructive expanding and invasive lesion. A triangle may be adjacent to the tumor produced by elevated periosteum and subsequent tumor ossification. The lesion may contain calcification and violates the cortex of the bone. Femur, tibia, humerus, and other long bones are the sites usually affected.

Surgical excision (limb salvage) or amputation is indicated based on the extent of the tumor. The lesion is radioresistant and does not respond to radiation therapy. Adjuvant chemotherapy is routinely used prior to surgical excision. The prognosis is improving, with 60–70% long-term survival rates being reported in modern series. Death usually occurs as a result of lung metastasis.

DiCaprio MR, Friedlaender GE: Malignant bone tumors: Limb sparing versus amputation. J Am Acad Orthop Surg 2003;11:25 [PMID: 12699369].

EWING SARCOMA

In Ewing sarcoma, the presenting complaint is usually pain and tenderness. Fever and leukocytosis may also be present, which makes osteomyelitis the main differential diagnosis. The lesion may be multicentric. Ewing sarcoma is radiolucent and destroys the cortex, frequently in the diaphysial region. Reactive bone formation may occur about the lesion, seen as successive layers of so-called onion skin layering.

Treatment is with multiagent chemotherapy, radiation, and surgical resection. The prognosis is poor in patients with large tumor size, pelvic lesions, and poor response to chemotherapy.

▼ MISCELLANEOUS DISEASES OF BONE

FIBROUS DYSPLASIA

Dysplastic fibrous tissue replacement of the medullary canal is accompanied by the formation of metaplastic bone in fibrous dysplasia. Three forms of the disease are recognized:

monostotic, polyostotic, and polyostotic with endocrine disturbances (precocious puberty in females, hyperthyroidism, and hyperadrenalism [Albright syndrome]).

Clinical Findings

A. Symptoms and Signs

The lesion or lesions may be asymptomatic. Pain, if present, is probably due to pathologic fractures. In females, endocrine disturbances may be present in the polyostotic variety and associated with café-au-lait spots.

B. Laboratory Findings

Laboratory findings are normal unless endocrine disturbances are present, in which case secretion of gonadotropic, thyroid, or adrenal hormones may be increased.

C. Imaging

The lesion begins centrally within the medullary canal, usually of a long bone, and expands slowly. Pathologic fracture may occur. If metaplastic bone predominates, the contents of the lesion will be of the density of bone. The disease is often asymmetrical, and limb length disturbances may occur as a result of stimulation of epiphysial cartilage growth. Marked deformity of the bone may result, and a shepherd's crook deformity of the upper femur is a classic feature of the disease.

Differential Diagnosis

The differential diagnosis includes other fibrous lesions of bone as well as destructive lesions such as unicameral bone cyst, eosinophilic granuloma, aneurysmal bone cyst, nonossifying fibroma, enchondroma, and chondromyxoid fibroma.

Treatment & Prognosis

If the lesion is small and asymptomatic, no treatment is needed. If the lesion is large and produces or threatens pathologic fracture, curettage and bone grafting are indicated. Unless the lesions impair epiphysial growth, the prognosis for patients with fibrous dysplasia is good. Lesions tend to enlarge during the growth period but are stable during adult life. Malignant transformation is rare.

UNICAMERAL BONE CYST

Unicameral bone cyst occurs in the metaphysis of a long bone, usually in the femur or humerus. It begins within the medullary canal adjacent to the epiphysial cartilage. It probably results from some fault in enchondral ossification. The cyst is considered active as long as it abuts onto the metaphysial side of the epiphysial cartilage, and there is a risk of growth arrest with or without treatment.

When a border of normal bone exists between the cyst and the epiphysial cartilage, the cyst is inactive. The lesion is usually identified when a pathologic fracture occurs, producing pain. Laboratory findings are normal. On radiograph, the cyst is identified centrally within the medullary canal, producing expansion of the cortex and thinning over the widest portion of the cyst.

Treatment consists of curettage and bone grafting. The cyst may heal after a fracture.

Dormans JP, Pill SG: Fractures through bone cysts: Unicameral bone cysts, aneurysmal bone cysts, fibrous cortical defects, and nonossifying fibromas. Instr Course Lect 2002;51:457 [PMID: 12064135].

ANEURYSMAL BONE CYST

Aneurysmal bone cyst is similar to unicameral bone cyst, but it contains blood rather than clear fluid. It usually occurs in a slightly eccentric position in the long bone, expanding the cortex of the bone but not breaking the cortex. Involvement of the flat bones of the pelvis is less common. On radiographs, the lesion appears somewhat larger than the width of the epiphysial cartilage. This feature distinguishes it from unicameral bone cyst.

Chromosomal abnormalities have been associated with aneurysmal bone cyst. The lesion may appear aggressive histologically, and it is important to differentiate it from osteosarcoma or hemangioma. Treatment is by curettage and bone grafting. The prognosis is good.

INFANTILE CORTICAL HYPEROSTOSIS (CAFFEY SYNDROME)

Infantile cortical hyperostosis is a benign disease of unknown cause that has its onset before age 6 months and is characterized by irritability, fever, and nonsuppurating, tender, painful swellings. Swellings may involve almost any bone of the body and are frequently widespread. Classically, swellings of the mandible and clavicle occur in 50% of patients; swellings of the ulna, humerus, and ribs also occur. The disease is limited to the shafts of bones and does not involve subcutaneous tissues or joints. It is self-limited but may persist for weeks or months. Anemia, leukocytosis, an increased ESR, and elevation of the serum alkaline phosphatase concentration are usually present. Cortical hyperostosis is demonstrable by a typical radiographic appearance and may be diagnosed on physical examination by an experienced pediatrician.

Fortunately the disease appears to be decreasing in frequency. Indomethacin may be useful for treatment. The prognosis is good, and the disease usually terminates without deformity.

GANGLION

A ganglion is a smooth, small cystic mass connected by a pedicle to the joint capsule, usually on the dorsum of the wrist. It may also occur in the tendon sheath over the flexor surfaces of the fingers. These ganglia can be excised if they interfere with function or cause persistent pain.

BAKER CYST

A Baker cyst is a herniation of the synovium in the knee joint into the popliteal region. In children, the diagnosis may be made by aspiration of mucinous fluid, but the cyst nearly always disappears with time. Whereas Baker cysts may be indicative of intra-articular disease in the adult, they occur without internal derangement in children and rarely require excision.

Kocher MS et al: Meniscal disorders: Normal, discoid, and cysts. Orthop Clin North Am 2003;34:329 [PMID: 12974483].

25

Sports Medicine

Pamela E. Wilson, MD
K. Brooke Pengel, MD

Sports medicine as a separate discipline has grown since the 1980s in response to an expanding body of knowledge in the areas of exercise physiology, biomechanics, and musculoskeletal medicine. As more and more children participate in recreational and competitive activities, an understanding of sports medicine and developmental issues will be of major importance to pediatric health care providers.

▼ BASIC PRINCIPLES

The basic unit of the musculoskeletal system is the muscle fiber, which can be classified as slow twitch, fast twitch, or intermediate type. Slow twitch (type 1) fibers are usually smaller, are recruited in muscle contractions first, and are innervated by smaller motor neurons. Fast twitch (type 2) fibers make up white muscle and are usually larger. They are recruited when the body needs to produce rapid muscle tension. They produce more lactic acid than type 1 fibers. An intermediate (type 2a) fiber is called fast oxidative glycolytic, or FOG. Untrained individuals have a 50:50 proportion of type 1 to type 2 fibers. Elite long distance runners can have up to 90% type 1 fibers. This apparent adaptation raises a question as to whether an athlete is genetically programmed or can develop adaptations that allow success in sports.

Exercise generates cardiorespiratory system responses, including increased VO_2 max (maximum amount of oxygen that can be consumed), increased cardiac output, reduced resting heart rate, and improved blood pressure responses.

Biomechanics is the study of movement and how the forces generated by the neuromuscular system translate into movement. It integrates principles of both biology and physics. Through biomechanics we can understand the intricacies of movement and how these movements affect athletic performance and result in injuries.

Types of Muscle Contraction Associated with Exercise

Muscle contractions are divided into three types: isometric, isotonic, and isokinetic. An **isometric exercise** is exercise against a fixed load in which no movement is achieved. Isometric exercise improves strength at a given angle, but does not affect endurance. Isometric exercise is beneficial for therapy during the acute phase of an injury in which certain muscles or groups of muscles need strengthening. Isometric exercise can cause an increase in blood pressure and heart rate and should be used cautiously if a cardiac condition is present. **Isokinetic exercise** uses the concept of constant velocity and can provide maximal muscle contractions through full range of motion. This type of exercise generally requires special equipment. Lastly, **isotonic exercise** uses the principle of constant load and muscle length changes to strengthen muscles. It is the most common type of exercise and can be sport-specific. Isotonic exercises can be further classified as below:

A. Concentric Exercise

In concentric exercises, the force of muscle contraction overcomes an external resistance, which results in shortening of the muscle. These muscles accelerate a distal segment in the kinetic chain and are therefore referred to as open kinetic chain movements. An example of such an exercise is a biceps curl, during which the biceps is actively contracting or shortening to lift the weight.

B. Eccentric Exercise

In eccentric exercises, contractions increase muscle tension associated with lengthening of the muscle and are used to decelerate a distal segment in the kinetic chain. This type of exercise is exemplified by the squatting motion, in which the quadriceps lengthens under tension to control downward motion. If the terminal segment in the chain is fixed, this type of movement is called closed kinetic chain movement.

De Ste Croix M et al: Assessment and interpretation of isokinetic muscle strength during growth and maturation. Sports Med 2003;33:727 [PMID: 12895130].

Strength Training

Strength is defined as the peak force that can be generated during a single maximal contraction. Strength training uses progressive resistance to improve an athlete's ability to resist or exert force. This can be achieved by a variety of techniques, including body weight, free weight, or machine resistance. The benefits of weight training are improved performance, endurance, and muscular strength. Weight training can be started in prepubescent athletes and if designed appropriately can be done safely with minimal risk of injury. Tanner staging (see Chapter 32) helps to define readiness for progression to more strenuous programs. Power lifting and weight lifting should be restricted to athletes who have reached or passed Tanner stage V. Individuals at Tanner stage IV or less can safely participate in a strength training program that is specifically and carefully designed for younger athletes. These programs incorporate submaximal resistance with multiple repetitions. They can be generalized or sport-specific. Care should be taken to prevent injuries while using weight-training equipment at home. Children and adults with disabilities can benefit from weight-training programs modified to meet their specific needs.

Benjamin HJ, Glow KM: Strength training for children and adolescents: What physicians can recommend. Phys Sportsmed 2003;31:9.
Faigenbaum AD: Strength training for children and adolescents. Clin Sports Med 2000;19;4:593 [PMID: 11019731].
Guy JA, Micheli LJ: Strength training for children and adolescence. J Am Acad Orthop Surg 2001;9:29 [PMID: 11174161].

PREPARTICIPATION HISTORY & PHYSICAL EXAMINATION

The preparticipation medical examination evaluates and screens for potential medical problems that could occur during athletic participation. The objectives of this evaluation are to establish baseline medical information, detect any medical condition that might limit athletic participation, evaluate the athlete for preventable injuries, meet the legal or insurance requirements of most states, assess the athlete's maturity, and make recommendations for protective equipment. The ideal timing of the examination is at least 4–6 weeks before training starts. This allows time for any needed interventions by the physician.

Preparticipation History

The history is the most important part of the encounter. Many key elements need to be explored with the athlete. Standardized history forms are available both on the Internet and in monographs. Figure 25–1A is one example of the essential questions contained in a preparticipation history. The history must include the following areas:

A. Cardiovascular History

The physician should note any history of cardiac murmurs, chest pain at rest or with exertion, syncopal episodes or sudden fatigue, shortness of breath, or recent illnesses with chest pain. The family history should specifically ask about underlying cardiac diseases, including hypertrophic cardiomyopathy, prolonged QT syndrome, Marfan syndrome, arrhythmias, and sudden death in family members. These questions may help identify potentially life-threatening cardiac lesions. The most common causes of sudden death in young athletes on the playing field are hypertrophic cardiomyopathy and congenital heart lesions.

B. History of Hypertension

Any history of hypertension requires investigation. The current guidelines for the diagnosis of hypertension are blood pressure above 130/75 mm Hg in a child younger than age 10 years or blood pressure above 140/85 mm Hg in a child 10 years of age or older.

C. History of Chronic Diseases

Diseases such as reactive airway disease or exercise-induced asthma, diabetes, renal disease, liver disease, chronic infections, neurologic disorders, or hematologic diseases should be noted.

D. Musculoskeletal Limitations and Prior Injuries

The physician should explore limited range of motion and muscle weakness along with prior injuries that may affect future performance. Chronic pain or soreness long after activity may reflect overuse syndromes that should be evaluated.

E. Menstrual History in Females

The physician should pay particular attention to the so-called female athletic triad: amenorrhea, eating disorders, and osteoporosis.

F. Nutritional Issues

The physician should record methods the athlete uses to maintain, gain, or lose weight.

G. Medication History

This information will provide data on current medications whose side effects may suggest activity modifications. Also, documenting drug use may provide the opportunity to explore with the patient drawbacks of using performance-enhancing compounds such as anabolic steroids, creatine, stimulants, and narcotics.

PREPARTICIPATION HISTORY

Name _____ DOB _____ Age _____ Sex (M or F)

Primary Physician _____ Sports _____

Allergies (medications, latex, foods, bees, etc) _____

Medications (Include prescription, nonprescription, supplements and vitamins) _____

Answer questions by checking yes (Y)/no (N)/don't know (?)

	Y	N	?
General Health			
1. Have you had any injuries or illnesses?			
2. Have you ever been hospitalized?			
3. Do you think you are too thin or overweight?			
4. Have you ever used anything to gain or lose weight?			
5. Any problems exercising in the heat: heat cramps, heat exhaustion or heat stroke?			
6. Ever had frostbite?			
7. Any vision problems?			
8. Do you wear glasses, contact lens, or eye protection?			
9. Any dental appliances?			
10. Have you had any surgeries?			
11. Any organs missing?			
12. Immunizations (tetanus/hepatitis B) are they current?			
13. Any concerns about participating in sports?			
Cardiac/Respiratory History			
1. Has any family member died suddenly, had heart disease before age 50 or other heart problems?			
2. Do you have any dizziness, chest pain, a racing heart, or shortness of breath with exercise?			
3. Have you ever passed out?			
4. Do you have a heart murmur, high blood pressure, or any heart condition?			
5. Can you exercise as much as your friends?			
6. Any history of asthma, problems breathing, coughing with exercise?			
Neurologic History			
1. Any history of a head injury/concussion: being knocked out, dazed, or having memory loss?			
2. Have you ever had a seizure or convulsion?			
3. Any never problems: stingers, burners, pinched serves numbness?			
4. Any problems with headaches?			
Musculoskeletal History			
1. Do you have a history of sprains, strains or fractures?			
2. An hip, knee or ankle injuries?			
3. Any shoulder, elbow, wrist hand or finger injuries?			
4. Any back or neck problems?			
5. Ever have to be in a splint, east or use crutches?			
6. Do you use any special equipment when competing (braces, orthotics, pads etc)			
Females Only			
1. Any problems with menstruation: cramps, irregularity, etc.			
2. When was your last period? _____			

COMMENT ON YES ANSWERS

_____

_____

_____

_____

_____

▲ **Figure 25-1. A:** Preparticipation history.

PREPARTICIPATION PHYSICAL EXAM

Name _____

Date of birth/age _____

Height _____ Weight _____ BP_____

Pulse R wrist _____ L wrist _____ other _____

Vision K 20/ _____ L 20/ _____ (was it corrected Y or N)

GENERAL EXAM *(circle normal or abnormal and record results or the form)*

APPEARANCE	normal abnormal	
HEENT	normal abnormal	
LUNGS	normal abnormal	
HEENT & PULSES	normal abnormal	
GU	normal abnormal	
SKIN & LYMPH NODES	normal abnormal	
NEURO	normal abnormal	

MUSCULOSKELETAL EXAM *(record ROM or instabilities if abnormal)*

NECK	normal abnormal	
BACK	normal abnormal	
SHOULDERS	normal abnormal	
ELBOW & WRIST	normal abnormal	
HANDS & FINGERS	normal abnormal	
HIP	normal abnormal	
KNEE	normal abnormal	
ANKLE & FOOT	normal abnormal	

Cleared for sports: YES or NO If not cleared for sport **WHY**?_____

Further evaluation/rehab or/secondary clearance: _____

Signature examinee: _____ **Date** _____

▲ **Figure 25-1. B:** Preparticipation examination.

Armsey TD, Hosey RG: Medical aspects of sports: Epidemiology of injuries, preparticipation examination, and drugs in sports. Clin Sports Med 2004;23:255 [PMID: 15183571].

Burrows M et al: The components of the female athlete triad do not identify all physically active females at risk. J Sports Sci 2007;25:12 [PMID: 17786682].

Kutscher EC et al: Anabolic steroids: A review for the clinician. Sports Med 2002;32:285 [PMID: 11929356].

Physical Examination

The physical examination should be focused on the needs of the athlete. It may be the only time that an athlete has contact with medical personnel and can be used to promote wellness along with screening for physical activity. Figure 25–1B is an example of a preparticipation physical exam form. The examination should include routine vital signs, including blood pressure measurements obtained in the upper extremity. The cardiovascular examination should include palpation of pulses, auscultation for murmurs in both sitting and standing, and evaluation of the effects of exercise on the individual. The musculoskeletal examination is used to determine strength, range of motion, flexibility, and previous injuries. Included is a quick guide that can be used to screen for abnormalities in this area (Table 25–1). The remainder of the examination should emphasize the following areas:

A. Skin

Are there any contagious lesions such as herpes or impetigo?

B. Vision

Are there any visual problems? Is there any evidence of retinal problems? Are both eyes intact?

C. Abdomen

Is there any evidence of hepatosplenomegaly?

D. Genitourinary System

Are any testicular abnormalities or hernias present?

E. Neurologic System

Are there any problems with coordination, gait, or mental processing?

F. Sexual Maturity

What is the individual's Tanner stage?

Recommendations for Participation

After completing the medical evaluation the physician can make recommendations about sports clearance. The options are unrestricted participation, limited participation, or no

Table 25–1. The screening sports examination.[a]

General evaluation	Have patient stand in front of examiner; evaluate both front and back along with posture.
	Look at general body habitus.
	Look for asymmetry in muscle bulk, scars, or unusual postures.
	Watch how patient moves when instructed.
Neck evaluation	Evaluate range of motion (ROM) by having patient bend head forward (chin to chest), rotate from side to side, and laterally bend (ear to shoulder).
	Observe for asymmetry, lack of motion, or pain with movement.
Shoulder and upper extremity evaluation	Observe clavicles, shoulder position, scapular position, elbow position, and fingers.
	ROM screening:
	Fully abduct arms with palms in jumping jack position.
	Internally and externally rotate shoulder.
	Flex and extend wrist, pronate and supinate wrist, flex and extend fingers.
	Do the following manual muscle testing:
	Have patient shrug shoulders (testing trapezius).
	Abduct to 90 degrees (testing deltoid).
	Flex elbow (testing biceps).
	Extend elbow over head (testing triceps).
	Test wrist flexion and extension.
	Have patient grasp fingers.
Back evaluation	General inspection to look for scoliosis or kyphosis.
	ROM screening:
	Bend forward touching toes with knees straight (spine flexion and hamstring range).
	Rotation, side bending, and spine extension.
Gait and lower extremity evaluation	General observation while walking.
	Have patient walk short distance normally (look at symmetry, heel-toe gait pattern, look at all joints involved in gait and leg lengths, any evidence of joint effusions or pain).
	Have patient toe-walk and heel-walk for short distance and check tandem walking (balance beam walking).

[a]If any abnormalities are found, a more focused evaluation is required.

participation. Table 25–2 is a composite of recommendations for sports participation organized by body system. In addition, recommendations for sports participation based on medical conditions can be found on the web site and in the journal of the American Academy of Pediatrics (AAP).

Ansved T: Muscular dystrophies: Influence of physical conditioning on the disease evolution. Curr Opin Clin Nutr Metab Care 2003;6:435 [PMID: 12806128].

Birrer RB, Sedaghat V: Exercise and diabetes mellitus: Optimizing performance in patients who have type 1 diabetes. Phys Sportsmed 2003;31:29.

Braith RW: Exercise for those with chronic heart failure. Phys Sportsmed 2002;30:29.

Committee on Sports Medicine and Fitness, American Academy of Pediatrics: Medical conditions affecting sports participation. Pediatrics 2001;107:1205 [PMID: 11331710].

Disabella V, Sherman C: Your guide to exercising with asthma. Phys Sportsmed 1998;26:85.

Draznin MB: Type 1 diabetes and sports participation: Strategies for training and competing safely. Phys Sportsmed 2000; 28:49.

Firoozi S et al: Risk of competitive sport in young athletes with heart disease. Heart 2003;89:710 [PMID: 12807837].

Howard GM et al: Epilepsy and sports participation. Curr Sports Med Rep 2004;3:15.

Howe WB: Preventing infectious disease in sports. Phys Sportsmed 2003;31:23.

MacKnight JM: Infectious mononucleosis: Ensuring safe return to sport. Phys Sportsmed 2002;30:27.

Maron BJ: Hypertrophic cardiomyopathy: Practical steps for preventing sudden death. Phys Sportsmed 2002a;30:19 [PMID: 11984027].

Maron BJ: The young competitive athlete with cardiovascular abnormalities: Causes of sudden death, detection by pre-participation screening, and standards for disqualification. Card Electrophysiol Rev 2002b;6:100.

Moeller JL: Contraindications to athletic participation: Spinal, systemic, dermatologic, paired-organ, and other issues. Phys Sportsmed 1996;24:56.

O'Kane JW: Upper respiratory infection. Phys Sportsmed 2002; 30:39.

Platt LS: Medical and orthopaedic conditions in Special Olympics athletes. J Athl Train 2001;36:74 [PMID: 16404438].

Primos WA: Sports and exercise during acute illness: Recommending the right course for patients. Phys Sportsmed 1996;24:44.

Salim MA, Alpert BS: Sports and Marfan syndrome. Phys Sportsmed 2001;29:80.

Tarnopolsky MS: Metabolic myopathies and physical activity: When fatigue is more than simple exertion. Phys Sportsmed 2002;30:37.

Terrell T et al: Blunt trauma reveals a single kidney: A disqualification dilemma. Phys Sportsmed 1997;25:75.

Vinger PF: A practical guide for sports eye protection. Phys Sportsmed 2000;28:49.

Winell J, Burke SW: Sports participation of children with Down syndrome. Orthop Clin North Am 2003;34:439 [PMID: 12975593].

REHABILITATION OF SPORTS INJURIES

Participation in sports can have great benefits. It provides physical activity, acquisition of motor skills, and social opportunities. All sports participation, however, carries an inherent risk of injuries. These injuries are classified as either acute or chronic. Chronic injuries occur over time and are related to repetitive stress. These injuries develop in response to overuse, repeated microtrauma, and inadequate repair of injured tissue. Acute injuries or macrotrauma are one-time events that can cause alterations in biomechanics and physiology.

Response to an acute injury occurs in two predictable phases. The first week is characterized by an acute inflammatory response. During this time initial vasoconstriction is followed by vasodilation. Chemical mediators of inflammation are released, resulting in the classical physical findings of local swelling, warmth, pain, and loss of function. This phase is essential in healing of the injury. The proliferative phase occurs over the next 2–4 weeks and involves repair and clean-up. Fibroblasts infiltrate and lay down new collagen. Lastly, the maturation phase allows for repair and regeneration of the damaged tissues.

The management of acute sports injuries is geared toward optimizing healing and restoring function. The goals of immediate care are to minimize the effects of the injury by reducing pain and swelling, to educate the athlete about the nature of the injury and how to take care of it, and to maintain the health of the rest of the body. The treatment for an acute injury is captured in the acronym **PRICE:**

- **P**rotect the injury from further damage (taping, splints, braces)
- **R**est the area
- **I**ce
- **C**ompression of the injury
- **E**levation immediately

Nonsteroidal anti-inflammatory drugs (NSAIDs) reduce the inflammatory response and reduce discomfort. These medications may be used immediately after the injury. Glucocorticoids should be administered judiciously. If administered inappropriately they may prolong the acute phase of recovery. Therapeutic use of physical modalities, including early cold and later heat, hydrotherapy, massage, electrical stimulation, iontophoresis, and ultrasound, can enhance recovery in the acute phase.

The recovery phase can be lengthy and requires athlete participation. Initial treatment is focused on joint range of motion and flexibility. Range-of-motion exercises should follow a logical progression of starting with passive motion, then moving to active assistive, and finally to active movement. Active range of motion is initiated once normal joint range has been reestablished. Flexibility exercises are sport-specific and aimed at reducing tight musculature. Strength training can begin early in this phase of rehabilitation. Initially only isometric exercises are encouraged. As recovery progresses and flexibility increases, isotonic and isokinetic exercises can be added to the program. These should be done at least three times per week.

Table 25–2. Recommendations and considerations for participation in sports.

Disorders	Considerations and Recommendations	References
Cardiac		
Anticoagulation treatment	Need to avoid all contact sports	
Aortic stenosis	Individualize treatment based on disease and systolic gradient: 　Mild: < 20 mm Hg, all sports if asymptomatic. 　Moderate: limited sports. 　Severe: no competitive sports.	
Arrhythmias	Consult with cardiologist as WPW and long QT syndrome can have serious consequences.	
Heart failure	Screen patient with LVEF < 30% for ischemia. Use AHA risk stratification criteria to define exercise capacity.	Braith 2002
Heart implants	No jumping, swimming, or contact sports.	
Hypertrophic cardiomyopathy	Single most common cause of cardiac death in young athletes. Athletes should not participate in sports except possibly low-intensity forms (eg, golf, bowling). Consult with cardiologist.	Maron 2002a, b
Marfan syndrome	Aortic root dilation is associated with mitral valve prolapse and regurgitation. Participate in sports with minimal physical demands.	Salim et al 2001
Mitral valve prolapse	Fairly common condition. No restrictions unless there is a history of syncope, positive family history of sudden death, arrhythmias with exercise, or moderate regurgitation.	
Syncope	Unexplained syncopal episodes during exercise must be evaluated by ECG, echocardiograph, Holter, and tilt test prior to resumption of any activities.	Firoozi 2002
Endocrine		
Diabetes mellitus type 1	No restrictions to activity, however: 　Short-term exercise = no insulin changes. 　Vigorous exercise = 25% reduction in insulin with 15–30 g of carbohydrates before and every 30 min during exercise. 　Strenuous exercise = may require up to an 80% reduction in insulin with extra carbohydrates. Generally monitor blood glucose closely.	Birrer et al 2003, Draznin 2000
Eye		
Detached retina	Do not participate in strenuous sports regardless of contact risk.	Moeller 1996
One eye	Consider avoiding contact sports, although if patient does participate use of eye protection is mandatory.	Vinger 2000
Gentitourinary		
One testicle	Need to wear protective cups in collision and contact sports.	
Solitary kidney	Advise not to participate in collision and contact sports.	Terrell 1997
Hematologic		
Hemophilia	Avoid contact and collision sports.	
Sickle cell trait	No restrictions if disorder is well controlled. Athletes should avoid dehydration and acclimate to altitude. There is, however, a known association between exercise and sudden death.	
Infectious disease		
General considerations	Fevers: should not participate in activities with moderate fevers; exercise affects fluid balance, immune system function, and temperature regulation. Intense exercise may worsen or prolong some viral illnesses.	Howe 2003, Primos 1996

(continued)

Table 25–2. Recommendations and considerations for participation in sports. *(Continued)*

Disorders	Considerations and Recommendations	References
Enterovirus	Coxsackievirus causes respiratory and GI symptoms but more importantly can cause myocarditis. Anyone with systemic symptoms such as fever or myalgias should avoid strenuous exercise.	Primos 1996
Herpes simplex, impetigo, tinea corpora	Close contact is required for transmission; use common-sense guidelines. For contact sports participation should not be allowed until lesions are crusted over or healed.	Moeller 1996
Infectious mononucleosis	Splenic rupture is most important consideration. Risk of spleen rupture highest during second and third weeks of illness. No athletic participation for a minimum of 21 days! Splenic ultrasounds should be considered in decision making. Too early a return to sports could cause EBV reactivation and relapse. First week of return to activity should be noncontact. Graded increases in intensity if fatigue tolerance is improved. Return to full activity if: no abdominal pain, normal spleen, and normal laboratory results.	MacKnight 2002
Sinusitis	Similar considerations as cold (see below) except diving should be restricted until symptoms resolve.	
Streptococcus A	Restrict from activity until afebrile and on antibiotics for > 24 h	O'Kane 2002
Upper respiratory infections (including common cold)	"Neck check," with symptoms (fevers, myalgias, arthralgias, etc) above the neck participation can be allowed; however, if they migrate below that level activity should be limited.	Primos 1996
Neurologic		
Epilepsy	Majority of sports are safe for those with good seizure control; contact sports are allowed with proper protection. Definitely wear a helmet. Fitness may reduce number of seizures. Swimming and water sports should be supervised. Sports such as free climbing, hang gliding, and scuba are not recommended.	Howard 2004
Herniated disk (with cord compression)	Avoid contact and collision sports.	
Muscle disease or myopathy	Exercise within physical limits. Low- to moderate-intensity activity is appropriate for patients with slow progressive disorders. Patients with disorders that are rapidly progressing should avoid high-resistance and eccentric muscle activity. Modification of exercise with intercurrent illness.	Tarnopolsky 2002, Ansved 2003
Spinal stenosis	Avoid contact and collision sports.	
Orthopedic		
Scoliosis	No restrictions unless severe.	
Spondylolisthesis	Grade 2 and above should avoid high-risk sports.	
Spondylolysis	Pars intra-articularis stress fracture. No restrictions if pain-free.	
Respiratory		
Asthma	No activity restrictions. Use common sense about when to use medications.	Disabella et al 1998
Pneumothorax	Can occur in sports, especially in males. Increased risk for recurrence; should consider not participating in strenuous and contact sports.	
Tuberculosis	Not allowed to participate because of exposure to other athletes.	

(continued)

Table 25–2. Recommendations and considerations for participation in sports. *(Continued)*

Disorders	Considerations and Recommendations	References
Other		
Cerebral palsy	Full participation with modifications.	
Developmental disabilities	Athletes with developmental disabilities often have associated medical problems including diabetes, obesity, and hypokinesia.	Platt 2001
Down syndrome	10–20% have atlantoaxial instability.	Platt 2001, Winell 2003
	All athletes need to be cleared with a lateral view radiograph including flexion and extension.	
	If abnormal no contact sports should be allowed.	
	Evaluation of underlying congenital heart disorders should be considered in this population.	
Spinal cord injury or spina bifida	Full participation.	
	Consider modification of equipment to accommodate activity or modification of activity to accommodate disability.	
	Consider how modification affects performance.	
	Be aware of thermoregulatory dysfunction, medications, and pressure areas.	

AHA, American Heart Association; EBV, Epstein-Barr virus; ECG, electrocardiogram; GI, gastrointestinal; LVEF, left ventricular ejection fraction; WPW, Wolff-Parkinson-White syndrome.

As the athlete approaches near-normal strength and is pain-free, the final maintenance phase can be introduced. During this phase the athlete continues to build strength and work on endurance. The biomechanics of sport-specific activity need to be analyzed and retraining incorporated into the exercise program. Generalized cardiovascular conditioning should continue during the entire rehabilitation treatment.

COMMON SPORTS MEDICINE ISSUES & INJURIES

INFECTIOUS DISEASES

Infectious diseases are common in both recreational and competitive athletes. These illnesses have an effect on basic physiologic function and athletic performance. Given this knowledge, physicians, parents, and coaches can adopt the common-sense guidelines listed in Table 25–3.

Rihn JA et al: Community-acquired methicillin-resistant *Staphylococcus aureus*: An emerging problem in the athletic population. Am J Sports Med 2005;33:1924 [PMID: 16314668].

HEAD & NECK INJURIES

Head and neck injuries occur most commonly in contact and individual sports. The sports with the highest incidences of brain injury are football, bicycling, baseball, horseback riding, and golf. The treatment of these injuries is controversial, and multiple guidelines have been developed. As a general rule, however, treatment of injuries in young chil-

dren should be as conservative as possible because of their developing central nervous systems.

1. Concussion

Concussion is a temporary and immediate impairment of neurologic function and may or may not have an associated period of unconscious. It is usually defined by the duration of the loss of consciousness (LOC), post-traumatic

Table 25–3. Sports participation guidelines: infectious diseases.

Athletes with temperatures > 100°F should not participate in sporting activities.

Athletes who have had recent infectious mononucleosis can return to noncontact training at 3 wk as long as there is no splenic enlargement. They may return to contact sports after 4 wk and a normal abdominal examination.

Athletes with a streptococcal pharyngitis can resume activity once treatment has been initiated and they are afebrile.

If a localized herpes gladiatorum or impetigo lesion is present, no contact sports are allowed until the lesions have resolved. Athletes with herpes zoster have the same restrictions. There are no restrictions for athletes with common warts. Athletes with molluscum contagiosum can compete if the affected areas are covered. Athletes with furuncles cannot be involved in contact sports or swimming until the lesions are healed.

Athletes with HIV infection may compete in all types of sports. Universal precautions should be used with all athletes who have sustained injuries.

amnesia (PTA), and confusion. The pathophysiology is related to alterations in brain metabolism and the release of neurotransmitters.

Concussions have been categorized by many different grading systems, but recent consensus recommends all athletes should be removed from play until symptoms have resolved. Once symptoms have resolved a six-step progression is outlined for return to play: (1) assess at rest; once asymptomatic progress to (2) light aerobic exercise, followed by (3) sport-specific exercise, then begin (4) noncontact drills followed by (5) contact drills, and finally (6) release to game play. If any symptoms are present, the athlete should not move to the next step.

Preseason testing may help practitioners in assessing acute concussive status. Among commonly used assessment tools are the Standardized Assessment of Concussion (SAC), Balance Error Scoring System (BESS), computerized testing, and symptoms checklist (Table 25–4). Neuropsychology testing is advocated for athletes with persistent symptoms. Recent findings related to multiple concussions in athletes indicate that one concussion episode places an athlete at a higher risk for a repeat concussion, and that children with repeat concussions may have more severe injuries with protracted recovery times. In general, conservative return to play guidelines should be used in children.

2. Second Impact Syndrome

Second impact syndrome is a rare but potentially deadly complication of head injuries. Athletes who have had a prior brain injury that has not healed and have a second injury are at risk for a loss of vascular autoregulation and subsequent malignant cerebral edema.

3. Atlantoaxial Instability

Atlantoaxial instability is common in children with Down syndrome because of underlying ligamentous laxity, including the annular ligament of C1, and hypotonia. Cervical neck films including flexion, extension, and neutral position eval-

Table 25–4. Concussion: symptom checklist.

Headache
Dizziness
Balance problems
Nausea
Vomiting
Light sensitivity
Noise sensitivity
Ringing in the ears
Fatigue or excessive sleepiness
Sleep abnormalities
Memory problems
Concentration difficulties
Irritability
Behavioral changes

uate the atlanto-dens interval (ADI). ADI is normally less than 2.5 mm, but up to 4.5 mm is acceptable in this population. Children with an ADI greater than 4.5 mm should be limited from contact and collision activities.

Dimberg EL: Management of common neurologic conditions in sports. Clin Sports Med 2005;24:637 [PMID: 16004923].
Patel DR: The pediatric athlete with disabilities. Pediatr Clin North Am 2002;49:803 [PMID: 12296534].
Winell J: Sports participation of children with Down syndrome. Orthop Clin North Am 2003;34:439 [PMID: 12974493].

4. Burners & Stingers

ESSENTIALS OF DIAGNOSIS & TYPICAL FEATURES

▶ Symptoms appear on the same side as an injury to the neck and shoulder.
▶ Burning pain or numbness in the shoulder and arm.
▶ Weakness may be present.

Burners and stingers are common injuries in contact sports, especially football. These types of cervical radiculopathies or brachial plexopathies occur when the head is laterally bent and the shoulder depressed. Symptoms include immediate burning pain and paresthesias down one arm generally lasting only minutes. Weakness in the muscles of the upper trunk—supraspinatus, deltoid, and biceps—can persist for weeks. The most important part of the workup is a thorough neurologic assessment to differentiate this injury from a serious cervical spine injury. The key distinguishing feature of the stinger is its unilateral nature. If symptoms persist, then a diagnostic evaluation should include cervical spine radiographs, magnetic resonance imaging (MRI) scans, and electromyography.

Treatment consists of removal from play and observation. The athlete can return to play once symptoms have resolved, neck and shoulder range of motion is pain-free, reflexes and strength are normal, and the Spurling test is negative. Preventative strategies include always wearing protective gear, proper blocking and tackling techniques, and maintaining neck and shoulder strength.

Weinberg, J et al: Etiology, treatment and prevention of athletic stingers. Clin Sports Med 2003;22:3 [PMID: 12852682].

SPINE INJURIES

Injuries to the spine are fairly common even in the pediatric population. As children have become more competitive in sports, the number of reported injuries has increased. Sports with a fairly high incidence of back injuries include golf, gymnastics, football, dance, wrestling, and weightlifting. Pain lasting more than 2 weeks indicates a possible structural problem and needs to be investigated.

Acute injury to the spine often results from an axial load injury. Patients present with focal tenderness of the thoracic or thoracolumbar spine. Evaluation includes plain radiography that may demonstrate mild wedging of the thoracic vertebra. When significant spinal tenderness or any neurological abnormalities are present, radiographs are often followed by computed tomography (CT) or MRI. Treatment of minor compression fractures includes pain control, bracing, rest from high-risk sports, and physical therapy. With appropriate rehabilitation, athletes can usually return to contact activity within 8 weeks.

1. Spondylolysis

ESSENTIALS OF DIAGNOSIS & TYPICAL FEATURES

▶ Injury to the pars interarticularis.
▶ Usually presents as back pain with extension.

Spondylolysis is an injury to the pars interarticularis. Pars defects are present in 4–6% of the population. The percentage of pars defects in athletes such as gymnasts, dancers, divers, and wrestlers is significantly increased. Repetitive overload results in stress fractures. Spondylolysis occurs at L5 in 85% of cases. The athlete presents with back pain that is aggravated by extension, such as arching the back in gymnastics. There may be palpable tenderness over the lower lumbar vertebrae, along with pain on the single leg hyperextension test. Tight hamstrings are another common physical examination finding. Evaluation includes anteroposterior (AP) and lateral radiographs of the lumbar spine. Although oblique radiographic views of the lumbar spine are helpful to look for the so-called Scottie dog sign, they are falling out of favor because they often fail to show the lesion. Single photon emission computed tomography scan, CT scan, and MRI can be useful to determine the presence of an active spondylolytic lesion.

Treatment includes refraining from hyperextension and high-impact sporting activities, stretching of the hamstrings, stabilization exercises, and lumbosacral bracing. Athletes can cross-train with low-impact activity and neutral or flexion-based physical therapy. Return to play is often delayed 6 weeks or longer based on clinical signs of healing. Surgery is reserved for refractory cases.

2. Spondylolisthesis

When a bilateral pars injury occurs, slippage of one vertebra over another causes a spondylolisthesis. These injuries are graded from 1 to 4 based on the percentage of slippage: grade 1 (0–25%), grade 2 (25–49%), grade 3 (50–74%), and grade 4 (75–100%). Patients present with hyperlordosis, kyphosis, pain with hyperextension, and in severe cases, a palpable step-off. Diagnosis is based on lateral radiographs.

Treatment is often symptom based. Asymptomatic athletes with less than 30% slippage have no restrictions and are followed on a routine basis. Slippage of 50% or more requires interventions of stretching hip flexors and hamstrings, working on core stability, along with bracing or surgery. If surgery is required, the athlete must understand that he or she cannot return to activities for at least a year and may not be able return to previous sporting activities.

3. Disk Herniation

Discogenic back pain accounts for a small percentage of back injuries in children. These injuries are almost unheard of in preadolescence. Back pain can originate from disk herniation, apophyseal injury, and disk degeneration. Most injuries occur at L4–L5 and L5–S1 vertebrae. Symptoms include back and leg pain. Pain may be increased with activities such as bending, sitting, and coughing. Pain often radiates down the lower extremity in a radicular pattern. Evaluation includes physical and neurologic examinations, including straight leg testing, sensory testing, and checking reflexes. If symptoms persist, evaluation includes electromyography, CT, and MRI scans.

Treatment usually is conservative as most back injuries improve spontaneously. The athlete can rest the back for a short period and then begin a structured exercise program of extension and isometrics followed by flexion exercises. If symptoms persist, a short course of steroids may be indicated. Surgery is recommended only if neurologic compromise persists.

Eddy D et al: A review of spine injuries and return to play. Clin J Sport Med 2005;15:453 [PMID: 16278551].
Herman MJ: Spondylolysis and spondylolisthesis in the child and adolescent athlete. Orthop Clin North Am 2003;34:461 [PMID: 12974495].

SHOULDER INJURIES

Shoulder injury is usually a result of acute trauma or chronic overuse. Acute injuries around the shoulder include contusions, fractures, sprains (or separations), and dislocations. The age of the patient affects the injury pattern, as younger patients are more likely to sustain fractures instead of sprains.

1. Fracture of the Clavicle

Clavicular fractures occur from a fall or direct trauma to the shoulder. Focal swelling and tenderness are present over the clavicle. Diagnosis is made by radiographs of the clavicle; the fractures are most common in the middle third of the bone.

Initial treatment is focused on pain control and protection with a sling and swathe. Early range of motion is permitted, based on pain level. Progressive rehabilitation is important. Athletes cannot return to contact sports for 8–10 weeks. Surgical indications for acute clavicular fractures include open fractures or neurovascular compromise. Fracture nonunion is unusual in young patients, but older adolescents with recurrent fractures or nonunion occasionally undergo surgical fixation.

2. Acromioclavicular Separation

A fall on the point of the shoulder is the most common cause of acromioclavicular separation. Tearing of the acromioclavicular joint capsule and possibly the coracoclavicular ligaments occurs. The injury is classified by the extent of the injuries to these ligaments. Athletes present with focal soft tissue swelling and tenderness over the acromioclavicular joint. More severe injuries are associated with deformity. Patients have a positive cross-arm test, in which pain is localized to the acromioclavicular joint. Radiographs are helpful to assess the degree of injury and to evaluate for a coexisting fracture.

Treatment is supportive, with rest and immobilization in a sling followed by progressive rehabilitation. Return to activity can be accomplished in 1–6 weeks depending on the severity of the injury. Full range of motion and full strength must be achieved.

3. Fracture of the Humerus

Fractures of the humerus occur from a severe blow or fall on the shoulder. Pain and swelling are localized to the proximal humeral region. The fractures can include the physes or may be extraphyseal. Some amount of displacement and angulation can be tolerated in this location because of the young athlete's potential for remodeling. Careful assessment of the brachial plexus and radial nerves are needed to rule out associated nerve damage.

Treatment consists of a sling for 4–6 weeks followed by progressive rehabilitation.

4. Acute Traumatic Anterior Shoulder Instability (Anterior Shoulder Dislocation/Subluxation)

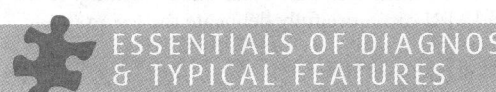

ESSENTIALS OF DIAGNOSIS & TYPICAL FEATURES

▶ Injury with an abducted and externally rotated arm.
▶ Severe pain in the shoulder.
▶ Squared-off shoulder on examination.
▶ Reduced range of motion of the shoulder

Acute traumatic anterior shoulder instability occurs from a significant force applied to the abducted and externally rotated shoulder. Most often, the humeral head is dislocated in an anterior and inferior direction. The patient has severe pain and a mechanical block to motion. Patients require immediate closed reduction. Radiographs are

helpful to confirm the position of the humeral head as well as to evaluate for coexisting fracture. MRI may be required for accurate visualization of fractures and cartilaginous injury.

Follow-up treatment for a glenohumeral dislocation in young athletes is controversial. Initially, the shoulder is immobilized for comfort. Range-of-motion exercises and progressive rehabilitation are initiated. Because of the high risk of recurrence, options for treatment should be individualized, with consideration given to both nonoperative and surgical management.

5. Rotator Cuff Injury

ESSENTIALS OF DIAGNOSIS & TYPICAL FEATURES

▶ Injury can be acute or chronic.
▶ Pain is described as diffuse or anterior and lateral.
▶ Overhead activities exacerbate the pain.

Numerous shoulder injuries are related to repetitive overuse and tissue failure. Rotator cuff injuries are common in sports requiring require repetitive overhead motions. Muscle imbalances and injury can cause the position of the humeral head to be abnormal, which may cause impingement of the supraspinatus tendon under the acromial arch. Patients with nontraumatic shoulder instability due to ligamentous and capsular laxity (also known as multidirectional instability) are prone to overuse rotator cuff injury. The athlete presents with a chronic history of pain in the anterior and lateral shoulder, which is increased with overhead activities. Diagnostic workup includes plain radiographs and an outlet view to look for anatomic variability.

The rehabilitation of this injury is geared toward reduction of inflammation, improved flexibility, core stabilization, and strengthening of the scapular stabilizers and rotator cuff muscles. A biomechanics evaluation can assist athletes in the recovery process by building sport-specific skills and eliminating substitution patterns.

6. Little League Shoulder

ESSENTIALS OF DIAGNOSIS & TYPICAL FEATURES

▶ Participation in a throwing sport.
▶ Pain with throwing.
▶ Pain in the lateral aspect of the humerus.
▶ Swelling around the shoulder.
▶ Widening of the proximal humeral physis on radiographs.

Proximal humeral epiphysitis, or "Little League shoulder," is an overuse injury that occurs in children aged 11–14 years who play overhead sports such as baseball. The patient presents with activity-related pain in the lateral aspect of the proximal humerus. Examination often shows tenderness over the proximal humerus. However, benign findings on office examination do not preclude this diagnosis. The hallmark feature is pain with throwing. Radiographs show widening, sclerosis, and irregularity of the proximal humeral physis. Comparison views are often helpful when considering this diagnosis.

Treatment consists of rest from throwing or other aggravating activity. Physical therapy is initiated during the rest period. Return to play can only be accomplished after a period of rest has significantly decreased the pain and the athlete has proceeded through a progressive throwing program. Healing can take several months. Signs of radiographic healing may lag behind the athlete's clinical progress, and normal radiographs are not necessarily required to return an athlete to play.

Sciascia A et al: The pediatric overhead athlete: What is the problem? Clin J Sports Med 2006;16:6 [PMID: 17119360].
Wasserlauf BF: Shoulder disorders in the skeletally immature throwing athlete. Orthop Clin North Am 2003;34:427 [PMID: 12974492].

ELBOW & FOREARM INJURIES

Injuries in the forearm are quite common with both chronic and acute etiologies (eg, the chronic overuse "Little League elbow" and the frequent childhood fracture typical of falls on an outstretched arm). When evaluating the elbow, consider dividing the examination into specific anatomic areas as discussed below.

1. Medial Epicondylitis

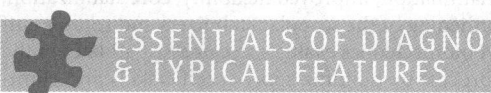

ESSENTIALS OF DIAGNOSIS & TYPICAL FEATURES

▶ Participation in a throwing sport.
▶ Pain over the medial condyles, especially with pitching.
▶ Swelling medial elbow.
▶ Elbow flexion contracture.

Medial epicondylitis, often called Little League elbow, encompasses a group of abnormalities that develop in young baseball pitchers secondary to the biomechanical forces generated around the elbow during throwing. These forces can result in shearing, inflammation, traction, and abnormal bone development. The symptoms are primarily swelling, pain, performance difficulties, and weakness. The pain localizes to the medial epicondyle, which may be tender to palpation. Wrist flexion and pronation increase symptoms. Workup includes a series of elbow radiographs, including comparison films, to look for widening of the epiphyseal lines and possibly MRI studies.

Treatment of the acute injury includes rest from throwing. It is not uncommon for a player to be benched for up to 6 weeks. Competition can be resumed once the player is asymptomatic. The key to treating this injury is prevention. Children should be properly conditioned and coached in correct throwing biomechanics. Guidelines for pitching limits in youth baseball have been developed. Little League limits 10- to 12-year-old children to 6 innings per week and 13- to 15-year-old children to 9 innings per week. Guidelines for limiting pitches per game are outlined in Table 25–5.

2. Panner Disease

Panner disease refers to variations in the normal ossification of the capitellum. This condition occurs in children aged 5–12 years who play sports that involve overhead throwing. The child may have dull aching in the lateral elbow that generally worsens when throwing. Swelling and reduced elbow extension usually are present. Radiographs show an abnormal capitellum, with fragmentation and areas of sclerosis.

Treatment is conservative, using rest, ice, and splinting. The child can return to play after radiographs normalize. The natural history of this condition is one of complete resolution of symptoms and ultimately normal ossification of the capitellum.

3. Osteochondritis Dissecans

Lateral elbow pain in a slightly older throwing athlete, usually aged 13–15 years, can be secondary to osteochondritis dissecans. Valgus compressive forces can lead to avascular necrosis of the capitellum, which can result in the formation of loose bodies. The athlete presents with lateral pain, swelling, lack of full extension, and occasionally locking. Radiographs and MRI can more fully delineate the lesion.

Table 25–5. Guidelines for pitching limits in youth baseball.

Age (years)	Pitches per Game[a]
8–10	52 ± 15
11–12	68 ± 18
13–14	76 ± 16
15–16	91 ± 16
16–17	106 ± 16

[a]Based on 2 games per week.

Treatment is based on classification and can be either conservative or surgical. The child should be seen by an orthopedic specialist with expertise in upper extremity injuries.

4. Lateral Epicondylitis

Lateral epicondylitis is common in skeletally mature athletes participating in racquet sports, particularly tennis. It is an overuse of the extensor muscle in the forearm and causes pain in the lateral elbow. Pain is increased by wrist extension.

Initial treatment is aimed at inflammation control. Stretching and strengthening of forearm muscles are the primary interventions during the subsequent phases. Stroke mechanics may need to be altered and a forearm brace used to decrease the forces in the extensor muscles.

5. Posterior Elbow Pain

Posterior elbow pain is uncommon. Etiologies include dislocations, fractures, triceps avulsions, olecranon apophysitis, and olecranon bursitis.

Benjamin HJ et al: Little League elbow. Clin Sports Med 2005;15:1 [PMID: 15654190].
Gerbino PG: Elbow disorders in throwing athletes. Orthop Clin North Am 2003;34:417 [PMID: 12974491].
Hang DW et al: A clinical and roentgenographic study of Little League elbow. Am J Sports Med 2004;32:79 [PMID: 14754727].

HAND & WRIST INJURIES

All hand and wrist injuries have the potential for long-term, serious disability and deserve a thorough evaluation.

1. Distal Phalanx Injury

Tuft injury requires splinting for 6 weeks or until the patient is pain-free. If there is significant displacement, then a K-wire can be used for reduction. **Nail bed injury** often requires splinting and drainage of subungual hematomas.

2. Distal Interphalangeal Injury

Mallet finger or **extensor tendon avulsion** occurs in ball-handling sports. The mechanism of injury is a force applied to an extended finger. Treatment is splinting in extension for 6 weeks for fractures and 8 weeks for tendon rupture.

3. Thumb Injury

Gamekeeper's thumb is an injury to the ulnar collateral ligament from forced abduction of the metacarpophalangeal joint. It is a common skiing injury. If a radiograph shows an avulsed fragment is displaced less than 2 mm, a thumb spica cast can be used. If there is no fragment and less than 35 degrees of lateral joint space opening, a spica cast for 6 weeks is indicated. Surgery is required for more serious injuries.

4. Fractures

Boxer's fracture is a neck fracture of the fifth digit. These fractures can be treated by closed reduction and casting for 3 weeks. A displaced fracture requires open reduction and internal fixation.

5. Wrist Injury

Most swollen wrists without evidence of instability can be splinted for several weeks. Radial and ulnar fractures, which are fairly common in children, must be ruled out. **Scaphoid fractures** are caused by a force applied to a hyperextended wrist. If evidence of snuffbox tenderness and swelling is present, the wrist must be immobilized for 10 days and then reassessed, even if radiographs are normal. A nondisplaced fracture requires at least 6 weeks of immobilization in a thumb spica cast. Nonunion can occur, particularly in fractures of the proximal pole of the scaphoid, and is related to the poor blood supply to this carpal bone. Displacement requires operative management.

Brook S et al: The management of scaphoid fractures. J Sci Med Sports 2005;8:181.
Geissler WB: Carpal fractures in athletes. Clin Sports Med 2001;20:167 [PMID: 11227704].
Wang QC, Johnson BA: Fingertip injuries. Am Fam Physician 2001;63:1961 [PMID: 11388710].

HIP INJURIES

Because the pelvis and hip articulate with both the lower extremities and the spine, this area is rich in ligaments, muscle attachments, and nerves. Injuries in young children are rare, but sprains, strains, and avulsion fractures are common. Additionally, athletes can be susceptible to overuse injury involving the hip.

1. Hip Avulsion Fractures

 ESSENTIALS OF DIAGNOSIS & TYPICAL FEATURES

▶ Fractures at apophyseal areas.
▶ Pain with weight bearing.
▶ Focal pain over the site of injury.

Avulsion fractures around the hip in adolescents occur at apophyseal regions such as the ischial tuberosity, anterior superior iliac spine, anterior inferior iliac spine, and iliac crest. The mechanism of injury is a forceful, unbalanced muscle contraction that causes avulsion of the muscle tendon insertion. The athlete presents with a history of an acute traumatic incident; often a "pop" is felt and the athlete is immediately unable to bear weight. Range of motion of the hip is limited secondary to pain, and focal tenderness is present over the apophysis.

Treatment is conservative. It is rare for surgery to be required even in displaced fractures. The athlete can progress to weight bearing as tolerated. The rehabilitation phase focuses on regaining motion, flexibility training, and pelvic and core strengthening. Progressive return to activity can often be accomplished in 4–6 weeks if full range of motion, full strength, and sport-specific skills have been achieved.

2. Slipped Capital Femoral Epiphysis

▸ Pain in the hip or knee, or both.
▸ Loss of internal rotation of the hip.
▸ Radiographs in the frog-leg position show widening of the physis and epiphyseal slippage.

Slipped capital femoral epiphysis can occur in children aged 11–16 years. The physis is weakened during times of rapid growing and is susceptible to shearing failure. Patients complain of groin, thigh, or knee pain and often have a limp. Examination shows painful range of motion of the hip, limited internal rotation, and obligatory external rotation when the hip is flexed. Radiographs include AP and frog-leg lateral films, which demonstrate widening of the physis and the epiphyseal slippage.

Treatment consists of immediate non–weight bearing and urgent referral to an orthopedic specialist for open reduction and internal fixation. Rehabilitation is a component of the postsurgical treatment, and return to activity is progressive over months. (See also Chapter 24.)

3. Acetabular Labral Tears

Acetabular labral tears cause anterior hip pain. The injury often occurs from a twisting injury of the hip that tears the fibrocartilaginous ring around the acetabulum. Athletes present with deep anterior hip or groin pain that worsens with activity and is resistant to treatment. Radiographic findings can be normal. An MRI arthrogram is used to demonstrate the tear. Treatment starts conservatively and requires rest. Arthroscopy is reserved for recalcitrant cases.

4. Adductor Strain

An adductor strain or a groin pull is generally caused by forced abduction as in running, falling, twisting, or tackling. Sports that require quick directional changes place the athlete at risk for these types of injuries. The associated pain is in the adductor muscle. There is often pain with adduction or hip flexion and tenderness over the adductor tubercle.

Treatment includes rest, ice, protection, and strengthening of the muscle when it heals. In severe cases the leg can be immobilized in a spica cast until the muscle has a chance to heal.

5. Hamstring Strain

Hamstring strain is a common injury in athletes. The mechanism of injury is forced extension of the knee or directional changes. The classic scenario is an athlete who suddenly stops play, grabbing the back of the knee. There are three grades of injury. Examination reveals pain on palpation of the muscle. Pain also occurs with knee flexion against resistance.

Initial treatment is focused on minimizing swelling, bruising, and pain. The thigh should be iced and compression applied. In moderate and severe injuries crutches may be needed for a short duration. The athlete can walk as soon as he or she can tolerate the activity. It is particularly important to stretch the hamstring because, as a two-joint muscle, it is more susceptible to injury than other types of muscle. Eccentric strengthening is an important component of rehabilitation.

6. Quadriceps Contusion

Quadriceps contusion is caused by a direct injury to the muscle, resulting in bruising, swelling, and pain. The amount of damage is directly related to the amount of force. The anterior and lateral thigh regions are most commonly injured often in contact sports such as football and lacrosse.

Treatment is rest, ice, and protection for the first 24 hours. The knee should be kept in a fully flexed position. Two to three days after the injury, range-of-motion exercises may begin in both flexion and extension. Once 120 degrees of motion has been established and movement does not cause pain, the athlete may return to competitive activity. If the muscle remains firm on examination after 2 weeks, then radiographs of the thigh should be obtained to rule out myositis ossificans. **Myositis ossificans** is an abnormal deposition of calcium in the muscle that may be induced by aggressive stretching of the muscle too early in the clinical course.

7. Hip Dislocation

▸ Usually produces posterior dislocation.
▸ Leg is flexed, adducted, and externally rotated.
▸ Hip pain is severe.
▸ This is an on-site emergency and must be treated quickly.

The hip joint can be dislocated in forceful injuries. Most hip dislocations occur in the posterior direction. Athletes with this injury classically present with hip flexion, adduction, and internal rotation. Hip dislocations in skeletally mature athletes are almost always associated with acetabular and femoral neck fracture. The preadolescent, skeletally immature competitor may have an isolated injury. Hip radiographs and CT scan may be needed to completely evaluate the injury.

This is a true on-field emergency, and the athlete should be transported to the nearest facility that has an orthopedic surgeon available. Severe bleeding, avascular necrosis, and nerve damage can result. Once reduction has been established in an uncomplicated case, protected weight bearing on crutches for 6 weeks is recommended followed by another 6 weeks of range-of-motion and strengthening exercises. An athlete may return gradually to competition after 3 months, when strength and motion are normal.

8. Pelvic Apophysitis

Pelvic apophysitis occurs in adolescent athletes who are typically competitive and are participating consistently, often year round, in their sport. Common locations are the ischial tuberosity and iliac crest. The athlete presents with pain over the apophysis and pain with resisted hip motion specific to the muscle insertion. Radiographs can show irregularity over the apophysis, or be normal. Treatment consists of relative rest, progressive rehabilitation focusing on flexibility, and pelvis and core stabilization.

9. Iliotibial Band Syndrome

Iliotibial band syndrome and associated trochanteric bursitis can cause pain when the hip is flexed, often as a result of reduced flexibility of the iliotibial band and gluteus medius tendons. The bursa is a structure that allows for improved motion by reducing friction. When a bursa becomes inflamed, movement is painful and may be limited. Other areas susceptible to inflammation, besides the hip, are the shoulder, elbow, and patella. Iliotibial band syndrome is best evaluated in a side-lying position, and pain is reproduced when the hip is actively flexed from a fully extended hip (Ober test).

Initial treatment is to alter the offending activity and then start a stretching program geared at the iliotibial band and hip abductors. Ultrasound is beneficial and corticosteroid injections may be used after conservative treatment has failed.

10. Femoral Neck Fractures

Femoral neck fractures (stress fractures) are generally the result of repetitive microtrauma. They commonly occur in running athletes who have increased their mileage. Athletes with this type of injury present with persistent pain in the groin and pain with internal and external rotation. Range of motion may be limited in hip flexion and internal rotation. If plain radiographs are negative, an MRI or a bone scan is indicated.

Treatment is based on the type of fracture. A transverse fracture generally requires internal fixation to prevent femoral displacement and the risk of avascular necrosis. A compression fracture is less likely to be displaced; treatment is conservative and involves resting the hip until it heals. Cardiovascular conditioning can be maintained easily through nonimpact exercises and activity.

Cooper DE: Severe quadriceps muscle contusions in athletes. Am J Sports Med 2004;32:820 [PMID: 15090402].
Maffulli N: Lower limb injuries in children in sports. Clin Sports Med 2000;19:637 [PMID: 11019733].

KNEE INJURIES

Knee injuries are one of the most common sports-related problems. The knee is stabilized through a variety of ligaments, tendons, and the menisci. Knee injuries can be divided into two groups: those resulting from acute or chronic causes. Acute injuries occur from a well-defined traumatic incident. The mechanism of injury is an important historical feature, although many young patients have difficulty describing the details of the inciting event. The onset of rapid swelling after a traumatic event indicates the presence of a hemarthrosis and likely internal derangement such as fracture, rupture of the anterior cruciate ligament (ACL), meniscal tear, or patellar dislocation.

1. Anterior Knee Pain

The most common knee complaint is anterior knee pain. This complaint can have multiple etiologies but should always include hip pathology as a possible source. Patellofemoral dysfunction is a common cause of anterior knee pain. The differential diagnosis is quite extensive and requires a thorough examination.

A. Patellofemoral Overuse Syndrome

Patellofemoral overuse syndrome occurs in runners and in athletes participating in sports that involve repetitive stress in the lower extremity. The athlete presents with activity-related pain in the anterior knee. Classically, pain is located over the medial surface and undersurface of the patella. In young athletes, it is infrequently associated with swelling and crepitus of the knee joint. The Q-angle often is increased. The Q-angle is measured by drawing a line from the antero-superior iliac spine down to the center of the patella and then through the tibial tubercle. The intersecting angle is the Q-angle. Normal is 14 degrees for males and 17 degrees for females. Q-angles greater than 20 degrees tend to cause the patella to track laterally, changing the knee biomechanics.

Treatment should be geared toward identifying the cause. Often athletes are overtraining and need to modify their current activities. Cross-training may help. Stretching and strengthening of the hamstrings and quadriceps are recommended. Use of braces providing proprioceptive feedback during competition is controversial.

B. Patellar Tendonitis ("Jumper's Knee")

This overuse injury is caused by repetitive loading of the quadriceps during running or jumping. This diagnosis is common in basketball and volleyball athletes. Tenderness is located directly over the patellar tendon.

C. Osgood-Schlatter Disease (Tibial Tubercle Apophysitis)

This condition is caused by the recurrent traction on the muscle-tendon unit that occurs in jumping and running sports. Fragmentation and microfractures of the tibial tubercle occur during its time of rapid growth. The condition occurs in the preteen and adolescent years and is most common in boys aged 12–15 years and girls aged 11–13 years. Pain usually is present at the tibial tubercle, and is aggravated by activities using eccentric quadriceps muscle movement. The pain can become so extensive that routine activity must be curtailed. Radiographs typically demonstrate fragmentation or irregular ossification of the tibial tubercle.

Typically the condition resolves on its own. In the interim, pain control using NSAIDs is indicated. Stretching the hamstrings and application of ice after workouts is helpful.

D. Sinding-Larsen-Johansson Disease (Apophysitis of the Inferior Pole of the Patella)

This condition involves a process similar to that in Osgood-Schlatter disease, but occurring in younger athletes, usually between ages 9 and 12 years. Traction from the patellar tendon results in fragmentation of the inferior patella that is often obvious on a lateral knee radiograph.

▶ Treatment

As with many injuries, control of pain and inflammation is essential. This begins with relative rest from offending activity and ice. Alignment problems and mechanics across the anterior knee can be improved with an effective rehabilitation program that includes flexibility and strengthening. Quadriceps, pelvic, and core strengthening are all important components of this program. Orthotics, in theory, can have an impact on mechanics across the knee joint if they correct excessive pronation or supination.

Knee bracing is controversial, and the major benefits are proprioceptive feedback and patellar tracking. Return to activity is often based on symptoms.

2. Posterior Knee Pain

Posterior knee pain usually results from an injury to the gastrocnemius-soleus complex caused by overuse. It can also include a Baker cyst, tibial stress fracture, or tendonitis of the hamstring. Treatment is rest, ice, and strengthening exercises after symptoms have improved.

3. Meniscal Injuries

ESSENTIALS OF DIAGNOSIS & TYPICAL FEATURES

▶ Posterior knee pain.
▶ Effusion and joint line tenderness.
▶ Feeling of locking or of the knee giving way.
▶ Positive McMurray test.

The meniscus of the knee cushions forces in the knee joint, increases nutrient supply to the cartilage, and stabilizes the knee. Most injuries are related to directional changes on a weight-bearing extremity. **Medial meniscus injuries** have a history of tibial rotation in a weight-bearing position. This happens frequently in ball-handling sports. **Lateral meniscus injuries** occur with tibial rotation with a flexed knee, as in exercises such as squatting or certain wrestling maneuvers. These injuries are uncommon in children younger than age 10 years.

▶ Clinical Findings

The athlete with such an injury has a history of knee pain, swelling, snapping, or locking or may report a feeling of the knee giving way. Physical examination often reveals swelling, joint line tenderness, and a positive McMurray hyperflexion-rotation test. The diagnostic test of choice is MRI of the knee, although standard knee radiographs should be included.

▶ Treatment

Treatment may be symptomatic for minor, isolated injuries of the meniscus that do not involve a mechanical block. Persistent loss of motion and other signs of meniscal damage suggest meniscal impingement and require more urgent referral for surgical management. Surgery is also indicated in failure of conservative care within 4–6 weeks of the injury. If surgery is needed, weight bearing may not be allowed, depending on the amount of meniscal damage and the type of repair required. Typically, however, range-of-motion and strengthening exercises can be resumed quickly, and return to play can be achieved within 4–6 weeks.

4. Medial & Lateral Collateral Ligament Injuries

ESSENTIALS OF DIAGNOSIS & TYPICAL FEATURES

▶ Pain on the medial or lateral portion of the knee.
▶ Tenderness along the ligament.
▶ Positive valgus stress test at 0 and 30 degrees.

The medial and lateral collateral ligaments are positioned along either side of the knee and act to stabilize the knee during varus and valgus stress. Medial injuries occur either with a blow to the lateral aspect of the knee, as seen in a football tackle, or with a noncontact rotational stress.

▶ Clinical Findings

The athlete may feel a "pop" or lose sensation along the medial aspect of the knee. The examination reveals an effusion and tenderness medially. A valgus stress test performed in 20–30 degrees of flexion reproduces pain.

Medial collateral ligament injuries are graded on a scale of 1 to 3. Grade 1 injuries represent a stretching injury. Grade 2 injury involves partial disruption of the ligament. Grade 3 injury is a complete disruption of the ligament. Radiographs are useful, especially in the skeletally immature athlete, to evaluate for distal femoral or proximal tibial bone injury. MRI scans are used if grade 3 injury or concomitant intra-articular derangement is suspected.

▶ Treatment

Treatment is almost always conservative. Initial injuries should be iced and elevated. A protective brace needs to be worn, and full knee motion in the brace can be permitted within a few days. Weight bearing is allowed, and a strengthening program can be started. The athlete should use the brace until the pain and range of motion have improved. The use of a functional brace is often required when a player returns to competition. Bracing is temporary, until the ligament heals properly and the athlete has no subjective feelings of instability.

5. Anterior Cruciate Ligament Injuries

ESSENTIALS OF DIAGNOSIS & TYPICAL FEATURES

- ▶ Pain and effusion of the knee.
- ▶ Pain along the anterior joint line.
- ▶ Positive Lachman test.

The ACL consists of three bands that prevent anterior subluxation of the tibia. It is injured by deceleration, twisting, and cutting motions. The mechanism of injury involves force applied to the knee during hyperextension, with excessive valgus stress and forced external rotation of the femur on a fixed tibia.

▶ Clinical Findings

The athlete often reports hearing or feeling a "pop," followed by swelling that occurs within hours of the injury. Evaluation of the knee begins with examination of the uninjured knee.

The Lachman test provides the most accurate information about knee stability in relation to the ACL. All other structures of the knee need to be examined to rule out concomitant injuries. Imaging of the knee includes plain radiographs along with an MRI scan. In skeletally immature athletes, a tibial spine avulsion is often seen on radiographs rather than a midsubstance ACL tear.

▶ Treatment

Initial treatment focuses on controlling swelling and pain management. Structured physical therapy can be instituted early to assist in regaining range of motion and strength. Treatment options include both conservative and surgical management. Conservative treatment includes bracing, strengthening, and restricting physical activity. Knee braces enhance proprioception and control terminal extension. Conservative management can be complicated by continued instability and damage to meniscal cartilage. Recent advances in surgical treatment of the skeletally immature athlete have been helpful in dealing with the complicated management of young athletes with ACL tears.

Surgical repair is typically indicated for young athletes in cutting sports and is also required for persistent instability. Surgery can be performed 2–6 weeks following the injury if the swelling and motion in the knee have improved. Rehabilitation of the knee starts immediately after surgery. A continuous passive range-of-motion machine is used postoperatively. Partial weight bearing is allowed in a brace that is set in full extension as the quadriceps strengthen. After 2 weeks, partial weight bearing and walking are started. The goals of the subsequent program are continued strength, muscle reeducation, endurance, agility, and coordination. Return to cutting and pivoting sports can be achieved by 6 months after surgery.

6. Posterior Cruciate Ligament Injuries

ESSENTIALS OF DIAGNOSIS & TYPICAL FEATURES

- ▶ Pain and swelling of the posterior knee.
- ▶ Increased pain with knee flexion.
- ▶ Positive posterior Drawer test.

The posterior cruciate ligament (PCL) runs from the medial femoral condyle to the posterior tibial plateau and has two parts. Its main function is to prevent posterior tibial subluxation. Injury to the PCL is uncommon; it occurs when the individual falls on a flexed knee with the ankle in plantarflexion or with forced hyperflexion of the knee. The most common sports in which PCL injuries are sustained are football and hockey.

Clinical Findings

The athlete presents with swelling and pain in the posterior and lateral knee. The examination begins with the uninjured knee and proceeds to the injured side. Confirmatory testing includes the posterior drawer test, performed with the patient supine, the knee flexed to 90 degrees, and the foot stabilized. Grading is based on the amount of translation. Grade 1 (mild) is up to 5 mm, grade 2 (moderate) is 5–10 mm, and grade 3 (severe) is more than 10 mm. Diagnostic imaging includes plain radiographs and MRI scan.

Treatment

Treatment can be determined as soon as the exact injury has been isolated. Treatment is controversial with respect to surgical versus nonsurgical management, although nonsurgical management is gaining popularity as outcomes tend to be similar for both groups.

Braces and a progressive rehabilitation program have been used successfully in athletes with grade 1 and 2 injuries. Athletes with grade 3 injuries and chronic instability may require surgery.

Andrish JT: Anterior cruciate ligament injuries in the skeletally immature patient. Am J Orthop 2001;30:103 [PMID: 11234936].

Guigliano DN et al: ACL tears in female athletes. Phys Med Rehabil Clin N Am 2007;18:3 [PMID: 17678760].

Kyist J: Rehabilitation following anterior cruciate ligament injury: Current recommendations for sports participation. Sports Med 2004;34:269 [PMID: 15049718].

FOOT & ANKLE INJURIES

Injuries in the lower leg, ankle, and foot are quite common in pediatric athletes. The types of injuries sustained tend to depend on the age group. Young children tend to have diaphyseal injuries, in contrast to older children in rapid growth, who tend to have epiphyseal and apophyseal injuries. Skeletally mature adolescents are prone to adult-pattern ligamentous injury.

Although fractures of the ankle are possible with inversion and eversion mechanisms, the most common acute injury involving the ankle is the ankle sprain.

1. Ankle Sprain

ESSENTIALS OF DIAGNOSIS
& TYPICAL FEATURES

▶ Mechanism is usually inversion and plantarflexion.

▶ Swelling and pain in the ankle over the ligament.

▶ Bruising over the ankle.

When a ligament is overloaded tearing occurs. These injuries are graded on a scale of 1 to 3. Grade 1 injury is a stretch without instability, grade 2 is a partial tear with some instability, and grade 3 is a total disruption of the ligament with instability of the joint. The ankle has three lateral ligaments (anterior talofibular, calcaneofibular, and posterior talofibular) and a medial deltoid ligament. Inversion of the foot generally damages the anterior talofibular ligament, whereas eversion injures the deltoid ligament. Lateral ankle sprains are far more common than medial ankle sprains because the deltoid ligament is stronger, mechanically, than the lateral ligaments.

Clinical Findings

Physical examination often reveals swelling, bruising, and pain. Diagnostic testing should be done when a bony injury is suspected. Obtaining radiographs is especially important when evaluating skeletally immature athletes who are more prone to growth plate injury.

The adult Ottawa criteria do not pertain to patients younger than age 18 years. Tenderness over the malleoli, tenderness beyond ligament attachments, and excessive swelling are reasons to obtain radiographs.

Differential Diagnosis

Other injuries to consider include injuries to the fifth metatarsal, which can occur with an inversion mechanism. In this injury, the athlete presents with localized swelling and tenderness over the base of the fifth metatarsal. Fractures at the base of the fifth metatarsal can be divided into avulsion, Jones, and diaphyseal fractures. Tibiofibular syndesmosis tear occurs with dorsiflexion and external rotation. Radiographs are required, and the squeeze teat is positive. Fractures of the malleoli, fibula, talar dome or calcaneus may also mimic ankle sprain.

Treatment

Appropriate treatment of ligamentous ankle injuries is imperative to ensure full recovery and should begin immediately after the injury. Phase 1 care involves immediate compressive wrapping and icing to control swelling and inflammation. Protected weight bearing is allowed in the early phase of rehabilitation. Phase 2 begins when the athlete can ambulate without pain. During this time ankle range of motion is emphasized, along with isometric contractions of the ankle dorsiflexors. Once 90% of strength has returned, active isotonic (eccentric and concentric exercises) and isokinetic exercises can be added. Phase 3 is designed to increase strength, improve proprioception, and add ballistic activity. The "foot alphabet" and "tilt board" are excellent methods to improve ankle proprioception. This program can be effective in returning athletes to activity within a few weeks, although up to 6 weeks may be required for return to full activity. The athlete should wear a protective brace for 3–4 months and continue to ice after exercising.

2. Sever Disease

Sever disease, or calcaneal apophysitis, occurs in athletes aged 9–12 years who are involved in high-impact activities such as gymnastics and soccer. Pain occurs at the point of muscle tendon insertion onto the growth center of the calcaneus. The athlete presents with activity-related heel pain, and examination reveals focal tenderness over the apophysis. Treatment consists of relative rest, heel cord stretching, ice massage and NSAIDS for pain control, and progression to activity as tolerated based on pain level.

3. Plantar Fasciitis

Plantar fasciitis is a common problem that manifests as heel pain in the adolescent or older athlete. It typically occurs in runners who log more than 30 miles per week and in athletes who have tight Achilles tendons or wear poorly fitting shoes. It is also common in people with cavus feet and in those who are overweight. The pain is worse upon first standing up in the morning and taking a few steps. A bone spur is often found on examination.

Treatment involves local massage, stretching of the gastrocsoleus, NSAIDs, arch supports, and local steroid injections. Runners may need to cut back on their weekly mileage until these measures eliminate pain.

Bahr R: Prevention of ankle sprains in adolescent athletes. Clin J Sports Med 2007;17:4 [PMID: 17620800].

Osborne MD, Rizzo TD Jr: Prevention and treatment of ankle sprains in athletes. Sports Med 2003;33:1145 [PMID: 14719982].

Verhagen E et al: The effects of a proprioceptive balance board training program for the prevention of ankle sprains: A proprioceptive controlled trial. Am J Sports Med 2004;32:1385 [PMID: 15310562].

PREVENTION

As in all activities, most sports-related injuries can be prevented by the use of protective equipment, common sense, and proper training. Protective equipment should be properly fitted and maintained by an individual with training and instruction. Helmets should be used in football, baseball, hockey, bicycling, skiing, in-line skating, skateboarding, or any sport with risk of head injury. Eye protection should be used in sports that have a high incidence of eye injuries. Proper protective padding should be identified and used, including chest pads for catchers; shin guards in soccer; shoulder, arm, chest, and leg padding in hockey; and wrist and elbow protectors in skating. A few common-sense concepts should be addressed by coaches, parents, and physicians in order to ensure the safety of children participating in sports. These include inspecting playing fields for potential hazards, adapting rules to the developmental level of the participants, and matching opponents equally.

The use of the preparticipation history and physical examination, described earlier, can identify potential problems and allow for prevention and early intervention. Proper training techniques reduce injuries by encouraging flexibility, promoting endurance, and teaching correct biomechanics. Sports education reinforces the concepts of fitness and a healthy lifestyle along with sport-specific training. Early identification of an injury allows the athlete to modify techniques and avoid micro- and macrotrauma. Once an injury has occurred, it needs to be identified properly and appropriate measures used to minimize inflammation. Rehabilitation of the injury starts as soon as it has been identified. Early and appropriate care offers the athlete an optimal chance for full recovery and return to full participation.

Rehabilitation Medicine

Pamela E. Wilson, MD

Gerald H. Clayton, PhD

Rehabilitation medicine is the multispecialty discipline involved in the diagnosis and therapy of individuals with congenital and acquired disabilities. The overarching goals are to maximize the patient's functional capabilities and improve quality of life. Disabilities are described using the World Health Organization's International Classification of Function, Health, and Disability. Three aspects require evaluation in every patient: (1) the impact of the disability on body structure and function, (2) the impact of the disability on activity and participation, and (3) the environmental factors with an impact on patient function. Evaluation of these three areas provides a common framework for discussing a disabling condition and the impact it has on the body and on the individual's ability to participate in society.

PEDIATRIC BRAIN INJURY

General Considerations

Every year there are an estimated 400,000 emergency department visits for brain injuries among children from birth through 14 years of age, with 3000 deaths and 29,000 hospitalizations. Children with brain injuries may have long-term deficits and disabilities that require identification and treatment. Brain injury is divided into primary and secondary injury.

Primary injury refers to the immediate injury causing focal or diffuse damage. *Focal damage* includes skull fracture, parenchymal bruising or contusion, extraparenchymal or intraparenchymal hemorrhage, blood clots, tearing of blood vessels, or penetrating injury. *Diffuse damage* includes diffuse axonal injury and edema. Consequences of primary injury, either focal or diffuse, include cellular disruption with release of excitatory amino acids, opiate peptides, and inflammatory cytokines.

Secondary injury refers to the loss of cellular function accompanying primary injury that results in loss of cerebrovascular regulation, altered cellular homeostasis, or cell death and functional dysregulation. A primary injury can initiate the processes of secondary programmed cell death (apoptosis), which further exacerbates the primary injury. Secondary injury may develop hours or days after the initial insult. It appears to be precipitated by elevated intracranial pressure, cerebral edema, and release of neurochemical mediators.

Clinical Classification & Severity Scores for Head Injury

Traumatic brain injury is usually categorized as open or closed. *Open* injuries are the result of penetration of the skull by missile or sharp object, or deformation of the skull with exposure of the underlying intracranial tissues. *Closed* injuries occur secondary to blunt trauma to the head, which causes movement (intracranial acceleration or deceleration and rotational forces) and compression of brain tissue. Brain contusions are referred to as *coup* (occurring at the site of injury) or *contra-coup* (occurring on the side of the brain opposite the injury). Measures for rating severity of injury and eventual outcomes are important in medical management. Included below are several common scales:

A. Glasgow Coma Scale

The Glasgow Coma Scale (GCS) is the most commonly used system to assess the depth and duration of impaired consciousness in the acute setting. The score is derived from three different areas of evaluation: motor responsiveness (maximum score 6), verbal performance (maximum score 5), and eye opening to stimuli (maximum score 6). The scale has been modified for use in infants and children younger than 5 years of age, allowing for their lack of verbal responsiveness and understanding (see Table 11–5). Cumulative scores on the GCS define injury as mild (13–15), moderate (9–12), and severe (≤ 8). The concept of post-traumatic amnesia is used to gauge severity of injury and is an adjunct to the GCS, termed the GCS-E (extended). Post-traumatic amnesia is defined as the period of time after an injury during which new memory cannot be incorporated and the person appears confused or disoriented. Amnesia can be retrograde, anterograde, or both.

B. Rancho Los Amigos Levels of Cognitive Function

The Rancho Los Amigos Levels of Cognitive Function (LCFS or "Rancho") is commonly used to gauge the overall severity of cognitive deficit and can be used serially during recovery as a rough gauge of improvement. The scale has 10 levels of functioning ranging from "no response" to "purposeful, appropriate."

C. Coma/Near Coma Score

The coma/near coma (CNC) score is a gauge of depth of coma for those with severe brain injury. It serves as a sensitive measure of clinical changes in sensory, perceptual, and primitive responses. Serial assessment of the patient's coma status with the CNC can provide a means to track recovery and assess the potential for active participation in therapy.

Common Sequelae of Brain Injury

Depending on the severity of brain injury, there may be deficits in cognition and behavior, and a variety of physical impairments. Injuries can also produce changes in sensory and motor function, emotional stability, social behavior, mental processing speed, memory, speech, and language. The consequences of mild brain injuries may be difficult to discern. Small intraparenchymal injuries, easily identified by computed tomography (CT) or magnetic resonance imaging (MRI) scans, may not cause obvious signs or symptoms. The following are common problems associated with brain injury.

A. Seizures

Seizures occurring in the first 24 hours after injury are referred to as *immediate seizures*. Those occurring during the first week are *delayed seizures,* and those starting more than 1 week after injury are referred to as *late seizures*. Seizure prophylaxis with medications is recommended in the first week after brain injury in children at high risk for seizures and in very young children, who are at higher risk for early seizures than are older children and adults. Seizure prophylaxis is also recommended for 1 week after any penetrating brain trauma. Seizure prophylaxis is probably not effective for prevention of late-onset seizures. Late-developing seizures may require long-term treatment.

B. Motor Function Deficits

Motor function deficits after brain injury include movement disorders, spasticity, paralysis, and weakness. These deficits can result in impaired ambulation, coordination, impaired ability to use upper extremities, and speech problems. Physical therapy is the primary modality of treatment for these problems.

C. Sensory or Perceptual Deficits

Sensory deficits after traumatic brain injury are most commonly the result of cranial nerve injuries or parenchymal brain damage. Abnormal sensation may result in swallowing problems, reduced self-protective mechanisms, neglect, visual processing dysfunction, and pain.

D. Paroxysmal Autonomic Instability Associated with Dystonia

Severe brain injuries can be associated with autonomic dysfunction of the thalamus and hypothalamus, which results in a constellation of symptoms known as paroxysmal autonomic instability associated with dystonia (PAID). PAID is manifested by tachycardia, tachypnea, sweating, hyperthermia, agitation, and posturing. Common medications used in the treatment of PAID include dopamine agonists such as bromocriptine, β-blockers such as propanolol, and α-agonists such as clonidine.

E. Cognitive and Behavioral Deficits

After brain injury, cognitive and behavioral deficits may be obvious immediately or develop gradually. They include decreased arousal, decreased attention, impaired executive function, and problems with memory and concentration. Emotional lability, depression, agitation, impulsivity, and aggression can emerge. Many of these behaviors improve spontaneously, but some require behavioral or pharmacologic intervention.

F. Hypothalamic-Pituitary-Adrenal Axis Dysfunction

Dysfunction of the hypothalamic-pituitary-adrenal axis is common after head injury. The syndrome of inappropriate antidiuretic hormone secretion (SIADH) and diabetes insipidus from a posterior pituitary injury can result in significant electrolyte and osmolality imbalance and must be monitored closely. Amenorrhea is common in females and typically resolves spontaneously. Injury near the onset of puberty can complicate normal development, and endocrine status should be monitored closely.

G. Cranial Nerve Injuries

The sensory and motor components of the cranial nerves are often damaged, resulting in a wide variety of deficits not centrally mediated. Sight, hearing, taste, and smell, as well as swallowing, are among the most commonly affected functions. The vestibulocochlear nerve (cranial nerve VII) is most often affected followed by the occulomotor nerve (cranial nerve III). Hyposmia or anosmia (cranial nerve I) can occur if the shearing forces at the cribriform plate disrupt the olfactory afferent nerves running centrally from the nose. Injury to cranial nerves III, IV, and VI can affect vision, causing diplopia and other deficits. Optic nerve (cranial nerve II) injury is relatively rare. If injury to the optic nerve occurs, it is usually apparent within 1 month of the initial traumatic event.

Developmental Considerations

Much of what we know of traumatic brain injury is based on experience in adults. The confounding effects of age and the etiologies unique to the pediatric population (eg, child abuse) make care of the pediatric head-injured patient very complex.

The assumption that younger children will fare better than older children or adults after a brain injury is a myth. The fact that, in a child, a significant amount of development and synaptic reorganization has yet to occur does not guarantee an improved chance for functional recovery. Indeed, disruption of developmental processes, especially in very young infants or neonates, may be catastrophic as these processes often cannot be resumed once disrupted.

The mechanism of injury plays an important role in determining the severity of brain injury in very young children. Mechanisms associated with nonaccidental injury such as shaking often result in global diffuse injury. The weak neck musculature, large head–to–body mass ratio, immature blood-brain barrier, and high intracranial fluid–to–brain mass ratio all contribute to widespread damage.

During puberty, major hormonal changes have an impact on the outcome of brain injury. Behavioral problems may be pronounced in brain-injured adolescents. Precocious puberty and precocious development of sexual activity may occur in preadolescents and should be carefully monitored.

Careful consideration should be given to the developmental progress of the brain-injured child and adolescent. Delays can be anticipated after moderate and severe brain injuries related to abnormalities of cognition and behavior. It is critical to identify developmental disabilities as early as possible so that appropriate therapy can be started in order to maximize the child's residual capabilities. Educational programs should include an individualized educational program (IEP) to support the child with significant remediation and assistance needs during their school years. Programs should also include a 504 plan (named for Section 504 of the Rehabilitation Act and the Americans with Disabilities Act) The 504 plan identifies the accommodations necessary in regular school settings for students with lesser disabilities so that they may be educated in a setting with their peers.

▶ Treatment

The primary goal of rehabilitation after childhood brain injury is to maximize functional independence. Rehabilitative care can be divided into three phases: acute, subacute, and long term. The acute and subacute phases typically occur in the inpatient setting while the long-term phase is an outpatient endeavor.

A. Acute Care

Therapy in the acute phase consists mainly of medical, surgical, and pharmacological measures to decrease brain edema, treat increased intracranial pressure, and normalize serum laboratory values. Nutrition is essential in the healing process and either parenteral nutrition or supplemental enteral feedings are employed. Current research suggests that transitioning to enteral nutrition (eg, nasogastric tube feeding) as soon as possible after brain injury is associated with improved outcomes. Placement of a gastrostomy tube for supplemental enteral feeding is often performed in patients with severe brain injuries when recovery will be protracted and swallowing function is inadequate for safe oral feeding.

B. Subacute Care

Therapy in the subacute phase is characterized by early, intensive participation in rehabilitative therapies promoting functional recovery. Treatment should be planned after consultation with physical therapy, occupational therapy, speech-language specialists, and neuropsychologists. Nursing staff members are a primary interface with the patient and often serve as educators for family-directed care. Most children and adolescents with brain injuries can be discharged home to continue with treatment on an outpatient basis.

C. Long-Term Care

Long-term follow-up starts immediately after discharge. Medical issues must be thoroughly and regularly reviewed to ensure that changing needs are met. Annual multidisciplinary evaluation is important, especially as the child approaches school age. Neuropsychological testing may be required to define cognitive and behavioral deficits and plan strategies to deal with them in the educational environment. Therapies should be flexible, providing strategies to maximize independence and facilitate the child's involvement in changing environments.

Medication is often required for cognitive and behavioral issues. Attention deficit, irritability, and fatigue associated with brain injury may be amenable to treatment with stimulants such as methylphenidate and modafinil. Dopaminergic agents such as amantadine, levodopa, and bromocriptine can be useful in improving cognition, processing speed, and agitation. Antidepressants such as selective serotonin reuptake inhibitors can be helpful in treating depression and mood lability. Anticonvulsants can be useful as mood stabilizers and in treating agitation and aggression. Tegretol and valproic acid are typical agents for this purpose.

Attention and arousal can also be successfully addressed by utilizing behavioral techniques to reinforce desired behaviors as well as identifying environmental situations that optimize those behaviors. Gains made in the behavioral realm often have a positive impact on therapies designed to address physical issues.

Prognosis & Outcomes

Directly after brain injury, poor pupillary reactivity, low blood pH, absence of deep tendon reflexes, and low GCS all correlate with poor outcome. An increased number of intra-cranial lesions and increased depth and duration of coma are also associated with poor functional recovery. Children younger than 1 year of age tend to have worse outcomes.

Functional outcome assessment is important for judging the efficacy of rehabilitation therapy. Global multidomain measures are used to provide a functional "snapshot in time" of select functions—motor function and mobility, self-care, cognition, socialization, and communication. Several of these measures are available; the WeeFIM is the one most commonly used in pediatrics.

Outcome associated with mild brain injury is often quite favorable. Most patients recover normal function within a short time frame. A small percentage will develop persistent problems such as chronic headache, poor focusing ability, altered memory, and vestibular abnormalities.

In children, recovery may not be fully achieved for many months or years after the initial injury. The impact of the injury on developmental processes, and its future conse-quences, are difficult to predict. Long-term follow-up is required, particularly as the child approaches school age.

Adelson PD et al: Guidelines for the acute medical management of severe traumatic brain injury in infants, children, and adoles-cents. Chapter 19. The role of anti-seizure prophylaxis follow-ing severe pediatric traumatic brain injury. Pediatr Crit Care Med 2003;4:S72 [PMID: 12847355].

Antiseizure prophylaxis for penetrating brain injury. J Trauma 2001;51:S41 [PMID: 11505199].

Atabaki SM: Pediatric head injury. Pediatr Rev 2007;28:215 [PMID: 17545333].

Blackman JA et al: Paroxysmal autonomic instability with dystonia after brain injury. Arch Neurol 2004;61:321 [PMID: 15023807].

Corwin B et al: Brain injury rehabilitation. In Braddom RL (editor): Physical Medicine & Rehabilitation. Saunders, 2000:1073.

Gordon WA et al: Traumatic brain injury rehabilitation: State of the science. Am J Phys Med Rehabil 2006;85:343 [PMID: 16554685].

Tenovuo O: Pharmacological enhancement of cognitive and behavioral deficits after traumatic brain injury. Curr Opin Neurol 2006;19:528 [PMID: 17102689].

SPINAL CORD INJURY

General Considerations

Epidemiologic studies of spinal cord injuries (SCI) suggest that there will be about 10,000 new injuries per year and that 20% will be in children younger than age 20 years. Motor vehicle accidents are the leading cause of SCI in all ages. Falls are common causes in young children. The phenomenon of SCI without obvious radiologic abnormality (SCIWORA) can be present in 20–40% of young children. Children from birth to 2 years tend to have high-level injuries to the cervical spine because of the anatomical features of the spine in this age group. The facets tend to be shallower and oriented horizontally, and the boney spine is more flexible than the spinal cord. In addition the head is disproportionately large and the neck muscles are weak.

SCI are classified using the American Spinal Injury Asso-ciation classification (ASIA class). This classification evalu-ates motor and sensory function, defines the neurologic level of the injury, and assesses the completeness of the deficit. The 72-hour ASIA examination is used in predicting recov-ery. A complete lesion identified on ASIA examination at 72 hours predicts a very poor recovery potential.

1. ASIA class A is a complete spinal cord injury, with no motor or sensory function in the lowest sacral segments.
2. ASIA class B is an incomplete injury, with preserved sensory function but no motor function in the sacral segments.
3. ASIA class C is an incomplete lesion in which the strength of more than 50% of key muscles below the injury level is graded less than 3/5 on manual muscle testing.
4. ASIA class D is an incomplete lesion in which the strength of more than 50% of key muscles below the injury level is graded greater than 3/5 on manual muscle testing.
5. ASIA class E is an injury in which full motor and sensory function is preserved.

Clinical Findings

A. Clinical Patterns of Spinal Cord Injury

1. Brown-Séquard injury—In this injury, the cord is hemi-sected, causing motor paralysis, loss of proprioception and vibration on the ipsilateral side and loss of pain and temper-ature on the contralateral side.

2. Central cord syndrome—Injury is to the central part of the cord and results in greater weakness in the arms than the legs.

3. Anterior cord syndrome—Disruption of the anterior spinal artery causes motor deficits and loss of pain and temperature sensation.

4. Conus medullaris syndrome—Injury or tumor of the conus causes minimal motor impairment but significant sensory and bowel and bladder abnormalities.

5. Cauda equina syndrome—Injury to the nerve roots produces flaccid bilateral weakness in the legs, sensory abnormalities in the perineum, and lower motor neuron bowel and bladder dysfunction.

B. Imaging

The diagnosis and anatomic description of SCI is made mainly through imaging techniques. Initial studies should include radiographs of the entire spine (including cervical spine) and special studies for boney structures. MRI imaging is required to evaluate soft tissues. CT scans, including three-dimensional reconstructions, may be used to further define the injured elements.

▶ Treatment

A. Initial Management

The two primary precepts of SCI treatment are early identification and immediate stabilization of the spine. The approach used to stabilize the spine is determined by the type of injury, location of injury, and underlying condition of the spinal cord. Stabilizing the spine may prevent further damage to the spinal cord. External traction devices such as halo traction and orthotics are often used. Some injuries require internal stabilization. The benefit of corticosteroid administration in pediatric SCI has not been established but treatment is usually initiated based on adult data from the National Acute Spinal Cord Injury Study. The initial loading dose is 30 mg/kg over 15 minutes, followed by 5.4 mg/kg for the next 23 hours if started within 3 hours of injury. If started within 3–8 hours of injury, corticosteroids should be continued for 48 hours.

B. Functional Expectations after Spinal Cord Injury

The lesions associated with SCI have a predictable impact on motor and sensory function. It is helpful to understand these concepts when discussing functional expectations with patients and parents (Table 26–1).

C. Special Clinical Problems Associated with Spinal Cord Injury

1. Autonomic hyperreflexia or dysreflexia—This condition occurs in spinal injuries above the level of T6. Noxious stimuli in the injured patient cause sympathetic vasoconstriction below the level of injury. Vasoconstriction produces hypertension and then a compensatory, vagally mediated bradycardia. Symptoms therefore include hypertension, bradycardia, headaches, and diaphoresis. This response may be severe enough to be life threatening. Treatment requires identification and relief of the underlying noxious stimulus. Bowel, bladder, and skin problems are the most common noxious stimuli causing this syndrome. The patient should be placed in an upright position and antihypertensive medication used if conservative measures fail. Nifedipine (oral or sublingual) has been used in treatment of this condition.

Table 26–1. Functional expectations related to spinal cord injury.

Level of Injury and Key Muscle Function	Functional Skills
C1–C4 (no upper extremity function)	Dependent for all skills, can use voice-activated computer, mouth stick; can drive power wheelchair with technology devices such as sip and puff, chin drive, or head array
C5 (biceps function)	Can assist with ADLs, power wheelchair with joy stick, push manual wheelchair short distances, use modified push rims
C6 (wrist extension)	More ADL skills; can push manual wheelchair indoors, perform level transfers; hand function augmented with adapted equipment
C7 (elbow extension)	ADLs independent; hand function augmented with adapted equipment; can push manual wheelchair indoor and outdoor
C8 (finger flexors)	ADLs independent; independent manual wheelchair skills; increased transfer skills
T1 (little finger abduction)	
T2–T12 (chest, abdominal and spinal extensors)[a]	ADLs independent; independent manual wheelchair skills; improved transfer; standing with braces
L1 and L2 (hip flexors)	Standing and walking with long leg braces, KAFO, and RGO; swing-through gait; manual wheelchair main form of mobility
L3 (knee extension)	Home and limited community ambulation; long leg or short leg braces
L4 (ankle dorsiflexion)	Community ambulation with short leg braces, AFO
L5 (long toe extensors)	Community ambulation; may be slower than peers and have some endurance issues
S1 (ankle plantar flexors)	

[a]Level defined by sensory dermatome.
ADLs, activities of daily living; AFO, ankle-foot orthosis; KAFO, braces named for the joints being supported (ie, knee-ankle-foot orthosis); RGO, reciprocal gait orthosis.

2. Hypercalcemia—Hypercalcemia often occurs in male adolescents within the first 2 months of becoming paraplegic or tetraplegic. The serum calcium level rises significantly in response to immobilization. Patients complain of abdominal pain and malaise. Behavioral problems may occur. Initial treatment is focused on hydration and forced diuresis using fluids and furosemide to increase urinary excretion of calcium. In severe cases, especially in older children, calcitonin and etidronate may be required.

3. Thermoregulation problems—These problems are most common and most severe in higher level injuries and usually result in a poikilothermic state. The ability to vasoconstrict and vasodilate below the injury level is impaired. The person with an SCI above T6 is particularly susceptible to environmental temperature and is at risk for hypothermia and hyperthermia.

4. Deep vein thrombosis—Thrombosis is a common complication of SCI, especially in postpubescent children. Deep vein thrombosis should be suspected in children with any unilateral extremity swelling, palpable cords in the calf muscles, fevers, erythema, or leg pain. Diagnosis is confirmed by Doppler ultrasound, and full evaluation may require spiral CT scan or ventilation-perfusion scan if pulmonary embolus is suspected. Preventative measures include elastic stockings and compression devices. Anticoagulation medications include heparin and low-molecular-weight heparin (0.5 mg/kg every 12 hours).

5. Heterotopic ossification—This complication occurs in both spinal cord and traumatic brain injuries. Ectopic calcium deposits usually appear around joints in the first 6 months after injury. They may cause swelling, decreased range of motion, pain with motion, palpable firm masses, fever, elevated sedimentation rate, and abnormal triple phase bone scan. Etidronate therapy should be started at the time of diagnosis. Surgical removal of ectopic deposits is controversial and usually performed only in cases of extreme loss of motion, pressure sores, or severe pain.

Bilston LE, Brown J: Pediatric spinal injury type and severity are age and mechanism dependent. Spine 2007;32:2339 [PMID: 17906576].

Bracken MB: Steroids for acute spinal cord injury. Cochrane Database Sys Rev 2002;(3):CD001046 [PMID: 12137616].

Hickey KJ et al: Prevalence and etiology of autonomic dysreflexia in children with spinal cord injuries. J Spinal Cord Med 2004;27(Suppl 1):S54 [PMID: 15503704].

Liao CC et al: Spinal cord injury without radiological abnormalities in preschool-aged children: correlation of magnetic resonance imaging findings and neurologic outcome. J Neurosurg 2005;103(Suppl 1):17 [PMID: 16122000].

BRACHIAL PLEXUS LESIONS

▶ General Considerations

The brachial plexus is the complex nervous connection between the spinal cord and the muscles of the upper extremity and scapular area. The nerve roots forming the plexus derive from the fifth cervical through the first thoracic nerves. These nerve roots form trunks that further divide into divisions and then into cords. The upper trunk (C5 and C6) is the most commonly injured, resulting in a symptom complex called **Erb palsy.** Injury to the lower trunk (C7–T1) produces **Klumpke palsy.** It is quite common for the entire brachial plexus to be involved. Mild brachial plexus injuries may produce only a nerve stretch or neurapraxia. Severe injury may cause complete avulsion of the nerve from the spinal cord.

▶ Clinical Findings

Erb palsy is characterized by shoulder weakness with internal rotation and adduction of the upper arm. The elbow is extended and the wrist flexed. There is good preservation of hand function. Klumpke palsy is characterized by good shoulder function but decreased or absent hand function. Brachial plexus injury may also cause Horner syndrome (unilateral miosis, ptosis and facial anhydrosis) due to disruption of cervical sympathetic nerves. Associated bony and nerve injuries are common in brachial plexus injury. The physical examination should include inspection of the humerus and clavicle for fractures. There may be injuries of the phrenic and facial nerves.

The diagnosis of a brachial plexus lesion should be based on the history and clinical examination. Diagnostic testing helps confirm, localize, and classify the lesion. Electromyography is helpful 3–4 weeks after the injury. This test not only is used diagnostically but can track recovery. MRI, myelography, and CT scan can help to locate the lesion and determine its extent.

▶ Treatment & Prognosis

Primary surgery to the nerves of the plexus is indicated for children who have no spontaneous recovery of biceps function by 6–9 months. Secondary procedures to maximize function include muscle transfers and orthopedic interventions. Physical therapy is the major treatment for brachial plexus injury and includes stretching, bracing, and functional training.

The currently accepted method of predicting recovery is based on the spontaneous recovery of the biceps. Children in whom antigravity function returns within 2 months of injury will probably have near-full recovery of function. If antigravity function is delayed until 6 months after injury, recovery will probably be limited. If antigravity function is absent at 6–9 months after injury, there will be no recovery of function and surgical options to transplant muscles and improve motor function should be considered.

Grossman JA: Early operative intervention for selected cases of brachial plexus birth injury. Arch Neurol 2006;63:1031 [PMID: 16831977].

O'Brien DF et al: Management of birth brachial plexus palsy. Childs Nerv Syst 2006;22:103 [PMID: 16320018].

Strombeck C et al: Long-term follow-up of children with obstetric brachial plexus palsy I: functional aspects. Devel Med Child Neurol 2007;49:198 [PMID: 17355476].

COMMON REHABILITATION PROBLEMS

1. Neurogenic Bladder

The function of the bladder is to hold and eventually expel urine. The muscles of the bladder include the detrusor and urethral sphincters. During the first year of life the bladder is a reflex-driven system that empties spontaneously. After the first year control begins to develop, and most children achieve continence by age 5 years. Children with damage to the central or peripheral nervous system may develop neurogenic bladder. Neurogenic bladder is usually classified as noted below.

1. *Uninhibited* neurogenic bladder occurs after upper motor neuron injuries at the level of the brain or SCI that result in failure to inhibit detrusor contractions. This results in a hyperreflexive voiding pattern.
2. *Reflex* neurogenic bladder results from damage to the sensory and motor nerves above the S3 and S4 level. The bladder empties reflexively but coordination may not be present and dyssynergia (contraction of the bladder musculature against a closed sphincter) can occur. Increased intravesicular pressure and vesicourethral reflux may be consequences of dyssynergia.
3. *Autonomous* neurogenic bladder is a flaccid bladder and is associated with lower motor neuron damage. Bladder volumes are usually increased and overflow incontinence can occur.
4. *Motor paralytic* neurogenic bladder results from injury to the motor nerves of the S2-4 roots. Sensation is intact but there is motor dysfunction. The child has the sensation to void but has difficulty with the voluntary contractions.
5. *Sensory paralytic* neurogenic bladder results when sensory roots are disrupted. Affected patients do not have sensation of the full bladder but are able to initiate voiding.

The diagnosis of neurogenic bladder requires a complete history and physical examination. The type of neurologic damage should be identified as this will help to predict anticipated voiding issues. The upper tracts should be assessed by several techniques, including ultrasound, intravenous pyelogram, and renogram (isotope) studies. Lower tract testing includes urinalysis, postvoid residuals, urodynamics, cystography, and cystoscopy.

▶ Treatment

Treatment is geared to the type of bladder dysfunction. The simplest methods are those employing behavioral strategies. Timed voiding can be effective for children with uninhibited bladders. In this technique, children are reminded verbally or use a cueing device (watch with a timer) to void every 2–3 hours before bladder capacity is reached. The Credé and Valsalva maneuvers are used in patients with an autonomous bladder to assist in draining a flaccid bladder. There is a risk of increasing intravesicular pressure during these maneuvers, which can provoke vesicoureteral reflux. These maneuvers should never be used in a patient with a reflex neurogenic bladder.

Medications are often employed to treat neurogenic bladder. Anticholinergics are commonly used to reduce detrusor contractions, decrease the sense of urgency, and increase bladder capacity. Medications include oxybutynin, tolterodine, and hyoscyamine. The side effects of these medications include sleepiness, nausea, and constipation. Families often find these effects unacceptable and frequently abandon treatment.

External methods are also used to improve continence and function. Absorbent pads and diapers, external catheters, internal catheters, and clean intermittent catheterization are some typical methods. Surgical procedures to protect the upper tracts from urinary reflux are often used. A young child with a high-pressure bladder is at particular risk for reflux and may need medication, clean intermittent catheterization, or vesicostomy to prevent hydrostatic renal damage and infection. An older child may require bladder augmentation or an intestinal conduit from bladder to skin surface to relieve bladder distention (Mitrofanoff procedure). If there is an incompetent urethral sphincter with urinary leakage, injections, slings, or implants may be used to increase the urethral barrier. Recently, electrical stimulation of sacral roots has been used to initiate voiding. Biofeedback training is also used to improve voiding.

2. Neurogenic Bowel

Control of bowel function depends on an intact autonomic (sympathetic and parasympathetic) and somatic nervous system. Interruption of any of these pathways can result in bowel control problems. Goals of treatment for patients with neurogenic bowel are to establish a predictable and reliable bowel habit, prevent incontinence, and prevent complications. There are two types of neurogenic bowel dysfunction: upper motor and lower motor dysfunction. The upper neuron bowel results from damage above the conus. Affected patients usually have reflex bowel contractions of high amplitude, absence of sensation, and no voluntary sphincter control. Patients with the lower motor neuron bowel have no sphincter control and no anocutaneous reflex. It has been described as a flaccid bowel. In general establishing a bowel program is much easier in patients with the upper motor neuron–type lesion.

▶ Treatment

Diet is extremely important in either type of bowel program. Fiber and fluids are critical elements. Stool consistency should be on the soft side, although some patients try to keep themselves constipated to prevent accidents. A predictable and scheduled bowel program is essential. Bowel movements should be scheduled to occur with meals, as the gastrocolic reflex can trigger defecation.

Laxative and stool softening medications are usually included in a comprehensive bowel program. Stool softeners such as docusate retain stool water. Mineral oil is another acceptable stool softener in patients not at risk for pulmonary aspiration. Bulking agents such as Metamucil increase fiber and water content of stool and reduce transit time. Stimulants such as senna fruit extract or bisacodyl increase peristalsis. Osmotic agents such as polyethylene glycol keep stools soft by retaining stool water.

Suppositories and enemas are often used when other methods have not been successful. Upper motor neuron bowel management may require digital rectal stimulation as part of the program. Newer surgical options include sacral nerve stimulators and techniques to provide flushing of the colon. Cecostomy button or antegrade continence enema is employed when other conservative methods have not been able to achieve desired goals.

3. Spasticity

Spasticity is a velocity-dependent increase in muscle tone and a loss of isolated muscle function. Whereas tone is the resistance felt in a muscle as it is moved in space, spasticity occurs when there is damage to the central nervous system from trauma or injury. It is included in the upper motor neuron syndrome (hyperactive and exaggerated reflexes, increased tone, clonus, positive Babinski sign). Spasticity is evaluated using the Ashworth Scale, with zero indicating no increase in muscle tone and 4 indicating complete rigidity of the extremity.

▶ Treatment

Treatment is goal directed and influenced by the functional status of the client. Spasticity has both positive and negative effects on quality of life. The positive aspects include the ability to use spasticity for functional tasks along with maintaining muscle strength. Negatively spasticity can interfere with positioning and hygiene, affect function, and can cause pain.

Options for therapy range from conservative to aggressive. A pyramidal approach starts from a base of prevention of nociceptive input and aggressive physical therapy. Children should be positioned properly and have appropriate equipment to support this strategy. Physical therapy is designed to reduce the long-term effects of spasticity by stretching and range-of-motion exercises. Heat and cold are useful in improving tone, but their effects are not long lived. Casting of both upper and lower extremities can decrease tone and increase range of motion. Constraint therapy can be used to try to improve upper extremity function.

The next step on the pyramid is the use of medications, mainly baclofen, diazepam, dantrolene, and tizanidine. Baclofen is a first-line medication, which produces effects at the spinal cord level. Side effects are mainly sleepiness and weakness. Seizure threshold may be reduced by baclofen. Baclofen can be delivered directly to the central nervous system through an intrathecal pump. It has been used successfully in children with brain injury, cerebral palsy, and SCI. Diazepam affects presynaptic GABA receptors in both the brain and the spinal cord. It can cause drowsiness and dependence. Dantrolene decreases the release of calcium in muscle. Side effects include weakness and, rarely, hepatotoxicity. Tizanidine is a newer agent and works at the α_2-adrenergic receptors presynaptically. It can cause dry mouth and sedation, and liver function tests can be elevated.

Relief of focal spasticity can be achieved by using chemodenervation techniques. Botulinum toxin A and B can be injected in selected muscles to improve range of motion, thus improving function and hygiene as well as reducing pain and deformity. More recently, botulinum toxins have been used to treat drooling, hyperhydrosis, and chronic pain. These toxins block the release of acetylcholine at the neuromuscular junction. The effects are temporary, lasting only 3–6 months, and repeat injections are often needed. Phenol injections are another option for treatment of local spasticity and are technically more challenging. Phenol denatures proteins in both myelinated and unmyelinated fibers and produces neurolysis or myolysis, depending on the site of injection. The effects may last longer than botulinum toxins. Injections carry a risk of sensory dysesthesia if mixed nerves are injected.

Surgical options include orthopedic procedures geared toward improving function and ambulation and alleviating deformities produced over time by spasticity. Contractures are common in the Achilles tendon, hamstrings, and adductors. Upper extremity contractures occur in the elbow, wrist, and finger flexors. Scoliosis is fairly common and bracing or surgery may be needed. Gait analysis may be helpful in evaluating the child with functional spasticity as a guide for the use of orthotics, therapy, and surgery. Neurosurgical techniques such as selective dorsal rhizotomy are used in a very select group of children to permanently alter spasticity patterns and improve ambulation.

Fowler CJ, O'Malley KJ: Investigation and management of neurogenic bladder dysfunction. J Neurol Neurosurg Psychiatry 2003;74(Suppl 4):iv27 [PMID: 14645464].

Lorenzo AJ et al: Minimally invasive approach for treatment of urinary and fecal incontinence in selected patients with spina bifida. Urology 2007;70:568 [PMID: 17905118].

Merenda LA, Hickey K: Key elements of bladder and bowel management for children with spinal cord injuries. SCI Nurs 2005;22:8 [PMID: 15794429].

Patki P et al: Long-term urological outcomes in paediatric spinal cord injury. Spinal Cord 2006;44:729 [PMID: 16446753].

Ronan S, Gold JT: Nonoperative management of spasticity in children. Childs Nerv Syst 2007;23:943 [PMID: 17646995].

Samson G, Cardenas DD: Neurogenic bladder in spinal cord injury. Phys Med Rehabil Clin North Am 2007;18:255 [PMID: 17543772].

Steinbok P: Selection of treatment modalities in children with spastic cerebral palsy. Neurosurg Focus 2006;15:21:2 [PMID: 16918225].

Rheumatic Diseases

Jennifer B. Soep, MD

J. Roger Hollister, MD

JUVENILE IDIOPATHIC ARTHRITIS

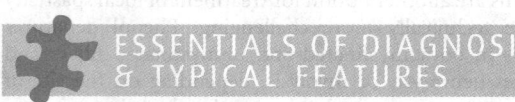

ESSENTIALS OF DIAGNOSIS & TYPICAL FEATURES

▶ Arthritis, involving pain, swelling, warmth, tenderness, morning stiffness, and decreased range of motion of one or more joints, lasting 6–12 weeks.

▶ May have associated systemic manifestations, including fever, rash, uveitis, serositis, anemia, fatigue, and growth failure.

▶ General Considerations

There are three classifications of juvenile chronic arthritis. These different systems of categorizing patients attempt to standardize the diagnosis and approach to patient care as well as assist in designing research protocols. Each classification contains three main subtypes: pauciarticular or oligoarticular, polyarticular, and systemic (Table 27–1). The exact cause of juvenile idiopathic arthritis (JIA) is not known, but there is substantial evidence that it is an autoimmune process with genetic susceptibility factors.

▶ Clinical Findings

A. Symptoms and Signs

The most common type of JIA is the pauciarticular/oligoarticular form, which affects 50% of patients and is characterized by arthritis of four or fewer joints. This type of JIA often affects medium to large joints. Because the arthritis is often asymmetrical, children may develop a leg-length discrepancy in which the involved leg grows longer due to increased blood flow and growth factors. The synovitis is usually mild and may be painless. Systemic features are uncommon except for inflammation in the eye. Up to 30% of children with this type of JIA develop insidious, asymptomatic uveitis, which may cause

blindness if untreated. The activity of the eye disease does not correlate with that of the arthritis. Therefore, routine ophthalmologic screening with slit-lamp examination must be performed at 3-month intervals if the antinuclear antibody (ANA) test is positive, and at 6-month intervals if the ANA test is negative, for 4 years after the onset of arthritis.

Polyarticular disease is defined as arthritis involving five or more joints. This type of JIA affects 35% of patients. Both large and small joints are involved, typically in a symmetrical pattern. Systemic features are not prominent, although low-grade fever, fatigue, rheumatoid nodules, and anemia may be present. This group is further divided into rheumatoid factor-positive (10%) and rheumatoid factor-negative (25%) disease. The former resembles adult rheumatoid arthritis with more chronic, destructive arthritis.

The systemic form, also known as Still disease, is the least common form, comprising 10–15% of patients with JIA. The arthritis can involve any number of joints and affects both large and small joints, but may be absent at disease onset. One of the classic features is a high fever, often as high as 39–40°C, typically occurring one to two times per day. In between fever spikes the temperature usually returns to normal or subnormal. Ninety percent of patients have a characteristic evanescent, salmon-pink macular rash that is most prominent on pressure areas and when fever is present. Other systemic features that may be present, but are not specific for JIA, include hepatosplenomegaly, lymphadenopathy, leukocytosis, and serositis.

B. Laboratory Findings

There is no diagnostic test for JIA. A normal erythrocyte sedimentation rate (ESR) does not exclude the diagnosis of JIA. However, patients with systemic JIA typically have significantly elevated markers of inflammation including ESR, C-reactive protein (CRP), white blood cell count, and platelets. Rheumatoid factor is positive in about 10–15% of patients, usually when onset of polyarticular disease occurs after age 8 years. A newer test, anti–cyclic citrullinated

Table 27–1. Classification of pediatric chronic arthritis.

American College of Rheumatology[a]	European League Against Rheumatism[b]	International League of Associations for Rheumatology[c]
Juvenile Rheumatoid Arthritis	Juvenile Chronic Arthritis	Juvenile Idiopathic Arthritis
Systemic	Systemic	Systemic
Polyarticular	Polyarticular, RF-negative	Polyarticular, RF-negative
	Juvenile rheumatoid arthritis (polyarticular, RF-positive)	Polyarticular, RF-positive
Pauciarticular	Pauciarticular	Oligoarthritis Persistent Extended
	Juvenile ankylosing spondylitis	Enthesitis-related arthritis
	Juvenile psoriatic arthritis	Psoriatic arthritis
		Undifferentiated arthritis Fits no other category Fits more than one category

Modified from a table that appears in Textbook of Pediatric Rheumatology, 4th Edition, page 215, Copyright Elsevier 2001.
[a]Brewer EJ Jr et al: Current proposed revision of JRA criteria. Arthritis Rheum 1977;20(Suppl):195.
[b]European League Against Rheumatism (EULAR) Bulletin No. 4: Nomenclature and classification of arthritis in children. National Zeitung AG, 1977.
[c]Petty RE et al: Revision of the proposed classification criteria for juvenile idiopathic arthritis: Durban 1997. J Rheumatol 1998;25:1991.
RF, rheumatoid factor.

peptide (CCP) antibody, may be detectable prior to the rheumatoid factor and has a very high specificity for rheumatoid arthritis. ANA are associated with an increased risk of iridocyclitis in patients with oligoarticular disease. A positive ANA test is also fairly common in patients with the late-onset rheumatoid factor-positive form of the disease.

Table 27–2 lists the general characteristics of joint fluid in various conditions. The main indication for joint aspiration and synovial fluid analysis is to rule out infection. A positive Gram stain or culture is the only definitive test for infection. A leukocyte count over 2000/μL suggests inflammation; this may be due to infection, any of the collagen-vascular diseases, leukemia, or reactive arthritis. A very low glucose concentration (< 40 mg/dL) or very high polymorphonuclear leukocyte count (> 60,000/μL) is highly suggestive of bacterial arthritis.

C. Imaging

In the early stages of the disease, only soft-tissue swelling and periarticular osteoporosis are seen. Magnetic resonance imaging (MRI) of involved joints may show early joint damage and if

Table 27–2. Joint fluid analysis.

Disorder	Cells/μL	Glucose[a]
Trauma	More red cells than white cells; usually < 2000 white cells	Normal
Reactive arthritis	3000–10,000 white cells, mostly mononuclear cells	Normal
Juvenile idiopathic arthritis and other inflammatory arthritides	5000–60,000 white cells, mostly neutrophils	Usually normal or slightly low
Septic arthritis	> 60,000 white cells, > 90% neutrophils	Low to normal

[a]Normal value is ≥ 75% of the serum glucose value.

obtained with gadolinium, can confirm the presence of synovitis. Later in the course of the disease, particularly in patients with rheumatoid factor-positive disease, plain films may demonstrate joint space narrowing due to cartilage thinning and erosive changes of the bone related to chronic inflammation.

▶ Differential Diagnosis

Table 27–3 lists the most common causes of limb pain in childhood. JIA is a diagnosis of exclusion; therefore, it is important to rule out other causes of the clinical signs and symptoms prior to settling on this diagnosis. The differential diagnosis is often quite broad, including orthopedic conditions, infectious diseases, and malignancies. A few key features can help distinguish these different entities, including the timing of the pain and associated signs and symptoms. In inflammatory conditions, patients frequently have increased symptoms in the morning with associated stiffness. In contrast, patients with an orthopedic abnormality typically have increased symptoms throughout the day and with activity. Growing pains, a common cause of leg pain in childhood, are characterized by poorly localized pain at night, which frequently wakes the child from sleep; no objective signs of inflammation; and no daytime symptoms. Patients with growing pains often ask to be massaged, which is not typical of those with arthritis.

It is particularly important to establish the diagnosis in the case of monoarticular arthritis. Bacterial arthritis is usually acute and monoarticular except for arthritis associated with gonorrhea, which may be associated with a migratory pattern. Fever, leukocytosis, and increased ESR with an acute process in a single joint demand synovial fluid examination and culture to identify the pathogen. Pain in the hip or lower extremity is a frequent symptom of childhood cancer, especially leukemia, neuroblastoma, and rhabdomyosarcoma. Infiltration of bone by tumor and a joint effusion may be seen. Radiographs of the affected site and examination of the blood smear for unusual cells and thrombocytopenia are necessary. An elevated lactate dehydrogenase value should

Table 27–3. Differential diagnosis of limb pain in children.

Orthopedic
Stress fracture
Chondromalacia patellae
Osgood-Schlatter disease
Slipped capital femoral epiphysis
Legg-Calvé-Perthes disease
Hypermobility syndrome
Reactive arthritis
Henoch-Schönlein purpura
Toxic synovitis of the hip
Transient synovitis following viral infection
Rheumatic fever
Post-streptococcal arthritis
Infections
Bacterial
Lyme arthritis
Osteomyelitis
Septic arthritis
Discitis
Viral
Parvovirus
Epstein-Barr virus
Hepatitis B arthritis
Rheumatologic
Juvenile idiopathic arthritis
Spondyloarthropathy
Systemic lupus erythematosus
Dermatomyositis
Neoplastic
Leukemia
Lymphoma
Neuroblastoma
Osteoid osteoma
Bone tumors (benign or malignant)
Pain syndromes
Growing pains
Fibromyalgia
Complex regional pain syndrome

also raise concern about an underlying neoplastic process. In doubtful cases, bone marrow examination is indicated.

In cases of reactive arthritis, a preceding illness is identified in approximately half of cases. Patients often have acute onset of arthritis, and there may be a migratory pattern. The duration of symptoms is a very important distinction between reactive arthritides and JIA. Symptoms associated with reactive arthritis typically resolve within 4–6 weeks. In contrast, to meet criteria for chronic arthritis, symptoms must be present for at least 6–12 weeks.

The arthritis of rheumatic fever is migratory, transient, and often more painful than that of JIA. Rheumatic fever is very rare in children younger than 5 years of age. In suspected cases, evidence of rheumatic carditis should be sought based on examination and electrocardiographic findings. Evidence of recent streptococcal infection is essential to the diagnosis. The fever pattern in rheumatic fever is low grade and persistent compared with the spiking fever that characterizes the systemic form of JIA. Lyme arthritis resembles oligoarticular JIA, but the former occurs as discrete, recurrent episodes of arthritis lasting 2–6 weeks. For patients suspected of having Lyme disease, testing for antibodies against *Borrelia burgdorferi* should be performed, with confirmatory testing by Western blot.

▶ Treatment

The objectives of therapy are to restore function, relieve pain, maintain joint motion, and prevent damage to cartilage and bone.

A. Nonsteroidal Anti-Inflammatory Medications

First-line therapy is nonsteroidal anti-inflammatory drugs (NSAIDs). A wide range of agents is available but only a few are approved for use in children, including naproxen (10 mg/kg per dose twice daily), ibuprofen (10 mg/kg per dose three to four times daily), and meloxicam (0.125 mg/kg once daily). NSAIDs are generally well tolerated in children, as long as they are taken with food. The average time to symptomatic improvement is 1 month, but in some patients a response is not seen for 8–12 weeks.

B. Disease-Modifying and Biologic Agents

For patients with JIA who fail to respond to NSAIDs, weekly methotrexate is the second-line medication of choice. Symptomatic response usually begins within 3–4 weeks. The low dosages used (5–10 mg/m^2/wk or 1 mg/kg/wk as a single dose) are generally well-tolerated. Potential side effects include nausea, vomiting, hair thinning, stomatitis, bone marrow suppression, and hepatotoxicity. A complete blood count and liver function tests should be obtained every 2–3 months. Several additional disease-modifying agents are available for use in patients with persistently active disease or those intolerant to methotrexate. Leflunomide is an antipyrimidine medication that has been shown to be as effective as methotrexate. Side effects may include diarrhea and alopecia. Medications that inhibit tumor necrosis factor, a cytokine known to play an important role in the pathogenesis of JIA, include etanercept, infliximab, and adalimumab. These drugs are generally quite effective in controlling disease and preventing cartilage and bone damage, and have been associated with healing based on radiologic changes. However, their potential long-term effects are unknown, and they are very expensive and require parenteral administration. Newer biologic agents, including anakinra, rituximab, and abatacept, have demonstrated some preliminary efficacy in patients who have not responded to other treatments.

C. Corticosteroids

Steroids are reserved for children with severe involvement, primarily patients with systemic disease. Local steroid joint injections may be helpful in patients who have arthritis in one or a few joints. Triamcinolone hexacetonide is a long-acting steroid that can be used for injections and is often associated with at least several months of disease control.

D. Uveitis

Iridocyclitis should be closely monitored by an ophthalmologist. Typically treatment is initiated with corticosteroid eye drops and dilating agents to prevent scarring between the iris and the lens. In patients who fail topical treatments, methotrexate, cyclosporine, and infliximab may be used.

E. Rehabilitation

Physical and occupational therapy are important to focus on range of motion, stretching, and strengthening. These exercises, as well as other modalities such as heat, water therapy, and ultrasound, can help control pain, maintain and restore function, and prevent deformity and disability. Young children with oligoarticular disease affecting asymmetrical lower extremity joints can develop a leg-length discrepancy, which may require treatment with a shoe lift on the unaffected side.

▶ Prognosis

The course and prognosis for JIA is variable, depending on the subtype of disease. Overall, the prognosis is good; 75–80% of patients remit without serious disability. In children with extended oligoarticular and polyarticular disease, more joints are involved; these patients may have more persistent and severe disease. Patients who are rheumatoid factor-positive are at highest risk for chronic, erosive arthritis that may continue into adulthood. The systemic features associated with systemic arthritis tend to remit within months to years. The prognosis in systemic disease is worse in patients with persistent systemic disease after six months, thrombocytosis and more extensive arthritis.

Goldmuntz EA, White PH: Juvenile idiopathic arthritis: A review for the pediatrician. Pediatr Rev 2006;27:e24 [PMID: 16581950].

Hashkes PJ, Laxer RM: Medical treatment of juvenile idiopathic arthritis. JAMA 2005;294:1671 [PMID: 16204667].

Ravelli A, Martini A: Juvenile idiopathic arthritis. Lancet 2007;369:767 [PMID: 17336654].

Tse SML, Laxer RM: Approach to acute limb pain in childhood. Pediatr Rev 2006;27:170 [PMID: 16651274].

ENTHESITIS-RELATED ARTHRITIS & SPONDYLOARTHROPATHY

Lower extremity arthritis, particularly in males older than 10 years of age, suggests a form of spondyloarthropathy. Inflammation of tendinous insertions (enthesopathy), such as the tibial tubercle or the heel, occurs in these diseases and not in JIA. Low back pain and sacroiliitis are commonly seen in this form of arthritis. Carriage of HLA-B27 antigen occurs in approximately 80% of patients with this disorder. No autoantibodies are found, but inflammatory indicators such as an elevated ESR or CRP may be present. Acute, not chronic, uveitis may occur.

NSAIDs, particularly indomethacin (2–4 mg/kg/d) and naproxen (15–20 mg/kg/d), are the first-line treatments for spondyloarthropathies. Refractory cases may respond to methotrexate, etanercept, or infliximab. Local corticosteroid injections are contraindicated in Achilles tendinitis. Unlike in adults, the disorder does not frequently progress to joint destruction or ankylosis in children.

Hofer M: Spondyloarthropathies in children—are they different from those in adults? Best Pract Res Clin Rheumatol 2006;20:315 [PMID: 16546059].

ENTEROPATHIC ARTHRITIS

Enteropathic arthritis includes several syndromes, such as Reiter syndrome, reactive arthritis, and the arthritis of inflammatory bowel disease and celiac disease. Their unifying feature is the association of arthritis with preceding or concurrent gastrointestinal symptoms. Reactive arthritis that follows diarrhea caused by *Salmonella, Shigella,* or *Yersinia* infection occurs with increased frequency in individuals who are HLA-B27–positive. The arthritis associated with Crohn disease and ulcerative colitis usually begins after or concurrent with active bowel disease. Other extraintestinal manifestations such as uveitis, stomatitis, hepatitis, and erythema nodosum may occur in these individuals.

Treatment for the musculoskeletal manifestations of inflammatory bowel disease, in addition to controlling the bowel disease, is primarily NSAIDs. Patients who have persistent disease may require treatment with second-line agents such as methotrexate or infliximab (or both).

SYSTEMIC LUPUS ERYTHEMATOSUS

ESSENTIALS OF DIAGNOSIS & TYPICAL FEATURES

▶ Multisystem inflammatory disease of the joints, serosal linings, skin, kidneys, blood, and central nervous system.

▶ Autoantibodies such as ANA, double-stranded DNA, and anti-Smith antibodies are present and related to the pathogenesis of disease.

▶ General Considerations

Systemic lupus erythematosus (SLE) is the prototype of immune complex diseases; its pathogenesis is related to the formation of antibody-antigen complexes that exist in the circulation and deposit in the involved tissues. The spectrum of symptoms is due to tissue-specific autoantibodies, as well as damage to the tissue by lymphocytes, neutrophils, and complement evoked by the deposition of immune complexes. Laboratory tests for these antibodies and complement components give an objective assessment of disease activity and response to therapy. Autoreactive T lymphocytes that have escaped clonal deletion and unregulated B-lymphocyte production of autoantibodies may initiate the disease.

▶ Clinical Findings

A. Symptoms and Signs

The onset of pediatric SLE is most common in girls between the ages of 9 and 15 years. Signs and symptoms depend on the organs affected by immune complex deposition. The American College of Rheumatology has established criteria to aid in the diagnosis of SLE; four of the following 11 criteria are necessary to establish the diagnosis:

1. Malar rash—photosensitive, so-called butterfly rash on the cheeks and nasal bridge.
2. Discoid rash—annular, scaly rash on the scalp, face, and extremities that can lead to scarring.
3. Photosensitivity—increased rash or other disease symptoms in response to sunlight exposure.
4. Mucous membrane ulcers—painless ulcers on the hard palate or nasal septum (or both).
5. Arthritis—nonerosive arthritis of large and small joints, typically in a symmetrical distribution.
6. Serositis—pericarditis or pleuritis (or both), often associated with chest pain and difficulty breathing.
7. Renal abnormalities—proteinuria (> 0.5 g/d) or cellular casts (or both).
8. Neurologic abnormalities—seizures or psychosis (or both).
9. Blood count abnormalities—low white blood cell count (< 4000/mm³), Coombs test–positive anemia and/or thrombocytopenia (< 100,000/mm³).
10. Positive ANA—seen in almost 100% of patients with SLE.
11. Autoantibodies—positive double-stranded DNA antibody, anti-Smith antibody, anticardiolipin antibodies, lupus anticoagulant, or false-positive blood test for syphilis.

Other common signs and symptoms include fever, fatigue, weight loss, anorexia, Raynaud phenomenon, myositis, vasculitis, chorea, neuropathies, depression, and cognitive changes.

B. Laboratory Findings

Complete blood count abnormalities are common, including leukopenia, anemia, and thrombocytopenia. Approximately 15% of patients are Coombs test–positive, but many patients develop anemia due to other causes, including chronic disease and blood loss. Patients with significant renal involvement may have electrolyte disturbances, elevated kidney function tests, and hypoalbuminemia. The ESR is frequently elevated

during active disease. In contrast, many patients with active SLE have a normal CRP. When the CRP is elevated, it is important to investigate possible infectious causes, particularly bacterial infections. It is critical to monitor the urinalysis in patients with SLE for proteinuria and hematuria, as the renal disease may be otherwise clinically silent. In immune complex diseases, complement is consumed; therefore, levels of C3 and C4 are depressed with active disease.

The ANA test is positive in almost 100% of patients, usually at titers of 1:320 or above. In patients with suspected SLE, it is important to obtain a full ANA profile—including antibodies directed against double-stranded DNA, Smith, ribonucleic protein, and SSA and SSB antibodies—to better characterize their serologic markers of disease. Because approximately 50–60% of pediatric SLE patients have antiphospholipid antibodies and are therefore at increased risk of thrombosis, it is important to screen all patients with SLE for anticardiolipin antibodies and lupus anticoagulant.

▶ Differential Diagnosis

Because there is such a wide spectrum of disease with SLE, the differential diagnosis is quite broad, including systemic JIA, mixed connective tissue disease (MCTD), rheumatic fever, vasculitis, malignancies, and bacterial and viral infections. A negative ANA test essentially excludes the diagnosis of SLE. Anti-double-stranded DNA and Smith antibodies are very specific for SLE. The preceding diagnostic criteria, which are very helpful in establishing the diagnosis of SLE, have a specificity and sensitivity of 96%.

MCTD, an overlap syndrome with features of several collagen-vascular diseases, shares many features with SLE. The symptom complex is diverse and often includes arthritis, fever, skin tightening, Raynaud phenomenon, muscle weakness, and rash. The ANA test is typically positive in very high titers. The ANA profile is negative except for antibodies directed against ribonucleicprotein.

▶ Treatment

The treatment of SLE should be tailored to the organ system involved so that toxicities may be minimized. Prednisone is the mainstay of treatment and has significantly lowered the mortality rate in SLE. Patients with severe, life-threatening, or organ-threatening disease are typically treated with intravenous pulse methylprednisolone, 30 mg/kg per dose (maximum of 1000 mg) daily for 3 days, and then switched to 2 mg/kg/d of prednisone. The dosage should be adjusted using clinical and laboratory parameters of disease activity, and the minimum amount of corticosteroid to control the disease should be used. Skin manifestations, arthritis, and fatigue may be treated with antimalarials such as hydroxychloroquine, 5–7 mg/kg/d orally. Pleuritic pain or arthritis can often be managed with NSAIDs.

If disease control is inadequate with prednisone or if the dose required produces intolerable side effects, a steroid-sparing agent, such as mycophenolate mofetil, azathioprine, or cyclophosphamide, should be added. More recently, rituximab, a monoclonal antibody directed against CD20, has been used for persistent active disease, particularly in patients with hematologic manifestations. Patients who have evidence of antiphospholipid antibodies should be treated with a baby aspirin every day to help prevent thrombosis. Thrombotic events due to these clotting antibodies require long-term anticoagulation.

The toxicities of the regimens must be carefully considered. Growth failure, osteoporosis, Cushing syndrome, adrenal suppression, and aseptic necrosis are serious side effects of chronic use of prednisone. When high doses of corticosteroids are used (> 2 mg/kg/d), there is a high risk of infection. Cyclophosphamide can cause bladder epithelial dysplasia, hemorrhagic cystitis, and sterility. Azathioprine has been associated with liver damage and bone marrow suppression. Immunosuppressant treatment should be withheld if the total white count falls below 3000/μL or the neutrophil count falls below 1000/μL. Retinal damage from hydroxychloroquine has not been observed with recommended dosages.

Course & Prognosis

The prognosis in SLE relates to the presence of renal involvement or infectious complications of treatment. Nonetheless, the survival rate has improved from 51% at 5 years in 1954 to 90% today. The disease has a natural waxing and waning cycle; the disease may flare at any time and spontaneous remission may occur.

Benseler SM, Silverman ED: Systemic lupus erythematosus. Pediatr Clin North Am 2005;52:443 [PMID: 15820375].
Ginzler EM, Dvorkina O: Newer therapeutic approaches for systemic lupus erythematosus. Rheum Dis Clin N Am 2005;31:315 [PMID: 15922148].
Gottlieb BS, Ilowite NT: Systemic lupus erythematosus in children and adolescents. Pediatr Rev 2006;27:323 [PMID: 16950937].
Ravelli A et al: Outcome in juvenile onset systemic lupus erythematosus. Curr Opin Rheumat 2005;17:568 [PMID: 16093835].

DERMATOMYOSITIS

ESSENTIALS OF DIAGNOSIS & TYPICAL FEATURES

▸ Pathognomonic skin rashes.
▸ Weakness of proximal muscles and occasionally of pharyngeal and laryngeal groups.
▸ Pathogenesis related to vasculitis.

General Considerations

Dermatomyositis is a rare autoimmune disease of muscle and skin. The cause is unknown, but there are likely genetic and environmental factors predisposing to the condition.

Small arteries and veins are involved, with infiltrates of neutrophils, lymphocytes, plasma cells, and histiocytes. The lesion progresses to intimal proliferation and thrombus formation. These vascular changes are found in the skin, muscle, kidney, retina, and gastrointestinal tract. Postinflammatory calcinosis may occur.

Clinical Findings

A. Symptoms and Signs

The predominant symptom is proximal muscular weakness, particularly affecting pelvic and shoulder girdle muscles. Tenderness, stiffness, and swelling may be found. Pharyngeal involvement, manifested as voice changes and difficulty swallowing, is associated with an increased risk of aspiration. Intestinal vasculitis can be associated with ulceration and perforation of involved areas. Flexion contractures and muscle atrophy may produce significant residual deformities. Calcinosis may follow the inflammation in muscle and skin.

Several characteristic rashes are seen in dermatomyositis. Patients often have a heliotrope rash with a reddish-purple hue on the upper eyelids, along with a malar rash that may be accompanied by edema of the eyelids and face. Gottron papules are shiny, erythematous, scaly plaques on the extensor surfaces of the knuckles, elbows, and knees. Nail-fold abnormalities, including dilation, thrombosis, and dropout of periungual capillaries, may identify patients with a worse prognosis.

B. Laboratory Findings

Determination of muscle enzyme levels, including aspartate aminotransferase, alanine aminotransferase, lactate dehydrogenase, creatine phosphokinase, and aldolase, is helpful in confirming the diagnosis, assessing disease activity, and monitoring the response to treatment. Even in the face of extensive muscle inflammation, the ESR and CRP are frequently normal. An MRI scan of the quadriceps muscle can be used in equivocal cases to confirm the presence of inflammatory myositis. Electromyography is useful to distinguish myopathic from neuropathic causes of muscle weakness. Muscle biopsy is indicated in doubtful cases of myositis without the pathognomonic rash.

Treatment

Treatment is aimed at suppression of the inflammatory response and prevention of the loss of muscle function and joint range of motion. Acutely, it is very important to assess the adequacy of the ventilatory effort and swallowing and to rule out intestinal vasculitis. Corticosteroids are the initial therapy of choice. Treatment is usually initiated with prednisone, 2 mg/kg/d, and continued until signs and symptoms of active disease are controlled; the dosage is then gradually tapered. In severe cases, intravenous pulse methylprednisolone for 3 days is indicated. Therapy is guided by the physical examination findings and muscle enzyme values. Steroid therapy is generally maintained at the lowest dose possible for at least 2 years to minimize the risk of exacerbations and calcinosis. If patients continue to have active disease, additional steroid-sparing agents such as methotrexate, cyclosporine, and in severe cases, cyclophosphamide, should be started.

Hydroxychloroquine and intravenous immunoglobulin are particularly helpful in managing the skin manifestations. As the rashes are photosensitive, sun protection is very important.

Physical and occupational therapy should be initiated early in the course of disease. Initially, passive range-of-motion exercises are performed to prevent loss motion. Later, once the muscle enzymes have normalized, a graduated program of stretching and strengthening exercises is introduced to restore normal strength and function.

► Course & Prognosis

Most patients have a monocyclic course; 10–20% of patients have more chronic or recurrent symptoms. Factors that influence the outcome include the rapidity of symptom onset, extent of weakness, presence of cutaneous or gastrointestinal vasculitis, timeliness of diagnosis, initiation of therapy, and response to treatment. Dermatomyositis in children is not associated with an increased risk of cancer as it is in adults.

Compeyrot-Lacassagne S, Feldman BM: Inflammatory myopathies in children. Pediatr Clin North Am 2005;52:493 [PMID: 15820377].
Lindsley CB: Juvenile dermatomyositis update. Curr Rheumatol Rep 2006;8:174 [PMID: 16901074].
McCann LJ et al: Juvenile Dermatomyositis Research Group. The Juvenile Dermatomyositis National Registry and Repository (UK and Ireland)—clinical characteristics of children recruited within the first 5 yr. Rheumatology (Oxford) 2006;45:1255 [PMID: 16567354].
Stringer E, Feldman BM: Advances in the treatment of juvenile dermatomyositis. Curr Opin Rheumatol 2006;18:503 [PMID: 16896290].

POLYARTERITIS NODOSA

Polyarteritis nodosa (PAN) is a rare disease, but a significant number of cases have been reported in childhood and infancy. No single cause has been found, but some series have reported an association with infectious triggers, including *Streptococcus,* hepatitis B, and parvovirus.

PAN is a multisystem disease that may manifest with fever, purpura, painful nodules, weight loss, myalgias, arthralgias, tingling, numbness, proteinuria or hematuria, hypertension, anorexia, and abdominal pain. Patients may also have central nervous system and cardiac involvement. Patients with isolated cutaneous disease present with painful nodules that have a predilection for the lower legs and feet. Diagnosis is confirmed by biopsies of involved tissues or arteriography demonstrating microaneurysms, stenosis, and dilation. Pathologically, the disease is a vasculitis of medium-sized arteries. Fibrosis of vessels and surrounding tissues accompanies the healing stages.

Treatment consists of prednisone and often requires other immunosuppressants, such as methotrexate, azathioprine, or cyclophosphamide. Isolated cutaneous disease can usually be managed with NSAIDs alone or with a short course of corticosteroids.

Kim S, Dedeoglu F: Update on pediatric vasculitis. Curr Opin Pediatr 2005;17:695 [PMID: 16282773].
Ozen S et al: Juvenile polyarteritis: Results of a multicenter survey of 110 children. J Pediatr 2004;145:517 [PMID: 15480378].

SCLERODERMA

Fortunately, the most common forms of scleroderma in childhood are localized morphea lesions and linear scleroderma, not the systemic disease. The skin disease begins as indurated, hyperpigmented or hypopigmented plaques (morphea) or linear bands (linear scleroderma) and ultimately leads to thickening and scarring of the involved areas. Patients may develop subcutaneous and muscular atrophy and joint contractures in underlying joints. Localized treatment with topical vitamin D analogues and ultraviolet light may be beneficial. Treatment with corticosteroids and methotrexate helps to limit extension of the disease and prevent the development of new lesions. Typically without treatment, the skin lesions progress over a 1–2-year period and then remit. No treatment is available to reverse the residual scarred areas; however, the skin tends to soften and develop more normal pigmentation over time.

In systemic sclerosis, the dermal process is generalized. Raynaud phenomenon is almost invariably present. Arthralgias, esophageal dysfunction, and renal disease are associated with systemic sclerosis. Involvement of the lungs, heart, and kidneys may lead to rapid deterioration. Supportive treatments should be initiated for the skin manifestations, Raynaud phenomenon, and gastrointestinal symptoms. Systemic immunosuppressant medications such as corticosteroids, methotrexate, and cyclophosphamide are used with variable response. Angiotensin-converting enzyme inhibitors are effective in preventing hypertensive renal crisis.

Zulian F et al; Juvenile Scleroderma Working Group of the Pediatric Rheumatology European Society (PRES): Juvenile localized scleroderma: Clinical and epidemiological features in 750 children. An international study. Rheumatology (Oxford) 2006;45:614 [PMID: 16368732].

RAYNAUD PHENOMENON

Raynaud phenomenon is an intermittent vasospastic disorder of the extremities. As much as 10% of the adult population has this disorder, and onset in childhood is not uncommon. The classic triphasic presentation is cold-induced pallor, then cyanosis, followed by hyperemia, but incomplete forms are frequent. In adults older than 35 years who are ANA-positive, Raynaud phenomenon may be a harbinger of rheumatic disease. This progression is rarely seen in childhood. Evaluation should include a detailed history with review of systems relevant to rheumatic disease and examination for nail-fold capillary abnormalities. In the absence of positive findings, Raynaud phenomenon is likely to be idiopathic.

Treatment involves education about keeping the extremities and core body warm and the role of stress, which may be a precipitant. In very symptomatic patients, treatment with calcium channel blockers such as nifedipine can be effective.

Nigrovic PA et al: Raynaud's phenomenon in children: A retrospective review of 123 patients. Pediatrics 2003;111:715 [PMID: 12671102].

Pavlov-Dolijanović S et al: The prognostic value of nailfold capillary changes for the development of connective tissue disease in children and adolescents with primary Raynaud phenomenon: A follow-up study of 250 patients. Pediatr Dermatol 2006;23:437 [PMID: 17014637].

NONINFLAMMATORY PAIN SYNDROMES

1. Complex Regional Pain Syndrome

Complex regional pain syndrome, previously known as reflex sympathetic dystrophy, is a painful condition that is frequently confused with arthritis. Prevalence and recognition of the condition appear to be increasing. Severe extremity pain leading to nearly complete loss of function is the hallmark of the condition. Evidence of autonomic dysfunction is demonstrated by pallor or cyanosis, temperature differences (with the affected extremity cooler than surrounding areas), and generalized swelling. On examination, marked cutaneous hyperesthesia to even the slightest touch is evident. Results of laboratory tests are normal, without evidence of systemic inflammation. Radiographic findings are normal except for late development of osteoporosis. Bone scans may be helpful and may demonstrate either increased or decreased blood flow to the painful extremity.

The cause of this condition remains elusive. Unlike adults with this disorder, children infrequently have a preceding history of trauma. Treatment includes physical therapy to focus on restoration of function, maintenance of range of motion, and pain relief. NSAIDs can be helpful for pain control, and in patients with more chronic disease, gabapentin is frequently effective. Persistent disease may respond to local nerve blocks. Counseling is helpful to identify potential psychosocial stressors and to assist with pain management. Long-term prognosis is good if recovery is rapid; recurrent episodes imply a less favorable prognosis.

Wilder RT: Management of pediatric patients with complex regional pain syndrome. Clin J Pain 2006;22:443 [PMID: 16772799].

2. Fibromyalgia

Fibromyalgia is a chronic pain syndrome characterized by diffuse musculoskeletal pain, fatigue, sleep disturbance, and chronic headaches. Weather changes, fatigue, and stress exacerbate symptoms. Patients have normal examination findings except for characteristic trigger points at the insertion of muscles, especially along the neck, spine, and pelvis.

Treatment centers on physical therapy, non-narcotic pain medications, improving sleep, and counseling. Low-dose amitriptyline or trazodone can help with sleep and may produce remarkable reduction in pain. Physical therapy should emphasize a graded rehabilitative approach to stretching and exercise and promote regular aerobic exercise. Pregabalin recently became the first medication to be approved by the Food and Drug Administration for the treatment of fibromyalgia. Use of the drug is associated with decreased pain in adults with fibromyalgia, and future studies are planned to test the safety and efficacy of its use in children with the condition. The prognosis for children with fibromyalgia is not clear, and long-term strategies may be necessary to enable them to cope with the condition.

Crofford LJ et al: Pregabalin for the treatment of fibromyalgia syndrome: Results of a randomized, double-blind, placebo-controlled trial. Arthritis Rheum 2005;52:1264 [PMID: 15818684].

Degotardi PJ et al: Development and evaluation of a cognitive-behavioral intervention for juvenile fibromyalgia. J Pediatr Psychol 2006;31:714 [PMID: 16120766].

3. Hypermobility Syndrome

Ligamentous laxity, which previously was thought to occur only in Ehlers-Danlos syndrome or Down syndrome, is now recognized as a common cause of joint pain. Patients with hypermobility present with episodic joint pain and occasionally with swelling that lasts a few days after increased physical activity. Depending on the activity, almost any joint may be affected. Five criteria have been established: (1) passive opposition of the thumb to the flexor surface of the forearm, (2) passive hyperextension of the fingers so that they are parallel to the extensor surface of the forearm, (3) hyperextension of the elbow, (4) hyperextension of the knee, and (5) palms on floor with knees extended. Results of laboratory tests are normal. The pain associated with the syndrome is produced by improper joint alignment caused by the laxity during exercise. Treatment consists of a graded conditioning program designed to provide muscular support of the joints to compensate for the loose ligaments and to train patients on how to protect their joints from hyperextension.

Adib N et al: Joint hypermobility syndrome in childhood. A not so benign multisystem disorder? Rheumatology (Oxford) 2005;44:744 [PMID: 15728418].

REFERENCES

Cassidy JT et al (editors): *Textbook of Pediatric Rheumatology.* Elsevier Saunders, 2005.

Laxer RM: Pediatric rheumatology. Pediatr Clin North Am 2005;52:xi-xii [PMID: 15820370].

Schaller JG: The history of pediatric rheumatology. Pediatr Res 2005;58:997 [PMID: 16183803].

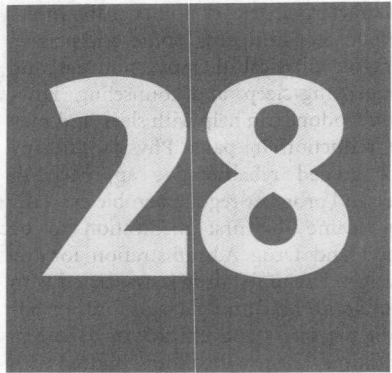

Hematologic Disorders

Daniel R. Ambruso, MD

Taru Hays, MD

Neil A. Goldenberg, MD

NORMAL HEMATOLOGIC VALUES

The normal ranges for peripheral blood counts vary significantly with age. Normal neonates show a relative polycythemia with a hematocrit concentration of 45–65%. The reticulocyte count at birth is relatively high at 2–8%. Within the first few days of life, erythrocyte production decreases, and the values for hemoglobin and hematocrit fall to a nadir at about 6–8 weeks. During this period, known as physiologic anemia of infancy, normal infants have hemoglobin values as low as 10 g/dL and hematocrits as low as 30%. Thereafter, the normal values for hemoglobin and hematocrit gradually increase until adult values are reached after puberty. Premature infants can reach a nadir hemoglobin level of 7–8 g/dL at 8–10 weeks.

Newborns have larger red cells than children and adults, with a mean corpuscular volume (MCV) at birth of more than 94 fL. The MCV subsequently falls to a nadir of 70–84 fL at about age 6 months. Thereafter, the normal MCV increases gradually until it reaches adult values after puberty.

The normal number of white blood cells is higher in infancy and early childhood than later in life. Neutrophils predominate in the differential white count at birth and in the older child. Lymphocytes predominate (up to 80%) between about ages 1 month and 6 years.

Normal values for the platelet count are 150,000–400,000/μL and vary little with age.

BONE MARROW FAILURE

Failure of the marrow to produce adequate numbers of circulating blood cells may be congenital or acquired and may cause pancytopenia (aplastic anemia) or involve only one cell line (single cytopenia). Constitutional and acquired aplastic anemias are discussed in this section and the more common single cytopenias in later sections. Bone marrow failure caused by malignancy or other infiltrative disease is discussed in Chapter 29. It is important to remember that

many drugs and toxins may affect the marrow and cause single or multiple cytopenias.

Suspicion of bone marrow failure is warranted in children with pancytopenia and in children with single cytopenias who lack evidence of peripheral red cell, white cell, or platelet destruction. Macrocytosis often accompanies bone marrow failure. Many of the constitutional bone marrow disorders are associated with a variety of congenital anomalies.

CONSTITUTIONAL APLASTIC ANEMIA (FANCONI ANEMIA)

ESSENTIALS OF DIAGNOSIS & TYPICAL FEATURES

▶ Progressive pancytopenia.

▶ Macrocytosis.

▶ Multiple congenital anomalies.

▶ Increased chromosome breakage in peripheral blood lymphocytes.

▶ General Considerations

Fanconi anemia is a syndrome characterized by defective DNA repair that is caused by a variety of genetic mutations. Inheritance is autosomal recessive, and the disease occurs in all ethnic groups. Hematologic manifestations usually begin with thrombocytopenia or neutropenia and subsequently progress over the course of months or years to pancytopenia. Typically the diagnosis is made between ages 2 and 10 years.

▶ Clinical Findings

A. Symptoms and Signs

Symptoms are determined principally by the degree of hematologic abnormality. Thrombocytopenia may cause purpura, petechiae, and bleeding; neutropenia may cause severe or recurrent infections; and anemia may cause weakness, fatigue, and pallor. Congenital anomalies are present in at least 50% of patients. The most common include abnormal pigmentation of the skin (generalized hyperpigmentation, café-au-lait or hypopigmented spots), short stature with delicate features, and skeletal malformations (hypoplasia, anomalies, or absence of the thumb and radius). More subtle anomalies are hypoplasia of the thenar eminence or a weak or absent radial pulse. Associated renal anomalies include aplasia, so-called horseshoe kidney, and duplication of the collecting system. Other anomalies are microcephaly, microphthalmia, strabismus, ear anomalies, and hypogenitalism.

B. Laboratory Findings

Thrombocytopenia or leukopenia typically occurs first, followed over the course of months to years by anemia and progression to severe aplastic anemia. Macrocytosis is virtually always present, is usually associated with anisocytosis and an elevation in fetal hemoglobin levels, and is an important diagnostic clue. The bone marrow reveals hypoplasia or aplasia. The diagnosis is confirmed by the demonstration of an increased number of chromosome breaks and rearrangements in peripheral blood lymphocytes. The use of diepoxybutane to stimulate these breaks and rearrangements provides a sensitive assay that is virtually always positive in children with Fanconi anemia, even before the onset of hematologic abnormalities.

Specific molecular markers or genes (Fanc-A, B, C, and others) found in different ethnic populations are identified in research laboratories and are not available as routine clinical tests.

▶ Differential Diagnosis

Because patients with Fanconi anemia frequently present with thrombocytopenia, the disorder must be differentiated from idiopathic thrombocytopenic purpura (ITP) and other more common causes of decreased platelets. In contrast to patients with ITP, those with Fanconi anemia usually exhibit a gradual fall in the platelet count. Counts less than 20,000/µL are often accompanied by neutropenia or anemia, along with phenotypical features. Fanconi anemia may also be manifested initially by pancytopenia, and must be differentiated from acquired aplastic anemia and other disorders, such as acute leukemia. Examination of the bone marrow and chromosome studies of peripheral blood lymphocytes (chromosomal breakage) will usually distinguish between these disorders.

▶ Complications

The most important complications of Fanconi anemia are those related to thrombocytopenia and neutropenia. Endocrine dysfunction may include growth hormone deficiency, hypothyroidism, or impaired glucose metabolism. In addition, persons with Fanconi anemia have a significantly increased risk of developing malignancies, especially acute

nonlymphocytic leukemia, head and neck cancers, genital cancers, and myelodysplastic syndromes. Death is usually the result of thrombocytopenic hemorrhage, overwhelming infection, or malignancy.

▶ Treatment

Attentive supportive care is a critical feature of management. Patients with neutropenia who develop fever require prompt evaluation and parenteral broad-spectrum antibiotics. Transfusions are important, but should be used judiciously, especially in the management of thrombocytopenia, which frequently becomes refractory to platelet transfusions as a consequence of alloimmunization. Transfusions from family members should be discouraged because of the negative effect on the outcome of bone marrow transplantation. At least 50% of patients with Fanconi anemia respond, albeit incompletely, to oxymetholone, and many recommend institution of androgen therapy before transfusions are needed. However, oxymetholone is associated with hepatotoxicity, hepatic adenomas, and masculinization, and is particularly troublesome for female patients.

Successful bone marrow transplantation cures the aplastic anemia and is an important treatment option for children with Fanconi anemia who have a human leukocyte antigen (HLA)–identical sibling donor. Before transplantation the prospective donor must be screened for Fanconi anemia by chromosome breakage testing.

▶ Prognosis

Many patients succumb to bleeding, infection, or malignancy in adolescence or early adulthood. The long-term outlook after successful bone marrow transplantation is uncertain, particularly with regard to the risk of subsequently developing malignancies.

Alter BP: Cancer in Fanconi anemia, 1927-2001. Cancer 2003;97:425 [PMID: 12518367].

Dufour C: Stem cell transplantation from HLA-matched related donor for Fanconi's anaemia: A retrospective review of the multicentric Italian experience on behalf of AIEOP-GITMO. Br J Haematol 2001;112:796 [PMID: 11260086].

Joenje H: The emerging genetic and molecular basis of Fanconi anemia. Nat Rev Genet 2001;2:446 [PMID: 11389461].

ACQUIRED APLASTIC ANEMIA

ESSENTIALS OF DIAGNOSIS & TYPICAL FEATURES

- ▶ Weakness and pallor.
- ▶ Petechiae, purpura, and bleeding.
- ▶ Frequent or severe infections.
- ▶ Pancytopenia with hypocellular bone marrow.

General Considerations

Acquired aplastic anemia is characterized by peripheral pancytopenia with a hypocellular bone marrow. Approximately 50% of cases in childhood are idiopathic. Other cases are secondary to idiosyncratic reactions to drugs such as phenylbutazone, sulfonamides, nonsteroidal anti-inflammatory drugs, and anticonvulsants. Toxic causes include exposure to benzene, insecticides, and heavy metals. Infectious causes include viral hepatitis (usually non-A, non-B, non-C), infectious mononucleosis, and human immunodeficiency virus (HIV). In immunocompromised children, aplastic anemia has been associated with human parvovirus B19. Immune mechanisms of marrow suppression are suspected in most cases.

Clinical Findings

A. Symptoms and Signs

Weakness, fatigue, and pallor result from anemia; petechiae, purpura, and bleeding occur because of thrombocytopenia; and fevers due to generalized or localized infections are associated with neutropenia. Hepatosplenomegaly and significant lymphadenopathy are unusual.

B. Laboratory Findings

Anemia is usually normocytic, with a low reticulocyte count. The white blood cell count is low, with a marked neutropenia. The platelet count is typically below 50,000/μL, and is frequently below 20,000/μL. Bone marrow aspiration and biopsy show hypocellularity, often marked.

Differential Diagnosis

Examination of the bone marrow usually excludes pancytopenia caused by peripheral destruction of blood cells or by infiltrative processes such as acute leukemia, storage diseases, and myelofibrosis. Many of these other conditions are associated with hepatosplenomegaly. Preleukemic conditions also may present with pancytopenia and hypocellular bone marrows. Cytogenetic analysis of the marrow is helpful, because a clonal abnormality may predict the subsequent development of leukemia. Since congenital anomalies may not be apparent in some children with Fanconi anemia, patients with newly diagnosed aplastic anemia should be studied for chromosome breaks and rearrangements in peripheral blood lymphocytes.

Complications

Acquired aplastic anemia is characteristically complicated by infection and hemorrhage, which are the leading causes of death. Other complications are those associated with therapy.

Treatment

Comprehensive supportive care is most important in the management of acute acquired aplastic anemia. Febrile illnesses require prompt evaluation and usually parenteral antibiotics. Red blood cell transfusions alleviate symptoms of anemia. Platelet transfusions may be lifesaving, but they should be used sparingly because many patients eventually develop platelet alloantibodies and become refractory to platelet transfusions.

Bone marrow transplantation is generally considered the treatment of choice for severe aplastic anemia when an HLA-compatible sibling donor is available. Because the likelihood of success with transplantation is influenced adversely by multiple transfusions, HLA typing of family members should be undertaken as soon as the diagnosis of aplastic anemia is made. Increasingly patients who lack HLA-matched siblings are able to find matched donors through cord blood banks or the National Marrow Donor Program.

An alternative to bone marrow transplantation from an HLA-matched sibling donor is immunomodulation, usually with antithymocyte globulin and cyclosporine. Responses are very good. Most patients show hematologic improvement and become transfusion-independent.

Prognosis

Children receiving early bone marrow transplantation from an HLA-identical sibling have a long-term survival rate of greater than 80%. Sustained, complete remissions may be seen in 65–80% of patients receiving immunosuppressive therapy. However, both therapies are associated with an increased risk of myelodysplastic syndromes, acute leukemia, and other malignancies in long-term survivors.

Brodsky R: Acquired severe aplastic anemia in children: Is there a standard of care? Pediatr Blood Cancer 2004;43:711 [PMID: 15503299].

Fouladi M: Improved survival in severe acquired aplastic anemia of childhood. Bone Marrow Transplant 2000;26:1149 [PMID: 11149724].

Goldenberg NA: Successful treatment of severe aplastic anemia in children using standardized immunosuppressive therapy with antithymocyte globulin and cyclosporine A. Pediatr Blood Cancer 2004;43:718 [PMID: 15390303].

Rosenfeld S: Antithymocyte globulin and cyclosporine for severe aplastic anemia: Association between hematologic response and long-term outcome. JAMA 2003;289:1130 [PMID: 12622583].

ANEMIAS

APPROACH TO THE CHILD WITH ANEMIA

Anemia is a relatively common finding, and identifying the cause is important. Even though anemia in childhood has many causes, the correct diagnosis can usually be established with relatively little laboratory cost. Frequently the cause is identified with a careful history. The possibility of nutritional causes should be addressed by inquiry about dietary intake; growth and development; and symptoms of chronic disease, malabsorption, or blood loss. Hemolytic disease may

▲ **Figure 28–1.** Investigation of anemia.

be associated with a history of jaundice (including neonatal jaundice) or by a family history of anemia, jaundice, gallbladder disease, splenomegaly, or splenectomy. The child's ethnic background may suggest the possibility of certain hemoglobinopathies or of deficiencies of red cell enzymes, such as glucose-6-phosphate dehydrogenase (G6PD). The review of systems may reveal clues to a previously unsuspected systemic disease associated with anemia. The patient's age is important because some causes of anemia are age-related. For example, patients with iron-deficiency anemia and β-globin disorders present more commonly at ages 6–36 months than at other times in life.

The physical examination may also reveal clues to the cause of anemia. Poor growth may suggest chronic disease or hypothyroidism. Congenital anomalies may be associated with constitutional aplastic anemia (Fanconi anemia) or with congenital hypoplastic anemia (Diamond-Blackfan anemia). Other disorders may be suggested by the findings of petechiae or purpura (leukemia, aplastic anemia, hemolytic-uremic syndrome), jaundice (hemolysis or liver disease), generalized lymphadenopathy (leukemia, juvenile rheumatoid arthritis, HIV infection), splenomegaly (leukemia, sickle hemoglobinopathy syndromes, hereditary spherocyto-

sis, liver disease, hypersplenism), or evidence of chronic or recurrent infections.

The initial laboratory evaluation of the anemic child consists of a complete blood count (CBC) with differential and platelet count, review of the peripheral blood smear, and a reticulocyte count. The algorithm in Figure 28–1 uses limited laboratory information, together with the history and physical examination, to reach a specific diagnosis or to focus additional laboratory investigations on a limited diagnostic category (eg, microcytic anemia, bone marrow failure, pure red cell aplasia, or hemolytic disease). This diagnostic scheme depends principally on the MCV to determine whether the anemia is microcytic, normocytic, or macrocytic, according to the percentile curves of Dallman and Siimes (Figure 28–2).

Although the incidence of iron deficiency in the United States has decreased significantly with improvements in infant nutrition, it remains an important cause of microcytic anemia, especially at ages 6–24 months. A trial of therapeutic iron is appropriate in such children, provided the dietary history is compatible with iron deficiency and the physical examination or CBC count does not suggest an alternative cause for the anemia. If

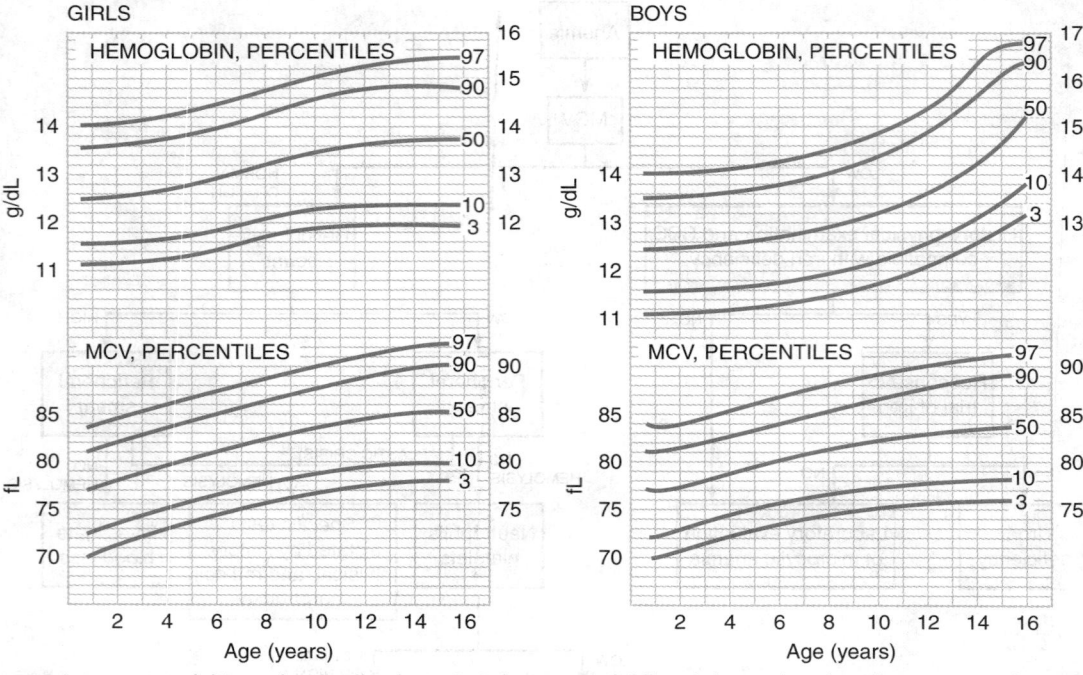

▲ **Figure 28–2.** Hemoglobin and red cell volume in infancy and childhood. (Reproduced, with permission, from Dallman PR, Siimes MA: Percentile curves for hemoglobin and red cell volume in infancy and childhood. J Pediatr 1979;94:26.)

this is not the case, or if a trial of therapeutic iron fails to correct the anemia and microcytosis, further laboratory evaluation is warranted.

Another key element of Figure 28–1 is the use of both the reticulocyte count and the peripheral blood smear to determine whether a normocytic or macrocytic anemia is due to hemolysis. Typically hemolytic disease is associated with an elevated reticulocyte count, but some children with chronic hemolysis initially present during a period of virus-induced aplasia when the reticulocyte count is not elevated. Thus, review of the peripheral blood smear for evidence of hemolysis (eg, spherocytes, red cell fragmentation, sickle forms) is important in the evaluation of children with normocytic anemias and low reticulocyte counts. When hemolysis is suggested, the correct diagnosis may be suspected by specific abnormalities of red cell morphology or by clues from the history or physical examination. Autoimmune hemolysis is usually excluded by direct antiglobulin testing. Review of blood counts and the peripheral blood smears of the mother and father may suggest genetic disorders such as hereditary spherocytosis. Children with normocytic or macrocytic anemias, with relatively low reticulocyte counts and no evidence of hemolysis on the blood smear, usually have anemias caused by inadequate erythropoiesis in the bone marrow. The presence of neutropenia or thrombocytopenia in such children suggests the possibility of aplastic anemia, malignancy, or severe folate or vitamin B_{12} deficiency, and usually dictates examination of the bone marrow.

Pure red cell aplasia may be congenital (Diamond-Black-fan anemia), acquired and transient (transient erythroblastopenia of childhood), a manifestation of a systemic disease such as renal disease or hypothyroidism, or due to malnutrition or mild deficiencies of folate or vitamin B_{12}.

Hermiston ML: A practical approach to the evaluation of the anemic child. Pediatr Clin North Am 2002;49:877 [PMID: 12430617].

PURE RED CELL APLASIA

Infants and children with normocytic or macrocytic anemia, a low reticulocyte count, and normal or elevated numbers of neutrophils and platelets should be suspected of having pure red cell aplasia. Examination of the peripheral blood smear in such cases is important because signs of hemolytic disease suggest chronic hemolysis complicated by an aplastic crisis due to parvovirus infection. Appreciation of this phenomenon is important because chronic hemolytic disease may not be diagnosed until the anemia is exacerbated by an episode of red cell aplasia and subsequent rapidly falling hemoglobin level. In such cases, cardiovascular compromise and congestive heart failure may develop quickly.

1. Congenital Hypoplastic Anemia (Diamond-Blackfan Anemia)

▶ Age: birth to 1 year.

▶ Macrocytic anemia with reticulocytopenia.

▶ Bone marrow with erythroid hypoplasia.

▶ Short stature or congenital anomalies in one third of patients.

General Considerations

Diamond-Blackfan anemia is a relatively rare cause of anemia that usually presents in infancy or early childhood. Early diagnosis is important because treatment with corticosteroids results in increased erythropoiesis in about two thirds of patients, thus avoiding the difficulties and complications of long-term chronic transfusion therapy. The cause is unclear; both autosomal dominant and autosomal recessive modes of inheritance occur.

Clinical Findings

A. Symptoms and Signs

Signs and symptoms are generally those of chronic anemia, such as pallor; congestive heart failure sometimes follows. Jaundice, splenomegaly, or other evidence of hemolysis is usually absent. Short stature or other congenital anomalies are present in one third of patients. A wide variety of anomalies have been described; those affecting the head, face, and thumbs are the most common.

B. Laboratory Findings

Diamond Blackfan anemia is characterized by severe macrocytic anemia and marked reticulocytopenia. The neutrophil count is usually normal or slightly decreased, and the platelet count is normal or elevated. The bone marrow usually shows a marked decrease in erythroid precursors but is otherwise normal. In older children, fetal hemoglobin levels are usually increased and there is evidence of persistent fetal erythropoiesis, such as the presence of the i antigen on erythrocytes. In addition, the level of adenosine deaminase in erythrocytes is elevated.

Differential Diagnosis

The principal differential diagnosis is transient erythroblastopenia of childhood. Children with Diamond-Blackfan anemia generally present at an earlier age, often have macrocytosis, and have evidence of fetal erythropoiesis and an elevated level of red cell adenosine deaminase. In addition,

short stature and congenital anomalies, are not associated with transient erythroblastopenia. Lastly, transient erythroblastopenia of childhood usually resolves within 6–8 weeks of diagnosis, whereas Diamond-Blackfan anemia is a lifelong affliction. Other disorders associated with decreased red cell production such as renal failure, hypothyroidism, and the anemia of chronic disease need to be considered.

Treatment

Oral corticosteroids should be initiated as soon as the diagnosis of Diamond-Blackfan anemia is made. Two thirds of patients will respond to prednisone, 2 mg/kg/d, and many of those who respond subsequently tolerate significant tapering of the dose. Patients who are unresponsive to prednisone require chronic transfusion therapy, which inevitably causes transfusion-induced hemosiderosis and the need for chelation with parenteral deferoxamine. Bone marrow transplantation is an alternative therapy that should be considered for transfusion-dependent patients who have HLA-matched siblings. Hematopoietic growth factors have been used in some cases with limited success. Unpredictable, spontaneous remissions occur in up to 20% of patients.

Prognosis

The prognosis for patients responsive to corticosteroids is generally good, particularly if remission is maintained with low doses of alternate-day prednisone. Patients dependent on transfusion are at risk for the complications of hemosiderosis, including death from congestive heart failure, cardiac arrhythmias, or hepatic failure. This remains a significant threat, particularly during adolescence, when compliance with nightly subcutaneous infusions of deferoxamine is often difficult to ensure.

Berndt A: Successful transplantation of CD34+ selected peripheral blood stem cells from an unrelated donor in an adult patient with Diamond-Blackfan anemia and secondary hemochromatosis. Bone Marrow Transplant 2005;35:99 [PMID: 15516941].

Vlachos A: Hematopoietic stem cell transplantation for Diamond-Blackfan anemia: A report from the Diamond–Blackfan Anemia Registry. Bone Marrow Transplant 2001;27:381 [PMID: 11313667].

2. Transient Erythroblastopenia of Childhood

▶ Age: 6 months to 4 years.

▶ Normocytic anemia with reticulocytopenia.

▶ Absence of hepatosplenomegaly or lymphadenopathy.

▶ Erythroid precursors initially absent from bone marrow.

General Considerations

Transient erythroblastopenia of childhood is a relatively common cause of acquired anemia in early childhood. The disorder is suspected when a normocytic anemia is discovered during evaluation of pallor or when a CBC is obtained for another reason. Because the anemia is due to decreased red cell production, and thus develops slowly, the cardiovascular system has time to compensate. Therefore, children with hemoglobin levels as low as 4–5 g/dL may look remarkably well. The disorder is thought to be autoimmune in most cases, because IgG from some patients has been shown to suppress erythropoiesis in vitro.

Clinical Findings

Pallor is the most common sign, and hepatosplenomegaly and lymphadenopathy are absent. The anemia is normocytic, and the peripheral blood smear shows no evidence of hemolysis. The platelet count is normal or elevated, and the neutrophil count is normal or, in some cases, decreased. Early in the course, no reticulocytes are identified. The Coombs test is negative, and there is no evidence of chronic renal disease, hypothyroidism, or other systemic disorder. Bone marrow examination shows severe erythroid hypoplasia initially; subsequently, erythroid hyperplasia develops along with reticulocytosis, and the anemia resolves.

Differential Diagnosis

Transient erythroblastopenia of childhood must be differentiated from Diamond-Blackfan anemia, particularly in infants younger than age 1 year. In contrast to Diamond-Blackfan anemia, transient erythroblastopenia is not associated with macrocytosis, short stature, or congenital anomalies, or with evidence of fetal erythropoiesis prior to the phase of recovery. Also in contrast to Diamond-Blackfan anemia, transient erythroblastopenia is associated with normal levels of red cell adenosine deaminase. Transient erythroblastopenia of childhood must also be differentiated from chronic disorders associated with decreased red cell production, such as renal failure, hypothyroidism, and other chronic states of infection or inflammation. As with other single cytopenias, the possibility of malignancy (ie, leukemia) should always be considered, particularly if fever, bone pain, hepatosplenomegaly, or lymphadenopathy is present. In such cases, examination of the bone marrow is generally diagnostic. Confusion may sometimes arise when the anemia of transient erythroblastopenia is first identified during the early phase of recovery when the reticulocyte count is high. In such cases, the disorder may be confused with the anemia of acute blood loss or with hemolytic disease. In contrast to hemolytic disorders, transient erythroblastopenia of childhood is not associated with jaundice or peripheral destruction of red cells.

Treatment & Prognosis

By definition, this is a transient disorder. Some children require red cell transfusions if cardiovascular compromise is present. Resolution of the anemia is heralded by an increase in the reticulocyte count, which generally occurs within 4–8 weeks of diagnosis. Transient erythroblastopenia of childhood is not treated with corticosteroids because of its short course.

NUTRITIONAL ANEMIAS

1. Iron-Deficiency Anemia

ESSENTIALS OF DIAGNOSIS & TYPICAL FEATURES

▶ Pallor and fatigue.
▶ Poor dietary intake of iron (ages 6–24 months).
▶ Chronic blood loss (age > 2 years).
▶ Microcytic hypochromic anemia.

General Considerations

Long considered the most common cause of anemia in pediatrics, iron deficiency has decreased substantially in incidence due to improved nutrition and the increased availability of iron-fortified infant formulas and cereals. Thus, the current approach to anemia in childhood must take into consideration a relatively greater likelihood of other causes.

Normal-term infants are born with sufficient iron stores to prevent iron deficiency for the first 4–5 months of life. Thereafter, enough iron needs to be absorbed to support the needs of rapid growth. For this reason, nutritional iron deficiency is most common between 6 and 24 months of life. A deficiency earlier than age 6 months may occur if iron stores at birth are reduced by prematurity, small birth weight, neonatal anemia, or perinatal blood loss or if there is subsequent iron loss due to hemorrhage. Iron-deficient children older than age 24 months should be evaluated for blood loss. Iron deficiency, in addition to causing anemia, has adverse effects on multiple organ systems. Thus, the importance of identifying and treating iron deficiency extends past the resolution of any symptoms directly attributable to a decreased hemoglobin concentration.

Clinical Findings

A. Symptoms and Signs

Symptoms and signs vary with the severity of the deficiency. Mild iron deficiency is usually asymptomatic. In infants with more severe iron deficiency, pallor, fatigue, irritability, and delayed motor development are common. Children whose iron deficiency is due in part to ingestion of unfortified cow's milk may be fat, with poor muscle tone. A history of pica is common.

B. Laboratory Findings

The severity of anemia depends on the degree of iron deficiency, and the hemoglobin level may be as low as 3–4 g/dL in severe cases. Red cells are microcytic and hypochromic, with a low MCV and low mean corpuscular hemoglobin. The red blood cell distribution width is typically elevated, even with mild iron deficiency. The reticulocyte count is usually normal or slightly elevated, but the reticulocyte index or absolute reticulocyte count is decreased. Iron studies show a decreased serum ferritin and a low serum iron, elevated total iron-binding capacity, and decreased transferrin saturation. These laboratory abnormalities are usually present with moderate to severe iron deficiency, but mild cases may be associated with variable laboratory results. The peripheral blood smear shows microcytic, hypochromic red blood cells with anisocytosis, and occasional target, teardrop, elliptical, and fragmented red cells. Leukocytes are normal, and very often platelet count is increased with normal morphology.

The bone marrow examination is not helpful in the diagnosis of iron deficiency in infants and small children because little or no iron is stored as marrow hemosiderin at these ages.

▶ Differential Diagnosis

The differential diagnosis is that of microcytic, hypochromic anemia. The possibility of thalassemia (α-thalassemia, β-thalassemia, and hemoglobin E disorders) should be considered, especially in infants of African, Mediterranean, or Asian ethnic background. In contrast to infants with iron deficiency, those with thalassemia generally have an elevated number of erythrocytes (the index of the MCV divided by the red cell number is usually less than 13) and are less likely, in mild cases, to have an elevated red blood cell distribution width. Thalassemias are associated with normal or increased levels of serum iron and ferritin and with normal iron-binding capacity. The hemoglobin electrophoresis in β-thalassemia minor typically shows an elevation of hemoglobin A_2 levels, but coexistent iron deficiency may lower the percentage of hemoglobin A_2 into the normal range. Hemoglobin electrophoresis will also identify children with hemoglobin E, a cause of microcytosis common in Southeast Asians. In contrast, the hemoglobin electrophoresis in α-thalassemia trait is normal. Lead poisoning has also been associated with microcytic anemia, but anemia with lead levels less than 40 mg/dL is often due to coexistent iron deficiency.

The anemia of chronic inflammation or infection is normocytic but in late stages may be microcytic. This anemia is usually suspected because of the presence of a chronic systemic disorder. The level of serum iron is low, but the iron-binding capacity is normal, and the serum ferritin level is normal or elevated. Relatively mild infections, particularly during infancy, may cause transient anemia. As a result, caution should be exercised when the diagnosis of mild iron deficiency is entertained in infants and young children who have had recent viral or bacterial infections. Ideally, screening tests for anemia should not be obtained within 3–4 weeks of such infections.

▶ Treatment

The recommended oral dose of elemental iron is 6 mg/kg/d in three divided daily doses. Mild cases may be treated with 2 mg/kg/d given once daily before breakfast. Parenteral administration of iron is rarely necessary. Iron therapy results in an increased reticulocyte count within 3–5 days, which is maximal between 5 and 7 days. The hemoglobin level begins to increase thereafter. The rate of hemoglobin rise is inversely related to the hemoglobin level at diagnosis. In moderate to severe cases, an elevated reticulocyte count 1 week after initiation of therapy confirms the diagnosis and documents compliance and response to therapy. When iron deficiency is the only cause of anemia, adequate treatment usually results in a resolution of the anemia within 4–6 weeks. Treatment is generally continued for a few additional months to replenish iron stores.

Hermiston ML: A practical approach to the evaluation of the anemic child. Pediatr Clin North Am 2002;49:877 [PMID: 12430617].

2. Megaloblastic Anemias

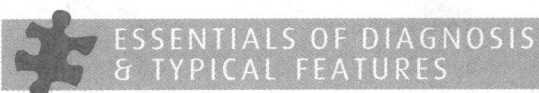

ESSENTIALS OF DIAGNOSIS & TYPICAL FEATURES

▶ Pallor and fatigue.
▶ Nutritional deficiency or intestinal malabsorption.
▶ Macrocytic anemia.
▶ Megaloblastic bone marrow changes.

▶ General Considerations

Megaloblastic anemia is a macrocytic anemia caused by deficiency of cobalamin (vitamin B_{12}), folic acid, or both. Cobalamin deficiency due to dietary insufficiency may occur in infants who are breast fed by mothers who are strict vegetarians or who have pernicious anemia. Intestinal malabsorption is the usual cause of cobalamin deficiency in children and occurs with Crohn disease, chronic pancreatitis, bacterial overgrowth of the small bowel, infection with the fish tapeworm (*Diphyllobothrium latum*), or after surgical resection of the terminal ileum. Deficiencies due to inborn errors of metabolism (transcobalamin II deficiency and methylmalonic aciduria) also have been described. Malabsorption of cobalamin due to deficiency of intrinsic factor (pernicious anemia) is rare in childhood.

Folic acid deficiency may be caused by inadequate dietary intake, malabsorption, increased folate requirements, or some combination of the three. Folate deficiency due to dietary deficiency alone is rare but occurs in severely malnourished infants and has been reported in infants fed goat's milk not fortified with folic acid. Folic acid is absorbed in the jejunum, and deficiencies are encountered in malabsorptive syndromes such as celiac disease. Anticonvulsion medications (eg, phenytoin and phenobarbital) and cytotoxic drugs (eg, methotrexate) also have been associated with folate deficiency, caused by interference with folate absorption or metabolism. Finally, folic acid deficiency is more likely to develop in infants and children with increased requirements. This occurs during infancy because of rapid growth and also in children with chronic hemolytic anemia. Premature infants are particularly susceptible to the development of the deficiency because of low body stores of folate.

Clinical Findings

A. Symptoms and Signs

Infants with megaloblastic anemia may show pallor and mild jaundice as a result of ineffective erythropoiesis. Classically, the tongue is smooth and beefy red. Infants with cobalamin deficiency may be irritable and may be poor feeders. Older children with cobalamin deficiency may complain of paresthesias, weakness, or an unsteady gait and may show decreased vibratory sensation and proprioception on neurologic examination.

B. Laboratory Findings

The laboratory findings of megaloblastic anemia include an elevated MCV and mean corpuscular hemoglobin. The peripheral blood smear shows numerous macro-ovalocytes with anisocytosis and poikilocytosis. Neutrophils are large and have hypersegmented nuclei. The white cell and platelet counts are normal with mild deficiencies, but may be decreased in more severe cases. Examination of the bone marrow typically shows erythroid hyperplasia with large erythroid and myeloid precursors. Nuclear maturation is delayed compared with cytoplasmic maturation, and erythropoiesis is ineffective. The serum indirect bilirubin concentration may be slightly elevated.

Children with cobalamin deficiency have a low serum vitamin B_{12} level, but decreased levels of serum vitamin B_{12} may also be found in about 30% of patients with folic acid deficiency. The level of red cell folate is a better reflection of folate stores than is the serum folic acid level. Serum levels of metabolic intermediates (methylmalonic acid and homocysteine) may help establish the correct diagnosis. Elevated methylmalonic acid levels are consistent with cobalamin deficiency, whereas elevated levels of homocysteine occur with both cobalamin and folate deficiency.

Differential Diagnosis

Most macrocytic anemias in pediatrics are not megaloblastic. Other causes of an increased MCV include drug therapy (eg, anticonvulsants, anti-HIV nucleoside analogues), Down syndrome, an elevated reticulocyte count (hemolytic anemias), bone marrow failure syndromes (Fanconi anemia, Diamond-Blackfan anemia), liver disease, and hypothyroidism.

Treatment

Treatment of cobalamin deficiency due to inadequate dietary intake is readily accomplished with oral supplementation. Most cases, however, are due to intestinal malabsorption and require parenteral treatment. In severe cases, parenteral therapy may induce life-threatening hypokalemia and require supplemental potassium. Folic acid deficiency is treated effectively with oral folic acid in most cases. Children at risk for the development of folic acid deficiencies, such as premature infants and those with chronic hemolysis, are often given folic acid prophylactically.

ANEMIA OF CHRONIC DISORDERS

Anemia is a common manifestation of many chronic illnesses in children. In some instances, causes may be mixed. For example, children with chronic disorders involving intestinal malabsorption or blood loss may have anemia of chronic inflammation in combination with nutritional deficiencies of iron, folate, or cobalamin. In other settings, the anemia is due to dysfunction of a single organ (eg, renal failure, hypothyroidism), and correction of the underlying abnormality resolves the anemia.

1. Anemia of Chronic Inflammation

Anemia is frequently associated with chronic infections or inflammatory diseases. The anemia is usually mild to moderate in severity, with a hemoglobin level of 8–12 g/dL. In general, the severity of the anemia corresponds to the severity of the underlying disorder, and there may be microcytosis, but not hypochromia. The reticulocyte count is low. The anemia is thought to be due to inflammatory cytokines that inhibit erythropoiesis, and shunting of iron into, and impaired iron release from, reticuloendothelial cells. Levels of erythropoietin are relatively low for the severity of the anemia. The serum iron concentration is low, but in contrast to iron deficiency, anemia of chronic inflammation is not associated with elevated iron-binding capacity and is associated with an elevated serum ferritin level. Treatment consists of correction of the underlying disorder, which, if controlled, generally results in improvement in hemoglobin level.

Hagar W: Diseases of iron metabolism. Pediatr Clin North Am 2002;49:893 [PMID: 12430618].

2. Anemia of Chronic Renal Failure

Severe normocytic anemia occurs in most forms of renal disease that have progressed to renal insufficiency. Although white cell and platelet production remain normal, the bone marrow shows significant hypoplasia of the erythroid series and the reticulocyte count is low. The principal mechanism is deficiency of erythropoietin, a hormone produced in the kidney, but other factors may contribute to the anemia. In the presence of significant uremia, a component of hemolysis may also be present. Recombinant human erythropoietin (epoetin alfa) corrects the anemia, largely eliminating the need for transfusions.

Seeherunvong W: Identification of poor responders to erythropoietin among children undergoing hemodialysis. J Pediatr 2001;138:710 [PMID: 11343048].
Yorgin PD: The clinical efficacy of higher hematocrit levels in children with chronic renal insufficiency and those undergoing dialysis. Semin Nephrol 2001;21:451 [PMID: 11559886].

3. Anemia of Hypothyroidism

Some patients with hypothyroidism develop significant anemia. Occasionally, anemia is detected before the diagnosis of the underlying disorder. A decreased growth velocity in an anemic child suggests hypothyroidism. The anemia is usually normocytic or macrocytic, but it is not megaloblastic and, hence not due to deficiencies of cobalamin or folate. Replacement therapy with thyroid hormone is usually effective in correcting the anemia.

CONGENITAL HEMOLYTIC ANEMIAS: RED CELL MEMBRANE DEFECTS

The congenital hemolytic anemias are divided into three categories: defects of the red cell membrane; hemoglobinopathies; and disorders of red cell metabolism. Hereditary spherocytosis and elliptocytosis are the most common red cell membrane disorders. The diagnosis is suggested by the peripheral blood smear, which shows characteristic red cell morphology (eg, spherocytes, elliptocytes). These disorders usually have an autosomal dominant inheritance, and the diagnosis may be suggested by a family history. The hemolysis is due to the deleterious effect of the membrane abnormality on red cell deformability. Decreased cell deformability leads to entrapment of the abnormally shaped red cells in the spleen. Many patients have splenomegaly, and splenectomy usually alleviates the hemolysis.

1. Hereditary Spherocytosis

ESSENTIALS OF DIAGNOSIS & TYPICAL FEATURES

▶ Anemia and jaundice.
▶ Splenomegaly.
▶ Positive family history of anemia, jaundice, or gallstones.
▶ Spherocytosis with increased reticulocytes.
▶ Increased osmotic fragility.
▶ Negative direct antiglobulin test (DAT).

▶ General Considerations

Hereditary spherocytosis is a relatively common inherited hemolytic anemia that occurs in all ethnic groups but is most common in persons of northern European ancestry, in whom the incidence is about 1:5000. The disorder is a heterogeneous one, marked by variable degrees of anemia, jaundice, and splenomegaly. In some persons, the disorder is mild and there is no anemia because erythroid hyperplasia fully compensates for hemolysis. Severe cases are transfusion-dependent prior to splenectomy. The hallmark of hereditary spherocytosis is the presence of microspherocytes in the peripheral blood. The disease is inherited in an autosomal dominant fashion in about 75% of cases; the remaining cases are thought to be autosomal recessive or to be caused by new mutations.

Hereditary spherocytosis is usually the result of a partial deficiency of spectrin, an important structural protein of the red cell membrane skeleton. Spectrin deficiency weakens the attachment of the cell membrane to the underlying membrane skeleton and causes the red cell to lose membrane surface area. This process creates spherocytes that are poorly deformable and have a shortened life span because they are trapped in the microcirculation of the spleen and engulfed by splenic macrophages. The extreme heterogeneity of hereditary spherocytosis is related directly to variable degrees of spectrin deficiency. In general, children who inherit spherocytosis in an autosomal dominant fashion have less spectrin deficiency and mild or moderate hemolysis. In contrast, those with nondominant forms of spherocytosis tend to have greater deficiency of spectrin and more severe anemia.

▶ Clinical Findings

A. Symptoms and Signs

Hemolysis causes significant neonatal hyperbilirubinemia in 50% of affected children. Splenomegaly subsequently develops in the majority and is often present by age 5 years. Jaundice is variably present and in many patients may be noted only during infection. Patients with significant chronic anemia may complain of pallor, fatigue, or malaise. Intermittent exacerbations of the anemia are caused by increased hemolysis or by aplastic crises, and may be associated with severe weakness, fatigue, fever, abdominal pain, or even heart failure.

B. Laboratory Findings

Most patients have mild chronic hemolysis with hemoglobin levels of 9–12 g/dL. In some cases, the hemolysis is fully compensated and the hemoglobin level is in the normal range. Rare cases of severe disease require frequent transfusions. The anemia is usually normocytic and hyperchromic, and many patients have an elevated mean corpuscular hemoglobin concentration. The peripheral blood smear shows numerous microspherocytes and polychromasia. The reticulocyte count is elevated, often higher than might be expected for the degree of anemia. White blood cell and platelet counts are usually normal. The osmotic fragility is increased, particularly after incubation at 37°C for 24 hours. Serum bilirubin usually shows an elevation in the unconjugated fraction. The DAT is negative.

Differential Diagnosis

Spherocytes are frequently present in persons with immune hemolysis. Thus, in the newborn, hereditary spherocytosis must be distinguished from hemolytic disease caused by ABO or other blood type incompatibilities. Older patients with autoimmune hemolytic anemia frequently present with jaundice and splenomegaly and with spherocytes on the peripheral blood smear. The DAT is positive in most cases of immune hemolysis and negative in hereditary spherocytosis. Occasionally, the diagnosis is confused in patients with splenomegaly from other causes, especially when hypersplenism increases red cell destruction and when some spherocytes are noted on the blood smear. In such cases, the true cause of the splenomegaly may be suggested by signs or symptoms of portal hypertension or by laboratory evidence of chronic liver disease. In contrast to children with hereditary spherocytosis, those with hypersplenism typically have some degree of thrombocytopenia or neutropenia.

Complications

Severe jaundice may occur in the neonatal period and, if not controlled by phototherapy, may occasionally require exchange transfusion. Splenectomy is associated with an increased risk of overwhelming bacterial infections, particularly with pneumococci. Gallstones occur in 60–70% of adults who have not undergone splenectomy and may form as early as age 5–10 years.

Treatment

Supportive measures include the administration of folic acid to prevent the development of red cell hypoplasia due to folate deficiency. Acute exacerbations of anemia, due to increased rates of hemolysis or to aplastic crises caused by infection with human parvovirus, may be severe enough to require red cell transfusions. Splenectomy is performed in many cases and always results in significant improvement. The procedure increases the survival of the spherocytic red cells and leads to complete correction of the anemia in most cases. Patients with more severe disease may show some degree of hemolysis after splenectomy. Except in unusually severe cases, the procedure should be postponed until the child is at least age 5 years because of the greater risk of post-splenectomy sepsis prior to

this age. All patients scheduled for splenectomy should be immunized with pneumococcal, *Haemophilus influenzae* type b, and meningococcal vaccines prior to the procedure, and some clinicians recommend penicillin prophylaxis afterward. Asplenic patients with fever should be promptly evaluated for severe infection. The need for splenectomy in mild cases is controversial. Splenectomy in the middle childhood years prevents the subsequent development of cholelithiasis and eliminates the need for the activity restrictions recommended for children with splenomegaly. However, these benefits must be weighed against the risks of the surgical procedure and the subsequent lifelong risk of post-splenectomy sepsis.

Prognosis

Splenectomy eliminates signs and symptoms in all but the most severe cases and reduces the risk of cholelithiasis. The abnormal red cell morphology and increased osmotic fragility persist without clinical consequence.

Delhommeau F: Natural history of hereditary spherocytosis during the first year of life. Blood 2000;95:393 [PMID: 10627440].

2. Hereditary Elliptocytosis

Hereditary elliptocytosis is a heterogeneous disorder that ranges in severity from an asymptomatic state with almost normal red cell morphology to severe hemolytic anemia. Most affected persons have numerous elliptocytes on the peripheral blood smear, but mild or no hemolysis. Those with hemolysis have an elevated reticulocyte count and may have jaundice and splenomegaly. These disorders are caused by mutations of red cell membrane skeletal proteins, and most have an autosomal dominant inheritance. Because most patients are asymptomatic, no treatment is indicated. Patients with significant degrees of hemolytic anemia may benefit from folate supplementation or from splenectomy.

Some infants with hereditary elliptocytosis present in the neonatal period with moderate to marked hemolysis and significant hyperbilirubinemia. This disorder has been termed transient infantile poikilocytosis because such infants exhibit bizarre erythrocyte morphology with elliptocytes, budding red cells, and small misshapen cells that defy description. The MCV is low, and the anemia may be severe enough to require red cell transfusions. Typically, one parent has hereditary elliptocytosis, usually mild or asymptomatic. The infant's hemolysis gradually abates during the first year of life, and the erythrocyte morphology subsequently becomes more typical of hereditary elliptocytosis.

CONGENITAL HEMOLYTIC ANEMIAS: HEMOGLOBINOPATHIES

The hemoglobinopathies are an extremely heterogeneous group of congenital disorders that occur in many different ethnic groups. The relatively high frequency of these genetic variants is related to the malaria protection afforded to

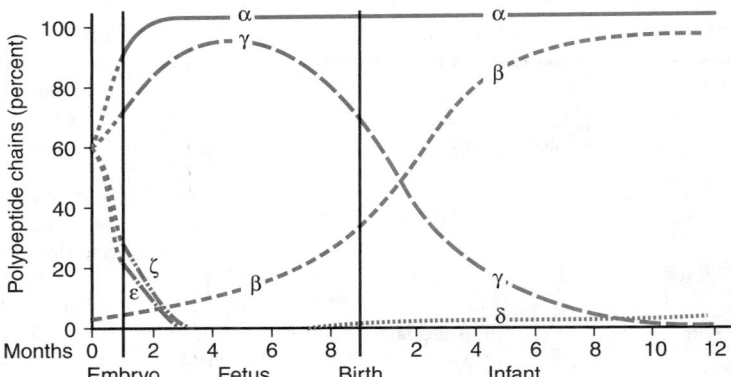

▲ **Figure 28–3.** Changes in hemoglobin polypeptide chains during human development. (Reproduced, with permission, from Miller DR, Baehner RL: *Blood Diseases of Infancy and Childhood,* 6th ed. Mosby, 1989.)

heterozygous individuals. The hemoglobinopathies are generally classified into two major groups. The first, the thalassemias, are caused by quantitative deficiencies in the production of globin chains. These quantitative defects in globin synthesis cause microcytic and hypochromic anemias. The second group of hemoglobinopathies consists of those caused by structural abnormalities of globin chains. The most important of these, hemoglobins S, C, and E, are all the result of point mutations and single amino acid substitutions in β-globin. Many, but not all, infants with hemoglobinopathies are identified by routine neonatal screening.

Figure 28–3 shows the normal developmental changes that occur in globin-chain production during gestation and the first year of life. At birth, the predominant hemoglobin is fetal hemoglobin (hemoglobin F), which is composed of two α-globin chains and two γ-globin chains. Subsequently, the production of γ-globin decreases and the production of β-globin increases so that adult hemoglobin (two α chains and two β chains) predominates after 2–4 months. Because α-globin chains are present in both fetal and adult hemoglobin, disorders of α-globin synthesis (α-thalassemia) are clinically manifest in the newborn as well as later in life. In contrast, patients with β-globin disorders such as β-thalassemia and sickle cell disease are generally asymptomatic during the first 3–4 months of age and present clinically after γ-chain production—and therefore fetal hemoglobin levels—have decreased substantially.

1. α-Thalassemia

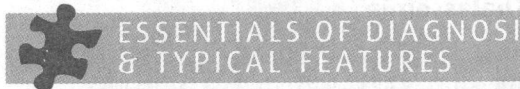

ESSENTIALS OF DIAGNOSIS
& TYPICAL FEATURES

▶ African, Mediterranean, Middle Eastern, Chinese, or Southeast Asian ancestry.

▶ Microcytic, hypochromic anemia of variable severity.

▶ Bart's hemoglobin detected by neonatal screening.

▶ General Considerations

Most of the α-thalassemia syndromes are the result of deletions of one or more of the α-globin genes on chromosome 16. Normal diploid cells have four α-globin genes; thus the variable severity of the α-thalassemia syndromes is related to the number of gene deletions (Table 28–1). The severity of the α-thalassemia syndromes varies among affected ethnic groups, depending on the genetic abnormalities prevalent in the population. In persons of African ancestry, α-thalassemia is usually caused by the deletion of only one of the two α-globin genes on each chromosome. Thus, in the African population, heterozygous individuals are silent carriers and homozygous individuals have α-thalassemia trait. In Asians, deletions of one or of both α-globin genes on the same chromosome are common; heterozygous individuals are either silent carriers or have α-thalassemia trait, and homozygous individuals or compound heterozygous individuals have α-thalassemia trait, hemoglobin H disease, or hydrops fetalis. Thus, the presence of α-thalassemia in a child of Asian ancestry may have important implications for genetic counseling, whereas this is not usually the case in families of African ancestry.

▶ Clinical Findings

The clinical findings depend on the number of α-globin genes deleted. Table 28–1 summarizes the α-thalassemia syndromes.

Persons with three α-globin genes (one-gene deletion) are asymptomatic and have no hematologic abnormalities. Hemoglobin levels and MCV are normal. Hemoglobin electrophoresis in the neonatal period shows 0–3% Bart's hemoglobin, which is a variant hemoglobin composed of four γ-globin chains. Hemoglobin electrophoresis after the first few months of life is normal. Thus, this condition is usually suspected only in the context of family studies or when a small amount of Bart's hemoglobin is detected by neonatal screening for hemoglobinopathies.

Table 28–1. The α-Thalassemias.

Usual Genotypes[a]	α-Gene Number	Clinical Features	Hemoglobin Electrophoresis[b]	
			Birth	> 6 mos
αα/αα	4	Normal	N	N
-α/αα	3	Silent carrier	0–3% Hb Bart's	N
-/αα or -α/-α	2	α-Thal trait	2–10% Hb Bart's	N
-/-α	1	Hb H disease	15–30% Hb Bart's	Hb; H present
-/-	0	Fetal hydrops	> 75% Hb Bart's	—

[a]α indicates presence of α-globin gene, – indicates deletion of α-globin gene.
[b]N = normal results, Hb = hemoglobin, Hb Bart's = γ_4, Hb H = β_4.

Persons with two α-globin genes (two-gene deletion) are typically asymptomatic. The MCV is usually less than 100 fL at birth. Hematologic studies in older infants and children show a normal or slightly decreased hemoglobin level with a low MCV and a slightly hypochromic blood smear with some target cells. The hemoglobin electrophoresis typically shows 2–10% Bart's hemoglobin in the neonatal period but is normal in older children and adults.

Persons with one α-globin gene (three-gene deletion) have a mild to moderately severe microcytic hemolytic anemia (hemoglobin level of 7–10 g/dL), which may be accompanied by hepatosplenomegaly and some bony abnormalities caused by the expanded medullary space. The reticulocyte count is elevated, and the red cells show marked hypochromia and microcytosis with significant poikilocytosis and some basophilic stippling. Hemoglobin electrophoresis in the neonatal period typically shows 15–30% Bart's hemoglobin. Later in life, hemoglobin H (composed of four β-globin chains) is present. Incubation of red cells with brilliant cresyl blue (hemoglobin H preparation) shows inclusion bodies formed by denatured hemoglobin H.

The deletion of all four α-globin genes causes severe intrauterine anemia and asphyxia and results in hydrops fetalis and fetal demise or neonatal death shortly after delivery. Extreme pallor and massive hepatosplenomegaly are present. Hemoglobin electrophoresis reveals a predominance of Bart's hemoglobin with a complete absence of normal fetal or adult hemoglobin.

▶ Differential Diagnosis

α-Thalassemia trait (two-gene deletion) must be differentiated from other mild microcytic anemias, including iron deficiency and β-thalassemia minor (see next section). In contrast to children with iron deficiency, children with α-thalassemia trait show normal or increased levels of ferritin and serum iron. In contrast to children with β-thalassemia minor, children with α-thalassemia trait have a normal hemoglobin electrophoresis after age 4–6 months. Finally, the history of a low MCV (96 fL) at birth or the presence of Bart's hemoglobin on the neonatal hemoglobinopathy screening test suggests α-thalassemia.

Children with hemoglobin H disease may have jaundice and splenomegaly, and the disorder must be differentiated from other hemolytic anemias. The key to the diagnosis is the decreased MCV and the marked hypochromia on the blood smear. With the exception of β-thalassemia, most other significant hemolytic disorders have a normal or elevated MCV and the red blood cells are not hypochromic. Infants with hydrops fetalis due to severe α-thalassemia must be distinguished from those with hydrops due to other causes of anemia, such as alloimmunization.

▶ Complications

The principal complication of α-thalassemia trait is the needless administration of iron, given in the belief that a mild microcytic anemia is due to iron deficiency. Persons with hemoglobin H disease may have intermittent exacerbations of their anemia in response to oxidant stress or infection, which occasionally require blood transfusions. Splenomegaly may exacerbate the anemia and may require splenectomy. Women pregnant with hydropic α-thalassemia fetuses are subject to increased complications of pregnancy, particularly toxemia and postpartum hemorrhage.

▶ Treatment

Persons with α-thalassemia trait require no treatment. Those with hemoglobin H disease should receive supplemental folic acid and avoid the same oxidant drugs that cause hemolysis in persons with G6PD deficiency, because exposure to these drugs may exacerbate their anemia. The anemia may also be exacerbated during periods of infection, and transfusions may be required. Hypersplenism may develop later in childhood and require surgical splenectomy. Genetic counseling and prenatal diagnosis should be offered to families at risk for hydropic fetuses.

Clarke GM: Laboratory investigation of hemoglobinopathies and thalassemias: Review and update. Clin Chem 2000;46:1284 [PMID: 10926923].

2. β-Thalassemia

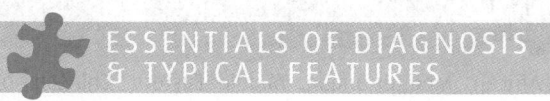

ESSENTIALS OF DIAGNOSIS & TYPICAL FEATURES

β-Thalassemia minor:

▶ Normal neonatal screening test.

▶ African, Mediterranean, Middle Eastern, or Asian ancestry.

- ► Mild microcytic, hypochromic anemia.
- ► No response to iron therapy.
- ► Elevated level of hemoglobin A_2.

β-Thalassemia major:

- ► Neonatal screening shows hemoglobin F only.
- ► Mediterranean, Middle Eastern, or Asian ancestry.
- ► Severe microcytic, hypochromic anemia with marked hepatosplenomegaly.

General Considerations

In contrast to the four α-globin genes, only two β-globin genes are present in diploid cells, one on each chromosome 11. Some β-thalassemia genes produce no β-globin chains and are termed β^0-thalassemia. Other β-globin genes produce some β-globin, but in diminished quantities, and are termed β^+-thalassemia. Persons affected by β-thalassemia may be heterozygous or homozygous. Individuals heterozygous for most β-thalassemia genes have β-thalassemia minor. Homozygous individuals have β-thalassemia major (Cooley anemia), a severe transfusion-dependent anemia, or a condition known as thalassemia intermedia, which is more severe than thalassemia minor but is not generally transfusion-dependent. β-Thalassemia major is the most common worldwide cause of transfusion-dependent anemia in childhood. In addition, β-thalassemia genes interact with genes for structural β-globin variants such as hemoglobin S and hemoglobin E to cause serious disease in compound heterozygous individuals. These disorders are discussed further in the sections dealing with sickle cell disease and with hemoglobin E disorders.

Clinical Findings

A. Symptoms and Signs

Persons with β-thalassemia minor are usually asymptomatic with a normal physical examination. Those with β-thalassemia major are normal at birth but develop significant anemia during the first year of life. If the disorder is not identified and treated with blood transfusions, such children grow poorly and develop massive hepatosplenomegaly and enlargement of the medullary space with thinning of the bony cortex. The skeletal changes cause characteristic facial deformities (prominent forehead and maxilla) and predispose the child to pathologic fractures.

B. Laboratory Findings

Children with β-thalassemia minor have normal neonatal screening results but subsequently develop a decreased MCV with or without mild anemia. The peripheral blood smear typically shows hypochromia, target cells, and sometimes basophilic stippling. Hemoglobin electrophoresis performed after 6–12 months of age is usually diagnostic when levels of hemoglobin A_2, hemoglobin F, or both are elevated. β-Thalassemia major is often initially suspected when hemoglobin A is absent on neonatal screening. Such infants are hematologically normal at birth, but develop severe anemia after the first few months of life. The peripheral blood smear typically shows a severe hypochromic, microcytic anemia with marked anisocytosis and poikilocytosis. Target cells are prominent, and nucleated red blood cells often exceed the number of circulating white blood cells. The hemoglobin level usually falls to 5–6 g/dL or less, and the reticulocyte count is elevated, but the reticulocyte index is normal to decreased. Platelet and white blood cell counts may be increased, and the serum bilirubin level is elevated. The bone marrow shows marked erythroid hyperplasia, but this finding is rarely needed for diagnosis. Hemoglobin electrophoresis shows only fetal hemoglobin and hemoglobin A_2 in children with homozygous β^0-thalassemia.

Those with β^+-thalassemia genes make some hemoglobin A but have a marked increase in fetal hemoglobin and hemoglobin A_2 levels. The diagnosis of homozygous β-thalassemia may also be suggested by the finding of β-thalassemia minor in both parents.

Differential Diagnosis

β-Thalassemia minor must be differentiated from other causes of mild microcytic, hypochromic anemias, principally iron deficiency and α-thalassemia. In contrast to patients with iron-deficiency anemia, those with β-thalassemia minor typically have an elevated number of red blood cells, and the index of the MCV divided by the red cell count is under 13. Generally, the finding of an elevated hemoglobin A_2 level is diagnostic; however, the A_2 level is lowered by coexistent iron deficiency. Thus, in children thought to be iron-deficient, hemoglobin electrophoresis with quantitation of hemoglobin A_2 is sometimes deferred until after a course of iron therapy.

β-Thalassemia major is rarely confused with other disorders. Hemoglobin electrophoresis and family studies readily distinguish it from hemoglobin E/β-thalassemia, which is the other important cause of transfusion-dependent thalassemia.

Complications

The principal complication of β-thalassemia minor is the unnecessary use of iron therapy in a futile attempt to correct the microcytic anemia. Children with β-thalassemia major who are inadequately transfused experience poor growth and recurrent infections and may have hepatosplenomegaly, thinning of the cortical bone, and pathologic fractures. Without treatment, most children die within the first decade of life. The principal complications of β-thalassemia major in transfused children are hemosiderosis, splenomegaly, and hypersplenism. Transfusion-related hemosiderosis requires chelation therapy with deferoxamine, given parentally, or deferasirox (Exjade), given orally, to prevent cardiac, hepatic, and endocrine dysfunction. Noncompliance with chelation in adolescents and young adults may lead to death from congestive heart failure, cardiac arrhythmias, or hepatic failure. Even with adequate transfusions, many patients develop splenomegaly and some degree of hypersplenism. This may require surgical splenectomy because of the increasing transfusion requirements, but the procedure increases the risk of thrombosis and overwhelming septicemia.

Treatment

β-Thalassemia minor requires no specific therapy, but diagnosis of the condition may have important genetic implications for the family. For patients with β-thalassemia major, two treatments are available: chronic transfusion with iron chelation and stem cell transplantation. Programs of blood transfusion are generally targeted to maintain a nadir hemoglobin level of 9–10 g/dL. This approach gives increased vigor and well-being, improved growth, and fewer overall complications. However, maintenance of good health currently requires iron chelation. Small doses of supplemental ascorbic acid may enhance the efficacy of iron chelation. Patients who undergo splenectomy to reduce transfusion requirements, and hence iron loading, should receive pneumococcal vaccine prior to the procedure and prophylactic penicillin and urgent treatment of all febrile illness after splenectomy.

Bone marrow or umbilical cord blood transplantation is an important therapeutic option for children with β-thalassemia major who have an HLA-identical sibling donor. The probability of hematologic cure is greater than 90% when transplantation is performed prior to the development of hepatomegaly or portal fibrosis.

Rund D: Medical progress: β-Thalassemia. N Engl J Med 2005;353:1135 [PMID: 16162884].

3. Sickle Cell Disease

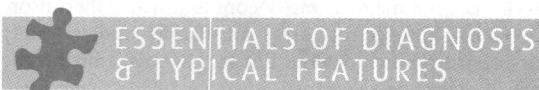

- ▶ Neonatal screening test with hemoglobins FS, FSC, or FSA.
- ▶ African, Mediterranean, Middle Eastern, Indian, or Caribbean ancestry.
- ▶ Anemia, elevated reticulocyte count, jaundice.
- ▶ Recurrent episodes of musculoskeletal or abdominal pain.
- ▶ Hemoglobin electrophoresis with hemoglobins S and F; hemoglobins S and C; or hemoglobins S, A, and F with S > A.
- ▶ Splenomegaly in early childhood with later disappearance.
- ▶ High risk of bacterial sepsis.

General Considerations

A high prevalence of sickle hemoglobin is found in persons of central African origin. It also occurs in other ethnic groups in Italy, Greece, Turkey, Saudi Arabia, and India. Sickle cell anemia is caused by homozygosity for the sickle gene and is the most common form of sickle cell disease. Other clinically important sickling disorders are compound heterozygous conditions in which the sickle gene interacts with genes for hemoglobins C, D_{Punjab}, O_{Arab}, C_{Harlem}, or β-thalassemia.

Overall, sickle cell disease occurs in about 1 of every 400 African American infants. Eight percent of African Americans are heterozygous carriers of the sickle gene and are said to have sickle cell trait.

The protean clinical manifestations of sickle hemoglobinopathies can be linked directly or indirectly to the propensity of deoxygenated hemoglobin S to polymerize. Polymerization of sickle hemoglobin distorts erythrocyte morphology, decreases red cell deformability, causes a marked reduction in red cell life span, increases blood viscosity, and predisposes to episodes of vaso-occlusion.

Neonatal screening for sickle hemoglobinopathies is now routine in most of the United States. The identification of affected infants at birth, when combined with follow-up programs of parental education, comprehensive medical care, and prophylactic penicillin, markedly reduces morbidity and mortality in early childhood.

Clinical Findings

A. Symptoms and Signs

These are related to the hemolytic anemia and to tissue ischemia and organ dysfunction caused by vaso-occlusion. Physical findings are normal at birth, and symptoms are unusual before age 3–4 months because high levels of fetal hemoglobin inhibit sickling. A moderately severe hemolytic anemia may be present by age 1 year. This causes pallor, fatigue, and jaundice, and predisposes to the development of gallstones during childhood and adolescence. Intense congestion of the spleen with sickled cells may cause splenomegaly in early childhood and results in functional asplenia as early as age 3 months. This places children at great risk for overwhelming infection with encapsulated bacteria, particularly pneumococci. Up to 30% of patients experience one or more episodes of acute splenic sequestration, characterized by sudden enlargement of the spleen with pooling of red cells, acute exacerbation of anemia, and, in severe cases, shock and death. Acute exacerbation of anemia also occurs with aplastic crises, usually caused by infection with human parvovirus, and other viruses.

Recurrent episodes of vaso-occlusion and tissue ischemia cause acute and chronic problems. Dactylitis, or hand-and-foot syndrome, is the most common initial symptom of the disease and occurs in up to 50% of children before age 3 years. Recurrent episodes of abdominal and musculoskeletal pain may occur throughout life. Strokes occur in about 8%

Table 28–2. Common clinical manifestations of sickle cell disease.

	Acute	Chronic

Children	Bacterial sepsis or meningitis[a]
	Splenic sequestration[a]
	Aplastic crisis
	Vaso-occlusive events
	  Dactylitis
	  Bone infarction
	  Acute chest syndrome[a]
	  Stroke[a]
	  Priapism
		Functional asplenia
		Delayed growth and development
		Avascular necrosis of the hip
		Hyposthenuria
		Cholelithiasis

Adults	Bacterial sepsis[a]
	Aplastic crisis
	Vaso-occlusive events
	  Bone infarction
	  Acute chest syndrome[a]
	  Stroke[a]
	  Priapism
	  Acute multiorgan failure syndrome[a]
		Leg ulcers
		Proliferative retinopathy
		Avascular necrosis of the hip
		Cholecystitis
		Chronic organ failure[a]
		  Liver
		  Lung
		  Kidney
		Decreased fertility

[a]Associated with significant mortality rate.

of children and tend to be recurrent. The so-called acute chest syndrome, characterized by fever, pleuritic chest pain, and acute pulmonary infiltrates with hypoxemia, is caused by pulmonary infection, infarction, or fat embolism from ischemic bone marrow. All tissues are susceptible to damage from vaso-occlusion, and multiple organ dysfunction is common by adulthood. Table 28–2 lists the common manifestations of sickle cell disease in children and adults.

B. Laboratory Findings

Children with sickle cell anemia (homozygous sickle cell disease) generally show a baseline hemoglobin level of 7–10 g/dL. This value may fall to life-threatening levels at the time of a sequestration or aplastic crisis. The baseline reticulocyte count is elevated markedly. The anemia is usually normocytic or macrocytic, and the peripheral blood smear typically shows the characteristic sickle cells as well as numerous target cells. Patients with sickle β-thalassemia also generally have a low MCV and hypochromia. Those with sickle β+-thalassemia tend to have less hemolysis and anemia. Persons with sickle hemoglobin C disease have fewer sickle forms and more target cells, and the hemoglobin level may be normal or only slightly decreased because the rate of hemolysis is much less than in sickle cell anemia.

Most infants with sickle hemoglobinopathies born in the United States are identified by neonatal screening. Results indicative of possible sickle cell disease require prompt confirmation with hemoglobin electrophoresis. Children

with sickle cell anemia and with sickle β0-thalassemia have only hemoglobins S and F. Persons with sickle β+-thalassemia have a preponderance of hemoglobin S with a lesser amount of hemoglobin A. Persons with sickle hemoglobin C disease have equal amounts of hemoglobins S and C. The use of solubility tests to screen for the presence of sickle hemoglobin should be avoided because a negative result is frequently encountered in infants with sickle cell disease, and because a positive result in an older child does not differentiate sickle cell trait from sickle cell disease. Thus, hemoglobin electrophoresis is always necessary to accurately identify a sickle disorder.

▶ Differential Diagnosis

Hemoglobin electrophoresis and sometimes hematologic studies of the parents are usually sufficient to confirm the correct diagnosis of a sickle cell disorder. Infants whose neonatal screening test shows only hemoglobins F and S occasionally have disorders other than sickle cell anemia or sickle β0-thalassemia. The most important of these disorders is a compound heterozygous condition of sickle hemoglobin and pancellular hereditary persistence of fetal hemoglobin. Such children, when older, typically have 30% fetal hemoglobin and 70% hemoglobin S, but they do not have significant anemia or develop vaso-occlusive episodes.

▶ Complications

Repeated tissue ischemia and infarction causes damage to virtually every organ system. Table 28–2 lists the most important complications. Patients who require multiple transfusions are at risk of developing transfusion-related hemosiderosis and red cell alloantibodies.

▶ Treatment

The cornerstone of treatment is enrollment in a program involving patient and family education, comprehensive outpatient care, and appropriate treatment of acute complications. Important to the success of such a program are psychosocial services, blood bank services, and the ready availability of baseline patient information in the setting in which acute illnesses are evaluated and treated. Management of sickle cell anemia and sickle β0-thalassemia includes prophylactic penicillin, which should be initiated by age 2 months and continued at least until age 5 years.

The routine use of penicillin prophylaxis in sickle hemoglobin C disease and sickle β+-thalassemia is controversial. Pneumococcal conjugate and polysaccharide vaccine should be administered to all children who have sickle cell disease. Other routine immunizations, including yearly vaccination against influenza, should be provided. All illnesses associated with fever greater than 38.5°C should be evaluated promptly, bacterial cultures performed, parenteral broad-spectrum antibiotics administered, and careful inpatient or outpatient observation conducted.

Treatment of painful vaso-occlusive episodes includes the maintenance of adequate hydration (with avoidance of over-hydration), correction of acidosis if present, administration of adequate analgesia, maintenance of normal oxygen saturation, and the treatment of any associated infections.

Red cell transfusions play an important role in management. Transfusions are indicated to improve oxygen-carrying capacity during acute severe exacerbations of anemia, as occurs during episodes of splenic sequestration or aplastic crisis. Red cell transfusions are not indicated for the treatment of chronic steady-state anemia, which is usually well tolerated, or for uncomplicated episodes of vaso-occlusive pain. Simple or partial exchange transfusion to reduce the percentage of circulating sickle cells is indicated for some severe acute vaso-occlusive events and may be lifesaving. These events include stroke, moderate to severe acute chest syndrome, and acute life-threatening failure of other organs. Transfusions may also be used prior to high-risk procedures such as surgery with general anesthesia and arteriograms with ionic contrast materials. Some patients who develop severe vaso-occlusive complications may benefit from chronic transfusion therapy. The most common indication for transfusion is stroke. Without transfusions, children with stroke have a 70–80% chance of recurrent stroke within a 2-year period. This risk of recurrent neurologic events is reduced markedly by the transfusion therapy.

Successful stem cell transplantation cures sickle cell disease, but to date its use has been limited because of the risks associated with the procedure, the inability to predict in young children the severity of future complications, and the paucity of HLA-identical sibling donors. Daily administration of oral hydroxyurea increases levels of fetal hemoglobin, decreases hemolysis, and reduces by 50% episodes of pain in severely affected adults with sickle cell anemia. The hematologic effects and short-term toxicity of hydroxyurea in children are similar to those in adults. Thus hydroxyurea is being used increasingly for selected children and adolescents who have frequent, severe complications.

▶ Prognosis

Early identification by neonatal screening of infants with sickle cell disease, combined with comprehensive care that includes prophylactic penicillin, has markedly reduced mortality in childhood. Most patients now live well into adulthood, but eventually succumb to complications.

Academy of Pediatrics, Section on Hematology/Oncology and Committee on Genetics: Health supervision for children with sickle cell disease. Pediatrics 2002;109:526 [PMID: 11875155].

Raphael RI: Pathophysiology and treatment of sickle cell disease. Clin Adv Hematol Oncol 2005;3:492 [PMID: 16167028].

Vichinsky EP: Causes and outcomes of the acute chest syndrome in sickle cell disease. N Engl J Med 2000;342:1855 [PMID: 10861320].

Walters MC: Bone marrow transplantation for sickle cell disease. N Engl J Med 1996;335:369 [PMID: 8663884].

4. Sickle Cell Trait

Individuals who are heterozygous for the sickle gene are said to have sickle cell trait. This genetic carrier state occurs in 8% of African Americans and is more common in some areas of Africa and the Middle East. Infants with sickle cell trait are identified by neonatal screening results that show hemoglobin FAS. Accurate identification of older persons with sickle cell trait depends on hemoglobin electrophoresis, which typically shows about 60% hemoglobin A and about 40% hemoglobin S. No anemia or hemolysis is present, and the physical examination is normal. Persons with sickle cell trait are generally healthy, and experience no illness attributable to the presence of sickle hemoglobin in their red cells. Life expectancy is normal.

Sickle trait erythrocytes are capable of sickling, particularly under conditions of significant hypoxemia, and several clinical abnormalities have been linked to this genetic carrier state. Exposure to environmental hypoxia (altitude > 3100 m [10,000 ft] above sea level) may precipitate splenic infarction. However, most persons with sickle cell trait who choose to visit such altitudes for skiing, hiking, or climbing do so without difficulty. Many develop some degree of hyposthenuria, and about 4% experience painless hematuria, usually microscopic but occasionally macroscopic. For the most part, these renal abnormalities are subclinical and do not progress to significant renal dysfunction. The incidence of bacteriuria and pyelonephritis may be increased during pregnancy, but overall rates of maternal and infant morbidity and mortality are not affected by the presence of sickle cell trait in the pregnant woman.

An epidemiologic study of army recruits in military basic training found a higher risk of sudden unexplained death following strenuous exertion in recruits with sickle cell trait than in those with normal hemoglobin. This study has raised concerns about exercise and exertion for persons with the trait. However, considerable evidence suggests that exercise is generally safe and that athletic performance is not adversely affected by sickle cell trait. Exercise tolerance is normal, and the incidence of sickle cell trait in black professional football players is similar to that of the general African-American population, suggesting no barrier to achievement in such a physically demanding profession. Thus, restrictions on athletic competition for children with sickle cell trait are not warranted. Sickle cell trait is most significant for its genetic implications.

5. Hemoglobin C Disorders

Hemoglobin C is detected by neonatal screening. Two percent of African Americans are heterozygous for hemoglobin C and are said to have hemoglobin C trait. Such individuals have no symptoms, anemia, or hemolysis, but the peripheral blood smear may show some target cells. Identification of persons with hemoglobin C trait is important for genetic counseling, particularly with regard to the possibility of sickle hemoglobin C disease in offspring.

Persons with homozygous hemoglobin C have a mild microcytic hemolytic anemia and may develop splenomegaly. The peripheral blood smear shows prominent target cells. As with other hemolytic anemias, complications of homozygous hemoglobin C include gallstones and aplastic crises.

Olson JF: Hemoglobin C disease in infancy and childhood. J Pediatr 1994;125:745 [PMID: 7965426].

6. Hemoglobin E Disorders

Hemoglobin E is the second most common hemoglobin variant worldwide, with a gene frequency greater than 10% in some areas of Thailand and Cambodia. In Southeast Asia, an estimated 30 million people have hemoglobin E trait. Persons heterozygous for hemoglobin E show hemoglobin FAE by neonatal screening and are asymptomatic and usually not anemic, but they may develop mild microcytosis. Persons homozygous for hemoglobin E are also asymptomatic but may have mild anemia; the peripheral blood smear shows microcytosis and some target cells.

Hemoglobin E is most important because of its interaction with β-thalassemia. Compound heterozygotes for hemoglobin E and β^0-thalassemia are normal at birth and, like infants with homozygous E, show hemoglobin FE on neonatal screening. Unlike homozygotes, they subsequently develop mild to severe microcytic hypochromic anemia. Such children may exhibit jaundice, hepatosplenomegaly, and poor growth if the disorder is not recognized and treated appropriately. In some cases, the anemia becomes severe enough to require lifelong transfusion therapy. In certain areas of the United States, hemoglobin E/β^0-thalassemia has become a more common cause of transfusion-dependent anemia than homozygous β-thalassemia.

7. Other Hemoglobinopathies

Hundreds of other human globin-chain variants have been described. Some, such as hemoglobins D and G, are relatively common. Heterozygous individuals, who are frequently identified during the course of neonatal screening programs for hemoglobinopathies, are generally asymptomatic and usually have no anemia or hemolysis. The principal significance of most hemoglobin variants is the potential for disease in compound heterozygous individuals who also inherit a gene for β-thalassemia or sickle hemoglobin. For example, children who are compound heterozygous for hemoglobins S and D_{Punjab} ($D_{Los\ Angeles}$) have sickle cell disease.

CONGENITAL HEMOLYTIC ANEMIAS: DISORDERS OF RED CELL METABOLISM

Erythrocytes depend on the anaerobic metabolism of glucose for the maintenance of adenosine triphosphate levels sufficient for homeostasis. Glycolysis also produces the 2,3-diphosphoglycerate levels needed to modulate the oxygen affinity of hemoglobin. Glucose metabolism via the hexose monophosphate shunt is necessary to generate sufficient reduced nicotinamide adenine dinucleotide phosphate (NADH) and reduced glutathione to protect red cells against oxidant damage. Congenital deficiencies of many glycolytic pathway enzymes have been associated with hemolytic anemias. In general, the morphologic abnormalities present on the peripheral blood smear are nonspecific, and the inheritance of these disorders is autosomal recessive or X-linked. Thus, the possibility of a red cell enzyme defect should be considered during the evaluation of a patient with a congenital hemolytic anemia in the following instances: when the peripheral blood smear does not show red cell morphology typical of membrane or hemoglobin defects (eg, spherocytes, sickle forms, target cells); when hemoglobin disorders are excluded by hemoglobin electrophoresis and by isopropanol precipitation tests; and when family studies do not suggest an autosomal dominant disorder. The diagnosis is confirmed by finding a low level of the deficient enzyme.

The two most common disorders of erythrocyte metabolism are G6PD deficiency and pyruvate kinase deficiency.

1. Glucose-6-Phosphate Dehydrogenase (G6PD) Deficiency

ESSENTIALS OF DIAGNOSIS & TYPICAL FEATURES

▶ African, Mediterranean, or Asian ancestry.
▶ Neonatal hyperbilirubinemia.
▶ Sporadic hemolysis associated with infection or with ingestion of oxidant drugs or fava beans.
▶ X-linked inheritance.

▶ General Considerations

Deficiency of G6PD is the most common red cell enzyme defect that causes hemolytic anemia. The disorder has X-linked recessive inheritance and occurs with high frequency among persons of African, Mediterranean, and Asian ancestry. Hundreds of different G6PD variants have been characterized. In most instances, the deficiency is due to enzyme instability; thus, older red cells are more deficient than younger ones, and are unable to generate sufficient NADH to maintain the levels of reduced glutathione necessary to protect the red cells against oxidant stress. Thus, most persons with G6PD deficiency do not have a chronic hemolytic anemia; instead, they have episodic hemolysis at times of exposure to the oxidant stress of infection or of certain drugs or food substances. The severity of the disorder varies among ethnic groups; G6PD deficiency in persons of African ancestry usually is less severe than in other ethnic groups.

Table 28–3. Some common drugs and chemicals that can induce hemolytic anemia in persons with G6PD deficiency.

Acetanilide	Niridazole
Doxorubicin	Nitrofurantoin
Furazolidone	Phenazopyridine
Methylene blue	Primaquine
Nalidixic acid	Sulfamethoxazole

Reproduced, with permission, from Beutler E: Glucose-6-phosphate dehydrogenase deficiency. N Engl J Med 1991;324:171.

▶ Clinical Findings

A. Symptoms and Signs

Infants with G6PD deficiency may have significant hyperbilirubinemia and require phototherapy or exchange transfusion to prevent kernicterus. The deficiency is an important cause of neonatal hyperbilirubinemia in infants of Mediterranean or Asian ancestry, but less so in infants of African ancestry. Older children with G6PD deficiency are asymptomatic and appear normal between episodes of hemolysis. Hemolytic episodes are often triggered by infection or by the ingestion of oxidant drugs such as antimalarial compounds and sulfonamide antibiotics (Table 28–3). Ingestion of fava beans may trigger hemolysis in children of Mediterranean or Asian ancestry but usually not in children of African ancestry. Episodes of hemolysis are associated with pallor, jaundice, hemoglobinuria, and sometimes cardiovascular compromise.

B. Laboratory Findings

The hemoglobin concentration, reticulocyte count, and peripheral blood smear are usually normal in the absence of oxidant stress. Episodes of hemolysis are associated with a variable fall in hemoglobin. "Bite" cells or blister cells may be seen, along with a few spherocytes. Hemoglobinuria is common, and the reticulocyte count increases within a few days. Heinz bodies may be demonstrated with appropriate stains. The diagnosis is confirmed by the finding of reduced levels of G6PD in erythrocytes. Because this enzyme is present in increased quantities in reticulocytes, the test is best performed at a time when the reticulocyte count is normal or near normal.

▶ Complications

Kernicterus is a risk for infants with significant neonatal hyperbilirubinemia. Episodes of acute hemolysis in older children may be life-threatening. Rare G6PD variants are associated with chronic hemolytic anemia; the clinical course of patients with such variants may be complicated by splenomegaly and by the formation of gallstones.

▶ Treatment

The most important treatment issue is avoidance of drugs known to be associated with hemolysis (see Table 28–3). For some patients of Mediterranean, Middle Eastern, or Asian ancestry, the consumption of fava beans must also be avoided. Infections should be treated promptly and antibiotics given when appropriate. Most episodes of hemolysis are self-limiting, but red cell transfusions may be lifesaving when signs and symptoms indicate cardiovascular compromise.

2. Pyruvate Kinase Deficiency

Pyruvate kinase deficiency is an autosomal recessive disorder observed in all ethnic groups but is most common in northern Europeans. The deficiency is associated with a chronic hemolytic anemia of varying severity. Approximately one third of those affected present in the neonatal period with jaundice and hemolysis that require phototherapy or exchange transfusion. Occasionally, the disorder causes hydrops fetalis and neonatal death. In older children, the hemolysis may require red cell transfusions or be mild enough to go unnoticed for many years. Jaundice and splenomegaly frequently occur in the more severe cases. The diagnosis of pyruvate kinase deficiency is occasionally suggested by the presence of echinocytes on the peripheral blood smear, but these findings may be absent prior to splenectomy. The diagnosis depends on the demonstration of low levels of pyruvate kinase activity in red cells.

Treatment of pyruvate kinase depends on the severity of the hemolysis. Blood transfusions may be required for significant anemia, and splenectomy may be beneficial. Although the procedure does not cure the disorder, it ameliorates the anemia and its symptoms. Characteristically, the reticulocyte count increases and echinocytes become more prevalent after splenectomy, despite the decreased hemolysis and increased hemoglobin level.

ACQUIRED HEMOLYTIC ANEMIA

1. Autoimmune Hemolytic Anemia

 ESSENTIALS OF DIAGNOSIS & TYPICAL FEATURES

▶ Pallor, fatigue, jaundice, and dark urine.

▶ Splenomegaly.

▶ Positive DAT.

▶ Reticulocytosis and spherocytosis.

▶ General Considerations

Acquired autoimmune hemolytic anemia is rare during the first 4 months of life but is one of the more common causes of acute anemia after the first year. It may arise as an isolated problem or may complicate an infection (hepatitis, upper respiratory tract infections, mononucleosis, or cytomegalovirus infection); systemic lupus erythematosus and other autoimmune syndromes;

immunodeficiency states, including autoimmune lympho-proliferative syndrome; or, rarely, malignancies.

▶ Clinical Findings

A. Symptoms and Signs

The disease usually has an acute onset manifested by weakness, pallor, dark urine, and fatigue. Jaundice is a prominent finding, and splenomegaly is often present. Some cases have a more chronic, insidious onset. Clinical evidence of an underlying disease may be present.

B. Laboratory Findings

The anemia is normochromic and normocytic and may vary from mild to severe (hemoglobin concentration < 5 g/dL). The reticulocyte count and index are usually increased but occasionally are normal or low. Spherocytes and nucleated red cells may be seen on the peripheral blood smear. Although leukocytosis and elevated platelet counts are a common finding, thrombocytopenia occasionally occurs. Other laboratory data consistent with hemolysis are present, such as increased indirect and total bilirubin, lactic dehydrogenase, aspartate aminotransferase, and urinary urobilinogen. Intravascular hemolysis is indicated by hemoglobinemia or hemoglobinuria. Examination of bone marrow shows marked erythroid hyperplasia and hemophagocytosis, but is seldom required for the diagnosis.

Serologic studies are helpful in defining pathophysiology, planning therapeutic strategies, and assessing prognosis (Table 28–4). In almost all cases, the direct and indirect antiglobulin (DAT and IAT) tests are positive. Further evaluation allows distinction into one of three syndromes. The presence of IgG on the patient's red blood cells, maximal in-vitro antibody activity at 37°C, and either no antigen specificity or an Rh-like specificity constitute warm autoimmune hemolytic anemia with extravascular destruction by the reticuloendothelial system. In contrast, the detection of complement alone on red blood cells, optimal reactivity in vitro at 4°C, and I or i antigen specificity are diagnostic of cold autoimmune hemolytic anemia with intravascular hemolysis. Although cold agglutinins are relatively common (~10%) in normal individuals, clinically significant cold antibodies exhibit in-vitro reactivity at 30°C or above.

Paroxysmal cold hemoglobinuria usually has a different cause. The laboratory evaluation is identical to cold autoimmune hemolytic anemia except for antigen specificity (P) and the exhibition of in-vitro hemolysis. Paroxysmal cold hemoglobinuria is almost always associated with significant infections, such as *Mycoplasma*, Epstein-Barr virus (EBV), and cytomegalovirus (CMV). Warm IgM antibodies are rare.

▶ Differential Diagnosis

Autoimmune hemolytic anemia must be differentiated from other forms of congenital or acquired hemolytic anemias. The DAT discriminates antibody-mediated hemolysis from other causes, such as hereditary spherocytosis. The presence of other cytopenias and antibodies to platelets or neutrophils suggests Evans syndrome.

Table 28–4. Classification of autoimmune hemolytic anemia (AIHA) in children.

Syndrome	Warm AIHA	Cold AIHA	Paroxysmal Cold Hemoglobinuria
Specific antiglobulin test IgG Complement	Strongly positive Negative or mildly positive	Negative Strongly positive	Negative Strongly positive
Temperature at maximal reactivity (in vitro)	37°C	4°C	4°C
Antigen specificity	May be panagglutinin or may have an Rh-like specificity	I or i	P
Other	. . .	. . .	Positive biphasic hemolysin test
Pathophysiology	Extravascular hemolysis, destruction by the RES (eg, spleen)	Intravascular hemolysis (may have extravascular component)	Intravascular hemolysis (may have extravascular component)
Prognosis	May be more chronic (> 3 mo) with significant morbidity and mortality. May be associated with a primary disorder (lupus, immunodeficiency, etc).	Generally acute (< 3 mo). Good prognosis: often associated with infection.	Acute, self-limited. Associated with infection.
Therapy	Responds to RES blockade, including steroids (prednisone, 2 mg/kg/d), IVIG (1 g/kg/d for 2 d), or splenectomy	May not respond to RES blockade. Severe cases may benefit from plasmapheresis.	Usually self-limited. Symptomatic management.

IVIG, intravenous immune globulin; RES, reticuloendothelial system.

► Complications

The anemia may be very severe and result in cardiovascular collapse, requiring emergency management. The complications of an underlying disease, such as disseminated lupus erythematosus or an immunodeficiency state, may be present.

► Treatment

Medical management of the underlying disease is important in symptomatic cases. Defining the clinical syndrome provides a useful guide to treatment. Most patients with warm autoimmune hemolytic anemia (in which hemolysis is mostly extravascular) respond to prednisone (2–4 mg/kg/d). After the initial treatment, the dose of corticosteroids may be decreased slowly. Patients may respond to 1 g of intravenous immune globulin (IVIG) per kilogram per day for 2 days, but fewer patients respond to IVIG than to prednisone. Although the rate of remission with splenectomy may be as high as 50%, particularly in warm autoimmune hemolytic anemia, this should be carefully considered in younger patients and withheld until other treatments have failed. In severe cases unresponsive to more conventional therapy, immunosuppressive agents such as cyclophosphamide, azathioprine, busulfan, and cyclosporine may be tried alone or in combination with corticosteroids. In refractory cases, rituximab may be a successful alternative, and transplantation has been used in a small number of cases.

Patients with cold autoimmune hemolytic anemia and paroxysmal cold hemoglobinuria are less likely to respond to corticosteroids or IVIG. Because these syndromes are most apt to be associated with infections and have an acute, self-limited course, supportive care may be sufficient. Plasma exchange may be effective in severe cold autoimmune (IgM) hemolytic anemia because the offending antibody has an intravascular distribution.

Supportive therapy is crucial. Patients with cold-reacting antibodies, particularly paroxysmal cold hemoglobinuria, should be kept in a warm environment. Transfusion may be necessary because of the complications of severe anemia but should be used only when there is no alternative. In most patients, cross-match compatible blood will not be found, and the least incompatible unit should be identified. Transfusion must be conducted carefully, beginning with a test dose (see Transfusion Medicine section, later in this chapter). Identification of the patient's phenotype for minor red cell alloantigens may be helpful in avoiding alloimmunization or in providing appropriate transfusions if alloantibodies arise after initial transfusions. Patients with severe intravascular hemolysis may have associated disseminated intravascular coagulation (DIC), and heparin therapy should be considered in such cases.

► Prognosis

The outlook for autoimmune hemolytic anemia in childhood usually is good unless associated diseases are present

(eg, congenital immunodeficiency, AIDS, lupus erythematosus), in which case hemolysis is likely to have a chronic course. In general, children with warm autoimmune hemolytic anemia are at greater risk for more severe and chronic disease with higher morbidity and mortality rates. Hemolysis and positive antiglobulin tests may continue for months or years. Patients with cold autoimmune hemolytic anemia or paroxysmal cold hemoglobinuria are more likely to have acute, self-limited disease (< 3 months). Paroxysmal cold hemoglobinuria is almost always associated with infection (eg, *Mycoplasma* infection, CMV, and EBV).

Naithani R: Autoimmune hemolytic anemia in children. Pediatr Hematol Oncol 2007;24:309 [PMID: 17613874].

Petz LD: Unusual problems regarding autoimmune hemolytic anemias. In Petz LD, Garratty G (editors): *Acquired Immune Hemolytic Anemias*, 2nd ed. Churchill Livingstone, 2004:341–344.

Shirey RS: Prophylactic antigen-matched donor blood for patients with warm autoantibodies: An algorithm for transfusion management. Transfusion 2002;42:1435 [PMID: 12421216].

Vaglio S: Autoimmune hemolytic anemia in childhood: Serologic features in 100 cases. Transfusion 2007;47:50 [PMID: 17207229].

Zecca M: Rituximab for the treatment of refractory autoimmune hemolytic anemia in children. Blood 2003;101:3857 [PMID: 12531800].

2. Nonimmune Acquired Hemolytic Anemia

Hepatic disease may alter the lipid composition of the red cell membrane. This usually results in the formation of target cells and is not associated with significant hemolysis.

Occasionally, hepatocellular damage is associated with the formation of spur cells and brisk hemolytic anemia. Renal disease may also be associated with significant hemolysis; hemolytic-uremic syndrome is one example. In this disorder, hemolysis is associated with the presence, on the peripheral blood smear, of echinocytes, helmet cells, fragmented red cells, and spherocytes.

A microangiopathic hemolytic anemia with fragmented red cells and some spherocytes may be observed in several conditions associated with intravascular coagulation and fibrin deposition within vessels. This occurs with DIC such as may complicate severe infection, but it may also occur when the intravascular coagulation is localized, as with giant cavernous hemangiomas (Kasabach-Merritt syndrome). Fragmented red cells may also be seen with mechanical damage (eg, associated with artificial heart valves).

▼ POLYCYTHEMIA & METHEMOGLOBINEMIA

CONGENITAL ERYTHROCYTOSIS (FAMILIAL POLYCYTHEMIA)

In pediatrics, polycythemia is usually secondary to chronic hypoxemia. However, several families with congenital erythrocytosis have been described. The disorder differs from polycythemia vera in that only red blood cells are affected; the white blood cell and platelet counts are normal. It occurs as an autosomal dominant or recessive disorder. There are usually no physical findings except for plethora and splenomegaly. The hemoglobin level may be as high as 27 g/dL. Patients usually have no symptoms other than headache and lethargy. Studies in a number of families have revealed (1) abnormal hemoglobin with altered oxygen affinity, (2) reduced red cell diphosphoglycerate, (3) autonomous increase in erythropoietin production, or (4) hypersensitivity of erythroid precursors to erythropoietin.

Treatment is not indicated unless symptoms are marked. Phlebotomy is the treatment of choice.

SECONDARY POLYCYTHEMIA

Secondary polycythemia occurs in response to hypoxemia. The most common cause of secondary polycythemia in children is cyanotic congenital heart disease. It also occurs in chronic pulmonary disease such as cystic fibrosis. Persons living at extremely high altitudes, as well as some with methemoglobinemia, develop polycythemia. It has on rare occasions been described without hypoxemia in association with renal tumors, brain tumors, Cushing disease, or hydronephrosis.

Polycythemia may occur in the neonatal period; it is particularly exaggerated in infants who are preterm or small for gestational age. In these infants, polycythemia is sometimes associated with other symptoms. It may occur in infants of diabetic mothers, in Down syndrome, and as a complication of congenital adrenal hyperplasia.

Iron deficiency may complicate polycythemia and aggravate the associated hyperviscosity. This complication should always be suspected when the MCV falls below the normal range. Coagulation and bleeding abnormalities, including thrombocytopenia, mild consumption coagulopathy, and elevated fibrinolytic activity, have been described in severely polycythemic cardiac patients. Bleeding at surgery may be severe.

The ideal treatment of secondary polycythemia is correction of the underlying disorder. When this cannot be done, phlebotomy may be necessary to control symptoms. Iron sufficiency should be maintained. Adequate hydration of the patient and phlebotomy with plasma replacement may be indicated prior to major surgical procedures. These measures prevent the complications of thrombosis and hemorrhage. Isovolumetric exchange transfusion is the treatment of choice in severe cases.

METHEMOGLOBINEMIA

Methemoglobin is continuously formed at a slow rate by the oxidation of heme iron to the ferric state. Normally, it is enzymatically reduced back to hemoglobin. Methemoglobin is unable to transport oxygen and causes a shift in the dissociation curve of the residual oxyhemoglobin. Cyanosis is produced with methemoglobin levels of approximately 15% or greater. Levels of methemoglobin increase by several mechanisms.

1. Hemoglobin M

The designation M is given to several abnormal hemoglobins associated with methemoglobinemia. Affected individuals are heterozygous for the gene, which is transmitted as an autosomal dominant disorder. The different types of hemoglobin M result from different amino acid substitutions in α-globin or β-globin. Hemoglobin electrophoresis at the usual pH will not always demonstrate the abnormal hemoglobin, and isoelectric focusing may be needed. The patient has cyanosis but is otherwise usually asymptomatic. Exercise tolerance may be normal, and life expectancy is not affected. This type of methemoglobinemia does not respond to any form of therapy.

2. Congenital Methemoglobinemia Due to Enzyme Deficiencies

Congenital methemoglobinemia is caused most frequently by congenital deficiency of the reducing enzyme diaphorase I (coenzyme factor I). It is transmitted as an autosomal recessive trait. Affected patients may have as much as 40% methemoglobin but usually have no symptoms, although a mild compensatory polycythemia may be present. Patients with methemoglobinemia associated with a deficiency of diaphorase I respond readily to treatment with ascorbic acid and methylene blue (see next section), but treatment is not usually indicated.

3. Acquired Methemoglobinemia

Several compounds activate the oxidation of hemoglobin from the ferrous to the ferric state, forming methemoglobin. These include the nitrites and nitrates (contaminated water), chlorates, and quinones. Drugs in this group are the aniline dyes, sulfonamides, acetanilid, phenacetin, bismuth subnitrate, and potassium chlorate. Poisoning with a drug or chemical containing one of these substances should be suspected in any infant or child who presents with sudden cyanosis. Methemoglobin levels in such cases may be extremely high and can produce anoxia, dyspnea, unconsciousness, circulatory failure, and death. Young infants and newborns are more susceptible to acquired methemoglobinemia because their red cells have difficulty reducing hemoglobin, probably because their NADH methemoglobin reductase is transiently deficient. Infants with metabolic acidosis from diarrhea and dehydration or other causes also may develop methemoglobinemia.

Patients with the acquired form of methemoglobinemia respond dramatically to methylene blue in a dose of 1–2 mg/kg intravenously. For infants and young children, a smaller dose (1–1.5 mg/kg) is recommended. Ascorbic acid administered orally or intravenously also reduces methemoglobin, but the response is slower.

DISORDERS OF LEUKOCYTES

NEUTROPENIA

 ESSENTIALS OF DIAGNOSIS
& TYPICAL FEATURES

▶ Increased frequency of infections.
▶ Ulceration of oral mucosa and gingivitis.
▶ Normal numbers of red cells and platelets.

▶ General Considerations

Neutropenia is an absolute neutrophil (granulocyte) count of less than 1500/μL in childhood, or below 1000/μL between ages 1 week and 2 years. During the first few days of life, an absolute neutrophil count of less than 3500 cells/μL may be considered neutropenia. Neutropenia results from absent or defective granulocyte stem cells, ineffective or suppressed myeloid maturation, decreased production of hematopoietic cytokines (eg, granulocyte colony-stimulating factor [G-CSF] or granulocyte-macrophage colony-stimulating factor [GM-CSF]), decreased marrow release, increased neutrophil destruction or consumption, or, in pseudoneutropenia, from an increased neutrophil marginating pool (Table 28–5).

The most severe types of congenital neutropenia include reticular dysgenesis (congenital aleukocytosis), Kostmann syndrome (severe neutropenia with maturation defect in the marrow progenitor cells), Shwachman syndrome (neutropenia with pancreatic insufficiency), neutropenia with immune deficiency states, cyclic neutropenia, and myelokathexis or dysgranulopoiesis. Genetic mutations for Chédiak-Higashi syndrome, Kostmann and Shwachman syndromes, and cyclic neutropenia have been identified. Neutropenia may also be associated with storage and metabolic diseases and immunodeficiency states. The most common causes of neutropenia are viral infection or drugs resulting in decreased neutrophil production in the marrow or increased destruction or both. Severe bacterial infections may be associated with neutropenia. Although rare, neonatal alloimmune neutropenia can be severe and associated with risk for infection. Autoimmune neutropenia in the mother can result in passive transfer of antibody to the fetus and neutropenia in the neonate. Malignancies, osteopetrosis, marrow failure syndromes, and hypersplenism usually are not associated with isolated neutropenia.

▶ Clinical Findings

A. Symptoms and Signs

Acute severe bacterial or fungal infection is the most significant complication of neutropenia. Although the risk is

Table 28–5. Classification of neutropenia of childhood.

Congenital neutropenia with stem cell abnormalities
  Reticular dysgenesis
  Cyclic neutropenia
Congenital neutropenia with abnormalities of committed myeloid progenitor cells
  Neutropenia with immunodeficiency disorders (T cells and B cells)
  Severe congenital neutropenia (Kostmann syndrome)
  Chronic idiopathic neutropenia of childhood
  Myelokathexis with dysmyelopoiesis
  Chédiak-Higashi syndrome
  Shwachman syndrome
  Cartilage-hair hypoplasia
  Dyskeratosis congenita
  Fanconi anemia
  Organic acidemias (eg, propionic, methylmalonic)
  Glycogenosis Ib
  Osteopetrosis
Acquired neutropenias affecting stem cells
  Malignancies (leukemia, lymphoma) and preleukemic disorders
  Drugs or toxic substances
  Ionizing radiation
  Aplastic anemia
Acquired neutropenias affecting committed myeloid progenitors or survival of mature neutrophils
  Ineffective granulopoiesis (vitamin B_{12}, folate, and copper deficiency
  Infection
  Immune (neonatal alloimmune or autoimmune; autoimmune or chronic benign neutropenia of childhood)
  Hypersplenism

increased when the absolute neutrophil count is less than 500/μL, the actual susceptibility is variable and depends on the cause of neutropenia, marrow reserves, and other factors. The most common types of infection include septicemia, cellulitis, skin abscesses, pneumonia, and perirectal abscesses. Sinusitis, aphthous ulcers, gingivitis, and periodontal disease also cause significant problems. In addition to local signs and symptoms, patients may have chills, fever, and malaise. In most cases, the spleen and liver are not enlarged. *Staphylococcus aureus* and gram-negative bacteria are the most common pathogens.

B. Laboratory Findings

Neutrophils are absent or markedly reduced in the peripheral blood smear. In most forms of neutropenia or agranulocytosis, the monocytes and lymphocytes are normal and the red cells and platelets are not affected. The bone marrow usually shows a normal erythroid series, with adequate megakaryocytes, but a marked reduction in the myeloid cells or a significant delay in maturation of this series may be noted. Total cellularity may be decreased.

In the evaluation of neutropenia (eg, persistent, intermittent, cyclic), attention should be paid to the duration and pattern of neutropenia, the types of infections and their frequency, and phenotypic abnormalities on physical examination. A careful family history and blood counts from the parents are useful. If an acquired cause, such as viral infection or drug, is not obvious and no other primary disease is present, white blood cell counts, white cell differential, and platelet and reticulocyte counts should be completed twice weekly for 4–6 weeks to determine the possibility of cyclic neutropenia. Bone marrow aspiration and biopsy are most important to characterize the morphologic features of myelopoiesis. Measuring the neutrophil counts in response to corticosteroid infusion may document the marrow reserves. Other tests that aid in the diagnosis include measurement of neutrophil antibodies, immunoglobulin levels, antinuclear antibodies, and lymphocyte phenotyping to detect immunodeficiency states. Cultures of bone marrow are important for defining the numbers of stem cells and progenitors committed to the myeloid series or the presence of inhibitory factors. Cytokine levels in plasma or mononuclear cells can be measured directly. Some neutropenia disorders have abnormal neutrophil function. Recent studies have documented abnormalities in an antiapoptotic gene, *HAX1,* and the elastase gene, *ELA2,* in Kostmann syndrome and *ELA2* mutations in cyclic neutropenia. A mutation for Shwachman syndrome has been described. Increased apoptosis in marrow precursors or circulating neutrophils has been described in several congenital disorders.

▶ Treatment

Identifiable toxic agents should be eliminated or associated diseases (eg, infections) treated. Prophylactic antimicrobial therapy is not indicated for afebrile, asymptomatic patients. Recombinant G-CSF and GM-CSF will increase neutrophil counts in most patients. Patients may be started on 3–5 mcg/kg/d of G-CSF (filgrastim) given subcutaneously or intravenously once a day. Depending on the counts, the dose may be adjusted. For patients with congenital neutropenia, the dose should be regulated to keep the absolute neutrophil count below 10,000/μL. Some patients maintain adequate counts with G-CSF given two to three times a week. Treatment will decrease infectious complications.

▶ Prognosis

The prognosis varies greatly with the cause and severity of the neutropenia. In severe cases with persistent agranulocytosis, the prognosis is poor in spite of antibiotic therapy; in mild or cyclic forms of neutropenia, symptoms may be minimal and the prognosis for normal life expectancy excellent. Up to 50% of patients with Shwachman syndrome may develop aplastic anemia, myelodysplasia, or leukemia during their lifetime. Patients with Kostmann syndrome also have a potential for leukemia.

Boxer LA: Strong evidence for autosomal dominant inheritance of severe congenital neutropenia associated with ELA2 mutations. J Pediatr 2006;148:633 [PMID: 16737875].

Dror Y: Update on childhood neutropenia: Molecular and clinical advances. Hematol Oncol Clin North Am 2004;18:1439 [PMID: 15511624].

Germeshausen M: Incidence of CSF3R mutations in severe congenital neutropenia and relevance for leukemogenesis: Results of a long-term survey. Blood 2007;109:93 [PMID: 16985178].

Grenda DS: Mutations of the ELA2 gene found in patients with severe congenital neutropenia induce the unfolded protein response and cellular apoptosis. Blood 2007;109:93 [PMID: 17761833].

Klein C: HAX1 deficiency causes autosomal recessive severe congenital neutropenia (Kostmann disease). Nat Genet 2007;39:86 [PMID: 17187068].

Sera Y: A comparison of the defective granulopoiesis in childhood cyclic neutropenia and in severe congenital neutropenia. Haematologica 2005;90:1032 [PMID: 16079102].

NEUTROPHILIA

Neutrophilia is an increase in the absolute neutrophil count in the peripheral blood to greater than 7500–8500 cells/μL for infants, children, and adults. To support the increased peripheral count, neutrophils may be mobilized from bone marrow storage or peripheral marginating pools. Neutrophilia occurs acutely in association with bacterial or viral infections, inflammatory diseases (eg, juvenile rheumatoid arthritis, inflammatory bowel disease, Kawasaki disease), surgical or functional asplenia, liver failure, diabetic ketoacidosis, azotemia, congenital disorders of neutrophil function (eg, chronic granulomatous disease, leukocyte adherence deficiency), and hemolysis. Drugs such as corticosteroids, lithium, and epinephrine increase the blood neutrophil count. Corticosteroids cause release of neutrophils from the marrow pool, inhibit egress from capillary beds, and postpone apoptotic cell death. Epinephrine causes release of the marginating pool. Acute neutrophilia has been reported after stress such as from electric shock, trauma, burns, surgery, and emotional upset. Tumors involving the bone marrow, such as lymphomas, neuroblastomas, and rhabdomyosarcoma, may be associated with leukocytosis and the presence of immature myeloid cells in the peripheral blood. Infants with Down syndrome have defective regulation of proliferation and maturation of the myeloid series and may develop neutrophilia. At times this process may affect other cell lines and mimic myeloproliferative disorders or acute leukemia.

The neutrophilias must be distinguished from myeloproliferative disorders such as chronic myelogenous leukemia and juvenile chronic myelogenous leukemia. In general, abnormalities involving other cell lines, the appearance of immature cells on the blood smear, and the presence of hepatosplenomegaly are important differentiating characteristics.

DISORDERS OF NEUTROPHIL FUNCTION

Neutrophils play a key role in host defenses. Circulating in capillary beds, they adhere to the vascular endothelium adjacent to sites of infection and inflammation. Moving between endothelial cells, the neutrophil migrates toward the offending agent. Contact with a microbe that is properly opsonized with complement or antibodies triggers ingestion, a process in which cytoplasmic streaming results in the formation of pseudopods that fuse around the invader, encasing it in a phagosome. During the ingestion phase, the oxidase enzyme system assembles and is activated, taking oxygen from the surrounding medium and reducing it to form toxic oxygen metabolites critical to microbicidal activity. Concurrently, granules from the two main classes (azurophil and specific) fuse and release their contents into the phagolysosome. The concentration of toxic oxygen metabolites (eg, hydrogen peroxide, hypochlorous acid, hydroxyl radical) and other compounds (eg, proteases, cationic proteins, cathepsins, defensins) increases dramatically, resulting in the death and dissolution of the microbe. Complex physiologic and biochemical processes support and control these functions. Defects in any of these processes may lead to inadequate cell function and an increased risk of infection.

Classification

Table 28–6 summarizes congenital neutrophil function defects. Recently described is a syndrome of severe neutrophil dysfunction and severe infections associated with a mutation in a GTPase signaling molecule, Rac2. New syndromes of innate immune dysfunction include defects in interferon and interleukin-12 receptor and signaling pathways, leading to monocyte and macrophage dysfunction and toll-like receptor signaling pathways (interleukin-1 receptor-associated [IRAK] deficiency) associated with recurrent bacterial infections. Other congenital or acquired causes of mild to moderate neutrophil dysfunction include metabolic defects (eg, glycogen storage disease, diabetes mellitus, renal disease, and hypophosphatemia), viral infections, and certain drugs. Neutrophils from newborn infants have abnormal adherence, chemotaxis, and bactericidal activity. Cells from patients with thermal injury, trauma, and overwhelming infection have defects in cell motility and bactericidal activity similar to those seen in neonates.

Clinical Findings

Recurrent bacterial or fungal infections are the hallmark of neutrophil dysfunction. Although many patients will have infection-free periods, episodes of pneumonia, sinusitis, cellulitis, cutaneous and mucosal infections (including perianal or peritonsillar abscesses), and lymphadenitis are frequent. As with neutropenia, aphthous ulcers of mucous membranes, severe gingivitis, and periodontal disease are also major complications. In general, S aureus or gram-negative organisms are commonly isolated from infected sites; other organisms may be specifically associated with a defined neutrophil function defect. In some disorders, fungi account

for an increasing number of infections. Deep or generalized infections, such as osteomyelitis, liver abscesses, sepsis, meningitis, and necrotic or gangrenous soft-tissue lesions, occur in specific syndromes (eg, leukocyte adherence deficiency or chronic granulomatous disease). Patients with severe neutrophil dysfunction may die in childhood from severe infections or associated complications. Table 28–6 summarizes pertinent laboratory findings.

▶ Treatment

The mainstays of management of these disorders are anticipation of infections and aggressive attempts to identify the foci and the causative agents. Surgical procedures to achieve these goals may be both diagnostic and therapeutic. Broad-spectrum antibiotics covering the range of possible organisms should be initiated without delay, switching to specific antimicrobial agents when the microbiologic diagnosis is made. When infections are unresponsive or they recur, granulocyte transfusions may be helpful.

Chronic management includes prophylactic antibiotics. Trimethoprim–sulfamethoxazole and some other antibiotics enhance the bactericidal activity of neutrophils from patients with chronic granulomatous disease. Some patients with Chédiak-Higashi syndrome improve clinically when given ascorbic acid. Recombinant γ-interferon decreases the number and severity of infections in patients with chronic granulomatous disease. Demonstration of this activity with one patient group raises the possibility that cytokines, growth factors, and other biologic response modifiers may be helpful in other conditions in preventing recurrent infections. Bone marrow transplantation has been attempted in most major congenital neutrophil dysfunction syndromes, and reconstitution with normal cells and cell function has been documented. Combining genetic engineering with autologous bone marrow transplantation may provide a future strategy for curing these disorders.

▶ Prognosis

For mild to moderate defects, anticipation and conservative medical management ensure a reasonable outlook. For severe defects, excessive morbidity and significant mortality exist. In some diseases, the development of noninfectious complications, such as the lymphoproliferative phase of Chédiak-Higashi syndrome or inflammatory syndromes in chronic granulomatous disease, may influence prognosis.

Ambruso DR: Human neutrophil immunodeficiency syndrome is associated with an inhibitory Rac2 mutation. Proc Natl Acad Sci U S A 2000;97:4654 [PMID: 10758162].

Ambruso DR, Johnston RB Jr: Chronic granulomatous disease of childhood. In Chernick V, Boat TF (editors): *Kendig's Disorders of the Respiratory Tract in Children.* WB Saunders, 2006:982–991.

Casanova JL: Primary immunodeficiencies: A field in its infancy. Science 2007;317:617 [PMID: 17673650].

Table 28–6. Classification of congenital neutrophil function deficits.

Disorder	Clinical Manifestations	Functional Defect	Biochemical Defect	Inheritance (Chromosome; Gene)
Chédiak-Higashi syndrome	Oculocutaneous albinism, photophobia, nystagmus, ataxia. Recurrent infections of skin, respiratory tract, and mucous membranes with gram-positive and gram-negative organisms. Many patients die during lymphoproliferative phase with hepatomegaly, fever. This may be a viral-associated hemophagocytic syndrome secondary to Epstein-Barr virus infection. Older patients may develop degenerative CNS disease.	Neutropenia. Neutrophils, monocytes, lymphocytes, platelets, and all granule-containing cells have giant granules. Most significant defect is in chemotaxis. Also milder defects in microbicidal activity and degranulation.	Gene deficit identified. Alterations in membrane fusion with formation of giant granules. Other biochemical abnormalities in cAMP and cGMP, microtubule assembly.	Autosomal recessive (1q42.1-.2; CHS1)
Leukocyte adherence deficiency I	Recurrent soft-tissue infections, including gingivitis, otitis, mucositis, periodontitis, skin infections. Delayed separation of the cord in newborn and problems with wound healing.	Neutrophilia. Diminished adherence to surfaces, leading to decreased chemotaxis.	Absence or partial deficiency of CD11/CD18 cell surface adhesive glycoproteins.	Autosomal recessive (12q22.3; ITGB2)
Leukocyte adherence deficiency II	Recurrent infections, mental retardation, craniofacial abnormalities, short stature.	Neutrophilia. Deficient "rolling" interactions with endothelial cells. Red cells have Bombay phenotype.	Deficient fucosyl transferase results in deficient sialyl Lewis X antigen, which interacts with P selectin on endothelial cell to establish neutrophil rolling, a prerequisite for adherence and diapedesis.	Autosomal recessive (11p11.2; SLC35C1)
Chronic granulomatous disease	Recurrent purulent infections with catalase-positive bacteria and fungi. May involve skin, mucous membranes. Patients also develop deep infections (lymph nodes, lung, liver, bones) and sepsis.	Neutrophilia. Neutrophils demonstrate deficient bactericidal activity but normal chemotaxis and ingestion. Defect in the oxidase enzyme system, resulting in absence or diminished production of oxygen metabolites toxic to microbes.	Several molecular defects in oxidase components. Absent cytochrome b_{558} with decreased expression of either (1) or (2): (1) gp91-phox (2) p22-phox Absent p47-phox or p67-phox (cytosolic components).	X-linked in 60–65% of cases (Xp21.1; CYBB) Autosomal recessive in < 5% of cases (16q24; CYBA) Autosomal recessive in 30% of cases (7q11.23; NCF1 and 1q25; NCF2, respectively)
Myeloperoxidase deficiency	Generally healthy. Fungal infections when deficiency associated with systemic diseases (eg, diabetes).	Diminished capacity to enhance hydrogen peroxide-mediated microbicidal activity.	Diminished or absent myeloperoxidase; post-translational defect in processing protein.	Autosomal recessive (17q22-23)
Specific granule deficiency	Recurrent skin and deep tissue infections.	Decreased chemotaxis and bactericidal activity.	Failure to produce specific granules or their contents during myelopoiesis. Defect in transcription factor.	Autosomal recessive (14q11.2; CEBPε)

cAMP, cyclic adenosine monophosphate; cGMP, cyclic guanosine monophosphate; CNS, central nervous system.

LYMPHOCYTOSIS

From the first week up to the fifth year of life, lymphocytes are the most numerous leukocytes in human blood. The ratio then reverses gradually to reach the adult pattern of neutrophil predominance. An absolute lymphocytosis in childhood is associated with acute or chronic viral infections, pertussis, syphilis, tuberculosis, and hyperthyroidism. Other noninfectious conditions, drugs, and hypersensitivity and serum sickness–like reactions cause lymphocytosis.

Fever, upper respiratory symptoms, gastrointestinal complaints, and rashes are clues in distinguishing infectious from noninfectious causes. The presence of enlarged liver, spleen, or lymph nodes is crucial to the differential diagnosis, which includes acute leukemia and lymphoma. Most cases of infectious mononucleosis are associated with hepatosplenomegaly or adenopathy. The absence of anemia and thrombocytopenia helps to differentiate these disorders. Evaluation of the morphology of lymphocytes on peripheral blood smear is crucial. Infectious causes, particularly infectious mononucleosis, are associated with atypical features in the lymphocytes such as basophilic cytoplasm, vacuoles, finer and less-dense chromatin, and an indented nucleus. These features are distinct from the characteristic morphology associated with lymphoblastic leukemia. Lymphocytosis in childhood is most commonly associated with infections and resolves with recovery from the primary disease.

EOSINOPHILIA

Eosinophilia in infants and children is an absolute eosinophil count greater than 300/µL. Marrow eosinophil production is stimulated by the cytokine interleukin-5. Allergies, particularly eczema, are the most common primary causes of eosinophilia in children. Eosinophilia also occurs in drug reactions, with tumors (Hodgkin and non-Hodgkin lymphomas and brain tumors), and with immunodeficiency and histiocytosis syndromes. Increased eosinophil counts are a prominent feature of many invasive parasitic infections. Gastrointestinal disorders such as chronic hepatitis, ulcerative colitis, Crohn disease, and milk precipitin disease may be associated with eosinophilia. Increased blood eosinophil counts have been identified in several families without association with any specific illness. Rare causes of eosinophilia include the hypereosinophilic syndrome, characterized by counts greater than 1500/µL and organ involvement and damage (hepatosplenomegaly, cardiomyopathy, pulmonary fibrosis, and central nervous system injury). This is a disorder of middle-aged adults and is rare in children. Eosinophilic leukemia has been described, but its existence as a distinct entity is controversial.

Eosinophils are sometimes the last type of mature myeloid cell to disappear after marrow ablative chemotherapy. Increased eosinophil counts are associated with graft-versus-host disease after bone marrow transplantation, and eleva-

tions are sometimes documented during rejection episodes in patients who have solid organ grafts.

▼ BLEEDING DISORDERS

Bleeding disorders may occur as a result of (1) quantitative or qualitative abnormalities of platelets, (2) quantitative or qualitative abnormalities in plasma procoagulant factors, (3) vascular abnormalities, or (4) accelerated fibrinolysis. The coagulation cascade and fibrinolytic system are shown in Figures 28–4 and 28–5.

The most critical aspect in evaluating the bleeding patient is obtaining detailed personal and family bleeding histories, including bleeding complications associated with dental interventions, surgeries, suture placement and removal, and trauma. Excessive mucosal bleeding is suggestive of a platelet disorder, von Willebrand disease, dysfibrinogenemia, or vasculitis. Bleeding into muscles and joints may be associated with a plasma procoagulant factor abnormality. In either scenario, the abnormality may be congenital or acquired. A thorough physical examination should be performed with

▲ **Figure 28–4.** The procoagulant system and formation of a fibrin clot. Vascular injury initiates the coagulation process by exposure of tissue factor (TF); the dashed lines indicate thrombin actions in addition to clotting of fibrinogen. The finely dotted lines indicate the feedback activation of the VII-TF complex by Xa and IXa. Ca⁺⁺, calcium; HK, high molecular weight kininogen; PK, prekallikrein; PL, phospholipid. (Reproduced, with permission, from Goodnight SH, Hathaway WE (editors): *Disorders of Hemostasis & Thrombosis: A Clinical Guide,* 2nd ed. McGraw-Hill, 2001.)

▲ **Figure 28–5.** The fibrinolytic system. Solid arrows indicate activation; dotted line arrows indicate inhibition. ECM, extracellular matrix; FDP, fibrinogen-fibrin degradation products; MMP, matrix metalloproteinases; PAI, plasminogen activator inhibitor; TAFI, t hrombin activatable fibrinolysis inhibitor; tPA, tissue plasminogen activator; uPA, urokinase; uPAR, cellular urokinase receptor. (Reproduced, with permission, from Goodnight SH, Hathaway WE (editors): *Disorders of Hemostasis & Thrombosis: A Clinical Guide,* 2nd ed. McGraw-Hill, 2001.)

special attention to the skin, oro- and nasopharynx, liver, spleen, and joints. Screening and diagnostic evaluation in patients with suspected bleeding disorders should initially include the following laboratory testing:

1. Prothrombin time (PT) to assess clotting function of factors VII, X, V, II, and fibrinogen.
2. Activated partial thromboplastin time (aPTT) to assess clotting function of high molecular weight kininogen, prekallikrein, XII, XI, IX, VIII, X, V, II, and fibrinogen.
3. Platelet count and size determined as part of a CBC.
4. Platelet functional assessment by platelet function analyzer-100 (PFA-100), or template bleeding time.
5. Fibrinogen functional level by clotting assay.

The following laboratory tests may also be useful:

1. Thrombin time to measure the generation of fibrin from fibrinogen following conversion of prothrombin to thrombin, as well as the antithrombin effects of fibrin-split products and heparin. The thrombin time may be prolonged in the setting of a normal fibrinogen concentration if the fibrinogen is dysfunctional (ie, dysfibrinogenemia).
2. Euglobulin lysis time (ELT), if available, to evaluate for accelerated fibrinolysis if the preceding workup is non-revealing despite documented history of pathologic bleeding. If the ELT is shortened, assessment of plasminogen activator inhibitor-1 and α_2-antiplasmin is warranted, as congenital deficiency in these fibrinolytic inhibitors may cause hyperfibrinolysis. In ill patients, measurement of fibrin degradation products may assist in the diagnosis of DIC.

Goodnight SH, Hathaway WE (editors): *Disorders of Hemostasis & Thrombosis: A Clinical Guide,* 2nd ed. New York: McGraw-Hill, 2001:41–51.

ABNORMALITIES OF PLATELET NUMBER OR FUNCTION

Thrombocytopenia in the pediatric age range is often immune-mediated (eg, idiopathic thrombocytopenic purpura, neonatal auto- or alloimmune thrombocytopenia, heparin-induced thrombocytopenia), but is also caused by consumptive coagulopathy (eg, DIC, Kasabach-Merritt syndrome), acute leukemias, rare disorders such as Wiskott-Aldrich syndrome and type IIb von Willebrand disease, and artifactually in automated cytometers (eg, Bernard-Soulier syndrome), where giant forms may not be enumerated as platelets by automated cell counters.

1. Idiopathic Thrombocytopenic Purpura

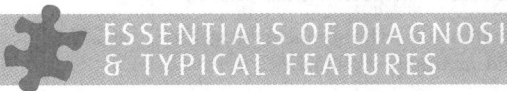

ESSENTIALS OF DIAGNOSIS & TYPICAL FEATURES

▶ Otherwise healthy child.
▶ Decreased platelet count.
▶ Petechiae, ecchymoses.

▶ General Considerations

Acute idiopathic thrombocytopenic purpura (ITP) is the most common bleeding disorder of childhood. It occurs most frequently in children aged 2–5 years and often follows infection with viruses, such as rubella, varicella, measles, parvovirus, influenza, or EBV. Most patients recover spontaneously within a few months. Chronic ITP (> 6 months' duration) occurs in 10–20% of affected patients. The thrombocytopenia results from clearance of circulating IgM- or IgG-coated platelets by the reticuloendothelial system. The spleen plays a predominant role in the disease by forming the platelet cross-reactive antibodies and sequestering the antibody-bound platelets.

▶ Clinical Findings

A. Symptoms and Signs

Onset of ITP is usually acute, with the appearance of multiple petechiae and ecchymoses. Epistaxis is also common at presentation. No other physical findings are usually present. Rarely, concurrent infection with EBV or CMV may cause hepatosplenomegaly or lymphadenopathy, simulating acute leukemia.

B. Laboratory Findings

1. Blood—The platelet count is markedly reduced (usually < 50,000/μL and often < 10,000/μL), and platelets frequently are of larger size on peripheral blood smear, suggesting accel-

Table 28–7. Common causes of thrombocytopenia.

	Increased Turnover		Decreased Production	
Antibody-Mediated	Coagulopathy	Other	Congenital	Acquired
Idiopathic thrombocyto-penic purpura	Disseminated intravascu-lar coagulopathy	Hemolytic-uremic syndrome	Fanconi anemia	Aplastic anemia
Infection	Sepsis	Thrombotic thrombocytopenic purpura	Wiskott-Aldrich syndrome	Leukemia and other malignancies
Immunologic diseases	Necrotizing enterocolitis Thrombosis Cavernous hemangioma	Hypersplenism Respiratory distress syndrome Wiskott-Aldrich syndrome	Thrombocytopenia with absent radii Metabolic disorders Osteopetrosis	Vitamin B_{12} and folate deficiencies

erated production of new platelets. The white blood count and differential are normal, and the hemoglobin concentration is preserved unless hemorrhage has been significant.

2. Bone marrow—The number of megakaryocytes is increased. Erythroid and myeloid cellularity is normal.

3. Other laboratory tests—Platelet-associated IgG or IgM, or both, may be demonstrated on the patient's platelets or in the serum. PT and aPTT are normal.

▶ Differential Diagnosis

Table 28–7 lists common causes of thrombocytopenia. ITP is a diagnosis of exclusion. Family history or the finding of predominantly giant platelets on the peripheral blood smear is helpful in determining whether thrombocytopenia is hereditary. Bone marrow examination should be performed if the history is atypical (ie, the child is not otherwise healthy, or if there is a family history of bleeding), if abnormalities other than purpura and petechiae are present on physical examination, or if other cell lines are affected on the CBC. The importance of performing a bone marrow examination prior to using corticosteroids in the treatment for ITP is controversial.

▶ Complications

Severe hemorrhage and bleeding into vital organs are the feared complications of ITP. Intracranial hemorrhage is the most serious (but rarely seen) complication, occurring in less than 1% of affected children. The most important risk factors for hemorrhage are a platelet count less than 10,000/μL and mean platelet volume less than 8 fL.

▶ Treatment
A. General Measures

Treatment is optional in most children in the absence of bleeding. Aspirin and other medications that compromise platelet function should be avoided. Bleeding precautions (eg, restriction from physical contact activities, use of helmets, etc)

should be observed. Platelet transfusion should be avoided except in circumstances of life-threatening bleeding, in which case emergent splenectomy is to be pursued. In this setting, administration of corticosteroids and IVIG is also advisable.

B. Corticosteroids

Patients with clinically significant but non–life-threatening bleeding (ie, epistaxis, hematuria, and hematochezia) and those with a platelet count of less than 10,000/μL may benefit from prednisone at 2–4 mg/kg orally per day for 3–5 days, decreasing to 1–2 mg/kg/d for a total of 14 days. The dosage is then tapered and stopped. No further prednisone is given regardless of the platelet count unless significant bleeding recurs, at which time prednisone is administered in the smallest dose that achieves resolution of bleeding episodes (usually 2.5–5 mg twice daily). Follow-up continues until the steroid can again be discontinued, spontaneous remission occurs, or other therapeutic measures are instituted.

C. Intravenous Immunoglobulin (IVIG)

IVIG is the treatment of choice for severe, acute bleeding, and may also be used as an alternative or adjunct to corticosteroid treatment in both acute and chronic ITP of childhood. IVIG may be effective even when the patient is resistant to corticosteroids; responses are prompt and may last for several weeks. Most patients receive 1 g/kg/d for 1–3 days. Infusion time is typically 4–6 hours. Platelets may be given simultaneously during life-threatening hemorrhage but are rapidly destroyed. Adverse effects of IVIG are common, including transient neurologic complications (eg, headache, nausea, and aseptic meningitis) in one third of patients. These symptoms may mimic those of intracranial hemorrhage and necessitate radiologic evaluation of the brain. A transient decrease in neutrophil number may also be seen.

D. Anti-Rho(D) Immunoglobulin

This polyclonal immunoglobulin binds to the D antigen on red blood cells. The splenic clearance of anti-D–coated red cells interferes with removal of antibody-coated platelets, resulting in improvement in thrombocytopenia. This approach is effective only in Rh(+) patients with a functional spleen. The time required for platelet increase is slightly longer than with IVIG. However, approximately 80% of Rh(+) children with acute or chronic ITP respond well. Significant hemolysis may occur transiently with an average hemoglobin concentration decrease of 0.8 g/dL. However, severe hemolysis occurs in 5% of treated children, and clinical and laboratory evaluation approximately 5 days following administration is warranted in all patients. Rho(D) immunoglobulin is less expensive and infused more rapidly than IVIG, but is more expensive than corticosteroids.

E. Splenectomy

Most children with chronic ITP have platelet counts greater than 30,000/μL. Up to 70% of such children spontaneously recover with a platelet count greater than 100,000/μL within 1 year. For the remainder, corticosteroids, IVIG, and anti-D immunoglobulin are typically effective treatment for acute bleeding. Splenectomy produces a response in 70–90%, but it should be considered only after persistence of significant thrombocytopenia for at least 1 year. Preoperative treatment with corticosteroids, IVIG, or anti-D immunoglobulin is usually indicated. Postoperatively, the platelet count may rise to 1 million/μL, but is not often associated with thrombotic complications in the pediatric age group. The risk of overwhelming infection (predominantly with encapsulated organisms) is increased after splenectomy, particularly in the young child. Therefore, the procedure should be postponed, if possible, until age 5 years. Administration of pneumococcal and *H influenzae* type b vaccines at least 2 weeks prior to splenectomy is recommended. Meningococcal vaccine, although controversial, may be considered. Penicillin prophylaxis should be started postoperatively and continued for 1–3 years.

F. Rituximab (Anti-CD20 Monoclonal Antibody)

The efficacy of treating childhood chronic ITP in several series and a phase I/II trial has been demonstrated; remission was observed in 40%. Because of significant adverse events, this therapy may be reserved for refractory cases with significant bleeding.

▶ Prognosis

Ninety percent of children with ITP will have a spontaneous remission. Features associated with the development of chronic ITP include female gender, age greater than 10 years at presentation, insidious onset of bruising, and the presence of other autoantibodies. Older child- and adolescent-onset ITP is associated with an increased risk of chronic autoimmune diseases. Appropriate screening by history and laboratory studies (eg, antinuclear antibody) is warranted.

Franchini M: Rituximab for the treatment of childhood chronic idiopathic thrombocytopenic purpura and hemophilia with inhibitors. Pediatr Blood Cancer 2007;49:6 [PMID: 17311349].

Imbach P: Childhood ITP: 12 months follow-up data from the prospective registry I of the Intercontinental Childhood ITP Study Group (ICIS). Pediatr Blood Cancer 2006;46:351 [PMID: 16086422].

Tarantino MD: The pros and cons of drug therapy for immune thrombocytopenic purpura in children. Hematol Oncol Clin North Am 2004;18:1301 [PMID: 15511617].

2. Thrombocytopenia in the Newborn

Thrombocytopenia is one of the most common causes of neonatal hemorrhage and should be considered in any newborn with petechiae, purpura, or other significant bleeding. Defined as a platelet count less than 150,000/μL, thrombocytopenia occurs in approximately 0.9% of unselected neonates. Several specific entities may be responsible (see Table 28–7); however, half of such neonates have alloimmune thrombocytopenia. Infection and DIC are the most common causes of thrombocytopenia in ill full-term newborns and in preterm newborns. In the healthy neonate, antibody-mediated thrombocytopenia (alloimmune or maternal autoimmune), viral syndromes, hyperviscosity, and major-vessel thrombosis are frequent causes of thrombocytopenia. Management is directed toward the underlying etiology.

A. Thrombocytopenia Associated with Platelet Alloantibodies (Neonatal Alloimmune Thrombocytopenia)

Platelet alloimmunization occurs in 1 in approximately 350 pregnancies. Unlike in Rh incompatibility, 30–40% of affected neonates are first-born. Thrombocytopenia is progressive over the course of gestation and worse with each subsequent pregnancy. Alloimmunization occurs when a platelet antigen of the infant differs from that of the mother and the mother is sensitized by fetal platelets that cross the placenta into the maternal circulation. In Caucasians, alloimmune thrombocytopenia is most often due to human platelet antigen (HPA)-1a incompatibility. Sensitization of a mother homozygous for HPA-1b to paternally acquired fetal HPA-1a antigen results in severe fetal thrombocytopenia in 1 in 1200 fetuses. Only 1 in 20 HPA-1a–positive fetuses of HPA-1a–negative mothers develop alloimmunization. The presence of antenatal maternal platelet antibodies on more than one occasion and their persistence into the third trimester is predictive of severe neonatal thrombocytopenia; a weak or undetectable antibody does not exclude thrombocytopenia. Severe intracranial hemorrhage occurs in 10–30% of affected neonates as early as 20 weeks' gestation. Petechiae or other bleeding manifestations are usually present shortly after birth. The disease is self-limited, and the platelet count normalizes within 4 weeks.

If alloimmunization is associated with clinically significant bleeding, transfusion of platelet concentrates harvested from the mother is more effective than random donor platelets in increasing the platelet count. Transfusion with HPA-matched platelets from unrelated donors or treatment with IVIG or methylprednisolone has also been successful in raising the platelet count and achieving hemostasis. If thrombocytopenia is not severe and bleeding is absent, observation alone is often appropriate.

Intracranial hemorrhage in a previous child secondary to alloimmune thrombocytopenia is the strongest risk factor for severe fetal thrombocytopenia and hemorrhage in a subsequent pregnancy. Amniocentesis or chorionic villus sampling to obtain fetal DNA for platelet antigen typing is sometimes performed if the father is heterozygous for HPA-1a. If alloimmunization has occurred with a previous pregnancy, irrespective of history of intracranial hemorrhage, screening cranial ultrasound for hemorrhage should begin at 20 weeks' gestation and be repeated regularly. In addition, cordocentesis should be performed at approximately 20 weeks' gestation, with prophylactic transfusion of irradiated, leukoreduced, maternal platelet concentrates. If the fetal platelet count is less than 100,000/μL, the mother should be treated with weekly IVIG. Delivery by elective cesarean section is recommended if the fetal platelet count is less than 50,000/μL, to minimize the risk of intracranial hemorrhage associated with birth trauma.

B. Thrombocytopenia Associated with Idiopathic Thrombocytopenic Purpura in the Mother (Neonatal Autoimmune Thrombocytopenia)

Infants born to mothers with ITP or other autoimmune diseases (eg, antiphospholipid antibody syndrome or systemic lupus erythematosus) may develop thrombocytopenia as a result of transfer of antiplatelet IgG from the mother to the infant. Unfortunately, maternal and fetal platelet counts and maternal antiplatelet antibody levels are unreliable predictors of bleeding risk. Antenatal corticosteroid administration to the mother is generally instituted once maternal platelet count falls below 50,000/μL, with or without a concomitant course of IVIG.

Most neonates with neonatal autoimmune thrombocytopenia do not develop clinically significant bleeding, and thus treatment for thrombocytopenia is not often required. The risk of intracranial hemorrhage is 0.2–2%. If diffuse petechiae or minor bleeding are evident, a 1- to 2-week course of oral prednisone, 2 mg/kg/d, may be administered. If the platelet count remains consistently less than 20,000/μL or if severe hemorrhage develops, IVIG should be given (1 g/kg daily for 1–3 days). Platelet transfusions are only indicated for life-threatening bleeding, and may only be effective after removal of antibody by exchange transfusion. The platelet nadir is typically between the fourth to sixth day of life and improves significantly by 1 month; full recovery may take 2–4 months. Platelet recovery may be delayed in breast-fed infants because of transfer of IgG to the milk.

C. Neonatal Thrombocytopenia Associated with Infections

Thrombocytopenia is commonly associated with severe generalized infections during the newborn period. Between 50% and 75% of neonates with bacterial sepsis are thrombocytopenic. Intrauterine infections such as rubella, syphilis, toxoplasmosis, CMV, herpes simplex, enteroviruses, and parvovirus are often associated with thrombocytopenia. In addition to specific treatment for the underlying disease, platelet transfusions may be indicated in severe cases.

D. Thrombocytopenia Associated with Kaposiform Hemangioendotheliomas (Kasabach-Merritt Syndrome)

A rare but important cause of thrombocytopenia in the newborn is kaposiform hemangioendotheliomas, a benign neoplasm with histopathology distinct from that of classic infantile hemangiomas. Intense platelet sequestration in the lesion results in peripheral thrombocytopenia and may rarely be associated with a DIC-like picture and hemolytic anemia. The bone marrow typically shows megakaryocytic hyperplasia in response to the thrombocytopenia. Corticosteroids, α-interferon, and vincristine are all useful for reducing the size of the lesion and are indicated if significant coagulopathy is present, the lesion compresses a vital structure, or the lesion is cosmetically unacceptable. If consumptive coagulopathy is present, heparin or aminocaproic acid may be useful. Depending on the site, embolization may be an option. Surgery is often avoided because of the high risk of hemorrhage.

Hall GW: Kasabach-Merritt syndrome: Pathogenesis and management. Br J Haematol 2001;112:851 [PMID: 11298580].

Kaplan RN: Differential diagnosis and management of thrombocytopenia in childhood. Pediatr Clin North Am 2004;51:1109 [PMID: 15275991].

3. Disorders of Platelet Function

Individuals with platelet function defects typically develop skin and mucosal bleeding similar to that occurring in persons with thrombocytopenia. Historically, platelet function has been screened by measuring the bleeding time. If this is prolonged, in-vitro platelet aggregation is studied using agonists, such as adenosine diphosphate, collagen, arachidonic acid, and ristocetin, and simultaneous comparison with a normal control subject. While labor-intensive, platelet aggregometry remains important in selected clinical situations. The PFA-100 has become available to evaluate platelet dysfunction and von Willebrand disease, and has replaced the template bleeding time in many clinical laboratories. Unfortunately, none of these tests of platelet function is uniformly predictive of clinical bleeding severity.

Platelet dysfunction may be inherited or acquired, with the latter being more common. Acquired disorders of platelet function may occur secondary to uremia, cirrhosis, sepsis, myeloproliferative disorders, congenital heart disease, and viral infections. Many pharmacologic agents decrease platelet function. The most common offending agents in the pediatric population are aspirin and other nonsteroidal anti-inflammatory drugs (NSAIDs), synthetic penicillins, and valproic acid. In acquired platelet dysfunction, the PFA-100 closure time is typically prolonged with collagen-epinephrine, but normal with collagen-ADP.

The inherited disorders are due to defects in platelet-vessel interaction, platelet-platelet interaction, platelet granule content or release (including defects of signal transduction), thromboxane and arachidonic acid pathway, and platelet-procoagulant protein interaction. Individuals with hereditary platelet dysfunction generally have a prolonged bleeding time with normal platelet number and morphology by light microscopy. PFA-100 closure time, in contrast to that in acquired dysfunction, is typically prolonged with both collagen-ADP and collagen-epinephrine.

Congenital causes of defective platelet–vessel wall interaction include Bernard-Soulier syndrome. This condition is characterized by increased platelet size and decreased platelet number. The molecular defect in this autosomal recessive disorder is a deficiency or dysfunction of glycoprotein Ib-V-IX complex on the platelet surface resulting in impaired von Willebrand factor (vWF) binding, and hence, impaired platelet adhesion to the vascular endothelium.

Glanzmann thrombasthenia is an example of platelet-platelet dysfunction. In this autosomal recessive disorder, glycoprotein IIb-IIIa is deficient or dysfunctional. Platelets do not bind fibrinogen effectively and exhibit impaired aggregation. As in Bernard-Soulier syndrome, acute bleeding is treated by platelet transfusion.

Disorders involving platelet granule content include storage pool disease and Quebec platelet disorder. In individuals with storage pool disease, platelet-dense granules lack adenosine dinucleotide phosphate and adenosine trinucleotide phosphate and are often found to be low in number by electron microscopy. These granules are also deficient in Hermansky-Pudlak, Chédiak-Higashi, and Wiskott-Aldrich syndromes. Whereas deficiency of α-granules results in the gray platelet syndrome, Quebec platelet disorder is characterized by a normal platelet α-granule number, but with abnormal proteolysis of α-granule proteins and deficiency of platelet α-granule multimerin. Epinephrine-induced platelet aggregation is markedly impaired.

Platelet dysfunction has also been observed in other congenital syndromes, such as Down and Noonan syndromes, without a clear understanding of the molecular defect.

▶ Treatment

Acute bleeding in many individuals with acquired or selected congenital platelet function defects responds to therapy with desmopressin acetate, likely due to an induced release of vWF from endothelial stores. If this therapy is ineffective, or if the patient has Bernard-Soulier syndrome or Glanzmann syndrome, the mainstay of treatment for bleeding episodes is platelet transfusion. Recombinant VIIa has variable efficacy and may be helpful in platelet transfusion-refractory patients.

Drachman JG: Inherited thrombocytopenia: When a low platelet count does not mean ITP. Blood 2004;103:390 [PMID: 14505084].

Sohal AS: Uremic bleeding: Pathophysiology and clinical risk factors. Thromb Res 2006;118:417 [PMID: 15993929].

INHERITED BLEEDING DISORDERS

Table 28–8 lists normal values for coagulation factors. The more common factor deficiencies are discussed in this section. Individuals with bleeding disorders should avoid exposure to medications that inhibit platelet function. Participation in contact sports should be considered in the context of the severity of the bleeding disorder.

1. Factor VIII Deficiency (Hemophilia A, Classic Hemophilia)

ESSENTIALS OF DIAGNOSIS & TYPICAL FEATURES

- ▶ Bruising, soft-tissue bleeding, hemarthrosis.
- ▶ Prolonged activated partial thromboplastin time (aPTT).
- ▶ Reduced factor VIII activity.

▶ General Considerations

Factor VIII activity is reported in units per milliliter, with 1 U/mL equal to 100% of the factor activity found in 1 mL of normal plasma. The normal range for factor VIII activity is 0.5–1.5 U/mL (50–150%). Hemophilia A occurs predominantly in males as an X- linked disorder. One third of cases are due to a new mutation. The incidence of factor VIII deficiency is 1:5000 male births.

▶ Clinical Findings

A. Symptoms and Signs

Patients with severe hemophilia A (< 1% plasma factor VIII activity) have frequent spontaneous bleeding episodes involving skin, mucous membranes, joints, muscles, and viscera. In contrast, patients with mild hemophilia A (5–40% factor VIII activity) bleed only at times of trauma or surgery. Those with moderate hemophilia A (1% to < 5% factor VIII activity) typically have intermediate bleeding manifestations. The most crippling aspect of factor VIII deficiency is the tendency to develop recurrent hemarthroses that incite joint destruction.

Table 28–8. Physiologic alterations in measurements of the hemostatic system.

Measurement	Normal Adults	Fetus (20 wk)	Preterm (25–32 wk)	Term Infant	Infant (6 mo)	Pregnancy (term)	Exercise (acute)	Aging (70–80 y)
Platelets								
Count µL/10³	250	107–297	293	332	—	260	↑18–40%	225
Size (fL)	9.0	8.9	8.5	9.1	—	9.6	↑	—
Aggregation ADP	N	+	↓	↓	—	↑	↓15%	—
Collagen	N	↓	↓	↓	—	N	↓60%	N
Ristocetin	N	—	↑	↑	—	—	↓10%	—
BT (min)	2–9	—	3.6±2	3.4±1.8	—	9.0±1.4	—	5.6
Procoagulant system								
PTT*	1	4.0	3	1.3	1.1	1.1	↓15%	↓
PT*	1.00	2.3	1.3	1.1	1	0.95	N	—
TCT*	1	2.4	1.3	1.1	1	0.92	N	—
Fibrinogen mg/dL	278 (0.61)	96 (50)	250 (100)	240 (150)	251 (160)	450 (100)	↓25%	↑15%
II, U/mL	1 (0.7)	0.16 (0.10)	0.32 (0.18)	0.52 (0.25)	0.88 (0.6)	1.15 (0.68-1.9)	—	N
V, U/mL	1.0 (0.6)	0.32 (0.21)	0.80 (0.43)	1.00 (0.54)	0.91 (0.55)	0.85 (0.40-1.9)	—	N
VII, U/mL	1.0 (0.6)	0.27 (0.17)	0.37 (0.24)	0.57 (0.35)	0.87 (0.50)	1.17 (0.87-3.3)	↑200%	↑25%
VIIIc, U/mL	1.0 (0.6)	0.50 (0.23)	0.75 (0.40)	1.50 (0.55)	0.90 (0.50)	2.12 (0.8-6.0)	↑250%	1.50
vWF, U/mL	1.0 (0.6)	0.65 (0.40)	1.50 (0.90)	1.60 (0.84)	1.07 (0.60)	1.7	↑75–200%	↑
IX, U/mL	1.0 (0.5)	0.10 (0.05)	0.22 (0.17)	0.35 (0.15)	0.86 (0.36)	0.81-2.15	↑25%	1.0-1.40
X, U/mL	1.0 (0.6)	0.19 (0.15)	0.38 (0.20)	0.45 (0.3)	0.78 (0.38)	1.30	—	N
XI, U/mL	1.0 (0.6)	0.13 (0.08)	0.2 (0.12)	0.42 (0.20)	0.86 (0.38)	0.7	—	N
XII, U/mL	1.0 (0.6)	0.15 (0.08)	0.22 (0.09)	0.44 (0.16)	0.77 (0.39)	1.3 (0.82)	—	↑16%
XIII, U/mL	1.04 (0.55)	0.30	0.4	0.61 (0.36)	1.04 (0.50)	0.96	—	—
PreK, U/mL	1.12 (0.06)	0.13 (0.08)	0.26 (0.14)	0.35 (0.16)	0.86 (0.56)	1.18	—	↑27%
HK, U/mL	0.92 (0.48)	0.15 (0.10)	0.28 (0.20)	0.64 (0.50)	0.82 (0.36)	1.6	—	↑32%
Anticoagulant system								
AT-U/mL	1.0	0.23	0.35	0.56	1.04	1.02	↑14%	N
α₂-MG, U/mL	1.05 (0.79)	0.18 (0.10)	—	1.39 (0.95)	1.91 (1.49)	1.53 (0.85)	—	—
C1IN, U/mL	1.01	—	—	0.72	1.41	—	—	—
PC, U/mL	1.0	0.10	0.29	0.50	0.59	0.99	N	N
Total PS, U/mL	1.0 (0.6)	0.15 (0.11)	0.17 (0.14)	0.24 (0.1)	0.87 (0.55)	0.89	—	N
Free, PS, U/mL	1.0 (0.5)	0.22 (0.13)	0.28 (0.19)	0.49 (0.33)	—	0.25	—	—
Heparin	1.01	0.10 (0.06)	0.25 (0.10)	0.49 (0.33)	0.97 (0.59)	—	—	↓15%
Cofactor II, U/mL	(0.73)							
TFPI, ng/mL	73	21	20.6	38	—	—	—	—
Fibrinolytic system								
Plasminogen U/mL	1.0	0.20	0.35 (0.20)	0.37 (0.18)	0.90	1.39	↓10%	N
t-PA, ng/mL	4.9	—	8.48	9.6	2.8	4.9	↑300%	N
α₂-AP, U/mL	1.0	1.0	0.74 (0.5)	0.83 (0.65)	1.11 (0.83)	0.95	N	N
PAI-1, U/mL	1.0	—	1.5	1.0	1.07	4.0	↓5%	N
Overall fibrinolysis	N	↑	↑	↑	—	↓	↑	↓

Except as otherwise indicated values are mean ±2 SD or values in parentheses are lower limits (–2 SD or lower range); +, positive or present; ↓, decreased; ↑, increased; N, normal or no change; *, values as ratio or subject/mean of reference range; α₂-MG, α₂-macroglobulin; α₂-AP, α₂-antiplasmin; ADP, adenosine diphosphate; AT, antithrombin; BT, bleeding time; C1IN, C1 esterase inhibitor; HK, high molecular weight kininogen; PAI, plasminogen activator inhibitor; PC, protein C; PreK, prekallikrein; PS, protein S; PT, prothrombin time; PTT, partial thromboplastin time; TCT, thrombin clotting time; TFPI, tissue factor pathway inhibitor; t-PA, tissue plasminogen activator; vWF, von Willebrand factor. Overall fibrinolysis is measured by euglobulin lysis time.

Adapted, with permission, from Goodnight SH, Hathaway WE (editors): *Disorders of Hemostasis & Thrombosis: A Clinical Guide,* 2nd ed. McGraw-Hill, 2001.

B. Laboratory Findings

Individuals with hemophilia A have a prolonged aPTT, except in some cases of mild deficiency. The prothrombin time (PT) is normal. The diagnosis is confirmed by finding decreased factor VIII activity with normal vWF activity. In two thirds of families of hemophilic patients, the females are carriers and some are mildly symptomatic. Carriers of hemophilia can be detected by determination of the ratio of factor VIII activity to vWF antigen and by molecular genetic techniques. In a male fetus or newborn with a family history of hemophilia A, cord blood sampling for factor VIII activity is accurate and important in subsequent care.

▶ Complications

Intracranial hemorrhage is the leading disease-related cause of death among patients with hemophilia. Most intracranial hemorrhages in moderate to severe deficiency are spontaneous (ie, not associated with trauma). Hemarthroses begin early in childhood and, if recurrent, result in joint destruction (ie, hemophilic arthropathy). Large intramuscular hematomas can lead to a compartment syndrome with resultant muscle and nerve death. Although these complications are most common in severe hemophilia A, they may be experienced by individuals with moderate or mild disease. A serious complication of hemophilia is the development of an acquired circulating antibody to factor VIII after treatment with factor VIII concentrate. Such factor VIII inhibitors develop in 15–25% of patients with severe hemophilia A, and may be amenable to desensitization with regular factor VIII infusion with or without immunosuppressive therapy. In recent years, recombinant factor VIIa has become a therapy of choice for treatment of acute hemorrhage in patients with hemophilia A and a high-titer inhibitor.

In prior decades, therapy-related complications in hemophilia A have included infection with the human immunodeficiency virus (HIV), hepatitis B virus (HBV), and hepatitis C virus (HCV). Through more stringent donor selection, the implementation of sensitive screening assays, the use of heat- or chemical viral inactivation methods, and the development of recombinant products, the risk of these infections is minimal. Inactivation methods do not eradicate viruses lacking a lipid envelope, however, so that transmission of parvovirus and hepatitis A remains a concern with the use of plasma-derived products. Immunization with hepatitis A and hepatitis B vaccines is recommended for all hemophilia patients.

▶ Treatment

The general aim of management is to raise the factor VIII activity to prevent or stop bleeding. Some patients with mild factor VIII deficiency may respond to desmopressin via release of endothelial stores of factor VIII and vWF into plasma; however, most patients require administration of exogenous factor VIII to achieve hemostasis. The in-vivo half-life of factor VIII is generally 8–12 hours but may

exhibit considerable variation among individuals depending on comorbid conditions. Non–life-threatening, non–limb-threatening hemorrhage is treated initially with 20–30 U/kg of factor VIII, to achieve a rise in plasma factor VIII activity to 40–60%. Large joint hemarthrosis and life- or limb-threatening hemorrhage is treated initially with approximately 50 U/kg of factor VIII, targeting a rise to 100% factor VIII activity. Subsequent doses are determined according to the site and extent of bleeding and the clinical response. Doses are rounded to the nearest whole vial size. In circumstances of suboptimal clinical response, recent change in bleeding frequency, or comorbid illness, monitoring the plasma factor VIII activity response may be warranted. For most instances of non–life-threatening hemorrhage in experienced patients with moderate or severe hemophilia A, treatment can be administered at home, provided adequate intravenous access exists and close contact is maintained with the hemophilia clinician team.

Prophylactic factor VIII infusions (eg, two or three times weekly) may prevent the development of arthropathy in severe hemophiliacs, and this approach is becoming more common in pediatric hemophilia care.

▶ Prognosis

The development of safe and effective therapies for hemophilia A has resulted in improved long-term survival in recent decades. In addition, more aggressive management and the coordination of comprehensive care through hemophilia centers have greatly improved quality of life and level of function.

Gouw SC: Treatment-related risk factors of inhibitor development in previously untreated patients with hemophilia A: The CANAL cohort study. Blood 2007;109:4648 [PMID: 17289808].

Manco-Johnson MJ: Prophylaxis versus episodic treatment to prevent joint disease in boys with severe hemophilia. N Engl J Med 2007;357:535 [PMID: 17687129].

2. Factor IX Deficiency (Hemophilia B, Christmas Disease)

The mode of inheritance and clinical manifestations of factor IX deficiency are the same as those of factor VIII deficiency. Hemophilia B is 15–20% as prevalent as hemophilia A. As in factor VIII deficiency, factor IX deficiency is associated with a prolonged aPTT, but the PT and thrombin time are normal. However, the aPTT is slightly less sensitive to factor IX deficiency than factor VIII deficiency. Diagnosis of hemophilia B is made by assaying factor IX activity, and severity is determined similarly to factor VIII deficiency. In general, clinical bleeding severity correlates less well with factor activity in hemophilia B than in hemophilia A.

The mainstay of treatment in hemophilia B is exogenous factor IX. Unlike factor VIII, about 50% of the administered dose of factor IX diffuses into the extravascular space. Therefore, 1 U/kg of plasma-derived factor IX concentrate or recombinant factor IX is expected to increase plasma factor IX activity by approximately 1%. Factor IX typically has a half-life of 20–22 hours in vivo, but due to variability, therapeutic monitoring may be warranted. As for factor VIII products, viral inactivation techniques for plasma-derived factor IX concentrates appear effective in eradicating HIV, HBV, and HCV. Only 1–3% of persons with factor IX deficiency develop an inhibitor to factor IX, but patients may be at risk for anaphylaxis when receiving exogenous factor IX. The prognosis for persons with factor IX deficiency is comparable to that of patients with factor VIII deficiency. Gene therapy research efforts are ongoing for both hemophilias.

Shapiro AD: Hemophilia B (factor IX deficiency). In Goodnight SH, Hathaway WE (editors): *Disorders of Hemostasis & Thrombosis: A Clinical Guide,* 2nd ed. McGraw-Hill, 2001:140–148.
Shapiro AD: The safety and efficacy of recombinant human blood coagulation factor IX in previously untreated patients with severe or moderately severe hemophilia B. Blood 2005;105:518 [PMID: 15383463].

3. Factor XI Deficiency (Hemophilia C)

Factor XI deficiency is a genetic, autosomally transmitted coagulopathy, typically of mild to moderate clinical severity. Cases of factor XI deficiency account for less than 5% of all hemophilia patients. Homozygotes generally bleed at surgery or following severe trauma, but do not commonly have spontaneous hemarthroses. In contrast to factor VIII and IX deficiencies, factor XI activity is least predictive of bleeding risk. Although typically mild, pathologic bleeding may be seen in heterozygous individuals with factor XI activity as high as 60%. The aPTT is often considerably prolonged. In individuals with deficiency of both plasma and platelet-associated factor XI, the PFA-100 may also be prolonged. Management typically consists of perioperative prophylaxis and episodic therapy for acute hemorrhage. Treatment includes infusion of fresh frozen plasma (FFP); platelet transfusion may also be useful for acute hemorrhage in patients with deficiency of platelet-associated factor XI. Desmopressin has been used in some cases. The prognosis for an average life span in patients with factor XI deficiency is excellent.

Salomon O: New observations on factor XI deficiency. Haemophilia 2004;10:184 [PMID: 15479396].

4. Other Inherited Bleeding Disorders

Other hereditary single clotting factor deficiencies are rare. Transmission is generally autosomal. Homozygous individuals with a deficiency or structural abnormality of prothrombin, factor V, factor VII, or factor X may have excessive bleeding.

Persons with dysfibrinogenemia (ie, structurally or functionally abnormal fibrinogen) may develop recurrent venous thromboembolic episodes or bleeding. Immunologic assay of fibrinogen is normal, but clotting assay may be low and the thrombin time prolonged. The PT and aPTT may be prolonged. Cryoprecipitate, which is rich in fibrinogen, is the treatment of choice, given the present lack of availability of a plasma-derived or recombinant fibrinogen product in the United States.

Afibrinogenemia resembles hemophilia clinically but has an autosomal recessive inheritance. Affected patients can experience a variety of bleeding manifestations, including mucosal bleeding, ecchymoses, hematomas, hemarthroses, and intracranial hemorrhage, especially following trauma. Fatal umbilical cord hemorrhage has been reported in neonates. The PT, aPTT, and thrombin time are all prolonged. A severely reduced fibrinogen concentration in an otherwise well child is confirmatory of the diagnosis. As in dysfibrinogenemia, cryoprecipitate infusion is used for surgical prophylaxis and for acute hemorrhage.

Acharya SS: Rare Bleeding Disorder Registry: Deficiencies of factors II, V, VII, X, XIII, fibrinogen and dysfibrinogenemias. J Thromb Haemost 2004;2:248 [PMID: 14995986].

VON WILLEBRAND DISEASE

ESSENTIALS OF DIAGNOSIS & TYPICAL FEATURES

► Easy bruising and epistaxis from early childhood.
► Menorrhagia.
► Prolonged PFA-100 (or bleeding time); normal platelet count; absence of acquired platelet dysfunction.
► Reduced activity or abnormal structure of vWF.

► General Considerations

von Willebrand disease (vWD) is the most common inherited bleeding disorder among Caucasians, with a prevalence of 1%. vWF is a protein present as a multimeric complex in plasma, which binds factor VIII and is a cofactor for platelet adhesion to the endothelium. An estimated 70–80% of all patients with vWD have classic vWD (type 1), which is caused by a partial quantitative deficiency of vWF. vWD type 2 involves a qualitative deficiency of (ie, dysfunctional) vWF, and vWD type 3 is characterized by a nearly complete deficiency of vWF. The majority (> 80%) of individuals with type 1 disease are asymptomatic. vWD is most often transmitted as an autosomal dominant trait, but can be autosomal recessive. The disease can also be acquired, developing in association with hypothyroidism, Wilms tumor, cardiac disease, renal disease, or systemic lupus erythematosus and in individuals receiving valproic acid. Acquired vWD is most often caused by the development of an antibody to vWF or increased turnover of vWF.

Clinical Findings

A. Symptoms and Signs

A history of increased bruising and excessive epistaxis is often present. Prolonged bleeding also occurs with trauma or at surgery. Menorrhagia is often a presenting finding in females.

B. Laboratory Findings

PT is normal, and aPTT is sometimes prolonged. Prolongation of the PFA-100 or bleeding time is usually present since vWF plays a role in platelet adherence to endothelium. Platelet number may be decreased in type 2b vWD. Factor VIII and vWF antigen are decreased in types 1 and 3, but may be normal in type 2 vWD. vWF activity (eg, ristocetin cofactor or collagen binding) is decreased in all types. Since normal vWF antigen levels vary by blood type (type O normally has lower levels), blood type must be determined. Complete laboratory classification requires vWF multimer assay. The diagnosis requires confirmation of laboratory testing and bleeding history is often helpful when present.

Treatment

The treatment to prevent or halt bleeding for most patients with vWD types 1 and 2 is desmopressin acetate, which causes release of vWF from endothelial stores. Desmopressin may be administered intravenously at a dose of 0.3 mcg/kg diluted in at least 20–30 mL of normal saline and given over 20–30 minutes. This dose typically elicits a three- to fivefold rise in plasma vWF. A high-concentration desmopressin nasal spray (150 mcg/spray), different than the preparation used for enuresis, may alternatively be used. Because response to vWF is variable among patients, factor VIII and vWF activities are typically measured before and 60 minutes after infusion, if no recent response has been measured. Desmopressin may cause fluid shifts, hyponatremia, and seizures in children younger than 2 years of age. Because release of stored vWF is limited, tachyphylaxis often occurs with desmopressin.

If further therapy is indicated, vWF-replacement therapy (eg, plasma-derived concentrate) is recommended; such therapy is also used in patients with type 1 or 2a vWD who exhibit suboptimal laboratory response to desmopressin, and for all individuals with type 2b or 3 vWD. Antifibrinolytic agents (eg, ε-aminocaproic acid) may be useful for control of mucosal bleeding. Topical thrombin and fibrin glue may also be of benefit, although antibodies that inhibit clotting proteins have been described. Estrogen-containing contraceptive therapy may be helpful for menorrhagia.

Prognosis

With the availability of effective treatment and prophylaxis for bleeding, life expectancy in vWD is normal.

Cox Gill J: Diagnosis and treatment of von Willebrand disease. Hematol Oncol Clin North Am 2004;18:1277 [PMID: 15511616].

Mannucci PM: Treatment of von Willebrand's disease. N Engl J Med 2004;351:683 [PMID: 15306670].

ACQUIRED BLEEDING DISORDERS

1. Disseminated Intravascular Coagulation (DIC)

ESSENTIALS OF DIAGNOSIS & TYPICAL FEATURES

▶ Presence of disorder known to trigger DIC.

▶ Evidence for consumptive coagulopathy (prolonged aPTT, PT, or thrombin time; increase in FSP (fibrin-fibrinogen split products); decreased fibrinogen or platelets).

General Considerations

DIC is an acquired pathologic process characterized by tissue factor–mediated diffuse coagulation activation in the host. DIC involves dysregulated, excessive thrombin generation, with consequent intravascular fibrin deposition and consumption of platelets and procoagulant factors. Microthrombi, composed of fibrin and platelets, may produce tissue ischemia and end-organ damage. The fibrinolytic system is frequently activated in DIC, leading to plasmin-mediated destruction of fibrin and fibrinogen; this results in fibrin-fibrinogen degradation products (FDPs) which exhibit anticoagulant and platelet-inhibitory functions. DIC commonly accompanies severe infection and other critical illnesses in infants and children. Conditions known to trigger DIC include endothelial damage (eg, endotoxin, virus), tissue necrosis (eg, burns), diffuse ischemic injury (eg, shock, hypoxia acidosis), and systemic release of tissue procoagulants (eg, certain cancers, placental disorders).

Clinical Findings

A. Symptoms and Signs

Signs of DIC may include (1) signs of shock, often including end-organ dysfunction, (2) diffuse bleeding tendency (eg, hematuria, melena, purpura, petechiae, persistent oozing from needle punctures or other invasive procedures), and (3) evidence of thrombotic lesions (eg, major vessel thrombosis, purpura fulminans).

B. Laboratory Findings

Tests that are most sensitive, easiest to perform, most useful for monitoring, and best reflect the hemostatic capacity of the patient are the PT, aPTT, platelet count, fibrinogen, and fibrin-fibrinogen split products. The PT and aPTT are typically prolonged and the platelet count and fibrinogen concentration may be decreased. However, in children, the fibrinogen level may be normal until late in the course. Levels of fibrin-fibrinogen split products are increased, and elevated levels of D-dimer, a cross-linked fibrin degradation byproduct, may be helpful in monitoring the degree of activation of both coagulation and fibrinolysis. However, D-dimer is nonspecific and may be elevated in the context of a triggering event (eg, severe infection) without concomitant DIC. Often, physiologic inhibitors of coagulation, especially antithrombin III and protein C, are consumed, predisposing to thrombosis. The specific laboratory abnormalities in DIC may vary with the triggering event and the course of illness.

▶ Differential Diagnosis

DIC can be difficult to distinguish from coagulopathy of liver disease (ie, hepatic synthetic dysfunction), especially when the latter is associated with thrombocytopenia secondary to portal hypertension and hypersplenism. Generally, factor VII activity is decreased markedly in liver disease (due to deficient synthesis of this protein, which has the shortest half-life among the procoagulant factors), but only mildly to moderately decreased in DIC (due to consumption). Factor VIII activity is often normal or even increased in liver disease, but decreased in DIC.

▶ Treatment

A. Therapy for Underlying Disorder

The most important aspect of therapy in DIC is the identification and treatment of the triggering event. If the pathogenic process underlying DIC is reversed, often no other therapy is needed for the coagulopathy.

B. Replacement Therapy for Consumptive Coagulopathy

Replacement of consumed procoagulant factors with FFP and of platelets via platelet transfusion is warranted in the setting of DIC with hemorrhagic complications, or as periprocedural bleeding prophylaxis. Infusion of 10–15 mL/kg FFP typically raises procoagulant factor activities by approximately 10–15%. Cryoprecipitate can also be given as a rich source of fibrinogen; one bag of cryoprecipitate per 3 kg in infants or one bag of cryoprecipitate per 6 kg in older children typically raises plasma fibrinogen concentration by 75–100 mg/dL.

C. Anticoagulant Therapy for Coagulation Activation

Continuous intravenous infusion of unfractionated heparin is sometimes given in order to attenuate coagulation activation and consequent consumptive coagulopathy. The rationale for heparin therapy is to maximize the efficacy of, and minimize the need for, replacement of procoagulants and platelets; however, clinical evidence demonstrating benefit of heparin in DIC is lacking. Heparin dosing is provided in the section on thrombosis treatment.

D. Specific Factor Concentrates

A nonrandomized pilot study of antithrombin concentrate in children with DIC and associated acquired antithrombin deficiency demonstrated favorable outcomes, suggesting that replacement of this consumed procoagulant may be of benefit. Protein C concentrate has also shown promise in two small pilot studies of meningococcal-associated DIC with purpura fulminans. Activated protein C has reduced mortality in septic adults in a large randomized multicenter trial; an international pediatric trial is ongoing.

2. Liver Disease

The liver is the major synthetic site of prothrombin, fibrinogen, high molecular weight kininogen, and factors V, VII, IX, X, XI, XII, and XIII. In addition, plasminogen and the physiologic anticoagulants (antithrombin III, protein C, and protein S) are hepatically synthesized. α_2-Antiplasmin, a regulator of fibrinolysis, is also produced in the liver. Deficiency of factor V and the vitamin K–dependent factors (II, VII, IX, and X) is most often a result of decreased hepatic synthesis and is manifested by a prolonged PT and often a prolonged aPTT. Extravascular loss and increased consumption of clotting factors may contribute to PT and aPTT prolongation. Fibrinogen production is often decreased, or an abnormal fibrinogen (dysfibrinogen) containing excess sialic acid residues may be synthesized, or both. Hypofibrinogenemia or dysfibrinogenemia is associated with prolongation of thrombin time and reptilase time. FDPs and D-dimers may be present because of increased fibrinolysis, particularly in the setting of chronic hepatitis or cirrhosis. Thrombocytopenia secondary to hypersplenism may occur. DIC and coagulopathy of liver disease also mimic vitamin K deficiency; however, vitamin K deficiency has normal factor V activity. Treatment of acute bleeding in the setting of coagulopathy of liver disease consists of replacement with FFP and platelets. Desmopressin may shorten the bleeding time and aPTT in patients with chronic liver disease, but its safety has not been well established. Recombinant VIIa also is efficacious for life-threatening hemorrhage.

3. Vitamin K Deficiency

The newborn period is characterized by physiologically depressed activity of the vitamin K–dependent factors (II, VII, IX, and X). If vitamin K is not administered at birth, a bleeding diathesis previously called hemorrhagic disease of the newborn, now termed vitamin K deficiency bleeding (VKDB), may develop. Outside of the newborn period, vitamin K deficiency may occur as a consequence of inadequate intake, excess loss, inadequate formation of active metabolites, or competitive antagonism.

One of three patterns is seen in the neonatal period:

1. Early VKDB of the newborn occurs within 24 hours of birth and is most often manifested by cephalohematoma, intracranial hemorrhage, or intra-abdominal bleeding. Although occasionally idiopathic, it is most often associated with maternal ingestion of drugs that interfere with vitamin K metabolism (eg, warfarin, phenytoin, isoniazid, and rifampin). Early VKDB occurs in 6–12% of neonates born to mothers who take these medications without receiving vitamin K supplementation. The disorder is often life-threatening.

2. Classic VKDB occurs at 24 hours to 7 days of age and usually is manifested as gastrointestinal, skin, or mucosal bleeding. Bleeding after circumcision may occur. Although occasionally associated with maternal drug usage, it most often occurs in well infants who do not receive vitamin K at birth and are solely breast fed.

3. Late neonatal VKDB occurs on or after day 8. Manifestations include intracranial, gastrointestinal, or skin bleeding. This disorder is often associated with fat malabsorption (eg, in chronic diarrhea) or alterations in intestinal flora (eg, with prolonged antibiotic therapy). Like classic VKDB, late VKDB occurs almost exclusively in breast-fed infants.

The diagnosis of vitamin K deficiency is suspected based on the history, physical examination, and laboratory results. The PT is prolonged out of proportion to the aPTT (also prolonged). The thrombin time becomes prolonged late in the course. The platelet count is normal. This laboratory profile is similar to the coagulopathy of acute liver disease, but with normal fibrinogen level and absence of hepatic transaminase elevation. The diagnosis of vitamin K deficiency is confirmed by a demonstration of noncarboxylated proteins in the absence of vitamin K in the plasma and by clinical and laboratory responses to vitamin K. Intravenous or subcutaneous treatment with vitamin K should be given immediately and not withheld while awaiting test results. In the setting of severe bleeding, additional acute treatment with FFP or recombinant factor VIIa may be indicated.

4. Uremia

Uremia is frequently associated with acquired platelet dysfunction. Bleeding occurs in approximately 50% of patients with chronic renal failure. The bleeding risk conferred by platelet dysfunction associated with metabolic imbalance may be compounded by decreased vWF activity and procoagulant deficiencies (eg, factor II, XII, XI, IX) due to increased urinary losses of these proteins in some settings of renal insufficiency. In accordance with platelet dysfunction, uremic bleeding is typically characterized by purpura, epistaxis, menorrhagia, or gastrointestinal hemorrhage. Acute bleeding may be managed with infusion of desmopressin acetate, factor VIII concentrates containing vWF, or cryoprecipitate with or without coadministration of FFP. Red cell transfusion may be required. Prophylactic administration of erythropoietin before the development of severe anemia appears to decrease the bleeding risk. Recombinant VIIa may be useful in refractory bleeding.

Goldenberg NA: Pediatric hemostasis and use of plasma components. Best Pract Res Clin Haematol 2006;19:143 [PMID: 16377547].

Hey E: Vitamin K—What, why, and when. Arch Dis Child Fetal Neonatal Ed 2003;88:F80 [PMID: 12598491].

VASCULAR ABNORMALITIES ASSOCIATED WITH BLEEDING

1. Henoch-Schönlein Purpura (Anaphylactoid Purpura)

ESSENTIALS OF DIAGNOSIS & TYPICAL FEATURES

▶ Purpuric cutaneous rash.
▶ Migratory polyarthritis or polyarthralgias.
▶ Intermittent abdominal pain.
▶ Nephritis.

▶ General Considerations

Henoch-Schönlein purpura (HSP), the most common type of small vessel vasculitis in children, primarily affects boys 2–7 years of age. Occurrence is highest in the spring and fall, and upper respiratory infection precedes the diagnosis in two thirds of children.

Leukocytoclastic vasculitis in HSP principally involves the small vessels of the skin, gastrointestinal tract, and kidneys, with deposition of IgA immune complexes. The most common and earliest symptom is palpable purpura, which results from extravasation of erythrocytes into the tissue surrounding the involved venules. Antigens from group A β-hemolytic streptococci and other bacteria, viruses, drugs, foods, and insect bites have been proposed as inciting agents.

▶ Clinical Findings

A. Symptoms and Signs

Skin involvement may be urticarial initially, progresses to a maculopapules, and coalesces to a symmetrical, palpable purpuric rash distributed on the legs, buttocks, and elbows. New lesions may continue to appear for 2–4 weeks, and may extend to involve the entire body. Two thirds of patients develop migratory polyarthralgias or polyarthritis, primarily of the ankles and knees. Intermittent, sharp abdominal pain occurs in approximately 50% of patients, and hemorrhage and edema of the small intestine can often be demonstrated. Intussusception may develop. From 25–50% of those affected develop renal involvement in the second or third week of illness with either a nephritic or, less commonly, nephrotic picture. Hypertension may accompany the renal involvement. In males, testicular torsion may also occur, and neurologic symptoms are possible due to small vessel vasculitis.

B. Laboratory Findings

The platelet count is normal or elevated, and other screening tests of hemostasis and platelet function are typically normal. Urinalysis frequently reveals hematuria, and sometimes proteinuria. Stool may be positive for occult blood. The anti-streptolysin O (ASO) titer is often elevated and the throat culture positive for group A β-hemolytic streptococci. Serum IgA may be elevated.

▷ Differential Diagnosis

The rash of septicemia (especially meningococcemia) may be similar to skin involvement in HSP, although the distribution tends to be more generalized. The possibility of trauma should be considered in any child presenting with purpura. Other vasculitides should also be considered. The lesions of thrombotic thrombocytopenic purpura are not palpable.

▷ Treatment

Generally, treatment is supportive. NSAIDs may be useful for the arthritis. Corticosteroid therapy may provide symptomatic relief for severe gastrointestinal or joint manifestations but does not alter skin or renal manifestations. If culture for group A β-hemolytic streptococci is positive or if the ASO titer is elevated, a therapeutic course of penicillin is warranted.

▷ Prognosis

The prognosis for recovery is generally good, although symptoms frequently (25–50%) recur over a period of several months. In patients who develop renal manifestations, microscopic hematuria may persist for years. Progressive renal failure occurs in less than 5% of patients with HSP, with an overall fatality rate of 3%.

Ronkainen J: Early prednisone therapy in Henoch-Schönlein purpura: A randomized, double-blind, placebo-controlled trial. J Pediatr 2006;149:241 [PMID: 16887443].

2. Collagen Disorders

Mild to life-threatening bleeding occurs with some types of Ehlers-Danlos syndrome, the most common inherited collagen disorder. Ehlers-Danlos syndrome is characterized by joint hypermobility, skin extensibility, and easy bruising. Coagulation abnormalities may sometimes be present, including platelet dysfunction and deficiencies of coagulation factors VIII, IX, XI, and XIII. However, bleeding and easy bruising, in most instances, relates to fragility of capillaries and compro-

mised vascular integrity. Individuals with Ehlers-Danlos syndrome types 4 and 6 are at risk for aortic dissection and spontaneous rupture of aortic aneurysms. Surgery should be avoided for patients with Ehlers-Danlos syndrome, as should medications that induce platelet dysfunction.

De Paepe A: Bleeding and bruising in patients with Ehlers-Danlos syndrome and other collagen vascular disorders. Br J Haematol 2004;127:491 [PMID: 15566352].

▼ THROMBOTIC DISORDERS

▷ General Considerations

Although uncommon in children, thrombotic disorders are being recognized with increasing frequency, particularly with heightened physician awareness and improved survival in pediatric intensive care settings. Several clinical conditions have a potential association with thrombotic events in childhood (see Clinical Risk Factors, below).

▷ Clinical Findings

Initial evaluation of the child who has thrombosis includes an assessment for potential triggering factors, as well as a family history of thrombosis and early cardiovascular or cerebrovascular disease.

A. Clinical Risk Factors

Clinical risk factors are present in more than 90% of children with acute venous thromboembolic events (VTEs). These conditions include the presence of an indwelling vascular catheter, cardiac disease, malignancy, infection, trauma, surgery, immobilization, collagen-vascular or chronic inflammatory disease, renal disease, and sickle cell anemia.

1. Inherited thrombophilia (hypercoagulability) states

A. PROTEIN C DEFICIENCY—Protein C is a vitamin K–dependent protein that is normally activated by thrombin bound to thrombomodulin and inactivates activated factors V and VIII. In addition, activated protein C promotes fibrinolysis. Two phenotypes of hereditary protein C deficiency exist. Heterozygous individuals with autosomal dominant protein C deficiency often present with VTEs as young adults, but the disorder may manifest during childhood or in later adulthood. In the absence of VTEs, prophylaxis is limited to periods of increased prothrombotic risk. Homozygous or compound heterozygous protein C deficiency is rare but phenotypically severe. Affected children generally present within the first 12 hours of life with purpura fulminans and/or VTEs. Retinal thrombosis may result in blindness. Prompt protein C replacement by infusion of FFP every 6–12 hours, or of protein C concentrate (if available), along with therapeutic heparin administration is recommended. Subsequent management requires chronic anticoagulation with warfarin or protein C concentrate. Recurrent VTEs are common, especially during periods of subtherapeutic anticoagulation or in the presence of conditions associated with increased prothrombotic risk.

B. Protein S deficiency—Protein S is a cofactor for protein C. Neonates with homozygous protein S deficiency have a course similar to those with homozygous or compound heterozygous protein C deficiency. Lifelong warfarin therapy is indicated in severe deficiency, or in heterozygous individuals who have experienced recurrent VTEs. Efforts must be made to distinguish from these conditions from acquired deficiency.

C. Antithrombin III (ATIII) deficiency—ATIII is the most important physiologic inhibitor of thrombin and inhibits activated factors IX, X, XI, and XII. ATIII deficiency is transmitted in an autosomal dominant pattern and is associated with VTEs, typically with onset in adolescence or young adulthood. Therapy for acute VTEs involves replacement with antithrombin concentrate (if available) and therapeutic anticoagulation. The efficiency of heparin may be significantly diminished in the setting of severe ATIII deficiency and anticoagulation with warfarin required. Patients with recurrent VTEs are maintained on lifelong warfarin.

D. Factor V Leiden mutation—An amino acid substitution in the gene coding for factor V results in factor V Leiden, a factor V polymorphism that is resistant to inactivation by activated protein C. The most common cause of activated protein C resistance in Caucasians, factor V Leiden is present in approximately 5% of the Caucasian population, 20% of Caucasian adults with deep vein thrombosis, and 40–60% of those with a family history of VTEs. VTEs occur in both heterozygous and homozygous individuals. In the former case, thrombosis is typically triggered by a clinical risk factor (or else develops in association with additional thrombophilia traits), whereas in the latter case, it is often spontaneous. Population studies suggest that the risk of VTEs is increased 7-fold in the setting of heterozygous factor V Leiden, 35-fold among heterozygous individuals taking the oral contraceptives, and 80-fold in those homozygous for factor V Leiden.

E. Prothrombin mutation—The 20210 glutamine to alanine mutation in the prothrombin gene is a relatively common polymorphism in Caucasians that enhances its activation to thrombin. In heterozygous form, prothrombin 20210 has been associated with a threefold increased risk for VTE.

F. Other inherited disorders—Qualitative abnormalities of fibrinogen (dysfibrinogenemias) are usually inherited in an autosomal dominant manner. Most individuals with dysfibrinogenemia are asymptomatic. Some patients experience bleeding, while others develop venous or arterial thrombosis. The diagnosis is suggested by a prolonged thrombin time with a normal fibrinogen concentration. Hyperhomocysteinemia can be an inherited or an acquired condition and is associated with an increased risk for both arterial and venous thromboses. In children, it may also serve as a risk factor for ischemic arterial stroke. However, hyperhomocysteinemia is quite uncommon in the setting of dietary folate supplementation (as in the United States), and is observed almost uniquely in cases of metabolic disease (eg, homocystinuria). Furthermore, methylene tetrahydrofolate reductase receptor mutations do not appear to constitute a risk factor for thrombosis in U.S. children when homocysteine is not elevated.

Lipoprotein(a) is a lipoprotein with homology to plasminogen. In-vitro studies suggest that lipoprotein(a) may both promote atherothrombosis and inhibit fibrinolysis. Case-control studies suggest that elevated plasma concentrations of lipoprotein(a) are associated with an increased odds of VTEs and ischemic arterial stroke in children.

Increased factor VIII may be demonstrated in patients with acute VTEs. This increase has been implicated as a risk factor for VTEs in adults and may be familial.

2. Acquired disorders

A. Antiphospholipid antibodies—The development of antiphospholipid antibodies is the most common form of acquired thrombophilia in children. Antiphospholipid antibodies, which include the lupus anticoagulant, anticardiolipin antibodies, and β_2-glycoprotein-1 antibodies, have become increasingly implicated in VTEs. The lupus anticoagulant is demonstrated in vitro by its inhibition of phospholipid-dependent coagulation assays (eg, aPTT and dilute Russell viper venom time), whereas immunologic techniques (eg, enzyme-linked immunosorbent assays) are often used to detect anticardiolipin and β_2-glycoprotein-1 antibodies. Although common in persons with autoimmune diseases such as systemic lupus erythematosus, antiphospholipid antibodies may also develop following certain drug exposures, infection, acute inflammation, and lymphoproliferative diseases. Sometimes VTEs and antiphospholipid antibodies may predate other signs of lupus for long periods of time. Viral illness is a common precipitant in children, and in many cases, the inciting infection may be asymptomatic.

If an antiphospholipid antibody persists for 6–12 weeks following the acute thrombotic event, the diagnosis of this syndrome is confirmed and anticoagulation should be continued at least until the antiphospholipid antibody becomes undetectable. In addition, consideration should be given to long-term anticoagulation.

B. Deficiencies of intrinsic anticoagulants—Acquired deficiencies of proteins C and S and ATIII may occur in the clinical context of excessive consumption, including sepsis, DIC, major-vessel or extensive VTE, and post–bone marrow transplant sinusoidal obstruction syndrome (formerly termed hepatic veno-occlusive disease). Pilot studies in children have suggested a possible therapeutic role for antithrombin or protein C concentrates in sepsis associated DIC and severe post-transplant sinusoidal obstruction syndrome.

C. Acute phase reactants—As part of the acute phase response, elevations in plasma fibrinogen concentration, plasma factor VIII, and platelet count may occur, all of which may contribute to an acquired prothrombotic state.

Reactive thrombocytosis is rarely associated with VTEs in children when the platelet count is less than 1 million/μL.

B. Symptoms and Signs

Presenting features of thrombosis vary with the anatomic site, extent of vascular involvement, degree of vaso-occlusion, and presence of end-organ dysfunction. The classic presentation of deep venous thrombosis of an upper or lower extremity is painful acute or subacute extremity swelling, while that for pulmonary embolism commonly involves dyspnea and pleuritic chest pain, and in cerebral sinovenous thrombosis often includes severe or persistent headache, with or without neurologic deficit. Arterial thrombosis of the lower extremity (eg, neonatal umbilical artery catheter–associated), as well as vasospasm without identified thrombosis, often manifests with diminished distal pulses and dusky discoloration of the limb.

C. Laboratory Findings

A comprehensive laboratory investigation for thrombophilia (ie, hypercoagulability) is recommended by the International Society on Thrombosis and Haemostasis in order to disclose possible underlying congenital or acquired abnormalities that may affect acute or long-term management. Testing for intrinsic anticoagulant deficiencies (proteins C and S and ATIII), procoagulant factor excesses or activators (eg, factor VIII and antiphospholipid antibodies), genetic mutations mediating enhanced procoagulant activity or reduced sensitivity to inactivation (factor V Leiden and prothrombin 20210 polymorphisms), biochemical mediators of endothelial damage (homocysteine and antiphospholipid antibodies), and markers or regulators of fibrinolysis (eg, D-dimer, plasminogen activator inhibitor-1, and lipoprotein[a]) should be completed. Interpretation of procoagulant factor and intrinsic anticoagulant levels should take into account the age dependence of normal values for these proteins. Among these VTE risk factors, antiphospholipid antibodies and elevated levels of homocysteine and lipoprotein(a) have also been well-demonstrated as risk factors for arterial thrombotic and ischemic events.

D. Imaging

Appropriate radiologic imaging is essential to objectively document the thrombus and to delineate the type (venous versus arterial), possible vaso-occlusion, and extent of thrombosis.

▶ Treatment

Current guidelines for the treatment of first-episode VTE in children have been largely based on adult experience and include therapeutic anticoagulation for at least 3 months. During the period of anticoagulation, bleeding precautions should be followed, as previously described (see treatment of Idiopathic Thrombocytopenic Purpura, earlier).

Initial therapy employs continuous intravenous unfractionated heparin or subcutaneous injections of low molecular weight heparin (LMWH) for at least 7 days, monitored by anti-Xa activity level to maintain anticoagulant levels of 0.3–0.7 or 0.5–1.0 IU/mL, respectively. Subsequent extended anticoagulant therapy is given with LMWH or daily oral warfarin, the latter agent monitored by the PT to maintain an international normalized ratio (INR) of 2.0–3.0 (2.5–3.5 in the presence of an antiphospholipid antibody). During warfarin treatment, the INR should be within the therapeutic range for two consecutive days before discontinuation of heparin. Warfarin pharmacokinetics are affected by acute illness, numerous medications, and changes in diet, and require frequent monitoring. LMWH offers the advantage of infrequent need for monitoring but is far more expensive than warfarin. In cases of limb- or life-threatening VTEs, including major proximal pulmonary embolus, and in cases of progressive VTE despite therapeutic anticoagulation, thrombolytic therapy (eg, tissue-type plasminogen activator) is often warranted. A recent cohort study has indicated that initial thrombolytic therapy may also reduce the risk of the post-thrombotic syndrome (PTS) in children with veno-occlusive deep venous thrombosis of the proximal lower extremities in whom adverse prognostic biomarkers (ie, elevated factor VIII and D-dimer levels) are present at diagnosis; however, the safety and efficacy of this approach must be evaluated in a subsequent clinical trial.

▶ Prognosis

Registries and cohort studies have suggested that recurrent VTE occurs in approximately 10% of children within 2 years. Persistent thrombosis is evident following completion of a standard therapeutic course of anticoagulation in up to 30% of children, with unclear clinical importance. At least 30% of children with deep venous thrombosis involving the extremities develop PTS, a condition of venous insufficiency of varying severity characterized by chronic skin changes, edema, and dilated collateral superficial venous formation, and often accompanied by functional limitation (pain with activities or at rest). The presence of homozygous anticoagulant deficiencies, multiple thrombophilia traits, or persistent antiphospholipid antibodies following VTE diagnosis has been associated with increased risk of recurrent VTE, leading to recommendation for extended anticoagulation in these instances. Recent evidence suggests that elevated plasma levels of factor VIII and D-dimer may be predictive of long-term post-thrombotic outcomes in children, including recurrent VTE, persistent thrombosis, and the development of PTS.

Goldenberg NA: Long-term outcomes of venous thrombosis in children. Curr Opin Hematol 2005;12:370 [PMID: 16093782].
Goldenberg NA: A thrombolytic regimen for high-risk deep venous thrombosis may substantially reduce the risk of postthrombotic syndrome in children. Blood 2007;110:45 [PMID: 17360940].

Table 28–9. Causes of chronic splenomegaly in children.

Cause	Associated Clinical Findings	Diagnostic Investigation
Congestive splenomegaly	History of umbilical vein catheter or neonatal omphalitis; signs of portal hypertension (varices, hemorrhoids, dilated abdominal wall veins); pancytopenia; history of hepatitis or jaundice	Complete blood count, platelet count, liver function tests, ultrasonography
Chronic infections	History of exposure to tuberculosis, histoplasmosis, coccidiomycosis, other fungal disease; chronic sepsis (foreign body in bloodstream; subacute infective endocarditis)	Appropriate cultures and skin tests, ie, blood cultures; PPD, fungal serology and antigen tests, chest film; HIV serology
Infectious mononucleosis	Fever, fatigue, pharyngitis, rash, adenopathy, hepatomegaly	EBV antibody titers
Leukemia, lymphoma, Hodgkin disease	Evidence of systemic involvement with fever, bleeding tendencies, hepatomegaly, and lymphadenopathy; pancytopenia	Blood smear, bone marrow examination, chest film, gallium scan, LDH, uric acid
Hemolytic anemia	Anemia, jaundice; family history of anemia, jaundice, and gallbladder disease in young adults	Reticulocyte count, Coombs test, blood smear, osmotic fragility test, hemoglobin electrophoresis
Reticuloendothelioses (histiocytosis X)	Chronic otitis media, seborrheic or petechial skin rashes, anemia, infections, lymphadenopathy, hepatomegaly, bone lesions	Skeletal radiographs for bone lesions; biopsy of bone, liver, bone marrow, or lymph node
Storages diseases	Family history of similar disorders, neurologic involvement, evidence of macular degeneration, hepatomegaly	Biopsy of liver or bone marrow in search for storage cells
Splenic cyst	Evidence of other infections (postinfectious cyst) or congenital anomalies; peculiar shape of spleen	Radionuclide scan, ultrasonography
Splenic hemangioma	Other hemangiomas, consumptive coagulopathy	Radionuclide scan, arteriography, platelet count, coagulation screen

EBV, Epstein-Barr virus; HIV, human immunodeficiency virus; LDH, lactic dehydrogenase; PPD, purified protein derivative.

Monagle P: Antithrombotic therapy in children: The Seventh ACCP Conference on Antithrombotic and Thrombolytic Therapy. Chest 2004;126(Suppl):645S [PMID: 15383489].

▼ SPLENIC ABNORMALITIES

SPLENOMEGALY & HYPERSPLENISM

The differential diagnosis of splenomegaly includes the general categories of congestive splenomegaly, chronic infections, leukemia and lymphomas, hemolytic anemias, reticuloendothelioses, and storage diseases (Table 28–9).

Splenomegaly due to any cause may be associated with hypersplenism and the excessive destruction of circulating red cells, white cells, and platelets. The degree of cytopenia is variable and, when mild, requires no specific therapy. In other cases, the thrombocytopenia may cause life-threatening bleeding, particularly when the splenomegaly is secondary to portal hypertension and associated with esophageal varices or the consequence of a storage disease. In such cases, treatment with surgical splenectomy or with splenic embolization may be warranted. Although more commonly associated with acute enlargement, rupture of an enlarged spleen can be seen in more chronic conditions such as Gaucher disease.

Stone DL: Life threatening splenic hemorrhage in two patients with Gaucher's disease. Am J Hematol 2000;64:140 [PMID: 10814997].

ASPLENIA & SPLENECTOMY

Children who lack normal splenic function are at risk for sepsis, meningitis, and pneumonia due to encapsulated bacteria such as pneumococci and *H influenzae*. Such infections are often fulminant and fatal because of inadequate antibody production and impaired phagocytosis of circulating bacteria.

Congenital asplenia is usually suspected when an infant is born with abnormalities of abdominal viscera and complex cyanotic congenital heart disease. Howell-Jolly bodies are usually present on the peripheral blood smear, and the absence of splenic tissue is confirmed by technetium radionuclide scanning. The prognosis depends on the underlying cardiac lesions, and many children die during the first few months. Prophylactic antibiotics, usually penicillin, and pneumococcal conjugate and polysaccharide vaccines are recommended.

The risk of overwhelming sepsis following surgical splenectomy is related to the child's age and to the underlying disorder. Because the risk is highest when the procedure is performed earlier in life, splenectomy is usually postponed until after age 5 years. The risk of postsplenectomy sepsis is also greater in children with malignancies, thalassemias, and reticuloendothelioses than in children whose splenectomy is performed for ITP, hereditary spherocytosis, or trauma. Prior to splenectomy, children should be immunized against *Streptococcus pneumoniae*, *H influenzae*, and *Neisseria meningitidis*. Additional management should include penicillin prophylaxis and prompt evaluation for fever 38.8°C or above or signs of severe infection.

Children with sickle cell anemia develop functional asplenia during the first year of life, and overwhelming sepsis is the leading cause of early deaths in this disease. Prophylactic penicillin reduces the incidence of sepsis by 84%.

Pickering L: American Academy of Pediatrics: Immunization in special circumstances. Red Book 2000;25:66.

TRANSFUSION MEDICINE

DONOR SCREENING & BLOOD PROCESSING: RISK MANAGEMENT

Minimizing the risks of transfusion begins by asking the donor questions that will protect the recipient from transmission of infectious agents as well as other risks of transfu-sions. In addition, information defining high-risk groups whose behavior increases the possible transmission of HIV, hepatitis, and other diseases is provided, with the request that persons in these groups not donate blood.

Before blood components can be released for transfusion, donor blood is screened for hepatitis B surface antigen; antibodies to hepatitis B, hepatitis C, HIV-1 and HIV-2, and human T-cell lymphotropic virus (HTLV) I and II; and a serologic test for syphilis (Table 28–10). Screening donor blood for viral genome (nucleic acid amplification [NAT] testing) was mandated for HIV, HCV, and West Nile virus. NAT testing for other viruses may be added in the future, and screening for Chagas disease was accepted in 2007. Positive tests are repeated.

Upon their confirmation, the unit in question is destroyed and the donor is notified and deferred from future dona-tions. Many of the screening tests used are very sensitive and have a high rate of false-positive results. As a result, confir-matory tests have been developed to check the initial screen-

Table 28–10. Transmission risks of infectious agents for which screening of blood products is routinely performed.

Disease Entity	Transmission	Screening and Processing Procedures	Approximate Risk of Transmission
Syphilis	Low risk: fresh blood drawn during spirochetemia can transmit infection. Organism not able to survive beyond 72 h during storage at 4°C.	Donor history. RPR or VDRL.	< 1:100,000
Hepatitis A	Units drawn during prodrome could transmit virus. Because of brief viremia during acute phase, absence of asymptomatic carrier phase, and fail-ure to detect transmission in multiple transfused individuals, infection by this agent is unlikely.	Donor history.	1:1,000,000
Hepatitis B	Prolonged viremia during various phases of the disease and asymptomatic carrier state make HBV infection a significant risk of transfusion. Incidence has markedly decreased with screen-ing strategies.	Donor history, education, and self-exclusion. Hepatitis B surface antigen (HBsAg). Surrogate tests for non-A, non-B hepatitis and screen for hepatitis C and retroviruses have helped screen out population at risk for transmitting HBV.	1:500,000– 1:200,000
Hepatitis C	Over two thirds of cases of non-A, non-B post-transfusion hepatitis may be due to this agent. Virus has characteristics similar to those of HBV which are responsible for risk from transfusion.	Donor history. Surrogate tests: hepatitis B core antibody (anti-HBc), anti-HCV. Nucleic acid testing for viral genome required.	1:2,000,000
Non-A, non-B, non-C hepatitis	Agents other than HAV, HBV, HCV, Epstein-Barr virus, and cytomegalovirus, which can cause post-transfusion hepatitis.	Donor history. Surrogate tests: anti-HBc.	Undefined.
Human immunodefi-ciency virus (HIV-1, HIV-2) infection	Retroviruses spread by sexual contact, parenteral (including transfusion) and vertical routes.	Donor history, education, and self-exclusion. Anti-HIV by EIA screening test. Western blot confirmatory, p24 antigen testing. Nucleic acid testing for viral genome required.	1:2,000,000
Human T-cell lymphotro-pic virus I and II (HTLV-I and II) infection	Retroviruses spread by sexual contact, parenteral (including transfusion) and vertical modes.	Donor history. Anti-HTLI-I and II by enzyme immunoassay screening test. Western blot confirmatory.	1:600,000

AIDS, acquired immunodeficiency syndrome; EIA, enzyme-linked immunosorbent assay; HAV, HBV, HCV, hepatitis A virus, hepatitis B virus, hepatitis C virus; HTLV, human T-cell lymphotropic virus; RPR, rapid plasma reagin; VDRL, syphilis test.

ing results and separate the false-positives from the true-positives. Recently, bacterial culture of platelet concentrates was added to the testing paradigm.

With these approaches, the risk of an infectious complication from blood components has been minimized (see Table 28–10), with the greatest risk being post-transfusion hepatitis (see sections on hepatitis C virus and non-A, non-B, non-C hepatitis in Chapter 21). Autologous donation is recognized by some centers as a safe alternative to homologous blood. Issues of donor size make the techniques of autologous donation difficult to apply to the pediatric population.

Primary CMV infections are significant complications of blood transfusion in transplant recipients, neonates, and immunodeficient individuals. Transmission of CMV can be avoided by using seronegative donors, apheresis platelet concentrates collected by techniques ensuring low numbers of residual white cells, or red cell or platelet products leukocyte-depleted by filtering (< 5 million white blood cells per packed red cell unit or apheresis platelet concentrate equivalent).

STORAGE & PRESERVATION OF BLOOD & BLOOD COMPONENTS

Whole blood is routinely fractionated into packed red cells, platelets, and FFP or cryoprecipitate for most efficient use of all blood components. The storage conditions and biologic characteristics of the fractions are summarized in Table 28–11. The conditions provide the optimal environment to maintain appropriate recovery, survival, and function and are different for each blood component. For example, red cells undergo dramatic metabolic changes during their 35–42-day storage, with a decrease in 2,3-diphosphoglycerate (DPG) by day 14 of storage, a decrease in adenosine triphosphate, and a gradual loss of intracellular potassium. Fortunately, these changes are reversed readily within hours to days after the red cells are transfused. However, in certain clinical conditions, these effects may define the type of components used. For example, blood less than 7–10 days old would be preferred for exchange transfusion in neonates or replacement of red cells in persons with severe cardiopulmonary disease to ensure adequate oxygen-carrying capacity. Storage time is not an issue when administering transfusions to those with chronic anemia.

If extracellular potassium in older packed red cells may present a problem, one may use blood less than 10 days old, making packed cells out of an older unit of whole blood, or washing blood stored as packed cells. Regardless of the blood's age, over 70% of the red cells will circulate after transfusion and approximate normal survival in the circulation.

Platelets are stored at 22°C for a maximum of 5 days; criteria for 7-day storage are being developed. At the extremes of storage, there should be at least a 60% recovery, a survival time that approximates turnover of fresh autologous platelets, and normalization of the bleeding time or PFA-100 in proportion to the peak platelet count. Frozen components, red cells, FFP, and cryoprecipitate are outdated at 10 years, 1 year, and 1 year, respectively. Frozen red cells retain the same biochemical and functional characteristics as the day they were frozen. FFP contains 80% or more of all of the clotting factors of fresh plasma. Factors VIII and XIII and fibrinogen are concentrated in cryoprecipitate.

PRETRANSFUSION TESTING

Both the donated blood and the recipient are tested for ABO and Rh(D) antigens and for auto- or alloantibodies in the plasma. The cross-match is required on any component that contains red cells. In the major cross-match, washed donor red cells are incubated with the serum from the patient, and agglutination is detected and graded. The antiglobulin phase of the test is then performed; Coombs reagent, which will detect the presence of IgG or complement on the surface of the red cells, is added to the mixture, and agglutination is evaluated. In the presence of a negative antibody screen in the recipient, a negative immediate spin cross-match test confirms the compatibility of the blood and antiglobulin phase is not required. Further testing is required if the antibody screen or the cross-match is positive, and blood should not be given until the nature of the reactivity is delineated. An incompatible cross-match is evaluated first with a DAT or Coombs test to detect IgG or complement on the surfaces of the recipient's red cells. The indirect antiglobulin test is also used to determine the presence of antibodies that will coat or activate complement, and additional studies are completed to define the antibody.

TRANSFUSION PRACTICE

General Rules

Several rules should be observed in administering any blood component:

1. In final preparation of the component, no solutions should be added to the bag or tubing set except for normal saline (0.9% sodium chloride for injection, USP), ABO-compatible plasma, or other specifically approved expanders. Hypotonic solutions cause hemolysis of red cells, and, if these are transfused, a severe reaction will occur. Any reconstitution should be completed by the blood bank.

2. Transfusion products should be protected from contact with any calcium-containing solution (eg, lactated Ringer); recalcification and reversal of the citrate effect will cause clotting of the blood component.

3. Blood components should not be warmed to a temperature greater than 37°C. If a component is incubated in a water bath, it should be enclosed in a watertight bag to prevent bacterial contamination of entry ports.

4. Whenever a blood bag is entered, the sterile integrity of the system is violated, and that unit should be discarded within 4 hours if left at room temperature or within 24 hours if the temperature is 4–6°C.

Table 28-11. Characteristics of blood and blood components.

Component	Storage Conditions	Composition and Transfusion Characteristics	Indications	Risks and Precautions	Administration
Whole blood	4°c for 35 days. RBC characteristics: • *Survival:* recovery decreases during storage, but is always > 70%. Cells that circulate approximate normal survival. • *Function:* 2,3-DPG levels fall to undetectable after second week of storage. This defect is repaired within 24 h of transfusion. • *Electrolytes:* with storage, potassium increases in plasma. This rises to high levels after 2 wk of storage.	Contains RBCs and many plasma compounds of whole blood. Leukocytes and platelets lose activity or viability after a few days under these conditions. Procoagulant clotting factors (particularly VIII and V) deteriorate rapidly during storage. Each unit has about 500 mL volume and Hct 36-40%.	Oxygen carrying capacity (anemia). Volume replacement for blood loss (> 15-20%) or severe shock.	Must be ABO-identical and cross-match-compatible. Infections. Febrile or hemolytic transfusion reactions. Alloimmunization to red cell, white cell, or platelet antigens.	During acute blood loss, as rapidly as tolerated. In other settings, 2-4 h. 10 mL/kg will raise Hct by 5% and support volume.
Packed red cells	Same as for whole blood. Special rejuvenating solutions allow storage for 42 d.	Contains RBCs; most plasma removed in preparation. Status of leukocytes, clotting factors, and platelets same as for whole blood. Hct about 70%, volume 200-250 mL. May request tighter pack to give Hct 80-90%.	Oxygen carrying capacity. Acute trauma or bleeding or situations requiring intensive cardiopulmonary support (Hct < 25-30%). Chronic anemia (Hct < 20%).	Same as for whole blood.	May be given as patient will tolerate, based on cardiovascular status over 2-4 h. Dose of 3 mL packed RBC/kg will raise Hct by 3%. If cardiovascular status is stable, give 10 mL/kg over 2-4 h. If unstable, use smaller volume or do packed RBC exchange.
Washed or filtered red cells	When cells are washed, there is a 24-h outdate. Up to that time, they have the same characteristics as for packed red cells.	Same as for packed red cells.	Same as for packed red cells. Depending on technique used and extent of reduction of white blood cells, washed red cells may achieve the following: • Avoid febrile reactions • Decrease transmission of CMV. • Decrease incidence of alloimmunization to white cell antigens.	Same as whole blood. Removal of white cells diminishes the risk of febrile reactions. Filtration with high-efficiency white cell filters may decrease rate of alloimmunization to white cell antigens and transmission of CMV.	Same as for packed red cells.
Frozen red cells	Packed red cells frozen in 40% glycerol solution at less than −65°C. After storage for 10 y, cells retain the same biochemical characteristics, function, and capacity for survival as on the day they were frozen; when thawed, 24-h outdate.	Same as for packed red cells.	Same as packed red cells. Useful for avoiding febrile reactions, decreasing transmission of CMV, autologous blood donation, and developing an inventory of rare red cell blood groups.	Same as for whole blood. Risk of CMV transmission is at same level as using seronegative components.	Same as for packed red cells.

Fresh frozen plasma	Plasma from whole blood stored at less than –18°C for up to 1 y.	Contains > 80% of all procoagulant and anticoagulant plasma proteins.	Replacement of plasma procoagulant and anticoagulant plasma proteins. May provide "other" factors, eg, treatment of TTP.	Need not be crossmatched; should be type-compatible. Volume overload, infectious diseases, allergic reactions. Solvent detergent-treated plasma or donor-retested plasma units have decreased risk for viral transmission.	As rapidly as tolerated by patient, but not > 4 h. Dose: 10–15 mL/kg will increase level of all clotting factors by 10–20%.
Cryoprecipitate	Produced by freezing fresh plasma to less than –65°C, then allowed to thaw 18 h at 4°C. After centrifugation, cryoprecipitate proteins are separated. May be stored at less than –18°C for up to 1 y.	Contains factor VIII, fibrinogen, and fibronectin at concentrations greater than those of plasma. Also contains factor XIII, VIII > 80 IU/pack, fibrinogen 100–350 mg/pack.	Treatment of acquired or congenital deficiencies of fibrinogen. Useful in making biologic glues that contain fibrinogen. Commercial clotting factor concentrates are the treatment of choice for factor VIII deficiency and von Willebrand disease because sterilization procedures further reduce the risk of viral transmission.	Same as for fresh frozen plasma. ABO agglutinogens may also be concentrated and can give positive direct agglutination test if not type-specific.	Cryoprecipitate can be given as a rapid infusion. Dose: $1/2$ pack/kg body weight will increase factor VIII level by 80–100% and fibrinogen by 200–250 mg/dL.
Platelet concentrates from whole blood donation	Separated from platelet-rich plasma and stored with gentle agitation at 22°C for 3–5 d. Containers currently in use are plastic and allow for gas exchange, diffusion of CO_2 helps keep pH > 6, a major factor in keeping platelets viable and functional.	Each unit contains about 5×10^{10} platelets. *Survival:* Although there may be some loss with storage, 60–70% recovery should be achieved, with stored platelets able to correct platelet function test in proportion to the peak counts reached.	Treatment of thrombocytopenia or platelet function defects.	No cross-match necessary. Should be ABO type-specific. Other risks as for whole blood.	Can be taken during rapid transfusion or as defined by cardiovascular status, not more than 4 h. Dose: 10 mL/kg should increase platelet count by at least 50,000/μL.
Platelet concentrates by apheresis techniques	Same as random donor units.	Platelet content is equivalent to 6–10 units of random donor concentrates. Depending on technique used, these may be relatively free of leukocytes, which is important for avoiding alloimmunization.	As above, particularly useful in treating patients who have insufficient production and also may have a problem with alloisoimmunization.	Same as above.	As above.
Granulocytes	Although they may be stored stationary at 20–24°C, transfuse as soon as possible after collection.	Contains at least 1×10^{10} granulocytes, but also platelets and red cells. When donors given 10 mcg/kg G-CSF subcutaneously and 8 mg Decadron orally 12–15 h before collection, yield increases to > 5×10^{10} granulocytes.	Severely neutropenic individuals (< 500/μL) with poor marrow reserves and suspected bacterial or fungal infections not responding to 48–72 h of parenteral antibiotics. Also in patients with neutrophil dysfunction.	Same as for platelets. Pulmonary leukostasis reactions. Severe febrile reactions.	Given in an infusion over 2–4 h. Dose: 1 unit daily for newborns and infants, 1×10^{9} granulocytes per kg.

CMV, cytomegalovirus; DPG, diphosphoglycerate; G-CSF, granulocyte colony-stimulating factor; Hct, hematocrit; RBC, red blood cell.

5. Transfusions of products containing red cells should not exceed 4 hours. Blood components in excess of what can be infused during this time period should be stored in the blood bank until needed.

6. Before transfusion, the blood component should be inspected visually for any unusual characteristics, such as the presence of flocculent material, hemolysis, or clumping of cells, and mixed thoroughly.

7. The unit and the recipient should be identified properly.

8. The administration set includes a standard 170–260 micron filter. Under certain clinical circumstances, an additional microaggregate filter may be used to eliminate small aggregates of fibrin, white cells, and platelets that will not be removed by the standard filter.

9. The patient should be observed during the entire transfusion and especially during the first 15 minutes. Any adverse symptoms or signs should be evaluated immediately and reactions to the transfusion reported promptly to the transfusion service.

10. When cross-match–incompatible red cells or whole blood unit(s) must be given to the patient (as with autoimmune hemolytic anemia), a test dose of 10% of the total volume (not to exceed 50 mL) should be administered over 15–20 minutes; the transfusion is then stopped and the patient observed. If no adverse effects are noted, the remainder of the volume can be infused carefully.

11. Blood for exchange transfusion in the newborn period may be cross-matched with either the infant's or the mother's serum. If the exchange is for hemolysis, 500 mL of whole blood stored for less than 7 days will be adequate. If replacement of clotting factors is a key issue, packed red cells (7 days old) reconstituted with FFP may be considered. Based on post-transfusion platelet counts, platelet transfusion may be considered. Other problems to be anticipated are acid-base derangements, hyponatremia, hyperkalemia, hypocalcemia, hypoglycemia, hypothermia, and hypervolemia or hypovolemia.

Choice of Blood Component

Several principles should be considered when deciding on the need for blood transfusion. Indications for blood or blood components must be well defined, and the patient's medical condition, not just the laboratory results, should be the basis for the decision. Specific deficiencies exhibited by the patient (eg, oxygen-carrying capacity, thrombocytopenia) should be treated with appropriate blood components and the use of whole blood minimized. Information about specific blood components is summarized in Table 28–11.

A. Whole Blood

Whole blood may be used in patients who require replacement of oxygen-carrying capacity and volume. More specifically, it should be considered when more than 15% of blood volume is lost. Doses vary depending on volume considerations (see Table 28–11). In acute situations, the transfusion may be completed rapidly to support blood volume.

B. Packed Red Cells

Packed red cells (which include leukocyte-poor, filtered, or frozen deglycerolized products) prepared from whole blood by centrifugal techniques are the appropriate choice for almost all patients with deficient oxygen-carrying capacity. Exact indications will be defined by the clinical setting, the severity of the anemia, the acuity of the condition, and any other factors affecting oxygen transport.

C. Platelets

The decision to transfuse platelets depends on the patient's clinical condition, the status of plasma phase coagulation, the platelet count, the cause of the thrombocytopenia, and the functional capacity of the patient's own platelets. In the face of decreased production and platelet counts less than 10,000–20,000/μL, the risk of severe, spontaneous bleeding is increased markedly, and—in the absence of antibody-mediated thrombocytopenia—transfusion should be considered. Under certain circumstances, especially with platelet dysfunction or treatment that inhibits the procoagulant system, transfusions at higher platelet counts may be necessary.

Transfused platelets are sequestered temporarily in the lungs and spleen before reaching their peak concentrations, 45–60 minutes after transfusion. A significant proportion of the transfused platelets never circulate but remain sequestered in the spleen. This phenomenon results in reduced recovery; only 60–70% of the transfused platelets are accounted for when peripheral platelet count increments are used as a measure of response.

In addition to cessation of bleeding, two variables indicate the effectiveness of platelet transfusions. The first is platelet recovery, as measured by the maximum number of platelets circulating in response to transfusion. The practical measure is the platelet count at 1 hour after transfusion. In the absence of immune or drastic nonimmune factors that markedly decrease platelet recovery, one would expect a 7000/μL increment for each random donor unit and a 40,000–70,000/μL increment for each single-donor apheresis unit in a large child or adolescent. For infants and small children, 10 mL/kg of platelets will increase the platelet count by at least 50,000/μL. The second variable is the survival of transfused platelets. Normally, if the recovery is great enough, transfused platelets will approach a normal half-life in the circulation. In the presence of increased platelet destruction, the life span may be shortened to a few days or a few hours. Frequent platelet transfusions may be required to maintain adequate hemostasis.

A particularly troublesome outcome in patients receiving long-term platelet transfusions is the development of a refractory state characterized by poor (< 30%) recovery or

Table 28-12. Adverse events following transfusions.

Event	Pathophysiology	Signs and Symptoms	Management
Acute hemolytic transfusion reaction	Preformed alloantibodies (most commonly to ABO) and occasionally autoantibodies cause rapid intravascular hemolysis of transfused cells with activation of clotting (DIC), activation of inflammatory mediators, and acute renal failure.	Fever, chills, nausea, chest pain, back pain, pain at transfusion site, hypotension, dyspnea, oliguria, hemoglobinuria.	The risk of this type of reaction overall is low (1:30,000), but the mortality rate is high (up to 40%). Stop the transfusion; maintain renal output with intravenous fluids and diuretics (furosemide or mannitol); treat DIC with heparin; and institute other appropriate supportive measures.
Delayed hemolytic transfusion reaction	Formation of alloantibodies after transfusion and resultant destruction of transfused red cells, usually by extravascular hemolysis.	Jaundice, anemia. A small percentage may develop chronic hemolysis.	Detection, definition, and documentation (for future transfusions). Supportive care. Risk, 1:2500.
Febrile reactions	Usually caused by leukoagglutinins in recipient, cytokines, or other biologically active compounds.	Fever. May also involve chills.	Supportive. Consider leukocyte-poor products for future. Risk per transfusion, 1:400-1:200.
Allergic reactions	Most causes not identified. In IgA-deficient individuals, reaction occurs as a result of antibodies to IgA.	Itching, hives, occasionally chills and fever. In severe reactions, may see signs of anaphylaxis: dyspnea, pulmonary edema.	Mild to moderate reactions: diphenhydramine. More severe reactions: epinephrine subcutaneously and steroids intravenously. Risk for mild to moderate allergic reactions, 1:1000. Severe anaphylactic reactions, 1:150,000.
Transfusion-related acute lung injury	Acute lung injury occurring within 6 h after transfusion. Two sets of factors interact to produce the syndrome. Patient factors: infection, surgery, cytokine therapy. Blood component factors: lipids, antibodies, cytokines. Two groups of factors interact during transfusion to result in lung injury indistinguishable from ARDS.	Tachypnea, dyspnea, hypoxia. Diffuse interstitial markings. Cardiac evaluation normal.	May consider younger products: packed red blood cells ≤ 2 weeks, platelets ≤ 3 days, washing components to prevent syndrome. Management: supportive care. Risk, 1:2000-1:3000 per transfusion. Current preventative procedures include avoiding donors at risk for alloimmunization: use of male-only FFP or white blood cell antibody-negative apheresis FFP or platelet products.
Dilutional coagulopathy	Massive blood loss and transfusion with replacement with fluids or blood components and deficient clotting factors.	Bleeding.	Replacement of clotting factors or platelets with appropriate blood components.
Bacterial contamination	Contamination of units results in growth of bacteria or production of clinically significant levels of endotoxin.	Chills, high fever, hypotension, other symptoms of sepsis or endotoxemia.	Stop transfusion; make aggressive attempts to identify organism; provide vigorous supportive medical care including antibiotics.
Graft-versus-host disease	Lymphocytes from donor transfused in an immunoincompetent host.	Syndrome can involve a variety of organs, usually skin, liver, gastrointestinal tract, and bone marrow.	Preventive management: irradiation (> 1500 cGy) of cellular blood components transfused to individuals with congenital or acquired immunodeficiency syndromes, intrauterine transfusion, very premature infants, and when donors are relatives of the recipient.
Iron overload	There is no physiologic mechanism to excrete excess iron. Target organs include liver, heart, and endocrine organs. In patients receiving red cell transfusions over long periods of time, there is an increase in iron burden.	Signs and symptoms of dysfunctional organs affected by the iron.	Chronic administration of iron chelator such as deferoxamine.

TFN:ARDS, adult respiratory distress syndrome; DIC, disseminated intravascular coagulation.

no response to platelet transfusion (as measured at 1 hour). Most (70–90%) of these refractory states result from the development of alloantibodies directed against HLA antigens on the platelet. Platelets have class I HLA antigens, and the antibodies are primarily against HLA A or B determinants. A smaller proportion of these alloantibodies (< 10%) may be directed against platelet-specific alloantigens. The most effective approach to prevent HLA sensitization is to use leukocyte-depleted components (< 5 million leukocytes per unit of packed red cells or per apheresis or 6–10 random donor unit concentrates). For the alloimmunized, refractory patient, the best approach is to provide HLA-matched platelets for transfusion. Reports have suggested that platelet cross-matching procedures using HLA-matched or unmatched donors may be helpful in identifying platelet concentrates most likely to provide an adequate response.

D. Fresh Frozen Plasma

The indication for FFP is replacement of plasma coagulation factors in clinical situations in which a deficiency of one or more clotting factors exists and associated bleeding manifestations are present. In some hereditary factor deficiencies, such as factor VIII deficiency or vWD, commercially prepared concentrates contain these factors in higher concentrations and, because of viral inactivation, impose less infectious risk and are more appropriate than plasma.

E. Cryoprecipitate

This component may be used for acquired or congenital disorders of hypofibrinogenemia or afibrinogenemia. Although cryoprecipitate is a rich source for factor VIII or vWF, commercial concentrates that contain these factors are more appropriate (see preceding section). The dose given depends on the protein to be replaced. Cryoprecipitate can be given in a rapid transfusion over 30–60 minutes.

F. Granulocytes

With better supportive care over the past 10 years, the need for granulocytes in neutropenic patients with severe bacterial infections has decreased. Indications still remain for severe bacterial or fungal infections unresponsive to vigorous medical therapy in either newborns or older children with bone marrow failure, or patients with neutrophil dysfunction. Newer mobilization schemes using G-CSF and steroids in donors result in granulocyte collections with at least 5×10^{10} neutrophils. This may provide a better product for patients requiring granulocyte support.

G. Apheresis Products and Procedures

Apheresis equipment allows one or more blood components to be collected from a donor while the rest are returned. Apheresis platelet concentrates, which have as many platelets as 6–10 units of platelet concentrates from whole blood donations, are one example; granulocytes are another. Apheresis techniques can also be used to collect hematopoietic stem cells that have been mobilized into the blood by cytokines (G-CSF or GM-CSF) given alone or after chemotherapy. These stem cells are used for allogeneic or autologous bone marrow transplantation. Blood cell separators can be used for the collection of single-source plasma or removal of a blood component that is causing disease. Examples include red cell exchange in sickle cell disease and plasmapheresis in Goodpasture syndrome or in Guillain-Barré syndrome.

Adverse Effects

The noninfectious complications of blood transfusions are outlined in Table 28–12. Most complications present a significant risk to the recipient.

Goodnough LT: Transfusion medicine. First of two parts—Blood transfusion. N Engl J Med 1999;340:438 [PMID: 9971869].

Goodnough LT: Transfusion medicine. Second of two parts—Blood conservation. N Engl J Med 1999;340:525 [PMID: 10021474].

Silliman CC: Transfusion-related acute lung injury. Blood 2005;105:2266 [PMID: 15572582].

Smith JW: Therapeutic apheresis: A summary of current indication categories endorsed by the AABB and the American Society for Apheresis. Transfusion 2003;43:820 [PMID: 12757535].

Stramer SL: Current risks of transfusion-transmitted agents: A review. Arch Pathol Lab Med 2007;131:702 [PMID: 17488155].

REFERENCES

Goodnight SH, Hathaway WE (editors): *Disorders of Hemostasis and Thrombosis: A Clinical Guide,* 2nd ed. McGraw-Hill, 2001.

Hillyer CD et al (editors): *Blood Banking and Transfusion Medicine, Basic Principles and Practice.* Churchill Livingstone, 2003.

Petz LD, Garratty G (editors): *Acquired Immune Hemolytic Anemias,* 2nd ed. Churchill Livingstone, 2004.

Vichinsky E et al (editors): Pediatric hematology/oncology, part I. Pediatr Clin North Am 2002.

Neoplastic Disease

Kelley Maloney, MD

Nicholas K. Foreman, MD

Roger H. Giller, MD

Brian S. Greffe, MD

Doug K. Graham, MD, PhD

Ralph R. Quinones, MD

Amy K. Keating, MD

Each year approximately 150 of every 1 million children younger than age 20 years are diagnosed with cancer. For children between the ages of 1 and 20 years, cancer is the fourth leading cause of death, behind unintentional injuries, homicides, and suicides. However, combined-modality therapy, including surgery, chemotherapy, and radiation therapy, has improved survival dramatically, such that the overall 5-year survival rate of pediatric malignancies is now greater than 75%. It is estimated that by the year 2020, 1 in 600 adults will be a survivor of childhood cancer.

Because pediatric malignancies are rare, cooperative clinical trials have become the mainstay of treatment planning and therapeutic advances. The Children's Oncology Group (COG), representing the amalgamation of four prior pediatric cooperative groups (Children's Cancer Group, Pediatric Oncology Group, Intergroup Rhabdomyosarcoma Study Group, and the National Wilms Tumor Study Group), offers current therapeutic protocols and strives to answer important treatment questions. A child or adolescent newly diagnosed with cancer should be enrolled in a cooperative clinical trial whenever possible. Because many protocols are associated with significant toxicities, morbidity, and potential mortality, treatment of children with cancer should be supervised by a pediatric oncologist familiar with the hazards of treatment, preferably at a multidisciplinary pediatric cancer center.

Advances in molecular genetics, cell biology, and tumor immunology have contributed and are crucial to the continued understanding of pediatric malignancies and their treatment. Continued research into the biology of tumors will lead to the identification of targeted therapy for specific tumor types with, it is hoped, fewer systemic effects.

Research in supportive care areas, such as prevention and management of infection, pain, and emesis, has improved the survival and quality of life for children undergoing cancer treatment. Long-term studies of childhood cancer survivors are yielding information that provides a rationale for modifying future treatment regimens to decrease morbidity. A guide for caring for childhood cancer survivors is now available to medical providers as well as families and details suggested examinations and late effects by type of chemotherapy received.

Cure Search. Children's Oncology Group. Available at: http://www.survivorshipguidelines.org.

Ries LAG et al: SEER Cancer Statistics Review, 1975–2000. Available at: http://seer.cancer.gov/csr/1975_2000.

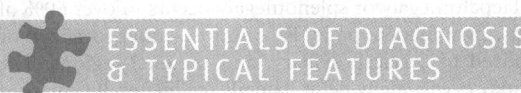

MAJOR PEDIATRIC NEOPLASTIC DISEASES

ACUTE LYMPHOBLASTIC LEUKEMIA

ESSENTIALS OF DIAGNOSIS & TYPICAL FEATURES

► Bone marrow aspirate or biopsy specimen shows more than 25% lymphoblasts.

► Pallor, petechiae, purpura (50%), bone pain (25%).

► Hepatosplenomegaly (60%), lymphadenopathy (50%).

► Single or multiple cytopenias: neutropenia, thrombocytopenia, anemia (99%).

► Leukopenia (15%) or leukocytosis (50%), often with lymphoblasts identifiable on blood smear.

► Diagnosis confirmed by bone marrow examination.

General Considerations

Acute lymphoblastic leukemia (ALL) is the most common malignancy of childhood, accounting for about 25% of all cancer diagnoses in patients younger than age 15 years. The worldwide incidence of ALL is about 1:25,000 children per year, including 3000 children per year in the United States. The peak age at onset is 4 years; 85% of patients are diagnosed between ages 2 and 10 years. Children with Down syndrome have a 14-fold increase in the overall rate of leukemia.

ALL results from uncontrolled proliferation of immature lymphocytes. Its cause is unknown, and genetic factors may play a role. Leukemia is defined by the presence of more than 25% malignant hematopoietic cells (blasts) on bone marrow aspirate. Leukemic blasts from the majority of cases of childhood ALL have an antigen on the cell surface called the common ALL antigen (CALLA). These blasts derive from B-cell precursors early in their development, called B-precursor ALL. Less commonly, lymphoblasts are of T-cell origin or of mature B-cell origin. Over 70% of children receiving aggressive combination chemotherapy and early presymptomatic treatment to the central nervous system (CNS) are now cured of ALL.

▶ Clinical Findings

A. Symptoms and Signs

Presenting complaints of patients with ALL include those related to decreased bone marrow production of red blood cells (RBCs), white blood cells (WBCs), or platelets and to leukemic infiltration of extramedullary (outside bone marrow) sites. Intermittent fevers are common, as a result of either cytokines induced by the leukemia itself or infections secondary to leukopenia. Many patients present due to bruising or pallor. About 25% of patients experience bone pain, especially in the pelvis, vertebral bodies, and legs. Physical examination at diagnosis ranges from virtually normal to highly abnormal. Signs related to bone marrow infiltration by leukemia include pallor, petechiae, and purpura. Hepatomegaly or splenomegaly occurs in over 60% of patients. Lymphadenopathy is common, either localized or generalized to cervical, axillary, and inguinal regions. The testes may occasionally be unilaterally or bilaterally enlarged secondary to leukemic infiltration. Superior vena cava syndrome is caused by mediastinal adenopathy compressing the superior vena cava. A prominent venous pattern develops over the upper chest from collateral vein enlargement. The neck may feel full from venous engorgement. The face may appear plethoric, and the periorbital area may be edematous.

A mediastinal mass can cause tachypnea, orthopnea, and respiratory distress. Leukemic infiltration of cranial nerves may cause cranial nerve palsies with mild nuchal rigidity. The optic fundi may show exudates of leukemic infiltration and hemorrhage from thrombocytopenia. Anemia can cause a flow murmur, tachycardia, and, rarely, congestive heart failure.

B. Laboratory Findings

A complete blood count (CBC) with differential is the most useful initial test because 95% of patients with ALL have a decrease in at least one cell type (single cytopenia): neutropenia, thrombocytopenia, or anemia. Most patients have decreases in at least two blood cell lines. The WBC count is low or normal (= 10,000/µL) in 50% of patients, but the differential shows neutropenia (absolute neutrophil count < 1000/µL) along with a small percentage of blasts amid normal lymphocytes. In 30% of patients the WBC count is between 10,000 and 50,000/µL; in 20% of patients it is over 50,000/µL, occasionally higher than 300,000/µL. Blasts are usually readily identifiable on peripheral blood smears from patients with elevated WBC counts. Peripheral blood smears also show abnormalities in RBCs, such as teardrops. Most patients with ALL have decreased platelet counts (< 150,000/µL) and decreased hemoglobin (< 11 g/dL) at diagnosis. In approximately 1% of patients diagnosed with ALL, CBCs and peripheral blood smears are entirely normal but patients have bone pain that leads to bone marrow examination. Serum chemistries, particularly uric acid and lactate dehydrogenase (LDH), are often elevated at diagnosis as a result of cell breakdown.

The diagnosis of ALL is made by bone marrow examination, which shows a homogeneous infiltration of leukemic blasts replacing normal marrow elements. The morphology of blasts on bone marrow aspirate can usually distinguish ALL from acute myeloid leukemia (AML). Lymphoblasts are typically small, with cell diameters of approximately two erythrocytes. Lymphoblasts have scant cytoplasm, usually without granules. The nucleus typically contains no nucleoli or one small, indistinct nucleolus. Immunophenotyping of ALL blasts by flow cytometry helps distinguish precursor B-cell ALL from T-cell ALL or AML. Histochemical stains specific for myeloblastic and monoblastic leukemias (myeloperoxidase and nonspecific esterase) distinguish ALL from AML. About 5% of patients present with CNS leukemia, which is defined as a cerebrospinal fluid (CSF) WBC count greater than 5/µL with blasts present on cytocentrifuged specimen.

C. Imaging

Chest radiograph may show mediastinal widening or an anterior mediastinal mass and tracheal compression secondary to lymphadenopathy or thymic infiltration, especially in T-cell ALL. Abdominal ultrasound may show kidney enlargement from leukemic infiltration or uric acid nephropathy as well as intra-abdominal adenopathy. Plain radiographs of the long bones and spine may show demineralization, periosteal elevation, growth arrest lines, or compression of vertebral bodies.

▶ Differential Diagnosis

The differential diagnosis, based on the history and physical examination, includes chronic infections by Epstein-Barr virus (EBV) and cytomegalovirus (CMV), causing lymphadenopathy, hepatosplenomegaly, fevers, and anemia. Prominent petechiae and purpura suggest a diagnosis of immune thrombocytopenic purpura. Significant pallor could be caused by transient erythroblastopenia of childhood, autoimmune hemolytic anemias, or aplastic anemia. Fevers and joint pains, with or without hepatosplenomegaly and lymphadenopathy, suggest juvenile rheumatoid arthritis (JRA). The diagnosis of leukemia usually becomes straightforward once the CBC reveals multiple cytopenias and leukemic blasts. Serum LDH levels may help distinguish JRA from leukemia, as the LDH is usually normal in JRA. An elevated WBC count with lymphocytosis is typical of pertussis; however, in pertussis the lymphocytes are mature, and neutropenia is rarely associated.

▶ Treatment

A. Specific Therapy

Intensity of treatment is determined by specific prognostic features present at diagnosis, the patient's response to therapy, and specific biologic features of the leukemia cells. The majority of patients with ALL are enrolled in clinical trials designed by clinical groups and approved by the National Cancer Institute; the largest group is COG. The first month of therapy consists of induction, at the end of which over 95% of patients exhibit remission on bone marrow aspirates by morphology. The drugs most commonly used in induction include oral prednisone or dexamethasone, intravenous vincristine and daunorubicin, intramuscular asparaginase, and intrathecal methotrexate. For T-cell ALL, intravenous cyclophosphamide may be added during induction.

Consolidation is the second phase of treatment, during which intrathecal chemotherapy along with continued systemic therapy and sometimes cranial radiation therapy are given to kill lymphoblasts "hiding" in the meninges. Several months of intensive chemotherapy follows consolidation. This intensification has led to improved survival in pediatric ALL.

Maintenance therapy can include daily oral mercaptopurine, weekly oral methotrexate, and, often, monthly pulses of intravenous vincristine and oral prednisone or dexamethasone. Intrathecal chemotherapy, either with methotrexate alone or combined with cytarabine and hydrocortisone, is usually given every 2–3 months.

These drugs have significant potential side effects. Patients need to be monitored closely to prevent drug toxicities and to ensure early treatment of complications. The duration of treatment ranges between 2.2 years for girls and 3.2 years for boys in COG trials. Treatment for ALL is tailored to prognostic, or risk, groups. A child aged 1–9 years with a WBC count below 50,000/μL at diagnosis and without poor biologic features [t(9;22) or t(4;11)] is considered to be at "standard risk" and receives less intensive therapy than a "high-risk" patient who has a WBC count at diagnosis over 50,000/μL or is older than age 10 years. Also important is the patient's response to treatment determined by minimal residual disease (MRD) monitoring. This risk-adapted treatment approach has significantly increased the cure rate among patients with less favorable prognostic features while minimizing treatment-related toxicities in those with favorable features. Bone marrow relapse is usually heralded by an abnormal CBC, either during treatment or following completion of therapy.

The CNS and testes are sanctuary sites of extramedullary leukemia. Currently, about one third of all ALL relapses are isolated to these sanctuary sites. Systemic chemotherapy does not penetrate these tissues as well as it penetrates other organs. Thus, presymptomatic intrathecal chemotherapy is a critical part of ALL treatment, without which many more relapses would occur in the CNS, with or without bone marrow relapse. The majority of isolated CNS relapses are diagnosed in an asymptomatic child at the time of routine intrathecal injection, when CSF cell count and differential shows an elevated WBC with leukemic blasts. Occasionally, symptoms of CNS relapse develop: headache, nausea and vomiting, irritability, nuchal rigidity, photophobia, and cranial nerve palsies. Currently, testicular relapse occurs in less than 5% of boys. The presentation of testicular relapse is usually unilateral painless testicular enlargement, without a distinct mass. Routine follow-up of boys both on and off treatment includes physical examination of the testes.

Bone marrow transplantation, now called hematopoietic stem cell transplantation (HSCT), is rarely used as initial treatment for ALL, because most patients are cured with chemotherapy alone. Patients whose blasts contain certain chromosomal abnormalities, such as t(9;22) or hypodiploidy (< 44 chromosomes), and patients with a very slow response to therapy may have a better cure rate with early HSCT from a human leukocyte antigen (HLA)-DR–matched sibling donor, or perhaps a matched unrelated donor, than with intensive chemotherapy alone. HSCT cures about 50% of patients who relapse, provided that a second remission is achieved with chemotherapy before transplant. Children who relapse more than 1 year after completion of chemotherapy (late relapse) may be cured with intensive chemotherapy without HSCT.

Several new biologic agents, including tyrosine kinase inhibitors and immunotoxins, are currently in various stages of research and development. Some of these therapies may prove relevant for future treatment of poor risk or relapsed ALL.

B. Supportive Care

Tumor lysis syndrome should be anticipated when treatment is started. Alkalinization of urine with intravenous sodium bicarbonate, maintaining brisk urine output, and treating with oral allopurinol are appropriate steps in managing tumor lysis syndrome. Serum levels of potassium, phosphorus, and uric acid should be monitored. If superior vena caval or superior mediastinal syndrome is present, general anesthesia is contraindicated temporarily. If hyperleukocytosis (WBC count > 100,000/μL) is accompanied by hyperviscosity and mental status changes, leukophoresis may be indicated to rapidly reduce the number of circulating blasts and minimize the potential thrombotic or hemorrhagic CNS complications. Throughout the course of treatment, all transfused blood and platelet products should be irradiated to prevent graft-versus-host disease from the transfused lymphocytes. Whenever possible, blood products should be leukodepleted to minimize CMV transmission, transfusion reactions, and sensitization to platelets.

Due to the immunocompromised state of the patient with ALL, bacterial, fungal, and viral infections are serious and can be life-threatening or fatal. During the course of treatment, fever (temperature = 38.3°C) and neutropenia (absolute neutrophil count < 500/μL) require prompt assessment, blood cultures from each lumen of a central line, and prompt treatment with empiric broad-spectrum antibiotics. Patients receiving ALL treatment must receive prophylaxis against *Pneumocystis jiroveci* (formerly *Pneumocystis carinii*). Trimethoprim–sulfamethoxazole given twice each day on 2 or 3 consecutive days per week is the drug of choice. Patients nonimmune to varicella are at risk for very serious—even fatal—infection. Such patients should receive varicella-zoster immune globulin (VZIG) within 72 hours after exposure and treatment with intravenous acyclovir for active infection.

▶ Prognosis

Cure rates depend on specific prognostic features present at diagnosis, biologic features of the leukemic blast, and the response to therapy. Two of the most important features are WBC count and age. Children aged 1–9 years whose diagnostic WBC count is less than 50,000/μL have a higher rate of cure than other patients (~85% event-free survival for these children). The rapidity of response to induction treatment has prognostic significance as well, reflecting leukemic blast sensitivity to chemotherapy. Patients are categorized as rapid early responders (RERs) or slow early responders (SERs) based on the percentage of blasts present in bone marrow aspirates within 7–14 days after induction begins. More intensive treatment regimens are given to SERs than RERs to increase their chance of cure.

Certain chromosomal abnormalities present in the leukemic blasts at diagnosis influence prognosis. Patients with t(9;22) generally have a very poor chance of cure even with intensive chemotherapy. Likewise, infants younger than age 6 months with t(4;11) have a poor chance of cure with conventional chemotherapy. In contrast, patients whose blasts are hyperdiploid (containing > 50 chromosomes instead of the normal 46) with trisomies of chromosomes 4, 10, and 17, and patients whose blasts have a t(12;21) and TEL-AML1 rearrangement have a greater chance of cure, approaching 90% survival, than do children without these characteristics.

Techniques based on leukemic blast immunophenotyping or immunoglobulin rearrangements have been developed to detect residual lymphoblasts in bone marrow (MRD), at the end of induction and during remission. Many groups have shown that even low levels of MRD predict an inferior outcome. In the current COG clinical trials, patients with levels of MRD above 0.1% at the end of remission induction will receive intensified therapy, in an attempt to improve their outcome.

Bostrom BC: Dexamethasone versus prednisone and daily oral versus weekly intravenous mercaptopurine for patients with standard-risk acute lymphoblastic leukemia: A report from the Children's Cancer Group. Blood 2003;101:3809 [PMID: 12531809].

Pearce JM et al: Childhood leukemia. Pediatr Rev 2005;26:96 [PMID: 15741325].

Peters C et al: Allogeneic haematopoitic stem cell transplantation in children with acute lymphoblastic leukaemia: The BFM/IBFM/EBMT concepts. Bone Marrow Transplant 2005;35:S9 [PMID: 15812540].

ACUTE MYELOID LEUKEMIA

ESSENTIALS OF DIAGNOSIS & TYPICAL FEATURES

▶ Bone marrow aspirate or biopsy shows 20% or more leukemic blasts.

▶ Fatigue, bleeding, or infection.

▶ Adenopathy, hepatosplenomegaly, skin nodules (M4 and M5 subtypes).

▶ Cytopenias: neutropenia (69%), anemia (44%), thrombocytopenia (33%).

▶ General Considerations

Approximately 500 new cases of acute myeloid leukemia (AML) occur per year in children and adolescents in the United States. Although AML accounts for only 25% of all leukemias in this age group, it is responsible for at least one third of deaths from leukemia in children and teenagers. Congenital conditions associated with an increased risk of AML include Diamond-Blackfan anemia; neurofibromatosis; Down syndrome; Wiskott-Aldrich, Kostmann, and Li-Fraumeni syndromes; as well as chromosomal instability syndromes such as Fanconi anemia. Acquired risk factors include exposure to ionizing radiation, cytotoxic chemotherapeutic agents, and benzenes. However, the vast majority of patients have no identifiable risk factors. Historically, the diagnosis of AML was based almost exclusively on morphology and immunohistochemical staining of the leukemic cells. AML has eight subtypes (M0–M7) according to the French-American-British (FAB) classification (Table 29–1). Immunophenotypic, cytogenetic, and molecular analyses are increasingly important in confirming the diagnosis of AML and subclassifying it into biologically distinct subtypes that have therapeutic and prognostic implications. Cytogenetic clonal abnormalities occur in 80% of patients with AML and are often predictive of outcome.

Aggressive induction therapy currently results in a 75–85% complete remission rate. However, long-term survival has improved only modestly to approximately 50%, despite

Table 29–1. FAB subtypes of acute myeloid leukemia.

FAB Classification	Common Name	Distribution in Childhood (Age)		Cytogenetic Associations	Clinical Features
		< 2 y	> 2 y		
M0	Acute myeloid leukemia, minimally differentiated	1%		inv (3q26), t(3;3)	
M1	Acute myeloblastic leukemia without maturation	17%	23%		
M2	Acute myeloblastic leukemia with maturation	26%		t(8;21), t(6;9); rare	Myeloblastomas or chloromas
M3	Acute promyelocytic leukemia	4%		t(15;17); rarely, t(11;17) or (5;17)	Disseminated intravascular coagulation
M4	Acute myelomonoblastic leukemia	30%	24%	11q23, inv 3, t(3;3), t(6;9)	Hyperleukocytosis, CNS involvement, skin and gum infiltration
M4Eo	Acute myelomonoblastic leukemia with abnormal eosinophils			inv16, t(16;16)	
M5	Acute monoblastic leukemia	46%	15%	11q23, t(9;11), t(8;16)	Hyperleukocytosis, CNS involvement, skin and gum infiltration
M6	Erythroleukemia	2%			
M7	Acute megakaryoblastic leukemia	7%	5%	t(1;22)	Down syndrome frequent (< age 2 y)

CNS, central nervous system; FAB, French-American-British classification.

the availability of several effective agents, improvements in supportive care, and increasingly intensive therapies.

Clinical Findings

The clinical manifestations of AML commonly include anemia (44%), thrombocytopenia (33%), and neutropenia (69%). Symptoms may be few and innocuous or may be life-threatening. The median hemoglobin value at diagnosis is 7 g/dL, and platelets usually number fewer than 50,000/μL. Frequently the absolute neutrophil count is under 1000/μL, although the total WBC count is over 100,000/μL in 25% of patients at diagnosis.

Hyperleukocytosis may be associated with life-threatening complications. Venous stasis and sludging of blasts in small vessels cause hypoxia, hemorrhage, and infarction, most notably in the lung and CNS. This clinical picture is a medical emergency requiring rapid intervention, such as leukophoresis, to decrease the leukocyte count. CNS leukemia is present in 5–15% of patients at diagnosis, a higher rate of initial involvement than in ALL. Certain subtypes, such as M4 and M5, have a higher likelihood of meningeal infiltration than do other subtypes. Additionally, clinically significant coagulopathy may be present at diagnosis in patients with M3, M4, or M5 subtypes. This problem manifests as bleeding or an abnormal disseminated intravascular coagulation screen and should be at least partially corrected prior to initiation of treatment, which may transiently exacerbate the coagulopathy.

▶ Treatment

A. Specific Therapy

AML is less responsive to treatment than ALL and requires more intensive chemotherapy. Toxicities from therapy are common and likely to be life-threatening; therefore, treatment should be undertaken only at a tertiary pediatric oncology center.

Current AML protocols rely on intensive administration of anthracyclines, cytarabine, and etoposide for induction of remission. After remission is obtained patients who have a matched sibling donor undergo allogeneic HSCT while those without an appropriate related donor are treated with additional cycles of aggressive chemotherapy for a total of 6–9 months. Inv16 and t(8;21) may herald a more responsive subtype of AML. In patients with a rapid response to induction, intensive chemotherapy alone may be curative. Trials with risk grouping are ongoing as more is understood about the varying biologic factors.

The biologic heterogeneity of AML is becoming increasingly important therapeutically. The M3 subtype, associated with t(15;17) demonstrated either cytogenetically or molecularly, is currently treated with all trans-retinoic acid in addition to chemotherapy with high-dose cytarabine and daunorubicin. All trans-retinoic acid leads to differentiation of promyelocytic leukemia cells and can induce remission, but cure requires conventional chemotherapy as well. The use of arsenic trioxide has also been investigated in the treatment of this subtype of AML with favorable results. This subtype has an increased event-free survival over other AML subtypes.

Another biologically distinct subtype of AML occurs in children with Down syndrome, M7, or megakaryocytic AML. Using less intensive treatment, remission induction rate and overall survival of these children are dramatically superior to non–Down syndrome children with AML. It is important that children with Down syndrome receive appropriate treatment specifically designed to be less intensive.

Biologic agents and new chemotherapeutic agents are increasingly being studied in the treatment of AML. The development and early success of antibody-targeted cytotoxic agents such as gemtuzumab ozogamicin (Mylotarg, a humanized anti-CD33 monoclonal antibody conjugated with calicheamicin) are encouraging steps in the quest for therapeutic agents that result in higher survival rates. Use of this agent as intensive chemotherapy for AML is now being evaluated in a randomized trial. Clofarabine, a newer nucleoside analogue, also has activity in AML and is currently undergoing trials in relapsed and refractory patients.

B. Supportive Care

Tumor lysis syndrome rarely occurs during induction treatment of AML. Nevertheless, when the diagnostic WBC cell count is greater than 100,000/μL or significant adenopathy or organomegaly is present, one should alkalinize urine with intravenous sodium bicarbonate, maintain brisk urine output, and follow potassium, uric acid, and phosphorous lab values closely. Hyperleukocytosis (WBC > 100,000/μL) is a medical emergency and, in a symptomatic patient, requires rapid intervention such as leukophoresis to rapidly decrease the number of circulating blasts and thereby decrease hyperviscosity. Delaying transfusion of packed RBCs until the WBC can be decreased to below 100,000/μL avoids exacerbating hyperviscosity. It is also important to correct the coagulopathy commonly associated with M3, M4, or M5 subtypes prior to beginning induction chemotherapy. As with the treatment of ALL, all blood products should be irradiated and leukodepleted; *Pneumocystis* prophylaxis must be administered during treatment and for several weeks afterward; and patients not immune to varicella must receive VZIG within 72 hours of exposure and prompt treatment with intravenous acyclovir for active infection.

Onset of fever (temperature ≥ 38.3°C) or chills associated with neutropenia requires prompt assessment, blood cultures from each lumen of a central venous line, other cultures such as throat or urine as appropriate, and prompt initiation of broad-spectrum intravenous antibiotics. Infections in this population of patients can rapidly become life-threatening. Because of the high incidence of invasive fungal infections, there should be a low threshold for initiating antifungal therapy. Filgrastim (granulocyte colony-stimulating factor) may be used to stimulate granulocyte recovery during the treatment of AML and results in shorter periods of neutropenia and hospitalization. It must be stressed that the supportive

care for this group of patients is as important as the leukemia-directed therapy and that this treatment should be carried out only at a tertiary pediatric cancer center.

▶ Prognosis

Published results from various centers show a 50–60% survival rate at 5 years following first remission for patients who do not have matched sibling hematopoietic stem cell donors. Patients with matched sibling donors fare slightly better, with 5-year survival rates of 60–70% after allogeneic HSCT.

As treatment becomes more sophisticated, outcome is increasingly related to the subtype of AML. Currently, AML in patients with t(8;21), t(15;17), inv 16, or Down syndrome has the most favorable prognosis, with 65–75% long-term survival using modern treatments, including chemotherapy alone. The least favorable outcome occurs in AML patients with monosomy 7 or 5, 7q, 5q–, or 11q23 cytogenetic abnormalities.

Alonzo TA et al: Postremission therapy for children with acute myeloid leukemia: The children's cancer group experience in the transplant era. Leukemia 2005;19:965 [PMID: 15830007].

Gibson BES et al: Treatment strategy and long-term results in paediatric patients treated in consecutive UK AML trials. Leukemia 2005;19:2130 [PMID:16304572].

Neudorf S et al: Allogeneic bone marrow transplantation for children with acute myelocytic leukemia in first remission demonstrates a role for graft versus leukemia in the maintenance of disease-free survival. Blood 2004;103:3655 [PMID: 14751924].

Sternherz PG, et al: Clofarabine induced durable complete remission in heavily pretreated adolescents with relapsed and refractory leukemia. J Pediatr Hematol Oncol 2007;29:656 [PMID: 17805046].

Tallman MS et al: Drug therapy for acute myeloid leukemia. Blood 2005;106:1154 [PMID: 15870183].

MYELOPROLIFERATIVE DISEASES

 ESSENTIALS OF DIAGNOSIS & TYPICAL FEATURES

▶ Leukocytosis with predominance of immature cells.

▶ Often indolent course.

▶ Fever, bone pain, respiratory symptoms.

▶ Hepatosplenomegaly.

Myeloproliferative diseases in children are relatively rare. They are characterized by ineffective hematopoiesis that results in excessive peripheral blood counts. The three most important types are chronic myelogenous leukemia (CML), which accounts for less than 5% of the childhood leukemias, transient myeloproliferative disorder in children with Down syndrome, and juvenile myelomonocytic leukemia (Table 29–2).

Table 29–2. Comparison of JMML, CML, and TMD.

	CML	TMD	JMML
Age at onset	> 3 y	< 3 mo	< 2 y
Clinical presentation	Nonspecific constitutional complaints, massive splenomegaly, variable hepatomegaly	DS features, often no or few symptoms; or hepatosplenomegaly, respiratory symptoms	Abrupt onset; eczematoid skin rash, marked lymphadenopathy, bleeding tendency, moderate hepatosplenomegaly, fever
Chromosomal alterations	t(9;22)	Constitutional trisomy 21, but usually no other abnormality	Monosomy or del (7q) in 20% of patients
Laboratory features	Marked leukocytosis (> 100,000/μL), normal to elevated platelet count, decreased to absent leukocyte alkaline phosphatase, usually normal muramidase	Variable leukocytosis, normal to high platelet count, large platelets, myeloblasts	Moderate leukocytosis (> 10,000/μL), thrombocytopenia, monocytosis (> 1000/μL), elevated fetal hemoglobin, normal to diminished leukocyte alkaline phosphatase, elevated muramidase

CML, chronic myelogenous leukemia; DS, Down syndrome; JMML, juvenile myelomonocytic leukemia; TMD, transient myeloproliferative disorder.

1. Chronic Myelogenous Leukemia

General Considerations

CML with translocation of chromosomes 9 and 22 (the Philadelphia chromosome, Ph⁺) is identical to adult Ph⁺CML. Translocation 9;22 results in the fusion of the *BCR* gene on chromosome 22 and the *ABL* gene on chromosome 9. The resulting fusion protein is a constitutively active tyrosine kinase that interacts with a variety of effector proteins and allows for deregulated cellular proliferation, decreased adherence of cells to the bone marrow extracellular matrix, and resistance to apoptosis. The disease usually progresses within 3 years to an accelerated phase and then to a blast crisis. It is generally accepted that Ph⁺ cells have an increased susceptibility to the acquisition of additional molecular changes that lead to the accelerated and blast phases of disease.

Clinical Findings

Patients with CML may present with nonspecific complaints similar to those of acute leukemia, including bone pain, fever, night sweats, and fatigue. However, patients can also be asymptomatic. Patients with a total WBC count of more than 100,000/μL may have symptoms of leukostasis, such as dyspnea, priapism, or neurologic abnormalities. Physical findings may include fever, pallor, ecchymoses, and hepatosplenomegaly. Anemia, thrombocytosis, and leukocytosis are frequent laboratory findings. The peripheral smear is usually diagnostic, with a characteristic predominance of myeloid cells in all stages of maturation and relatively few blasts.

Treatment & Prognosis

Historically, hydroxyurea or busulfan has been used to reduce or eliminate Ph⁺ cells. However, HSCT is the only consistently curative intervention. Reported survival rates for patients younger than age 20 years transplanted in the chronic phase from matched related donors are 70–80%. Unrelated stem cell transplants result in survival rates of 50–65%.

The understanding of the molecular mechanisms involved in the pathogenesis of CML has led to the rational design of molecularly targeted therapy. Imatinib mesylate (Gleevec) is a tyrosine kinase inhibitor that has had dramatic success in the treatment of CML, with most adults and children achieving cytogenetic remission. The durability of the remission for children is unclear but is now the accepted upfront therapy. However, some patients are resistant to imatinib, and its role in the long-term management of children with CML awaits further studies.

2. Transient Myeloproliferative Disorder

Transient myeloproliferative disorder is unique to patients with trisomy 21 or mosaicism for trisomy 21. It is characterized by uncontrolled proliferation of blasts, usually of megakaryocytic origin, during early infancy and spontaneous resolution. The pathogenesis of this process is not well understood, although mutations in the *GATA1* gene have recently been implicated as initial events.

Although the true incidence is unknown, it is estimated to occur in up to 10% of patients with Down syndrome. Despite the fact that the process usually resolves by 3 months of age, organ infiltration may cause significant morbidity and mortality.

Patients can present with hydrops fetalis, pericardial or pleural effusions, or hepatic fibrosis. More frequently, they are asymptomatic or only minimally ill. Therefore, treatment is primarily supportive. Patients without symptoms are not treated, and those with organ dysfunction receive low doses of chemotherapy or leukophoresis (or both) to reduce peripheral blood blast counts. Although patients with transient myeloproliferative disorder have apparent resolution of the process, approximately 30% go on to develop acute megakaryoblastic leukemia (AML M7) within 3 years.

3. Juvenile Myelomonocytic Leukemia

Juvenile myelomonocytic leukemia (JMML), accounts for approximately one third of the myelodysplastic and myeloproliferative disorders in childhood. Patients with neurofibromatosis type 1 (NF-1) are at higher risk of JMML than the general population. It typically occurs in infants and very young children and is occasionally associated with monosomy 7 or a deletion of the long arm of chromosome 7.

Patients with JMML present similarly to those with other hematopoietic malignancies, with lymphadenopathy, hepatosplenomegaly, skin rash, or respiratory symptoms. Patients may have stigmata of NF-1 with neurofibromas or café-au-lait spots. Laboratory findings include anemia, thrombocytopenia, leukocytosis with monocytosis, and elevated fetal hemoglobin.

The results of chemotherapy for children with JMML have been disappointing, with estimated survival rates of less than 30%. Approximately 40–45% of patients are projected to survive long term using HSCT, although optimizing conditioning regimens and donor selection may improve these results.

Crispino JD: GATA1 mutations in Down syndrome: Implications for biology and diagnosis of children with transient myeloproliferative disorder and acute megakaryoblastic leukemia. Pediatr Blood Cancer 2005;44:40 [PMID: 15390312].

Cwynarski K et al: Stem cell transplantation for chronic myeloid leukemia in children. Blood 2003;102:1224 [PMID: 12714525].

Gassas A, et al: A basic classification and a comprehensive examination of pediatric myeloproliferative syndromes. J Pediatr Hematol Oncol 2005;27:192 [PMID: 15838389].

Goldman JM, Melo JV: Chronic myeloid leukemia—Advances in biology and new approaches to treatment. N Engl J Med 2003;349:1451 [PMID: 14534339].

Mundschau G et al: Mutagenesis of GATA1 is an initiating event in Down syndrome leukemogenesis. Blood 2003;101:4298 [PMID: 12560215].

Passmore SJ et al: Paediatric myelodysplastic syndromes and juvenile myelomonocytic leukaemia in the UK: A population-based study of incidence and survival. Br J Haematol 2003;121:758 [PMID: 12780790].

Pulsipher MA: Treatment of CML in pediatric patients: Should imatinib mesylate (STI-571, Gleevec) or allogeneic hematopoietic cell transplant be front-line therapy? Pediatr Blood Cancer 2004;43:523 [PMID: 15382266].

Thornley I et al: Treating children with chronic myeloid leukemia in the imatinib era: A therapeutic dilemma? Med Pediatr Oncol 2003;41:115 [PMID: 12825214].

BRAIN TUMORS

ESSENTIALS OF DIAGNOSIS & TYPICAL FEATURES

▶ Classic triad: morning headache, vomiting, and papilledema.

▶ Increasing head circumference, cranial nerve palsies, dysarthria, ataxia, hemiplegia, papilledema, hyperreflexia, macrocephaly, cracked pot sign.

▶ Seizures, personality change, blurred vision, diplopia, weakness, decreased coordination, precocious puberty.

▶ General Considerations

The classic triad of morning headache, vomiting, and papilledema is present in fewer than 30% of children at presentation. School failure and personality changes are common in older children. Irritability, failure to thrive, and delayed development are common in very young children with brain tumors. Recent-onset head tilt can result from a posterior fossa tumor.

Brain tumors are the most common solid tumors of childhood, accounting for 1500–2000 new malignancies in children each year in the United States and for 25–30% of all childhood cancers. In general, children with brain tumors have a better prognosis than do adults. Favorable outcome occurs most commonly with low-grade and fully resectable tumors. Unfortunately, cranial irradiation in young children can have significant neuropsychological, intellectual, and endocrinologic sequelae.

Brain tumors in childhood are biologically and histologically heterogeneous, ranging from low-grade localized lesions to high-grade tumors with neuraxis dissemination. High-dose systemic chemotherapy is used frequently, especially in young children with high-grade tumors, in an effort to delay, decrease, or completely avoid cranial irradiation. Such intensive treatment may be accompanied by autologous HSCT or peripheral stem cell reconstitution.

The causes of pediatric brain tumors are unknown. The risk of developing astrocytomas is increased in children with neurofibromatosis or tuberous sclerosis. Several studies show that some childhood brain tumors occur in families with increased genetic susceptibility to childhood cancers in general, brain tumors, or leukemia and lymphoma. A higher incidence of seizures has been observed in relatives of children with astrocytoma. Certain pediatric brain tumors such as ependymoma have been linked to polyomavirus, but the exact relationship is unknown. The risk of developing a brain tumor is increased in children who received cranial irradiation for treatment of meningeal leukemia.

Because pediatric brain tumors are rare, they are often misdiagnosed or diagnosed late; most pediatricians see no more than two children with brain tumors during their careers.

▶ Clinical Findings

A. Symptoms and Signs

Clinical findings at presentation vary depending on the child's age and the tumor's location. Children younger than age 2 years more commonly have infratentorial tumors. Children with such tumors usually present with nonspecific symptoms such as vomiting, unsteadiness, lethargy, and irritability. Signs may be surprisingly few or may include macrocephaly, ataxia, hyperreflexia, and cranial nerve palsies. Because the head can expand in young children, papilledema is often absent. Measuring head circumference and observing gait are essential in evaluating a child for possible brain tumor. Eye findings and apparent visual disturbances such as difficulty tracking can occur in association with optic pathway tumors such as optic glioma. Optic glioma occurring in a young child is often associated with neurofibromatosis.

Older children more commonly have supratentorial tumors, which are associated with headache, visual symptoms, seizures, and focal neurologic deficits. Initial presenting features are often nonspecific. School failure and personality changes are common. Vaguely described visual disturbance is often present, but the child must be directly asked. Headaches are common, but they often will not be predominantly in the morning. The headaches may be confused with migraine.

Older children with infratentorial tumors characteristically present with symptoms and signs of hydrocephalus, which include progressively worsening morning headache and vomiting, gait unsteadiness, double vision, and papilledema. Cerebellar astrocytomas enlarge slowly, and symptoms may worsen over several months. Morning vomiting may be the only symptom of posterior fossa ependymomas, which originate in the floor of the fourth ventricle near the vomiting center. Children with brainstem tumors may present with facial and extraocular muscle palsies, ataxia, and hemiparesis; hydrocephalus occurs in approximately 25% of these patients at diagnosis.

B. Imaging and Staging

In addition to the tumor biopsy, neuraxis imaging studies are obtained to determine whether dissemination has occurred. It is unusual for brain tumors in children and adolescents to disseminate outside the CNS.

Magnetic resonance imaging (MRI) has become the preferred diagnostic study for pediatric brain tumors. MRI provides better definition of the tumor and delineates indolent gliomas that may not be seen on computed tomography (CT) scan. In contrast, a CT scan can be done in less than 10 minutes—as opposed to the 30 minutes required for an MRI scan—and is still useful if an urgent diagnostic study is necessary or to detect calcification of a tumor. Both scans are generally done with and without contrast enhancement. Contrast enhances regions where the blood-brain barrier is disrupted. Postoperative scans to document the extent of tumor resection should be obtained within 48 hours after surgery to avoid postsurgical enhancement.

Imaging of the entire neuraxis and CSF cytologic examination should be part of the diagnostic evaluation for patients with tumors such as medulloblastoma, ependymoma, and pineal region tumors. Diagnosis of neuraxis drop metastases (tumor spread along the neuraxis) can be accomplished by gadolinium-enhanced MRI incorporating sagittal and axial views. MRI of the spine should be obtained preoperatively in all children with midline tumors of the fourth ventricle or cerebellum. A CSF sample should be obtained during the diagnostic surgery. Lumbar CSF is preferred over ventricular CSF for cytologic examination. Levels of biomarkers in the blood and CSF, such as human chorionic gonadotropin and α-fetoprotein, may be helpful at diagnosis and in follow-up. Both human chorionic gonadotropin and α-fetoprotein should be obtained from the blood preoperatively for all pineal and suprasellar tumors.

The neurosurgeon should discuss staging and sample collection with an oncologist before surgery in a child newly presenting with a scan suggestive of brain tumor.

C. Classification

About 50% of the common pediatric brain tumors occur above the tentorium and 50% in the posterior fossa. In the very young child, posterior fossa tumors are more common. Most childhood brain tumors can be divided into two categories according to the cell of origin: (1) glial tumors, such as astrocytomas and ependymomas, or (2) nonglial tumors, such as medulloblastoma and other primitive neuroectodermal tumors. Some tumors contain both glial and neural elements (eg, ganglioglioma). A group of less common CNS tumors does not fit into either category (ie, craniopharyngiomas, germ cell tumors, choroid plexus tumors, and meningiomas). Low-grade and high-grade tumors are found in most categories. Table 29–3 lists the locations and frequencies of the common pediatric brain tumors.

Astrocytoma is the most common brain tumor of childhood. Most are juvenile pilocytic astrocytoma (WHO grade I) found in the posterior fossa with a bland cellular morphol-

Table 29–3. Location and frequency of common pediatric brain tumors.

Location	Frequency of Occurrence (%)
Hemispheric	**37**
Low-grade astrocytoma	23
High-grade astrocytoma	11
Other	3
Posterior fossa	**49**
Medulloblastoma	15
Cerebellar astrocytoma	15
Brainstem glioma	15
Ependymoma	4
Midline	**14**
Craniopharyngioma	8
Chiasmal glioma	4
Pineal region tumor	2

Table 29–4. Prognostic factors in children with medulloblastoma.

Factor	Favorable	Unfavorable
Extent of disease	Nondisseminated	Disseminated
Size of primary tumor after surgery	≤ 3 cm (completely resected)	> 3 cm
Histologic features	Undifferentiated	Foci of glial, ependymal, or neuronal differentiation
Age	≥ 4 y	< 4 y

ogy and few or no mitotic figures. Low-grade astrocytomas are in many cases curable by complete surgical excision alone. Chemotherapy is effective in low-grade astrocytomas.

Medulloblastoma and related primitive neuroectodermal tumors are the most common high-grade brain tumors in children. These tumors usually occur in the first decade of life, with a peak incidence between ages 5 and 10 years and a female-to-male ratio of 2.1:1.3. The tumors typically arise in the midline cerebellar vermis, with variable extension into the fourth ventricle. Neuraxis dissemination at diagnosis affects from 10–46% of patients. Prognostic factors are outlined in Table 29–4.

Brainstem tumors are third in frequency of occurrence in children. They are frequently of astrocytic origin and often are high-grade. Children with tumors that diffusely infiltrate the brainstem and involve primarily the pons have a long-term survival rate of less than 15%. Brainstem tumors that occur above or below the pons and grow in an eccentric or cystic manner have a somewhat better outcome. Exophytic tumors in this location may be amenable to surgery. Generally, brainstem tumors are treated without a tissue diagnosis.

Other brain tumors such as ependymomas, germ cell tumors, choroid plexus tumors, and craniopharyngiomas are less common, and each is associated with unique diagnostic and therapeutic challenges.

▶ Treatment

A. Supportive Care

Dexamethasone should be started prior to initial surgery (0.5–1.0 mg/kg initially, then 0.25–0.5 mg/kg/d in four divided doses). Anticonvulsants (usually phenytoin, 4–8 mg/kg/d) should be started if the child has had a seizure or if the surgical approach is likely to induce seizures. Because postoperative treatment of young children with high-grade brain tumors incorporates increasingly more intensive systemic chemotherapy, consideration should also be given to the use of prophylaxis for prevention of oral candidiasis and *Pneumocystis* infection. Dexamethasone and phenytoin potentially reduce the effectiveness of chemotherapy and should be discontinued as soon after surgery as possible.

Optimum care for the pediatric patient with a brain tumor requires a multidisciplinary team including subspecialists in pediatric neurosurgery, neurooncology, neurology, endocrinology, neuropsychology, radiation therapy, and rehabilitation medicine, as well as highly specialized nurses, social workers, and staff in physical therapy, occupational therapy, and speech and language science.

B. Specific Therapy

The goal of treatment is to eradicate the tumor with the least short- and long-term morbidity. Long-term neuropsychological morbidity becomes an especially important issue related to deficits caused by the tumor itself and the sequelae of treatment. Meticulous surgical removal of as much tumor as possible is generally the preferred initial approach. Technologic advances in the operating microscope, the ultrasonic tissue aspirator, and the CO_2 laser (which is less commonly used in pediatric brain tumor surgery); the accuracy of computerized stereotactic resection; and the availability of intraoperative monitoring techniques such as evoked potentials and electrocorticography have increased the feasibility and safety of surgical resection of many pediatric brain tumors. Second-look surgery after chemotherapy is increasingly being used when tumors are incompletely resected at initial surgery.

Radiation therapy for pediatric brain tumors is in a state of evolution. For tumors with a high probability of neuraxis dissemination (eg, medulloblastoma), craniospinal irradiation is still standard therapy in children older than age 3 years. In others (eg, ependymoma), craniospinal irradiation has been abandoned because neuraxis dissemination at first relapse is rare. Approaches to the delivery of radiation to minimize the adverse effects on normal brain tissue are being explored and include stereotactic irradiation and the use of three-dimensional treatment planning.

Chemotherapy is effective in treating low-grade and malignant astrocytomas and medulloblastomas. A series of brain tumor protocols for children younger than age 3 years involved administering intensive chemotherapy after tumor resection and delaying or omitting radiation therapy. The results of these trials have generally been disappointing but have taught valuable lessons regarding the varying responses to chemotherapy of different tumor types. Future trials may give shorter courses of more intense chemotherapy followed by conformal radiotherapy. Conformal techniques allow the delivery of radiation to strictly defined fields and may limit side effects.

In older children with malignant glioma, the current approach is surgical resection of the tumor and combined-modality treatment with irradiation and intensive chemotherapy. In patients with glioblastoma, the use of high-dose chemotherapy and autologous bone marrow or peripheral stem cell reconstitution is being studied. Initial results have been mixed, but the toxicity of such therapy remains a concern. Surgery is not indicated for diffuse brainstem

gliomas. Traditional treatment of these tumors has been local irradiation. Hyperfractionation to increase the dose from the conventional 54 Gy to 72–78 Gy showed no apparent benefit in a recent Children's Cancer Group (CCG) study. New approaches are needed for this prognostically poor tumor.

The treatment of low-grade astrocytomas is evolving. Increasing numbers of young children are receiving antitumor chemotherapeutic agents such as carboplatin and vincristine after incomplete resection of these tumors. The role of irradiation after subtotal resection even in older children is being questioned.

▶ **Prognosis**

Despite improvements in surgery and radiation therapy, the outlook for cure remains poor for children with high-grade glial tumors. For children with high-grade gliomas, an early CCG study showed a 45% progression-free survival rate for children who received radiation therapy and chemotherapy. A follow-up CCG study in which all patients had chemotherapy and radiation therapy showed a 5-year progression-free survival rate of 36%. There is a possibility of effective salvage therapy with high-dose chemotherapy for children who relapse. In addition, the extent of resection appeared to correlate positively with prognosis, with a 3-year progression-free survival rate of 17% for patients receiving biopsy only, 29–32% for patients receiving partial or subtotal resections, and 54% for those receiving 90% resections. Biologic factors that may affect survival are being increasingly recognized. The prognosis for diffuse pontine gliomas remains very poor, with no benefit from high-dose chemotherapy plus radiation therapy versus radiation alone.

The 5- and even 10-year survival rate for low-grade astrocytomas of childhood is 60–90%. However, prognosis depends on both site and grade. A child with a pilocytic astrocytoma of the cerebellum has a considerably better prognosis than a child with a fibrillary astrocytoma of the cerebral cortex. Recently, a new entity of low-grade tumor of childhood, the pilomyxoid astrocytoma has been recognized. Pilomyxoid astrocytomas seem to have a worse prognosis than juvenile pilocytic astrocytomas. For recurrent or progressive low-grade astrocytoma of childhood, relatively moderate chemotherapy may improve the likelihood of survival.

Conventional craniospinal irradiation for children with low-stage medulloblastoma results in survival rates of 60–90%. Ten-year survival rates are lower (40–60%). Chemotherapy allows a reduction in the craniospinal radiation dose while preserving survival rates for average-risk patients (86% survival at 5 years on the most recent COG average-risk protocol). However, even reduced-dose craniospinal irradiation has an adverse effect on intellect, especially in children younger than age 7 years. Five-year survival rates for high-risk medulloblastoma have been 25–40%, but a recent trial reported at the American Society of Clinical Oncology (ASCO) conference in 2007 suggests a dramatically improved prognosis for patients receiving intensive chemotherapy and irradiation. Children with supratentorial primitive neuroectodermal tumors also benefit from the addition of chemotherapy to craniospinal irradiation.

Major challenges remain in treating brain tumors in children younger than age 3 years and in treating brainstem gliomas and malignant gliomas. The increasing emphasis is on the quality of life of survivors, not just the survival rate.

Foreman NK et al: A study of sequential high dose cyclophosphamide and high dose carboplatin with peripheral stem cell rescue in resistant or recurrent pediatric brain tumors. J Neurooncol 2005;71:181 [PMID: 15690136].

Jakacki R et al: Outcome for metastatic (M+) medulloblastoma (MB) treated with carboplatin during craniospinal radiotherapy (CSRT) followed by cyclophosphamide (CPM) and vincristine: Preliminary results of COG 99701. J Clin Oncol 2007;25:A2017.

Komotar RJ et al: Pilomyxoid astrocytoma: A review. MedGenMed 2004;6:42 [PMID: 15775869].

Packer RJ et al: Long-term neurologic and neurosensory sequelae in adult survivors of a childhood brain tumor: Childhood cancer survivor study. J Clin Oncol 2003;21:3255 [PMID: 12947060].

Packer RJ et al: Phase III study of craniospinal radiation therapy followed by adjuvant chemotherapy for newly diagnosed average-risk medulloblastoma. J Clin Oncol 2006;24:4202 [PMID: 16943538].

Pollack IF et al: Association between chromosome 1p and 19q loss and outcome in pediatric malignant gliomas: Results from the CCG-945 cohort. Pediatr Neurosurg 2003;39:114 [PMID: 12876389].

LYMPHOMAS & LYMPHOPROLIFERATIVE DISORDERS

The term *lymphoma* refers to a malignant proliferation of lymphoid cells, usually in association with and arising from lymphoid tissues (ie, lymph nodes, thymus, spleen). In contrast, the term *leukemia* refers to a malignancy arising from the bone marrow, which may include lymphoid cells. Because lymphomas can involve the bone marrow, the distinction between the two can be confusing. The diagnosis of lymphoma is a common one among childhood cancers, accounting for 10–15% of all malignancies. The most common form is Hodgkin disease, which represents nearly half of all cases. The remaining subtypes, referred to collectively as non-Hodgkin lymphoma, are divided into four main groups: lymphoblastic, small noncleaved cell, large B-cell, and anaplastic large cell lymphomas.

In contrast to lymphomas, lymphoproliferative disorders (LPDs) are quite rare in the general population. Most are polyclonal, nonmalignant (though often life-threatening) accumulations of lymphocytes that occur when the immune system fails to control virally transformed lymphocytes. However, a malignant monoclonal proliferation can also arise. The post-transplant LPDs arise in patients who are immunosuppressed to prevent solid organ or bone marrow transplant rejection, particularly liver and heart transplant patients. Spontaneous LPDs occur in immunodeficient individuals and, less commonly, in immunocompetent persons.

1. Hodgkin Disease

► General Considerations

Children with Hodgkin disease have a better response to treatment than do adults, with a 75% overall survival rate at more than 20 years following diagnosis. Although adult therapies are applicable, the management of Hodgkin disease in children younger than age 18 years frequently differs. Because excellent disease control can result from several different therapeutic approaches, selection of staging procedures (radiographic, surgical, or other procedures to determine additional locations of disease) and treatment are often based on the potential long-term toxicity associated with the intervention.

Although Hodgkin disease represents 50% of the lymphomas of childhood, only 15% of all cases occur in children aged 16 years or younger. Children younger than age 5 years account for 3% of childhood cases. There is a 4:1 male predominance in the first decade. Notably, in underdeveloped countries the age distribution is quite different, with a peak incidence in younger children.

Hodgkin disease is subdivided into four histologic groups, and the distribution in children parallels that of adults: lymphocyte-predominant (10–20%); nodular sclerosing (40–60%) (increases with age); mixed cellularity (20–40%); and lymphocyte-depleted (5–10%). Prognosis is independent of subclassification, with appropriate therapy based on stage (see later discussion of staging).

► Clinical Findings

A. Symptoms and Signs

Children with Hodgkin disease usually present with painless cervical adenopathy. The lymph nodes often feel firmer than inflammatory nodes and have a rubbery texture. They may be discrete or matted together and are not fixed to surrounding tissue. The growth rate is variable, and involved nodes may wax and wane in size over weeks to months.

As Hodgkin disease nearly always arises in lymph nodes and spreads to contiguous nodal groups, a detailed examination of all nodal sites is mandatory. Lymphadenopathy is common in children, so the decision to perform biopsy is often difficult or delayed for a prolonged period. Indications for consideration of early lymph node biopsy include lack of identifiable infection in the region drained by the enlarged node, a node greater than 2 cm in size, supraclavicular adenopathy or abnormal chest radiograph, and lymphadenopathy increasing in size after 2 weeks or failing to resolve within 4–8 weeks.

Constitutional symptoms occur in about one third of children at presentation. Symptoms of fever greater than 38.0°C, weight loss of 10% in the previous 6 months, and drenching night sweats are defined by the Ann Arbor staging criteria as B symptoms. The A designation refers to the absence of these symptoms. B symptoms are of prognostic value, and more aggressive therapy is usually required for cure. Generalized pruritus and pain with alcohol ingestion may also occur.

Half of patients have asymptomatic mediastinal disease (adenopathy or anterior mediastinal mass), although symptoms due to compression of vital structures in the thorax may occur. A chest radiograph should be obtained when lymphoma is being considered. The mediastinum must be evaluated thoroughly before any surgical procedure is undertaken to avoid airway obstruction or cardiovascular collapse during anesthesia and possible death. Splenomegaly or hepatomegaly is generally associated with advanced disease.

B. Laboratory Findings

The CBC is usually normal, although anemia, neutrophilia, eosinophilia, and thrombocytosis may be present. The erythrocyte sedimentation rate and other acute-phase reactants are often elevated and can serve as markers of disease activity. Immunologic abnormalities occur, particularly in cell-mediated immunity, and anergy is common in patients with advanced-stage disease at diagnosis. Autoantibody phenomena such as hemolytic anemia and an idiopathic thrombocytopenic purpura–like picture have been reported.

C. Staging

Staging of Hodgkin disease determines treatment and prognosis. The most common staging system is the Ann Arbor classification that describes extent of disease by I–IV and symptoms by an A or a B suffix (eg, stage IIIB). A systematic search for disease includes chest radiography; CT scan of the chest, abdomen, and pelvis; and bilateral bone marrow aspirates and biopsies. Technetium bone scanning may show bony involvement and is usually reserved for patients with bone pain, as bone involvement is rare. Gallium scanning defines gallium-avid tumors and is most useful in evaluating residual mediastinal disease at the completion of treatment. Positron emission tomography is increasingly used in the staging and follow-up of patients with Hodgkin disease, often replacing gallium scanning.

The staging laparotomy in pediatrics is rarely performed because almost all patients are given systemic chemotherapy rather than radiation therapy. This shift in favored therapy is due to the toxicities of high-dose, extended-field radiation in children and the complications of laparotomy, including post-splenectomy sepsis.

D. Pathologic Findings

The diagnosis of Hodgkin disease requires the histologic presence of the Reed-Sternberg cell or its variants in tissue. Reed-Sternberg cells are germinal-center B cells that have undergone malignant transformation. Nearly 20% of these tumors in developed countries are positive for EBV, and there is building evidence to implicate EBV in the development of Hodgkin disease.

▶ Treatment & Prognosis

To achieve long-term disease-free survival while minimizing treatment toxicity, Hodgkin disease is increasingly treated by chemotherapy alone—and less often by radiation therapy.

Several combinations of chemotherapeutic agents are effective, and treatment times are relatively short compared with pediatric oncology protocols for leukemia. A current COG study is addressing whether only 9 weeks of therapy with AV-PC (Adriamycin [doxorubicin], vincristine, prednisone, and cyclophosphamide) is sufficient to induce a complete response in patients with low-risk Hodgkin disease. Two additional drugs, bleomycin and etoposide, are currently added in the treatment of intermediate-risk patients for a total of 4–6 months of therapy for patients with intermediate-risk disease. The removal of involved field irradiation in patients with intermediate-risk Hodgkin disease who respond early to chemotherapy is being investigated. Combined-modality therapy with chemotherapy and irradiation is used in advanced disease.

Current treatment gives children with stage I and stage II Hodgkin disease at least a 90% disease-free likelihood of survival 5 years after diagnosis, which generally equates with cure. Two thirds of all relapses occur within 2 years after diagnosis, and relapse rarely occurs beyond 4 years. In more advanced disease (stages III and IV), 5-year event-free survival rates range from over 60% to 90%. With more patients being long-term survivors of Hodgkin disease, the risk of secondary malignancies, both leukemias and solid tumors, is becoming more apparent and is higher in patients receiving radiation therapy. Therefore, elucidating the optimal treatment strategy that minimizes such risk should be the goal of future studies.

Patients with relapsed Hodgkin disease are often salvageable using chemotherapy and radiation therapy. An increasingly popular alternative is autologous HSCT, which may improve survival rates. Allogeneic HSCT is also used, but carries increased risks of complications and may not offer added survival benefit.

Buglio D: Novel small-molecule therapy of Hodgkin lymphoma. Expert Rev Anticancer Ther 2007;7:735 [PMID: 17492936].

Hodgkin's lymphoma in younger patients: Lessons learned on the road to success. Oncology 2007;21:434 [PMID: 17474345].

Lin HM: Second malignancy after treatment of pediatric Hodgkin disease. J Pediatr Hematol Oncol 2005;27:28 [PMID: 15654275].

Schwartz CL: Special issues in pediatric Hodgkin's disease. Eur J Haematol 2005;Suppl 66:55 [PMID: 16007870].

2. Non-Hodgkin Lymphoma

▶ Cough, dyspnea, orthopnea, swelling of the face, lymphadenopathy, mediastinal mass, pleural effusion.

▶ Abdominal pain, abdominal distention, vomiting, constipation, abdominal mass, ascites, hepatosplenomegaly.

▶ Adenopathy, fevers, neurologic deficit, skin lesions.

▶ General Considerations

Non-Hodgkin lymphomas (NHLs) are a diverse group of cancers accounting for 5–10% of malignancies in children younger than age 15 years. About 500 new cases arise per year in the United States. The incidence of NHLs increases with age. Children aged 15 years or younger account for only 3% of all cases of NHLs, and the disease is uncommon before age 5 years. There is a male predominance of approximately 3:1. In equatorial Africa, NHLs cause almost 50% of pediatric malignancies.

Most children who develop NHL are immunologically normal. However, children with congenital or acquired immune deficiencies (eg, Wiskott-Aldrich syndrome, severe combined immunodeficiency syndrome, X-linked lymphoproliferative syndrome, HIV infection, immunosuppressive therapy following solid organ or marrow transplantation) have an increased risk of developing NHLs. It has been estimated that their risk is 100–10,000 times that of age-matched control subjects.

Animal models suggest a viral contribution to the pathogenesis of NHL, and there is evidence of viral involvement in human NHL as well. In equatorial Africa, 95% of Burkitt lymphomas contain DNA from the Epstein-Barr virus. But in North America, less than 20% of Burkitt tumors contain the EBV genome. The role of other viruses (eg, human herpesviruses 6 and 8), disturbances in host immunologic defenses, chronic immunostimulation, and specific chromosomal rearrangements as potential triggers in the development of NHL is under investigation.

Unlike adult NHL, virtually all childhood NHLs are rapidly proliferating, high-grade, diffuse malignancies. These tumors exhibit aggressive behavior but are usually very responsive to treatment. Nearly all pediatric NHLs are histologically classified into four main groups: lymphoblastic lymphoma (LL), small noncleaved cell lymphoma (Burkitt lymphoma [BL] and Burkitt-like lymphoma [BLL]), large B-cell lymphoma (LBCL), and anaplastic large cell lymphoma (ALCL). Immunophenotyping and cytogenetic features, in addition to clinical presentation, are increasingly important in the classification, pathogenesis, and treatment of NHLs. Comparisons of pediatric NHLs are summarized in Table 29–5.

Table 29–5. Comparison of pediatric non-Hodgkin lymphomas.

	Lymphoblastic Lymphoma	Small Noncleaved Cell Lymphoma (BL and BLL)	Large B-Cell Lymphoma	Anaplastic Large Cell Lymphoma
Incidence (%)	30–40	35–50	10–15	10–15
Histopathologic features	Indistinguishable from ALL lymphoblasts	Large nucleus with prominent nucleoli surrounded by very basophilic cytoplasm that contains lipid vacuoles	Large cells with cleaved or noncleaved nuclei	Large pleomorphic cells
Immunophenotype	Immature T cell	B cell	B cell	T cell or null cell
Cytogenetic markers	Translocations involving chromosome 14q11 and chromosome 7; interstitial deletions of chromosome 1	t(8;14), t(8;22), t(2;8)	Many	t(2;5)
Clinical presentation	Intrathoracic tumor, mediastinal mass (50–70%), lymphadenopathy above diaphragm (50–80%)	Intra-abdominal tumor (90%), jaw involvement (10–20% sporadic BL, 70% endemic BL), bone marrow involvement	Abdominal tumor most common; unusual sites: lung, face, brain, bone, testes, muscle	Lymphadenopathy, fever, weight loss, night sweats, extranodal sites including viscera and skin
Treatment	Similar to ALL therapy; 24 mos duration	Intensive administration of alkylating agents and methotrexate; CNS prophylaxis; 3–9 mo duration	Similar to therapy for BL/BLL	Similar to therapy for lymphoblastic lymphoma or BL/BLL

ALL, acute lymphoblastic leukemia; BL, Burkitt lymphoma; BLL, Burkitt-like lymphoma.

▶ Clinical Findings

A. Symptoms and Signs

Childhood NHLs can arise in any site of lymphoid tissue, including lymph nodes, thymus, liver, and spleen. Common extralymphatic sites include bone, bone marrow, CNS, skin, and testes. Signs and symptoms at presentation are determined by the location of lesions and the degree of dissemination. Because NHL usually progresses very rapidly, the duration of symptoms is quite brief, from days to a few weeks. Nevertheless, children present with a limited number of syndromes, most of which correlate with cell type.

Children with LL often present with symptoms of airway compression (cough, dyspnea, orthopnea) or superior vena cava obstruction (facial edema, chemosis, plethora, venous engorgement), which are a result of mediastinal disease. *These symptoms are a true emergency necessitating rapid diagnosis and treatment.* Pleural or pericardial effusions may further compromise the patient's respiratory and cardiovascular status. CNS and bone marrow involvement are not common at diagnosis. When bone marrow contains more than 25% lymphoblasts, patients are diagnosed with ALL.

Most patients with BL and BLL present with abdominal disease. Abdominal pain, distention, a right lower quadrant mass, or intussusception in a child older than age 5 years suggests the diagnosis of BL. Bone marrow involvement is common (~65% of patients). BL is the most rapidly prolifer-

ating tumor known and has a high rate of spontaneous cell death as it outgrows its blood supply. Consequently, children presenting with massive abdominal disease frequently have tumor lysis syndrome (hyperuricemia, hyperphosphatemia, and hyperkalemia). These abnormalities can be aggravated by tumor infiltration of the kidney or urinary obstruction by tumor. Although similar histologically, numerous differences exist between cases of BL occurring in endemic areas of equatorial Africa and the sporadic cases of North America (Table 29–6).

Table 29–6. Comparison of endemic and sporadic Burkitt lymphoma.

	Endemic	Sporadic
Incidence	10 per 100,000	0.9 per 100,000
Cytogenetics	Chromosome 8 breakpoint upstream of c-*myc* locus	Chromosome 8 breakpoint within c-*myc* locus
EBV association	≥ 95%	≤ 20%
Disease sites at presentation	Jaw (58%), abdomen (58%), CNS (19%), orbit (11%), marrow (7%)	Jaw (7%), abdomen (91%), CNS (14%), orbit (1%), marrow (20%)

CNS, central nervous system; EBV, Epstein-Barr virus.

Large cell lymphomas are similar clinically to the small noncleaved cell lymphomas, although unusual sites of involvement are quite common, particularly with ALCL. Skin lesions, focal neurologic deficits, and pleural or peritoneal effusions without an obvious associated mass are frequently seen.

B. Diagnostic Evaluation

Diagnosis is made by biopsy of involved tissue with histology, immunophenotyping, and cytogenetic studies. If mediastinal disease is present, general anesthesia must be avoided if the airway or vena cava is compromised by tumor. In these cases samples of pleural or ascitic fluid, bone marrow, or peripheral nodes obtained under local anesthesia may confirm the diagnosis. Major abdominal surgery and intestinal resection should be avoided in patients with an abdominal mass that is likely to be BL, as the tumor will regress rapidly with the initiation of chemotherapy. The rapid growth of these tumors and the associated life-threatening complications demand that further studies be done expeditiously so that specific therapy is not delayed.

After a thorough physical examination, a CBC, liver function tests, and a biochemical profile (electrolytes, calcium, phosphorus, uric acid, renal function) should be obtained. An elevated LDH reflects tumor burden and can serve as a marker of disease activity. Imaging studies should include a chest radiograph and chest CT scan, an abdominal ultrasound or CT scan, and possibly a gallium or positron emission tomography scan. Bone marrow and CSF examinations are also essential.

▶ Treatment

A. Supportive Care

The management of life-threatening problems at presentation is critical. The most common complications are superior mediastinal syndrome and acute tumor lysis syndrome. Patients with airway compromise require prompt initiation of specific therapy. Because of the risk of general anesthesia in these patients, it is occasionally necessary to initiate corticosteroids or low-dose emergency radiation therapy until the mass is small enough for a biopsy to be undertaken safely. Response to steroids and radiation therapy is usually prompt (12–24 hours).

Tumor lysis syndrome should be anticipated in all patients who have NHL with a large tumor burden. Maintaining a brisk urine output (> 5 mL/kg/h) with intravenous fluids and diuretics is the key to management. Allopurinol will reduce serum uric acid, and alkalinization of urine will increase its solubility. Rasburicase is an effective intravenous alternative to allopurinol. Because phosphate precipitates in alkaline urine, alkali administration should be discontinued if hyperphosphatemia occurs. Renal dialysis is occasionally necessary to control metabolic abnormalities. Every attempt should be made to correct or minimize metabolic abnormalities before initiating chemotherapy;

however, this period of stabilization should not exceed 24–48 hours.

B. Specific Therapy

Systemic chemotherapy is the mainstay of therapy for NHLs. Nearly all patients with NHL require intensive intrathecal chemotherapy for CNS prophylaxis. Surgical resection is not indicated unless the entire tumor can be resected safely, which is rare. Partial resection or debulking surgery has no role. Radiation therapy does not improve outcome, so its use is confined to exceptional circumstances.

Therapy for LL is generally based on treatment protocols designed for ALL and involves dose-intensive, multiagent chemotherapy. The duration of therapy is 2 years. Treatment of BL and BLL using alkylating agents and intermediate- to high-dose methotrexate administered intensively but for a relatively short time produce the highest cure rates. LBCL is treated similarly, whereas ALCL has been treated with both BL and LL protocols.

Monoclonal antibodies such as rituximab (anti-CD20) allow for more targeted therapy of lymphomas and have been successful in improving outcomes in adults. Studies employing this type of therapy in children are underway in those with newly diagnosed as well as relapsed or refractory B-cell NHL.

▶ Prognosis

A major predictor of outcome in NHL is the extent of disease at diagnosis. Ninety percent of patients with localized disease can expect long-term, disease-free survival. Patients with extensive disease on both sides of the diaphragm, CNS involvement, or bone marrow involvement in addition to a primary site have a 70–80% failure-free survival rate. Relapses occur early in NHL; patients with LL rarely have recurrences after 30 months from diagnosis, whereas patients with BL and BLL very rarely have recurrences beyond 1 year. Patients who experience relapse may have a chance for cure by autologous or allogeneic HSCT.

Cairo MS et al: Childhood and adolescent non-Hodgkin lymphoma: New insights in biology and critical challenges for the future. Pediatr Blood Cancer 2005;45:753 [PMID: 15929129].

Jacobsen E et al: Update on the therapy of highly aggressive non-Hodgkin's lymphoma. Expert Opin Biol Ther 2006;6:699 [PMID: 16805709].

Shukla NN et al: Non-Hodgkin's lymphoma in children and adolescents. Curr Oncol Rep 2006;8:387 [PMID: 16901400].

Yuston JT et al: Biology and treatment of Burkitt's lymphoma. Curr Opin Hematol 2007;14:375 [PMID: 17534164].

3. Lymphoproliferative Disorders

LPDs can be thought of as a part of a continuum with lymphomas. Whereas LPDs represent inappropriate, often polyclonal proliferations of nonmalignant lymphocytes, lymphomas represent the development of malignant clones, sometimes arising from recognized LPDs.

A. Post-Transplantation Lymphoproliferative Disorders

Post-transplantation lymphoproliferative disorders (PTLDs) arise in patients who have received substantial immuno-suppressive medications for solid organ or bone marrow transplantation. In these patients, reactivation of latent EBV infection in B cells drives a polyclonal proliferation of these cells that is fatal if not halted. Occasionally a true lymphoma develops, often bearing a chromosomal translocation.

LPDs are an increasingly common and significant complication of transplantation. The incidence of PTLD ranges from approximately 2% to 15% of transplant recipients, depending on the organ transplanted and the immunosuppressive regimen.

Treatment of these disorders is a challenge for transplant physicians and oncologists. The initial treatment is reduction in immunosuppression, which allows the patient's own immune cells to destroy the virally transformed lymphocytes. However, this is only effective in approximately half of the patients. For those patients who do not respond to reduced immune suppression, chemotherapy of various regimens may succeed. The use of anti-B-cell antibodies, such as rituximab (anti-CD20), for the treatment of PTLDs has been promising in clinical trials.

B. Spontaneous Lymphoproliferative Disease

Immunodeficiencies in which LPDs occur include Bloom syndrome, Chédiak-Higashi syndrome, ataxia-telangiectasia, Wiskott-Aldrich syndrome, X-linked lymphoproliferative syndrome, congenital T-cell immunodeficiencies, and HIV infection. Treatment depends on the circumstances, but unlike PTLD, few therapeutic options are often available. Castleman disease is an LPD occurring in pediatric patients without any apparent immunodeficiency. The autoimmune lymphoproliferative syndrome (ALPS) is characterized by widespread lymphadenopathy with hepatosplenomegaly, and autoimmune phenomena. ALPS results from mutations in the Fas ligand pathway that is critical in regulation of apoptosis.

Gheorghe G et al: Posttransplant Hodgkin lymphoma preceded by polymorphic posttransplant lymphoproliferative disorder: Report of a pediatric case and review of the literature. J Pediatr Hematol Oncol 2007;29:112 [PMID: 17279008].

Gottschalk S et al: Post-transplant lymphoproliferative disorders. Annu Rev Med 2005;56:29 [PMID: 15660500].

Giulina LB et al: Treatment with rituximab in benign and malignant hematologic disorders in children. J Pediatr 2007;150:338 [PMID: 17382107].

Gross TG: Post-transplant lymphoproliferative disease in children following solid organ transplant and rituximab—the final answer? Pediatr Transplant 2007;11:575 [PMID: 17663676].

NEUROBLASTOMA

ESSENTIALS OF DIAGNOSIS & TYPICAL FEATURES

► Bone pain, abdominal pain, anorexia, weight loss, fatigue, fever, irritability.
► Abdominal mass (65%), adenopathy, proptosis, periorbital ecchymosis, skull masses, subcutaneous nodules, hepatomegaly, spinal cord compression.

► General Considerations

Neuroblastoma arises from neural crest tissue of the sympathetic ganglia or adrenal medulla. It is composed of small, fairly uniform cells with little cytoplasm and hyperchromatic nuclei that may form rosette patterns. Pathologic diagnosis is not always easy, and neuroblastoma must be differentiated from the other "small, round, blue cell" malignancies of childhood (Ewing sarcoma, rhabdomyosarcoma, peripheral neuroectodermal tumor, and lymphoma).

Neuroblastoma accounts for 7–10% of pediatric malignancies and is the most common solid neoplasm outside the CNS. Fifty percent of neuroblastomas are diagnosed before age 2 years and 90% before age 5 years.

Neuroblastoma is a biologically diverse disease with varied clinical behavior ranging from spontaneous regression to progression through very aggressive therapy. Unfortunately, despite significant advances in our understanding of this tumor at the cellular and molecular level, the overall survival rate in advanced disease has changed little in 20 years, with 3-year event-free survival being less than 15%.

► Clinical Findings

A. Symptoms and Signs

Clinical manifestations vary with the primary site of malignant disease and the neuroendocrine function of the tumor. Many children present with constitutional symptoms such as fever, weight loss, and irritability. Bone pain suggests metastatic disease, which is present in 60% of children older than 1 year of age at diagnosis. Physical examination may reveal a firm, fixed, irregularly shaped mass that extends beyond the midline. The margins are often poorly defined. Although most children have an abdominal primary tumor (40% adrenal gland, 25% paraspinal ganglion), neuroblastoma can arise wherever there is sympathetic tissue. In the posterior mediastinum, the tumor is usually asymptomatic and discovered on a chest radiograph obtained for other reasons. Patients with cervical neuroblastoma present with a neck mass, which is often misdiagnosed as infection. Horner syndrome (unilateral ptosis, myosis, and anhydrosis) or heterochromia iridis (differently colored irises) may accompany cervical neuroblastoma. Paraspinous tumors can extend through the spinal foramina, causing cord compression. Patients may present with paresis, paralysis, and bowel or bladder dysfunction.

The most common sites of metastases are bone, bone marrow, lymph nodes (regional as well as disseminated), liver, and subcutaneous tissue. Neuroblastoma has a predilection for metastasis to the skull, in particular the sphenoid bone and retrobulbar tissue. This causes periorbital ecchymosis and proptosis. Liver metastasis, particularly in the newborn, can be massive. Subcutaneous nodules are bluish in color and associated with an erythematous flush followed by blanching when compressed, probably secondary to catecholamine release.

Neuroblastoma may also be associated with unusual paraneoplastic manifestations. Perhaps the most striking example is opsoclonus-myoclonus, also called dancing eyes/dancing feet syndrome. This phenomenon is characterized by the acute onset of rapid and chaotic eye movements, myoclonic jerking of the limbs and trunk, ataxia, and behavioral disturbances. This process, which often persists after therapy is complete, is thought to be secondary to cross-reacting antineural antibodies. Intractable, chronic watery diarrhea is associated with tumor secretion of vasoactive intestinal peptides. Both of these paraneoplastic syndromes are associated with favorable outcomes.

B. Laboratory Findings

Anemia is present in 60% of children with neuroblastoma and can be due to chronic disease or marrow infiltration. Occasionally, thrombocytopenia is present, but thrombocytosis is a more common finding, even with metastatic disease in the marrow. Urinary catecholamines (vanillylmandelic acid and homovanillic acid) are elevated in at least 90% of patients at diagnosis and should be measured prior to surgery.

C. Imaging

Plain radiographs of the primary tumor may show stippled calcifications. Metastases to bone appear irregular and lytic. Periosteal reaction and pathologic fractures may also be seen. CT scanning provides more information, including the extent of the primary tumor, its effects on surrounding structures, and the presence of liver and lymph node metastases. Classically, in tumors originating from the adrenal gland, the kidney is displaced inferolaterally, which helps to differentiate neuroblastoma from Wilms tumor. MRI is useful in determining the presence of spinal cord involvement in tumors that appear to invade neural foramina.

Technetium bone scanning is obtained for the evaluation of bone metastases, because the tumor usually takes up technetium Metaiodobenzyl-guanidine (MIBG) scanning is also performed to detect metastatic disease.

D. Staging

Staging of neuroblastoma is performed according to the International Neuroblastoma Staging System (INSS) (Table

Table 29–7. International Neuroblastoma Staging System.

Stage	Description
1	Localized tumor with complete gross excision, with or without microscopic residual disease; representative ipsilateral lymph nodes negative for tumor microscopically.
2A	Localized tumor with incomplete gross excision; representative ipsilateral nonadherent lymph nodes negative for tumor microscopically.
2B	Localized tumor with or without complete gross excision, with ipsilateral nonadherent lymph nodes positive for tumor. Enlarged lymph nodes must be negative microscopically.
3	Unresectable unilateral tumor infiltrating across the midline, with or without regional lymph node involvement; or localized unilateral tumor with contralateral regional lymph node involvement; or midline tumor with bilateral extension by infiltration (unresectable) or by lymph node involvement. The midline is defined as the vertebral column. Tumors originating on one side and crossing the midline must infiltrate to or beyond the opposite side of the vertebral column.
4	Any primary tumor with dissemination to distant lymph nodes, bone, bone marrow, liver, skin, or other organs, except as defined for stage 4S.
4S	Localized primary tumor, as defined for stage 1, 2A, or 2B, with dissemination limited to skin, liver, or bone marrow, and limited to infants younger than age 1 y. Marrow involvement should be < 10% of nucleated cells.

29–7). A biopsy of the tumor is performed to determine the biologic characteristics of the tumor. In addition, bilateral bone marrow aspirates and biopsies must be performed to evaluate marrow involvement.

Tumors are classified as favorable or unfavorable based on histologic characteristics. Amplification of the *MYCN* protooncogene is a reliable marker of aggressive clinical behavior with rapid disease progression. Tumor cell DNA content is also predictive of outcome. Hyperdiploidy is a favorable finding, whereas diploid DNA content is associated with a worse outcome.

▶ Treatment & Prognosis

Patients are treated based on a risk stratification system adopted by the COG based on INSS stage, age, *MYCN* status, histology, and DNA index. The mainstay of therapy is surgical resection coupled with chemotherapy. The usually massive size of the tumor often makes primary resection impossible. Under these circumstances, only a biopsy is performed. Following chemotherapy, a second surgical procedure may allow for resection of the primary tumor. Radiation therapy is sometimes also necessary. Effective chemotherapeutic agents in the treatment of neuroblastoma include cyclophosphamide, doxorubicin, etoposide, cisplatin, vincristine, and topotecan. About 80% of patients achieve complete or partial remission, although in advanced disease, remission is seldom durable.

For low-risk disease (stage 1 and 2, with good biologic features), surgical resection alone may be sufficient to affect a cure. Infants younger than 1 year with stage 4S disease may need little if any therapy, although chemotherapy may be initiated because of bulky disease causing mechanical complications. In intermediate-risk neuroblastoma (subsets of patients with stage 3 and 4 disease) the primary treatment approach is surgical combined with chemotherapy. High-risk patients (the majority with stage 3 and 4 disease) require multimodal therapy, including surgery, irradiation, chemotherapy, and autologous HSCT. The administration of *cis*-retinoic acid, a differentiating agent, can prolong disease-free survival in advanced-stage neuroblastoma when administered in the setting of minimal residual disease (MRD) after HSCT.

Cooperative clinical trials are underway in high-risk patients using ch14.18 (a monoclonal antibody specific for the predominant antigen on neuroblastoma cells) and cytokines to eradicate MRD. A phase II study is underway using fenretinide, a synthetic retinoid, and radiolabeled MIBG is also being investigated.

For children with stage 1, 2, or 4S disease, the 5-year survival rate is 70–90%. Infants younger than 460 days old have a greater than 80% likelihood of long-term survival. Children older than age 1 year with stage 3 disease have an intermediate prognosis (approximately 40–70%). Older patients with stage 4 disease have a poor prognosis (5–50% survival 5 years from diagnosis), although patients 12–18 months old with hyperdiploidy and nonamplified *MYCN* have an excellent prognosis.

George RE et al: Hyperdiploidy plus nonamplified *MYCN* confers a favorable prognosis in children 12–18 months old with disseminated neuroblastoma: A Pediatric Oncology Group Study. J Clin Oncol 2005;23:6466 [PMID: 16116152].

London WB et al: Evidence for an age cutoff greater than 365 days for neuroblastoma risk group stratification in the children's oncology group. J Clin Oncol 2005;23:6459 [PMID: 16116153].

Matthay KK et al: Opsoclonus myoclonus syndrome in neuroblastoma: A report from a workshop on the dancing eyes syndrome at the advances in neuroblastoma meeting in Genoa, Italy, 2004. Cancer Lett 2005;228:275 [PMID: 15922508].

National Cancer Institute: http://www.cancer.gov/cancertopics/types/neuroblastoma.

Schmidt ML et al: Favorable prognosis for patients 12–18 months of age with stage 4 nonamplified *MYCN* neuroblastoma: A Children's Cancer Group Study. J Clin Oncol 2005;23:6474 [PMID: 16116154].

WILMS TUMOR (NEPHROBLASTOMA)

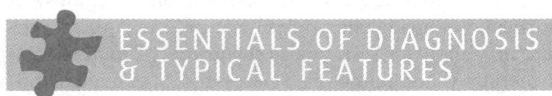

ESSENTIALS OF DIAGNOSIS & TYPICAL FEATURES

▸ Asymptomatic abdominal mass or swelling (83%).

▸ Fever (23%), hematuria (21%).

▸ Hypertension (25%), genitourinary malformations (6%), aniridia, hemihypertrophy.

General Considerations

Approximately 460 new cases of Wilms tumor occur annually in the United States, representing 5–6% of cancers in children younger than age 15 years. After neuroblastoma, this is the second most common abdominal tumor in children. The majority of Wilms tumors are of sporadic occurrence. However, in a few children, Wilms tumor occurs in the setting of associated malformations or syndromes, including aniridia, hemihypertrophy, genitourinary malformations (eg, cryptorchidism, hypospadias, gonadal dysgenesis, pseudohermaphroditism, and horseshoe kidney), Beckwith-Wiedemann syndrome, Denys-Drash syndrome, and WAGR syndrome (Wilms tumor, aniridia, ambiguous genitalia, mental retardation).

The median age at diagnosis is related both to gender and laterality, with bilateral tumors presenting at a younger age than unilateral tumors, and males being diagnosed earlier than females. Wilms tumor occurs most commonly between ages 2 and 5 years; it is unusual after age 6 years. The mean age at diagnosis is 4 years.

Clinical Findings

A. Symptoms and Signs

Most children with Wilms tumor present with increasing size of the abdomen or an asymptomatic abdominal mass incidentally discovered by a parent. The mass is usually smooth and firm, well demarcated, and rarely crosses the midline, though it can extend inferiorly into the pelvis. About 25% of patients are hypertensive at presentation. Gross hematuria is an uncommon presentation, although microscopic hematuria occurs in approximately 25% of patients.

B. Laboratory Findings

The CBC is usually normal, but some patients have anemia secondary to hemorrhage into the tumor. Blood urea nitrogen and serum creatinine are usually normal. Urinalysis may show some blood or leukocytes.

C. Imaging and Staging

Ultrasonography or CT of the abdomen should establish the presence of an intrarenal mass. It is also essential to evaluate the contralateral kidney for presence and function as well as synchronous Wilms tumor. The inferior vena cava needs to be evaluated by ultrasonography for the presence and extent of tumor propagation. The liver should be imaged for the presence of metastatic disease. A plain chest radiograph (four views) or chest CT scans (or both) should be obtained to determine whether pulmonary metastases are present.

Approximately 10% of patients will have metastatic disease at diagnosis. Of these, 80% will have pulmonary disease and 15% liver metastases. Bone and brain metastases are extremely uncommon and usually associated with different, more aggressive renal tumors, such as clear cell sarcoma or rhabdoid tumor; hence, bone scans and brain imaging are not routinely performed. The clinical stage is ultimately decided at surgery and confirmed by the pathologist.

▶ Treatment & Prognosis

In the United States, treatment of Wilms tumor begins with surgical exploration of the abdomen via an anterior surgical approach to allow for inspection and palpation of the contralateral kidney. The liver and lymph nodes are inspected and suspicious areas biopsied or excised. En bloc resection of tumor is performed. Every attempt is made to avoid tumor spillage at surgery as this may change staging and treatment. Because therapy is tailored to tumor stage, it is imperative that a surgeon familiar with the staging requirements perform the operation.

In addition to the staging, the histologic type has implications for therapy and prognosis. Favorable histology (FH; see later discussion) refers to the classic triphasic Wilms tumor and its variants. Unfavorable histology (UH) refers to the presence of diffuse anaplasia (extreme nuclear atypia) and is present in 5% of Wilms tumors. Only a few small foci of anaplasia in a Wilms tumor give a worse prognosis to patients with stage II, III, or IV tumors. Loss of heterozygosity of chromosomes 1p and 16q are adverse prognostic factors in those with favorable histology. Following excision and pathologic examination, the patient is assigned a stage that defines further therapy.

Improvement in the treatment of Wilms tumor has resulted in an overall cure rate of approximately 90%. The National Wilms Tumor Study Group's fourth study (NWTS-4) demonstrated that survival rates were improved by intensifying therapy during the initial treatment phase while shortening overall treatment duration (24 weeks vs 60 weeks of treatment).

Table 29–8 provides an overview of the current treatment recommendations in NWTS-5. Patients with stage III or IV Wilms tumor require radiation therapy to the tumor bed and to sites of metastatic disease. Chemotherapy is optimally begun within 5 days after surgery, whereas radiation therapy should be started within 10 days. Stage V (bilateral Wilms tumor) disease dictates a different approach, consisting of possible bilateral renal biopsies followed by chemotherapy and second-look renal-sparing surgery. Radiation therapy may also be necessary.

Using these approaches, 4-year overall survival rates through NWTS-4 are as follows: stage I FH, 96%; stage II–IV FH, 82–92%; stage I–III UH (diffuse anaplasia), 56–70%; stage IV UH, 17%. Patients with recurrent Wilms tumor have a salvage rate of approximately 50% with surgery, radiation therapy, and chemotherapy (singly or in combina-

Table 29–8. Treatment of Wilms tumor.

Stage/Histologic Subtype	Treatment
I–II FH and I UH	18 weeks (dactinomycin and vincristine)
III–IV FH and II–IV focal anaplasia	24 weeks (dactinomycin, vincristine, and doxorubicin) with radiation
II–IV UH (diffuse anaplasia)	24 weeks (vincristine, doxorubicin, etoposide, and cyclophosphamide with radiation

FH, favorable histology; UH, unfavorable histology.

tion). HSCT is also being explored as a way to improve the chances of survival after relapse.

Future Considerations

Although progress in the treatment of Wilms tumor has been extraordinary, important questions remain to be answered. Questions have been raised regarding the role of prenephrectomy chemotherapy in the treatment of Wilms tumor. Presurgical chemotherapy seems to decrease tumor rupture at resection but may unfavorably affect outcome by changing staging. Future studies will be directed at minimizing acute and long-term toxicities for those with low-risk disease and improving outcomes for those with high-risk and recurrent disease.

Grundy PE et al: Loss of heterozygosity for chromosomes 1p and 16q is an adverse prognostic factor in favorable-histology Wilms tumor: A report from the National Wilms Tumor Study Group. J Clin Oncol 2005;23:7312 [PMID: 16129848].

Kalapurakal JA et al: Management of Wilms' tumour: Current practice and future goals. Lancet Oncol 2004;5:37 [PMID: 14700607].

National Cancer Institute: http://www.cancer.gov/cancertopics/types/wilms

Rivera MN, Haber DA: Wilms' tumour: Connecting tumorigenesis and organ development in the kidney. Natl Rev Cancer 2005;5:699 [PMID: 16110318].

BONE TUMORS

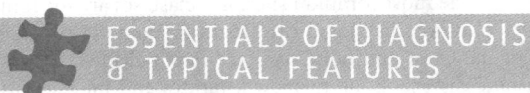

ESSENTIALS OF DIAGNOSIS & TYPICAL FEATURES

▶ Bone pain.

▶ Mass lesion noted on examination.

Primary malignant bone tumors are uncommon in childhood with only 650–700 new cases per year. Osteosarcoma accounts for 60% of cases and occurs mostly in adolescents and young adults. Ewing sarcoma is the second most common malignant tumor of bony origin and occurs in toddle to young adults. Both tumors have a male predominance

The cardinal signs of bone tumor are pain at the site of involvement, often following slight trauma, mass formation, and fracture through an area of cortical bone destruction.

1. Osteosarcoma

General Considerations

Although osteosarcoma is the sixth most common malignancy in childhood, it ranks third among adolescents and young adults. This peak occurrence during the adolescent growth spurt suggests a causal relationship between rapid bone growth and malignant transformation. Further evidence for this relationship is found in epidemiologic data showing patients with osteosarcoma to be taller than their peers, osteosarcoma occurring most frequently at sites where the greatest increase in length and size of bone occurs, and osteosarcoma occurring at an earlier age in girls than boys, corresponding to their earlier growth spurt. The metaphyses of long tubular bones are primarily affected. The distal femur accounts for more than 40% of cases, with the proximal tibia, proximal humerus, and mid and proximal femur following in frequency.

Clinical Findings

A. Symptoms and Signs

Pain over the involved area is the usual presenting symptom with or without an associated soft tissue mass. Patients generally have symptoms for several months prior to diagnosis. Systemic symptoms (fever, weight loss) are rare. Laboratory evaluation may reveal elevated serum alkaline phosphatase or LDH levels.

B. Imaging and Staging

Radiographic findings show permeative destruction of the normal bony trabecular pattern with indistinct margins. In addition, periosteal new bone formation and lifting of the bony cortex may create a Codman triangle. A soft tissue mass plus calcifications in a radial or sunburst pattern are frequently noted. MRI is more sensitive in defining the extent of the primary tumor and in many centers has replaced CT scanning. The most common sites of metastases are the lung ($\leq$ 20% of newly diagnosed cases) and the bone (10%). CT scan of the chest and bone scan are essential for detecting metastatic disease. Bone marrow aspirates and biopsies are not indicated.

Despite the rather characteristic radiographic appearance, a tissue sample is needed to confirm the diagnosis. Placement of the incision for biopsy is of critical importance. A misplaced incision could preclude a limb salvage procedure and necessitate amputation. The surgeon who will carry out the definitive surgical procedure should perform the biopsy. A staging system for osteosarcoma based on local tumor extent and presence or absence of distant metastasis has been proposed, but it has not been validated.

Treatment & Prognosis

Historical studies showed that over 50% of patients receiving surgery alone developed pulmonary metastases within 6 months after surgery. This suggests the presence of micrometastatic disease at diagnosis. Adjuvant chemotherapy trials showed improved disease-free survival rates of 55–85% in patients followed for 3–10 years.

Osteosarcomas are highly radioresistant lesions; for this reason, radiation therapy has no role in its primary management. Chemotherapy is often administered prior to definitive surgery (neoadjuvant chemotherapy). This permits an early attack on micrometastatic disease and may also shrink the tumor, facilitating a limb salvage procedure. Preoperative chemotherapy also makes detailed histologic evaluation of tumor response to the chemotherapy agents possible. If the histologic response is poor (> 10% viable tumor tissue), postoperative chemotherapy can be changed accordingly. Chemotherapy may be administered intra-arterially or intravenously, although the benefits of intra-arterial chemotherapy are disputed. Agents having efficacy in the treatment of osteosarcoma include doxorubicin, cisplatin, high-dose methotrexate, and ifosfamide.

Definitive cure requires en bloc surgical resection of the tumor with a margin of uninvolved tissue. Amputation and limb salvage are equally effective in achieving local control of osteosarcoma. Contraindications to limb-sparing surgery include major involvement of the neurovascular bundle by tumor; immature skeletal age, particularly for lower extremity tumors; infection in the region of the tumor; inappropriate biopsy site; and extensive muscle involvement that would result in a poor functional outcome.

Postsurgical chemotherapy is generally continued until the patient has received 1 year of treatment. Relapses are unusual beyond 3 years, but late relapses do occur. Histologic response to neoadjuvant chemotherapy is an excellent predictor of outcome. Patients with localized disease having 90% tumor necrosis have a 70–85% long-term, disease-free survival rate. Other favorable prognostic factors include distal skeletal lesions, longer duration of symptoms, age older than 20 years, female gender, and near-diploid tumor DNA index. Patients with metastatic disease at diagnosis or multifocal bone lesions do not fair well, despite advances in chemotherapy and surgical techniques.

2. Ewing Sarcoma

General Considerations

Ewing sarcoma accounts for only 10% of primary malignant bone tumors; fewer than 200 new cases occur each year in the United States. It is a disease primarily of white males, almost never affects blacks, and occurs mostly in the second decade of life. Ewing sarcoma is considered a "small, round, blue cell" malignancy. The differential diagnosis includes rhabdomyosarcoma, lymphoma, and neuroblastoma. Although most commonly a tumor of bone, it may also occur in soft tissue (extraosseous Ewing sarcoma or peripheral neuroectodermal tumor [PNET]).

Clinical Findings

A. Symptoms and Signs

Pain at the site of the primary tumor is the most common presenting sign, with or without swelling and erythema. No specific laboratory findings are characteristic of Ewing sarcoma, but an elevated LDH may be present and is of prognostic significance.

B. Imaging and Staging

The radiographic appearance of Ewing sarcoma overlaps with osteosarcoma, although Ewing sarcoma usually involves the diaphyses of long bones. The central axial skeleton gives rise to 40% of Ewing tumors. Evaluation of a patient diagnosed as having Ewing sarcoma should include CT scan or MRI (or both) of the primary lesion to define the extent of local disease as precisely as possible. This is imperative for planning future surgical procedures or radiation therapy. Metastatic disease is present in 25% of patients at diagnosis. The lung (38%), bone (particularly the spine) (31%), and the bone marrow (11%) are the most common sites for metastasis. CT scan of the chest, bone scanning, and bilateral bone marrow aspirates and biopsies are all essential to the staging workup.

A biopsy is essential in establishing the diagnosis. Histologically, Ewing sarcoma consists of sheets of undifferentiated cells with hyperchromatic nuclei, well-defined cell borders, and scanty cytoplasm. Necrosis is common. Electron microscopy, immunocytochemistry, and cytogenetics may be necessary to confirm the diagnosis. A generous tissue biopsy specimen is often necessary for diagnosis but should not delay starting chemotherapy.

A consistent cytogenetic abnormality, t(11;22), has been identified in Ewing sarcoma and PNET and is present in 85–90% of tumors. These tumors also express the protooncogene c-*myc*, which may be helpful in differentiating Ewing sarcoma from neuroblastoma, in which c-*myc* is not expressed.

Treatment & Prognosis

Therapy usually commences with the administration of chemotherapy after biopsy and is followed by local control measures. Depending on many factors, including the primary site of the tumor and the response to chemotherapy, local control could be achieved by surgery, radiation therapy, or a combination of these methods. Following local control, chemotherapy continues for approximately 1 year. Effective treatment for Ewing sarcoma uses combinations of dactinomycin, vincristine, doxorubicin, cyclophosphamide, etoposide, and ifosfamide. Patients with small localized primary tumors have a 50–70% long-term, disease-free survival rate. For patients with metastatic disease and large pelvic primary

tumors, survival is poor. Autologous HSCT is being investigated for the treatment of these high-risk patients.

Bernstein M et al: Ewing's sarcoma family of tumors: Current management. Oncologist 2006;11:503 [PMID: 16720851].

Burdach S et al: High-dose therapy for patients with primary multifocal and early relapsed Ewing's tumors: Results of two consecutive regimens assessing the role of total-body irradiation. J Clin Oncol 2003;21:3072 [PMID: 12915596].

Goorin AM et al: Presurgical chemotherapy compared with immediate surgery and adjuvant chemotherapy for nonmetastatic osteosarcoma: Pediatric Oncology Group Study POG-8651. J Clin Oncol 2003;15:1574 [PMID: 12697883].

Goyal S et al: Symptom interval in young people with bone cancer. Eur J Cancer 2004;40:2280 [PMID: 15454254].

Grimer RJ et al: Surgical options for children with osteosarcoma. Lancet Oncol 2005;6:85 [PMID: 15683817].

Marec-Berard P, Philip T: Ewing sarcoma: The pediatrician's point of view. Pediatr Blood Cancer 2004;42:477 [PMID: 15049024].

Marina N et al: Biology and therapeutic advances for pediatric osteosarcoma. Oncologist 2004;19:422 [PMID: 15266096].

RHABDOMYOSARCOMA

ESSENTIALS OF DIAGNOSIS & TYPICAL FEATURES

▶ Painless, progressively enlarging mass; proptosis; chronic drainage (nasal, aural, sinus, vaginal); cranial nerve palsies.

▶ Urinary obstruction, constipation, hematuria.

General Considerations

Rhabdomyosarcoma is the most common soft tissue sarcoma occurring in childhood and accounts for 10% of solid tumors in childhood. The peak incidence is at ages 2–5 years; 70% of children are diagnosed before age 10 years. A second smaller peak is seen in adolescents with extremity tumors. Males are affected more commonly than females.

Rhabdomyosarcoma can occur anywhere in the body. When rhabdomyosarcoma imitates striated muscle and cross-striations are seen by light microscopy, the diagnosis is straightforward. Immunohistochemistry, electron microscopy, or chromosomal analysis is sometimes necessary to make the diagnosis. Rhabdomyosarcoma is further classified into subtypes based on pathologic features: embryonal (60–80%), of which botryoid is a variant; alveolar (about 15–20%); undifferentiated sarcoma (8%); pleomorphic, which is seen in adults (1%); and other (11%). These subtypes occur in characteristic locations and have different metastatic potentials and outcomes.

Although the pathogenesis of rhabdomyosarcoma is unknown, in rare cases a genetic predisposition has been determined. Li-Fraumeni syndrome is an inherited mutation of the *p53* tumor suppressor gene that results in a high risk

Table 29–9. Characteristics of rhabdomyosarcoma.

Primary Site	Frequency (%)	Symptoms and Signs	Predominant Pathologic Subtype
Head and neck	35		Embryonal
Orbit	9	Proptosis	
Parameningeal	16	Cranial nerve palsies; aural or sinus obstruction with or without drainage	
Other	10	Painless, progressively enlarging mass	
Genitourinary	22		Embryonal (botryoid variant in bladder and vagina)
Bladder and prostate	13	Hematuria, urinary obstruction	
Vagina and uterus	2	Pelvic mass, vaginal discharge	
Paratesticular	7	Painless mass	
Extremities	18	Adolescents, swelling of affected body part	Alveolar (50%), undifferentiated
Other	25	Mass	Alveolar, undifferentiated

of bone and soft tissue sarcomas in childhood plus breast cancer and other malignant neoplasms before age 45 years. Two characteristic chromosomal translocations [t(2;13) and t(1;13)] have been described in alveolar rhabdomyosarcoma. The t(1;13) translocation appears to be a favorable prognostic feature in patients with metastatic alveolar rhabdomyosarcoma, whereas t(2;13) is associated with poor outcomes.

Clinical Findings

A. Symptoms and Signs

The presenting symptoms and signs of rhabdomyosarcoma result from disturbances of normal body function due to tumor growth (Table 29–9). For example, patients with orbital rhabdomyosarcoma present with proptosis, whereas patients with rhabdomyosarcoma of the bladder can present with hematuria, urinary obstruction, or a pelvic mass.

B. Imaging

A plain radiograph and a CT or MRI scan should be obtained to determine the extent of the primary tumor and to assess regional lymph nodes. A lung CT scan is obtained to rule out pulmonary metastasis, the most common site of metastatic disease at diagnosis. A skeletal survey and a bone scan are obtained to determine whether bony metastases are present. Bilateral bone marrow biopsies and aspirates are obtained to rule out bone marrow infiltration. Additional studies may be warranted in certain sites. For example, in parameningeal primary tumors, a lumbar puncture is performed to evaluate CSF for tumor cells.

Treatment

Optimal management and treatment of rhabdomyosarcoma is complex and requires combined modality therapy. When

feasible, the tumor should be excised, but this is not always possible because of the site of origin and size of tumor. When only partial tumor resection is feasible, the operative procedure is usually limited to biopsy and sampling of lymph nodes. Debulking of unresectable tumor may improve outcomes. Chemotherapy can often convert an inoperable tumor to a resectable one. A second-look procedure to remove residual disease and confirm the clinical response to chemotherapy and radiation therapy is generally performed at about week 20 of therapy.

Radiation therapy is an effective method of local tumor control for both microscopic and gross residual disease. It is generally administered to all patients, the only exception being those with a localized tumor that has been completely resected. All patients with rhabdomyosarcoma receive chemotherapy, even when the tumor is fully resected at diagnosis. The exact regimen and duration of chemotherapy are determined by primary site, group, and tumor node metastasis classification. Vincristine, dactinomycin, and cyclophosphamide have shown the greatest efficacy in the treatment of rhabdomyosarcoma.

Prognosis

The age of the patient, the extent of tumor at diagnosis, the primary site, the pathologic subtype, and the response to treatment all influence the long-term, disease-free survival rate from the time of diagnosis. Children with localized disease at diagnosis have a 70–75% 3-year disease-free survival rate, whereas children with metastatic disease at presentation have a worse outcome (39% 3-year disease-free survival).

Newer treatment strategies for high-risk patients include different drug combinations and dosing schedules with hematopoietic growth factor support, hyperfractionated radiation therapy, and autologous HSCT.

Joshi D et al: Age is an independent prognostic factor in rhabdomyosarcoma: A report from the Soft Tissue Sarcoma Committee of the Children's Oncology Group. Pediatr Blood Cancer 2004;42:64 [PMID: 14752797].

National Cancer Institute: http://www.cancer.gov/cancertopics/types/childrhabdomyosarcoma

Raney RB et al: Results of treatment of fifty-six patients with localized retroperitoneal and pelvic rhabdomyosarcoma: A report from the Intergroup Rhabdomyosarcoma Study-IV, 1991–1997. Pediatr Blood Cancer 2004;42:618 [PMID: 15127417].

Stevens MCG: Treatment for childhood rhabdomyosarcoma: The cost of cure. Lancet Oncol 2005;6:77 [PMID: 15683816].

RETINOBLASTOMA

▶ General Considerations

Retinoblastoma is a neuroectodermal malignancy arising from embryonic retinal cells that accounts for 3% of malignant disease in children younger than age 15 years. It is the most common intraocular tumor in pediatric patients and causes 5% of cases of childhood blindness. In the United States, 200–300 new cases occur per year. This is a malignancy of early childhood, with 90% of the tumors diagnosed before age 5 years. Bilateral involvement occurs in 20–30% of children and typically is diagnosed at a younger age (median age 14 months) than unilateral disease (median age 23 months).

Retinoblastoma is the prototype of hereditary cancers due to a mutation in the retinoblastoma gene (*RB1*), which is located on the long arm of chromosome 13 (13q14). This gene is a tumor-suppressor gene that normally controls cellular growth. When the gene is inactivated, as in retinoblastoma, cellular growth is uncontrolled. Uncontrolled cell growth leads to tumor formation. Inactivation of both *RB1* alleles within the same cell is required for tumor formation.

Retinoblastoma is known to arise in heritable and nonheritable forms. Based on the different clinical characteristics of the two forms, Knudson proposed a "two-hit" hypothesis for retinoblastoma tumor development. He postulated that two independent events were necessary for a cell to acquire tumor potential. Mutations at the *RB1* locus can be inherited or arise spontaneously. In heritable cases, the first mutation arises during gametogenesis, either spontaneously (90%) or through transmission from a parent (10%). This mutation is present in every retinal cell and in all other somatic and germ cells. Ninety percent of persons who carry this germline mutation will develop retinoblastoma. For tumor formation, the loss of the second *RB1* allele within a cell must occur; loss of only one allele is insufficient for tumor formation. The second mutation occurs in a somatic (retinal) cell. In nonheritable cases (60%), both mutations arise in a somatic cell after gametogenesis has taken place.

▶ Clinical Findings

A. Symptoms and Signs

Children with retinoblastoma generally come to medical attention while the tumor is still confined to the globe. Although present at birth, retinoblastoma is not usually detected until it has grown to a considerable size. Leukocoria (white pupillary reflex) is the most common sign (found in 60% of patients). Parents may note an unusual appearance of the eye or asymmetry of the eyes in a photograph. The differential diagnosis of leukocoria includes *Toxocara canis* granuloma, astrocytic hamartoma, retinopathy of prematurity, Coats disease, and persistent hyperplastic primary vitreous. Strabismus (in 20% of patients) is seen when the tumor involves the macula and central vision is lost. Rarely (in 7% of patients), a painful red eye with glaucoma, a hyphema, or proptosis is the initial manifestation. A single focus or multiple foci of tumor may be seen in one or both eyes at diagnosis. Bilateral involvement occurs in 20–30% of children.

B. Diagnostic Evaluation

Suspected retinoblastoma requires a detailed ophthalmologic examination under general anesthesia. An ophthalmologist makes the diagnosis of retinoblastoma by the appearance of the tumor within the eye without pathologic confirmation. A white to creamy pink mass protruding into the vitreous matter suggests the diagnosis; intraocular calcifications and vitreous seeding are virtually pathognomonic of retinoblastoma. A CT scan of the orbits detects intraocular calcification, evaluates the optic nerve for tumor infiltration, and detects extraocular extension of tumor. A single focus or multiple foci of tumor may be seen in one or both eyes at diagnosis. Metastatic disease of the marrow and meninges can be ruled out with bilateral bone marrow aspirates and biopsies plus CSF cytology.

▶ Treatment

Each eye is treated according to the potential for useful vision, and every attempt is made to preserve vision. The choice of therapy depends on the size, location, and number of intraocular lesions. Absolute indications for enucleation include no vision, neovascular glaucoma, inability to examine the treated eye, and inability to control tumor growth with conservative treatment. External beam irradiation has been the mainstay of therapy. A total dose of 35–45 Gy is administered. However, many centers are investigating the role of systemic chemotherapy for the treatment of retinoblastoma confined to the globe and the elimination of external beam radiotherapy is now accepted. Cryotherapy, photocoagulation, and radioactive plaques can be used for local tumor control. Patients with metastatic disease receive chemotherapy.

Children with retinoblastoma confined to the retina (whether unilateral or bilateral) have an excellent prognosis, with 5-year survival rates greater than 90%. Mortality is correlated directly with extent of optic nerve involvement, orbital extension of tumor, and massive choroid invasion. Patients who have disease in the optic nerve beyond the lamina cribrosa have a 5-year survival rate of only 40%. Patients with meningeal or metastatic spread rarely survive, although intensive chemotherapy and autologous HSCT have produced long-term survivors.

Patients with the germline mutation (heritable form) have a significant risk of developing second primary tumors. Osteosarcomas account for 40% of such tumors. Second malignant neoplasms occur in both patients who have and those who have not received radiation therapy. The 30-year cumulative incidence for a second neoplasm is 35% in patients who received radiation therapy and 6% in those who did not receive radiation therapy. The risk continues to increase over time. Although radiation contributes to the risk, it is the presence of the retinoblastoma gene itself that is responsible for the development of nonocular tumors in these patients.

Abramson DH, Sxhefler AC: Update on retinoblastoma. Retina 2004;24:828 [PMID: 15579980].

Antoneli CB et al: Extraocular retinoblastoma: A 13-year experience. Cancer 2003;15:1292 [PMID: 12973854].

Brichard B et al: Combined chemotherapy and local treatment in the management of intraocular retinoblastoma. Med Pediatr Oncol 2002;38:411 [PMID: 11984802].

Deegan WF: Emerging strategies for the treatment of retinoblastoma. Curr Opin Ophthamol 2003;14:291 [PMID: 14502057].

Nahum MP et al: Long-term follow-up of children with retinoblastoma. Pediatr Hematol Oncol 2001;18:173 [PMID: 11293284].

Rodriguez-Galindo C et al: Treatment of intraocular retinoblastoma with vincristine and carboplatin. J Clin Oncol 2003;15:2019 [PMID: 12743157].

Shields C et al: Continuing challenges in the management of retinoblastoma with chemotherapy. Retina 2004;24:849 [PMID: 15579981].

HEPATIC TUMORS (SEE ALSO CHAPTER 21)

Two thirds of liver masses found in childhood are malignant. Ninety percent of hepatic malignancies are either hepatoblastoma or hepatocellular carcinoma. Hepatoblastoma accounts for the vast majority of liver tumors in children younger than age 5 years, hepatocellular carcinoma for the majority in children aged 15–19 years. The features of these hepatic malignancies are compared in Table 29–10. Of the benign tumors, 60% are hamartomas or vascular tumors such as hemangiomas. There is mounting evidence for a strong association between prematurity and the risk of hepatoblastoma.

Children with hepatic tumors usually come to medical attention because of an enlarging abdomen. Approximately 10% of hepatoblastomas are first discovered on routine examination. Anorexia, weight loss, vomiting, and abdominal pain are associated more commonly with hepatocellular carcinoma. Serum α-fetoprotein is often elevated and is an excellent marker for response to treatment.

Imaging studies should include abdominal ultrasound, CT scan, or MRI. Malignant tumors have a diffuse hyperechoic pattern on ultrasonography, whereas benign tumors are usually poorly echoic. Vascular lesions contain areas with varying degrees of echogenicity. Ultrasound is also useful for imaging the hepatic veins, portal veins, and inferior vena cava. CT scanning and, in particular, MRI are important for defining the extent of tumor within the liver. CT scanning of the chest and bone scan should be obtained to evaluate for metastatic spread. Because bone marrow involvement is extremely rare, bone marrow aspirates and biopsies are not indicated.

The prognosis for children with hepatic malignancies depends on the tumor type and the resectability of the

Table 29–10. Comparison of hepatoblastoma and hepatocellular carcinoma in childhood.

	Hepatoblastoma	Hepatocellular Carcinoma
Median age at presentation	1 y (0–3 y)	12 y (5–18 y)
Male-to-female ratio	1.7:1	1.4:1
Associated conditions	Hemihypertrophy, Beckwith-Wiedemann syndrome, prematurity, Gardner syndrome	Hepatitis B virus infection, hereditary tyrosinemia, biliary cirrhosis, α_1-antitrypsin deficiency
Pathologic features	Fetal or embryonal cells; mesenchymal component (30%)	Large pleomorphic tumor cells and tumor giant cells
Solitary hepatic lesion	80%	20–50%
Unique features at diagnosis	Osteopenia (20–30%), isosexual precocity (3%)	Hemoperitoneum, polycythemia
Laboratory features		
Hyperbilirubinemia	5%	25%
Elevated AFP	> 90%	50%
Abnormal liver function tests	15–30%	> 30–50%

AFP, α-fetoprotein.

tumor. Complete resectability is essential for survival. Chemotherapy can decrease the size of most hepatoblastomas. Following biopsy of the lesion, neoadjuvant chemotherapy is administered prior to attempting complete surgical resection. Chemotherapy can often convert an inoperable tumor to a completely resectable one and can also eradicate metastatic disease. Approximately 50–60% of hepatoblastomas are fully resectable, whereas only one third of hepatocellular carcinomas can be completely removed. Even with complete resection, only one third of patients with hepatocellular carcinoma are long-term survivors. A recent CCG/Pediatric Oncology Group trial has shown cisplatin, fluorouracil, and vincristine to be as effective as but less toxic than cisplatin and doxorubicin in treating hepatoblastoma. Other drug combinations that have demonstrated benefit include carboplatin plus etoposide and doxorubicin plus ifosfamide. Radiation as well as liver transplantation is being investigated for patients whose tumors cannot be completely resected following chemotherapy.

Feusner J, Plaschkes J: Hepatoblastoma and low birth weight: A trend or chance observation? Med Pediatr Oncol 2002;39:508 [PMID: 12228908].
Katzenstein HM et al: Hepatocellular carcinoma in children and adolescents: Results from the Pediatric Oncology Group and the Children's Cancer Group intergroup study. J Clin Oncol 2002;12:2789 [PMID: 12065555].
Katzenstein HM et al: Treatment of unresectable and metastatic hepatoblastoma: A Pediatric Oncology Group Phase II study. J Clin Oncol 2002;20:3438 [PMID: 12177104].
Malogolowkin MH et al: Intensified platinum therapy is an ineffective strategy for improving outcome in pediatric patients with advanced hepatoblastoma. J Clin Oncol 2006;24:2879 [PMID: 16782927].
Myers RL: Tumors of the liver in children. Surg Oncol 2007;16:195 [PMID: 17714939].

LANGERHANS CELL HISTIOCYTOSIS

ESSENTIALS OF DIAGNOSIS & TYPICAL FEATURES

▶ Seborrheic skin rashes.
▶ Diaper rash.
▶ Draining ears.
▶ Bone pain.

▶ General Considerations

Langerhans cell histiocytosis (LCH; formerly called histiocytosis X) is a rare and poorly understood spectrum of disorders. It can occur as an isolated lesion or as widespread systemic disease involving virtually any body site. Eosinophilic granuloma, Hand-Schüller-Christian disease, and Letterer-Siwe disease are all syndromes encompassed by this disorder. LCH is not a true malignancy, but instead is a clonal, reactive proliferation of normal histiocytic cells, perhaps resulting from an immunoregulatory defect.

The distinctive pathologic feature is proliferation of histiocytic cells beyond what would be seen in a normal inflammatory process. Langerhans histiocytes have typical features: on light microscopy, the nuclei are deeply indented (coffee bean–shaped) and elongated, and the cytoplasm is pale, distinct, and abundant. Additional diagnostic characteristics include Birbeck granules on electron microscopy, expression of CD1 on the cell surface, and positive immunostaining for S-100 protein.

▶ Clinical Findings

Because LCH encompasses a broad spectrum of diseases, its presentation can be variable, from a single asymptomatic lesion to widely disseminated disease.

Patients with localized disease present primarily with lesions limited to bone. Occasionally found incidentally on radiographs obtained for other reasons, these lesions are well-demarcated and frequently found in the skull, clavicles, ribs, and vertebrae. These lesions can be painful. Patients can also present with localized disease of the skin, often as a diaper rash that does not resolve.

Bony lesions, fever, weight loss, otitis media, exophthalmos, and diabetes insipidus occur in a small number of children with the disease. Children with this multifocal disease, formerly called Hand-Schüller-Christian disease, commonly present with generalized symptoms and organ dysfunction.

Children with disseminated LCH (formerly called Letterer-Siwe disease) typically present before age 2 years with a seborrheic skin rash, fever, weight loss, lymphadenopathy, hepatosplenomegaly, and hematologic abnormalities.

Diagnosis is made with biopsy of the involved organ. The workup should include a CBC, liver and kidney function tests, a skeletal survey or technetium bone scan, and a urinalysis with specific gravity to rule out diabetes insipidus.

▶ Treatment & Prognosis

The outcome in LCH is extremely variable, but the process usually resolves spontaneously. Isolated lesions may need no therapy at all. Intralesional corticosteroids, curettage, and low-dose radiation therapy are useful local treatment measures for symptomatic focal lesions. Patients with localized disease have an excellent prognosis.

Multifocal disease is often treated with systemic chemotherapy. Prednisone with vinblastine or etoposide can be given repeatedly or continuously until lesions heal; the drugs can then be reduced and finally stopped. HSCT can also be used with success in refractory cases.

Multifocal disease is less predictable, but most cases resolve without sequelae. Age, degree of organ involvement, and response to therapy are the most important prognostic factors. Infants with disseminated disease tend to do poorly, with mortality rates approaching 50%. New treatment approaches for patients who do not respond to conventional chemotherapy have been evaluated in small studies. 2-Chlorodeoxyadenosine (2-CDA) has been used with some success. Therapeutic strategies targeting the dysregulated immune response using interferon-α or etanercept (anti–tumor necrosis factor-α) have also been reported.

Bernstrand C: Long-term follow-up of Langerhans cell histiocytosis: 39 years' experience at a single centre. Acta Paediatr 2005;94:1073 [PMID: 16188852].

Henter JI et al: Successful treatment of Langerhan's cell histiocytosis with etanercept. N Engl J Med 2001;345:1577 [PMID: 11794238].

Jubran RF et al: Predictors of outcome in children with Langerhans cell histiocytosis. Pediatr Blood Cancer 2005;45:37 [PMID: 15768381].

Kilborn TN et al: Paediatric manifestations of Langerhans cell histiocytosis: A review of the clinical and radiological findings. Clin Radiol 2003;58:269 [PMID: 12662947].

Kiss C et al: Interferon-alpha therapy in children with malignant diseases: Clinical experience in twenty-four patients treated in a single pediatric oncology unit. Med Pediatr Oncol 2002;39:115 [PMID: 12116059].

Rodriquez-Galindo C et al: Treatment of children with Langerhans cell histiocytosis with 2-chlorodeoxyadenosine. Am J Hematol 2002;69:179 [PMID: 11891804].

HEMATOPOIETIC STEM CELL TRANSPLANTATION

Amy K. Keating, MD, Roger H. Giller, MD,
& Ralph R. Quinones, MD

INDICATIONS & RATIONALE

Hematopoietic stem cell transplantation (HSCT), often referred to as bone marrow transplantation, involves the intravenous infusion of stem cells to reestablish normal hematopoiesis following marrow ablative or subablative chemotherapy, or radiation therapy (or both). HSCT is considered standard therapy for a variety of malignancies, hematopoietic disorders (aplastic anemia, hemoglobinopathies), storage diseases, and severe immunodeficiencies. It is considered first-line therapy in illnesses such as JMML and severe combined immunodeficiency, as no other curative therapy exists, but most often it is recommended only in high-risk situations or when conventional treatment fails. For example, HSCT is used in sickle cell disease for patients with significant complications and in leukemia patients who have very high-risk cytogenetic features.

The rationale for HSCT in patients with nonmalignant disorders is that the transplanted stem cells replace the absent or defective hematopoietic or lymphoid elements. In patients with storage disorders, such as Hurler disease, HSCT provides enzyme-making donor macrophages that populate host tissues.

In children with oncologic disorders, HSCT is multidimensional. Because marrow function is rescued with hematopoietic stem cells, higher doses of chemotherapy or radiation (or both) can be administered, which may overcome cancer cell resistance and achieve optimal tumor cell kill. Additionally, in patients who receive an allogeneic HSCT (stem cells from another person), the donor lymphoid cells may recognize the cancer as foreign and provide an immunologic attack on the malignancy, a concept known as the graft-versus-tumor (GVT) effect.

PREPARATION FOR HSCT

The selection of the stem cell source for transplantation is an important first step. There are a variety of stem cell sources to consider, and their utility is dependent on the disease process. HSCT sources can be divided into two main categories: autologous (ie, infusion of the patient's own hematopoietic stem cells) and allogeneic (ie, infusion of another individual's hematopoietic stem cells). Stem cells can be obtained from bone marrow, peripheral blood, or umbilical cord blood.

Autologous transplantation, often referred to as "stem cell rescue" is restricted to the treatment of selected pediatric malignancies, such as neuroblastoma, lymphoma, certain brain tumors, and Ewing sarcoma. Autologous transplantation offers the ability to deliver large doses of chemotherapy followed by hematopoietic rescue using an infusion of the patients own stem cells. Relapse of the original disease continues to be the greatest obstacle to successful autologous transplantation, likely due to limitations in achieving systemic cancer control prior to transplant, collecting sufficient progenitor cells that are not contaminated by tumor cells, and lack of GVT effect.

The selection of a suitable donor for allogeneic transplantation is critical and remains a major challenge. The principle genes known to encode for allogeneic recognition reside within the major histocompatibility complex (MHC) located on chromosome 6. The MHC class I antigens, HLA-A, HLA-B, and HLA-C, and the class II antigens, HLA-DR and HLA-DQ, can mediate graft rejection or graft-versus-host disease (GVHD). Each child expresses one set of paternal and one set of maternal HLA antigens. Thus, the probability of one child inheriting any specific combination and matching another sibling for an allogeneic transplant is 1 in 4. Large worldwide registries for bone marrow and umbilical cord blood donors have been developed; however, finding a closely matched unrelated donor can still be difficult, especially in underrepresented minority populations.

TRANSPLANT FUNDAMENTALS

Transplantation has four major treatment phases: preparative therapy, lymphohematopoietic rescue, supportive care, and long-term follow-up. The preparative phase is designed to be both myeloablative and antineoplastic. In the allogeneic transplant recipient, the preparative treatment also provides the necessary immunosuppression for successful donor engraftment. Preparative regimens use one or more chemotherapy drugs, often in combination with total body irradiation.

Lymphohematopoietic rescue is accomplished by the intravenous infusion of bone marrow, peripheral blood progenitor cells, or umbilical cord blood. Graft failure after allogeneic transplantation is rare in patients receiving stem cells from genotypically identical related donors but may be as high as 5–15% if the donor and patient are mismatched or unrelated. In allogeneic transplantation, marrow processing prior to infusion may include removal of contaminating RBCs for ABO incompatibility or T-cell depletion to reduce the risk of GVHD. In autologous transplantation, tumor purging or stem cell enrichment procedures can be performed for selected indications.

Supportive care in the initial months after transplantation includes transfusions, infection prophylaxis and treatment, and nutritional support. Immunosuppression for GVHD prophylaxis is necessary in allogeneic transplants. All blood products should be leukocyte-depleted to reduce the risk of CMV transmission. In addition, blood products must be irradiated to prevent GVHD from contaminating lymphocytes that remain even in leukocyte reduced blood products.

Successful engraftment usually occurs 10–28 days following transplantation. Peripheral blood stem cell transplant patients usually recover neutrophil counts earlier than patients receiving bone marrow or cord blood transplants. Platelet recovery generally occurs 6 or more weeks after HSCT. Hematopoietic growth factors such as granulocyte colony-stimulating factor may be used to hasten myeloid recovery.

INFECTIOUS COMPLICATIONS

Infections from bacteria, viruses, fungi, and protozoa account for significant morbidity and mortality in HSCT patients. Certain infections are typically seen at different time intervals after transplantation. During the early phase (0–1 month after transplant), when profound neutropenia and mucosal disruption occur, bacteria from the patient's aerodigestive tract are common culprits in bacteremia. Empiric antibiotic coverage and intravenous immune globulin decrease the risk of bacterial sepsis immediately following transplant. The presence of central venous catheters makes antibiotic coverage against gram-positive bacteria an important consideration in infection management. Reactivation of herpes simplex virus may occur in as many as 70% of seropositive patients; thus, acyclovir prophylaxis is commonly employed. Fungal infections, particularly with Candida and Aspergillus, have made antifungal prophylaxis routine.

In the intermediate post-HSCT phase (1–6 months after transplant), the patient often has reduced T-lymphocyte numbers and function and thus is susceptible to viral pathogens, including CMV from endogenous reactivation, as well as common viruses found in the general population. The heightened potential of community acquired viral pathogens, such as respiratory syncytial virus, adenovirus, influenza, parainfluenza, and human metapneumovirus, to result in life-threatening illness in HSCT recipients is critical to recognize. Reducing acquisition of these infections through careful handwashing and contact restriction is important until immune competence returns. If infection develops, prompt diagnosis and use of available antiviral therapies, such as inhaled ribavirin, can be lifesaving. Prophylactic administration of acyclovir or ganciclovir helps limit CMV and other herpesvirus (herpes simplex virus, varicella-zoster virus) infections. Protozoal infections such as Pneumocystis jiroveci pneumonia, also a risk in this intermediate phase, can be prevented by prophylaxis with trimethoprim–sulfamethoxazole, dapsone, or pentamidine.

The late phase (6–12 months after transplant), is characterized by infections from encapsulated bacteria such as Pneumococcus due to dysfunction of the reticuloendothelial system. Reactivation of varicella-zoster virus as shingles is also common. Patients on prolonged immunosuppressive treatment for chronic GVHD have increased and protracted risk of all types of infections.

GRAFT-VERSUS-HOST DISEASE

Despite the use of immunosuppressive agents, anti–T-cell antibodies, and T-cell depletion of the donor graft, approximately 20–70% of allogeneic HSCT patients experience some degree of acute GVHD. Factors influencing GVHD risk include the degree of HLA match, stem cell source, patient age, and donor sex. Acute GVHD occurs within the first 100 days after transplantation. The first manifestation typically is a maculopapular skin rash. Skin biopsies may be done to confirm the diagnosis. Intestinal involvement results in secretory diarrhea, and hepatic involvement leads to cholestatic jaundice. Chronic GVHD occurs after day 100 and may involve multiple organ systems. Sclerotic skin, malabsorption, weight loss, keratoconjunctivitis sicca, oral mucositis, chronic lung disease, and cholestatic jaundice are common manifestations. Treatment of GVHD consists of further use of immunosuppressive agents.

LONG-TERM COMPLICATIONS

Long-term follow-up of HSCT patients is essential. Patients are at risk for numerous complications, including pulmonary disease, cataracts, endocrine dysfunction affecting growth and fertility, cardiac dysfunction, avascular necrosis of bone, developmental delay, and secondary malignancies.

Although HSCT has many challenges, it represents an important advance in curative treatment for a variety of serious pediatric illnesses.

Bollard CM et al: Hematopoietic stem cell transplantation in pediatric oncology. In Pizzo PA, Poplack DG (editors): Principles and Practice of Pediatric Oncology. Lippincott Williams & Wilkins, 2006.

Talano JM et al: Recent molecular and cellular advances in pediatric bone marrow transplantation. Pediatr Clin North Am 2006;53:685 [PMID: 16872999].

LATE EFFECTS OF PEDIATRIC CANCER THERAPY

Late effects of treatment by surgery, radiation, and chemotherapy have been identified in survivors of pediatric cancer. Current estimates are that 1 in every 900 adults younger than age 45 years is a pediatric cancer survivor. One recent study found that 60% of survivors of pediatric cancer diagnosed between 1970 and 1986 have at least one chronic condition. Virtually any organ system can demonstrate sequelae related to previous cancer therapy. This has necessitated the creation of specialized oncology clinics whose function it is to identify and provide treatment to these patients.

The Childhood Cancer Survivor Study, a pediatric multiinstitutional collaborative project, was designed to investigate the various aspects of late effects of pediatric cancer therapy in a cohort of over 14,000 survivors of childhood cancer.

GROWTH COMPLICATIONS

Children who have received cranial irradiation are at highest risk of developing growth complications. Growth complications of cancer therapy in the pediatric survivor are generally secondary to direct damage to the pituitary gland, resulting in growth hormone deficiency. However, new evidence in children treated for ALL suggests that chemotherapy alone may result in an attenuation of linear growth without evidence of catch-up growth once therapy is discontinued. Up to 90% of patients who receive more than 30 Gy of radiation to the CNS will show evidence of growth hormone deficiency within 2 years. Approximately 50% of children receiving 24 Gy will have growth hormone problems. The effects of cranial irradiation appear to be age-related, with children younger than age 5 years at the time of therapy being particularly vulnerable. These patients usually benefit from growth hormone therapy. Currently, there is no evidence that such therapy causes a recurrence of cancer.

Spinal irradiation inhibits vertebral body growth. In 30% of treated children, standing heights may be less than the fifth percentile. Asymmetrical exposure of the spine to radiation may result in scoliosis.

Growth should be monitored closely, particularly in young survivors of childhood cancer. Follow-up studies should include height, weight, growth velocity, scoliosis examination, and, when indicated, growth hormone testing.

ENDOCRINE COMPLICATIONS

Thyroid dysfunction, manifesting as hypothyroidism, is common in children who received total body irradiation, cranial irradiation, or local radiation therapy to the neck. Particularly at risk are children with brain tumors who received more than 3000 cGy and those who received more than 4000 cGy to the neck region. The average time to develop thyroid dysfunction is 12 months after exposure, but the range is wide. Therefore, individuals at risk should be monitored yearly for at least 7 years from the completion of therapy. Although signs and symptoms of hypothyroidism may be present, most patients will have a normal thyroxine level with an elevated thyroid-stimulating hormone level. These individuals should be given thyroid hormone replacement because persistent stimulation of the thyroid from an elevated thyroid-stimulating hormone level may predispose to thyroid nodules and carcinomas. In a recent report from the Childhood Cancer Survivor Study, thyroid cancer occurred at 18 times the expected rate for the general population in pediatric cancer survivors who received radiation to the neck region. Hyperthyroidism, although rare, also occurs in patients who have received neck irradiation.

Precocious puberty, delayed puberty, and infertility are all potential consequences of cancer therapy. Precocious puberty, more common in girls, is usually a result of cranial irradiation causing premature activation of the hypothalamic-pituitary axis. This results in premature closure of the epiphysis and decreased adult height. Luteinizing hormone analogue and growth hormone are used to halt early puberty and facilitate continued growth.

Gonadal dysfunction in males is usually the result of radiation to the testes. Patients who receive testicular irradiation as part of their therapy for ALL, abdominal irradiation for Hodgkin disease, or total body irradiation for HSCT are at highest risk. Radiation damages both the germinal epithelium (producing azoospermia) and Leydig cells (causing low testosterone levels and delayed puberty). Alkylating agents such as ifosfamide and cyclophosphamide can also interfere with male gonadal function, resulting in oligospermia or azoospermia, low testosterone levels, and abnormal follicle-stimulating hormone (FSH) and luteinizing hormone (LH) levels. Determination of testicular size, semen analysis, and measurement of testosterone, FSH, and LH levels will help identify abnormalities in patients at risk. When therapy is expected to result in gonadal dysfunction, pretherapy sperm banking should be offered to adolescent males.

Exposure of the ovaries to abdominal radiation may result in delayed puberty with a resultant increase in FSH and LH and a decrease in estrogen. Girls receiving total body irradiation as preparation for HSCT and those receiving craniospinal irradiation are at particularly high risk for delayed puberty as well as premature menopause. In patients at high risk for development of gonadal complications, a detailed menstrual history should be obtained, and LH, FSH, and estrogen levels should be monitored if indicated.

No studies to date have confirmed an increased risk of spontaneous abortions, stillbirths, premature births, congenital malformations, or genetic diseases in the offspring of childhood cancer survivors. Women who have received abdominal irradiation may develop uterine vascular insufficiency or fibrosis of the abdominal and pelvic musculature or uterus, and their pregnancies should be considered high-risk.

CARDIOPULMONARY COMPLICATIONS

Pulmonary dysfunction generally manifests as pulmonary fibrosis. Therapy-related factors known to cause pulmonary toxicities include certain chemotherapeutic agents, such as bleomycin, the nitrosoureas, and busulfan, as well as lung or total body irradiation. Pulmonary toxicity due to chemotherapy is related to the total cumulative dose received. Pulmonary function tests in patients with therapy-induced toxicity show restrictive lung disease, with decreased carbon monoxide diffusion and small lung volumes. Individuals exposed to these risk factors should be counseled to refrain from smoking and to give proper notification of the treatment history if they should require general anesthesia.

Cardiac complications usually result from exposure to anthracyclines (daunorubicin, doxorubicin, and mitoxantrone), which destroy myocytes and lead to inadequate myocardial growth as the child ages, and eventually result in congestive heart failure. The incidence of anthracycline cardiomyopathy increases in a dose-dependent fashion. At least 5% of patients who have received a cumulative dose of more than 550 mg/m^2 of anthracyclines experience cardiac dysfunction. In a recent study, complications from these agents appeared 6–19 years following administration of the drugs. Pregnant women who have received anthracyclines should be followed closely for signs and symptoms of congestive heart failure, as peripartum cardiomyopathy has been reported.

Radiation therapy to the mediastinal region, which is a common component of therapy for Hodgkin disease, has been linked to an increased risk of coronary artery disease; chronic restrictive pericarditis may also occur in these patients.

Current recommendations include an exercise echocardiogram and electrocardiogram every 1–5 years, depending on the age at therapy, total cumulative dose received, and presence or absence of mediastinal irradiation. Selective monitoring with various modalities is indicated for those who were treated with anthracyclines when they were younger than age 4 years or received more than 500 mg/m^2 of these drugs. Measurement of serum levels of cardiac troponin-T or atrial natriuretic peptide may be useful in assessing early cardiotoxicity of anthracyclines.

RENAL COMPLICATIONS

Long-term renal side effects stem from therapy with cisplatin, alkylating agents (ifosfamide and cyclophosphamide), or pelvic irradiation. Patients who have received cisplatin may develop abnormal creatinine clearance, which may or may not be accompanied by abnormal serum creati-

nine levels, as well as persistent tubular dysfunction with hypomagnesemia. Alkylating agents can cause hemorrhagic cystitis, which may continue after chemotherapy has been terminated and has been associated with the development of bladder carcinoma. Ifosfamide can also cause Fanconi syndrome, which may result in clinical rickets if adequate phosphate replacement is not provided. Pelvic irradiation may result in abnormal bladder function with dribbling, frequency, and enuresis.

Patients seen in long-term follow-up who have received nephrotoxic agents should be monitored with urinalysis, appropriate electrolyte profiles, and blood pressure. Urine collection for creatinine clearance or renal ultrasound may be indicated in individuals with suspected renal toxicity.

NEUROPSYCHOLOGICAL COMPLICATIONS

Pediatric cancer survivors who have received cranial irradiation for ALL or brain tumors appear to be at greatest risk for neuropsychological sequelae. The severity of cranial irradiation effects varies among individual patients and depends on the dose and dose schedule, the size and location of the radiation field, the amount of time elapsed after treatment, the child's age at therapy, and the child's gender. Girls may be more susceptible than boys to CNS toxicity because of more rapid brain growth and development during childhood.

The main effects of CNS irradiation appear to be related to attention capacities, ability with nonverbal tasks and mathematics, and short-term memory. Recent studies support the association between treatment with high-dose systemic methotrexate, triple intrathecal chemotherapy, and, more recently, dexamethasone and more significant cognitive impairment.

Additionally, pediatric cancer patients have been reported as having more behavior problems and as being less socially competent than a sibling control group. Adolescent survivors of cancer demonstrate an increased sense of physical fragility and vulnerability manifested as hypochondriasis or phobic behaviors.

Finally, childhood cancer survivors are more likely to report symptoms of depression and somatic distress in adulthood. Pediatric cancer survivors may require ongoing counseling or other psychological interventions once they have completed therapy.

SECOND MALIGNANCIES

Approximately 3–12% of children receiving cancer treatment will develop a new cancer within 20 years of their first diagnosis. This is a tenfold increased incidence when compared with age-matched control subjects. Particular risk factors include exposure to alkylating agents, epipodophyllotoxins (VP-16), and radiation therapy, primary diagnosis of retinoblastoma or Hodgkin disease, or the presence of an inherited genetic susceptibility syndrome (Li-Fraumeni syndrome or NF). In a recent report, the cumulative estimated incidence of second malignant neoplasms for the cohort of the Childhood Cancer Survivor Study was 3.2% at 20 years from diagnosis.

Second hematopoietic malignancies (acute myelogenous leukemia) occur as a result of therapy with epipodophyllotoxins or alkylating agents. It is unclear whether the schedule of drug administration and the total dose are related to the development of this secondary leukemia.

Children receiving radiation therapy are at risk for developing second malignancies, such as sarcomas, carcinomas, or brain tumors, in the field of radiation. A recent report examining the incidence of second neoplasms in a cohort of pediatric Hodgkin disease patients showed the cumulative risk of a second neoplasm to be as high as 8% at 15 years from diagnosis. The most common solid tumor was breast cancer (the majority located within the radiation field) followed by thyroid cancer. Girls aged 10–16 years when they received radiation therapy were at highest risk and had an actuarial incidence that approached 35% by age 40 years.

Bassal M et al: Risk of selected subsequent carcinomas in survivors of childhood cancer: A report from the Childhood Cancer Survivor Study. J Clin Oncol 2006;24:476 [PMID: 16421424].

Chow EJ et al: Decreased adult height in survivors of childhood acute lymphoblastic leukemia: A report from the Childhood Cancer Survivor Study. J Pediatr 2007;150:370 [PMID: 17382112].

Henderson TO et al: Secondary sarcomas in childhood cancer survivors: A report from the Childhood Cancer Survivor Study. J Natl Cancer Inst 2007;99:300 [PMID: 17312307].

Oeffinger KC et al: Chronic health conditions in adult survivors of childhood cancer. N Engl J Med 2006;355:1572 [PMID: 17035650].

Poutanen T et al: Long-term prospective follow-up of cardiac function after cardiotoxic therapy for malignancy in children. J Clin Oncol 2003;21:2349 [PMID: 12805337].

Schultz KA et al: Behavioral and social outcomes in adolescent survivors of childhood cancer: A report from the Childhood Cancer Survivor Study. J Clin Oncol 2007;25:3649 [PMID: 17704415].

Zebrack BJ et al: Psychological distress in long-term survivors of solid tumors diagnosed in childhood: A report from the Childhood Cancer Survivor Study. Pediatr Blood Cancer 2007;49:47 [PMID: 16755550].

Pain Management & Palliative Care

Brian S. Greffe, MD

Jeffrey L. Galinkin, MD

Nancy A. King, MSN, RN, CPNP

Children experience pain to at least the same level as adults. Multiple studies have shown that neonates and infants perceive pain and remember these painful experiences. Frequently, opioid and nonopioid analgesics are underprescribed and underdosed in children owing to excessive concerns about respiratory depression or incomplete understanding of the need for pain medications in children, or both. Few data are available to guide the dosing of many pain medications, and the majority of pain medications available on the market today are unlabeled for use in pediatric patients.

Taddio A, Katz J: The effects of early pain experience in neonates on pain responses in infancy and childhood. Paediatr Drugs 2005;7:245 [PMID: 16118561].

PAIN MANAGEMENT

PAIN ASSESSMENT

Pain Scales

Standardizing pain measurements requires the use of appropriate pain scales. At most institutions, pain scales are stratified by age (Table 30–1) and are used throughout the institution from operating room to medical floor to clinic, creating a common language around a patient's pain. Pain assessment using such scales has become the "fifth vital sign" in hospital settings and is documented at least as frequently as heart rate and blood pressure at many pediatric centers around the world. Many pain scales are available (see Figures 30–1 and 30–2, and Table 30–2, for examples). The type of scale used is less important than its use on a consistent basis.

Special Populations

Noncommunicative patients such as neonates and the cognitively impaired are often difficult to assess for pain. In these patient populations, use of an appropriate assessment tool (see Table 30–1) on a frequent basis is essential to assure adequate pain control. An increasing pain score trend is often a sign of discomfort.

ACUTE PAIN

▶ General Considerations

Acute pain is caused by an identifiable source. In most cases it is self-limiting, and treatment is a reflection of severity and type of injury. In children the majority of acute pain is cased by trauma or, if in a hospital setting, an iatrogenic source such as surgery.

▶ Treatment

Treatment of acute pain depends on the disposition of the individual patient. For outpatient care the mainstay of treatment is nonsteroidal anti-inflammatory drugs (NSAIDs; Table 30–3). Acetaminophen is the most commonly used NSAID. Acetaminophen is administered via oral or rectal routes but is more predictable in its effects as an oral dose. Round-the-clock administration has been proved to be more effective than as-needed (PRN) dosing for minor pain or as an adjunct for major pain. The toxicity of acetaminophen is low in clinically used doses; however, liver damage or failure can occur with doses exceeding 200 mg/kg/d. Other oral analgesics available in suspension are ibuprofen and naproxen (see Table 30–3 for dosing).

When pain is more severe oral opioids can be added for short-term use (Table 30–4). Many of these drugs are formulated with an NSAID, for example, oxycodone plus acetaminophen (Percocet) and hydrocodone plus acetaminophen (Lortab). When using combination drugs, the dose of drug is based on the opioid component. Other concomitantly administered similar NSAIDs should be discontinued. The most commonly used oral opioids are oxycodone, hydrocodone, and codeine. Codeine is the least recommended because of its metabolism, which involves conversion of the

Table 30–1. Commonly used pain scales and their age-appropriate use.

Scale	Type	Description	Age Group
Numeric	Self-report	0–10 scale; 0 = no pain, 10 = worst pain you could ever imagine	Children who understand the concept of numbers, rank, and order; generally > 8 y
Bieri and Wong-Baker scales	Self-report	6 faces that range from no pain to the worst pain you can imagine (see Figures 30–1 and 30–2)	Younger children who have difficulty with numeric scale; cognitive age 3–7 y
FLACC[a]	Behavioral observer	5 categories: face, legs, activity, cry, and consolability; range of total score is 0–10; score ≥ 7 is severe pain (see Table 30–2)	Nonverbal children > 1 y
CRIES,[b] NIPS, PIPP	Behavioral observer	Rates a set of standard criteria and gives a score	Nonverbal infant < 1 y

[a]FLACC is an acronym derived from the categories assessed by the scale: face, legs, activity, cry, consolability.
[b]CRIES is an acronym for Crying Requires O_2 saturation, Increased vital signs, Expression and Sleeplessness.
NIPS, Neonatal Infant Pain Scale; PIPP, Premature Infant Pain Profile.

parent drug to morphine via the cytochrome P-450 2D6 isoenzyme. Between 1% and 10% of people (Asians, 1–2%; African Americans, 1–3%; Caucasians, 5–10%) have a genetic polymorphism that makes them poor metabolizers of codeine. These patients obtain no effect from this drug. A very small percentage of patients (primarily from East Africa) are ultrarapid metabolizers. These patients convert 10–15 times the amount of parent drug to the active compound, which can result in clinical toxicity. Morphine, oxycodone, and hydrocodone are all available as suspensions, are active as administered, and are metabolized by multiple routes.

For severe pain not amenable to oral analgesics, an intravenous opioid can be titrated to effect; options for pain relief are dependent on the severity and location of pain, and the patient's age. Often the NSAID ketorolac (0.5–1.0 mg/kg) is used as an adjunct for severe pain. Side effects of ketorolac are the same as for adults: renal insufficiency, gastric irritability and prolonged bleeding times due to decreased platelet adhesiveness. Patients with bleeding concerns should not receive ketorolac.

Patient-controlled analgesia (PCA) pumps can be used in children as young as age 6 years with proper instruction and coaching (Table 30–5). Morphine and hydromorphone are the most commonly used drugs for PCA management in the United States. Whenever PCA is used it is imperative to assess patients frequently (at least hourly) to assure adequate pain relief.

Andersson T et al: Drug-metabolizing enzymes: Evidence for clinical utility of pharmacogenomic tests. Clin Pharmacol Ther 2005;78:559 [PMID: 16338273].

CHRONIC PAIN

▶ General Considerations

Chronic pain is pain that persists past the usual course of an acute illness or beyond the time that is expected for an acute injury. In children this is an increasingly recognized problem; it is estimated that chronic pain may affect up to 10–15% of children in the United States. Among the conditions commonly producing chronic pain in children are headache, abdominal pain, myofascial pain, fibromyalgia, juvenile rheumatoid arthritis, complex regional pain syndrome, phantom limb pain, and pain associated with cancer. Multiple contributing factors, including psychosocial issues and family dynamics, often contribute to chronic pain in children. Associating pain with a single physical cause can lead the physician to order repeated invasive laboratory and diagnostic tests,

| 0 | 2 | 4 | 6 | 8 | 10 |

▲ **Figure 30–1.** Bieri Faces Pain Scale, revised. (Reproduced, with permission, from Bieri D et al: The Faces Pain Scale for the self-assessment of the severity of pain experienced by children: Development, initial validation, and preliminary investigation for ratio scale properties. Pain 1990;41:139.)

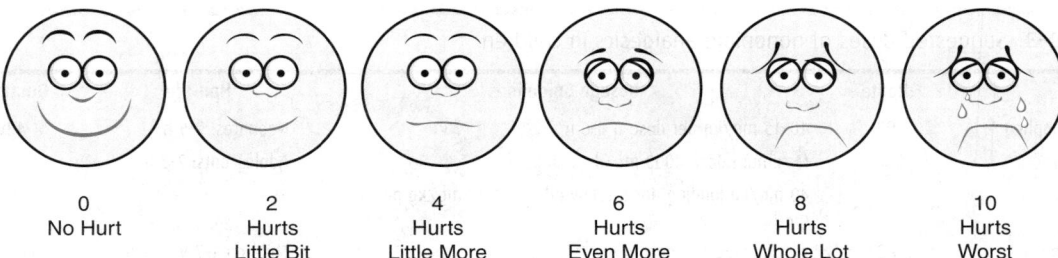

0	2	4	6	8	10
No Hurt	Hurts Little Bit	Hurts Little More	Hurts Even More	Hurts Whole Lot	Hurts Worst

▲ **Figure 30–2.** Wong-Baker pain scale. (Reproduced, with permission, from Wong DL, Baker CM: Smiling faces as anchor for pain intensity scales. Pain 2001;89:295.)

and to overprescribe medications. A multidimensional assessment to chronic pain is optimal and often required.

McGrath PA, Ruskin, DA: Caring for children with chronic pain: Ethical considerations. Paediatr Anaesth 2007;17:505 [PMID: 17498011].

Pediatric chronic pain. A position statement from the American Pain Society. Available at: http://www.ampainsoc.org/advocacy/pediatric.htm.

Weisman SJ, Rusy LM: Pain management in infants and children. In Motoyama EK, Davis PJ (editors): *Smith's Anesthesia for Infants and Children*, 7th ed. Mosby/Elsevier, 2006:436.

▶ Treatment

A multidisciplinary team approach is standard of care for treating chronic pain in children. All children evaluated for chronic pain should be seen on their initial visit by all primary members of the team to establish a management strategy. Team members should include a physician specializing in pain management, a pediatric psychologist or psychiatrist (or both), occupational and physical therapists, advanced pain nurses (APNs), and a social worker. The majority of pediatric chronic pain management programs in the United States base their approach on combined intensive rehabilitation and intensive psychotherapy, relying minimally on invasive procedures and pharmacotherapy.

A. Tolerance, Dependence, and Addiction

Adults and children are similar in their physiologic and psychological responses to opioids. A consensus paper by the American Academy of Pain Medicine, American Pain Society, and American Society of Addiction Medicine defined important differences between normal and pathologic responses to opioids. The definitions of tolerance, dependence, and addiction are listed below.

1. Tolerance—A state of adaptation in which exposure to a drug induces changes that result in a diminution of one or more of the drug's effects over time. Tolerance develops at different rates for different opioid effects (ie, tolerance develops to sleepiness and respiratory depression before it develops to constipation and analgesia).

2. Dependence—A state of adaptation manifested by a drug class–specific withdrawal syndrome that can be produced by abrupt cessation, rapid dose reduction, or decreasing blood level of the drug; by administration of an antagonist; or by a combination of these actions.

Table 30–2. FLACC pain assessment tool.[a]

Categories	Score 0	Score 1	Score 2
Face	No particular expression or smile	Occasional grimace or frown, withdrawn, disinterested	Frequent to constant frown, clenched jaw, quivering chin
Legs	Normal position or relaxed	Uneasy, restless, tense	Kicking, or legs drawn up
Activity	Lying quietly, normal position, moves easily	Squirming, shifting back and forth, tense	Arched, rigid, or jerking
Cry	No cry (awake or asleep)	Moans or whimpers, occasional complaint	Crying steadily, screams or sobs, frequent complaints
Consolability	Content, relaxed	Reassured by occasional touching, hugging, or being talked to, distractible	Difficult to console or comfort

[a]FLACC is an acronym derived from the categories assessed by the scale: face, legs, activity, cry, consolability.
Reproduced, with permission, from Merkel SI et al: The FLACC: A behavioral scale for scoring postoperative pain in young children. Pediatr Nurs 1997;23:293.

Table 30–3. Suggested doses of nonopioid analgesics in children.

	Route	Dosage Guidelines	Half-life	Duration
Acetaminophen	PO	10–15 mg/kg per dose q 4–6 h	Neonates: 2–5 h	4 h
		Maximum dose 4000 mg/d	Adolescents: 2–3 h	
	PR	40 mg/kg loading dose, followed by 10–20 mg/kg per dose q 6 h	—	—
Ibuprofen	PO	4–10 mg/kg per dose q 6–8 h	Children 1–7 y: 1–2 h	6–8 h
		Maximum dose 40 mg/kg/d, not to exceed 2400 mg/d	Adolescents: 2–4 h	
Ketorolac	IV	0.5 mg/kg per dose q 6 h	Children: ~ 6 h	4–6 h
		Maximum of 30 mg per dose; maximum course of 8 doses	Adolescents: ~ 5 h	

IV, intravenous; PO, by mouth; PR, by rectum.

3. Addiction—A primary, chronic, neurobiologic disease, the development and manifestations of which are influenced by genetic, psychosocial, and environmental factors. Addiction is characterized by behaviors that include one or more of the following (the 3 Cs):

- Loss of **C**ontrol over use of drug
- **C**raving and compulsive use of drug
- Use despite adverse **C**onsequences

Addiction is rare when opioids are used appropriately for acute pain in inpatient and outpatient settings. It should be emphasized that tolerance and dependence are not synonymous with addiction.

Heit HA: Addiction, physical dependence, and tolerance: Precise definitions to help clinicians evaluate and treat chronic pain patients. J Pain Palliat Care Pharmacother 2003;17:15 [PMID: 14640337].

B. Withdrawal

1. Recognition—Withdrawl symptoms can be expected to occur for all patients after 1 week of opioid treatment. Signs of withdrawal in older children include agitation, irritability, dysphoria, tachycardia, tachypnea, nasal congestion, temperature instability, and feeding intolerance. In neonates with withdrawal (neonatal abstinence syndrome), common symptoms include neurologic excitability, gastrointestinal dysfunction, autonomic signs (increased sweating, nasal stuffiness, fever, mottling, poor weight gain), and skin excoriation caused by excessive rubbing.

2. Treatment protocol—To minimize withdrawal symptoms in patients being weaned from opioid medications, clinicians should devise a schedule for dose reduction in conjunction with the patient and family. The duration of opioid therapy must be taken into consideration. Standard protocols involve switching to an opioid that can be administered once a day (eg, methadone) and decreasing the dose by 10–25% every 1–2 days. The patient should be monitored for signs of withdrawal over this period. If symptoms develop, consider lorazepam, 0.05–0.1 mg/kg every 6–8 hours or a clonidine patch, 0.1 mg/d (changed every fifth day).

Berens RJ et al: A prospective evaluation of opioid weaning in opioid-dependent pediatric critical care patients. Anesth Analg 2006;102:1045 [PMID: 16551896].

PEDIATRIC PALLIATIVE & END-OF-LIFE CARE

It has been estimated that almost 55,000 children die each year in the United States. At least half of these children die during the newborn period or within the first year of life. Many of these children, particularly those older than 1 year of age, suffer from illnesses that are clearly life-limiting. Thousands more are diagnosed with life-limiting illnesses resulting in chronic conditions that may last for many years, even decades. Children who are diagnosed with life-threatening illnesses that may be curable (eg, cancer) continue to live with the potential of a recurrence of their malignancy for many years. In all of these populations palliative and end-of-life care can play an important role during patients' illnesses.

Although commonly used interchangeably, *palliative care* and *end-of-life care* are not synonymous terms. Palliative care aims to prevent, relieve, reduce, or soothe the symptoms produced by potential life-limiting illnesses or their treatments and to maintain the patient's quality of life along the entire continuum of treatment. Provision of palliative care does not imply imminent death nor does it prohibit aggressive curative treatment modalities. Rather, it acknowledges the uncertainty and potential for suffering inherent in a potentially life-limiting condition such as cancer. Understanding how a family defines quality of life and suffering for their child is imperative and provides a framework for decision making between care providers and the family throughout treatment.

While a child is responding well to treatment, the primary focus is on achieving cure of the disease. Palliative care

Table 30–4. Suggested doses of oral and intravenous opioids in infants and children.

Drug	Route	Dosage Guidelines	Onset	Duration
Intravenous Opioids				
Fentanyl	IV intermittent	0.5–1 mcg/kg per dose (best for intermittent short-duration analgesia; titrate to effect)	1–3 min	30–60 min
Hydromorphone	IV	Children: 0.015 mg/kg per dose q 3–6 h Adolescent: 1–4 mg q 3–6 h	15 min	4–5 h
Methadone	IV	0.1 mg/kg per dose q 4 h for 2–3 doses, then q 6–12 h	10–20 min	6–8 h (22–48 h after repeated doses)
Morphine	IV intermittent	0.05–0.1 mg/kg per dose q 2–4 h	Neonates: 7–8 h 1–3 mo: 6 h 6 mo–2.5 y: 3 h 3–19 y: 1–2 h	2–4 h
Oral Opioids				
Codeine	PO	0.5–1 mg/kg per dose q 4–6 h, maximum of 60 mg per dose	30–60 min	4–6 h
Hydrocodone (in Vicodin, Lortab elixir)	PO	Children: 0.15–0.2 mg/kg per dose q 4–6 h Adolescents: 1–2 tabs q 4–6 h (limited due to acetaminophen content; see acetaminophen recommendations in text)	10–20 min	3–6 h
Hydromorphone	PO	Children: 0.03–0.1 mg/kg per dose q 4–6 h Adolescents: 1–4 mg q 3–4 h	15–30 min	4–5 h
Methadone	PO	0.1 mg/kg per dose q 4–6 h for 2–3 doses, then q 6–12 h	30–60 min	6–8 h (22–48 h after repeated doses)
Morphine	PO-IR	0.2–0.5 mg/kg per dose q 4–6 h	15–60 min	3–5 h
	PO-ER	0.3–0.6 mg/kg per dose q 12 h	1–2 h	8–12 h
Oxycodone	PO	0.05–0.2 mg/kg q 4–6 h	10–15 min	3 h

ER, extended release; IR, immediate release; IV, intravenous; PO, by mouth (orally).
Based on information in Polaner DM: Acute pain management in infants and children. In Perkins RM et al (editors): *Pediatric Hospital Medicine,* 2nd ed. Lippincott Williams & Wilkins, 2008:743.

goals at this time focus on promoting quality of life in preparation for survivorship in the face of a potentially life-limiting illness. Some of these goals include helping a family come to terms with the diagnosis, addressing issues of treatment-related pain and distress, facilitating reintegration into the social realms of school and community, and promoting as much normalcy in the child's life as possible. When it becomes clear that the chances for cure are poor or present an unreasonable cost to the child's quality of life, the goals of palliative care shift. The focus is still on promoting quality of life but now in preparation for a comfortable and dignified end of life with increasingly less attention given to the treatment or cure of the disease itself.

Palliative care not only comprises support in the pain and symptom management of the disease but also addresses equally the psychosocial, emotional, and spiritual needs of patients with a potential life-limiting illness and their family.

CHILDREN WHO MAY BENEFIT FROM PALLIATIVE CARE

Four groups of conditions have been identified for which palliative care is appropriate:

1. Conditions for which curative treatment is possible but may fail, such as advanced or progressive cancer and complex and severe congenital or acquired heart disease.

2. Conditions requiring intensive long-term treatment aimed at maintaining the quality of life such as HIV/AIDS, cystic fibrosis, and muscular dystrophy.

3. Progressive conditions in which treatment is exclusively palliative after diagnosis, such as progressive metabolic disorders and certain chromosomal abnormalities.

4. Conditions involving severe, nonprogressive disability, causing extreme vulnerability to health complications, such as severe cerebral palsy and anoxic brain injury.

Table 30–5. Patient-controlled analgesia dosing recommendations.

	Morphine	Fentanyl	Hydromorphone
Solution	1 mg/mL	10 mcg/mL	0.1 mg/mL or 1 mg/mL
Initial dose	15–20 mcg/kg (maximum 1.5 mg)	0.25 mcg/kg	3–4 mcg/kg (maximum 0.3 mg)
Lockout time	8–10 min	8–10 min	8–10 min
Basal infusion	0–20 mcg/kg/h	0–1 mcg/kg/h	0–4 mcg/kg/h
Maximum starting dose	100 mcg/kg/h	1–2 mcg/kg/h	20 mcg/kg/h

PAIN MANAGEMENT IN PALLIATIVE CARE

Optimal pain management is critical when providing pediatric palliative care. (See the section on Pain Management, earlier, for definitions and guidelines for treatment.) Children who are opioid-naïve will usually respond very well to conventional dosing of narcotics. Children who have been receiving a long-term narcotic such as codeine for pain management may need a dosage at the higher end of the spectrum when switching to an opioid such as morphine. Adjunctive medications such as NSAIDs can be extremely helpful as well and may help reduce the frequency of narcotic dose escalations. However, children at the end of life may need ongoing upward dose adjustments, which at times may exceed normal dose recommendations. When given with the intent to achieve comfort in the dying child, these escalations are ethically and morally appropriate.

QUALITY-OF-LIFE ADJUNCTS & SYMPTOM MANAGEMENT

Certain nonpain symptoms and signs may develop more quickly in children at the end of life as compared with the adult population. A thorough and complete history and physical examination should be obtained. It is critical to determine how much distress the symptom causes the child and how much it interferes with the child's and family's routine. Areas of management should include pharmacologic intervention, nursing care, and psychosocial support. Symptoms that commonly occur during disease progression and at the end of life in children with a life-limiting condition are listed in Table 30–6, along with suggestions for management.

PSYCHOSOCIAL ASPECTS OF PALLIATIVE CARE

Pediatric palliative care is unique in that caregivers must be familiar with children's normal emotional and spiritual development. Working with a child at his or her level of development through the use of both oral and expressive communication allows the child to be more open with respect to hopes, dreams, and fears. A child's understanding of death depends on his or her stage of cognitive development. Children generally understand death as a changed state by age 3 years, universality by 5–6 years, and personal mortality by 8–9 years.

As end of life approaches, psychosocial support is invaluable to the child and family. Children may need someone to talk to outside of the family unit who can respond to their questions and concerns open and honestly. Parents may need guidance and support in initiating discussions with or responding to questions from their child about death and dying. Children and adolescents may have specific tasks they wish to complete before they die. Some want to have input into funeral and memorial service plans and disposition of their body. Parents often need support in making funeral arrangements, handling financial concerns, talking with siblings and other family members, and coping with their own grief.

It is important to recognize that grief is not an illness but a normal, multidimensional, unique, and dynamic process presenting as pervasive distress due to a perceived loss. Once parents have accepted the reality of the loss of the child, they must then complete the other tasks of grief, such as experiencing the pain of their loss and adjusting to an environment without their child, in order to move on with their lives. Parents who lose a child are at high risk for complicated grief reactions such as absent grief, delayed grief, and prolonged or unresolved grief. Siblings are also at risk for complicated grief and require special attention.

SPIRITUAL & CULTURAL SUPPORT

Health care decisions are often intertwined with a family's culture and belief system. Understanding the influences of a family's beliefs and culture allows the practitioner to provide sensitive, appropriate care, particularly at the end of life. Interaction with members of the family's faith and cultural communities can often be instrumental in helping both the care team and the community support of the family. Allowance for specific prayers, rituals, or other activities may help facilitate procedures and discussions.

Families who speak a foreign language are at risk for inadequate support. They may have fewer opportunities to express their concerns and fears, ask questions, and validate their understanding due to language and cultural constraints. Every effort should be made to find and utilize a qualified interpreter, particularly for any discussion that involves delivering difficult news or making critical decisions. Many times, the role of interpreter is imposed on a bilingual family member or friend who may not understand

Table 30–6. Symptom management in pediatric palliative care.

Symptom	Causes	Management
Nausea and vomiting	Chemotherapy, narcotics, metabolic imbalances	Consider diphenhydramine; hydroxyzine; 5-HT$_3$ inhibitors; prokinetic agents for GI motility
Anorexia	Cancer, pain, abnormal taste, GI alterations, metabolic changes, drugs, psychological factors	Treat underlying condition; encourage exercise; arrange dietary consultation; consider appetite stimulants (dronabinol, megestrol, steroids)
Constipation and diarrhea	Narcotics, chemotherapy, malabsorption, drug-related	Laxatives (must be initiated whenever starting narcotics); loperamide for diarrhea
Dyspnea	Airway obstruction; decrease in functional lung tissue due to effusion, infection, metastases; impaired chest wall movement; anemia	Treat specific cause (eg, surgery to alleviate obstruction, red blood cell transfusion, chemotherapy or radiation therapy for metastatic disease); nonpharmacologic management (reassurance, position of comfort, improvement of air circulation using electric fan, oxygen, and relaxation therapy); pharmacologic management with opioids given IV or SQ as continuous infusion; nebulized morphine in older patients; concomitant use of anxiolytics (lorazepam, midazolam) if agitation
Terminal respiratory congestion	Airway or oral secretions at end of life, resulting in rattling, noisy, gurgling breath sounds	Repositioning; anticholinergics such as hycosine IV, SQ, or PO, or transdermal scopolamine
Pressure sores	Direct tissue damage; tissue fragility; immobility; diminished response to pain or irritation	Prevention (avoidance of trauma, pressure relief, good hygiene); treatment with local hygiene, debridement, use of appropriate wound dressings, antibiotics, analgesics
Bone pain	Bony metastases; leukemic infiltration of bone marrow	Palliative radiation; bone-seeking isotopes; bisphosphonates; chemotherapy; analgesics
Agitation	Present in conjunction with pain, dyspnea, terminal phase of illness	Benzodiazepines (midazolam); barbiturates to achieve complete sedation in terminal restlessness
Pruritus	Urticaria, postherpetic neuralgia, cholestasis, uremia, opioids	Antihistamines (cholestasis, uremia, opioids); 5-HT$_3$ receptor antagonists (cholestasis, opioids)
Fatigue	Marrow infiltration by malignant cells (leukemia)	Transfusions (red blood cells, platelets) to relieve symptoms; hemostatics (eg, aminocaproic acid)

GI, gastrointestinal; 5-HT$_3$, 5-hydroxytryptamine 3; IV, intravenous; PO, by mouth (orally); SQ, subcutaneous.

medical terminology well enough to translate clearly or who may deliberately translate the information inaccurately in an attempt to protect the family.

ADVANCE CARE PLANNING

Advance care planning allows patients and families to make known their wishes about what to do in care of serious or life-threatening problems. Advance care planning has been described as a four-step process. First, individuals considered decision makers are identified and included in the process. Second, an assessment of the patient's and family's understanding of the illness and prognosis is made and the impending death is described in terms the child and family can understand. Third, on the basis of their understanding of the illness and prognosis, the goals of care are determined regarding current and future intervention—curative, uncertain, or primarily focused on providing comfort. Finally, shared decisions about the current and future use or abandonment of life-sustaining techniques and aggressive medi-

cal interventions are made. If a disagreement exists between parents or between parents and patient regarding these techniques or interventions, it may be prudent to involve the hospital's ethics committee to aid in resolving these issues.

Some states permit parents to sign an advanced directive that asserts their decision not to have resuscitative attempts made in the event of a cardiac or respiratory arrest outside of the hospital. When an advanced directive is in place, emergency responders are not required to provide cardiopulmonary resuscitation if called to the scene. Some school districts will respect an advanced directive on school property, many will not. If a child with an advanced directive in place wishes to attend school, a discussion between the medical team and school officials should be arranged to determine the best plan should the child have a cardiac or respiratory arrest at school.

Parents, and occasionally the child, may bring up the possibility of donating organs or body tissues after death. Although the tissues that may be donated by a child may be limited in some instances by the type of disease (eg, cancer), some parents find immense comfort in knowing their child was able to benefit another. If the parents have not discussed donation with the physician by the time of death and donation is possible, the physician should offer the opportunity to the family.

Autopsy is another subject many physicians find difficult to approach with a family, but it is an important option to discuss. In cases of anticipated death from natural causes, autopsies are generally not mandatory; however, information obtained from an autopsy may be useful for parental peace of mind or medical research. If death at home is to be followed by an autopsy, special arrangements for transporting and receiving the body will need to be made with the mortuary or the coroner.

REFERENCES

Goldman A et al (editors): *Oxford Textbook of Palliative Care for Children.* Oxford University Press, 2006.

Himelstein B et al: Pediatric palliative care. N Engl J Med 2004;350:1752 [PMID: 15103002].

Kang T et al (editors): Pediatric palliative care. Pediatr Clin North Am 2007;54(5).

Romesberg TL: Building a case for neonatal palliative care. Neonatal Netw 2007;26:111 [PMID: 17402603].

Storey P, Knight C: Alleviating psychological and spiritual pain in the terminally ill. In: *Hospice/Palliative Care Training for Physicians: A Self-Study Program.* American Academy of Hospice and Palliative Care Medicine, Mary Ann Liebert, Inc, 2003.

Woodruff R (editor): *Palliative Medicine: Evidence-Based Symptoms and Supportive Care for Patients with Advanced Cancer,* 4th ed. Oxford University Press, 2005.

Web Resources

Education on Palliative and End-of-Life Care (the EPEC Project; adult-focused information for health care providers): http://www.epec.net

Initiative for Pediatric Palliative Care (IPPC): http://www.ippcweb.org

National Hospice and Palliative Care Organization (NHPCO): Children's Project on Palliative/Hospice Services (ChiPPs): http://www.nhpco.org

Immunodeficiency

Lora J. Stewart, MD

Richard B. Johnston, Jr., MD

Andrew H. Liu, MD

The immune deficiencies of childhood comprise numerous rare disorders that have been well characterized by a combination of clinical patterns, immunologic laboratory evidence, and often molecular identification of the mutant gene. Children with primary immunodeficiency (PID) commonly present with recurrent or severe infections, but most children with frequent minor infections (eg, otitis media or sinusitis) do not have an underlying immune disorder. Immunodeficiency should be considered when infections are severe, persistent, resistant to standard treatment, or caused by opportunistic organisms. Clinical patterns and recurring infections with certain types of microbes are indicative of specific immune deficiencies. Because delay in the diagnosis of PIDs is common, heightened diagnostic suspicion is warranted.

Host immunity can be divided into four main groups for the purpose of categorizing PIDs: antibody immunity (B lymphocytes), combined immunity (T and B lymphocytes), phagocytic immunity (neutrophil or mononuclear cells), and complement (bactericidal proteins also involved in opsonization). Understanding the role each category plays in host defense allows critical evaluation for possible immunodeficiency as the cause of recurrent infections.

IMMUNODEFICIENCY EVALUATION: PRIMARY CONSIDERATIONS

Before evaluating for a defined primary immunodeficiency, consider conditions that increase susceptibility to infection, such as allergic rhinitis (causing sinusitis), cystic fibrosis (causing failure to thrive, pneumonia, and sinus disease), asthma (causing chronic cough and pneumonia), foreign bodies, and conditions that interfere with skin integrity. Also exclude common causes of secondary immunodeficiency such as HIV infection, malnutrition, drugs, and protein loss via gastroenteropathy or kidney disease. If a single site is involved, exclude anatomic defects and foreign bodies. Figure 31–1 outlines the approach to considering PIDs.

Key clinical patterns can indicate the likelihood of a PID, the category of immune impairment (Table 31–1), and sometimes the specific PID. The frequency and severity of infections can be helpful when considering a PID. The Modell Foundation warning signs for PID are found in Figure 31–2. Children who meet two or more of these signs should be screened for PID. Age at the onset of infections can be a helpful clue, as defects in different arms of the immune system will present at typical ages. For instance, defects of phagocytes and cellular immunity typically present during the first months of life, whereas maternal antibody protects infants with antibody deficiency for 3–6 months. The type of infections should guide initial investigation, as antibody, complement, and phagocyte defects predispose mainly to bacterial infections; but diarrhea, superficial candidiasis, opportunistic infections, and severe herpesvirus infections are more characteristic of T-lymphocyte immunodeficiency. Combined immunodeficiency syndromes will present with a combination of infections typical for B-lymphocyte and T-lymphocyte deficiencies. Table 31–1 classifies PID into four main host immunity categories based on differences in these revealing clinical parameters of age of onset, specific pathogens, affected organs, and other special features. Finally, male gender increases the likelihood of an X-linked PID, while consanguinity increases the likelihood of an autosomal recessive form of PID.

The level of laboratory investigation should be based on the clinical presentation and the suspected category of host immunity impairment. A complete blood count and quantitative immunoglobulin measurement will identify the majority of those with PID, as antibody deficiencies account for at least 50% of PIDs (Figure 31–3). Table 31–2 summarizes the approach to laboratory evaluation of PID.

Cunningham-Rundles C: Immune deficiency: Office evaluation and treatment. Allergy Asthma Proc 2003;24:409 [PMID: 14763242].

Woroniecka M, Ballow M: Primary immune deficiencies: Presentation, diagnosis, and management. Pediatr Clin 2000;47:1211 [PMID: 11130993].

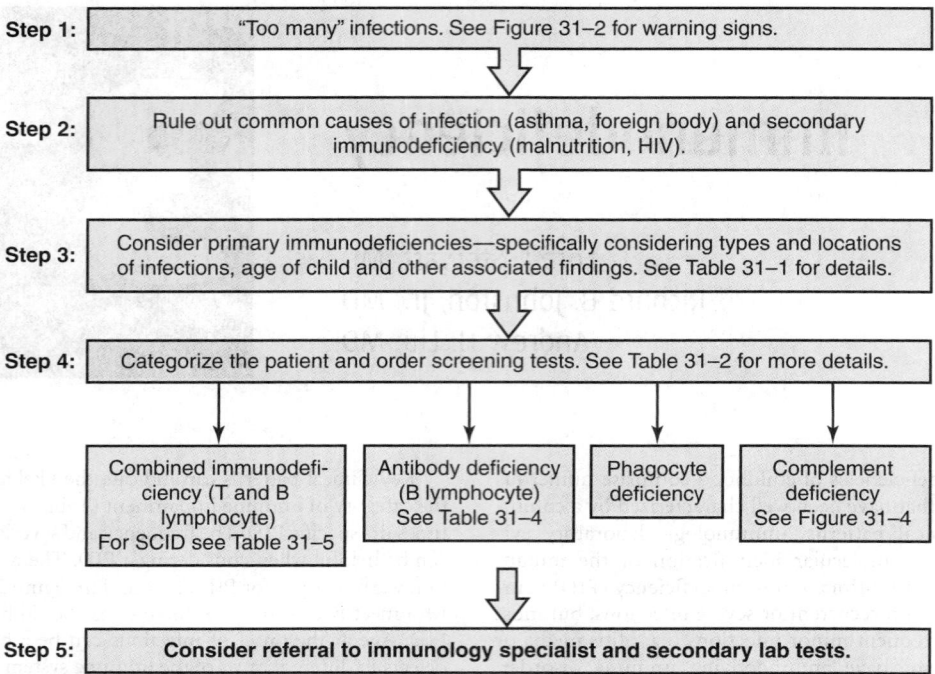

Step 1: "Too many" infections. See Figure 31–2 for warning signs.

Step 2: Rule out common causes of infection (asthma, foreign body) and secondary immunodeficiency (malnutrition, HIV).

Step 3: Consider primary immunodeficiencies—specifically considering types and locations of infections, age of child and other associated findings. See Table 31–1 for details.

Step 4: Categorize the patient and order screening tests. See Table 31–2 for more details.

Combined immunodeficiency (T and B lymphocyte) For SCID see Table 31–5

Antibody deficiency (B lymphocyte) See Table 31–4

Phagocyte deficiency

Complement deficiency See Figure 31–4

Step 5: **Consider referral to immunology specialist and secondary lab tests.**

▲ **Figure 31–1.** General approach to primary immunodeficiencies.

Antibodies & Immunoglobulins

Initial laboratory screening for antibody deficiency measures serum immunoglobulins (IgG, IgM and IgA, but not IgD). The normal ranges of IgG, IgM, and IgA vary by age as the production by B lymphocytes matures (see Table 31–3 for normal ranges). Some patients may have normal immunoglobulin levels but do not make protective specific antibodies; other patients have abnormal immunoglobulin levels but make protective specific antibodies. When interpreting immunoglobulin concentrations, remember that infants have lower normal values compared with adults. Evaluation of specific antibodies includes isohemagglutinins, which are naturally occurring antibodies (except in patients with blood group AB) and are detectable by age 6 months. Additional testing options include tetanus, diphtheria, *Haemophilus*, rubella, and mumps antibody levels following immunization. Assessing antibody response to pneumococcal polysaccharide can be helpful in the face of repeated pneumococcal infections, but as a screening tool it is often difficult to interpret, as the normal immune response to unconjugated polysaccharide vaccines may be weak or difficult to measure. The gold standard is preimmunization and postimmunization titers, with at least a threefold increase in titers 3 weeks postimmunization. Obtaining T- and B-lymphocyte counts is recommended if an initial screen revealed very low immunoglobulin concentrations for all classes, as certain hypogammaglobuline-

mic syndromes have low levels of or absent B lymphocytes (such as X-linked Bruton agammaglobulinemia). Protein electrophoresis can help identify the monoclonal increases seen in the oligoclonal gammopathy of Epstein-Barr virus (EBV) infections in X-linked lymphoproliferative syndrome, and in heavy-chain diseases. Serum albumin should be measured in patients with hypogammaglobulinemia to exclude secondary deficiencies due to protein loss through bowel or kidneys. IgG or IgA subclass measurements may be abnormal in patients with varied immunodeficiency syndromes, but they are rarely helpful in an initial evaluation.

Ballow M: Primary immunodeficiency disorders: Antibody deficiency. J Allergy Clin Immunol 2002;109:581 [PMID: 11941303].

T Lymphocytes

Initial laboratory screening for T lymphocytes includes a complete blood cell count with differential to evaluate for a decreased absolute lymphocyte count (< 1000/µL). Delayed hypersensitivity skin tests (such as *Candida*, tetanus, or mumps) give good evidence for antigen-specific T-lymphocyte immunity, but a negative or anergic result is not helpful, as it may be due to young age, chronic illness, or poor test technique. Even T-lymphocyte deficiencies will often not manifest anergy until the impairment is severe (eg, AIDS). When T-lymphocyte abnormalities are

Table 31–1. Categorical clinical features of primary immunodeficiencies.

Characteristic	Combined Deficiency (T- and B-Lymphocyte Defect)	Antibody Deficiency (B-Lymphocyte Defect)	Phagocyte Defect	Complement Defect
Age at onset of infections	Early onset, usually before 6 mo	Onset after maternal antibodies decline, usually after 3–6 mo; some later childhood or adult	Early onset	Any age
Specific pathogens	**Bacteria:** *Streptococcus pneumonia, Campylobacter fetus, Staphylococcus aureus, Haemophilus influenzae, Pseudomonas aeruginosa, Mycoplasma hominis, Ureaplasma urealyticum, Listeria monocytogenes, Salmonella typhi,* enteric flora, atypical mycobacteria, and BCG **Viruses:** CMV, EBV, varicella, RSV, enterovirus, rotavirus **Fungi/protozoa:** *Candida albicans, Aspergillus fumigatus* **Opportunistic:** *Pneumocystis carinii, cryptosporidium, Toxoplasma gondii*	**Bacteria:** *S pneumonia, C fetus, H influenzae, P aeruginosa, U urealyticum, S aureus, M hominis* **Viruses:** enteroviruses **Fungi/protozoa:** *Giardia lamblia* **Opportunistic:** none	**Bacteria:** *S aureus,* enteric flora, *P aeruginosa, S typhi, Serratia* spp, *Nocardia asteroides, Klebsiella* spp, atypical mycobacteria, and BCG **Viruses:** none **Fungi/protozoa:** *C albicans, A fumigatus* **Opportunistic:** none	**Bacteria:** especially *Neisseria* spp, *S pneumoniae, S aureus, P aeruginosa, H influenzae, U urealyticum* **Viruses:** none **Fungi/protozoa:** none **Opportunistic:** none
Affected organs	**General:** failure to thrive **Infectious:** severe infection (meningitis, septicemia, sinopulmonary), recurrent candidiasis, protracted diarrhea	**Infections:** recurrent sinopulmonary, pneumonia, meningitis **GI:** chronic malabsorption and IBD-like symptoms **Other:** arthritis	**Skin:** dermatitis, impetigo, cellulitis **Lymph nodes:** suppurative adenitis **Oral cavity:** periodontitis, ulcers **Lungs:** pneumonia, pneumatoceles **Other:** abscesses, osteomyelitis	**Infections:** meningitis, arthritis, septicemia, recurrent sinopulmonary
Special features	GVHD: maternal T cells or blood product transfusion Postvaccination: disseminated BCG or polio Absent lymphoid tissue Absent thymic shadow on chest radiograph	Autoimmunity Lymphoreticular malignancy Postvaccination paralytic polio Chronic enteroviral encephalitis	Poor wound healing; "cold" abscesses	**Autoimmune disorders:** SLE, vasculitis, dermatomyositis, scleroderma, glomerulonephritis, angioedema

BCG, bacille Calmette-Guérin; CMV, cytomegalovirus; EBV, Epstein-Barr virus; GVHD, graft-versus-host disease; IBD, inflammatory bowel disease; RSV, respiratory syncytial virus; SLE, systemic lupus erythematosus.
Adapted, with permission, from Woroniecka M, Ballow M: Presentation, diagnosis, and management. Pediatr Clin North Am 2000;47:1211.

suspected, it is important to check for specific antibody production and absolute numbers of T and B lymphocytes and their subsets (including CD3, CD4, CD8, CD19/CD20, and CD16/CD56). Because proper B-lymphocyte function and antibody production is dependent on T-lymphocyte function, most T-lymphocyte deficiencies manifest as combined impairments. Tests of T-lymphocyte proliferation and cytokine production can be supportive for characterizing immunodeficiency detected by initial tests, but they are not useful screening tests for children with chronic illness, recurrent infections, or young age; additionally, borderline function is often interpreted based on clinical correlation.

Phagocytic Immunity

Initial laboratory screening should include an evaluation for neutropenia with a complete blood count and differen-

10 Warning Signs of Primary Immunodeficiency

Primary Immunodeficiency (PI) causes children and young adults to have infections that come back frequently or are unusually hard to cure. In America alone, up to 1/2 million people suffer from one of the 100 known primary immunodeficiency diseases. If you or someone you know are affected by two or more of the following warning signs, speak to a physician about the possible presence of an underlying primary immunodeficiency.

1	Eight or more new ear infections in one year.	6	Recurrent, deep skin or organ abscesses.
2	Two or more serious sinus infections within 1 year.	7	Persistent thrush in mouth or elsewhere on skin, after age 1.
3	Two or more months on antibiotics with little effect.	8	Need for intravenous antibiotics to clear infections.
4	Two or more pneumonias within 1 year.	9	Two or more deep-seated infections.
5	Failure of an infant to gain weight or grow normally.	10	A family history of primary immunodeficiency.

▲ **Figure 31–2.** Warning signs of primary immunodeficiency. (Adapted, with permission, from the Jeffrey Modell Foundation.)

tial. A blood smear can be done to exclude Howell-Jolly bodies of asplenia and to look for normal lysosomal granules in neutrophils. The respiratory burst and generation of bactericidal factors can be tested by nitroblue tetrazolium reduction, but this test has generally been replaced by assessment of reduced nicotinamide adenine dinucleotide phosphate (NADPH) oxidase activity using flow cytometry (dihydrorhodamine flow cytometry assay). Leukocyte adhesion molecules are also screened by flow cytometry methods, although the difference in symptoms of suspected phagocyte defects should dictate which tests are used. Quantification of bacterial ingestion and microbicidal activity may be available.

Rosenzweig SD, Holland SM: Phagocyte immunodeficiencies and their infections. J Allergy Clin Immunol 2004;113:620 [PMID: 15100664].

Complement Pathways (Figure 31–4)

Deficiency of classic complement pathway components can be excluded by a normal hemolytic complement titer (CH50), for which the patient's serum must be separated and frozen to −70°C within 30 minutes of collection to prevent autodegradation of complement components. Alternative complement pathway deficiencies are similarly identified by AH50. Measuring individual complement component levels is not necessary if both CH50 and AH50 are normal. If the CH50 and AH50 are both low, the deficiency must be in their shared terminal pathway (C3, C5, C6, C7, C8, or C9). If CH50 is low, but AH50 is normal, the deficiency must be C1, C4, or C2; if AH50 is low and CH50 is normal, the deficiency must be factor D or B or properdin.

Wen L et al: Clinical and laboratory evaluation of complement deficiency. J Allergy Clin Immunol 2004;113:585 [PMID: 15100659].

Combined cellular and antibody deficiencies 15%

Cellular deficiencies 5%

Phagocytic deficiencies 10%

Complement deficiencies 5%

Antibody deficiencies 65%

▲ **Figure 31–3.** Relative frequencies of primary immunodeficiencies. (Adapted, with permission, from Stiehm ER et al (editors): *Immunologic Disorders in Infants and Children*, 5th ed. Elsevier, 2004.)

Table 31–2. Laboratory evaluation for primary immunodeficiency.

Suspected Defect	Screening Evaluation	Secondary Evaluation	Advanced Evaluation
B-lymphocyte defect	Quantitative immunoglobulins (IgG, IgM, and IgA)	B-lymphocyte enumeration panel (CD19/20)	Screen for specific genetic mutations
		Antibody response to prior or repeat immunizations (tetanus, diphtheria, Hib)	Screen for memory B cells (IgM-IgD-CD27+)
		Isohemagglutinins	
Combined T- and B-lymphocyte defect	Absolute lymphocyte count HIV testing	T- and B-lymphocyte enumeration panel (T = CD3, CD4 and CD8; B = CD19/20)	DNA analysis for specific genetic mutations
		Lymphocyte proliferation assay to mitogens and antigens	ADA or PNP levels of RBC
		Delayed-type hypersensitivity	Cytotoxicity studies
Phagocyte defect	WBC count with differential IgE level	Dihydrorhodamine flow cytometry	Bacteriocidal assays
		Nitroblue tetrazolium reduction assay	Chemotaxis assay
Complement defect	CH50	AH50	Individual complement levels and function

ADA, adenosine deaminase; Hib, *Haemophilus influenzae* type 1; HIV, human immunodeficiency virus; PNP, purine nucleoside phosphorylase; RBC, red blood cell; WBC, white blood cell.
Adapted, with permission, from Cunningham-Rundles C: Immune deficiency: Office evaluation and treatment. Allergy Asthma Proc 2000;24:409.

ANTIBODY DEFICIENCY SYNDROMES

 ESSENTIALS OF DIAGNOSIS & TYPICAL FEATURES

▶ Recurrent bacterial infections, typically encapsulated bacteria.

▶ Low immunoglobulin levels (usually).

▶ Inability to make specific antibody to vaccinations or infections.

General Considerations

Antibody deficiencies include both congenital and acquired forms that result in low (hypogammaglobulinemia) or very low (agammaglobulinemia) levels of immunoglobulins (IgM, IgG, and IgA). Deficiencies result in recurrent bacterial infections, specifically with encapsulated bacteria, including pneumonia, otitis, sinusitis, meningitis, cellulitis, and sepsis. As a group, antibody deficiencies represent nearly half of all pri-

Table 31–3. Normal values for immunoglobulins by age.

Age	IgG (mg/dL)	IgM (mg/dL)	IgA (mg/dL)
Newborn	1031 ± 200	11 ± 7	2 ± 3
1–3 mo	430 ± 119	30 ± 11	21 ± 13
4–6 mo	427 ± 186	43 ± 17	28 ± 18
7–12 mo	661 ± 219	55 ± 23	37 ± 18
13–24 mo	762 ± 209	58 ± 23	50 ± 24
25–36 mo	892 ± 183	61 ± 19	71 ± 34
3–5 y	929 ± 228	56 ± 18	93 ± 27
6–8 y	923 ± 256	65 ± 25	124 ± 45
9–11 y	1124 ± 235	79 ± 33	131 ± 60
12–16 y	946 ± 124	59 ± 20	148 ± 63
Adults	1158 ± 305	99 ± 27	200 ± 61

Adapted, with permission, from Stiehm ER et al: *Immunologic Disorders of Infants and Children*, 5th ed. Elsevier, 2004.

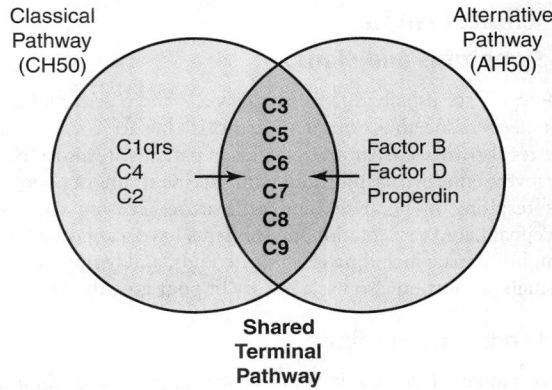

▲ **Figure 31–4.** Complement proteins and laboratory test pathways.

mary immunodeficiencies. Table 31–4 outlines primary antibody deficiency syndromes, laboratory findings, and genetic inheritance in these disorders. Patients who are unable to make specific antibody to vaccinations or infections are candidates for replacement gamma globulin therapy (ie, intravenous immunoglobulin [IVIG]). In contrast, those with secondary or transient hypogammaglobulinemia (ie, low total serum IgG level) who are able to make specific antibodies generally do not need or benefit from replacement IVIG.

1. X-Linked Agammaglobulinemia

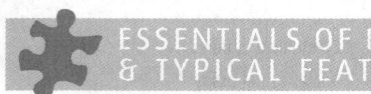

ESSENTIALS OF DIAGNOSIS
& TYPICAL FEATURES

- ▶ Child presents with infections early, usually after age 4 months.
- ▶ Typical bacterial infections include *Haemophilus influenzae* and *Streptococcus pneumonia.*
- ▶ Risk for severe enteroviral infections with vaccine strains of poliovirus.
- ▶ Failure to thrive and absent lymphoid tissue on examination.
- ▶ Very low levels of immunoglobulins and B lymphocytes.

▶ General Considerations

Children with X-linked agammaglobulinemia (XLA) typically present with infections after 4 months of age, when maternally derived IgG levels have declined. XLA is caused by a mutation on the X chromosome that results in low to absent circulating B lymphocytes and affects male patients. Early detection and diagnosis allow lifesaving replacement therapy with IVIG to be started prior to a potentially life-threatening infection.

▶ Clinical Findings

A. Symptoms and Signs

Infections are usually due to *H influenzae* and *S pneumoniae,* but deep tissue infections and arthritis due to *Ureaplasma* species also are seen. Antibody-deficient patients are also at risk for severe enterovirus infections with vaccine strains of poliovirus resulting in paralysis, and echoviruses causing chronic encephalitis. At presentation, male infants have scant or absent lymphoid tissue including tonsils, adenoids, and lymph nodes. A small proportion also has a history of poor growth.

B. Laboratory Findings

Most patients have low levels of or absent immunoglobulins (IgM, IgG, and IgA) and, despite a normal leukocyte count, have low numbers of or absent B lymphocytes. XLA accounts

for 85% of congenital hypogammaglobulinemia and occurs in about 1:200,000 male births. It results from mutations in the gene encoding the B lymphocyte tyrosine kinase (BTK), which is important for B-lymphocyte maturation. A BTK mutation by molecular analysis confirms the diagnosis of XLA.

▶ Differential Diagnosis

The differential diagnosis includes other causes of antibody deficiency as well as combined immunodeficiencies. Children with XLA are male and typically present at a young age with serious or recurrent bacterial infections, often with encapsulated species. Additionally, compared with other causes of antibody deficiency, XLA patients have the lowest or even absent numbers of B lymphocytes, but normal numbers of T lymphocytes. The normal T-lymphocyte number and function in XLA differ from findings in combined immunodeficiency. Additional causes of recurrent infections and low immunoglobulin levels include protein loss through renal or gastrointestinal disease, but patients with these disorders present with normal numbers of B lymphocytes and, typically, an isolated IgG deficiency.

▶ Treatment

Current therapy is with lifelong replacement IgG. In addition to preventing infections, IVIG replacement usually results in resolution of inflammatory arthritis and improves growth. Because the severity of infections varies and antibiotics are widely used, diagnosis is often delayed for years, but XLA must be considered in males with recurrent infections regardless of severity.

2. Autosomal Recessive Congenital Agammaglobulinemia

▶ General Considerations

Autosomal recessive congenital agammaglobulinemia is rare, accounting for less than 15% of all congenital hypogammaglobulinemia. It occurs in both male and female children and is caused by an abnormality in the immunoglobulin chain expressed on the surface of B lymphocytes. In the most common form, defects of the μ heavy-chain gene result in abnormal or absent IgM.

▶ Clinical Findings

A. Symptoms and Signs

Children present with recurrent infections, but the infections tend to have a very early onset, typically before age 6 months. Infections are bacterial and include pneumonia, otitis, sinusitis, meningitis, cellulitis, and sepsis.

B. Laboratory Findings

Patients usually have low numbers of circulating B lymphocytes and low levels of or absent immunoglobulins. Specific

Table 31–4. Antibody deficiency disorders.

Disease	Serum Ig	Circulating B Cells	Genetic Mutation	Mode of Inheritance
XLA	All isotypes very low or absent	< 2%	Mutations in BTK	X linked
Autosomal recessive congenital hypogammaglobulinemia				
Igα defect	All isotypes low or absent	< 2%	Defect in Igα molecule	AR
Surrogate light chain	All isotypes low or absent	< 2%	Mutations in λ5/14.1	AR
BLNK defect	All isotypes low or absent	< 2%	Mutations BLNK	?
μ Heavy chain	All isotypes low or absent	< 2%	Mutations in μ heavy chain	AR
Common variable immunodeficiency	Variable, some or all isotypes decreased	Normal or decreased	Unknown, likely not a single gene, AD form is TACI	Variable
Autosomal recessive forms of hyper-IgM syndrome	Normal or increased IgM, other isotypes decreased	IgM-bearing B cells only	Mutations in *AID* or *UNG* genes	AR
Transient hypogammaglobulinemia of infancy	IgG and IgA decreased, but IgM usually normal	Normal	Defect unknown	?
IgA deficiency	Very low or absent IgA	Normal	Defect unknown	Variable
IgG subclass deficiency	IgG subclasses decreased	Normal	Defect unknown	?

AD, autosomal dominant; AR, autosomal recessive; TACI, transmembrane activator and calcium-modulator and cyclophilin ligand interactor; XLA, X-linked agammaglobulinemia.

Adapted, with permission, from Ballow M: Primary immunodeficiency disorders: Antibody deficiency. J Allergy Clin Immunol 2002;109:581.

antibody function is poor. When diagnosis is suspected, detection of a mutation in the μ heavy chain can confirm the most common type. Additional mutations include mutations of the Igα molecule, the BLNK adaptor protein, and the λ5 surrogate light chain.

▶ Differential Diagnosis

The differential diagnosis is similar that of XLA, and includes XLA for male patients.

▶ Treatment

Treatment and prognosis are similar to those outlined for XLA.

3. Common Variable Immunodeficiency

ESSENTIALS OF DIAGNOSIS & TYPICAL FEATURES

▶ Recurrent infections, often with *Giardia lamblia* and *Campylobacter jejuni.*

▶ Decreased levels of IgG and IgA; poor specific antibody responses.

▶ Often associated with autoimmune diseases.

▶ General Considerations

Common variable immunodeficiency (CVID) is a diagnosis of exclusion after other causes of hypogammaglobulinemia have been eliminated. Onset may be at any age, and the incidence approaches 1:30,000. Many cases are sporadic, but a small percentage of patients have autosomal dominant or recessive inheritance and some cases are associated with HL-DR/DQ alleles.

▶ Clinical Findings

A. Symptoms and Signs

Patients have recurrent infections, most often of the sinopulmonary tract, but chronic gastrointestinal infections may manifest with recurrent diarrhea. Patients with CVID are at risk for developing bronchiectasis, autoimmune diseases (idiopathic thrombocytopenic purpura, autoimmune hemolytic anemia, rheumatoid arthritis, and inflammatory bowel disease), and malignancies (especially gastric carcinoma and lymphoma).

B. Laboratory Findings

Laboratory findings are variable but typically reveal low levels of IgG and IgA, normal numbers of B lymphocytes, low numbers of memory B lymphocytes (evaluated by flow cytometry), and abnormal specific antibody levels and responses. Some patients have evidence of T-lymphocyte abnormalities as well. Chronic gastrointestinal tract infections are often due to *G lamblia* or *C jejuni*.

Although CVID is typically a diagnosis of exclusion, recent research has yielded multiple specific mutations that have previous been labeled simply as CVID. One example is a mutation in a member of the tumor necrosis factor receptor family, identified as transmembrane activator and calcium-modulator and cyclophilin ligand interactor (TACI), which mediates isotype switching in B lymphocytes. TACI mutations were recently found in 10–15% of patients with CVID, as well as in some relatives of CVID patients with IgA deficiency. The mutations appear to be autosomal dominant with variable penetrance of clinical immunodeficiency and disease.

▶ **Differential Diagnosis**

When a patient presents with recurrent infections, low immunoglobulin levels, and potentially autoimmune symptoms, many different diagnoses must be considered, including other causes of low immunoglobulin levels (loss and abnormal production) and autoimmune diseases. CVID patients have normal numbers of B lymphocytes despite their poor specific antibody responses, which differentiates them from patients with XLA and autosomal recessive agammaglobulinemia. Patients with CVID also lack the specific mutations responsible for those disorders.

▶ **Treatment**

Treatment includes lifelong replacement therapy with IgG and routine assessment for bronchiectasis, autoimmune disorders, and malignancies. Prognosis depends on time to diagnosis and implementation of IgG replacement therapy, and can be good. Other complications include B-cell hyperplasia in the gut that may be severe enough to resemble Crohn disease, and gastric atrophy with achlorhydria, sometimes followed by pernicious anemia. Lymphoreticular proliferation can occur after EBV infection and is not always malignant.

Abonia JP et al: Common variable immunodeficiency. Allergy Asthma Proc 2002;23:53 [PMID: 11894736].

Castigli E, Geha RS: Molecular basis of common variable immunodeficiency. J Allergy Clin Immunol 2006;117:740 [PMID: 16630927].

Kokron CM et al: Clinical and laboratory aspects of common variable immunodeficiency. Ann Braz Acad Sci 2004;76:707 [PMID: 15558152].

4. Autosomal Recessive Hyper-IgM Immunodeficiency

Autosomal recessive forms of hyper-IgM immunodeficiency differ from the X-linked form (see section on Other Combined Immunodeficiency Disorders, later), as affected patients have normal expression and function of CD40 ligand.

Patients have mutations in activation-induced cytidine deaminase (AID) or uracil glycosylase (UNG). AID is required for B lymphocytes to switch from producing IgM to production of IgG, IgA, or IgE. UNG is also important for isotype class switching. The clinical presentation of AID- and UNG-deficient patients is less severe than that of X-linked hyper-IgM syndrome and also lacks opportunistic infections. Affected patients often have associated lymphoid hyperplasia compared with the paucity of lymphoid tissue seen in X-linked hyper-IgM syndrome. Treatment with IVIG replacement decreases infections and often normalizes IgM levels.

Etzioni A, Ochs HD: The hyper-IgM syndrome—an evolving story. Pediatr Res 2004;56:519 [PMID: 15319456].

5. Acquired Hypogammaglobulinemia

Acquired forms of hypogammaglobulinemia are common and may develop at any age. Causes of secondary hypogammaglobulinemia (nephrotic syndrome and protein-losing enteropathy) should be excluded by measuring serum albumin. Generally, acquired forms are not treated with IVIG because, although immunoglobulin levels are low, antibody function is adequately protective. Morphologic disorders or associated syndromes may point to a specific diagnosis.

Conley ME: Early defects in B cell development. Curr Opin Allergy Clin Immunol 2002;2:517 [PMID: 14752335].

6. Transient Hypogammaglobulinemia

Serum IgG levels normally decrease during an infant's first 4–5 months of life as maternal IgG acquired in utero is metabolized. Transient hypogammaglobulinemia represents a delay in the onset of immunoglobulin synthesis that results in a prolonged nadir. Symptomatic patients present with recurrent infections, including upper respiratory tract infections, otitis, and sinusitis. Diagnosis is suspected in infants with low levels of IgG and IgA (usually two standard deviations below normal for age), but normal levels of IgM and normal numbers of circulating B lymphocytes. Importantly, infants have normal specific antibody responses and T-lymphocyte function. Apart from appropriate antibiotics, no treatment is required. Infants with severe infection and hypogammaglobulinemia could be given IVIG replacement, but benefits and risk must be considered and this is rarely necessary. Recovery occurs between 18 and 30 months of age and the prognosis for affected infants is excellent provided infections are treated promptly and appropriately.

7. Selective Immunoglobulin Deficiencies

Selective IgA deficiency is the most common immune abnormality, found in approximately 1:700 persons. It is defined by a serum IgA level less than 7 mg/dL. Serum IgM, IgG, specific antibodies, and B- and T-lymphocyte numbers and function are normal. Most people with low serum IgA are without symptoms, but when symptoms are present, they include upper respiratory tract infections or diarrhea (or both). Associations also exist with inflammatory bowel disease, allergic disease, asthma, and autoimmune disorders (thyroiditis, arthritis, vitiligo, thrombocytopenia, and diabetes). IgA is primarily effective in its secreted form on mucosal surfaces.

IgA replacement is currently not feasible. For the majority of symptomatic IgA-deficient patients, antibiotics and appropriate autoimmune therapies are sufficient, but some patients have been treated with IVIG replacement. Caution must be exercised, as IgA-deficient patients are at risk for developing anti-IgA antibodies with blood product exposure, and the administration of blood products can result in anaphylaxis. Therefore when blood products are needed, washed packed red blood cells and volume expanders without blood products are recommended.

The possibility that deficiency of an IgG subclass (ie, abnormally low serum IgG2, IgG3, or IgG4) might predispose to recurrent upper respiratory tract infections in patients with normal total serum immunoglobulin levels is not well established. Normally, IgG1 comprises over 60% of total IgG and IgG2 over 10%. IgG3 accounts for about 5%, and IgG4 may be undetectable in up to 20% of healthy persons. Additionally, serum levels are age-related. It has been difficult to establish a link between IgG subclass deficiencies and any consistent pattern of infections. IgG replacement should be reserved for patients with defects in specific antibody production, which is rarely seen in patients with selective IgA or IgG subclass deficiencies.

Treatment of Hypogammaglobulinemia

The mainstay of therapy for hypogammaglobulinemia is replacement IgG, but management of infections is also important. Additional treatment modalities have included the use of cytokine therapy such as interleukin (IL)-2, hormone replacement, and vitamin supplementation. Curative therapy with bone marrow transplantation (BMT) has been successful in patients with XLA. Gene therapy is not yet available outside a research setting. Replacement IgG is usually given by intravenous infusions at a dose of 400–600 mg/kg every 3–4 weeks to maintain trough serum IgG levels above 500–800 mg/dL (a higher trough level is targeted for patients with established pulmonary disease). Subcutaneous replacement is available but requires more frequent injections and may limit maximum dosing. The aim of treatment is to *prevent* future infections and minimize any progression of chronic lung disease (bronchitis or bronchiectasis). Despite the passive immunity provided by replacement IgG, infection remains a persistent risk and prognosis additionally depends on timely and appropriate antibiotics. Typical infecting organisms include encapsulated bacteria, but *Ureaplasma* and *Mycoplasma* species must also be considered. Infusions are generally well tolerated, with most reactions being mild, including headache, back and limb pain, anxiety,

and tightness of the chest. Rare systemic reactions can occur, including tachycardia, shivering, fever, and in severe cases, anaphylactoid shock. For patients with congenital hypogammaglobulinemia, replacement therapy is currently lifelong.

Durandy A et al: Immunoglobulin replacement therapy in primary antibody deficiency diseases—maximizing success. Int Arch Allergy Immunol 2005;136:217 [PMID: 15713984].

SEVERE COMBINED IMMUNODEFICIENCY DISEASES

ESSENTIALS OF DIAGNOSIS & TYPICAL FEATURES

▶ Onset in first year of life.
▶ Recurrent infections caused by bacteria, viruses, fungi, and opportunistic pathogens.
▶ Chronic diarrhea and failure to thrive.
▶ Absent lymphoid tissue.

▶ General Considerations

Combined T- and B-lymphocyte diseases include severe combined immunodeficiency diseases (SCID) that encompass congenital diseases caused by different genetic mutations that result in severe deficiency of T and B lymphocytes. Despite differences in underlying mutations, affected patients present similarly, with recurrent infections caused by bacteria, viruses, fungi, and opportunistic pathogens. Additionally, patients often suffer from chronic diarrhea and failure to thrive. Without treatment, all patients with SCID typically die within the first years of life. SCID must be considered in the differential diagnosis in any infant with diarrhea and hypogammaglobulinemia.

▶ Clinical Findings

A. Symptoms and Signs

Common presentations include persistent cough, tachypnea or hypoxia secondary to underlying *Pneumocystis carinii* infection, or persistent oral or diaper candidiasis. Physical examination is notable for a lack of lymphoid tissue including tonsils and lymph nodes. A chest radiograph usually demonstrates an absent thymic shadow.

B. Laboratory Findings

Laboratory evaluation often reveals lymphopenia and some degree of hypogammaglobulinemia. Occasionally, an infant with SCID will present with normal numbers of lymphocytes resulting from transfusion-related engraftment or maternal T-lymphocyte engraftment via peripartum transfusion. Natural killer (NK) cells and B-lymphocyte numbers may be decreased, normal, or elevated. Additionally, in-vitro lymphocyte assays show poor response to mitogens, and specific antibodies are absent. Antenatal diagnosis is possible. Once the diagnosis of SCID is suspected, genetic testing should be pursued to confirm the diagnosis and the mutation present for both prognostic and genetic counseling purposes. Nine genes with mutations that result in SCID have been described to date. Clinical presentation and treatment is generally similar. The variants of SCID can be organized by the presence or absence of specific lymphocytes, including T, B, and NK cells (Table 31–5).

Differential Diagnosis

The differential diagnosis of SCID includes other causes of recurrent and severe infections and abnormal immune responses, most notably HIV disease. Other causes of hypogammaglobulinemia or agammaglobulinemia may be considered but will be ruled out due to abnormal T-lymphocyte function. The infection spectrum and severity of presentation in children with SCID is more severe and of earlier onset than that seen with CVID. Symptoms of congenital abnormalities with combined immunodeficiency features are discussed later in this chapter (see section on Genetic Syndromes Associated with Immunodeficiency).

Treatment

When SCID is suspected, *Pneumocystis* prophylaxis with trimethoprim-sulfamethoxazole and replacement IgG therapy should be initiated. *Patients with suspected SCID should only be transfused with irradiated blood products and should not receive any live vaccines.* Confirmation of the diagnosis should include screening for SCID subtypes listed in Table 31–5. BMT offers the best possibility of cure, with use of a human leukocyte antigen (HLA)-matched sibling offering the highest chance of success. In affected patients without HLA-identical donors, T-lymphocyte–depleted HLA haploidentical grafts or umbilical cord stem cells are used. For most patients, myeloablation is not necessary as the patient is without T lymphocytes. Additionally, most patients do not require graft-versus-host disease (GVHD) prophylaxis unless the donor is unrelated. T-lymphocyte reconstitution takes approximately 4 months, but only about 50% of patients regain full B-lymphocyte function, with the majority requiring long-term IVIG replacement. For months post-transplantation, patients are susceptible to many serious infections and prophylaxis is usually continued. Additionally, any signs or symptoms of infection must be promptly investigated and aggressively treated. The highest rate of success is in the youngest patients prior to developing infections (> 95% survival), but overall rates of survival range from 50–100% depending on the underlying mutation. Regarding gene therapy, X-linked SCID has been treated with autologous bone marrow in which normal function was transduced to lymphocytes by retroviral gene transfer. Unfortunately, two patients developed leukemia due to insertion of the retroviral vector near an oncogene. At this time, safer vectors are being sought.

Buckley RH: Molecular defects in human severe combined immunodeficiency and approaches to immune reconstitution. Annu Rev Immunol 2004;22:625 [PMID: 15032591].

Chinen J, Puck JM: Success and risks of gene therapy in primary immunodeficiencies. J Allergy Clin Immunol 2004;113:595 [PMID: 15100660].

Table 31–5. Severe combined immunodeficiency (SCID) variants.

Gene	Locus	Gene Product and Function	Presence of			Inheritance
			T Cell	B Cell	NK Cell	
IL2RG	xq13.1	Common γ chain of IL-2, 4, 7, 9, 15, 21 cytokine receptors; necessary to activate JAK3 for intracellular signaling	–	+	–	XLR
ADA	20q13.11	Part of the purine salvage pathway; necessary for removal of toxic metabolites that inhibit all lymphoid cells	–	–	–	AR
JAK3	19p13.1	A tyrosine kinase important for differentiation of lymphoid cells	–	+	–	AR
IL7R	5p13	IL-7 receptor is necessary for T-cell development and activates JAK3	–	+	+	AR
RAG1/RAG2	11p13	DNA recombinases, which mediate DNA recombination during B- and T-cell development	–	–	+	AR
CD3δ	11q23	Essential for T-cell development	–	+	+	AR
CD45	1q31-q32	Tyrosine kinase, important for regulation of other kinases in T- and B-cell antigen receptor development	–	+	+	AR
Artemis	20q13.11	Involved in repairing DNA double-strand breaks that occur during recombination	–	–	+	AR

–, absent; +, present; AR, autosomal recessive; IL, interleukin; NK, natural killer; XLR, X-linked recessive.
Adapted, with permission, from Kalman et al: Mutations in genes for T-cell development: IL7R, CD45, IL2RG, JAK3, RAG1, RAG2, ARTEMIS, and ADA and severe combined immunodeficiency: HuGE review. Genet Med 2004;6:16.

1. X-Linked Severe Combined Immunodeficiency

X-linked SCID, the most common form (40%) of SCID, results from mutations in *IL2RG* (IL-2 receptor gene) that encodes the common γ chain. The γ-chain protein is shared by multiple cell surface receptors for cytokines that are essential for T-lymphocyte maturation, including IL-2, IL-4, IL-7, IL-9, IL-15, and IL-21. Within the first 3 months of life, male infants present with diarrhea, cough, and rash. Laboratory evaluation reveals low T-lymphocyte numbers, normal numbers of B lymphocytes (which do not produce functional antibody), and absent NK cells.

2. Adenosine Deaminase Deficiency

Adenosine deaminase deficiency (ADA) is an autosomal recessive form of SCID caused by absence of adenosine deaminase, which is important for removal of toxic metabolites formed in T lymphocytes, including adenosine, 2' deoxyadenosine, and 2'O-methyladeosine. Increased levels of these metabolites result in T-lymphocyte death. Subsequently, affected patients develop complete absence of T-lymphocyte function. ADA SCID is distinguished from other variants of SCID by the following findings: the most profound lymphopenia ($< 500/mm^3$); skeletal abnormalities, including chondro-osseous dysplasia (flared costochondral junctions and bone-in-bone anomalies in vertebrae); and deficiency of all types of lymphocytes. Diagnosis is suspected in patients with profound lymphopenia and recurrent infections. The diagnosis is confirmed with a red blood cell assay for ADA activity. The genetic mutation is on chromosome 20q13.2–13.11. In addition to BMT, restoration of immune competence can occur in some patients with weekly infusions of polyethylene glycol–stabilized ADA enzyme conjugate. Gene therapy of stem cells with an ADA-incorporating retroviral vector has been successful, but the vector had oncogenic adverse effects. The development of safer vectors is yet to come.

3. Janus Kinase 3 Deficiency

Another form of autosomal recessive SCID is due to mutations in the gene encoding janus kinase 3, which is important for intracellular signaling through the common γ chain. The clinical presentation and lymphocyte phenotype most closely resembles X-linked SCID, with low T and NK lymphocytes, and elevated, nonfunctional B lymphocytes.

4. Interleukin-7-Receptor-Alpha-Chain Deficiency

IL-7-receptor-alpha-chain (IL-7Rα) deficiency SCID is transmitted by autosomal recessive inheritance. The IL-7 receptor is important for T-lymphocyte maturation and mutations result in low T-lymphocyte numbers, but normal numbers of dysfunctional B lymphocytes and NK cells.

5. Recombinase-Activating Gene Deficiencies

Another form of autosomal recessive SCID is due to mutations in recombinase activating genes (*RAG1* and *RAG2*), which encode proteins critical for assembling antigen receptor genes for both T and B lymphocytes. Several mutations in these genes have been described. The clinical presentation is similar to that of other forms of SCID, but the lymphocyte phenotype differs, as patients with SCID due to *RAG1* or *RAG2* mutations lack both T and B lymphocytes, but maintain normal or elevated numbers of NK cells.

Omenn syndrome is an autosomal recessive syndrome characterized by SCID, eczematoid rash, hepatosplenomegaly, lymphadenopathy, and alopecia. The disease is caused by mutations in *RAG1*, *RAG2*, or Artemis (see below). Laboratory evaluation reveals absent B lymphocytes, normal to elevated T-lymphocyte numbers with restricted function, and normal functional NK cells. Additionally, affected patients often have eosinophilia and elevated levels of IgE. The syndrome is typically fatal, although BMT has been used.

Ege M et al: Ommen syndrome due to ARTEMIS mutations. Blood 2005;105:4179 [PMID: 15731174].

6. CD3-Delta-Chain Deficiency

CD3-delta-chain (CD3δ) deficiency is a rare form of autosomal recessive SCID. Homozygous defects in the CD3δ chain halt T-lymphocyte maturation. Clinical presentation and lymphocyte phenotype are similar to IL-7Rα deficiency, but CD3δ-chain deficiency differs from other forms of SCID in that these patients have a normal appearing thymic silhouette on chest radiograph.

Dadi H et al: Effect of CD3δ deficiency on maturation of alpha/beta and gamma/delta T-cell lineages in severe combined immunodeficiency. N Engl J Med 2003;349:1821 [PMID: 14602880].

7. CD45 Deficiency

Another rare form of autosomal recessive SCID is due to mutations in the gene for CD45. CD45 is a tyrosine phosphatase important for regulating signal transduction. Affected patients have a similar presentation to other forms of SCID and a lymphocyte phenotype with low to absent T and NK cells, but elevated B lymphocytes.

8. Artemis Deficiency

Artemis is a DNA repair factor important for repairing cuts in the double-stranded DNA essential for the assembly of antigen receptors for T and B lymphocytes. Inheritance is autosomal recessive, and clinical presentation and lymphocyte phenotype are similar to those seen in *RAG1* and *RAG2* deficiencies.

9. ZAP-70 Deficiency

Deficiency of zeta-chain–associated protein (ZAP)-70 results in a rare form of autosomal recessive combined immunodeficiency. ZAP-70 is a tyrosine kinase critical for T-lymphocyte signaling and activation. Clinical presentation is similar to that of other forms of SCID, but most affected patients have palpable lymph nodes and visible thymic silhouette. Lymphocyte evaluation reveals absence of CD8$^+$ T lymphocytes, normal but nonfunctional CD4$^+$ T lymphocytes, normal numbers of poorly functioning B lymphocytes, and normal numbers and function of NK cells.

Elder M: SCID due to ZAP-70 deficiency. Pediatr Hematol Oncol 1997;19:546 [PMID: 9407944].

OTHER COMBINED IMMUNODEFICIENCY DISORDERS

Combined immunodeficiencies include defects that directly impair both T and B lymphocytes, as well as T-lymphocyte–specific defects, because proper B-lymphocyte function and antibody production are dependent on T-lymphocyte function. Therefore, most T-lymphocyte deficiencies manifest as combined impairments.

1. Wiskott-Aldrich Syndrome

> ### ESSENTIALS OF DIAGNOSIS & TYPICAL FEATURES

- ▶ Immunodeficiency with recurrent infections.
- ▶ Microplatelet thrombocytopenia.
- ▶ Eczema.
- ▶ Occurs only in males.

▶ General Considerations

Wiskott-Aldrich syndrome (WAS) is an X-linked recessive disease characterized by immunodeficiency, microplatelet thrombocytopenia, and eczema. The syndrome results from mutations of the gene encoding WASP at X11p. WASP is a protein involved in the rearrangement of actin and is important in interactions between T lymphocytes and antigen-presenting cells.

▶ Clinical Findings

A. Symptoms and Signs

Common presenting symptoms include bloody diarrhea, cerebral hemorrhage, and severe infections with polysaccharide-encapsulated bacteria, but clinical presentation can vary from classic severe WAS to mild thrombocytopenia without immunodeficiency, or X-linked thrombocytopenia (XLT), depending on the mutation. Early deaths are due to bleeding and infections,

but malignancies and autoimmune syndromes can develop over time. Survival beyond adolescence is rare in patients not receiving treatment, although XLT is sometimes diagnosed in adults.

B. Laboratory Findings

Laboratory findings that suggest the diagnosis are a low platelet count, low or absent isohemagglutinins, and reduced antibody responses to polysaccharide antigens (*S pneumoniae* and *H influenzae*). IgM may be low; IgA and IgE are often high.

▶ Differential Diagnosis

In addition to WAS and XLT, the differential diagnosis in a patient with a low platelet count must include other causes of platelet consumption, destruction, and abnormal production, such as idiopathic thrombocytopenic purpura, leukemia or myelodysplasia, drug adverse effect, and infection. WAS can be differentiated from these other conditions by small-sized platelets on smear evaluation, the presence of eczema (and atopy), and documented immune dysfunction. Additionally, there is a continuum between WAS and XLT that lacks immunodeficiency. Subsequently, a scoring system has been developed to help clinicians distinguish WAS from XLT.

▶ Treatment

Treatment includes infection prophylaxis with antibiotics (including trimethoprim–sulfamethoxazole for *P carinii* pneumonia) and IgG replacement therapy for patients with deficient antibody responses. Splenectomy to reduce thrombocytopenia has been helpful in some patients with XLT but must be followed by antibiotic prophylaxis because of the increased risk of septicemia and sudden death. Platelet transfusions should be avoided unless severe bleeding has occurred. Finally, BMT using the best-matched donor offers the possibility of a definitive cure, but is associated with morbidity and mortality.

Dupuis Girod S et al: Autoimmunity in Wiskott-Aldrich syndrome: Risk factors, clinical features, and outcome in a single-center cohort of 55 patients. Pediatrics 2003;111:e622 [PMID: 12728121].
Ochs HD, Notarangelo LD: X-linked immunodeficiencies. Curr Allergy Asthma Rep 2004;4:339 [PMID: 15283872].

2. 22q11.2 Deletion Syndrome (DiGeorge Syndrome)

> ### ESSENTIALS OF DIAGNOSIS & TYPICAL FEATURES

- ▶ Congenital heart defects.
- ▶ Hypocalcemia.
- ▶ Distinctive craniofacial features.
- ▶ Thymic hypoplasia.

General Considerations

DiGeorge syndrome or 22q11.2 deletion syndrome is an autosomal dominant syndrome resulting in defective development of the third and fourth pharyngeal pouches. There is considerable variability in phenotype based on the location and extent of microdeletion. Overlapping syndromes include velocardiofacial syndrome and Shprintzen syndrome. The incidence is about 1:4000 births, and the abnormal chromosome is usually inherited from the mother. The associated immunodeficiency is secondary to the aplastic or hypoplastic thymus, where T-lymphocyte maturation occurs. Surprisingly, most patients have no or only mild immune defects. The term *partial DiGeorge syndrome* is commonly applied to these patients with impaired rather than absent thymus function.

Clinical Findings

A. Symptoms and Signs

Clinical characteristics include congenital heart defects, hypocalcemia due to hypoparathyroidism, distinctive craniofacial features, renal anomalies, and thymic hypoplasia. Presentation usually results from cardiac failure, or from hypocalcemia 24–48 hours postpartum. The diagnosis is sometimes made during the course of cardiac surgery when no thymus is found in the mediastinum. Additional important clinical issues include delayed speech and behavioral problems.

B. Laboratory Findings

Laboratory evaluation typically reveals normal to decreased numbers of T lymphocytes with preserved T-lymphocyte function and normal B-lymphocyte function. In the rare patient with absent or dysfunctional T lymphocytes, B-lymphocyte function and antibody production may be abnormal as well. Over time, T-lymphocyte numbers normalize in the majority of patients who have low numbers of T lymphocytes at presentation. Diagnosis is confirmed via fluorescence in situ hybridization chromosomal analysis for the microdeletion on chromosome 22.

Treatment

Treatment of the 22q11.2 deletion syndrome may require surgery for cardiac defects, and vitamin D, calcium, or parathyroid hormone replacement to correct hypocalcemia. Transfusion products should be irradiated. Both thymic grafts and BMT have been used successfully in patients with absent T-lymphocyte immunity.

Sediva A et al: Early development of immunity in DiGeorge syndrome. Med Sci Monit 2005;11:CR182 [PMID: 15795698].

3. Ataxia-Telangiectasia

Ataxia-telangiectasia (A-T) is an autosomal recessive disorder characterized by progressive cerebellar ataxia (due to degeneration of Purkinje cells), telangiectasia, and variable immunodeficiency. Ataxia develops by age 5 years, followed by the appearance of telangiectasias of the conjunctivae and exposed areas (ie, nose, ears, and shoulders). The mutated A-T protein kinase is encoded on chromosome 11 and is required for cell cycle regulation and DNA repair. The Nijmegen breakage syndrome is probably a variant of A-T with more severe clinical features, including microcephaly and birdlike facies. Abnormal findings in A-T include elevated serum α-fetoprotein levels (useful diagnostically); thymic hypoplasia and lymphopenia; immunoglobulin deficiencies, including low levels of IgA, IgE, or IgG; and defective ability to repair radiation-induced DNA fragmentation. Clinically, the most important symptom is progressive loss of motor coordination, followed by weakness. Respiratory tract infections and many types of malignancy (including carcinomas and lymphomas) are the major causes of death. There is no definitive treatment, although IVIG and aggressive antibiotics have been used with limited success. Heterozygotes may have a small increased risk for breast cancer.

Nowak-Wegrzyn A et al: Immunodeficiency and infections in ataxia-telangiectasia. J Pediatr 2004;144:505 [PMID: 15069401].
Perlman S et al: Ataxia-telangiectasia: Diagnosis and treatment. Semin Pediatr Neurol 2003;10:173 [PMID: 14653405].

4. X-Linked Hyper-IgM Syndrome

X-linked hyper-IgM or CD40 ligand deficiency is the most common form of hyper-IgM and involves a defect in CD40 ligand (CD154) on T lymphocytes. Unlike the autosomal recessive forms of hyper-IgM, the mutation results in both antibody and cell-mediated deficiencies, as the interaction between CD40L (on T cells) and CD40 (on antigen-presenting cells) is important for both antibody production and T-cell activation. Affected males have low levels of IgG and IgA, but normal or elevated levels of IgM and normal numbers of B lymphocytes. Typically, male infants present with recurrent bacterial and opportunistic infections such as *P carinii* pneumonia or *Cryptosporidium* diarrhea. Additionally, affected males have a high frequency of sclerosing cholangitis, increased liver and biliary tract carcinomas, neutropenia, and autoimmune syndromes, including thrombocytopenia, arthritis, and inflammatory bowel disease. Conservative treatment includes IVIG and antibiotic prophylaxis, but because prognosis is still quite poor, BMT has been used with preliminary success.

Etzioni A, Ochs HD: The hyper-IgM syndrome—an evolving story. Pediatr Res 2004;56:519 [PMID: 15319456].
Jacobsohn DA et al: Nonmyeloablative hematopoietic stem cell transplant for X-linked hyper-immunoglobulin M syndrome with cholangiopathy. Pediatrics 2004;113:e122 [PMID: 14754981].

5. Immunodeficiency Due to Mutations of Nuclear Factor-κB–Essential Modulator

Immunodeficiency due to mutations in the gene for nuclear factor-κB–essential modulator (NEMO) is an X-linked syndrome in which male patients manifest ectodermal dysplasia (abnormal teeth, fine sparse hair, and abnormal or absent sweat glands) and defects of T- and B-lymphocytes. Many mutations are fatal in utero for male infants. Female carriers may have incontinentia pigmenti. The mutation results in abnormal immunoreceptor signaling. Surviving males present with early serious infections, including opportunistic infections such as *Pneumocystis* and atypical mycobacteria. Laboratory evaluation reveals hypogammaglobulinemia and poor specific antibody production, but normal numbers of T and B lymphocytes. Functional evaluation of lymphocytes demonstrates variable response. Because patients with confirmed NEMO mutations are quite rare, the best treatment course is unknown, but aggressive antibiotic therapy in combination with IVIG as well as BMT has been used. Prognosis is dependent on the severity of immunodeficiency, with most deaths due to infection.

Orange JS et al: The presentation and natural history of immunodeficiency caused by nuclear factor kappaB essential modulator mutation. J Allergy Clin Immunol 2004;113:725 [PMID: 15100680].

6. Combined Immunodeficiency with Defective Expression of Major Histocompatibility Complex Types I & II

Major histocompatibility complex class I (MHC I) deficiency or bare lymphocyte syndrome type I is an autosomal recessive combined immunodeficiency. Affected patients have abnormal TAP proteins important for intracellular transport and expression of MHC I on cell surfaces. Patients with bare lymphocyte syndrome type I present with recurrent sinopulmonary and skin infections. The diagnosis is confirmed by demonstrating an absence of MHC I expression.

Major histocompatibility complex class II (MHC II) deficiency or bare lymphocyte syndrome type II is a rare autosomal recessive combined immunodeficiency in which cells lack MHC II expression. Clinical presentation includes recurrent viral, bacterial, and fungal infections. Patients with bare lymphocyte syndrome type II have normal numbers of T and B lymphocytes, but low CD4$^+$ lymphocyte numbers, abnormal lymphocyte function, and hypogammaglobulinemia. They also have a high incidence of sclerosing cholangitis. When this diagnosis is suspected, demonstration of absent MHC class II molecules confirms the disorder. Severe cases are fatal without BMT, but milder phenotypes may be managed with IVIG replacement and aggressive use of antibiotics.

Nekrep N et al: When the lymphocyte loses its clothes. Immunity 2003:18;453 [PMID: 12705848].

7. Diseases Due to Defective Interferon Gamma & Interleukin-12 Pathways

The interferon-γ and IL-12 pathways are critical for macrophage, T-lymphocyte, and NK cell immunity toward mycobacterial infections. Multiple defects have been described in both the receptors for these cytokines and the receptors for signal transducer and activator of transcription molecules, with affected patients variably susceptible to atypical mycobacteria or infection after bacille Calmette-Guérin vaccination. Age of onset is variable, and symptoms can manifest in early adulthood. Treatment with supplemental interferon-γ is effective for some patients in combination with appropriate antibiotics. Most patients should also receive long-term mycobacterial prophylaxis.

Fieschi C, Casanova JL: The role of interleukin-12 in human infectious diseases: Only a faint signature. Eur J Immunol 2003;33:1461 [PMID: 2778462].

8. Purine Nucleoside Phosphorylase Deficiency

Purine nucleoside phosphorylase (PNP) deficiency is an immunodeficiency due to defects in the gene encoding PNP, which is important in the purine salvage pathway. Deficiency of PNP causes toxic metabolites that result in T-lymphocyte death, but in many patients B lymphocytes are spared. This autosomal recessive disease not only results in recurrent and serious infections, but affected patients have concomitant neurologic (developmental delay, ataxia, and spasticity) and autoimmune disorders. Infections present at variable ages. Laboratory evaluation reveals low numbers of or absent T lymphocytes and a variable B-lymphocyte deficiency. Without BMT, this disease is fatal due to infection or malignancy.

Dror Y et al: Purine nucleoside phosphorylase deficiency associated with a dysplastic marrow morphology. Pediatr Res 2004;55:472 [PMID: 14711904].

Myers LA et al: Purine nucleoside phosphorylase deficiency presenting with lymphopenia and developmental delay: Successful correction with umbilical cord blood transplantation. J Pediatr 2004;145:710 [PMID: 15520787].

PHAGOCYTIC DEFECTS

Phagocytic defects include abnormalities of both numbers (neutropenia) and function of polymorphonuclear leukocytes (neutrophils, eosinophils, and basophils). Functional defects consist of impairments in adhesion, chemotaxis, or bacterial killing.

1. Neutropenia

Evaluation for the presence of neutropenia should be included when considering recurrent infections. The diagnosis and treatment of neutropenia is discussed in Chapter 28. Additionally, some primary immunodeficiency syndromes are associated with neutropenia (eg, XLA).

Dror Y, Sung L: Update on childhood neutropenia: Molecular and clinical advances. Hematol Oncol Clin North Am 2004;18:1439 [PMID: 15511624].

2. Chronic Granulomatous Disease

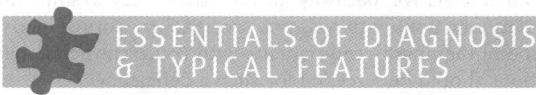

ESSENTIALS OF DIAGNOSIS & TYPICAL FEATURES

▶ Recurrent infections with catalase-positive bacteria and fungi.

▶ X-linked and autosomal recessive forms.

▶ Caused by abnormal superoxide generation within phagocytes.

▶ General Considerations

Chronic granulomatous disease is a rare immunodeficiency caused by defective superoxide generation; specifically, defects are seen in NADPH oxidase. Most cases (65%) are inherited as X-linked recessive diseases, but autosomal recessive forms also exist.

▶ Clinical Findings

A. Symptoms and Signs

Clinical presentation is characterized by recurrent and serious infections of skin, lungs, and liver with catalase-positive bacteria, fungi, and subsequent granuloma formation. Patients also typically have lymphadenopathy, hepatosplenomegaly, and signs of chronic and recurrent skin infections.

B. Laboratory Findings

Patients typically present with serious infection, positive cultures, and normal numbers of white blood cells. The five most common infecting organisms are *Staphylococcus aureus*, *Burkholderia cepacia*, *Serratia marcescens*, *Nocardia* species, and *Aspergillus* species. Patients also present with granuloma development from past infections, including granulomas of the skin, liver, and genitourinary tract. Patients may have an elevated erythrocyte sedimentation rate, even between obvious infections. Diagnosis is confirmed by demonstrating lack of superoxide production via dihydrorhodamine flow cytometry. This test, unlike the nitroblue tetrazolium test, allows differentiation between X-linked and autosomal recessive forms and also demonstrates carrier status of X-linked disease.

▶ Differential Diagnosis

The differential diagnosis includes other phagocytic cell abnormalities or deficiencies described in this section. Additionally, other immunodeficient states leading to recurrent bacterial or fungal infections, such as hypogammaglobinemia, CVID, SCID,

and other combined immunodeficiencies, should be considered. Notably, in contrast to these disorders, chronic granulomatous disease is defined by the absence of the superoxide burst.

▶ Treatment

Treatment includes prophylactic and symptomatic use of antibiotics and antifungals in combination with interferon-γ. Additionally, BMT has been successful.

Jurkowska M et al: Genetic and biochemical background of chronic granulomatous disease. Arch Immunol Ther Exp (Warsz) 2004;52:113 [PMID: 15179325].

3. Leukocyte Adhesion Deficiencies Types I & II

ESSENTIALS OF DIAGNOSIS & TYPICAL FEATURES

▶ Recurrent serious infections.

▶ "Cold" abscesses without pus formation.

▶ Poor wound healing.

▶ Gingival or periodontal disease (or both).

▶ General Considerations

The ability of white blood cells to travel to peripheral sites of infections is critical for effectiveness of phagocytic immunity. In leukocyte adhesion deficiency (LAD), defects in molecules required for leukocyte adherence and migration prevent these cells from arriving at the sites of infections. LAD I is an autosomal recessive disease caused by mutations in the common chain of the β_2 integrin family (CD18) located on chromosome 21q22.3. These mutations result in impaired neutrophil migration in addition to poor adherence, phagocytosis, and antibody-dependent immunity.

▶ Clinical Findings

A. Symptoms and Signs

Clinically, patients present with variable phenotypes, including recurrent serious infections, lack of pus formation, poor wound healing, and gingival and periodontal disease. The hallmark feature is little inflammation and absent neutrophils on histopathologic evaluation of infected sites (ie, "cold" abscesses) especially when concurrent with peripheral blood neutrophilia. The most severe phenotype manifests with infections in the neonatal period, including delayed separation of the umbilical cord with associated omphalitis.

B. Laboratory Findings

Laboratory evaluation often demonstrates a striking leukocytosis. Diagnosis of suspected cases is confirmed by flow cytometry analysis for CD18.

Treatment

Treatment includes aggressive antibiotic therapy. LAD II is a rare autosomal recessive disease caused by an inborn error in fucose metabolism that results in abnormal expression of sialyl-Lewis X (CD15s), which functions as a selectin ligand. The resulting phenotype is similar to LAD I, characterized by recurrent infections, lack of pus formation, poor wound healing, and periodontal disease, but additionally, LAD II patients have developmental delays, short stature, dysmorphic facies, and the Bombay (hh) blood group. Diagnosis is confirmed by flow cytometry analysis for CD15s, and treatment is usually limited to antibiotics, although fucose supplementation has been reported with some success.

4. Glucose-6-Phosphate Dehydrogenase Deficiency

Severe forms of X-linked glucose-6-phosphate dehydrogenase deficiency result in recurrent infections and increased risk of severe malarial infection due to abnormal neutrophil respiratory burst. Glucose-6-phosphate dehydrogenase–associated immunodeficiency is much less common than the associated hemolytic anemia.

5. Myeloperoxidase Deficiency

Leukocyte myeloperoxidase is important for intracellular destruction of *Candida albicans*. Although deficiency is quite common, few patients present with recurrent or chronic candidal infections. Diagnosis can be confirmed with assays measuring myeloperoxidase levels in leukocytes. Symptomatic and prophylactic antifungal therapy is often necessary in patients with recurrent infections. The myeloperoxidase gene has been localized to chromosome 17.

COMPLEMENT DEFECTS

As a component of the innate immune system, complement works through opsonization, lysis of target cells, and recruitment of phagocytic cells, and by facilitating antibody-mediated immunity. The complement system includes three pathways of enzymatic reactions: classical, alternative, and lectin (see Figure 31–4). All three pathways share C3 cleavage and result in promotion of inflammation, elimination of pathogens, and enhancement of the immune system response. Activation of the complement system occurs through bacterial proteins and surface-bound IgG and IgM antibodies.

1. Complement Factor Deficiencies

Rare deficiencies of individual complement factors (C1–C9) are inherited by autosomal recessive transmission. Deficiencies of factors C1, C2, and C4 do not predispose to increased infections, but are associated with autoimmune disorders such as systemic lupus erythematosus. Primary C3 deficiency presents with severe pyogenic infections, as C3 is critical for opsonization in both the classical and alternative pathways. There are also acquired forms of C3 deficiency that predispose patients to similar infectious risks. Terminal complement factor deficiency (C5, C6, C7, C8, and C9) or properdin (an alternative pathway factor) deficiency results in recurrent infections with *Neisseria* species. Survivors of meningococcal meningitis and patients with recurrent neisserial infections should be screened for such a deficiency.

Deficiency of mannose-binding lectin has been linked to increased risk of infections, but recent studies have been unable to confirm deficiency as a risk factor.

Dahl M et al: A population-based study of morbidity and mortality in mannose-binding lectin deficiency. J Exp Med 2004;199:1391 [PMID: 15148337].
Wen L et al: Clinical and laboratory evaluation of complement deficiency. J Allergy Clin Immunol 2004;113:585 [PMID: 15100659].

2. Hereditary Angioedema Due to C1 Esterase Inhibitor Deficiency

ESSENTIALS OF DIAGNOSIS & TYPICAL FEATURES

► Recurrent episodes of angioedema.
► No associated urticaria or pruritus.
► Onset at any age.

General Considerations

Hereditary angioedema is a rare autosomal dominant disorder caused by C1 esterase inhibitor (C1-INH) deficiency in which susceptibility to infection is not increased. There is also an acquired form associated with angiotensin-converting enzyme inhibitor medication use or some B-lymphocyte malignancies.

Clinical Findings

A. Symptoms and Signs

Affected patients can experience edema of skin and bowel and potentially life-threatening edema of the airway. Typical sites of swelling include the face, extremities, and genitals. Trauma, accidental or intentional (eg, due to surgery, childbirth, or dental work), may induce edema. Typical problems include episodic intestinal obstruction and dental procedure-induced upper airway obstruction. The edema is usually nonpainful (unless it involves the bowel) and lasts 48–72 hours. There is no associated urticaria (ie, redness) or pruritus. Age of onset is quite variable, and there is often a positive family history.

B. Laboratory Findings

Initial screening tests for complement that show decreased CH50 or low levels of C4 suggest the diagnosis. Confirmation comes from demonstration of low or absent levels of C1-INH or poor or absent C1-INH function. Additionally, C2 and C4 levels are low, and C1q is normal.

▶ Differential Diagnosis

Other causes of acquired angioedema, including that associated with certain medications (most notably angiotensin-converting enzyme modifying drugs), autoimmune diseases, and lymphoproliferative diseases, should be considered. Hereditary angioedema is distinguished from the acquired form of the disorder by normal levels of C1q.

▶ Treatment

Intravenous C1-INH concentrate is the treatment of choice for the emergency management of acute edema (eg, laryngeal or diffuse facial edema, severe abdominal attacks). Volume replacement is often needed due to fluid loss from edema. Fresh-frozen plasma may be used if C1-INH concentrate is not available. Long-term prophylaxis is a consideration when attacks occur monthly or have been life-threatening. The synthetic androgen danazol prevents attacks by increasing C1-INH levels. Antifibrinolytic agents (eg, tranexamic acid) may have a preferable adverse effects profile to androgens. For short-term prophylaxis prior to dental or surgical procedures, C1-INH concentrate is preferred; tranexamic acid, danazol, or fresh-frozen plasma can also be used.

Bowen T et al: Canadian 2003 international consensus algorithm for the diagnosis, therapy and management of hereditary angioedema. J Allergy Clin Immunol 2004;114:629 [PMID: 15356569].

Farkas H et al: Management of hereditary angioedema in pediatric patients. Pediatrics 2007;120:e713 [PMID: 17724112].

3. Paroxysmal Nocturnal Hemoglobinuria

Paroxysmal nocturnal hemoglobinuria is a rare X-linked disorder with variable disease expression in which affected patients have intravascular hemolysis, bone marrow failure, and thrombosis, but no associated immune defect. Paroxysmal nocturnal hemoglobinuria is caused by a mutation in phosphatidylinositol-glycan complementation class A, which is critical for certain erythrocyte surface proteins. Without these surface proteins, erythrocytes are highly susceptible to complement-mediated lysis. Thrombotic events, particularly intra-abdominal, are the major cause of death. Additional morbidity and mortality is due to bone marrow failure and associated bone marrow malignancies.

Meletis J, Terpos E: Recent insights into the pathophysiology of paroxysmal nocturnal hemoglobinuria. Med Sci Monit 2003;9: RA161 [PMID: 12883466].

OTHER WELL-DEFINED IMMUNODEFICIENCY SYNDROMES

1. Hyper-IgE Syndrome

Hyper-IgE syndrome (HIES), also known as Job syndrome, is a rare primary immunodeficiency characterized by elevated levels of IgE (> 2000 IU/mL), neonatal eczematoid rash, recurrent infections with *S aureus*, recurrent pneumonia with pneumatocele formation, and typical facies. Inheritance appears to be sporadic, although autosomal dominant and recessive cases have been reported. Additional clinical findings include retained primary teeth, scoliosis, hyperextensibility, high palate, and osteoporosis. In addition to staphylococcal infections, affected patients also have increased incidence of infections due to *Streptococcus* spp, *Pseudomonas* spp, *C albicans*, and even opportunistic infections with *Pneumocystis carinii*. Laboratory evaluation reveals normal to profoundly elevated levels of IgE and occasionally an associated eosinophilia. However, elevated IgE levels themselves are not a risk factor for HIES, as atopic dermatitis and parasite infection are much more common causes of elevated IgE. Diagnosis is often difficult due to variable presentation, which may become progressively severe with increasing age. Subsequently, diagnosis is often only made over time and evolving syndrome characteristics. The underlying cause of HIES is unknown. The mainstay of treatment is prophylactic and symptomatic antibiotic use in combination with good skin care. IVIG has been used with some success to decrease infections and possibly modify IgE levels.

Grimbacher B et al: Hyper-IgE syndromes. Immunol Rev 2005;203:244 [PMID: 15661034].

2. Immune Dysregulation, Polyendocrinopathy, Enteropathy, X-Linked Syndrome

Immune dysregulation, polyendocrinopathy, enteropathy, X-linked (IPEX) syndrome is a rare disease that usually manifests with severe diarrhea and insulin-dependent diabetes mellitus within the first months of life. Affected males also have severe eczema, food allergy, autoimmune cytopenias, lymphadenopathy, splenomegaly, and recurrent infections. Most die before 2 years of age due to malnutrition or sepsis. IPEX syndrome results from mutations in the *FOXP3* gene that encodes a protein essential for developing regulatory T lymphocytes. Leukocyte counts and immunoglobulin levels are generally normal. Immunosuppression and nutritional supplementation produce temporary improvements, but the prognosis is poor and most cases result in early death. BMT has been attempted with variable success.

Chatila TA et al: JM2, encoding a fork head-related protein, is mutated in X-linked autoimmunity-allergic dysregulation syndrome. J Clin Invest 2000;106:R75 [PMID: 11120765].

Nieves DS et al: Dermatologic and immunologic findings in the immune dysregulation, polyendocrinopathy, enteropathy, X-linked syndrome. Arch Dermatol 2004;140:466 [PMID: 15096376].

3. X-Linked Lymphoproliferative Syndrome

X-linked lymphoproliferative syndrome is an immunodeficiency that develops following EBV infection. Affected males develop fulminant infectious mononucleosis with hemophagocytic syndrome, multiple organ system failure, and bone marrow aplasia. The mutated gene encodes a signaling protein used by T lymphocytes and NK cells called SLAM-adapter protein. Affected boys are immunologically normal prior to EBV infection, and during acute infection they produce antibody to EBV. In most instances, infection with EBV is fatal. Patients who survive the initial episode or who are never infected with EBV in childhood develop lymphomas, vasculitis, hypogammaglobulinemias (with elevated IgM) or common variable immunodeficiency in later life. Antenatal diagnosis is possible.

Latour S, Veilette A: Molecular and immunological basis of X-linked lymphoproliferative disease. Immunol Rev 2003;192: 221 [PMID: 12670406].

4. Chronic Mucocutaneous Candidiasis

There are two forms of chronic mucocutaneous candidiasis (CMC). The first type is an autosomal dominant disorder that is characterized by isolated candidal infections of the skin, nails, and mucous membranes, and is not due to other causes. Systemic disease is not characteristic, but case reports of intracranial mycotic aneurysms exist. Primary CMC most commonly occurs as an isolated syndrome, but can be associated with endocrine or autoimmune disorders. The underlying defect is unknown, but the prognosis is quite good with antifungal therapy.

An autosomal recessive form of CMC with associated autoimmunity, also known as autoimmune polyendocrinopathy, candidiasis, ectodermal dysplasia (APECED) syndrome, is characterized by recurrent candidal infections, abnormal T-lymphocyte response to *Candida,* autoimmune endocrinopathies, and ectodermal dystrophies. APECED is caused by mutations in the gene for an important transcription regulator protein called autoimmune regulator that is critical for normal thymocyte development. Treatment includes antifungal therapy in combination with therapy for associated endocrinopathies.

Lawrence T et al: Autosomal-dominant primary immunodeficiencies. Cur Opin Hematol 2004;12:22 [PMID: 15604887].
Soderbergh A et al: Prevalence and clinical associations of 10 defined autoantibodies in autoimmune polyendocrine syndrome type 1. J Clin Endocrinol Metab 2004;89:557 [PMID: 14764761].

5. Autoimmune Lymphoproliferative Syndrome

Autoimmune lymphoproliferative syndrome (ALPS) results from mutations of genes important for regulating programmed lymphocyte death (apoptosis). Most commonly, the defect is in Fas (CD95) or Fas ligand, but other defects in the Fas pathway have also been described (eg, caspase 10). Clinical presentation includes lymphadenopathy, splenomegaly, and autoimmune disorders (autoimmune hemolytic anemia, neutropenia, thrombocytopenia, and sometimes arthritis). Occasionally, patients have frequent infections. The diagnosis is suspected when T-lymphocyte subsets by flow cytometry demonstrate elevated numbers of $CD3^+CD4^-CD8^-$ (double negative) T lymphocytes. Several different types of ALPS are distinguished by the response of lymphocytes to Fas-induced apoptosis. Patients are often heterozygous, and inheritance is mostly autosomal dominant. Treatment with prednisone often controls the lymphadenopathy. Infections should be treated appropriately. In some cases, BMT has been curative. Affected patients are also at risk for lymphoma. Mutations affecting another apoptosis-related protein, caspase 8, cause an ALPS variant syndrome in which the susceptibility to infection by herpes simplex virus also increases.

Bleesing JJH: Autoimmune lymphoproliferative syndrome: A genetic disorder of abnormal lymphocyte apoptosis. Immunol Allergy Clin North Am 2002;22:339 [PMID: 11269222].
Rieux-Laucat F et al: Cell-death signaling and human disease. Curr Opin Immunol 2003;15:325 [PMID: 12787759].

GENETIC SYNDROMES ASSOCIATED WITH IMMUNODEFICIENCY

Several described genetic syndromes have associated immunodeficiency that is often identified after the syndrome has been diagnosed. Usually, the immune defect is not the major presenting clinical problem.

Ming JE et al: Genetic syndromes associated with immunodeficiency. Immunol Allergy Clin North Am 2002;22:261.
Ming JE, Stiehm ER: Syndromic immunodeficiencies with humoral defects. Immunol Allergy Clin North Am 2001;21:91.

1. Bloom Syndrome

Characteristics of Bloom syndrome include growth retardation, sun sensitivity, and telangiectasias of the face. The syndrome results from mutations in a DNA helicase that lead to excess sister chromatid exchanges. Affected patients have an increased risk of malignancy and life-threatening infections. Serum IgA and IgM are variably low, and T-lymphocyte function is abnormal.

2. Transcobalamin 2 Deficiency

Transcobalamin 2 deficiency is due to defective cellular transport of cobalamin and results in megaloblastic anemia, diarrhea, and poor growth. Affected patients have hypogammaglobulinemia and poor specific antibody production.

3. Immunodeficiency, Centromeric Instability, Facial Anomalies Syndrome

Immunodeficiency, centromeric instability, facial anomalies (ICF) syndrome is a rare condition caused by abnormal DNA methyltransferase. Unlike other chromosome instability syndromes, ICF syndrome does not have an associated hypersensitivity to sunlight. Affected patients have severe respiratory, gastrointestinal, and skin infections due to low or absent immunoglobulins and abnormal T-lymphocyte numbers and function.

4. Trisomy 21

Patients with trisomy 21 or Down syndrome have increased susceptibility to respiratory infection. Immunodeficiency is variable, and abnormal numbers and function of T and B lymphocytes have been reported. Additionally, patients have an increased incidence of autoimmune diseases.

5. Turner Syndrome

Turner syndrome (partial or complete absence of one X chromosome) is associated with increased risk of otitis media, respiratory infections, and malignancies. Immune defects are variable but may include abnormal T-lymphocyte numbers and function and hypogammaglobulinemia.

6. Chédiak-Higashi Syndrome

Chédiak-Higashi syndrome is a rare autosomal recessive disease caused by mutations in a lysosomal trafficking gene. The neutrophils of affected individuals have giant lysosomes, impaired chemotaxis, neutropenia, and abnormal NK-cell cytotoxicity. Patients present with recurrent infections (particularly periodontitis), partial oculocutaneous albinism, and neuropathy. Most patients progress to generalized lymphohistiocytic infiltration syndrome, which is a common cause of death. Treatment strategies address infections and neuropathy and the use of immunosuppression attempts to slow lymphoproliferative progression.

7. Griscelli Syndrome

Characterized by partial albinism, neutropenia, thrombocytopenia, and lymphohistiocytosis, Griscelli syndrome is a rare autosomal recessive syndrome resulting from mutations in the myosin VA gene. Affected patients have recurrent and serious infections caused by fungi, viruses, and bacteria. Immunologic evaluation demonstrates variable immunoglobulin levels and antibody function with impaired T-lymphocyte function. BMT can correct the immunodeficiency. Griscelli syndrome is distinguished from Chédiak-Higashi syndrome by the lack of granules in white blood cells.

8. Netherton Syndrome

Patients with the autosomal recessive Netherton syndrome present with trichorrhexis (brittle hair), ichthyosiform rash, and allergic diseases. A subset of patients develops recurrent infections. Immune function is variable but may include hypo- or hypergammaglobulinemia, abnormal T-lymphocyte function, or abnormal phagocyte function. The disease results from mutations in a serine protease inhibitor encoded on the *SPINK5* gene.

9. Cartilage-Hair Hypoplasia

Cartilage-hair hypoplasia is an autosomal recessive form of chondrodysplasia manifesting with short-limbed short stature, hypoplastic hair, defective immunity, and poor erythrogenesis. The immune defect is characterized by mild to moderate lymphopenia and abnormal lymphocyte function, but normal antibody function. Affected patients have increased susceptibility to infections and increased risk of lymphoma. The disorder results from mutation in the *RMRP* gene that encodes the RNA component of an RNase MRP complex. BMT can restore cell-mediated immunity but does not correct the cartilage or hair abnormalities.

Ridanpaa M et al: The major mutation in the *RMRP* gene causing CHH among the Amish is the same as that found in most Finnish cases. Am J Med Genet C Semin Med Genet 2003;121:81 [PMID: 12888988].

GRAFT-VERSUS-HOST DISEASE

Graft-versus-host disease (GVHD) occurs when immunologically competent donor T lymphocytes are grafted into a host who is unable to reject them. The immunocompetent donor T lymphocytes recognize the host as foreign, leading to significant morbidity and potentially death. In addition to BMT-associated disease, GVHD can also occur in immunodeficient patients who receive nonirradiated blood products (ie, containing liver donor T lymphocytes) or engraftment of maternally derived T lymphocytes during birth. A progressive skin rash followed by diarrhea, hepatitis, nephritis, pulmonary infiltrates, fever, and marrow damage characterize GVHD. Laboratory evaluation reveals eosinophilia and leukocytosis, and diagnosis is confirmed by biopsy. Prevention is the most successful approach to GVHD. With BMT, GVHD prophylactic immunosuppressant regimens include methotrexate, cyclosporine, and mycophenolate mofetil. Treatment of GVHD includes similar regimens in addition to antithymocyte serum, corticosteroids, and monoclonal antibodies directed against T lymphocytes.

Jaksh M, Mattsson J: The pathophysiology of acute graft-versus-host disease. Scand J Immunol 2005:61:398.

REFERENCES

Ballow M: Primary immunodeficiency disorders: Antibody deficiency. J Allergy Clin Immunol 2002;109:581 [PMID: 11941303].

Bonilla FA, Geha RS: Primary immunodeficiency diseases. J Allergy Clin Immunol 2003;111:S571 [PMID: 12592303].

Rosenzweig SD, Holland SM: Phagocyte immunodeficiencies and their infections. J Allergy Clin Immunol 2004;113:620 [PMID: 15100664].

Stiehm ER et al (editors): *Immunologic Disorders in Infants and Children,* 5th ed. Elsevier, 2004.

Endocrine Disorders

Philip S. Zeitler, MD, PhD

Sharon H. Travers, MD

Francis Hoe, MD

Kristen Nadeau, MD

Michael S. Kappy, MD, PhD

GENERAL CONCEPTS

The classic concept that hormones are secreted substances affecting distant target cells has been updated to account for other mechanisms of hormonal action. Some hormones stimulate or inhibit metabolic processes in neighboring, not distant cells (eg, pancreatic islets or cartilage). This mechanism is termed *paracrine* activity. Other hormones affect the cells that produce them, a mechanism termed *autocrine*. Recognition that insulin, glucagon, ghrelin, somatostatin, cholecystokinin, and other hormones are synthesized by the brain and gut supports the concept of paracrine and autocrine processes in these tissues.

Another concept of modern endocrine physiology is that specific hormone receptors in target tissues are required for hormonal action. For example, in the complete androgen insensitivity syndrome, androgen receptors are defective and affected males have varying degrees of undervirilization of the external genitalia and wolffian duct system despite having both testes (the end organ) and adequate testosterone (the hormone). Similarly, in nephrogenic diabetes insipidus or pseudohypoparathyroidism, affected children have defective antidiuretic hormone or parathyroid hormone receptor function, respectively, and have diabetes insipidus or hypoparathyroidism, despite adequate hormone secretion. Alternatively, abnormal *activation* of a hormone receptor leads to the effects of the hormone in the absence of excessive hormone secretion. Examples of this phenomenon are the McCune-Albright syndrome (precocious puberty and hyperthyroidism), testotoxicosis (familial male precocious puberty), and hypercalciuric hypocalcemia.

HORMONE TYPES

Hormones are of three main chemical types: peptides and proteins, steroids, and amines. The peptide hormones include those released by the anterior and posterior pituitary, pancreatic islet cells, parathyroids, lungs (angiotensin II), heart and brain (atrial and brain natriuretic hormones), and hypothalamus (releasing hormones), as well as many local growth factors (insulin-like growth factor-1). Steroid hormones are secreted primarily by the adrenal cortex, gonads, and kidney (active vitamin D [$1,25(OH)_2 D3$]). The amine hormones are secreted by the adrenal medulla (epinephrine) and the thyroid gland (triiodothyronine [T_3] and thyroxine [T_4]).

As a rule, the peptide hormones and epinephrine act rapidly and bind to specific receptors on the surface of their target cell. The metabolic effects of these hormones are usually stimulation or inhibition of the activity of cellular enzymes or transport proteins (*post-translational effects*). The steroid hormones, thyroid hormone, and active vitamin D, in contrast, act more slowly and bind to specific cytoplasmic receptors in the target cell and subsequently to specific regions (genes) on nuclear DNA, where they direct a readout of specific protein(s). Their metabolic effects are generally stimulation or inhibition of the synthesis of enzymes or transport proteins (*transcriptional effects*), which increases or decreases the amount rather than the activity of these proteins in the target cell.

Metabolic processes that must be regulated rapidly such as blood glucose or calcium are usually under the control of the peptide hormones and epinephrine, whereas processes regulated more slowly such as pubertal development and metabolic rate are under the control of steroid hormones and thyroid hormone. Control of electrolyte homeostasis is intermediate and is regulated by a combination of peptide and steroid hormones (Table 32–1).

FEEDBACK CONTROL OF HORMONE SECRETION

An understanding of feedback control of hormonal secretion is fundamental to the understanding of endocrine disorders of childhood and their treatment. Hormone secretion is generally regulated by feedback in response to changes in the internal environment (see Table 32–1). When the metabolic imbalance

Table 32–1. Hormonal regulation of metabolic processes.

First Level (Most Direct)			
Metabolite or Other Parameter	**Stimulus**	**Endocrine Gland**	**Hormone**
Glucose	Hyperglycemia	Pancreatic beta cell	Insulin
Glucose	Hypoglycemia	Pancreatic alpha cell	Glucagon
Glucose	Hypoglycemia	Adrenal medulla	Epinephrine
Calcium	Hypercalcemia	Thyroid C cell	Calcitonin (?)
Calcium	Hypocalcemia	Parathyroid	PTH
Sodium/plasma osmolality	Hypernatremia/hyperosmolality	Hypothalamus with posterior pituitary gland as reservoir	ADH
Plasma volume	Hypervolemia	Heart	ANH
Second Level: Sodium and Potassium Balance			
Metabolite or Other Parameter	**Abnormality**	**Endocrine Gland**	**Hormone**
Sodium/potassium	Hyponatremia	Kidney	Renin (an enzyme)
	Hyperkalemia	Liver and others	Angiotensin I
	Hypovolemia	Lung	Angiotensin II
		Adrenal cortex	Aldosterone
Third Level (Most Complex)			
Hypothalamic Releasing Hormone	**Tropic Hormone (Pituitary Gland)**	**Endocrine Target Tissue**	**Endocrine Gland Hormone**
CRH	ACTH	Adrenal cortex	Cortisol
GHRH	GH	Liver et al tissues	IGF-1
GnRH	LH	Testis	Testosterone
GnRH	FSH/LH	Ovary	Estradiol/progesterone
TRH	TSH	Thyroid gland	T_4 and T_3

ACTH, corticotropin; ADH, antidiuretic hormone; ANH, atrial natriuretic hormone; CRH, corticotropin-releasing hormone; FSH, follicle-stimulating hormone; GH, growth hormone; GHRH, growth hormone-releasing hormone; GnRH, gonadotropin-releasing hormone; IGF-1, insulin-like growth factor-1; LH, luteinizing hormone; PTH, parathyroid hormone; T_3, triiodothyronine; T_4, thyroxine; TRH, thyrotropin-releasing hormone; TSH, thyroid-stimulating hormone.

is corrected, the stimulus for the hormone's secretion ceases or is inhibited. Overcorrection of the imbalance stimulates secretion of a counterbalancing hormone or hormones.

Hypothalamic-pituitary control of hormone secretion is also regulated by feedback, so that end-organ failure (endocrine gland insufficiency) causing decreased circulating endocrine gland hormones results in increased secretion of their respective hypothalamic releasing and pituitary hormones (Table 32–1 and Figure 32–1). If restoration of normal circulating concentrations of hormones occurs, feedback inhibition at the pituitary and hypothalamus results in cessation of the previously stimulated secretion of releasing and pituitary hormones and restoration of their circulating concentrations to normal. Similarly, if there is autonomous endocrine gland hyperfunction (eg, McCune-Albright syndrome, Graves disease, or adrenal tumor), the specific hypothalamic releasing and pituitary hormones are suppressed (see Figure 32–1).

DISTURBANCES OF GROWTH

Disturbance of growth and development is the most common problem evaluated by a pediatric endocrinologist. While most cases represent normal developmental variants, it is critical to identify abnormal growth patterns, as deviations from the norm can be the first or only manifestation of many endocrine disorders. Determination of height velocity is the most critical factor in evaluating a child's growth. A persistent increase or decrease in height percentiles between age 2 years and the onset of puberty always warrants evaluation. It is more difficult to distinguish normal from abnormal growth in the first 2 years of life, as infants may have catch-up or catch-down growth during this period.

Appropriate standards must be used to evaluate growth. The National Center for Health Statistics provides standard growth charts for North American children (see Chapter 1). Specific growth charts are also available for some ethnic

▲ Figure 32–1. General scheme of the hypothalamus-pituitary-endocrine gland axis. Releasing hormones synthesized in the hypothalamus are secreted into the hypophysial portal circulation. Trophic hormones are secreted by the pituitary gland in response, and they in turn act on specific endocrine glands to stimulate the secretion of their respective hormones. The endocrine gland hormones exert their respective effects on various target tissues (end organs) and exert a negative feedback (feedback inhibition) on their own secretion by acting at the level of the pituitary and hypothalamus. This system is characteristic of those hormones listed in Table 32–1 (third level).

groups. Normal values can vary by country of origin. In addition, growth charts are available for children with specific growth disturbances, such as Turner syndrome and Down syndrome.

TARGET HEIGHT & SKELETAL MATURATION

A child's growth and height potential is determined largely by genetic factors. The target (midparental) height of a child is calculated from the mean parental height plus or minus 6.5 cm for boys and girls, respectively. This calculation helps identify a child's genetic growth potential. Most children achieve an adult height within 8 cm of this number. Another parameter to determine growth potential is skeletal maturation or bone age. Beyond the neonatal period, bone age is evaluated by comparing a radiograph of the child's left hand and wrist with the standards of Greulich and Pyle. Delayed or advanced bone age is not diagnostic of any specific disease, but the extent of skeletal maturation is used to determine remaining growth potential as a percentage of total height and allows prediction of ultimate height.

SHORT STATURE

Short stature has many causes. It is important to distinguish normal variants of growth (familial short stature and constitutional growth delay) and pathologic conditions (Table 32–2). Pathologic short stature is more likely in children whose growth velocity is abnormal (crossing major height percentiles on the growth curve) or who are significantly short for their family. Children with chronic illness or nutritional deficiencies may have poor linear growth, but this is typically associated with inadequate weight gain. In contrast, endocrine causes of short stature are usually associated with normal or excessive weight gain.

1. Familial Short Stature & Constitutional Growth Delay

Children with familial short stature typically have normal birth weight and length. In the first 2 years of life their linear growth velocity decelerates as they near their genetically determined percentile. Once this target percentile is reached, the child has normal linear growth parallel to the growth curve. Skeletal maturation and timing of puberty are consistent with chronologic age. The height percentile the child follows is maintained, and final height is short but appropriate for the family (Figure 32–2). For example, an infant boy of a mother who is 5'0" and father who is 5'5" (calculated midparental height 5'5") may have a birth length at the 50th percentile. However, this child's length percentile will drift downward during the first 2 years of life and will settle in at the fifth percentile where it will stay.

Children with constitutional growth delay do not necessarily have short parents but have a growth pattern similar to those with familial short stature. The difference is that children with constitutional growth delay have a delay in skeletal maturation and a delay in the onset of puberty. In these children, growth continues beyond the time the average child stops growing, and final height is appropriate for target height (Figure 32–3). There is often a history of other family members being "late bloomers."

2. Growth Hormone Deficiency

Human growth hormone (GH) is produced by the anterior pituitary gland under the stimulation of growth hormone–releasing hormone (GHRH) and the inhibition of somatostatin. GH is secreted in a pulsatile pattern in response to sleep, exercise, and hypoglycemia and has direct growth-promoting and metabolic effects (Figure 32–4). GH also promotes growth indirectly by stimulating production of insulin-like growth factors, primarily IGF-1.

Table 32–2. Causes of short stature.

A. Genetic-familial short stature
B. Constitutional growth delay
C. Endocrine disturbances
  1. Growth hormone (GH) deficiency
    a. Hereditary
      (1) Growth hormone–releasing hormone (GHRH) receptor mutation
      (2) GH gene deletion
      (3) GH resistance
      (4) Congenital hypopituitarism—GH deficiency in combination with deficiency of other anterior pituitary hormones
    b. Idiopathic—with and without associated abnormalities of midline structures of the central nervous system
      (1) Isolated GH deficiency
      (2) Combined pituitary hormone deficiency
    c. Acquired
      (1) Transient—eg, psychosocial short stature
      (2) Organic—tumor, irradiation of the central nervous system, infection, or trauma
  2. Insulin-like growth factor 1 (IGF-1) deficiency
  3. Hypothyroidism
  4. Excess cortisol—Cushing disease and Cushing syndrome (including iatrogenic causes)
  5. Precocious puberty
  6. Diabetes mellitus (poorly controlled)
  7. Pseudohypoparathyroidism
  8. Rickets
D. Intrauterine growth restriction
  1. Intrinsic fetal abnormalities—chromosomal disorders
  2. Syndromes (eg, Russell-Silver, Noonan, Bloom, de Lange, Cockayne)
  3. Congenital infections
  4. Placental abnormalities
  5. Maternal abnormalities
    a. Hypertension/toxemia
    b. Drug use
    c. Malnutrition
E. Inborn errors of metabolism
  1. Mucopolysaccharidosis
  2. Other storage diseases
F. Intrinsic diseases of bone
  1. Defects of growth of tubular bones or spine (eg, achondroplasia, metatropic dwarfism, diastrophic dwarfism, metaphyseal chondrodysplasia)
  2. Disorganized development of cartilage and fibrous components of the skeleton (eg, multiple cartilaginous exostoses, fibrous dysplasia with skin pigmentation)
G. Short stature associated with chromosomal defects
  1. Autosomal (eg, Down syndrome, Prader-Willi syndrome)
  2. Sex chromosomal (eg, Turner syndrome–XO)
H. Chronic systemic diseases, congenital defects, and cancers (eg, chronic infection and infestation, inflammatory bowel disease, hepatic disease, cardiovascular disease, hematologic disease, central nervous system disease, pulmonary disease, renal disease, malnutrition, cancers, collagen-vascular disease)
I. Psychosocial short stature (deprivation dwarfism)

Growth hormone deficiency (GHD) is characterized by decreased growth velocity and delayed skeletal maturation in the absence of other explanations. Laboratory tests indicate subnormal GH secretion or action. GHD may be isolated or coexist with other pituitary hormone deficiencies. GHD may be congenital (septo-optic dysplasia or ectopic posterior pituitary), genetic (GH or GHRH gene mutation), or acquired (craniopharyngioma, germinoma, histiocytosis, or cranial irradiation). Idiopathic GHD is more common than any other cause, with an incidence of about 1:4000 children. GH resistance syndrome (Laron dwarfism) is caused by a mutation in the GH receptor. Presentation is similar to GHD, but short stature is severe and there is a distinctive facial appearance. Additional forms of GH resistance are caused by mutations in other molecular components of the GH signaling pathway.

Infants with GHD have normal birth weight with only slightly reduced length, suggesting that GH is a minor contributor to intrauterine growth. GH-deficient infants classically present as newborns with hypoglycemia or other pituitary deficiencies such as central hypothyroidism or adrenal insufficiency. Micropenis is a feature of newborn males with gonadotropin and GH deficiency. Because GH promotes lipolysis, many GH-deficient children have truncal adiposity. Growth retardation begins in infancy or may be delayed until later childhood. Regardless of onset, the primary manifestation of idiopathic or acquired GHD is subnormal growth velocity (Figure 32–5).

Laboratory tests to assess GH status may be difficult to interpret. Children with normal and short stature have a broad range of GH secretion patterns, and significant overlap exists between normal and GH-deficient children. Provocative studies are performed using such agents as insulin-induced hypoglycemia, arginine, levodopa, clonidine, or glucagon. Serum concentrations of IGF-1 and IGF-binding protein 3 may give reasonable estimations of GH secretion in the adequately nourished child (see Figure 32–4). When results of GH tests are equivocal, a trial of GH treatment can help determine whether an abnormally short child will benefit from GH. Current treatment for GHD is subcutaneous recombinant GH given 6 or 7 days per week with total weekly dose of 0.15–0.3 mg/kg.

GH therapy is approved by the U.S. Food and Drug Administration (FDA) for children with GHD and growth restriction associated with chronic renal failure, for girls with Turner syndrome, children with Prader-Willi syndrome, and children born small for gestational age (SGA) who fail to demonstrate catch-up growth by age 4. GH therapy has also been approved for children with idiopathic short stature whose current height is more than 2.25 standard deviations below the norm for age. Final height improvement may be 5–7 cm in this population. This last indication is controversial and the role of GH for idiopathic short stature is still unclear. Side effects of recombinant GH are uncommon but include benign intracranial hypertension and slipped capital femoral epiphysis. With early diagnosis and treatment, children with GHD reach normal or near-normal adult height. Recombinant IGF-1 is available for use in children with GH resistance or IGF-1 deficiency.

Mother's Stature _____ **Father's Stature** _____

Date	Age	Weight	Stature	BMI*

To Calculate BMI: Weight (kg) ÷ Stature (cm) ÷ Stature (cm)
× 10,000 **or** Weight (lb) ÷ Stature (in) ÷ Stature (in) × 703

Target Ht

Predicted Ht

AGE (YEARS)

▲ **Figure 32–2.** Typical pattern of growth in a child with familial short stature. After attaining an appropriate percentile during the first 2 years of life, the child will have normal linear growth parallel to the growth curve. Skeletal maturation and the timing of puberty are consistent with chronologic age. The height percentile the child has been following is maintained, and final height is short but appropriate for the family.

▲ **Figure 32–3.** Typical pattern of growth in a child with constitutional growth delay. Growth slows during the first 2 years of life, similarly to children with familial short stature. Subsequently the child will have normal linear growth parallel to the growth curve. However, skeletal maturation and the onset of puberty are delayed. Growth continues beyond the time the average child has stopped growing, and final height is appropriate for target height.

▲ **Figure 32–4.** The GHRH/GH/IGF-1 system. The effects of growth hormone (GH) on growth are partly due to its direct anabolic effects in muscle, liver, and bone. In addition, GH stimulates many tissues to produce insulin-like growth factor 1 (IGF-1) locally, which stimulates the growth of the tissue itself (paracrine effect of IGF-1). The action of GH on the liver results in the secretion of IGF-1 (circulating IGF-1), which stimulates growth in other tissues (endocrine effect of IGF-1). The action of growth hormone on the liver also enhances the secretion of IGF-binding protein 3 (IGFBP-3) and acid-labile subunit (ALS), which form a high-molecular-weight complex with IGF-1. The function of this complex is to transport IGF-1 to its target tissues, but the complex also serves as a reservoir and possible inhibitor of IGF-1 action. In various chronic illnesses, the direct metabolic effects of GH are inhibited; the secretion of IGF-1 in response to GH is blunted, and in some cases IGFBP-3 synthesis is enhanced, resulting in marked inhibition in the growth of the child. GHRH, growth hormone–releasing hormone.

3. Small for Gestational Age/Intrauterine Growth Restriction

Small-for-gestational-age (SGA) infants have birth weights below the 10th percentile for the population's birth weight/gestational age relationship. SGA infants include constitutionally small infants growing at their potential and infants with intrauterine growth restriction (IUGR). IUGR refers to a heterogeneous group of patients who fail to grow at a normal rate in utero.

SGA/IUGR is a result of poor maternal environment, intrinsic fetal abnormalities, congenital infections, or other fetal malnutrition. Intrinsic fetal abnormalities causing SGA/IUGR (often termed primordial short stature) include Russell-Silver, Seckel, Noonan, Bloom, and Cockayne syndromes, and progeria. Many children with mild SGA/IUGR (except those with intrinsic fetal abnormalities) exhibit catch-up growth during the first 3 years. However, 15–20% remain short throughout life, particularly those whose in-utero growth restriction occurred over several months rather than just the last 2–3 months gestation. Catch-up growth

may also be inadequate in preterm SGA/IUGR infants with inadequate postnatal nutrition. Children who do not show catch-up growth may have normal growth velocity, but they will follow a lower height percentile than expected for the family. In contrast to children with constitutional growth delay, those with SGA/IUGR have skeletal maturation that corresponds to chronologic age or is only mildly delayed.

GH therapy for SGA/IUGR children with growth delay is FDA approved and appears to be effective in increasing growth velocity and final adult height.

4. Disproportionate Short Stature

Skeletal dysplasias cause disproportionate short stature. There are more than 200 types of sporadic and genetic skeletal dysplasias. Measurements of arm span and upper-to-lower body segment ratio are helpful in determining whether a child has normal body proportions. If disproportionate short stature is found, a skeletal survey may be useful because specific radiographic features characterize certain disorders. Because skeletal dysplasias are rare, the effect of GH on most types is unknown.

Mother's Stature _____ **Father's Stature** _____

Date	Age	Weight	Stature	BMI*

***To Calculate BMI:** Weight (kg) + Stature (cm) + Stature (cm)
× 10,000 **or** Weight (lb) + Stature (in) + Stature (in) × 703

AGE (YEARS)

Target Ht
Predicted Ht

GH
Treatment

▲ **Figure 32–5.** Typical pattern of growth in a child with acquired growth hormone deficiency. Children with acquired growth hormone deficiency have an abnormal growth velocity and fail to maintain height percentile during childhood. Other phenotypic features (central adiposity and immaturity of facies) may be present. Children with congenital growth hormone deficiency will cross percentiles during the first 2 years of life, similarly to the pattern seen in familial short stature and constitutional delay, but will fail to attain a steady height percentile subsequently.

5. Short Stature Associated with Syndromes

Short stature is associated with many syndromes, including Turner, Down, and Prader-Willi. Girls with Turner syndrome often have recognizable features such as micrognathia, webbed neck, low posterior hairline, edema of hands and feet, multiple pigmented nevi, and an increased carrying angle. In some girls, however, short stature is the only obvious manifestation. Consequently, any girl with unexplained short stature should have a chromosomal evaluation. Although girls with Turner syndrome are not usually GH-deficient, GH therapy can improve final height by an average of 6.0 cm. Duration of GH therapy is a significant predictor of long-term height gain; consequently, it is important that Turner syndrome be diagnosed early and GH started as soon as possible.

GH is also approved for growth failure in Prader-Willi syndrome. Many of these individuals are GH-deficient. GH improves growth, body composition, and physical activity in these patients. A few deaths have been reported in Prader-Willi children receiving GH. All of the deaths were in very obese children, children with respiratory impairments, sleep apnea, or unidentified respiratory infections. The role of GH, if any, in these deaths is unknown. As a precaution, it is recommended that all Prader-Willi patients be evaluated for upper airway obstruction and sleep apnea prior to starting GH therapy.

Children with Down syndrome should be evaluated for GHD only if their linear growth is abnormal compared with the Down syndrome growth chart.

6. Psychosocial Short Stature (Psychosocial Dwarfism)

Psychosocial short stature refers to growth retardation in association with emotional deprivation. Undernutrition probably contributes to growth retardation in some children. Other symptoms include bizarre eating and drinking habits, bowel and bladder incontinence, social withdrawal, and delayed speech. GH secretion in children with psychosocial short stature is diminished, but GH therapy is usually not beneficial. Foster home placement or a change in the psychological environment at home usually results in improved growth and normalization of GH secretion, personality, and eating behaviors.

Clinical Evaluation

Laboratory investigation should be guided by the history and physical examination. Data included in history and physical include size at birth, pattern of growth since birth, familial growth patterns, pubertal stage, dysmorphic features, body segment proportion, and psychological health. In a child with poor weight gain as the primary disturbance, history of chronic illness and nutritional assessment are indicated. The following laboratory tests may be useful:

1. Radiograph of left hand and wrist for bone age
2. Complete blood count (to detect chronic anemia or infection)

3. Erythrocyte sedimentation rate (often elevated in collagen-vascular disease, cancer, chronic infection, and inflammatory bowel disease)
4. Urinalysis, blood urea nitrogen, and serum creatinine (occult renal disease)
5. Serum electrolytes, calcium, and phosphorus (renal tubular disease and metabolic bone disease)
6. Stool examination for fat, serum endomysial antibody (malabsorption or celiac disease)
7. Karyotype (in girls)
8. Thyroid function tests: free thyroxine (FT4) and thyroid-stimulating hormone (TSH)
9. IGF-1 and IGF-binding protein 3

Hardin DS et al: Twenty years of recombinant human growth hormone in children: Relevance to pediatric care providers. Clin Pediatr (Phila) 2007;46:279 [PMID: 17475983].

Kemp SF et al: Efficacy and safety results of long-term growth hormone treatment of idiopathic short stature. J Clin Endocrinol Metab 2005;90:5247 [PMID: 15998780].

Rosenbloom AL: The role of recombinant insulin-like growth factor I in the treatment of the short child. Curr Opin Pediatr 2007;19:458 [PMID: 17630612].

TALL STATURE

Although we usually think of growth disturbances as producing short stature, potentially serious pathologic conditions may be associated with tall stature and excessive growth (Table 32–3). Excessive GH secretion is rare and is generally associated with a functioning pituitary adenoma. GH excess leads to gigantism if the epiphyses are open and to acromegaly if the epiphyses are closed. Affected children present with an accelerated growth velocity. The diagnosis is confirmed by elevated GH and IGF-1 levels and failure of GH suppression during a standard oral glucose tolerance test.

Constitutional tall stature may be a concern to adolescent girls. However, the upper limit of acceptable height in both sexes is increasing, and concerns about excessive growth for girls are becoming less frequent. When such concerns arise, the family history, growth curve, pubertal stage, and assessment of skeletal maturation allow assessment of predicted

Table 32–3. Causes of tall stature.

A. Constitutional (familial)
B. Endocrine causes
1. Growth hormone excess (pituitary gigantism)
2. Precocious puberty
3. Hypogonadism
C. Nonendocrine causes
1. Klinefelter syndrome
2. XYY males
3. Marfan syndrome
4. Cerebral gigantism (Soto syndrome)
5. Homocystinuria

final adult height. Reassurance, counseling, and education may alleviate the family's concerns. Rarely, when the predicted height is excessive and unacceptable, estrogen therapy may accelerate bone maturation and shorten the growth period.

Iughetti L et al: Diagnostic approach and therapy of overgrowth and tall stature in childhood. Minerva Pediatr 2003;55:563 [PMID: 14676728].

DISORDERS OF THE POSTERIOR PITUITARY GLAND

The posterior pituitary (neurohypophysis) is an extension of the ventral hypothalamus. Its two principal hormones—oxytocin and arginine vasopressin—are synthesized in the supraoptic and paraventricular nuclei of the ventral hypothalamus. After synthesis, these peptide hormones are packaged in granules with specific neurophysins and transported via the axons to their storage site in the posterior pituitary. Vasopressin is essential for water balance; it acts primarily on the kidney to promote reabsorption of water from urine. Oxytocin is most active during parturition and breast feeding and is not discussed further here.

ARGININE VASOPRESSIN (ANTIDIURETIC HORMONE) PHYSIOLOGY

Vasopressin release is controlled primarily by serum osmolality and intravascular volume. Release is stimulated by minor increases in plasma osmolality (detected by osmoreceptors in the anterolateral hypothalamus) and large decreases in intravascular volume (detected by baroreceptors in the cardiac atria). Disorders of vasopressin release and action include (1) central (neurogenic) diabetes insipidus, (2) nephrogenic diabetes insipidus (see Chapter 22), and (3) the syndrome of inappropriate secretion of antidiuretic hormone (see Chapter 43).

CENTRAL DIABETES INSIPIDUS

ESSENTIALS OF DIAGNOSIS & TYPICAL FEATURES

▸ Polydipsia, polyuria (> 2 L/m^2/d), nocturia, dehydration, and hypernatremia.

▸ Inability to concentrate urine after fluid restriction (urine specific gravity < 1.010; urine osmolality < 300 mOsm/kg).

▸ Plasma osmolality > 300 mOsm/kg with urine osmolality < 600 mOsm/kg.

▸ Low plasma vasopressin with antidiuretic response to exogenous vasopressin.

▸ General Considerations

Central diabetes insipidus (DI) is an inability to synthesize and release vasopressin. Without vasopressin the kidneys cannot concentrate urine, causing excessive urinary water loss. Genetic causes of central DI are rare and include mutations in the vasopressin gene (mostly in the neurophysin portion of the vasopressin precursor) and the WFS1 gene that causes DI, diabetes mellitus, optic atrophy, and deafness (Wolfram or DIDMOAD syndrome). Midline brain abnormalities, such as septo-optic dysplasia and holoprosencephaly are also associated with central DI. Traumatic brain injury or neurosurgery in or near the hypothalamus or pituitary can cause transient or permanent DI. Traumatic DI often has three phases. Initially, transient DI is caused by edema in the hypothalamus or pituitary area. In 2–5 days, unregulated release of vasopressin from dying neurons causes the syndrome of inappropriate secretion of antidiuretic hormone (SIADH). Finally, permanent DI occurs if a sufficient number of vasopressin neurons are destroyed.

Tumors and infiltrative diseases of the hypothalamus and pituitary may cause DI. In children with craniopharyngioma, DI usually develops after neurosurgical intervention. In contrast, germinomas often present with DI. Germinomas may be undetectable for several years; consequently, children with unexplained DI should have regularly repeated magnetic resonance imaging (MRI). Infiltrative diseases such as histiocytosis and lymphocytic hypophysitis can cause DI. In these conditions, as in germinomas, MRI scans characteristically show thickening of the pituitary stalk. Infections involving the base of the brain also cause transient DI.

▸ Clinical Findings

Onset of DI is often abrupt, characterized by polyuria, nocturia, enuresis, and intense thirst. Children with DI typically crave cold water. Hypernatremia, hyperosmolality, and dehydration occur if insufficient fluid intake due to lack of access or impaired thirst mechanism does not keep up with urinary losses. In infants, symptoms may also include failure to thrive, vomiting, constipation, and unexplained fevers. Some infants may present with severe dehydration, circulatory collapse, and seizures. Vasopressin deficiency may be masked in patients with panhypopituitarism due to the impaired excretion of free water associated with adrenal insufficiency. Treating these patients with glucocorticoids may unmask their DI.

DI is confirmed when serum hyperosmolality is associated with urine hypo-osmolarity. If the history indicates that the child can go through the night comfortably without drinking, outpatient testing is appropriate. Oral fluid intake is prohibited after midnight. Osmolality, sodium, and specific gravity of the first morning void are obtained. If urine specific gravity is greater than 1.015, DI is excluded. If urine is not concentrated, a blood sample is obtained within a few minutes of the urine collection for osmolality, sodium, creatinine, and calcium concentration.

If screening results are unclear or if symptoms preclude safely withholding fluids at home, a water deprivation test performed in the hospital is indicated. In this test, fluid is withheld and the child is monitored. Serum osmolality greater than 290 mOsm/kg associated with inappropriately dilute urine; osmolality less than 600 mOsm/kg is diagnostic for DI. Low serum vasopressin concentration and an antidiuretic response to vasopressin administration at the end of the test distinguishes central from nephrogenic DI. Children with central DI should have a head MRI scan with contrast to look for tumors or infiltrative processes. The posterior pituitary "bright spot" on MRI is often absent in DI.

Decreased ability to concentrate urine also occurs in hypercalcemic disorders and renal tubular abnormalities (eg, Fanconi syndrome). Primary polydipsia must be distinguished from DI. Children with primary polydipsia tend to have lower serum sodium levels and usually can concentrate their urine with overnight fluid deprivation. Some may have secondary nephrogenic DI due to dilution of the renal medullary interstitium and decreased renal concentrating ability, but this resolves with restriction of fluid intake.

▶ Treatment

Central DI is treated with oral or intranasal desmopressin acetate (DDAVP). The aim of therapy is to provide antidiuresis that allows uninterrupted sleep and approximately 1 hour of diuresis before the next dose. Children hospitalized with acute-onset DI can be managed with intravenous vasopressin. Due to the amount of antidiuresis, intravenous fluids will need to be restricted to two-thirds the maintenance rate and electrolytes closely monitored to avoid water intoxication. Infants with DI should not be treated with DDAVP. Treatment with DDAVP in association with the volume of formula or breast milk needed to ensure adequate caloric intake could cause water intoxication. For this reason, infants are treated with extra free water, rather than DDAVP, to maintain normal hydration. A formula with a low renal solute load and chlorothiazides may be helpful in infants with central DI.

Cheetham T, Baylis PH: Diabetes insipidus in children: Pathophysiology, diagnosis and management. Paediatr Drugs 2002;4:785 [PMID: 12431131].

Ghirardello S et al: The diagnosis of children with central diabetes insipidus. J Pediatr Endocrinol Metab 2007;20:359 [PMID: 17451074].

Rivkees SA et al: The management of central diabetes insipidus in infancy: Desmopressin, low renal solute load formula, thiazide diuretics. J Pediatr Endocrinol Metab 2007;20:459 [PMID: 17550208].

Wise-Faberowski L et al: Perioperative management of diabetes insipidus in children. J Neurosurg Anesthesiol 2004;16:14 [PMID: 14676564].

▼ THYROID GLAND

FETAL DEVELOPMENT OF THE THYROID

The fetal thyroid synthesizes thyroid hormone as early as the 10th week of gestation. Thyroid hormone appears in fetal serum by the 11th week of gestation and increases throughout gestation. The fetal pituitary-thyroid axis functions largely independently of the maternal pituitary-thyroid axis because maternal thyroid-stimulating hormone (TSH) cannot cross the placenta. However, maternal thyroid hormone can cross the placenta in limited amounts.

A TSH surge occurs at birth, peaking at about 70 mU/L within 30–60 minutes. The surge causes thyroid hormone levels to increase rapidly in the first days of life. TSH level decreases to childhood levels within a few weeks. This physiologic neonatal TSH surge can cause a false-positive newborn screen for hypothyroidism (ie, high TSH) if the blood sample is collected on the first day of life.

PHYSIOLOGY

Hypothalamic thyrotropin-releasing hormone (TRH) stimulates the anterior pituitary gland to release TSH. In turn, TSH stimulates the thyroid gland to take up iodine, and to synthesize and release the active hormones, thyroxine (T_4) and triiodothyronine (T_3). This process is regulated by negative feedback involving the hypothalamus, pituitary, and thyroid (see Figure 32–1).

T_4 is the predominant thyroid hormone secreted by the thyroid gland. Most circulating T_3 and T_4 is bound to thyroxine-binding globulin (TBG), albumin, and prealbumin. Less than 1% of T_3 and T_4 exists as free T_3 (FT_3) and free T_4 (FT_4). T_4 is deiodinated in the tissues to either T_3 (active) or reverse T_3 (inactive). In peripheral tissues, T_3 binds to high-affinity nuclear thyroid hormone receptors in the cytoplasm and translocates to the nucleus, exerting its biologic effects by modifying gene expression.

The T_4 level is low in hypothyroidism. It may also be low in premature infants, malnutrition, severe illness, and following therapy with T_3. It is not clear whether premature infants with low T_4 benefit from treatment. T_4 is also low in situations that affect TBG. TBG levels are decreased in familial TBG deficiency, nephrosis, and in patients receiving androgens. In sepsis, TBG cleavage is increased. Treatment with certain medications (heparin, furosemide, salicylates, and phenytoin) results in abnormal binding to TBG. However, since these effects involve primarily TBG levels, and not thyroid function per se, TSH and FT_4 levels remain in the normal range.

T_3 and T_4 levels are high in hyperthyroidism and may be elevated in conditions associated with increased TBG levels (congenital TBG excess, pregnancy, estrogen therapy) and increased thyroid hormone binding to transport proteins.

HYPOTHYROIDISM (CONGENITAL & ACQUIRED HYPOTHYROIDISM)

ESSENTIALS OF DIAGNOSIS & TYPICAL FEATURES

▶ Growth retardation, decreased physical activity, weight gain, constipation, dry skin, cold intolerance, and delayed puberty.

▶ Neonates with congenital hypothyroidism often look normal but may have thick tongue, large fontanels, poor muscle tone, hoarseness, umbilical hernia, jaundice, and intellectual retardation.

▶ T_4, FT_4, and T_3 resin uptake are low; TSH levels are elevated in primary hypothyroidism.

▶ General Considerations

Thyroid hormone deficiency may be congenital or acquired (Table 32–4). It can be due to defects in the thyroid gland (primary hypothyroidism) or in the hypothalamus or pituitary (central hypothyroidism).

Congenital hypothyroidism occurs in about 1:3000–1:4000 infants. Untreated, it causes severe neurocognitive impairment. Most cases are sporadic resulting from hypoplasia or aplasia of the thyroid gland or failure of the gland to migrate to its normal anatomic location (ie, lingual or sublingual thyroid gland). Another cause of congenital hypothyroidism is dyshormonogenesis due to enzymatic defects in thyroid hormone synthesis. Since antithyroid drugs, including propylthiouracil (PTU) and methimazole, freely cross the placenta, goitrous hypothyroid newborns may be born to hyperthyroid mothers treated with these drugs during pregnancy.

Low T_4 levels may also be caused by decreased TSH secretion associated with prolonged glucocorticoid use, dopamine, or somatostatin. Cabbage, soybeans, aminosalicylic acid, thiourea derivatives, resorcinol, phenylbutazone, cobalt, and excessive iodine intake can cause goiter and hypothyroidism during pregnancy. Many of these agents cross the placenta and should be used with caution during pregnancy. Iodine deficiency also causes hypothyroidism. In severe maternal iodine deficiency, both the fetus and the mother are T_4-deficient, with irreversible brain damage in the fetus.

Juvenile hypothyroidism, particularly if goiter is present, is usually a result of chronic lymphocytic (Hashimoto) thyroiditis.

Several hundred patients with resistance to thyroid hormone have been described. These syndromes are generally familial and are classified on the basis of the site of resistance (eg, generalized, pituitary, or peripheral tissue).

▶ Clinical Findings

A. Symptoms and Signs

Even when the thyroid gland is completely absent, most newborns with congenital hypothyroidism appear normal at

Table 32–4. Causes of hypothyroidism.

> **A. Congenital**
> 1. Aplasia, hypoplasia, or maldescent of thyroid
>   a. Embryonic defect of thyroid development
> 2. Inborn errors of thyroid hormone synthesis, secretion, or recycling (due to autosomal recessive mutations)
>   a. Iodide transport defect
>   b. Organification defect
>   (1) Mutation in iodine peroxidase
>   (2) Mutation in pendrin: Pendred syndrome, associated with congenital sensorineural deafness
>   c. Coupling defect
>   d. Iodotyrosine deiodinase defect
>   e. Abnormal iodinated polypeptide (thyroglobulin)
>   f. Inability to convert T_4 to T_3
> 3. Maternal antibody-mediated (inhibit TSH binding to receptor)
> 4. TSH receptor defect
> 5. Thyroid hormone receptor defect
> 6. In utero exposures
>   a. Radioiodine
>   b. Goitrogens (propylthiouracil, methimazole)
>   c. Iodine excess
> 7. Iodide deficiency (endemic cretinism)
>
> **B. Acquired (juvenile hypothyroidism)**
> 1. Autoimmune (lymphocytic) thyroiditis
> 2. Thyroidectomy or radioiodine therapy for
>   a. Thyrotoxicosis
>   b. Thyroid cancer
> 3. Irradiation to the thyroid
> 4. Thyrotropin deficiency
>   a. Isolated
>   b. Associated with other anterior pituitary hormone deficiencies
> 5. TRH deficiency due to hypothalamic injury or disease
> 6. Medications
>   a. Iodides
>   (1) Excess (eg, amiodarone)
>   (2) Deficiency
>   b. Lithium
>   c. Cobalt
> 7. Large hemangiomas
> 8. Idiopathic

T_3, triiodothyronine; T_4, thyroxine; TRH, thyrotropin-releasing hormone.

birth and gain weight normally for the first few months of life without treatment. Since congenital hypothyroidism must be treated as early as possible to prevent intellectual impairment, the diagnosis should be based on the newborn screening test and not on signs or symptoms. Jaundice associated with an unconjugated hyperbilirubinemia may be present in newborns with congenital hypothyroidism. Some infants may have obvious findings of thick tongue, hypotonia, large fontanelles, constipation, umbilical hernia, hoarse cry, and dry skin.

Juvenile hypothyroidism often presents with short stature and abnormal weight gain. Other findings include delayed epiphyseal development, delayed closure of fontanels, and retarded dental eruption. The skin may be dry, thick, scaly, coarse, pale, cool, or mottled, or have a yellowish tinge. The hair may be dry, coarse, or brittle. Lateral thinning of the eyebrows may occur. Musculoskeletal findings include hypotonia and a slow relaxation component of deep tendon reflexes (best appreciated in the ankles). Muscular hypertrophy (Kocher-Debré-Sémélaigne syndrome) is not commonly seen in congenital hypothyroidism. Other findings include physical and mental sluggishness, nonpitting myxedema, constipation, large tongue, hypothermia, bradycardia, hoarse voice or cry, umbilical hernia, and transient deafness. Puberty may be delayed. Metromenorrhagia may occur in older girls. Sometimes, hypothyroidism induces pseudopuberty. Galactorrhea can also occur, due to stimulation of prolactin secretion.

In hypothyroidism resulting from enzymatic defects, ingestion of goitrogens, or chronic lymphocytic thyroiditis, the thyroid gland may be enlarged. Thyroid enlargement in children is usually symmetrical, and the gland is moderately firm and not nodular. In chronic lymphocytic thyroiditis, however, the thyroid frequently has a cobblestone surface.

B. Laboratory Findings

Total T_4 and FT_4 levels are decreased. T_3 resin uptake (T_3RU) is low. In primary hypothyroidism, the serum TSH level is elevated. In central hypothyroidism, the TSH level may be low or inappropriately normal. Circulating autoantibodies to thyroid peroxidase and thyroglobulin may be present. Serum prolactin may be elevated, resulting in galactorrhea. Serum GH may be decreased, with subnormal GH response to stimulation in children with severe primary hypothyroidism, as well as low IGF-1 or IGF-binding protein 3 levels, or both.

C. Imaging

Thyroid imaging, while helpful in establishing the cause of congenital hypothyroidism, is not usually obtained, as it does not affect the treatment plan. Bone age is delayed. Centers of ossification, especially of the hip, may show multiple small centers or a single stippled, porous, or fragmented center (epiphyseal dysgenesis). Cardiomegaly is common. Long-standing primary hypothyroidism may be associated with thyrotrophic hyperplasia characterized by an enlarged sella or pituitary gland.

D. Screening Programs for Neonatal Hypothyroidism

All newborns should be screened for congenital hypothyroidism shortly after birth as most do not have suggestive physical findings. Depending on the state, the newborn screen either measures the total T_4 or TSH level. Abnormal newborn screening results should be confirmed immediately with a T_4 and TSH level. Treatment should be started as soon as possible. Initiation of treatment in the first month of life and good compliance during infancy usually results in a normal neurocognitive outcome.

▶ Differential Diagnosis

Primary hypothyroidism due to intrinsic defects of the thyroid gland must be differentiated from central hypothyroidism due to pituitary or hypothalamic hormone deficiencies of TSH or TRH. TSH and T_4 levels in combination are the most useful tests. When central hypothyroidism is diagnosed, evaluation for other pituitary hormone deficiencies and head MRI imaging are required.

▶ Treatment

Levothyroxine (75–100 mcg/m²/d) is the drug of choice for acquired hypothyroidism. In neonates with congenital hypothyroidism, the initial dose is 10–15 mcg/kg/d. Serum total T_4 or FT_4 concentrations are used to monitor the adequacy of initial therapy because the normally high neonatal TSH may not normalize for several days to weeks. Subsequently, T_4 and TSH are used in combination, as elevations of serum TSH are sensitive early indicators of the need for increased medication or better compliance.

American Academy of Pediatrics et al: Update of newborn screening and therapy for congenital hypothyroidism. Pediatrics. 2006;117:2290 [PMID: 16740880].

Kempers MJ et al: Intellectual and motor development of young adults with congenital hypothyroidism diagnosed by neonatal screening. J Clin Endocrinol Metab 2006;91:418 [PMID: 16303842].

Mitchell ML, Klein RZ: The sequelae of untreated maternal hypothyroidism. Eur J Endocrinol 2004;151(Suppl 3):U45 [PMID: 15554886].

Obregon MJ et al: The effects of iodine deficiency on thyroid hormone deiodination. Thyroid 2005;15:917 [PMID: 16131334].

Park SM, Chatterjee VK: Genetics of congenital hypothyroidism. J Med Genet 2005;42:379 [PMID: 15863666].

Rovet JF: Children with congenital hypothyroidism and their siblings: Do they really differ? Pediatrics 2005;115:e52 [PMID: 15629966].

Selva KA et al: Neurodevelopmental outcomes in congenital hypothyroidism: Comparison of initial T4 dose and time to reach target T4 and TSH. J Pediatr 2005;147:775 [PMID: 16356430].

THYROIDITIS

1. Chronic Lymphocytic Thyroiditis (Chronic Autoimmune Thyroiditis, Hashimoto Thyroiditis)

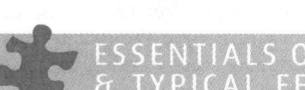

ESSENTIALS OF DIAGNOSIS & TYPICAL FEATURES

▶ Firm, freely movable, nontender, diffusely enlarged thyroid gland.

▶ Thyroid function is usually normal but may be elevated or decreased depending on the stage of the disease.

General Considerations

Chronic lymphocytic thyroiditis is the most common cause of goiter and acquired hypothyroidism in childhood. It is more common in girls, and the incidence peaks during puberty. The disease is caused by an autoimmune attack on the thyroid. Susceptibility to thyroid autoimmunity (and other endocrine autoimmune disorders) is associated with certain histocompatibility alleles.

Clinical Findings

A. Symptoms and Signs

The thyroid is characteristically enlarged, firm, freely movable, nontender, and symmetrical. It may also be nodular. Onset is usually insidious. Occasionally patients note a sensation of tracheal compression or fullness, hoarseness, and dysphagia. No local signs of inflammation or systemic infection are present. Most patients are euthyroid. Some patients are symptomatically hypothyroid, and few patients are symptomatically hyperthyroid.

B. Laboratory Findings

Laboratory findings vary. Serum concentrations of TSH, T_4, FT_4, and T_3RU are usually normal. Some patients are hypothyroid with an elevated TSH and low thyroid hormone levels. Few patients are hyperthyroid with a suppressed TSH and elevated thyroid hormone levels. Thyroid antibodies (antithyroglobulin, antithyroid peroxidase) are frequently elevated. Thyroid uptake scan adds little to the diagnosis. Surgical or needle biopsy is diagnostic but seldom indicated.

Treatment

The treatment of chronic lymphocytic thyroiditis with normal thyroid function is controversial. Full replacement doses of thyroid hormone may decrease the size of the thyroid, but may also result in hyperthyroidism. Hypothyroidism commonly develops over time. Consequently, patients require lifelong surveillance. Children with documented hypothyroidism should receive thyroid hormone replacement.

2. Acute (Suppurative) Thyroiditis

Acute thyroiditis is rare. The most common causes are group A streptococci, pneumococci, *Staphylococcus aureus,* and anaerobes. Oropharyngeal organisms are thought to reach the thyroid via a patent foramen cecum and thyroglossal duct remnant. Thyroid abscesses may form. The patient is always toxic with fever and chills. The thyroid gland is enlarged and exquisitely tender with associated erythema, hoarseness, and dysphagia. Thyroid function tests are typically normal. Patients have a leukocytosis, "left shift," and elevated erythrocyte sedimentation rate. Specific antibiotic therapy should be administered.

3. Subacute (Nonsuppurative) Thyroiditis

Subacute thyroiditis (de Quervain thyroiditis) is rare. It is thought to be caused by viral infection with mumps, influenza, echovirus, coxsackievirus, Epstein-Barr virus, or adenovirus. Presenting features are similar to acute thyroiditis: fever, malaise, sore throat, dysphagia, and thyroid pain that may radiate to the ear. The thyroid is firm and enlarged. Sedimentation rate is elevated. In contrast to acute thyroiditis, the onset is generally insidious and serum thyroid hormone concentrations may be elevated.

HYPERTHYROIDISM

ESSENTIALS OF DIAGNOSIS & TYPICAL FEATURES

► Nervousness, emotional lability, hyperactivity, fatigue, tremor, palpitations, excessive appetite, weight loss, increased perspiration, and heat intolerance.

► Goiter, exophthalmos, tachycardia, widened pulse pressure, systolic hypertension, weakness, and smooth, moist, warm skin.

► TSH is suppressed. Thyroid hormone levels (T_4, FT_4, T_3, T_3RU) are elevated.

General Considerations

In children, most cases of hyperthyroidism are due to Graves disease, caused by antibodies directed at the TSH receptor that stimulate thyroid hormone production. Hyperthyroidism may also be due to acute, subacute, or chronic thyroiditis; autonomous functioning thyroid nodules; tumors producing TSH; McCune-Albright syndrome; exogenous thyroid hormone excess; and acute iodine exposure.

Clinical Findings

A. Symptoms and Signs

Hyperthyroidism is more common in females than males. In children, it most frequently occurs during adolescence. The course of hyperthyroidism tends to be cyclic, with spontaneous remissions and exacerbations. Symptoms include worsening school performance, poor concentration, fatigue, hyperactivity, emotional lability, nervousness, personality disturbance, insomnia, weight loss (despite increased appetite), palpitations, heat intolerance, increased perspiration, diarrhea, polyuria, and irregular menses. Signs include tachycardia, systolic hypertension, increased pulse pressure, tremor, proximal muscle weakness, and moist, warm, skin. Accelerated growth and development may occur. Thyroid storm is a rare condition characterized by fever, cardiac failure, emesis, delirium, coma, and death. Most cases of Graves disease are associated with a diffuse firm goiter. A thyroid bruit and thrill may be present. Many cases are associated with exophthalmos, but severe ophthalmopathy is rare.

B. Laboratory Findings

TSH is suppressed. T_4, FT_4, T_3, FT_3, and T_3RU are elevated except in rare cases in which only the serum T_3 is elevated (T_3 thyrotoxicosis). The presence of thyroid-stimulating immunoglobulin (TSI) confirms the diagnosis of Graves disease. TSH receptor binding antibodies (TRaB) are usually elevated.

C. Imaging

In Graves disease, radioactive iodine uptake by the thyroid is increased, whereas in subacute and chronic thyroiditis it is decreased. An autonomous hyperfunctioning nodule takes up iodine and appears as a "hot nodule" while the surrounding tissue has decreased iodine uptake. In children with hyperthyroidism, bone age may be advanced. In infants, accelerated skeletal maturation may be associated with premature fusion of the cranial sutures. Long-standing hyperthyroidism causes osteoporosis.

▶ Differential Diagnosis

Hypermetabolic states (severe anemia, chronic infections, pheochromocytoma, and muscle-wasting disease) may resemble hyperthyroidism clinically but differ in thyroid function tests.

▶ Treatment

A. General Measures

In untreated hyperthyroidism, strenuous physical activity should be avoided. Bed rest may be required in severe cases.

B. Medical Treatment

1. β-Adrenergic blocking agents—These agents are adjuncts to therapy. They can rapidly ameliorate symptoms such as nervousness, tremor, and palpitations, and are indicated in severe disease with tachycardia and hypertension. $β_1$-Specific agents such as atenolol are preferred because they are more cardioselective.

2. Antithyroid agents (propylthiouracil [PTU] and methimazole)—Antithyroid agents are frequently used in the initial treatment of childhood hyperthyroidism. These drugs interfere with thyroid hormone synthesis. PTU also inhibits the peripheral conversion of T_4 to T_3. It usually takes a few weeks to produce a clinical response and adequate control is usually achieved within a few months. If medical therapy is unsuccessful, more definitive therapy, such as radioablation of the thyroid or thyroidectomy, should be considered.

A. INITIAL DOSAGE—Methimazole is initiated at a dose of 10–60 mg/d (0.5-1 mg/kg/d) given once a day. PTU is started

at a dose of 150–600 mg/d (5-10 mg/kg/d) in three divided doses. Initial dosing is continued until FT_4 or T_4 have normalized and signs and symptoms have subsided.

B. MAINTENANCE—The optimal dose of maintenance medication remains unclear. Recent studies suggest that 10–15 mg/d of methimazole or 100–150 mg/d of PTU provide adequate long-term control in most patients with a minimum of side effects. If the TSH level becomes elevated, many providers decrease the dose of the antithyroid agent. Some providers continue the same dose of antithyroid agent and add exogenous thyroid hormone replacement.

C. TOXICITY—If rash, vasculitis, arthralgia or arthritis, granulocytopenia, or hepatitis occur, the drug must be discontinued.

3. Iodide—Large doses of iodide usually produce a rapid but short-lived blockade of thyroid hormone synthesis and release. This approach is recommended only for acute management of severely thyrotoxic patients.

C. Radiation Therapy

Radioactive iodine ablation of the thyroid is usually reserved for children whose Graves disease is unresponsive to medications, who develop adverse effects from medications, who fail to remit after several years of medical therapy, or who are poorly adherent with therapy. Some pediatric endocrinologists advocate radioablation as first-line therapy for children with Graves disease. Antithyroid agents should be discontinued 4–7 days prior to radioablation to allow resumption of radioiodine uptake by the thyroid. [131]I administered orally concentrates in the thyroid and results in gradual ablation of the gland. In the first 2 weeks following radioablation, hyperthyroidism may worsen as thyroid tissue is destroyed and thyroid hormone is released. Therapy with a β-adrenergic antagonist may be necessary for a few months until FT_4 and T_4 normalize. In most cases, hypothyroidism develops and thyroid hormone replacement is needed. Long-term follow-up studies have not shown any increased incidence of thyroid cancer, leukemia, infertility, or birth defects in patients who receive ablative doses of [131]I.

D. Surgical Treatment

Subtotal and total thyroidectomy are infrequently used in children with Graves disease. Surgery is indicated for extremely large goiters, goiters with a suspicious nodule, very young or pregnant patients, or patients refusing radioiodine ablation. Before surgery, a β-adrenergic blocking agent should be given to treat symptoms and antithyroid agents should be given for several weeks to minimize the surgical risks associated with hyperthyroidism. Iodide (eg, Lugol's solution, 1 drop every 8 hours, or saturated solution of potassium iodide, 1–2 drops daily) should be given for 1–2 weeks prior to surgery to reduce thyroid vascularity and inhibit release of thyroid hormone. Surgical complications include hypoparathyroidism, recurrent laryngeal nerve damage, and rarely, death. An experienced thyroid surgeon is crucial to good surgical outcome. After thyroidectomy, patients become hypothyroid and need thyroid hormone replacement.

▶ Course & Prognosis

Partial remissions and exacerbations may continue for several years. Treatment with an antithyroid agent results in prolonged remissions in one third to two thirds of children.

Beck-Peccoz P et al: Safety of medications and hormones used in the treatment of pediatric thyroid disorders. Pediatr Endocrinol Rev 2004;(Suppl 1):124 [PMID: 16456491].

Dotsch J et al: Graves disease in childhood: A review of the options for diagnosis and treatment. Paediatr Drugs 2003;5:95 [PMID: 12529162].

Lee JA et al: The optimal treatment for pediatric Graves' disease is surgery. J Clin Endocrinol Metab 2007;92:80 [PMID: 17341575].

Rivkees SA, Dinauer C: An optimal treatment for pediatric Graves' disease is radioiodine. J Clin Endocrinol Metab 2007;92:797 [PMID: 17341574].

Neonatal Graves Disease

Transient congenital hyperthyroidism (neonatal Graves disease) occurs in about 1% of infants born to mothers with Graves disease. It occurs when maternal TSH receptor antibodies cross the placenta and stimulate excess thyroid hormone production in the fetus and newborn. Neonatal Graves disease can be associated with irritability, IUGR, poor weight gain, flushing, jaundice, hepatosplenomegaly, and thrombocytopenia. Severe cases may result in cardiac failure and death. Hyperthyroidism may develop several days after birth, especially if the mother was treated with PTU (which crosses the placenta). Symptoms develop as PTU levels decline in the newborn after birth. Thyroid studies should be obtained at birth and repeated within the first week. Immediate management should focus on the cardiac manifestations. Temporary treatment may be necessary with iodide, antithyroid agents, β-adrenergic antagonists, or corticosteroids. Hyperthyroidism gradually resolves over 1–3 months as maternal antibodies decline. As TSH receptor antibodies may still be present in the serum of previously hyperthyroid mothers after thyroidectomy or radioablation, neonatal Graves disease should be considered in all infants of mothers with a history of hyperthyroidism.

Polak M et al: Fetal and neonatal thyroid function in relation to maternal Graves' disease. Best Pract Res Clin Endocrinol Metab 2004;18:289 [PMID: 15157841].

Radetti G et al: Fetal and neonatal thyroid disorders. Minerva Pediatr 2002;54:383 [PMID: 12244277].

THYROID CANCER

Thyroid cancer is rare in childhood. Children usually present with a thyroid nodule or an asymptomatic asymmetrical neck mass. Dysphagia and hoarseness are unusual but may

occur. Thyroid function tests are usually normal. A "cold" nodule is often seen on a technetium or radioiodine uptake scan of the thyroid. Fine-needle aspiration biopsy of the nodule assists in the diagnosis.

The most common thyroid cancer is papillary thyroid carcinoma, a well-differentiated carcinoma arising from the thyroid follicular cell. Children frequently present with local metastases to the cervical lymph nodes and occasionally with pulmonary metastasis. Despite its aggressive presentation, children with papillary thyroid carcinoma have a relatively good prognosis, with a 20-year survival rate greater than 90%. Treatment consists of total thyroidectomy and removal of all involved lymph nodes, usually followed by radioiodine ablation to destroy residual thyroid remnant and metastatic tissue left behind after surgery. Thyroid hormone replacement is then started to suppress TSH to prevent stimulation of residual thyroid tissue. Since papillary thyroid carcinoma in children is associated with a high recurrence rate, regular follow-up with serum thyroglobulin levels (a tumor marker), neck ultrasound, and radioiodine whole body scan are required.

Follicular thyroid carcinoma, medullary thyroid carcinoma, anaplastic carcinoma, and lymphoma are less common thyroid malignancies. Medullary thyroid carcinoma, due to autosomal dominant mutations in the RET proto-oncogene, arises from the thyroid C cells, which secrete calcitonin. It can occur sporadically or can be inherited in multiple endocrine neoplasia (MEN) type 2 and familial medullary thyroid carcinoma. It is associated with elevated serum calcitonin levels. In affected families, all members should be screened for the mutation, and those identified with the mutation should be treated with prophylactic thyroidectomy in early childhood.

Halac I, Zimmerman D: Thyroid nodules and cancers in children. Endocrinol Metab Clin North Am 2005;34:725 [PMID: 16085168].

Hung W, Sarlis NJ: Current controversies in the management of pediatric patients with well-differentiated nonmedullary thyroid cancer: A review. Thyroid 2002;12:683 [PMID: 12225637].

Leboulleux S et al: Follicular cell-derived thyroid cancer in children. Horm Res 2005;63:145 [PMID: 15802922].

Rachmiel M et al: Evidence-based review of treatment and follow up of pediatric patients with differentiated thyroid carcinoma. J Pediatr Endocrinol Metab 2006;19:1377 [PMID: 17252690].

▼ DISORDERS OF CALCIUM & PHOSPHORUS METABOLISM

Serum calcium concentration is tightly regulated by the coordinated actions of the parathyroid glands, kidney, liver, and small intestine. Low serum calcium concentrations, detected by calcium-sensing receptors on the surface of parathyroid cells, stimulate parathyroid hormone (PTH) release. PTH in turn promotes release of calcium and phosphorus from bone, reabsorption of calcium from urinary filtrate, and excretion of phosphorus in the urine. Another essential cofactor in calcium homeostasis is 1,25-dihydroxy vitamin D (calcitriol). The first step in production of this active form of vitamin D occurs in the liver where dietary vitamin D is hydroxylated to 25-hydroxy vitamin D. The final step in formation of calcitriol is 1-hydroxylation, which takes place in the kidney under control of PTH. The primary effect of calcitriol is to promote the absorption of calcium from the intestines. In concert with PTH, it also facilitates calcium and phosphorus mobilization from bones. Deficiencies or excesses of PTH or calcitriol, abnormalities in their receptors, or abnormalities of vitamin D metabolism lead to clinically significant aberrations in calcium homeostasis. Although calcitonin, released from the thyroid gland C cells, also reduces serum calcium concentration, changes in its serum concentration rarely cause clinically relevant disease.

HYPOCALCEMIC DISORDERS

A normal serum calcium concentration is approximately 8.9–10.2 mg/dL, depending on the laboratory. The normal concentration of ionized calcium is approximately 1.1–1.3 mmol/L. Levels in newborns are slightly lower, and in premature infants may be as low as 7 mg/dL. Fifty to 60% of calcium in the serum is protein-bound and metabolically fairly inactive. Thus, measurement of ionized serum calcium, the metabolically active form, is helpful if serum proteins are low or in conditions such as acidosis that cause abnormal calcium binding to protein.

ESSENTIALS OF DIAGNOSIS & TYPICAL FEATURES

▶ Tetany with facial and extremity numbness, tingling, cramps, spontaneous muscle contractures, carpopedal spasm, positive Trousseau and Chvostek signs, loss of consciousness, and convulsions.

▶ Diarrhea, prolongation of electrical systole (QT interval), and laryngospasm.

▶ In hypoparathyroidism or pseudohypoparathyroidism: defective nails and teeth, cataracts, and ectopic calcification in the subcutaneous tissues and basal ganglia.

▶ General Considerations

Hypocalcemia is a consistent feature of conditions such as hypoparathyroidism, pseudohypoparathyroidism, transient tetany of the newborn, and severe vitamin D deficiency rickets and may be present in rare disorders of vitamin D action (receptor defects). Hypocalcemia may also occur in intestinal malabsorption of calcium, chronic renal disease, tumor lysis syndrome, or rhabdomyolysis, or as the result of an activating mutation in the calcium-sensing receptor of the

parathyroid glands and kidneys (hypercalciuric hypocalcemia). (See Table 32–5.)

Deficient PTH *secretion* may due to deficient parathyroid tissue (DiGeorge syndrome), autoimmunity, or sometimes, magnesium deficiency. Decreased PTH *action* may be due to magnesium deficiency, vitamin D deficiency, or defects in the PTH receptor (pseudohypoparathyroidism). Occasionally, PTH deficiency is idiopathic. Table 32–6 summarizes the characteristics of disorders of PTH secretion and action. Autoimmune parathyroid destruction with subsequent hypoparathyroidism may be isolated, or associated with other autoimmune disorders in the APECED syndrome (autoimmune polyendocrinopathy–candidiasis–ectodermal dystrophy, or APS-1). Hypoparathyroidism may also result from unavoidable surgical removal in patients with thyroid cancer. Other features of the DiGeorge syndrome (a deletion of 22.q11) include congenital absence of the thymus (with thymus-dependent immunologic deficiency) and cardiovascular anomalies, especially coarctation of the aorta.

Autosomal dominant hypocalcemia (also called familial hypercalciuric hypocalcemia) is associated with a gain-of-function mutation in the calcium receptor, which causes a low serum PTH despite hypocalcemia, and excessive urinary loss of calcium. A family history of hypocalcemia may be the clue that differentiates this condition from other causes of hypocalcemia.

Transient neonatal hypoparathyroidism (transient tetany of the newborn) is caused both by a relative deficiency of PTH secretion and PTH action (see Table 32–6). The early form of this condition (first 2 weeks of life) occurs in newborns with birth asphyxia. In mothers with hyperparathyroidism, maternal hypercalcemia may suppress fetal PTH secretion and cause early transient neonatal hypoparathyroidism. Likewise, women with gestational diabetes may have relative hyperparathyroidism in the third trimester and their infants may experience transient hypoparathyroidism. Associated hypomagnesemia often aggravates the symptoms associated with hypocalcemia. The late form of neonatal hypoparathyroidism (after 2 weeks of age) occurs in infants receiving high-phosphate formulas (whole cow's milk is a well-known example). Phosphate binds calcium and produces functional hypocalcemia.

Tumor lysis syndrome and rhabdomyolysis cause cellular destruction that liberates large amounts of intracellular phosphate that complex with serum calcium, producing functional hypocalcemia. Malabsorption states such as celiac disease impair the absorption of calcium, vitamin D and magnesium, all of which cause hypocalcemia (see Table 32–6). Hypomagnesemia, due to losses from the gastrointestinal tract or kidney, may cause or augment the severity of hypocalcemia by impairing the release of PTH.

Rickets is a term describing the characteristic clinical and bony radiologic features associated with vitamin D deficiency (see Chapter 10). Vitamin D deficiency caused by lack of sunlight exposure or dietary deficiency is the most com-

Table 32–5. Hypocalcemia associated with rickets and other disorders.

Condition	Pathogenesis	Disease States/Inheritance	Clinical Features	Initial Biochemical Findings			
				Serum Calcium	Serum Phosphorus	Serum Alkaline Phosphatase	Other
Malabsorption	Impairment in intestinal absorption in any or all of the following: calcium, vitamin D, and magnesium	Cystic fibrosis, celiac disease, Shwachman syndrome	Failure to thrive, poor weight gain, steatorrhea, superimposed vitamin D deficiency rickets	Low or normal	Low or normal	Variable: usually high in vitamin D deficiency, but may be low with concomitant zinc deficiency	Potentially low magnesium levels, potentially low 25-OH vitamin D
Chronic renal insufficiency	Decreased renal phosphate excretion, decreased 1-OHase activity	Obstruction, glomerulonephritis, dysplastic kidneys	Uremia, growth failure, acidosis	Low or normal	Elevated	Elevated or normal	Elevated PTH levels in long-standing cases, low 1,25-OH vitamin D
Rhabdomyolysis	Muscle damage with liberation of large amounts of intracellular phosphate	Crush injuries of muscles, Pompe disease, carnitine deficiency	Hypocalcemic tetany, cardiac arrhythmia, risk of renal failure	Low	Elevated	Normal	Myoglobinuria
Tumor lysis syndrome	Release of intracellular phosphate and potassium	Initiation of chemotherapy for ALL, Burkitt lymphoma, or other malignancies	Hypocalcemic tetany, cardiac arrhythmia, risk of renal failure	Low	Elevated	Normal	Hyperkalemia, elevated uric acid
Vitamin D–deficiency rickets	Deficient dietary vitamin D intake, vitamin D malabsorption; other risk factors include dark skin and lack of sunlight exposure	May cluster in families due to shared risk factors	Characteristic skeletal changes appear early, poor growth, symptomatic hypocalcemia is a late finding	Normal until late in course	Low or normal	Elevated	Elevated PTH levels, low 25-OH vitamin D
Vitamin D–dependent rickets	Mutation in 1-hydroxylase enzyme required for synthesis of fully active 1,25-OH vitamin D	Autosomal recessive inheritance	Skeletal changes of rickets, symptomatic hypocalcemia	Low	Low or normal	Elevated	Elevated PTH, low 1,25-OH vitamin D
Vitamin D–resistant rickets	Mutation in 1,25-OH vitamin D receptor	Autosomal recessive inheritance	Severe skeletal changes of rickets, total alopecia, symptomatic hypocalcemia	Low	Low or normal	Elevated	Elevated PTH, elevated 1,25-OH vitamin D
Hypophosphatemic rickets	Excessive loss of phosphate in the urine (? due to abnormal humoral factor)	X-linked dominant	Skeletal changes primarily in the lower extremities—genu varum or valgus, short stature	Normal or low	Very low	Usually high	Normal PTH levels initially, abnormally high urinary phosphate excretion

ALL, acute lymphoblastic leukemia; PTH, parathyroid hormone.

Table 32-6 Hypocalcemia associated with disorders of parathyroid hormone secretion or action.

Condition	Pathogenesis	Inheritance Pattern	Clinical Features	Initial Biochemical Findings[a]			
				Serum Calcium	Serum Phosphorus	Serum Alkaline Phosphatase	Serum PTH
Isolated hypoparathyroidism	Trauma, surgical destruction, isolated autoimmune destruction, rare familial forms	None; reports in familial forms of inheritance as X-linked recessive, autosomal recessive, or autosomal dominant	Symptoms of hypocalcemia	Low	High	Normal/Low	Low
DiGeorge syndrome	Deletion in chromosome 22	Majority represent new mutations	Symptoms of hypocalcemia, cardiac anomalies, immune disorder	Low	High	Normal/Low	Low
APS type 1	Autoimmune destruction	Autosomal recessive	Mucocutaneous candidiasis, Addison disease; potential for autoimmune destruction in other endocrine glands	Low	High	Normal/Low	Low
PHP type IA	Mutation in stimulatory G protein; resistance to PTH action	Autosomal dominant	AHO phenotype, variable hypocalcemia, may have resistance to other hormones using G protein signaling	Low or normal	Elevated or normal	Variable	Elevated
PPHP	Mutation in stimulatory G protein	Autosomal dominant—frequently found within same families with PHP type IA	AHO phenotype, biochemical parameters are normal	Normal	Normal	Normal	Normal
Transient tetany of the newborn-late onset	Deficiency in PTH secretion or action	Sporadic—associated with difficult deliveries, infants of diabetic mothers, or maternal hyperparathyroidism	Onset of symptoms of hypocalcemia within 2 wk of birth	Low	Normal or low	Normal or low	Normal or low
Transient tetany of the newborn-early onset	Deficiency in PTH secretion or action	Sporadic—associated with infant formulas that have a high phosphate content	Onset of symptoms of hypocalcemia after 2 wk of age	Low	Normal or low	Normal or low	Normal or low
Familial hypercalciuric hypocalcemia	Gain of functional mutation of calcium-sensing receptor	Autosomal dominant	Symptoms of hypocalcemia, family history	Low	High	Normal/Low	Low

[a]Urinary calcium excretion (calcium/creatinine ratio) is low in all but familial hypercalciuric hypocalcemia.
AHO, Albright hereditary osteodystrophy; APS, autoimmune polyglandular syndrome; PHP, pseudohypoparathyroidism; PPHP, pseudopseudohypoparathyroidism; PTH, parathyroid hormone.

mon cause of rickets. Occult vitamin D deficiency is probably more common than is presently recognized. This concern forms the basis for the recommendation by the American Association of Pediatrics that breast-fed infants receive vitamin D supplementation of 200 IU/d. Rickets can also be caused by defects in the metabolism of vitamin D (see Table 32–5), including liver disease (impaired 25-hydroxylation), kidney disease (impaired 1-hydroxylation of 25-(OH) vitamin D), genetic deficiency of 1α-hydroxylase (vitamin D–dependent rickets), or end-organ resistance to vitamin D (vitamin D–resistant rickets).

Familial hypophosphatemic rickets has skeletal findings similar to those of vitamin D–related rickets. The defect in this condition is abnormal renal phosphate loss. Dietary deficiency of calcium may also cause rickets but more often causes osteopenia.

Clinical Findings

A. Symptoms and Signs

Prolonged hypocalcemia from any cause is associated with tetany, photophobia, blepharospasm, and diarrhea. The symptoms of tetany are numbness, muscle cramps, twitching of the extremities, carpopedal spasm, and laryngospasm. Tapping the face in front of the ear causes facial spasms (Chvostek sign). Some patients with hypocalcemia exhibit bizarre behavior, irritability, loss of consciousness, and convulsions. Retarded physical and mental development may be present. Headache, vomiting, increased intracranial pressure, and papilledema may occur. In early infancy, respiratory distress may be a presenting finding.

B. Laboratory Findings

In rickets, calcium levels may be low or normal (see Tables 32–5 and 32–6). Phosphate levels in hypocalcemia disorders may be low, normal, or high depending on the cause of the hypocalcemia. Magnesium levels may also be low. PTH levels are reduced in many hypocalcemic conditions, but may be elevated in pseudohypoparathyroidism or severe vitamin D deficiency. Measurement of urinary excretion of calcium as the calcium-to-creatinine ratio can assist in diagnosis and monitoring of therapy in children on calcitriol therapy.

C. Imaging

Soft tissue and basal ganglia calcification may occur in idiopathic hypoparathyroidism and pseudohypoparathyroidism. Various skeletal changes are associated with rickets, including cupped and irregular long bone metaphyses. Torsional deformities can result in genu varum (bowleg). Accentuation of the costochondral junction gives the rachitic rosary appearance seen on the chest wall.

Differential Diagnosis

Tables 32–5 and 32–6 outline the features of disorders associated with hypocalcemia. In individuals with hypoalbu-minemia, the total serum calcium may be low and yet the functional serum ionized calcium is normal. Ionized calcium is the test of choice for hypocalcemia in patients with low serum albumin.

Treatment

A. Acute or Severe Tetany

Hypocalcemia is corrected acutely by administration of intravenous calcium gluconate or calcium chloride; 10 mg/kg is the usual dose in acute treatment. Intravenous calcium infusions should not exceed 50 mg/min because of possible cardiac arrhythmia. Cardiac monitoring should be performed during calcium infusion.

B. Maintenance Management of Hypoparathyroidism or Chronic Hypocalcemia

The objective of treatment is to maintain the serum calcium and phosphate at near normal levels without excess urinary calcium excretion.

1. Diet—Diet should be high in calcium with added calcium supplements starting at a dose of 50–75 mg of elemental calcium per kilogram of body weight per day divided in three to four doses. The dose may be changed based on response of serum level and urinary calcium excretion. Therapy should be monitored to prevent hypercalcemia. Supplemental calcium can often be discontinued in patients with rickets after vitamin D therapy has stabilized.

2. Vitamin D supplementation—Various vitamin D preparations are available. Ergocalciferol (vitamin D_2) and calcitriol (1,25-dihydroxyvitamin D_3) are used in most cases. Ergocalciferol is preferred for treatment of vitamin D deficiency. However, impaired metabolism of vitamin D to its active end product, 1,25-$(OH)_2$ vitamin D, or impaired PTH function requires supplementation with calcitriol. Selection and dosage of vitamin D supplements varies with the underlying condition and the response to therapy. Monitoring of therapy is essential to avoid toxicity.

3. Monitoring—Dosages of calcium and vitamin D must be tailored for each patient. Monitoring serum calcium, urine calcium, and serum alkaline phosphatase levels at 1–3-month intervals is necessary to ensure adequate therapy and to prevent hypercalcemia and nephrocalcinosis.

The major goals of monitoring are to ensure (1) maintenance of serum calcium and phosphorus concentrations within normal ranges, (2) normalization of alkaline phosphatase activity for age, (3) regression of skeletal changes, and (4) maintenance of an age-appropriate urine calcium-to-creatinine ratio. The ratio should be less than 0.8 in newborns, 0.3–0.6 in children, and less than 0.25 in adolescents (creatine and calcium measured in mg/dL).

Monitoring goals are somewhat different in hypophosphatemic rickets. Serum calcium and alkaline phosphatase should be maintained within normal limits. Phosphorus levels should be corrected only to the low normal range. Monitoring of serum PTH is necessary to ensure that secondary hyperparathyroidism does not develop from excessive phosphate treatment or inadequate calcitriol replacement.

PSEUDOHYPOPARATHYROIDISM (RESISTANCE TO PARATHYROID HORMONE ACTION)

In pseudohypoparathyroidism (PHP), PTH production is adequate, but target organs (renal tubule, bone, or both) fail to respond because of receptor resistance. Resistance to PTH action is due to a heterozygous inactivating mutation in the stimulatory G protein subunit associated with the PTH receptor, which leads to impaired signaling. Resistance to other G protein–dependent hormones such as TSH, GHRH, and follicle-stimulating hormone (FSH)/luteinizing hormone (LH), may also be present.

There are several types of PHP with variable biochemical and phenotypic features (see Table 32–6). Biochemical abnormalities in PHP (hypocalcemia and hyperphosphatemia) are similar to those seen in hypoparathyroidism, but the PTH levels are elevated. PHP may be accompanied by a characteristic phenotype known as Albright hereditary osteodystrophy (AHO), which includes short stature; round, full facies; irregularly shortened fourth metacarpal; a short, thick-set body; delayed and defective dentition; and mild mental retardation. Corneal and lenticular opacities and ectopic calcification of the basal ganglia and subcutaneous tissues (osteoma cutis) may occur with or without abnormal serum calcium levels. Treatment is the same as for hypoparathyroidism.

Pseudopseudohypoparathyroidism (PPHP) describes individuals with the AHO phenotype, but normal calcium homeostasis. PHP and PPHP can occur in the same cohort. Genomic imprinting is probably responsible for the different phenotypic expression of disease. Heterozygous loss of the maternal allele causes PHP and heterozygous loss of the paternal allele causes PPHP.

Gelfand IM, DiMeglio LA: Hypocalcemia as a presenting feature of celiac disease in a patient with DiGeorge syndrome. J Ped Endocrinol Metab 2007;20:253 [PMID: 17396443].

Iyer P, Diamond F: Shedding light on hypovitaminosis D and rickets. Adv Pediatr 2007;54:115 [PMID: 17918469].

Koo WWK: Neonatal calcium, magnesium and phosphorus disorders. In Lifshitz F (editor): Pediatric Endocrinology, 5th ed. Informa Healthcare, 2007:497.

Levine M, Kappy MS, Zapalowski C: Disorders of calcium, phosphate parathyroid hormone and vitamin D. In Kappy MS, Allen DB, Geffner ME (editors): Principles and Practice of Pediatric Endocrinology. Charles C Thomas, 2007:695.

HYPERCALCEMIC STATES

Hypercalcemia is defined as a serum level above 11 mg/dL. Severe hypercalcemia is a level above 13.5 mg/dL.

ESSENTIALS OF DIAGNOSIS & TYPICAL FEATURES

▶ Abdominal pain, polyuria, polydipsia, hypertension, nephrocalcinosis, failure to thrive, renal stones, intractable peptic ulcer, constipation, uremia, and pancreatitis.

▶ Bone pain or pathologic fractures, subperiosteal bone resorption, renal parenchymal calcification or stones, and osteitis fibrosa cystica.

▶ Impaired concentration, altered mental status, mood swings, and coma.

▶ General Considerations

More than 80% of hypercalcemic children or adolescents have either hyperparathyroidism or a malignant tumor. Table 32–7 summarizes the differential diagnosis of childhood hypercalcemia.

Hyperparathyroidism is rare in childhood and may be primary or secondary. The most common cause of primary hyperparathyroidism is parathyroid adenoma. Diffuse parathyroid hyperplasia or multiple adenomas may occur in families. Familial hyperparathyroidism may be an isolated disease, or it may be associated with MEN type 1, or rarely type 2A. Hypercalcemia of malignancy is associated with

Table 32–7. Hypercalcemic states.

A. Primary hyperparathyroidism
1. Parathyroid hyperplasia
2. Parathyroid adenoma
3. Familial, including MEN types 1 and 2
4. Ectopic PTH secretion
B. Hypercalcemic states other than primary hyperparathyroidism associated with increased intestinal or renal absorption of calcium
1. Hypervitaminosis D (including idiopathic hypercalcemia of infancy)
2. Familial hypocalciuric hypercalcemia
3. Lithium therapy
4. Sarcoidosis
5. Phosphate depletion
6. Aluminum intoxication
C. Hypercalcemic states other than hyperparathyroidism associated with increased mobilization of bone minerals
1. Hyperthyroidism
2. Immobilization
3. Thiazides
4. Vitamin A intoxication
5. Malignant neoplasms
a. Ectopic PTH secretion or PTH-related protein (PTHRP)
b. Prostaglandin-secreting tumor and perhaps prostaglandin release from subcutaneous fat necrosis
c. Tumors metastatic to bone
d. Myeloma

MEN, multiple endocrine neoplasia; PTH, parathyroid hormone.

solid and hematologic malignancies and is due either to local destruction of bone by tumor or to ectopic secretion of PTH-related protein. When ectopic PTH-related protein is present, calcium is elevated, serum PTH is suppressed, and serum PTH-related protein is elevated. Chronic renal disease with impaired phosphate excretion is the most common secondary cause of hyperparathyroidism.

Kollars J et al: Primary hyperparathyroidism in pediatric patients. Pediatrics 2005;115:974 [PMID: 15805373].

► Clinical Findings

A. Symptoms and Signs

1. Due to hypercalcemia—Manifestations include hypotonicity and muscle weakness; apathy, mood swings, and bizarre behavior; nausea, vomiting, abdominal pain, constipation, and weight loss; hyperextensibility of joints; and hypertension, cardiac irregularities, bradycardia, and shortening of the QT interval. Coma occurs rarely. Calcium deposits occur in the cornea or conjunctiva (band keratopathy) and are detected by slitlamp examination. Intractable peptic ulcer and pancreatitis occur in adults but rarely in children.

2. Due to increased calcium and phosphate excretion—Loss of renal concentrating ability causes polyuria, polydipsia, and calcium phosphate deposition in renal parenchyma or as urinary calculi with progressive renal damage.

3. Due to changes in the skeleton—Initial findings include bone pain, osteitis fibrosa cystica, subperiosteal bone absorption in the distal clavicles and phalanges, absence of lamina dura around the teeth, spontaneous fractures, and moth-eaten appearance of the skull on radiographs. Later, there is generalized demineralization with high risk of subperiosteal cortical bone.

B. Imaging

Bone changes may be subtle in children. Technetium sestamibi scintigraphy is preferred over conventional procedures (ultrasound, computed tomography [CT], and MRI) for localizing parathyroid tumors.

► Treatment

A. Symptomatic Management

Initial management is vigorous hydration with normal saline and forced calcium diuresis with a loop diuretic such as furosemide (1 mg/kg given every 6 hours). If response is inadequate, glucocorticoids or calcitonin may be used. Bisphosphonates, standard agents for the management of acute hypercalcemia in adults, are being used more often in refractory pediatric hypercalcemia.

B. Chronic Hypercalcemia

Treatment options vary with the underlying cause. Resection of parathyroid adenoma or subtotal removal of hyperplastic parathyroid glands is the preferred treatment. Postoperatively, hypocalcemia due to the rapid remineralization of chronically calcium-deprived bones may occur. A diet high in calcium and vitamin D is recommended immediately postoperatively and is continued until serum calcium concentrations are normal and stable. Treatment of secondary hyperparathyroidism from chronic renal disease is primarily directed at controlling serum phosphorus levels with phosphate binders. Pharmacologic doses of calcitriol are used to suppress PTH secretion. Long-term therapy for hypercalcemia of malignancy is the treatment of the underlying disorder.

► Course & Prognosis

The prognosis after resection of a single adenoma is excellent. The prognosis following subtotal parathyroidectomy for diffuse hyperplasia or removal of multiple adenomas is usually good and depends on correction of the underlying defect. In patients with multiple sites of parathyroid adenoma or hyperplasia, MEN is likely, and other family members may be at risk. Genetic counseling and DNA analysis to determine the specific gene defect are indicated.

FAMILIAL HYPOCALCIURIC HYPERCALCEMIA (FAMILIAL BENIGN HYPERCALCEMIA)

Familial hypocalciuric hypercalcemia is distinguished by low to normal urinary calcium excretion as a result of high renal reabsorption of calcium. PTH is normal or slightly elevated. In most cases, the genetic defect is a mutation in the membrane-bound calcium-sensing receptor expressed on parathyroid and renal tubule cells. It is inherited as an autosomal dominant trait with high penetrance. There is a low rate of new mutations. Most patients are asymptomatic, and treatment is unnecessary. A severe form of symptomatic neonatal hyperparathyroidism may occur in infants homozygous for the receptor mutation.

HYPERVITAMINOSIS D

Vitamin D intoxication is almost always the result of ingestion of excessive amounts of vitamin D. Signs, symptoms, and treatment of vitamin D–induced hypercalcemia are the same as those in other hypercalcemic conditions. Treatment depends on the stage of hypercalcemia. Severe hypercalcemia requires hospitalization and aggressive intervention. Due to the storage of vitamin D in the adipose tissue, several months of a low-calcium, low–vitamin D diet may be required.

IDIOPATHIC HYPERCALCEMIA OF INFANCY (WILLIAMS SYNDROME)

Williams syndrome is an uncommon disorder of infancy characterized by elfin-appearing facies and hypercalcemia in infancy. Other features include failure to thrive, mental and motor retardation, cardiovascular abnormalities (primarily supravalvular aortic stenosis), irritability, purposeless movements, constipation, hypotonia, polyuria, polydipsia, and hypertension. A gregarious and affectionate personality is the rule in children with the syndrome. Hypercalcemia may not appear until several months after birth. Treatment consists of restriction of dietary calcium and vitamin D (Calcilo formula) and, in severe cases, moderate doses of glucocorticoids.

A defect in the metabolism of, or responsiveness to, vitamin D is postulated as the cause of Williams syndrome. Elastin deletions localized to chromosome 7 have been identified in more than 90% of patients. Fluorescent in-situ hybridization analysis (FISH) may be the best initial diagnostic tool. The risk of hypercalcemia generally resolves by age 4 years and dietary restrictions can be relaxed.

IMMOBILIZATION HYPERCALCEMIA

Abrupt immobilization, particularly in a rapidly growing adolescent, may cause hypercalcemia and hypercalciuria. Abnormalities often appear 1–3 weeks after immobilization. Medical or dietary intervention may be required in severe cases.

HYPOPHOSPHATASIA

Hypophosphatasia is a rare autosomal recessive condition characterized by deficiency of alkaline phosphatase activity in serum, bone, and tissues. Enzyme deficiency leads to poor skeletal mineralization with clinical and radiographic features similar to rickets. Six different clinical forms are identified. The perinatal form is characterized by severe skeletal deformity and death within a few days of birth. The infantile form includes failure to thrive, hypotonia, and craniosynostosis. The childhood form manifests with variable skeletal findings, reduced bone mineral density, and premature loss of deciduous teeth. Serum calcium levels may be elevated. The diagnosis of hypophosphatasia is made by demonstrating elevated urinary phosphoethanolamine associated with low serum alkaline phosphatase. Therapy is generally supportive. Children who survive the neonatal period may experience gradual improvement. Calcitonin may be of value for the acute treatment of hypercalcemia.

Diaz R: Calcium disorders in children and adolescents. In Lifshitz F (editor): *Pediatric Endocrinology*, 5th ed. Informa Healthcare, 2007:475.

Potts JT Jr.: Diseases of the parathyroid glands and other hyper- and hypocalcemic disorders. In Lameson JL (editor): *Harrison's Endocrinology*. McGraw-Hill, 2006:431.

Zajickova K et al: Identification and functional characterization of a novel mutation in the calcium-sensing receptor gene in familial hypocalciuric hypercalcemia. J Clin Endocrinol Metab 2007;92:2616 [PMID: 17473068].

▶ GONADS (OVARIES & TESTES)

DEVELOPMENT & PHYSIOLOGY

The fetal gonads develop from bipotential anlagen in the genital ridge. The genital ridge contains gonadal tissue, and

müllerian and wolffian structures with the potential to differentiate into components of the internal reproductive structures. Table 32–8 summarizes the male and female structures arising from müllerian and wolffian ducts. The *SRY* gene region of the Y chromosome, promotes testicular differentiation of the bipotential gonads. WT1 and other transcription factors, such as SF1, DAX1, WNT4, and SOX9, are also important in gonadal differentiation. Once testicular differentiation has been determined, the fetal testis produces two substances critical for male differentiation. Antimüllerian hormone promotes the regression of müllerian structures, and testosterone stimulates growth of wolffian-based internal structures. Dihydrotestosterone (DHT), formed by 1α-reductase action on testosterone, is primarily responsible for virilization of the external genitalia. In the absence of both antimüllerian hormone and testosterone, differentiation into female internal and external genitalia occurs.

AMBIGUOUS GENITALIA

Ambiguous genitalia is the result of incomplete or disordered genital or gonadal development that causes a discordance between genetic sex, gonadal sex, and phenotypic sex. When an infant is born with ambiguity, immediate consultation with pediatric endocrinology, urology, and if possible psychiatry is required. Disorders of sexual differentiation stem from alterations in three main processes: gonadal differentiation, steroidogenesis, or androgen action.

1. Disorders of Gonadal Differentiation

These abnormalities include XY sex reversal, XX sex reversal, XY gonadal dysgenesis, true hermaphroditism, vanishing testes, and Leydig cell hypoplasia. Patients with XY sex reversal usually have pure gonadal dysgenesis. They have completely normal female external genitalia and present as girls with delayed puberty and amenorrhea. XX sex reversal, characterized by masculine or ambiguous genital development in an XX individual, can be caused by translocation of the *SRY* gene to the X chromosome. A true hermaphrodite must have both ovarian and testicular tissue and typically has a karyotype of 46,XX. Individuals with XY gonadal dysgenesis usually have a mosaic karyotype in which some cell lines are 45,XO and others are 46,XY. These individuals may present with normal male phenotype or ambiguity. Dysgenetic gonads have an increased risk for neoplastic transformation. Because of decreased testosterone production in utero, 46,XY individuals with vanishing testes or Leydig cell hypoplasia will have some degree of undervirilization.

2. Disorders of Steroidogenesis

These disorders generally present as micropenis, genital ambiguity, or complete absence of male external genitalia in an XY individual (Figure 32–6). Testicular tissue is present and produces antimüllerian hormone. Thus, internal struc-

Table 32–8. Sexual differentiation in the female and male.

Internal Duct Derivatives			
Müllerian Duct Derivatives		**Wolffian Duct Derivatives**[a]	
Fallopian tubes (oviducts) and fimbriae		Epididymis	
		Vas deferens	
Uterus		Seminal vesicles	
Cervix		Ejaculatory duct	
Vagina (posterior two thirds)		Prostatic urethra	
External Genitalia Homologues			
Primitive Structure	**Female Genitalia**	**Male Genitalia**[b]	
Genital tubercle	Clitoris	Glans penis	
Genital swelling	Labia majora	Scrotum	
Genital/urethral fold	Labia minora	Penile urethra/corpora	

[a]Normal wolffian duct development is dependent on the local production of testosterone by Leydig cells of the adjacent testis and on testosterone's diffusion into the surrounding embryonic tissues. Thus, females with congenital adrenal hyperplasia who are virilized as the result of circulating androgens do not have wolffian duct development. Normal male development is also dependent on regression of müllerian duct derivatives through the local action of müllerian inhibiting factor elaborated by the Sertoli cells of the adjacent testis.

[b]Normal development of male external genitalia depends on an adequate circulating concentration of testosterone, which is converted to dihydrotestosterone in the target tissues by 5α-reductase. Elevated concentrations of other (adrenal) androgens, as occurs in females with congenital adrenal hyperplasia, can virilize the genital tubercle, and cause genital swelling and genital/urethral folds, resulting in varying degrees of ambiguity.

tures are wolffian. Disorders in this category include enzymatic defects in testosterone synthesis (12-ketoreductase deficiency) or defects in conversion of testosterone to DHT (5α-reductase deficiency). If the enzyme defect is incomplete, the external genitalia may masculinize at puberty when testosterone production increases. Since the gonads and adrenal gland share common enzymes of steroid hormone production, some of the enzymatic defects associated with male genital ambiguity may also affect production of cortisol and aldosterone, leading to cortisol deficiency and salt wasting (see later section on the Adrenal Cortex). In an XX individual, the most common disorder in this category is congenital adrenal hyperplasia secondary to 21-hydroxylase deficiency. In the classic salt-losing form of this disorder, infant girls present with genital ambiguity but have normal uterus and ovaries.

3. Disorders of Androgen Action

Defects in testosterone action result from absent or defective androgen receptors (androgen insensitivity). Depending on the degree of abnormality in androgen binding, the genital phenotype can range from relatively mild male ambiguity to complete female external development.

4. Miscellaneous Syndromes

Syndromes such as VATER (vertebral defects, anal atresia, tracheoesophageal fistula with esophageal atresia, and radial

and renal anomalies), WAGR (Wilms tumor, aniridia, genitourinary malformations, and mental retardation), Denys-Drash, and Smith-Lemli-Opitz produce a wide variety of congenital anomalies, including genital ambiguity. Maternal exposure to androgens or androgen antagonists is a rare cause of genital ambiguity in newborns.

Brown J, Warne G: Practical management of the intersex infant. J Pediatr Endocrinol Metab 2005;18:3 [PMID: 15679065].

MacLaughlin DR, Donahoe PK: Sex determination and differentiation. N Engl J Med 2004;350:367 [PMID: 14736929].

MacGillivray MH, Mazur T: Intersex. Adv Pediatr 2005;52:295 [PMID: 16124345].

ABNORMALITIES IN FEMALE PUBERTAL DEVELOPMENT & OVARIAN FUNCTION

1. Precocious Puberty in Girls

Precocious puberty is defined as pubertal development occurring below the age limit set for normal onset of puberty. Puberty is considered precocious in girls if the onset of secondary sexual characteristics occurs before age 8 years. Precocious puberty is more common in girls than in boys. This disparity is explained by the large number of girls with central idiopathic precocity, a rare condition in boys. Girls between 6 and 8 years of age may also show signs of puberty but it can be a benign, slowly progressing form that requires no intervention. The age of pubertal onset may be advanced by obesity.

▲ **Figure 32–6.** The corticosteroid hormone synthetic pathway. The pathways illustrated are present in differing amounts in the steroid-producing tissues: adrenal glands, ovaries, and testes. In the adrenal glands, mineralocorticoids from the zona glomerulosa, glucocorticoids from the zona fasciculata, and androgens (and estrogens) from the zona reticularis are produced. The major adrenal androgen is androstenedione, because the activity of 17-ketoreductase is relatively low. The adrenal gland does secrete some testosterone and estrogen, however. The pathways leading to the synthesis of mineralocorticoids and glucocorticoids are not present to any significant degree in the gonads; however, the testes and ovaries each produce both androgens and estrogens. Further metabolism of testosterone to dihydrotestosterone occurs in target tissues of the action of the enzyme 5α-reductase. DHEA, dehydroepiandrosterone.

Central (gonadotropin-releasing hormone [GnRH]-dependent) precocious puberty involves activation of the hypothalamic GnRH pulse generator, an increase in gonadotropin secretion, and a resultant increase in production of sex steroids (Table 32–9). The sequence of hormonal and physical events in central precocious puberty is identical to that of normal puberty. Central precocious puberty in girls is generally idiopathic but may be secondary to central nervous system (CNS) abnormality that disrupts the prepubertal restraint on the GnRH pulse generator. Such CNS abnormalities include, but are not limited to, hypothalamic hamartomas, CNS tumors, cranial irradiation, hydrocephalus, and trauma. Peripheral precocious puberty (GnRH-independent) occurs independent of gonadotropin secretion. In girls, peripheral precocious puberty is caused by ovarian or adrenal tumors, ovarian cysts, congenital adrenal hyperplasia, McCune-Albright syndrome, or exogenous estrogen. Estrogen-secreting ovarian or adrenal tumors are rare. Girls with these tumors typically present with markedly elevated estrogen levels and rapidly progressive pubertal changes.

Table 32–9. Causes of precocious pubertal development.

A. **Central (GnRH-dependent) precocious puberty**
 1. Idiopathic
 2. Central nervous system abnormalities
  a. Acquired—abscess, chemotherapy, radiation, surgical trauma
  b. Congenital—arachnoid cyst, hydrocephalus, hypothalamic hamartoma, septo-optic dysplasia, suprasellar cyst
  c. Tumors—astrocytoma, craniopharyngioma, glioma
B. **Peripheral (GnRH-independent) precocious puberty**
 1. Congenital adrenal hyperplasia
 2. Adrenal tumors
 3. McCune-Albright syndrome
 4. Familial male-limited gonadotropin independent precocious puberty
 5. Gonadal tumors
 6. Exogenous estrogen—oral (contraceptive pills) or topical
 7. Ovarian cysts (females)
 8. HCG-secreting tumors (eg, hepatoblastomas, choriocarcinomas) (males)

GnRH, gonadotropin-releasing hormone; HCG, human chorionic gonadotropin.

McCune-Albright syndrome is a triad of irregular café-au-lait lesions, polyostotic fibrous dysplasia, and GnRH-independent precocious puberty. It is caused by an activating mutation in the gene encoding the α-subunit of G_s, the G protein that stimulates adenyl cyclase. Endocrine cells with this mutation have autonomous hyperfunction and secrete excess amounts of their respective hormones.

▶ Clinical Findings

A. Symptoms and Signs

Female central precocious puberty usually starts with breast development, followed by pubic hair growth and menarche. The order may vary. Girls with ovarian cysts or tumors generally have signs of estrogen excess such as breast development and possibly vaginal bleeding. Adrenal tumors or congenital adrenal hyperplasia produce signs of adrenarche (ie, pubic hair, axillary hair, acne, and sometimes, increased body odor). Children with precocious puberty usually have accelerated growth and may temporarily be tall for age. However, because skeletal maturation advances at a more rapid rate than linear growth, final adult stature may be compromised.

B. Laboratory Findings

One of the first steps in evaluating a child with early pubertal development is obtaining a radiograph of the left hand and wrist to determine skeletal maturity (bone age). If the bone age is advanced, further evaluation is warranted. In central precocious puberty, the basal serum concentrations of FSH and LH may still be in the prepubertal range. Thus, documentation of the maturity of the hypothalamic-pituitary axis depends on demonstrating a pubertal LH response after stimulation with a GnRH agonist. In peripheral precocious puberty, basal serum FSH and LH are low, and the LH response to GnRH stimulation is suppressed by feedback inhibition of the hypothalamic-pituitary axis by the autonomously secreted gonadal steroids (see Figure 32–1). In girls with an ovarian cyst or tumor, estradiol levels will be markedly elevated. In girls with signs of adrenarche and an advanced bone age, androgen levels (testosterone, androstenedione, dehydroepiandrosterone) and possible adrenal intermediate metabolites (such as 17-hydroxyprogesterone) should be measured.

C. Imaging

When a diagnosis of central precocious puberty is made, an MRI of the brain should be done to evaluate for CNS lesions. It is unlikely that an abnormality will be found in girls 6–8 years of age, so the need for an MRI in this age group should be individually assessed. In girls whose laboratory tests suggest peripheral precocious puberty, an ultrasound of the ovaries and adrenal gland is indicated.

▶ Treatment

Girls with central precocious puberty can be treated with GnRH analogues, such as leuprolide. GnRH analogues downregulate pituitary GnRH receptors and thus decrease gonadotropin secretion. With treatment, physical changes of puberty regress or cease to progress, and linear growth slows to a prepubertal rate. Projected final heights often increase as a result of slowing of skeletal maturation. Usually, GnRH analogues are given as a monthly depot intramuscular injection and side effects are rare. After stopping therapy, pubertal progression resumes, and ovulation and pregnancy have been documented. Therapy is instituted for both psychosocial and final height considerations.

Treatment of peripheral precocious puberty is dependent on the underlying cause. In a girl with an ovarian cyst, intervention is generally not necessary, as the cyst usually regresses spontaneously. Treatment with glucocorticoids is indicated for congenital adrenal hyperplasia. Surgical resection is indicated for the rare adrenal or ovarian tumor.

In McCune-Albright syndrome, therapy with antiestrogens (eg, tamoxifen), agents that block estrogen synthesis (ketoconazole), or aromatase inhibitors (eg, letrozole) may be effective. Regardless of the cause of precocious puberty or the medical therapy selected, attention to the psychological needs of the patient and family is essential.

2. Benign Variants of Precocious Puberty

Premature thelarche (benign early breast development) occurs most commonly at 12–36 months. It is often bilateral but may begin or remain unilateral. In the absence of other signs of pubertal development (accelerated growth rate or skeletal maturation, pubic hair, vaginal mucosal maturation), no laboratory evaluation is necessary. Treatment is parental reassurance regarding the self-limited nature of the condition. Observation of the child every few months is also indicated. Onset of thelarche after age 36 months or in association with other signs of puberty requires evaluation.

Premature adrenarche (benign early adrenal maturation) is manifested by development of pubic hair and body odor, and less commonly, axillary hair and can occur before age 8 years. No increase in growth rate or skeletal maturation occurs, and no abnormal virilization (eg, clitoromegaly) is present. No treatment is required, although girls with premature adrenarche are at risk for developing polycystic ovarian syndrome during puberty.

de Sanctis C et al: Pubertal development in patients with McCune-Albright syndrome or pseudohypoparathyroidism. J Pediatr Endocrinol Metab 2003;16(Suppl 2):293 [PMID: 12729407].

Nathan BM, Palmert MR: Regulation and disorders of pubertal timing. Endocrinol Metab Clin North Am 2005;34:617 [PMID: 16085163].

Partsch CJ et al: Management and outcome of central precocious puberty. Clin Endocrinol (Oxf) 2002;56:129 [PMID: 11874402].

3. Delayed Puberty

Delayed puberty in girls should be evaluated if there are no pubertal signs by age 13 years or menarche by 16 years. Failure to complete pubertal development to Tanner stage V within 4 years of onset is considered delay. Primary amenorrhea refers to the absence of menarche, and secondary amenorrhea refers to the cessation of established menses for at least 6 months.

The most common cause of delayed puberty is constitutional growth delay (Table 32–10). This growth pattern, characterized by short stature, normal growth velocity, and a delay in skeletal maturation, is described in detail earlier in this chapter. The timing of puberty is related to the bone age, not the chronologic age. Girls may also have delayed puberty from any condition that delays growth and skeletal maturation, such as hypothyroidism and growth hormone deficiency.

Primary hypogonadism in girls refers to a primary abnormality of the ovaries. The most common diagnosis in this category is Turner syndrome, in which the lack of or an abnormal second X chromosome leads to early loss of oocytes and accelerated stromal fibrosis. Other types of primary ovarian insufficiency are less common, including 46,XY gonadal dysgenesis, 46,XX gonadal dysgenesis, galactosemia, and autoimmune ovarian failure. Radiation and chemotherapy can also cause primary ovarian insufficiency.

Central hypogonadism refers to a hypothalamic or pituitary deficiency of GnRH or FSH/LH, respectively. Central hypogonadism can be functional (reversible), or caused by stress, undernutrition, prolactinemia, excessive exercise, or chronic illness. Permanent central hypogonadism is typically associated with conditions that cause multiple pituitary hormone deficiencies, such as congenital hypopituitarism, CNS tumors, or cranial irradiation. Isolated gonadotropin deficiency is rare but may occur in Kallmann syndrome, which is also characterized by hyposmia or anosmia. In either primary or central hypogonadism, signs of adrenarche are generally present.

Delayed menarche or secondary amenorrhea may result from primary ovarian failure or central hypogonadism, or may be the consequence of hyperandrogenism, anatomic obstruction precluding menstrual outflow, or müllerian agenesis. This latter disorder is called Mayer-Rokitansky-Küster-Hauser syndrome and is characterized by an absent vagina and various uterine abnormalities, with or without renal and skeletal anomalies.

Girls with complete androgen insensitivity syndrome (androgen receptor defect) typically present with primary amenorrhea, breast development, and absence of sexual hair. The affected individual (46,XY) has functioning testes that produce müllerian-inhibiting hormone during fetal life. Thus no müllerian duct (oviduct or uterus) development occurs. External genitalia are female because of the lack of androgen action. At puberty, testosterone produced in the testes is aromatized to estrogen resulting in breast development.

▶ Clinical Evaluation

The history should ascertain whether and when puberty commenced, level of exercise, nutritional intake, stressors, sense of smell, symptoms of chronic illness, and family history of delayed puberty. Past growth records should be assessed to determine if height and weight velocity have been appropriate. Physical examination includes body proportions, breast and genital development, and stigmata of Turner syndrome. Pelvic examination or pelvic ultrasonography should be considered, especially in girls with primary amenorrhea.

A bone age radiograph should be obtained first. If the bone age is lower than that consistent with pubertal onset (< 12 years in girls), evaluations should focus on finding the cause of the bone age delay. If short stature and normal growth velocity are present, constitutional growth delay is likely. If growth rate is abnormal, laboratory studies may include a complete blood count, erythrocyte sedimentation rate, chemistry panel, and renal and liver function tests to look for unsuspected chronic medical illness. Evaluation for hypothyroidism and growth hormone deficiency may also be indicated. Measurement of FSH and LH may not be helpful in the setting of delayed bone age since prepubertal levels are normally low. Determination of a karyotype should be considered if there is short stature, or any stigmata of Turner syndrome.

If the patient has attained a bone age of more than 12 years consistent with onset of puberty and there are minimal or no signs of puberty on physical examination, FSH and LH levels will distinguish between primary ovarian failure and central hypogonadism. Primary ovarian failure is also called hypergonadotropic hypogonadism, as there is lack of estrogen feedback to the brain with elevated FSH and LH. If gonadotropins are elevated, a karyotype is the next step, as

Table 32–10. Cause of delayed puberty or amenorrhea.

A. Constitutional growth delay
B. Hypogonadism
  1. Primary ovarian insufficiency
    a. Gonadal dysgenesis (Turner syndrome, true gonadal dysgenesis)
    b. Premature ovarian failure
      (1) Autoimmune disease
      (2) Surgery, radiation, chemotherapy
    c. Galactosemia
  2. Central hypogonadism
    a. Hypothalamic or pituitary tumor, infection, irradiation
    b. Congenital hypopituitarism
    c. Kallmann syndrome
    d. Functional (chronic illness, undernutrition, exercise, hyperprolactinemia
C. Anatomic
  1. Müllerian agenesis (Mayer-Rokitansky-Küster-Hauser syndrome)
  2. Complete androgen resistance

Turner syndrome is the most common cause of female hypergonadotropic hypogonadism. Central hypogonadism is characterized by low gonadotropin levels, and evaluation is geared toward determining if the hypogonadism is functional or permanent. Laboratory tests should be directed toward identifying chronic disease and hyperprolactinemia. Cranial MRI may be helpful.

In girls with adequate breast development and amenorrhea, a progesterone challenge may be helpful to determine if sufficient estrogen is being produced. Girls who are producing estrogen have a withdrawal bleed after 5–10 days of oral progesterone, whereas those who are estrogen-deficient have little or no bleeding. The exception is girls with an absent uterus (androgen insensitivity or Mayer-Rokitansky-Küster-Hauser syndrome). They have sufficient estrogen but cannot have withdrawal bleeding. The most common cause of amenorrhea in girls with sufficient estrogen is polycystic ovarian syndrome. Girls who are estrogen-deficient should be evaluated similarly to those who have delayed puberty.

► Treatment

Replacement therapy in hypogonadal girls begins with estrogen alone at the lowest available dosage. Oral preparations such as estradiol or topical patches are used. Cyclic estrogen–progesterone therapy is started 12–18 months later, and eventually the patient may be switched over to a birth control pill for convenience. Progesterone therapy is needed to counteract the effects of estrogen on the uterus, as unopposed estrogen promotes endometrials hyperplasia. Estrogen is also necessary to promote bone mineralization and prevent osteoporosis.

Hoffman B, Bradshaw KD: Delayed puberty and amenorrhea. Semin Reprod Med 2003;21:353 [PMID: 14724768].
Kaplowitz P: Precocious puberty: Update on secular trends, definitions, diagnosis, and treatment. Adv Pediatr 2004;51:37 [PMID: 15366770].
Sybert VP, McCauley E: Turner's syndrome. N Engl J Med 2004;351:1227 [PMID: 15371580].

4. Secondary Amenorrhea

See discussion of amenorrhea in Chapter 3.

ABNORMALITIES IN MALE PUBERTAL DEVELOPMENT & TESTICULAR FUNCTION

1. Precocious Puberty in Boys

Puberty is considered precocious in boys if secondary sexual characteristics appear before age 9 years. While the frequency of central precocious puberty is much lower in boys than girls, boys are more likely to have an associated CNS abnormality (see Table 32–9).

Several types of gonadotropin-independent (peripheral) precocious puberty occur in boys (see Table 32–9). Increased adrenal androgen production from an adrenal tumor or from a virilizing form of congenital adrenal hyperplasia (CAH) will cause pubertal changes in boys. Familial male-limited gonadotropin-independent puberty (testotoxicosis) is a condition in which a mutated LH receptor on the Leydig cell is autonomously activated, resulting in testicular production of testosterone despite prepubertal LH levels. McCune-Albright syndrome can also occur in boys. Leydig cell tumors of the testis cause rapid onset of unilateral testicular enlargement and physical signs of testosterone excess. Human chorionic gonadotropin (HCG)–secreting tumors such as teratomas, CNS germinomas, and hepatoblastomas also cause early puberty in boys as HCG can stimulate the Leydig cells to produce testosterone.

► Clinical Findings

A. Symptoms and Signs

In precocious development, increased growth rate and growth of pubic hair are the most common presenting signs. Testicular size may differentiate central precocity, in which the testes enlarge, from gonadotropin-independent causes in which the testes usually remain small (< 2 cm in the longitudinal axis). Tumors of the testis are associated with either asymmetrical or unilateral testicular enlargement.

B. Laboratory Findings

Elevated testosterone levels verify early pubertal status but do not differentiate the source. As in girls, basal serum LH and FSH concentrations may not be in the pubertal range in boys with central precocious puberty, but the LH response to GnRH stimulation testing is pubertal. Sexual precocity caused by CAH is usually associated with abnormal plasma dehydroepiandrosterone, androstenedione, 17-hydroxyprogesterone (in CAH due to 21-hydroxylase deficiency), 11-deoxycortisol (in CAH due to 11-hydroxylase deficiency), or a combination of these steroids (see later section on the Adrenal Cortex). Serum β-HCG concentrations can signify the presence of an HCG-producing tumor (eg, CNS dysgerminoma or hepatoma) in boys who present with apparent true isosexual precocity (ie, accompanied by testicular enlargement) but suppressed gonadotropins following GnRH testing.

C. Imaging

In all boys with central precocious puberty, cranial MRI should be obtained to evaluate for a CNS abnormality. Ultrasonography may be useful in detecting hepatic, adrenal, and testicular tumors.

► Treatment

Treatment of central precocious puberty in boys is similar to that in girls. Treatment of McCune-Albright syndrome or familial Leydig cell hyperplasia with agents that block steroid synthesis (ketoconazole), with antiandrogens (spironolactone), or a combination of the two has been successful. Estrogen receptor blockers (tamoxifen) or aromatase inhibitors (anastrazole or letrozole) have been used to delay skeletal maturation and early epiphyseal closure.

2. Delayed Puberty

Boys should be evaluated for delayed puberty if they have no secondary sexual characteristics by 14 years of age or if more than 5 years have elapsed since the first signs of puberty without completion of genital growth.

The most common cause of delayed puberty in boys, as in girls, is constitutional growth delay, a normal variant of growth that is described in detail earlier in this chapter. Testicular failure or insufficiency may be a primary, due to absence, malfunction, or destruction of testicular tissue, or central, due to pituitary or hypothalamic insufficiency. Primary testicular failure may be due to anorchia, Klinefelter syndrome (47,XXY) or other sex chromosome abnormalities, enzymatic defects in testosterone synthesis, or inflammation or destruction of the testes following infection (mumps), autoimmune disorders, radiation, trauma, or tumor.

Central hypogonadism may accompany panhypopituitarism, Kallmann syndrome (GnRH deficiency with anosmia), or isolated LH or FSH deficiencies. Destructive lesions in or near the anterior pituitary (especially craniopharyngioma and glioma) or infection may also result in hypothalamic or pituitary dysfunction. Prader-Willi syndrome and Laurence-Moon syndrome (Bardet-Biedl syndrome) are frequently associated with LH and FSH deficiency secondary to GnRH deficiency. Deficiencies in gonadotropins may be partial or complete. Functional or reversible gonadotropin may occur with chronic illness, malnutrition, hyperprolactinemia, hypothyroidism, or excessive exercise.

▶ Clinical Evaluation

The history should focus on whether and when puberty has started, testicular descent, symptoms of chronic illness, nutritional intake, sense of smell, and family history of delayed puberty. Physical examination should include body proportions, height and weight, pubertal stage, and testicular location, size, and consistency. Testes less than 2 cm in length are prepubertal; testes more than 2.5 cm in length suggests early pubertal growth.

A radiograph of the left hand and wrist to assess bone age should be the first step in evaluating a boy with delayed puberty. If bone age is delayed (< 11–12 years) and growth velocity is normal, constitutional growth delay is the most likely diagnosis.

Laboratory evaluation includes LH and FSH levels (especially if bone age is > 12 years). Elevated gonadotropin levels indicate primary hypogonadism or testicular failure. The most common cause of primary hypogonadism in boys is Klinefelter syndrome; however, the usual presentation of this

disorder is not delayed puberty but failure to complete puberty with a discrepancy noted between testicular size (small) and degree of virilization. If gonadotropin values are low, the working diagnosis is central hypogonadism and further evaluation should focus on looking for pituitary hormone deficiencies, chronic disease or undernutrition (or both), hyperprolactinemia, and CNS abnormalities.

▶ Treatment

Boys with simple constitutional delay may be offered a short (4–6 months) course of low-dose depot testosterone (50–75 mg per month) to stimulate their pubertal appearance and "jump-start" their endogenous development. In adolescents with permanent hypogonadism, treatment with depot testosterone, beginning with 50–75 mg intramuscularly each month, may be used until growth is complete. Thereafter, adult dosing (150–200 mg every 2–3 weeks) may be used. An alternative to intramuscular injections is testosterone gel, either in single-dose packets or in a pump set to dispense a preset dose. Gel is applied daily after showering. Specific therapy for GnRH deficiency with pulsatile subcutaneous GnRH may promote fertility in patients with hypothalamic-pituitary insufficiency. However, the inconvenience of treatment and the need for repeated doses for long periods of time have limited its application in pediatrics.

3. Cryptorchidism

Cryptorchidism (undescended testis) is common. It is most often unilateral and right-sided. At birth, approximately 4% of full-term male newborns have an undescended testis, with a higher proportion among premature infants (9–30%). In over 50% of these patients, the cryptorchid testis descends by the third month. By age 1 year, the prevalence of cryptorchidism is about 1%. Further descent may occur through puberty, perhaps stimulated by endogenous gonadotropins.

Infertility and testicular malignancy are major risks of cryptorchidism. The exact incidence of impaired fertility is unknown and incidence figures vary. However, histologic changes clearly occur as early as age 6 months in children with undescended testes. The reported malignancy rate in men with a cryptorchid testis is 48.9 per 100,000, 22 times the rate in the general population. In addition, tumors may develop in the contralateral testis, indicating that abnormal testicular development (dysgenesis) may be bilateral in unilateral cryptorchidism. In most cases, true cryptorchidism is thought to be the result of testicular dysgenesis. Cryptorchid testes frequently have a short spermatic artery and or poor blood supply. Although early scrotal positioning of undescended testes (orchidopexy) obviates further damage related to the intra-abdominal location, the testes generally remain abnormal, spermatogenesis is rare, and the risk of malignant neoplasm is increased.

Cryptorchidism can occur in an isolated fashion or associated with other findings. Abnormalities in the hypothalamic-pituitary-gonadal axis predispose to cryptorchidism. Androgen biosynthesis or receptor defects also predispose to cryptorchidism and undervirilization.

The diagnosis of bilateral cryptorchidism in an apparently normal male newborn should never be made until the possibility that the child is actually a fully virilized female with potentially fatal salt-losing CAH has been considered.

▶ Clinical Findings

In infants younger than 3–4 months of age, LH, FSH, and testosterone levels help determine whether testes are present. After this time, an HCG stimulation test is done to confirm the presence or absence of abdominal testes. Ultrasonography, CT scanning, and MRI may detect testes in the inguinal region, but these studies are not completely reliable in finding abdominal testes.

▶ Differential Diagnosis

In palpating the testis, the cremasteric reflex that causes the testis to retract into the inguinal canal or abdomen (pseudocryptorchidism) may be elicited. To prevent retraction during examination, the fingers first should be placed across the abdominal ring and the upper portion of the inguinal canal to obstruct testicular ascent. Examination while the child is in the squatting position or in a warm bath is helpful. No treatment for retractile testes is necessary, and the prognosis for testicular descent and function is excellent.

▶ Treatment

A. Surgical Treatment

The current recommendation for treatment of cryptorchidism is that surgical orchidopexy be performed by an experienced surgeon if descent has not occurred by 1 year of age.

B. Hormonal Treatment

HCG at doses ranging from 250–1000 IU twice weekly for 5 weeks has been used for treatment. Such therapy generally causes descent of retractile testes, but is rarely successful in treating cryptorchidism. Androgen treatment (depot testosterone) is indicated as replacement therapy in the male child who lacks functional testes beyond the normal age of puberty.

4. Gynecomastia

Gynecomastia is a common, self-limited condition that may occur in up to 75% of normal pubertal boys. Adolescent gynecomastia typically resolves within 2 years but may not totally resolve if the degree of gynecomastia is extreme. Gynecomastia may sometimes occur as part of Klinefelter syndrome, or it may occur in boys who are taking drugs such as antidepressants or marijuana. Therapy, either medical (antiestrogens or aromatase inhibitors) or surgical, should be considered in prolonged or severe cases (see Chapter 3).

TESTICULAR TUMORS

Most malignant tumors of the testis are seminomas and teratomas. Seminomas are rare in childhood; they may be hormone-producing. The major hormone-producing tumor of the testis is the Leydig cell tumor. It is often associated with sexual precocity. Other testicular tumors (choriocarcinomas and dysgerminomas) have been reported in association with sexual precocity. Treatment of testicular tumors is surgical removal; chemotherapy and radiation therapy are not used in childhood unless there is high-grade malignancy or metastases. The prognosis in patients with Leydig cell tumors is generally good.

Grumbach MM: The neuroendocrinology of human puberty revisited. Horm Res 2002;57(Suppl 2):2 [PMID: 12065920].

Kaplowitz P: Precocious puberty: Update on secular trends, definitions, diagnosis, and treatment. Adv Pediatr 2004;51:37 [PMID: 15366770].

Leung AK, Robson WL: Current status of cryptorchidism. Adv Pediatr 2004;51:351 [PMID: 15366780].

▼ ADRENAL CORTEX

The adult adrenal cortex has a regional distribution of terminal steroid production. The outermost zona glomerulosa is the predominant source of aldosterone. The middle zona fasciculata makes cortisol and small amounts of mineralocorticoids. The innermost zona reticularis produces mainly androgens and estrogens. A fetal zone, or provisional cortex, that predominates during fetal development produces glucocorticoids, mineralocorticoids, androgens, and estrogens. The fetal zone is relatively deficient in 3β-ol dehydrogenase (see Figure 32–6); hence placentally produced progesterone is the major precursor used in fetal adrenal production of cortisol and aldosterone.

The adrenal cortical production of cortisol is under the control of pituitary adrenocorticotropic hormone (ACTH; see Figure 32–1 and Table 32–1), which is in turn regulated by the hypothalamic peptide, corticotropin-releasing hormone (CRH). The complex interaction of CNS influences on CRH secretion, coupled with negative feedback of serum cortisol, leads to a diurnal pattern of ACTH and cortisol release. ACTH concentration is greatest during the early morning hours with a smaller peak in the late afternoon and a nadir at night. The pattern of serum cortisol concentration follows this pattern with a lag of a few hours. In the absence of cortisol feedback, there is dramatic CRH and ACTH hypersecretion.

Glucocorticoids are critical for gene expression in a many cell types. In excess, glucocorticoids are both catabolic and antianabolic; that is, they promote the release of amino acids from muscle and increase gluconeogenesis while decreasing incorporation of amino acids into muscle protein. They also antagonize insulin activity and facilitate lipolysis. Glucocorticoids help maintain blood pressure by promoting peripheral vascular tone and sodium and water retention.

Mineralocorticoids (primarily aldosterone in humans) promote sodium retention and stimulate potassium excretion in the distal renal tubule. Although ACTH can stimulate aldosterone production, the predominant regulator of aldosterone secretion is the volume-and sodium-sensitive renin-angiotensin-aldosterone system. Elevations of serum potassium also directly influence aldosterone release from the cortex.

Androgen (dehydroepiandrosterone and androstenedione) production by the zona reticularis is insignificant before puberty. At the onset of puberty, androgen production increases and may be an important factor in the dynamics of puberty in both sexes. The adrenal gland is a major source of androgen in the pubertal and adult female.

ADRENOCORTICAL INSUFFICIENCY (ADRENAL CRISIS, ADDISON DISEASE)

The leading causes of adrenal insufficiency are hereditary enzyme defects (congenital adrenal hyperplasia), autoimmune destruction of the glands (Addison disease), central adrenal insufficiency caused by intracranial neoplasm or its treatment, or congenital midline defects associated with optic nerve hypoplasia (septo-optic dysplasia). A rare form of familial adrenal insufficiency occurs in association with cerebral sclerosis and spastic paraplegia (adrenoleukodystrophy). Addison disease may be familial and has been described in association with hypoparathyroidism, candidiasis, hypothyroidism, pernicious anemia, hypogonadism, and diabetes mellitus as one of the polyglandular autoimmune syndromes. Less commonly, the gland is destroyed by tumor, calcification, or hemorrhage (Waterhouse-Friderichsen syndrome). Adrenal disease secondary to opportunistic infections (fungal or tuberculous) is reported in AIDS. In children, central adrenal insufficiency due to anterior pituitary tumor is rare. A temporary salt-losing disorder resulting from partial mineralocorticoid deficiency or renal underresponsiveness (pseudohypoaldosteronism) may occur during infancy or with pyelonephritis.

Acute illness, surgery, trauma, or hyperthermia may precipitate an adrenal crisis in patients with adrenal insufficiency. Patients with primary adrenal insufficiency are at greater risk for life-threatening crisis than patients with central ACTH deficiency because mineralocorticoid secretion and low-level autonomous cortisol secretion remain intact in central ACTH deficiency.

▶ Clinical Findings

A. Symptoms and Signs

1. Acute form (adrenal crisis)—Manifestations include nausea, vomiting, diarrhea, abdominal pain, dehydration, fever (sometimes followed by hypothermia), weakness, hypotension, circulatory collapse, confusion and coma. In-creased pigmentation may be associated with primary adrenal insufficiency caused by melanocyte-stimulating activity of the hypersecreted parent molecule, ACTH.

2. Chronic form—Manifestations include fatigue, hypotension, weakness, failure to gain, weight loss, salt craving (primary insufficiency), vomiting, and dehydration. Diffuse tanning with increased pigmentation over pressure points, scars, and mucous membranes may be present in primary adrenal insufficiency. A small heart may be seen on chest radiograph.

B. Laboratory Findings

1. Suggestive of adrenocortical insufficiency—In primary adrenal insufficiency, serum sodium and bicarbonate levels, arterial partial pressure of carbon dioxide, blood pH, and blood volume are decreased. Serum potassium and urea nitrogen levels are increased. Urinary sodium level and the ratio of urinary sodium to potassium are inappropriate for the degree of hyponatremia. In central adrenal insufficiency, serum sodium levels may be mildly decreased as a result of impaired water excretion. Eosinophilia and moderate lymphopenia occur in both forms of insufficiency.

2. Confirmatory tests

A. ACTH (COSYNTROPIN) STIMULATION TEST—In primary adrenal insufficiency (originating in the gland itself), plasma cortisol and aldosterone concentrations do not increase significantly over baseline 60 minutes after an intravenous dose of ACTH (250 mcg). To diagnose central adrenal insufficiency, a low dose of ACTH is given (1 mcg).

B. BASELINE SERUM ACTH CONCENTRATION—Values are elevated in primary adrenal failure and low in central adrenal insufficiency.

C. URINARY FREE CORTISOL AND 17-HYDROXYCORTICOSTEROID EXCRETION—Values are decreased.

D. CRH TEST—This test assesses responsiveness of the entire hypothalamic-pituitary-adrenal axis. After administration of ovine CRH, serum concentrations of ACTH and cortisol are measured over 2 hours. Verification of an intact axis or localization of the site of impairment is possible with careful interpretation of results.

▶ Differential Diagnosis

Acute adrenal insufficiency must be differentiated from severe acute infections, diabetic coma, various disturbances of the CNS, and acute poisoning. In the neonatal period, adrenal insufficiency may be clinically indistinguishable from respiratory distress, intracranial hemorrhage, or sepsis. Chronic adrenocortical insufficiency must be differentiated from anorexia nervosa, certain muscular disorders (myasthenia gravis), salt-losing nephritis, and chronic debilitating infections, and must be considered in cases of recurrent spontaneous hypoglycemia.

▶ Treatment

A. Acute Insufficiency (Adrenal Crisis)

1. Hydrocortisone sodium succinate—Hydrocortisone sodium succinate is given initially at a dose of 50 mg/m² intravenously over 2–5 minutes or intramuscularly; thereafter, it is given intravenously, 12.5 mg/m², every 4–6 hours until stabilization is achieved and oral therapy can be tolerated.

2. Fluids and electrolytes—In primary adrenal insufficiency, 5–10% glucose in normal saline, 10–20 mL/kg intravenously, is given over the first hour and repeated if necessary to reestablish vascular volume. Normal saline is continued thereafter at 1½–2 times the maintenance fluid requirements. Intravenous boluses of glucose (10% glucose, 2 mL/kg) may be needed every 4–6 hours to treat hypoglycemia. In central adrenal insufficiency, routine fluid management is generally adequate after restoration of vascular volume and institution of cortisol replacement.

3. Fludrocortisone—When oral intake is tolerated, fludrocortisone, 0.05–0.15 mg daily, is started and continued as necessary every 12–24 hours for primary adrenal insufficiency.

4. Inotropic agents—Rarely, inotropic agents such as dopamine and dobutamine are needed. However, adequate cortisol replacement is critical because pressor agents may be ineffective in adrenal insufficiency.

5. Waterhouse-Friderichsen syndrome with fulminant infections—The use of adrenocorticosteroids and norepinephrine in the treatment or prophylaxis of fulminant infections remains controversial. Corticosteroids may augment the generalized Shwartzman reaction in fatal cases of meningococcemia. However, corticosteroids should be considered if there is possible adrenal insufficiency, particularly if there is hypotension and circulatory collapse.

B. Maintenance Therapy

Following initial stabilization, the most effective substitution therapy is hydrocortisone, combined with fludrocortisone in primary adrenal insufficiency. Overtreatment should be avoided as it causes obesity, growth retardation, and other cushingoid features. Additional hydrocortisone, fludrocortisone, or sodium chloride, singly or in combination, may be necessary with acute illness, surgery, trauma, or other stress reactions. Supportive adrenocortical therapy should be given whenever surgical operations are performed in patients who have at some time received prolonged therapy with adrenocorticosteroids.

1. Glucocorticoids—A maintenance dosage of 6–10 mg/m²/d of hydrocortisone (or equivalent) is given orally in two or three divided doses. The dosage of all glucocorticoids is increased to 30–50 mg/m²/d during intercurrent illnesses or other times of stress.

2. Mineralocorticoids—In primary adrenal insufficiency, fludrocortisone is given, 0.05–0.15 mg orally daily as a single dose or in two divided doses. Periodic monitoring of blood pressure is recommended to avoid overdosing.

3. Salt—The child should be given ready access to table salt. Frequent blood pressure determinations in the recumbent position should be made to check for hypertension. In the infant, supplementation of 3–5 mEq Na⁺/kg/d by adding the injectable solution (4 mg/mL) to formula or breast milk is generally required until table foods are introduced.

C. Corticosteroids in Patients with Adrenocortical Insufficiency Who Undergo Surgery

1. Before operation—Hydrocortisone sodium succinate, 30–50 mg/m²/d intravenously 1 hour before surgery.

2. During operation—Hydrocortisone sodium succinate, 25–100 mg intravenously with 5–10% glucose in saline throughout surgery.

3. During recovery—Hydrocortisone sodium succinate, 12.5 mg/m² intravenously every 4–6 hours until oral doses are tolerated. The oral dose of three to five times the maintenance dose is continued until the acute stress is over, at which time the patient can be returned to the maintenance dose.

▶ Course & Prognosis

The course of acute adrenal insufficiency is rapid, and death may occur within a few hours, particularly in infants, unless adequate treatment is given. Spontaneous recovery is unlikely. Patients who have received long-term treatment with adrenocorticosteroids may exhibit adrenal collapse if they undergo surgery or other acute stress. Pharmacologic doses of glucocorticoids during these episodes may be needed throughout life. In all forms of acute adrenal insufficiency, the patient should be observed carefully once the crisis has passed and evaluated with laboratory tests to assess the degree of permanent adrenal insufficiency.

Patients with chronic adrenocortical insufficiency who receive adequate therapy can lead normal lives.

Eisenbarth GS, Gottlieb PA: Autoimmune polyendocrine syndromes. N Engl J Med 2004;350:2068 [PMID: 15141045].

CONGENITAL ADRENAL HYPERPLASIAS

ESSENTIALS OF DIAGNOSIS & TYPICAL FEATURES

▶ Genital virilization in females, with labial fusion, urogenital sinus, enlargement of the clitoris, or other evidence of androgen action.

▶ Salt-losing crises in infant males or isosexual precocity in older males with infantile testes.

▶ Increased linear growth and advanced skeletal maturation.

▶ Elevation of plasma 17-hydroxyprogesterone concentrations in the most common form; may be associated with hyponatremia, hyperkalemia, and metabolic acidosis, particularly in newborns.

General Considerations

Autosomal recessive mutations in the enzymes of adrenal steroidogenesis in the fetus cause abnormal cortisol biosynthesis with increased ACTH secretion. ACTH excess subsequently results in adrenal hyperplasia with increased production of adrenal hormone precursors, including androgens. Increased pigmentation, especially of the scrotum, labia majora, and nipples, is common with excessive ACTH secretion. Congenital adrenal hyperplasia (CAH) is most commonly (> 80% of patients) the result of homozygous 21-hydroxylase (cytochrome P-450 C21) deficiency (see Figure 32–6). In its severe form, excess adrenal androgen production starting in the first trimester of fetal development causes virilization of the female fetus and life-threatening hypovolemic, hyponatremic shock (adrenal crisis) in the newborn. Other enzyme defects that less commonly result in CAH include 11-hydroxylase, 3β-ol dehydrogenase, 20,22-desmolase, 18-hydroxylase-17, and 22-desmolase deficiencies. The clinical syndromes associated with these defects are shown in Figure 32–6 and Table 32–11.

Studies of patients with 21-hydroxylase deficiency indicate that the clinical type (salt-wasting or non–salt-wasting) is usually consistent within a kindred and that a close genetic linkage exists between the 21-hydroxylase gene and the human leukocyte antigen complex on chromosome 6. The latter finding has allowed more precise heterozygote detection and prenatal diagnosis. Population studies indicate that the defective gene is present in 1:250–1:100 people and that the incidence of the disorder is 1:15,000–1:5000. Mass screening for this enzyme defect, using a microfilter paper technique to measure serum 17-hydroxyprogesterone, has been established in some U.S. states.

Nonclassic presentations of 21-hydroxylase deficiency have been reported with increasing frequency. Affected persons have a normal phenotype at birth but develop evidence of virilization during later childhood, adolescence, or early adulthood. In these cases, previously referred to as late-onset or acquired enzyme deficiency, results of hormonal studies are characteristic of 21-hydroxylase deficiency. An asymptomatic form has also been identified in which individuals have none of the phenotypic features of the disorder, but have hormonal study results identical to patients with nonclassic 21-hydroxylase deficiency. The nonclassic form appears to be less severe than the classic form. Because members of the same family may have classic, nonclassic, and asymptomatic forms, the disorders may be due to allelic variations of the same enzyme.

Table 32–11. Clinical and laboratory findings in adrenal enzyme defects resulting in congenital adrenal hyperplasia.

Enzyme Deficiency[a]	Urinary 17-Ketosteroids	Elevated Plasma Metabolite	Plasma Androgens	Aldosterone	Hypertension/Salt Loss	External Genitalia
20,22-Desmolase	↓↓↓	—	↓↓↓	↓↓↓	−/+	Males: ambiguous Females: normal
3β-ol Dehydrogenase	↑↑ (DHEA)	17-OH pregnenolone (DHEA)	↑ (DHEA)	↓↓↓	−/+	Males: ambiguous Females: possibly virilized
17-Hydroxylase	↓↓↓	Progesterone	↓↓	Normal to ↑	+/−	Males: ambiguous Females: normal
21-Hydroxylase[a]	↑↑↑	17-OHP	↑↑	↓↓	−/+	Males: normal Females: virilized
11-Hydroxylase	↑↑	11-Deoxycortisol	↑↑↓↓	(↑ Deoxycorticosterone)	+/−	Males: normal Females: virilized
17,20-Desmolase	↓↓↓	17-Hydroxysteroids (?)	↓↓	Normal	−/−	Males: ambiguous Females: normal

[a]Children with "simple virilizing (non–salt-wasting)" forms of 21-hydroxylase deficiency congenital adrenal hyperplasia (CAH) may have normal aldosterone production and serum electrolytes, but some children have normal aldosterone production and serum electrolytes at the expense of elevated plasma renin activity and are, by definition, compensated salt-wasters. These children usually receive mineralocorticoid as well as glucocorticoid treatment. Children with 21-hydroxylase deficiency CAH should therefore have documented normal plasma renin activity in addition to normal serum electrolytes before they are considered non–salt-wasters.

DHEA, dehydroepiandrosterone; 17-OHP, 17-hydroxyprogestrone.

▶ Clinical Findings

A. Symptoms and Signs

1. In females—Abnormality of the external genitalia varies from mild enlargement of the clitoris to complete fusion of the labioscrotal folds, forming a scrotum, a penile urethra, a penile shaft, and with clitoral enlargement sufficient to form a normal-sized glans (see Table 32–8). Signs of adrenal insufficiency (salt loss) may occur in the first days of life but more typically appear in the first or second week. Rarely, adrenal insufficiency does not occur for months or years. With milder enzyme defects, salt loss may not occur, and virilization predominates (simple virilizing form). In untreated non–salt-losing 21-hydroxylase or 11-hydroxylase deficiency, growth rate and skeletal maturation are accelerated and patients appear muscular. Pubic hair appears early (often before the second birthday), acne may be excessive, and the voice may deepen. Excessive pigmentation may develop. Final adult height is often compromised.

2. In males—The male infant usually appears normal at birth but may present with salt-losing crisis in the first 2–4 weeks of life. In milder forms, salt-losing crises may not occur. In this circumstance, enlargement of the penis and increased pigmentation may be noted during the first few months. Other symptoms and signs are similar to those of affected females. The testes are not enlarged except in the rare male in whom aberrant adrenal cells (adrenal rests) are present in the testes, producing unilateral or asymmetrical bilateral enlargement. In the rare isolated defect of 17,20-desmolase activity, ambiguous genitalia may be present because of impaired androgen production (see Figure 32–6).

B. Laboratory Findings

1. Blood—Hormonal studies are essential for accurate diagnosis. Findings characteristic of the enzyme deficiencies are shown in Table 32–11.

2. Genetic studies—Rapid chromosomal diagnosis should be obtained in any newborn with ambiguous genitalia.

C. Imaging

Adrenal ultrasonography, CT scanning, and MRI may be useful in defining pelvic anatomy or enlarged adrenals or in localizing an adrenal tumor. Contrast-enhanced radiographs of the vagina and pelvic ultrasonography may be helpful in delineating the internal anatomy in a newborn with ambiguous genitalia.

▶ Treatment

A. Medical Treatment

Treatment goals in CAH are normalization of growth velocity and skeletal maturation with the smallest dose of glucocorticoid that can suppress adrenal function. Excessive glu-cocorticoids cause the undesirable side effects of Cushing syndrome. Mineralocorticoid replacement sustains normal electrolyte homeostasis, but excessive mineralocorticoids cause hypertension.

1. Glucocorticoids—Initially, parenteral or oral hydrocortisone (30–50 mg/m^2/d) suppresses abnormal adrenal steroidogenesis within 2 weeks. When adrenal suppression has been accomplished, as evidenced by normalization of serum 17-hydroxyprogesterone, patients are placed on maintenance doses of 15–20 mg/m^2/d in two or three divided doses. Between 50% and 60% of the daily dose should be given in the late evening to suppress early morning ACTH rise. Dosage is adjusted to maintain normal growth rate and skeletal maturation. Various serum and urine androgens have been used to monitor therapy, including 17-hydroxyprogesterone, androstenedione, and urinary pregnanetriol. No one test is universally accepted. In adolescent girls, normal menses are a sensitive index of the adequacy of therapy. Therapy should be continued throughout life in both males and females because of the possibility of malignant degeneration of the hyperplastic adrenal gland. In pregnant females with CAH, suppression of adrenal androgen secretion is critical to avoid virilization of the fetus, particularly a female fetus.

2. Mineralocorticoids—Fludrocortisone, 0.05–0.15 mg, is given orally once a day or in two divided doses. Periodic monitoring of blood pressure and plasma renin is recommended to adjust dosing.

B. Surgical Treatment

For affected females, consultation with a urologist experienced in female genital reconstruction should be arranged as soon as possible during infancy.

▶ Course & Prognosis

When therapy is initiated in early infancy, abnormal metabolic effects and progression of masculinization can be avoided. Treatment with glucocorticoids permits normal growth, development, and sexual maturation. If not adequately controlled, CAH results in sexual precocity and masculinization throughout childhood. Affected individuals will be tall as children but short as adults because of a rapid rate of skeletal maturation and premature closure of the epiphyses. If treatment is delayed or inadequate until somatic development is completed (12–14 years as determined by bone age), true central sexual precocity may occur in males and females.

Patient education stressing lifelong therapy is important to ensure compliance in adolescence and later life. Virilization and multiple surgical genital reconstructions are associated with a high risk of psychosexual disturbances in female patients. Ongoing psychological evaluation and support is a critical component of care.

Merke DP, Bornstein SR: Congenital adrenal hyperplasia. Lancet 2005;365:2135 [PMID: 15964450].

Speiser PW, White PC: Congenital adrenal hyperplasia. N Engl J Med 2003;349:776 [PMID: 12930931].

ADRENOCORTICAL HYPERFUNCTION (CUSHING DISEASE, CUSHING SYNDROME)

ESSENTIALS OF DIAGNOSIS & TYPICAL FEATURES

▶ Truncal adiposity, thin extremities, moon facies, muscle wasting, weakness, plethora, easy bruising, purple striae, decreased growth rate, and delayed skeletal maturation.

▶ Hypertension, osteoporosis, and glycosuria.

▶ Elevated serum corticosteroids, low serum potassium, eosinopenia, and lymphopenia.

▶ General Considerations

Cushing syndrome may result from excessive secretion of adrenal steroids autonomously (adenoma or carcinoma), excess pituitary ACTH secretion (Cushing disease), ectopic ACTH secretion, or chronic exposure to exogenous glucocorticoid medications. In children younger than 12 years, Cushing syndrome is usually iatrogenic (secondary to exogenous ACTH or glucocorticoids). It may rarely be due to adrenal tumor, adrenal hyperplasia, pituitary adenoma, or extrapituitary ACTH-producing tumor.

▶ Clinical Findings

A. Symptoms and Signs

1. Excess glucocorticoid—Manifestations include adiposity, most marked on the face, neck, and trunk (a fat pad in the interscapular area is characteristic); fatigue; plethoric facies; purplish striae; easy bruising; osteoporosis; hypertension; glucose intolerance; back pain; muscle wasting and weakness; and marked retardation of growth and skeletal maturation.

2. Excess mineralocorticoid—Patients have hypokalemia, mild hypernatremia with water retention, increased blood volume, edema, and hypertension.

3. Excess androgen—Hirsutism, acne, and varying degrees of virilization are present. Menstrual irregularities occur in older girls.

B. Laboratory Findings

1. Blood

A. PLASMA CORTISOL—Values are elevated, with loss of normal diurnal variation. Determination of cortisol level between midnight and 2 AM may be a sensitive indicator of the loss of diurnal variation.

B. SERUM CHLORIDE AND POTASSIUM—Both values are usually low, but serum sodium and bicarbonate concentrations may be elevated with metabolic alkalosis.

C. SERUM ACTH—ACTH concentration is decreased in adrenal tumor and increased with ACTH-producing pituitary or extrapituitary tumors.

D. CBC—Polymorphonuclear leukocytosis with lymphopenia and eosinopenia are common. Polycythemia occurs.

2. Salivary cortisol—This is a less invasive means by which to measure serial cortisol values, and the tests may be performed at home. Salivary cortisol obtained at midnight is a highly specific and sensitive test for hypercortisolism.

3. 24-Hour urinary free cortisol excretion—This value is elevated. It is considered the most useful initial test to document hypercortisolism, although midnight salivary cortisol is considered a reasonable and more practical alternative.

4. Response to dexamethasone suppression testing—The suppression of adrenal function by a small dose (0.5 mg) of dexamethasone is reduced in adrenal hyperfunction; larger doses (4–16 mg/d in four divided doses) of dexamethasone cause suppression of adrenal activity when the disease is due to ACTH hypersecretion, whereas hypercortisolism due to adenomas and adrenal carcinomas is rarely suppressed.

5. CRH test—The CRH stimulation test, in conjunction with petrosal sinus sampling, is effective in distinguishing pituitary and ectopic sources of ACTH excess and for lateralization of pituitary sources prior to surgery.

C. Imaging

Pituitary imaging may demonstrate a pituitary adenoma. Adrenal imaging by CT scan may demonstrate adenoma or bilateral hyperplasia. Radionuclide studies of the adrenals may be useful in complex cases. Osteoporosis, evident first in the spine and pelvis, with compression fractures may occur in advanced cases. Skeletal maturation is usually delayed.

▶ Differential Diagnosis

Children with exogenous obesity accompanied by striae and hypertension are often suspected of having Cushing syndrome. The child's height, growth rate, and skeletal maturation are helpful in differentiating the two. Children with Cushing syndrome have a poor growth rate, relatively short stature, and delayed skeletal maturation, while those with exogenous obesity usually have a normal or slightly increased growth rate, normal to tall stature, and advanced skeletal maturation. The color of the striae (purplish in Cushing syndrome, pink in obesity) and the distribution of the obesity assist in differentiation. The urinary free cortisol excretion (in milligrams per gram of creatinine) may be mildly elevated in obesity, but midnight salivary cortisol is normal.

Treatment

In all cases of primary adrenal hyperfunction due to tumor, surgical removal, is indicated if possible. Glucocorticoids should be administered parenterally in pharmacologic doses during and after surgery until the patient is stable. Supplemental oral glucocorticoids, potassium, salt, and mineralocorticoids may be necessary until the suppressed contralateral adrenal gland recovers, sometimes over a period of several months. The use of mitotane, a DDT derivative that is toxic to the adrenal cortex, and aminoglutethimide, an inhibitor of steroid synthesis, have been suggested, but their efficacy in children with adrenal tumors has not been determined. Pituitary microadenomas may respond to pituitary surgery or irradiation.

Prognosis

If the tumor is malignant, the prognosis is poor if it cannot be completely removed. If it is benign, cure is to be expected following proper preparation and surgery.

Raff H, Findling JW: A physiologic approach to diagnosis of the Cushing syndrome. Ann Intern Med 2003;138:980 [PMID: 12809455].

Yehuda R et al: Relationship between 24-hour urinary-free cortisol excretion and salivary cortisol levels sampled from awakening to bedtime in healthy subjects. Life Sci 2003;73:349 [PMID: 12757842].

PRIMARY HYPERALDOSTERONISM

Primary hyperaldosteronism may be caused by an adrenal adenoma or adrenal hyperplasia. It is characterized by paresthesias, tetany, weakness, nocturnal enuresis, periodic paralysis, low serum potassium and elevated serum sodium levels, hypertension, metabolic alkalosis, and production of large volume, alkaline urine with low specific gravity. The specific gravity does not respond to vasopressin. Glucose tolerance test is frequently abnormal. Plasma and urinary aldosterone are elevated. In contrast to renal disease or Bartter syndrome, plasma renin activity is suppressed, creating a high aldosterone-to-renin ratio. In patients with adrenal tumor, ACTH may further increase the excretion of aldosterone. Marked improvement after the administration of an aldosterone antagonist such as spironolactone may be of diagnostic value.

Treatment is with glucocorticoids (glucocorticoid remediable hyperaldosteronism or familial hyperaldosteronism type 1), spironolactone (familial hyperaldosteronism type 2), or subtotal or total adrenalectomy for hyperplasia, and surgical removal if a tumor is present.

Hood S et al: Prevalence of primary hyperaldosteronism assessed by aldosterone/renin ratio and spironolactone testing. Clin Med 2005;5:55 [PMID: 15745200].

Mulatero P et al: Diagnosis of primary aldosteronism: From screening to subtype differentiation. Trends Endocrinol Metab 2005;16:114 [PMID: 15808809].

Young WF Jr: Minireview: Primary aldosteronism—Changing concepts in diagnosis and treatment. Endocrinology 2003;144: 2208 [PMID: 12746276].

USES OF GLUCOCORTICOIDS & ADRENOCORTICOTROPIC HORMONE IN TREATMENT OF NONENDOCRINE DISEASES

Glucocorticoids are used for their anti-inflammatory and immunosuppressive properties in a variety of conditions in childhood. Pharmacologic doses are necessary to achieve these effects, and side effects are common.

Numerous synthetic preparations possessing variable ratios of glucocorticoid to mineralocorticoid activity are available (Table 32–12).

Table 32–12. Potency equivalents for adrenocorticosteroids.

Adrenocorticosteroid	Trade Names	Potency/mg Compared with Cortisol (Glucocorticoid Effect)	Potency/mg Compared with Cortisol (Sodium-Retaining Effect)
Glucocorticoids			
Hydrocortisone (cortisol)	Cortef	1	1
Cortisone	Cortone Acetate	0.8	1
Prednisone	Meticorten, others	4–5	04
Methylprednisolone	Medrol, Meprolone	5–6	Minimal
Triamcinolone	Aristocort, Kenalog Kenacort, Atolone	5–6	Minimal
Dexamethasone	Decadron, others	25–40	Minimal
Betamethasone	Celestone	25	Minimal
Mineralocorticoid			
Fludrocortisone	Florinef	15–20	300–400

Actions

Glucocorticoids exert a direct or permissive effect on virtually every tissue of the body; major known effects include the following:

1. Gluconeogenesis in the liver
2. Stimulation of fat breakdown (lipolysis) and redistribution of body fat
3. Catabolism of protein with an increase in nitrogen and phosphorus excretion
4. Decrease in lymphoid and thymic tissue and a decreased cellular response to inflammation and hypersensitivity
5. Alteration of CNS excitation
6. Retardation of connective tissue mitosis and migration; decreased wound healing
7. Improved capillary tone and increased vascular compartment volume and pressure

Side Effects of Therapy

When prolonged use of pharmacologic doses of glucocorticoids is necessary, clinical manifestations of Cushing syndrome are common. Side effects may occur with the use of synthetic exogenous agents by any route, including inhalation and topical administration, or with the use of ACTH. Use of a larger dose of glucocorticoids given once every 48 hours (alternate-day therapy) lessens the incidence and severity of some of the side effects (Table 32–13).

Tapering of Pharmacologic Doses of Steroids

Prolonged use of pharmacologic doses of glucocorticoids causes suppression of ACTH secretion and consequent adrenal atrophy. The abrupt discontinuation of glucocorticoids may result in adrenal insufficiency. ACTH secretion generally does not restart until the administered steroid has been given in subphysiologic doses (< 6 mg/m²/d orally) for several weeks.

If pharmacologic glucocorticoid therapy has been given for less than 10–14 days, the drug can be discontinued abruptly (if the condition for which it was prescribed allows) because adrenal suppression will be short-lived. However, it is advisable to educate the patient and family about the signs and symptoms of adrenal insufficiency in case problems arise.

If tapering is necessary in treating the condition for which the glucocorticoid is prescribed, a reduction of 25–50% every 2–7 days is sufficiently rapid to permit observation of clinical symptomatology. An alternate-day schedule (single dose given every 48 hours) will allow for a 50% decrease in the total 2-day dosage while providing the desired pharmacologic effect. If tapering is not required for the underlying disease, the dosage can be rapidly decreased safely to the physiologic range. Although a rapid decrease in dose to the physiologic range will not lead to frank adrenal insufficiency (because adequate exogenous cortisol is being provided), some patients may experience a steroid withdrawal syn-

Table 32–13. Side effects of glucocorticoid use.

A. Endocrine and metabolic effects
 1. Hyperglycemia and glycosuria (chemical diabetes)
 2. Cushing syndrome
 3. Persistent suppression of pituitary-adrenal responsiveness to stress with resultant hypoadrenocorticism
B. Effects on electrolytes and minerals
 1. Marked retention of sodium and water, producing edema, increased blood volume, and hypertension (more common in endogenous hyperadrenal states)
 2. Potassium loss with symptoms of hypokalemia
 3. Hypocalcemia, tetany
C. Effects on protein metabolism and skeletal maturation
 1. Negative nitrogen balance, with loss of body protein and bone protein, resulting in osteoporosis, pathologic fractures, and aseptic bone necrosis
 2. Suppression of growth, retarded skeletal maturation
 3. Muscular weakness and wasting
 4. Osteoporosis
D. Effects on the gastrointestinal tract
 1. Excessive appetite and intake of food
 2. Activation or production of peptic ulcer
 3. Gastrointestinal bleeding from ulceration or from unknown cause (particularly in children with hepatic disease)
 4. Fatty liver with embolism, pancreatitis, nodular panniculitis
E. Lowering of resistance to infectious agents; silent infection; decreased inflammatory reaction
 1. Susceptibility to fungal infections; intestinal parasitic infections
 2. Activation of tuberculosis; false-negative tuberculin reaction
 3. Stimulation of activity of herpes simplex virus
F. Neuropsychiatric effects
 1. Euphoria, excitability, psychotic behavior, and status epilepticus with electroencephalographic changes
 2. Increased intracranial pressure with pseudotumor cerebri syndrome
G. Hematologic and vascular effects
 1. Bleeding into the skin as a result of increased capillary fragility
 2. Thrombosis, thrombophlebitis, cerebral hemorrhage
H. Miscellaneous effects
 1. Myocarditis, pleuritis, and arteritis following abrupt cessation of therapy
 2. Cardiomegaly
 3. Nephrosclerosis, proteinuria
 4. Acne (in older children), hirsutism, amenorrhea, irregular menses
 5. Posterior subcapsular cataracts; glaucoma

drome, characterized by malaise, insomnia, fatigue, and loss of appetite. These symptoms may necessitate a two- or three-step decrease in dose to the physiologic range.

Once a physiologic equivalent dose (8–10 mg/m²/d hydrocortisone or equivalent) is achieved and the patient's underlying disease is stable, the dose can be decreased to 4–5 mg/m²/d given only in the morning. This will allow the adrenal axis to recover. After this dose has been given for 4–6 weeks, assessment of endogenous adrenal activity is estimated by obtaining fasting plasma cortisol concentrations between 7 and 8 AM prior to the morning steroid dose or by a low-dose ACTH stimulation test (1 mcg cosyntropin followed by measurement of cortisol after 45–60 minutes). When an alternate-day schedule is followed, plasma cortisol is measured the morning before treatment. Plasma cortisol concentration in the physiologic range (> 10 mg/dL) indicates return of basal physiologic adrenal rhythm. Exogenous steroids may then be discontinued safely, although it is advisable to continue giving stress doses of glucocorticoids when appropriate until recovery of the response to stress has been documented.

After basal physiologic adrenal function returns, the adrenal reserve or capacity to respond to stress and infection can be estimated by the low-dose ACTH stimulation test, in which 1 mcg of synthetic ACTH (cosyntropin) is administered intravenously. Plasma cortisol is measured prior to (zero time) and at 45–60 minutes after the infusion. A plasma cortisol concentration greater than 18 mg/dL at 60 minutes indicates a satisfactory adrenal reserve.

Even if the results of testing are normal, patients who have received prolonged treatment with glucocorticoids may develop signs and symptoms of adrenal insufficiency during acute stress, infection, or surgery for months to years after treatment has been stopped. Careful monitoring, and the use of stress doses of glucocorticoids, should be considered during severe illnesses and surgery.

Allen DB: Inhaled steroids for children: Effects on growth, bone, and adrenal function. Endocrinol Metab Clin North Am 2005;34:555 [PMID: 16085159].

Gulliver T, Eid N: Effects of glucocorticoids on the hypothalamic-pituitary-adrenal axis in children and adults. Immunol Allergy Clin North Am 2005;25:541 [PMID: 16054542].

National Asthma Education and Prevention Program: Long-term management of asthma in children: Safety of inhaled corticosteroids. J Allergy Clin Immunol 2002;110(Suppl):S160 [PMID: 12542074].

ADRENAL MEDULLA PHEOCHROMOCYTOMA

Pheochromocytoma is uncommon and only 10% of the reported cases occur in pediatric patients. The tumor can be located wherever chromaffin tissue (adrenal medulla, sympathetic ganglia, or carotid body) is present, possibly from decreased apoptosis of neural crest cells during development. It may be multiple, recurrent, and sometimes malignant. Familial forms include pheochromocytomas associated with the dominantly inherited neurofibromatosis type 1, MEN type 2, and von Hippel-Lindau syndromes, as well as mutations of the succinate dehydrogenase genes. Neuroblastomas, ganglioneuromas, and other neural tumors, as well as carcinoid tumors may secrete pressor amines and mimic pheochromocytoma.

The symptoms of pheochromocytoma are generally caused by excessive secretion of epinephrine or norepinephrine and most commonly include headache, sweating, tachycardia, and hypertension. Other symptoms are anxiety, hypertension, dizziness, weakness, nausea and vomiting, diarrhea, dilated pupils, blurred vision, abdominal and precordial pain, and vasomotor instability (flushing and postural hypotension). Sustained symptoms may lead to cardiac, renal, optic, or cerebral damage.

Laboratory diagnosis is possible in more than 90% of cases. Serum and urine catecholamines are elevated, but abnormalities may be limited periods of symptomatology or paroxysm. Plasma free metanephrine level (phenoxybenzamine, tricyclic antidepressants, and β-adrenoreceptor blockers can create false-positive results) is the most sensitive test and the gold standard for diagnosis. Levels three times the normal range are diagnostic. Intermediate values may require additional testing, with urinary vanillylmandelic acid and urinary total metanephrines providing the highest specificity. Provocative tests using histamine, tyramine, or glucagon and the phentolamine tests may be abnormal but are dangerous and are rarely necessary. After demonstrating a tumor biochemically, imaging methods including CT or MRI are used to localize the tumor. When available, functional ligands such as (123)I-MIBG, [18F]DA positron emission tomography scanning and somatostatin receptor scintigraphy (with either [123I]Tyr3-octreotide or [111In]DTPA-octreotide) are useful in further diagnostic evaluation.

Laparoscopic tumor removal is the treatment of choice; however, the procedure must be undertaken with great caution and with the patient properly stabilized. Oral phenoxybenzamine or intravenous phentolamine is used preoperatively. Profound hypotension may occur as the tumor is removed but may be controlled with an infusion of norepinephrine, which may have to be continued for 1–2 days.

Unless irreversible secondary vascular changes have occurred, complete relief of symptoms is to be expected after recovery from removal of a benign tumor. However, prognosis is poor in patients with metastases, which occur more commonly with large, extra-adrenal pheochromocytomas.

Ilias I, Pacak K: Current approaches and recommended algorithm for the diagnostic localization of pheochromocytoma. J Clin Endocrinol Metab 2004;89:479 [PMID: 14764749].

Kinney MA et al: Perioperative management of pheochromocytoma. J Cardiothorac Vasc Anesth 2002;16:359 [PMID: 12073213].

Maxwell PH: A common pathway for genetic events leading to pheochromocytoma. Cancer Cell 2005;8:91 [PMID: 16098460].

Pozo J et al: Sporadic phaeochromocytoma in childhood: Clinical and molecular variability. J Pediatr Endocrinol Metab 2005; 18:527 [PMID: 16042317].

Diabetes Mellitus

H. Peter Chase, MD
George S. Eisenbarth, MD, PhD

ESSENTIALS OF DIAGNOSIS & TYPICAL FEATURES

▶ Polyuria, polydipsia, and weight loss.

▶ Hyperglycemia and glucosuria with or without ketonuria.

GENERAL CONSIDERATIONS

Type 1 diabetes or immune-mediated diabetes (previously called juvenile diabetes or insulin-dependent diabetes mellitus [IDDM]) is the most common type of diabetes in people younger than age 40 years. It is associated with islet cell antibodies (immunologic markers), diminished insulin production, and being ketosis-prone.

Type 2 diabetes (non–insulin-dependent diabetes mellitus [NIDDM], non–immune-mediated) is the most common type in persons older than age 40 years; it is associated with being overweight, insensitivity to insulin, and not being prone to ketosis. Type 2 diabetes is increasing in frequency in children and is found in up to half of black and Hispanic children and in over two thirds of American Indian children who develop diabetes. It occurs most frequently in overweight teenagers.

Maturity-onset diabetes of youth (MODY) is much less common and comprises several forms of diabetes in non-obese children with identified genetic mutations (eg, mutations of glucokinase or hepatic nuclear factor 1 or 2 genes). It presents as a nonketotic form of diabetes without islet cell antibodies and often is associated with a family history of diabetes in several generations.

Neonatal diabetes, which is rare, is associated with several distinct etiologies that require specialty evaluation and specific therapies. For example, some children have transient neonatal diabetes. Others have specific mutations and are best treated with sulfonylurea medications after receiving initial insulin therapy.

▶ Pathogenesis

A. Type 1 Diabetes

Type 1 diabetes results from immunologic damage to the insulin-producing β-cells of the pancreatic islets. This damage occurs gradually—over months or years in most people—and symptoms do not appear until about 90% of the pancreatic islets have been destroyed. The immunologic damage requires a genetic predisposition and is probably influenced by environmental factors.

The importance of genetics is shown by the fact that among identical twins, more then 50% of second twins develop diabetes after the first twin develops the disease. About 6% of siblings or offspring of persons with type 1 diabetes also develop diabetes (compared with prevalence in the general population of 0.2–0.3%). The condition is more common in white children but occurs in all racial groups. There is an association with human leukocyte antigen (HLA)-DR3 and HLA-DR4, and about 95% of white diabetic children have at least one of these HLA types. Forty percent have both HLA-DR3 and HLA-DR4 (one from each parent), compared with only 3% of the general population.

The importance of environmental factors is suggested because not all second identical twins develop diabetes. Important environmental factors may be viral infections or factors in the diet.

The immunologic basis of diabetes is demonstrated by the ability of cyclosporin, a potent immunosuppressive agent, to preserve islet tissue for 1–2 years when given to newly diagnosed patients. However, renal damage from cyclosporin precludes its use. White blood cells are found in the islets of newly diagnosed patients and may release toxic products (free radicals, interleukin-1, and tumor necrosis factor) that injure the islets. Antibodies to islet cells, insulin, glutamic acid decarboxylase, ICA512 (IA-2), and other antigens are present for months to years prior to diagnosis in the serum of over 90% of patients who will develop type 1 diabetes. These antibodies are probably the effect and not the cause of islet β-cell destruction.

B. Type 2 Diabetes

Type 2 diabetes has a strong genetic component, although the inherited defects vary in different families. Obesity (particularly central) and lack of exercise are often major environmental contributing factors. Insulin insensitivity results from all of these circumstances. The prevalence is increased among females, which may be related to its association with the polycystic ovary syndrome. Acanthosis nigricans, a thickening and darkening of the skin over the posterior neck, armpits, or elbows, may aid in the diagnosis of type 2 diabetes.

▶ Prevention

A. Type 1 Diabetes

Free antibody screening is now available for families having a relative with type 1 diabetes (1-800-425-8361). Intervention trials on antibody-positive first-degree relatives have begun in an effort to try to prevent type 1 diabetes.

B. Type 2 Diabetes

The prevention of type 2 diabetes was evaluated in a large study, the Diabetes Prevention Program. The study found that 30 minutes of exercise per day (5 days/wk) and a low-fat diet reduced the risk of diabetes by 58%. Taking metformin also reduced the risk of type 2 diabetes by 31%.

▶ Clinical Findings

The classic symptoms of polyuria, polydipsia, and weight loss are now so well recognized that friends or family members often suspect the diagnosis of type 1 diabetes in affected individuals. Other cases may be detected by finding glucosuria on routine office urinalysis. Up to 50% of new cases of diabetes used to be diagnosed in patients presenting in coma, but most are now diagnosed before the individuals develop severe ketonuria, ketonemia, and secondary acidosis. Children often have a preceding minor illness, such as a flulike episode. Blood or urine glucose levels can be checked in a few seconds, which could be life-saving. No disease other than diabetes (mellitus or insipidus) presents with continued frequent urination in spite of a dry tongue. An oral glucose tolerance test is rarely necessary in children. A random blood glucose level above 300 mg/dL (16.6 mmol/L) or a fasting blood glucose level above 200 mg/dL (11 mmol/L) is sufficient to make the diagnosis of diabetes. The 1997 revised guidelines for the diagnosis of diabetes (see references) are a fasting plasma glucose level over 126 mg/dL (7 mmol/L) or a plasma glucose level above 200 mg/dL (11.1 mmol/L) taken randomly (with symptoms of diabetes) or 2 hours after an oral glucose load (1.75 g glucose/kg up to a maximum of 75 g). Confirmation of such abnormalities on more than one occasion is recommended as transient hyperglycemia can occur, particularly with illness. Impaired (not yet diabetic) fasting glucose values are 100–125 mg/dL (5.5–6.9 mmol/L) and impaired 2-hour values are 140–200 mg/dL (7.8–11.1 mmol/L). If the presentation is mild, hospitalization is usually not necessary.

▶ Treatment

Most children have type 1 diabetes. The five major variables in treatment are (1) insulin type and dosage, (2) diet, (3) exercise, (4) stress management, and (5) blood glucose and ketone monitoring. All must be considered to obtain safe and effective metabolic control. Although teenagers can be taught to perform many of the tasks of diabetes management, they do better when supportive—not overbearing—parents continue to be involved in management of their disease. Children younger than age 10 or 11 years cannot reliably administer insulin without adult supervision because they lack fine motor control and may not understand the importance of accurate dosage.

A. Patient and Family Education

Education about diabetes for all family members is essential for the home management of diabetes. The use of an educational book (see *Understanding Diabetes* in the references) can be very helpful to the family. All caregivers need to learn about diabetes, how to give insulin injections, perform home blood glucose monitoring, and handle acute complications. The stress imposed on the family around the time of initial diagnosis may lead to feelings of shock, denial, sadness, anger, fear, and guilt. Meeting with a counselor to express these feelings at the time of diagnosis helps with long-term adaptation.

A. Insulin

Insulin has three key functions: (1) it allows glucose to pass into the cell; (2) it decreases the physiologic production of glucose, particularly in the liver; and (3) it turns off ketone production.

1. Treatment of new-onset diabetes—The greater the acidemia and ketone production, the greater the amount of insulin needed. If ketonemia is significant, venous blood pH is low (< 7.30), and the patient is dehydrated, intravenous insulin and fluid therapy should be given (see later discussion of ketonuria, ketonemia, and ketoacidosis). If the child is adequately hydrated and has a normal venous blood pH, one or two intramuscular or subcutaneous injections of 0.1–0.2 U/kg of regular insulin—or preferably of insulin lispro (Humalog, [H]) or insulin aspart (NovoLog, [NL])—1 hour apart will help shut down ketone production. If ketone production is insignificant or absent, this regimen is not necessary, and routine subcutaneous injections can be started.

When ketones are not present, the child is usually more responsive to insulin, and a total daily dosage of 0.25–0.5 U/kg/24 h (by subcutaneous injection) can be used. If ketones are or were present, the child usually does not produce as much insulin and will require 0.5–1 U/kg of total insulin per 24 hours.

Children usually receive mixtures of a rapid-acting insulin (to cover food intake or high blood glucose) and a longer-acting insulin (to suppress endogenous hepatic glucose production). This is achieved by combining insulins of different formulations with the desired properties (Table 33–1). The dosages are adjusted with each injection during the first week. In the past, most physicians began treatment of newly diagnosed children with two injections per day of an intermediate-acting insulin (eg, NPH) and a rapid-acting insulin such as Humalog or NovoLog (H or NL). About two thirds of the total dosage is usually given before breakfast and the remainder before dinner. If human regular insulin is used, the injections are given 30–60 minutes before meals; when using H or NL as the rapid-acting insulin, the injections are given 10–15 minutes before eating. In young children who eat irregular amounts of food, it is often helpful to wait until after the meal to give the injection and decide on the appropriate dose of H or NL. Children younger than age 4 years usually need 1 or 2 units of rapid-acting insulin to cover meals; the remainder of the dosage is NPH insulin. Children aged 4–10 years may require up to 4 units of rapid-acting insulin to cover breakfast and dinner, whereas proportionately higher doses (usually 4–10 units) of H or NL or regular insulin are used for older children.

An alternative approach using one of two basal insulins, insulin glargine (Lantus) or insulin Detemir (Levemir), is now available, and many physicians initiate therapy with one of these insulins. The basal insulin is given once or twice daily in the morning, or at dinner, or at bedtime depending on patient and family wishes. The dose is adjusted up or down depending on the morning fasting glucose levels. The most physiologic insulin regimen is then to add H/NL prior to each meal and snack. Children who are unable to consistently receive H or NL at lunch or with snacks can receive H/NL with NPH at breakfast. The main advantage of Lantus or Levemir over two injections of NPH daily is that severe hypoglycemic episodes (particularly at night) are greatly reduced with their use.

2. Continuing insulin dosage—The total daily insulin dosage may need to be increased gradually to 1 U/kg (especially if ketones are present at onset). When gluconeogenesis and glycolysis are suppressed by insulin, a honeymoon or grace period is a common phenomenon. There is often a temporary decrease in the insulin dose during this period. This occurs 1–4 weeks after diagnosis in over 50% of children and tends to last longer in older children.

In helping families with day-to-day dosing of regular insulin or H or NL, some physicians initially use sliding scales, more recently referred to as "thinking" scales, to emphasize that the family must always be thinking about food recently eaten, or to be eaten, and recent or forthcoming exercise in addition to the blood glucose level. Examples of thinking scales are included in *Understanding Diabetes* (see references).

After the appropriate dosage of intermediate (eg, NPH) or long-acting (Lantus or Levemir) insulin is achieved, daily adjustments usually are not needed. However, small decreases may be made for heavy activity (eg, afternoon sports or overnight events). Many families gradually learn to make small (0.5–1 unit) weekly adjustments in insulin dosage based on home blood glucose testing. Understanding the onset, peak, and duration of insulin activity is essential (see Table 33–1).

As noted earlier, when one of the more physiologic (closer to human insulin output) basal insulins, Lantus or Levemir, is used, it must be given alone in the syringe or pen. When changing a patient from two injections per day of NPH insulin to Lantus or Levemir, the total 24-hour dose of NPH is divided in half to use as the initial dose. The dose of Lantus or Levemir is then increased or decreased 1 or 2 units every few days based on the fasting morning blood glucose levels. Common glucose level goals are 70–180 mg/dL (3.9–10 mmol/L) for preteens and 70–150 mg/dL (3.9–8.3 mmol/L) for teens. A rapid-acting insulin (H or NL) is then given before meals and snacks or a mixture of H or NL and NPH is given in the morning and H or NL at dinner. The dosages of H or NL may initially be based on a "thinking" scale (see previous discussion), and may later be based on carbohydrate-counting as the family becomes more knowledgeable (see discussion of diet, later).

Continuous subcutaneous insulin (insulin pump) therapy is being used more often in children, particularly for emotionally mature teens who are willing to do frequent blood glucose monitoring and to count carbohydrates. Basal insulin doses (usually H/NL) are chosen by the physician, with bolus doses prior to meals selected by the patient (or an appropriate adult) depending on the carbohydrate content of the food to be eaten. Insulin pump therapy is discussed in depth in Chapter 26 of *Understanding Diabetes* (see references).

Table 33–1. Kinetics of insulin action.

Type of Insulin	Begins Working	Main Effect	All Gone
Rapid-acting			
Regular	30 min	2–4 h	6–9 h
Humalog or NovoLog	10–15 min	30–80 min	4 h
Intermediate-acting			
NPH	2–4 h	6–8 h	12–15 h
Long-acting			
Lantus or Levemir	1–2 h	2–23 h	24–26 h
Premixed			
NPH/Regular	30 min	Variable[a]	12–18 h
NPH/75/25[b]	15 min	1–8 h	12–15 h

[a]Available in various combinations to fit individual needs.
[b]A mixture of 75% NPH and 25% Humalog.
NPH, neutral protamine Hagedorn insulin.

The following regimen constitutes intensive diabetes management: (1) three or more insulin injections per day, or insulin pump therapy; (2) four or more blood glucose determinations per day; (3) careful attention to dietary intake; and (4) frequent contact with the health care provider. This approach was shown in the Diabetes Control and Complications Trial (DCCT; see section on diet) to result in improved glucose control and to reduce the risk for retinal, renal, cardiovascular, and neurologic complications of diabetes. All teenagers with suboptimal glucose control who are willing to comply should be considered for intensive diabetes management.

3. Treatment of type 2 diabetes—The treatment of type 2 diabetes in children varies with the severity of the disease. If the glycosylated hemoglobin (HbA_{1c}) fraction is still normal (or near normal) and ketone levels are not moderately or significantly increased, modification of lifestyle (preferably for the entire family) is the first line of therapy. This must include reducing caloric intake and increasing exercise. If the HbA_{1c} fraction is mildly elevated (6.2–9.0%) and ketone levels are not moderately or significantly increased, an oral hypoglycemia agent can be tried. Metformin is usually tried along with modification of lifestyle, starting with a dose of 250–500 mg once daily. If needed, and if gastrointestinal adaptation has occurred, the dose can be gradually increased to 1 g twice daily. If the presentation is more severe, with moderately or significantly increased urine ketone levels, or blood β-hydroxybutyrate is more than 1.0 mmol/L, the initial treatment is similar to that of type 1 diabetes (including intravenous or subcutaneous insulin). Oral hypoglycemic agents may be tried at a later date, particularly if weight loss has been successful.

B. Diet

The mainstays of dietary treatment are discussed in detail in *Understanding Diabetes* (see references). The American Diabetes Association no longer recommends any one diabetic diet. Instead, nutrition therapy for diabetics should be individualized, with consideration given to the patient's customary cultural eating habits and other lifestyle circumstances. Some families and children (particularly those with weight problems) find exchange diets helpful initially while they are learning food categories. Most centers now just use exchanges of carbohydrates, referred to below as carbohydrate-counting or "carb-counting."

The DCCT found that four nutrition factors contributed to better glucose control (lower HbA_{1c} levels): (1) adherence to a meal plan, (2) avoidance of extra snacks, (3) avoidance of overtreatment of low blood glucose levels (hypoglycemia), and (4) prompt treatment of high blood glucose levels. Two other nutritional factors include adjusting insulin levels for meals and maintaining a consistent schedule of nighttime snacks. The DCCT popularized the carb-counting dietary plan in which the dosage of H/NL or regular insulin is altered with each injection to adjust for the amount of carbohydrate to be eaten and the amount of exercise contemplated. One

carbohydrate count is 15 g of glucose in the United States (10 g in the United Kingdom). A common formula is to use 1 unit of H/NL for each 15 g of carbohydrate eaten, although this ratio must be adjusted (using blood glucose levels 2 hours after meals) for each person.

C. Exercise

Regular aerobic exercise—at least 30 minutes a day—is important for children with diabetes. Exercise fosters a sense of well-being; helps increase insulin sensitivity; and helps maintain proper weight, blood pressure, and blood fat levels. Exercise may also help maintain normal peripheral circulation in later years. It is particularly important for children with type 2 diabetes.

Hypoglycemia during exercise or in the 2–12 hours after exercise (delayed hypoglycemia) can be prevented by careful monitoring of blood glucose before, during, and after exercise; sometimes by reducing the dosage of the insulin active at the time of (or after) the exercise; and by providing extra snacks. Children using insulin pumps should reduce preexercise bolus insulin dosages as well as the basal dosages during (and sometimes after) the exercise. In general, the longer and more vigorous the activity, the greater the reduction in insulin dose. Extra snacks should also be eaten. Fifteen grams of glucose usually covers about 30 minutes of exercise. The use of drinks containing 5–10% dextrose, such as Gatorade, during the period of exercise is often beneficial.

D. Stress Management

Management of stress is important on a short-term basis because stress hormones increase blood glucose levels. Chronic emotional upsets may lead to missed injections or other compliance problems. When this happens, counseling for the family and child becomes an important part of diabetes management.

E. Home Blood Glucose Measurements

All families must be able to monitor blood glucose levels three or four times daily—and more frequently in small infants and patients who have glucose control problems or intercurrent illnesses. Blood glucose levels can be monitored using any of the available meters, which generally have an accuracy of 90% or better. Target levels when no food has been eaten for 2 or more hours vary according to age (Table 33–2).

Blood glucose results should be recorded even if the meter has a memory feature. This allows the family to look for patterns and make changes in insulin dosage. If more than 50% of the values are above the desired range for age or more than 14% below the desired range, the insulin dosage usually needs to be adjusted. Some families are able to make these changes independently (particularly after the first year), whereas others need help from the health care provider. Children with diabetes should be evaluated by a clinician every 3 months. This provides an opportunity to

Table 33–2. Ideal glucose levels after 2 or more hours of fasting.[a]

Age (y)	Glucose Level
4 or younger	80–200 mg/dL (4.6–11 mmol/L)
5–11	70–180 mg/dL (3.9–10 mmol/L)
12 or older	70–150 mg/dL (3.9–8.3 mmol/L)

[a]At least half of the values must be below the upper limit to have a good HbA$_{1c}$ value. The values should also be below the upper limits for age when tested 2 h after a meal.

adjust insulin dosages according to changes in growth and blood glucose levels as well as to check for changes noted on physical examination (eg, eyes and thyroid). Continuous glucose monitoring (CGM) is now being used in some children and adolescents. Subcutaneous glucose levels are obtained every 1–5 minutes from a sensor placed under the skin. As with insulin pump therapy, additional education, usually at a specialty diabetes center, is required.

F. Laboratory Evaluations

In addition to home measurements of blood glucose and blood or urine ketone levels, the HbA$_{1c}$ level should be measured every 3 months. This test reflects the frequency of elevated blood glucose levels over the previous 3 months. Normal values vary among laboratories but are usually below 6.2% HbA$_{1c}$. The desired ranges are based on age. For the HbA$_{1c}$ method, these ranges are as follows: 12–19 years, less than 7.5%; 6–11 years, less than 8.0%; and younger than 5 years, 7.5–8.5%. Higher levels are allowed in younger children to reduce the risk of hypoglycemia because their brains are still developing and they may not relate symptoms of hypoglycemia to a need for treatment. Low HbA$_{1c}$ values are generally associated with a greater risk for hypoglycemia (see the following section). Using either method, longitudinal averages more than 33% above the upper limit of normal are associated with a higher risk for later renal and retinal complications. In the intensive treatment group of the DCCT, the lower HbA$_{1c}$ values resulted in greater than 50% reductions in the retinal, renal, cardiovascular, and neurologic complications of diabetes.

Since atherosclerosis is the major cause of death in older patients with diabetes it is important to measure serum cholesterol, low-density lipoprotein cholesterol, and high-density lipoprotein cholesterol levels once yearly. Cholesterol levels should be below 200 mg/dL and low-density lipoprotein cholesterol levels below 100 mg/dL in postpubertal patients with diabetes.

When puberty is reached and the individual has had diabetes for 3 years or longer, the urinary excretion of albumin should be measured (as microalbumin) in two separate urine samples once yearly (see discussion of chronic compli-

cations, later). This can be done using timed overnight urine collections or first-morning voids (expressed per milligram of creatinine). Normal values differ with the methodology of the laboratory but are generally below 20 mcg/min (or 30 mcg/mg creatinine). People with type 2 diabetes should have this test done soon after diagnosis and then annually.

If the thyroid is enlarged (about 20% of patients with type 1 diabetes), the thyroid-stimulating hormone level should be measured yearly. This is usually the first test to become abnormal in the autoimmune thyroiditis commonly associated with type 1 diabetes.

In recent years antiendomysial and transglutaminase antibodies, reliable predictors of celiac disease, have been shown to be more common in children with diabetes as well as in their siblings. Risk of celiac disease is associated with HLA-DR3 and is more frequent in children with diabetes (celiac disease occurring in about 5%). The celiac antibodies should be checked in diabetic children with poor growth (especially when not related to poor glucose control) or those who present with gastrointestinal symptoms. The 21-hydroxylase autoantibody, a marker of increased risk of Addison disease, is present in approximately 1.3% of patients with type 1 diabetes, although Addison disease develops in only about one third of these antibody-positive individuals.

Type 2 diabetes is not an autoimmune disease, and the islet antibody tests are negative. An elevated insulin or C-peptide level is also helpful, indicating that insulin production is normal or elevated.

A checklist of the physician's contributions to good diabetes care is presented in Table 33–3.

▶ Acute Complications

A. Hypoglycemia

Hypoglycemia (or insulin reaction) is defined as a blood glucose level below 60 mg/dL (or 3.3 mmol/L). For preschool

Table 33–3. Physician's checklist of good diabetes management.

Variable	Frequency of Measurement	Tests and Values
Blood glucose	3–4 times daily	See Table 33–2
Hemoglobin A$_{1c}$	Every 3 mo	See text
Urine microalbumin	Annually after 3 y of diabetes (pubertal patients)	< 20 mcg/min
Ophthalmology referral	Annually after 3 y of diabetes (age 10 y or older)	Retinal photographs
Signs of other endocrinopathy	Evaluate at least annually (eg, thyroid enlargement)	(eg: TSH: 0.5–5.0 IU/mL)
Blood lipid panel	Annually	Cholesterol < 200 mg/dL; LDL < 100

TSH, thyroid-stimulating hormone.

children, values below 70 mg/dL (3.9 mmol/L) should be cause for concern. The common symptoms of hypoglycemia are hunger, weakness, shakiness, sweating, drowsiness (at an unusual time), headache, and behavioral changes. Children learn to recognize hypoglycemia at different ages but can often report "feeling funny" as young as age 4–5 years. If low blood glucose is not treated immediately with simple sugar, the hypoglycemia may result in loss of consciousness or convulsions. If hypoglycemia is left untreated for several hours, brain damage or death can occur.

Consistency in daily routine, correct insulin dosage, regular blood glucose monitoring, controlled snacking, compliance of patients and parents, and good education are all important in preventing severe hypoglycemia. In addition, insulin should not be injected prior to getting into a hot tub, bath, or shower. The heat will increase circulation to the skin and cause more rapid insulin uptake. The use of H/NL insulin and of Lantus insulin has also helped to reduce the occurrence of hypoglycemia.

The treatment of mild hypoglycemia involves giving 4 oz of juice, a sugar-containing soda drink, or milk, and waiting 10 minutes. If the blood glucose level is still below 60 mg/dL (3.3 mmol/L), the liquids are repeated. If the glucose level is above 60 mg/dL, solid foods are given. Moderate hypoglycemia, in which the person is conscious but incoherent, is treated by squeezing one-half tube of concentrated glucose (eg, Insta-Glucose or cake frosting) between the gums and lips and stroking the throat to encourage swallowing.

In the DCCT study, 10% of patients with standard management and 25% of those with intensive insulin management—insulin pumps or three or more insulin shots per day—had one or more severe hypoglycemic reactions each year. Families are advised to have glucagon in the home and to treat hypoglycemia by giving subcutaneous or intramuscular injections of 0.3 mL (30 units in an insulin syringe) for children younger than age 5 years and 0.5 mL (50 units) to those older than age 5 years. Some patients (usually those who have had diabetes for more than 10 years) fail to recognize the symptoms of low blood glucose (hypoglycemic unawareness). For these individuals, glucose control must be liberalized to prevent severe hypoglycemic reactions. School personnel, sports coaches, and babysitters must be trained to recognize and treat hypoglycemia.

B. Ketonuria, Ketonemia, and Ketoacidosis

Families must be educated to check blood or urine ketone levels during any illness (including vomiting even once) or any time a fasting blood glucose level is above 240 mg/dL (13.3 mmol/L), or a randomly measured glucose level is above 300 mg/dL (16.6 mmol/L). If moderate or significant ketonuria is detected, or the blood ketone (β-hydroxybutyrate—using the Precision Xtra meter) is above 1.0 mmol/L, the health care provider must be called. Usually 10–20% of the total daily insulin dosage is given subcutaneously as H or NL (or regular) insulin every 2–3 hours until the elevated ketones are gone. This prevents ketonuria and ketonemia

from progressing to ketoacidosis and allows most patients to receive treatment at home by telephone management. Juices and other fluids to help wash out the ketones and to prevent dehydration are encouraged. If deep breathing (Kussmaul respirations) or excessive weakness occurs, the patient should be evaluated promptly by a physician.

Acidosis (venous blood pH < 7.30) is now present in fewer than 25% of newly diagnosed children. Acidosis may also occur in those with known diabetes who do not check blood or urine ketone levels or fail to call the health care provider when ketones levels are elevated. Repeated episodes of ketoacidosis usually result from missed insulin injections and signify that counseling may be indicated, and that a responsible adult must take over the diabetes management. If for any reason this is not possible, a change in the child's living situation may be necessary.

Treatment of diabetic ketoacidosis (DKA) is based on four physiologic principles: (1) restoration of fluid volume, (2) inhibition of lipolysis and return to glucose utilization, (3) replacement of body salts, and (4) correction of acidosis. Laboratory tests at the start of treatment should include venous blood pH, blood glucose, and an electrolyte panel. Mild DKA is defined as a venous blood pH of 7.2–7.3; moderate DKA, a pH of 7.10–7.19; and severe DKA, a pH below 7.10. Patients with severe DKA should be hospitalized in a pediatric intensive care unit, if available in the area. More severe cases may benefit from determination of osmolality, calcium and phosphorus, and blood urea nitrogen levels. Severe and moderate episodes of DKA generally require hourly determinations of serum glucose, electrolytes, and venous pH levels, whereas these parameters can be measured every 2 hours if the pH level is 7.20–7.30.

1. Restoration of fluid volume—Dehydration is judged by (1) acute loss of body weight (if a recent weight is known), (2) dryness of oral mucous membranes, (3) low blood pressure, and (4) tachycardia. Initial treatment is with physiologic saline (0.9%), 10–20 mL/kg during the first hour. If indicated by continued signs of dehydration, this is repeated during the second hour. The total volume of fluid in the first 4 hours of treatment should not exceed 40 mL/kg because of the danger of cerebral edema (see later discussion). Human albumin, 10 mL/kg of 5% solution, can be given over 30 minutes if the patient is in shock. After initial reexpansion, half-physiologic (0.45%) saline usually is given at 1.5 times maintenance. Maintenance fluids are as discussed in Chapter 43.

2. Inhibition of lipolysis and return to glucose utilization—Insulin turns off fat breakdown and ketone formation. Regular insulin is usually given intravenously at a rate of 0.1 U/kg/h. The insulin solution should be administered by pump and can be made by diluting 30 units of regular insulin in 150 mL of 0.9% saline (1 U/5 mL). If the glucose level falls below 250 mg/dL (13.9 mmol/L), 5% dextrose is added to the intravenous fluids. If the glucose level continues to decrease below 120 mg/dL (6.6 mmol/L), 10% dextrose can be added. If necessary, the insulin dosage can be reduced to 0.05 U/kg/h, but it should not be discontinued before the venous blood pH reaches 7.30. The half-life of intravenous insulin is 6 minutes, whereas subcutaneous H or NL insulin takes 10–15 minutes, and regular insulin takes 30–60 minutes, to begin activity. Thus it is often better to continue intravenous insulin until subcutaneous insulin can begin acting.

3. Replacement of body salts—In patients with DKA, both sodium and potassium pass into the urine with the ketones and are depleted. In addition to body depletion, serum sodium concentrations may be falsely lowered by hyperglycemia, causing water to be drawn into the intravenous space, and by hyperlipidemia if fat replaces some of the water in the serum used for electrolyte analysis. Sodium is usually replaced adequately by the use of physiologic and half-physiologic saline in the rehydration fluids, as discussed earlier.

Serum potassium levels may be elevated initially because of inability of potassium to stay in the cell in the presence of acidosis (even though total body potassium is low). Potassium should not be given until the serum potassium level is known to be low or normal and the pH is above 7.10. It is then usually given at a concentration of 40 mEq/L, with half of the potassium (20 mEq/L) either as potassium acetate or potassium chloride and the other half as potassium phosphate (20 mEq/L). Hypocalcemia can occur if all of the potassium is given as the phosphate salt; hypophosphatemia occurs if none of the potassium is of the phosphate salt.

4. Correction of acidosis—Acidosis is corrected as the fluid volume and aerobic glycolysis are restored and as insulin is administered to inhibit ketogenesis. As noted earlier, measurement of the venous blood pH (identical to arterial blood pH) reveals the severity of acidosis. Bicarbonate is usually not given, even with severe DKA.

5. Management of cerebral edema—Some degree of cerebral edema has been shown by computed tomography scan to be common in DKA. Associated clinical symptoms are rare, unpredictable, and may be associated with demise. Cerebral edema may be related to overhydration with hypotonic fluids, although the cause is not well understood. It is now recommended that no more than 40 mL/kg of fluids be given in the first 4 hours of treatment. Cerebral edema is more common with a pH lower than 7.1, an arterial partial carbon dioxide pressure lower than 20 mm Hg, or when the serum sodium is noted to be falling rather than rising. Early neurologic signs may include headache, excessive drowsiness, and dilated pupils. Prompt initiation of therapy should include elevation of the head of the bed, hyperventilation, mannitol (1 g/kg over 30 minutes), and fluid restriction. If the cerebral edema is not recognized and treated early, over 50% of patients will die or have permanent brain damage.

▶ Chronic Complications

In the past, about 30–40% of persons with type 1 diabetes eventually developed renal failure or loss of vision. Factors that greatly reduce this likelihood are maintenance of longitudinal HbA$_{1c}$ levels in a good range, maintenance of blood pressure below the 90th percentile for age, and abstinence from smoking or chewing tobacco. Annual retinal examinations and urine microalbumin measurements are important for children aged 10 years or older who have had diabetes for 3 years or longer (see section on laboratory evaluations, earlier). Data now show that the use of angiotensin-converting enzyme inhibitors may reverse or delay kidney damage when it is detected in the microalbuminuria stage (20–300 mcg/min). Similarly, laser treatment to coagulate proliferating capillaries prevents bleeding and leakage of blood into the vitreous fluid or behind the retina. This treatment helps to prevent retinal detachment and to preserve useful vision for many people with proliferative diabetic retinopathy.

REFERENCES

American Diabetes Association: Clinical practice recommendations. Diabetes Care 2007;30(Suppl 1):524.

American Diabetes Association: Type 2 diabetes in children and adolescents. Diabetes Care 2000;23:381 [PMID: 10868870].

Chase HP et al: Continuous subcutaneous glucose monitoring in children with type 1 diabetes. Pediatrics 2001;107:222 [PMID: 11158450].

Chase HP et al: The impact of the diabetes control and complications trial and Humalog insulin on glycohemoglobin levels and severe hypoglycemia in type 1 diabetes. Diabetes Care 2001;24:430 [PMID: 11289463].

Chase HP: *Understanding Diabetes*, 11th ed. SFI, 2006. Available from Children's Diabetes Foundation, 777 Grant Street, Suite 302, Denver, CO 80203 for $25.00 (phone: 1-800-695-2873; web site: http://www.barbaradaviscenter.org).

Diabetes Control and Complications Trial Research Group: The effect of intensive treatment of diabetes on the development and progression of long-term complications in insulin-dependent diabetes mellitus. N Engl J Med 1993;329:977 [PMID: 8366922].

Diabetes Prevention Program Research Group: Reduction in the incidence of type 2 diabetes with lifestyle intervention or metformin. N Engl J Med 2002;346:393 [PMID: 11832527].

Glaser N et al: Risk factors for cerebral edema in children with diabetic ketoacidosis. The Pediatric Emergency Medicine Collaborative Research Committee of the American Academy of Pediatrics. N Engl J Med 2001;344:264 [PMID: 11172153].

Maniatis AK et al: Continuous subcutaneous insulin infusion therapy for children and adolescents: An option for routine diabetes care. Pediatrics 2001;107:351 [PMID: 11158469].

Report of the Expert Committee on the Diagnosis and Classification of Diabetes Mellitus. Diabetes Care 1997;20:1183 [PMID: 9203460].

Roberts MD et al: Diabetic ketoacidosis with intracerebral complications. Pediatr Diabetes 2001;2:109 [PMID: 15016193].

Inborn Errors of Metabolism

Janet A. Thomas, MD

Johan L.K. Van Hove, MD, PhD, MBA

Disorders in which single gene defects cause clinically significant blocks in metabolic pathways are called inborn errors of metabolism. For many years after Garrod first described them in 1908, these conditions were considered rare. Because the number of recognized inborn errors has increased, they are now acknowledged to be important causes of disease in children (estimated incidence 1:1500 children). Many of these disorders can now be treated effectively. Even when treatment is not available, correct diagnosis permits parents to make informed decisions about future offspring.

The pathology is almost always due either to accumulation of enzyme substrate behind a metabolic block or to deficiency of the reaction product. In some cases, the accumulated enzyme substrate is diffusible and has adverse effects on distant organs; in other cases, as in lysosomal storage diseases, the substrate primarily accumulates locally.

The clinical manifestations of inborn errors vary widely with both mild and severe forms of virtually every disorder. Many patients do not match the classic phenotype because mutations are not identical in different patients, even though they occur in the same gene.

A first treatment strategy is to enhance the reduced enzyme activity. Gene replacement is a long-term goal, but problems of gene delivery to target organs and control of gene action make this an unrealistic option at present. Enzyme replacement therapy using intravenously administered recombinant enzyme has been developed as an effective strategy in lysosomal storage disorders. Organ transplantation (liver or bone marrow) can provide a source of enzyme for some conditions. Pharmacologic doses of a cofactor such as a vitamin can sometimes be effective in restoring enzyme activity. Alternatively, some strategies are designed to cope with the consequences of enzyme deficiency. Strategies used to avoid substrate accumulation include restriction of precursor in the diet (eg, low-phenylalanine diet for phenylketonuria), avoidance of catabolism, inhibition of an enzyme in the synthesis of the precursor (eg, NTBC in tyrosinemia type I), or removal of accumulated substrate pharmacologically (eg, glycine therapy for isovaleric acidemia) or by dialysis. An inadequately produced metabolite can also be supplemented (eg, glucose administration for glycogen storage disease type I).

Inborn errors can manifest at any time, can affect any organ system, and can mimic many common pediatric problems. This chapter focuses on when to consider metabolic disorder in the differential diagnosis of common pediatric problems. A few of the more important disorders are then discussed in detail.

DIAGNOSIS

SUSPECTING INBORN ERRORS

Inborn errors must be considered in the differential diagnosis of critically ill newborns, children with seizures, neurodegeneration, mental retardation, developmental delay, recurrent vomiting, Reye-like syndrome, parenchymal liver disease, cardiomyopathy, unexplained metabolic acidosis, hyperammonemia, and hypoglycemia. Inborn errors should be suspected when (1) symptoms accompany changes in diet, (2) the child's development regresses, (3) the child shows specific food preferences or aversions, or (4) the family has a history of parental consanguinity or problems suggestive of inborn error such as retardation or unexplained deaths in first- and second-degree relatives.

Physical findings associated with inborn errors include alopecia or abnormal hair, retinal cherry-red spot or retinitis pigmentosa, cataracts or corneal opacity, hepatomegaly or splenomegaly, coarse features, skeletal changes (including gibbus), neurologic regression, and intermittent or progressive ataxia or dystonia. Other features that may be important in the context of a suspicious history include failure to thrive, microcephaly, rash, jaundice, hypotonia, and hypertonia.

Finding an immediate cause of symptoms does not rule out an underlying inborn error. For example, renal tubular acidosis and cirrhosis may be due to an underlying inborn error. Acute crises may be brought on by intercurrent infections in some inborn errors. Some inborn errors suggest a diagnosis of nonaccidental trauma (eg, glutaric acidemia type I) or poisoning (eg, methylmalonic acidemia). In addition, children with inborn errors may be at higher risk for child abuse or neglect because of their frustrating irritability.

LABORATORY STUDIES

Table 34–1 lists common clinical and laboratory features of different groups of inborn errors. Table 34–2 lists the most common laboratory tests used to diagnose these diseases and offers suggestions about their use.

Laboratory studies are almost always needed for the diagnosis of inborn errors. Serum electrolytes and pH should be used to estimate anion gap and acid-base status. Serum lactate, pyruvate, and ammonia levels are available in most hospitals but care is needed in obtaining samples appropriately. Amino acid and organic acid studies must be performed at specialized facilities to ensure accurate analysis and interpretation. An increasing number of inborn errors are diagnosed with DNA sequencing, but interpretation of private mutations can be problematic.

The physician should know what conditions a test can detect and when it can detect them. For example, urine organic acids may be normal in patients with medium-chain acyl-CoA dehydrogenase deficiency or biotinidase deficiency; glycine may be elevated only in cerebrospinal fluid (CSF) in patients with glycine encephalopathy. A result that is normal in one physiologic state may be abnormal in another. For instance, the urine of a child who becomes hypoglycemic upon prolonged fasting should be positive for ketones. In such a child, the absence of ketones in the urine suggests a defect in fatty acid oxidation.

Samples used to diagnose metabolic disease may be obtained at autopsy. Samples must be obtained in a timely fashion and may be analyzed directly or stored frozen until a particular analysis is justified by the results of postmortem examination, new clinical information, or developments in the field. Studies of other family members may help establish the diagnosis of a deceased patient. It may be possible to demonstrate that parents are heterozygous carriers of a particular disorder or that a sibling has the condition.

COMMON CLINICAL SITUATIONS

1. Mental Retardation

Some inborn errors can cause mental retardation without other distinguishing characteristics. Measurements of serum amino acids, urine organic acids, and serum uric acid should be obtained in every patient with nonspecific mental retardation. Urine screens for mucopolysaccharides and succinylpurines, and serum testing for carbohydrate-deficient glycoproteins are useful because these disorders do not always have specific physical findings. Absent speech can point to disorders of creatine. Abnormalities of the brain detected by magnetic resonance imaging can suggest specific groups of disorders (eg, cortical migrational abnormalities in peroxisomal biogenesis disorders).

2. Acute Presentation in the Neonate

Acute metabolic disease in the neonate is most often a result of disorders of protein or carbohydrate metabolism and may be clinically indistinguishable from sepsis. Prominent symptoms include poor feeding, vomiting, altered mental status or muscle tone, jitteriness, seizures, and jaundice. Acidosis or altered mental status out of proportion to systemic symptoms should increase suspicion of a metabolic disorder. Laboratory measurements should include electrolytes, ammonia, lactate, glucose, blood pH, and urine ketones and reducing substances. Glycine in CSF should be measured if glycine encephalopathy is suspected. Serum and urine amino acid, urine organic acid, and serum acylcarnitine analysis should be performed on samples collected before oral intake is discontinued and sent later for analysis if indicated by the results of initial studies. Neonatal cardiomyopathy or ventricular arrhythmias should be investigated with serum acylcarnitine analysis.

3. Vomiting & Encephalopathy in the Infant or Older Child

Electrolytes, ammonia, glucose, urine pH, urine reducing substances, and urine ketones should be measured in all patients with vomiting and encephalopathy before any treatment affects the results. Samples for serum amino acids, serum acylcarnitine profile, and urine organic acid analysis should be obtained early and frozen pending the results of initial studies. In the presentation of a Reye-like syndrome (ie, vomiting, encephalopathy, and hepatomegaly), amino acids, acylcarnitines, carnitine levels, and organic acids should be assessed immediately. Hypoglycemia with inappropriately low urine or serum ketones suggests the diagnosis of fatty acid oxidation defects.

4. Hypoglycemia

Duration of fasting, presence or absence of hepatomegaly, and Kussmaul breathing provide clues to the differential diagnosis of hypoglycemia. Serum insulin, cortisol, and growth hormone should be obtained on presentation. Urine ketones, urine organic acids, plasma lactate, serum acylcarnitine profile, carnitine levels, ammonia, and uric acid should be measured. Ketone body production is usually not efficient in the neonate, and ketonuria in a hypoglycemic or acidotic neonate suggests an inborn error. In the older child, inappropriately low urine ketone levels suggest an inborn error of fatty acid oxidation. Assessment of ketone generation requires simultaneous measurements of quantitative serum 3-hydroxybutyrate, acetoacetate, and free fatty acids

Table 34–1. Presenting clinical and laboratory features of inborn errors.

	Defects of Carbohydrate Metabolism	Defects of Amino Acid Metabolism[a]	Organic Acid Disorders[b]	Defects of Fatty Acid Oxidation	Defects of Purine Metabolism	Lysosomal Storage Diseases	Disorders of Peroxisomes	Disorders of Energy Metabolism
Neurodevelopmental								
Mental/developmental retardation	+	+++	+++	+	++	+++	+++	+++
Developmental regression	–	–	+	–	+	+++	+++	+++
Acute encephalopathy	+++	+++	+++	+++	–	–	–	+
Seizures	+	+++	+++	+	–	+++	++	+++
Ataxia/movement disorder	–	+	++	–	+++	–	–	+++
Hypotonia	+	++	++	+++	–	+	+++	+++
Hypertonia	–	++	+++	–	++	+	–	+
Abnormal behavior	–	++	++	–	++	++	–	+
Growth								
Failure to thrive	+++	+++	+++	+	–	+	–	++
Short stature	++	–	+	–	–	++	–	++
Macrocephaly	–	–	+	–	–	++	++	–
Microcephaly	+	++	+++	–	–	+	–	++
General								
Vomiting/anorexia	++	+++	+++	+++	–	–	++	+
Food aversion or craving	++	+++	+++	+++	–	–	–	–
Odor	–	++	++	–	–	–	–	–
Dysmorphic features	–	+	+	–	–	++	++	–
Congenital malformations	–	++	++	–	–	–	++	+
Organ-specific								
Hepatomegaly	+++	–	++	+++	–	+++	+++	+
Liver disease/cirrhosis	++	+	–	+	–	–	+	++
Splenomegaly	–	–	–	–	–	++	+	–
Skeletal dysplasia	–	–	–	–	–	++	++	–
Cardiomyopathy	+	–	+	+++	–	++	–	+++
Tachypnea/hyperpnea	++	++	++	++	–	–	–	+
Rash	–	++	++	–	–	–	–	–
Alopecia or abnormal hair	–	+	++	–	–	–	+	–
Cataracts or corneal opacity	++	–	–	–	–	++	–	+
Retinal abnormality	–	+	+	+	–	++	++	++
Frequent infections	++	–	++	–	++	–	–	–
Deafness	–	–	+	–	–	++	–	+++

(continued)

Table 34–1. Presenting clinical and laboratory features of inborn errors. *(Continued)*

	Defects of Carbohydrate Metabolism	Defects of Amino Acid Metabolism[a]	Organic Acid Disorders[b]	Defects of Fatty Acid Oxidation	Defects of Purine Metabolism	Lysosomal Storage Diseases	Disorders of Peroxisomes	Disorders of Energy Metabolism
Laboratory								
Hypoglycemia	+++	+	++	++	–	–	–	+
Hyperammonemia	–	++	++	++	–	–	–	–
Metabolic acidosis	++	++	+++	++	–	–	–	+++
Respiratory alkalosis	–	++	–	–	–	–	–	–
Elevated lactate/ pyruvate	++	–	+++	++	–	–	–	+++
Elevated liver enzymes	++	++	++	+++	–	+	+	+
Neutropenia or thrombocytopenia	+	–	+	–	++	+	–	+
Ketosis	+++	++	+++	–	–	–	–	+
Hypoketosis	–	–	+	+++	–	–	–	–

[a]Includes disorders of the urea cycle but not maple syrup urine disease.
[b]Includes maple syrup urine disease and disorders of pyruvate oxidation.
+++, most conditions in group; ++, some; +, one or few; –, not found.

in relation to a sufficient duration of fasting and age. Metabolites obtained during the acute episode can be very helpful and avoid the need for a formal fasting test.

5. Hyperammonemia

Symptoms of hyperammonemia may appear and progress rapidly or insidiously. Decreased appetite, irritability, and behavioral changes appear first with vomiting, ataxia, lethargy, seizures, and coma appearing as ammonia levels increase. Tachypnea is also characteristic and is due to a direct effect on respiratory drive. Physical examination cannot exclude the presence of hyperammonemia, and serum ammonia should be measured whenever hyperammonemia is possible.

Severe hyperammonemia may be due to urea cycle disorders, organic acidemias, or fatty acid oxidation disorders (such as carnitine-acylcarnitine translocase deficiency) or, in the premature infant, transient hyperammonemia of the newborn. The cause can usually be ascertained by measuring quantitative serum amino acids (eg, citrulline), plasma carnitine and acylcarnitine esters, and urine organic acids and orotic acid. Respiratory alkalosis is usually present in urea cycle defects and transient hyperammonemia of the newborn, while acidosis is characteristic of hyperammonemia due to organic acidemias.

6. Acidosis

Inborn errors may cause chronic or acute acidosis at any age, with or without an increased anion gap. Inborn errors should be considered when acidosis occurs with recurrent vomiting or hyperammonemia and when acidosis is out of proportion to the clinical status. Acidosis due to an inborn error can be difficult to correct. The main causes of anion gap metabolic acidosis are lactic acidosis, ketoacidosis (including abnormal ketone body production such as in β-ketothiolase deficiency), methylmalonic acidemia or other organic acidurias, intoxication (ethanol, methanol, ethylene glycol, and salicylate), and uremia. Causes of non–anion gap metabolic acidosis include loss of base in diarrhea or renal tubular acidosis (isolated renal tubular acidosis or renal Fanconi syndrome). If renal bicarbonate loss is found, then a distinction must be made between isolated renal tubular acidosis and a more generalized renal tubular disorder or renal Fanconi syndrome by testing for renal losses of phosphorus and amino acids. Inborn errors associated with renal tubular acidosis or renal Fanconi syndrome include cystinosis, tyrosinemia type I, carnitine palmitoyltransferase I, and mitochondrial diseases. Serum glucose and ammonia levels and urinary pH and ketones should be examined. Samples for amino acids and organic acids should be obtained at once and may be evaluated immediately or frozen for later analysis, depending on how strongly an inborn error is suspected. It is useful to test blood lactate and pyruvate levels in the chronically acidotic patient even if urine organic acid levels are normal. Lactate and pyruvate levels are difficult to interpret in the acutely ill patient, but in the absence of shock, high levels of lactic acid suggest primary lactic acidosis.

Table 34–2. Obtaining and handling samples to diagnose inborn errors.

Test	Comments
Acid-base status	Accurate estimation of anion gap must be possible. Samples for blood gases should be kept on ice and analyzed immediately.
Blood ammonia	Sample should be kept on ice, and analyzed immediately.
Blood lactic acid and pyruvic acid	Sample should be collected without a tourniquet, kept on ice, and analyzed immediately. Conversion of lactic acid into pyruvic acid must be prevented. Normal literature values are for the fasting, rested state.
Amino acids	Blood and urine should be examined. CSF glycine should be measured if nonketotic hyperglycinemia is to be ruled out. Normal literature values are for the fasting state. Growth of bacteria in urine should be prevented.
Organic acids	Urine preferred for analysis. Serum or CSF organic acids are rarely indicated and often miss diagnoses.
Carnitine and acylcarnitine profile	Blood or plasma may be analyzed for total, free, and esterified carnitine; normal values are for the healthy, nonfasted state. Acylcarnitine profile in blood identifies compounds esterified to carnitine. Rarely urine and bile studies may be needed for certain conditions. Profiling in cultured fibroblasts after fat loading can be helpful in diagnosis of certain conditions.
Urine mucopolysaccharides	Variations in urine concentration may cause errors in screening tests. Diagnosis requires knowing which mucopolysaccharides are increased. Some patients with Morquio disease and many with Sanfilippo disease do not have abnormal mucopolysacchariduria.
Enzyme assays	Specific assays must be requested. Exposure to heat may cause loss of enzyme activity. Enzyme activity in whole blood may become normal after transfusion or vitamin therapy. Leukocyte or fibroblast pellets should be kept frozen prior to assays. Fibroblasts may be grown from skin biopsies taken up to 72 h after death. Tissues such as liver and kidney should be taken as soon as possible after death, frozen immediately, and kept at –70°C until assayed.

CSF, cerebrospinal fluid.

MANAGEMENT OF METABOLIC EMERGENCIES

Patients with severe acidosis, hypoglycemia, and hyperammonemia may be very ill; initially mild symptoms may worsen quickly, and coma and death may ensue within hours. With prompt and vigorous treatment, however, patients can recover completely, even from deep coma. All oral intake should be stopped. Sufficient glucose should be given intravenously to avoid or minimize catabolism in a patient with a known inborn error who is at risk for crisis. Most conditions respond favorably to glucose administration, although a few (eg, primary lactic acidosis due to pyruvate dehydrogenase deficiency) do not. After exclusion of fatty acid oxidation disorders, immediate institution of intravenous fat emulsions (eg, intralipid) can provide crucial caloric input. Severe or increasing hyperammonemia should be treated pharmacologically or with dialysis, and severe acidosis should be treated with bicarbonate. More specific measures can be instituted when a diagnosis is established.

NEWBORN SCREENING

Criteria for screening newborns for a disorder include its frequency, its consequences if untreated, the ability of therapy to mitigate consequences, the cost of testing, and the cost of treatment. All states in the United States screen newborns for phenylketonuria and hypothyroidism. In most states newborns are screened for galactosemia. Other metabolic disorders for which newborns are frequently screened include maple syrup urine disease, homocystinuria due to cystathionine β-synthase deficiency, and biotinidase deficiency. Expanded newborn screening using tandem mass spectrometry detects several disorders of amino acid, organic acid, and fatty acid metabolism.

Some screening tests measure a metabolite (eg, phenylalanine) that becomes abnormal with time and exposure to diet. In such instances the disease cannot be detected reliably until intake of the substrate is established. Other tests (eg, for biotinidase deficiency) measure enzyme activity and can be performed at any time. Transfusions may cause false-negative results in this instance, and exposure of the sample to heat may cause false-positive results. Technologic advances have extended the power of newborn screening but have brought additional challenges. For example, although tandem mass spectrometry can detect many more disorders in the newborn period, consensus on diagnosis and treatment for some conditions is still under development.

Screening tests are not diagnostic, and diagnostic tests must be undertaken when an abnormal screening result is obtained. Further, because false-negative results occur, a normal newborn screening test does not rule out a condition.

The timing of newborn screening recommended by the American Academy of Pediatrics (between 24 and 72 hours of life) is appropriate for the detection of phenylketonuria, but hypothyroidism, for instance, can be missed when screening is carried out at the same time. Early discharge of neonates causes significant problems in newborn screening, with both false-negative and false-positive results. Nevertheless, all infants should be screened before discharge from the hospital.

The appropriate response to an abnormal screening test depends on the condition in question and the predictive value of the test. For example, when screening for galactosemia by enzyme assay, complete absence of enzyme activity is highly predictive of classic galactosemia. Failure to treat may rapidly lead to death. In this case, treatment must be initiated immediately while diagnostic studies are pending. In phenylketonuria, however, a diet restricted in phenylalanine is harmful to the infant whose screening test is a false-positive, while diet therapy produces an excellent outcome in the truly affected infant if treatment is established within the first weeks of life. Therefore, treatment for phenylketonuria should only be instituted when the diagnosis is confirmed. Physicians should combine current American Academy of Pediatrics recommendations, state laws and regulations, and consultation with their local metabolic center to arrive at appropriate strategies for each hospital and practice.

Carroll AE, Downs SM: Comprehensive cost-utility analysis of newborn screening strategies. Pediatrics 2006;117:S287 [PMID: 16735255].

Chace DH, Kalas TA: A biochemical perspective on the use of tandem mass spectrometry for newborn screening and clinical testing. Clin Biochem 2005;38:296 [PMID: 15766731].

Claudius I et al: The emergency department approach to newborn and childhood metabolic crisis. Emerg Med Clin North Am 2005;23:843 [PMID: 15982549].

Frazier DM et al: The tandem mass spectrometry newborn screening experience in North Carolina: 1997–2005. J Inherit Metab Dis 2006;29:76 [PMID: 16601872].

Gelb MH et al: Direct multiplex assay of enzymes in dried blood spots by tandem mass spectrometry for the newborn screening of lysosomal storage disorders. J Inherit Metab Dis 2006;29:397 [PMID: 16763908].

Hardelid P, Dezateux C: Neonatal screening for inborn errors of metabolism. Lancet 2005;365:2176 [PMID: 15978919].

Horster F et al: Disorders of intermediary metabolism: toxic leukoencephalopathies. J Inherit Metab Dis 2005;28:345 [PMID: 15868467].

Kaye CI et al: Introduction to the newborn screening fact sheets. Pediatrics 2006;118:1304 [PMID: 16960984].

Kaye CI et al: Newborn screening fact sheets. Pediatrics 2006;118:e934 [PMID: 16950973].

Kayton A: Newborn screening: A literature review. Neonatal Netw 2007;26:85 [PMID: 17402600].

Pasquali M et al: Biochemical findings in common inborn errors of metabolism. Am J Med Genet C Semin Med Genet 2006;142:64 [PMID: 16602099].

Raghuveer TS et al: Inborn errors of metabolism in infancy and early childhood: An update. Am Fam Physician 2006;73:1981 [PMID: 16770930].

Saudubray JM et al: Clinical approach to treatable inborn metabolic diseases: An introduction. J Inherit Metab Dis 2006;29:261 [PMID: 16763886].

Tarini BA et al: State newborn screening in the tandem mass spectrometry era: More tests, more false-positive results. Pediatrics 2006;118:448 [PMID: 16882794].

Tran K et al: Clinical efficacy and cost-effectiveness of newborn screening for medium chain acyl-CoA dehydrogenase deficiency using tandem mass spectrometry. Clin Biochem 2007;40:235 [PMID: 17222812].

Turecek F et al: Tandem mass spectrometry in the detection of inborn errors of metabolism for newborn screening. Methods Mol Bio 2007;359:143 [PMID: 17484116].

Wilcken B: Recent advances in newborn screening. J Inherit Metab Dis 2007;30:129 [PMID: 17342450].

DISORDERS OF CARBOHYDRATE METABOLISM

GLYCOGEN STORAGE DISEASES

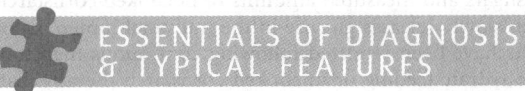

ESSENTIALS OF DIAGNOSIS & TYPICAL FEATURES

▶ Types 0, I, III, VI, and IX manifest with hypoglycemia in infants.

▶ Types II, V, and VII manifest with rhabdomyolysis or muscle weakness.

Glycogen is a highly branched polymer of glucose that is stored in liver and muscle. Different enzyme defects affect its biosynthesis and degradation. The hepatic forms of the glycogenoses cause growth failure, hepatomegaly, and severe fasting hypoglycemia. They include glucose-6-phosphatase deficiency (type I; von Gierke disease), debrancher enzyme deficiency (type III), hepatic phosphorylase deficiency (type VI), and phosphorylase kinase deficiency (type IX), which normally regulates hepatic phosphorylase activity. There are two forms of glucose-6-phosphatase deficiency: in type Ia, the catalytic glucose-6-phosphatase is deficient, and in type Ib, the glucose-6-phosphate transporter is deficient. The latter form also has neutropenia. Glycogenosis type IV, brancher enzyme deficiency, usually presents with progressive liver cirrhosis.

The myopathic forms of glycogenosis affect skeletal muscle. Skeletal myopathy with weakness or rhabdomyolysis may be seen in muscle phosphorylase deficiency (type V), phosphofructokinase deficiency (type VII), and acid maltase deficiency (type II; Pompe disease). The infantile form of Pompe disease also has hypertrophic cardiomyopathy and macroglossia. The gluconeogenetic disorder fructose-1,6-bisphosphatase deficiency presents with major lactic acidosis and delayed hypoglycemia on fasting.

▶ Diagnosis

Initial tests include glucose, lactate, triglycerides, cholesterol, uric acid, transaminases, and creatine kinase. Functional testing includes responsiveness of blood glucose to fasting and glucagon; for myopathic forms, an ischemic exercise test is helpful. Diagnostic confirmation requires enzyme assays of leukocytes, liver, or muscle. Disorders diagnosable from analysis of red or white blood cells include deficiency of debrancher enzyme (type III) and phosphorylase kinase (type IX). Pompe disease can usually be diagnosed by assaying acid maltase in a blood spot with confirmation in fibroblasts. Glycogenosis type I can often be diagnosed by molecular analysis.

▶ Treatment

Treatment is designed to prevent hypoglycemia and avoid secondary metabolite accumulations such as elevated lactate in glycogenosis type I. In the most severe hepatic forms, the special diet must be strictly monitored with restriction of free sugars and measured amounts of uncooked cornstarch, which slowly releases glucose in the intestinal lumen. Good results have been reported following continuous nighttime carbohydrate feeding or uncooked cornstarch therapy. Late complications even after years of treatment include focal segmental glomerulosclerosis, hepatic adenoma or carcinoma, and gout. Enzyme replacement therapy in Pompe disease corrects the cardiomyopathy, but the response in skeletal myopathy is variable with optimal results seen in patients treated early and who have some cross-reacting material present.

Belingheri M et al: Combined liver-kidney transplantation in glycogen storage disease 1a: A case beyond the guidelines. Liver Transpl 2007;13:762 [PMID: 17457869].

Hagemans ML et al: Clinical manifestation and natural course of late-onset Pompe's disease in 54 Dutch patients. Brain 2005;128:671 [PMID: 15659425].

Kishnani PS et al: Recombinant human acid [alpha]-glucosidase: Major clinical benefits in infantile-onset Pompe disease. Neurology 2007;68:99 [PMID: 17151339].

Koeberl DD et al: Glycogen storage disease types I and II: Treatment updates. J Inherit Metab Dis 2007;30:159 [PMID: 17308886].

Moraru E et al: Glycogen storage disease type 1—between chronic ambulatory follow-up and pediatric emergency. J Gastrointestin Liver Dis 2007;16:47 [PMID: 17410288].

Nogales-Gadea G et al: Molecular genetics of McArdle's disease. Curr Neurol Neurosci Rep 2007;7:84 [PMID: 17217859].

Ollivier K et al: Exercise tolerance and daily life in McArdle's disease. Muscle Nerve 2005;31:637 [PMID: 15614801].

Ozen H: Glycogen storage diseases: New perspectives. World J Gastroenterol 2007;13:2541 [PMID: 17552001].

Rake JP et al: Guidelines for management of glycogen storage disease type I—European Study on Glycogen Storage Disease Type I (ESGSD I). Eur J Pediatr 2002;161(Suppl 1):S112 [PMID: 12373584].

Shin YS: Glycogen storage disease: Clinical, biochemical, and molecular heterogeneity. Semin Pediatr Neurol 2006;13:115 [PMID: 17027861].

Visser G et al: Consensus guidelines for management of glycogen storage disease type 1b—European Study on Glycogen Storage Disease Type 1. Eur J Pediatr 2002;161(Suppl 1):S120 [PMID: 12373585].

GALACTOSEMIA

ESSENTIALS OF DIAGNOSIS & TYPICAL FEATURES

▶ Severely deficient neonates present with vomiting, jaundice and hepatomegaly on initiation of lactose-containing feedings.

▶ Renal Fanconi syndrome, cataracts of the ocular lens, hepatic cirrhosis, and sepsis occur in untreated children.

▶ Developmental delay, tremor, and ataxia occur in untreated or partially treated children.

▶ Delayed speech and ovarian failure occur even with treatment.

Classic galactosemia is caused by almost total deficiency of galactose-1-phosphate uridyltransferase. Accumulation of galactose-1-phosphate in liver and renal tubules causes hepatic parenchymal disease and renal Fanconi syndrome. Onset of the severe disease is marked in the neonate by vomiting, jaundice (both direct and indirect), hepatomegaly, and rapid onset of liver insufficiency after initiation of milk feeding. Hepatic cirrhosis is progressive. Without treatment, death frequently occurs within a month, often from *Escherichia coli* sepsis. Cataracts, caused by accumulation of galactitol in the lens, usually develop within 2 months in untreated cases, but usually reverse with treatment. With prompt institution of a galactose-free diet, the prognosis for survival without liver disease is excellent. Even when dietary restriction is instituted early, patients with galactosemia are at increased risk for speech and language deficits and ovarian failure. Some patients develop progressive mental retardation, tremor, and ataxia. Milder variants of galactosemia with better prognosis exist in all populations.

The disorder is autosomal recessive with an incidence of approximately 1:40,000 live births. Because disease in infancy may be severe, newborn screening is common. Screening is accomplished by demonstrating enzyme deficiency in red cells with the Beutler test or by demonstrating increased serum galactose.

▶ Diagnosis

In infants receiving foods containing galactose, laboratory findings include galactosuria and hypergalactosemia together with proteinuria and aminoaciduria. Absence of urine-reducing substances does not exclude the diagnosis. Galactose-1-phosphate is elevated in red blood cells. When the diagnosis is suspected, galactose-1-phosphate uridyltransferase should be assayed in erythrocytes. Blood transfusions give false-negative results and sample deterioration false-positive results.

▶ Treatment

A galactose-free diet should be instituted as soon as the diagnosis is made. Compliance with the diet must be monitored by following galactose-1-phosphate levels in red blood cells. Appropriate diet management requires not only the exclusion of milk but an understanding of the galactose content of foods. Avoidance of galactose should be life-long with appropriate calcium replacement.

Bosch AM: Classical galactosaemia revisited. J Inherit Metab Dis 2006;29:516 [PMID: 16838075].

Forges T et al: Pathophysiology of impaired ovarian function in galactosaemia. Hum Reprod Update 2006;12:573 [PMID: 16835432].

Panis B et al: Effect of calcium, vitamins K1 and D3 on bone in galactosemia. Bone 2006;39:1123 [PMID: 16782422].

Ridel KR et al: An updated review of the long-term neurological effects of galactosemia. Pediatr Neurol 2005;33:153 [PMID: 16087312].

Rubio-Gozalbo ME et al: The endocrine system in treated patients with classical galactosemia. Mol Genet Metab 2006;89:316 [PMID: 16935538].

Segal S et al: Pathways of galactose metabolism by galactosemics: Evidence for galactose conversion to hepatic UDPglucose. Mol Genet Metab 2006;87:92 [PMID: 16260165].

Zaffanello M et al: Neonatal screening, clinical features and genetic testing for galactosemia. Genet Med 2005;7:211 [PMID: 15775761].

Patient and parent support group web site with useful information for families: http://www.galactosemia.org

HEREDITARY FRUCTOSE INTOLERANCE

Hereditary fructose intolerance is an autosomal recessive disorder in which deficient activity of fructose-1-phosphate aldolase causes hypoglycemia and tissue accumulation of fructose-1-phosphate on fructose ingestion. Other abnormalities include failure to thrive, vomiting, jaundice, hepatomegaly, proteinuria, and generalized aminoaciduria. The untreated condition can progress to death from liver failure.

▶ Diagnosis

The diagnosis is suggested by finding fructosuria or an abnormal transferrin glycoform in the untreated patient. The appearance of hypoglycemia and hypophosphatemia after a closely monitored intravenous fructose loading test (200 mg/kg) is diagnostic. The diagnosis is confirmed by finding reduced enzyme activity of fructose-1-phosphate aldolase in the liver. Some patients may be diagnosed by identification of one of the common mutations on DNA analysis, but their absence does not exclude the diagnosis.

▶ Treatment

Treatment consists of strict dietary avoidance of fructose. Vitamin supplementation is usually needed. Management is complicated by the fact that many drugs and vitamins are dispensed in a sucrose base. Treatment monitoring can be done with transferrin glycoform analysis. If diet compliance is poor, physical growth retardation may occur. Growth will resume when more stringent dietary restrictions are reinstituted. If the disorder is recognized early, the prospects for normal development are good. As affected individuals grow up, they may recognize the association of nausea and vomiting with ingestion of fructose-containing foods and selectively avoid them.

Wong D: Hereditary fructose intolerance. Mol Genet Metab 2005; 85:165 [PMID: 16086449].

▼ DISORDERS OF ENERGY METABOLISM

The most common disorders of central mitochondrial energy metabolism are pyruvate dehydrogenase deficiency and deficiencies of respiratory chain components. Disorders of the Krebs cycle include deficiencies in fumarase, 2-ketoglutarate dehydrogenase, and succinyl-CoA ligase. In many, but not all patients, lactate is elevated in either blood or CSF. In pyruvate dehydrogenase deficiency, the lactate:pyruvate ratio is normal, whereas in respiratory chain disorders, the ratio is increased. Care must be taken to distinguish an elevated lactate level that is due to these conditions (called primary lactic acidoses) from elevated lactate that is a consequence of hypoxia, ischemia, or sampling problems. Table 34–3 lists some causes of primary lactic acidosis.

Patients with a defect in the pyruvate dehydrogenase complex often have agenesis of the corpus callosum or Leigh syndrome (lesions in the globus pallidus, dentate nucleus, and periaqueductal gray matter). They can have mild facial

Table 34–3. Causes of primary lactic acidosis in childhood.

Defects of the pyruvate dehydrogenase complex
E_1 (pyruvate decarboxylase) deficiency
E_2 (dihydrolipoyl transacetylase) deficiency
E_3 (lipoamide dehydrogenase) deficiency
Pyruvate decarboxylase phosphate phosphatase deficiency
Abnormalities of gluconeogenesis
Pyruvate carboxylase deficiency
Isolated
Biotinidase deficiency
Holocarboxylase synthetase deficiency
Fructose-1,6-diphosphatase deficiency
Glucose-6-phosphatase deficiency (von Gierke disease)
Defects in the mitochondrial respiratory chain
Complex I deficiency
Complex IV deficiency (cytochrome C oxidase deficiency; frequent cause of Leigh disease)
ATPase deficiency (frequent cause of Leigh disease)
Complex II deficiency
Complex III deficiency
Combined deficiencies
Coenzyme Q10 deficiency
Other respiratory chain disorders
Defects in the Krebs cycle
Succinyl-CoA ligase deficiency

dysmorphism. Recurrent altered mental status, recurrent ataxia, and recurrent acidosis are typical of many disturbances of pyruvate metabolism. The most common genetic defect is in the X-linked E_1 component, with males carrying milder mutations and females carrying severe mutations leading to cystic brain lesions.

The respiratory chain disorders are frequent (1:5000), and involve a heterogenous group of genetic defects that produce a variety of clinical syndromes (now > 50) of varying severity and presentation. The disorders can affect multiple organs. The following set of symptoms (not intended as a comprehensive listing) can indicate a respiratory chain disorder:

1. General: failure to thrive
2. Brain: progressive neurodegeneration, Leigh syndrome, myoclonic seizures, brain atrophy, and subcortical leukodystrophy
3. Eye: optic neuropathy, retinitis pigmentosa, and progressive external ophthalmoplegia
4. Ears: nerve deafness
5. Muscle: myopathy with decreased endurance or rhabdomyolysis
6. Kidney: renal Fanconi syndrome
7. Endocrine: diabetes mellitus and hypoparathyroidism
8. Intestinal: pancreatic or liver insufficiency or pseudoobstruction
9. Skin: areas of hypopigmentation
10. Heart: cardiomyopathy, conduction defects, and arrhythmias.

Respiratory chain disorders are among the more common causes of static, progressive, or self-limited neurodevelopmental problems in children. Patients may present with nonspecific findings such as hypotonia, failure to thrive, or renal tubular acidosis, or with more specific features such as ophthalmoplegia or cardiomyopathy. Symptoms are often combined in recognizable clinical syndromes with ties to specific genetic causes. Ragged red fibers and mitochondrial abnormalities may be noted on histologic examination of muscle. Thirteen of the more than 100 genes that control activity of the respiratory chain are part of the mitochondrial genome. Therefore inheritance of defects in the respiratory chain may be mendelian or maternal.

▶ Diagnosis

Pyruvate dehydrogenase deficiency is diagnosed by enzyme assay in leukocytes or fibroblasts. Confirmation can be obtained by molecular analysis. Diagnosis of respiratory chain disorders is based on a convergence of clinical, biochemical, morphologic, enzymatic, and molecular data. Classic pathologic features of mitochondrial disorders are the accumulation of mitochondria, which produces ragged red fibers in skeletal muscle biopsy, and abnormal shapes and inclusions on electron microscopy. However, these findings are only present in 5% of children. Enzyme analysis on skeletal muscle or liver tissue is complicated by an overlap between normal and affected range. Mitochondrial DNA analysis in blood or tissue may identify a diagnostic mutation. A rapidly increasing number of nuclear genes causing respiratory chain defects are being recognized. Children with defects in mtDNA maintenance often present with liver disease and neurodegeneration and are diagnosed by sequencing the causative nuclear genes. Although diagnostic criteria have been published, the cause of lactic acidemia still cannot be defined in many patients. In some instances, the genetics and prognosis may be clear, but in many cases neither prognosis nor genetic risk can be predicted.

▶ Treatment

A ketogenic diet is useful in pyruvate dehydrogenase deficiency. In rare patients with primary coenzyme Q deficiency, coenzyme Q treatment is very effective. Other treatments are of theoretical value, with little data on efficacy. Thiamine and lipoic acid have been tried in patients with pyruvate dehydrogenase complex deficiencies, and coenzyme Q and riboflavin have been helpful in some patients with respiratory chain defects. Dichloroacetic acid has been tried in pyruvate dehydrogenase complex deficiencies and in respiratory chain disorders, with limited clinical response and adverse effects.

Blok MJ et al: Mutations in the ND5 subunit of complex I of the mitochondrial DNA are a frequent cause of oxidative phosphorylation disease. J Med Genet 2007;44:e74 [PMID: 17400793].

Brown GK: Congenital brain malformations in mitochondrial disease. J Inherit Metab Dis 2005;28:393 [PMID: 15868471].

Chaturvedi S et al: Mitochondrial encephalomyopathies: Advances in understanding. Med Sci Monit 2005;11:RA238 [PMID: 15990701].

Debray FG et al: Long-term outcome and clinical spectrum of 73 patients with mitochondrial diseases. Pediatrics 2007;119:722 [PMID: 17403843].

DiMauro S: Mitochondrial myopathies. Curr Opin Rheumatol 2006;18:636 [PMID: 17053512].

DiMauro S, Gurgel-Giannetti J: The expanding phenotype of mitochondrial myopathy. Curr Opin Neurol 2005;18:538 [PMID: 16155436].

DiMauro S, Hirano M: Mitochondrial encephalomyopathies: An update. Neuromuscul Disord 2005;15:276 [PMID: 15792866].

DiMauro S, Mancuso M: Mitochondrial diseases: therapeutic approaches. Biosci Rep 2007;27:125 [PMID: 17486439].

DiMauro S et al: Approaches to the treatment of mitochondrial diseases. Muscle Nerve 2006;34:265 [PMID: 16810684].

Filosto M, Mancuso M: Mitochondrial diseases: A nosological update. Acta Neurol Scand 2007;115:211 [PMID: 17376118].

Huntsman RJ et al: Atypical presentations of Leigh syndrome: a case series and review. Pediatr Neurol 2005;32:334 [PMID: 15866434].

Garcia-Cazorla A et al: Mitochondrial respiratory chain deficiencies expressing the enzymatic deficiency in the hepatic tissue: A study of 31 patients. J Pediatr 2006;149:401 [PMID: 16939756].

Garcia-Cazorla A et al: Pyruvate carboxylase deficiency: Metabolic characteristics and new neurological aspects. Ann Neurol 2006;59:121 [PMID: 16278852].

Lee WS, Sokol RJ: Mitochondrial hepatopathies: Advances in genetics and pathogenesis. Hepatology 2007;45:1555 [PMID: 17538929].

Lerman-Sagie T et al: White matter involvement in mitochondrial diseases. Mol Genet Metab 2005;84:127 [PMID: 15670718].

Maceluch JA, Niedziela M: The clinical diagnosis and molecular genetics of Kearns-Sayre syndrome: A complex mitochondrial encephalomyopathy. Pediatr Endocrinol Rev 2006;4:117 [PMID: 17342029].

Morava E et al: Mitochondrial disease criteria: Diagnostic applications in children. Neurology 2006;67:1823 [PMID: 17130416].

Mordekar SR et al: The significance of reduced respiratory chain enzyme activities: Clinical, biochemical and radiological associations. Eur J Paediatr Neurol 2006;10:78 [PMID: 16567117].

Pithukpakorn M: Disorders of pyruvate metabolism and the tricarboxylic acid cycle. Mol Genet Metab 2005;85:243 [PMID: 16156009].

Sarzi E et al: Mitochondrial DNA depletion is a prevalent cause of multiple respiratory chain deficiency in childhood. J Pediatr 2007;150:531 [PMID: 17452231].

Taylor RW, Turnbull DM: Mitochondrial DNA mutations in human disease. Nat Rev Genet 2005;6:389 [PMID: 15861210].

Wong LJ: Diagnostic challenges of mitochondrial DNA disorders. Mitochondrion 2007;7:45 [PMID: 17276740].

Yaplito-Lee J et al: Cardiac manifestations in oxidative phosphorylation disorders of childhood. J Pediatr 2007;150:407 [PMID: 17382120].

Zhang Y et al: Clinical and molecular survey in 124 Chinese patients with Leigh or Leigh-like syndrome. J Inherit Metab Dis 2007;30:265 [PMID: 17323145].

Patient and parent support group web site with useful information for families: http://www.umdf.org

DISORDERS OF AMINO ACID METABOLISM

DISORDERS OF THE UREA CYCLE

Ammonia is mostly derived from the catabolism of amino acids and is converted to an amino group in urea by enzymes of the urea cycle. Patients with severe defects (often those enzymes early in the urea cycle) usually present in infancy with severe hyperammonemia, vomiting, and encephalopathy, which is rapidly fatal. In patients with milder genetic defects, the course may be milder with vomiting and encephalopathy after protein ingestion or infection. Although defects in argininosuccinic acid synthetase (citrullinemia) and argininosuccinic acid lyase (argininosuccinic acidemia) may cause severe hyperammonemia in infancy, the usual clinical course is chronic with mental retardation. Ornithine transcarbamylase deficiency is X-linked. The rest of the urea cycle disorders are autosomal recessive. Age at onset of symptoms varies with residual enzyme activity, protein intake, growth, and stresses such as infection. Even within a family, males with ornithine transcarbamylase deficiency may differ by decades in the age of symptom onset. Many female carriers of ornithine transcarbamylase deficiency have protein intolerance. Some develop migraine-like symptoms after protein loads, and others develop potentially fatal episodes of vomiting and encephalopathy after protein ingestion, infections, or during labor and delivery. Trichorrhexis nodosa is common in patients with the chronic form of argininosuccinic acidemia.

▶ **Diagnosis**

Blood ammonia should be measured in any acutely ill newborn in whom a cause is not obvious. In urea cycle defects, early hyperammonemia is associated with respiratory alkalosis. Serum citrulline is low or undetectable in carbamoyl phosphate synthetase and ornithine transcarbamylase deficiency, high in argininosuccinic acidemia, and very high in citrullinemia. Large amounts of argininosuccinic acid are found in the urine of patients with argininosuccinic acidemia. Urine orotic acid is increased in infants with ornithine transcarbamylase deficiency. Citrullinemia and argininosuccinic acidemia can be diagnosed in utero by appropriate enzyme assays, but carbamoyl phosphate synthetase and ornithine transcarbamylase deficiency can be diagnosed in utero only by molecular methods.

▶ **Treatment**

During treatment of acute hyperammonemic crisis, protein intake should be stopped, and glucose and lipids should be given to reduce endogenous protein breakdown from catabolism. Arginine should be given intravenously, both because it is an essential amino acid for patients with urea cycle defects and because it increases the excretion of waste nitrogen in patients with citrullinemia and argininosuccinic acidemia. Sodium benzoate, either alone or with sodium phenylacetate, can be given intravenously to treat hyperammonemic coma. Additionally, hemodialysis or hemofiltration is indicated for severe or persistent hyperammonemia, as is usually the case in the newborn. Peritoneal dialysis and double-volume exchange transfusion are insufficiently effective in this setting.

Long-term treatment includes oral administration of arginine (or citrulline), adherence to a low-protein diet, and administration of sodium benzoate and sodium phenylbutyrate (a prodrug of sodium phenylacetate), to increase excretion of nitrogen as hippuric acid and phenylacetylglutamine. Symptomatic heterozygous female carriers of ornithine transcarbamylase deficiency should also receive such treatment. Liver transplantation may be curative and is indicated for patients with severe disorders.

The outcome of urea cycle disorders depends on the genetic severity of the condition (residual activity) and the severity and prompt treatment of hyperammonemic episodes. Many patients with urea cycle defects, no matter what the enzyme defect, develop permanent neurologic and intellectual impairments, with cortical atrophy and ventricular dilation seen on computed tomographic scan. Rapid identification and treatment of the initial hyperammonemic episode improves outcome.

Bachmann C: Outcome and survival of 88 patients with urea cycle disorders: A retrospective evaluation. Eur J Pediatr 2003;162:410 [PMID: 12684900].

Enns GM et al: Survival after treatment with phenylacetate and benzoate for urea cycle disorders. N Engl J Med 2007;356:2282 [PMID: 17538087].

Gropman AL, Batshaw ML: Cognitive outcome in urea cycle disorders. Mol Genet Metab 2004;81(Suppl 1):S58 [PMID: 15050975].

Lee B et al: Considerations in the difficult-to-manage urea cycle disorder patient. Crit Care Clin 2005;21:S19 [PMID: 16227112].

Nassogne MC et al: Urea cycle defects: Management and outcome. J Inherit Metab Dis 2005;28:407 [PMID: 15868473].

Nicolaides P et al: Neurological outcome in patients with ornithine carbamoyltransferase deficiency. Arch Dis Child 2002;86:54 [PMID: 11806886].

Scaglia F, Lee B: Clinical, biochemical, and molecular spectrum of hyperargininemia due to arginase I deficiency. Am J Med Genet C Semin Med Genet 2006;142:113 [PMID: 16602094].

Singh RH et al: Nutritional management of urea cycle disorders. Crit Care Clin 2005;21:S27 [PMID: 16227113].

Smith W et al: Urea cycle disorders: Clinical presentation outside the newborn period. Crit Care Clin 2005;21:S9 [PMID: 16227115].

Summar ML et al: Unmasked adult-onset urea cycle disorders in the critical care setting. Crit Care Clin 2005;21:S1 [PMID: 16227111].

Patient and parent support group web site with useful information for families: http://www.nucdf.org

Urea Cycle Disorders Consortium: http://rarediseasesnetwork.epi.usf.edu/ucdc/about/index.htm

PHENYLKETONURIA & THE HYPERPHENYLALANINEMIAS

ESSENTIALS OF DIAGNOSIS & TYPICAL FEATURES

▶ Mental retardation, hyperactivity, seizures, light complexion, and eczema characterize untreated patients.

▶ Newborn screening for elevated serum phenylalanine identifies most infants.

▶ Disorders of cofactor metabolism also produce elevated serum phenylalanine level.

▶ Early diagnosis and treatment with phenylalanine-restricted diet prevents mental retardation.

Probably the best-known disorder of amino acid metabolism is the classic form of phenylketonuria caused by decreased activity of phenylalanine hydroxylase, the enzyme that converts phenylalanine to tyrosine. In classic phenylketonuria, there is little or no phenylalanine hydroxylase activity. In the less severe hyperphenylalaninemias there may be significant residual activity. Rare variants can be due to deficiency of dihydropteridine reductase or defects in biopterin synthesis.

Phenylketonuria is an autosomal recessive trait, with an incidence in Caucasians of approximately 1:10,000 live births. On a normal neonatal diet, affected patients develop hyperphenylalaninemia. Patients with untreated phenylketonuria exhibit severe mental retardation, hyperactivity, sei-

zures, a light complexion, and eczema. The patient's urine has a "mouse-like" odor.

Success in preventing severe mental retardation in phenylketonuric children by restricting phenylalanine starting in early infancy led to screening programs to detect the disease early. Because the outcome is best when treatment is begun in the first month of life, infants should be screened during the first few days. A second test is necessary when newborn screening is done before 24 hours of age. In such cases the second test should be completed by the third week of life.

▶ Diagnosis & Treatment

The diagnosis of phenylketonuria in a severely mentally retarded older child with typical biochemical and physical characteristics is straightforward, but in the newborn period, especially when there is no family history, the condition must be differentiated from other forms of hyperphenylalaninemia. This is usually done by determining serum phenylalanine and tyrosine levels on a normal diet and by examining pterins in blood and urine.

Prenatal diagnosis of phenylketonuria is possible using molecular methods. Molecular approaches are replacing serum measurements of phenylalanine and tyrosine to determine carrier status. Prenatal diagnosis of defects in pterin metabolism can often be made.

A. Classic Phenylketonuria

Findings include persistently elevated serum levels of phenylalanine (> 20 mg/dL or 1200 μM on a regular diet), normal or low serum levels of tyrosine, and normal pterins. Poor phenylalanine tolerance persists throughout life. Restriction of dietary phenylalanine intake is indicated, and a favorable outcome is the rule.

Treatment of classic phenylketonuria is to limit dietary phenylalanine intake to amounts that permit normal growth and development. Dietary goals usually aim for a phenylalanine level less than 360 μM (6 mg/dL). Metabolic formulas deficient in phenylalanine are available but must be supplemented with normal milk and other foods to supply enough phenylalanine to permit normal growth and development. Serum phenylalanine concentrations must be monitored frequently while ensuring that growth, development, and nutrition are adequate. This monitoring is best done in experienced clinics. Although dietary treatment is most effective when initiated during the first months of life, it may also be of benefit in reversing behaviors such as hyperactivity, irritability, and distractibility when started later in life.

Phenylalanine restriction should continue throughout life, both because of subtle changes in intellect and behavior in persons receiving treatment early who later stop the diet, and because of the risk of late development of potentially irreversible neurologic damage after stopping the diet. Counseling should be given during adolescence, and women's diets should be monitored closely prior to conception and throughout pregnancy.

Children with classic phenylketonuria who receive treatment promptly after birth and achieve phenylalanine and tyrosine homeostasis will develop well physically and can be expected to have normal or near-normal intellectual development.

Treatment with R-tetrahydrobiopterin results in improved phenylalanine tolerance in up to 60% of patients with a deficiency in phenylalanine hydroxylase, with best results seen in patients with hyperphenylalaninemia. Provision of high doses of large neutral amino acids results in a moderate reduction in phenylalanine and is used as an adjunctive treatment in some adults with phenylketonuria.

B. Persistent Hyperphenylalaninemia

In infants receiving a normal protein intake, serum phenylalanine levels are usually 240–1200 μM (4–20 mg/dL), and pterins are normal. Phenylalanine restriction is indicated if phenylalanine levels consistently exceed 600 μM (10 mg/dL).

C. Transient Hyperphenylalaninemia

Serum phenylalanine levels are elevated early but progressively decline toward normal. Dietary restriction is only temporary, if required at all.

D. Dihydropteridine Reductase Deficiency

Serum phenylalanine levels vary. The pattern of pterin metabolites is abnormal. Seizures and psychomotor regression occur even with diet therapy, probably because the enzyme defect also causes neuronal deficiency of serotonin and dopamine. These deficiencies require treatment with levodopa, carbidopa, 5-hydroxytryptophan, and folinic acid.

E. Defects in Biopterin Biosynthesis

Serum phenylalanine levels vary. Total pterins are low, and their pattern may suggest the specific defect, which can be at one of several steps in the biosynthetic pathway. Clinical findings include myoclonus, tetraplegia, dystonia, oculogyric crises, and other movement disorders. Treatment is the same as for dihydropteridine reductase deficiency. Tetrahydrobiopterin may be added.

F. Tyrosinemia of the Newborn

Serum phenylalanine levels are lower than those associated with phenylketonuria and are accompanied by marked hypertyrosinemia. Tyrosinemia of the newborn usually occurs in premature infants and is due to immaturity of 4-hydroxyphenylpyruvic acid oxidase. The condition resolves spontaneously within 3 months, almost always without sequelae.

G. Maternal Phenylketonuria

Offspring of phenylketonuric mothers may have transient hyperphenylalaninemia at birth. Elevated maternal phenylalanine causes mental retardation, microcephaly, growth retardation, and often congenital heart disease or other malformations in the offspring. The risk to the fetus is lessened considerably by maternal phenylalanine restriction with maintenance of phenylalanine levels below 360 μM (6 mg/dL) throughout pregnancy and optimally started before conception.

Channon S et al: Effects of dietary management of phenylketonuria on long-term cognitive outcome. Arch Dis Child 2007;92:213 [PMID: 17068073].

Fiege B, Blau N: Assessment of tetrahydrobiopterin (BH4) responsiveness in phenylketonuria. J Pediatr 2007;150:627 [PMID: 17517248].

Fiege B et al: Extended tetrahydrobiopterin loading test in the diagnosis of cofactor-responsive phenylketonuria: A pilot study. Mol Genet Metab 2005;86(Suppl 1):S91 [PMID: 16290003].

Gambol PJ: Maternal phenylketonuria syndrome and case management implications. J Pediatr Nurs 207;22:129 [PMID: 17382850].

Gassio R et al: Cognitive functions in classic phenylketonuria and mild hyperphenylalaninaemia: Experience in a paediatric population. Dev Med Child Neurol 2005;47:443 [PMID: 15991863].

Giovannini M et al: Phenylketonuria: Dietary and therapeutic challenges. J Inherit Metab Dis 2007;30:145 [PMID: 17347911].

Koch R: Maternal phenylketonuria: The importance of early control during pregnancy. Arch Dis Child 2005;90:114 [PMID: 15665159].

Lee PJ et al: Maternal phenylketonuria: Report from the United Kingdom Registry 1978–97. Arch Dis Child 2005;90:143 [PMID: 15665165].

Leuzzi V et al: The pathogenesis of the white matter abnormalities in phenylketonuria. A multimodal 3.0 tesla MRI and magnetic resonance spectroscopy (1H MRS) study. J Inherit Metab Dis 2007;30:209 [PMID: 17245558].

Matalon R et al: Double blind placebo control trial of large neutral amino acids in treatment of PKU: Effect on blood phenylalanine. J Inherit Metab Dis 2007;30:153 [PMID: 17334706].

Matalon R et al: Large neutral amino acids in the treatment of phenylketonuria (PKU). J Inherit Metab Dis 2006;29:732 [PMID: 16988900].

Santos LL et al: The time has come: A new scene for PKU treatment. Genet Mol Res 2006;5:33 [PMID: 16755495].

Schindeler S et al: The effects of large neutral amino acid supplements in PKU: An MRS and neuropsychological study. Mol Genet Metab 2007;91:48 [PMID: 17368065].

Patient and parent support group web site with useful information for families: http://www.pkunews.org and www.pkunetwork.org

HEREDITARY TYROSINEMIA

Type 1 hereditary tyrosinemia is caused by deficiency of fumarylacetoacetase. It presents with acute or progressive hepatic parenchymal damage, renal tubular dysfunction with generalized aminoaciduria, hypophosphatemic rickets, or neuropathic crises. Tyrosine and methionine are increased in blood and tyrosine metabolites and δ-aminolevulinic acid in urine. The key diagnostic metabolite is elevated succinylacetone in urine. Liver failure may be rapidly fatal in infancy or somewhat more chronic, with liver cell carcinoma almost invariable in long-term survivors. The condition is autosomal recessive and is especially common in Scandinavia and in the Chicoutimi–Lac St. Jean region of Quebec. Prenatal diagnosis is possible. Tyrosinemia type II presents with corneal ulcers and keratotic lesions on palms and soles and very high serum tyrosine levels (> 600 μM).

▶ Diagnosis

Similar clinical and biochemical findings may occur in other liver diseases such as galactosemia and hereditary fructose intolerance. Increased succinylacetone occurs only in fumarylacetoacetase deficiency, and is diagnostic. Enzyme assay in liver biopsy or mutation analysis can provide further diagnostic confirmation. Diagnostic confirmation of tyrosinemia type II is by molecular methods.

▶ Treatment

A diet low in phenylalanine and tyrosine is indicated and can ameliorate liver disease, but does not prevent carcinoma development. Pharmacologic therapy to inhibit 4-hydroxyphenylpyruvate dehydrogenase using 2-(2-nitro-4-trifluoromethylbenzoyl)-1,3-cyclohexanedione (NTBC) decreases the production of toxic metabolites, maleylacetoacetate and fumarylacetoacetate. It improves the liver disease and renal disease, prevents acute neuronopathic attacks, and greatly reduces the risk of hepatocellular carcinoma. Liver transplantation is effective therapy for these children. Tyrosinemia type II symptoms respond to treatment with dietary tyrosine restriction.

Ashorn M et al: Current strategies for the treatment of hereditary tyrosinemia type 1. Paediatr Drugs 2006;8:47 [PMID: 16494511].

Held PK: Disorders of tyrosine catabolism. Mol Genet Metab 2006;88:103 [PMID: 16773741].

Magera MJ et al: Quantitative determination of succinylacetone in dried blood spots for newborn screening of tyrosinemia type I. Mol Genet Metab 2006;88:16 [PMID: 16448836].

McKiernan PJ: Nitisinone in the treatment of hereditary tyrosinaemia type 1. Drugs 2006;66:743 [PMID: 16706549].

Scott CR: The genetic tyrosinemias. Am J Med Genet C Semin Med Genet 2006;142:121 [PMID: 16602095].

Viglizzo GM et al: Richner-Hanhart syndrome (tyrosinemia II): Early diagnosis of an incomplete presentation with unusual findings. Pediatr Dermatol 2006;23:259 [PMID: 16780475].

MAPLE SYRUP URINE DISEASE (BRANCHED-CHAIN KETOACIDURIA)

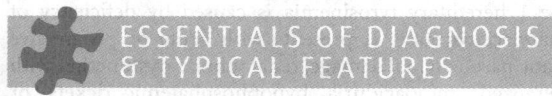

ESSENTIALS OF DIAGNOSIS & TYPICAL FEATURES

▶ Typical presentation is infantile encephalopathy.

Maple syrup urine disease is due to deficiency of the enzyme catalyzing oxidative decarboxylation of the branched-chain keto acid derivatives of leucine, isoleucine, and valine. Accumulated keto acids of leucine and isoleucine cause the characteristic odor. Only leucine and its corresponding keto acid have been implicated in causing central nervous system dysfunction. Many variants of this disorder have been described, including mild, intermittent, and thiamin-dependent forms. All are autosomal recessive traits.

Patients with classic maple syrup urine disease are normal at birth but after about 1 week develop feeding difficulties, coma, and seizures. Unless diagnosis is made and dietary restriction of branched-chain amino acids is begun, most will die in the first month of life. Nearly normal growth and development may be achieved if treatment is begun before about age 10 days.

▶ Diagnosis

Amino acid analysis shows marked elevations of branched-chain amino acids including alloisoleucine in serum and urine. Alloisoleucine, a transamination product of the keto acid of isoleucine, is almost pathognomonic. Urine organic acids demonstrate the characteristic keto acids. The magnitude and consistency of amino acid and organic acid changes are altered in mild and intermittent forms of the disease. Prenatal diagnosis is possible.

▶ Treatment

Metabolic formulas deficient in branched-chain amino acids are available but must be supplemented with normal milk and other foods to supply enough branched-chain amino acids to permit normal growth and development. Serum levels of branched-chain amino acids must be monitored frequently in the first months of life to deal with changing protein requirements. Acute episodes must be aggressively treated to prevent catabolism and negative nitrogen balance.

Heldt K et al: Diagnosis of MSUD by newborn screening allows early intervention without extraneous detoxification. Mol Genet Metab 2005;84:313 [PMID: 15781191].

Hoffmann B et al: Impact of longitudinal plasma leucine levels on the intellectual outcome in patients with classic MSUD. Pediatr Res 2006;59:17 [PMID: 16326996].

Le Roux C et al: Neuropsychometric outcome predictors for adults with maple syrup urine disease. J Inherit Metab Dis 2006;29:201 [PMID: 16601892].

Simon E et al: Maple syrup urine disease: Favourable effect of early diagnosis by newborn screening on the neonatal course of the disease. J Inherit Metab Dis 2006;29:532 [PMID: 16817013].

Simon E et al: Social outcome in adults with maple syrup urine disease (MSUD). J Inherit Metab Dis 2007;30:264 [PMID: 17310329].

Simon E et al: Variant maple syrup urine disease (MSUD)—the entire spectrum. J Inherit Metab Dis 2006;29:716 [PMID: 17063375].

Strauss KA et al: Elective liver transplantation for the treatment of classical maple syrup urine disease. Am J Transplant 2006;6:557 [PMID: 16468966].

HOMOCYSTINURIA

ESSENTIALS OF DIAGNOSIS & TYPICAL FEATURES

▶ Consider in a child of any age with a marfanoid habitus, dislocated lenses, or thrombosis.

▶ Identification through newborn screening is essential to ensure early treatment and a normal outcome.

Homocystinuria is most often due to deficiency of cystathionine β-synthase (CBS), but may also be due to deficiency of methylenetetrahydrofolate reductase (MTHR) or to defects in the biosynthesis of methyl-B_{12}, the coenzyme for N^5-methyltetrahydrofolate methionine S-methyltransferase (methionine synthase). All known inherited forms of homocystinuria are transmitted as autosomal recessive traits and can be diagnosed in the fetus.

About 50% of patients with untreated CBS deficiency are mentally retarded, and most have arachnodactyly, osteoporosis, and a tendency to develop dislocated lenses and thromboembolic phenomena. Mild variants of CBS deficiency present with thromboembolic events. Milder elevations of homocysteine are increasingly recognized as a factor in the etiology of vascular disease leading to myocardial infarction and stroke. These mild elevations are often caused by mutations leading to heat-sensitive defects in MTHR. Patients with remethylation defects usually exhibit failure to thrive and a variety of neurologic symptoms, including brain atrophy, microcephaly, and seizures in infancy and early childhood.

▶ Diagnosis

Diagnosis is made by demonstrating homocystinuria in a patient who is not severely deficient in vitamin B_{12}. Serum methionine levels are usually high in patients with CBS deficiency and often low in patients with remethylation defects. When the remethylation defect is due to deficiency of methyl-B_{12}, megaloblastic anemia or hemolytic uremic syndrome may be present, and an associated deficiency of adenosyl-B_{12} may cause methylmalonic aciduria. Studies of cultured fibroblasts may be necessary to make a specific diagnosis.

▶ Treatment

About 50% of patients with CBS deficiency respond to large oral doses of pyridoxine. Early treatment of pyridoxine nonresponders is by dietary methionine restriction. Oral administration of betaine increases methylation of homocysteine to methionine in patients with CBS deficiency or with remethylation defects and improves neurologic function. Early treatment prevents mental retardation, lens dislocation, and thromboembolic manifestations, which justifies the screening of newborn infants. Large doses of vitamin B_{12} (eg, 1–5 mg hydroxocobalamin administered daily intramus-cularly or subcutaneously) are indicated in some patients with defects in cobalamin metabolism.

Finkelstein JD: Inborn errors of sulfur-containing amino acid metabolism. J Nutr 2006;136:1750S [PMID: 16702350].

Lawson-Yuen A, Levy HL: The use of betaine in the treatment of elevated homocysteine. Mol Genet Metab 2006;88:201 [PMID: 16545978].

NONKETOTIC HYPERGLYCINEMIA

ESSENTIALS OF DIAGNOSIS & TYPICAL FEATURES

▶ Severely affected newborns have apnea, hypotonia, lethargy, myoclonic seizures, and hiccups.

▶ Mental and motor retardation in most patients.

▶ Children may present with developmental delay, mild chorea, and seizures.

▶ EEG shows burst suppression.

▶ Cerebrospinal fluid (CSF) glycine is elevated.

Inherited deficiency of various subunits of the glycine cleavage enzyme causes nonketotic hyperglycinemia. Glycine accumulation in the brain disturbs neurotransmission of the glycinergic receptors and the N-methyl-D-aspartate receptor. In its most severe form, also termed glycine encephalopathy, the condition presents in the newborn as hypotonia, lethargy proceeding to coma, myoclonic seizures, and hiccups, with a burst suppression pattern on electroencephalography. Apnea spells may develop requiring ventilator assistance in the first 2 weeks, followed by spontaneous recovery. The majority of patients develop severe mental retardation and seizures. Some patients have agenesis of the corpus callosum or posterior fossa malformations. Some patients present with seizures, developmental delay, and mild chorea later in infancy or in childhood. All forms of the condition are autosomal recessive.

▶ Diagnosis

Nonketotic hyperglycinemia should be suspected in any neonate or infant with seizures and is confirmed by demonstrating a large increase in glycine in nonbloody CSF, with the ratio of CSF glycine to serum glycine being abnormally high. CSF glycine should be measured in any infant with neonatal apnea and a burst suppression pattern on electroencephalography. Enzyme analysis in a liver sample can confirm the diagnosis and can distinguish between defects in the T-protein or the P- and H-proteins. Molecular analysis is diagnostic in many cases. Prenatal diagnosis is possible only by assaying the enzyme in uncultured chorionic villus samples or by molecular analysis if both mutations are known in advance.

Treatment

In patients with mild disease, treatment with sodium benzoate (to normalize serum glycine levels) and dextromethorphan or ketamine (to block N-methyl-D-aspartate receptors) controls seizures and improves outcome. Treatment of severely affected patients is generally unsuccessful. High-dose benzoate therapy can aid in seizure control but does not prevent severe mental retardation.

Applegarth DA, Toone JR: Glycine encephalopathy (nonketotic hyperglycinaemia): Review and update. J Inherit Metab Dis 2004;27:417 [PMID: 15272469].

Chien YH et al: Poor outcome for neonatal-type nonketotic hyperglycinemia treated with high-dose sodium benzoate and dextromethorphan. J Child Neurol 2004;19:39 [PMID: 15032382].

Dinopoulos A et al: Atypical variants of nonketotic hyperglycinemia. Mol Genet Metab 2005;86:61 [PMID: 16157495].

Hoover-Fong JE et al: Natural history of nonketotic hyperglycinemia in 65 patients. Neurology 2004;63:1847 [PMID: 15557500].

Van Hove JLK et al: Benzoate treatment and the glycine index in nonketotic hyperglycinaemia. J Inherit Metab Dis 2005;28:651 [PMID: 16151895].

ORGANIC ACIDEMIAS

ESSENTIALS OF DIAGNOSIS & TYPICAL FEATURES

▶ Consider in any child presenting with metabolic acidosis and ketosis in early infancy.

Organic acidemias are disorders of amino and fatty acid metabolism in which nonamino organic acids accumulate in serum and urine. These conditions are usually diagnosed by examining organic acids in urine, a complex procedure that requires considerable interpretive expertise and is usually performed only in specialized laboratories. Table 34–4 lists the clinical features of organic acidemias, together with the urine organic acid patterns typical of each. Additional details about some of the more important organic acidemias are provided in the sections that follow.

PROPIONIC & METHYLMALONIC ACIDEMIA (KETOTIC HYPERGLYCINEMIAS)

Idiopathic hyperglycinemia was first reported in 1961 as a syndrome of mental retardation and episodic ketoacidosis, neutropenia, thrombocytopenia, osteoporosis, and hyperglycinemia induced by protein intake or infection. It was then renamed ketotic hyperglycinemia to distinguish it from nonketotic hyperglycinemia, described in the preceding section. It is now known that the syndrome is almost always due to propionic or methylmalonic acidemia.

The oxidation of threonine, valine, methionine, and isoleucine results in propionyl-CoA, which propionyl-CoA carboxylase converts into L-methylmalonyl-CoA, which is metabolized through methylmalonyl-CoA mutase to succinyl-CoA. Gut bacteria and the breakdown of odd-chain-length fatty acids also substantially contribute to propionyl-CoA production. Propionic acidemia is due to a defect in the biotin-containing enzyme propionyl-CoA carboxylase, and methylmalonic acidemia is due to a defect in methylmalonyl-CoA mutase. In most cases the latter is due to a defect in the mutase apoenzyme, but in others it is due to a defect in the biosynthesis of its adenosyl-B_{12} coenzyme. In some of these defects, only the synthesis of adenosyl-B_{12} is blocked; in others, the synthesis of methyl-B_{12} is also blocked.

Clinical symptoms in propionic and methylmalonic acidemia vary according to the location and severity of the enzyme block. Children with severe blocks present with acute, life-threatening metabolic acidosis, hyperammonemia, and bone marrow depression early in infancy or with metabolic acidosis, vomiting, and failure to thrive during the first few months of life. Most patients with severe disease have mild or moderate mental retardation. Late complications include pancreatitis, cardiomyopathy, and basal ganglia stroke, and in methylmalonic aciduria, interstitial nephritis.

All known forms of propionic and methylmalonic acidemia are transmitted as autosomal recessive traits and can be diagnosed in utero.

Diagnosis

Laboratory findings consist of increases in urinary organic acids derived from propionyl-CoA or methylmalonic acid (see Table 34–4). Hyperglycinemia can be present. In some forms of abnormal B_{12} metabolism homocysteine can be elevated.

Treatment

Patients with enzyme blocks in B_{12} metabolism usually respond to massive doses of vitamin B_{12} given intramuscularly. Vitamin B_{12} nonresponsive methylmalonic acidemia and propionic acidemia require amino acid restriction, strict prevention of catabolism, and carnitine supplementation to enhance propionylcarnitine excretion. Intermittent metronidazole can help reduce the propionate load from the gut. In the acute setting, hemodialysis or hemofiltration may be needed. Combined liver-renal transplantation is an option for patients with renal insufficiency, and liver transplantation has shown promise for patients with life-threatening cardiomyopathy.

Barshes NR et al: Evaluation and management of patients with propionic acidemia undergoing liver transplantation: A comprehensive review. Pediatr Transplant 2006;10:773 [PMID: 17032422].

Deodato F et al: Methylmalonic and propionic aciduria. Am J Med Genet C Semin Med Genet 2006;142:104 [PMID: 16602092].

Dionisi-Vici C et al: 'Classical' organic acidurias, propionic aciduria, methylmalonic aciduria and isovaleric aciduria: Long-term outcome and effects of expanded newborn screening using tandem mass spectrometry. J Inherit Metab Dis 2006;29:383 [PMID: 16763906].

Table 34–4. Clinical and laboratory features of organic acidemias.

Disorder	Enzyme Defect	Clinical and Laboratory Features
Isovaleric acidemia	Isovaleryl-CoA dehydrogenase	Acidosis and odor of sweaty feet in infancy, or growth retardation and episodes of vomiting, lethargy, and acidosis. Isovalerylglycine always present in urine, with 3-hydroxyisovaleric acid during acute episodes.
3-Methylcrotonyl-CoA carboxylase deficiency	3-Methylcrotonyl-CoA carboxylase	Acidosis and feeding problems in infancy, or Reye-like episodes in older child. 3-Methylcrotonylglycine in urine, usually with 3-hydroxyisovaleric acid.
Combined carboxylase deficiency	Holocarboxylase synthetase	Hypotonia and lactic acidosis in infancy. 3-Hydroxyisovaleric acid in urine, often with small amounts of 3-hydroxypropionic and methylcitric acids. Often biotin-responsive.
Biotinidase deficiency	Biotinidase	Alopecia, seborrheic rash, and ataxia in infancy or childhood. Urine organic acids as above. Always biotin-responsive.
3-Hydroxy-3-methylglutaric acidemia	3-Hydroxy-3-methylglutaryl-CoA lyase	Hypoglycemia and acidosis in infancy; Reye-like episodes with nonketotic hypoglycemia or leukodystrophy in older children. 3-Hydroxy-3-methylglutaric, 3-methylglutaconic, and 3-hydroxyisovaleric acids in urine.
3-Ketothiolase deficiency	3-Ketothiolase	Ketotic hyperglycinemia syndrome in infancy, or episodes of vomiting, severe metabolic acidosis (hyperketosis), and encephalopathy. 2-Methyl-3-hydroxybutyric and 2-methylacetoacetic acids and tiglylglycine in urine, especially after isoleucine load.
Propionic acidemia	Propionyl-CoA carboxylase	Hyperammonemia and metabolic acidosis in infancy; ketotic hyperglycinemia syndrome later. 3-Hydroxypropionic and methylcitric acids in urine, with 3-hydroxy- and 3-ketovaleric acids during ketotic episodes.
Methylmalonic acidemia	Methylmalonyl-CoA mutase	Clinical features same as in propionic acidemia. Methylmalonic acid in urine, often with 3-hydroxypropionic and methylcitric acids.
	Defects in B_{12} biosynthesis	Clinical features same as above when only adenosyl-B_{12} synthesis is decreased; early neurologic features prominent when accompanied by decreased synthesis of methyl-B_{12}. In latter instance, hypomethioninemia and homocystinuria accompany methylmalonic aciduria.
Pyroglutamic acidemia	Glutathione synthetase	Acidosis and hemolytic anemia in infancy; chronic acidosis later. Pyroglutamic acid in urine.
Glutaric acidemia type I	Glutaryl-CoA dehydrogenase	Progressive extrapyramidal movement disorder in childhood, with episodes of acidosis, vomiting, and encephalopathy. Glutaric acid and 3-hydroxyglutaric acid in serum and urine.
Glutaric acidemia type II	Electron transfer flavoprotein (ETF) ETF:ubiquinone oxidoreductase (ETF dehydrogenase)	Hypoglycemia, acidosis, hyperammonemia, and odor of sweaty feet in infancy, often with polycystic and dysplastic kidneys. Later onset may be with episodes of hypoketotic hypoglycemia, liver dysfunction, or slowly progressive skeletal myopathy. Glutaric, ethylmalonic, 3-hydroxyisovaleric, isovalerylglycine, and 2-hydroxyglutaric acids in urine, often with sarcosine in serum and urine.
4-Hydroxybutyric acidemia	Succinic semialdehyde dehydrogenase	Seizures and developmental retardation. 4-Hydroxybutyric acid in urine.

CoA, coenzyme A.

Kanaumi T et al: Neuropathology of methylmalonic acidemia in a child. Pediatr Neurol 2006;34:156 [PMID: 16458832].

Kasahara M et al: Current role of liver transplantation for methylmalonic acidemia: A review of the literature. Pediatr Transplant 2006;10:943 [PMID: 17096763].

Morel CF et al: Combined methylmalonic aciduria and homocystinuria (cblC): Phenotype-genotype correlations and ethnic-specific observations. Mol Genet Metab 2006;88:315 [PMID: 16714133].

Tanpaiboon P: Methylmalonic acidemia (MMA). Mol Genet Metab 2005;85:2 [PMID: 15959932].

Touati G et al: Methylmalonic and propionic acidurias: Management without or with a few supplements of specific amino acid mixture. J Inherit Metab Dis 2006;29:288 [PMID: 16763890].

Yang Y et al: Clinical and biochemical studies on Chinese patients with methylmalonic aciduria. J Child Neurol 2006;21:1020 [PMID: 17156691].

Yannicelli S: Nutrition therapy of organic acidaemias with amino acid-based formulas: Emphasis on methylmalonic and propionic acidaemia. J Inherit Metab Dis 2006;29:281 [PMID: 16763889]. Patient and parent support group web site with useful information for families: http://www.oaanews.org

ISOVALERIC ACIDEMIA

Isovaleric acidemia, caused by deficiency of isovaleryl-CoA dehydrogenase in the leucine oxidative pathway, was the first organic acidemia to be described in humans. Patients with this disorder usually present with poor feeding, metabolic acidosis, seizures, and an odor of sweaty feet during the first few days of life, with coma and death occurring if the condition is not recognized and treated. Other patients have a more chronic course, with episodes of vomiting and lethargy, hair loss, and pancreatitis precipitated by intercurrent infections or increased protein intake. The condition is autosomal recessive and can be diagnosed in utero.

▶ Diagnosis

Isovalerylglycine is consistently detected in the urine by organic acid chromatography.

▶ Treatment

Providing a low-protein diet or a diet low in leucine is effective. Conjugation with either glycine or carnitine helps in maintaining metabolic stability. Outcome is usually good.

Vockley J, Ensenauer R: Isovaleric acidemia: New aspects of genetic and phenotypic heterogeneity. Am J Med Genet C Semin Med Genet 2006;142:95 [PMID: 16602101].

CARBOXYLASE DEFICIENCY

Isolated pyruvate carboxylase deficiency presents with lactic acidosis and hyperammonemia in early infancy. Even if biochemically stabilized, the neurologic outcome is dismal. Isolated 3-methylcrotonyl-CoA carboxylase deficiency is frequently recognized on newborn screening using tandem mass spectrometric analysis of acylcarnitines. It is usually a benign condition that only rarely causes symptoms of acidosis and neurologic depression. All carboxylases require biotin as a cofactor. Holocarboxylase synthetase and biotinidase are two enzymes of biotin metabolism in mammals. Holocarboxylase synthetase covalently binds biotin to the apocarboxylases for pyruvate, 3-methylcrotonyl-CoA, and propionyl-CoA; and biotinidase releases biotin from these proteins and from proteins in the diet. Recessively inherited deficiency of either enzyme causes deficiency of all three carboxylases (ie, multiple carboxylase deficiency). Patients with holocarboxylase synthetase deficiency usually present as neonates with hypotonia, skin problems, and massive acidosis. Those with biotinidase deficiency more often present somewhat later with a syndrome of ataxia, seizures, sebor-

rhea, and alopecia. Newborn screening for the condition is justified because many patients with biotinidase deficiency do not have typical symptoms, but do develop preventable neurologic sequelae.

▶ Diagnosis

This diagnosis should be considered in patients with typical symptoms or in those with primary lactic acidosis. Urine organic acids are usually but not always abnormal (see Table 34–4). Diagnosis is made by enzyme assay. Biotinidase can be assayed in serum, and holocarboxylase synthetase in leukocytes or fibroblasts.

▶ Treatment

Oral administration of biotin in large doses often reverses the organic aciduria within days and the clinical symptoms within days to weeks. Hearing loss can occur in patients with biotinidase deficiency despite treatment.

Grunewald S et al: Biotinidase deficiency: A treatable leukoencephalopathy. Neuropediatrics 2004;35:211 [PMID: 15328559].
Sivri HS et al: Hearing loss in biotinidase deficiency: Genotype-phenotype correlation. J Pediatr 2007;150:439 [PMID: 17382128].
Weber P et al: Outcome in patients with profound biotinidase deficiency: Relevance of newborn screening. Dev Med Child Neurol 2004;46:481 [PMID: 15230462].
Wolf B: Biotinidase deficiency: New directions and practical concerns. Curr Treat Options Neurol 2003;5:321 [PMID: 12791199].

GLUTARIC ACIDEMIA TYPE I

ESSENTIALS OF DIAGNOSIS & TYPICAL FEATURES

▶ Suspect in children with acute basal ganglia necrosis and macrocrania with subdural bleeds.

▶ Presymptomatic diagnosis by newborn screening and treatment reduces the incidence of acute encephalopathic crises.

Glutaric acidemia type I is due to deficiency of glutaryl-CoA dehydrogenase. Patients have frontotemporal atrophy with enlarged sylvian fissures and macrocephaly. Sudden or chronic neurodegeneration secondary to neuronal degeneration in the caudate and putamen causes a progressive extrapyramidal movement disorder in childhood with dystonia and athetosis. Children with glutaric acidemia type I may present with retinal hemorrhages and intracranial bleeding and may thus be considered victims of child abuse. Severely debilitated children often die in the first decade, but several reported patients have had only mild neurologic abnormalities. Most patients develop symptoms in the first 6 years of life. The condition is autosomal recessive and prenatal diagnosis is possible.

Diagnosis

Glutaric acidemia type I should be suspected in patients with acute or progressive dystonia in the first 6 years of life. Magnetic resonance imaging of the brain is highly suggestive. The diagnosis is supported by finding glutaric, 3-hydroxyglutaric acid, and glutarylcarnitine in urine or serum. Demonstration of deficiency of glutaryl-CoA dehydrogenase in fibroblasts, leukocytes, or a mutation in the *GCDH* gene confirms the diagnosis. Prenatal diagnosis is by enzyme assay, quantitative metabolite analysis in amniotic fluid, or mutation analysis.

Treatment

Aggressive management of catabolism during intercurrent illness and supplementation with large amounts of carnitine may prevent degeneration of the basal ganglia. Dietary lysine and tryptophan are frequently restricted in young patients. Neurologic symptoms, once present, do not resolve. Symptomatic treatment of severe dystonia is important for affected patients.

Funk CB et al: Neuropathological, biochemical and molecular findings in a glutaric acidemia type 1 cohort. Brain 2005;128(Pt 4):711 [PMID: 15689364].

Gordon N: Glutaric aciduria types I and II. Brain Dev 2006;28:136 [PMID: 16368216].

Hedlund GL et al: Glutaric acidemia type 1. Am J Med Genet C Semin Med Genet 2006;142:86 [PMID: 16602100].

Kölker S et al: Decline of acute encephalopathic crises in children with glutaryl-CoA dehydrogenase deficiency identified by newborn screening in Germany. Pediatr Res 2007;62:357 [PMID:17622945].

Kölker S et al: Guideline for the diagnosis and management of glutaryl-CoA dehydrogenase deficiency (glutaric aciduria type I). J Inherit Metab Dis 2007;30:5 [PMID: 17203377].

Kölker S et al: Natural history, outcome, and treatment efficacy in children and adults with glutaryl-CoA dehydrogenase deficiency. Pediatr Res 2006;59:840 [PMID: 16641220].

Lindner M et al: Neonatal screening for glutaric aciduria type I: Strategies to proceed. J Inherit Metab Dis 2006;29:378 [PMID: 16763905].

DISORDERS OF FATTY ACID OXIDATION & CARNITINE

FATTY ACID OXIDATION DISORDERS

ESSENTIALS OF DIAGNOSIS & TYPICAL FEATURES

▶ Obtain an acylcarnitine profile for any child with hypoglycemia to evaluate for a fatty acid oxidation defect.

▶ Early diagnosis and treatment can prevent cardiomyopathy in affected children.

Deficiencies of very-long-chain and medium-chain acyl-CoA dehydrogenase (VLCAD, MCAD) and long-chain 3-hydroxyacyl-CoA dehydrogenase (LCHAD), three enzymes of fatty acid β-oxidation, usually cause Reye-like episodes of hypoketotic hypoglycemia, mild hyperammonemia, hepatomegaly, and encephalopathy. Sudden death in infancy is a less common presentation. The long-chain defects, which also include carnitine palmitoyltransferase deficiency I and II and carnitine-acylcarnitine translocase deficiency, often also cause skeletal myopathy with hypotonia and cardiomyopathy, and ventricular arrhythmias. Less severe defects present with recurrent episodes of rhabdomyolysis. LCHAD deficiency may produce progressive liver cirrhosis, peripheral neuropathy, and retinitis pigmentosa. Mothers of affected infants can have acute fatty liver of pregnancy or HELLP syndrome (hemolysis, elevated liver enzymes, and low platelets). Mild carnitine palmitoyltransferase I deficiency may cause renal tubular acidosis and hypertriglyceridemia. MCAD deficiency is common, occurring in perhaps 1:9000 live births. Reye-like episodes may be fatal or cause residual neurologic damage. Episodes tend to become less frequent and severe with time. After the diagnosis is made and treatment instituted, morbidity decreases and mortality is avoided in MCAD deficiency.

Short-chain acyl-CoA dehydrogenase (SCAD) deficiency is characterized by the presence of ethylmalonic acid in the urine, and although some patients have symptoms similar to those in MCAD deficiency, many are asymptomatic. Glutaric acidemia type II results from defects in the transfer of electrons from fatty acid oxidation and some amino acid oxidation into the respiratory chain. Some patients with glutaric acidemia type II have a clinical presentation resembling MCAD deficiency. Patients with a severe neonatal presentation also have renal cystic disease and dysmorphic features. The least affected patients can present with late-onset myopathy and be riboflavin responsive. Some develop cardiomyopathy or leukodystrophy. These conditions are autosomal recessive.

Diagnosis

The hypoglycemic presentation of the Reye episode is associated with a lack of an appropriate ketone response to fasting. Patients with MCAD deficiency may excrete hexanoylglycine, suberylglycine, and phenylpropionylglycine in the urine organic acids. Urine and blood findings in glutaric acidemia type II and SCAD deficiency are often diagnostic. The finding of normal urine organic acids does not exclude these conditions, because excretion of dicarboxylic acids and other products of microsomal and peroxisomal oxidation of fatty acids can be intermittent.

The analysis of acylcarnitine esters is currently the first-line diagnostic test and shows diagnostic metabolites regardless of clinical status. MCAD deficiency is characterized by elevated octanoylcarnitine. A similar typical pattern can be recognized in deficiencies of VLCAD, LCHAD, carnitine acylcarnitine translocase, and severe carnitine palmitoyl-transferase. This is used in neonatal screening. Further confirmation can be obtained from analysis of fatty acid oxidation in fibroblasts. A common mutation in MCAD and in LCHAD deficiency is useful in confirming the diagnosis. Molecular sequencing is available for each defect, and enzyme assays for each enzyme can be done in fibroblasts in specialized laboratories.

▶ **Treatment**

Acutely, management involves prevention of hypoglycemia by avoiding prolonged fasting (> 8–12 hours). Chronic therapy includes providing carbohydrate snacks before bedtime and vigorous treatment of fasting associated with intercurrent infections. Because fatty acid oxidation can be compromised by associated carnitine deficiency, patients with MCAD deficiency usually receive oral carnitine. Carnitine use in VLCAD and LCHAD deficiency is less clear. Restriction of dietary long-chain fats is controversial in MCAD deficiency, but is required for VLCAD and LCHAD deficiencies. Medium-chain triglycerides are contraindicated in MCAD deficiency but are an essential energy source for patients with VLCAD and LCHAD deficiencies or carnitine acylcarnitine translocase deficiency. Riboflavin may be beneficial in some patients with glutaric acidemia type II. Outcome in MCAD deficiency is excellent but is more guarded in patients with the other disorders.

Alonso EM: Acute liver failure in children: The role of defects in fatty acid oxidation. Hepatology 2005;41:696 [PMID: 15789368].

Angelini C et al: Task force guidelines handbook: EFNS guidelines on diagnosis and management of fatty acid mitochondrial disorders. Eur J Neurol 2006;13:923 [PMID: 16930355].

Derks TG et al: The natural history of medium-chain acyl CoA dehydrogenase deficiency in the Netherlands: Clinical presentation and outcome. J Pediatr 2006;148:665 [PMID: 16737882].

Derks TG et al: Safe and unsafe duration of fasting for children with MCAD deficiency. Eur J Pediatr 2007;166:5 [PMID: 16788829].

Jamerson PA: The association between acute fatty liver of pregnancy and fatty acid oxidation disorders. J Obstet Gynecol Neonatal Nurs 2005;34:87 [PMID: 15673650].

Mayell SJ et al: Late presentation of medium-chain acyl-CoA dehydrogenase deficiency. J Inherit Metab Dis 2007;30:104 [PMID: 17143576].

Rhead WJ: Newborn screening for medium-chain acyl-CoA dehydrogenase deficiency: A global perspective. J Inherit Metab Dis 2006;29:370 [PMID: 16763904].

Schymik I et al: Pitfalls of neonatal screening for very-long-chain acyl-CoA dehydrogenase deficiency using tandem mass spectrometry. J Pediatr 2006;149:128 [PMID: 16860141].

Shekhawat PS et al: Fetal fatty acid oxidation disorders, their effect on maternal health and neonatal outcome: Impact of expanded newborn screening on their diagnosis and management. Pediatr Res 2005;57(5 Pt 2):78R [PMID: 15817498].

van Maldegem BT et al: Clinical, biochemical, and genetic heterogeneity in short-chain acyl-coenzyme A dehydrogenase deficiency. JAMA 2006;296:943 [PMID: 16926354].

Waddell L et al: Medium-chain acyl-CoA dehydrogenase deficiency: Genotype-biochemical phenotype correlations. Mol Genet Metab 2006;87:32 [PMID: 16291504].

Wilcken B et al: Outcome of neonatal screening for medium-chain acyl-CoA dehydrogenase deficiency in Australia: A cohort study. Lancet 2007;369:37 [PMID: 17208640].

Patient and parent support group web site with useful information for families: http://www.fodsupport.org

CARNITINE

Carnitine is an essential nutrient found in highest concentration in red meat. Its primary function is to transport long-chain fatty acids into mitochondria for oxidation. Primary defects of carnitine transport may manifest as Reye syndrome, cardiomyopathy, or skeletal myopathy with hypotonia. These disorders are rare compared with secondary carnitine deficiency, which may be due to diet (especially intravenous alimentation or ketogenic diet), renal losses, drug therapy (especially valproic acid), and other metabolic disorders (especially disorders of fatty acid oxidation and organic acidemias). The prognosis depends on the cause of the carnitine abnormality. Primary carnitine deficiency is one of the most treatable causes of dilated cardiomyopathy in children.

Free and esterified carnitine can be measured in blood. Muscle carnitine may be low despite normal blood levels, particularly in respiratory chain disorders. If carnitine insufficiency is suspected, the patient should be evaluated to rule out disorders that might cause secondary carnitine deficiency.

Oral or intravenous L-carnitine is used in carnitine deficiency or insufficiency in doses of 25–100 mg/kg/d or higher. Treatment is aimed at maintaining normal carnitine levels. Carnitine supplementation in patients with some disorders of fatty acid oxidation and organic acidosis may also augment excretion of accumulated metabolites. Supplementation may not prevent metabolic crises in such patients.

Amat di San Filippo C et al: Pharmacological rescue of carnitine transport in primary carnitine deficiency. Hum Mutat 2006;27:513 [PMID: 16652335].

Deschauer M et al: Muscle carnitine palmitoyltransferase II deficiency: Clinical and molecular genetic features and diagnostic aspects. Arch Neurol 2005;62:37 [PMID: 15642848].

Kilfoyle D et al: Recurrent myoglobinuria due to carnitine palmitoyltransferase II deficiency: Clinical, biochemical, and genetic features of adult-onset cases. N Z Med J 2005;118:U1320 [PMID: 15776096].

Korman SH et al: Novel metabolic and molecular findings in hepatic carnitine palmitoyltransferase I deficiency. Mol Genet Metab 2005;86:337 [PMID: 16146704].

Longo N et al: Disorders of carnitine transport and the carnitine cycle. Am J Med Genet C Semin Med Genet 2006;142:77 [PMID: 16602102].

Rubio-Gozalbo ME et al: Carnitine-acylcarnitine translocase deficiency, clinical, biochemical and genetic aspects. Mol Aspects Med 2004;25:521 [PMID: 15363639].

PURINE METABOLISM DISORDERS

Hypoxanthine-guanine phosphoribosyltransferase is an enzyme that converts the purine bases hypoxanthine and guanine to inosine monophosphate and guanosine monophosphate, respectively. Hypoxanthine-guanine phosphoribosyltransferase deficiency (Lesch-Nyhan syndrome) is an X-linked recessive disorder. The complete deficiency is characterized by central nervous system dysfunction and purine overproduction with hyperuricemia and hyperuricuria. Depending on the residual activity of the mutant enzyme, male hemizygous individuals may be severely disabled by choreoathetosis, spasticity, and compulsive, mutilating lip and finger biting, or they may have only gouty arthritis and urate ureterolithiasis. Enzyme deficiency can be measured in erythrocytes, fibroblasts, and cultured amniotic cells; this disorder can thus be diagnosed in utero. Adenylosuccinate lyase deficiency involves a defect in the synthesis of purines. Patients present with static mental retardation, hypotonia, and seizures.

Diagnosis

Diagnosis of Lesch-Nyhan syndrome is made by demonstrating an elevated uric acid:creatinine ratio in urine, followed by demonstration of enzyme deficiency in red blood cells or fibroblasts. Screening for adenylosuccinate lyase deficiency is by measurement of succinylpurines using the Bratton-Marshal colorimetric test, with confirmation by further metabolite and molecular assays.

Treatment

Hyperhydration and alkalinization are essential to prevent kidney stones and urate nephropathy. Allopurinol and probenecid may be given to reduce hyperuricemia and prevent gout but do not affect the neurologic status. Physical restraints are often more effective than neurologic medications for automutilation. No effective treatment exists for adenylosuccinate lyase deficiency.

Deutsch SI et al: Hypothesized deficiency of guanine-based purines may contribute to abnormalities of neurodevelopment, neuromodulation, and neurotransmission in Lesch-Nyhan syndrome. Clin Neuropharmacol 2005;28:28 [PMID: 15711436].

Nyhan WL: Inherited hyperuricemic disorders. Contrib Nephrol 2005;147:22 [PMID: 15604603].

Nyhan WL: Lesch-Nyhan disease. J Hist Neurosci 2005;14:1 [PMID: 15804753].

LYSOSOMAL DISEASES

Lysosomes are cellular organelles in which complex macromolecules are degraded by specific acid hydrolases. Deficiency of a lysosomal enzyme causes its substrate to accumulate in the lysosomes of tissues that degrade it, resulting in a characteristic clinical picture. These storage disorders are classified as mucopolysaccharidoses, lipidoses, or mucolipidoses, depending on the nature of the stored material. Two additional disorders, cystinosis and Salla disease, are caused by defects in lysosomal proteins that normally transport material from the lysosome to the cytoplasm. Table 34–5 lists clinical and laboratory features of these conditions. Most are inherited as autosomal recessive traits, and all can be diagnosed in utero.

Diagnosis

The diagnosis of mucopolysaccharidosis is suggested by certain clinical and radiologic findings (dysostosis multiplex). Urine screening tests can detect increased mucopolysaccharides and further identify which specific mucopolysaccharides are present. Diagnosis must be confirmed by enzyme assays of leukocytes or cultured fibroblasts. Analysis of urinary oligosaccharides indicates a specific disorder prior to enzymatic testing. Lipidoses present with visceral symptoms or neurodegeneration. The pattern of the leukodystrophy associated with many lipidoses can indicate a specific condition. Diagnosis is made by appropriate enzyme assays of peripheral leukocytes or cultured skin fibroblasts. Molecular analysis is also available for most conditions.

Treatment

Most conditions cannot be treated effectively, but new avenues have given hope in many conditions. Hematopoietic stem cell transplantation can greatly improve the course of some lysosomal diseases and is first-line treatment in some, such as infantile Hurler syndrome. Several disorders are treated with infusions of recombinant modified enzyme. Treatment of Gaucher disease is very effective and long-term data suggest excellent outcome. Similar treatments have been developed for Fabry disease, several mucopolysaccharidoses, and Pompe disease. Substantial improvements in these conditions have been reported but with limitations. New avenues for treatment under development are offered through substrate inhibition and chaperone therapy. Treatment of cystinosis with cysteamine results in depletion of stored cystine and prevention of complications including renal disease.

Aerts JM et al: Substrate reduction therapy of glycosphingolipid storage disorders. J Inherit Metab Dis 2006;29:449 [PMID: 16763917].

Boelens JJ: Trends in haematopoietic cell transplantation for inborn errors of metabolism. J Inherit Metab Dis 2006;29:413 [PMID: 16763911].

Brady RO: Enzyme replacement for lysosomal diseases. Annu Rev Med 2006;57:283 [PMID: 16409150].

Clarke JT: Narrative review: Fabry disease. Ann Intern Med 2007;146:425 [PMID: 17371887].

Cox TM: Substrate reduction therapy for lysosomal storage disease. Acta Paediatr Suppl 2005;94:69 [PMID: 15895716].

Cox-Brinkman J et al: Haematopoietic cell transplantation (HCT) in combination with enzyme replacement therapy (ERT) in patients with Hurler syndrome. Bone Marrow Transplant 2006;38:17 [PMID: 16715104].

Table 34–5. Clinical and laboratory features of lysosomal storage diseases.

Disorder	Enzyme Defect	Clinical and Laboratory Features
I. Mucopolysaccharidoses		
Hurler syndrome	α-Iduronidase	Autosomal recessive. Mental retardation, hepatosplenomegaly, umbilical hernia, coarse facies, corneal clouding, dorsolumbar gibbus, severe heart disease. Heparan sulfate and dermatan sulfate in urine.
Scheie syndrome	α-Iduronidase (incomplete)	Autosomal recessive. Corneal clouding, stiff joints, normal intellect. Clinical types intermediate between Hurler and Scheie common. Heparan sulfate and dermatan sulfate in urine.
Hunter syndrome	Sulfoiduronate sulfatase	X-linked recessive. Coarse facies, hepatosplenomegaly, mental retardation variable. Corneal clouding and gibbus not present. Heparan sulfate and dermatan sulfate in urine.
Sanfilippo syndrome:		Autosomal recessive. Severe mental retardation and hyperactivity, with comparatively mild skeletal changes, visceromegaly, and facial coarseness. Types cannot be differentiated clinically. Heparan sulfate in urine.
Type A	Sulfamidase	
Type B	α-N-Acetylglucosaminidase	
Type C	Acetyl-CoA: α-glucosaminide-N-acetyltransferase	
Type D	α-N-acetylglucosamine-6-sulfatase	
Morquio syndrome	N-Acetylgalactosamine-6-sulfatase	Autosomal recessive. Severe skeletal changes, platyspondylisis, corneal clouding. Keratan sulfate in urine.
Maroteaux-Lamy syndrome	N-Acetylgalactosamine-4-sulfatase	Autosomal recessive. Coarse facies, growth retardation, dorsolumbar gibbus, corneal clouding, hepatosplenomegaly, normal intellect. Dermatan sulfate in urine.
β-Glucuronidase deficiency	β-Glucuronidase	Autosomal recessive. Varies from mental retardation, dorsolumbar gibbus, corneal clouding, and hepatosplenomegaly to mild facial coarseness, retardation, and loose joints. Hearing loss common. Dermatan sulfate or heparan sulfate in urine.
II. Mucolipidoses		
Mannosidosis	α-Mannosidase	Autosomal recessive. Varies from severe mental retardation, coarse facies, short stature, skeletal changes, and hepatosplenomegaly to mild facial coarseness and loose joints. Hearing loss common. Abnormal oligosaccharides in urine.
Fucosidosis	α-Fucosidase	Autosomal recessive. Variable: coarse facies, skeletal changes, hepatosplenomegaly, occasional angiokeratomas. Abnormal oligosaccharides in urine.
I-cell disease (mucolipidosis II)	N-Acetylglucosaminyl-phospho-transferase	Autosomal recessive; severe and mild forms known. Very short stature, mental retardation, early facial coarsening, clear cornea, and stiffness of joints. Increased lysosomal enzymes in serum. Abnormal sialyl oligosaccharides in urine.
Sialidosis	N-Acetylineuraminidase (sialidase)	Autosomal recessive. Mental retardation, coarse facies, skeletal dysplasia, myoclonic seizures, macular cherry-red spot. Abnormal sialyl oligosaccharides in urine.
III. Lipidoses		
Niemann-Pick disease	Sphingomyelinase	Autosomal recessive. Acute and chronic forms known. Acute neuronopathic form common in eastern European Jews. Accumulation of sphingomyelin in lysosomes of RE system and CNS. Hepatosplenomegaly, developmental retardation, macular cherry-red spot. Death by 1–4 y in severe type A; mild type B develops respiratory insufficiency usually in adulthood.
Metachromatic leukodystrophy	Arylsulfatase A	Autosomal recessive. Late infantile form, with onset at 1–4 y, most common. Accumulation of sulfatide in white matter with central leukodystrophy and peripheral neuropathy. Gait disturbances (ataxia), motor incoordination, absent deep tendon reflexes, and dementia. Death usually in first decade.
Krabbe disease (globoid cell leukodystrophy)	Galactocerebroside α-galactosidase	Autosomal recessive. Globoid cells in white matter. Onset at 3–6 mo with seizures, irritability, retardation, and leukodystrophy. Death by 1–2 y. Juvenile and adult forms are rare.

(continued)

Table 34–5. Clinical and laboratory features of lysosomal storage diseases. *(Continued)*

Disorder	Enzyme Defect	Clinical and Laboratory Features
Fabry disease	α-Galactosidase A	X-linked recessive. Storage of trihexosylceramide in endothelial cells. Pain in extremities, angiokeratoma corporis diffusum and (later) poor vision, hypertension, and renal failure.
Farber disease	Ceramidase	Autosomal recessive. Storage of ceramide in tissues. Subcutaneous nodules, arthropathy with deformed and painful joints, and poor growth and development. Death within first year.
Gaucher disease	Glucocerebroside β-glucosidase	Autosomal recessive. Acute neuronopathic form: Accumulation of glucocerebroside in lysosomes of RE system and CNS. Retardation, hepatosplenomegaly, macular cherry-red spot, and Gaucher cells in bone marrow. Death by 1–2 y. Chronic form common in eastern European Jews. Accumulation of sphingomyelin in lysosomes of RE system. Hepatosplenomegaly and flask-shaped osteolytic bone lesions. Consistent with normal life expectancy.
G_{M1} gangliosidosis	G_{M1} ganglioside β-galactosidase	Autosomal recessive. Accumulation of G_{M1} ganglioside in lysosomes of RE system and CNS. Infantile form: Abnormalities at birth with dysostosis multiplex, hepatosplenomegaly, macular cherry-red spot, and death by 2 y. Juvenile form: normal development to 1 y of age, then ataxia, weakness, dementia, and death by 4–5 y. Occasional inferior beaking of vertebral bodies of L1 and L2.
G_{M2} gangliosidoses Tay-Sachs disease Sandhoff disease	 β-N-Acetylhexosaminidase A β-N-Acetylhexosaminidase A and B	Autosomal recessive. Tay-Sachs disease common in eastern European Jews; Sandhoff disease is panethnic. Clinical phenotypes are identical, with accumulation of G_{M2} ganglioside in lysosomes of CNS. Onset at age 3–6 mo, with hypotonia, hyperacusis, retardation, and macular cherry-red spot. Death by 2–3 y. Juvenile and adult onset forms of Tay-Sachs disease are rare.
Wolman disease	Acid lipase	Autosomal recessive. Accumulation of cholesterol esters and triglycerides in lysosomes of reticuloendothelial system. Onset in infancy with gastrointestinal symptoms and hepatosplenomegaly, and death by 3–6 mo. Adrenals commonly enlarged and calcified.
Niemann-Pick disease type C	NPC1 gene (95%), NPC2 gene (5%)	Autosomal recessive. Blocked transport of lipids and cholesterol from late endosomes to lysosomes. Infantile cholestatic liver disease, or later neurodegeneration with vertical supranuclear gaze palsy, ataxia, seizures, spasticity and loss of speech. Some have splenomegaly.

CNS, central nervous system; RE, reticuloendothelial.

Eng CM et al: Fabry disease: Guidelines for the evaluation and management of multiorgan system involvement. Genet Med 2006;8:539 [PMID: 16980809].

Hoffmann B, Mayatepek E: Neurological manifestations in lysosomal storage disorders—from pathology to first therapeutic possibilities. Neuropediatrics 2005;36:285 [PMID: 16217702].

Iturriaga C et al: Niemann-Pick C disease in Spain: Clinical spectrum and development of a disability scale. J Neurol Sci 2006;249:1 [PMID: 16814322].

Kaplan P et al: The clinical and demographic characteristics of nonneuronopathic Gaucher disease in 887 children at diagnosis. Arch Pediatr Adolesc Med 2006;160:603 [PMID: 16754822].

Millington DS: Newborn screening for lysosomal storage disorders. Clin Chem 2005;51:808 [PMID: 15855665].

Montano AM et al: International Morquio A Registry: Clinical manifestation and natural course of Morquio A disease. J Inherit Metab Dis 2007;30:165 [PMID: 17347914].

Reuser AJ, Drost MR: Lysosomal dysfunction, cellular pathology and clinical symptoms: Basic principles. Acta Paediatr Suppl 2006;95:77 [PMID: 16720471].

Ries M et al: Enzyme-replacement therapy with agalsidase alfa in children with Fabry disease. Pediatrics 2006;118:924 [PMID: 16950982].

Ries M et al: Pediatric Fabry disease. Pediatrics 2005;115:e344 [PMID: 15713906].

Sifuentes M et al: A follow-up study of MPS I patients treated with laronidase enzyme replacement therapy for 6 years. Mol Genet Metab 2007;90:171 [PMID: 17011223].

Vedder AC et al: The Dutch Fabry cohort: Diversity of clinical manifestations and Gb3 levels. J Inherit Metab Dis 2007;30:68 [PMID: 17206462].

Vellodi A: Lysosomal storage disorders. Br J Haematol 2005; 128:413 [PMID: 15686451].

Verot L et al: Niemann-Pick C disease: Functional characterization of three NPC2 mutations and clinical and molecular update on patients with NPC2. Clin Genet 2007;71:320 [PMID: 17470133].

Wraith JE et al: Enzyme replacement therapy in patients who have mucopolysaccharidosis I and are younger than 5 years: Results of a multinational study of recombinant human alpha-L-iduronidase (laronidase). Pediatrics 2007;120:e37 [PMID: 17606547].

Patient and parent support group web site with useful information for families: http://www.mpssociety.org and www.ulf.org

PEROXISOMAL DISEASES

Peroxisomes are intracellular organelles that contain a large number of enzymes, many of which are oxidases linked to catalase. Among the enzyme systems in peroxisomes is one for β-oxidation of unusual very-long-chain fatty acids, phytanic acid, and bile acids, and one for plasmalogen biosynthesis. In addition, peroxisomes contain oxidases for D- and L-amino acids, pipecolic acid, and phytanic acid, and an enzyme (alanine-glyoxylate aminotransferase) that effects transamination of glyoxylate to glycine.

In some peroxisomal diseases, many enzymes are deficient. Zellweger (cerebrohepatorenal) syndrome, the best known among these, is caused by several defects in organelle assembly. Patients present in infancy with seizures, hypotonia, characteristic facies with a large forehead, and cholestatic hepatopathy. At autopsy renal cysts and absent peroxisomes are seen. Patients with a similar but milder biochemical and clinical phenotype have neonatal adrenoleukodystrophy or neonatal Refsum disease. They often have detectable peroxisomes.

In other peroxisomal diseases, only a single enzyme is deficient. Primary hyperoxaluria (alanine-glyoxylate aminotransferase deficiency) causes renal stones and nephropathy. Mutations in the X-linked very-long-chain fatty acid transporter gene, *ABCD1*, cause either a rapid leukodystrophy with loss of function (adrenoleukodystrophy), slow progressive spasticity and neuropathy (adrenomyeloneuropathy), or adrenal insufficiency. Defective phytanic acid oxidation in adult Refsum disease causes ataxia, leukodystrophy, cardiomyopathy, neuropathy, and cataracts. Other isolated enzyme deficiencies can mimic Zellweger syndrome.

Abnormalities of plasmalogen synthesis are clinically associated with rhizomelic chondrodysplasia punctata. Except for adrenoleukodystrophy, all peroxisomal diseases are autosomal recessive and can be diagnosed in utero.

▷ Diagnosis

The best screening test for Zellweger syndrome and other biogenesis disorders is determination of very-long-chain fatty acids in serum or plasma. Urine bile acids are abnormal in other peroxisomal disorders. Phytanic acid and plasmalogens can also be measured. Together, these studies identify most peroxisomal diseases. Tissue biopsy and appropriate enzyme assays are needed for confirmation, especially when the parents plan further pregnancies.

▷ Treatment

Bone marrow transplantation may be an effective treatment at the early stages of adrenoleukodystrophy. Lorenzo's oil, in combination with a very-low-fat diet and essential fatty acid supplementation, is ineffective in patients with established symptoms, but shows promise in prevention of neurologic symptoms in presymptomatic males with adrenoleukodystrophy. Dietary treatment is used for adult Refsum disease. Liver transplantation protects the kidneys in severe primary hyperoxaluria.

Crane DI et al: PEX1 mutations in the Zellweger spectrum of the peroxisome biogenesis disorders. Hum Mutat 2005;26:167 [PMID: 16086329].

Faust PL et al: Peroxisome biogenesis disorders; the role of peroxisomes and metabolic dysfunction in developing brain. J Inherit Metab Dis 2005;28:369 [PMID: 15868469].

Ferdinandusse S, Houten SM: Peroxisomes and bile acid biosynthesis. Biochim Biophys Acta 2006;1763:1427 [PMID: 17034878].

Ferdinandusse S et al: Clinical and biochemical spectrum of D-bifunctional protein deficiency. Ann Neurol 2006;59:92 [PMID: 16278854].

Ferri R, Chance PF: Lorenzo's oil: Advances in the treatment of neurometabolic disorders. Arch Neurol 2005;62:1045 [PMID: 16009756].

Moser HW et al: X-linked adrenoleukodystrophy. Nat Clin Pract Neurol 2007;3:140 [PMID: 17342190].

Moser HW et al: Adrenoleukodystrophy: New approaches to a neurodegenerative disease. JAMA 2005;294:3131 [PMID: 16380594].

Moser HW et al: Follow-up of 89 asymptomatic patients with adrenoleukodystrophy treated with Lorenzo's oil. Arch Neurol 2005;62:1073 [PMID: 16009761].

Oglesbee D: An overview of peroxisomal biogenesis disorders. Mol Genet Metab 2005;84:299 [PMID: 15875330].

Shimozawa N: Molecular and clinical aspects of peroxisomal diseases. J Inherit Metab Dis 2007;30:193 [PMID: 17347916].

Shimozawa N et al: Molecular and neurologic findings of peroxisome biogenesis disorders. J Child Neurol 2005;20:326 [PMID: 15921234].

Steinberg SJ et al: Peroxisome biogenesis disorders. Biochim Biophys Acta 2006;1763:1733 [PMID: 17055079].

Wanders RJ, Waterham HR: Peroxisomal disorders I: Biochemistry and genetics of peroxisome biogenesis disorders. Clin Genet 2005;67:107 [PMID: 15679822].

Wanders RJ, Waterham HR: Peroxisomal disorders: The single peroxisomal enzyme deficiencies. Biochim Biophys Acta 2006;1763:1707 [PMID: 17055078].

CONGENITAL DISORDERS OF GLYCOSYLATION

Many proteins, including many enzymes, require glycosylation with carbohydrate moieties for normal function. The carbohydrate-deficient glycoprotein syndromes are a family of disorders that result from failure of glycosylation. Children with type Ia disease usually present with prenatal growth disturbance, often with abnormal fat distribution, cerebellar hypoplasia, typical facial dysmorphic features, and mental retardation. The typical course includes chronic liver disease, peripheral neuropathy, endocrinopathies, retinopathy, and in some patients, acute life-threatening events.

Patients with type Ib disease have a variable combination of liver fibrosis, protein-losing enteropathy, and hypoglycemia. More than a dozen other forms are characterized by additional key symptoms, including coloboma, cutis laxa, severe epilepsy, ichthyosis, and Dandy-Walker malformation. Biochemical differences and variations in clinical course (eg, the absence of peripheral neuropathy) characterize the other types. Pathophysiology probably relates to defects of those biochemical pathways that require glycosylated proteins. The syndromes appear so far to be inherited in an autosomal recessive manner, and frequency was initially estimated to be as high as 1:20,000 in northern Europe.

▶ Diagnosis

Diagnosis is supported by finding altered levels of glycosylated enzymes or other proteins such as transferrin, thyroxine-binding globulin, lysosomal enzymes, and clotting factors (IX, XI, antithrombin III, and proteins C and S). However, these levels may be normal in carbohydrate-deficient glycoprotein syndromes or abnormal in other conditions. Diagnosis is confirmed by finding typical patterns of altered isoelectric focusing of selected proteins. Most diagnostic laboratories examine serum transferrin to screen for N-linked defects and apoC1 for O-linked defects. Follow-up diagnosis is by assaying enzyme activity, analysis of lipid-linked oligosaccharides in fibroblasts, and mutation analysis.

▶ Treatment

Treatment is supportive, with opportunity to monitor and provide early treatment for expected clinical features. Mannose treatment is curative for patients with type Ib deficiency only.

Eklund EA, Freeze HH: The congenital disorders of glycosylation: A multifaceted group of syndromes. NeuroRx 2006;3:254 [PMID: 16554263].

Leroy JG: Congenital disorders of N-glycosylation including diseases associated with O- as well as N-glycosylation defects. Pediatr Res 2006;60:643 [PMID: 17065563].

Sparks SE: Inherited disorders of glycosylation. Mol Genet Metab 2006;87:1 [PMID: 16511948].

SMITH-LEMLI-OPITZ SYNDROME & DISORDERS OF CHOLESTEROL SYNTHESIS

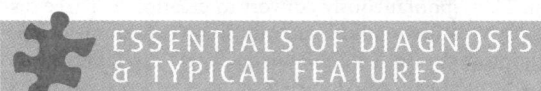

ESSENTIALS OF DIAGNOSIS & TYPICAL FEATURES

▶ Two- or three-toe syndactyly, facial dysmorphism, cardiac and genitourinary anomalies.

▶ Developmental delay, hypotonia, microcephaly, and poor growth in neonates with Smith-Lemli-Opitz (SLO) syndrome.

▶ Symptoms range from mild to life threatening.

▶ Elevated 7- and 8-dehydrocholesterol in serum and other tissue is diagnostic in SLO syndrome; serum cholesterol is usually low, but may be within normal range.

Several defects of cholesterol synthesis are associated with malformations and neurodevelopmental disability. Smith-Lemli-Opitz (SLO) syndrome is an autosomal recessive disorder caused by a deficiency of the enzyme 7-dehydrocholesterol δ^7-reductase. It is characterized by microcephaly, poor growth, mental retardation, typical dysmorphic features of face and extremities (particularly two- to three-toe syndactyly), and often malformations of the heart and genitourinary system. Severity ranges from moderate to severe mental retardation to early death. Although deficient synthesis of cholesterol leads directly to deficiency of some hormones and bile acids, the pathophysiology of the malformations is unclear. Frequency is estimated to be between 1:40,000 and 1:20,000. Other cholesterol synthetic defects are seen in Conradi Hünnermann syndrome with chondrodysplasia punctata and atrophic skin. Cholestanolosis (cerebrotendinous xanthomatosis) manifests with progressive ataxia and cataracts.

▶ Diagnosis

In SLO, elevated 7- and 8-dehydrocholesterol in serum or other tissues, including amniotic fluid, is diagnostic. Serum cholesterol levels may be low or in the normal range. Enzymes of cholesterol synthesis may be assayed in cultured fibroblasts or amniocytes, and mutation analysis is possible.

▶ Treatment

Although postnatal treatment does not resolve prenatal injury, supplementation with cholesterol in SLO improves growth and behavior. The role of supplemental bile acids is controversial. Simvastatin reduces 7- and 8-dehydrocholesterol and increases cholesterol levels by induction of its synthetic enzymes, but its effect on clinical symptoms is unclear.

Correa-Cerro LS, Porter FD: 3beta-hydroxysterol Delta7-reductase and the Smith-Lemli-Opitz syndrome. Mol Genet Metab 2005;84:112 [PMID: 15670717].

Haas D et al: Effects of cholesterol and simvastatin treatment in patients with Smith-Lemli-Opitz syndrome. J Inherit Metab Dis 2007;30:375 [PMID: 17497248].

Hennekam RC: Congenital brain anomalies in distal cholesterol biosynthesis defects. J Inherit Metab Dis 2005;28:385 [PMID: 15868470].

Rossi M et al: Characterization of liver involvement in defects of cholesterol biosynthesis: Long-term follow-up and review. Am J Med Genet A 2005;132:144 [PMID: 15580635].

Sikora DM et al: The near universal presence of autism spectrum disorders in children with Smith-Lemli-Opitz syndrome. Am J Med Genet A 2006;140:1511 [PMID: 16761297].

Yu H, Patel SB: Recent insights into the Smith-Lemli-Opitz syndrome. Clin Genet 2005;68:383 [PMID: 16207203].

DISORDERS OF NEUROTRANSMITTER METABOLISM

ESSENTIALS OF DIAGNOSIS & TYPICAL FEATURES

- ▶ Movement disorder, especially dystonia and oculogyric crises.
- ▶ Severe seizures, abnormal tone, ataxia, and mental retardation occur in severely affected infants.
- ▶ Mildly affected patients have dopa-responsive dystonia with diurnal variability.
- ▶ Deficient serine synthesis causes microcephaly, seizures and failure of myelination in neonates.

Abnormalities of neurotransmitter metabolism are increasingly recognized as causes of significant neurodevelopmental disabilities. Affected patients may present with movement disorders (especially dystonia and oculogyric crises), seizures, abnormal tone, ataxia, or mental retardation. Patients may be mildly affected (eg, dopa-responsive dystonia with diurnal variation) or severely affected (eg, intractable seizures with profound mental retardation). Deficient serine synthesis leads to congenital microcephaly, infantile seizures, and failure of myelination.

Pyridoxine-dependent epilepsy manifests as a severe seizure disorder in the neonatal or early infantile period that responds to high doses of pyridoxine. The disorder is caused by deficient activity of the enzyme α-amino adipic semialdehyde dehydrogenase resulting from mutations in the antiquitin (*ALDH7A1*) gene. Pyridoxal-phosphate–responsive encephalopathy manifests as a severe seizure disorder in infancy that responds to pyridoxal-phosphate. This disorder is caused by mutations in the *PNPO* gene encoding pyridox(am)ine oxidase, which is necessary for activation of pyridoxine.

▶ Diagnosis

Although some disorders can be diagnosed by examining serum amino acids or urine organic acids (eg, 4-hydroxybutyric aciduria), in most cases, diagnosis requires analysis of CSF. Spinal fluid samples for neurotransmitter analysis require special collection and handling, as the neurotransmitter levels are graduated along the axis of the central nervous system and are highly unstable once the sample is collected. A phenylalanine loading test can be diagnostic for mild defects in GTP-cyclohydrolase deficiency, in which neurotransmitter analysis may be insufficiently sensitive. Analysis of CSF amino acids shows elevated threonine in pyridoxal-phosphate–responsive disease and decreased serine and glycine in serine biosynthetic defects.

▶ Treatment

For some conditions, such as pyridoxine-responsive seizures, pyridoxal-phosphate–responsive encephalopathy, or dopa-

responsive dystonia, response to treatment can be dramatic. For others, response to therapy is less satisfactory in part because of poor penetration of the blood-brain barrier. Supplementation with serine and glycine can substantially improve outcome in serine deficiency.

Abeling NG et al: Sepiapterin reductase deficiency an autosomal recessive DOPA-responsive dystonia. Mol Genet Metab 2006;89:116 [PMID: 16650784].

Clayton PT: B6-responsive disorders: A model of vitamin dependency. J Inherit Metab Dis 2006;29:317 [PMID: 16763894].

Coman DJ et al: Seizures, ataxia, developmental delay and the general paediatrician: Glucose transporter 1 deficiency syndrome. J Paediatr Child Health 2006;42:263 [PMID: 16712556].

de Koning TJ, Klomp LW: Serine-deficiency syndromes. Curr Opin Neurol 2004;17:197 [PMID: 15021249].

Echenne B et al: Sepiapterin reductase deficiency: Clinical presentation and evaluation of long-term therapy. Pediatr Neurol 2006;35:308 [PMID: 17074599].

Hoffmann et al: Pyridoxal-5'-phosphate may be curative in early-onset epileptic encephalopathy. J Inherit Metab Dis 2007;30:96 [PMID: 17216302].

Pearl PL et al: Inherited disorders of neurotransmitters in children and adults. Clin Biochem 2005;38:1051 [PMID: 16298354].

Pearl PL et al: Diagnosis and treatment of neurotransmitter disorders. Curr Treat Options Neurol 2006;8:441 [PMID: 17032564].

Pearl PL et al: The pediatric neurotransmitter disorders. J Child Neurol 2007;22:606 [PMID: 17690069].

Ramaekers VT, Blau N: Cerebral folate deficiency. Dev Med Child Neurol 2004;46:843 [PMID: 15581159].

Sedel F et al: Dihydropteridine reductase deficiency: Levodopa's long-term effectiveness without dyskinesia. Neurology 2006;67:2243 [PMID: 17190955].

Tanaka Y et al: Early initiation of L-dopa therapy enables stable development of executive function in tetrahydrobiopterin (BH4) deficiency. Dev Med Child Neurol 2007;49:372 [PMID: 17489812].

Van Hove JLK et al: Expanded motor and psychiatric phenotype in autosomal dominant Segawa syndrome due to GTP cyclohydrolase deficiency. J Neurol Neurosurg Psychiatry 2006;77:18 [PMID: 16361586].

Wang D et al: Glut-1 deficiency syndrome: Clinical, genetic, and therapeutic aspects. Ann Neurol 2005;57:111 [PMID: 15622525].

CREATINE SYNTHESIS DISORDERS

Creatine and creatine phosphate are essential for storage and transmission of phosphate-bound energy in muscle and brain. They spontaneously convert to creatinine. Three disorders of creatine synthesis are now known: arginine:glycine amidinotransferase (AGAT) deficiency, guanidinoacetate methyltransferase (GAMT) deficiency, and creatine transporter (CrT1) deficiency. GAMT and AGAT deficiencies are autosomal recessive disorders, whereas CrT1 deficiency is X-linked. All patients demonstrate developmental delay, mental retardation, autistic behavior, seizures, and severe expressive language disturbance. Patients may also show developmental regression and brain atrophy. Patients with GAMT deficiency have more severe seizures and an extrapyramidal movement disorder. The seizure disorder is milder in CrT1-deficient patients. Some female heterozygotes of CrT1 deficiency may also show developmental delay or learning disabilities.

Diagnosis

The common feature of all creatine synthesis defects is a severe depletion of creatine and phosphocreatine in the brain demonstrable by reduction to absence of signal on magnetic resonance spectroscopy. In GAMT deficiency, guanidinoacetate accumulates, whereas in AGAT deficiency, guanidinoacetate is decreased, particularly in urine. Guanidinoacetate seems to be responsible for the severe seizures and movement disorder found in GAMT deficiency. Blood, urine, and CSF creatine levels are decreased in GAMT deficiency but normal in AGAT deficiency. Urine excretion of creatine and creatinine is elevated in CrT1 deficiency. Enzyme and molecular analyses are available for diagnostic confirmation.

Treatment

Treatment with oral creatine supplementation is in part successful in GAMT and AGAT deficiencies. It is not beneficial in CrT1 deficiency. Treatment by combined arginine restriction and ornithine substitution in GAMT deficiency can decrease guanidinoacetate concentrations and improve the clinical course.

Battini R et al: Arginine:glycine amidinotransferase (AGAT) deficiency in a newborn: Early treatment can prevent phenotypic expression of the disease. J Pediatr 2006;148:828 [PMID: 16769397].

Lion-Francois L et al: High frequency of creatine deficiency syndromes in patients with unexplained mental retardation. Neurology 2006;67:1713 [PMID: 17101918].

Mercimek-Mahmutoglu S et al: GAMT deficiency: Features, treatment, and outcome in an inborn error of creatine synthesis. Neurology 2006;67:480 [PMID: 16855203].

Schulze A et al: Presymptomatic treatment of neonatal guanidinoacetate methyltransferase deficiency. Neurology 2006;67:719 [PMID: 16924036].

Verhoeven NM et al: Laboratory diagnosis of defects of creatine biosynthesis and transport. Clin Chim Acta 2005;361:1 [PMID: 16169544].

Genetics & Dysmorphology

Ellen R. Elias, MD

Anne Chun-Hui Tsai, MD, MSc

David K. Manchester, MD

Genetics is an exciting and rapidly evolving field that has significant relevance to the understanding of human embryology, physiology, and disease processes. Tremendous advances in molecular biology and biochemistry are allowing more comprehensive understanding of mechanisms inherent in genetic disorders, as well as improved diagnostic tests and management options. Many of the newer technologies and terms may be unfamiliar to the clinician in practice. Thus, the topics in the first part of the chapter serve as an introduction and review of the basic principles of genetics, including basic knowledge of cytogenetics and molecular biology. The principles of inherited human disorders are reviewed, encompassing different causes of genetic disorders, with a discussion of dysmorphology and teratology. The topics in the second part of the chapter focus on common clinical disorders including descriptions of the diseases, with a discussion of their pathogenesis, diagnosis, and management.

FOUNDATIONS OF GENETIC DIAGNOSIS

CYTOGENETICS

Cytogenetics is the study of genetics at the chromosome level. Chromosomal anomalies occur in 0.4% of all live births and are a common cause of mental retardation and congenital anomalies. The prevalence of chromosomal anomalies is much higher among spontaneous abortions and stillbirths.

Chromosomes

Human chromosomes consist of DNA (the blueprint of genetic material), specific proteins forming the backbone of the chromosome (called histones), and other chromatin structural and interactive proteins. Chromosomes contain most of the genetic information necessary for growth and differentiation. The nuclei of all normal human cells, with the exception of gametes, contain 46 chromosomes, consisting of 23 pairs (Figure 35–1). Of these, 22 pairs are called autosomes. They are numbered according to their size; chromosome 1 is the largest and chromosome 22 the smallest. In addition, there are two sex chromosomes: two X chromosomes in females and one X and one Y chromosome in males. The two members of a chromosome pair are called homologous chromosomes. One homolog of each chromosome pair is maternal in origin (from the egg); the second is paternal (from the sperm). The egg and sperm each contain 23 chromosomes (haploid cells). During formation of the zygote, they fuse into a cell with 46 chromosomes (diploid cell).

Cell Division

Cells undergo cycles of growth and division that are controlled according to their needs and functions.

Mitosis is a kind of cell division, occurring in stages, during which DNA replication takes place and two daughter cells, genetically identical to the original parent cells, are formed. This cell division is typical for all somatic cells (cells other than the sperm or egg, which are called germline cells). There are four phases of mitosis: interphase, prophase, metaphase, and anaphase (Figure 35–2). In interphase, chromosomes are long, thin, and nonvisible. At this time, the genetic material is replicated. In prophase, the chromosomes are more condensed. During metaphase (the phase following DNA replication but preceding cell division), individual chromosomes can be visualized. Each arm consists of two identical parts, called chromatids. Chromatids of the same chromosome are called sister chromatids. In anaphase, the genetic material is separated into two cells.

Meiosis (Figure 35–3), during which eggs and sperm are formed, is cell division limited to gametes. During meiosis, three unique processes take place:

1. Crossing over of genetic material between two homologous chromosomes. This is preceded by the pairing of both members of each chromosome pair, which facilitates the physical exchange of homologous genetic material.

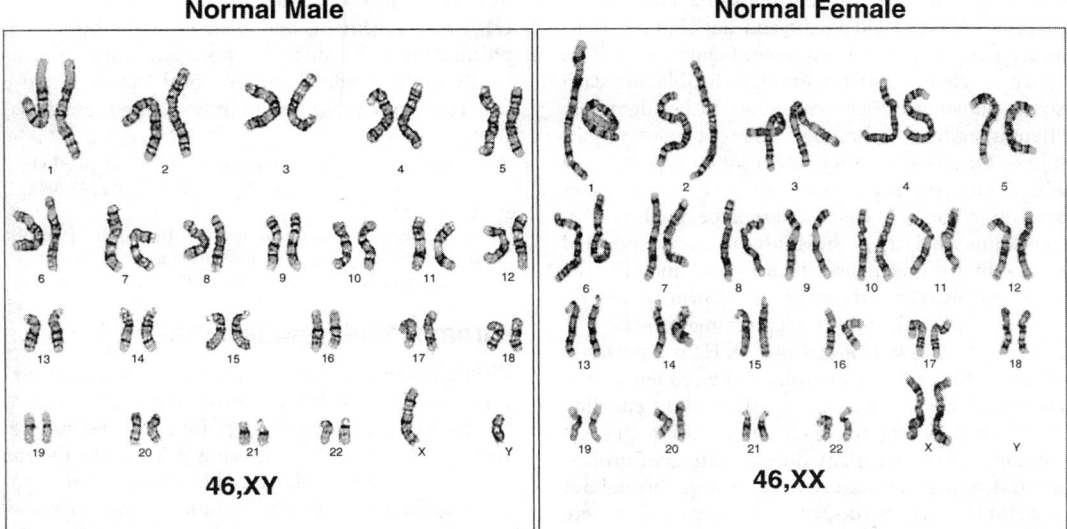

▲ **Figure 35-1.** Normal male and female human karyotype. (Courtesy of Billie Carstens at CGL.)

2. Random assortment of maternally and paternally derived homologous chromosomes into the daughter cells. The distribution of maternal or paternal chromosomes to a particular daughter cell occurs independently in each cell.

3. Two cell divisions, the first of which is a reduction division—that is, separation between the homologous chromosomes. The second meiotic division is like mitosis, separating two sister chromatids into two genetically identical daughter cells.

Chromosome Preparation & Analysis

Chromosome structure is visible only during mitosis, most often achieved in the laboratory by stimulating a blood lymphocyte culture with a mitogen for 3 days. Other tissues used for this purpose include skin, products of conception,

cartilage, and bone marrow. Chorionic villi or amniocytes are used for prenatal diagnosis. Spontaneously dividing cells without a mitogen are present in bone marrow, and historically, bone marrow biopsy was done when immediate identification of a patient's chromosome constitution was necessary for appropriate management (eg, to rule out trisomy 13 in a newborn with a complex congenital heart disease). However, this invasive test has been replaced by the availability of the FISH technique (see following discussion).

▲ **Figure 35-2.** Stages of mitotic division.

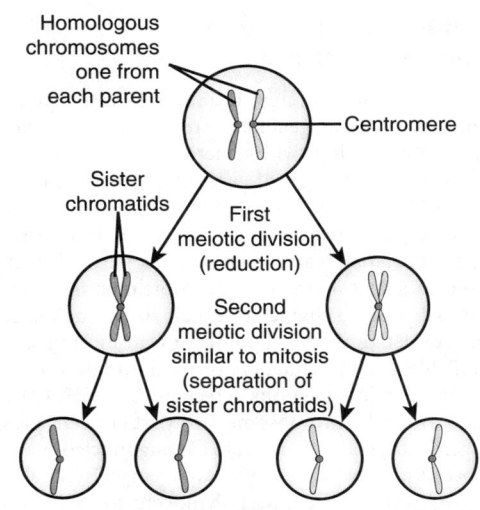

▲ **Figure 35-3.** Meiosis—demonstrating conversion from the diploid somatic cell to the haploid gamete.

Cells processed for routine chromosome analysis are stained on glass slides to yield a light-and-dark band pattern across the arms of the chromosomes (see Figure 35–1). This band pattern is characteristic and reproducible for each chromosome, allowing the chromosomes to be identified. Using different staining techniques, different banding patterns result: G, Q, and R banding. The most commonly used is G banding. The layout of chromosomes on a sheet of paper in a predetermined order is called a karyotype. High-resolution chromosome analysis is the study of more elongated chromosomes in prometaphase. In such an analysis, the bands can be visualized in greater detail, allowing detection of smaller, more subtle chromosomal rearrangements.

Fluorescence in situ hybridization (FISH) is a powerful technique that labels a known chromosome sequence with DNA probes attached to fluorescent dyes, thus enabling visualization of specific regions of chromosomes by fluorescent microscopy. There are many different kinds of probes, including paint probes (a mixture of sequences throughout one chromosome), sequence-specific probes, centromere probes, and telomere probes. A cocktail of differently colored probes, one color for each chromosome, called multicolor FISH, or M-FISH, can detect complex rearrangements between chromosomes. FISH can detect submicroscopic structural rearrangements undetectable by classic cytogenetic techniques and can identify marker chromosomes. (For pictures of FISH studies, go to http://www.kumc.edu/gec/prof/cytogene.html.)

FISH also allows interphase cells (lymphocytes, amniocytes) to be screened for numerical abnormalities such as trisomy 13, 18, or 21, and sex chromosome anomalies. However, because of the possible background or contamination of the signal, the abnormality must be confirmed by conventional chromosome analysis.

Array-Based Comparative Genomic Hybridization

Advances in computer chip technology have led to the development of new genetic testing using comparative genomic hybridization with microarray technique. This technique allows detection of very small genetic imbalances anywhere in the genome. Its usefulness has been well documented in cancer research and more recently in assessing small chromosomal rearrangements. In particular, it has been used to detect interstitial and subtelomeric submicroscopic imbalances, to characterize their size at the molecular level, and to define the breakpoints of translocations. Clinically available arrays include (1) focused interest arrays that can pick up all microdeletions detectable by FISH, (2) 1-mb bacterial artificial chromosome arrays that can pick up rearrangements greater than 1 mb, (3) oligonucleotide arrays using special probes that can pick up changes as small as 80 kb, and (4) single nucleotide polymorphism (SNP) arrays, which are used more widely in research settings. Although

this powerful new technology can identify extremely subtle DNA rearrangements and changes, many human polymorphisms, including small deletions and duplications, are not totally understood. Therefore, special caution and parental studies are often required in interpreting these data.

Bejjani BA et al: Array-based comparative genomic hybridization in clinical diagnosis. Exp Rev Mol Diagn 2005;5:421 [PMID: 15934818].

Slater HR et al: High-resolution identification of chromosomal abnormalities using oligonucleotide arrays containing 116,204 SNPs. Am J Hum Genet 2005;77:709 [PMID: 16252233].

Chromosome Nomenclature

Visible under the microscope is a constriction site on the chromosome called the centromere, which separates the chromosome into two arms: p, for petite, refers to the short arm, and q, the letter following p, refers to the long arm. Each arm is further subdivided into numbered bands visible using different staining techniques. Centromeres are positioned at different sites on different chromosomes and are used to differentiate the chromosome structures seen during mitosis as **metacentric** (p arm and q arm of almost equal size), **submetacentric** (p arm shorter than q arm), and **acrocentric** (almost no p arm). The use of named chromosome arms and bands provides a universal method of chromosome description. Common symbols include *del* (deletion), *dup* (duplication), *inv* (inversion), *ish* (in situ hybridization), *i* (isochromosome), *pat* (paternal origin), *mat* (maternal origin), and *r* (ring chromosome). These terms are further defined under Chromosomal Abnormalities, below.

Chromosomal Abnormalities

There are two types of chromosomal anomalies: numerical and structural.

A. Abnormalities of Chromosomal Number

When a human cell has 23 chromosomes, such as human ova or sperm, it is in the haploid state (n). After conception, in cells other than the reproductive cells, 46 chromosomes are present in the diploid state (2n). Any number that is an exact multiple of the haploid number—for example, 46(2n), 69(3n), or 92(4n)—is referred to as euploid. Polyploid cells are those that contain any number other than the usual diploid number of chromosomes. Polyploid conceptions are usually not viable except in a "mosaic state," with the presence of more than one cell line in the body (see later text for details).

Cells deviating from the multiple of the haploid number are called aneuploid, meaning not euploid, indicating an abnormal number of chromosomes. Trisomy, an example of aneuploidy, is the presence of three of a particular chromosome rather than two. It results from unequal division, called nondisjunction, of chromosomes into daughter cells. Trisomies are the most common numerical chromosomal anomalies found in humans (eg, trisomy 21 [Down syndrome], trisomy 18, and trisomy 13). Monosomies, the presence of only one member of a chromosome pair, may be complete or partial. Complete monosomies may result from nondisjunction or anaphase lag. All complete autosomal monosomies appear to be lethal early in development and only survive in mosaic forms. Sex chromosome monosomy, however, can be viable.

B. Abnormalities of Chromosomal Structure

Many different types of structural chromosomal anomalies exist. Figure 35–4 displays the formal nomenclature as well as the ideogram demonstrating chromosomal anomalies. In clinical context, the sign (+) or (–) *preceding* the chromo-some number indicates increased or decreased number, respectively, of that particular whole chromosome in a cell. For example, 47, XY+21 designates a male with three copies of chromosome 21. The sign (+) or (–) *after* the chromo-some number signifies extra material or missing material, respectively, on one of the arms of the chromosome. For example, 46,XX,8q– denotes a deletion on the long arm of chromosome 8. Detailed nomenclature, such as 8q11, is required to further demonstrate a specific missing region so that genetic counseling can be provided.

1. Deletion (del) (see Figure 35–4A)—This refers to an absence of normal chromosomal material. It may be termi-nal (at the end of a chromosome) or interstitial (within a chromosome). The missing part is described using the

▲ **Figure 35–4.** Examples of structural chromosomal abnormalities: deletion, duplication, inversion, ring chromosome, translocation, and insertion.

code "del," followed by the number of the chromosome involved in parentheses, and a description of the missing region of that chromosome, also in parentheses, for example, 46,XX,del(1)(p36.3). This chromosome nomenclature describes the loss of genetic material from band 36.3 of the short arm of chromosome 1, which results in 1p36.3 deletion syndrome. Some more common deletions result in clinically recognizable conditions associated with mental handicaps and characteristic facial features. (See descriptions of common genetic disorders caused by chromosomal deletions later in the chapter.)

2. Duplication (dup) (see Figure 35–4B)—An extra copy of a chromosomal segment can be tandem (genetic material present in the original direction) or inverted (genetic material present in the opposite direction). A well-described duplication of chromosome 22q11 causes cat eye syndrome, resulting in iris coloboma and anal or ear anomalies.

3. Inversion (inv) (see Figure 35–4C)—In this aberration, a rearranged section of a chromosome is inverted. It can be paracentric (not involving the centromere) or pericentric (involving the centromere).

4. Ring chromosome (r) (see Figure 35–4D)—Deletion of the normal telomeres (and possibly other subtelomeric sequences) leads to subsequent fusion of both ends to form a circular chromosome. Ring chromosomal anomalies often cause growth retardation and mental handicap.

5. Translocation (trans) (see Figure 35–4E)—This interchromosomal rearrangement of genetic material may be balanced (the cell has a normal content of genetic material arranged in a structurally abnormal way) or unbalanced (the cell has gained or lost genetic material as a result of chromosomal interchange). Balanced translocations may further be described as reciprocal, the exchange of genetic material between two nonhomologous chromosomes, or robertsonian, the fusion of two acrocentric chromosomes.

6. Insertion (ins) (see Figure 35–4F)—Breakage within a chromosome at two points and incorporation of another piece of chromosomal material is called insertion. This requires three breakpoints and may occur between two chromosomes or within the same chromosome. The clinical presentation or phenotype depends on the origin of the inserted materials.

C. Sex Chromosomal Anomalies

Abnormalities involving sex chromosomes, including aneuploidy and mosaicism, are relatively common in the general population. The most common sex chromosome anomalies include 45,X (Turner syndrome), 47,XXX, 47,XXY (Klinefelter syndrome), 47,XYY, and different mosaic states. (See later text for clinical discussion.)

D. Mosaicism

Mosaicism is the presence of two or more different chromosome constitutions in different cells of the same individual.

For example, a patient may have some cells with 47 chromosomes and others with 46 chromosomes (46,XX/47,XX,+21 indicates mosaicism for trisomy 21; similarly, 45,X/46,XX/47,XXX indicates mosaicism for a monosomy and a trisomy X). Mosaicism should be suspected if clinical symptoms are milder than expected in a nonmosaic patient with the same chromosomal abnormality, or if the patient's skin shows unusual pigmentation. The prognosis is frequently better for a patient with mosaicism than for one with a corresponding chromosomal abnormality without mosaicism. In general, the smaller the proportion of the abnormal cell line, the better the prognosis. In the same patient, however, the proportion of normal and abnormal cells in various tissues, such as skin, brain, internal organs, and peripheral blood, may be significantly different. Therefore, the prognosis for a patient with chromosomal mosaicism can seldom be assessed reliably based on the karyotype in peripheral blood alone.

E. Uniparental Disomy

Under normal circumstances, one member of each homologous pair of chromosomes is of maternal origin from the egg and the other is of paternal origin from the sperm (Figure 35–5A). In uniparental disomy (UPD), both copies of a particular chromosome pair originate from the same parent. If UPD is caused by an error in the first meiotic division, both homologous chromosomes of that parent will be present in the gamete—a phenomenon called heterodisomy (see Figure 35–5B). If the disomy is caused by an error in the second meiotic division, two copies of the same chromosome will be present through the mechanism of rescue, duplication, and complementation (see Figure 35–5C–E)—a phenomenon called isodisomy. Isodisomy may also occur as a postfertilization error (see Figure 35–5F).

A chromosomal analysis would not reveal an abnormality, but DNA analysis would reveal that the child inherited two copies of DNA of a particular chromosome from one parent without the contribution from the other parent. Possible mechanisms for the adverse effects of UPD include homozygosity for deleterious recessive genes and the consequences of imprinting (see later discussion in the Imprinting section). It is suspected that UPD of some chromosomes is lethal.

UPD has been documented for certain human chromosomes, including chromosomes 7, 11, 15, and X, and has been found in patients with Prader-Willi, Angelman, and Beckwith-Wiedemann syndromes. In addition, cystic fibrosis with only one carrier parent (caused by maternal isodisomy) has been reported. UPD may cause severe prenatal and postnatal growth retardation.

F. Contiguous Gene Syndromes

Contiguous gene syndromes result when a deletion causes the loss of genes adjacent to each other on a chromosome. Although many genes may be missing, the deletion may still

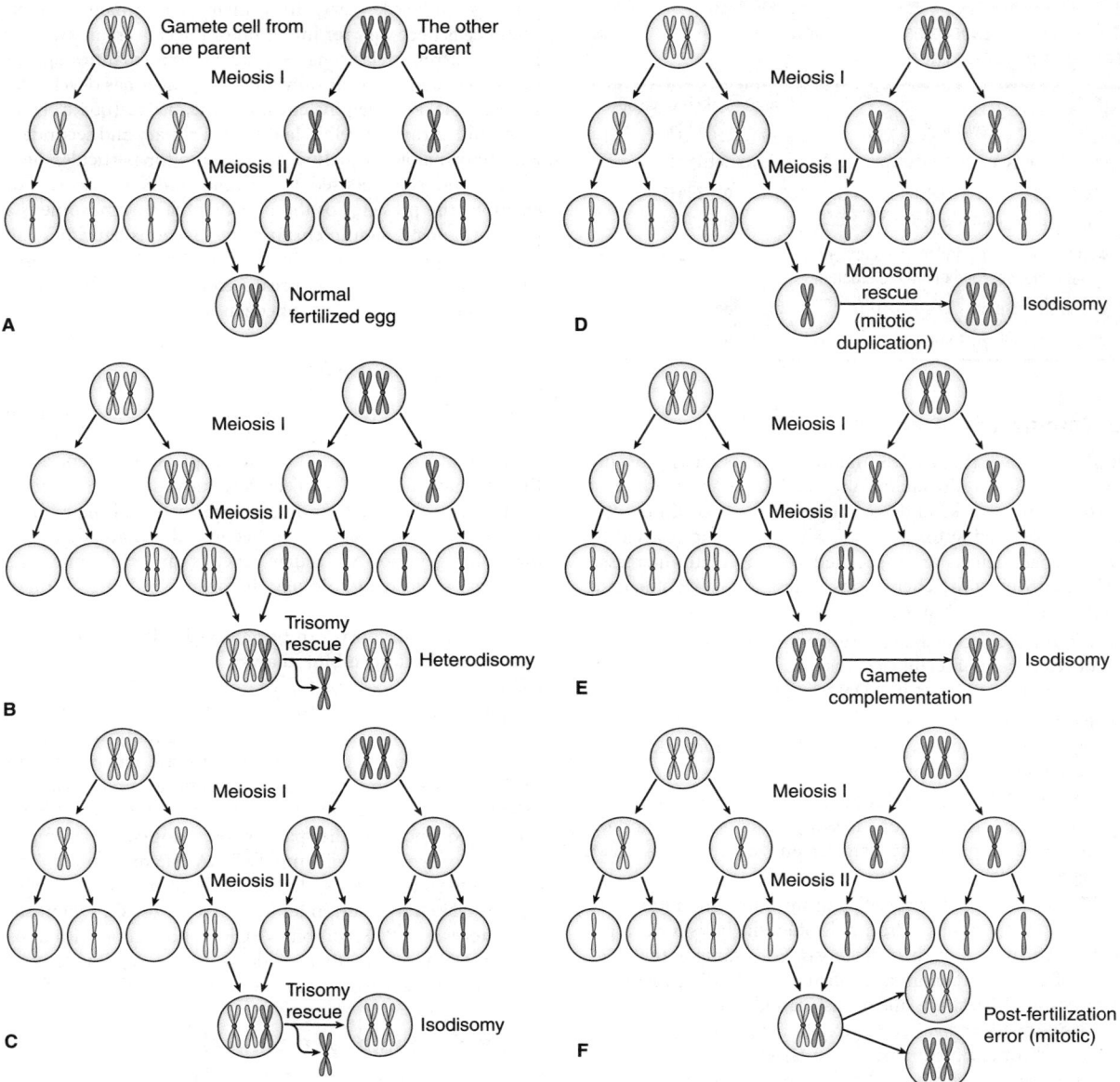

▲ **Figure 35–5.** The assortment of homologous chromosomes during normal gametogenesis and uniparental disomy. **A:** Fertilization of normal gametes. **B:** Heterodisomy by trisomy rescue. **C:** Isodisomy by trisomy rescue. **D:** Isodisomy by monosomy rescue (mitotic duplication). **E:** Gamete complementation. **F:** Postfertilization error.

be too small to be detected by routine karyotype. Therefore, contiguous gene syndromes are sometimes called "microdeletion syndromes." The genes involved in these syndromes are related only through their linear placement on the same chromosome segments and may not influence each other's functions directly. Table 35–1 lists examples of some cur-

rently known contiguous gene syndromes and their associated chromosomal abnormalities. These deletions may be familial (passed on by a parent), or occur de novo. The deletions may be diagnosed by high-resolution chromosome analysis in some affected individuals, or may be submicroscopic and detectable only with FISH or DNA analysis.

Table 35–1. Examples of common contiguous gene syndromes.

Syndrome	Abnormal Chromosome Segment
Prader-Willi/Angelman syndrome	del 15q11
Shprintzen/DiGeorge spectrum	del 22q11
Miller-Dieker syndrome	del 17p13
Wilms tumor with aniridia, genitourinary malformations, and mental retardation	del 11p13
Williams syndrome	del 7q11
Smith-Magenis syndrome	del 17p11

G. Chromosome Fragility

It is well known that environmental factors such as exposure to radiation, certain chemicals, and viruses contribute to chromosome breaks and rearrangements. In addition, several well-defined autosomal recessive syndromes caused by DNA repair defects are associated with a greatly increased risk of chromosome aberrations. These are called chromosome instability or breakage syndromes. Examples are:

- **Bloom syndrome,** characterized by small stature and development of telangiectasias on exposure to sunlight. It is caused by a defect in a DNA helicase.

- **Fanconi anemia,** often associated with radial ray defect, pigmentary changes, mild mental retardation, and development of pancytopenia.

- **Ataxia-telangiectasia** (Louis-Bar syndrome), characterized by telangiectasia of the skin and eyes, immunodeficiency, and progressive ataxia; and caused by a DNA repair defect.

The knowledge that specific chromosome aberrations are associated with these syndromes is often the basis for cytogenetic confirmation of their diagnosis. For example, the diagnosis of Fanconi anemia is confirmed by finding increased chromosomal breakage and translocations between nonhomologous quadriradii after diepoxy-butane treatment. Assessment of chromosome breaks and sister chromatid exchanges requires special techniques that lead to enhancement of the breaks, or special staining that allows visualization of the exchanged chromatids.

Levran O et al: The BRCA 1-interacting helicase BRIP1 is deficient in Fanconi anemia. Nat Genet 2005;37:931 [PMID: 16116424].

H. Chromosomal Abnormalities in Cancer

Numerical and structural chromosomal abnormalities are often identified in hematopoietic and solid-tumor neoplasms in individuals with otherwise normal chromosomes. These cytogenetic abnormalities have been categorized as primary and secondary. In primary abnormalities, their presence is necessary for initiation of the cancer; an example is 13q– in retinoblastoma. Secondary abnormalities appear de novo in somatic cells only after the cancer has developed, for example, Philadelphia chromosome, t(9;22)(q34;q11), in acute and chronic myeloid leukemia. Primary and secondary chromosomal abnormalities are specific for particular neoplasms and can be used for diagnosis or prognosis. For example, the presence of the Philadelphia chromosome is a good prognostic sign in chronic myelogenous leukemia and indicates a poor prognosis in acute lymphoblastic leukemia. The sites of chromosome breaks coincide with the known loci of oncogenes and anti-oncogenes.

MOLECULAR GENETICS

Advances in molecular biology have revolutionized human genetics, as they allow for the localization, isolation, and characterization of genes that encode protein sequences. As the Human Genome Project has moved into the postcloning era, the function of gene products and their interaction with one another has become the main theme of molecular genetics. Molecular genetics can help explain the complex underlying biology involved in many human diseases.

Molecular diagnosis can be achieved using the following technology. **Southern blot analysis** is the molecular genetic technique used to look for changes in genomic DNA. A similar technique, called **Northern blot analysis,** is used to look for RNA abnormalities. **Western blot analysis** is used to look for protein changes. The **polymerase chain reaction (PCR)** replicates fragments of DNA between predetermined primers so that sufficient DNA is obtained for characterization or sequencing in the space of a few hours. For example, 20 cycles of synthesis will amplify DNA one millionfold. The disadvantage of PCR is that a small contamination with foreign DNA can result in an incorrect diagnosis. **Quantitative fluorescent PCR** combines PCR amplification with fluorescent DNA probes to provide real-time replication and rapid determination of gene copy number and dosage effects.

Molecular Biology in Clinical Genetics & Genetic Diagnosis

Genetic diagnosis can be performed by direct detection of a mutant gene or by indirect methods. Direct detection is possible only when the gene causing the disease and the nature of the mutation are known. The advantage of a diagnostic study using the direct detection of a mutant gene is that it requires the affected individual only and need not involve the testing of other family members. The methods of direct DNA diagnosis include restriction analysis, single strand conformational polymorphism analysis, direct sequencing with assistance of PCR, heteroduplex assay, and protein truncation assay. The molecular mechanisms causing human diseases include point mutations, deletions, and insertions, and the unstable expansion of trinucleotide repeats, which leads to genetic anticipation. Some disorders that may be diagnosed via direct DNA mutational analysis include Duchenne muscular dystrophy, hemophilia, some forms of craniosynostosis, cystic fibrosis, and fragile X syndrome.

Indirect detection of abnormal genes is used when the gene is known but there is extensive heterogeneity of the molecular defect between families, or when the gene responsible for a disease is unknown but its chromosome location is known.

One form of indirect analysis is the linkage method. Linkage traces the inheritance of the abnormal gene between members in a kindred. This method requires that the affected individual be studied, as well as parents and other relatives, both affected and unaffected. Linkage analysis, is performed by using markers such as a restriction fragment length polymorphisms. Another method uses flanking microsatellite polymorphisms. An increase in density of polymorphisms discovered over the past few years allows the presence or absence of an abnormal copy of a gene in an individual to be predicted with a high degree of confidence, if the relatives have informative polymorphisms. Microsatellite polymorphisms are being used in sibling research studies to identify the multiple genes that contribute to polygenic traits such as diabetes and obesity. They are also used increasingly to identify gene changes in tumors.

Neurofibromatosis is an example of a disorder in which both the direct and indirect assay may be used. An estimated 90–95% of patients with neurofibromatosis type 1 have a mutation or deletion that can be identified using a direct assay of the neurofibromin gene (*NF1*). The other cases must rely on indirect methods such as linkage analysis for prenatal diagnosis.

Molecular Biology in Prevention & Treatment of Human Diseases

Recombinant DNA technology has the potential to prevent genetic disease by facilitating the detection of carriers of defective genes and permitting prenatal diagnosis. Family studies can also clarify the mode of inheritance, thus allowing more accurate determination of recurrence risks and appropriate options. For example, differentiation of gonadal mosaicism from decreased penetrance of a dominant gene has important implications for genetic counseling. In the past, the diagnosis of a genetic disease characterized by late onset of symptoms (eg, Huntington disease) could not be made prior to the appearance of clinical symptoms. In some inborn errors of metabolism, diagnostic tests (eg, measurement of enzyme activities) could be conducted only on inaccessible tissues. Gene identification (mutation analysis) techniques can enormously enhance the ability to diagnose both symptomatic and presymptomatic individuals, heterozygous carriers of gene mutations, and affected fetuses.

However, presymptomatic DNA testing is associated with psychological, ethical, and legal implications and therefore should be used only with informed consent. Formal genetic counseling is indicated to best interpret the results of molecular testing.

A normal gene introduced into an individual affected with a serious inherited disorder during embryonic life (germline therapy) in principle has the potential to be transmitted to future generations, whereas its introduction into somatic cells (somatic therapy) affects only the recipient. Experimental gene therapy by bone marrow transplantation is being tried for adenosine deaminase deficiency. Recombinant enzyme replacement has been successfully applied in treating the non-neurologic form of Gaucher disease, Fabry disease, Pompe disease, mucopolysaccharidosis types I and II, and some types of lysosomal storage disease.

▼ PRINCIPLES OF INHERITED HUMAN DISORDERS

MENDELIAN INHERITANCE

Traditionally, autosomal single gene disorders follow the principles explained by Mendel's observations. To summarize, the inheritance of genetic traits through generations relies on segregation and independent assortment. **Segregation** is the process through which gene pairs are separated during gamete formation. Each gamete receives only one copy of each gene (allele). **Independent assortment** refers to the idea that the segregation of different alleles occurs independently.

Victor McKusick's catalog, *Mendelian Inheritance in Man,* lists more than 10,000 entries in which the mode of inheritance is presumed to be autosomal dominant, autosomal recessive, X-linked dominant, X-linked recessive, and Y-linked. Single genes at specific loci on one or a pair of chromosomes cause these disorders. An understanding of inheritance terminology is helpful in approaching mendelian disorders. Analysis of the pedigree and the pattern of transmission in the family, identification of a specific condition, and knowledge of that condition's mode of inheritance usually allow for explanation of the inheritance pattern.

Terminology

The following terms are important in understanding heredity patterns.

1. Dominant and recessive—As defined by Mendel, concepts for dominant and recessive refer to the **phenotypic expression** of alleles and are not intrinsic characteristics of gene loci. Therefore, it is inappropriate to discuss "a dominant locus."

2. Genotype—Genotype means the genetic status, that is, the alleles an individual carries.

3. Phenotype—Phenotype is the expression of an individual's genotype including appearance, physical features, organ structure, and biochemical and physiologic nature. It may be modified by environment.

4. Pleiotropy—Pleiotropy refers to the phenomenon whereby a single mutant allele can have widespread effects or expression in different tissues or organ systems. In other words, an allele may produce more than one effect on the phenotype. For example, Marfan syndrome has manifestations in different organ systems (skeletal, cardiac, ophthalmologic, etc) due to a single mutation within the *fibrillin* gene.

5. Penetrance—Penetrance refers to the proportion of individuals with a particular genotype that express the same phenotype. Penetrance is a proportion that ranges between 0 and 1.0 (or 0 and 100%). When 100% of mutant individuals express the phenotype, penetrance is **complete.** If some mutant individuals do not express the phenotype, penetrance is said to be **incomplete,** or **reduced.** Dominant conditions with incomplete penetrance, therefore, are characterized by "skipped" generations with unaffected, obligate gene carriers.

6. Expressivity—Expressivity refers to the variability in degree of phenotypic expression (severity) seen in different individuals with the same mutant genotype. Expressivity may be extremely variable or fairly consistent, both within and between families. Intrafamilial variability of expression may be due to factors such as epistasis, environment, genetic anticipation, presence of phenocopies, mosaicism, and chance (stochastic factors). Interfamilial variability of expression may be due to the previously mentioned factors, but may also be due to allelic or locus genetic heterogeneity.

7. Genetic heterogeneity—Several different genetic mutations may produce phenotypes that are identical or similar enough to have been traditionally considered as one diagnosis. "Anemia" or "mental retardation" are examples of this. There are two types of genetic heterogeneity, locus heterogeneity and allelic heterogeneity.

A. Locus heterogeneity—Locus heterogeneity describes a phenotype caused by mutations at more than one genetic locus; that is, mutations at different loci cause the same phenotype or a group of phenotypes that appear similar enough to have been previously classified as a single disease, clinical "entity," or diagnostic spectrum. An example would be Sanfilippo syndrome (mucopolysaccharidosis types IIIA, B, C, and D), in which the same phenotype is produced by four different enzyme deficiencies.

B. Allelic heterogeneity—This term is applied to a phenotype causing different mutations at a single gene locus. As an example, cystic fibrosis may be caused by many different genetic changes, such as homozygosity for the common ΔF508 mutation, or ΔF508 and an R117H mutation. The latter example represents **compound heterozygosity.**

8. Phenotypic heterogeneity or "clinical heterogeneity"—This term describes the situation in which more than one phenotype is caused by different allelic mutations at a single locus. For example, different mutations in the *FGFR2* gene can cause different craniosynostosis disorders, including Crouzon syndrome, Jackson-Weiss syndrome, Pfeiffer syndrome, and Apert syndrome. These syndromes are clinically distinguishable and are due to the presence of a variety of genetic mutations within single genes.

9. Homozygous—A cell or organism that has identical alleles at a particular locus is said to be homozygous. For example, a cystic fibrosis patient with a ΔF508 mutation on both alleles would be called homozygous for that mutation.

10. Heterozygous—A cell or organism that has nonidentical alleles at a genetic locus is said to be heterozygous. In autosomal dominant conditions, a mutation of only one copy of the gene pair is all that is necessary to result in a disease state. However, an individual who is heterozygous for a recessive disorder will not manifest symptoms (see next section).

Online Mendelian Inheritance in Man: http://www.ncbi.nlm.nih.gov/entrez/query.fcgi?db=OMIM

Hereditary Patterns

A. Autosomal Dominant Inheritance

Autosomal dominant inheritance has the following characteristics:

1. Affected individuals in the same family may experience variable expressivity.
2. Nonpenetrance is common, and the penetrance rate varies for each dominantly inherited condition.
3. Both males and females can pass on the abnormal gene to children of either sex, although the manifestations may vary according to sex. For example, pattern baldness is a dominant trait but affects only males. In this case, the trait is said to be sex-limited.
4. Dominant inheritance is typically said to be vertical, that is, the condition passes from one generation to the next in a vertical fashion (Figure 35–6).
5. In some cases, the family history seems to be completely negative, and the patient appears to be the first affected individual. This spontaneous appearance may be caused by a new mutation. In more severe disorders, where there is a decrease in reproductive fitness, there is a high rate of new mutations. The mutation rate increases with advancing paternal age (particularly after age 40 years). Several other explanations for a negative family history are possible, however, including:
   a. Nonpaternity.
   b. Decreased penetrance or mild manifestations in one of the parents.

LEGEND:

☐ Male   ◐ Scoliosis   ◨ Café-au-lait spots

○ Female   ◐ Neurofibromata   ◨ Mental retardation

▲ **Figure 35–6.** Autosomal dominant inheritance. Variable expressivity in neurofibromatosis type 1.

c. Germline mosaicism (ie, mosaicism in the germ cell line of either parent), in which case the risk of recurrence increases. Germline mosaicism may mimic autosomal recessive inheritance, because it leads to situations in which two children of completely normal parents are affected with a genetic disorder. The best example of this is osteogenesis imperfecta type II. Laboratory studies have documented germline mosaicism by finding that only one allele of the paired collagen genes is abnormal in the severe form instead of both, as would be expected in a recessive disease. The recurrence risk in this form of osteogenesis imperfecta is 7%.

d. The abnormality present in the patient may be a phenocopy, or it may be a similar but genetically different abnormality with a different mode of inheritance.

6. As a general rule, dominant traits are more often related to structural abnormalities of protein, as for example in Marfan syndrome.

7. If a parent is affected, the risk for each offspring of inheriting the abnormal dominant gene is 50%, or 1:2. This is true whether the gene is penetrant or not in the parent.

8. The severity of the condition in the offspring is not related to the severity in the affected parent. In some disorders, it may be related to the sex of the parent transmitting the gene. For example, if the gene for myotonic dystrophy is passed through the mother, there is a 10–20% chance that the child (regardless of sex) may have a severe congenital form of the disease. Conversely, if the gene for Huntington disease is passed through the father, the probability is 5–10% that the offspring may have the severe, rigid juvenile form. In these two conditions the inheritance of the gene is associated with expansion of the triplet repeats (see section on Genetic Anticipation, later).

9. If an abnormality represents a new mutation of a dominant trait, the parents of the affected individual run a low risk during subsequent pregnancies, but the risk for the offspring of the affected individual is 50%. Although a mutation is thought to be new because the parents are not affected, the risk for an affected sibling is still slightly increased over the general population, because of the possibility of germline mosaicism.

10. Prevention options available for future pregnancies include prenatal diagnosis, artificial insemination, and egg or sperm donation, depending on which parent has the abnormal gene.

B. Autosomal Recessive Inheritance

Autosomal recessive inheritance also has some distinctive characteristics:

1. There is less variability among affected persons. Parents are carriers and are clinically normal. (There are, however, exceptions to this rule. For example, carriers of sickle cell trait may become symptomatic if they become hypoxic.)

2. Males and females are affected equally.

3. Inheritance is horizontal; siblings may be affected (Figure 35–7).

4. Recessive conditions are usually rare; the rarer the condition, the more likely it is that consanguinity is present. Conversely, if a child whose parents are related presents with an unrecognized abnormality, a recessive condition must be suspected.

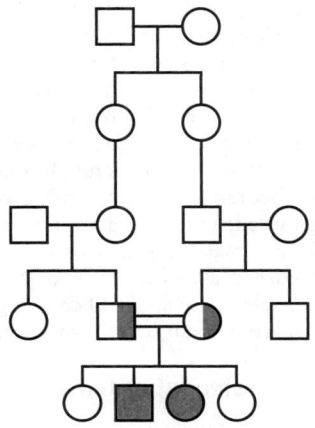

LEGEND:

■ Affected (Cystic fibrosis)   ☐—○ Consanguineous marriage

◐ Carrier

▲ **Figure 35–7.** Autosomal recessive inheritance: cystic fibrosis.

5. The family history is usually negative, with the exception of siblings. However, in common conditions such as cystic fibrosis, a second- or third-degree relative may be affected.

6. Recessive conditions are frequently associated with enzyme defects.

7. The recurrence risk for parents of an affected child is 25%, or 1:4 for each pregnancy. The gene carrier frequency in the general population can be used to assess the risk of having an affected child with a new partner, for unaffected siblings, and for the affected individuals themselves.

8. In rare instances, a child with a recessive disorder and a normal karyotype may have inherited both copies of the abnormal gene from one parent and none from the other. This uniparental disomy (UPD) was first described in a girl with cystic fibrosis and growth retardation. This phenomenon is of unknown frequency, but it is more likely to be present in a child with more than one autosomal recessive condition, or in a patient with unexpected and seemingly unrelated abnormalities or severe growth retardation. Molecular testing can confirm the presence of UPD. The recurrence risk is obviously lower in such a situation, although the factors predisposing to UPD are unknown. Maternal age may play a role in these situations.

9. Options available for future pregnancies include prenatal diagnosis, adoption, artificial insemination, and egg or sperm donation.

C. X-Linked Inheritance

When a gene for a specific disorder is on the X chromosome, the condition is said to be X-linked, or sex-linked. Females may be either homozygous or heterozygous, because they have two X chromosomes. Males, by contrast, have only one X, and a male is said to be hemizygous for any gene on his X chromosome. The severity of any disorder is greater in males than in females (within a specific family). According to the Lyon hypothesis, because one of the two X chromosomes in each cell is inactivated, and this inactivation is random, the clinical picture in females depends on the percentage of mutant versus normal alleles inactivated. The X chromosome is not inactivated until about 14 days of gestation, and parts of the short arm remain active throughout life.

D. X-Linked Recessive Inheritance

The following features are characteristic of X-linked recessive inheritance:

1. Males are affected, and heterozygous females are either normal or have mild manifestations.

2. Inheritance is diagonal through the maternal side of the family (Figure 35–8A).

3. A female carrier has a 50% chance that each daughter will be a carrier and a 50% chance that each son will be affected.

4. All of the daughters of an affected male are carriers, and none of his sons are affected. Because a father can give only his Y chromosome to his sons, male-to-male transmission excludes X-linked inheritance except in the rare case of UPD, in which a son receives both the X and the Y from his father.

5. The mutation rate is high in some X-linked disorders, particularly when the affected male dies or is so incapacitated by the disorder that reproduction is unlikely. In such instances, the mutation is thought to occur as a new mutation in the affected male, and in the mother, each one third of the time and to be present in earlier generations one third of the time. For this reason, genetic counseling may be difficult in families with an isolated case.

6. On rare occasions, a female may be fully affected. Several possible mechanisms may account for a fully affected female: (a) unfavorable lyonization; (b) 45,X karyotype; (c) homozygosity for the abnormal gene; (d) an X-autosome translocation, or other structural abnormality of one X chromosome, in which the X chromosome of normal structure is preferentially inactivated; (e) UPD; and (f) nonrandom inactivation, which may be controlled by an autosomal gene.

E. X-Linked Dominant Inheritance

The X-linked dominant inheritance pattern is much less common than the X-linked recessive type. Examples include incontinentia pigmenti and hypophosphatemic or vitamin D–resistant rickets.

1. The heterozygous female is symptomatic, and the disease is twice as common in females because they have two X chromosomes that can have the mutation.

2. Clinical manifestations are more variable in females than in males.

3. The risk for the offspring of heterozygous females to be affected is 50% regardless of sex.

4. All of the daughters but none of the sons of affected males will have the disorder (see Figure 35–8B).

5. Although a homozygous female is possible (particularly in an inbred population), she would be severely involved. All of her children would also be affected but more mildly.

6. Some disorders (eg, incontinentia pigmenti) are lethal in males (and in homozygous females). Affected women have twice as many daughters as sons and an increased incidence of miscarriages, because affected males will be spontaneously aborted. A 47,XXY karyotype has allowed affected males to survive.

F. Y-Linked Inheritance

In Y-linked inheritance, also known as "holandric" inheritance, a disorder is caused by genes located on the Y chromo-

LEGEND:

■ Duchenne-muscular dystrophy

◐ Carrier

† Deceased

LEGEND:

■ Affected male

● Affected female

▲ **Figure 35–8.** **A:** X-linked recessive inheritance. **B:** X-linked dominant inheritance.

some. These conditions are relatively rare with only about 40 entries listed in McKusick's catalog. Male-to-male transmission is seen in this category, with all sons of affected males being affected and no daughters or females being affected.

MULTIFACTORIAL INHERITANCE

Many common attributes, such as height, are familial, and are the result of the actions of multiple rather than single genes. Inheritance of these traits is described as **polygenic** or **multifactorial.** The latter term recognizes that environmental factors such as diet also contribute to these traits. Geneticists are now finding that multiple genes are often expressed

in hierarchies, in which the action of a small number of genes, two or three, explains much of the variation observed within affected populations.

Studies of twins have proven useful in determining the relative importance of genetic versus environmental factors in the expression of polygenic traits. If genetic factors are of little or no importance, then the concordance between monozygotic and dizygotic twins should be the same. (Dizygotic twins are no more genetically similar to each other than to other siblings.) If an abnormality is completely genetic, the concordance between identical twins should be 100%. In polygenic conditions, the concordance rate for identical twins is usually higher than that seen in dizygotic twins but is still not 100%, indicating that both genetic and environmental factors are playing a role.

Many disorders and congenital abnormalities that are clearly familial but do not segregate as mendelian traits (eg, autosomal dominant, recessive, etc) show polygenic inheritance. For the most part, these conditions become manifest when thresholds of additive gene actions or contributing environmental factors are exceeded. Many common disorders ranging from hypertension, stroke, and thrombophlebitis to behavioral traits such as alcoholism demonstrate multifactorial (polygenic) inheritance. Some common birth defects, including isolated congenital heart disease, cleft lip and palate, and neural tube defects, also demonstrate polygenic inheritance. Neural tube defects provide a good model illustrating how identification of both environmental and genetic contributions to multifactorial traits can lead to preventive measures.

Polygenic or multifactorial inheritance has several distinctive characteristics:

1. The risk for relatives of affected persons is increased. The risk is higher for first-degree relatives (those who have 50% of their genes in common) and lower for more distant relations, although the risk for the latter is higher than for the general population (Table 35–2).

2. The recurrence risk varies with the number of affected family members. For example, after one child is born with a neural tube defect, the recurrence risk is 2–3%. If a second affected child is born, the risk for any future child increases to 10–12%. This is in contrast to single gene disorders, in which the risk is the same no matter how many family members are affected.

3. The risk is higher if the defect is more severe. In Hirschsprung disease, another polygenic condition, the longer the aganglionic segment, the higher is the recurrence risk.

4. Sex ratios may not be equal. If a marked discrepancy exists, the recurrence risk is higher if a child of the less commonly affected sex has the disorder. This assumes that more genetic factors are required to raise the more resistant sex above the threshold. For example, pyloric stenosis is more common in males. If the first affected child is a female, the recurrence risk is higher than if the child is a male.

5. The risk for the offspring of an affected person is approximately the same as the risk for siblings, assuming that the spouse of the affected person has a negative family history. For many conditions, however, assortative mating, "like marrying like," adds to risks in offspring.

NONMENDELIAN INHERITANCE

Epigenetic Regulation

Although development is regulated by genes, it is initiated and sustained by nongenetic processes. Epigenetic events are points

Table 35–2. Empiric risks for some congenital disorders.

Anencephaly and spina bifida: incidence (average) 1:1000	
One affected child: 2–3%	
Two affected children: 10–12%	
One affected parent: 4–5%	
Hydrocephalus: incidence 1:2000 newborns	
Occasional X-linked recessive	
Often associated with neural tube defect	
Some environmental etiologies (eg, toxoplasmosis)	
Recurrence risk, one affected child	
Hydrocephalus: 1%	
Some central nervous system abnormality: 3%	
Nonsyndromic cleft lip and/or palate: incidence (average) 1:1000	
One affected child: 2–4%	
One affected parent: 2–4%	
Two affected children: 10%	
One affected parent, one affected child: 10–20%	
Nonsyndromic cleft palate: incidence 1:2000	
One affected child: 2%	
Two affected children: 6–8%	
One affected parent: 4–6%	
One affected parent, one affected child: 15–20%	
Congenital heart disease: incidence 8:1000	
One affected child: 2–3%	
One affected parent, one affected child: 10%	
Clubfoot: incidence 1:1000 (male: female = 2:1)	
One affected child: 2–3%	
Congenital dislocated hip: incidence 1:1000	
(female > male) with marked regional variation	
One child affected: 2–14%	
Pyloric stenosis: Incidence, males: 1:200; females: 1:1000	
Male index patient	
Brothers	3.2%
Sons	6.8%
Sisters	3.0%
Daughters	1.2%
Female index patient	
Brothers	13.2%
Sons	20.5%
Sisters	2.5%
Daughters	11.1%

of interaction between developmental programs and the physicochemical environments in differentiating cells. Genetic imprinting and DNA methylation are examples of epigenetic processes that affect development. Certain genes important in regulation of growth and differentiation are themselves regulated by chemical modification that occurs in specific patterns in gametes. For example, genes that are methylated are "turned off" and not transcribed. The pattern of which genes are methylated may be determined or affected by the sex of the parent of origin (see next section). Expression of imprinted genes may sometimes be limited to specific organs (eg, the brain), and imprinting may be relaxed and methyl groups lost as development progresses. Disruption of imprinting is now recognized as contributing to birth defect syndromes (described later in this chapter). Certain techniques developed to assist infertile couples (advanced reproductive technology) may affect epigenetic processes and lead to genetic disorders in the offspring conceived via these methods.

Niemitz EL, Feinberg AP: Epigenetics and assisted reproductive technology: A call for investigation. Am J Hum Genet 2004;74:599 [PMID: 14991528].

Imprinting

Although the homologs of chromosome pairs may appear identical on routine karyotype analysis, it is now known that the parental origin of each homolog can affect which genes are actually transcribed and which are inactivated. The term *imprinting* refers to the process by which preferential transcription of certain genes takes place, depending on the parental origin, that is, which homolog (maternal or paternal) the gene is located on. Certain chromosomes, particularly chromosome X, and the autosomes 15, 11, and 7, have imprinted regions where certain genes are only read from one homolog (ie, either the maternal or paternal allele) under normal circumstances, and the gene on the other homolog is normally inactivated. Errors in imprinting may arise because of UPD (in which a copy from one parent is missing), by a chromosomal deletion causing loss of the gene normally transcribed, or by mutations in the imprinting genes that normally code for transcription or inactivation of other genes downstream. A good example of how imprinting may affect human disease is Beckwith-Wiedemann syndrome, the gene for which is located on chromosome 11p15.

Cohen MM et al: *Overgrowth Syndromes*. Oxford University Press, 2002.

Genetic Anticipation

Geneticists coined the term "anticipation" to describe an unusual pattern of inheritance in which symptoms became manifest at earlier ages and with increasing severity as traits are passed to subsequent generations. Mapping of the genes responsible for these disorders led to the discovery that certain repeat sequences of DNA at disease loci were not stable when passed through meiosis. Repeated DNA sequences, in particular triplets (eg, CGG and CAG), tended to increase their copy number. As these runs of triplets

expanded, they eventually affected the expression of genes and produced symptoms. Curiously, all the disorders undergoing triplet repeat expansion detected thus far produce neurologic symptoms. Most are progressive. In general, the size of the triplet expansion is roughly correlated with the timing and severity of symptoms. The reasons for the meiotic instability of these sequences are not yet understood. The mechanisms appear to involve interactions between DNA structure (eg, formation of hairpin loops) and replication enzymes (DNA polymerase complexes) during meiosis.

Triplet repeat instability can modify the inheritance of autosomal dominant, autosomal recessive, and X-linked traits. Autosomal dominant disorders include several spinal cerebellar atrophies, Huntington disease, and myotonic dystrophy. Unstable triplet repeat expansion contributes to at least one autosomal recessive disorder, Friedreich ataxia. The most common X-linked disorder demonstrating triplet repeat instability and expansion is fragile X syndrome.

Mitochondrial Inheritance

Mitochondrial DNA is double-stranded, circular, and smaller than nuclear DNA, and is found in the cytoplasm. It codes for enzymes involved in oxidative phosphorylation, which generates adenosine triphosphate. Since the 1990s, enormous advances in technology and improved clinical documentation have led to a better understanding of the interesting disorders caused by mutations in mitochondrial DNA (mtDNA).

Mitochondrial disorders have been associated with deletions or duplications in mtDNA. Large deletions are usually sporadic, but smaller deletions may be secondary events due to defects in dominantly inherited nuclear genes. Mitochondrial dysfunction may also be caused by mutations in nuclear genes encoding mitochondrial proteins and can be inherited as dominant, recessive, or X-linked traits. Because of the difficulty in diagnosing mitochondrial disorders and the variability of the clinical course, it is often difficult to calculate specific recurrence risks.

Mitochondrial disorders have the following characteristics:

1. They show remarkable phenotypic variability.

2. They are maternally inherited, because only the egg has any cytoplasmic material, and during early embryogenesis any sperm-born mitochondrial material will be eliminated.

3. In most mitochondrial disorders, cells are heteroplasmic (Figure 35–9). That is, all cells contain both normal and mutated or abnormal mtDNA. The proportion of normal to abnormal mtDNA in the mother's egg seems to determine the severity of the offspring's disease and the age at onset in most cases.

4. Those tissues with the highest adenosine triphosphate requirements—specifically, central nervous system (CNS) and skeletal muscle—seem to be most susceptible to mutations in mtDNA.

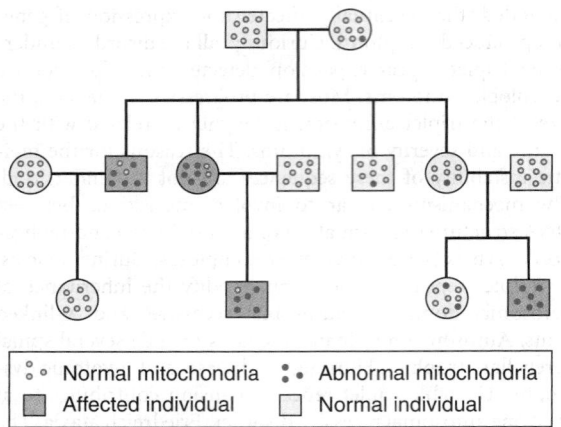

° ° Normal mitochondria	• • Abnormal mitochondria
▨ Affected individual	☐ Normal individual

▲ **Figure 35–9.** Mitochondrial inheritance. Mutations are transmitted through the maternal line.

5. Somatic cells show an increase in mtDNA mutations and a decline in oxidative phosphorylation function with age. This explains the later onset of some of these disorders and may indeed be a clue to the whole aging process.

Hayashida K et al: The sperm mitochondria—Specific translocator has a key role in maternal mitochondrial inheritance. Cell Biol Int 2005;29:472 [PMID: 15979907].

FAMILY HISTORY & PEDIGREE

The first step in the collection of information regarding the genetics of a syndromic diagnosis is the construction of a family tree or pedigree. Underused by most medical personnel, the pedigree is a valuable record of genetic and medical information, which is much more useful in visual form than in list form. Tips for pedigree preparation include the following:

- Start with the proband—the patient's siblings and parents, and obtain a three-generational history if possible.
- Always ask about consanguinity.
- Obtain data from both sides of the family.
- Ask about spontaneous abortions, stillbirths, infertility, children relinquished for adoption, and deceased individuals.

In the course of taking the family history, one may find information that is not relevant in elucidating the cause of the patients' problem but may indicate a risk for other important health concerns. Such information should be appropriately followed and addressed. Such conditions that may arise are an overwhelming family history of early-onset breast and ovarian cancer, or multiple pregnancy losses necessitating chromosome analyses.

Dysmorphology & Human Embryology

Birth defects are the leading cause of death in the first year of life. They are evident in 2–3% of newborn infants and in up to 7% of adults. Many are now detected by ultrasound prior to birth. Clinical investigation of the causes and consequences of birth defects is called dysmorphology.

MECHANISMS

Developmental Genetics

Most birth defects are multifactorial: They result from imbalances between genetic processes regulating development and the environments in which they unfold. Specific causes of maldevelopment can be identified in about 35% of cases, but advances in developmental biology and human genetics promise better understanding. So far, single gene mutations and chromosomal abnormalities account for at least 25% of birth defects, with the numbers of specific genes and chromosome loci now being associated with recurring phenotypes, or syndromes, rapidly increasing.

Genes for the fundamental processes regulating cell division, or proliferation, and those that program cell death, or apoptosis, are now being described. Both cellular proliferation and apoptosis are very active in embryogenesis and the balance between these processes is easily disrupted. Imbalances in the regulation of cell cycles are an important determinant of birth defects and may contribute to such commonly occurring problems as neural tube defects, branchial arch anomalies, limb reductions, and congenital heart disease.

Morphogenic processes and the genes that regulate them have been highly conserved through evolution. Thus, experiments in lower organisms such as *Drosophila* (fruit flies) can identify candidate genes for human birth defects. For example, mutations in *pax* genes, which are involved in eye development in *Drosophila* produce "small eye" in mice, and aniridia and other abnormalities of the anterior chamber of the eyes of humans.

Embryology and developmental biology have recently and rapidly moved from descriptive to experimental disciplines that use tools such as in situ hybridization to visualize the expression of genes in embryos, and transgenic animals in which developmentally active genes are "knocked out" to determine the contributions of specific genes to organ development. These investigations have uncovered, for example, important regulatory interactions such as the hedgehog signaling pathway, which affects morphogenesis in organs as diverse as limbs, the heart, and the CNS. Human mutations in one evolutionarily conserved gene, sonic hedgehog (*SHH*), can result in holoprosencephaly, a severe birth defect in which the CNS fails to complete its normal hemispheric division.

Cellular Interactions

The picture emerging from experimental studies of morphogenesis is one of a hierarchy of gene expression during development. Morphogenesis begins with expression of genes encoding transcription factors. These proteins bind to DNA in undifferentiated embryonic cells and recruit them into developmental fields, groups of cells primed to respond to specific signals later in development. This recruitment also establishes spatial relationships and orients cells with respect to their neighbors. As fields differentiate into identifiable tissues (eg, ectoderm, mesoderm, and endoderm), cellular proliferation, migration, and further differentiation are mediated through genes encoding cell signaling proteins.

Signaling proteins include growth factors and their receptors, cellular adhesion molecules, and extracellular matrix proteins that both provide structure and position signals within developing structures. During morphogenesis groups of primed cells repeatedly proliferate, migrate, and then differentiate in response to locally expressed growth factors or signaling proteins. Within these interactions are keys to understanding not only many human birth defects but also cancer. The genes that organize cell proliferation and differentiation during development are often precisely those that mutate during carcinogenesis.

Environmental Factors

The effects of exogenous agents during development are also mediated through genetically regulated pathways. At the cellular level, xenobiotics (compounds foreign to nature) cause birth defects either because they disrupt cell signaling and thereby misdirect morphogenesis, or because they are cytotoxic and lead to cell death in excess of the usual developmental program.

In general, drug receptors expressed in embryos and fetuses are the same molecules that mediate pharmacologic effects in adults. However, effector systems may be different, reflecting incomplete morphogenesis and differences between fetal and postnatal physiology. These circumstances allow prediction of dose-response relationships during development on the one hand, but call for caution about predicting effects on the other.

Xenobiotics must traverse the placenta to affect embryonic and fetal tissues. The human placenta is a relatively good barrier against microorganisms, but it is ineffective at excluding drugs and many chemicals. The physicochemical properties (eg, molecular size, solubility, and charge) that allow foreign chemicals to be absorbed into the maternal circulation also allow them to cross the placenta. The placenta can metabolize some xenobiotics but it is far more active against steroid hormones and low-level environmental contaminants than drugs.

The timing of xenobiotic exposures is an important determinant of their effects. Morphogenic processes express so-called critical periods, during which the organs they produce are particularly susceptible to maldevelopment. Figure 35–10 shows critical periods of development for the major organs of the fetus. Periods of susceptibility are not all confined to early gestation. Note, in particular, that the developing brain is susceptible to toxicity throughout pregnancy.

As discussed, over-the-counter, prescribed, and abused drugs that are pharmacologically active in mothers will, in general, equilibrate to the same levels across the placenta. Agents known to produce cytotoxicity at these levels in adults are therefore likely to be teratogenic (ie, cause birth defects). Abused substances such as alcohol that are toxic to adults are predictably toxic to embryos and fetuses. Drugs generally safe in adults will be generally safe for fetuses. However, keeping in mind that embryonic and fetal physiology may differ from that of an adult in response to pharmacologic agents, some risk for abnormal development must always be considered. Risk assessment requires continuous monitoring of populations exposed to drugs during pregnancy.

Effects of toxic environmental contaminants on the embryo and fetus are also dose-dependent. Thus, the level of exposure to a toxin frequently becomes the primary determinant of its risk. Exposures producing symptoms in mothers can be assumed to be potentially toxic to the fetus.

Environmental mutagens present a special problem. Animal experiments indicate that high levels of exposure to mutagenic agents are also teratogenic. Most effects are mediated through increased apoptosis responding to DNA damage. This is especially true for the developing brain. At lower doses attempts to repair DNA damage in embryonic or fetal cells may lead to somatic mutations that can contribute to carcinogenesis or be expressed as mosaic organ dysgenesis.

Not all transplacental pharmacologic effects are toxic. The potential for therapeutic uses of drugs during pregnancy is increasing. For example, folic acid supplementation can lower risks for birth defects such as spina bifida, and maternally administered corticosteroids can induce fetal synthesis and secretion of pulmonary surfactants prior to delivery.

MECHANICAL FACTORS

Much of embryonic development and all of fetal growth occurs normally within the low pressure and space provided by amniotic fluid. Loss or inadequate production of amniotic fluid can have disastrous effects, as can disruption of placental membranes. When this occurs early in gestation, for whatever reason, major, often lethal, distortion of the embryo (early amnion disruption sequence) results. Later, deformation or even amputation of fetal extremities (amniotic band sequence) can occur.

Movement is also important for morphogenesis. Fetal movement is necessary for normal development of joints and is the principal determinant of folds and creases present at birth in the face, hands, feet, and other areas of the body. Clubfoot is an etiologically heterogeneous condition in which the foot is malpositioned at birth. It more often results from mechanical constraint secondary to intrauterine crowding, weak fetal muscles, or abnormal neurologic function than from primary skeletal maldevelopment.

Lung and kidney development are particularly sensitive to mechanical forces. Constriction of the chest through maldevelopment of the ribs, lack of surrounding amniotic fluid, or lack of movement (fetal breathing) leads to varying degrees of pulmonary hypoplasia in which lungs are smaller than normal and develop fewer alveoli. Mechanically induced pulmonary hypoplasia is a common cause of respiratory distress at birth and may be lethal.

Cystic renal dysplasia commonly accompanies birth defects that obstruct ureters or outflow from the bladder. As urinary pressure within obstructed collecting systems increases it distorts cell surface interactions in developing tissues and alters

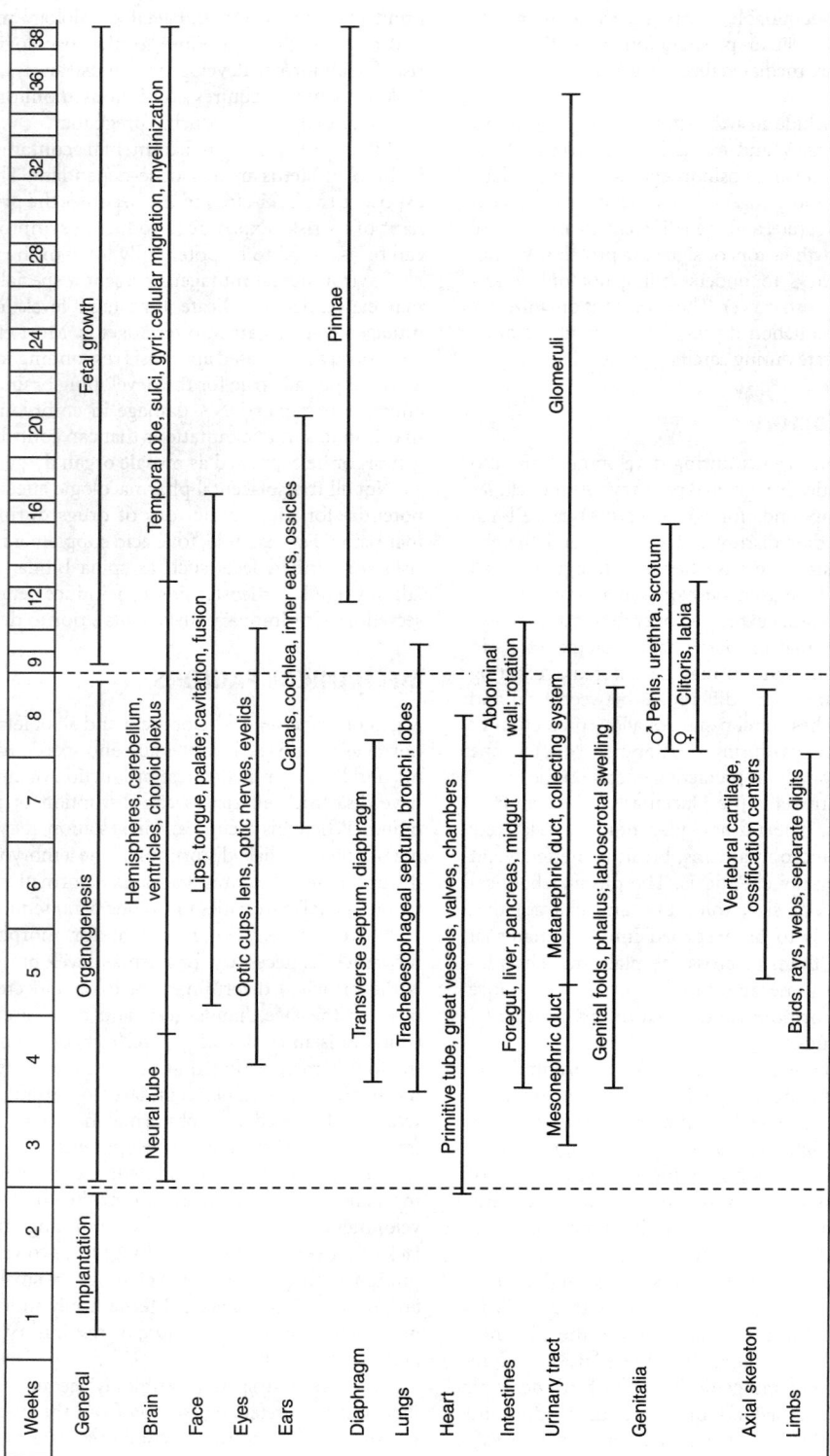

▲ **Figure 35–10.** Critical periods in human gestation.

histogenesis. Developing kidneys exposed to increased internal pressures for long periods eventually become nonfunctional.

CLINICAL DYSMORPHOLOGY

Terminology

Classification of dysmorphic features strives to reflect mechanisms of maldevelopment. However, much of the terminology that describes abnormal development in humans remains historical and documents recognition of patterns prior to understanding of their biology. For example, birth defects are referred to as **malformations** when they result from altered genetic or developmental processes. When physical forces interrupt or distort morphogenesis, their effects are termed **disruptions** and **deformations,** respectively. The term **dysplasia** is used to denote abnormal histogenesis. Malformations occurring together more frequently than would be expected by chance alone may be classified as belonging to **associations.** Those in which the order of maldevelopment is understood may be referred to as **sequences.** For example, Robin sequence (or Pierre Robin anomalad) is used to describe cleft palate that has occurred because poor growth of the jaw (retrognathia) has displaced the tongue and prevented posterior closure of the palate. **Syndromes** are simply recurrent patterns of maldevelopment.

Evaluation of the Dysmorphic Infant

Physicians caring for infants with birth defects frequently must seek accurate diagnoses and provide care under conditions of great stress. The extent of an infant's abnormalities may not be immediately apparent, and parents who feel grief and guilt are often desperate for information. As with any medical problem, however, the history and physical examination provide most of the clues to diagnosis. Special aspects of these procedures are outlined in the following sections.

A. History

Pregnancy histories nearly always contain important clues to the diagnosis. Parental recall after delivery of an abnormal infant is better than recall after a normal birth. An obstetric wheel can help document gestational age and events of the first trimester: the last menstrual period, the onset of symptoms of pregnancy, the date of diagnosis of the pregnancy, the date of the first prenatal visit, and the physician's impressions of fetal growth at that time. Family histories should always be reviewed. Environmental histories should include descriptions of parental habits and work settings in addition to medications and use of drugs, tobacco, and alcohol.

B. Physical Examination

Meticulous physical examination is crucial for accurate diagnosis in dysmorphic infants and children. In addition to the routine procedures described in Chapter 1, special attention should be paid to the neonate's physical measurements (Figure 35–11). Photographs are helpful and should include a ruler for reference.

C. Imaging and Laboratory Studies

Radiologic and ultrasonographic examinations can be extremely helpful in the evaluation of dysmorphic infants. Films of infants with apparent limb or skeletal anomalies should include views of the skull and all of the long bones in addition to frontal and lateral views of the axial skeleton. Chest and abdominal films should be obtained when indicated. The pediatrician should consult a radiologist for further workup. Computed tomography (CT), magnetic resonance imaging (MRI), and ultrasonography are all useful diagnostic tools, but their interpretation in the face of birth defects may require considerable experience.

Cytogenetic analysis provides specific diagnoses in approximately 5% of dysmorphic infants who survive the newborn period. Chromosomal abnormalities are recognized in 10–15% of infants who die. Common disorders such as trisomies 21 and 18 can be determined rapidly through use of FISH, but this technique is limited and should always be accompanied by a complete karyotype. A normal karyotype does not rule out the presence of significant genetic disease. Any case requiring rapid diagnosis should be discussed with an experienced clinical geneticist.

D. Perinatal Autopsy

When a dysmorphic infant dies, postmortem examination can provide important diagnostic information. The pediatrician should discuss the case thoroughly with the pathologist, and photographs should always be taken. Radiologic imaging should be included whenever limb anomalies or disproportionate growth is present. Tissue, most often skin, should be submitted for cytogenetic analysis. The pediatrician and the pathologist should also consider whether samples of blood, urine, or other tissue should be obtained for biochemical analyses. Placental as well as fetal tissue can be used for viral culture.

CHROMOSOMAL DISORDERS: ABNORMAL NUMBER

TRISOMIES

1. Trisomy 21 (Down Syndrome)

ESSENTIALS OF DIAGNOSIS & TYPICAL FEATURES

▶ Small, brachycephalic head; characteristic facies of upslanting palpebral fissures, epicanthal folds, midface hypoplasia, and small, dysplastic pinnae.

▶ Generalized hypotonia.

Measurement	Range (cm)	
	Term (38–40 week)	Preterm (38–40 week)
1 Head circumference	32–37	27–32
2 Anterior fontanelle $\left(\dfrac{L-W}{2}\right)$	0.7–3.7	. . .
3 Interpupillary distance	3.3–4.5	3.1–3.9
4 Palpebral fissure	1.5–2.1	1.3–1.6
5 Inner canthal distance	1.5–2.5	1.4–2.1
6 Outer canthal distance	5.3–7.3	3.9–5.1
7 Philtrum	0.6–1.2	0.5–0.9
8 Ear length	3–4.3	2.4–3.5
9 Chest circumference	28–38	23–29
10 Internipple distance*	6.5–10	5–6.5
11 Height	47–55	39–47
12 Ratio $\dfrac{\text{Upper body segment}}{\text{Lower body segment}}$ 13	1.7	. . .
14 Hand (palm to middle finger)	5.3–7.8	4.1–5.5
15 Ratio of middle finger to hand	0.38–0.48	0.38–0.5
16 Penis (pubic bone to tip of glans)	2.7–4.3	1.8–3.2

*Internipple distance should not exceed 25% of chest circumference.

▲ **Figure 35–11.** Neonatal measurements.

- Cognitive disabilities (mild to severe).
- Associated with congenital heart disease and gastrointestinal anomalies.

Down syndrome occurs in about 1:600 newborns; however, the incidence is greater if the mother is older than age 35 years. Cognitive disabilities are characteristic of Down syndrome, with typical intelligence quotients (IQs) between 20 and 80 (mostly between 45 and 55). Generalized hypotonia is common. Sexual development is delayed, especially in males, who are usually sterile. The affected newborn may have prolonged physiologic jaundice, polycythemia, and a transient leukemoid reaction. Later, there is an increased tendency for thyroid dysfunction, hearing loss, celiac disease, and atlanto-occipital instability. Leukemia is 12–20 times more common in Down syndrome patients than in unaffected children.

Clinical Findings

The principal physical findings include a small, brachycephalic head, characteristic facies (up-slanting palpebral fissures, epicanthal folds, midface hypoplasia, and small, dysplastic pinnae), and minor limb abnormalities. About one third to one half of children with Down syndrome have congenital heart disease, most often endocardial cushion defects or other septal defects. Anomalies of the gastrointestinal tract, including esophageal and duodenal atresias, are seen in about 15% of cases.

Information regarding health care guidelines for patients with Down syndrome can be found at http://www.downsyn.com/guidelines/healthcare.html.

2. Trisomy 18 Syndrome

The incidence of trisomy 18 syndrome is about 1:4000 live births, and the ratio of affected males to females is approximately 1:3. Trisomy 18 is characterized by prenatal and postnatal growth retardation that is often severe, and hypertonicity. Complications are related to associated birth defects. Death is often caused by heart failure or pneumonia and usually occurs in infancy or early childhood, although a small percentage of patients reach adulthood. Surviving children show significant developmental delay.

Clinical Findings

Infants with trisomy 18 are often small for gestational age and have dysmorphic features including a characteristic facies and extremities (overlapping fingers and rockerbottom feet), and congenital heart disease (often ventricular septal defect or patent ductus arteriosus). To see clinical pictures of patients with trisomy 18, go to the following web site: http://medgen.genetics.utah.edu/photographs/pages/trisomy_18.htm.

3. Trisomy 13 Syndrome

The incidence of trisomy 13 is about 1:12,000 live births, and 60% of affected individuals are female. Most infants with trisomy 13 have congenital anomalies that are incompatible with survival. Surviving children demonstrate failure to thrive, developmental retardation, apneic spells, seizures, and deafness. Death usually occurs in early infancy or by the second year of life, commonly as a result of heart failure or infection.

Clinical Findings

The symptoms and signs include prenatal and postnatal growth deficiency (although, unlike trisomy 18, infants may have a normal birth weight), CNS malformations, arrhinencephaly, eye malformations (anophthalmia, colobomas), cleft lip and palate, polydactyly or syndactyly, and congenital heart disease (usually ventricular septal defect). The facies of an infant with trisomy 13 can be viewed at the following web site: http://medgen.genetics.utah.edu/photographs/pages/trisomy_13.htm.

Treatment of Trisomies

A. Medical Therapy

No convincing documentation is available relative to the merit of any of the forms of alternative therapy that have been attempted in Down syndrome, ranging from megadoses of vitamins to amino acid solutions. However, interventions for specific issues such as surgery or medications for heart problems, antibiotics for infections and thyroid function tests, infant stimulation programs, special education, and physical, occupational, and speech therapies are all indicated. The goal of treatment is to help affected children develop to their full potential. Parents' participation in support groups such as the local chapter of the National Down Syndrome Congress should be encouraged. See the following web site: http://www.ndss.org/.

There is no treatment, other than general supportive care, for trisomy 13 or 18. Because it is sometimes necessary to decide immediately after birth how extensive therapy should be for a severely malformed infant, trisomies 13 and 18 can be screened for in interphase nuclei of blood lymphocytes by FISH and confirmed by direct chromosome analysis of blood or bone marrow mitoses. A support group for families of children with trisomies 13 and 18 who survive beyond infancy is called SOFT. See the following web site: http://www.trisomy.org/.

B. Genetic Counseling

Most parents of trisomic infants have normal karyotypes. The risk of having a child affected with a trisomy varies with maternal age. For trisomy 21, age-specific risks are 1:2000 for mothers younger than 25 years; 1:200 for mothers 35 years of age; and 1:100 for mothers at age 40. The recurrence risk for trisomy in future pregnancies is equal to 1:100 plus the age-specific maternal risk; for example, a 40-year-old mother who has already given birth to a child with Down syndrome would have a risk of 1:100 for her age, plus 1:100 for her prior history, or 1:50.

If the child has a trisomy resulting from a translocation, and the parent has an abnormal karyotype, the risks are increased. When the mother is the carrier of a balanced 14/21 translocation, there is a 10–15% chance that the child will be affected and a 33% chance that the child will be a balanced translocation carrier. When the father is the carrier, there is a smaller than 0.5% chance of having another affected child. If the child has a 21/21 translocation and one parent has the translocation, the recurrence risk is 100%.

The recurrence risks in other trisomies are analogous to those for Down syndrome. The mother's age at the time of conception and the nature of the chromosomal abnormality are important in genetic counseling, which is indicated for prevention of all chromosomal abnormalities. Prenatal diagnosis is available.

SEX CHROMOSOME ABNORMALITIES

1. Turner Syndrome (Monosomy X, Gonadal Dysgenesis)

ESSENTIALS OF DIAGNOSIS & TYPICAL FEATURES

▶ Webbed neck, triangular facies, short stature, wide-set nipples, amenorrhea, and absence of secondary sex characteristics.

▶ Associated with coarctation of the aorta and genitourinary malformations.

▶ IQ is usually normal but learning disabilities are common.

▶ Mosaic individuals may manifest only short stature and amenorrhea.

The incidence of Turner syndrome is 1:10,000 females. However, it is estimated that 95% of conceptuses with monosomy X are miscarried and only 5% are liveborn.

▶ Clinical Findings

Newborns with Turner syndrome may have webbed neck, edema of the hands and feet, coarctation of the aorta, and a characteristic triangular facies. Later symptoms include short stature, a shield chest with wide-set nipples, streak ovaries, amenorrhea, absence of secondary sex characteristics, and infertility. Some affected girls, particularly those with mosaicism, have only short stature and amenorrhea, without dysmorphic features.

Complications relate primarily to coarctation of the aorta, when present. Rarely, the dysgenetic gonads may become neoplastic (gonadoblastoma). The incidence of malformations of the urinary tract is increased. Learning disabilities are common, secondary to difficulties in perceptual motor integration. Patients with pseudohypoparathyroidism and Noonan syndrome have a similar phenotype to patients with Turner syndrome, but have normal chromosomes.

▶ Treatment

In Turner syndrome the identification and treatment of perceptual difficulties before they become problematic is very important. Teenage patients need counseling to cope with the stigma of their condition and to understand the need for hormone therapy. Estrogen replacement therapy will permit development of secondary sex characteristics and normal menstruation and prevent osteoporosis. Growth hormone therapy has been used to increase the height of affected girls. Females with 45,X or 45,X mosaicism have a low fertility rate, and those who become pregnant have a high risk of fetal wastage (spontaneous miscarriage, ~30%; stillbirth, 6–10%). Furthermore, their liveborn offspring have an increased frequency of chromosomal abnormalities involving either sex chromosomes or autosomes, and congenital malformations. Thus, prenatal ultrasonography and chromosome analysis are indicated for the offspring of females with sex chromosome abnormalities.

2. Klinefelter Syndrome (XXY)

ESSENTIALS OF DIAGNOSIS & TYPICAL FEATURES

▶ Diagnosis is rarely made before puberty.

▶ Key findings include microorchidism; lack of libido; minimal facial hair; and tall, eunuchoid build.

▶ IQ can vary (normal to borderline or even severely retarded, depending on karyotype).

The incidence of Klinefelter syndrome in the newborn population is roughly 1:1000, but it is about 1% among mentally retarded males and about 3% among males seen at infertility clinics. The maternal age at birth is often advanced. Unlike Turner syndrome, Klinefelter syndrome is rarely the cause of spontaneous abortions. The diagnosis is seldom made before puberty except as a result of prenatal diagnosis, because prepubertal boys have a normal phenotype.

▶ Clinical Findings

The characteristic findings after puberty include microorchidism associated with otherwise normal external genitalia, azoospermia, sterility, gynecomastia, normal to borderline IQ, diminished facial hair, lack of libido and potency, and a tall, eunuchoid build. In chromosome variants with three or four X chromosomes (XXXY and XXXXY), mental retardation may be severe, and radioulnar synostosis may be present as well as anomalies of the external genitalia and cryptorchidism. In the XXXXY cases, these findings are especially prominent, and microcephaly, short stature, and dysmorphic features also occur. In general, the physical and mental abnormalities associated with Klinefelter syndrome increase as the number of sex chromosomes increases.

▶ Treatment

Males with Klinefelter syndrome require testosterone replacement therapy. The presence of the extra X chromosome may allow expression of what might normally be a lethal X-linked disorder to occur.

3. XYY Syndrome

Newborns with XYY syndrome in general are normal. Affected individuals may on occasion exhibit an abnormal behavior pattern from early childhood and may have mild retardation. Fertility may be normal. Many males with an XYY karyotype are normal. There is no treatment. Long-term problems may relate to low IQ and environmental stress.

4. XXX Syndrome

The incidence of females with an XXX karyotype is approximately 1:1000. Females with XXX are phenotypically normal. However, they tend to be taller than usual and to have lower IQs than their normal siblings. Learning and behavioral issues are relatively common. This is in contrast to individuals with XXXX, a much rarer condition causing more severe developmental issues, and a dysmorphic phenotype reminiscent of Down syndrome.

Jones KL: *Smith's Recognizable Patterns of Human Malformation*, 6th ed. Elsevier, 2006.

Chromosomal Abnormalities: Abnormal Structure

Chromosomal abnormalities most often present in newborns as multiple congenital anomalies in association with intrauterine growth retardation. In addition to trisomies as just described, other more subtle chromosomal abnormalities are also common. In some cases, the karyotype is normal, but a subtle chromosomal rearrangement can be detected by FISH. Another new technology, called comparative genomic hybridization array, enables screening for multiple submicroscopic chromosomal abnormalities (ie, microdeletions) simultaneously, and may be a very helpful tool in evaluating the child with a suspected chromosomal abnormality.

Although most cases of severe chromosomal abnormality such as trisomy are lethal, some individuals may survive if the abnormality exists in mosaic form. Two examples of this include trisomy 8 and cat eye syndrome, caused by extra genetic material, which is derived from a portion of chromosome 22.

Vissers LE et al: Array-based comparative genomic hybridization for genome-wide detection of submicroscopic chromosomal abnormalities. Am J Hum Genet 2003;73:1261 [PMID: 14628292].

CHROMOSOME DELETION DISORDERS

Three common chromosomal deletion disorders that are often detected on routine karyotype analysis, and easily confirmed via FISH assay are 1p36– syndrome, Wolf-Hirschhorn syndrome (4p–), and cri du chat syndrome (5p–).

1. Deletion 1p36 Syndrome

Microcephaly and a large anterior fontanelle are characteristic features of 1p36– syndrome. Cardiac defects are common, and

dilated cardiomyopathy may present in infancy. Mental retardation, hypotonia, hearing loss, and seizures are usually seen.

2. Wolf-Hirschhorn Syndrome

Also known as 4p– (deletion of 4p16), this syndrome is characterized by microcephaly and unusual development of the nose and orbits that produces an appearance suggesting an ancient Greek warrior's helmet. Other anomalies commonly seen include cleft lip and palate, and cardiac and renal defects. Seizure disorders are common, and the majority of patients have severe mental retardation.

3. Cri du Chat Syndrome

Also known as 5p– (deletion of terminal chromosome 5p), this disorder is characterized by unique facial features, growth retardation, and microcephaly. Patients have an unusual catlike cry. Most patients have major organ anomalies and significant developmental delay.

CHROMOSOME MICRODELETION DISORDERS

Four common contiguous gene disorders (microdeletion disorders), which are usually suspected on the basis of an abnormal phenotype and then confirmed by FISH assay, are Williams syndrome, Miller-Dieker syndrome, Smith-Magenis syndrome, and velocardiofacial syndrome.

1. Williams Syndrome

Williams syndrome is a contiguous gene disorder involving the elastin gene and other neighboring genes at 7q11.2. It is characterized by short stature; congenital heart disease (supravalvular aortic stenosis); coarse, elfin-like facies with prominent lips; hypercalcemia or hypercalciuria in infancy; developmental delay; and neonatal irritability evolving into an overly friendly personality. Calcium restriction may be necessary in early childhood to prevent nephrocalcinosis. The hypercalcemia often resolves during the first year of life. The natural history includes progression of cardiac disease and predisposition to hypertension and spinal osteoarthritis in adults. Most patients have mild to moderate intellectual deficits.

2. Miller-Dieker Syndrome

A contiguous gene syndrome involving 17p13, this abnormality is characterized by microcephaly and severe CNS dysgenesis. The most commonly seen CNS malformation is termed *lissencephaly* ("smooth brain" as the brain is lacking its normal convolutions and gyri). An unusually developed face and forehead reflect abnormal migration of neuronal germinal matrix cells. Mutations in the gene *MDS1*, which is located in the critical region, can cause isolated lissencephaly, without the full picture of Miller-Dieker. Severe cognitive and developmental delay and seizure disorders are common.

3. Smith-Magenis Syndrome

This syndrome is associated with microdeletion of 17p11 and is characterized by prominent forehead, deep-set eyes, cupid-shaped upper lip, self-mutilating behavior (pulling nails and hair, putting objects into body orifices), sleep disturbance, and developmental delay. Some patients also have seizure disorders. Some individuals with larger deletions involving *PMP22* can present with peripheral neuropathy.

4. Velocardiofacial Syndrome (Deletion 22q11 Syndrome)

Also known as DiGeorge syndrome, this abnormality was originally described in newborns presenting with cyanotic congenital heart disease, usually involving great vessel abnormalities; thymic hypoplasia leading to immunodeficiency; and hypocalcemia due to absent parathyroid glands. This chromosomal abnormality is associated with a highly variable phenotype. Characteristics include mild microcephaly, palatal clefting or incompetence, speech and language delays, and congenital heart disease (ventricular or atrial septal defect). Midline defects such as umbilical hernia and hypospadias can be associated anomalies. In some cases, individuals have an apparent predisposition to psychosis.

MENDELIAN DISORDERS

AUTOSOMAL DOMINANT DISORDERS

Neurofibromatosis, Marfan syndrome, achondroplasia, osteogenesis imperfecta, and the craniosynostoses are among the most well known autosomal dominant disorders. There are many other common autosomal dominant disorders, including Treacher Collins syndrome, associated with a distinct craniofacial phenotype including malar and mandibular hypoplasia, and Noonan syndrome, which has a phenotype similar to Turner syndrome and is characterized by short stature and a webbed neck. Two other common genetic disorders whose causative genes were recently identified and found to be dominant mutations are CHARGE syndrome and Cornelia de Lange syndrome.

1. Neurofibromatosis Type 1

Neurofibromatosis type 1 (NF-1) is one of the most common autosomal dominant disorders, occurring in 1:3000 births and seen in all races and ethnic groups. In general, the disorder is progressive, with new manifestations appearing over time. Neurofibromatosis type 2 (NF-2), characterized by bilateral acoustic neuromas, with minimal or no skin manifestations, is a different disease caused by a different gene.

The gene for NF-1 is on the long arm of chromosome 17 and seems to code for a protein similar to a tumor suppresser factor. NF results from many different mutations of this gene. Approximately half of all NF cases are caused by new mutations. Careful evaluation of the parents is necessary to provide accurate genetic counseling. Recent evidence suggests that pene-

trance is close to 100% in those who carry the gene if individuals are examined carefully.

Café-au-lait macules may be present at birth, and about 80% of individuals with NF-1 will have more than six by age 1 year. Neurofibromas are benign tumors consisting of Schwann cells, nerve fibers, and fibroblasts; they may be discrete or plexiform. The incidence of Lisch nodules, which can be seen with a slit lamp, also increases with age. Affected individuals commonly have a large head, bony abnormalities on radiographic studies, scoliosis, and a wide spectrum of developmental problems. Although the average IQ is within the normal range, it is lower than in unaffected family members. (For more details of medical evaluation and treatment, see Chapter 23 of this book.) Useful information is provided on the following web site: http://www.nfinc.org.

Hyperpigmented macules can occur in other conditions such as Albright, Noonan, and Leopard syndromes, but the lesions are either single or different in character.

2. Marfan Syndrome

ESSENTIALS OF DIAGNOSIS & TYPICAL FEATURES

▶ Skeletal abnormalities (Ghent criteria).
▶ Lens dislocation.
▶ Dilation of the aortic root.
▶ Dural ectasia.
▶ Positive family history.

▶ Clinical Findings

Genetic testing is available for mutations causing Marfan syndrome, but the diagnosis remains largely clinical and is based on the Ghent criteria (available at http://www.genetests.org). Children most often present with a positive family history, suspicious skeletal findings, or ophthalmologic complications. Motor milestones are frequently delayed due to joint laxity and mild myopathy. Adolescents are prone to spontaneous pneumothorax. Dysrhythmias may be present. Aortic and valvular complications are not common in children but are more likely in sporadic cases. The characteristic facies is long and thin, with down-slanting palpebral fissures. The palate is high arched, and dentition is often crowded. The uvula may be bifid.

Marfan syndrome is genetically heterogeneous. Mutations in the gene for fibrillin1 proteins (*FBN1*) are most common but mutations in (*FBN2*) and in transforming growth factor β receptors (*TGFBR1* and *2*) can also produce phenotypes that fit criteria for a clinical diagnosis of Marfan syndrome.

▶ Differential Diagnosis

Homocystinuria should be excluded through metabolic testing in all individuals with marfanoid skeletal features. An

X-linked recessive disorder, **Lujan syndrome**, combines marfanoid habitus with mental retardation. Other connective tissue disorders, **Ehlers-Danlos syndrome,** and **Stickler syndrome** should also be considered.

Genes mutated in Marfan syndrome can also be mutated in related disorders: **Beal syndrome** (*FBN2*), **Shprintzen-Goldberg Syndrome** (*FBN1*) and the recently described **Loeys-Dietz syndrome** (*TGFBR1* and *2*). The reader is referred to reviews available at http://www.genetests.org for descriptions of these disorders.

Complications

The skeletal problems including scoliosis are progressive. Astigmatism and myopia are very common and surveillance for lens dislocation is necessary.

The most serious associated medical problems involve the heart. Although many patients with Marfan syndrome have mitral valve prolapse, the most serious concern is progressive aortic root dilation, which may lead to aneurysmal rupture and death, and progressive or acute valvular (aortic more frequently than mitral) incompetency.

Families and practitioners seeking additional information about Marfan syndrome can be referred to the National Marfan Foundation (http://www.marfan.org).

Treatment

A. Medical Therapy

Medical treatment for patients with Marfan syndrome includes surveillance for and appropriate management of the ophthalmologic, orthopedic, and cardiac issues. Serial echocardiograms are indicated to diagnose and follow the degree of aortic root enlargement, which can be managed medically or surgically, in more severe cases. Prophylactic β-adrenergic blockade can slow the rate of aortic dilation and reduce the development of aortic complications.

Interest in the effects of deficient extracellular fibrillin-1 has led to the discovery that the mild myopathy in Marfan syndrome reflects excessive signaling by transforming growth factor β (TGFβ), an inhibitor of myoblast differentiation. Animal studies suggest that aortic aneurysm can be prevented by TGFβ antagonists, including blockers of angiotensin II type 1 receptors. Research studies are currently underway using this approach in human patients.

B. Genetic Counseling

Genetic testing for mutations in *FBN1* and *2* and in *TGFBR1* and *2* should be considered in all individuals with Marfan syndrome as penetrance is variable and apparently unaffected family members can carry and pass on mutations.

3. Achondroplasia

Achondroplasia, the most common form of skeletal dysplasia, is caused by a mutation in *FGFR3*.

Clinical Findings

The classic phenotype includes relative macrocephaly, midface hypoplasia, short-limbed dwarfism, and trident-shaped hands. The phenotype is apparent at birth. Individuals with achondroplasia are cognitively normal.

Treatment

A. Medical Therapy

Orthopedic intervention is necessary for spinal problems including severe lumbar lordosis and gibbus deformity. Long bone lengthening surgery, such as the Ilizarov procedure, is used in some centers to increase height and upper extremity function, but its use is controversial.

Head circumference during infancy must be closely monitored and plotted on a diagnosis-specific head circumference chart. Bony overgrowth at the level of the foramen magnum may lead to progressive hydrocephalus and brainstem compression, and may warrant neurosurgical intervention.

Many patients find support through organizations such as the Little People of America, at the following web site: http://www.lpaonline.org.

B. Genetic Counseling

The vast majority of cases (approximately 90%) represent a new mutation. Two hemizygous parents with achondroplasia have a 25% risk of having a child homozygous for *FGFR3* mutations, which is a lethal disorder.

4. Osteogenesis Imperfecta

Osteogenesis imperfecta (OI), or brittle bone disease, is a relatively common disorder, caused by mutations in type I collagen. Most patients with more severe disease represent new mutations for this disorder.

Clinical Findings

There are four main types of OI.

- Type I is a mild form, with increased incidence of fracturing and blue sclerae.
- Type II is generally lethal in the newborn period with multiple congenital fractures and severe lung disease.
- Type III is the severe form causing significant bony deformity secondary to multiple fractures (many of which are congenital), blue sclerae, short stature, and mild restrictive lung disease.
- Type IV is a mild form with increased incidence of fracturing (*not* usually congenital); dentinogenesis imperfecta is common.

Treatment

A. Medical Therapy

A major advancement in the treatment of OI patients has been the use of pamidronate, a bisphosphonate compound, which has been reported to lead to a reduced incidence of fracture and improvement in bone density. Patients should be followed by an experienced orthopedist, as rodding of long bones and surgery to correct scoliosis are often required. Hearing assessments are indicated, because of the association between OI and deafness. Close dental follow-up is also necessary.

B. Genetic Counseling

All four types of OI are associated with mutations in the gene coding for type I collagen. Collagen analysis is usually performed in skin fibroblasts to confirm the diagnosis. DNA analysis in blood is also possible. The milder forms may be seen as the result of dominant inheritance, while the more severe forms of OI generally result from new mutations.

5. Craniosynostoses Syndromes

The craniosynostoses disorders are common dominant disorders associated with premature fusion of cranial sutures. This class of disorders is now known to be caused by mutations in *FGFR* genes.

Crouzon syndrome is the most common of these disorders and is associated with multiple suture fusions, but with normal limbs. Other craniosynostosis disorders have limb as well as craniofacial anomalies, and include Pfeiffer, Apert, Jackson-Weiss, and Saethre-Chotzen syndromes.

Facial features associated with craniosynostosis include shallow orbits leading to proptosis, midface narrowing that may result in upper airway obstruction, and hydrocephalus that may require shunting. Children with craniosynostosis undergo multiple staged craniofacial and neurosurgical procedures to address these issues.

6. CHARGE Syndrome

CHARGE syndrome affects structures derived from rostral neural crest cells but also includes abnormal development of the eyes and midbrain. The acronym CHARGE serves as a mnemonic for associated abnormalities that include **c**olobomas, congenital **h**eart disease, choanal **a**tresia, growth **r**etardation, **g**enital abnormalities (hypogenitalism), and **e**ar abnormalities, with deafness. Facial asymmetry is a common finding. CHARGE is now known to be caused by mutations in the *CHD7* gene on chromosome 8q. A web site with information on CHARGE syndrome is available at http://www.chargesyndrome.org/.

Vissers LE et al: Mutations in a new member of the chromodomain gene family cause CHARGE syndrome. Nat Genet 2004;36:955 [PMID: 15300250].

7. Cornelia de Lange Syndrome

Cornelia de Lange syndrome is characterized by severe growth retardation; limb, especially hand, reduction defects (50%); congenital heart disease (25%); and stereotypical facies with hirsutism, medial fusion of eyebrows (synophrys), and thin, down-turned lips. The course and severity are variable, but the prognosis for survival and normal development is poor. Muta-

tions of the *NIBPL* gene are present in the majority of patients; however, a mutation of *SMC1* on the X chromosome is responsible for a subset of patients with the syndrome.

Jones KL: *Recognizable Patterns of Human Malformation,* 6th ed. Elsevier, 2006.

8. Noonan Syndrome

Noonan syndrome is an autosomal dominant disorder characterized by short stature, congenital heart disease, abnormalities of cardiac conduction and rhythm, occasional bleeding diatheses, webbed neck, down-slanting palpebral fissures, hearing loss, and low-set ears. Affected children may be large at birth and have mild subcutaneous edema. The phenotype evolves with age and may be difficult to recognize in older relatives. Mild developmental delays are often present. Mutations in the *PTPN11* gene cause most cases of Noonan syndrome, but others are the result of mutations in other proto-oncogenes. Products of these genes help control cell cycling through RAS-MAPK signal transduction pathways. Cell cycling controls are also affected by mutations in other genes that produce more complicated Noonan-like disorders (ie, Costello and cardiofaciocutaneous syndromes) in which cardiomyopathies are prominent. Because mutations causing NF-1 also affect RAS proto-oncogene signaling, it is not surprising that there is an NF-1 subtype with a so-called Noonan phenotype.

AUTOSOMAL RECESSIVE DISORDERS

1. Cystic Fibrosis

The gene for cystic fibrosis, *CFTR*, is found on the long arm of chromosome 7. Approximately 1 in 22 persons are carriers. Over 600 different mutations have been identified: the most common in the Caucasian population, known as $\Delta F508$, is a three-base deletion coding for phenylalanine.

Cloning of the gene for cystic fibrosis and identification of the mutation in the majority of cases have completely changed genetic counseling and prenatal diagnosis for this disorder, although the sweat chloride assay is still important in confirming the diagnosis. The American College of Medical Genetics recommends the 25-mutation assay using PCR-based techniques, which can cover 85–90% of the mutations.

The identification of the mutation in the cystic fibrosis gene has also raised the issue of mass newborn screening, because of the high frequency of this gene in the Caucasian population. Some states, such as Colorado, have offered newborn screening by trypsinogen assay, which can detect 70% of patients with cystic fibrosis. Although early detection can ensure good nutritional status starting at birth, newborn screening is controversial as there is no cure for cystic fibrosis. (For more details of medical management, see Chapters 18 and 21 in this text.)

2. Smith-Lemli-Opitz Syndrome

Smith-Lemli-Opitz syndrome is caused by a metabolic error in the final step of cholesterol production, resulting in low cholesterol levels and accumulation of the precursor 7-dehydrocholesterol (7-DHC). (See also Chapter 34.)

Clinical Findings

Patients with Smith-Lemli-Opitz syndrome present with a characteristic phenotype, including dysmorphic facial features (Figure 35–12), multiple congenital anomalies (including defects of the CNS, heart, cleft palate, cardiac system, kidneys, genitalia, and limbs), hypotonia, growth failure, and mental retardation. The diagnosis can be confirmed via a simple blood test looking for the presence of the precursor, 7-DHC, which is not detectible in an unaffected individual. This blood test can only be done in special laboratories. Prenatal testing is available.

Treatment

Treatment with cholesterol can ameliorate the growth failure and lead to improvement in behavior and developmental course, although treatment does not cure this complex disorder.

3. Sensorineural Hearing Loss

Although there is marked genetic heterogeneity in causes of sensorineural hearing loss, including dominant, recessive, and X-linked patterns, nonsyndromic, recessively inherited deafness is the predominant form of severe inherited childhood deafness. Several hundred genes are known to cause hereditary hearing loss and deafness. The hearing loss may be conductive, sensorineural, or a combination of both; syndromic or nonsyndromic; and prelingual (before language develops) or postlingual (after language develops). The genetic forms of hearing loss are diagnosed by otologic, audiologic, and physical examination; family history; ancillary testing (such as CT examination of the temporal bone); and molecular genetic testing. Molecular genetic tests are available for many types of syndromic and nonsyndromic deafness, but often only on a research basis. In the clinical setting, molecular genetic testing is available for some recessive conditions including Usher syndrome types 2A (USH2A gene) and 3 (one mutation in USH3A), and at least six other rare forms of genetically caused deafness.

Testing for deafness-causing mutations in two more common genes, GJB2 (which encodes the protein connexin 26) and GJB6 (which encodes the protein connexin 30), plays a prominent role in diagnosis and genetic counseling. Mutations in connexin 26 are present in 49% of cases of prelingual deafness.

Nance WE: The genetics of deafness. Ment Retard Dev Disabil Res Rev 2003;9:109 [PMID: 12784229].

4. Spinal Muscular Atrophy

Spinal muscular atrophy (SMA) is an autosomal recessive neuromuscular disorder in which anterior horn cells in the spinal cord degenerate. The mechanism for the loss of cells

▲ **Figure 35–12.** Child with Smith-Lemli-Opitz syndrome, featuring bitemporal narrowing, upturned nares, ptosis, and small chin.

appears to involve apoptosis of neurons in the absence of the product of the SMN1 (survival motor neuron) gene located on chromosome 5q. Loss of anterior horn cells leads to progressive atrophy of skeletal muscle. The disorder has an incidence of approximately 1 in 12,000, with the majority of the cases presenting in infancy. Carrier frequencies approach 1 in 50 in populations with European ancestry.

Clinical Findings

Three clinical subtypes are recognized based on age of onset and rate of progression. SMA I is the most devastating. Mild weakness may be present at birth but is clearly evident by 3 months and is accompanied by loss of reflexes and fasciculations in affected muscles. Progression of the disorder leads to eventual respiratory failure, usually by age 1 year. Symptoms of SMA II begin later, with weakness and decreased reflexes generally apparent by age 2 years. Children affected with SMA III begin to become weak as they approach adolescence.

Homozygous deletion of exon 7 of SMN1 is detectable in approximately 95–98% of cases of all types of SMA and confirms the diagnosis. The SMN1 region on chromosome 5q is complex and variability in presentation appears to involve expression of neighboring genes, including a more centromeric *SMN2* pseudogene. Approximately 2–5% of patients affected with SMA will be compound heterozygotes in whom there is one copy of *SMN1* with exon 7 deleted and a second copy with a point mutation.

Prenatal diagnosis is available through genetic testing, but careful molecular analysis of the proband and demonstration of carrier status in parents is advised since, in addition to the problem of potential compound heterozygosity, 2% of cases occur as a result of a de novo mutation in one *SMN1* allele. In this case one of the parents is not a carrier and recurrence risks are low. Carrier testing is further complicated by a duplication of *SMN1* in 4% of the population that results in there being two *SMN1* genes on one of their chromosomes. Hence reproductive risk assessment, carrier testing and prenatal diagnosis of SMA are best undertaken in the context of careful genetic counseling.

5. Metabolic Disorders

Most inborn errors of metabolism are inherited in an autosomal recessive pattern. (See Chapter 34 in this text for detailed explanations of these disorders.)

X-LINKED DISORDERS

1. Duchenne & Becker Muscular Dystrophies

Duchenne muscular dystrophy (DMD) results from failure of synthesis of the muscle cytoskeletal protein dystrophin, the gene for which is located on the X chromosome, Xp12. Approximately 1 in 4000 male children are affected. Mutations in the same gene that result in partial expression of the dystrophin protein produce a less severe phenotype, Becker muscular dystrophy (BMD). In both DMD and BMD, progressive degeneration of skeletal and cardiac muscle occurs. Boys with DMD exhibit proximal muscle weakness and pseudo-hypertrophy of calf muscles by age 5–6 years. Patients become nonambulatory by age 13. Serum creatine kinase levels are markedly elevated. Boys with DMD frequently die in their 20s of respiratory failure and cardiac dysfunction. The prognosis for BMD is more variable. Although corticosteroids are useful in maintaining strength, they do not slow progression of the disorder.

The gene for dystrophin is very large and a common target for mutation. Large deletions or duplications can be detected in the gene for dystrophin in 65% of cases. Methods for detecting small and even point mutations have now been developed. Mutation testing and careful clinical assessment are replacing muscle biopsies in making the diagnosis of DMD.

One third of DMD cases presenting with a negative family history are likely to be new mutations. Genetic counseling is complicated by the fact that germline mosaicism for mutations in the dystrophin gene occur in approximately 15–20% of families. Therefore, if a mutation has been detected in a proband, prenatal diagnosis is routinely offered to his mother regardless of her apparent carrier status. It is also necessary to look for mutations in all sisters of affected boys. Since mutations are now detected in the great majority of DMD cases, there is considerably less need for estimating carrier risks based on creatine kinase levels or using genetic linkage for prenatal diagnosis. Nonetheless, counseling and prenatal diagnosis remain difficult in some families. (Additional information about muscular dystrophies is included in Chapter 23.)

2. Hemophilia

Hemophilia A is an X-linked, recessive, bleeding disorder caused by a deficiency in the activity of coagulation factor VIII. Affected individuals develop a variable phenotype of hemorrhage into joints and muscles, easy bruising, and prolonged bleeding from wounds. The disorder is caused by heterogeneous mutations in the factor VIII gene, which maps to Xq28. Carrier detection and prenatal diagnosis can be done by direct detection of selected mutations, especially the inversions, the most common gene change, as well as indirectly by linkage analysis. Replacement of factor VIII is done using a variety of preparations derived from human plasma or recombinant techniques. Although replacement therapy is effective in most cases, 10–15% of treated individuals develop neutralizing antibodies that decrease its effectiveness. (See Chapter 28 in this text for additional discussion.)

3. Metabolic Disorders

Some important inborn errors are inherited as X-linked disorders, such as adrenoleukodystrophy. (See Chapter 32 in this text for more detailed descriptions.)

NONMENDELIAN DISORDERS

DISORDERS OF IMPRINTING

1. Beckwith-Wiedemann Syndrome

The association of macrosomia (enlarged body size), macroglossia (enlarged tongue), and omphalocele constitutes the Beckwith-Wiedemann syndrome (BWS), now known to be related to abnormal expression of genes located at chromosome 11p15. Other associated findings include mild facial dysmorphism (hypertelorism, unusual ear creases), infantile hypoglycemia due to transient hyperinsulinemia, multiple congenital anomalies (cleft palate and genitourinary anomalies common), and increased risk for certain malignancies, especially Wilms tumor (7–10%).

A growth factor gene, *IGF2*, is imprinted such that the maternal allele is ordinarily not expressed during intrauterine development. Chromosomal abnormalities affecting expression of this gene, such as duplication of the paternal 11p15 region, or paternal UPD, are associated with BWS. Paternal UPD may also lead to loss of expression of a tumor suppressor gene (*H19*), normally read from the maternal homolog, contributing to the increased predisposition to cancer seen in this disorder. Supporting evidence for the role of imprinting in BWS is that paternal imprinting has been documented in about 10% of BWS patients, and that about 70% of Wilms tumors from patients with BWS show loss of imprinting of the genes coding for *IGF2* and *H19*. Children affected with BWS should undergo tumor surveillance protocols, including an abdominal ultrasound every 3 months until they reach age 7 years, as diagnosing malignancy at early stages leads to a significant improvement in outcome.

2. Prader-Willi Syndrome

Prader-Willi syndrome results from lack of expression of several imprinted genes, including *SNRPn,* located on chromosome 15q11. Clinical characteristics include severe hypotonia in infancy that often necessitates placement of a feeding gastrostomy tube. In older children, characteristic facies evolve over time, including almond-shaped eyes, along with frequent strabismus. Short stature, obesity, hypogenitalism, and small hands and feet with tapering fingers are now believed to be associated with growth hormone deficiency. Obsessive hyperphagia (usual onset 3–4 years) and type 2 (adult-onset) diabetes mellitus are common features.

Multiple chromosomal rearrangements and mutations have been reported to disrupt expression of the genes that contribute to this syndrome. Of these, deletion of the paternally inherited allele of chromosome 15q11 (detected by FISH) is the most common chromosomal abnormality causing Prader-Willi syndrome, followed by maternal UPD, diagnosed by DNA methylation studies.

3. Angelman Syndrome

Angelman syndrome also involves imprinting and results from a variety of mutations that inactivate a ubiquitin-protein ligase gene, *UBE3A,* located in the same region of chromosome 15 as *SNRPn,* the maternally imprinted gene involved in Prader-Willi syndrome (see preceding section). *UBE3A* is paternally imprinted, and during normal development the maternal allele is expressed only in the brain. The classic phenotype includes severe mental retardation with prognathism, seizures, and marked delay in motor milestones, abnormal puppet-like gait and posturing, poor language development, and paroxysmal laughter and tongue thrusting.

Angelman syndrome is most commonly caused when sequences detectable by FISH on 15q11 are deleted from the maternal homolog. Uniparental paternal disomy 15 is the least common cause. Mutations in *UBE3A* cause the disorder in about one fourth of cases. Imprinting errors, which may be associated with advanced reproductive techniques, may also result in Angelman syndrome.

Niemitz EL, Feinberg AP: Epigenetics and assisted reproductive technology: A call for investigation. Am J Hum Genet 2004;74:599 [PMID: 14991528].

4. Uniparental Disomy for Chromosome 7

Certain genes on chromosome 7 are now known to be imprinted. UPD7 has been reported to cause cystic fibrosis in a child who inherited two copies of the ΔF508 deletion from one parent. That child also had Russell-Silver syndrome, a syndrome associated with intrauterine growth failure and dwarfism. Imprinting abnormalities and UPD may prove to be associated with growth abnormalities.

DISORDERS ASSOCIATED WITH ANTICIPATION

1. (Autosomal Dominant) Myotonic Dystrophy

Most myotonic dystrophy, an autosomal dominant condition characterized by muscle weakness and tonic muscle spasms (myotonia) along with hypogonadism, frontal balding, cardiac conduction abnormalities, and cataracts, presents in adults. This disorder occurs when a CTG repeat in the *DMPK* gene on chromosome 19 expands to 50 or more copies. Normal individuals have from 5–35 CTG repeat copies. Individuals carrying 35–49 repeats are generally asymptomatic, but repeat copies greater than 35 are meiotically unstable and tend to further expand when passed to subsequent generations. Individuals with 50–100 copies may be only mildly affected (eg, cataracts). Most individuals with repeat copies greater than 100 will have symptoms or electrical myotonia as adults.

As unstable alleles continue to expand and copy numbers approach 400, symptoms become evident in children. Expansion greater than 1000 copies produces fetal and neonatal disease that can be lethal. Expansion from approximately 200–400 repeat copies produces mild, often clinically undetected symptoms, while very large copy numbers (800–2000) are associated with fetal manifestations (polyhydramnios and arthrogryposis). This occurs most frequently when the unstable repeats are passed through an affected mother. Therefore, an important component in the workup of the floppy or weak infant is a careful neurologic assessment of both parents for evidence of weakness or myotonia. Molecular testing that measures the number of CTG repeats is diagnostic clinically and prenatally. (See Chapter 23 for additional discussion.)

2. (Autosomal Recessive) Friedreich Ataxia

Symptoms of Friedreich ataxia include loss of coordination (cerebellar dysfunction) with both motor and sensory findings beginning in preadolescence and typically progressing through the teenage years. The gene involved, *FDRA,* is located on chromosome 9. Normal individuals carry 7–33 GAA repeats at this locus. Close to 96% of affected patients are homozygous for repeat expansions that exceed 66 copies. However, point mutations in the gene also occur. Meiotic instability for GAA repeats is more variable than for others and contractions occur more frequently than do expansions. Relationships between genotype and phenotype are also more complex. Molecular diagnostic testing requires careful interpretation with respect to prognosis and reproductive risks. (See Chapter 23 for additional discussion.)

3. (X-Linked) Fragile X Syndrome

Fragile X syndrome, present in approximately 1 in 1000 males, is the most common cause of cognitive disabilities (mental retardation) in males. The responsible gene is *FMR1*, which has unstable CGG repeats at the 5' end. Normal individuals have up to 50 CGG repeats. Individuals with 51–200 CGG repeats have a premutation and may manifest symptoms including developmental, behavioral, and physical traits, premature ovarian failure in a subset of females; and a progressive, neurologic deterioration in older males called FXTAS (fragile X–associated tremor-ataxia syndrome). Affected individuals with fragile X syndrome (full mutation) have more than 200 CGG repeats and also have hypermethylation of both the CGG expansion and an adjacent CpG island. This methylation turns off the FMR1 gene. DNA analysis, rather than cytogenetic testing, is the method of choice for confirming the diagnosis of fragile X syndrome.

▶ Clinical Features

Most males with fragile X syndrome present with intellectual disabilities, oblong facies with large ears, and large testicles, especially after puberty. Other physical signs include symptoms suggestive of a connective tissue disorder (eg, hyperextensible joints or mitral valve prolapse). Many affected individuals are hyperactive and exhibit infantile autism or autistic-like behavior.

About half of females with the fragile X full mutation show normal intelligence, but may evidence mild learning disabilities and behavioral problems. Unlike other X-linked disorders where female heterozygotes are asymptomatic, half of females with the full mutation have lower IQs in the range of mental retardation and more severe behavioral problems. Females have more mild phenotypic changes than the males. Clinical expression of fragile X differs in male and female offspring depending on which parent is transmitting the gene. The premutation can change into the full mutation only when passed through a female. Identification of the abnormal DNA amplification by direct DNA analysis can confirm the diagnosis of fragile X in an affected individual and can detect asymptomatic gene carriers of both sexes. Therefore, DNA analysis is a reliable test for prenatal and postnatal diagnosis of fragile X syndrome and facilitates genetic counseling. (Management considerations for patients with fragile X syndrome are described in Chapter 2.)

Hagerman PJ, Hagerman RJ: The fragile-X premutation: A maturing perspective. Am J Hum Genet 2004;74:805 [PMID: 15052536].

DISORDERS ASSOCIATED WITH MITOCHONDRIAL INHERITANCE

More than 100 point mutations and rearrangements of mtDNA have been identified, which are associated with a large number of human diseases. Symptoms of mitochondrial disorders are secondary to deficiency in the respiratory chain enzymes of oxidative phosphorylation, which supply energy to all cells. Mitochondrial diseases are usually progressive disorders with neurologic dysfunction including hypotonia, developmental delay, and seizures. Ophthalmologic issues, hearing loss, gastrointestinal tract dysfunction with growth failure, renal, endocrine, cardiac, and autonomic dysfunction are some of the many issues which can affect patients with mitochondrial diseases. The following disorders are three of the more common ones.

1. MELAS

MELAS is an acronym for **m**itochondrial **e**ncephalopathy, **l**actic **a**cidosis, and **s**trokelike episodes. Symptoms occur in the pediatric age group and include recurrent episodes resembling stroke (blindness, paralysis), headache, vomiting, weakness of proximal muscles, and elevated blood lactate. (***Note:*** Lactate may be falsely elevated secondary to technical difficulties in obtaining a free-flowing blood specimen or delay in laboratory measurement.) The most common mutation causing MELAS is in the tRNA^{Leu} gene (*A3243G*).

2. MERRF

MERRF is an acronym for **m**yoclonus **e**pilepsy with **r**agged **r**ed **f**ibers. Children with MERRF present with a variety of neurologic symptoms, including myoclonus, deafness, weakness of muscles, and seizures. Eighty percent of cases are due to a missense mutation in the mitochondrial tRNA^{Lys} gene (*A8344G*).

3. Leigh Subacute Necrotizing Encephalomyelopathy

Multiple different abnormalities in respiratory chain function lead to Leigh disease, a very severe disorder associated with progressive loss of developmental milestones, along with extrapyramidal symptoms and brainstem dysfunction. Episodes of deterioration are frequently associated with an intercurrent febrile illness. Symptoms include hypotonia, unusual choreoathetoid hand movements, feeding dysfunction with failure to thrive, and seizures. Focal necrotic lesions of the brainstem and thalamus are hallmarks on MRI scan. Mitochondrial mutations affecting the respiratory chain, especially complexes I, II, and IV, and nuclear DNA mutations affecting complex II have been identified as causing Leigh disease.

Kahler SG, Fahey MC: Metabolic disorders and mental retardation. Am J Med Genet C Semin Med Genet 2003;117:31 [PMID: 12561056].

DISORDERS OF MULTIFACTORIAL INHERITANCE

CLEFT LIP & CLEFT PALATE

ESSENTIALS OF DIAGNOSIS & TYPICAL FEATURES

▶ Cleft lip is more common in males, cleft palate in females.

▶ Cleft lip and palate may be isolated defects (nonsyndromic) or associated with other anomalies as part of a genetic disorder (syndromic).

▶ Pierre Robin anomalad, the association of cleft palate, micrognathia, and glossoptosis may lead to severe airway complications in young infants, necessitating tracheostomy.

▶ General Considerations

From a genetic standpoint, cleft lip with or without cleft palate is distinct from isolated cleft palate. Although both can occur in a single family, particularly in association with certain syndromes, this pattern is unusual. Racial background is a factor in the incidence of facial clefting. Among Asians, Caucasians, and blacks, the incidence is 1.61, 0.9, and 0.31, respectively, per 1000 live births.

▶ Clinical Findings

A cleft lip may be unilateral or bilateral and complete or incomplete. It may occur with a cleft of the entire palate or just the primary (anterior and gingival ridge) or secondary (posterior) palate. An isolated cleft palate can involve only the soft palate or both the soft and hard palates. It can be a V-shaped or a wide horseshoe, U-shaped cleft. When the cleft palate is associated with micrognathia and glossoptosis (a tongue that falls back and causes respiratory or feeding problems), it is called the **Pierre Robin sequence** or **anomalad.** Among individuals with facial clefts—more commonly those with isolated cleft palate—the incidence of other congenital abnormalities is increased, with up to a 60% association with other anomalies or syndromes. The incidence of congenital heart disease, for example, is 1–2% in liveborn infants, but among those with Pierre Robin sequence it can be as high as 15%. Associated abnormalities should be looked for in the period immediately after birth and before surgery.

▶ Differential Diagnosis

A facial cleft may occur in many different circumstances. It may be an isolated abnormality or part of a more generalized syndrome. Prognosis, management, and accurate determi-

nation of recurrence risks all depend on accurate diagnosis. In evaluating a child with a facial cleft, the physician must determine if the cleft is nonsyndromic or syndromic.

A. Nonsyndromic

In the past, nonsyndromic cleft lip or cleft palate was considered a classic example of polygenic or multifactorial inheritance. More recently, however, this mode of inheritance has been questioned, and several studies have suggested one or more major autosomal loci, both recessive and dominant (or co-dominant). Empirically, however, the recurrence risk is still in the range of 2–3% because of nonpenetrance or the presence of other contributing genes.

B. Syndromic

Cleft lip, with or without cleft palate, and isolated cleft palate may occur in a variety of syndromes that may be environmental, chromosomal, single gene, or of unknown origin (Table 35–3). Prognosis and accurate recurrence risks depend on the correct diagnosis.

▶ Complications

Problems associated with facial clefts include early feeding difficulties, which may be severe; airway obstruction necessitating tracheostomy; recurrent serous otitis media associated with fluctuating hearing and language delays; speech problems, including language delay, hypernasality, and articulation errors; and dental and orthodontic complications.

▶ Treatment

A. Medical Therapy

Long-term management ideally should be provided through a multidisciplinary cleft palate clinic.

Table 35–3. Syndromic isolated cleft palate (CP) and cleft lip with or without cleft palate (CL/CP).

Environmental
Maternal seizures, anticonvulsant usage (CL/CP or CP)
Fetal alcohol syndrome (CL/CP)
Amniotic band syndrome (CL/CP)
Chromosomal
Trisomies 13 and 18 (CL/CP)
Wolf-Hirschhorn or 4p- syndrome (CL/CP)
Shprintzen or 22q11.2 deletion syndrome (CP)
Single-gene disorders
Treacher Collins syndrome, AD (CP)
Stickler syndrome, AD (CP)
Smith-Lemli-Opitz, AR (CP)
Unknown cause
Moebius syndrome (CP)

AD, autosomal dominant; AR, autosomal recessive.

B. Genetic Counseling

Accurate counseling depends on accurate diagnosis and the differentiation of syndromic from nonsyndromic clefts. A complete family history must be taken, and the patient and both parents must be examined. The choice of laboratory studies is guided by the presence of other abnormalities and clinical suspicions, and may include chromosome analysis, FISH, eye examination, and radiologic studies. Clefts of both the lip and the palate can be detected on detailed prenatal ultrasound.

NEURAL TUBE DEFECTS

ESSENTIALS OF DIAGNOSIS & TYPICAL FEATURES

▶ Various defects, ranging from anencephaly to open or skin-covered lesions of the spinal cord, may occur in isolation or as part of a syndrome.

▶ Myelomeningocele is usually associated with hydrocephalus, neurogenic bladder and bowel, and congenital paralysis in the lower extremities.

▶ Anomalies of the CNS, heart, and kidneys may also be seen.

▶ MRI helps determine the extent of the anatomic defect in skin covered lesions.

General Considerations

Neural tube defects comprise a variety of malformations, including anencephaly, encephalocele, spina bifida (myelomeningocele), sacral agenesis, and other spinal dysraphisms. Evidence suggests that the neural tube develops via closure at multiple rather than just two closure sites and that each closure site is mediated by different genes and affected by different teratogens. Hydrocephalus associated with the Arnold-Chiari type II malformation commonly occurs with myelomeningocele. Sacral agenesis, also called the caudal regression syndrome, occurs more frequently in infants of diabetic mothers.

Clinical Findings

At birth, neural tube defects can present as an obvious rachischisis (open lesion), or as a more subtle skin-covered lesion. In the latter case, MRI should be conducted to better define the anatomic defect. The extent of neurologic deficit depends on the level of the lesion and may include clubfeet, dislocated hips, or total flaccid paralysis below the level of the lesion. Hydrocephalus may be apparent at birth or may develop after the back has been surgically repaired. Neurogenic bladder and bowel are commonly seen. Other anomalies of the CNS may be present, as well as anomalies of the heart or kidneys.

Differential Diagnosis

Neural tube defects may occur in isolation (nonsyndromic) or as part of a genetic syndrome. They may result from teratogenic exposure to alcohol or the anticonvulsant valproate. Any infant with dysmorphic features or other major anomalies in addition to a neural tube defect should be evaluated by a geneticist, and a chromosome analysis should be performed.

Treatment

A. Neurosurgical Measures

Infants with an open neural tube defect should be placed in prone position, and the lesion kept moist with sterile dressing. Neurosurgical closure should occur within 24–48 hours after birth to reduce risk of infection. The infant should be monitored closely for signs of hydrocephalus. Shunts are required in about 85% of cases of myelomeningocele and are associated with complications including malfunction and infection. Symptoms of the Arnold-Chiari II malformation include feeding dysfunction, abducens nerve palsy, vocal cord paralysis with stridor, and apnea. Shunt malfunction may cause an acute worsening of Arnold-Chiari symptoms that may be life-threatening.

B. Orthopedic Measures

The child's ability to walk varies according to the level of the lesion. Children with low lumbar and sacral lesions walk with minimal support, while those with high lumbar and thoracic lesions are rarely functional walkers. Orthopedic input is necessary to address foot deformities and scoliosis. Physical therapy services are indicated.

C. Urologic Measures

Neurogenic bladders have variable presentations. Urodynamic studies are recommended early on to define bladder function, and management is guided by the results of these studies. Continence can often be achieved by the use of anticholinergic or sympathomimetic agents, clean intermittent catheterization, and a variety of urologic procedures. Renal function should be monitored regularly, and an ultrasound examination should be periodically repeated. Symptomatic infections should be treated.

Symptoms of neurogenic bowel include incontinence and chronic constipation and are managed with a combination of dietary modifications, laxatives, stool softeners, and rectal stimulation. A surgical procedure called ACE (antegrade continence enema) may be recommended for patients with severe constipation that is unresponsive to conservative management.

D. Genetic Counseling

Most isolated neural tube defects are polygenic, with a recurrence risk of 2–3% in future pregnancies. The recurrence risk for siblings of the parents and siblings of the patients is 1–2%. A patient with spina bifida has a 5% chance of having an affected child. Prenatal diagnosis is possible. In fetuses with open neural tube defects, maternal serum α-fetoprotein levels measured at 16–18 weeks' gestation are elevated. α-Fetoprotein and acetylcholine esterase levels in amniotic fluid are also elevated. Ultrasound studies alone will detect approximately 90% of neural tube defects.

Prophylactic folic acid can significantly lower the incidence and recurrence rate of neural tube defects, if the intake of the folic acid starts at least 3 months prior to conception and continues for the first month of pregnancy, at a dose of 4 mg/d for women at increased risk. For women of childbearing age without a family history of neural tube defects, the dose is 0.4 mg of folic acid daily. Folic acid supplementation prior to conception may also lower the incidence of other congenital malformations such as conotruncal heart defects.

▶ Special Issues & Prognosis

All children requiring multiple surgical procedures (ie, patients with spina bifida or urinary tract anomalies) have a significant risk for developing hypersensitivity type I (IgE-mediated) allergic reactions to latex. For this reason, nonlatex medical products are now routinely used when caring for patients with neural tube defects.

Most individuals with spina bifida are cognitively normal, but learning disabilities are common. Individuals with encephalocele or other CNS malformations generally have a much poorer intellectual prognosis. Individuals with closed spinal cord abnormalities (eg, sacral lipomas) have more mild issues in general, and intelligence is usually normal. Problems in older patients include the development of spinal cord tethering, which usually presents with back pain, progressive scoliosis, and changes in bowel or bladder function. This often requires neurosurgical intervention.

Individuals with neural tube defects have lifelong medical issues, requiring the input of a multidisciplinary medical team. A good support for families is the national Spina Bifida Association, at the following web site: http://www.sbaa.org.

COMMON RECOGNIZABLE DISORDERS WITH VARIABLE OR UNKNOWN CAUSE

The text that follows describes several important and common human malformation syndromes. The best illustrations of these syndromes are found in *Smith's Recognizable Patterns of Human Malformation*. An excellent Internet site at the University of Kansas Medical Center can be consulted for further information: http://www.kumc.edu/gec/support.

1. Arthrogryposis Multiplex

Arthrogryposis multiplex is due to lack of fetal movement. Causes most often involve constraint, CNS maldevelopment or

injury, and neuromuscular disorders. Polyhydramnios is often present as a result of lack of fetal swallowing. Pulmonary hypoplasia may also be present, reflecting lack of fetal breathing. The workup includes brain imaging, careful consideration of metabolic disease, neurologic consultation, and, in some cases, electrophysiologic studies and muscle biopsy. The parents should be examined, and a family history reviewed carefully for findings such as muscle weakness or cramping, cataracts, and early-onset heart disease, suggesting myotonic dystrophy.

2. Goldenhar Syndrome

Goldenhar syndrome, also known as vertebro-auriculo-facial syndrome, is an association of multiple anomalies involving the head and neck. The classic phenotype includes hemifacial microsomia (one side of the face smaller than the other), and abnormalities of the pinna on the same side with associated deafness. Ear anomalies may be quite severe and include anotia. A characteristic benign fatty tumor in the outer eye, called an epibulbar dermoid, is frequently present, as are preauricular ear tags. Vertebral anomalies, particularly of the cervical vertebrae, are common. The Arnold-Chiari type I malformation (herniation of the cerebellum into the cervical spinal canal) is a common associated anomaly. Cardiac anomalies and hydrocephalus are seen in more severe cases. Most patients with Goldenhar syndrome have normal intelligence. The cause is unknown; however, there is significant overlap with the Townes-Brocks syndrome, now known to be caused by mutations in the *SALL1* gene.

3. Kabuki Syndrome

Kabuki syndrome is a disorder of unknown cause characterized by a distinctive facial appearance (hypertelorism with long palpebral fissures, large pinnae), developmental delay, and hearing loss. Most cases are sporadic, although a few cases with dominant transmission have been reported. Anomalies of the heart and genitourinary system are occasionally seen.

4. Oligohydramnios Sequence (Potter Sequence)

This condition presents in newborns as severe respiratory distress due to pulmonary hypoplasia in association with positional deformities of the extremities, usually bilateral clubfeet, and typical facies consisting of suborbital creases, depressed nasal tip and low-set ears, and retrognathia. The sequence may be due to prolonged lack of amniotic fluid. Most often it is due to leakage, renal agenesis, or severe obstructive uropathy.

5. Opitz G/BBB Syndrome

Disrupted development of midline structures is a feature of several overlapping malformation syndromes, a number of them heritable. Hypertelorism (wide set eyes), midbrain anomalies (agenesis of the corpus callosum), cardiac septal defects, and genitourinary tract anomalies (hypospadias) are the most common features. Current clinical genetic terminology refers to these conditions as Opitz G/BBB syndrome. Hypotonia and problems with swallowing and gastroesophageal reflux are hallmark symptoms. Mentation is usually subnormal. Both autosomal dominant and X-linked inheritance have been documented. Linkage studies have recently identified a candidate gene dubbed *M101* on the X chromosome. Several patients with Opitz G/BBB syndrome have also been shown by FISH to have deletions of 22q11. Additional resources include the Opitz Family Network and the Opitz G/BBB Family Network and the following web site: http://www.opitznet.org/joinus.html.

6. Overgrowth Syndromes

Overgrowth syndromes are becoming increasingly recognized as important childhood conditions. They may present at birth and are characterized by macrocephaly, motor delays (cerebral hypotonia), and, in many cases, asymmetry of extremities. Bone age may be advanced. The most common overgrowth syndrome is **Sotos syndrome**. Patients with Sotos syndrome have a characteristic facies with a prominent forehead and down-slanting palpebral features. The cause of the syndrome is unknown. Patients have a small but increased risk of cancer.

Other overgrowth syndromes include **Beckwith-Wiedemann syndrome** (BWS), described earlier, and two single gene disorders, Simpson-Golabi-Behmel syndrome and Bannayan-Riley-Ruvalcaba syndrome. Patients with **Simpson-Golabi-Behmel syndrome** exhibit a BWS-like phenotype, but with additional anomalies, including polydactyly and more severe facial dysmorphism. Unlike patients with BWS, who have normal intelligence, patients with Simpson-Golabi-Behmel syndrome often have developmental delay. It is inherited as an X-linked disorder. Patients with **Bannayan-Riley-Ruvalcaba syndrome** have macrosomia, macrocephaly, and unusual freckling of the penis. They have mild developmental issues and may present with autism. They may develop hemangiomatous or lymphangiomatous growths and have a predisposition to intestinal malignancies. The cause of Bannayan-Riley-Ruvalcaba syndrome was recently found to be a mutation of the *PTEN* gene implicated in Cowden syndrome, the association of intestinal polyposis with malignant potential.

7. Rubinstein-Taybi Syndrome

Rubinstein-Taybi syndrome is a genetic disorder of unknown cause, characterized by developmental delay, growth failure, and a distinctive facial dysmorphology comprising microcephaly, prominent nose, and small chin. Feeding problems are common. About 25% of patients have been found with a microdeletion of chromosome 16 detectable by FISH, but most patients have a normal karyotype.

8. Syndromic Short Stature

Short stature is an important component of numerous syndromes, or it may be an isolated finding. In the absence of nutritional deficiencies, endocrine abnormalities, evidence of skeletal dysplasia (disproportionate growth with abnormal skeletal films), or a positive family history, intrinsic short stature can be due to UPD. The phenotype of Russell-Silver syndrome—short stature with normal head growth (pseudohydrocephalus), normal development, and minor dysmorphic features (especially fifth finger clinodactyly)—has been associated in some cases with maternal UPD7.

9. VACTERL Association

ESSENTIALS OF DIAGNOSIS & TYPICAL FEATURES

VACTERL association is described by an acronym denoting the association of:

▶ **V**ertebral defects (segmentation anomalies).

▶ Imperforate **a**nus.

▶ **C**ardiac malformation (most often ventricular septal defect).

▶ **T**racheo-**e**sophageal fistula.

▶ **R**enal anomalies.

▶ **L**imb (most often radial ray) anomalies.

The disorder is sporadic, and some of the defects may be life-threatening. The prognosis for normal development is good. The cause is unknown, but a high association with monozygotic twinning suggests a mechanism dating back to events perhaps as early as blastogenesis. Recently, disturbance of the sonic hedgehog pathway was suggested to be part of the mechanism for VACTERL, based on a mouse model.

Careful examination and follow-up are important, because numerous other syndromes have overlapping features, such as the *SALL4* mutation that leads to Okihiro syndrome, Duane-Radial ray syndrome, and IVIC syndrome, which has a recurrence risk of 50%. In addition, Feingold syndrome, which is caused by mutation in the *MYCN* gene, and a newly described STAR syndrome due to a novel gene identified on the X chromosome need to be excluded. Chromosomal studies and genetic consultation are warranted.

Paradisi I, Arias S: IVIC syndrome is caused by a c.2607delA mutation in the SALL4 locus. Am J Med Genet 2007;143A:326 [PMID: 17256792].

EVALUATION OF THE DEVELOPMENTALLY DELAYED CHILD

Cognitive disabilities or developmental delays affect 8% of the population. Disorders associated with symptoms of delayed development are heterogeneous but frequently include heritable components. Evaluation should be multidisciplinary; Table 35–4 lists the main features of developmental delay, emphasizing the major clinical and genetic considerations. (See Chapter 2 for additional information about developmental delay and intellectual disability/mental retardation.)

Obtaining a detailed history, including pertinent prenatal and perinatal events, is critical. Feeding issues and slow growth velocity are seen in many genetic disorders causing developmental delay. Rate of developmental progress and particularly a history of loss of skills are important clues, as the latter might suggest a metabolic disorder with a neurodegenerative component. Family history can provide clues to suggest possible genetic etiologies, particularly if there is a history of consanguinity or a family pattern of other affected individuals.

Physical examination provides helpful clues. Referral to a clinical geneticist is indicated whenever unusual features are encountered. Neurologic, ophthalmologic, and audiologic consultation should be sought when indicated. Brain imaging should be requested in cases involving unexplained deviations from normal head growth. Neuroimaging and skeletal studies may also be indicated when dysmorphic features are present.

Metabolic and genetic testing procedures other than those listed in the Table 35–4 may also be indicated.

Interpretation & Follow-Up

Clinical experience indicates that specific diagnoses can be made in approximately half of patients evaluated according to the protocol presented here. With specific diagnosis comes prognosis, ideas for management, and insight into recurrence risks. Prenatal diagnosis may also become possible.

Follow-up is important both for patients in whom diagnoses have been made and for those patients initially lacking a diagnosis. Genetic information is accumulating rapidly and can be translated into new diagnoses and better understanding with periodic review of clinical cases.

Autism

Autism is a developmental disorder comprising abnormal function in three domains: language development, social development, and behavior. The majority of patients with autism also have cognitive disabilities and might be appropriately evaluated according to the recommendations above. However, given the enormous increase in prevalence of autism in the past decade, it is worth discussing the genetic evaluation of autism separately.

There are multiple known genetic causes of autism. Advances in molecular diagnosis, understanding of metabolic derangements, and technologies such as FISH are allowing more patients with autism to be identified with specific genetic disorders. This allows more accurate genetic counseling for recurrence risk, as well as diagnosis-specific interventions which may improve prognosis.

With this in mind, recommendations for the genetic evaluation of a child with autism include the following:

1. Genetic referral if dysmorphic features or cutaneous abnormalities are present (ie, hypopigmented spots such as those seen in patients with **tuberous sclerosis**).

Table 35–4. Evaluation of the child with developmental delay.

History
  Pregnancy history
  Growth parameters at birth
  Neonatal complications
  Feeding history
  History of somatic growth
  Motor, language, and psychosocial milestones
  Seizures
  Loss of skills
  Abnormal movements
  Results of previous tests and examinations
Family history
  Developmental and educational histories
  Psychiatric disorders
  Pregnancy outcomes
  Medical history
  Consanguinity
Physical examination
  General pediatric examination, including growth parameters
  Focused dysmorphologic evaluation including measurement of facial features and limbs
  Complete neurologic examination
  Parental growth parameters (especially head circumferences) and dysmorphic features should also be assessed
Imaging studies
  See text
Laboratory assessment[a]
  Chromosomes (high-resolution analysis)
  Fragile X testing (analysis of *FMR1* gene for triplet repeats)
  FISH analyses guided by dysmorphic features
  Comparative genomic hybridization (CGH) microarray
  Other blood analyses: complete blood count, electrolytes, liver function tests, creatinine kinase (CK), lactate, pyruvate
  Serum amino acid analysis
  Urine amino and organic acid analyses
  Urine analysis for mucopolysaccharides (if coarse features and organomegaly)

[a]In many cases, negative results may be important.
FISH, fluorescence in situ hybridization.

2. Laboratory testing to include the following:
   a. Chromosomes with high-resolution banding.
   b. Molecular testing for **fragile X syndrome.**
   c. FISH testing for 22q deletions and 15q derangements.
   d. Methylation testing for UPD15 if phenotype is suggestive of **Angelman syndrome.**
   e. Measurement of cholesterol and 7-dehydrocholesterol if syndactyly is present between the second and third toes, to rule out mild form of **Smith-Lemli-Opitz syndrome.**
   f. *MECP2* testing if clinical course is suggestive of **Rett syndrome** (ie, neurodegenerative course, progressive microcephaly, and seizures in a female patient).

Autism spectrum disorders are discussed in more detail in Chapter 2 of this text.

▼ PERINATAL GENETICS

TERATOGENS

1. Drug Abuse & Fetal Alcohol Syndrome

Fetal alcohol syndrome results from excessive exposure to alcohol during gestation and affects 30–40% of offspring of mothers whose daily intake of alcohol exceeds 3 ounces. Features of the syndrome include short stature, poor head growth (may be postnatal in onset), developmental delay, and midface hypoplasia characterized by a poorly developed long philtrum, narrow palpebral fissures, and short nose with anteverted nares. Facial findings may be subtle, but careful measurements and comparisons with standards (see Figure 35–11) are helpful. Structural abnormalities occur in half of affected children. Cardiac anomalies and neural tube defects are commonly seen. Genitourinary tract anomalies are frequent. Neurobehavioral effects also occur and may be stereotypic with poor judgment and inappropriate social interactions such as lack of stranger anxiety in toddlers commonly found. Behavioral problems may occur without other classic features of fetal alcohol syndrome.

Maternal abuse of drugs and other psychoactive substances is also associated with increased risks for adverse perinatal outcomes including miscarriage, preterm delivery, growth retardation, and increased risk for injury to the developing CNS. Methamphetamine and crack cocaine appear to be particularly dangerous. Maternal abuse of inhalants such as glue appears to be associated with findings similar to those of fetal alcohol syndrome. For most abused substances, the link between exposures and specific adverse outcomes is less well demonstrated than with alcohol. Multiple factors are probably involved, and it should be recognized that substance abuse often involves more than one drug.

Careful evaluation for other syndromes and chromosomal disorders should be included in the workup of exposed infants. Behavioral abnormalities in older children may be the result of maternally abused substances but they may also reflect evolving psychiatric disorders. Psychiatric disorders, many recognized as heritable, affect large numbers of men and women with substance abuse problems. Fetal alcohol spectrum disorders are discussed in more detail in Chapter 2.

2. Maternal Anticonvulsant Effects

Anticonvulsant exposure during pregnancy is associated with adverse outcomes in approximately 10% of children born to women treated with these agents. A syndrome characterized by small head circumference, anteverted nares, cleft lip and palate (occasionally), and distal digital hypoplasia was first described in association with maternal use of phenytoin but also occurs with other anticonvulsants including carbamazepine. Risks for spina bifida are increased, especially in pregnancies exposed to valproic acid.

3. Retinoic Acid Embryopathy

Vitamin A and its analogs are potent morphogens that have considerable teratogenic potential. Developmental toxicity occurs in approximately one third of pregnancies exposed in the first trimester to the synthetic retinoid isotretinoin, commonly prescribed to treat acne. Exposure disrupts migration of rostral neural crest cells and produces CNS maldevelopment, especially of the posterior fossa; ear anomalies (often absence of pinnae); congenital heart disease (great vessel anomalies); and tracheoesophageal fistula. These findings constitute a partial phenocopy of DiGeorge syndrome and demonstrate the continuum of contributing genetic and epigenetic factors in morphogenesis. It is now recognized that vitamin A itself, when taken as active retinoic acid in doses exceeding 25,000 IU/d during pregnancy, can produce similar fetal anomalies. For safety, vitamin A intake is therefore limited to 10,000 IU/d of retinoic acid. Maternal ingestion of large amounts of vitamin A taken as retinol during pregnancy, however, does not increase risks, because conversion of this precursor to active retinoic acid is internally regulated.

ASSISTED REPRODUCTION

Assisted reproductive technologies including in vitro fertilization now contribute significantly to human reproduction. Although healthy live births are accepted as the usual outcomes resulting from successful application of these procedures, questions about the risks of adverse effects on development are beginning to be raised. Increased rates of twinning, both monozygotic and dizygotic, are well recognized while the possibility of increased rates of birth defects remains controversial. Abnormal imprinting appears to be associated with in-vitro fertilization. Evidence supports increased prevalence of Beckwith-Wiedemann and Angelman syndromes among offspring of in vitro pregnancies.

PRENATAL DIAGNOSIS

Prenatal screening for birth defects is now routinely offered to pregnant women of all ages. Prenatal diagnosis for specific genetic disorders is indicated in 7–8% of pregnancies. Prenatal diagnosis introduces options for management including termination of abnormal pregnancies, preparation for specialized perinatal care, and, in some cases, fetal therapies.

Prenatal assessment of the fetus includes techniques that screen maternal blood, image the conceptus, and sample fetal and placental tissues (Table 35–5).

Maternal Blood Analysis

Elevated levels of maternal serum α-fetoprotein correlate with open neural tube defects but low levels are associated with Down syndrome and other chromosomal abnormalities. First trimester measurements of PAPA (pregnancy-

Table 35–5. Prenatal diagnostic techniques.

Maternal blood screening such as α-fetoprotein, estriol, human
   chorionic gonadotropin (hCG), and inhibin-A ("quad screen")
     Trisomies 21 and 18
     Neural tube defects
     Smith-Lemli-Opitz syndrome
Fetal cells in maternal blood (research only)
Fetal ultrasound
     Structural defects
     Fetal hydrops
     Poly- or oligohydramnios
Fetal radiograph
     Skeletal defects
Fetal MRI
Amniocentesis
     Karyotyping
     Fetal cells for molecular or metabolic studies
     Amniotic fluid α-fetoprotein level for neural tube defects
     Biochemical studies on fluid
Chorionic villus sampling
     Karyotyping
     Fetal cells for molecular or metabolic studies
Fetal tissues
     Blood by percutaneous umbilical blood sampling
     Biopsy of other fetal tissues
Direct fetal visualization via fetoscopy (rarely used today because of
   the advances in fetal visualization by ultrasound and MRI)

hCG, human chorionic gonadotropin; MRI, magnetic resonance imaging.

associated plasma protein A) and the free β-subunit of human chorionic gonadotropin screen for trisomies 21 and 18. In the second trimester maternal α-fetoprotein, human chorionic gonadotropin, unconjugated estradiol, and inhibin combine to estimate risks for trisomies 21 and 18. Low estradiol levels can also predict cases of Smith-Lemli-Opitz syndrome, a devastating autosomal recessive disorder discussed earlier.

Fetal cells, including lymphocytes, trophoblasts, and nucleated red blood cells, circulate at low frequency in maternal blood and may eventually provide access to direct information about the conceptus.

Analysis of Fetal Samples

A. Amniocentesis

Whereas maternal blood levels are screened for fetal abnormalities, genetic amniocentesis is applied to make specific diagnoses. This procedure samples fluid surrounding the fetus; the cells obtained are cultured for cytogenetic, molecular, or metabolic analyses. α-Fetoprotein and other chemical markers can also be measured. This is a safe procedure with a complication rate (primarily for miscarriage) of less than 1% in experienced hands.

B. Chorionic Villus Sampling (Placental)

Chorionic villus sampling is now available in most perinatal centers and is generally performed at 11–12 weeks' gestation. Tissue obtained by chorionic villus sampling provides DNA for molecular analysis and contains dividing cells (cytotrophoblasts) that can be rapidly karyotyped. However, direct cytogenetic preparations may be of poor quality. In addition, chromosomal abnormalities detected by this technique may be confined to the placenta (**confined placental mosaicism**). Cultured preparations may be more relevant.

C. Fetal Blood and Tissue

Fetal blood can be sampled directly in late gestation through ultrasound-guided percutaneous umbilical blood sampling. A wide range of diagnostic tests ranging from biochemical to cytogenetic can be applied. Fetal urine sampled from the bladder or dilated proximal structures can provide important information about fetal renal function.

It is occasionally necessary to obtain biopsy specimens of fetal tissues such as liver or muscle for accurate prenatal diagnosis; however, these procedures are available in only a few perinatal centers.

D. Embryo Biopsy

With the advent of single-cell PCR techniques as well as interphase FISH it is now possible to make genetic diagnoses in preimplantation human embryos by removing and analyzing blastocyst cells. How useful and accepted this technique will become remains to be seen.

Fetal Imaging

Fetal ultrasonography and MRI imaging are becoming increasingly common during pregnancy while radiographs are seldom employed. Ultrasonography has joined maternal blood sampling as a screening technique for common chromosomal aneuploidies, neural tube defects, and other structural anomalies. Pregnancies at increased risk for CNS anomalies, skeletal dysplasias, and structural defects of the heart and kidneys should be monitored by careful ultrasound examinations. Although MRI has had limited use to date, it appears that there will be a definite place for it in defining abnormalities of the fetal brain.

Rimoin DL et al: *Emery and Rimoin's Principles and Practice of Medical Genetics*, 3rd ed. Churchill Livingstone, 2002.

Allergic Disorders

Mark Boguniewicz, MD
Ronina A. Covar, MD
David M. Fleischer, MD

Allergic disorders are among the most common problems seen by pediatricians and primary care physicians, affecting over 25% of the population in developed countries. In the most recent National Health and Nutrition Examination Survey conducted in the United States between 1988 and 1994, 54% of the population had positive test responses to one or more allergens. In children, the increased prevalence of asthma, allergic rhinitis, and atopic dermatitis has been accompanied by significant morbidity and school absenteeism, with adverse consequences for school performance and quality of life, as well as economic burden measured in billions of dollars. Understanding the language of allergy and the basic mechanisms involved may help physicians when treating these disorders. In this chapter, atopy refers to a genetically determined predisposition to develop IgE antibodies found in patients with asthma, allergic rhinitis, and atopic dermatitis. This chapter discusses the major allergic disorders seen in pediatric practice.

ASTHMA

 ESSENTIALS OF DIAGNOSIS & TYPICAL FEATURES

▶ Episodic symptoms of airflow obstruction including wheezing, cough, and chest tightness.

▶ Airflow obstruction at least partially reversible.

▶ Exclusion of alternative diagnoses.

▶ General Considerations

Asthma is the most common chronic disease of childhood, affecting over 6 million children in the United States, and almost two of every three children affected have had at least one attack due to asthma in the past year. Despite advances in the understanding of asthma, associated morbidity and mortality rates are still historically high. Recent data suggest that death rates appear to have stabilized, yet the rate has not declined for black children. Although asthma prevalence in children increases with age, health care utilization is most marked among the very young. The prevalence, morbidity, and mortality rates for asthma are higher among minority and inner city populations. The reasons for this are unclear but may be related to a combination of more severe disease, poor access to health care, lack of asthma education, delay in prescribing appropriate controller therapy, and environmental factors (eg, irritants including smoke and air pollutants, and perennial allergen exposure).

Up to 80% of children with asthma develop symptoms before their fifth birthday. Atopy (personal or familial) is the strongest identifiable predisposing factor. Exposure to tobacco smoke, especially from the mother, is also a risk factor for asthma. About 40% of infants and young children who have wheezing with viral infections in the first few years of life will have continuing asthma through childhood. Sensitization to inhalant allergens increases over time and is found in the majority of children with asthma. The principal allergens associated with asthma are perennial aeroallergens such as dust mite, animal dander, cockroach, and *Alternaria* (a soil mold). Rarely, foods may provoke isolated asthma symptoms. Other triggers include exercise, cold air, cigarette smoke, pollutants, strong chemical odors, and rapid changes in barometric pressure. Aspirin sensitivity is uncommon in children. Psychological factors may precipitate asthma exacerbations and place the patient at high risk from the disease.

Pathologic features of asthma include shedding of airway epithelium, edema, mucus plug formation, mast cell activation, and collagen deposition beneath the basement membrane. The inflammatory cell infiltrate includes eosinophils, lymphocytes, and neutrophils, especially in fatal asthma exacerbations. Airway inflammation contributes to airway hyperresponsiveness, airflow limitation, and disease chronicity. Persistent airway inflammation can lead to airway wall remodeling and irreversible changes.

▶ Clinical Findings

A. Symptoms and Signs

Wheezing is the most characteristic sign of asthma, although some children may have recurrent cough and shortness of breath. Complaints may include "chest congestion," prolonged cough, exercise intolerance, dyspnea, and recurrent bronchitis or pneumonia. If symptoms are absent or mild, chest auscultation during forced expiration may reveal prolongation of the expiratory phase and wheezing. As the obstruction becomes more severe, wheezes become more high-pitched and breath sounds diminished. With severe obstruction, wheezes may not be heard because of poor air movement. Flaring of nostrils, intercostal and suprasternal retractions, and use of accessory muscles of respiration are signs of severe obstruction. Flushed, moist skin may be noted, and mucous membranes may be dry. Cyanosis of the lips and nail beds may be seen with underlying hypoxia. Tachycardia and pulsus paradoxus also occur. Agitation and lethargy may be signs of impending respiratory failure.

B. Laboratory Findings

Airway hyperresponsiveness to nonspecific stimuli is a hallmark of asthma. These include inhaled pharmacologic agents such as histamine and methacholine as well as physical stimuli such as exercise and cold air. Airways may exhibit hyperresponsiveness or twitchiness even when pulmonary function tests are normal. Giving increasing amounts of a bronchoconstrictive agent to induce a decrease in lung function (usually a 20% drop in forced expiratory volume in 1 second [FEV_1]) is the most common method of testing airway responsiveness. Hyperresponsiveness in normal children younger than age 5 years is greater than in older children. The level of airway hyperresponsiveness usually correlates with the severity of asthma.

During acute asthma exacerbations, FEV_1 is diminished and the flow-volume curve shows a "scooping out" of the distal portion of the expiratory portion of the loop (Figure 36–1). The residual volume, functional residual capacity, and total lung capacity are usually increased, while the vital capacity is decreased. Reversal or significant improvement of these abnormalities in response to inhaled bronchodilator therapy alone or with anti-inflammatory therapy is observed. Increased airway resistance also results in a decreased peak expiratory flow rate (PEFR). Diurnal variation in PEFR (ie, the difference between morning and evening measurements) of greater than 15–20% has been used as a defining feature of asthma. Significant changes in PEFR may occur before symptoms become evident. In more severe cases, PEFR monitoring enables earlier recognition of suboptimal asthma control. Exercise, cold air, and methacholine or histamine challenges may help to establish a diagnosis of asthma when the history, examination, and pulmonary function tests are not definitive. Alternatively, a diagnostic trial of inhaled bronchodilators and anti-inflammatory medications may be helpful, especially in infants and young children in whom underdiagnosis and undertreatment are common. Infant pulmonary function can be measured in sedated children with compression techniques. The forced oscillation technique can be used to measure airway resistance in younger children.

Hypoxemia is present early with a normal or low P_{CO_2} level and respiratory alkalosis. Hypoxemia may be aggravated

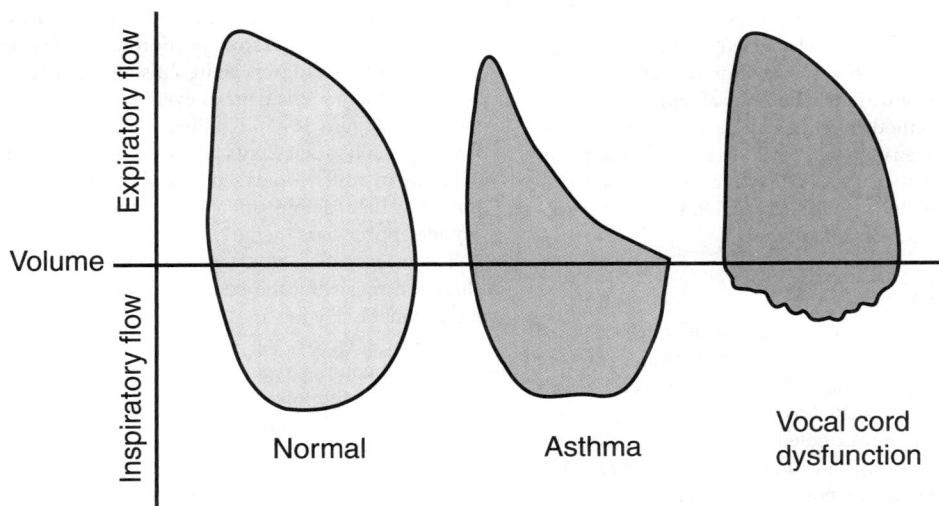

▲ **Figure 36–1.** Representative flow-volume loops in persons with normal lung function, asthma, and vocal cord dysfunction.

during treatment with a β_2-agonist due to ventilation-perfusion mismatch. Oxygen saturation less than 91% is indicative of significant obstruction. Respiratory acidosis and increasing CO_2 tension may ensue with further airflow obstruction and signal impending respiratory failure. Hypercapnia is usually not seen until the FEV_1 falls below 20% of predicted value. Metabolic acidosis has also been noted in combination with respiratory acidosis in children with severe asthma and indicates imminent respiratory failure. PaO_2 less than 60 mm Hg despite oxygen therapy and $PaCO_2$ over 60 mm Hg and rising more than 5 mm Hg per hour are relative indications for mechanical ventilation in a child in status asthmaticus.

Pulsus paradoxus may be present with moderate or severe asthma exacerbation. In moderate asthma exacerbation in a child, this may be between 10 and 25 mm Hg, and in severe asthma exacerbation between 20 and 40 mm Hg. Absence of pulsus paradoxus in a child with severe asthma exacerbation may signal respiratory muscle fatigue.

Clumps of eosinophils on sputum smear and blood eosinophilia are frequent findings. Their presence tends to reflect disease activity and does not necessarily mean that allergic factors are involved. Leukocytosis is common in acute severe asthma without evidence of bacterial infection and may be more pronounced after epinephrine administration. Hematocrit can be elevated with dehydration during prolonged exacerbations or in severe chronic disease. Potential noninvasive measures of airway inflammation include serum eosinophil cationic protein levels, exhaled nitric oxide, and induced sputum. Each test has its strengths and weaknesses.

C. Imaging

On chest radiographs, bilateral hyperinflation with flattening of the diaphragms, peribronchial thickening, prominence of the pulmonary arteries, and areas of patchy atelectasis may be present. Atelectasis may be misinterpreted as the infiltrates of pneumonia. High-resolution computed tomography has been used to quantify hyperinflation and bronchial wall thickening as a marker of airway remodeling in children with severe asthma and define peripheral airways disease and is useful in ruling out certain diagnoses in patients with difficult to manage asthma.

Allergy testing is discussed in the general measures section under Treatment, Chronic Asthma.

▶ Differential Diagnosis

Diseases that may be mistaken for asthma are often related to the patient's age (Table 36–1). Congenital abnormalities must be excluded in infants and young children. Asthma can be confused with croup, acute bronchiolitis, pneumonia, and pertussis. Immunodeficiency may be associated with cough and wheezing. Foreign bodies in the airway may cause dyspnea or wheezing of sudden onset, and on auscultation wheezing may be unilateral. Asymmetry of the lungs secondary to air trapping may be seen on a chest radiograph, especially with forced expiration. Cystic fibrosis can be associated with or mistaken for asthma.

Table 36–1. Differential diagnosis of asthma in infants and children.

Viral bronchiolitis
Aspiration
Laryngotracheomalacia
Vascular rings
Airway stenosis or web
Enlarged lymph nodes
Mediastinal mass
Foreign body
Bronchopulmonary dysplasia
Obliterative bronchiolitis
Cystic fibrosis
Vocal cord dysfunction
Cardiovascular disease

Vocal cord dysfunction is an important masquerader of asthma, although the two can coexist. It is characterized by the paradoxic closure of the vocal cords that can result in dyspnea and wheezing. Diagnosis is made by direct visualization of the vocal cords. In normal individuals, the vocal cords abduct during inspiration and may adduct slightly during expiration. Asthmatic patients may have narrowing of the glottis during expiration as a physiologic adaptation to airway obstruction. In contrast, patients with isolated vocal cord dysfunction typically show adduction of the anterior two thirds of their vocal cords during inspiration, with a small diamond-shaped aperture posteriorly. Because this abnormal vocal cord pattern may be intermittently present, a normal examination does not exclude the diagnosis. Exercise or methacholine challenges can often precipitate symptoms of vocal cord dysfunction. The flow-volume loop may provide additional clues to the diagnosis of vocal cord dysfunction. Truncation of the inspiratory portion can be demonstrated in most patients during an acute episode, and some patients continue to show this pattern even when they are asymptomatic (see Figure 36–1). Children with vocal cord dysfunction, especially adolescents, tend to be overly competitive, primarily in athletics and scholastics. A psychiatric consultation may help define underlying psychological issues and provide appropriate therapy.

Treatment of isolated vocal cord dysfunction includes education regarding the condition and appropriate breathing exercises. Hypnosis, biofeedback, and psychotherapy have been effective for some patients. During an acute episode, a helium–oxygen mixture (heliox) can be administered because the low density of the gas mixture facilitates movement of air through the adducted vocal cords.

▶ Conditions That May Increase Asthma Severity

Chronic hyperplastic sinusitis is frequently found in association with asthma. Upper airway inflammation has been shown to contribute to the pathogenesis of asthma, and asthma may improve after treatment of sinusitis. However, sinus surgery is usually not indicated for initial treatment of chronic mucosal disease associated with allergy.

A significant correlation has been observed between nocturnal asthma and gastroesophageal reflux. Patients may not complain of burning epigastric pain or have other reflux symptoms—cough may be the only sign. For patients with poorly controlled asthma, particularly with a nocturnal component, investigation for gastroesophageal reflux may be warranted even in the absence of suggestive symptoms.

The risk factors for death from asthma include psychological and sociological factors. They are probably related to the consequences of illness denial as well as to nonadherence with prescribed therapy. Recent studies have shown that less than 50% of inhaled asthma medications are taken as prescribed and that compliance does not improve with increasing severity of illness. Moreover, children requiring hospitalization for asthma, or their caregivers, have often failed to institute appropriate home treatment.

▶ Complications

With acute asthma, complications are primarily related to hypoxemia and acidosis and can include generalized seizures. Pneumomediastinum or pneumothorax can be a complication in status asthmaticus. With chronic asthma, recent studies point to airway wall remodeling and loss of pulmonary function with persistent airway inflammation. Childhood asthma independent of any corticosteroid therapy has been shown to be associated with delayed maturation and slowing of prepubertal growth velocity. However, attainment of final predicted adult height does not appear to be compromised.

▶ Treatment

A. Chronic Asthma

1. General measures—Management of asthma should include identification of precipitating factors and comorbid conditions that may worsen asthma, evaluation of the patient's and family's knowledge and skills for self-management, and assessment of asthma severity and control. Patients should avoid exposure to tobacco smoke and allergens to which they are sensitized, exertion outdoors when levels of air pollution are high, β-blockers, and sulfite-containing foods. Patients with persistent asthma should be given the inactivated influenza vaccine yearly unless they have a contraindication.

For patients with persistent asthma, the clinician should use the patient's history to assess sensitivity to seasonal allergens and *Alternaria* mold; use skin testing or in-vitro testing to assess sensitivity to perennial indoor allergens; assess the significance of positive tests in the context of the patient's history; and identify relevant allergen exposures. For dust mite–allergic children, important environmental control measures include encasing the pillow and mattress in an allergen-impermeable cover and washing the sheets and blankets on the patient's bed weekly in hot water. Other measures include keeping indoor humidity below 50%, minimizing the number of stuffed toys, and washing such toys weekly in hot water. Children allergic to furred animals or feathers should avoid indoor exposure to pets, especially for prolonged periods of time. If removal of the pet is not possible, the animal should be kept out of the bedroom with the door closed. Carpeting and upholstered furniture should be removed. While a high-efficiency particle-arresting filter unit in the bedroom may reduce allergen levels, clinical symptoms may persist if the pet remains indoor. For cockroach-allergic children, control measures need to be instituted when infestation is present in the home. Poison baits, boric acid, and traps are preferred to chemical agents, which can be irritating if inhaled by asthmatic individuals. Indoor molds are especially prominent in humid or damp environments. Measures to control dampness or fungal growth in the home may be of benefit. Patients can reduce exposure to outdoor allergens by staying in an air-conditioned environment. Allergen immunotherapy may be useful for implicated aeroallergens that cannot be avoided. However, it should be administered only in facilities staffed and equipped to treat life-threatening reactions.

The patient and family must understand the role of asthma triggers, the importance of disease activity even without obvious symptoms, how to use objective measures to gauge disease activity, and the importance of airway inflammation—and they must learn to recognize the warning signs of worsening asthma, allowing for early intervention. A stepwise care plan should be developed for all patients with asthma. This educational process extends to school personnel and all those who care for children with asthma.

Because the degree of airflow limitation is poorly perceived by many patients, peak flow meters can aid in the assessment of airflow obstruction and day-to-day disease activity. Peak flow rates may provide early warning of worsening asthma. They are also helpful in monitoring the effects of medication changes. Spacer devices optimize delivery of medication from metered-dose inhalers to the lungs and, with inhaled steroids, minimize side effects. Large-volume spacers are preferred.

Patients should be treated for rhinitis, sinusitis, or gastroesophageal reflux, if present. Treatment of upper respiratory tract symptoms is an integral part of asthma management. Intranasal corticosteroids are recommended to treat chronic rhinosinusitis in patients with persistent asthma because they reduce lower airway hyperresponsiveness and asthma symptoms. Intranasal cromolyn reduces asthma symptoms during the ragweed season but less so than intranasal corticosteroids. Treatment of rhinosinusitis includes medical measures to promote drainage and the use of antibiotics for acute bacterial infections (see Chapter 17). Medical management of gastroesophageal reflux includes avoiding eating or drinking 2 hours before bedtime, elevating the head of the bed with 6- to 8-inch blocks, and using appropriate pharmacologic therapy.

2. Pharmacologic therapy—A revised stepwise approach to pharmacologic therapy, broken down by age categories, is recommended in the National Asthma Education and Prevention Program's *Expert Panel Report 3* (http://www.nhlbi.nih. gov) (Tables 36–2 through 36–10). This approach is based on the concepts of asthma severity, asthma control, and responsiveness to therapy. A separate set of recommendations for younger children is provided given the lack of tools which can be used to assess lung function and quality of life otherwise available for older children. Treatment recommendations for older children and adults are better supported by stronger evidence from available clinical trials, whereas those for younger children have been extrapolated from studies in older children and adults.

Asthma severity is the intrinsic intensity of disease, and assessment is generally most accurate in patients not receiving controller therapy. Hence, assessing asthma severity directs the level of initial therapy. The two general categories are intermittent and persistent asthma, the latter further subdivided into mild, moderate, and severe. In contrast, asthma control refers to the degree to which symptoms, ongoing functional impairments and risk of adverse events are minimized and goals of therapy are met. Assessment of asthma control is important in adjusting therapy and is categorized as well controlled, not well controlled, and very poorly controlled. Responsiveness to therapy is the ease with which asthma control is attained by treatment. It can also encompass monitoring for adverse effects related to medication use.

Classification of asthma severity and control is premised on the domains of current impairment and risk, recognizing that these domains may respond differently to treatment. The level of asthma severity or control is based on the most severe impairment or risk category. Generally, the assessment is symptom based, except for the use of lung function for school-aged children and youths. Impairment includes an assessment of the patient's recent symptom frequency and intensity and functional limitations (ie, nighttime awakenings, need for short-acting β_2-agonists for quick relief, work or school days missed, ability to engage in normal or desired activities, and quality of life assessments) and airflow compromise using

Table 36–2. Classifying asthma severity and initiating treatment in children aged 0–4 years: assessing severity and initiating treatment for patients who are not currently taking long-term control medications.

Components of Severity		Classification of Asthma Severity (0–4 y)			
				Persistent	
		Intermittent	Mild	Moderate	Severe
Impairment	Symptoms	≤ 2 d/wk	> 2 d/wk but not daily	Daily	Throughout the day
	Nighttime awakenings	0	1–2×/mo	3–4×/mo	> 1×/wk
	SABA use for symptoms (not EIB pretreatment)	≤ 2 d/wk	> 2 d/wk but not daily	Daily	Several times per day
	Interference with normal activity	None	Minor limitation	Some limitation	Extremely limited
Risk	Exacerbations requiring systemic corticosteroids	0–1/y	≥ 2 exacerbations in 6 mo requiring systemic corticosteroids, or ≥ 4 wheezing episodes/1y lasting > 1 d AND risk factors for persistent asthma		
		Consider severity and interval since last exacerbation. Frequency and severity may fluctuate over time. Exacerbations of any severity may occur in patients in any severity category.			
Recommended step for initiating therapy		Step 1	Step 2	Step 3 and consider short course of oral systemic corticosteroids	
		In 2–6 wk, depending on severity, evaluate level of asthma control that is achieved. If no clear benefit is observed within 4–6 wk, stop treatment and consider adjusting therapy or alternative diagnoses.			

Notes:
- The stepwise approach is meant to assist, not replace, the clinical decision making required to meet individual patient needs.
- Level of severity is determined by both impairment and risk. Assess impairment domain by caregiver's recall of previous 2-4 weeks. Assign severity to the most severe category in which any feature occurs.
- At present, there are inadequate data to correspond frequencies of exacerbations with different levels of asthma severity. In general, more frequent and severe exacerbation (eg, requiring urgent, unscheduled care, hospitalizion, or ICU admission) indicate greater underlying disease severity. For treatment purposes, patients who had ≥ 2 exacerbations requiring oral systemic corticosteroids in the past 6 months, or ≥ 4 wheezing episodes in the past year, and who have risk factors for persistent asthma may be considered the same as patients who have persistent asthma, even in the absence of impairment levels consistent with persistent asthma. EIB, exercise-induced bronchospasm; SABA, short-acting β_2-agonist use.
Adapted from the National Asthma Education and Prevention Program: Expert Panel Report 3 (EPR 3): Guidelines for the Diagnosis and Management of Asthma—Summary Report 2007. J Allergy Clin Immunol 2007;120(Suppl):S94-138. Available at: http://www.nhlbi.nih.gov/guidelines/asthma/asthgdln.htm.

preferably spirometry. On the other hand, risk refers to an evaluation of the patient's likelihood of developing asthma exacerbations, reduced lung growth in children (or progressive decline in lung function in adults), or risk of untoward effects from medications.

The choice of initial therapy is based on assessment of asthma severity, and for patients who are already on controller therapy, revision of treatment is based on assessment of asthma control and responsiveness to therapy. The goals of therapy are to reduce the components of both impairment (eg, preventing chronic and troublesome symptoms, allowing infrequent need of quick relief medications, maintaining

"normal" lung function, maintaining normal activity levels including physical activity and school attendance, meeting families' expectations and satisfaction with asthma care) and risk (eg, preventing recurrent exacerbations, reduced lung growth, and medication adverse effects).

1. The stepwise approach is meant to assist, not replace, the clinical decision making required to meet individual patient needs.
2. In the absence of persistent symptoms, the new clinical guidelines recommend considering initiation of long-term controller therapy for infants and younger children who

Table 36–3. Classifying asthma severity and initiating treatment in children aged 5–11 years: assessing severity and initiating treatment for patients who are not currently taking long-term control medications.

Components of Severity		Classification of Asthma Severity (5–11 y)			
			Persistent		
		Intermittent	Mild	Moderate	Severe
Impairment	Symptoms	≤ 2 d/wk	> 2 d/wk but not daily	Daily	Throughout the day
	Nighttime awakenings	≤ 2×/mo	3–4×/mo	> 1×/wk but not nightly	Often 7×/wk
	SABA use for symptoms (not EIB pretreatment)	≤ 2 d/wk	> 2 d/wk but not daily	Daily	Several times per day
	Interference with normal activity	None	Minor limitation	Some limitation	Extremely limited
	Lung function	Normal FEV_1 between exacerbations			
		FEV_1 > 80% predicted	FEV_1 > 80% predicted	FEV_1 = 60–80% predicted	FEV_1 < 60% predicted
		FEV_1/FVC > 85%	FEV_1/FVC > 80%	FEV_1/FVC = 75–80%	FEV_1/FVC < 75%
Risk	Exacerbations requiring systemic corticosteroids	0–1/y (see note)	≥ 2/y (see note)		
		Consider severity and interval since last exacerbation. Frequency and severity may fluctuate over time.			
		Relative annual risk of exacerbations may be related to FEV_1.			
Recommended step for initiating therapy		Step 1	Step 2	Step 3, medium-dose ICS option	Step 3, medium-dose ICS option, or Step 4
				Consider short course of oral systemic corticosteroids	
		In 2–6 wk, evaluate level of asthma control that is achieved, and adjust therapy accordingly.			

Notes:
• The stepwise approach is meant to assist, not replace, the clinical decision making required to meet individual patient needs.
• Level of severity is determined by both impairment and risk. Assess impairment domain by patient's or caregiver's recall of previous 2–4 weeks and spirometry. Assign severity to the most severe category in which any feature occurs.
• At present, there are inadequate data to correspond frequencies of exacerbations with different levels of asthma severity. In general, more frequent and intense exacerbations (eg, requiring urgent, unscheduled care, hospitalization, or ICU admission) indicate greater underlying disease severity. For treatment purposes, patients who had ≥ 2 exacerbations requiring oral systemic corticosteroids in the past year may be considered the same as patients who have persistent asthma, even in the absence of persistent levels consistent with persistent asthma.
EIB, exercise-induced bronchospasm; SABA, short-acting β_2-agonist use; FEV_1, forced expiratory volume in 1 second; FVC, forced vital capacity; ICS, inhaled corticosteroids.
Adapted from the National Asthma Education and Prevention Program: Expert Panel Report 3 (EPR 3): Guidelines for the Diagnosis and Management of Asthma—Summary Report 2007. J Allergy Clin Immunol 2007;120(Suppl):S94–138. Available at: http://www.nhlbi.nih.gov/guidelines/asthma/asthgdln.htm.

Table 36–4. Classifying asthma severity and initiating treatment in children 12 years and older and adults: assessing severity and initiating treatment for patients who are not currently taking long-term control medications.

		Classification of Asthma Severity (>12 y)			
			Persistent		
Components of Severity		Intermittent	Mild	Moderate	Severe
Impairment	Symptoms	≤ 2 d/wk	> 2 d/wk but not daily	Daily	Throughout the day
	Nighttime awakenings	≤ 2×/mo	3–4×/mo	> 1×/wk but not nightly	Often 7×/wk
	SABA use for symptoms (not EIB pretreatment)	≤ 2 d/wk	> 2 d/wk but not daily and not more than 1× on any day	Daily	Several times per day
	Interference with normal activity	None	Minor limitation	Some limitation	Extremely limited
	Lung function	Normal FEV$_1$ between exacerbations			
	Normal FEV$_1$/FVC: 8–19 y, 85%	FEV$_1$ >80% predicted	FEV$_1$ > 80% predicted	FEV$_1$ = 60–80% predicted	FEV$_1$ < 60% predicted
	20–39 y, 80%	FEV$_1$/FVC normal	FEV$_1$/FVC normal	FEV$_1$/FVC reduced 5%	FEV$_1$/FVC reduced > 5%
	40–59 y, 75%				
	60–80 y, 70%				
Risk	Exacerbations requiring systemic corticosteroids	0–1/y (see note)		≥ 2/y	
		Consider severity and interval since last exacerbation. Frequency and severity may fluctuate over time for patients in any severity category.			
		Relative annual risk of exacerbations may be related to FEV$_1$.			
Recommended step for initiating therapy		Step 1	Step 2	Step 3	Step 4 or 5
					Consider short course of oral systemic corticosteroids
		In 2–6 wk, evaluate level of asthma control that is achieved and adjust therapy accordingly.			

Notes:
• The stepwise approach is meant to assist, not replace, the clinical decision making required to meet individual patient needs.
• Level of severity is determined by assessment of both impairment and risk. Assess impairment domain by patient's or caregiver's recall of previous 2–4 weeks and spirometry. Assign severity to the most severe category in which any feature occurs.
• At present, there are inadequate data to correspond frequencies of exacerbations with different levels of asthma severity. In general, more frequent and intense exacerbations (eg, requiring urgent, unscheduled care, hospitalization, or ICU admission) indicate greater underlying disease severity. For treatment purposes, patients who had ≥ 2 exacerbations requiring oral systemic corticosteroids in the past year may be considered the same as patients who have persistent asthma, even in the absence of impairment levels consistent with persistent asthma.
EIB, exercise-induced bronchospasm; SABA, short-acting β$_2$-agonist use; FEV$_1$, forced expiratory volume in 1 second; FVC, forced vital capacity; ICU, intensive care unit.
Adapted from the National Asthma Education and Prevention Program: Expert Panel Report 3 (EPR 3): Guidelines for the Diagnosis and Management of Asthma—Summary Report 2007. J Allergy Clin Immunol 2007;120(Suppl):S94–138. Available at: http://www.nhlbi.nih.gov/guidelines/asthma/asthgdln.htm.

have risk factors for asthma (ie, modified asthma predictive index: parental history of asthma, physician-diagnosed atopic dermatitis, or sensitization to aeroallergens or two of the following: wheezing apart from colds, sensitization to foods, or peripheral eosinophilia *and* four or more episodes of wheezing over the past year that lasted longer than 1 day and affected sleep or two or more exacerbations in 6 months requiring systemic corticosteroids.

3. Inhaled corticosteroids, either as monotherapy or in combination with adjunctive therapy, are preferred treatment for all levels of persistent asthma.
4. Along with medium-dose inhaled corticosteroids, combination therapy with inhaled corticosteroids plus any of the following adjunctive therapies—long-acting inhaled β$_2$-agonists (LABAs), leukotriene modifying agents, cromones, and theophylline—is recommended as step 3

Table 36–5. Assessing asthma control and adjusting therapy in children aged 0–4 years.

Components of Control		Classification of Asthma Control (0–4 y)		
		Well Controlled	Not Well Controlled	Very Poorly Controlled
Impairment	Symptoms	≤ 2 d/wk	> 2 d/wk	Throughout the day
	Nighttime awakenings	≤ 1×/mo	> 1×/mo	> 1×/wk
	SABA use for symptoms (not EIB pretreatment)	≤ 2 d/wk	> 2 d/wk	Several times per day
	Interference with normal activity	None	Some limitation	Extremely limited
Risk	Exacerbations requiring oral systemic corticosteroids	0–1/y	2–3/y	> 3 y
	Treatment-related adverse effects	Medication side effects can vary in intensity from none to very troublesome and worrisome. The level of intensity does not correlate to specific levels of control but should be considered in the overall assessment of risk.		
Recommended action for treatment		Maintain current treatment. Regular follow up every 1–6 mo. Consider step down if well controlled for at least 3 mo.	Step up (1 step) and Reevaluate in 2–6 wk. If no clear benefit in 4–6 wk, consider alternative diagnoses or adjusting therapy. For side effects, consider alternative treatment options.	Consider short course of oral systemic corticosteroids. Step up (1–2 steps), and Reevaluate in 2 wk. If no clear benefit in 4–6 wk, consider alternative diagnoses or adjusting therapy. For side effects, consider alternative treatment options.

Notes:
• The stepwise approach is meant to assist, not replace, the clinical decision making required to meet individual patient needs.
• The level of control is based on the most severe impairment or risk category. Assess impairment domain by caregiver's recall of previous 2–4 weeks. Symptom assessment for longer periods should reflect a global assessment such as inquiring whether the patient's asthma is better or worse since the last visit.
• At present, there are inadequate data to correspond frequencies of exacerbations with different levels of asthma control. In general, more frequent and intense exacerbations (eg, requiring urgent, unscheduled care, hospitalization, or ICU admission) indicate poorer disease control. For treatment purposes, patients who had ≥ 2 exacerbations requiring oral systemic corticosteroids in the past year may be considered the same as patients who have not-well-controlled asthma, even in the absence of impairment levels consistent with not-well-controlled asthma.
• Before step-up therapy:
  a. Review adherence to medications, inhaler technique, and environmental control.
  b. If alternative treatment option was used in a step, discontinue it and use preferred treatment for that step.
EIB, exercise-induced bronchospasm.
Adapted from the National Asthma Education and Prevention Program: Expert Panel Report 3 (EPR 3): Guidelines for the Diagnosis and Management of Asthma—Summary Report 2007. J Allergy Clin Immunol 2007(Suppl);120:S94–138. Available at: http://www.nhlbi.nih.gov/guidelines/asthma/asthgdln.htm.

treatment for moderate persistent asthma, or as step-up therapy for uncontrolled persistent asthma for school-aged children and youths. In children aged 0–4 years, medium-dose inhaled corticosteroids as monotherapy remain the step 3 therapy, and combination therapy to be initiated only as a step 4 treatment. A rescue course of systemic corticosteroids may be necessary at any step.

Asthma medications are classified as long-term controller medications and quick-relief medications. The former include anti-inflammatory agents, long-acting bronchodila-tors, and leukotriene modifiers. Unlike the other asthma controller medications, LABAs cannot be administered as monotherapy.

Inhaled corticosteroids are the most potent inhaled anti-inflammatory agents currently available. Different inhaled corticosteroids are not equivalent on a per puff or microgram basis (Table 36–11). Early intervention with inhaled corticosteroids can improve asthma control and prevent exacerbations during treatment, but they do not prevent the development of persistent asthma nor do they alter its natural history. Inhaled corticosteroids may be

Table 36–6. Assessing asthma control and adjusting therapy in children aged 5–11 years.

Components of Control		Classification of Asthma Control (5–11 y)		
		Well Controlled	**Not Well Controlled**	**Very Poorly Controlled**
Impairment	Symptoms	≤ 2 d/wk but not more than once on each day	> 2 d/wk or multiple times on ≤ 2 d/wk	Throughout the day
	Nighttime awakenings	≤ 1×/mo	≥ 2×/mo	≥ 2×/wk
	SABA use for symptoms (not EIB pretreatment)	≤ 2 d/wk	> 2 d/wk	Several times per day
	Interference with normal activity	None	Some limitation	Extremely limited
	Lung function	FEV$_1$ or peak flow > 80% predicted or personal best FEV$_1$/FVC > 80%	FEV$_1$ or peak flow = 60–80% predicted or personal best FEV$_1$/FVC = 75–80%	FEV$_1$ or peak flow < 60% predicted or personal best FEV$_1$/FVC < 75%
Risk	Exacerbations requiring oral systemic corticosteroids	0–1/y	≥ 2/y	≥ 2/y
		Consider severity and interval since last exacerbation.		
	Reduction in lung growth	Evaluation requires long-term follow-up.		
	Treatment-related adverse effects	Medication side effects can vary in intensity from none to very troublesome and worrisome. The level of intensity does not correlate to specific levels of control but should be considered in the overall assessment of risk.		
Recommended action for treatment		Maintain current treatment step. Regular follow up every 1–6 mo. Consider step down if well controlled for at least 3 mo.	Step up at least 1 step and Reevaluate in 2–6 wk. For side effects, consider alternative treatment options.	Consider short course of oral systemic corticosteroids. Step up (1–2 steps), and Reevaluate in 2 wk. For side effects, consider alternative treatment options.

Notes:
• The stepwise approach is meant to assist, not replace, the clinical decision making required to meet individual patient needs.
• The level of control is based on the most severe impairment or risk category. Assess impairment domain by patient's or caregiver's recall of previous 2–4 weeks and by spirometry or peak flow measures. Symptom assessment for longer periods should reflect a global assessment such as inquiring whether the patient's asthma is better or worse since the last visit.
• At present, there are inadequate data to correspond frequencies of exacerbations with different levels of asthma control. In general, more frequent and intense exacerbations (eg, requiring urgent, unscheduled care, hospitalization, or ICU admission) indicate poorer disease control. For treatment purposes, patients who had ≥ 2 exacerbations requiring oral systemic corticosteroids in the past year may be considered the same as patients who have not-well-controlled asthma, even in the absence of impairment levels consistent with not-well-controlled asthma.
• Before step-up therapy:
  a. Review adherence to medications, inhaler technique, environmental control, and comorbid conditions.
  b. If alternative treatment option was used in a step, discontinue it and use preferred treatment for that step.
EIB, exercise-induced bronchospasm; FEV$_1$, forced expiratory volume in 1 second; FVC, forced vital capacity.
Adapted from the National Asthma Education and Prevention Program: Expert Panel Report 3 (EPR 3): Guidelines for the Diagnosis and Management of Asthma—Summary Report 2007. J Allergy Clin Immunol 2007;120(Suppl):S94-138. Available at: http://www.nhlbi.nih.gov/guidelines/asthma/asthgdln.htm.

associated with slowing of growth velocity in children, although a study of asthmatic children treated with budesonide (mean dose, 412 mcg/d) for a mean of 9.2 years showed no adverse effect on final adult height. Possible risks from inhaled corticosteroids need to be weighed against the risks from undertreated asthma. The adverse effects from inhaled corticosteroids are generally dose and duration dependent, so that greater risks for systemic adverse effects are expected with high doses. The various inhaled corticosteroids are delivered in different devices such as metered dose inhaler (MDI) (beclomethasone, fluticasone, flunisolide and triamcinolone), dry powder inhaler (DPI) (Flovent Diskus, Pulmicort Flexhaler or Turbohaler, and Asmanex Twisthaler) and nebulized aerosol suspensions (Pulmicort respules). Except for triamcinolone, the inhaled corticosteroids delivered in MDI now use the more ozone friendly hydrofluoroalkane (HFA) propellant, which has replaced chlorofluorocarbons (CFC).

Table 36–7. Assessing asthma control and adjusting therapy in youths aged 12 years or older and adults.

Components of Control		Classification of Asthma Control (≥ 12 y)		
		Well Controlled	Not Well Controlled	Very Poorly Controlled
Impairment	Symptoms	≤ 2 d/wk	> 2 d/wk	Throughout the day
	Nighttime awakenings	≤ 2×/mo	1–3×/wk	≥ 4×/wk
	SABA use for symptoms (not EIB pretreatment)	≤ 2 d/wk	> 2 d/wk	Several times per day
	Interference with normal activity	None	Some limitation	Extremely limited
	Lung function	FEV$_1$ or peak flow > 80% predicted or personal best	FEV$_1$ or peak flow = 60–80% predicted or personal best	FEV$_1$ or peak flow < 60% predicted or personal best
	Validated questionnaires			
	ATAQ	0	1–2	3–4
	ACQ	≤ 0.75[a]	≥ 1.5	N/A
	ACT	≥ 20	16–19	≤ 15
Risk	Exacerbations requiring oral systemic corticosteroids	0–1/y	≥ 2/y	≥ 2/y
		Consider severity and interval since last exacerbation.		
	Progressive loss of lung function	Evaluation requires long-term follow-up.		
	Treatment-related adverse effects	Medication side effects can vary in intensity from none to very troublesome and worrisome. The level of intensity does not correlate to specific levels of control but should be considered in the overall assessment of risk.		
Recommended action for treatment		Maintain current treatment step. Regular follow up every 1–6 mo to maintain control. Consider step down if well controlled for at least 3 mo.	Step up (1 step) and Reevaluate in 2–6 wk. For side effects, consider alternative treatment options.	Consider short course of oral systemic corticosteroids. Step up (1–2 steps), and Reevaluate in 2 wk. For side effects, consider alternative treatment options.

[a]ACQ values of 0.76–1.40 are indeterminate regarding well-controlled asthma.

Notes:

• The stepwise approach is meant to assist, not replace, the clinical decision making required to meet individual patient needs.

• The level of control is based on the most severe impairment or risk category. Assess impairment domain by patient's recall of previous 2–4 weeks and by spirometry or peak flow measures. Symptom assessment for longer periods should reflect a global assessment, such as inquiring whether the patient's asthma is better or worse since the last visit.

• At present, there are inadequate data to correspond frequencies of exacerbations with different levels of asthma control. In general, more frequent and intense exacerbations (eg, requiring urgent, unscheduled care, hospitalization, or ICU admission) indicate poorer disease control. For treatment purposes, patients who had ≥ 2 exacerbations requiring oral systemic corticosteroids in the past year may be considered the same as patients who have not-well-controlled asthma, even in the absence of impairment levels consistent with not-well-controlled asthma.

Validated questionnaires for the impairment domain (the questionnaires do not assess lung function or the risk domain):

  a. ATAQ= Asthma Therapy Assessment Questionnaire

  b. ACQ= Asthma Control Questionnaire

  c. ACT= Asthma Control Test

Minimal Important Difference: 1.0 for ATAQ; 0.5 for the ACQ; not determined for ACT

• Before step-up therapy:

  a. Review adherence to medications, inhaler technique, environmental control, and comorbid conditions.

  b. If alternative treatment option was used in a step, discontinue it and use preferred treatment for that step.

EIB, exercise-induced bronchospasm; FEV$_1$, forced expiratory volume in 1 second; FVC, forced vital capacity.

Adapted, with permission, from the National Asthma Education and Prevention Program: Expert Panel Report 3 (EPR 3): Guidelines for the Diagnosis and Management of Asthma—Summary Report 2007. J Allergy Clin Immunol 2007;120(Suppl):S94–138. Available at: http://www.nhlbi.nih.gov/guidelines/asthma/asthgdln.htm.

Table 36–8. Stepwise approach for managing asthma in children aged 0–4 years.

Intermittent Asthma	Persistent Asthma: Daily Medication[a] Consult with asthma specialist if step 3 or higher is required. Consider consultation at step 2.					
Step 1 Preferred SABA prn	**Step 2** Preferred Low-dose ICS Alternative: cromolyn or montelukast	**Step 3** Preferred Medium-dose ICS	**Step 4** Preferred Medium-dose ICS + either LABA or montelukast	**Step 5** Preferred High-dose ICS + either LABA or montelukast	**Step 6** Preferred High-dose ICS + either LABA or montelukast Oral systemic corticosteroids	Step up if needed (first check adherence, inhaler technique, and environmental control) **Assess Control** Step down if possible (and asthma is well controlled at least 3 mo)

Patient Education and Environmental Control at Each Step

Quick-Relief Medication for All Patients

- SABA as needed for symptoms. Intensity of treatment depends on severity of symptoms.
- With viral respiratory infection: SABA q 4–6 h up to 24 h (longer with physician consult). Consider short course of systemic corticosteroids if exacerbation is severe or patient has history of previous severe exacerbations.
- Caution: frequent use of SABA may indicate the need to step up treatment.

[a]Alphabetical order is used when more than one treatment option is listed within either preferred or alternative therapy.

Notes:
- The stepwise approach is meant to assist, not replace, the clinical decision making required to meet individual patient needs.
- If alternative treatment is used and response is inadequate, discontinue it and use the preferred treatment before stepping up.
- If clear benefit is not observed within 4-6 weeks and patient/family medication technique and adherence are satisfactory, consider adjusting therapy or an alternative diagnosis.
- Studies on children aged 0–4 years are limited. Step 2 preferred therapy is based on Evidence A. All other recommendations are based on expert opinion and extrapolation from studies in older children.
ICS, inhaled corticosteroid; LABA, inhaled long-acting β_2-agonist; prn, as needed; SABA, inhaled short acting β_2-agonist.
Adapted from the National Asthma Education and Prevention Program: Expert Panel Report 3 (EPR 3): Guidelines for the Diagnosis and Management of Asthma—Summary Report 2007. J Allergy Clin Immunol 2007;120(Suppl):S94–138. Available at: http://www.nhlbi.nih.gov/guidelines/asthma/asthgdln.htm.

Only inhaled corticosteroids have been shown to be effective in long-term clinical studies with infants. Nebulized budesonide is approved for children as young as 12 months. The suspension (available in quantities of 0.25 mg/2 mL, 0.5 mg/2 mL, and 1.0 mg/2 mL) is usually administered either once or twice daily in divided doses. Notably, this drug should not be given by ultrasonic nebulizer. Limited data suggest that inhaled corticosteroids may be effective even in very young children when delivered by metered-dose inhaler with a spacer and mask.

Fewer data are available with nedocromil, although data from the Childhood Asthma Management Program study showed that an inhaled corticosteroid was superior to nedocromil with respect to several efficacy parameters, including rate of hospitalization, symptom-free days, need for albuterol rescue, and longer time to treatment with prednisone, when each was compared to a placebo.

Sustained-release theophylline, an alternative long-term control medication for older children, may have particular risks of adverse effects in infants, who frequently have febrile illnesses that increase theophylline concentrations. Hence, theophylline use requires monitoring of serum concentration to prevent numerous dose-related acute toxicities.

Salmeterol and formoterol (both LABAs) can be used as adjunctive therapy with anti-inflammatory medications for long-term symptom control. They should not be used for treatment of acute symptoms, nor should they be used without any inhaled corticosteroid therapy, even if the patient feels better. Salmeterol is available as an inhalation powder (1 inhalation twice daily for patients aged 4 years and older). It is also available combined with fluticasone (50 mcg salmeterol with 100, 250, or 500 mcg fluticasone in a DPI or 21 mcg salmeterol with 45, 115, or 230 mcg fluticasone in an MDI).

Table 36–9. Stepwise approach for managing asthma in children aged 5–11 years.

Intermittent Asthma	Persistent Asthma: Daily Medication[a] Consult with asthma specialist if step 4 or higher is required. Consider consultation at step 3.					
Step 1 Preferred SABA prn	Step 2 Preferred Low-dose ICS Alternative: cromolyn, LTRA, nedocromil, or theophylline	Step 3 Preferred Either Low dose ICS + either LABA, LTRA, or theophylline Or: Medium-dose ICS	Step 4 Preferred Medium-dose ICS + LABA Alternative Medium-dose ICS + either LTRA or theophylline	Step 5 Preferred High dose ICS + LABA Alternative: High-dose ICS + either LTRA or theophylline	Step 6 Preferred High dose ICS + LABA + oral systemic corticosteroid Alternative: High-dose ICS + either LTRA or theophylline + oral systemic corticosteroid	Step up if needed (first check adherence, inhaler technique, and environmental control, and comorbid conditions) **Assess Control** Step down if possible (and asthma is well controlled at least 3 mo)

Patient Education, Environmental Control, and Management of Comorbidities at Each Step

Steps 2–4: consider subcutaneous allergen immunotherapy for patients who have persistent allergic asthma.

Quick-Relief Medication for All Patients

- SABA as needed for symptoms. Intensity of treatment depends on severity of symptoms: up to 3 treatments at 20-min intervals as needed. Short course of oral systemic corticosteroids may be needed.
- Caution: Increasing use of SABA or use > 2 d/wk for symptom relief (not prevention of EIB) generally indicates inadequate control and the need to step up treatment.

[a]Alphabetical order is used when more than one treatment option is listed within either preferred or alternative therapy.
Notes:
- The stepwise approach is meant to assist, not replace, the clinical decision making required to meet individual patient needs.
- If alternative treatment is used and response is inadequate, discontinue it and use the preferred treatment before stepping up.
- Theophylline is a less desirable alternative due to the need to monitor serum concentration levels.
- Step 1 and 2 medications are based on Evidence A. Step 3 ICS and ICS plus adjunctive therapy are based on Evidence B for efficacy of each treatment and extrapolation from comparator trials in older children and adults—comparator trials are not available for this age group; steps 4–6 are based on expert opinion and extrapolation from studies in older children and adults.
- Immunotherapy for steps 2–4 is based on Evidence B for house dust mites, animal danders, and pollens; evidence is weak or lacking for molds and cockroaches. Evidence is strongest for immunotherapy with single allergens. The role of allergy in asthma is greater in children than in adults. Clinicians who administer immunotherapy should be prepared and equipped to identify and treat anaphylaxis that may occur.
ICS, inhaled corticosteroid; LABA, inhaled long-acting β₂-agonist; LTRA, leukotriene receptor antagonist; prn, as needed; SABA, inhaled short-acting β₂-agonist
Adapted from the National Asthma Education and Prevention Program: Expert Panel Report 3 (EPR 3): Guidelines for the Diagnosis and Management of Asthma—Summary Report 2007. J Allergy Clin Immunol 2007;120(Suppl):S94-138. Available at: http://www.nhlbi.nih.gov/guidelines/asthma/asthgdln.htm.

For children 12 years and older, 1 inhalation DPI or 2 inhalations MDI, can be taken twice daily. (**Note:** The 100/50 fluticasone/salmeterol combination is approved in children aged 4 and older.) It can also be used 30 minutes before exercise (but not in addition to regularly used LABAs). Formoterol has a more rapid onset of action and is available singly as a DPI (Aerolizer, 12 mcg) or combined with an inhaled corticosteroid (formoterol fumarate, 4.5 mcg, with budesonide, 80 or 160 mcg, in an MDI). Formoterol DPI is approved for use in children 5 years and older, 1 inhalation (12 mcg) twice daily, while the combination product is approved for children 12 years and older, 2 inhalations twice

daily. For long-term control, formoterol should be used in combination with an anti-inflammatory agent. It can be used for exercise-induced bronchospasm in patients 5 years and older, 1 inhalation at least 15 minutes before exercise (but not in addition to regularly used LABAs). Of note, the U.S. Food and Drug Administration (FDA) has requested the manufacturers of Advair Diskus and HFA (salmeterol and fluticasone), Serevent Diskus (salmeterol xinafoate), Foradil Aerolizer (formoterol fumarate), Symbicort HFA, and Brovana (arformoterol tartrate inhalation solution, a LABA approved for chronic obstructive pulmonary disease) to update their product information warning sections regarding an increase in severe

Table 36–10. Stepwise approach for managing asthma in youths aged 12 years and older and adults.

Intermittent Asthma	Persistent Asthma: Daily Medication[a] Consult with asthma specialist if step 4 or higher is required. Consider consultation at step 3.					
Step 1 *Preferred* SABA prn	**Step 2** *Preferred* Low-dose ICS *Alternative:* cromolyn, LTRA, nedocromil, or theophylline	**Step 3** *Preferred* *Either* Low dose ICS + LABA *Or* Medium-dose ICS *Alternative:* Low-dose ICS + either LTRA, theophylline, or zileuton	**Step 4** *Preferred* Medium dose ICS + LABA *Alternative:* Medium-dose ICS + either LTRA, theophylline, or zileuton	**Step 5** *Preferred* High dose ICS + LABA *And* Consider omalizumab for patients who have allergies	**Step 6** *Preferred* High dose ICS + LABA + oral systemic corticosteroid *And* Consider omalizumab for patients who have allergies	Step up if needed (first check adherence, inhaler technique, and environmental control, and comorbid conditions) **Assess Control** Step down if possible (and asthma is well controlled at least 3 mo)

Patient Education, Environmental Control, and Management of Comorbidities

Steps 2–4: Consider subcutaneous allergen immunotherapy for patients who have allergic asthma.

Quick-Relief Medication for All Patients

- SABA as needed for symptoms. Intensity of treatment depends on severity of symptoms: up to 3 treatments at 20-min intervals as needed. Short course of oral systemic corticosteroids may be needed.

- Use of SABA > 2 d/wk for symptom relief (not prevention of EIB) generally indicates inadequate control and the need to step up treatment.

[a]Alphabetical order is used when more than one treatment option is listed within either preferred or alternative therapy.

Notes:

- The stepwise approach is meant to assist, not replace, the clinical decision making required to meet individual patient needs.
- If alternative treatment is used and response is inadequate, discontinue it and use the preferred treatment before stepping up.
- Theophylline requires monitoring of serum concentration levels.
- Zileuton is less desirable alternative due to limited studies as adjunctive therapy and the need to monitor liver function.
- In step 6, before oral systemic corticosteroids are introduced, a trial of high-dose ICS + LABA + either LTRA, theophylline, or zileuton may be considered, although this approach has not been studied in clinical trials.
- Step 1, 2 and 3 preferred therapies are based on Evidence A; step 3 alternative therapy is based on Evidence A for LTRA, Evidence B for theophylline, and Evidence D for zileuton. Step 4 preferred therapy is based on Evidence B, and alternative therapy is based on Evidence B for LTRA and theophylline and Evidence D for zileuton. Step 5 preferred therapy is based on Evidence B. Step 6 preferred therapy is based on (EPR-1 1997) and Evidence B for omalizumab.
- Immunotherapy for steps 2–4 is based on Evidence B for house dust mite, animal dander, and pollens; evidence is weak or lacking for molds and cockroaches. Evidence is strongest for immunotherapy with single allergens. The role of allergy in asthma is greater in children than in adults.
- Clinicians who administer immunotherapy or omalizumab should be prepared and equipped to identify and treat anaphylaxis that may occur.

ICS, inhaled corticosteroid; LABA, inhaled long-acting β_2-agonist; LTRA, leukotriene receptor antagonist; prn, as needed; SABA, inhaled short-acting β_2-agonist. Adapted from the National Asthma Education and Prevention Program: Expert Panel Report 3 (EPR 3): Guidelines for the Diagnosis and Management of Asthma—Summary Report 2007. J Allergy Clin Immunol 2007;120(Suppl):S94–138. Available at: http://www.nhlbi.nih.gov/guidelines/asthma/asthgdln.htm.

asthma episodes associated with these agents. This action is in response to data showing an increased number of asthma-related deaths in patients receiving LABA therapy in addition to their usual asthma care as compared with patients not receiving LABAs. This notice is also intended to reinforce the appropriate use of LABAs in the management of asthma. Specifically, LABA products should not be initiated as first-line asthma therapy, used with worsening wheezing, or used for acute control of bronchospasm. No data are available regarding safety concerns in patients using these products for

Table 36–11. Estimated comparative inhaled corticosteroid doses.

Drug	Low Daily Dose Child 0–4 y	Child 5–11 y	Adult	Medium Daily Dose Child 0–4 y	Child 5–11 y	Adult	High Daily Dose Child 0–4 y	Child 5–11 y	Adult
Beclomethasone HFA, 40 or 80 mcg/puff	NA	80–160 mcg	80–240 mcg	NA	> 160–320 mcg	> 240–480 mcg	NA	> 320 mcg	> 480 mcg
Budesonide DPI 90, 180, or 200 mcg/inhalation	NA	180–400 mcg	180–600 mcg	NA	> 400–800 mcg	> 600–1200 mcg	NA	> 800 mcg	> 1200 mcg
Budesonide inhaled suspension for nebulization, 0.25-, 0.5-, and 1.0-mg dose	0.25–0.5 mg	0.5 mg	NA	> 0.5–1.0 mg	1.0 mg	NA	> 1.0 mg	2.0 mg	NA
Flunisolide, 250 mcg/puff	NA	500–750 mcg	500–1000 mcg	NA	1000–1250 mcg	> 1000–2000 mcg	NA	> 1250 mcg	> 2000 mcg
Flunisolide HFA, 80 mcg/puff	NA	160 mcg	320 mcg	NA	320 mcg	> 320–640 mcg	NA	≥ 640 mcg	> 640 mcg
Fluticasone HFA/MDI, 44, 110, or 220 mcg/puff	176 mcg	88–176 mcg	88–264 mcg	> 176–352 mcg	> 176–352 mcg	> 264–440 mcg	> 352 mcg	> 352 mcg	> 440 mcg
Fluticasone DPI, 50, 100, or 250 mcg/inhalation	NA	100–200 mcg	100–300 mcg	NA	>200–400 mcg	>300–500 mcg	NA	> 400 mcg	> 500 mcg
Mometasone DPI, 220 mcg/inhalation	NA	NA	220 mcg	NA	NA	440 mcg	NA	NA	> 440 mcg
Triamcinolone acetonide, 75 mcg/puff	NA	300–600 mcg	300–750 mcg	NA	> 600–900 mcg	> 750–1500 mcg	NA	> 900 mcg	> 1500 mcg

DPI, dry powder inhaler; HFA, hydrofluoroalkane; MDI, metered-dose inhaler; NA, not available (either not approved or no data available or safety and efficacy not established for this age group).

Adapted from the National Asthma Education and Prevention Program: Expert Panel Report 3 (EPR 3): Guidelines for the Diagnosis and Management of Asthma—Summary Report 2007. J Allergy Clin Immunol 2007;120(Suppl):S94–138. Available at: http://www.nhlbi.nih.gov/guidelines/asthma/asthgdln.htm.

exercise-induced bronchoconstriction. Additional information, including copies of the Patient and Healthcare Professional information sheets, can be found at: http://www.fda.gov/cder/drug/infopage/LABA/default.htm.

Montelukast and zafirlukast are leukotriene-receptor antagonists available in oral formulations. Montelukast is given once daily and has been approved for treatment of chronic asthma in children aged 1 year and older. It is also indicated for seasonal allergic rhinitis in patients 2 years and older, and for perennial allergic rhinitis in patients 6 months and older. To date, no drug interactions have been noted. The dosage is 4 mg for children 1–5 years (oral granules are available for children aged 12–23 months), 5 mg for children aged 6–14 years, and 10 mg for those aged 15 years and older. The drug is given without regard to mealtimes, preferably in the evening. Zafirlukast is approved for patients aged 5 years and older. The dose is 10 mg twice daily for those 5–11 years and 20 mg twice daily for those 12 years and older. It should be taken 1 hour before or 2 hours after meals. Zileuton is a 5-lipoxygenase inhibitor indicated for chronic treatment in children 12 years of age and older, 600 mg four times a day. Patients need to have hepatic transaminase levels evaluated at

initiation of therapy, then once a month for the first 3 months, every 2–3 months for the remainder of the first year, and periodically thereafter if receiving long-term zileuton therapy. Rare cases of Churg-Strauss syndrome have been reported in adult patients with severe asthma whose steroid dosage was being tapered during concomitant treatment with leukotriene-receptor antagonists (as well as inhaled corticosteroids), but no causal link has been established. Both zafirlukast and zileuton are microsomal P450 enzyme inhibitors that can inhibit the metabolism of drugs such as warfarin and theophylline. Of note, in a study of children with mild to moderate persistent asthma that looked at whether responses to an inhaled corticosteroid and a leukotriene-receptor antagonist are concordant for individuals or whether asthmatic patients who do not respond to one medication respond to the other, response to fluticasone and montelukast were found to vary considerably. Children with low pulmonary function or high levels of markers associated with allergic inflammation responded better to the inhaled corticosteroid.

Quick-relief medications include short-acting inhaled β_2-agonists (SABAs) such as albuterol, levalbuterol, pirbuterol, or terbutaline. Albuterol can be given by nebulizer, 0.05 mg/kg (with a minimal dose of 0.63 mg and a maximum of 5 mg) in 2–3 mL saline (although it is also available in a 0.63 mg/3 mL and 1.25 mg/3 mL dosing) or by MDI. It is better to use SABAs as needed rather than on a regular basis. Increasing use, including more than one canister per month, may signify inadequate asthma control and the need to intensify anti-inflammatory therapy. Levalbuterol, the (R)-enantiomer of racemic albuterol, is available in solution for nebulization in patients aged 6–11 years, 0.31 mg every 8 hours, and in patients 12 years and older, 0.63–1.25 mg every 8 hours. It has recently become available in an HFA formulation for children 4 years and older, 2 inhalations (90 mcg) every 4–6 hours as needed. Anticholinergic agents such as ipratropium, 1–3 puffs or 0.25–0.5 mg by nebulizer every 6 hours, may provide additive benefit when used together with an inhaled SABA. Systemic corticosteroids such as prednisone, prednisolone, and methylprednisolone can be given in a dosage of 1–2 mg/kg, usually up to 60 mg/d in single or divided doses for 3–10 days. There is no evidence that tapering the dose following a "burst" prevents relapse.

Anti-IgE (omalizumab) is a recombinant DNA-derived humanized IgG_1 monoclonal antibody that selectively binds to human IgE. It inhibits the binding of IgE to the high-affinity IgE receptor (FcɛRI) on the surface of mast cells and basophils. Reduction in surface-bound IgE on FcɛRI-bearing cells limits the degree of release of mediators of the allergic response. Treatment with omalizumab also reduces the number of FcɛRI receptors on basophils in atopic patients. Omalizumab is indicated for patients 12 years of age and older with moderate to severe persistent asthma who have a positive skin test or in-vitro reactivity to a perennial aeroallergen with serum IgE of 700 IU/mL or less, and whose symptoms are inadequately controlled with inhaled corticosteroids. Omalizumab has been shown to decrease the incidence of asthma exacerbations in these patients. Dosing is based on the patient's weight and serum IgE level and is given subcutaneously every 2–4 weeks. The FDA has ordered a black box warning to the label because of new reports of serious and life-threatening anaphylactic reactions (bronchospasm, hypotension, syncope, urticaria, and angioedema of the throat or tongue) in patients after treatment with Xolair (omalizumab). Based on reports from approximately 39,500 patients, anaphylaxis following Xolair treatment occurred in at least 0.1% of treated people. Although these reactions occurred within 2 hours of receiving a Xolair subcutaneous injection, they also included reports of serious delayed reactions 2–24 hours or even longer after receiving the injections. Anaphylaxis occurred after any dose of Xolair (including the first dose), even in patients with no allergic reaction to previous doses. Omalizumab-treated patients should be observed in the facility for an extended period after the drug is given, and medical providers who administer the injection should be prepared to manage life-threatening anaphylactic reactions. Patients who receive omalizumab should be fully informed about the signs and symptoms of anaphylaxis, their chance of developing delayed anaphylaxis following each injection, and how to treat it, including the use of autoinjectable epinephrine.

Continual monitoring is necessary to ensure that control of asthma is achieved and sustained. Once control is established, gradual reduction in therapy is appropriate and may help determine the minimum amount of medication necessary to maintain control. Regular follow-up visits with the clinician are important to assess the degree of control and consider appropriate adjustments in therapy. At each step, patients should be instructed to avoid or control exposure to allergens, irritants, or other factors that contribute to asthma severity.

Referral to an asthma specialist for consultation or co-management is recommended if there are difficulties in achieving or maintaining control. For children younger than age 5 years, referral is recommended for moderate persistent asthma or if the patient requires step 3 or 4 care and should be considered if the patient requires step 2 care (see Table 36–8). For children 5 years and older, consultation with a specialist is recommended if the patient requires step 4 care or higher and should be considered at step 3 (see Tables 36–9 and 36–10). Referral is also recommended if allergen immunotherapy or anti-IgE therapy is being considered.

3. Exercise-induced bronchospasm—Exercise-induced bronchospasm should be anticipated in all asthma patients. It typically occurs during or minutes after vigorous activity, reaches its peak 5–10 minutes after stopping the activity, and usually resolves over the next 20–30 minutes. Participation in physical activity should be encouraged in children with asthma, although the choice of activity may need to be modified based on the severity of illness, presence of other triggers such as cold air, and, rarely, confounding factors such as osteoporosis. Treatment immediately prior to vigorous activity or exercise is usually effective. SABAs, cromolyn, or nedocromil can be used before exercise. The combination of a SABA with either cromolyn or nedocromil is more effective than either drug alone. Salmeterol and formoterol may block exercise-induced bronchospasm for up to 12 hours (as discussed earlier). However, decreased duration of protection against exercise-induced bronchospasm can be expected with regular use. Montelukast may be effective up to 24 hours. Occasionally an extended warm-up period may induce a refractory state, allowing patients to exercise without a need for repeat medications. If symptoms occur during usual play activities, a step-up in long-term therapy is warranted. Poor endurance or exercise-induced bronchospasm can be an indication of poorly controlled persistent asthma.

B. Acute Asthma

1. General measures—The most effective strategy in managing asthma exacerbations involves early recognition of warning signs and early treatment. For patients with moderate or severe persistent asthma or a history of severe exacerbations, this should include a written action plan. The latter usually defines the patient's peak flow zones and steps to take if peak flows are between 50% and 80% or below 50% of personal best. The child, parents, and other caregivers must be able to assess asthma severity accurately. Prompt communication with the clinician is indicated with severe symptoms or a drop in peak flow or with decreased response to SABAs. At such times, intensification of therapy may include a short course of oral corticosteroids. The child should be removed from exposure to any irritants or allergens that could be contributing to the exacerbation.

2. Management at home—Early treatment of asthma exacerbations may prevent progression to severe disease. Initial treatment should be with a SABA such as albuterol or levalbuterol; 2–6 puffs from an MDI can be given every 20 minutes up to three times, or a single treatment can be given by nebulizer (0.05 mg/kg [minimum dose, 1.25 mg; maximum, 2.5 mg] of 0.5% solution of albuterol in 2–3 mL saline; or 0.075 mg/kg [minimum dose, 1.25 mg; maximum, 5 mg] of levalbuterol). If the response is good as assessed by sustained symptom relief or improvement in PEFR to over 80% of the patient's best, the SABA can be continued every 3–4 hours for 24–48 hours. Patients should be advised to seek medical care once excessive doses of bronchodilator therapy are used or for prolonged periods (eg, > 12 puffs/d for more than 24 hours). Doubling the dose of inhaled corticosteroids is not proven sufficient to prevent worsening of exacerbations. If the patient does not completely improve from the initial therapy or PEFR falls between 50% and 80% predicted or personal best, the SABA should be continued, an oral corticosteroid should be added, and the patient should contact the physician urgently. If the child experiences marked distress or if PEFR persists at 50% or less, the patient should repeat the SABA immediately and go to the emergency department or call 911 or another emergency number for assistance.

3. Management in the office or emergency department—Functional assessment of the patient includes obtaining objective measures of airflow limitation with PEFR or FEV_1 and monitoring the patient's response to treatment; however, very severe exacerbations may prevent the execution of lung function measurements using maximal expiratory maneuver. Flow-volume loops should be obtained to differentiate upper and lower airway obstruction, especially in patients with atypical presentation. Other tests may include oxygen saturation and blood gases. Chest radiographs are not recommended routinely but should be considered to rule out pneumothorax, pneumomediastinum, pneumonia, or lobar atelectasis. If the initial FEV_1 or PEFR is over 40%, initial treatment can be with a SABA by inhaler (albuterol, 4–8 puffs) or nebulizer (0.15 mg/kg of albuterol 0.5% solution; minimum dose, 2.5 mg), up to three doses in the first hour. Oxygen should be given to maintain oxygen saturation at greater than 90%. Oral corticosteroids (1–2 mg/kg/d in divided doses; maximum of 60 mg/d for children ≤ age 12 years and 80 mg/d for those > 12 years) should be instituted if the patient responds poorly to therapy or if the patient has

recently been on oral corticosteroids. Sensitivity to adrenergic drugs may improve after initiation of corticosteroids. If the initial FEV_1 or PEFR is under 40%, initial treatment should be with a high-dose SABA plus ipratropium bromide (0.25–0.5 mg every 20 minutes) by nebulizer or continuously for the first hour (0.5 mg/kg/h). Oxygen should be given to maintain oxygen saturation at greater than 90%, and systemic corticosteroids should be administered. For patients with severe exacerbation having no response to initial aerosolized therapy, or for those who cannot cooperate with or who resist inhalation therapy, adjunctive therapies such as intravenous magnesium sulfate (25–75 mg/kg up to 2 g in children) and heliox-driven albuterol nebulization should be considered. Epinephrine 1:1000 or terbutaline 1 mg/mL (both 0.01 mg/kg up to 0.3–0.5 mg) may be administered subcutaneously every 20 minutes for three doses; although the use of intravenous β_2-agonists is still unproven. For impending or ongoing respiratory arrest, patients should be intubated and ventilated with 100% oxygen, given intravenous corticosteroids, and admitted to an intensive care unit (ICU). Potential indications for ICU admission also include any FEV_1 or PEFR less than 25% of predicted that improves less than 10% after treatment or values that fluctuate widely. (See Asthma [life-threatening] in Chapter 13.) Further treatment is based on clinical response and objective laboratory findings. Hospitalization should be considered strongly for any patient with a history of respiratory failure.

4. Hospital management—For patients who do not respond to outpatient and emergency department treatment, admission to the hospital becomes necessary for more aggressive care and support. The decision to hospitalize should also be based on presence of risk factors for mortality from asthma, duration and severity of symptoms, severity of airflow limitation, course and severity of previous exacerbations, medication use at the time of the exacerbation, access to medical care, and home and psychosocial conditions. Fluids should be given at maintenance requirements unless the patient has poor oral intake secondary to respiratory distress or vomiting, because overhydration may contribute to pulmonary edema associated with high intrapleural pressures generated in severe asthma. Potassium requirements should be kept in mind because both corticosteroids and β_2-agonists can cause potassium loss. Moisturized oxygen should be titrated by oximetry to maintain oxygen saturation above 90%. Inhaled β_2-agonist should be continued by nebulization in single doses as needed or by continuous therapy, along with systemic corticosteroids (as discussed earlier). Ipratropium is no longer recommended during hospitalization. In addition, the role of methylxanthines in hospitalized children remains controversial. Antibiotics may be necessary to treat coexisting bacterial infection. Sedatives and anxiolytic agents are contraindicated in severely ill patients owing to their depressant effects on respiration. Chest physiotherapy is usually not recommended for acute exacerbations.

5. Patient discharge—Criteria for discharging patients home from the office or emergency department should include a sustained response of at least 1 hour to bronchodilator therapy with FEV$_1$ or PEFR greater than 70% of predicted or personal best and oxygen saturation greater than 90% in room air. Prior to discharge, the patient's or caregiver's ability to continue therapy and assess symptoms appropriately needs to be considered. Patients should be given an action plan for management of recurrent symptoms or exacerbations, and instructions about medications should be reviewed. The inhaled SABA and oral corticosteroids should be continued, the latter for 3–10 days. Finally, the patient or caregiver should be instructed about the follow-up visit, typically within 1 week. Hospitalized patients should receive more intensive education prior to discharge. Referral to an asthma specialist should be considered for all children with severe exacerbations or multiple emergency department visits or hospitalizations.

▶ Prognosis

Since the 1970s, morbidity rates for asthma have increased, and mortality rates may have stabilized. Mortality statistics indicate that a high percentage of deaths have resulted from under-recognition of asthma severity and undertreatment, particularly in labile asthmatic patients and in asthmatic patients whose perception of pulmonary obstruction is poor. Long-term outcome studies suggest that children with mild symptoms generally outgrow their asthma, while patients with more severe symptoms, marked airway hyperresponsiveness, and a greater degree of atopy tend to have persistent disease. In a recently published report of an unselected birth cohort from New Zealand, more than one in four children had wheezing that persisted from childhood to adulthood or that relapsed after remission. Recent evidence suggests that early intervention with anti-inflammatory therapy does not alter the development of persistent asthma, and it is also unclear if such intervention or environmental control measures influence the natural history of childhood asthma. Nonetheless, the pediatrician or primary care provider together with the asthma specialist has the responsibility to optimize control and, it is hoped, reduce the severity of asthma in children. Interventions that can have long-term effects such as halting progression or inducing remission are necessary to decrease the public health burden of this common condition.

Resources for health care providers, patients, and families include:

Asthma and Allergy Foundation of America
1233 20th St NW, Suite 402
Washington, DC 20036; (800) 7-ASTHMA
http://www.aafa.org/

Asthma and Allergy Network/Mothers of Asthmatics
2751 Prosperity Avenue, Suite 150
Fairfax, VA 22031; (800) 878-4403
http://www.aanma.org/

Lung Line (800) 222-LUNG

Akinbami LJ; Centers for Disease Control and Prevention, National Center for Health Statistics: The state of childhood asthma. Adv Data 2006;381:1.

Bacharier LB et al: Classifying asthma severity in children. Mismatch between symptoms, medication use, and lung function. Am J Respir Crit Care Med 2004;170:426 [PMID: 15172893].

Bisgaard H et al: Intermittent inhaled corticosteroids in infants with episodic wheezing. N Engl J Med. 2006;354:1998 [PMID: 16687712].

Guilbert T et al: Long-term inhaled corticosteroids in preschool children at high risk for asthma. N Engl J Med 2006;354:1985 [PMID: 16687711].

National Asthma Education and Prevention Program: Expert Panel Report 3 (EPR 3): Guidelines for the Diagnosis and Management of Asthma—Summary Report 2007. J Allergy Clin Immunol 2007;120(Suppl):S94 [PMID: 17983880]. Available at: http://www.nhlbi.nih.gov/guidelines/asthma/asthgdln.htm.

Sears MR et al: A longitudinal, population-based, cohort study of childhood asthma followed to adulthood. N Engl J Med 2003;349:1414 [PMID: 14523172].

Smith AD et al: Use of exhaled nitric oxide measurements to guide treatment in chronic asthma. N Engl J Med 2005;352:2163 [PMID: 15914548].

Spahn JD et al: Is forced expiratory volume in one second the best measure of severity in childhood asthma? Am J Respir Crit Care Med 2004;169:784 [PMID: 14754761].

Szefler SJ et al: Characterization of within-subject responses to fluticasone and montelukast in childhood asthma. J Allergy Clin Immunol 2005;115:233 [PMID: 15696076].

ALLERGIC RHINOCONJUNCTIVITIS

ESSENTIALS OF DIAGNOSIS & TYPICAL FEATURES

After exposure to allergen:

▶ Sneezing.

▶ Itching of nose and eyes.

▶ Clear rhinorrhea or nasal congestion.

▶ General Considerations

Allergic rhinoconjunctivitis is the most common allergic disease and significantly affects quality of life as well as school performance and attendance. It frequently coexists with asthma and is a risk factor for subsequent development of asthma. Prevalence of this disease increases during childhood, peaking at 15% in the postadolescent years. Although allergic rhinoconjunctivitis is more common in boys during early childhood, there is little difference in incidence between the sexes after adolescence. Race and socioeconomic status are not considered to be important factors.

The pathologic changes in allergic rhinoconjunctivitis are chiefly hyperemia, edema, and increased serous and mucoid secretions caused by mediator release, all of which lead to variable degrees of nasal obstruction, pruritus, and rhinorrhea. This process may involve the eyes and other structures, including the sinuses and possibly the middle ear. Inhalant allergens are primarily responsible for symptoms, but food allergens can cause symptoms as well. Children with allergic rhinitis seem to be more susceptible to—or at least may experience more symptoms from—upper respiratory infections, which, in turn, may aggravate the allergic rhinitis.

Allergic rhinoconjunctivitis has been classified as perennial, seasonal (hay fever), or episodic; however, there are areas where pollens and soil molds may be present year round while exposure to typical perennial allergens such as indoor furred animals may be intermittent. For this reason, the preferred terms are *intermittent* (ie, symptoms present < 4 days a week or for < 4 weeks) and *persistent* (ie, symptoms present > 4 days a week and for > 4 weeks). In addition, severity should be noted as *mild* (ie, without impairment or disturbance of sleep, daily activities, leisure, sport, school, or work, or the presence of troublesome symptoms) or *moderate-severe* (ie, presence of one or more of the aforementioned). The major pollen groups in the temperate zones include trees (late winter to early spring), grasses (late spring to early summer), and weeds (late summer to early fall), but seasons can vary significantly in different parts of the country. Mold spores also cause seasonal allergic rhinitis, principally in the summer and fall. Seasonal allergy symptoms may be aggravated by coincident exposure to perennial allergens.

▶ Clinical Findings

A. Symptoms and Signs

Patients may complain of itching of the nose, eyes, palate, or pharynx and loss of smell or taste. Nasal itching can cause paroxysmal sneezing and epistaxis. Repeated rubbing of the nose (so-called allergic salute) may lead to a horizontal crease across the lower third of the nose. Nasal obstruction is associated with mouth breathing, nasal speech, allergic salute, and snoring. Nasal turbinates may appear pale blue and swollen, with dimpling, or injected, with minimal edema. Typically, clear and thin nasal secretions are increased, with anterior rhinorrhea, sniffling, postnasal drip, and congested cough. Nasal secretions often cause poor appetite, fatigue, and pharyngeal irritation. Conjunctival injection, tearing, periorbital edema, and infraorbital cyanosis (so-called allergic shiners) are frequently observed. Increased pharyngeal lymphoid tissue ("cobblestoning") from chronic drainage and enlarged tonsillar and adenoidal tissue may be present.

B. Laboratory Findings

Eosinophilia often can be demonstrated on smears of nasal secretions or blood. This is a frequent but nonspecific finding and may occur in nonallergic conditions. Although serum IgE may be elevated, measurement of total IgE is a poor screening tool owing to the wide overlap between atopic and nonatopic subjects. Skin testing to identify allergen-specific IgE is the most sensitive and specific test for inhalant allergies; alternatively, the Phadia ImmunoCAP assay, radioallergosorbent test (RAST), or other in-vitro tests can be done for suspected allergens.

▶ Differential Diagnosis

Disorders that need to be differentiated from allergic rhinitis include infectious rhinosinusitis. Foreign bodies and structural abnormalities such as choanal atresia, marked septal deviation, nasal polyps, and adenoidal hypertrophy may cause chronic symptoms. Overuse of topical nasal decongestants may result in rhinitis medicamentosa (rebound congestion). Use of medications such as propranolol, clonidine, and some psychoactive drugs may cause nasal congestion. Illicit drugs such as cocaine can cause rhinorrhea. Spicy or hot foods may cause gustatory rhinitis. Nonallergic rhinitis with eosinophilia syndrome is usually not seen in young children. Vasomotor rhinitis is associated with persistent symptoms but without allergen exposure. Less common causes of symptoms that may be confused with allergic rhinitis include pregnancy, congenital syphilis, hypothyroidism, tumors, and cerebrospinal fluid rhinorrhea.

▶ Complications

Sinusitis may accompany allergic rhinitis. Allergic mucosal swelling of the sinus ostia can obstruct sinus drainage, interfering with normal sinus function and predisposing to chronic mucosal disease. Nasal polyps due to allergy are unusual in children, and cystic fibrosis should be considered if they are present.

▶ Treatment

A. General Measures

The value of identification and avoidance of causative allergens cannot be overstated. Reducing indoor allergens through environmental control measures as discussed in the section on asthma can be very effective. Nasal saline irrigation may be useful.

B. Pharmacologic Therapy

Pharmacologic management of mild intermittent rhinitis includes oral or intranasal H_1 antihistamines and intranasal decongestants (for < 10 days and not to be repeated more than twice a month). Oral decongestants are not usually recommended in children. Options for moderate-severe intermittent rhinitis are oral or intranasal antihistamines, oral H_1 antihistamines and decongestants, intranasal corticosteroids, and cromones. The same medication options are available for persistent rhinitis, but a stepwise approach is proposed both for treatment of mild and moderate-severe persistent rhinitis. For mild persistent rhinitis, reassessment after 2–4 weeks is recommended and treatment should be continued, with a possible reduction in intranasal corticosteroids, even if the symptoms have abated. If, however, the patient has persistent mild symptoms while on H_1 antihistamines or cromones, an intranasal corticosteroid is appropriate. For moderate-severe persistent disease, use of intranasal corticosteroids as first-line therapy is recommended. For severe nasal congestion, either a short 1- to 2-week course of an oral corticosteroid or an intranasal decongestant for less than 10 days may be added. If the patient improves, the treatment should last for at least 3 months or until the pollen season is over. If the patient does not improve within 2–4 weeks despite adequate compliance and use of medications, comorbidities such as nasal polyps, sinusitis, and significant allergen exposure, should be considered, as well as the possibility of misdiagnosis. Once these are ruled out, options include increasing the dose of the intranasal corticosteroid, combination therapy with an H_1 antihistamine (particularly if major symptoms are sneezing, itching, or rhinorrhea), ipratropium bromide (if major symptom is rhinorrhea), or an oral H_1 antihistamine and decongestant. Referral to a specialist may be considered if the treatment is not sufficient.

1. Antihistamines—Antihistamines help control itching, sneezing, and rhinorrhea. Sedating antihistamines include diphenhydramine, chlorpheniramine, hydroxyzine, and clemastine. Sedating antihistamines may cause daytime somnolence and negatively affect school performance and other activities, especially driving. Second-generation antihistamines include loratadine, desloratadine, cetirizine, and fexofenadine. Cetirizine is approved for use in children aged 6–23 months (2.5 mg daily), 2–5 years (2.5–5.0 mg/d or 2.5 mg twice a day), and 6 years or older (5–10 mg/d). It is now available without a prescription. Loratadine is approved for use in children aged 2–5 years (5 mg/d) and 6 years or older (10 mg/d), and is available without prescription in tablet, rapidly disintegrating tablet, and liquid formulations. Desloratadine is approved for use in children aged 6–11 months (1 mg/d), 1–5 years (1.25 mg/d), and for 12 years and older (5 mg/d). Fexofenadine is approved for children aged 6–23 months (15 mg twice a day), 2–11 years (30 mg twice a day), and 12 years or older (60 mg twice a day or 180 mg once daily). Levocetirizine (5 mg/d) is approved for children aged 6 years and older. Loratadine, fexofenadine, and cetirizine are available in combination with pseudoephedrine for patients aged 12 years or older. Azelastine is available in a nasal spray and levocabastine and emedastine as ophthalmic preparations.

2. Decongestants—α-Adrenergic agents help to relieve nasal congestion. Topical decongestants such as phenylephrine and oxymetazoline should not be used for more than 4 days for severe episodes because prolonged use may be associated with rhinitis medicamentosa. Oral decongestants, including pseudoephedrine, phenylephrine, and phenylpropanolamine, are often combined with antihistamines or expectorants and cough suppressants in over-the-counter (OTC) cold medications, but there are no convincing data to support the use of OTC decongestants for upper respiratory illnesses in children. They may cause insomnia, agitation, tachycardia, and, rarely, cardiac arrhythmias. Of note, the FDA has recommended the

removal of phenylpropanolamine from all drug products due to a public health advisory concerning the risk of hemorrhagic stroke associated with its use.

3. Corticosteroids—Intranasal corticosteroid sprays are effective in controlling allergic rhinitis if used chronically. They are minimally absorbed in usual doses and are available in pressurized nasal inhalers and aqueous sprays. Mometasone and fluticasone furoate nasal sprays have been approved for use in children as young as age 2 years (1 spray in each nostril once daily) and in children 12 years or older (2 sprays/nostril once daily). Fluticasone propionate nasal spray is approved for children 4 years or older, and budesonide and triamcinolone nasal sprays are approved for those 6 years or older (1–2 sprays/nostril once daily). Flunisolide is approved for ages 6–14 years (1 spray/nostril three times a day or 2 sprays/nostril twice a day). Side effects include nasal irritation, soreness, and bleeding, although epistaxis occurs commonly in patients with allergic rhinitis if corticosteroids are used chronically. Rarely, these drugs can cause septal perforation. Excessive doses may produce systemic effects, especially if used together with orally inhaled steroids for asthma. Onset of action is within hours, although clinical benefit is usually not observed for a week or more. They may be effective alone or together with antihistamines.

4. Other pharmacologic agents—Montelukast is approved for perennial allergic rhinitis in children aged 6 months and older (4 mg/d for ages 6–23 months) and seasonal allergic rhinitis in children 2 years and older in doses as discussed in the preceding section, under pharmacologic therapy for chronic asthma. Intranasal ipratropium can be used as adjunctive therapy for rhinorrhea. Intranasal cromolyn may be used alone or in conjunction with oral antihistamines and decongestants. It is most effective when used prophylactically, 1–2 sprays/nostril, four times a day. This dose may be tapered if symptom control is achieved. Rarely, patients complain of nasal irritation or burning. Most patients find complying with four-times-daily dosing difficult. Cromolyn is also available in an ophthalmic solution. (See also Chapter 15.) Other ophthalmic mast cell stabilizers include lodoxamide 0.1% solution, 1–2 drops four times a day, and nedocromil, 1–2 drops two times a day. Olopatadine 0.1%, epinastine 0.05%, and ketotifen 0.025% ophthalmic solutions have antihistamine and mast cell–stabilizing actions and can be given to children older than age 3 years as 1 drop twice a day (8 hours apart) apart for olopatadine and every 8–12 hours for ketotifen, respectively. Olopatadine 0.2% is the first once-daily ophthalmic medication available for the treatment of ocular pruritus associated with allergic conjunctivitis.

C. Surgical Therapy

Surgical procedures, including turbinectomy, polypectomy, and functional endoscopic sinus surgery, are rarely indicated in allergic rhinitis or chronic hyperplastic sinusitis.

D. Immunotherapy

Allergen immunotherapy should be considered when symptoms are severe and due to unavoidable exposure to inhalant allergens, especially if symptomatic measures have failed. Immunotherapy is the only form of therapy that may alter the course of the disease. It should not be prescribed by sending the patient's serum to a laboratory where extracts based on in-vitro tests are prepared for the patient (ie, the remote practice of allergy). Subcutaneous immunotherapy should be done in a facility where a physician prepared to treat anaphylaxis is present. Patients with concomitant asthma should not receive an injection if their asthma is not under good control (ie, peak flows preinjection are below 80% of personal best), and the patient should wait for 25–30 minutes after an injection before leaving the facility. Outcomes with single allergen immunotherapy show success rates of approximately 80%. The optimal duration of therapy is unknown, but data suggest that immunotherapy for 3–5 years may have lasting benefit.

▶ Prognosis

Allergic rhinoconjunctivitis associated with sensitization to indoor allergens tends to be protracted unless specific allergens can be identified and eliminated from the environment. In seasonal allergic rhinoconjunctivitis, symptoms are usually most severe from adolescence through mid-adult life. After moving to a region devoid of problem allergens, patients may be symptom-free for several years, but they can develop new sensitivities to local aeroallergens.

Bousquet J et al; Aria Workshop Group; World Health Organization: Allergic rhinitis and its impact on asthma. J Allergy Clin Immunol 2001;108(Suppl):S147 [PMID: 11707753].
Simons FER: Advances in H1-antihistamines. N Engl J Med 2004; 351:2203 [PMID: 15548781].

ATOPIC DERMATITIS

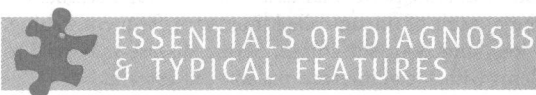

ESSENTIALS OF DIAGNOSIS & TYPICAL FEATURES

▶ Pruritus.

▶ Facial and extensor involvement in infants and young children.

▶ Flexural lichenification in older children and adolescents.

▶ Chronic or relapsing dermatitis.

▶ Personal or family history of atopic disease.

▶ General Considerations

Atopic dermatitis is a chronically relapsing inflammatory skin disease typically associated with respiratory allergy.

Over half of patients with atopic dermatitis will develop asthma and allergic rhinitis—often as they outgrow their atopic dermatitis. A subset of patients with atopic dermatitis has been shown to have mutations in the gene encoding filaggrin, a protein essential for normal epidermal barrier function. These patients have early-onset, more severe and persistent disease. Mutations in filaggrin have also been associated with increased risk for asthma, but only in patients with atopic dermatitis. Atopic dermatitis may result in significant morbidity, leading to school absenteeism, occupational disability, and emotional stress. The disease presents in early childhood, with onset prior to age 5 years in approximately 90% of patients.

▶ Clinical Findings

A. Symptoms and Signs

Atopic dermatitis has no pathognomonic skin lesions or laboratory parameters. Diagnosis is based on the clinical features, including severe pruritus, a chronically relapsing course, and typical morphology and distribution of the skin lesions. Acute atopic dermatitis is characterized by intensely pruritic, erythematous papules associated with excoriations, vesiculations, and serous exudate; subacute atopic dermatitis by erythematous, excoriated, scaling papules; and chronic atopic dermatitis by thickened skin with accentuated markings (lichenification) and fibrotic papules. Patients with chronic atopic dermatitis may have all three types of lesions present concurrently. Patients usually have dry, "lackluster" skin. During infancy, atopic dermatitis involves primarily the face, scalp, and extensor surfaces of the extremities. The diaper area is usually spared. When involved, it may be secondarily infected with *Candida*. In older patients with long-standing disease, the flexural folds of the extremities are the predominant location of lesions.

B. Laboratory Findings

Identification of allergens involves taking a careful history and performing selective immediate hypersensitivity skin tests or in-vitro tests when appropriate. Negative skin tests with proper controls have a high predictive value for ruling out a suspected allergen. Positive skin tests have a lower correlation with clinical symptoms in suspected food allergen–induced atopic dermatitis and should be confirmed with double-blind, placebo-controlled food challenges unless there is a coincidental history of anaphylaxis to the suspected food. Alternatively, specific IgE levels to milk, egg, peanut, and fish proteins have been established with the Phadia ImmunoCAP assay correlating with a greater than 95% chance of a clinical reaction.

Elevated serum IgE levels can be demonstrated in 80–85% of patients with atopic dermatitis, and a similar number have positive immediate skin tests or in-vitro tests with food and inhalant allergens. Several well-controlled studies suggest that specific allergens can influence the course of this disease. However, triggers for clinical disease cannot be predicted simply by performing allergy testing. Double-blind, placebo-controlled food challenges show that food allergens can cause exacerbations in a subset of patients with atopic dermatitis. Although lesions induced by single positive challenges are usually transient, repeated challenges, more typical of real-life exposure, can result in eczematous lesions. Furthermore, elimination of food allergens results in amelioration of skin disease and a decrease in spontaneous basophil histamine release. Exacerbation of atopic dermatitis can occur with exposure to aeroallergens such as house dust mites, and environmental control measures have been shown to result in clinical improvement. Patients can make specific IgE directed at *Staphylococcus aureus* toxins secreted on the skin, and this correlates with clinical severity better than total serum IgE levels. Eosinophilia may occur. Routine skin biopsy does not differentiate atopic dermatitis from other eczematous processes and is not usually indicated.

▶ Differential Diagnosis

Scabies can present as a pruritic skin disease. However, distribution in the genital and axillary areas and the presence of linear lesions as well as skin scrapings may help to distinguish it from atopic dermatitis. Seborrheic dermatitis may be distinguished by a lack of significant pruritus; its predilection for the scalp (so-called cradle cap); and its coarse, yellowish scales. Allergic contact dermatitis may be suggested by the distribution of lesions with a greater demarcation of dermatitis than in atopic dermatitis. Occasionally, allergic contact dermatitis superimposed on atopic dermatitis may appear as an acute flare of the underlying disease. Nummular eczema is characterized by coin-shaped plaques. Although unusual in children, mycosis fungoides or cutaneous T-cell lymphoma has been described and is diagnosed by skin biopsy. Eczematous rash has been reported in patients with HIV infection. Other disorders that may resemble atopic dermatitis include Wiskott-Aldrich syndrome, severe combined immunodeficiency disease, hyper-IgE syndrome, IPEX (immune dysregulation, polyendocrinopathy, enteropathy, X-linked) syndrome, zinc deficiency, phenylketonuria, and Letterer-Siwe disease.

▶ Complications

Ocular complications associated with atopic dermatitis can lead to significant morbidity. Atopic keratoconjunctivitis is always bilateral, and symptoms include itching, burning, tearing, and copious mucoid discharge. It is frequently associated with eyelid dermatitis and chronic blepharitis, and may result in visual impairment from corneal scarring. Vernal conjunctivitis is a severe bilateral recurrent chronic inflammatory process of the upper eyelid conjunctiva, occurring primarily in younger patients. (See Chapter 15.) It has a marked seasonal incidence, often in the spring. The associated intense pruritus is exacerbated by exposure to

irritants, light, or perspiration. Examination of the eye reveals a papillary hypertrophy or cobblestoning of the upper inner eyelid surface. Keratoconus in atopic dermatitis is believed to result from persistent rubbing of the eyes in patients with atopic dermatitis and allergic rhinitis. Anterior subcapsular cataracts may develop during adolescence or early adult life.

Patients with atopic dermatitis have increased susceptibility to infection or colonization with a variety of organisms. These include viral infections with herpes simplex, molluscum contagiosum, and human papillomavirus. Of note, even a past history of atopic dermatitis is considered a contraindication for receiving the current smallpox (vaccinia) vaccine. Superimposed dermatophytosis may cause atopic dermatitis to flare. *S aureus* can be cultured from the skin of more than 90% of patients with atopic dermatitis, compared with only 5% of normal subjects. Patients with atopic dermatitis often have toxin-secreting *S aureus* cultured from their skin and can make specific IgE antibodies against the toxins found on their skin. *S aureus* toxins can act as superantigens, contributing to persistent inflammation or exacerbations of atopic dermatitis. Patients without obvious superinfection may show a better response to combined antistaphylococcal and topical corticosteroid therapy than to corticosteroids alone. Although recurrent staphylococcal pustulosis can be a significant problem in atopic dermatitis, invasive *S aureus* infections occur rarely and should raise the possibility of an immunodeficiency such as hyper-IgE syndrome. Patients with atopic dermatitis may be predisposed to colonization and infections by microbial organisms due to decreased synthesis of antimicrobial peptides in the skin, which may be mediated by increased levels of TH2-type cytokines.

Patients with atopic dermatitis often have a nonspecific hand dermatitis. This is frequently irritant in nature and aggravated by repeated wetting.

Nutritional disturbances may result from unwarranted and unnecessarily vigorous dietary restrictions imposed by physicians and parents.

Poor academic performance and behavioral disturbances may be a result of uncontrolled intense or frequent itching, sleep loss, and poor self-image. Severe disease may lead to problems with social interactions and self-esteem.

▶ Treatment

A. General Measures

Patients with atopic dermatitis have a lowered threshold of irritant responsiveness. Avoidance of irritants such as detergents, chemicals, and abrasive materials as well as extremes of temperature and humidity is important in managing this disease. New clothing should be washed to reduce the content of formaldehyde and other chemicals. Because residual laundry detergent in clothing may be irritating, using a liquid rather than a powder detergent and adding an extra rinse cycle is beneficial. Occlusive clothing should be avoided in favor of cotton or cotton blends. Temperature in the home and work environments should be controlled to minimize sweating. Swimming is usually well tolerated; however, because swimming pools are treated with chlorine or bromine, patients should shower and use a mild cleanser to remove these chemicals, then apply a moisturizer or occlusive agent. Sunlight may be beneficial to some patients with atopic dermatitis, but nonsensitizing sunscreens should be used to avoid sunburn. Prolonged sun exposure can cause evaporative losses, overheating, and sweating, all of which can be irritating.

In children who have undergone controlled food challenges, eggs, milk, peanuts, soy, wheat, and fish account for approximately 90% of the food allergens that exacerbate atopic dermatitis. Avoidance of foods implicated in controlled challenges can lead to clinical improvement. Extensive elimination diets, which can be nutritionally unsound and burdensome, are almost never warranted because even patients with multiple positive skin tests rarely react to more than three foods on blinded challenges.

In patients who demonstrate specific IgE to dust mite allergen, environmental control measures aimed at reducing the dust mite load improve atopic dermatitis. These include use of dust mite–proof covers on pillows and mattresses, washing linens weekly in hot water, decreasing indoor humidity levels, and in some cases removing bedroom carpeting.

Counseling may be of benefit when dealing with the frustrations associated with atopic dermatitis. Relaxation, behavioral modification, or biofeedback training may help patients with habitual scratching. Patients with severe or disfiguring disease may require psychotherapy.

Clinicians should provide the patient and family with both general information and specific written skin care recommendations. The patient or parent should demonstrate an appropriate level of understanding to help ensure a good outcome. Educational pamphlets and a video about atopic dermatitis can be obtained from the National Eczema Association, a national nonprofit, patient-oriented organization, at: (800) 818-7546; http://www.nationaleczema.org.

B. Hydration

Patients with atopic dermatitis have evaporative losses due to a defective skin barrier, so soaking the affected area or bathing for 10–15 minutes in warm water, then applying an occlusive agent to retain the absorbed water, is an essential component of therapy. Oatmeal or baking soda added to the bath may feel soothing to certain patients but does not improve water absorption. Atopic dermatitis of the face or neck can be treated by applying a wet facecloth or towel to the involved area. The washcloth may be more readily accepted by a child if it is turned into a mask and also allows the older patient to remain functional. Lesions limited to the hands or feet can be treated by soaking in a basin. Daily baths may be needed and increased to several times daily during flares of atopic dermatitis, while showers may be adequate for

patients with mild disease. It is important to use an occlusive preparation within a few minutes after soaking the skin to prevent evaporation, which is both drying and irritating.

C. Moisturizers and Occlusives

An effective emollient combined with hydration therapy will help skin healing and can reduce the need for topical corticosteroids. Moisturizers are available as lotions, creams, and ointments. Because lotions contain more water than creams, they are more drying because of their evaporative effect. Preservatives and fragrances in lotions and creams may cause skin irritation. Moisturizers often need to be applied several times daily on a long-term basis and should be obtained in the largest size available. Crisco shortening can be substituted as an inexpensive alternative. Petroleum jelly (Vaseline) is an effective occlusive agent when used to seal in water after bathing. Topical nonsteroidal creams approved as medical devices (thus, currently requiring prescriptions) for relief and management of signs and symptoms of dermatoses include Atopiclair and MimyX.

D. Corticosteroids

Corticosteroids reduce the inflammation and pruritus in atopic dermatitis. Topical corticosteroids can decrease *S aureus* colonization. Systemic corticosteroids, including oral prednisone, should be avoided in the management of this chronic relapsing disease. The dramatic improvement observed with systemic corticosteroids may be associated with an equally dramatic flaring of atopic dermatitis following their discontinuation.

Topical corticosteroids are available in a wide variety of formulations, ranging from extremely high-potency to low-potency preparations (see Table 14–3). Choice of a particular product depends on the severity and distribution of skin lesions. Patients need to be counseled regarding the potency of their corticosteroid preparation and its potential side effects. In general, the least potent agent that is effective should be used. However, choosing a preparation that is too weak may result in persistence or worsening of the atopic dermatitis. Side effects include thinning of the skin, telangiectasias, bruising, hypopigmentation, acne, and striae, although these occur infrequently when low- to medium-potency topical corticosteroids are used appropriately. In contrast, use of potent topical corticosteroids for prolonged periods—especially under occlusion—may result in significant atrophic changes as well as systemic side effects. The face (especially the eyelids) and intertriginous areas are especially sensitive to corticosteroid side effects, and only low-potency preparations should be used routinely on these areas. Because topical corticosteroids are commercially available in a variety of bases, including ointments, creams, lotions, solutions, gels, and sprays, there is no need to compound them. Ointments are most occlusive and in general provide better delivery of the medication while preventing evaporative losses. However, in a humid environment, creams may be better tolerated than ointments because the increased occlusion may cause itching or even folliculitis. Creams and lotions, while easier to spread, can contribute to skin dryness and irritation. Solutions can be used on the scalp and hirsute areas, although they can be irritating, especially to open lesions. With clinical improvement, a less potent corticosteroid should be prescribed and the frequency of use decreased. Topical corticosteroids can be discontinued when inflammation resolves, but hydration and moisturizers need to be continued. Several topical steroids including fluticasone 0.05% cream and desonide 0.05% hydrogel have been approved in infants as young as 3 months of age for up to 28 days.

E. Topical Calcineurin Inhibitors

Tacrolimus and pimecrolimus are immunomodulatory agents that inhibit the transcription of proinflammatory cytokines as well as other allergic mediators and target key cells in allergic inflammation. They are available in topical formulations, and long-term studies up to 12 months have confirmed both efficacy and safety. Local burning at the site of application, which occurs more frequently with tacrolimus ointment, has been the most common side effect, although this is usually a transient problem. Tacrolimus ointment—0.03% for children 2–15 years of age and 0.1% for older patients—is approved for twice daily short-term and intermittent long-term use in moderate-to-severe atopic dermatitis. Pimecrolimus 1% cream is approved for patients 2 years of age or older who have mild-to-moderate atopic dermatitis. As a precaution, patients should wear sunscreen with both drugs. More recently, several studies in children as young as 3 months of age with all disease severities have been performed for up to 12 months with pimecrolimus 1% cream used at the earliest sign of disease activity (eg, erythema and pruritus). With this early intervention approach, the need for topical corticosteroid rescue was significantly decreased.

Although there is no evidence of a causal link between cancer and the use of topical calcineurin inhibitors, the FDA has issued a boxed warning for pimecrolimus cream and tacrolimus ointment because of a lack of long-term safety data (see U.S. package inserts for Elidel [Novartis], and Protopic [Astellas]). The new labeling states that these drugs are recommended as second-line treatments and that their use in children under the age of 2 years is currently not recommended.

F. Tar Preparations

Tar preparations are used primarily in shampoos and rarely as bath additives. Side effects associated with tar products include skin dryness or irritation, especially if applied to inflamed skin, and, less commonly, photosensitivity reactions and folliculitis.

G. Wet Dressings

Wet dressings are used together with hydration and topical corticosteroids primarily for the treatment of severe atopic dermatitis. They can also serve as an effective barrier against the persistent scratching that often undermines therapy. Total body dressings can be applied by using wet pajamas or long underwear with dry pajamas or a sweat suit on top. Hands and feet can be covered by wet tube socks with dry tube socks on top. Alternatively, wet gauze with a layer of dry gauze over it can be used and secured in place with an elastic bandage. Dressings can be removed when they dry out, usually after several hours, and are often best tolerated at bedtime. Incorrect use of wet dressings can result in chilling, maceration of the skin, or secondary infection.

H. Anti-Infective Therapy

Systemic antibiotic therapy may be important when treating atopic dermatitis secondarily infected with *S aureus*. For limited areas of involvement, a topical antibiotic such as mupirocin or retapamulin ointment may be effective. A first- or second-generation cephalosporins or semisynthetic penicillin is usually the first choice for oral therapy, as erythromycin-resistant organisms are fairly common. Maintenance antibiotic therapy is rarely indicated and may result in colonization by methicillin-resistant bacteria. Some pediatric dermatologists have recommended bleach baths (6% sodium hypochlorite, $^{1}/_{4}$–$^{1}/_{2}$ cup in a full tub of water) for 10–15 minutes two or three times per week for patients with recurrent methicillin-resistant *S aureus*.

Disseminated eczema herpeticum usually requires treatment with systemic acyclovir. Patients with recurrent cutaneous herpetic lesions can be given prophylactic oral acyclovir. Superficial dermatophytosis and *Malassezia sympodialis* infection can be treated with topical or (rarely) systemic antifungal agents.

I. Antipruritic Agents

Pruritus is usually the least well-tolerated symptom of atopic dermatitis. Oral antihistamines and anxiolytics may be effective owing to their tranquilizing and sedating effects and can be taken mostly in the evening to avoid daytime somnolence. Nonsedating antihistamines may be less effective in treating pruritus, although beneficial effects have been reported in blinded studies. Use of topical antihistamines and local anesthetics should be avoided because of potential sensitization.

J. Recalcitrant Disease

Patients who are erythrodermic or who appear toxic may need to be hospitalized. Hospitalization may also be appropriate for those with severe disease who fail outpatient management. Marked clinical improvement often occurs when the patient is removed from environmental allergens or stressors. In the hospital, compliance with therapy can be monitored, the patient and family can receive intense education, and controlled provocative challenges can be conducted to help identify triggering factors.

Ultraviolet light therapy can be useful for chronic recalcitrant atopic dermatitis in a subset of patients under the supervision of a specialist. Photochemotherapy with oral methoxypsoralen therapy followed by UVA (ultraviolet A) has been used in a limited number of children with severe atopic dermatitis unresponsive to other therapy, and significant improvement has been noted. However, the increased long-term risk of cutaneous malignancies from this therapy prevents its widespread use.

Limited published data are available on use of the systemic immunosuppressive agent cyclosporine in children. In an open study, children given oral cyclosporine, 5 mg/kg daily for 6 weeks, improved significantly and tolerated the treatment well. Unfortunately, discontinuation of treatment resulted in relapse, although the relapse rate was variable. Patients treated with this agent should have their dose titrated to the lowest effective dose after the disease is brought under control with appropriate monitoring, under the care of a specialist familiar with the drug.

K. Experimental and Unproved Therapies

Several uncontrolled trials have suggested that desensitization to specific allergens may improve atopic dermatitis; however, controlled trials with standardized extracts of relevant allergens in atopic dermatitis are needed before this form of therapy can be recommended. Treatment of atopic dermatitis with high-dose intravenous immunoglobulin and omalizumab is currently investigational. Although disturbances in the metabolism of essential fatty acids have been reported in patients with atopic dermatitis, controlled trials with fish oil and evening primrose have shown no clinical benefit.

▶ Prognosis

Although it has been held that most children outgrow atopic dermatitis by adolescence, recent studies present less optimistic outcomes. In one study, atopic dermatitis had disappeared in only 18% of children followed from infancy until age 13 years, although the symptoms had become less severe in 65%. In a prospective study from Finland, 77–91% of adolescent patients receiving treatment for moderate or severe atopic dermatitis had persistent or frequently relapsing dermatitis as adults, although only 6% had severe disease. More than half of adolescents receiving treatment for mild dermatitis experienced a relapse of disease as adults. Adults whose childhood atopic dermatitis has been in remission for a number of years may present with hand dermatitis, especially if daily activities require repeated hand wetting.

Akdis CA et al: Diagnosis and treatment of atopic dermatitis in children and adults: European Academy of Allergology and Clinical Immunology/American Academy of Allergy, Asthma and Immunology/PRACTALL Consensus Report. J Allergy Clin Immunol 2006;118:152 [PMID: 16815151].

Boguniewicz M: Atopic dermatitis: Beyond the itch that rashes. Immunol Allergy Clin North Am 2005;25:333 [PMID: 15878459].

Boguniewicz M et al: Clinical pearls: Atopic dermatitis. J Allergy Clin Immunol 2006;118:40 [PMID: 16815136].

Fonacier L et al: Report of the Topical Calcineurin Task Force of the American College of Allergy, Asthma and Immunology and the American Academy of Allergy, Asthma and Immunology. J Allergy Clin Immunol 2005;115:1249 [PMID: 15940142].

Paul C et al: Safety and tolerability of 1% pimecrolimus cream among infants: Experience with 1133 patients treated for up to 2 years. Pediatrics 2006;117:e118 [PMID: 16361223].

URTICARIA & ANGIOEDEMA

ESSENTIALS OF DIAGNOSIS & TYPICAL FEATURES

▶ Urticaria: erythematous, blanchable, circumscribed, pruritic, edematous papules ranging from 1–2 mm to several centimeters in diameter and involving the superficial dermis. Individual lesions can coalesce.

▶ Angioedema: edema extending into the deep dermis or subcutaneous tissues.

▶ Both resolve without sequelae—urticaria usually within hours (individual lesions rarely lasting up to 24 hours), angioedema within 72 hours.

▶ General Considerations

Urticaria and angioedema are common dermatologic conditions, occurring at some time in up to 25% of the population. About half of patients will have concomitant urticaria and angioedema, whereas 40% will have only urticaria and 10% only angioedema. Urticarial lesions are arbitrarily designated as acute, lasting less than 6 weeks, or chronic, lasting more than 6 weeks. Acute versus chronic urticaria can also be distinguished by differences in histologic features. A history of atopy is common with acute urticaria or angioedema. In contrast, atopy does not appear to be a factor in chronic urticaria.

Mast cell degranulation, dilated venules, and dermal edema are present in most forms of urticaria or angioedema. The dermal inflammatory cells may be sparse or dense depending on the chronicity of the lesions. Mast cells are thought to play a critical role in the pathogenesis of urticaria or angioedema through release of a variety of vasoactive mediators. Mast cell activation and degranulation can be triggered by different stimuli, including cross-linking of Fc receptor-bound IgE by allergens or anti-FcεRI antibodies. Non–IgE-mediated mechanisms have also been identified, including complement anaphylatoxins (C3a, C5a), radio-contrast dyes, and physical stimuli. Chronic urticarial lesions have greater numbers of perivascular mononuclear cells, consisting primarily of T cells. There is also a marked increase in cutaneous mast cells. The cause of acute disease can be identified in about half of patients and includes allergens such as foods, aeroallergens, latex, drugs, and insect venoms. Infectious agents, including streptococci, mycoplasmas, hepatitis B virus, and Epstein-Barr virus, can cause acute urticaria. Urticaria or angioedema can occur after the administration of blood products or immunoglobulin. This results from immune complex formation with complement activation, vascular alterations, and triggering of mast cells by anaphylatoxins. Opiate analgesics, polymyxin B, tubocurarine, and radiocontrast media can induce acute urticaria by direct mast cell activation. These disorders can also occur following ingestion of aspirin or nonsteroidal anti-inflammatory agents (see later section on Adverse Reactions to Drugs & Biologicals).

Physical urticarias represent a heterogeneous group of disorders in which urticaria or angioedema is triggered by physical stimuli, including pressure, cold, heat, water, or vibrations. Dermographism is the most common form of physical urticaria, affecting up to 4% of the population and occurring at skin sites subjected to mechanical stimuli. Many physical urticarias are considered to be acute because the lesions are usually rapid in onset, with resolution within hours. However, symptoms can recur for months to years.

The cause of chronic urticaria is usually not due to allergies and typically cannot be determined. It can be associated with an underlying systemic disease such as thyroid disease. Some studies have demonstrated IgG autoantibodies directed at the high-affinity receptor for IgE or at IgE, suggesting that chronic urticaria may be an autoimmune disease.

► Clinical Findings

A. Symptoms and Signs

Cold-induced urticaria or angioedema can occur within minutes of exposure to a decreased ambient temperature or as the skin is warmed following direct cold contact. Systemic features include headache, wheezing, and syncope. If the entire body is cooled, as may occur during swimming, hypotension and collapse can occur. Two forms of dominantly inherited cold urticaria have been described. The immediate form is known as familial cold urticaria, in which erythematous macules appear rather than wheals, along with fever, arthralgias, and leukocytosis. The delayed form consists of erythematous, deep swellings that develop 9–18 hours after local cold challenge without immediate lesions.

In solar urticaria, which occurs within minutes after exposure to light of appropriate wavelength, pruritus is followed by morbilliform erythema and urticaria.

Cholinergic urticaria occurs after increases in core body and skin temperatures and typically develops after a warm bath or shower, exercise, or episodes of fever. Occasional episodes are triggered by stress or the ingestion of certain foods. The eruption appears as small punctate wheals surrounded by extensive areas of erythema. Rarely the urticarial lesions become confluent and angioedema develops. Associated features can include one or more of the following: headache, syncope, bronchospasm, abdominal pain, vomiting, and diarrhea. In severe cases, systemic anaphylaxis may develop. In pressure urticaria or angioedema, red, deep, painful swelling occurs immediately or 4–6 hours after the skin has been exposed to pressure. The immediate form is often associated with dermographism. The delayed form, which may be associated with fever, chills, and arthralgias, may be accompanied by elevated erythrocyte sedimentation rate and leukocytosis. Lesions are frequently diffuse, tender, and painful rather than pruritic. They typically resolve within 48 hours.

B. Laboratory Findings

Laboratory tests are selected on the basis of the history and physical findings. Testing for specific IgE antibody to food or inhalant allergens may be helpful in implicating a potential cause. Specific tests for physical urticarias, such as an ice cube test or a pressure test, may be indicated. Intradermal injection of methacholine reproduces clinical symptoms locally in about one third of patients with cholinergic urticaria. A throat culture for streptococcal infection may be warranted with acute urticaria. In chronic urticaria, selected screening studies to look for an underlying disease may be indicated, including a complete blood count, erythrocyte sedimentation rate, biochemistry panel, and urinalysis. Antithyroid antibodies may be considered. Intradermal testing with the patient's serum has been suggested as a method of detecting histamine-releasing activity, including autoantibodies. Other tests should be done based on suspicion of a specific underlying disease. If the history or appearance of the urticarial lesions suggests vasculitis, a skin biopsy for immunofluorescence is indicated. Patient diaries occasionally may be helpful to determine the cause of recurrent hives. A trial of food or drug elimination may be considered.

► Differential Diagnosis

Urticarial lesions are usually easily recognized—the major dilemma is the etiologic diagnosis. Lesions of urticarial vasculitis typically last for more than 24 hours. "Papular urticaria" is a term used to characterize multiple papules from insect bites, found especially on the extremities, and is not true urticaria. Angioedema can be distinguished from other forms of edema because it is transient, asymmetrical, and nonpitting and does not occur predominantly in dependent areas. Hereditary angioedema is a rare autosomal dominant disorder caused by a quantitative or functional deficiency of C1-esterase inhibitor and characterized by episodic, frequently severe, nonpruritic angioedema of the skin, gastrointestinal tract, or upper respiratory tract. Life-threatening laryngeal angioedema may occur.

Complications

In severe cases of cholinergic urticaria, systemic anaphylaxis may develop. In cold-induced disease, sudden cooling of the entire body as can occur with swimming can result in hypotension and collapse.

Treatment

A. General Measures

The most effective treatment is identification and avoidance of the triggering agent. Underlying infection should be treated appropriately. Patients with physical urticarias should avoid the relevant physical stimulus. Epinephrine can be used for treatment of acute episodes, especially when laryngeal edema complicates an attack (see next section on Anaphylaxis). Intubation may be indicated for life-threatening laryngeal edema.

B. Antihistamines

For the majority of patients, H_1 antihistamines given orally or systemically are the mainstay of therapy. Antihistamines are more effective when given on an ongoing basis rather than after lesions appear. For breakthrough symptoms, the dose may need to be increased. In the case of cold urticaria, the best treatment appears to be cyproheptadine. Cholinergic urticaria can be treated with hydroxyzine and dermographism with hydroxyzine or diphenhydramine. The addition of H_2 antihistamines may benefit some patients who fail to respond to H_1-receptor antagonists alone. Second-generation antihistamines (discussed previously under Allergic Rhinoconjunctivitis) are long acting, show good tissue levels, are non- or minimally sedating at usual dosing levels, and lack anticholinergic effects.

C. Corticosteroids

Although corticosteroids are usually not indicated in the treatment of acute or chronic urticaria, severe recalcitrant cases may require alternate-day therapy in an attempt to diminish disease activity and facilitate control with antihistamines. Systemic corticosteroids may also be needed in the treatment of urticaria or angioedema secondary to necrotizing vasculitis, an uncommon occurrence in patients with serum sickness or collagen-vascular disease.

D. Other Pharmacologic Agents

Limited studies suggest that some patients may benefit from treatment with a leukotriene-receptor antagonist. The tricyclic antidepressant doxepin blocks both H_1 and H_2 histamine receptors and may be particularly useful in chronic urticaria, although its use may be limited by the sedating side effect. A limited number of patients—including euthyroid patients—with chronic urticaria and antithyroid antibodies have improved when given thyroid hormone. Treatment of chronic urticaria with hydroxychloroquine,

nifedipine, colchicine, dapsone, sulfasalazine, cyclosporine, or intravenous immune globulin should be considered investigational.

Prognosis

Spontaneous remission of urticaria and angioedema is frequent, but some patients have a prolonged course. Reassurance is important, because this disorder can cause significant frustration. Periodic follow-up is indicated, particularly for patients with laryngeal edema, to monitor for possible underlying cause.

Boguniewicz M: Chronic urticaria in children. Allergy Asthma Proc 2005;26:13 [PMID: 15813283].

ANAPHYLAXIS

ESSENTIALS OF DIAGNOSIS & TYPICAL FEATURES

- ▶ Serious allergic reaction that is rapid in onset and may cause death after exposure to allergen in a previously sensitized person.
- ▶ Generalized pruritus, anxiety, urticaria, angioedema, throat fullness, wheezing, dyspnea, hypotension, and collapse.

General Considerations

Anaphylaxis is an acute life-threatening clinical syndrome that occurs when large quantities of inflammatory mediators are rapidly released from mast cells and basophils after exposure to an allergen in a previously sensitized patient. Anaphylactoid reactions mimic anaphylaxis but are not mediated by IgE antibodies. They may be mediated by anaphylatoxins such as C3a or C5a or through nonimmune mast cell degranulating agents. Some of the common causes of anaphylaxis or anaphylactoid reactions are listed in Table 36–12. Idiopathic anaphylaxis by definition has no recognized external cause. The clinical history is the most important tool in making the diagnosis of anaphylaxis.

Clinical Findings

A. Symptoms and Signs

The symptoms and signs of anaphylaxis or anaphylactoid reactions depend on the organs affected. Onset typically occurs within minutes after exposure to the offending agent and can be short-lived, protracted, or biphasic, with recurrence after several hours despite treatment.

Table 36–12. Common causes of systemic allergic and pseudoallergic reactions.

Causes of anaphylaxis
Drugs
Antibiotics
Anesthetic agents
Foods
Peanuts, tree nuts, shellfish, and others
Biologicals
Latex
Insulin
Allergen extracts
Antisera
Blood products
Enzymes
Monoclonal antibodies (eg omalizumab)
Insect venoms
Causes of anaphylactoid reactions
Radiocontrast media
Aspirin and other nonsteroidal anti-inflammatory drugs
Anesthetic agents

Anaphylaxis is highly likely when any one of the following three criteria are fulfilled:

1. Acute onset of an illness (minutes to several hours) with involvement of the skin, mucosal tissue, or both (eg, generalized hives, pruritus or flushing, swollen lips-tongue-uvula) *and at least one of the following:*
   a. Respiratory compromise (eg, dyspnea, wheeze-bronchospasm, stridor, reduced peak expiratory flow, hypoxemia)
   b. Reduced blood pressure or associated symptoms of end-organ dysfunction (eg, hypotonia [collapse], syncope, incontinence)
2. Two or more of the following that occur rapidly after exposure to a *likely* allergen for that patient (minutes to several hours):
   a. Involvement of the skin-mucosal tissue (eg, generalized urticaria, itch-flush, swollen lips-tongue-uvula)
   b. Respiratory compromise (eg, dyspnea, wheeze-bronchospasm, stridor, reduced PEFR, hypoxemia)
   c. Reduced blood pressure or associated symptoms (eg, hypotonia [collapse], syncope, incontinence)
   d. Persistent gastrointestinal symptoms (eg, crampy abdominal pain, vomiting)
3. Reduced blood pressure after exposure to a *known* allergen for that patient (minutes to several hours)
   a. Infants and children: low systolic blood pressure (age specific) or greater than 30% decrease in systolic pressure
   b. Low systolic blood pressure in children, defined as less than 70 mm Hg in those aged from 1 month to 1 year, less than (70 mm Hg + [2 × age]) in those 1–10 years of age, and less than 90 mm Hg in those 11–17 years

B. Laboratory Findings

Tryptase released by mast cells can be measured in the serum and may be helpful when the diagnosis of anaphylaxis is in question. The blood sample should be obtained within 3 hours of onset of the reaction, although tryptase levels are often normal, particularly in individuals with food-induced anaphylaxis. The complete blood count may show an elevated hematocrit due to hemoconcentration. Elevation of serum creatine kinase, aspartate aminotransferase, and lactic dehydrogenase may be seen with myocardial involvement. Electrocardiographic abnormalities may include ST-wave depression, bundle branch block, and various arrhythmias. Arterial blood gases may show hypoxemia, hypercapnia, and acidosis. The chest radiograph may show hyperinflation.

▶ Differential Diagnosis

Although shock may be the only sign of anaphylaxis, other diagnoses should be considered, especially in the setting of sudden collapse without typical allergic findings. Other causes of shock along with cardiac arrhythmias must be ruled out. (See Chapters 11 and 13.) Respiratory failure associated with asthma may be confused with anaphylaxis. Mastocytosis, hereditary angioedema, scombroid poisoning, vasovagal reactions, vocal cord dysfunction, and anxiety attacks may cause symptoms mistaken for anaphylaxis.

▶ Complications

Depending on the organs involved and the severity of the reaction, complications may vary from none to aspiration pneumonitis, acute tubular necrosis, bleeding diathesis, or sloughing of the intestinal mucosa. With irreversible shock, heart and brain damage can be terminal. Risk factors for fatal or near-fatal anaphylaxis include age (adolescents and young adults), reactions to peanut or tree nuts, associated asthma, strenuous exercise, and ingestion of medications such as β-blockers.

▶ Prevention

Strict avoidance of the causative agent is extremely important. An effort to determine its cause should be made, beginning with a thorough history. Typically there is a strong temporal relationship between exposure and onset of symptoms. Testing for specific IgE to allergen with either in-vitro or skin testing may be indicated. With exercise-induced anaphylaxis, patients should be instructed to exercise with another person and to stop exercising at the first sign of symptoms. If prior ingestion of food has been implicated, eating within 4 hours—perhaps up to 12 hours—before exercise should be avoided. Patients with a history of anaphylaxis should carry epinephrine for self-administration (eg, EpiPen or Twinject in 0.15-mg and 0.3-mg doses), and they and all caregivers should be instructed on its use. They should also carry an oral antihistamine such as diphenhydramine, preferably in liquid or fast-melt preparation to hasten absorption, and wear a medical alert bracelet. Patients with idiopathic anaphylaxis may require prolonged treatment with oral corticosteroids. Specific measures for dealing with food, drug, latex, and insect venom allergies as well as radiocontrast media reactions are discussed in the next sections.

► Treatment

A. General Measures

Anaphylaxis is a medical emergency that requires rapid assessment and treatment. Exposure to the triggering agent should be discontinued. Airway patency should be maintained and blood pressure and pulse monitored. The patient should be placed in a supine position with the legs elevated unless precluded by shortness of breath or emesis. Oxygen should be delivered by mask or nasal cannula with pulse oximetry monitoring. If the reaction is secondary to a sting or injection into an extremity, a tourniquet may be applied proximal to the site, briefly releasing it every 10–15 minutes.

B. Epinephrine

Epinephrine is the treatment of choice for anaphylaxis. Epinephrine 1:1000, 0.01 mg/kg to a maximum of 0.5 mg, should be injected intramuscularly, without delay. This dose may be repeated at intervals of 5–15 minutes as necessary for controlling symptoms and maintaining blood pressure. If the precipitating allergen has been injected intradermally or subcutaneously, absorption may be delayed by giving 0.1 mL of epinephrine subcutaneously at the injection site unless the site is a digit. There is no precisely established dosing regimen for intravenous epinephrine in anaphylaxis, but a 5–10-mcg intravenous bolus for hypotension and 0.1–0.5 mg intravenously for cardiovascular collapse have been suggested.

C. Antihistamines

Diphenhydramine, an H_1-blocker, 1–2 mg/kg up to 50 mg, can be given intramuscularly or intravenously. Intravenous antihistamines should be infused over a period of 5–10 minutes to avoid inducing hypotension. Addition of ranitidine, an H_2-blocker, 1 mg/kg up to 50 mg intravenously, may be more effective than an H_1-blocker alone, especially for hypotension, but histamine blockers should be considered second-line treatment for anaphylaxis.

D. Fluids

Treatment of persistent hypotension despite epinephrine requires restoration of intravascular volume by fluid replacement, initially with a crystalloid solution, 20–30 mL/kg in the first hour.

E. Bronchodilators

Nebulized β_2-agonists such as albuterol 0.5% solution, 2.5 mg (0.5 mL) diluted in 2–3 mL saline, or levalbuterol, 0.63 mg or 1.25 mg, may be useful for reversing bronchospasm. Intravenous methylxanthines are generally not recommended because they provide little benefit over inhaled β_2-agonists and may contribute to toxicity.

F. Corticosteroids

Although corticosteroids do not provide immediate benefit, when given early they may prevent protracted or biphasic anaphylaxis. Intravenous methylprednisolone, 1–2 mg/kg, or hydrocortisone, 5 mg/kg, can be given every 4–6 hours. Oral prednisone, 1 mg/kg up to 50 mg, might be sufficient for less severe episodes.

G. Vasopressors

Hypotension refractory to epinephrine and fluids should be treated with intravenous vasopressors such as noradrenaline, vasopressin, or dopamine. (See Chapter 13.)

H. Observation

The patient should be monitored after the initial symptoms have subsided, because biphasic or protracted anaphylaxis can occur despite ongoing therapy. Biphasic reactions occur in 1–20% of anaphylactic reactions, but no reliable clinical predictors have been identified. Observation periods should be individualized based on the severity of the initial reaction, but a reasonable time for observation is 4–6 hours in most patients, with prolonged observation or admission for severe or refractory symptoms.

► Prognosis

Anaphylaxis can be fatal. In two reports describing children, adolescents, and adults who died from food-induced anaphylaxis (eg, from peanuts, tree nuts, fish, shellfish, and milk) over the past 12 years, treatment with epinephrine was delayed for more than 1 hour after onset as it was not readily accessible in the majority of subjects. The prognosis, however, is good when signs and symptoms are recognized promptly and treated aggressively, and the offending agent is subsequently avoided. Exercise-induced and idiopathic anaphylaxis may be recurrent. Because accidental exposure to the causative agent may occur, patients, parents, and caregivers must be prepared to recognize and treat anaphylaxis (emergency action plan).

Sampson HA et al: Second symposium on the definition and management of anaphylaxis: Summary report—second National Institute of Allergy and Infectious Disease/Food Allergy and Anaphylaxis Network symposium. J Allergy Clin Immunol 2006;117:391 [PMID: 16461139].

Simons FE et al: Risk assessment in anaphylaxis: Current and future approaches. J Allergy Clin Immunol 2007;120:S2 [PMID: 17602945].

ADVERSE REACTIONS TO DRUGS & BIOLOGICALS

ESSENTIALS OF DIAGNOSIS & TYPICAL FEATURES

► Most adverse drug reactions are not allergic although patients or caregivers often report them as a drug allergy.

► Antibiotics constitute the most frequent cause of allergic drug reactions.

► Reliable testing for most drugs other than penicillins and a few large protein molecules is not available.

The majority of adverse drug reactions are not immunologically mediated and may be due to idiosyncratic reactions, overdosage, pharmacologic side effects, nonspecific release of pharmacologic effector molecules, or drug interactions.

Patients or caregivers often describe an adverse drug reaction as being allergic in nature, and clinicians may document a drug allergy in the patient's medical record based solely on this history. Adverse drug reactions are any undesirable and unintended response elicited by a drug. Allergic or hypersensitivity drug reactions are adverse reactions involving immune mechanisms. Although hypersensitivity reactions account for only 5–10% of all adverse drug reactions, they are the most serious, with 1:10,000 resulting in death.

1. Antibiotics

Antibiotics constitute the most frequent cause of allergic drug reactions. Amoxicillin, trimethoprim–sulfamethoxazole, and ampicillin are the most common causes of cutaneous drug reactions.

Most antibiotics and their metabolites are low-molecular-weight compounds that do not stimulate immunity until they have become covalently bound to a carrier protein. The penicillins and other β-lactam antibiotics, including cephalosporins, carbacephems, carbapenems, and monobactams, share a common β-lactam ring structure and a marked propensity to couple to carrier proteins. Penicilloyl is the predominant metabolite of penicillin and is called the major determinant. The other penicillin metabolites are present in low concentrations and are referred to as minor determinants. Sulfonamide reactions are mediated presumably by a reactive metabolite (hydroxylamine) produced by cytochrome P-450 oxidative metabolism. Slow acetylators appear to be at increased risk. Other risk factors for drug reactions include previous exposure, previous reaction, age (20–49 years), route (parenteral), and dose of administration (high, intermittent). Atopy does not predispose to development of a reaction, but atopic individuals have more severe reactions.

Immunopathologic reactions to antibiotics include type I (IgE-mediated) reactions resulting from a drug or metabolite interaction with preformed specific IgE bound to the surfaces of tissue mast cells or circulating basophils. Release of mediators such as histamine and leukotrienes contributes to the clinical development of angioedema, urticaria, bronchospasm, or anaphylaxis. Type II (cytotoxic) reactions involve IgG or IgM antibodies that recognize drug bound to cell membranes. In the presence of serum complement, the antibody-coated cell is either cleared or destroyed, causing drug-induced hemolytic anemia or thrombocytopenia. Type III (immune complex) reactions are caused by soluble complexes of drug or metabolite with IgG or IgM antibody. If the immune complex is deposited on blood vessel walls and activates the complement cascade, serum sickness may result. Type IV (T-cell–mediated) reactions require activated T lymphocytes that recognize a drug or its metabolite as seen in allergic contact dermatitis. Sensitization usually occurs via the topical route of administration. Immunopathologic reactions not fitting into the type I–IV classification include Stevens-Johnson syndrome, exfoliative dermatitis, and the maculopapular rash associated with penicillin or ampicillin. The prevalence of morbilliform rashes in patients given ampicillin is between 5.2% and 9.5% of treatment courses. However, patients given ampicillin during Epstein-Barr virus and cytomegalovirus infections or with acute lymphoblastic anemia have a 69–100% incidence of non-IgE-mediated rash. Serum sickness–like reactions resemble type III reactions, although immune complexes are not documented; β-lactams, especially cefaclor, and sulfonamides, have been implicated most often. They may result from an inherited propensity for hepatic biotransformation of drug into toxic or immunogenic metabolites. The incidence of "allergic" cutaneous reactions to trimethoprim–sulfamethoxazole in patients with AIDS has been reported to be as high as 70%. The mechanism is thought to relate to the severe immune dysregulation, although it may be due to glutathione deficiency resulting in toxic metabolites.

► Clinical Findings

A. Symptoms and Signs

Allergic reactions can result in pruritus, urticaria, angioedema, or anaphylaxis. Serum sickness is characterized by fever, rash, lymphadenopathy, myalgias, and arthralgias. Cytotoxic drug reactions can result in symptoms and signs associated with the underlying anemia or thrombocytopenia. Delayed-type hypersensitivity may cause contact dermatitis.

B. Laboratory Findings

Skin testing is the most rapid, useful, and sensitive method of demonstrating the presence of IgE antibody to a specific allergen. Skin testing to nonpenicillin antibiotics may be difficult, however, because many immunologic reactions are due to metabolites rather than to the parent drug and because the relevant metabolites for most drugs other than penicillin have not been identified. Because metabolites are usually low-molecular-weight haptens, they must combine with carrier proteins to be useful for diagnosis. In the case of contact sensitivity reactions to topical antibiotics, a 48-hour patch test can be useful.

Solid-phase in-vitro immunoassays for IgE to penicillins are available for identification of IgE to penicilloyl but are considerably less sensitive and give less information than skin testing. Assays for specific IgG and IgM have been shown to correlate with a drug reaction in immune cytopenias, but in most other instances such assays are not clinically useful. Skin testing for immediate hypersensitivity is helpful only in predicting reactions caused by IgE antibodies. Most nonpruritic maculopapular rashes will not be predicted by skin testing.

Approximately 80% of patients with a history of penicillin allergy will have negative skin tests. Penicillin therapy in patients with a history of an immediate hypersensitivity reaction to penicillin, but with negative skin tests to both penicilloyl and the minor determinant mixture, is accompanied by a 1–3% chance of urticaria or other mild allergic reactions at some time during therapy, with anaphylaxis occurring in less than 0.1% of patients. In contrast, the predictive value of a positive skin test is approximately 60%. Testing with penicilloyl linked to polylysine (PPL) alone has a sensitivity of about 76%; use of both PPL and penicillin G (used as a minor determinant) increases sensitivity to about 95%. Not using the minor determinant mixture in skin testing can result in failure to predict potential anaphylactic reactions. Unfortunately the minor determinant mixture is still not commercially available, although most academic allergy centers make their own. Approximately 4% of subjects tested who have no history of penicillin allergy have positive skin tests, and most fatalities occur in patients with no prior history of reaction. Rarely, patients may have skin test reactivity only to a specific semisynthetic penicillin. Resensitization in skin test–negative children occurs infrequently (< 1%) after a course of oral antibiotic.

The degree of cross-reactivity of determinants formed from cephalosporins with IgE to other β-lactam drugs remains unresolved, especially because haptens that may be unique to cephalosporin metabolism remain unknown. The degree of clinical cross-reactivity is much lower than the in-vitro cross-reactivity. A clinical adverse reaction rate of 3–7% for cephalosporins may be expected in patients with positive histories of penicillin allergy. Antibodies to the second- and third-generation cephalosporins appear to be directed at the unique side chains rather than at the common ring structure. The present literature suggests that a positive skin test to a cephalosporin used at a concentration of 1 mg/mL would place the patient at increased risk for an allergic reaction to that antibiotic. However, a negative skin test would not exclude sensitivity to a potentially relevant metabolite. One review concluded that there is no increased incidence of allergy to second- and third-generation cephalosporins in patients with penicillin allergy and that penicillin skin testing does not identify patients who develop cephalosporin allergy. However, another study suggested that although only 2% of penicillin-allergic patients would react to a cephalosporin, they would be at risk for anaphylaxis.

Carbacephems (loracarbef) are similar to cephalosporins, although the degree of cross-reactivity is undetermined. Carbapenems (imipenem) represent another class of β-lactam antibiotics with a bicyclic nucleus and a high degree of cross-reactivity with penicillin. In contrast, monobactams (aztreonam) contain a monocyclic rather than bicyclic ring structure, and limited data suggest that aztreonam can be safely administered to most penicillin-allergic subjects.

Skin testing for non–β-lactam antibiotics is less reliable, because the relevant degradation products are for the most part unknown or multivalent reagents are unavailable.

▶ Treatment

A. General Measures

Withdrawal of the implicated drug is usually a central component of management. Acute IgE-mediated reactions such as anaphylaxis, urticaria, and angioedema are treated according to established therapeutic guidelines that include the use of epinephrine, H_1- and H_2-receptor blocking agents, volume replacement, and systemic corticosteroids (see previous sections). Antibiotic-induced immune cytopenias can be managed by withdrawal of the offending agent or reduction in dose. Drug-induced serum sickness can be suppressed by drug withdrawal, antihistamines, and corticosteroids. Contact allergy can be managed by avoidance and treatment with antihistamines and topical corticosteroids. Reactions such as toxic epidermal necrolysis and Stevens-Johnson syndrome require immediate drug withdrawal and supportive care.

B. Alternative Therapy

If possible, subsequent therapy should be with an alternative drug that has therapeutic actions similar to the drug in question but with no immunologic cross-reactivity.

C. Desensitization

Administering gradually increasing doses of an antibiotic either orally or parentally over a period of hours to days may be considered if alternative therapy is not acceptable. This should be done only by a physician familiar with desensitization, typically in an intensive care setting. Of note, desensitization is only effective for the course of therapy for which the patient was desensitized, unless maintained on a chronic prophylactic dose of the medication as patients revert from a desensitized to allergic state after the drug is discontinued. In addition, desensitization does not reduce or prevent non–IgE-mediated reactions. Patients with Stevens-Johnson syndrome should not be desensitized because of the high mortality rate.

Prognosis

The prognosis is good when drug allergens are identified early and avoided. Stevens-Johnson syndrome and toxic epidermal necrolysis may be associated with a high mortality rate.

2. Latex Allergy

General Considerations

Allergic reactions to latex and rubber products have become increasingly common since the institution of universal precautions for exposure to bodily fluids. Children with spina bifida appear to have a unique sensitivity to latex, perhaps because of early and frequent latex exposure as well as altered neuroimmune interactions. Atopy—especially symptomatic latex allergy—appears to be significantly increased in patients with spina bifida experiencing anaphylaxis during general anesthesia. Other conditions requiring chronic or recurrent exposure to latex such as urogenital anomalies and ventriculoperitoneal shunt have also been associated with latex hypersensitivity. The combination of atopy and frequent exposure seems to synergistically increase the risk of latex hypersensitivity.

Latex is the milky fluid obtained by tapping the cultivated rubber tree, *Hevea brasiliensis*. During manufacture of latex products, various antioxidants and accelerators such as thiurams, carbamates, and mercaptobenzothiazoles are added. Latex products are typically produced by dipping a porcelain mold into a tank of latex and then vulcanizing it to enhance mechanical stability. The product is washed or "leached" of excess proteins, then dry-lubricated with a powder such as corn starch.

Latex is a complex biologic mixture composed of rubber particles in a phospholipoprotein envelope and a serum containing sugars, lipids, nucleic acids, minerals, and various proteins. The protein component is thought to contain the allergenic properties. Extra leaching steps may reduce the protein content and hence the allergenicity of the final product. IgE from latex-sensitized individuals reacts with different protein components, supporting the notion that more than one clinically important latex antigen exists. New allergenic epitopes are generated during the manufacturing process. Thus, polypeptides from latex glove extracts vary both quantitatively and qualitatively with different brands and lots of gloves. Identification of the causative antigens is important because it may be possible to alter the manufacturing process to reduce the final allergen content.

Latex is ubiquitous in medical settings, and many sources may be inconspicuous. Synthetic alternatives to some latex products—including gloves, dressings, and tape—are available. Avoidance of contact with latex-containing items, however, may be insufficient to prevent allergic reactions, because lubricating powders may serve as vehicles for aerosolized latex antigens. The use of powder-free latex gloves is an important control measure for airborne latex allergen.

Nonmedical sources of latex are also common and include balloons, toys, rubber bands, erasers, condoms, and shoe soles. Pacifiers and bottle nipples have also been implicated as sources of latex allergen, although these products are molded rather than dipped, and allergic reactions to molded products are less common. Latex-allergic patients and their caregivers must be continuously vigilant for hidden sources of exposure.

Clinical Findings

A. Symptoms and Signs

The clinical manifestations of IgE-mediated reactions to latex can involve the full spectrum of symptoms associated with mast cell degranulation. Localized pruritus and urticaria occur after cutaneous contact; conjunctivitis and rhinitis can result from aerosol exposure or direct facial contact. Systemic reactions, including bronchospasm, laryngospasm and hypotension, may occur with more substantial exposure or in extremely sensitive individuals. Finally, vascular collapse and shock leading to fatal cardiovascular events may occur. Intraoperative anaphylaxis represents a common and serious manifestation of latex allergy.

Allergic contact dermatitis to rubber products typically appears 24–48 hours after contact. The primary allergens include accelerators and antioxidants used in the manufacturing process. The diagnosis is established by patch testing. Shoe soles are an important source of exposure. The skin lesions appear primarily as a patchy eczema on exposed surfaces, although reactions can become generalized.

B. Laboratory Findings

Epicutaneous prick testing is a rapid, inexpensive, and sensitive test that detects the presence of latex-specific IgE on skin mast cells. Obstacles to its use include lack of a standardized antigen. Reports of life-threatening anaphylactic events have been associated with skin testing to latex, and intradermal testing may be especially dangerous. A commercially available extract is pending FDA approval.

Immunoassay testing involves the in-vitro measurement of specific IgE, which binds latex antigens. Antigen sources used for testing have included native plant extracts, raw latex, and finished products. When compared with a history of latex-induced symptoms or positive skin tests, the sensitivity of immunoassays testing for latex antigens ranges from 50–100% with specificity between 63% and 100%. These broad ranges may reflect the patient population studied and the source of latex antigen as well as the assay employed. A positive immunoassay test to latex in the presence of a highly suggestive latex allergy history is useful and may circumvent the potential concerns associated with prick skin testing in certain patients.

Cross-reactivity has been demonstrated between latex and a number of other antigens such as foods. Banana, avocado, and chestnut have been found to be antigenically similar to latex both immunologically and clinically.

▶ Complications

Complications may be similar to those caused by other allergens. Prolonged exposure to aerosolized latex may lead to persistent asthma. Chronic allergic contact dermatitis, especially on the hands, can lead to functional disability.

▶ Treatment

Avoidance remains the cornerstone of treatment for latex allergy. Prevention and supportive therapy are the most common methods for managing this problem. Patients identified as being allergic to latex may need to have a personal supply of vinyl or latex-free gloves for use when visiting a physician or dentist. "Hypoallergenic gloves" are poorly classified with respect to their ability to induce IgE-mediated reactions; the FDA currently uses this term to designate products that have a reduced capacity to induce contact dermatitis. Gloves made from synthetic materials include Neolon (Becton-Dickinson), Tactyl 1 (Smart Practice), and Elastyren (Hermal). Autoinjectable epinephrine and medical identification bracelets may be prescribed for latex-allergic patients along with avoidance counseling.

Prophylactic premedication of latex-allergic individuals has been used in some surgical patients at high risk for latex allergy. The rationale for this therapy is derived from the pretreatment protocols developed for iodinated radio-contrast media and anesthetic reactions. Although there has been some success using this regimen, anaphylaxis has occurred despite pretreatment. This approach should not substitute for careful avoidance measures.

▶ Prognosis

Owing to the ubiquitous nature of natural rubber, the prognosis is guarded for patients with severe latex allergy. Chronic exposure to airborne latex particles may lead to chronic asthma. Chronic dermatitis can lead to functional disability.

3. Vaccines

Mumps-measles-rubella (MMR) vaccine has been shown to be safe in egg-allergic patients (although rare reactions to gelatin or neomycin can occur). The ovalbumin content in influenza vaccine is variable, and skin testing with the specific vaccine lot is warranted in patients with egg allergy. (*Note:* Some patients who tolerate cooked egg, that is, denatured protein, may still react to the vaccine.) In addition, the newly introduced live intranasal influenza vaccine is contraindicated in egg-allergic children.

4. Radiocontrast Media

Non–IgE-mediated anaphylactoid reactions may occur with radiocontrast media with up to a 30% reaction rate on reexposure. Management involves using a low-molarity agent and premedication with prednisone, diphenhydramine, and possibly an H_2-blocker.

5. Insulin

Approximately 50% of patients receiving insulin have positive skin tests, but IgE-mediated reactions occur rarely. Insulin resistance is mediated by IgG. If less than 24 hours has elapsed after an allergic reaction to insulin, do not discontinue insulin but rather reduce the dose by one third, then increase by 2–5 units per injection. Skin testing and desensitization are necessary if the interval between the allergic reaction and subsequent dose is greater than 24 hours.

6. Local Anesthetics

Less than 1% of reactions to local anesthetics are IgE-mediated. Management involves selecting a local anesthetic from another class. Esters of benzoic acid include benzocaine and procaine; amides include lidocaine and mepivacaine. Alternatively, the patient can be skin tested with the suspected agent, followed by a provocative challenge. To rule out paraben sensitivity, skin testing can be done with 1% lidocaine from a multidose vial.

7. Aspirin & Other Nonsteroidal Anti-Inflammatory Drugs

Adverse reactions to aspirin and nonsteroidal anti-inflammatory drugs (NSAIDs) include urticaria and angioedema; rhinosinusitis, nasal polyps, and asthma; anaphylactoid reactions; and NSAID-related hypersensitivity pneumonitis. After a systemic reaction, a refractory period of 2–7 days occurs. Most aspirin-sensitive patients tolerate sodium salicylate. All NSAIDs inhibiting cyclooxygenase (COX) cross-react with aspirin. Cross-reactivity between aspirin and tartrazine (yellow dye No. 5) has not been substantiated in controlled trials. No skin test or in-vitro test is available to diagnose aspirin sensitivity. Oral challenge can induce severe bronchospasm. Desensitization and cross-desensitization to NSAIDs can be achieved in most patients and maintained long-term. Leukotriene-receptor antagonists or 5-lipoxygenase inhibitors attenuate the reaction to aspirin challenge and may be beneficial adjunct treatment in aspirin-sensitive asthmatic patients. Preliminary studies suggest that COX-2 inhibitors may be tolerated by patients with ASA-induced asthma.

8. Biological Agents

In recent years, a growing number of biological agents have become available for the treatment of autoimmune, neoplastic, cardiovascular, infectious, and allergic diseases, among others. Their use may be associated with a variety of adverse reactions including hypersensitivity reactions. The FDA issued a boxed warning regarding risk of anaphylaxis and need for patient monitoring with use of omalizumab (see pharmacologic therapy section under Treatment, Chronic Asthma, earlier).

Bohlke K et al: Risk of anaphylaxis after vaccination of children and adolescents. Pediatrics 2003;112:815 [PMID: 12952113].

Centers for Disease Control and Prevention, National Immunization Program: http://www.cdc.gov/nip

Chiu AM et al: Anaphylaxis: Drug allergy, insect stings, and latex. Immunol Allergy Clin North Am 2005;25:389 [PMID: 15878462].

Lee SJ et al: Adverse reactions to biologic agents: Focus on autoimmune disease therapies. J Allergy Clin Immunol 2005;116:900 [PMID: 16210067].

Limb SL et al: Delayed onset and protracted progression of anaphylaxis after omalizumab administration in patients with asthma. J Allergy Clin Immunol 2007;120:1378 [PMID: 17936893].

Offit PA: Addressing parents' concerns: Do vaccines contain harmful preservatives, adjuvants, additives, or residuals? Pediatrics 2003;112:1394 [PMID: 14654615].

Pichichero ME: A review of evidence supporting the American Academy of Pediatrics recommendation for prescribing cephalosporin antibiotics for penicillin-allergic patients. Pediatrics 2005;115:1048 [PMID: 15805383].

Zeiger RS: Current issues with influenza vaccination in egg allergy. J Allergy Clin Immunol 2002;110:834 [PMID: 12373275].

FOOD ALLERGY

ESSENTIALS OF DIAGNOSIS & TYPICAL FEATURES

► Temporal relationship between ingestion of a suspected food and onset of allergic symptoms.

► For IgE-mediated reactions, positive prick skin test or in-vitro test to a suspected food allergen confirmed by a double-blind, placebo-controlled food challenge (except in cases of anaphylaxis).

► General Considerations

Food allergy, defined as an adverse immune response to food proteins, affects 6% of young children and 3–4% of adults. The most common IgE-associated food allergens in children are egg (1.3%), milk (2.5%), peanut (0.8%), soy (0.4%), wheat (0.4%), tree nuts (0.2%), fish (0.2%), and shellfish (0.1%). In older patients, fish (0.4%), shellfish (2%), peanut (0.6%) and tree nuts (0.5%) are most often involved in allergic reactions, and may be lifelong allergies. The highest prevalence of food allergy is found in children with moderate-to-severe atopic dermatitis, with approximately 35% affected, whereas chronic conditions such as urticaria and asthma are much less likely due solely to food allergy. Of note, food allergy can be caused by non-IgE (cell)–mediated mechanisms, in conditions such as food-protein–induced enterocolitis or proctocolitis. It can also be caused by mixed IgE- and cell-mediated mechanisms, as in allergic eosinophilic esophagitis and gastroenteritis.

Some adverse reactions diagnosed by patients or physicians as food allergy involve pharmacologic or metabolic mechanisms and reactions to food toxins. Foods containing significant amounts of vasoactive amines such as chocolate, cheese, and some wines and beers may precipitate migraine headaches in some patients. Claims that dyes, sugar, and food additives may contribute to hyperactivity in children with attention-deficit/hyperactivity disorder are controversial. In the occasional case in which a child appears to benefit from a restricted diet, there is no evidence for an IgE-mediated etiology. Anaphylactoid reactions can occur after ingestion of foods such as certain fish containing high amounts of histamine.

► Clinical Findings

A. Symptoms and Signs

Most reactions to foods occur minutes to 2 hours after ingestion. A history of a temporal relationship between the ingestion of a suspected food and onset of a reaction—as well as the nature and duration of symptoms observed—is important in establishing the diagnosis of food allergy. With chronic atopic dermatitis or persistent urticaria, the association with food may be less obvious (see earlier sections on Atopic Dermatitis and Urticaria). At times, acute symptoms may occur, but the cause may not be obvious because of hidden food allergens. A symptom diary kept for 7–14 days may be helpful in establishing an association between ingestion of foods and symptoms and also provides a baseline observation for the pattern of symptom expression. It is important to record both the form in which the food was ingested and the foods ingested concurrently.

Hives, flushing, facial angioedema, and mouth or throat itching are common. In severe cases, angioedema of the tongue, uvula, pharynx, or upper airway can occur. Contact urticaria can occur without systemic symptoms in some children. Gastrointestinal symptoms include abdominal discomfort or pain, nausea, vomiting, and diarrhea. Children with food allergy may occasionally have isolated rhinoconjunctivitis or wheezing. Rarely, anaphylaxis to food may involve only cardiovascular collapse (see section on Anaphylaxis).

B. Laboratory Findings

Typically, fewer than 50% of histories of food allergy will be confirmed by blinded challenge (although this percentage is much higher in food-induced anaphylaxis). Prick skin testing is useful to rule out a suspected food allergen, because the predictive value is high for a properly performed negative test with an extract of good quality (negative predictive accuracy of greater than 95%). In contrast, the predictive value for a positive test is approximately 50%. RAST and other in-vitro tests have lower specificity and positive predictive values. In contrast, specific IgE levels to milk, egg, peanut, and fish proteins have been established with the Phadia ImmunoCAP assay correlating with a greater than 95% chance of a clinical reaction. Measurement of IgG to foods is not clinically useful as IgG responses are a reflection of normal immune recognition of foreign food proteins.

The double-blind, placebo-controlled food challenge is considered the gold standard for diagnosing food allergy except in severe reactions. If there is high suspicion of possible allergic reactivity to a food with a negative skin test or undetectable ImmunoCAP level (or both), a food challenge may be necessary to confirm the presence or absence of allergy. Even when multiple food allergies are suspected, most patients will test positive to three or fewer foods on blinded challenge. Therefore, extensive elimination diets are almost never indicated. Elimination without controlled challenge is a less desirable but at times more practical approach for suspected food allergy. Elimination diets and food challenges may also be the only tools for evaluation of suspected non-IgE-mediated food reactions.

Differential Diagnosis

Repeated vomiting in infancy may be due to pyloric stenosis or gastroesophageal reflux. With chronic gastrointestinal symptoms, enzyme deficiency (eg, lactase), cystic fibrosis, celiac disease, chronic intestinal infections, gastrointestinal malformations, and irritable bowel syndrome should be considered.

Treatment

Treatment consists of eliminating and avoiding foods that have been documented to cause allergic reactions. This involves educating the patient, parent, and caregivers regarding hidden food allergens, the necessity for reading labels, and the signs and symptoms of food allergy and its appropriate management (emergency action plan). New food labeling laws went into effect in January 2006 requiring simple terms to indicate the presence of the major food allergens listed previously (eg, milk instead of casein). Consultation with a dietitian familiar with food allergy may be helpful, especially when common foods such as milk, egg, peanut, soy, or wheat are involved All patients with a history of IgE-mediated food allergy should carry self-injectable epinephrine (see section on Anaphylaxis) and a fast-acting antihistamine, and consider wearing medical identification jewelry. Monoclonal anti-IgE, Chinese herbal formula, oral and sublingual immunotherapy, and vaccines have shown promise as possible future treatments of food allergy.

Prognosis

The prognosis is good if the offending food can be identified and avoided. Unfortunately, accidental exposure to food allergens in severely allergic patients can result in death. Most children outgrow their food allergies to milk, egg, wheat, and soy but not to peanut or tree nuts (only 20% and 10% of children may outgrow peanut and tree nut allergy, respectively). The natural history of food allergy can be followed by measuring food-specific IgE levels by Immuno-CAP assay, as discussed earlier, and performing food challenges when indicated. Approximately 2% of children will have food allergy as adults. Resources for food-allergic patients include the Food Allergy and Anaphylaxis Network, at: (800) 929-4040; http://www.foodallergy.org.

Sicherer SH et al: Food Allergy. J Allergy Clin Immunol 2006;117:S470 [PMID: 16455349].

INSECT ALLERGY

ESSENTIALS OF DIAGNOSIS
& TYPICAL FEATURES

▶ Local or systemic allergic signs and symptoms after insect sting.

Allergic reactions to insects include symptoms of respiratory allergy as a result of inhalation of particulate matter of insect origin, local cutaneous reactions to insect bites, and anaphylactic reactions to stings. The latter are almost exclusively caused by Hymenoptera and result in approximately 40 deaths each year in the United States. The order Hymenoptera includes honey bees, yellow jackets, yellow hornets, white-faced hornets, wasps, and fire ants. Africanized honey bees, also known as killer bees, are a concern because of their aggressive behavior and excessive swarming, not because their venom is more toxic. Rarely, patients sensitized to reduviid bugs (also known as kissing bugs) may have episodes of nocturnal anaphylaxis. Lepidopterism refers to adverse effects secondary to contact with larval or adult butterflies and moths. Salivary gland antigens are responsible for immediate and delayed skin reactions in mosquito-sensitive patients.

Clinical Findings

A. Symptoms and Signs

Insect bites or stings can cause local or systemic reactions ranging from mild to fatal responses in susceptible persons. The frequency increases in the summer months and with outdoor exposure. Local cutaneous reactions include urticaria as well as papulovesicular eruptions and lesions that resemble delayed hypersensitivity reactions. Papular urticaria is almost always the result of insect bites, especially of mosquitoes, fleas, and bedbugs. Toxic systemic reactions consisting of gastrointestinal symptoms, headache, vertigo, syncope, convulsions, or fever can occur following multiple stings. These reactions result from histamine-like substances in the venom. In children with hypersensitivity to fire ant venom, sterile pustules occur at sting sites on a nonimmunologic basis due to the inherent toxicity of piperidine alkaloids in the venom. Mild systemic reactions include itching, flushing, and urticaria. Severe systemic reactions may include dyspnea, wheezing, chest tightness, hoarseness, fullness in the throat, hypotension, loss of consciousness, incontinence, nausea, vomiting, and abdominal pain. Delayed systemic reactions occur from 2 hours to 3 weeks following the sting and include serum sickness, peripheral neuritis, allergic vasculitis, and coagulation defects.

B. Laboratory Findings

Skin testing is indicated for children with systemic reactions. Venoms of honeybee, yellow jacket, yellow hornet, white-faced hornet, and wasp are available for skin testing and treatment. Fire ant venom is not yet commercially available, but an extract made from fire ant bodies appears adequate to establish the presence of IgE antibodies to fire ant venom. Of note, venom skin test results can be negative in patients with systemic allergic reactions, especially in the first few weeks after a sting, and the tests may need to be repeated. The presence of a positive skin test denotes prior sensitization but does not predict whether a reaction will occur with the patient's next sting, nor does it differentiate between local and systemic reactions. It is common for children who have had an allergic reaction to have positive skin tests to more than one venom. This might reflect sensitization from prior stings that did not result in an allergic reaction or cross-reactivity between closely related venoms. In-vitro testing (compared with skin testing) has not substantially improved the ability to predict anaphylaxis. With venom RAST, there is a 15–20% incidence of both false-positive and false-negative results. Tests for mosquito saliva antigens or other insect allergy are not commercially available.

▶ Complications

Secondary infection can complicate allergic reactions to insect bites or stings. Serum sickness, nephrotic syndrome, vasculitis, neuritis, and encephalopathy may be seen as late sequelae of reactions to stinging insects.

▶ Treatment

For cutaneous reactions caused by biting insects, symptomatic therapy includes cold compresses, antipruritics (including antihistamines), and occasionally potent topical corticosteroids. Treatment of stings includes careful removal of the stinger, if present, by flicking it away from the wound and not by grasping in order to prevent further envenomation. Topical application of monosodium glutamate, baking soda, or vinegar compresses is of questionable efficacy. Local reactions can be treated with ice, elevation of the affected extremity, oral antihistamines, and NSAIDs as well as potent topical corticosteroids. Large local reactions, in which swelling extends beyond two joints or an extremity, may require a short course of oral corticosteroids. Anaphylactic reactions following Hymenoptera stings should be managed essentially the same as anaphylaxis (see section on Anaphylaxis). Children who have had severe or anaphylactic reactions to Hymenoptera stings—or their parents and caregivers—should be instructed in the use of epinephrine. Patients at risk for anaphylaxis from an insect sting should also wear a medical alert bracelet indicating their allergy. Children at risk from insect stings should avoid wearing bright-colored clothing and perfumes when outdoors and should wear long pants and shoes when walking in the grass. Patients who experience severe systemic reactions and have a positive skin test should receive venom immunotherapy. Immunotherapy is not indicated for children with only urticarial or local reactions.

▶ Prognosis

Children generally have milder reactions than adults after insect stings, and fatal reactions are extremely rare. Patients aged 3–16 years with reactions limited to the skin, such as urticaria and angioedema, appear to be at low risk for more severe reactions with subsequent stings.

Golden D: Outcomes of allergy to insect stings in children, with and without venom immunotherapy. N Engl J Med 2004;351:668 [PMID: 15306668].

Antimicrobial Therapy

John W. Ogle, MD

PRINCIPLES OF ANTIMICROBIAL THERAPY

Antimicrobial therapy of infections is arguably the most important scientific development of 20th-century medicine. It contributes significantly to the quality of life of many people and reduces the morbidity and mortality due to infectious disease. The remarkable success of antimicrobial therapy has been achieved with comparatively little toxicity and expense. The relative ease of administration and the widespread availability of these drugs have led many to adopt a philosophy of broad-spectrum empiric antimicrobial therapy for many common infections.

Unfortunately this era of cheap, safe, and reliable therapy may be coming to a close owing to the increasing frequency of antimicrobial resistance in previously susceptible microorganisms. The problem of antimicrobial resistance is certainly not new—resistance was recognized for sulfonamides and penicillins shortly after their introduction. What is new is the worldwide dissemination of resistant clones of microorganisms, such as *Streptococcus pneumoniae* and *Staphylococcus aureus,* which are inherently virulent and commonly cause serious infections, not only among hospitalized patients but also among outpatients.

Until recently the recognition of new resistant clones was balanced by the promise of newer and more potent antimicrobial agents. Today, because fewer new agents are under development, clinicians are beginning to encounter limitations in their ability to treat some serious bacterial infections. Many factors contribute to the selection of resistant clones. Our success in treating chronic diseases and immune-compromising conditions, which has resulted in additional years of life for patients, has increased opportunities for selection of resistant strains in inpatient units and chronic care facilities. Overuse of antimicrobial agents also contributes to the selection of resistant strains. Examples include medications for mildly ill patients with self-limited conditions such as viral infections, and administration of broad-spectrum antimicrobials for patients whose conditions can be treated with

narrow-spectrum agents. Similarly, failure to document infection with cultures obtained prior to starting therapy limits our willingness to stop or narrow the spectrum of antimicrobials. Insufficient research has been conducted to determine the optimal duration of therapy, with the result that we probably often treat longer than is necessary. Prophylactic strategies, as used for prevention of recurrent otitis media or urinary tract infection, create a selection pressure for antibiotic resistance.

The decision-making process for choosing an appropriate antimicrobial agent is summarized in Table 37–1. Accurate clinical diagnosis is based on the history, physical examination, and initial laboratory tests. The clinical diagnosis then leads to a consideration of the organisms most commonly associated with the clinical condition, the usual pattern of antimicrobial susceptibility of these organisms, and past experience with successful treatment regimens.

Cultures should be obtained in potentially serious infections. Empiric antimicrobial therapy may be initiated, then modified according to the patient's response and the culture results. Often several equally safe and efficacious antimicrobials are available. In this circumstance, the relative cost and ease of administration of the different choices should be considered.

Other important considerations include the patient's age, immune status, and exposure history. Neonates and young infants may present with nonspecific signs of infection, making the differentiation of serious disease from mild illness difficult. In older children, clinical diagnosis is more precise, which may permit therapy to be avoided or allow use of a narrower-spectrum antibiotic. Immune deficiency may increase the number and types of potential infecting organisms that need to be considered, including organisms that are usually avirulent but may cause infections that are serious and difficult to treat. An abnormal immune response may also diminish the severity of the clinical signs and symptoms of infection and thus lead to underestimation of the severity of illness. The exposure history may suggest greater likelihood of certain types of infecting organisms.

Table 37–1. Steps in decision making for use of antimicrobial agents.

Step	Action	Example
1	Determine diagnosis	Septic arthritis
2	Consider age and preexisting condition	Previously healthy 2-year-old child
3	Consider common organisms	*Staphylococcus aureus, Kingella kingae*
4	Consider organism susceptibility	Penicillin- or ampicillin-resistant, frequency MRSA[a] in community
5	Obtain proper cultures[b]	Blood, joint fluid
6	Initiate empiric therapy based on above considerations and past experience (eg, personal, literature)	Nafcillin and cefotaxime, substitute vancomycin for nafcillin if obviously ill or MRSA prevalent.
7	Modify therapy based on culture results and patient response	*S aureus* isolated. Discontinue cefotaxime. Substitute nafcillin for vancomycin if susceptible.
8	Follow clinical response	Interval physical examination
9	Stop therapy	Clinically improved or well, minimum 3-4 weeks

[a]Methicillin-resistant *S aureus*.
[b]Indicated for serious or unusual infections or those with unpredictable clinical response to empiric therapy.

This history includes exposures from family members, classmates, and day care environments and exposure to unusual organisms by virtue of travel, diet, or contact with animals.

Final important considerations are the pace and seriousness of the illness. A rapidly progressive and severe illness should be treated initially with broad-spectrum antimicrobials until a specific etiologic diagnosis is made. A mildly ill outpatient should receive treatment preferentially with narrow-spectrum antimicrobials.

Antimicrobial susceptibility, antimicrobial families, and dosing recommendations are listed in Tables 37–2 to 37–6.

ANTIMICROBIAL SUSCEPTIBILITY TESTING

Cultures and other diagnostic material must be obtained prior to initiating antimicrobial therapy—especially when the patient has a serious infection, initial attempts at therapy have failed, or multiagent therapy is anticipated. Whenever cultures identify the causative organism, therapy can be narrowed or optimized according to susceptibility results. Antimicrobial susceptibility testing should be done in a laboratory using carefully defined procedures (Clinical and Laboratory Standards Institute).

There are several ways to test antimicrobial susceptibility. Identification of an antibiotic-destroying enzyme (eg, β-

lactamase) implies resistance to β-lactam–containing antimicrobial agents. Tube or microtiter broth dilution techniques can be used to determine the minimum inhibitory concentration (MIC) of antibiotic, which is the amount of antibiotic (in mcg/mL) necessary to inhibit the organism under specific laboratory conditions. Disk susceptibility testing (also performed under carefully controlled conditions) yields similar results. The E-test is a standardized test for some organisms that correlates well with MICs. Clinical laboratories usually define antimicrobial susceptibility (susceptible, intermediate, and resistant) in relation to levels of the test antibiotic achievable in the blood or another body fluid (cerebrospinal fluid [CSF] or urine).

Organisms are usually considered susceptible to an antibiotic if the MIC of the antibiotic for the organism is significantly lower than levels of that agent achieved in the blood using appropriate parenteral dosages. This assumption of susceptibility should be reconsidered whenever the patient has a focus of infection (eg, meningitis, osteomyelitis, or abscess) in which poor antibiotic penetration might occur, because the levels of antibiotic in such areas might be lower than the MIC. Conversely, although certain organisms may be reported to be resistant to an antibiotic because sufficiently high blood concentrations cannot be achieved, urine concentrations may be much higher. If so, a urinary tract infection might respond to an antibiotic that would not be adequate for treatment of septicemia.

Thus, antimicrobial susceptibility testing, although a very important part of therapeutic decision making, reflects assumptions that the clinician must understand, especially for serious infections. Ultimately the true test of the efficacy of therapy is patient response. Patients who do not respond to seemingly appropriate therapy may require reassessment, including reconsidering the diagnosis, reculturing, and repeat susceptibility testing, to determine whether resistant strains have evolved or superinfection with a resistant organism is present. Antimicrobial therapy cannot be expected to cure some infections unless additional supportive treatment (usually surgical) is undertaken.

ALTERATION OF DOSE & MEASUREMENT OF BLOOD LEVELS

Certain antimicrobial agents have not been approved (and often not tested) for use in newborns. For those that have been approved, it is important to recognize that both dose and frequency of administration may need to be altered (see Tables 37–4 and 37–5), especially in young (7 days or younger) or low-birth-weight neonates (≤ 2000 g).

Antimicrobial agents are excreted or metabolized through various physiologic mechanisms (eg, renal, hepatic). It is important to consider these routes of excretion and alter the antimicrobial dosage appropriately in any patient with some degree of organ dysfunction. (See Chapter 43.) As indicated in Table 37–4, an assessment of renal or hepatic

Table 37–2. Susceptibility of some common pathogenic microorganisms to various antimicrobial drugs.

Organism	Potentially Useful Antibiotics[a]
Bacteria	
Anaerobic bacteria[b]	Cefotetan,[c] cefoxitin,[c] clindamycin, ertapenem,[c] imipenem,[c] meropenem, metronidazole, penicillins with or without β-lactamase inhibitor, tigecycline[c]
Bacillus anthracis	Amoxicillin, ciprofloxacin, clindamycin, doxycycline, rifampin, vancomycin
Bartonella henselae	Azithromycin, ciprofloxacin, clarithromycin, doxycycline, erythromycin, rifampin
Bordetella pertussis	Amoxicillin, azithromycin, clarithromycin, erythromycin, trimethoprim–sulfamethoxazole
Borrelia burgdorferi	Amoxicillin, cefuroxime, cephalosporins (III),[d] clarithromycin, doxycycline
Campylobacter spp	Azithromycin, carbapenems, erythromycin, fluoroquinolones,[c,e] tetracyclines
Clostridium spp	Clindamycin, metronidazole, penicillins, tetracyclines
Clostridium difficile	Bacitracin (PO), metronidazole, vancomycin (PO)
Corynebacterium diphtheriae	Clindamycin, erythromycin, penicillins
Enterobacteriaceae[f]	Aminoglycosides,[g] ampicillin, aztreonam, cefepime, cephalosporins, ertopenem, fluoroquinolones,[c,e] imipenem, meropenem, tigecycline, trimethoprim–sulfamethoxazole
Enterococcus	Ampicillin (with aminoglycoside), carbapenems (not *E faecium*), linezolid, quinupristin–dalfopristin[c] (*E faecium* only), tigecycline, vancomycin,
Haemophilus influenzae	Amoxicillin-clavulanate, ampicillin (if β-lactamase–negative),[h] cephalosporins (II and III),[d] chloramphenicol, fluoro-quinolones,[c,e] rifampin, trimethoprim–sulfamethoxazole
Listeria monocytogenes	Ampicillin with aminoglycoside, trimethoprim–sulfamethoxazole, vancomycin
Moraxella catarrhalis	Amoxicillin-clavulanate, ampicillin (if β-lactamase–negative),[h] cephalosporins (II, III),[d] erythromycin, fluorquinolones, trimethoprim–sulfamethoxazole
Neisseria gonorrhoeae	Ampicillin (if β-lactamase–negative),[h] cephalosporins (II and III),[d] penicillins, selected fluoroquinolones (only if known susceptible),[c,e] spectinomycin
Neisseria meningitidis	Ampicillin, cephalosporins (II and III),[d] fluoroquinolones,[c,e] penicillins, rifampin
Nocardia asteroides	Tetracycline, trimethoprim–sulfamethoxazole (+ amikacin for severe infections)
	Meropenem or cephalosporins (II, III)[d] for brain abscess
Pasteurella multocida	Amoxicillin–clavulanate, ampicillins, penicillins, tetracyclines
Pseudomonas aeruginosa	Aminoglycosides,[g] anti-*Pseudomonas* penicillins,[c] aztreonam, cefepime, ceftazidime, ciprofloxacin,[c] imipenem, meropenem
Salmonella spp	Ampicillin, azithromycin, cephalosporins (III),[d] fluoroquinolones,[c,e] trimethoprim–sulfamethoxazole
Shigella spp	Ampicillin, azithromycin, cephalosporins (III),[d] fluoroquinolones,[c,e] tetracyclines, trimethoprim–sulfamethoxazole
Staphylococcus aureus	Antistaphylococcal penicillins,[i] cefepime, cephalosporins (I and II), ciprofloxacin, clindamycin, erythromycin, rifampin, trimethoprim–sulfamethoxazole, vancomycin
S aureus (methicillin-resistant)	Clindamycin, daptomycin,[c] linezolid, quinupristin–dalfopristin,[c] tigecycline,[c] trimethoprim–sulfamethoxazole, vanco-mycin
Staphylococci (coagulase-negative)	Cephalosporins (I and II),[j] clindamycin, rifampin, vancomycin
Streptococci (most species)	Ampicillin, cephalosporins, clindamycin, enhanced fluoroquinolones,[c,k] erythromycin, meropenem, penicillins, vancomycin
Streptococcus pneumoniae[l]	Ampicillin, cephalosporins, enhanced fluoroquinolones,[c,k] erythromycin, meropenem, penicillin, vancomycin
Intermediate organisms	
Chlamydia spp	Clarithromycin, erythromycin, levofloxacin,[c] ofloxacin,[c] tetracyclines
Mycoplasma spp	Azithromycin, clarithromycin, erythromycin, fluoroquinolones,[c,e] tetracyclines
Rickettsia spp	Fluoroquinolones,[c,e] tetracyclines

(continued)

Table 37–2. Susceptibility of some common pathogenic microorganisms to various antimicrobial drugs. *(Continued)*

Organism	Potentially Useful Antibiotics[a]
Fungi	
Candida spp	Amphotericin B, caspofungin, fluconazole, flucytosine, itraconazole, ketoconazole, micafungin, posaconazole, voriconazole
Fungi, systemic[b]	Amphotericin B, caspofungin, fluconazole, itraconazole,[c] ketoconazole, micafungin, posaconazole, voriconazole
Dermatophytes	Butenafine, ciclopirox olamine, clotrimazole, econazole, fluconazole, griseofulvin, itraconazole,[c] ketoconazole, miconazole, naftifine, oxiconazole, terbinafine
Pneumocystis jiroveci	Atovaquone, clindamycin–primaquine, dapsone, pentamidine, trimethoprim–sulfamethoxazole
Viruses	
Herpes simplex	Acyclovir, penciclovir,[c] famciclovir,[c] foscarnet, trifluridine, valacyclovir[c]
Human immunodeficiency virus	Five classes: (1) nucleoside reverse transcriptase inhibitors, (2) non-nucleoside reverse transcriptase inhibitors, (3) protease inhibitors, (4) fusion inhibitors, (5) integrase inhibitors; optimally combinations of ≥ 3 drugs should be used (see Chapter 39)
Influenza virus	Amantadine,[m] oseltamivir, rimantidine,[m] zanamivir
Respiratory syncytial virus	Ribavirin[n]
Varicella-zoster virus	Acyclovir, famciclovir,[c] valacyclovir[c]
Cytomegalovirus	Cidofovir, fomivirsen (topical or intravitreal), foscarnet, ganciclovir, valganciclovir
Hepatitis B[c]	Adefovir, interferon alfa, lamivudine
Hepatitis C[c]	Interferon alfa, ribavirin

[a]In alphabetical order. Selection depends on patient's age, diagnosis, site of infection, severity of illness, antimicrobial susceptibility of suspected organism, and drug risk.
[b]Species-dependent.
[c]Not FDA-approved for use in children.
[d]Refer to second- (II) or third- (III) generation cephalosporins.
[e]Includes ciprofloxacin, levofloxacin, lomefloxacin, norfloxacin, ofloxacin, moxifloxacin, gatifloxacin, gemifloxacin.
[f]Includes *E coli, Klebsiella* spp, *Enterobacter* spp, and others; antimicrobial susceptibilities should always be measured.
[g]Amikacin, gentamicin, kanamycin, tobramycin.
[h]Also applies to amoxicillin and related compounds.
[i]Cloxacillin, dicloxacillin, methicillin, nafcillin, oxacillin.
[j]Only if the coagulase-negative *Staphylococcus* is also methicillin- or oxacillin-sensitive.
[k]Includes levofloxacin, lomefloxacin, moxifloxacin, gatifloxacin, gemifloxacin.
[l]Because of increasing frequency of *S pneumoniae* strains resistant to penicillin and cephalosporins, presumptive therapy for severe infections (eg, meningitis) should include vancomycin until susceptibility studies are available.
[m]Influenza A only. Resistance is common, not currently recommended in the United States.
[n]FDA-approved for therapy of respiratory syncytial virus by aerosol, but clinical studies show variable efficacy.

function may be routinely necessary for patients receiving certain drugs (eg, renal function for aminoglycosides, hepatic function for erythromycin or clindamycin); otherwise, harmful drug levels may accumulate. If significant organ dysfunction is present, drug clearance may be delayed and dosage modification may be necessary (see detailed descriptions in individual drug information packets), and measurement of drug levels may be indicated.

Serum levels of drugs posing a high risk of toxicity (eg, aminoglycosides) are ordinarily measured, and measurement of other drugs (eg, vancomycin) may be useful in selected circumstances (see following discussion). For certain other serious bacterial infections (eg, bacterial endocar-

ditis), measurement of the serum concentration of an antimicrobial may be important to deliver optimal therapy.

Certain drug interactions may require modification of drug dosage or other therapeutic alterations. (See Chapter 43.) For example, rifampin stimulates the metabolism of warfarin, birth control pills, prednisone, and anticonvulsants by stimulating the cytochrome P-450 (CYP-450) metabolic pathway. Dosage adjustments or alternative medications may be necessary to avoid significant adverse events. Another common example is erythromycin, which may inhibit the metabolism of theophylline, resulting in toxic theophylline levels. Although many drug interactions are known and well documented, it may be difficult to predict

Table 37–3. Groups of common antibacterial agents.

Group	Examples	Some Common Susceptible Organisms[a]	Common Resistant Organisms	Common or Unique Adverse Reactions
Penicillin group				
Penicillins	Penicillin G, V	*Streptococcus, Neisseria*	*Staphylococcus, Haemophilus,* Enterobacteriaceae	Rash, anaphylaxis, drug fever, bone marrow suppression
Ampicillins	Ampicillin, amoxicillin	(Same as penicillins), plus *Haemophilus* (β-lactamase negative), *Escherichia coli, Enterococcus*	*Staphylococcus,* many Enterobacteriaceae	Diarrhea
Anti-staphylococcal penicillins	Cloxacillin, dicloxacillin, methicillin, nafcillin, oxacillin	*Streptococcus, Staphylococcus aureus*	Gram-negative, *Staphylococcus* (coagulase-negative), *Enterococcus*	Renal (interstitial nephritis)
Anti-*Pseudomonas* penicillins	Azlocillin, piperacillin, ticarcillin	(Same as ampicillins), plus *Pseudomonas*	(Same as ampicillins)	Decreased platelet adhesiveness, hypokalemia, hypernatremia
Penicillin with β-lactamase inhibitor combination	Amoxicillin–clavulanate, ampicillin–sulbactam, ticarcillin–clavulanate	Broad-spectrum	Some Enterobacteriaceae, *Pseudomonas*	Diarrhea
Carbapenems	Imipenem–cilastatin meropenem, ertapenem	Broad-spectrum, gram-negative rods, anaerobes, *Pseudomonas*	MRSA,[b] many enterococci	Central nervous system (CNS), seizures
Cephalosporin group				
First-generation (I)	Cefazolin, cephalexin, cephalothin, cephapirin, cephradine	Gram-positive	Gram-negative, *Enterococcus,* some *Staphylococcus* (coagulase-negative)	Rash; anaphylaxis, drug fever
Second-generation (II)	Cefaclor, cefamandole, cefprozil, cefonicid, cefuroxime, loracarbef	Gram-positive, some *Haemophilus,* some Enterobacteriaceae	*Enterococcus, Pseudomonas,* some *Staphylococcus* (coagulase-negative)	Serum sickness (cefaclor)
	Cefoxitin, cefotetan	Same as second-generation plus anaerobes		
Third-generation (III)	Cefotaxime, ceftizoxime, ceftriaxone, cefpodoxime, ceftibuten, cefdinir	*Streptococcus, Haemophilus,* Enterobacteriaceae, *Neisseria*	*Pseudomonas, Staphylococcus*	Biliary sludging (ceftriaxone) rash
	Ceftazidime, cefepime[c]	(Same as other third-generation cephalosporins), plus *Pseudomonas Staphylococcus*		
Other drugs				
Clindamycin	Clindamycin	Gram-positive, anaerobes, some MRSA	Gram-negative, *Enterococcus*	Nausea, vomiting, hepatotoxicity
Vancomycin	Vancomycin	Gram-positive	Gram-negative	"Red man" syndrome, shock, ototoxicity, renal
Macrolides and azilides	Erythromycin, clarithromycin, azithromycin	Gram-positive *Bordetella, Haemophilus, Mycoplasma, Chlamydia, Legionella, Salmonella, Shigella*	Some Gram-negative	Nausea and vomiting
Monobactams	Aztreonam	Gram-negative aerobes, *Pseudomonas*	Gram-positive cocci	Rash, diarrhea

(continued)

Table 37–3. Groups of common antibacterial agents. *(Continued)*

Group	Examples	Some Common Susceptible Organisms[a]	Common Resistant Organisms	Common or Unique Adverse Reactions
Oxazolidinones	Linezolid	Gram-positive aerobes	Gram-negative aerobes	Diarrhea, thrombocytopenia
Streptogramins	Quinupristin–dalfopristin	Gram-positive aerobes	Gram-negative aerobes	Arthralgia, myalgia
Fluoroquinolones[d]	Ciprofloxacin, ofloxacin	Gram-negative, *Chlamydia*, *Mycoplasma*, *Pseudomonas* (ciprofloxacin)	*Enterococcus, Streptococcus, S pneumoniae*, anaerobes, *Staphylococcus*	Gastrointestinal (GI), rash, CNS
	Gatifloxacin, levofloxacin, moxifloxacin	Gram-negative, streptococci, *S pneumoniae*, staphylococci	Some *Enterococcus*	GI, rash, CNS
Tetracyclines	Chlortetracycline, tetracycline, doxycycline, minocycline	Anaerobes, *Mycoplasma*, *Chlamydia*, *Rickettsia*, *Ehrlichia*	Many Enterobacteriaceae, *Staphylococcus*	Teeth stained,[e] rash, flora overgrowth, hepatotoxicity, pseudotumor cerebri
Sulfonamides	Many	Gram-negative (urine)	Gram-positive	Rash, renal, bone marrow suppression, Stevens-Johnson syndrome
Trimethoprim–sulfamethoxazole	Trimethoprim–sulfamethoxazole	*S aureus*, gram-negative, *S pneumoniae*, *Haemophilus influenzae*	*Streptococcus, Pseudomonas*, anaerobes	Rash, renal, bone marrow suppression, Stevens-Johnson syndrome
Rifampin	Rifampin	*Neisseria, Haemophilus, Staphylococcus, Streptococcus*	Resistance develops rapidly if used as sole agent	Rash, GI, hepatotoxicity, CNS, bone marrow suppression, alters metabolism of other drugs
Aminoglycosides	Amikacin, gentamicin, kanamycin, streptomycin, tobramycin	Gram-negative, including *Pseudomonas aeruginosa*	Gram-positive, anaerobes, some pseudomonads	Nephrotoxicity, ototoxicity, potentiates neuromuscular blocking agents

[a]Not all strains susceptible; always obtain antimicrobial susceptibility tests on significant isolates.
[b]MRSA = methicillin-resistant *S aureus*.
[c]Safety and efficacy are not established in children younger than age 2 months.
[d]Not approved for children.
[e]Dose-dependent in children younger than age 9 years.

interactions that result from a combination of four, five, or more different medications. A high level of suspicion regarding adverse clinical events should be maintained.

THE USE OF NEW ANTIMICROBIAL AGENTS

New antibiotics are introduced frequently, often with claims about unique features that distinguish these usually more expensive products from existing compounds. Often these drugs share many properties with existing drugs. The role that any new antimicrobial will play can only be determined over time, during which new or previously unrecognized side effects might be described and the clinical efficacy established. Clinical trials may not be confirmed in the larger number of patients subsequently treated in practice. Because this may take many years, a conservative approach to using new antibiotics seems fitting, especially because their costs are often higher, and appropriate antimicrobial choices for most common infections already exist. It is appropriate to ask if a new antimicrobial has been proved to be as effective as (or

more effective than) the current drug of choice, and whether its side effects are comparable (or less common) and its cost reasonable. The withdrawal of moxalactam and caution regarding use of trovafloxacin due to unexpected serious side effects, which were not anticipated despite extensive premarket testing, highlight the caution necessary before using new antimicrobials. The heavy marketing of new cephalosporins and fluoroquinolones, which are very similar to existing drugs, is typical of the difficulty in evaluating antimicrobials.

The development of new antibiotics is important as a response to the emergence of resistant organisms and for treatment of infections that are clinically difficult to treat (eg, viruses, fungi, and some resistant bacteria). Fortunately these infections are either rare or (usually) self-limited in immunocompetent hosts.

PROPHYLACTIC ANTIMICROBIAL AGENTS

Antimicrobials can be used to decrease the incidence of postoperative infections (Table 37–7). A dose of an antimi-

Table 37–4. Guidelines for use of common parenteral antibacterial agents[a] in children age 1 month or older.

Agent	Route	Dose[b] (mg/kg/d)	Maximum Daily Dose	Interval (hours)	Adjustment[c]	Blood Levels[d] (mcg/mL) Peak	Trough
Amikacin	IM, IV	15–22.5	1.5 g	8	R	15–25	< 10
Ampicillin	IM, IV	100–400	12 g	4–6	R		
Aztreonam	IM, IV	90–120	6 g	6–8	R		
Cefazolin	IM, IV	50–100	6 g	8	R		
Cefepime[e]	IM, IV	100–150	4–6 g	8–12	R		
Cefotaxime	IM, IV	100–200	12 g	6–8	R		
Cefoxitin	IM, IV	80–160	12 g	4–6	R		
Ceftazidime	IM, IV	100–150	6 g	8	R		
Ceftizoxime	IM, IV	150–200	12 g	6–8	R		
Ceftriaxone	IM, IV	50–100	4 g	12–24	R		
Cefuroxime	IM, IV	100–150	6 g	6–8	R		
Cephalothin	IM, IV	75–125	12 g	4–6	R		
Cephradine	IM, IV	50–100	8 g	6	R		
Clindamycin	IM, IV	25–40	4 g	6–8	R, H		
Gentamicin	IM, IV	3–7.5	300 mg	8	R	5–10	< 2
Linezolid	IV, PO	20	1.2 g	12	R		
Meropenem	IV	60–120	2 g	8	R		
Metronidazole	IV	30	4 g	6	H		
Nafcillin	IM, IV	150	12 g	6	H		
Penicillin G	IM, IV	100,000–250,000 units/kg	20 million units	4–6	H, R		
Penicillin G (benzathine)	IM	50,000 units/kg	2.4 million units	Single dose	None		
Penicillin G (procaine)	IM	25,000–50,000 units/kg	4.8 million units	12–24	R		
Tetracycline[f]	IV[f]	20–30	2 g	12	R		
Ticarcillin	IV	200–300	24 g	4–6	R		
Tobramycin	IM, IV	3–6	300 mg	8	R	5–10	< 2
Vancomycin	IV	40–60	2 g	6	R	20–40[g]	< 5–10[g]

[a]Not including some newly released drugs, ones not recommended for use in children, or ones not widely used.

[b]Always consult package insert for complete prescribing information. Dosage may differ for alternative routes, newborns (see Table 37-6), or patients with liver or renal failure (see Adjustment column) and may not be recommended for use in pregnant women or newborns. Maximum dosage may be indicated only in severe infections or by parenteral routes.

[c]Mode of excretion (R = renal, H = hepatic) of antimicrobial agent should be assessed at the onset of therapy and dosage modified or levels determined as indicated in package insert.

[d]Suggested levels to reduce toxicity.

[e]Safety and efficacy are not established in children younger than age 2 months.

[f]Use with caution in children younger than age 9 years because of tooth staining with repeated doses.

[g]Target peak and trough vancomycin levels are not well correlated with either toxicity or outcome. Measure selectively in meningitis, impaired or changing renal function, or altered volume of distribution.

Table 37–5. Guidelines for use of common oral antibacterial agents in children age 1 month or older.

Agent[a]	Dose[b] (mg/kg/d)	Interval (hours)	Other Considerations
Amoxicillin	40	8–12	Gastrointestinal (GI) side effects
Amoxicillin[c] (high dose)	80–90	12	GI side effects
Amoxicillin–clavulanate	45	12	GI side effects
Ampicillin	50	6	GI side effects
Azithromycin	10 (first dose) then 5; 12 for pharyngitis	24	GI side effects
Cefaclor	40	8	Serum sickness-like illness
Cefadroxil	30	12	
Cefpodoxime	10	12	Taste (suspension)
Cefprozil	30	12	GI side effects
Ceftibuten	9	24	GI side effects
Cefuroxime	30–40	12	GI side effects
Cephalexin	25–50	6	
Cephradine	25–50	6	
Clarithromycin	15	12	GI side effects
Clindamycin	20–30	6	GI side effects
Cloxacillin	50–100	6	GI side effects
Dicloxacillin	12–25	6	GI side effects
Doxycycline[d]	2–4	12–24	Teeth stained < 9 years
Erythromycin[e]	20–50	6–12	GI side effects
Erythromycin–sulfisoxazole	40 (erythromycin)	6–8	
Furazolidone	5–8	6	
Linezolid	20	12	GI side effects
Loracarbef	15; 30 for otitis	12	
Metronidazole	15–35	8	
Nitrofurantoin	5–7	6	
Oxacillin	50–100	6	
Penicillin V	25–50	6	Taste (suspension)
Rifampin	10–20	12–24	
Sulfisoxazole	120–150	6	
Tetracycline[d]	25–50[c]	6	Teeth stained < 9 years
Trimethoprim–sulfamethoxazole	8–12 (TMP)	12	Stevens-Johnson syndrome

[a]Not including some newly released drugs, ones not recommended for use in children, or ones not widely used.
[b]Always consult package insert for complete prescribing information. Dosage may differ for alternative routes, newborns (see Table 37- 6), or patients with liver or renal failure (see Table 37-4, Adjustment column) and may not be recommended for use in pregnant women or newborns. Maximum dosage may be indicated only in severe infections or by parenteral routes.
[c]Higher dose amoxicillin indicated for therapy of otitis media in regions where rates of penicillin-resistant *Streptococcus pneumoniae* are high.
[d]Use with caution in children younger than age 9 years because of tooth staining with repeated doses.
[e]Preparation-dependent.

crobial given 30 minutes to 2 hours prior to surgery can reduce postoperative wound infection. The goal is to achieve high levels in the serum at the time of incision and by this means—along with good surgical technique—to minimize viable bacterial contamination of the wound. During a lengthy procedure, a second dose may be given. No evidence exists that multiple subsequent doses of antimicrobials confer additional benefit. The antimicrobial(s) used for prophylaxis are directed toward the flora that most commonly cause postoperative infection at a given anatomic site. Gram-

Table 37–6. Guidelines for use of selected antimicrobial agents in newborns.

	Route	Body Wt (g)	Maximum Dosage (mg/kg/d) [Frequency]				Blood Levels (mcg/mL)	
			< 7	Days	8–30	Days	Peak	Trough
Amikacin[a]	IV, IM	< 2000	15	[q12h]	22.5	[q8h]	15–25	5–10
		> 2000	20	[q12h]	30	[q8h]		
Ampicillin	IV, IM	< 2000	100	[q12h]	150	[q8h]		
		> 2000	150	[q8h]	200	[q6h]		
Cefotaxime	IV, IM		100	[q12h]	150	[q8h]		
Ceftazidime	IV, IM	< 2000	100	[q12h]	150	[q8h]		
		> 2000	100	[q8h]	150	[q8h]		
Clindamycin	IV, IM, PO	< 2000	10	[q12h]	15	[q8h]		
		> 2000	15	[q8h]	20	[q6h]		
Erythromycin	PO		20	[q12h]	30	[q8h]		
Gentamicin[a]	IV, IM		5	[q12–18h]	7.5	[q8h]	5–10	< 2
Nafcillin	IV	< 2000	50	[q12h]	75	[q8h]		
		> 2000	75	[q8h]	150	[q6h]		
Oxacillin	IV, IM	< 2000	100	[q12h]	150	[q8h]		
		> 2000	50	[q8h]	200	[q6h]		
Penicillin G[b]	IV	< 2000	100,000	[q12h]	150,000	[q8h]		
		> 2000	150,000	[q8h]	200,000	[q6h]		
Ticarcillin	IV, IM	< 2000	150	[q12h]	225	[q8h]		
		> 2000	225	[q8h]	300	[q6h]		
Tobramycin[a]	IV, IM		5	[q12–18h]	7.5	[q8h]	5–10	< 2
Vancomycin[c]	IV		20	[q12h]	30	[q8h]	20–40	5–10

[a]Neonates weighting < 1200 g may require even smaller doses. Antibiotic levels should be closely monitored.
[b]Penicillin dosages are in units/kg/d. Other preparations (eg, benzathine penicillin) may be given IM. See specific diseases for dosage.
[c]Target peak and trough vancomycin levels are not well correlated with either toxicity or outcome.

positive cocci such as *S aureus* are usually targeted, and a first-generation cephalosporin (eg, cefazolin) is a cost-effective choice. Third-generation cephalosporins and other broad-spectrum agents are more expensive and offer less benefit because they are less active than cefazolin against *S aureus*. Cefoxitin or cefotetan is useful for procedures such as colorectal surgery, although cefazolin is appropriate for most gynecologic patients. In colorectal surgery, orally administered antimicrobials such as neomycin and erythromycin may be as effective as parenteral antimicrobials.

In hospitals where the predominant *S aureus* strains are methicillin-resistant or in cases where the patient is allergic to penicillin and cephalosporins, vancomycin can be considered. However, prophylactic vancomycin has caused hypotension at the time of induction of general anesthesia. Frequent use of vancomycin as a prophylactic antimicrobial will contribute to the development of vancomycin-resistant strains such as *Enterococcus faecalis*. For these reasons, vancomycin should generally not be used for prophylaxis,

although it might prove useful for individual patients at extremely high risk.

Prophylactic antimicrobials are given in several other circumstances. Endocarditis prophylaxis is indicated during dental and colorectal or genitourinary procedures in patients with high-risk heart lesions, such as prosthetic cardiac valves, surgically corrected systemic pulmonary shunts, and mitral valve prolapse with regurgitation. Patients with indwelling vascular catheters, such as Broviac catheters, should receive prophylaxis during similar procedures, which are likely to induce a transient bacteremia. Prophylaxis against infection with group A streptococci reduces the recurrence rate for acute rheumatic fever. Postexposure prophylaxis is given after exposure to pertussis, *Haemophilus influenzae* type b (Hib) infection (depending on age), meningococcus, gonococcus, tuberculosis (household exposure), plague, aerosolized tularemia or anthrax, and other high-risk infections. Family or close contacts of patients with severe invasive streptococcal disease may benefit from prophylaxis. Silver nitrate, erythromycin, povidone–iodine, and tetra-

Table 37–7. Antimicrobial prophylaxis and preferred prophylactic agents: Selected conditions and pathogens.[a]

Pathogen (Indication)	Prophylactic Agent
Bacillus anthracis[b]	Amoxicillin (if proved susceptible), ciprofloxacin, doxycycline
Bacterial endocarditis[c]	Ampicillin, ampicillin and gentamicin, amoxicillin, or other approved regimens
Bordetella pertussis (exposure to respiratory secretions)	Azithromycin, clarithromycin, erythromycin
Chlamydia trachomatis (genital contact)	Erythromycin
Haemophilus influenzae type b[d] (household exposure)	Rifampin
Mycobacterium tuberculosis (household exposure)	Isoniazid
Neisseria meningitidis (household exposure)	Rifampin, sulfadiazine,[e] ciprofloxacin
Neisseria gonorrhoeae (ophthalmia neonatorum)	Erythromycin, silver nitrate ophthalmic
N gonorrhoeae (sexual contact)	Ceftriaxone, cefixime, cefpodoxime
Treponema pallidum (sexual contact)	Penicillin
Streptococcus pneumoniae (sickle cell disease, asplenia)	Penicillin
Postoperative wound infection[f]	Cefazolin, other regimens[f]
Group A streptococci (rheumatic fever)[g]	Benzathine penicillin G, penicillin, sulfadiazine
Group B streptococcal sepsis	Ampicillin to mother prior to delivery
Pneumonic *Yersinia pestis*[h] (exposure)	Tetracycline[i]
Francisella tularensis[h] (aerosolized exposure)	Tetracycline[i]
Vibrio cholera	Tetracycline,[i] trimethoprim–sulfamethoxazole
Recurrent urinary tract infection	Nitrofurantoin, trimethoprim–sulfamethoxazole
Pneumocystis jiroveci (formerly *Pneumocystis carinii*)— (HIV, some immunocompromised patients)	Atovaquone, clindamycin-primaquine, dapsone, trimethoprim–sulfamethoxazole, pentamidine

[a]Decisions for prophylaxis must take a number of factors into account, including the evidence for efficacy of therapy, the degree of the exposure to an infecting agent, the risk and consequences of infection, the susceptibility of the infecting agent to antimicrobials, and the patient's ability to tolerate and comply with the antimicrobial agent. See individual chapters of the text for discussion.

[b]Decisions for prophylaxis should be made in accordance with the responsible public health department recommendations.

[c]See discussion in Chapter 19 (Cardiovascular Diseases).

[d]Prophylaxis provided to family if contacts include children younger than age 4 years. Some experts provide prophylaxis in day care settings after one case and some after two cases of *H influenzae* type B infection.

[e]Only for known sulfadiazine-susceptible strains.

[f]Alternative regimens may be used, depending on the site of surgery and the degree of contamination.

[g]Oral prophylaxis may be indicated in some patients. Alternative regimens indicated for penicillin-allergic patients. See discussion in chapter.

[h]Prophylaxis not well established. Carefully assess risk on a case-by-case basis.

[i]Usually not indicated for children younger than age 9 years because of tooth staining with repeated doses.

cycline can be used in ophthalmic preparations for prevention of gonococcal ophthalmia neonatorum. Children with asplenia or sickle cell disease receive prophylactic penicillin to protect against overwhelming *S pneumoniae* sepsis, usually started immediately with the onset of fever.

Prophylactic antimicrobials are sometimes used for some children at high risk for recurrent urinary tract infection, but the rate of infection is not decreased in recent studies.

INITIAL EMPIRIC ANTIMICROBIAL CHOICES FOR SELECTED CONDITIONS

General recommendations for specific conditions are as follows. A specific selection depends on the patient's age, diagno-sis, site of infection, severity of illness, antimicrobial suscepti-bility of bacterial isolates, and history of drug allergy. Always consult the package insert for detailed prescribing informa-tion. Tables 37–2 to 37–6 include further information.

Neonatal Sepsis & Meningitis

The newborn with sepsis may have signs of focal infection, such as pneumonia or respiratory distress syndrome, or may have subtle nonfocal signs. Group B streptococci, *Escherichia coli*, other gram-negative rods, and *Listeria monocytogenes* are com-monly encountered. Ampicillin and gentamicin (or another aminoglycoside) are preferred. If meningitis is present, many clinicians substitute a third-generation cephalosporin for the aminoglycoside. *S pneumoniae* is an uncommon cause of meningitis in neonates. However, if the Gram stain shows gram-positive cocci suggesting *S pneumoniae,* substitution of vancomycin for ampicillin should be considered. In the newborn with cellulitis, *S aureus* including methicillin-resistant *S aureus* (MRSA) and group A streptococci are additional considerations. Nafcillin, oxacillin, or a first-generation cephalosporin is usually added. Vancomycin is added if MRSA is common. Omphalitis is often polymicrobial, and *Enterococcus* species, gram-negative aerobes, and anaerobes may be causative. Clindamycin, ampicillin, and an aminoglycoside or cefotaxime cover the most likely organisms; early surgical intervention is indicated.

Sepsis in an Infant

S pneumoniae and *Neisseria meningitidis* are most commonly encountered in infants. Hib infection may occur in unimmunized children. A third-generation cephalosporin is appropriate. Intermediate-level penicillin and cephalosporin resistance in *S pneumoniae* usually do not cause therapy to fail unless meningitis or another difficult-to-treat infection, such as endocarditis or osteomyelitis is present.

Occult bacteremia may be encountered in young infants with high fever. Prior to immunization with vaccines effective against Hib, persistent bacteremia and complications including meningitis were seen in approximately 50% of children infected with occult Hib bacteremia. With widespread use of Hib vaccine, Hib is a very uncommon cause of occult bacteremia in young children with fever. Similarly, prior to the introduction of the 7-valent conjugate pneumococcal (PCV7) vaccine, *S pneumonia* bacteremia was demonstrated in 3–5% of infants aged 3–36 months with fever of 39°C or greater, no identified source for fever on examination, and white blood cell count (WBC) of 15,000/mm^3. The risk of bacteremia increased to 6–10% in younger children with progressively high fever and high WBCs. The risk of developing meningitis due to persistent *S pneumoniae* is estimated at 3% of those who are known to be bacteremic. The risk of *S pneumoniae* bacteremia and its complications is significantly reduced in children immunized with the PCV7 vaccine. In clinical trials and subsequent nationally surveillance for the incidence of disease, this vaccine reduced the incidence of invasive pneumococcal diseases by approximately 90%. Observation without antimicrobials, but with appropriate plans for follow-up examinations, is appropriate for most febrile young children who are fully immunized.

Nosocomial Sepsis

Many bacterial pathogens can cause infection in hospitalized patients. Recent local experience is usually the best guide to etiologic diagnosis. For example, some intensive care units experience frequent infections due to *Enterobacter cloacae,* whereas in other units *Klebsiella pneumoniae* is the most common nosocomial isolate. Initial therapy should include antibiotics effective for MRSA and resistant *Pseudomonas*

aeruginosa if these are frequent isolates. *E faecalis* is a common cause of nosocomial bacteremia in patients with central catheters, particularly in units where cephalosporins are heavily used. Coagulase-negative staphylococci are commonly isolated from patients with indwelling central catheters. In seriously ill patients, when the local experience suggests that *Enterococcus* species or coagulase-negative staphylococci are common, the initial regimen should include vancomycin. Because *Enterococcus* species and coagulase-negative staphylococci commonly cause fever without significant morbidity or mortality, initial regimens without vancomycin are appropriate, with adjustment of treatment after susceptibility is known. If *P aeruginosa* or other resistant gram-negative rods are common, ceftazidime or cefepime should be included in initial therapy.

Meningitis

Bacterial meningitis in neonates is usually caused by infection with group B streptococci, *E coli*, other gram-negative rods, or *L monocytogenes*. A combination of ampicillin and gentamicin or another aminoglycoside—or ampicillin and a third-generation cephalosporin—is started initially. In an infant or older child, *S pneumoniae* or *N meningitidis* are the most common isolates. As previously noted, Hib is uncommon now because of widespread immunization. Increasingly, *S pneumoniae* with multiple resistances to penicillin, cephalosporins, and other drugs is isolated. In many communities, 30–40% of *S pneumoniae* isolates have intermediate susceptibility to penicillin (MIC between 0.1 and 2 mcg/mL), and 5–10% of isolates may be highly resistant to penicillin (MIC > 2 mcg/mL). Resistance to a third-generation cephalosporin (MIC > 2 mcg/mL) may occur in 3–5% of isolates.

In bacterial meningitis, peak CSF antimicrobial concentrations 10 or more times greater than the MIC of the organism are desirable, but this may be difficult to achieve if organisms are resistant. The therapeutic problem is complicated if dexamethasone, which reduces the entry of some antimicrobials into the CSF, is also given.

Initial therapy of bacterial meningitis in an older child thus should include vancomycin and a third-generation cephalosporin. Alternatively, meropenem has also been successful. A lumbar puncture should be considered 24–48 hours after the start of therapy to assess the sterility of the CSF. Rifampin should be added if the Gram stain or cultures of CSF are positive on repeated lumbar puncture, if the child has failed to improve, or if an organism with a very high MIC to ceftriaxone is isolated. The optimal therapy of highly resistant *S pneumoniae* meningitis is not well established by clinical data.

Meningitis in a child with a ventriculoperitoneal shunt is most commonly caused by coagulase-negative staphylococci, many of which are methicillin-resistant, and *Corynebacterium* species, which are resistant to many antimicrobials. In many of these patients who are not seriously ill, therapy should be postponed while awaiting the appropriate shunt fluid for Gram stain and culture. Seriously ill patients should initially be given vancomycin and a third-generation cephalosporin, because *S aureus* and gram-negative rods are also possible and can cause serious infection.

Urinary Tract Infection

E coli is the most common isolate from the urinary tract. Outpatients with symptoms of lower urinary tract disease or with mild illness can be given ampicillin, cephalexin, or trimethoprim–sulfamethoxazole (TMP–SMX). Local experience and resistance rates should guide initial therapy. In selected patients with pyelonephritis, outpatient therapy is effective using parenteral aminoglycosides or ceftriaxone once per day. Oral cefixime has been used in place of ceftriaxone for outpatient therapy. Ciprofloxacin has been approved by the U.S. Food and Drug Administration (FDA) for therapy of urinary tract infection in children older than 1 year, but it should be reserved for complicated cases. For hospitalized patients with genitourinary tract infection and suspected bacteremia, ampicillin and gentamicin or a third-generation cephalosporin is appropriate. Gram stain should be used to guide the initial choice. For patients with known or suspected resistant organisms, such as *P aeruginosa,* or for patients with urosepsis, an aminoglycoside and ceftazidime, cefepime, or ticarcillin may be started. Unit-specific data on typical bacterial species and their patterns of susceptibility should guide the antimicrobial choice for nosocomial urinary tract infections.

Bacterial Pneumonia

Bacterial pneumonia in newborns generally should be treated with the same antimicrobial choices as sepsis. Infants and older children are frequently infected with *S pneumoniae.* Ampicillin and amoxicillin are effective in most patients eligible for outpatient therapy. Children who require hospitalization may benefit from a second- or third-generation cephalosporin. The broader initial coverage is indicated because of the greater severity of disease. A rapidly progressive pneumonia, with pneumatoceles or large pleural effusions, may be due to MRSA or group A streptococci, Hib, or another gram-negative rod. Vancomycin should be used in addition to a third-generation cephalosporin.

Children aged 6 years and older frequently have infection with *Mycoplasma pneumoniae, Chlamydia pneumoniae,* or *S pneumoniae.* Erythromycin, clarithromycin, or azithromycin is usually indicated for initial empiric therapy.

Skin & Soft Tissue Infections

S aureus and *Streptococcus pyogenes* are the most common causes of skin and soft tissue infections (SSTIs) in children. Community-acquired MRSA infections are common in many communities and complicate clinical decision making. Culture and susceptibility testing of abscesses, cellulitis, and more serious SSTIs is very important for optimal clinical management. Children with cellulitis more commonly have infection with group A streptococci, and empiric outpatient therapy with cephalexin or dicloxacillin is preferred. Children with small (< 5 cm) abscesses usually are effectively treated with incision

and drainage without an antimicrobial. Outpatient therapy of large (> 5 cm) abscesses includes incision and drainage and empiric clindamycin or TMP–SMX depending on local susceptibility patterns. Group A streptococcal infections are not adequately treated with TMP–SMX. However, in many communities, 50% or more of MRSA isolates are also resistant to clindamycin, fluoroquinolones, and erythromycin. Adequate cultures, the thoroughness of drainage procedures, and careful outpatient follow-up are needed to ensure optimal outcomes.

SPECIFIC ANTIMICROBIAL AGENTS

PENICILLINS

Aminopenicillins

Penicillin remains the drug of choice for streptococcal infections, acute rheumatic fever prophylaxis, syphilis, oral anaerobic infections, dental infections, *N meningitidis* infection, leptospirosis, rat-bite fever, actinomycosis, and infections due to *Clostridium* and *Bacillus* species. For oral therapy of minor infections, amoxicillin or ampicillin is usually equivalent. For systemic therapy, aqueous penicillin G is preferable. For treatment of streptococcal pharyngitis, some experts recommend a first-generation cephalosporin. Amoxicillin is preferred for oral therapy of Lyme disease in children. For dog or cat bites, where *Pasteurella multocida* is commonly encountered, amoxicillin–clavulanate provides good coverage of *Pasteurella* as well as *Staphylococcus.* An alternative is separate prescriptions for penicillin and an antistaphylococcal drug such as cephalexin, or clindamycin and TMP–SMX in penicillin-allergic patients. For human bites, amoxicillin–clavulanate provides adequate therapy for *Eikenella corrodens* and other mixed oral aerobes and anaerobes. The β-lactamase inhibitor sulbactam combined with ampicillin is given parenterally for human and animal bites, and some other infections due to organisms from the oral flora, in which mixed aerobic and anaerobic bacteria may be resistant to ampicillin due to β-lactamase production.

Penicillinase-Resistant Penicillins

S aureus is usually resistant to penicillin and amoxicillin owing to penicillinase production. Nafcillin, oxacillin, methicillin, and first- and second-generation cephalosporins are stable to penicillinase and are usually equivalent for intravenous therapy. Methicillin is associated with more frequent interstitial nephritis. Oxacillin and methicillin are renally excreted, whereas nafcillin is excreted through the biliary tract. These properties are occasionally considered in children with renal or liver failure. Cost should usually be the deciding factor for choosing an agent. Often both *S aureus* and *S pyogenes* are suspected initially (eg, in cellulitis or postoperative wound infections). The penicillinase-resistant penicillins (PRPs) and first- and second-generation cephalosporins are efficacious for most streptococcal infections, although penicillin remains the drug of choice.

MRSA is an increasingly common and serious community-acquired infection in children and may cause nosocomial infection. MRSA infections are also resistant to other PRPs and to other cephalosporins. Vancomycin is effective against MRSA and coagulase-negative staphylococci. S aureus infections range in severity from minor infections treated on an outpatient basis to life-threatening infections. Severe infections due to MRSA are a serious concern in many communities. It is important to culture and determine antimicrobial susceptibility of suspected S aureus infections. In communities with frequent MRSA infections in children, initial therapy of seriously ill children should include vancomycin. MRSA may also be resistant to macrolides and clindamycin by alteration in the bacterial 23S ribosomal RNA. Many strains reported as clindamycin-susceptible and erythromycin-resistant are truly resistant to clindamycin. This inducible resistance to clindamycin may be detected in erythromycin-resistant MRSA that demonstrates a D-zone in disk susceptibility testing to clindamycin. Community-acquired MRSA is more likely to be susceptible to TMP–SMX, clindamycin, and gentamicin than hospital-acquired infections.

For outpatient therapy, cloxacillin, dicloxacillin, and first- or second-generation cephalosporins are usually equally effective for infections due to susceptible S aureus. Cost may determine the choice between drugs.

Anti-*Pseudomonas* Penicillins

Ticarcillin, mezlocillin, and piperacillin are active intravenously against streptococci, ampicillin-susceptible enterococci, H influenzae, gram-negative rods (including more resistant gram-negative rods such as Enterobacter, Proteus, and Pseudomonas aeruginosa), and gram-negative anaerobes such as Bacteroides fragilis. P aeruginosa is inherently resistant to most antimicrobials, and high levels of these drugs are usually required. The combination of ticarcillin and an aminoglycoside is synergistic against P aeruginosa and many other enteric gram-negative rods. Ticarcillin in a fixed combination with clavulanic acid that has activity against β-lactamase–producing strains of Klebsiella, S aureus, and Bacteroides. Piperacillin is more active in vitro against many gram-negative enteric infections and may be advantageous in some circumstances, but it is not FDA-approved in children. Piperacillin–tazobactam is another combination antimicrobial and β-lactamase inhibitor that has enhanced activity against many β-lactamase producers.

Antipseudomonal penicillins cause the same toxicities as penicillin and therefore are usually very safe. Carbenicillin, ticarcillin, and piperacillin contain large amounts of sodium, which may cause problems for some patients with cardiac or renal disease.

GLYCOPEPTIDE AGENTS

Vancomycin and teicoplanin are glycopeptide antimicrobial agents active against the cell wall of gram-positive organisms. Only vancomycin is licensed in the United States. Vancomycin is useful for parenteral therapy of resistant gram-positive cocci such as penicillin- and cephalosporin-resistant S pneumoniae, MRSA, methicillin-resistant coagulase-negative staphylococci, and ampicillin-resistant enterococci. Vancomycin is also used orally for therapy of colitis due to Clostridium difficile, although it should not be used as the drug of first choice.

The empiric use of vancomycin has increased tremendously over the last several years. As a result, vancomycin-resistant enterococci (VRE) and coagulase-negative staphylococci have become problems, particularly in inpatient units, intensive care units, and oncology wards. S aureus with increased MICs to vancomycin has been reported in the United States and Japan. This resistance is of concern because of the inherent virulence of many S aureus strains. Vancomycin use should be monitored carefully in hospitals and their intensive care units. It should not be used empirically when an infection is mild or when other antimicrobial agents are likely to be effective. Vancomycin should be stopped promptly if infection is found to be due to organisms susceptible to other antimicrobials. Infection control guidelines for prevention of spread of VRE are published by the Centers for Disease Control and Prevention.

Rapid infusion of vancomycin is associated with the "red man syndrome," characterized by diffuse red flushing, at times pruritus, and occasionally tachycardia and hypotension. As a result, vancomycin is infused slowly over 1 hour or longer in some cases. Diphenhydramine or hydrocortisone (or both) may also be used as premedication.

Measurement of peak-and-trough serum vancomycin concentrations is not necessary in most clinical situations, because the levels achieved with standard dosing are usually predictable and nontoxic. Measurement of serum concentrations is helpful in patients with abnormal or unpredictable renal function; in those with altered volume of distribution, as occurs in nephrotic syndrome or shock; and in those receiving higher-dose therapy (eg, for meningitis or other difficult-to-treat infections). For patients receiving antimicrobials for weeks to months, weekly monitoring of clinical signs and symptoms and of urinalysis, creatinine, and complete blood count will allow detection of toxicity.

OXAZOLIDINONES

Linezolid is the first drug in this new class of antimicrobials which have a distinct new mechanism of action; they bind to the 50s-ribosomal RNA subunit and prevent initiation of protein synthesis. Because of this unique mechanism, there is no cross-resistance with other classes of antimicrobials. The in-vitro development of resistance has also been uncommon.

Linezolid is active against aerobic gram-positive organisms, including streptococci, staphylococci, enterococci, and pneumococci. Because linezolid is active against gram-positive organisms resistant to other antimicrobials (eg, MRSA, methicillin-resistant, coagulase-negative staphylococci, VRE, and penicillin-resistant S pneumoniae), it is useful for these difficult-to-treat infections.

Linezolid is safe and well tolerated in children. Gastrointestinal symptoms are the most commonly encountered side effect. Neutropenia and thrombocytopenia have been reported, and linezolid should therefore be used with monitoring in patients at increased risk for these problems or in patients receiving therapy for 2 weeks or longer. Linezolid is an inhibitor of monoamine oxidase (MAO) and should not be used in patients taking MAO inhibitors, or in patients taking phenylpropanolamine or pseudoephedrine.

Linezolid should be used only for infections due to a proven gram-positive pathogen that is known or strongly suspected to be resistant to other available agents.

QUINUPRISTIN-DALFOPRISTIN

Quinupristin and dalfopristin are two antimicrobials of the streptogramin class, which individually are bacteriostatic, but in combination are synergistic and bacteriocidal. These drugs are combined in a fixed ratio of 70:30, known as Synercid. Streptogramins inhibit protein synthesis by binding to the 50s ribosomal subunit. The streptogramins were discovered many years ago, but interest has increased only recently due to the activity of these agents against some very difficult-to-treat gram-positive infections.

The quinupristin–dalfopristin combination has activity against staphylococci, streptococci, pneumococci, and some enterococci. Quinupristin–dalfopristin is primarily indicated for serious infections due to vancomycin-resistant *Enterococcus faecium* and MRSA. Quinupristin–dalfopristin is not active against *E faecalis* and, therefore, differentiation of these strains from *E faecium* is important prior to initiating therapy.

Quinupristin–dalfopristin is not approved for therapy in children. Nonetheless, therapy has been initiated under a compassionate release program in some pediatric patients seriously ill with difficult-to-treat infections due to resistant organisms.

Arthralgias and myalgias have at times been severe in adult patients. Other significant side effects include elevated bilirubin and inflammation at intravenous sites.

Quinupristin–dalfopristin is a significant inhibitor of CYP-450 3A4 and, therefore, must be used with caution in patients receiving drugs metabolized by this mechanism (eg, clarithromycin, itraconazole, erythromycin, and many others).

The use of quinupristin–dalfopristin should be limited to serious infections due to proven *E faecium* or *S aureus* infections, or infections due to proven gram-positive cocci that are resistant to other agents.

CEPHALOSPORINS

Cephalosporin agents make up a large and often confusing group of antimicrobials. Many of these drugs are similar in antibacterial spectrum and side effects and may have similar names. Clinicians should learn well the properties of one or two drugs in each class. Cephalosporins are often grouped as "generations" to signify their similar antimicrobial activity. First-generation cephalosporins such as cefazolin intrave-

nously and cephalexin orally are useful mainly for susceptible *S aureus* infection and urinary tract infection due to susceptible *E coli*. Second-generation cephalosporins, such as cefuroxime intravenously and cefprozil and cefuroxime orally, have somewhat reduced, but acceptable, activity against gram-positive cocci, and greater activity against some gram-negative rods compared with first generation cephalosporins. They are active against *H influenzae* and *Moraxella catarrhalis,* including strains that produce β-lactamase capable of inactivating ampicillin. Third-generation cephalosporins have substantially less activity against gram-positive cocci, such as *S aureus,* but greatly augmented activity against aerobic gram-negative rods. Cefotaxime and ceftriaxone are examples of intravenous drugs, whereas cefpodoxime and ceftibuten are representative oral drugs. Cefepime is a new antimicrobial often described as fourth-generation because of its broad activity against gram-positive and gram-negative organisms, including *P aeruginosa.* Cefepime is stable to β-lactamase degradation and is a poor inducer of β-lactamase. Cefepime will be most useful for organisms resistant to other drugs. Cefepime is not approved for use in children younger than age 2 months.

No cephalosporin agent has substantial activity against *L monocytogenes,* enterococci, or MRSA. The only cephalosporins useful for treating anaerobic infections are cefoxitin and cefotetan, which are second-generation cephalosporins with excellent activity against *B fragilis.* Ceftazidime is a third-generation cephalosporin with appreciable activity against *P aeruginosa.*

Allergy to β-lactam antimicrobials is reported commonly by parents. Immediate hypersensitivity reactions, including anaphylaxis or hives, most commonly predict true allergy. In contrast, many delayed reactions and nonspecific rashes are likely due to the underlying infection or nonallergic reactions. (See Chapter 36.) Cephalosporins should be used with caution in children with immediate hypersensitivity reactions to penicillins or cephalosporins.

Resistance to cephalosporins is common among aerobic gram-negative rods. The presence of inducible cephalosporinases in some gram-negative rod organisms, such as *P aeruginosa, Serratia marcescens, Citrobacter,* and *Enterobacter,* has led to clinical failures because of the emergence of resistance during therapy. Extended-spectrum β-lactamases mediate broad resistance to all penicillins, aminopenicillins, cephalosporins, and monobactams. Carbapenems, fluoroquinolones, or combinations including these drugs are used for serious infections due to gram-negative organisms with these enzymes. Active laboratory-based surveillance is necessary to detect resistance in these gram-negative organisms.

AZTREONAM

Aztreonam is the only monobactam antimicrobial agent approved in the United States. Although it is not approved for use in children younger than age 9 months, there is considerable pediatric experience with its use, including in neonates and premature infants. Aztreonam is active against aerobic gram-negative rods, including *P aeruginosa*. Aztreonam has activity against *H influenzae* and *M catarrhalis*, including those that are β-lactamase producers. Most patients with allergy to penicillin or cephalosporins are not sensitized to aztreonam, except that children with prior reactions to ceftazidime may have reactions to aztreonam because aztreonam and ceftazidime have a common side chain.

CARBAPENEMS

Meropenem, ertapenem, and imipenem are broad-spectrum β-lactam antimicrobials. Imipenem–cilastatin is a combination of an active antibiotic and cilastatin, which inhibits the metabolism of imipenem in the kidney and thereby results in high serum and urine levels of imipenem. These carbapenems are also active against *S pneumoniae*, including many penicillin-resistant and cephalosporin-resistant strains. Carbapenems have been used successfully to treat meningitis and may be considered if vancomycin is not tolerated. An increased frequency of seizures is encountered when central nervous system infections are treated with carbapenems. These agents are broadly active against streptococci, MRSA, some enterococci, and gram-negative rods such as *P aeruginosa*, β-lactamase–producing *H influenzae*, and gram-negative anaerobes. Ertapenem has less activity against *P aeruginosa*, *Acinetobacter* species, and *Enterococcus* species than meropenem and imipenem. Because carbapenems are active against so many species of bacteria, there is a strong temptation to use them as single-drug empiric therapy. Units that have used carbapenems heavily have encountered resistance in many different species of gram-negative rods.

MACROLIDES & AZILIDES

Erythromycin was once the most commonly used macrolide antimicrobial agent but now azithromycin and clarithromycin are often preferred because of decreased side effects. It is active against many bacteria that are resistant to cell wall–active antimicrobials and is the drug of choice for *Bordetella pertussis, Legionella pneumophila, C pneumoniae, M pneumoniae,* and *Chlamydia trachomatis* infections (in children in whom tetracycline is not an option). Erythromycin is used for outpatient therapy of streptococcal and staphylococcal infections in patients with penicillin allergy. More serious infections due to streptococci and staphylococci are usually treated with penicillins, clindamycin, PRPs, or cephalosporins because of a significant incidence of erythromycin resistance in both species. *S pneumoniae* resistant to erythromycin and the related macrolides are now frequent in many communities. This limits the ability of macrolide antimicrobials for therapy of otitis media and sinusitis. Gastrointestinal side effects are common. Interactions with theophylline, carbamazepine, terfenadine, cycloserine, and other drugs may require dosage modifications of erythromycin and clarithromycin. Significant interactions with azithromycin are less common. Erythromycin exposure is associated with

pyloric stenosis in newborns, so azithromycin is preferred in most neonates.

Erythromycin is available in many formulations, including the base, estolate, ethyl succinate, and stearate. Transient hepatic toxicity occurs in adults, but is much less common in children. Erythromycin base and stearate should be taken with meals for best absorption.

Clarithromycin and azithromycin, macrolide and azalide antimicrobials, respectively, are much less likely than erythromycin to cause nausea, vomiting, and diarrhea. These agents are useful in children who cannot tolerate erythromycin. Clarithromycin is more active than erythromycin against *H influenzae, M catarrhalis,* and *Neisseria gonorrhoeae* and is the drug of choice, usually in combination, for some nontuberculous mycobacterial infections. Azithromycin has a prolonged tissue half-life that achieves a prolonged antimicrobial effect. Azithromycin is dosed once daily for 5 days, but must be taken 1 hour before or 2 hours after meals because food interferes with absorption. Although azithromycin is active against *H influenzae*, some authors report poor eradication of *H influenzae* from the middle ear. Azithromycin can be used for single-dose therapy of *C trachomatis* infections. It is beneficial in adolescents when compliance with erythromycin or tetracycline is a concern. Azithromycin is useful for therapy of *Shigella* and *Salmonella* infections, including typhoid fever resistant to ampicillin and TMP–SMX. Alternatives include third-generation cephalosporins and fluoroquinolones. Clarithromycin is effective against Lyme disease, but 7 days of azithromycin for that indication was inferior to amoxicillin. Clarithromycin and azithromycin are alternative drugs for toxoplasmosis in sulfonamide-allergic patients and as alternatives to erythromycin in legionellosis. In-vitro and limited clinical experience in providing treatment to contacts of pertussis patients suggests efficacy equal to that of erythromycin. Clarithromycin and azithromycin are considerably more expensive than most erythromycin formulations, which for that reason are usually preferred, but they are advantageous by virtue of their twice-daily and once-daily dosing, respectively. Some failures of the newer macrolides have occurred in *S pneumoniae* sepsis and meningitis, perhaps because of low serum levels despite the high tissue levels achieved. High rates of resistance to macrolides and azalides have been encountered in some communities. The frequent use of azithromycin for respiratory infections and acute otitis media has contributed to selection of resistant strains.

CLINDAMYCIN

Clindamycin is active against *S aureus,* some MRSA, *S pyogenes,* other streptococcal species except enterococci, and both gram-positive and gram-negative anaerobes. Clindamycin or metronidazole is frequently combined with other antimicrobials for empiric therapy of suspected anaerobic or mixed anaerobic and aerobic infections. Empiric use of clindamycin is justified in suspected anaerobic infections because cultures frequently cannot be obtained and, if obtained, may be slow in confirming anaerobic infection. Examples are pelvic inflammatory disease, necrotizing enterocolitis, other infections in which the integrity of the gastrointestinal or genitourinary tracts is compromised, and sinusitis. Clindamycin does not achieve high levels in CSF, but brain abscesses, toxoplasmosis, and other central nervous system infections, where disruption of the blood-brain barrier occurs, may be successfully treated with clindamycin. Clindamycin should be added to regimens for treatment of serious streptococcal and staphylococcal infections, such as necrotizing fasciitis and toxic shock syndrome. Both in-vitro and clinical data suggest increased bactericidal killing and improved outcomes occur with clindamycin. For most oral anaerobes (eg, in a dental abscess), penicillin is more active than clindamycin. Clindamycin has been associated with the occurrence of *C difficile*–related pseudomembranous colitis. Although diarrhea is a frequent side effect, pseudomembranous colitis is uncommonly due to clindamycin in children.

SULFONAMIDES

Sulfonamides—the oldest class of antimicrobials—remain useful for treatment of urinary tract infections. They are used also for other infections due to *E coli* and for *Nocardia*. Although useful for rheumatic fever prophylaxis in penicillin-allergic patients, sulfonamides fail to eradicate group A streptococci and cannot be used for treatment of acute infections.

TMP–SMX is a fixed combination that is more active than either drug alone. Gram-positive cocci, including some *S pneumoniae*, many staphylococci, *Haemophilus*, and many gram-negative rods, are susceptible. Unfortunately, resistance to TMP–SMX has become more common. *S pneumoniae* resistant to penicillin and cephalosporins is often also resistant to TMP–SMX and erythromycin. In some communities, *Shigella* and *Salmonella enteritidis* strains remain susceptible, as do most *E coli*. TMP–SMX is therefore very useful for treatment of urinary tract infections and bacterial dysentery. TMP–SMX is also the drug of choice for treatment or prophylaxis against *Pneumocystis jiroveci* infection. Dermatologic and myelosuppressive side effects limit the use of TMP–SMX in some children infected with HIV.

Sulfonamide is associated with several cutaneous reactions, including urticaria, photosensitivity, Stevens-Johnson syndrome, purpura, and maculopapular rashes. Hematologic side effects such as leukopenia, thrombocytopenia, and hemolytic anemia are uncommon. Common gastrointestinal side effects are nausea and vomiting. The dermatologic and hematologic side effects are thought to be more common and more severe with TMP–SMX than with sulfonamide alone.

TETRACYCLINES

Tetracyclines, which are effective against a broad range of bacteria, are not commonly used in children because alternative effective drugs are available. Many different tetracycline formulations are available. Tetracyclines are effective against *B pertussis* and *E coli* and many species of *Rickettsia*, *Chlamydia*, and *Mycoplasma*. Doxycycline or minocycline is the drug of choice for eradication of *C trachomatis* in pelvic inflammatory disease and nongonococcal urethritis.

Staining of permanent teeth was noted in young children given repeated courses of tetracyclines. As a result, tetracyclines are generally not given to children younger than age 9 years unless alternative drugs are unavailable. A single course of tetracycline does not pose a significant risk of tooth staining. Mucous membrane candidiasis, photosensitivity, nausea, and vomiting are other common side effects. Tetracycline should be taken on an empty stomach, either 1 hour before or 2 hours after a meal. Doxycycline is well absorbed even in the presence of food; administration with food may minimize gastrointestinal side effects. Doxycycline is often preferred because it is better tolerated than tetracycline, and twice-daily administration is convenient.

Tetracycline is used for therapy of rickettsial infections such as Rocky Mountain spotted fever, ehrlichiosis, rickettsialpox, murine typhus, and Q fever; as an alternative to erythromycin for *M pneumoniae* and *C pneumoniae* infections; and for treatment of psittacosis, brucellosis, *P multocida* infection, and relapsing fever.

Tigecycline is a new polyketide antimicrobial that is an analogue of tetracycline and a bacteriostatic inhibitor of protein synthesis. Tigecycline is active against gram-negative aerobes, anaerobes, and many gram-positive cocci including MRSA. It is approved for intravenous therapy of adults with complicated SSTIs and complicated intra-abdominal infections.

AMINOGLYCOSIDES

The aminoglycosides bind to ribosomal subunits and inhibit protein synthesis. They are active against aerobic gram-negative rods, including *P aeruginosa*. Streptomycin was the first drug in this class, but today it is used only to treat tuberculosis and the occasional cases of plague and tularemia.

Aminoglycosides are used to treat serious gram-negative infections and are given intravenously or intramuscularly. They are also used to treat pyelonephritis, suspected gram-negative sepsis, and in other settings where *P aeruginosa* infections are common, such as cystic fibrosis and burns. Aminoglycosides have activity against gram-positive organisms and, combined with penicillin or ampicillin, may achieve synergistic killing of *L monocytogenes* and group B streptococci. Penicillin, ampicillin, or vancomycin combined with gentamicin is indicated for therapy of serious enterococcal infections, such as sepsis or endocarditis because of more rapid clinical improvement with combined therapy. Aminoglycosides have activity against *S aureus* but are always used in combination with other antistaphylococcal antibiotics.

Aminoglycosides are not active in an acidic environment and may not be effective against abscesses. Aminoglycosides diffuse poorly into the CSF and achieve only about 10% of serum concentrations. As a result, a third-generation cephalosporin is preferred for treatment of bacillary meningitis.

Aminoglycosides kill bacteria in a concentration-dependent manner. They also have a prolonged suppressive effect on the regrowth of susceptible organisms (postantibiotic effect). These principles have led some investigators to establish guidelines for once-daily dosing of aminoglycosides, using larger initial doses given every 24 hours. Although aminoglycosides are associated with both renal and eighth nerve toxicity, the entry of the drug into renal and cochlear cells is saturable. It therefore was predicted that once-daily dosing would result in less toxicity than traditional twice-daily or three-times-daily dosing. Studies in adult patients confirm that once-daily dosing is as efficacious as traditional dosing and is associated with less toxicity. Although there is extensive experience with dosing intervals of 18–36 hours in premature infants, small total daily doses are customarily used (2.0–2.5 mg/kg per dose of gentamicin or tobramycin). A convenient and cost-effective approach in children is based on the experience with adult patients and uses larger daily doses (4–7 mg/kg per dose every 24 hours). Nevertheless, traditional twice-daily or three-times-daily dosing regimens of aminoglycosides, with monitoring of serum levels, are still widely used. Careful monitoring is necessary, particularly in children with abnormal or changing renal function, premature infants, and infants with rapidly changing volumes of distribution. Aminoglycosides are usually infused over 30–45 minutes, and the peak serum concentration is measured 30–45 minutes after the end of the infusion. A trough serum concentration is measured prior to the next dose. The efficacious and nontoxic serum concentrations for gentamicin and tobramycin are trough less than 2 mcg/mL and peak 5–10 mcg/mL; for amikacin, trough less than 10 mcg/mL and peak 15–25 mcg/mL (see Table 37–4). Aminoglycoside levels and creatinine levels should be measured in children expected to receive more than 3 days of therapy, and repeated weekly in children on long-term therapy, even when renal function is normal and stable.

FLUOROQUINOLONES

Modification of the quinolone structure of nalidixic acid has led to many new compounds called fluoroquinolones, which are well absorbed after oral administration and possess excellent antibacterial activity against resistant gram-negative pathogens. The seven currently available fluoroquinolones vary in their activity against specific organisms. Fluoroquinolones are active against most of the Enterobacteriaceae, including *E coli, Enterobacter, Klebsiella*, in some cases *P aeruginosa*, and many other gram-negative bacteria such as *H influenzae, M catarrhalis, N gonorrhoeae*, and *N meningitidis*. Some fluoroquinolones (ofloxacin and levofloxacin) are active against *C trachomatis* and *Mycoplasma*. The fluoroquinolones are active against some enterococci, *S aureus*, MRSA, and coagulase-negative staphylococci. The newer quinolones have good activity against penicillin and cephalosporin-resistant *S pneumoniae*, but clinical experience in children is limited.

Ciprofloxacin and its otic and ophthalmic preparations are the only fluoroquinolone antimicrobials currently FDA-approved for use in children older than 1 year, although fluoroquinolones offer very attractive alternatives to approved agents. The objection to quinolones is based on the recognition that nalidixic acid and other quinolones cause arthropathy when tested experimentally in newborn animals of many species. The fear that children would also be more susceptible than adults to cartilage injury has not been realized in clinical experience. Both retrospective long-term follow-up studies of children given nalidixic acid and prospective studies of children receiving treatment under protocols with fluoroquinolones have shown similar rates of toxicity compared with adult patients. Arthropathy occurs uncommonly, although tendon rupture is a reported rare, serious complication. For these reasons, quinolones should be considered for use in children when the benefit clearly outweighs the risk, when no alternative drug is available, and after discussion with the parents.

Ciprofloxacin is useful for oral therapy of resistant gram-negative urinary tract infections, such as those caused by *P aeruginosa*. Ofloxacin, levofloxacin, ciprofloxacin, and gatifloxacin are useful for single-dose therapy of uncomplicated gonorrhea, and ofloxacin and levofloxacin are an alternative therapy for treating *Chlamydia* infections and pelvic inflammatory disease. Ciprofloxacin and ofloxacin are used as therapy of resistant cases of shigellosis. Levofloxacin and ciprofloxacin are usually the drugs of choice for treatment of traveler's diarrhea. Ciprofloxacin is useful for treatment of *P aeruginosa* infection in patients with cystic fibrosis, and as therapy for chronic suppurative otitis media. Several quinolones are used as therapy for pneumonia due to *Legionella, Mycoplasma*, or *Chlamydia pneumoniae*, although a macrolide is often preferred, and as prophylactic therapy of meningococcal infection. Ofloxacin and levofloxacin are used for treatment of some cases of *Mycobacterium tuberculosis* and some atypical mycobacterial infections.

METRONIDAZOLE

Metronidazole has excellent activity against most anaerobes, particularly gram-negative anaerobes, such as *Bacteroides* and *Fusobacterium*, and against gram-positive anaerobes such as *Clostridium, Prevotella*, and *Porphyromonas*. Gram-positive anaerobic cocci such as *Peptococcus* and *Peptostreptococcus* are often more susceptible to penicillin or to clindamycin. Because metronidazole lacks activity against aerobic organisms, it is usually given with one or more other antibiotics. Metronidazole is well absorbed after oral administration and has excellent penetration into the central nervous system. Metronidazole is the drug of choice for bacterial vaginosis and for *C difficile* enterocolitis. It is active against many parasites, including *Giardia lamblia* and *Entamoeba histolytica*.

DAPTOMYCIN

Daptomycin has broad bactericidal activity against gram-positive cocci. Daptomycin is a lipopeptide that binds to bacterial cell membranes, resulting in membrane depolarization and cell death. Daptomycin is active against methicillin-sensitive and -resistant *S aureus, S pyogenes,* and *Streptococcus agalactiae,* as well as *E faecium* (including vancomycin-resistant strains), and *E faecalis* (vancomycin-sensitive strains). Daptomycin is given as a once-daily intravenous infusion of 4 mg/kg and is approved for therapy of complicated SSTIs, but has not been sufficiently studied in children younger than 18 years to make recommendations for dosing and use. Daptomycin therapy of pneumonia was unsuccessful in a large percentage of cases, and should not be used. Daptomycin is excreted renally, so a modification of dosing is needed in patients with impaired renal function. Nausea, constipation, and headache are the most common side effects of therapy. In patients with muscle pain, monitoring creatinine phosphokinase levels should be done.

REFERENCES

Bradley JS, Nelson JB: *Nelson's Pocketbook of Pediatric Antimicrobial Therapy,* 16th ed. Lippincott Williams & Wilkins, 2006–2007.

Conway et al: Recurrent urinary tract infections: Risk factors and association with prophylactic antimicrobials. JAMA 2007;298:179 [PMID: 17622599].

Fortunav et al: Evaluation and treatment of community-acquired *Staphylococcus aureus* infections in term and late-preterm, previously healthy neonates. Pediatrics 2007;120:937 [PMID: 17974729].

Gilbert DN et al: *The Sanford Guide to Antimicrobial Therapy,* 35th ed. Antimicrobial Therapy, Inc., 2007.

Web Resources

Alliance for the Prudent Use of Antibiotics: http://www.tufts.edu/med/apua

CDC Antibiotic and Antimicrobial Resistance page: http://www.cdc.gov/drugresistance

National Center for Preparedness, Detection, and Control of Infectious Diseases: http://www.cdc.gov/ncpdcid/

Infections: Viral & Rickettsial

Myron J. Levin, MD

Adriana Weinberg, MD

▼ VIRAL INFECTIONS

Viruses cause most pediatric infections. Mixed viral or viral-bacterial infections of the respiratory and intestinal tracts are rather common, as is prolonged asymptomatic shedding of some viruses in childhood. Thus the detection of a virus is not always proof that it is the cause of a given illness. Viruses are often a predisposing factor for bacterial respiratory infections (eg, otitis, sinusitis, and pneumonia).

Many respiratory and herpes viruses can now be detected within 24–48 hours by combining culture and monoclonal antibody techniques ("rapid culture technique"). Diagnosis of many viral illnesses is also possible through antigen or nucleic acid detection techniques. These techniques are more rapid than isolation of viruses in tissue culture and in most cases are equally sensitive or more so. Polymerase chain reaction (PCR) amplification of viral genes has led to recognition of previously undetected infections. New diagnostic tests have changed some basic concepts about viral diseases and made diagnosis of viral infections both more certain and more complex. Only laboratories with excellent quality-control procedures should be used, and the results of new tests must be interpreted cautiously. The availability of specific antiviral agents increases the value of early diagnosis for some serious viral infections. Table 38–1 lists viral agents associated with common clinical signs, and Table 38–2 lists diagnostic tests. The viral diagnostic laboratory should be contacted for details regarding specimen collection, handling, and shipping. Table 38–3 lists common causes of red rashes in children that should be considered in the differential diagnosis of certain viral illnesses.

RESPIRATORY INFECTIONS

Many viral infections cause upper or lower respiratory tract signs and symptoms. Those that produce a predominance of these signs and symptoms are described in the text that follows. Many so-called respiratory viruses can also produce distinct nonrespiratory disease (eg, enteritis or cystitis caused by adenoviruses; parotitis caused by parainfluenza viruses). Respiratory viruses can cause disease in any area of the respiratory tree. Thus they can cause coryza, pharyngitis, sinusitis, tracheitis, bronchitis, bronchiolitis, and pneumonia—although certain viruses tend to be closely associated with one anatomic area (eg, parainfluenza with croup, respiratory syncytial virus [RSV] with bronchiolitis) or discrete epidemics (eg, influenza, RSV, parainfluenza). Nevertheless it is impossible on clinical grounds to be certain of the viral cause of an infection in a given child. This information is provided by the virology laboratory and is often important for epidemiologic, therapeutic, and preventive reasons. In immunocompromised patients these annoying, but otherwise benign, viruses can cause severe pneumonia.

VIRUSES CAUSING THE COMMON COLD

The common cold syndrome (also called upper respiratory infection) is characterized by combinations of runny nose, nasal congestion, sore throat, tearing, cough, and sneezing. Low-grade fever may be present. The causal agent is usually not sought or determined. Epidemiologic studies indicate that rhinoviruses, which are the most common cause (30–40%), are present throughout the year but are more prevalent in the colder months in temperate climates. Adenoviruses also cause colds in all seasons, but epidemics are common. Respiratory syncytial, parainfluenza, and influenza viruses cause the cold syndrome during epidemics from late fall through winter. Coronaviruses, including the recently identified strains NL63 and HKU1, account for 5–10% of colds in winter. Equally prevalent are other newly identified respiratory viruses such as the human bocavirus, a parvovirus, and the KI polyomavirus. Enteroviruses cause the "summer cold." One outcome of these infections is morbidity continuing for 5–7 days. It is likely also that changes in respiratory epithelium, local obstruction, and altered local immunity are sometimes the precursors of more severe illnesses such as otitis

Table 38–1. Some viral causes of clinical syndromes.

Rash	**Adenopathy**	**Arthritis (Arthralgia)**
Enterovirus	Epstein-Barr virus	Parvovirus B19
Adenovirus	Cytomegalovirus	Rubella
Measles	Rubella[e]	Hepatitis B
Rubella	HIV	Dengue
Human herpes virus type 6[a] or 7[a]	**Croup**	**Congenital or perinatal infection**
Varicella	Parainfluenza	Adenovirus
Parvovirus B19[b]	Influenza	Cytomegalovirus
Epstein-Barr virus	Adenovirus	Hepatitis B
Dengue	Other respiratory viruses	Hepatitis C[l]
Human immunodeficiency virus (HIV), acute syndrome	**Bronchiolitis**	Rubella
	Respiratory syncytial virus[f]	HIV
Fever	Adenovirus	Parvovirus B19
Enterovirus	Parainfluenza	Enterovirus
Epstein-Barr virus	Influenza	Varicella
Human herpes virus type 6[a] or 7	Human metapneumovirus	Herpes simplex virus
Cytomegalovirus	**Pneumonia**	**Meningoencephalitis**
Influenza	Respiratory syncytial virus	Enterovirus
Rhinovirus	Adenovirus	Mumps
Most others	Parainfluenza	Other Arthropod-borne viruses
Conjunctivitis	Hantavirus	Herpes simplex virus
Adenovirus	Measles	Cytomegalovirus
Enterovirus 70	Varicella[g]	Lymphocytic choriomeningitis virus
Measles	Cytomegalovirus[h,i]	Measles
Herpes simplex virus[c]	Influenza	Varicella
Parotitis	**Enteritis**	Adenovirus
Mumps	Rotavirus	HIV
Parainfluenza	Enteric adenovirus	Epstein-Barr virus
Enterovirus	Enterovirus	Influenza
Cytomegalovirus	Astrovirus	West Nile virus
Epstein-Barr virus	Calicivirus	
HIV	Novovirus	
Pharyngitis	Cytomegalovirus	
Adenovirus	**Hepatitis**	
Enterovirus	Hepatitis A,[j] B, C, D, E	
Epstein-Barr virus	Epstein-Barr virus	
Herpes simplex virus[d]	Adenovirus	
Influenza	Cytomegalovirus	
Other respiratory viruses	Varicella[k]	
	Parvovirus B19	

[a]Roseola agent.
[b]Erythema infectiosum agent.
[c]Conjunctivitis rare, only in primary infections; keratitis in older patients.
[d]May cause isolated pharyngeal vesicles at any age.
[e]May cause adenopathy without rash; especially post-auricular.
[f]Over 70% of cases.
[g]Immunosuppressed, pregnant, rarely other adults.
[h]Usually only in young infants.
[i]Severely immunosuppressed at risk.
[j]Anicteric cases more common in children; these may resemble viral gastroenteritis.
[k]Common, but only mild laboratory abnormalities.
[l]Especially when the mother is HIV-positive.

Table 38–2. Diagnostic tests for viral infections.

Agent	Rapid Antigen Detection (Specimen)	Tissue Culture Mean Days to Positive (Range)	Acute	Paired	PCR[a]	Comments
Adenovirus	+ (respiratory and enteric)	10 (1–21)	–	+	+	"Enteric" strains detected by culture on special cell line, antigen detection, or PCR
Arboviruses	–	–	+	+	+	Acute serum may diagnose many forms
Astrovirus	–	–	–	–	+	Diagnosis by electron microscopy
Calicivirus	–	–	–	–	+	Diagnosis by electron microscopy
Colorado tick virus	On RBC	–	–	RL, CDC	+	
Coronavirus	–	RL	–	+	+	
Cytomegalovirus	+ (tissue biopsy, urine, blood, respiratory secretions)	2 (2–28)	+	+	+	Diagnosis by presence of IgM antibody
Enterovirus	–	2 (2–14)	–	+	+	
Epstein-Barr virus	–	–	+	+	+	Single serologic panel defines infection status; heterophil antibodies less sensitive
Hantavirus	–	–	+	ND	RL	Diagnosis by presence of IgM antibody
Hepatitis A virus	–	–	+	ND	RL	Diagnosis by presence of IgM antibody
Hepatitis B virus	+ (blood)	–	+	ND	+	Diagnosis by presence of surface antigen or anti-core IgM antibody
Hepatitis C virus	–	–	+	ND	+	Positive serology suggests that hepatitis C may be the causative agent. PCR is confirmatory.
Herpes simplex virus	+ (mucosa, tissue biopsy, respiratory secretions, skin)	1 (1–7)	+	+	+	Serology rarely used for herpes simplex. IgM antibody used in selected cases.
Human herpesvirus-6 and 7	–	2	+	+	+	Roseola agent
Human immunodeficiency virus	+ (blood) (acid dissociation of immune complexes)	15 (5–28)	+	ND	+	Antibody proves infection unless passively acquired (< age 15 mo); culture not widely available; PCR definitive for early diagnosis in infant
Human metapneumovirus	+	2	–	+	+	
Influenza virus	+ (respiratory secretions)	2 (2–14)	–	+	+	Antigen detection 70–90% sensitive
Lymphocytic choriomeningitis virus	–	–	–	+	RL	Can be isolated in suckling mice
Measles virus	+ (respiratory secretions)	–	+	+	+	Difficult to grow; IgM serology diagnostic
Mumps virus	–	> 5	+	+	+	IgM ELISA antibody may allow single-specimen diagnosis
Parvovirus B19	–	–	+	ND	+	Erythema infectiosum agent
Parainfluenza virus	+ (respiratory secretions)	2 (2–14)	–	+	+	
Rabies virus	+ (skin, conjunctiva, suspected animal source tissue biopsy)	–	+	+	CDC	Usually diagnosed by antigen detection
Respiratory syncytial virus	+ (respiratory secretions)	2 (2–21)	–	+	+	Rapid antigen detection; 90% sensitive

(continued)

Table 38–2. Diagnostic tests for viral infections. *(Continued)*

Agent	Rapid Antigen Detection (Specimen)	Tissue Culture Mean Days to Positive (Range)	Serology			Comments
			Acute	Paired	PCR[a]	
Rhinovirus	–	4 (2–7)	–	–	+	Too many strains to type serologically
Rotavirus	+ (feces)	–	–	–	+	Electron microscopy useful for many enteric viruses
Rubella virus	–	> 10	+	+	+	Recommended that paired sera be tested simultaneously
Varicella-zoster virus	+ (skin scraping)	3 (3–21) RL	+	+	+	
West Nile virus	–	RL	+	+	+	

[a]Useful only when performed on selected specimens by qualified laboratories.

Key:

Plus signs signify commercially or widely available; **minus signs** signify not commercially available. ***Note:*** Results from some commercial laboratories are unreliable.
RL, CDC: Specific antibody titers or PCR available by arrangement with individual research laboratories or the Centers for Disease Control and Prevention.
ND: Not done.
ELISA, enzyme-linked immunosorbent assay; PCR, polymerase chain reaction; RBC, red blood cell.

media, pneumonia, and sinusitis. During and following a cold the bacterial flora change, and bacteria are found in normally sterile areas of the upper airway. Asthma attacks are frequently provoked by viruses that cause the common cold. There is no evidence that antibiotics will prevent these complications, and the unjustified widespread use of antibiotics for cold symptoms has contributed to the emergence of antibiotic-resistant respiratory flora.

In 5–10% of children, symptoms from these virus infections persist for more than 10 days. This overlap with the symptoms of bacterial sinusitis presents a difficult problem for clinicians, especially because colds can produce an abnormal computed tomography (CT) scan of the sinuses. Viruses that cause a minor illness in immunocompetent children, such as rhinoviruses, can cause severe lower respiratory disease in immunologically or anatomically compromised children.

There is no evidence that symptomatic relief for children can be achieved with oral antihistamines, decongestants, or cough suppressants. Topical decongestants provide temporary improvement in nasal symptoms. Zinc and vitamin C have not been shown to have a significant preventative or therapeutic role.

Allander T et al: Human bocavirus and acute wheezing in children. Clin Infect Dis 2007;44:904 [PMID: 17342639].

Bialasiewicz S et al: A newly reported human polyomavirus, KI virus, is present in the respiratory tract of Australian children. J Clin Virol 2007;40:15 [PMID: 17706457].

Greenberg SB: Rhinovirus and coronavirus infections. Semin Respir Crit Care Med 2007;28:182 [PMID: 17458772].

Lau SK et al: Coronavirus HKU1 and other coronavirus infections in Hong Kong. J Clin Microbiol 2006;44:2063 [PMID: 16757599].

Sutter AI et al: Antihistamines for the common cold. Cochrane Database Syst Rev 2003;(3)CD001267 [PMID: 12917904].

Taverner D et al: Nasal decongestants for the common cold. Cochrane Database Syst Rev 2007;(1)CD001953 [PMID: 17253470].

Winther B et al: Temporal relationships between colds, upper respiratory viruses detected by polymerase chain reaction, and otitis media in young children followed through a typical cold season. Pediatrics 2007;119:1069 [PMID: 17545372].

INFECTIONS DUE TO ADENOVIRUSES

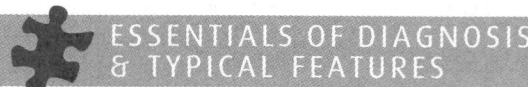

ESSENTIALS OF DIAGNOSIS & TYPICAL FEATURES

▶ Multiple syndromes, depending on the type of adenovirus.

▶ Upper respiratory infections; most notable is severe pharyngitis with tonsillitis and cervical adenopathy.

▶ Conjunctivitis.

▶ Pneumonia.

▶ Enteric adenoviruses cause mild diarrheal illnesses.

▶ Definitive diagnosis by antigen detection, PCR, or culture.

There are over 50 types of adenoviruses, which account for 5–10% of all respiratory illnesses in childhood, usually pharyngitis or tracheitis. Adenoviral infections are common early in life. Enteric adenoviruses are an important cause of childhood diarrhea. Epidemic respiratory disease occurs in winter and spring, especially in closed environments such as day care centers and institutions. Because of latent infection in lymphoid tissue, asymptomatic shedding from the respiratory or intestinal tract is common.

Table 38-3. Red rashes in children.

Condition	Incubation Period (days)	Prodrome	Rash	Laboratory Tests	Comments, Other Diagnostic Features
Adenovirus	4–5	URI; cough; fever	Morbilliform (may be petechial)	Normal; may see leukopenia or lymphocytosis	Upper or lower respiratory symptoms are prominent. No Koplik spots. No desquamation.
Drug allergy	—	None, or fever alone, or with myalgia, pruritus	Macular, maculopapular, urticarial, or erythroderma	Leukopenia, eosinophilia	Rash variable. Severe reactions may resemble measles, scarlet fever; Kawasaki disease; marked toxicity possible.
Enterovirus	2–7	Variable fever, chills, myalgia, sore throat	Usually macular, maculopapular on trunk or palms, soles; vesicles or petechiae also seen	Variable	Varied rashes may resemble those of many other infections. Pharyngeal or hand-foot-mouth vesicles may occur.
Ehrlichiosis (monocytic)	5–21	Fever; headache; flulike; myalgia; GI symptoms	Variable; maculopapular, petechial, scarlatiniform, vasculitic	Leukopenia, thrombocytopenia, abnormal liver function. Serology for diagnosis; morulae in monocytes.	Geographic distribution is a clue; seasonal; tick exposure; rash present in only 45%.
Erythema multiforme	—	Usually none or related to underlying cause	Discrete, red maculopapular lesions; symmetrical, distal, palms and soles; target lesions classic	Normal or eosinophilia	Reaction to drugs (especially sulfonamides), or infectious agents (mycoplasma; herpes simplex virus). Urticaria, arthralgia also seen.
Kawasaki disease	Unknown	Fever, cervical adenopathy, irritability	Polymorphous (may be erythroderma) on trunk and extremities; red palms and soles, conjunctiva, lips, tongue, pharynx. Desquamation is common.	Leukocytosis, thrombocytosis, elevated ESR or C-reactive protein; pyuria; decreased albumin; negative cultures and streptococcal serology; resting tachycardia	Swollen hands, feet; prolonged illness; uveitis; aseptic meningitis; no response to antibiotics. Vasculitis and aneurysms of coronary and other arteries occur (cardiac ultrasound).
Leptospirosis	4–19	Fever (biphasic), myalgia, chills	Variable erythroderma	Leukocytosis; hematuria, proteinuria; hyperbilirubinemia	Conjunctivitis; hepatitis, aseptic meningitis may be seen. Rodent, dog contact.
Measles	9–14	Cough, rhinitis, conjunctivitis	Maculopapular; face to trunk; lasts 7–10 d; Koplik spots in mouth	Leukopenia	Toxic. Bright red rash becomes confluent, may desquamate. Fever falls after rash appears. Inadequate measles vaccination.
Parvovirus (erythema infectiosum)	10–17 (rash)	Mild (flulike)	Maculopapular on cheeks ("slapped cheek"), forehead, chin; then down limbs, trunk, buttocks; may fade and reappear for several weeks	IgM-EIA; PCR	Purpuric stocking-glove rash is rare, but distinctive; aplastic crisis in patients with chronic hemolytic anemia. May cause arthritis or arthralgia.
Rocky Mountain spotted fever	3–12	Headache (retro-orbital); toxic; GI symptoms; high fever; flulike	Onset 2–6 d after fever; palpable maculopapular on palms, soles, extremities, with spread centrally; petechial	Leukopenia; thrombocytopenia; abnormal liver function; CSF pleocytosis; Serology positive at 7–10 d of rash; biopsy will give earlier diagnosis	Eastern seaboard and southeastern United States; April–September; tick exposure.

(continued)

Table 38-3. Red rashes in children. (*Continued*)

Condition	Incubation Period (days)	Prodrome	Rash	Laboratory Tests	Comments, Other Diagnostic Features
Roseola (exanthem subitum) (HHV-6)	10–14	Fever (3–4 d)	Pink, macular rash occurs at end of febrile period; transient	Normal	Fever often high; disappears when rash develops; child appears well. Usually occurs in children 6 mo–3 y of age. Seizures may complicate.
Rubella	14–21	Usually none	Mild maculopapular; rapid spread face to extremities; gone by day 4	Normal or leukopenia	Postauricular, occipital adenopathy common. Polyarthralgia in some older girls. Mild clinical illness. Inadequate rubella vaccination.
Staphylococcal scalded skin	Variable	Irritability, absent to low fever	Painful erythroderma, followed in 1–2 d by cracking around eyes, mouth; bullae form with friction (Nikolsky sign)	Normal if only colonized by staphylococci; leukocytosis and sometimes bacteremia if infected	Normal pharynx. Look for focal staphylococcal infection. Usually occurs in infants.
Staphylococcal scarlet fever	1–7	Variable fever	Diffuse erythroderma; resembles streptococcal scarlet fever except eyes may be hyperemic, no "strawberry" tongue, pharynx spared	Leukocytosis is common because of infected focus	Focal infection usually present.
Stevens-Johnson syndrome	—	Pharyngitis, conjunctivitis, fever, malaise	Bullous erythema multiforme; may slough in large areas; hemorrhagic lips; purulent conjunctivitis	Leukocytosis	Classic precipitants are drugs (especially sulfonamides), *Mycoplasma pneumoniae* and herpes simplex infections. Pneumonitis and urethritis also seen.
Streptococcal scarlet fever	1–7	Fever, abdominal pain, headache, sore throat	Diffuse erythema, "sandpaper" texture; neck, axillae, inguinal areas; spreads to rest of body; desquamates 7–14 d	Leukocytosis; positive group A *Streptococcus* culture of throat or wound; positive streptococcal antigen test in pharynx	Strawberry tongue, red pharynx with or without exudate. Eyes, perioral and periorbital area, palms, and soles spared. Pastia lines. Cervical adenopathy. Usually occurs in children 2–10 y of age.
Toxic shock syndrome	Variable	Fever, myalgia, headache, diarrhea, vomiting	Nontender erythroderma; red eyes, palms, soles, pharynx, lips	Leukocytosis; abnormal liver enzymes and coagulation tests; proteinuria	*Staphylococcus aureus* infection; toxin-mediated multiorgan involvement. Swollen hands, feet. Hypotension or shock.

CSF, cerebrospinal fluid; EIA, enzyme immunoassay; ESR, erythrocyte sedimentation rate; GI, gastrointestinal; HHV-6, human herpesvirus 6; IFA, immunofluorescent assay; PCR, polymerase chain reaction; URI, upper respiratory infection.

Specific Adenoviral Syndromes

A. Pharyngitis

Pharyngitis is the most common adenoviral disease in children. Fever and adenopathy are common. Tonsillitis may be exudative. Rhinitis and an influenza-like systemic illness may be present. Laryngotracheitis or bronchitis may accompany pharyngitis.

B. Pharyngoconjunctival Fever

Conjunctivitis may occur alone and be prolonged, but most often is associated with preauricular adenopathy, fever, pharyngitis, and cervical adenopathy. Foreign body sensation and other symptoms last less than a week. Lower respiratory symptoms are uncommon.

C. Epidemic Keratoconjunctivitis

Symptoms are severe conjunctivitis with punctate keratitis and occasionally visual impairment. A foreign body sensation, photophobia, and swelling of conjunctiva and eyelids are characteristic. Preauricular adenopathy and subconjunctival hemorrhage are common.

D. Pneumonia

Severe pneumonia may occur at all ages. It is especially common in young children (younger than age 3 years). Chest radiographs show bilateral peribronchial and patchy ground-glass interstitial infiltrates in the lower lobes. Symptoms persist for 2–4 weeks. Adenoviral pneumonia can be necrotizing and cause permanent lung damage, especially bronchiectasis. A pertussis-like syndrome with typical cough and lymphocytosis can occur with lower respiratory tract infection. A new variant of adenovirus serotype 14, which appeared in 2006 in the United States, can cause unusually severe, sometimes fatal pneumonia in children and adults.

E. Rash

A diffuse morbilliform (rarely petechial) rash resembling measles, rubella, or roseola may be present. Koplik spots are absent.

F. Diarrhea

Enteric adenoviruses (types 40 and 41) cause 3–5% of cases of short-lived diarrhea in afebrile children.

G. Mesenteric Lymphadenitis

Fever and abdominal pain may mimic appendicitis. Pharyngitis is often associated. Adenovirus-induced adenopathy may be a factor in appendicitis and intussusception.

H. Other Syndromes

Immunosuppressed patients, including neonates, may develop severe or fatal pulmonary or gastrointestinal infections or multisystem disease. Other rare complications include encephalitis, hepatitis, and myocarditis. Adenoviruses have been implicated in the syndrome of idiopathic myocardiopathy. Hemorrhagic cystitis can be a serious problem in immunocompromised children.

▶ Laboratory & Diagnostic Studies

Diagnosis is by culture of conjunctival, respiratory, or stool specimens. Several days to weeks are required for growth in conventional cultures. Viral culture using the rapid culture technique with immunodiagnostic reagents detects virus in 48 hours. Adenovirus infection can also be diagnosed using these reagents directly on respiratory secretions. This is quicker but less sensitive than the culture methods. PCR is an important, relatively rapid diagnostic method for adenovirus infections. Special cells are needed to isolate enteric adenoviruses. Enzyme-linked immunosorbent assay (ELISA) tests rapidly detect enteric adenoviruses in diarrheal specimens. Respiratory adenovirus infections can be detected retrospectively by comparing acute and convalescent sera, but this is not helpful during an acute illness.

▶ Treatment

There is no specific treatment for adenovirus infections. Intravenous immune globulin (IVIG) may be tried in immunocompromised patients with severe pneumonia. There are anecdotal reports of successful treatment of immunocompromised patients with ribavirin or cidofovir, but only cidofovir inhibits adenovirus in vitro.

Castro-Rodriguez JA et al. Adenovirus pneumonia in infants and factors for developing bronchiolitis obliterans. Pediatr Pulmonol 2006;41:947 [PMID: 16871594].

Centers for Disease Control and Prevention (CDC): Acute respiratory disease associated with adenovirus serotype 14—four states, 2006–2007. MMWR Morb Mortal Wkly Rep 2007;56:1181 [PMID: 18004235].

Chuang YY et al: Severe adenovirus infection in children. J Microbiol Immunol Infect 2003;36:37 [PMID: 22626563].

INFLUENZA

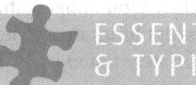

ESSENTIALS OF DIAGNOSIS & TYPICAL FEATURES

- ▶ Fever, cough, pharyngitis, malaise, congestion.
- ▶ Pneumonia.
- ▶ Encephalitis.
- ▶ Seasonal: late fall through mid-spring.
- ▶ Detection of virus, viral antigens, or nucleic acid in respiratory secretions.

Symptomatic infections are common in children because they lack immunologic experience with influenza viruses. Infection rates in children are greater than in adults and are instrumental in initiating community outbreaks. Epidemics occur in fall and winter. Three main types of influenza viruses (A/H1N1, A/H3N2, B) cause most human epidemics, with antigenic drift ensuring a supply of susceptible hosts of all ages. Recently, avian influenza A/H5N1 caused human outbreaks in Asia.

▶ Clinical Findings

Spread of influenza occurs by way of airborne respiratory secretions. The incubation period is 2–7 days.

A. Symptoms and Signs

Influenza infection in older children and adults produces a characteristic syndrome of sudden onset of high fever, severe myalgia, headache, and chills. These symptoms overshadow the associated coryza, pharyngitis, and cough. Usually absent are rash, marked conjunctivitis, adenopathy, exudative pharyngitis, and dehydrating enteritis. Fever, diarrhea, vomiting, and abdominal pain are common in young children. Infants may develop a sepsis-like illness and apnea. Chest examination is usually unremarkable. Unusual clinical findings or variants include croup (most severe with type A influenza), exacerbation of asthma, myositis (especially calf muscles), myocarditis, parotitis, encephalopathy (distinct from Reye syndrome), nephritis, and a transient maculopapular rash. Acute illness lasts 2–5 days. Cough and fatigue may last several weeks. Viral shedding may persist for several weeks in young children.

B. Laboratory Findings

The leukocyte count is normal to low, with variable shift. Influenza infections may be more difficult to recognize in children than in adults even during epidemics, and therefore a specific laboratory test is highly recommended. The virus may be found in respiratory secretions by direct fluorescent antibody staining of nasopharyngeal epithelial cells, ELISA, optic immunoassay (OIA), or PCR. It can also be cultured within 3–7 days from pharyngeal swabs or throat washings. Many laboratories use the rapid culture technique by centrifuging specimens onto cultured cell layers and detecting viral antigen after 48 hours. Other body fluids or tissues (except lung) rarely yield the virus in culture and are more appropriately tested by PCR, which, due to its high sensitivity, can increase influenza detection in respiratory specimens. A late diagnosis may be made with paired serology, using hemagglutination inhibition assays.

C. Imaging

The chest radiograph is nonspecific; it may show hyperaeration, peribronchial thickening, diffuse interstitial infiltrates, or bronchopneumonia in severe cases. Hilar nodes are not enlarged. Pleural effusion is rare in uncomplicated influenza.

▶ Differential Diagnosis

The following may be considered: all other respiratory viruses, *Mycoplasma pneumoniae* or *Chlamydia pneumoniae* (longer incubation period, prolonged illness), streptococcal pharyngitis (pharyngeal exudate or petechiae, adenitis, no cough), bacterial sepsis (petechial or purpuric rash may occur), toxic shock syndrome (rash, hypotension), and rickettsial infections (rash, different season, insect exposure). High fever, the nature of preceding or concurrent illness in family members, and the presence of influenza in the community are distinguishing features from parainfluenza or RSV infections.

▶ Complications & Sequelae

Lower respiratory tract symptoms are most common in children younger than age 5 years. Hospitalization rates are highest in children younger than 2 years. Influenza can cause croup in these children. Secondary bacterial infections (classically staphylococcal) of the middle ear, sinuses, or lungs are most common. Of the viral infections that precede Reye syndrome, varicella and influenza (usually type B) are most notable. During an influenza outbreak, ill children who develop protracted vomiting or irrational behavior should be evaluated for Reye syndrome. Influenza can also cause viral or postviral encephalitis, with cerebral symptoms much more prominent than those of the accompanying respiratory infection. Although the myositis is usually mild and resolves promptly, severe rhabdomyolysis and renal failure have been reported.

Children with underlying cardiopulmonary, metabolic, neuromuscular, or immunosuppressive disease may develop severe viral pneumonia.

▶ Prevention

The inactivated influenza vaccine is moderately protective in older children (see Chapter 9). A new, live-attenuated influenza vaccine (FluMist) is significantly more efficacious in children and is currently recommended for immunocompetent children 2 years of age or older. It is currently recommended that all children 6–59 months of age should be immunized and that two doses be administered during the first year of immunization. New recommendations include immunization of all children older than age 6 months to 18 years of age. Medical staff and family members should also be immunized to protect high-risk patients. Due to the increase in type A influenza virus resistance to adamantanes, when indicated, chemoprophylaxis should be done with a neuraminidase inhibitor such as zanamivir (2 inhalations twice daily if older than age 7 years) or oseltamivir (children < 15 kg, 30 mg twice daily; those 15–23 kg, 45 mg twice daily; those 23–40 kg, 60 mg twice daily; and those > 40 kg, 75 mg twice daily). For outbreak prophylaxis, therapy should be maintained for 2 weeks or more and for 1 week after the last case of influenza is diagnosed. Chemoprophylaxis should be considered during an epidemic for high-risk children who cannot be immunized or who have not yet developed immunity (about 6 weeks after primary vaccination or 2 weeks after a booster dose).

Treatment & Prognosis

Treatment consists of general support and management of pulmonary complications, especially bacterial superinfections. Antivirals are of some benefit in immunocompetent hosts if begun within 48 hours after symptom onset. Studies in lung transplant patients indicate that oseltamivir might be useful for treatment of influenza in this immunocompromised population.

Recovery is usually complete unless severe cardiopulmonary or neurologic damage has occurred. Fatal cases occur in immunodeficient and anatomically compromised children.

Effective treatment or prophylaxis of influenza in children markedly reduces the incidence of acute otitis media and antibiotic usage during the flu season.

Belshe RB et al: Live attenuated versus inactivated influenza vaccine in infants and young children. N Engl J Med 2007;356:685 [PMID: 17301299].

Deyde VM et al: Surveillance of resistance of to adamantanes among influenza A(H3N2) and A(H1N1) viruses isolated worldwide. J Infect Dis 2007;196:249 [PMID: 17570112].

Fiore A et al: Prevention and control of influenza. Recommendations of the Advisory Committee on Immunization Practices (ACIP). MMWR Recomm Rep 2007;56:RR-6:1 [PMID: 12755288].

PARAINFLUENZA

ESSENTIALS OF DIAGNOSIS & TYPICAL FEATURES

▶ Fever, nasal congestion, sore throat, cough.

▶ Croup.

▶ Detection of live virus, antigens, or nucleic acid in respiratory secretions.

Parainfluenza viruses (types 1–4) are the most important cause of croup. Most infants are infected with type 3 within the first 3 years of life, often in the first year. Infection with types 1 and 2 is experienced gradually over the first 5 years of life. Types 1 and 2 occur in the fall; type 3 appears annually, with a peak in the spring or summer. Most primary infections are symptomatic and frequently involve the lower respiratory tract.

Clinical Findings

A. Symptoms and Signs

Clinical diseases include febrile upper respiratory infection (especially in older children with re-exposure), laryngitis, tracheobronchitis, croup, and bronchiolitis (second most common cause after RSV). The relative incidence of these manifestations is type-specific. Parainfluenza viruses (especially type 1) cause 65% of cases of croup in young children, 25% of tracheobronchitis, and 50% of laryngitis. Types 1 and 2 are more likely to cause bronchiolitis. Pneumonia occurs in infants and immunodeficient children, and it leads to particularly high mortality among stem cell recipients. Onset is acute. Most children are febrile. Symptoms of upper respiratory tract infection often accompany croup.

B. Laboratory Findings

Diagnosis is often based on clinical findings. These viruses can be identified by conventional or rapid culture techniques (48 hours), by direct immunofluorescence on nasopharyngeal epithelial cells in respiratory secretions (< 3 hours), or by PCR (< 48 hours).

Differential Diagnosis

Parainfluenza-induced respiratory syndromes are difficult to distinguish from those caused by other respiratory viruses. Croup must be distinguished from epiglottitis caused by *Haemophilus influenzae* (abrupt onset, toxicity, drooling, dyspnea, little cough, left shift of blood smear, and a history of inadequate immunization).

Treatment

No specific therapy or vaccine is available. Croup management is discussed in Chapter 18. Ribavirin is active in vitro and has been used in immunocompromised children, but its efficacy is unproved.

Fry AM et al: Seasonal trends of human parainfluenza viral infections: United States, 1990–2004. Clin Infect Dis 2006;43: 1016 [PMID: 16983614].

RESPIRATORY SYNCYTIAL VIRUS DISEASE

ESSENTIALS OF DIAGNOSIS & TYPICAL FEATURES

▶ Diffuse wheezing and tachypnea following upper respiratory symptoms in an infant (bronchiolitis).

▶ Epidemics in late fall to early spring (January–February peak).

▶ Hyperinflation on chest radiograph.

▶ Detection of RSV antigen in nasal secretions.

General Considerations

RSV is the most important cause of lower respiratory tract illness in young children, accounting for more than 70% of cases of bronchiolitis and 40% of cases of pneumonia. Outbreaks occur annually, and attack rates are high; 60% of children are infected in the first year of life, and 90% by age 2 years. During peak season (cold weather in temperate climates), the clinical diagnosis of RSV infection in infants with bronchiolitis is as accurate as most laboratory tests. Despite the presence of serum antibody, reinfection is common. Distinct genotypes predominate in a community. Yearly shift in these is a partial explanation for reinfection. However, reinfection generally causes only upper respiratory symptoms in anatomically normal children. No vaccine is available. Immunosuppressed patients may develop progressive severe pneumonia. Children with congenital heart disease with increased pulmonary blood flow, children with chronic lung disease (eg, cystic fibrosis), and premature infants younger than age 6 months are also at higher risk for severe illness.

▶ Clinical Findings

A. Symptoms and Signs

Initial symptoms are those of upper respiratory infection. Low-grade fever may be present. The classic disease is bronchiolitis, characterized by diffuse wheezing, variable fever, cough, tachypnea, difficulty feeding, and, in severe cases, cyanosis. Hyperinflation, crackles, prolonged expiration, wheezing, and retractions are present. The liver and spleen may be palpable because of lung hyperinflation, but are not enlarged. The disease usually lasts 3–7 days in previously healthy children. Fever is present for 2–4 days; it does not correlate with pulmonary symptoms and may be absent during the height of lung involvement.

Apnea may be the presenting manifestation, especially in premature infants, in the first few months of life; it usually resolves after a few days, often being replaced by obvious signs of bronchiolitis. No explanation for apnea has been found.

RSV infection in subsequent years is more likely to cause tracheobronchitis or upper respiratory tract infection. Exceptions are immunocompromised hosts and children with severe chronic lung or heart disease, who may have especially severe or prolonged primary infections and are subject to additional attacks of severe pneumonitis.

B. Laboratory Findings

Rapid detection of RSV antigen in nasal or pulmonary secretions by fluorescent antibody staining or ELISA requires only several hours and is more than 90% sensitive and specific. Rapid tissue culture methods take 48 hours and have comparable sensitivity.

C. Imaging

Diffuse hyperinflation and peribronchiolar thickening are most common; atelectasis and patchy infiltrates also occur in uncomplicated infection, but pleural effusions are rare. Consolidation (usually subsegmental) occurs in 25% of children with lower respiratory tract disease.

▶ Differential Diagnosis

Although almost all cases of bronchiolitis are due to RSV during an epidemic, other viruses, particularly human metapneumovirus, cannot be excluded. Mixed infections with other viruses, chlamydiae, or bacteria can occur. Wheezing may be due to asthma, a foreign body, or other airway obstruction. RSV infection may closely resemble chlamydial pneumonitis when fine crackles are present and fever and wheezing are not prominent. The two may also coexist. Cystic fibrosis may resemble RSV infection; a positive family history or failure to thrive associated with hyponatremia or hypoalbuminemia should prompt a sweat chloride test. Pertussis should also be considered in this age group, especially if cough is prominent and if the infant is younger than age 6 months. A markedly elevated leukocyte count should suggest bacterial superinfection (neutrophilia) or pertussis (lymphocytosis).

▶ Complications

RSV commonly infects the middle ear. Symptomatic otitis media is more likely when secondary bacterial infection is present (usually due to pneumococci or *H influenzae*). This is the most common complication (10–20%). Bacterial pneumonia complicates only 0.5–1% of hospitalized patients. Sudden exacerbations of fever and leukocytosis should suggest bacterial infection. Respiratory failure or apnea may require mechanical ventilation, but occurs in less than 2% of hospitalized previously healthy full-term infants. Cardiac failure may occur as a complication of pulmonary disease or myocarditis. RSV—as well as parainfluenza and influenza viruses—commonly causes exacerbations of asthma. Nosocomial infection is so common during outbreaks that elective hospitalization or surgery, especially for those with underlying illness, should be postponed. Well-designed hospital programs to prevent nosocomial spread are imperative (see next section).

▶ Prevention & Treatment

Children who are very hypoxic or cannot feed because of respiratory distress must be hospitalized and given humidified oxygen and tube or intravenous feedings. Antibiotics, decongestants, and expectorants are of no value in routine infections. Such children should be kept in respiratory isolation. Cohorting ill infants in respiratory isolation during peak season (with or without rapid diagnostic attempts) and emphasizing good hand-washing may greatly decrease nosocomial transmission.

The utility of bronchodilator therapy has not been consistently demonstrated. Often a trial of bronchodilator therapy is given to determine response and is subsequently discontinued if there is no improvement. Racemic epinephrine occasionally works when albuterol fails. The use of corticosteroids is also controversial. A meta-analysis of numerous studies indicates a significant effect on hospital stay, especially in those most ill at the time of treatment. The use of a single dose of corticosteroids has no lasting effect on respiratory status and does not prevent hospitalization.

Ribavirin is the only licensed antiviral therapy used for RSV infection. It is given by continuous aerosolization. There is great controversy about its efficacy, and its use is infrequent in infants without significant anatomic or immunologic defects. At best, there is a very modest effect on disease severity in immunocompetent infants with no underlying anatomic abnormality. Even in high-risk infants, clinical response to ribavirin therapy was not demonstrated in several studies. Nevertheless, ribavirin is sometimes used in severely ill children who are immunologically or anatomically compromised, in those with severe cardiac disease, and in those with evidence of severe RSV infection.

Monthly intramuscular administration of humanized RSV monoclonal antibody is now recommended to prevent severe disease in high-risk patients during epidemic periods. Monthly administration should be considered during the RSV season for high-risk children, as described in Chapter 9.

Use of passive immunization for immunocompromised children is logical, but not established. RSV antibody is not effective for treatment of established infection.

Prognosis

Although mild bronchiolitis does not produce long-term problems, 30–40% of patients hospitalized with this infection will wheeze later in childhood, and RSV infection in infancy may be one important precursor to asthma. Chronic restrictive lung disease and bronchiolitis obliterans are rare sequelae.

Corneli HM et al: A multicenter, randomized, controlled trial of dexamethasone for bronchiolitis. N Eng J Med 2007;357:331 [PMID: 17652648].

Lukacs NW et al: Respiratory syncytial virus-induced pulmonary disease and exacerbation of allergic asthma. Contributions to microbiology. 2007;14:68 [PMID: 17684333].

Simoes EA et al: Palivizumab prophylaxis, respiratory syncytial virus, and subsequent recurrent wheezing. J Pediatr 2007;151:34 [PMID: 17586188].

HUMAN METAPNEUMOVIRUS INFECTION

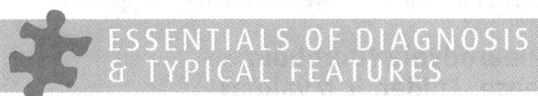

ESSENTIALS OF DIAGNOSIS & TYPICAL FEATURES

► Cough, coryza, sore throat.
► Bronchiolitis.
► Detection of viral antigens or nucleic acid in respiratory secretions.

General Considerations

After its discovery in 2001, human metapneumovirus (hMPV) was identified as a common agent of respiratory tract infections that is very similar to RSV in epidemiologic and clinical characteristics. Like RSV, parainfluenza, mumps, and measles, hMPV belongs to the paramyxovirus family. Humans are its only known reservoir. Seroepidemiologic surveys indicate that the virus has worldwide distribution. More than 90% of children contract hMPV infection by age 5 years, typically during late autumn through early spring outbreaks. hMPV accounts for 15–25% of the cases of bronchiolitis and pneumonia in children younger than 2 years of age. Older children and adults can also develop symptomatic infection.

Clinical Findings

A. Symptoms and Signs

The most common symptoms are fever, cough, rhinorrhea, and sore throat. Bronchiolitis and pneumonia occur in 40–70% of the children who acquire hMPV before the age of 2 years. Asymptomatic infection is uncommon. Other manifestations include otitis, conjunctivitis, diarrhea, and myalgia. Acute wheezing has been associated with hMPV in children of all ages, raising the possibility that this virus, like RSV, might trigger reactive airway disease. Dual infection with hMPV and RSV or other respiratory viruses seems to be a common occurrence and may increase morbidity and mortality.

B. Laboratory Findings

The virus has very selective tissue culture tropism, which accounts for its late discovery in spite of its presence in archived specimens from the mid-1900s. The preferred method of diagnosis is PCR performed on respiratory specimens. Rapid shell vial culture is an acceptable, albeit less sensitive, alternative. Antibody tests are available, but are most appropriately used for epidemiologic studies.

C. Imaging

Lower respiratory tract infection frequently shows hyperinflation and patchy pneumonitis on chest radiographs.

Treatment & Prognosis

No antiviral therapies are available to treat hMPV. Children with lower respiratory tract disease may require hospitalization and ventilatory support, but less frequently than with RSV-associated bronchiolitis. Duration of hospitalization in hMPV is typically shorter than in RSV.

Percivalle E et al: Rapid detection of human metapneumovirus strains in nasopharyngeal aspirates and shell vial cultures by monoclonal antibodies. J Clin Microbiol 2005;43:3443 [PMID: 16000473].

Williams JV et al: The role of human metapneumovirus in upper respiratory tract infections in children: A 20-year experience. J Infect Dis 2006;193:387 [PMID: 16388486].

INFECTIONS DUE TO ENTEROVIRUSES

ESSENTIALS OF DIAGNOSIS & TYPICAL FEATURES

▶ Acute febrile illness with headache and sore throat.

▶ Summer–fall epidemics.

▶ Other common features: rash, nonexudative pharyngitis.

▶ Common cause of aseptic meningitis.

▶ Complications: myocarditis, neurologic damage, life-threatening illness in newborns.

Enteroviruses are a major cause of illness in young children. The multiple types are physically and biochemically similar and may produce identical syndromes. The multiplicity of types makes vaccine development impractical and has hindered development of antigen detection and serologic tests. However, common RNA sequences and group antigens have led to diagnostic tests for viral nucleic acid and proteins. A PCR assay is available in many medical centers, but tissue culture is still used in some centers as a diagnostic method for echoviruses, polioviruses, and coxsackie B viruses. Although cultures may turn positive in 2–4 days, the relatively rapid answer obtained with PCR facilitates clinical decisions, particularly in cases of meningoencephalitis and severe unexplained illness in neonates.

Transmission is fecal-oral or from upper respiratory secretions. Multiple enteroviruses circulate in the community at any one time; summer–fall outbreaks are common in temperate climates, but infections are seen year-round. After poliovirus, coxsackie B virus is most virulent, followed by echovirus. Neurologic, cardiac, and overwhelming neonatal infections are the most severe forms of illness.

ACUTE FEBRILE ILLNESS

Accompanied by nonspecific upper respiratory or enteric symptoms, sudden onset of fever and irritability in infants or young children is often enteroviral in origin, especially in late summer and fall. More than 90% of enteroviral infections are not distinctive. Occasionally a petechial rash is seen; more often a diffuse maculopapular or morbilliform eruption (often prominent on palms and soles) occurs on the second to fourth day of fever. Rapid recovery is the rule. More than one febrile enteroviral illness can occur in the same patient in one season. The leukocyte count is usually normal. Infants, because of fever and irritability, may undergo an evaluation for bacteremia or meningitis and be hospitalized to rule out sepsis. Approximately half of these infants have aseptic meningitis. In the summer months enterovirus infection is more likely than human herpesvirus 6 to cause an acute medical visit for fever. Duration of illness is 4–5 days.

Sawyer MH: Enterovirus infections: Diagnosis and treatment. Semin Pediatr Infect Dis 2002;13:40 [PMID: 12118843].

Stalkup JR, Chilukuri S: Enterovirus infections: A review of clinical presentation, diagnosis, and treatment. Dermatol Clin 2002;20: 217 [PMID: 12120436].

RESPIRATORY TRACT ILLNESSES

1. Febrile Illness with Pharyngitis

This syndrome is most common in older children, who complain of headache, sore throat, myalgia, and abdominal discomfort. The usual duration is 3–4 days. Vesicles or papules may be seen in the pharynx. There is no exudate. Occasionally, enteroviruses are the cause of croup, bronchitis, or pneumonia. They may also exacerbate asthma.

2. Herpangina

Herpangina is characterized by an acute onset of fever and posterior pharyngeal grayish white vesicles that quickly form ulcers (< 20 in number), often linearly arranged on the posterior palate, uvula, and tonsillar pillars. Bilateral faucial ulcers may also be seen. Dysphagia, vomiting, abdominal pain, and anorexia also occur and, rarely, parotitis or vaginal ulcers. Symptoms disappear in 4–5 days. The epidemic form is due to a variety of coxsackie A viruses; coxsackie B viruses and echoviruses cause sporadic cases.

The differential diagnosis includes primary herpes simplex gingivostomatitis (ulcers are more prominent anteriorly, and gingivitis is present), aphthous stomatitis (fever absent, recurrent episodes, anterior lesions), trauma, hand-foot-and-mouth disease (see later discussion), and Vincent angina (painful gingivitis spreading from the gum line, underlying dental disease). If the enanthema is missed, tonsillitis might be incorrectly diagnosed.

3. Acute Lymphonodular Pharyngitis

Coxsackievirus A10 has been associated with a febrile pharyngitis characterized by nonulcerative yellow-white posterior pharyngeal papules in the same distribution as herpangina. The duration is 1–2 weeks; therapy is supportive.

4. Pleurodynia (Bornholm Disease, Epidemic Myalgia)

Caused by coxsackie B virus (epidemic form) or many nonpolio enteroviruses (sporadic form), pleurodynia is associated with an abrupt onset of unilateral or bilateral spasmodic pain of variable intensity over the lower ribs or upper abdomen. Associated symptoms include headache, fever, vomiting, myalgias, and abdominal and neck pain. Physical findings include fever, chest muscle tenderness, decreased thoracic excursion, and occasionally a friction rub. The chest radiograph is normal. Hematologic tests are nondiagnostic. The illness generally lasts less than 1 week.

This is a disease of muscle, but the differential diagnosis includes bacterial pneumonia, empyema, tuberculosis, and endemic fungal infections (all excluded radiographically and by auscultation), costochondritis (no fever or other symptoms), and a variety of abdominal problems, especially those causing diaphragmatic irritation.

There is no specific therapy. Potent analgesic agents and chest splinting alleviate the pain.

RASHES (INCLUDING HAND-FOOT-AND-MOUTH DISEASE)

The rash may be macular, maculopapular, urticarial, scarlatiniform, petechial, or vesicular. One of the most characteristic is that of hand-foot-and-mouth disease (caused by coxsackieviruses, especially types A5, A10, and A16), in which vesicles or red papules are found on the tongue, oral mucosa, hands, and feet. Often they appear near the nails and on the heels. Associated fever, sore throat, and malaise are mild. The rash may appear when fever abates, simulating roseola.

1. Cardiac Involvement

Myocarditis and pericarditis may be caused by a number of nonpolio enteroviruses, particularly type B coxsackieviruses. Most commonly, upper respiratory symptoms are followed by substernal pain, dyspnea, and exercise intolerance. A friction rub or gallop may be detected. Ultrasound will define ventricular dysfunction, and electrocardiography may show pericarditis or ventricular irritability. Creatine phosphokinase may be elevated. The disease may be mild or fatal; most children recover completely. In infants, other organs may be involved at the same time; in older patients, cardiac disease is usually the sole manifestation (see Chapter 19 for therapy). Enteroviral RNA is present in cardiac tissue in some cases of dilated cardiomyopathy or myocarditis; the significance of this finding is unknown. Epidemics of enterovirus 71, which occur in Asia, as well as sporadic cases in the United States, are associated with severe left ventricular dysfunction and pulmonary edema following typical mucocutaneous manifestations of enterovirus infection. Enterovirus 71 also can cause isolated severe neurologic disease or neurologic disease in combination with myocardial disease.

2. Severe Neonatal Infection

Sporadic and nosocomial nursery cases of severe systemic enteroviral disease occur. Clinical manifestations include combinations of fever, rash, pneumonitis, encephalitis, hepatitis, gastroenteritis, myocarditis, pancreatitis, and myositis. The infants, usually younger than 1 week old, may appear septic, with cyanosis, dyspnea, and seizures. The differential diagnosis includes bacterial and herpes simplex infections, necrotizing enterocolitis, other causes of heart or liver failure, and metabolic diseases. Diagnosis is suggested by the finding of cerebrospinal fluid (CSF) mononuclear pleocytosis and confirmed

by the isolation of virus or detection of enteroviral RNA in urine, stool, CSF, or pharynx. Therapy is supportive. IVIG is often administered, but its value is uncertain. Passively acquired maternal antibody may protect newborns from severe disease. For this reason, labor should not be induced in pregnant women near term who have suspected enteroviral disease.

Huang F-L et al: Left ventricular dysfunction in children with fulminant enterovirus 71 infection: An evaluation of the clinical course. Clin Infect Dis 2002;34:1020 [PMID: 11880970].

Pérez-Vélez CM et al: Outbreak of neurologic enterovirus type 71 disease: A diagnostic challenge. Clin Infect Dis 2007;45:950 [PMID: 17879907].

CENTRAL NERVOUS SYSTEM ILLNESSES

1. Poliomyelitis

ESSENTIALS OF DIAGNOSIS & TYPICAL FEATURES

▶ Inadequate immunization or underlying immune deficiency.

▶ Headache, fever, muscle weakness.

▶ Aseptic meningitis.

▶ Asymmetrical, flaccid paralysis; muscle tenderness and hyperesthesia; intact sensation; late atrophy.

▶ General Considerations

Poliovirus infection is subclinical in 90–95% of cases; it causes nonspecific febrile illness in about 5% of cases and aseptic meningitis, with or without paralytic disease, in 1–3%. In endemic areas, most older children and adults are immune because of prior inapparent infections. Occasional cases in the United States occur in patients who travel to foreign countries. Most recent cases were in immunodeficient patients who received the oral poliovirus vaccine (OPV) or were exposed to recent vaccinees. Severe poliovirus infection was a rare complication of OPV vaccination as a result of reversion of the vaccine virus. The incidence of vaccine-associated paralytic poliomyelitis (VAPP) in the United States was 1:750,000 and 1:2.4 million doses for the first and second dose of OPV, respectively. Although rare, VAPP became more common than wild-type poliomyelitis in the United States in the 1980s. This led to change in the recommended immunization regimen, substituting inactivated polio vaccine (IPV) for OPV (see Chapter 9).

▶ Clinical Findings

A. Symptoms and Signs

The initial symptoms are fever, myalgia, sore throat, and headache for 2–6 days. In less than 10% of infected children, several symptom-free days are followed by recurrent fever and signs of aseptic meningitis: headache, stiff neck, spinal rigidity, and nausea. Mild cases resolve completely. In only 1–2% of these children does high fever, severe myalgia, and anxiety portend progression to loss of reflexes and subsequent flaccid paralysis. Sensation remains intact, although hyperesthesia of skin overlying paralyzed muscles is common and pathognomonic.

Paralysis is usually asymmetrical. Proximal limb muscles are more often involved than distal, and lower limb involvement is more common than upper. Bulbar involvement affects swallowing, speech, and cardiorespiratory function and accounts for most deaths. Bladder distention and marked constipation characteristically accompany lower limb paralysis. Paralysis is usually complete by the time the temperature normalizes. Weakness often resolves completely. Atrophy is usually apparent by 4–8 weeks. Most improvement of muscle paralysis occurs within 6 months.

B. Laboratory Findings

In patients with meningeal symptoms, the CSF contains up to several hundred leukocytes (mostly lymphocytes) per microliter; the glucose level is normal, and protein concentration is mildly elevated. Poliovirus is easy to grow in cell culture and can be readily differentiated from other enteroviruses. It is rarely isolated from spinal fluid but is often present in the throat and stool for several weeks following infection. Paired serology is also diagnostic. Laboratory methods are available to differentiate wild from attenuated vaccine isolates.

▶ Differential Diagnosis

Aseptic meningitis due to poliovirus is indistinguishable from that due to other viruses. Paralytic disease in the United States is usually due to nonpolio enteroviruses. Polio may resemble Guillain-Barré syndrome (variable sensory loss, symmetrical loss of function; minimal pleocytosis, high protein concentration in spinal fluid), polyneuritis (sensory loss), pseudoparalysis due to bone or joint problems (eg, trauma, infection), botulism, or tick paralysis.

▶ Complications & Sequelae

Complications are the result of the acute and permanent effects of paralysis. Respiratory, pharyngeal, bladder, and bowel malfunction are most critical. Deaths are usually due to complications arising from respiratory dysfunction. Limbs injured near the time of infection, such as by intramuscular injections, excessive prior use, or trauma, tend to be most severely involved and have the worst prognosis for recovery (provocation paralysis). Postpolio muscular atrophy occurs in 30–40% of paralyzed limbs 20–30 years later, characterized by increasing weakness and fasciculations in previously affected, partially recovered limbs.

▶ Treatment & Prognosis

Therapy is supportive. Bed rest, fever and pain control (heat therapy is helpful), and careful attention to progression of weakness (particularly of respiratory muscles) are important. No intramuscular injections should be given during the acute phase. Intubation or tracheostomy for secretion control and catheter drainage of the bladder may be needed. Assisted ventilation and enteral feeding may also be needed. Pleconaril, which is an antiviral drug active against most enteroviruses, has no effect on polioviruses. Postpolio paralysis is mild in about 30%, permanent in 15%, and results in death in 5–10%. Disease is worse in adults and pregnant women than in children.

2. Nonpolio Viral Meningitis

Nonpolio enteroviruses cause over 80% of cases of aseptic meningitis at all ages. In the summer and fall, multiple cases may be seen associated with circulation of neurotropic strains. Nosocomial outbreaks also occur.

▶ Clinical Findings

The usual enteroviral incubation period is 4–6 days. Because many enteroviral infections are subclinical or not associated with CNS symptoms, a history of contact with a patient with meningitis is unusual. Neonates may acquire infection from maternal blood, vaginal secretions, or feces at birth; occasionally the mother has had a febrile illness just prior to delivery.

A. Symptoms and Signs

Onset is usually acute with variable fever, marked irritability, and lethargy in infants. Incidence is much greater in children younger than age 1 year. Older children also describe frontal headache, photophobia, and myalgia. Abdominal pain, diarrhea, and vomiting may occur. The incidence of rash varies with the infecting strain. If rash occurs, it is usually seen after several days of illness and is diffuse, macular or maculopapular, occasionally petechial, but not purpuric. Oropharyngeal vesicles and rash on the palms and soles suggest an enterovirus. The anterior fontanelle may be full. Meningismus may be present. The illness may be biphasic, with nonspecific symptoms and signs preceding those related to the CNS. In older children, it is easier to demonstrate meningeal signs. Seizures are unusual, and focal neurologic findings, which are rare, should lead to a search for an alternative cause. Frank encephalitis, which is also uncommon at any age, occurs most often in neonates. Because of the overall frequency of enteroviral disease in children, 10–20% of all cases of encephalitis of proved viral origin are caused by enteroviruses. Enterovirus 71 infections that begin with typical mucocutaneous manifestations of enteroviruses can be complicated by severe brainstem encephalitis and polio-like flaccid paralysis. Enterovirus 70 outbreaks have resulted in hemorrhagic conjunctivitis together with paralytic poliomyelitis. Very pathogenic enteroviruses are now appearing in the United States. Other nonpolio enteroviruses cause sporadic cases of acute motor weakness similar to that seen with poliovirus infection. Children with congenital immune deficiency, especially agammaglobulinemia, are subject to chronic enteroviral meningoencephalitis that is often fatal or associated with severe sequelae.

B. Laboratory Findings

Blood leukocyte counts are nonspecific and often normal. The spinal fluid leukocyte count is 100–1000/μL. Early in the illness, polymorphonuclear cells predominate; a shift to mononuclear cells occurs within 8–36 hours. In about 95% of cases, spinal fluid parameters include a total leukocyte count less than 3000/μL, protein less than 80 mg/dL, and glucose more than 60% of serum values. Marked deviation from any of these findings should prompt consideration of another diagnosis (see following section). The syndrome of inappropriate secretion of antidiuretic hormone may occur but is rarely clinically significant.

Culture of CSF may yield an enterovirus within a few days (< 70%). However, PCR for enteroviruses is the most useful diagnostic method in many centers (sensitivity > 90%) and can give an answer within 24–48 hours. Virus may be detected in acellular CSF. Detection of an enterovirus from throat or stool suggests, but does not prove, enteroviral meningitis. Vaccine poliovirus present in feces in infants being evaluated for aseptic meningitis (outside of the United States) may confuse the diagnosis but can usually be distinguished by growth characteristics.

C. Imaging

Cerebral imaging is not often indicated; if done, it is usually normal. Subdural effusions, infarcts, edema, or focal abnormalities seen in bacterial meningitis are absent except for the rare case of focal encephalitis.

► Differential Diagnosis

In the prevaccine era, mumps and polio were leading causes of aseptic meningitis, but now this is usually caused by enteroviruses, especially in the summer and fall. Other causative viruses are mosquito-borne viruses (flavivirus, bunyavirus). These are usually considered during an investigation of encephalitis, but many of them are more likely to cause isolated meningitis and should be considered when seasonal clusters of viral meningitis occur. Primary herpes simplex infection can cause aseptic meningitis in adolescents who have a genital herpes infection. In neonates, early herpes simplex meningoencephalitis may mimic enteroviral disease (see next section on Infections Due to Herpesviruses). This is an important alternative diagnosis to exclude because of the need for urgent specific therapy. Lymphocytic choriomeningitis virus causes meningitis in children in contact with rodents (pet or environmental exposure).

Meningitis occurs in some patients at the time of infection with human immunodeficiency virus (HIV).

Other causes of aseptic meningitis that may resemble enteroviral infection include partially treated bacterial meningitis (recent antibiotic treatment, CSF parameters resembling those seen in bacterial disease and bacterial antigen sometimes present); parameningeal foci of bacterial infection such as brain abscess, subdural empyema, mastoiditis (predisposing factors, glucose level in CSF may be lower, focal neurologic signs, and characteristic imaging); tumors or cysts (malignant cells detected by cytologic examination, a history of neurologic symptoms, higher protein concentration or lower glucose level in CSF); trauma (presence, without exception, of red blood cells, which may be erroneously assumed to be due to traumatic lumbar puncture, but are crenated and fail to clear); vasculitis (other systemic or neurologic signs, found in older children); tuberculous or fungal meningitis (see Chapters 40 and 41); cysticercosis; parainfectious encephalopathies (*M pneumoniae*, cat-scratch disease, respiratory viruses [especially influenza]); Lyme disease; leptospirosis; and rickettsial diseases.

► Prevention & Treatment

No specific therapy exists. Infants are usually hospitalized, isolated, and treated with fluids and antipyretics. Moderately to severely ill infants are given appropriate antibiotics for bacterial pathogens until cultures are negative for 48–72 hours. This practice is changing somewhat, and hospital stay shortened, in areas where the PCR assay for enteroviruses is available. If patients—especially older children—are mildly ill, antibiotics may be withheld and the child observed. The illness usually lasts less than 1 week. Codeine compounds or other strong analgesics may be needed. C-reactive protein and lactate levels are usually low in the CSF of children with viral meningitis; both may be elevated with bacterial infection. With clinical deterioration, repeat lumbar puncture, cerebral imaging, neurologic consultation, and more aggressive diagnostic tests should be considered. Herpesvirus encephalitis is an important consideration in such cases, particularly in infants younger than age 1 month, and this may warrant empiric acyclovir therapy until an etiologic diagnosis is made.

Measures to prevent enteroviral infection include good hygiene, scrupulous hand washing, and proper isolation in the hospital.

► Prognosis

In general, enteroviral meningitis has no significant short-term neurologic or developmental sequelae. Developmental delay may follow severe neonatal infections. Unlike mumps, enterovirus infections rarely cause hearing loss.

King RL al: Routine cerebrospinal fluid enterovirus polymerase chain reaction testing reduces hospitalization and antibiotic use for infants 90 days of age or younger. Pediatrics 2007;120:489 [PMID: 17766520].

Rittichier KR et al: Diagnosis and outcomes of enterovirus infections in young infants. Ped Infect Dis J 2005;24:546 [PMID: 15933567].

Romero JR, Newland JG: Viral meningitis and encephalitis: Traditional and emerging viral agents. Semin Pediatr Infect Dis 2003;14:72 [PMID: 12881794].

INFECTIONS DUE TO HERPESVIRUSES

HERPES SIMPLEX INFECTIONS

ESSENTIALS OF DIAGNOSIS & TYPICAL FEATURES

▶ Grouped vesicles on an erythematous base, typically in or around the mouth or genitals.

▶ Tender regional adenopathy, especially with primary infection.

▶ Fever and malaise with primary infection.

▶ Recurrent episodes in many patients.

▶ General Considerations

There are two types of herpes simplex viruses. Type 1 (HSV-1) causes most cases of oral, skin, and cerebral disease. Type 2 (HSV-2) causes most (80–85%) genital and congenital infections. Latent infection in sensory ganglia routinely follows primary infection. Recurrences may be spontaneous or induced by external events (eg, fever, menstruation, or sunlight) or immunosuppression. Transmission is by direct contact with infected secretions. Herpes simplex viruses are very susceptible to antiviral drugs.

Primary infection with HSV-1 often occurs early in childhood, although many adults (20–50%) have never been infected. Primary infection with HSV-1 is subclinical in 80% of cases and causes gingivostomatitis in the remainder. HSV-2, which is transmitted sexually, is also usually (65%) subclinical or produces mild, nonspecific symptoms. Infection with one type of HSV may prevent or attenuate clinically apparent infection with the other type, but individuals can be infected at different times with both HSV-1 and HSV-2. Recurrent episodes are due to reactivation of latent HSV.

▶ Clinical Findings

The source of primary infection is usually an asymptomatic excreter. Most previously infected individuals shed HSV at irregular intervals. At any one time (point prevalence), more than 5% of normal seropositive adults excrete HSV-1 in the saliva; the percentage is higher in recently infected children. HSV-2 shedding in genital secretions occurs with a point prevalence exceeding 10%, depending on the method of detection (viral isolation vs PCR) and the interval since the initial infection. A history of contact with an active HSV infection is unusual.

A. Symptoms and Signs

1. Gingivostomatitis—High fever, irritability, and drooling occur in infants. Multiple oral ulcers are seen on the tongue and on the buccal and gingival mucosa, occasionally extending to the pharynx. Pharyngeal ulcers may predominate in older children and adolescents. Diffusely swollen red gums that are friable and bleed easily are typical. Cervical nodes are swollen and tender. Duration is 7–14 days. Herpangina, aphthous stomatitis, thrush, and Vincent angina should be excluded.

2. Vulvovaginitis or urethritis—Genital herpes (especially HSV-2) in a prepubertal child should suggest sexual abuse. Vesicles or painful ulcers on the vulva, vagina, or penis and tender adenopathy are seen. Systemic symptoms (fever, flulike illness, myalgia) are common with the initial episode. Painful urination may cause retention. Primary infections last 10–14 days before healing. Lesions may resemble trauma, syphilis (ulcers are painless), or chancroid (ulcers are painful and nodes are erythematous and fluctuant) in the adolescent, and bullous impetigo, trauma, and severe chemical irritation in younger children.

3. Cutaneous infections—Direct inoculation onto cuts or abrasions may produce localized vesicles or ulcers. A deep HSV infection on the fingers (called herpetic whitlow) may be mistaken for a bacterial felon or paronychia; surgical drainage is of no value and is contraindicated. HSV infection of eczematous skin may result in extensive areas of vesicles and shallow ulcers (eczema herpeticum), which may be mistaken for impetigo or varicella.

4. Recurrent mucocutaneous infection—Recurrent oral shedding is usually asymptomatic. Perioral recurrences often begin with a prodrome of tingling or burning limited to the vermilion border, followed by vesiculation, scabbing, and crusting around the lips over the next 3–5 days. Intraoral lesions rarely recur. Fever, adenopathy, and other symptoms are absent. Recurrent cutaneous herpes most closely resembles impetigo, but the latter is often outside the perinasal and perioral region, responds to antibiotics, yields a positive result on Gram stain, and *Streptococcus pyogenes* or *Staphylococcus aureus* can be isolated. Recurrent genital disease is common after the initial infection with HSV-2. It is shorter (5–7 days) and milder (mean, four lesions) than primary infection and is not associated with systemic symptoms.

5. Keratoconjunctivitis—Keratoconjunctivitis may be part of a primary infection due to spread from infected saliva. Most cases are caused by reactivation of virus latent in the ciliary ganglion. Keratoconjunctivitis produces photophobia, pain, and conjunctival irritation. With recurrences, dendritic corneal ulcers may be demonstrable with fluorescein staining. Stromal invasion may occur. Corticosteroids should never be used for unilateral keratitis without ophthalmologic consultation. Other causes of these symptoms include trauma, bacterial infections, and other viral infections (especially adenovirus if pharyngitis is present; bilateral involvement makes HSV unlikely) (see Chapter 15).

6. Encephalitis—Although unusual in infants outside the neonatal period, encephalitis may occur at any age, usually without cutaneous herpes lesions. In older children, HSV encephalitis can follow a primary infection, but often represents reactivation of latent virus. HSV is the most common cause of sporadic severe encephalitis. It is the most important because it can be treated with specific antiviral therapy. Fever, headache, behavioral changes, and neurologic deficits or focal seizures occur. Mild mononuclear pleocytosis is typically present along with an elevated protein concentration, which continues to rise on repeat lumbar punctures. In older children hypodense areas with a medial and inferior temporal lobe predilection are seen on CT scan, especially after 3–5 days, but the findings in infants may be more diffuse. Magnetic resonance imaging (MRI) is more sensitive and is positive sooner. Periodic focal epileptiform discharges are seen on electroencephalograms, but are not diagnostic of HSV infection. Viral cultures of CSF are rarely positive. The PCR assay to detect HSV DNA in CSF is a sensitive and specific rapid test. Without early antiviral therapy, the prognosis is poor. The differential diagnosis includes mumps, mosquito-borne and other viral encephalitides, parainfectious and postinfectious encephalopathy, brain abscess, acute demyelinating syndromes, and bacterial meningoencephalitis.

7. Neonatal infections—Infection is acquired by ascending spread prior to delivery (5–10% of cases) or most often at the time of vaginal delivery from a mother with genital infection. Occasionally the infection is acquired in the postpartum period from oral secretions of family members or hospital personnel. A history of genital herpes in the mother is usually absent. Within a few days and up to 4 weeks, skin vesicles appear (especially at sites of trauma, such as where scalp monitors were placed). Some infants have infections limited to the skin, eye, or mouth. Other infants are acutely ill, presenting with jaundice, shock, bleeding, or respiratory distress. Some infants appear well initially, but dissemination of the infection to the brain or other organs becomes evident during the ensuing week if it is untreated. HSV infection (and empiric therapy) should be considered in newborns with the sepsis syndrome who are unresponsive to antibiotic therapy and have negative bacterial cultures. Skin lesions may be absent at the time of presentation. Some infected infants exhibit only neurologic symptoms at 2–3 weeks after delivery: apnea, lethargy, fever, poor feeding, or persistent overt seizures. The brain infection in these children is often diffuse and is best diagnosed by MRI. The skin lesions may resemble impetigo, bacterial scalp abscesses, or miliaria; some children may fail to develop skin lesions. Skin lesions may recur over weeks or months after recovery from the acute illness. Progressive culture-negative pneumonitis is another manifestation of neonatal HSV.

B. Laboratory Findings

With multisystem disease, abnormalities in platelets, clotting factors, and liver function tests are often present. A finding of lymphocytic pleocytosis and elevated CSF protein indicates aseptic meningitis or encephalitis. Virus may be cultured from infected epithelial sites (vesicles, ulcers, or conjunctival scrapings) and from infected tissue (skin, brain) obtained by biopsy. Cultures of CSF yield positive results in about 50% of neonatal cases, but are uncommon in older children. HSV will be detected within 2 days by rapid tissue culture methods, but PCR is the preferred diagnostic method. Isolation from throat, eye, urine, or stool of a newborn is diagnostic. Vaginal culture of the mother may offer circumstantial evidence for the diagnosis, but may be negative.

Rapid diagnostic tests include immunofluorescent stains or ELISA to detect viral antigen in skin or mucosal scrapings. The PCR assay for HSV DNA is positive (> 95%) in the CSF when there is brain involvement. Serum is often positive in the presence of multisystem disease.

▶ Complications, Sequelae, & Prognosis

Gingivostomatitis may result in dehydration due to dysphagia; severe chronic oral disease and esophageal involvement may occur in immunosuppressed patients. Primary vulvovaginitis may be associated with aseptic meningitis, paresthesias, autonomic dysfunction due to neuritis (urinary retention, constipation), and secondary candidal infection. HIV transmission from and acquisition by individuals who are seropositive for HSV infection is increased. Extensive cutaneous disease (as in eczema) may be associated with dissemination, and with bacterial superinfection. Keratitis may result in corneal opacification or perforation. Untreated encephalitis is fatal in 70% of patients and causes severe damage in most of the remainder. When acyclovir treatment is instituted early, 20% of patients die and 40% are neurologically impaired. Disseminated neonatal infection is often fatal in spite of therapy, and survivors are often impaired.

▶ Treatment

A. Specific Measures

HSV is sensitive to antiviral therapy.

1. Topical antivirals—Antiviral agents are effective for corneal disease and include 1% trifluridine, 5% acyclovir, and 3% vidarabine. Trifluridine appears superior; cure rates over 95% are reported. These agents should be used with the guidance of an ophthalmologist.

2. Mucocutaneous HSV infections—These infections respond to administration of oral nucleoside analogues (acyclovir, valacyclovir, or famciclovir). The main indications are severe genital HSV infection in adolescents (see Chapter 42) and severe gingivostomatitis in young children. Antiviral therapy is beneficial for primary disease when begun early. Recurrent disease rarely requires therapy. Frequent genital recurrences may be suppressed by oral administration of nucleoside analogues, but this approach should be used sparingly. Other forms of severe cutaneous disease, such as eczema herpeticum, respond to these antivirals. Intravenous acyclovir may be required when disease is extensive in immunocompromised children (500 mg/m^2 every 8 hours). Oral acyclovir, which is available in suspension, is also used within 72–96 hours for severe primary gingivostomatitis in immunocompetent young children (10 mg/kg per dose four times a day for 5–7 days). Antiviral therapy does not alter the incidence or severity of subsequent recurrences of oral or genital infection. Development of resistance to antivirals is very rare after treating immunocompetent patients, but it is reported in immunocompromised patients who receive frequent and prolonged therapy.

3. Encephalitis—Treatment consists of intravenous acyclovir, 500 mg/m^2 every 8 hours for 21 days.

4. Neonatal infection—Newborns receive intravenous acyclovir, 20 mg/kg every 8 hours for 21 days (14 days if infection is limited to skin, eye, or mouth).

B. General Measures

1. Gingivostomatitis—Gingivostomatitis is treated with pain relief and temperature control measures. Maintaining hydration is important because of the long duration of illness (7–14 days). Nonacidic, cool fluids are best. Topical anesthetic agents (eg, viscous lidocaine or an equal mixture of kaolin–attapulgite [Kaopectate], diphenhydramine, and viscous lidocaine) may be used as a mouthwash for older children who will not swallow it; ingested lidocaine may be toxic to infants or may lead to aspiration. Antiviral therapy is indicated in normal hosts with severe disease. Antibiotics are not helpful.

2. Genital infections—Genital infections require pain relief, assistance with voiding (warm baths, topical anesthetics, rarely catheterization), and psychological support. Lesions should be kept clean; drying may shorten the duration of symptoms. Sexual contact should be avoided during the interval from prodrome to crusting stages. Because of the frequency of asymptomatic shedding, the only effective way to prevent spread is the use of condoms.

3. Cutaneous lesions—Skin lesions should be kept clean, dry, and covered if possible to prevent spread. Systemic analgesics may be helpful. Secondary bacterial infection is uncommon in patients with lesions on the mucosa or involving small areas. Secondary infection should be considered and treated if necessary (usually with an antistaphylococcal agent) in patients with more extensive lesions. Candidal superinfection occurs in 10% of women with primary genital infections.

4. Recurrent cutaneous disease—Recurrent disease is usually milder than primary infection. Sun block lip balm helps prevent labial recurrences after intense sun exposure. There is no evidence that the many popular topical or vitamin therapies are efficacious.

5. Keratoconjunctivitis—An ophthalmologist should be consulted regarding the use of cycloplegics, anti-inflammatory agents, local debridement, and other therapies.

6. Encephalitis—Extensive support will be required for obtunded or comatose patients. Rehabilitation and psychological support are often needed for survivors.

7. Neonatal infection—The affected infant should be isolated and given acyclovir. Cesarean delivery is indicated if the mother has obvious cervical or vaginal lesions, especially if these represent primary infection (35–50% transmission rate). With infants born vaginally to mothers who have active lesions, appropriate cultures should be obtained at 24–48 hours after birth, and the infants should be observed closely. Treatment is given to infants whose culture results are positive or who have suggestive signs or symptoms. Infants born to mothers with obvious primary genital herpes should receive therapy before the culture results are known. For women with a history of genital herpes infection, but no genital lesions, vaginal delivery with peripartum cultures of maternal cervix is the standard. Clinical follow-up of the newborn is recommended when maternal culture results are positive. Repeated cervical cultures during pregnancy are not useful.

Baker DA: Consequences of herpes simplex virus in pregnancy and their prevention. Curr Opinions in Infect Dis 2007;20:73 [PMID: 17197885].

Fatahzadeh M, Schwartz RA: Human herpes simplex virus infections: Epidemiology, pathogenesis, symptomatology, diagnosis, and management. J Am Acad Dermatol 2007;57:737 [PMID: 17939933].

Kimberlin DW: Herpes simplex virus infections of the newborn. Semin Perinatol 2007;19:19 [PMID: 17317423].

VARICELLA & HERPES ZOSTER

ESSENTIALS OF DIAGNOSIS & TYPICAL FEATURES

▶ Varicella (chickenpox):

- Exposure to varicella or herpes zoster 10–21 days previously; no prior history of varicella.
- Widely scattered red macules and papules concentrated on the face and trunk, rapidly progressing to clear vesicles on an erythematous base, pustules, and then crusting, over 5–6 days.
- Variable fever and nonspecific systemic symptoms.

▶ Herpes zoster (shingles):

- History of varicella.
- Dermatomal paresthesias and pain prior to eruption (more common in older children).
- Dermatomal distribution of grouped vesicles on an erythematous base.

General Considerations

Primary infection with varicella-zoster virus results in varicella, which almost always confers lifelong immunity; the virus remains latent in sensory ganglia. Herpes zoster, which represents reactivation of this latent virus, occurs in 20% of individuals some time in their life. The incidence of herpes zoster is highest in elderly individuals and in immunosuppressed patients. Spread of varicella from a contact is by respiratory secretions or fomites from vesicles or pustules, with a greater than 90% infection rate in susceptible persons. Exposure to herpes zoster is about one third as likely to cause varicella in a susceptible host. Over 95% of young adults with a history of varicella are immune, as are 90% of native-born Americans who are unaware of having had varicella. Many individuals from tropical or subtropical areas never have childhood exposure and remain susceptible through early adulthood. Humans are the only reservoir.

Clinical Findings

Exposure to varicella or herpes zoster has usually occurred 14–16 days previously (range, 10–21 days). Contact may not have been recognized, since the index case of varicella is infectious 1–2 days before rash appears. Although varicella is the most distinctive childhood exanthem, inexperienced observers may mistake other diseases for varicella. A 1- to 3-day prodrome of fever, respiratory symptoms, and headache may occur, especially in older children. The preeruptive pain of herpes zoster may last several days and be mistaken for other illnesses.

A. Symptoms and Signs

1. Varicella—The usual case consists of mild systemic symptoms followed by crops of red macules that rapidly become small vesicles with surrounding erythema (described as a "dew drop on a rose petal"), form pustules, become crusted, and then scab over and leave no scar. The rash appears predominantly on the trunk and face. Lesions occur in the scalp, and sometimes occur in the nose, mouth (where they are nonspecific ulcers), conjunctiva, and vagina. The magnitude of systemic symptoms usually parallels skin involvement. Up to five crops of lesions may be seen. New crops usually stop forming after 5–7 days. Pruritus is often intense. If varicella occurs in the first few months of life, it is often mild as a result of persisting maternal antibody. Once crusting begins, the patient is no longer contagious.

2. Herpes zoster—The eruption of shingles involves a single dermatome, usually truncal or cranial. The rash does not cross the midline. Ophthalmic zoster may be associated with corneal involvement. The closely grouped vesicles, which resemble a localized version of varicella or herpes simplex, often coalesce. Crusting occurs in 7–10 days. Postherpetic neuralgia is rare in children. A few vesicles are occasionally seen outside the involved dermatome. Herpes zoster is a common problem in HIV-infected or other immunocompromised children. Herpes zoster is also common in children who had varicella in early infancy or whose mothers had varicella during pregnancy.

B. Laboratory Findings

Leukocyte counts are normal or low. Leukocytosis suggests secondary bacterial infection. The virus can be identified by fluorescent antibody staining of a lesion smear. Rapid culture methods take 48 hours. Diagnosis made with paired serology is not clinically useful. Serum aminotransferase levels may be modestly elevated during normal varicella.

C. Imaging

Varicella pneumonia classically produces numerous bilateral nodular densities and hyperinflation. This is very rare in immunocompetent children. Abnormal chest radiographs are seen more frequently in adults.

Differential Diagnosis

Varicella is usually distinctive. Similar rashes include those of coxsackievirus infection (fewer lesions, lack of crusting), impetigo (fewer lesions, smaller area, no classic vesicles, positive Gram stain, perioral or peripheral lesions), papular urticaria (insect bite history, nonvesicular rash), scabies (burrows, no typical vesicles; failure to resolve), parapsoriasis (rare in children younger than age 10 years, chronic or recurrent, often a history of prior varicella), rickettsialpox (eschar where the mite bites, smaller lesions, no crusting), dermatitis herpetiformis (chronic, urticaria, residual pigmentation), and folliculitis. Herpes zoster is sometimes confused with a linear eruption of herpes simplex or a contact dermatitis (eg, *Rhus* dermatitis).

Complications & Sequelae

A. Varicella

Secondary bacterial infection with staphylococci or group A streptococci is most common, presenting as impetigo, cellulitis or fasciitis, abscesses, scarlet fever, or sepsis. Bacterial superinfection occurs in 2–3% of children. Before a vaccine became available, hospitalization rates associated with varicella were 1:750–1:1000 cases in children and 10-fold higher in adults.

Protracted vomiting or a change in sensorium suggests Reye syndrome or encephalitis. Because Reye syndrome usually occurs in patients who are also using salicylates, these should be avoided in patients with varicella. Encephalitis occurs in less than 0.1% of cases, usually in the first week of illness, and is usually limited to cerebellitis with ataxia, which resolves completely. Diffuse encephalitis can be severe.

Varicella pneumonia usually afflicts immunocompromised children (especially those with leukemia or lymphoma or those receiving high doses of corticosteroids or chemotherapy) and adults; pregnant women may be at special risk. Cough, dyspnea, tachypnea, rales, and cyanosis occur several days after onset of rash. Varicella may be life-threatening in immunosuppressed patients. In addition to pneumonitis, their disease may be complicated by hepatitis and encephalitis. Varicella exposure in such patients must be evaluated immediately for postexposure prophylaxis (see Chapter 9).

Hemorrhagic varicella lesions may be seen without other complications. This is most often caused by autoimmune thrombocytopenia, but hemorrhagic lesions can occasionally represent idiopathic disseminated intravascular coagulation (purpura fulminans).

Neonates born to mothers who develop varicella from 5 days before to 2 days after delivery are at high risk for severe or fatal (5%) disease and must be given varicella-zoster immune globulin (VZIG) and followed closely (see Chapter 9).

Varicella occurring during the first 20 weeks of pregnancy may cause (2% incidence) congenital infection associated with cicatricial skin lesions, associated limb anomalies, and cortical atrophy.

Unusual complications of varicella include optic neuritis, myocarditis, transverse myelitis, orchitis, and arthritis.

B. Herpes Zoster

Complications of herpes zoster include secondary bacterial infection, motor or cranial nerve paralysis (cases in adults), encephalitis, keratitis, and dissemination in immunosuppressed patients. These complications are rare in immunocompetent children, and they do not develop prolonged pain. Postherpetic neuralgia does occur in immunocompromised children.

▷ Prevention

VZIG is available for postexposure prevention of varicella in high-risk susceptible persons (see Chapter 9). Postexposure prophylaxis with acyclovir is effective when it is started at 8 or 9 days after exposure and is continued for 7 days. Varicella vaccine is also useful for postexposure prophylaxis when given within 3–5 days of the exposure. Two doses of the live attenuated varicella vaccine are now part of routine childhood immunization, and "catch-up" immunization is recommended for all other susceptible children and adults.

▷ Treatment

A. General Measures

Supportive measures include maintenance of hydration, administration of acetaminophen for discomfort, cool soaks or antipruritics for itching (diphenhydramine, 1.25 mg/kg every 6 hours, or hydroxyzine, 0.5 mg/kg every 6 hours), and observance of general hygiene measures (keep nails trimmed and skin clean). Care must be taken to avoid overdosage with antihistaminic agents. Topical or systemic antibiotics may be needed for bacterial superinfection.

B. Specific Measures

Although acyclovir is more active against herpes simplex, it is the preferred drug for varicella and herpes zoster infections. Recommended parenteral acyclovir dosage for severe disease is 10 mg/kg (500 mg/m^2) intravenously every 8 hours, each dose infused over 1 hour. Parenteral therapy should be started early in immunosuppressed patients or high-risk infected neonates. VZIG is of no value for established disease. The effect of oral acyclovir (80 mg/kg/d, divided in four doses) on varicella in immunocompetent children was modestly beneficial and nontoxic, but only when administered within 24 hour after the onset of varicella. Oral acyclovir should be used selectively in immunocompetent children (eg, when intercurrent illness is present; possibly when second attacks occur in the household or when the patient is an adolescent—both of which are associated with more severe disease) and in children with underlying chronic illnesses. Valacyclovir and famciclovir are superior antiviral agents because of better absorption; only acyclovir is available as a pediatric suspension. Herpes zoster in an immunocompromised child should be treated with intravenous acyclovir when it is severe, but oral valacyclovir or famciclovir can be used in immunocompromised children when the nature of the illness and the immune status support this decision.

▷ Prognosis

Except for secondary bacterial infections, serious complications are rare and recovery complete in immunocompetent hosts.

Marin M et al; Centers for Disease Control and Prevention (CDC): Prevention of varicella: Recommendations of the Advisory Committee on Immunization Practices (ACIP). MMWR Recomm Rep 2007;56(RR-4):1 [PMID: 17585291].

ROSEOLA INFANTUM (EXANTHEM SUBITUM)

ESSENTIALS OF DIAGNOSIS & TYPICAL FEATURES

▶ High fever in a child aged 6–36 months.
▶ Minimal toxicity.
▶ Rose-pink maculopapular rash appears when fever subsides.

▷ General Considerations

Roseola infantum is a benign illness caused by human herpesviruses 6 (HHV-6) or 7 (HHV-7). HHV-6 is a major cause of acute febrile illness in young children. Its significance is its ability to mimic more serious causes of high fever and its role in inciting febrile seizures.

Clinical Findings

The most prominent historical feature is the abrupt onset of fever, often reaching 40.6°C, which lasts up to 8 days (mean, 4 days) in an otherwise mildly ill child. The fever then ceases abruptly, and a characteristic rash may appear. Roseola occurs predominantly in children aged 6 months to 3 years, with 90% of cases occurring before the second year. HHV-7 infection tends to occur somewhat later in childhood. These viruses are the most common recognized cause of exanthematous fever in this age group and are responsible for 20% of emergency department visits by children aged 6–12 months.

A. Symptoms and Signs

Mild lethargy and irritability may be present, but generally there is a dissociation between systemic symptoms and the febrile course. The pharynx, tonsils, and tympanic membranes may be injected. Conjunctivitis and pharyngeal exudate are notably absent. Diarrhea and vomiting occur in one third of patients. Adenopathy of the head and neck often occurs. The anterior fontanelle is bulging in one quarter of HHV-6-infected infants. If rash appears (20–30% incidence), it begins on the trunk and spreads to the face, neck, and extremities. Rose-pink macules or maculopapules, 2–3 mm in diameter, are nonpruritic, tend to coalesce, and disappear in 1–2 days without pigmentation or desquamation. Rash may occur without fever.

B. Laboratory Findings

Leukopenia and lymphocytopenia are present early. Laboratory evidence of hepatitis occurs in some patients, especially adults.

Differential Diagnosis

The initial high fever may require exclusion of serious bacterial infection. The relative well-being of most children and the typical course and rash soon clarify the diagnosis. The erythrocyte sedimentation rate is normal. If the child has a febrile seizure, it is important to exclude bacterial meningitis. The CSF is normal in children with roseola. In children who receive antibiotics or other medication at the beginning of the fever, the rash may be attributed incorrectly to drug allergy.

Complications & Sequelae

Febrile seizures occur in 10% of patients (even higher percentages in those with HHV-7 infections). There is evidence that HHV-6 can directly infect the central nervous system, causing meningoencephalitis or aseptic meningitis. Multiorgan disease (pneumonia, hepatitis, bone marrow suppression, encephalitis) may occur in immunocompromised patients.

Treatment & Prognosis

Fever is managed readily with acetaminophen and sponge baths. Fever control should be a major consideration in

children with a history of febrile seizures. Roseola infantum is otherwise entirely benign.

Dyer JA: Childhood viral exanthems. Pediatr Ann 2007;36:21 [PMID: 17269280].

War KN: The natural history and laboratory diagnosis of human herpesviruses-6 and -7 infections in the immunocompetent. J Clin Virol 2005;32:183 [PMID: 15722023].

CYTOMEGALOVIRUS INFECTIONS

ESSENTIALS OF DIAGNOSIS & TYPICAL FEATURES

▶ Primary infection:
- Asymptomatic or minor illness in young children.
- Mononucleosis-like syndrome without pharyngitis in postpubertal individuals.

▶ Congenital infection:
- Intrauterine growth retardation.
- Microcephaly with intracerebral calcifications and seizures.
- Retinitis and encephalitis.
- Hepatosplenomegaly with thrombocytopenia.
- "Blueberry muffin" rash.
- Sensorineural deafness.

▶ Immunocompromised hosts:
- Retinitis and encephalitis.
- Pneumonitis.
- Enteritis and hepatitis.
- Bone marrow suppression.

General Considerations

Cytomegalovirus (CMV) is a ubiquitous herpesvirus transmitted by many routes. It can be acquired in utero following maternal viremia or postpartum from birth canal secretions or maternal milk. Young children are infected by the saliva of playmates; older individuals are infected by sexual partners (eg, from saliva, vaginal secretions, or semen). Transfused blood products and transplanted organs can be a source of CMV infection. Clinical illness is determined largely by the patient's immune competence. Immunocompetent individuals usually develop a mild self-limited illness, whereas immunocompromised children can develop severe, progressive, often multiorgan disease. In-utero infection can be teratogenic.

1. In-Utero Cytomegalovirus Infection

Approximately 0.5–1.5% of children are born with CMV infections acquired during maternal viremia. CMV infection is asymptomatic in over 90% of these children, who are usually born to mothers who had experienced reactivation of latent CMV infection during the pregnancy. Symptomatic infection occurs predominantly in infants born to mothers with primary CMV infection but can also result from recurrent, most likely, reinfection during pregnancy. Even when exposed to a primary maternal infection, less than 50% of fetuses are infected, and in only 10% of those infants is the infection symptomatic at birth. Primary infection in the first half of pregnancy poses the greatest risk for severe fetal damage.

▶ Clinical Findings

A. Symptoms and Signs

Severely affected infants are born ill; they are often small for gestational age, floppy, and lethargic. They feed poorly and have poor temperature control. Hepatosplenomegaly, jaundice, petechiae, seizures, and microcephaly are common. Characteristic signs are a distinctive chorioretinitis and periventricular calcification. A purpuric (so-called blueberry muffin) rash similar to that seen with congenital rubella may be present. The mortality rate is 10–20%. Survivors usually have significant sequelae, especially mental retardation, neurologic deficits, retinopathy, and hearing loss. Isolated hepatosplenomegaly or thrombocytopenia may occur. Even mildly affected children may subsequently manifest mental retardation and psychomotor delay. However, most infected infants (90%) are born to mothers with preexisting immunity who had a reactivation of latent CMV during pregnancy. These children have no clinical manifestations at birth. Of these, 10–15% develop sensorineural hearing loss, which is often bilateral and may appear several years after birth.

B. Laboratory Findings

In severely ill infants, anemia, thrombocytopenia, hyperbilirubinemia, and elevated aminotransferase levels are common. Lymphocytosis occurs occasionally. Pleocytosis and an elevated protein concentration are found in CSF. The diagnosis is readily confirmed by isolation of CMV from urine or saliva within 48 hours, using rapid culture methods combined with immunoassay. The presence in the infant of IgM-specific CMV antibodies suggests the diagnosis. Some commercial ELISA kits are 90% sensitive and specific for these antibodies.

C. Imaging

Head radiologic examinations may show microcephaly, periventricular calcifications, and ventricular dilation. These findings strongly correlate with neurologic sequelae and retardation. Long bone radiographs may show the "celery stalk" pattern characteristic of congenital viral infections. Interstitial pneumonia may be present.

▶ Differential Diagnosis

CMV infection should be considered in any newborn who is seriously ill shortly after birth, especially once bacterial sepsis, metabolic disease, intracranial bleeding, and cardiac disease have been excluded. Other congenital infections to be considered in the differential diagnosis include toxoplasmosis (serology, more diffuse calcification of the CNS, specific type of retinitis, macrocephaly), rubella (serology, specific type of retinitis, cardiac lesions, eye abnormalities), enteroviral infections (time of year, maternal illness, severe hepatitis), herpes simplex (skin lesions, cultures, severe hepatitis), and syphilis (serology for both infant and mother, skin lesions, bone involvement).

▶ Prevention & Treatment

Support is rarely required for anemia and thrombocytopenia. Most children with symptoms at birth have significant neurologic, intellectual, visual, or auditory impairment. Ganciclovir, 5 mg/kg every 12 hours, is recommended for children with severe, life- or sight-threatening disease, or if end-organ disease recurs or progresses. Duration is 2–3 weeks or until symptoms resolve. This approach decreases viral shedding and limits progression of symptoms, including hearing loss, during treatment. However, the therapeutic advantage is progressively lost over time after treatment is discontinued. Children who are asymptomatic at birth have a 6–23% incidence of hearing loss. Children with positive CMV blood PCR results during the first month of life are more likely to develop hearing loss. Studies are currently ongoing to determine if early treatment prevents late-onset hearing loss.

Recent developments in the diagnosis of primary CMV infection during pregnancy using anti-CMV IgM and low-avidity IgG assays followed by quantitative CMV PCR testing of the amniotic fluid at 20–24 weeks' gestation have made possible the diagnosis of congenital CMV infection before birth. Many pregnant women elect to terminate gestation under these circumstances, but a recent study has also shown that passive immunoprophylaxis with hyperimmune CMV IgG may prevent development of congenital disease.

2. Perinatal Cytomegalovirus Infection

CMV infection can be acquired from birth canal secretions or shortly after birth from maternal milk. In some socioeconomic groups, 10–20% of infants are infected at birth and excrete CMV for many months. Infection can also be acquired in the postnatal period from unscreened transfused blood products.

▶ Clinical Findings

A. Symptoms and Signs

Ninety percent of immunocompetent infants infected by their mothers at birth develop subclinical illness (ie, virus excretion only) or a minor illness within 1–3 months. The remainder develop an illness lasting several weeks and characterized by hepatosplenomegaly, lymphadenopathy, and interstitial pneumonitis in various combinations. The severity of the pneumonitis may be increased by the simultaneous presence of *Chlamydia trachomatis*. Infants who receive blood products are often premature and immunologically impaired. If they are born to CMV-negative mothers and subsequently receive CMV-containing blood, they frequently develop severe infection and pneumonia after a 2- to 6-week incubation period.

B. Laboratory Findings

Lymphocytosis, atypical lymphocytes, anemia, and thrombocytopenia may be present, especially in premature infants. Liver function is abnormal. CMV can be isolated from urine and saliva. Secretions obtained at bronchoscopy contain CMV and epithelial cells bearing CMV antigens. Serum levels of CMV antibody rise significantly.

C. Imaging

Chest radiographs show a diffuse interstitial pneumonitis in severely affected infants.

▶ Differential Diagnosis

CMV infection should be considered as a cause of any prolonged illness in early infancy, especially if hepatosplenomegaly, lymphadenopathy, or atypical lymphocytosis is present. This must be distinguished from granulomatous or malignant diseases and from congenital infections (syphilis, toxoplasmosis, hepatitis B) not previously diagnosed. Other viruses (Epstein-Barr virus [EBV], HIV, adenovirus) can cause this syndrome. CMV is a recognized cause of viral pneumonia in this age group. Because asymptomatic CMV excretion is common in early infancy, care must be taken to establish the diagnosis and to rule out concomitant pathogens such as *Chlamydia* and RSV. Severe CMV infection in early infancy may indicate that the child has a congenital or acquired immune deficiency.

▶ Prevention & Treatment

The self-limited disease of normal infants requires no therapy. Severe pneumonitis in premature infants requires oxygen administration and often intubation. Very ill infants should receive ganciclovir (6 mg/kg every 12 hours). CMV infection acquired by transfusion can be prevented by excluding CMV-seropositive blood donors. Milk donors should also be screened for prior CMV infection. It is likely that high-risk infants receiving large doses of IVIG for other reasons will be protected against severe CMV disease.

3. Cytomegalovirus Infection Acquired in Childhood & Adolescence

Young children are readily infected by playmates, especially because CMV continues to be excreted in saliva and urine for

many months after infection. The cumulative annual incidence of CMV excretion by children in day care centers exceeds 75%. In fact, young children in a family are often the source of primary CMV infection of their mothers during subsequent pregnancies. An additional peak of CMV infection takes place when adolescents become sexually active. Sporadic acquisition of CMV occurs after blood transfusion and transplantation.

▶ Clinical Findings

A. Symptoms and Signs

Most young children who acquire CMV are asymptomatic or have a minor febrile illness, occasionally with adenopathy. They provide an important reservoir of virus shedders that facilitates spread of CMV. Occasionally a child may have prolonged fever with hepatosplenomegaly and adenopathy. Older children and adults, many of whom are infected during sexual activity, are more likely to be symptomatic in this fashion and can present with a syndrome that mimics the infectious mononucleosis syndrome that follows EBV infection (1–2 weeks of fever, malaise, anorexia, splenomegaly, mild hepatitis, and some adenopathy; see next section). This syndrome can also occur 2–4 weeks after transfusion of CMV-infected blood.

B. Laboratory Findings

In the CMV mononucleosis syndrome, lymphocytosis and atypical lymphocytes are common, as is a mild rise in aminotransferase levels. CMV is present in saliva and urine, and CMV DNA can be uniformly detected in plasma or blood.

▶ Differential Diagnosis

In older children, CMV infection should be included as a possible cause of fever of unknown origin, especially when lymphocytosis and atypical lymphocytes are present. CMV infection is distinguished from EBV infection by the absence of pharyngitis, the relatively minor adenopathy, and the absence of serologic evidence of acute EBV infection. Mononucleosis syndromes also are caused by *Toxoplasma gondii*, rubella virus, adenovirus, hepatitis A virus, and HIV.

▶ Prevention

Screening of transfused blood or filtering blood (thus removing CMV-containing white blood cells) prevents cases related to this source.

4. Cytomegalovirus Infection in Immunocompromised Children

In addition to symptoms experienced during primary infection, immunocompromised hosts develop symptoms with reinfection or reactivation of latent CMV. This is clearly seen in children with acquired immunodeficiency syndrome (AIDS), after transplantation, or with congenital immunodeficiencies. However, in most immunocompromised patients, primary infection is more likely to cause severe symptoms than is reactivation or reinfection. The severity of the resulting disease is generally proportionate to the degree of immunosuppression.

Clinical Findings

A. Symptoms and Signs

A mild febrile illness with myalgia, malaise, and arthralgia may occur, especially with reactivation disease. Severe disease often includes subacute onset of dyspnea and cyanosis as manifestations of interstitial pneumonitis. Auscultation reveals only coarse breath sounds and scattered rales. A rapid respiratory rate may precede clinical or radiographic evidence of pneumonia. Hepatitis without jaundice or hepatomegaly is common. Diarrhea, which can be severe, occurs with CMV colitis, and CMV can cause esophagitis with symptoms of odynophagia or dysphagia. These enteropathies are most common in AIDS, as is the presence of a retinitis that often progresses to blindness. Encephalitis and polyradiculitis also occur in AIDS.

B. Laboratory Findings

Neutropenia and thrombocytopenia are common. Atypical lymphocytosis is infrequent. Serum aminotransferase levels are often elevated. The stools may contain occult blood if enteropathy is present. CMV is readily isolated from saliva, urine, buffy coat, and bronchial secretions. Results are available in 48 hours. Interpretation of positive cultures is made difficult by asymptomatic shedding of CMV in saliva and urine in many immunocompromised patients. CMV disease correlates more closely with the presence of CMV in the blood or lung lavage fluid. Monitoring for the appearance of CMV DNA in plasma or CMV antigen in blood mononuclear cells is used as a guide to early antiviral ("preemptive") therapy.

C. Imaging

Bilateral interstitial pneumonitis is present on chest radiographs.

Differential Diagnosis

The initial febrile illness must be distinguished from treatable bacterial or fungal infection. Similarly the pulmonary disease must be distinguished from intrapulmonary hemorrhage; drug-induced or radiation pneumonitis; pulmonary edema; and bacterial, fungal, parasitic, and other viruses infection in this population. CMV infection is seen bilaterally and interstitially on chest radiographs, cough is nonproductive, chest pain is absent, and the patient is not usually toxic. *Pneumocystis jiroveci* (formerly *Pneumocystis carinii*) infection may have a similar presentation. These patients may have polymi-

crobial disease. It is suspected that bacterial and fungal infections are enhanced by the neutropenia that can accompany CMV infection. Infection of the gastrointestinal tract is diagnosed by endoscopy. This will exclude candidal, adenoviral, and herpes simplex infections and allows tissue confirmation of CMV-induced mucosal ulcerations.

Prevention & Treatment

Blood donors should be screened to exclude those with prior CMV infection, or blood should be filtered. Ideally, seronegative transplant recipients should receive organs from seronegative donors. Severe symptoms, most commonly pneumonitis, often respond to early therapy with intravenous ganciclovir (5 mg/kg every 12 hours for 14–21 days). Neutropenia is a frequent side effect of this therapy. Foscarnet and cidofovir are alternative therapeutic agents recommended for patients with ganciclovir-resistant virus. Prophylactic use of oral or intravenous ganciclovir or foscarnet may prevent CMV infections in organ transplant recipients. A new drug with an excellent safety profile, maribavir, has shown efficacy in hematopoietic stem cell recipients. Additional studies are being conducted in solid organ transplant recipients. Preemptive therapy can be used in transplant recipients by monitoring CMV blood PCR and instituting therapy when the results reach a certain threshold regardless of clinical signs or symptoms. CMV-seropositive children with AIDS and low CD4 counts (< 50/μL) should have funduscopic examinations and plasma CMV DNA measurements every 3 months.

Bradford RD et al: Detection of cytomegalovirus (CMV) DNA by polymerase chain reaction is associated with hearing loss in newborns with symptomatic congenital CMV infection involving the central nervous system. J Infect Dis 2005;191:227 [PMID: 15609232].

Fowler KB, Boppana SB: Congenital cytomegalovirus (CMV) infection and hearing deficit. J Clin Virol 2006;35:226 [PMID: 16386462].

Nigro G et al: Passive immunization during pregnancy for congenital cytomegalovirus infection. N Engl J Med 2005;353:1350 [PMID: 16192480].

INFECTIOUS MONONUCLEOSIS (EPSTEIN-BARR VIRUS)

ESSENTIALS OF DIAGNOSIS & TYPICAL FEATURES

► Prolonged fever.

► Exudative pharyngitis.

► Generalized adenopathy.

► Hepatosplenomegaly.

► Atypical lymphocytes.

► Heterophil antibodies.

General Considerations

Mononucleosis is the most characteristic syndrome produced by EBV infection. Young children infected with EBV have either no symptoms or a mild nonspecific febrile illness. As the age of the host increases, EBV infection is more likely to produce the typical features of the mononucleosis syndrome in 20–25% of infected adolescents. EBV is acquired readily from asymptomatic carriers (15–20% of whom excrete the virus in saliva on any given day) and from recently ill patients, who excrete virus for many months. Young children are infected from the saliva of playmates and family members. Adolescents may be infected through sexual activity. EBV can also be transmitted by blood transfusion and organ transplantation.

Clinical Findings

A. Symptoms and Signs

After an incubation period of 1–2 months, a 2- to 3-day prodrome of malaise and anorexia yields, abruptly or insidiously, to a febrile illness with temperatures exceeding 39°C. The major complaint is pharyngitis, which is often (50%) exudative. Lymph nodes are enlarged, firm, and mildly tender. Any area may be affected, but posterior and anterior cervical nodes are almost always enlarged. Splenomegaly is present in 50–75% of patients. Hepatomegaly is common (30%), and the liver is frequently tender. Five percent of patients have a rash, which can be macular, scarlatiniform, or urticarial. Rash is almost universal in patients taking penicillin or ampicillin. Soft palate petechiae and eyelid edema are also observed.

B. Laboratory Findings

1. Peripheral blood—Leukopenia may occur early, but an atypical lymphocytosis (comprising over 10% of the total leukocytes at some time in the illness) is most notable. Hematologic changes may not be seen until the third week of illness and may be entirely absent in some EBV syndromes (eg, neurologic ones).

2. Heterophil antibodies—These nonspecific antibodies appear in over 90% of older patients with mononucleosis but in fewer than 50% of children younger than age 5 years. They may not be detectable until the second week of illness and may persist for up to 12 months after recovery. Rapid screening tests (slide agglutination) are usually positive if the titer is significant; a positive result strongly suggests but does not prove EBV infection.

3. Anti-EBV antibodies—It may be necessary to measure specific antibody titers when heterophil antibodies fail to appear, as in young children. Acute EBV infection is established by detecting IgM antibody to the viral capsid antigen (VCA) or by detecting a fall over several weeks of IgG anti-VCA titers (IgG antibody peaks by the time symptoms appear).

4. EBV PCR—This assay detects EBV DNA. It is the method of choice for the diagnosis of CNS and ocular infections. Quantitative EBV PCR in peripheral blood mononuclear cells has been used to detect EBV-related lymphoproliferative disorders in transplant patients.

Differential Diagnosis

Severe pharyngitis may suggest group A streptococcal infection. Enlargement of only the anterior cervical lymph nodes, a neutrophilic leukocytosis, and the absence of splenomegaly suggest bacterial infection. Although a child with a positive throat culture result for streptococcus usually requires therapy, up to 10% of children with mononucleosis are asymptomatic streptococcal carriers. In this group, penicillin therapy is unnecessary and often causes a rash. Severe primary herpes simplex pharyngitis, occurring in adolescence, may also mimic infectious mononucleosis. In this type of pharyngitis, some anterior mouth ulcerations should suggest the correct diagnosis. EBV infection should be considered in the differential diagnosis of any perplexing prolonged febrile illness. Similar illnesses that produce atypical lymphocytosis include rubella (pharyngitis not prominent, shorter illness, less adenopathy and splenomegaly), adenovirus (upper respiratory symptoms and cough, conjunctivitis, less adenopathy, fewer atypical lymphocytes), hepatitis A or B (more severe liver function abnormalities, no pharyngitis, no lymphadenopathy), and toxoplasmosis (negative heterophil test, less pharyngitis). Serum sickness-like drug reactions and leukemia (smear morphology is important) may be confused with infectious mononucleosis. CMV mononucleosis is a close mimic except for minimal pharyngitis and less adenopathy; it is much less common. Serologic tests for EBV and CMV should clarify the correct diagnosis. The acute initial manifestation of HIV infection is a mononucleosis-like syndrome in many patients.

Complications

Splenic rupture is a rare complication, which usually follows significant trauma. Hematologic complications, including hemolytic anemia, thrombocytopenia, and neutropenia, are more common. Neurologic involvement can include aseptic meningitis, encephalitis, isolated neuropathy such as Bell palsy, and Guillain-Barré syndrome. Any of these may appear prior to or in the absence of the more typical signs and symptoms of infectious mononucleosis. Rare complications include myocarditis, pericarditis, and atypical pneumonia. Recurrence or persistence of EBV-associated symptoms for 6 months or longer characterizes chronic active EBV. This disease is due to continuous viral replication and warrants specific antiviral therapy. Rarely EBV infection becomes a progressive lymphoproliferative disorder characterized by persistent fever, multiple organ involvement, neutropenia or pancytopenia, and agammaglobulinemia. Hemocytophagia is often present in the bone marrow. An X-linked genetic defect in immune response has been inferred for some patients (Duncan syndrome, X-linked lymphoproliferative disorder). Children with other congenital immunodeficiencies or chemotherapy-induced immunosuppression can also develop progressive EBV infection, EBV-associated lymphoproliferative disorder or lymphoma, and other malignancies.

▶ Treatment & Prognosis

Bed rest may be necessary in severe cases. Acetaminophen controls high fever. Potential airway obstruction due to swollen pharyngeal lymphoid tissue responds rapidly to systemic corticosteroids. Corticosteroids may also be given for hematologic and neurologic complications, although no controlled trials have proved their efficacy in these conditions. Fever and pharyngitis disappear by 10–14 days. Adenopathy and splenomegaly can persist several weeks longer. Some patients complain of fatigue, malaise, or lack of well-being for several months. Although corticosteroids may shorten the duration of fatigue and malaise, their long-term effects on this potentially oncogenic viral infection are unknown, and indiscriminate use is discouraged. Patients with splenic enlargement should avoid contact sports for 6–8 weeks. Acyclovir, valacyclovir, penciclovir, ganciclovir, and foscarnet are active against EBV and are indicated in the treatment of chronic active EBV.

Management of EBV-related lymphoproliferative disorders relies primarily on decreasing the immunosuppression whenever possible. Adjunctive therapy with acyclovir, ganciclovir, or another antiviral active against EBV as well as CMV hyperimmune globulin has been used without scientific evidence of efficacy.

Higgins CD et al: A study of risk factors for acquisition of Epstein-Barr virus and its subtypes. J Infect Dis 2007;195:474 [PMID: 17230406].
Nystad TW, Myrmel H: Prevalence of primary versus reactivated Epstein-Barr virus infection in patients with VCA IgG-, VCA IgM- and EBNA-1-antibodies and suspected infectious mononucleosis. J Clin Virol 2007;38:292 [PMID: 17336144].

VIRAL INFECTIONS SPREAD BY INSECT VECTORS

In the United States, mosquitoes are the most common insect vectors that spread viral infections (Table 38–4). As a consequence, these infections—and others that are spread by ticks—tend to occur as summer–fall epidemics that coincide with the seasonal breeding and feeding habits of the vector, and the etiologic agent varies by region. Thus a careful travel and exposure history is critical for correct diagnostic workup.

ENCEPHALITIS

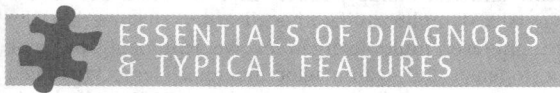

ESSENTIALS OF DIAGNOSIS & TYPICAL FEATURES

▶ Fever and headache.

▶ Change in mental status or behavior (or both), with or without focal neurologic deficits.

▶ CSF shows a mononuclear cell pleocytosis, elevated protein level, and normal glucose level.

Encephalitis is a common severe manifestation of many infections spread by insects (see Table 38–4). With many viral pathogens, the infection is most often subclinical, or mild CNS disease such as meningitis is present. These infections have some distinguishing features in terms of subclinical infection rate, unique neurologic syndromes, associated non-neurologic symptoms, and prognosis. The diagnosis is generally made clinically during recognized outbreaks and is confirmed by virus-specific serology. Prevention consists of control of mosquito vectors and precautions with proper clothing and insect repellents to minimize mosquito and tick bites.

West Nile Virus Encephalitis

This flavivirus is the most important arbovirus infection in the United States. Since it was described in 1999 in New York, it has spread to 47 states. In 2007, West Nile virus caused more than 3300 clinically apparent infections, more than 1000 nervous system infections, and 95 deaths. Its reservoir includes more than 160 species of birds whose migration explain the rapid growth of the epidemic. During summer–fall epidemics most infected individuals are asymptomatic. Approximately 20% develop West Nile fever, which is characterized by fever, headache, retro-orbital pain, nausea and vomiting, lymphadenopathy, and a maculopapular rash (20–50%). Less than 1% of infected patients develop meningitis or encephalitis, but 10% of these cases are fatal (0.1% of all infections). The major risk factor for severe disease is age older than 50 years and immune compromise, although children develop West Nile fever and occasionally have neurologic disease. The neurologic manifestations are most often those found with other encephalitides. However, distinguishing atypical features include polio-like flaccid paralysis, movement disorders (parkinsonism, tremor, myoclonus), brainstem symptoms, polyneuropathy, and optic neuritis. Muscle weakness, facial palsy, and hyporeflexia are common (20% of each finding). Diagnosis is best made by detecting IgM antibody (EIA) to the virus in CSF. This will be present by 2–3 days (95%) after onset. PCR is a specific diagnostic tool but is less sensitive than antibody detection. Antibody rise in serum can also be used for diagnosis.

Treatment is supportive, although various antivirals and specific immune globulin are being studied. The infection is not spread between contacts, but is spread by donated organs and blood and breast milk and transplacentally. The coming years will indicate if this virus will become a serious endemic problem in the United States.

Truemper EJ, Romero JR: West Nile virus. Pediatr Ann 2007;36:414 [PMID: 17691625].

Table 38–4. Some viral diseases spread by insects in the United States.

Disease	Natural Reservoir (Vector)	Geographic Distribution	Incubation Period	Clinical Presentations	Laboratory Findings	Complications, Sequelae	Diagnosis, Therapy, Comments
Flaviviruses							
St. Louis encephalitis (SLE)	Birds (Culex mosquitoes)	Southern Canada, central and southern United States, Caribbean, South America	2–5 d (up to 3 wk)	Abrupt onset of fever, chills, headache, nausea, vomiting; may develop generalized weakness, seizures, coma, ataxia, cranial nerve palsies. Aseptic meningitis is common in children.	Modest leukocytosis, neutrophilia, elevated liver enzymes. CSF: 100–200 WBCs/μL (PMNs predominate early).	Mortality rate 2–5% at age < 5 or > 50 years. Neurologic sequelae in 1–20%.	~35 cases/y, < 2% symptomatic. (Worse in elderly.) Therapy: supportive. Diagnosis: serology. Specific antibody often present within 5 d.
Dengue	Humans (Aedes mosquitoes)	Asia, Africa, Central and South America, Caribbean; observed in Texas/Mexico border area	4–7 d (range, 3–14 d)	Fever, headache, myalgia, joint and bone pain, retroocular pain, nausea and vomiting; maculopapular or petechial rash in 50%, sparing palms and soles; adenopathy. Meningoencephalitis in 5–10% of children.	Leukopenia, thrombocytopenia. CSF: 100–500 mononuclear cells/μL if neurologic signs are present.	Hemorrhagic fever, shock syndrome, prolonged weakness.	High infection rate. 50–150 cases occur in U.S. travelers to endemic areas. Biphasic course may occur. Therapy: supportive. Diagnosis: serology; IgM-EIA antibody by day 6.
West Nile	Birds (Culex mosquitoes); small mammals	North Africa, Middle East, parts of Asia, Europe, continental United States	3–12 d	Abrupt onset of fever, headache, sore throat, myalgia, retroocular pain, conjunctivitis; 20–50% with rash; adenopathy. Encephalitis may be accompanied by muscle weakness, flaccid paralysis, or movement disorders.	Mild leukocytosis; 10–15% lymphopenic; moderate CSF pleocytosis.	Mortality rate 10%, of those with CNS symptoms, especially in elderly; weakness and myalgia may persist for an extended period.	Most important mosquito-borne encephalitis in the United States. Diagnosis: IgM-EIA serology; cross-reacts with St. Louis encephalitis; positive by 2–3 d after onset of CNS symptoms. Diagnosis by PCR is less sensitive. Therapy: supportive.
Alpha toga viruses							
Eastern equine encephalitis	Birds (Culisata mosquitoes)	Eastern seaboard United States, Caribbean, South America	2–5 d	Similar to that of St. Louis encephalitis but more severe. Progresses rapidly in one third to coma and death.	Leukocytosis with neutrophilia. CSF: 500–2000 WBCs/μL; PMNs predominate early.	Mortality rate 20–50%; neurologic sequelae in over 50% of children.	Fewer than 10 cases/y. Only 3–10% of cases are symptomatic. Therapy: supportive. Diagnosis: serology. Titers often positive in first week. Equine deaths may signal an outbreak.

(continued)

Table 38–4. Some viral diseases spread by insects in the United States. (*Continued*)

Disease	Natural Reservoir (Vector)	Geographic Distribution	Incubation Period	Clinical Presentations	Laboratory Findings	Complications, Sequelae	Diagnosis, Therapy, Comments
Western equine encephalitis	Birds (*Culisata* mosquitoes)	Canada, Mexico, and United States west of Mississippi River	2–5 d	Similar to that of St. Louis encephalitis. Most infections are subclinical.	Variable white counts. CSF: 10–300 WBCs/µL.	Permanent brain damage, 10% overall; most severe in older adults.	No reported cases in United States in recent years. Case/infection is 1:1000 for older adults and 1:1 for infants. Equine illness precedes human outbreaks. Diagnosis: IgM antibody in first week. Therapy: supportive.
Venezuelan equine encephalitis	Horses (10 species of mosquitoes)	South and Central America, Texas	1–6 d	Similar to that of St. Louis encephalitis.	Lymphopenia, mild thrombocytopenia, abnormal liver function tests. CSF: 50–200 mononuclear cells/µL.	Severe disease more common in infants; 20% fatality rate for encephalitis.	Most infections do not cause encephalitis. No cases in United States in recent years. Vaccination of horses will stop epidemic. Therapy: supportive. Diagnosis: IgM antibody (EIA).
Bunyavirus							
California encephalitis (LaCrosse, Jamestown Canyon, California)	Chipmunks and other small mammals (*Aedes* mosquitoes)	Northern and mid-central United States, southern Canada	3–7 d	Similar to that of St. Louis encephalitis; sore throat and respiratory symptoms are common; focal neurologic signs in up to 25%. Seizures prominent. Prepubertal children are most likely to have severe disease. Can mimic HSV encephalitis.	Variable white counts. CSF: 30–200 (up to 600) WBCs/µL; variable PMNs; protein often normal.	Mortality rate < 1%. Seizure disorder may begin during acute illness.	About 150 cases/y in United States, 5% symptomatic. > 10% with sequelae. Therapy: supportive. Diagnosis: serology. Up to 90% have specific IgM antibody in first week; 25% of population in certain regions has IgG antibody.
Coltivirus							
Colorado tick fever	Small mammals (*Dermacentor andersoni*, or wood tick)	Rocky Mountain region of United States and Canada	3–4 d (range, 2–14 d)	Fever, chills, myalgia, conjunctivitis, headache, retroorbital pain; rash in < 10%. No respiratory symptoms. Biphasic fever in 50%.	Leukopenia (maximum at 4–6 d), mild thrombocytopenia.	Rare encephalitis, coagulopathy.	Patient may have no known tick bite. Acute illness lasts 7–10 d; prolonged fatigue in adults. Therapy: supportive. Diagnosis: serology, direct FA staining of red cells for viral antigen, PCR.

CNS, central nervous system; CSF, cerebrospinal fluid; EIA, enzyme immunoassay; FA, fluorescent antibody; HSV, herpes simplex virus; PCR, polymerase chain reaction; PMN, polymorphonuclear neutrophil; WBC, white blood cell.

DENGUE

▶ Travel or residence in an endemic area.

▶ First infection (first episode) results in nonspecific rash and fever; retro-orbital pain, severe myalgia, and arthralgia may occur.

▶ Subsequent infection with a different (heterotypic) serotype of dengue results in dengue hemorrhagic fever (thrombocytopenia, bleeding, plasma leak syndrome); this may progress to shock (dengue shock syndrome).

In endemic areas 50–100 million cases of dengue occur each year, often in severe forms. In the United States, 50–150 cases are diagnosed, most often in travelers from the Caribbean or Asia and less often in those visiting Central and South America, making it the most common arboviral disease in travelers. Dengue occurs in Mexico, and Texas has sporadic indigenous outbreaks. The spread of dengue requires the requisite species of mosquito, which transmits virus from a reservoir of viremic humans in endemic areas. Most patients have mild disease, especially young children, who may have a nonspecific fever and rash. Severity is a function of age, and prior infection with other serotypes of dengue virus is a prerequisite for severe hemorrhagic complications.

▶ Clinical Findings

A. Symptoms and Signs

Dengue fever begins abruptly 4–7 days after transmission (range, 3–14 days) with fever, chills, severe retro-orbital pain, severe muscle and joint pain, nausea, and vomiting. Erythema of the face and torso may occur early. After 3–4 days a centrifugal maculopapular rash appears in half of patients. The rash can become petechial, and mild hemorrhagic signs (epistaxis, gingival bleeding, microscopic blood in stool or urine) may be noted. The illness lasts 5–7 days, although rarely fever may reappear for several additional days.

B. Laboratory Findings

Leukopenia and a mild drop in platelets are common. Liver function tests are usually normal. Diagnosis is made by viral culture of plasma (50% sensitive up to the fifth day), by detecting IgM-specific ELISA antibodies (90% sensitive at the sixth day), or by detecting a rise in type-specific antibody. PCR testing is available for diagnosis in some areas.

▶ Differential Diagnosis

This diagnosis should be considered for any traveler to an endemic area who has symptoms suggestive of a systemic viral illness, although less than 1 in 1000 travelers to these areas develop dengue. Often the areas visited have other unique pathogens circulating (eg, malaria, typhoid fever, leptospirosis, and measles). EBV, influenza, enteroviruses, and acute HIV infection may produce a similar illness. An illness that starts 2 weeks after the trip ends or that lasts longer than 2 weeks is not dengue.

▶ Complications

Rarely dengue fever is associated with meningoencephalitis (5–10%) or hepatic damage. More common in endemic areas is the appearance of dengue hemorrhagic fever, which is defined by significant thrombocytopenia (<100,000 platelets/μL), bleeding, and a plasma leak syndrome [hemoconcentration = hematocrit >20% higher than baseline), hypoalbuminemia, and pleural or peritoneal effusions]. This is the consequence of circulating antibody and other immune responses acquired from a prior heterotypic dengue virus infection; thus it is rarely seen in typical travelers. Failure to recognize and treat this complication may lead to dengue shock syndrome, which is defined by signs of circulatory failure and hypotension or shock, and has a high fatality rate (10%).

▶ Prevention

Prevention of dengue fever involves avoiding high-risk areas and using conventional mosquito avoidance measures. The main vector is a daytime feeder. A vaccine to prevent dengue is being tested.

▶ Treatment

Dengue fever is treated by oral replacement of fluid lost from gastrointestinal symptoms. Analgesic therapy, which is often necessary, should not include drugs that affect platelet function. Recovery is complete without sequelae. The hemorrhagic syndrome requires prompt fluid therapy with plasma expanders and isotonic saline.

Ligon BL: Dengue fever and dengue hemorrhagic fever: A review of the history, transmission, treatment, and prevention. Semin Pediatr Infect Dis 2005;16:60 [PMID: 15685151].

Wichmann O et al: Severe dengue virus infection in travelers: Risk factors and laboratory indicators. J Infect Dis 2007;195:1089 [PMID: 17357044].

COLORADO TICK FEVER

▶ Travel in endemic area; tick bite.

▶ Fever, chills, headache, retro-orbital pain, myalgia.

▶ Biphasic fever curve.

▶ Leukopenia early in the illness.

Colorado tick fever, a tick-borne illness, is endemic in the high plains and mountains of the central and northern Rocky Mountains and northern Pacific coast of the United States. The reservoir of the virus consists of squirrels and chipmunks. Many hundreds of cases of Colorado tick fever occur each year in visitors or laborers entering this region, primarily from May through July.

Clinical Findings

A. Symptoms and Signs

After a 3- to 4-day incubation period (maximum, 14 days) fever begins suddenly together with chills, lethargy, headache, ocular pain, myalgia, abdominal pain, and nausea and vomiting. Conjunctivitis may be present. A nondistinctive maculopapular rash occurs in 5–10% of patients. The illness lasts 7–10 days, and half of patients have a biphasic fever curve with several afebrile days in the midst of the illness.

B. Laboratory Findings

Leukopenia is characteristic early in the illness. Platelets are modestly decreased. Specific ELISA testing is available, but 3–4 weeks may elapse before seroconversion. Fluorescent antibody staining will detect virus-infected erythrocytes during the illness and for weeks after recovery.

Differential Diagnosis

Early findings, especially if rash is present, may suggest enterovirus, measles, or rubella infection. Enteric fever may be an early consideration because of the presence of leukopenia and thrombocytopenia. A history of tick bite, which is often obtained; information about local risk; and the biphasic fever pattern will help with the diagnosis. Because of the wilderness exposure, diseases such as leptospirosis, borreliosis, tularemia, ehrlichiosis, and Rocky Mountain spotted fever will be considerations.

Complications

Meningoencephalitis occurs in 3–7% of patients. Cardiac and pulmonary complications are rare.

Prevention & Treatment

Prevention involves avoiding endemic areas and using conventional means to avoid tick bite. Therapy is supportive. Do not use analgesics that modify platelet function.

Gunther G, Haglund M: Tick-borne encephalopathies: Epidemiology, diagnosis, treatment and prevention. CNS Drugs 2005;19:1009-32 [PMID: 16332143].

OTHER MAJOR VIRAL CHILDHOOD EXANTHEMS

See the earlier section on Infections Due to Herpesvirus for a discussion of varicella and roseola, two other major childhood exanthems.

ERYTHEMA INFECTIOSUM

ESSENTIALS OF DIAGNOSIS & TYPICAL FEATURES

▶ Fever and rash with "slapped-cheek" appearance, followed by a symmetrical, full-body maculopapular rash.

▶ Arthritis in older children.

▶ Profound anemia in patients with impaired erythrocyte production.

▶ Nonimmune hydrops fetalis following infection of pregnant women.

General Considerations

This benign exanthematous illness of school-aged children is caused by the human parvovirus designated B19. Spread is respiratory, occurring in winter–spring epidemics. A nonspecific mild flulike illness may occur during the initial viremia at 7–10 days; the characteristic rash occurring at 10–17 days represents an immune response. The patient is viremic and contagious prior to—but not after—the onset of rash.

Approximately half of infected individuals have a subclinical illness. Most cases (60%) occur in children between ages 5 and 15 years, with an additional 40% occurring later in life. Forty percent of adults are seronegative. The disease is mildly contagious; the secondary attack rate in a school or household setting is 50% among susceptible children and 20–30% among susceptible adults.

Clinical Findings

Owing to the nonspecific nature of the exanthem and the many subclinical cases, a history of contact with an infected individual is often absent or unreliable. Recognition of the illness is easier during outbreaks.

A. Symptoms and Signs

Typically the first sign of illness is the rash, which begins as raised, fiery red maculopapular lesions on the cheeks that coalesce to give a "slapped-cheek" appearance. The lesions are warm, nontender, and sometimes pruritic. They may be scattered on the forehead, chin, and postauricular areas, but the circumoral region is spared. Within 1–2 days, similar lesions appear on the proximal extensor surfaces of the extremities and spread distally in a symmetrical fashion. Palms and soles are usually spared. The trunk, neck, and buttocks are also commonly involved. Central clearing of confluent lesions produces a characteristic lacelike pattern. The rash fades in several days to several weeks but frequently reappears in response to local irritation, heat (bathing), sunlight, and stress. Nearly 50% of infected children have some rash remaining (or recurring) for 10 days. Fine desquamation may be present. Mild systemic symptoms occur in up to 50% of children. These symptoms include low-grade fever, mild malaise, sore throat, and coryza. They appear for 2–3 days and are followed by a week-long asymptomatic phase before the rash appears.

Purpuric stocking-glove rashes, neurologic disease, and severe disorders resembling hemolytic-uremic syndrome have also been described in association with parvovirus B19.

B. Laboratory Findings

A mild leukopenia occurs early in some patients, followed by leukocytosis and lymphocytosis. Specific IgM and IgG serum antibody tests are available, but care must be used in choosing a reliable laboratory for this test. Nucleic acid detection tests are often definitive. The disease is not diagnosed by routine viral culture.

▶ Differential Diagnosis

In children immunized against measles and rubella, parvovirus B19 is the most frequent agent of morbilliform and rubelliform rashes. The characteristic rash and the mild nature of the illness distinguish erythema infectiosum from other childhood exanthems. It lacks the prodromal symptoms of measles and the lymphadenopathy of rubella. Systemic symptoms and pharyngitis are more prominent with enteroviral infections and scarlet fever.

▶ Complications & Sequelae

A. Arthritis

Arthritis is more common in older patients, beginning with late adolescence. Approximately 10% of children have severe joint symptoms. Girls are affected more commonly than boys. Pain and stiffness occur symmetrically in the peripheral joints. Arthritis usually follows the rash and may persist for 2–6 weeks but resolves without permanent damage.

B. Aplastic Crisis

Parvovirus B19 replicates primarily in erythroid progenitor cells. Consequently, reticulocytopenia occurs for approximately 1 week during the illness. This goes unnoticed in individuals with a normal erythrocyte half-life but results in severe anemia in patients with chronic hemolytic anemia. The rash of erythema infectiosum follows the hemolysis in these patients.

Pure red cell aplasia, leukopenia, pancytopenia, idiopathic thrombocytopenic purpura, and a hemophagocytic syndrome have also been described. Patients with AIDS and other immunosuppressive illnesses may develop prolonged anemia or pancytopenia. Patients with hemolytic anemia and aplastic crisis, or with immunosuppression, may be contagious and should be isolated while in the hospital.

C. Other End-Organ Infections

Parvovirus is under study as a potential cause of a variety of collagen-vascular diseases, neurologic syndromes, hepatitis, and myocarditis.

D. In-Utero Infections

Infection of susceptible pregnant women may produce fetal infection with hydrops fetalis. Fetal death occurs in about 6% of cases, and most fatalities occur in the first 20 weeks; this is higher than the rate of fetal loss expected in typical pregnancies. The risk of fetal infection is unknown. Congenital anomalies have not been associated with parvovirus B19 infection during pregnancy.

▶ Treatment & Prognosis

Erythema infectiosum is a benign illness for immunocompetent individuals. Patients with aplastic crisis may require blood transfusions. It is unlikely that this complication can be prevented by quarantine measures, because acute parvovirus infection in contacts is often unrecognized and is most contagious prior to the rash. Pregnant women who are exposed to erythema infectiosum or who work in a setting in which an epidemic occurs should be tested for evidence of prior infection. Susceptible pregnant women should then be followed up for evidence of parvovirus infection. Approximately 1.5% of women of childbearing age are infected during pregnancy. If maternal infection occurs, the fetus should be followed by ultrasonography for evidence of hydrops and distress. In-utero transfusion or early delivery may salvage some fetuses. Pregnancies should not be terminated because of parvovirus infection. The risk of fetal death among exposed pregnant women of unknown serologic status is less than 2.5% for homemakers and less than 1.5% for schoolteachers.

Intramuscular immune globulin is not protective. High-dose IVIG has stopped viremia and led to marrow recovery in some cases of prolonged aplasia. Its role in immunocompetent patients and pregnant women is unknown.

Dyer JA: Childhood viral exanthems. Pediatr Ann 2007;36:21 [PMID: 17269280].

Servey JT et al: Clinical presentation of parvovirus B19 infection. Am Fam Physician 2007;75:373 [PMID: 17304869].

MEASLES (RUBEOLA)

ESSENTIALS OF DIAGNOSIS & TYPICAL FEATURES

▶ Exposure to measles 9–14 days previously.

▶ Prodrome of fever, cough, conjunctivitis, and coryza.

▶ Koplik spots (few to many small white papules on a diffusely red base on the buccal mucosa) 1–2 days prior to and after onset of rash.

▶ Maculopapular rash spreading down from the face and hairline to the trunk over 3 days and later becoming confluent.

▶ Leukopenia.

▶ General Considerations

This childhood exanthem is rarely seen in the United States because of universal vaccination (64 cases in first half of 2008, all of which were imported or related to imported cases). Sporadic clusters of cases are the result of improper immunization more so than of vaccine failures, and are usually related to imported cases. It is recommended that all children be revaccinated on entrance into primary or secondary school (see Chapter 9). The attack rate in susceptible individuals is extremely high; spread is via respiratory droplets. Morbidity and mortality rates in the developing world are substantial because of underlying malnutrition and secondary infections. Because humans are the sole reservoir of measles, there is the potential to eliminate this disease worldwide.

▶ Clinical Findings

A history of contact with a suspected case may be absent because airborne spread is efficient and patients are contagious during the prodrome. Contact with an imported case may not be recognized. In temperate climates, epidemic measles is a winter–spring disease. Many suspected cases are misdiagnoses of other viral infections.

A. Symptoms and Signs

High fever and lethargy are prominent. Sneezing, eyelid edema, tearing, copious coryza, photophobia, and harsh cough ensue and worsen. Koplik spots are white macular lesions on the buccal mucosa, typically opposite the lower molars. These are almost pathognomonic for rubeola, although they may be absent. A discrete maculopapular rash begins when the respiratory symptoms are maximal and spreads quickly over the face and trunk, coalescing to a bright red. As it involves the extremities, it fades from the face and is completely gone within 6 days; fine desquamation may occur. Fever peaks when the rash appears and usually falls 2–3 days thereafter.

B. Laboratory Findings

Lymphopenia is characteristic. Total leukocyte counts may fall to 1500/μL. The diagnosis is usually made by detection of measles IgM antibody in serum drawn at least 3 days after the onset of rash or later by detection of a significant rise in antibody. Direct detection of measles antigen by fluorescent antibody staining of nasopharyngeal cells is a useful rapid method. PCR testing of oropharyngeal secretions or urine is extremely sensitive and specific and can detect infection up to 5 days before symptoms.

C. Imaging

Chest radiographs often show hyperinflation, perihilar infiltrates, or parenchymal patchy, fluffy densities. Secondary consolidation or effusion may be visible.

▶ Differential Diagnosis

Table 38–3 lists other illnesses that may resemble measles.

▶ Complications & Sequelae

A. Respiratory Complications

These complications occur in up to 15% of patients. Bacterial superinfections of lung, middle ear, sinus, and cervical nodes are most common. Fever that persists after the third or fourth day of rash suggests such a complication, as does leukocytosis. Bronchospasm, severe croup, and progressive viral pneumonia or bronchiolitis (in infants) also occur. Immunosuppressed patients are at much greater risk for fatal pneumonia than are immunocompetent patients.

B. Cerebral Complications

Encephalitis occurs in 1 in 2000 cases. Onset is usually within a week after appearance of rash. Symptoms include combativeness, ataxia, vomiting, seizures, and coma. Lymphocytic pleocytosis and a mildly elevated protein concentration are usual CSF findings, but the fluid may be normal. Forty percent of patients so affected die or have severe neurologic sequelae.

Subacute sclerosing panencephalitis (SSPE) is a slow measles virus infection of the brain that becomes symptomatic years later in about 1 in 100,000 previously infected children. This progressive cerebral deterioration is associated with myoclonic jerks and a typical electroencephalographic pattern. It is fatal in 6–12 months. High titers of measles antibody are present in serum and CSF.

C. Other Complications

These include hemorrhagic measles (severe disease with multiorgan bleeding, fever, cerebral symptoms), thrombocytopenia, appendicitis, keratitis, myocarditis, and premature delivery or stillbirth. Mild liver function test elevation has been detected in up to 50% of cases in young adults; frank jaundice may also occur. Measles causes transient immunosuppression; thus, reactivation or progression of tuberculosis (including transient cutaneous anergy) occurs in untreated children.

▶ Prevention

The current two-dose active vaccination strategy is successful. Vaccine should not be withheld for concurrent mild acute illness, tuberculosis or positive tuberculin skin test, breast feeding, or exposure to an immunodeficient contact. The vaccine is recommended for HIV-infected children without severe HIV complications and adequate CD4 cells (≥ 15%).

Treatment & Prognosis

Vaccination prevents the disease in susceptible exposed individuals if given within 72 hours (see Chapter 9). Immune globulin (0.25 mL/kg intramuscularly; 0.5 mL/kg if immunocompromised) will prevent or modify measles if given within 6 days. Suspected cases should be diagnosed promptly and reported to the local health department.

Recovery generally occurs 7–10 days after onset of symptoms. Therapy is supportive: eye care, cough relief (avoid opioid suppressants in infants), and fever reduction (acetaminophen, lukewarm baths; avoid salicylates). Secondary bacterial infections should be treated promptly; antimicrobial prophylaxis is not indicated. Ribavirin is active in vitro and may be useful in infected immunocompromised children. High-dose intravenous ribavirin in combination with intrathecal interferon-α has been successfully used in the management of SSPE. In malnourished children, vitamin A supplementation should be given to attenuate the illness.

Hosoya M et al: Pharmacokinetics and effects of ribavirin following intraventricular administration for treatment of subacute sclerosing panencephalitis. Antimicrob Agents Chemother 2004;48:4631 [PMID: 15561836].

Orenstein W et al: Measles elimination in United States. J Infect Dis 2004;189(Suppl):S1 [PMID: 15106120].

RUBELLA

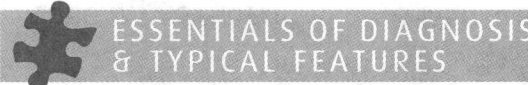

ESSENTIALS OF DIAGNOSIS & TYPICAL FEATURES

▸ History of rubella vaccination usually absent.

▸ Prodromal nonspecific respiratory symptoms and adenopathy (postauricular and occipital).

▸ Maculopapular rash beginning on face, rapidly spreading to the entire body, and disappearing by fourth day.

▸ Few systemic symptoms.

▸ Congenital infection.

  • Retarded growth, development.

  • Cataracts, retinopathy.

  • Purpuric "blueberry muffin" rash at birth.

  • Jaundice, thrombocytopenia.

  • Deafness.

  • Congenital heart defect.

General Considerations

If it were not teratogenic, rubella would be of little clinical importance. Clinical diagnosis is difficult in some cases because of its variable expression. In one study, over 80% of infections were subclinical. Because of inadequate vaccination, outbreaks now occur in adolescents or adults. Rubella is transmitted by aerosolized respiratory secretions. Patients are infectious 5 days before until 5 days after the rash. Endemic rubella is absent in the US and congenital rubella, in infants both of unimmunized women and of women who have apparently been reinfected in pregnancy, is now very rare.

Clinical Findings

The incubation period is 14–21 days. The nondistinctive signs may make exposure history unreliable. A history of immunization makes rubella unlikely but still possible. Congenital rubella usually follows maternal infection in the first trimester.

A. Symptoms and Signs

1. Infection in children—Young children may only have rash. Older patients often have a nonspecific prodrome of low-grade fever, ocular pain, sore throat, and myalgia. Postauricular and suboccipital adenopathy (sometimes generalized) is characteristic. This often precedes the rash or may occur without rash. The rash consists of erythematous discrete maculopapules beginning on the face. A "slapped-cheek" appearance or pruritus may occur. Scarlatiniform or morbilliform rash variants may occur. The rash spreads quickly to the trunk and extremities after it fades from the face; it is gone by the fourth day. Enanthema is usually absent.

2. Congenital infection—More than 80% of women infected in the first 4 months of gestation are delivered of affected infants; congenital disease occurs in less than 5% of women infected later in pregnancy. Later infections can result in isolated defects, such as deafness. The main manifestations are as follows:

A. GROWTH RETARDATION—Between 50% and 85% of infants are small at birth and remain so.

B. CARDIAC ANOMALIES—Pulmonary artery stenosis, patent ductus arteriosus, ventricular septal defect.

C. OCULAR ANOMALIES—Cataracts, microphthalmia, glaucoma, retinitis.

D. DEAFNESS—Sensorineural (> 50% of cases).

E. CEREBRAL DISORDERS—Chronic encephalitis; retardation.

F. HEMATOLOGIC DISORDERS—Thrombocytopenia, dermal nests of extramedullary hematopoiesis or purpura ("blueberry muffin" rash), lymphopenia.

G. OTHERS—Hepatitis, osteomyelitis, immune disorders, malabsorption, diabetes.

B. Laboratory Findings

Leukopenia is common, and platelet counts may be low. Congenital infection is associated with low platelet counts, abnormal liver function tests, hemolytic anemia, pleocytosis, and very high rubella IgM antibody titers. Total serum IgM is elevated, and IgA and IgG levels may be depressed.

Virus may be isolated from throat or urine from 1 week before to 2 weeks after onset of rash. Children with congenital infection are infectious for months. The virus laboratory must be notified that rubella is suspected. Serologic diagnosis is best made by demonstrating a fourfold rise in antibody titer between specimens drawn 1–2 weeks apart. The first should be drawn promptly, because titers increase rapidly after onset of rash. Both specimens must be tested simultaneously by a single laboratory. Specific IgM antibody can be measured by immunoassay. Because the decision to terminate a pregnancy is usually based on serologic results, testing must be done carefully.

C. Imaging

Pneumonitis and bone metaphyseal longitudinal lucencies may be present in radiographs of children with congenital infection.

▶ Differential Diagnosis

Rubella may resemble infections due to enterovirus, adenovirus, measles, EBV, roseola, parvovirus, *T gondii,* and *Mycoplasma.* Drug reactions may also mimic rubella. Because public health implications are great, sporadic suspected cases should be confirmed serologically or virologically.

Congenital rubella must be differentiated from congenital CMV infection, toxoplasmosis, and syphilis.

▶ Complications & Sequelae

A. Arthralgia and Arthritis

Both occur more often in adult women. Polyarticular involvement (fingers, knees, wrists), lasting a few days to weeks, is typical. Frank arthritis occurs in a small percentage of patients. It may resemble acute rheumatoid arthritis.

B. Encephalitis

With an incidence of about 1:6000, this is a nonspecific parainfectious encephalitis associated with a low mortality rate. A syndrome resembling SSPE (see Measles section, earlier) has also been described in congenital rubella.

C. Rubella in Pregnancy

Infection in the mother is self-limited and not severe.

▶ Prevention

Rubella is one of the infections that could be eradicated. See Chapter 9 for the indication and efficacy of rubella vaccine. Standard prenatal care should include rubella antibody testing. Seropositive mothers are at no risk; seronegative mothers are vaccinated after delivery.

A pregnant woman possibly exposed to rubella should be tested immediately; if seropositive, she is immune and need

not worry. If she is seronegative, a second specimen should be drawn in 4 weeks, and both specimens should be tested simultaneously. Seroconversion in the first trimester suggests high fetal risk; such women require counseling regarding therapeutic abortion.

When pregnancy termination is not an option, some experts recommend intramuscular administration of 20 mL of immune globulin within 72 hours after exposure in an attempt to prevent infection. (This negates the value of subsequent antibody testing.) The efficacy of this practice is unknown.

▶ Treatment & Prognosis

Symptomatic therapy is sufficient. Arthritis may improve with administration of anti-inflammatory agents. The prognosis is excellent in all children and adults but poor in congenitally infected infants, in whom most defects are irreversible or progressive. The severe cognitive defects seem to correlate closely in these infants with the degree of growth failure.

Reef SE, Cochi SL: The evidence for elimination of rubella and congenital rubella syndrome in United States: A public health achievement. Clin Infect Dis 2006;43(Suppl 3):S123 [PMID: 16998770].

INFECTIONS DUE TO OTHER VIRUSES

HANTAVIRUS CARDIOPULMONARY SYNDROME

ESSENTIALS OF DIAGNOSIS & TYPICAL FEATURES

▶ Influenza-like prodrome (fever, myalgia, headache, cough).

▶ Rapid onset of unexplained pulmonary edema and myocardiopathy.

▶ Residence or travel in endemic area; exposure to aerosols from deer mouse droppings or secretions.

▶ General Considerations

Hantavirus cardiopulmonary syndrome is the first native bunyavirus infection endemic in the United States. This syndrome is distinctly different in mode of spread (no arthropod vector) and clinical picture from other bunyavirus diseases.

▶ Clinical Findings

The initial cases of hantavirus cardiopulmonary syndrome involved travel to or residence in a limited area in the southwestern United States where there was a potential for exposure to the reservoir, the deer mouse. This and many other related rodents live in many other locales, and the disease has been confirmed in more than 30 other states, with additional cases in Canada. Epidemics occur when environmental conditions favor large increases in the rodent population and increased prevalence of virus in this reservoir.

A. Symptoms and Signs

After an incubation period of 2–3 weeks, onset is sudden, with a nonspecific virus-like prodrome: fever; back, hip, and leg pain; chills; headache; and nausea and vomiting. Abdominal pain may be present. Sore throat, conjunctivitis, rash, and adenopathy are absent, and respiratory symptoms are absent or limited to a dry cough. After 1–10 days (usually 3–7), dyspnea, tachypnea, and evidence of a pulmonary capillary leak syndrome appear. This often progresses rapidly over a period of hours. Hypotension is common not only from hypoxemia, but also from myocardial dysfunction. Copious, amber-colored, nonpurulent secretions are common. Decreased cardiac output due to myocardiopathy and elevated systemic vascular resistance distinguish this disease from early bacterial sepsis.

B. Laboratory Findings

The hemogram shows leukocytosis with a prominent left shift and immunoblasts, thrombocytopenia, and hemoconcentration. Lactate dehydrogenase (LDH) is elevated, as are liver function tests; serum albumin is low. Creatinine is elevated in some patients, and proteinuria is common. Lactic acidosis and low venous bicarbonate are poor prognostic signs. A serum IgM ELISA test is positive early in the illness. Otherwise the diagnosis is made by specific staining of tissue or PCR, usually at autopsy.

C. Imaging

Initial chest radiographs are normal. Subsequent radiographs show bilateral interstitial infiltrates with the typical butterfly pattern of acute pulmonary edema, bibasilar airspace disease, or both. Significant pleural effusions are often present. These findings contrast with those of other causes of acute respiratory distress syndrome.

▶ Differential Diagnosis

In some geographic areas, plague and tularemia may be possibilities. Infections with viral respiratory pathogens and *Mycoplasma* have a slower tempo, do not elevate the LDH level, and do not cause the hematologic changes seen in this syndrome. Q fever, psittacosis, toxin exposure, legionellosis, and fungal infections are possibilities, but the history, tempo of the illness, and blood findings, as well as the exposure history, should be distinguishing features. Hantavirus cardiopulmonary syndrome is a consideration in previously healthy persons with a febrile illness associated with unexplained pulmonary edema.

▶ Treatment & Prognosis

Ribavirin, to which hantaviruses and other bunyaviruses are susceptible, has not been demonstrated to alter the course of the illness. Management should concentrate on oxygen therapy and mechanical ventilation as required. Because of capillary leakage, Swan-Ganz catheterization to monitor cardiac output and inotropic support—rather than fluid therapy—should be used to maintain perfusion. Venoarterial extracorporeal membrane oxygenation can provide short-term support for selected patients. The virus present in North America is not spread by person-to-person contact. No isolation is required. The case fatality rate is 30–40%. Guidelines are available for reduction of exposure to the infectious agent.

Chang B et al: Hantavirus cardiopulmonary syndrome. Semin Respir Crit Care Med 2007;28:193 [PMID: 17458773].

MUMPS

ESSENTIALS OF DIAGNOSIS & TYPICAL FEATURES

- ▶ No prior mumps immunization.
- ▶ Parotid gland swelling.
- ▶ Aseptic meningitis with or without parotitis.

▶ General Considerations

Mumps was one of the classic childhood infections; virus spread by the respiratory route attacked almost all unimmunized children (asymptomatically in 30–40% of cases), and produced lifelong immunity. The vaccine is so efficacious that clinical disease is rare in immunized children. As a result of subclinical infections or childhood immunization, 95% of adults are immune. Infected patients can spread the infection from 1–2 days prior to the onset of symptoms and for 5 additional days. The incubation period is 14–21 days.

A history of exposure to a child with parotitis is not proof of mumps exposure. In an adequately immunized individual, parotitis is usually due to another cause. Currently in the United States less than 1 case is reported per 100,000 population.

▶ Clinical Findings

A. Symptoms and Signs

1. Salivary gland disease—Tender swelling of one or more glands, variable fever, and facial lymphedema are typical. Parotid involvement is most common; signs are bilateral in 70% of patients. The ear is displaced upward and outward; the mandibular angle is obliterated. Systemic toxicity is usually absent. Parotid stimulation with sour foods may be quite painful. The orifice of the Stensen duct may be red and swollen; yellow secretions may be expressed, but pus is absent. Parotid swelling dissipates after 1 week.

2. Meningoencephalitis—Prior to widespread immunization, mumps was the most common cause of aseptic meningitis, which is usually manifested by mild headache or asymptomatic mononuclear pleocytosis. Fewer than 10% of patients have clinical meningitis or encephalitis. Cerebral symptoms do not correlate with parotid symptoms, which are absent in many patients with meningoencephalitis. Although neck stiffness, nausea, and vomiting can occur, encephalitic symptoms are rare (1:4000 cases of mumps); recovery in 3–10 days is the rule.

3. Pancreatitis—Abdominal pain may represent transient pancreatitis. Because salivary gland disease may elevate serum amylase, specific markers of pancreatic function (lipase, amylase isoenzymes) are required for assessing pancreatic involvement.

4. Orchitis, oophoritis—Involvement of the gonads is associated with fever, local tenderness, and swelling. Epididymitis is usually present. Orchitis is unusual in young children but occurs in up to one third of affected postpubertal males. Usually it is unilateral and resolves in 1–2 weeks. Although one third of infected testes atrophy, bilateral involvement and sterility are rare.

5. Other—Thyroiditis, mastitis (especially in adolescent females), arthritis, and presternal edema (occasionally with dysphagia or hoarseness) may be seen.

B. Laboratory Findings

Peripheral blood leukocyte count is usually normal. Up to 1000 cells/μL (predominantly lymphocytes) may be present in the CSF, with mildly elevated protein and normal to slightly decreased glucose. Viral culture or PCR tests of saliva, throat, urine, or spinal fluid may be positive for at least 1 week after onset. Paired sera assayed by ELISA are currently used for diagnosis. Complement-fixing antibody to the soluble antigen disappears in several months; its presence in a single specimen thus indicates recent infection.

▶ Differential Diagnosis

Mumps parotitis may resemble the following conditions: cervical adenitis (the jaw angle may be obliterated, but the ear does not usually protrude; the Stensen duct orifice is normal; leukocytosis and neutrophilia are observed); bacterial parotitis (pus in the Stensen duct, toxicity, exquisite tenderness); recurrent parotitis (idiopathic or associated with calculi); tumors or leukemia; and tooth infections. Many viruses, including parainfluenza, enteroviruses, EBV, CMV, and influenza virus, can cause parotitis. Parotid swelling in HIV infection is less painful and tends to be bilateral and chronic, but bacterial parotitis occurs in some children with HIV infection.

Unless parotitis is present, mumps meningitis resembles that caused by enteroviruses or early bacterial infection. An elevated amylase level is a useful clue in this situation. Isolated pancreatitis is not distinguishable from many other causes of epigastric pain and vomiting. Mumps is a classic cause of orchitis, but torsion, bacterial or chlamydial epididymitis, *Mycoplasma* infection, other viral infections, hematomas, hernias, and tumors must also be considered.

▶ Complications

The major neurologic complication is nerve deafness (usually unilateral), which can result in inability to hear high tones. It may occur without meningitis. Permanent damage is rare, occurring in less than 0.1% of cases of mumps. Aqueductal stenosis and hydrocephalus (especially following congenital infection), myocarditis, transverse myelitis, and facial paralysis are other rare complications.

▶ Treatment & Prognosis

Treatment is supportive and includes provision of fluids, analgesics, and scrotal support for orchitis. Systemic corticosteroids have been used for orchitis, but their value is anecdotal. Surgery is not recommended.

Peltola H et al: Mumps outbreaks in Canada and the United States: Time for new thinking on mumps vaccines. Clin Infect Dis 2007;45:459 [PMID: 17638194].

RABIES

ESSENTIALS OF DIAGNOSIS & TYPICAL FEATURES

▶ History of animal bite 10 days to 1 year (usually < 90 days) previously.

▶ Paresthesias or hyperesthesia in bite area.

▶ Progressive limb and facial weakness in some patients (dumb rabies; 30%).

▶ Irritability followed by fever, confusion, combativeness, muscle spasms (especially pharyngeal with swallowing) in all patients (furious rabies).

▶ Rabies antigen detected in corneal scrapings or tissue obtained by brain or skin biopsy; Negri bodies seen in brain tissue.

▶ General Considerations

Rabies remains a potentially serious public health problem wherever animal immunization is not widely practiced or when humans play or work in areas with sylvan rabies. Although infection does not always follow a bite by a rabid animal (about 40% infection rate following rabid dog bites), infection is almost invariably fatal. Any warm-blooded animal may be infected, but susceptibility and transmissibility vary with different species. Bats often carry and excrete the virus in saliva or feces for prolonged periods; they are the major cause of rabies in the United States. Dogs and cats are usually clinically ill within 10 days after becoming contagious (the standard quarantine period for suspect animals). Valid quarantine periods or signs of illness are not fully known for many species. Rodents rarely transmit infection. Animal vaccines are very effective when properly administered, but a single inoculation may fail to produce immunity in up to 20% of dogs.

The risk is assessed according to the type of animal (bats always considered rabid; raccoons, skunks, foxes in many areas); wound extent and location (infection more common after head or hand bites, or if wounds have extensive salivary contamination or are not quickly and thoroughly cleaned); geographic area (urban rabies is rare to nonexistent in U.S. cities; rural rabies is possible, especially outside the United States); and animal vaccination history (risk low if documented). Most rabies in the United States is with genotypes found in bats, yet a history of bat bite is rarely obtained. Aerosolized virus in caves inhabited by bats has caused infection.

Clinical Findings

A. Symptoms and Signs

Paresthesias at the bite site are usually the first symptoms. Nonspecific anxiety, excitability, or depression follows, then muscle spasms, drooling, hydrophobia, delirium, and lethargy. Swallowing or even the sensation of air blown on the face may cause pharyngeal spasms. Seizures, fever, cranial nerve palsies, coma, and death follow within 7–14 days after onset. In a minority of patients, the spastic components are initially absent and the symptoms are primarily flaccid paralysis and cranial nerve defects. The furious components appear subsequently.

B. Laboratory Findings

Leukocytosis is common. CSF is usually normal or may show elevation of protein and mononuclear cell pleocytosis. Cerebral imaging and electroencephalography are not diagnostic.

Infection in an animal may be determined by use of the fluorescent antibody test to examine brain tissue for antigen. Rabies virus is excreted in the saliva of infected humans, but the diagnosis is usually made by antigen detection in scrapings or tissue samples of richly innervated epithelium, such as the cornea or the hairline of the neck. Classic Negri cytoplasmic inclusion bodies in brain tissue are not always present. Seroconversion occurs after 7–10 days.

Differential Diagnosis

Failure to elicit the bite history in areas where rabies is rare may delay diagnosis. Other disorders to be considered include parainfectious encephalopathy; encephalitis due to herpes simplex, mosquito-borne viruses, other viruses; and Guillain-Barré syndrome.

Prevention

See Chapter 9 for information regarding vaccination and postexposure prophylaxis. Rabies immune globulin and diploid cell vaccine have made prophylaxis more effective and minimally toxic; however, rare cases of prophylaxis failure are still being reported. Because rabies is almost always fatal, presumed exposures must be managed carefully.

Treatment & Prognosis

Survival is rare but has been reported in patients receiving meticulous intensive care. No antiviral preparations are of proved benefit. Early diagnosis is important for the protection and prophylaxis of individuals exposed to the patient.

Willoughby RE et al: Survival after treatment of rabies with induction of coma. N Engl J Med 2005;352:2508 [PMID: 15958806].

RICKETTSIAL INFECTIONS

Rickettsiae are pleomorphic, gram-negative coccobacilli that are obligate intracellular parasites. Rickettsial diseases are often included in the differential diagnosis of febrile rashes, although some (notably Q fever) are not characterized by rash. Severe headache is a prominent symptom. The endothelium is the primary target tissue, and the ensuing vasculitis is responsible for severe illness.

All rickettsioses except Q fever are transmitted by cutaneous arthropod contact, either by bite or contamination of skin breaks with tick feces. Evidence of such contact by history or physical examination may be completely lacking, especially in young children. The geographic distribution of the vector is often the primary determinant for suspicion of these infections. Therapy often must be empiric. Many new broad-spectrum antimicrobials are inactive against these cell wall–deficient organisms; tetracycline is usually effective.

HUMAN EHRLICHIOSIS

ESSENTIALS OF DIAGNOSIS & TYPICAL FEATURES

- ▶ Residing or travel in endemic area when ticks are active.
- ▶ Tick bite noted (~75%).
- ▶ Fever, headache, rash (~67%), gastrointestinal symptoms.
- ▶ Leukopenia, thrombocytopenia, elevated serum transaminases, hypoalbuminemia.
- ▶ Definitive diagnosis by specific serology.

Ehrlichia species are responsible for febrile pancytopenia in animals. In humans, *Ehrlichia sennetsu* is responsible for a mononucleosis-like syndrome seen in Japan and Malaysia. One agent of North American human ehrlichiosis has been identified as *Ehrlichia chaffeensis*. The reservoir hosts are probably wild rodents, deer, and sheep; ticks are the vectors. Most cases caused by this agent are reported in the south-central, southeastern, and middle Atlantic states. Arkansas, Missouri, Kentucky, Tennessee, and North Carolina are high-prevalence areas. Almost all cases occur between March and October, when ticks are active.

A second ehrlichiosis syndrome, seen in the upper Midwest and Northeast (Connecticut, Wisconsin, Minnesota, and New York are high-prevalence areas, is caused by *Anaplasma phagocytophilum* and *E ewingii*.

E chaffeensis has a predilection for mononuclear cells, whereas *A phagocytophilum* and *E ewingii* infect and produce intracytoplasmic inclusions in granulocytes. Hence diseases caused by these agents are referred to as human monocytic ehrlichiosis or human granulocytic ehrlichiosis, respectively. Ehrlichiosis, Lyme disease, and babesiosis share some tick vectors; thus dual infections are common and should be considered in patients who fail to respond to therapy.

▶ Clinical Findings

In approximately 75% of patients, a history of tick bite can be elicited. The majority of the remaining patients report having been in a tick-infested area. The usual incubation period is 5–21 days.

A. Symptoms and Signs

Fever is universally present and headache is common (less so in children). Gastrointestinal symptoms (abdominal pain, anorexia, nausea and vomiting) are reported in most pediatric patients. Distal limb edema may also occur in children. Chills, photophobia, conjunctivitis, and myalgia occur in more than half of patients. Rash occurs in two thirds of children with monocytic ehrlichiosis but is less common (~50%) in granulocytic ehrlichiosis. Rash may be erythematous, macular, papular, petechial, scarlatiniform, or vasculitic. Meningitis occurs. Interstitial pneumonitis, acute respiratory distress syndrome, and renal failure occur in severe cases. Physical examination reveals rash (not usually palms and soles), mild adenopathy, and hepatomegaly. In children without a rash, infection may present as a case of fever of unknown origin.

B. Laboratory Findings

Laboratory abnormalities include leukopenia with left shift, lymphopenia, thrombocytopenia, and elevated aminotransferase levels. Hypoalbuminemia is common. Disseminated intravascular coagulation can occur in severe cases. Anemia occurs in one third of patients. The definitive diagnosis is made serologically, either by a single high titer or a fourfold rise in titer. The Centers for Disease Control and Prevention uses appropriate antigens in an immunofluorescent antibody test in order to distinguish between the etiologic agents. Intracytoplasmic inclusions (morulae) may occasionally be observed in mononuclear cells in monocytic ehrlichiosis, and are usually observed in polymorphonuclear cells from the peripheral blood or bone marrow in granulocytic ehrlichiosis. Specific PCR testing is available for diagnosis.

▶ Differential Diagnosis

Erlichiosis should be included in the differential diagnosis of children in regions where these infections exist who present during tick season with fever, leucopenia or thrombocytopenia (or both), and increased serum transaminase levels. Patients should be treated concurrently with attempts to establish the diagnosis. The differential diagnosis includes septic or toxic shock, other rickettsial infections (especially Rocky Mountain spotted fever), Colorado tick fever, leptospirosis, Lyme borreliosis, relapsing fever, EBV, CMV, viral hepatitis and other viral infections, Kawasaki disease, systemic lupus erythematosus, and leukemia.

▶ Treatment & Prognosis

Asymptomatic or clinically mild and undiagnosed infections are common in some endemic areas. The disease may last several weeks if untreated. One quarter of hospitalized children require intensive care. Meningoencephalitis and persisting neurologic deficits occur in 5–10% of patients. Doxycycline, 2–4 mg/kg/d divided every 12 hours (maximum 100 mg per dose) for 7–10 days, is the treatment of choice. Response to therapy should be evident in 24–48 hours. Deaths are uncommon but do occur in children. Immune compromise is a risk factor for severe disease.

Dumler J et al: Ehrlichiosis in humans: Epidemiology, clinical presentation, diagnosis, and treatment. Clin Infect Dis 2007;45(Suppl 1):S45 [PMID: 17582569].

Schutze GE et al: Human monocytic ehrlichiosis in children. Pediatr Infect Dis J 2007;26:475 [PMID: 17529862].

ROCKY MOUNTAIN SPOTTED FEVER

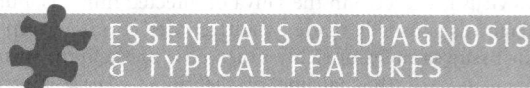

ESSENTIALS OF DIAGNOSIS
& TYPICAL FEATURES

▶ Residing or travel in endemic area when ticks are active.

▶ Fever, rash (palms and soles), gastrointestinal symptoms, headache.

▶ Tick bite (50%).

▶ Thrombocytopenia, hyponatremia.

▶ Definitive diagnosis by specific serology.

Rickettsia rickettsii causes one of many similar tick-borne illnesses characterized by fever and rash that occur worldwide. Most are named for their geographic area. In all except Rocky Mountain spotted fever and murine typhus, there is a characteristic eschar at the bite site, called the *tache noire*. Dogs and rodents are reservoirs of *R rickettsii*.

Rocky Mountain spotted fever is the most severe of these infections and the most important (500–1000 cases per year) in the United States. It occurs predominantly along the eastern seaboard; in the southeastern states; and in Arkansas, Texas, Missouri, Kansas, and Oklahoma. It is much less common in the west. Most cases occur in children exposed in rural areas from April to September. Because tick attachment lasting 6 hours or longer is needed, frequent tick removal is a preventive measure.

▶ Clinical Findings

A. Symptoms and Signs

After the incubation period of 3–12 days (mean, 7 days), there is high fever (> 40°C, often hectic), usually of abrupt onset, myalgia, severe and persistent headache (retro-orbital; less obvious in infants), toxicity, photophobia, vomiting, and diarrhea. A rash occurs in more than 95% of patients and appears 2–6 days after fever onset as macules and papules; most characteristic (65%) is involvement of the palms, soles, and extremities. The rash becomes petechial and spreads centrally. Conjunctivitis, splenomegaly, edema, meningismus, irritability, and confusion may occur.

B. Laboratory Findings

Laboratory findings are nonspecific and reflect diffuse vasculitis: thrombocytopenia, hyponatremia, early mild leukopenia, proteinuria, mildly abnormal liver function tests, hypoalbuminemia, and hematuria. CSF pleocytosis is common. Serologic diagnosis is achieved with indirect fluorescent or latex agglutination antibody methods, but generally only 7–10 days after onset of the illness. Skin biopsy with specific fluorescent staining may give the diagnosis within the first week of the illness.

▶ Differential Diagnosis

The differential diagnosis includes meningococcemia, measles, meningococcal meningitis, staphylococcal sepsis, enteroviral infection, leptospirosis, Colorado tick fever, scarlet fever, murine typhus, Kawasaki disease, and ehrlichiosis.

▶ Treatment & Prognosis

To be effective, therapy for Rocky Mountain spotted fever must be started early and is often based on a presumptive diagnosis in endemic areas prior to rash onset. It is important to remember that atypical presentations, such as the absence of pathognomonic rash, often lead to delay in appropriate therapy. Doxycycline is the agent of choice for children,

regardless of age. Treatment should be continued for 2 or 3 days after the temperature has returned to normal for a full day. A minimum of 10 days of therapy is recommended.

Complications and death result from severe vasculitis, especially in the brain, heart, and lung. The mortality rate is 5–7%. Persistent neurologic deficits occur. Delay in therapy is an important determinant of mortality.

Alvarez AC et al: Fever and rash in a child: When to worry? Pediatr Ann 2007;36:30 [PMID: 17269281].

Buckingham SC et al: Clinical and laboratory features, hospital course, and outcome of Rocky Mountain spotted fever. J Pediatr 2007;150:180 [PMID: 17236897].

Masters EJ et al: Rocky Mountain spotted fever: A clinician's dilemma. Arch Intern Med 2003;163:769 [PMID: 12695267].

ENDEMIC TYPHUS (MURINE TYPHUS)

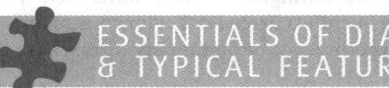

ESSENTIALS OF DIAGNOSIS & TYPICAL FEATURES

- ▶ Residing in endemic area.
- ▶ Fever for 10–14 days.
- ▶ Headache, chills, myalgia.
- ▶ Maculopapular rash spreading from trunk to extremities (not on palms and soles) 3–7 days after fever onset.
- ▶ Definitive diagnosis by serology.

Endemic typhus is present in the southern United States, mainly in southern Texas, and in Southern California. The disease is transmitted by fleas from infected rodents, from their feces in scratches, or by inhalation. Domestic cats, dogs, and opossums may play a role in the transmission of suburban cases. No eschar appears at the inoculation site, which may go unnoticed. The incubation period is 6–14 days. Headache, myalgia, and chills slowly worsen. Fever may last 10–14 days. After 3–8 days, a rash appears. Truncal macules and papules spread to the extremities; the rash is rarely petechial. The location of the rash in typhus, with sparing of the palms and soles, helps distinguish the disease from Rocky Mountain spotted fever. Rash may be absent in 20–40% of patients. Hepatomegaly may be present. Intestinal and respiratory symptoms may occur. Mild thrombocytopenia and elevated liver enzymes may be present. The illness is usually self-limited and milder than epidemic typhus. More prolonged neurologic symptoms have been described. Therapy is usually not needed. Doxycycline is the drug of choice. Therapy for 3 days is usually sufficient. Fluorescent antibody and ELISA tests are available.

Purcell K et al: Murine typhus in children, south Texas. Emerg Infect Dis 2007;13:926 [PMID: 17553239].

Q FEVER

► Exposure to farm animals (sheep, goats, cattle) and pets.

► Flulike illness (fever, severe headache, myalgia).

► Cough; atypical pneumonia.

► Hepatomegaly and hepatitis.

► Diagnosis by serology.

Coxiella burnetii is transmitted by inhalation rather than by an arthropod bite. The birth tissues and excreta of domestic animals and of some rodents are a major infectious source. Unpasteurized milk from infected animals may also transmit disease. Q fever is also distinguished from other rickettsial diseases by the infrequent occurrence of cutaneous manifestations and by the prominence of pulmonary disease.

► Clinical Findings

A. Symptoms and Signs

Many patients have a self-limited flulike syndrome of chills, fever, severe headache, and myalgia of abrupt onset occurring 10–30 days after exposure. Abdominal pain, vomiting, chest pain, and dry cough are prominent in children. Examination of the chest may produce few findings, as in other atypical pneumonias. Hepatosplenomegaly is common. The illness lasts 1–4 weeks and frequently is associated with weight loss.

B. Laboratory Findings

Leukopenia with left shift is characteristic. Thrombocytopenia is unusual and another distinction from other symptomatic rickettsial diseases. Aminotransferase and γ-glutamyl transferase levels are elevated. Diagnosis is made by finding a complement-fixing antibody response (fourfold rise or single high titer) to the phase II organism. Chronic infection is indicated by antibody against the phase I organism. IgM ELISA and specific PCR tests are also available.

C. Imaging

Pneumonitis occurs in 50% of patients. Multiple segmental infiltrates are common, but the radiographic appearance is not pathognomonic. Consolidation and pleural effusion are rare.

► Differential Diagnosis

In the appropriate epidemiologic setting, Q fever should be considered in evaluating causes of atypical pneumonias such as from *M pneumoniae*, viruses, *Legionella*, and *C pneumoniae*. It should also be included among the causes of mild to moderate hepatitis without rash or adenopathy in children with exposure to farm animals.

► Treatment & Prognosis

Typically the illness lasts 1–2 weeks without therapy. One complication is chronic disease, which often implies myocarditis or granulomatous hepatitis. Meningoencephalitis is also a rare complication.

C burnetii is also one of the causes of so-called culture-negative endocarditis. Endocarditis is difficult to treat; mortality approaches 50%. The course of the uncomplicated illness is shortened with tetracycline; doxycycline is preferred. Therapy is continued for several days after the patient becomes afebrile. Quinolones are also effective.

Cutler SJ et al: Q fever. J Infect 2007;54:313 [PMID:17147957].

Terheggen U, Leggat PA: Clinical manifestations of Q fever in adults and children. Travel Med Infect Dis 2007;5:159 [PMID: 17448942].

Human Immunodeficiency Virus Infection

39

Elizabeth J. McFarland, MD

ESSENTIALS OF DIAGNOSIS & TYPICAL FEATURES

Children younger than age 18 months:

▶ Definitive diagnosis:

- Positive results on two separate determinations on blood or tissue (excluding cord blood) for one or more of the following HIV detection tests: HIV nucleic acid detection (DNA or RNA), HIV antigen (p24), HIV culture.

▶ Presumptive clinical diagnosis (in settings lacking access to HIV virologic diagnostic tests):

- HIV-seropositive by repeatedly reactive enzyme-linked immunosorbent assay (ELISA) and confirmatory test.

  and

- Meets criteria for AIDS diagnosis based on the 1987 Centers for Disease Control and Prevention (CDC) AIDS surveillance case (see Table 39–1 and CDC case definition, MMWR Morb Mortal Wkly Rep, 1994) *or* has evidence of cellular and humoral immunodeficiency (without another cause) and symptoms compatible with HIV infection.

Children older than age 18 months:

▶ HIV-seropositive on two separate determinations on blood by ELISA and confirmatory test.

  or

▶ Meets any of the criteria listed for children younger than age 18 months.

General Considerations

Human immunodeficiency virus (HIV) is a retrovirus that primarily infects cells of the immune system, including helper T lymphocytes (CD4 T lymphocytes), monocytes, and macrophages. The function and number of CD4 T lymphocytes and other affected cells are diminished by HIV infection, with profound effects on both humoral and cell-mediated immunity. In the absence of treatment, HIV infection causes generalized immune incompetence, leading to conditions that meet the definition of acquired immunodeficiency syndrome (AIDS), and eventually death. The clinical diagnosis of AIDS is made when an HIV-infected child develops any of the opportunistic infections, malignancies, or conditions listed in category C of the Centers for Disease Control and Prevention (CDC) disease staging criteria (Table 39–1). In adults and adolescents, the criteria for a diagnosis of AIDS also include absolute CD4 lymphocyte counts of 200/μL or less.

Combination antiretroviral treatment, available in resource-rich settings since 1996, can forestall disease progression for 10 years or longer in many patients. The full duration of the favorable outcome of therapy is not yet defined, and it is not known whether adverse effects from the medications will affect mortality or limit use. Nevertheless, HIV infection can be considered a chronic rather than acutely terminal disease for people with access to treatment.

▶ Transmission & Epidemiology

HIV is transmitted by sexual contact, percutaneous exposure to contaminated blood (eg, injecting drug use or transfusion with contaminated blood products), and mother-to-child (vertical) transmission. Vertical transmission may occur in utero, at the time of delivery, or via breast feeding. Risk factors associated with mother-to-child transmission include high maternal plasma HIV RNA, advanced maternal disease stage, low CD4 lymphocyte count, premature delivery, and factors related to increased exposure to maternal blood or cervical secretions at the time of delivery (eg, duration of rupture of membranes, presence of blood in the infant's gastric secretions, and first-born twin delivery). Without intervention, 15–30% of infants born to HIV-infected women will be infected.

Table 39–1. Clinical categories of children with human immunodeficiency virus (HIV) infection.

Category N: Not symptomatic
No signs or symptoms or only one of the conditions listed in category A

Category A: Mildly symptomatic
Having two or more of the following conditions:
  Lymphadenopathy
  Hepatomegaly
  Splenomegaly
  Dermatitis
  Parotitis
  Recurrent or persistent upper respiratory infection, sinusitis, or otitis media

Category B: Moderately symptomatic
Having symptoms attributed to HIV infection other than those in category A or C
Examples:
  Anemia, neutropenia, thrombocytopenia
  Bacterial meningitis, pneumonia, sepsis (single episode)
  Candidiasis, oropharyngeal, persisting more than 2 mo
  Cardiomyopathy
  Cytomegalovirus infection with onset < age 1 mo
  Diarrhea, recurrent or chronic
  Hepatitis
  Herpes simplex virus recurrent stomatitis, bronchitis, pneumonitis, esophagitis at < 1 month of age
  Herpes zoster, two or more episodes or more than one dermatome
  Leiomyosarcoma
  Lymphoid interstitial pneumonia
  Nephropathy
  Nocardiosis
  Persistent fever
  Toxoplasmosis with onset < age 1 mo
  Varicella, complicated

Category C: Severely symptomatic
  Serious bacterial infections, multiple or recurrent
  Candidiasis, esophageal or pulmonary
  Coccidioidomycosis, disseminated
  Cryptosporidiosis or isosporiasis with diarrhea > age 1 mo
  Cytomegalovirus infection with onset > age 1 mo
  Encephalopathy
  Herpes simplex virus: persistent oral lesions, or bronchitis, pneumonitis, esophagitis at > age 1 mo
  Histoplasmosis
  Kaposi sarcoma
  Lymphoma
  Mycobacterium tuberculosis, extrapulmonary
  Mycobacterium infection, other species, disseminated
  Pneumocystis jiroveci pneumonia
  Progressive multifocal leukoencephalopathy
  Salmonella septicemia, recurrent
  Toxoplasmosis of the brain with onset > age 1 mo
  Wasting syndrome

Adapted from MMWR Recomm Rep 1994;43(RR-12):6, 8.

The rate of vertical transmission can be reduced to less than 2% by providing combination antiretroviral treatment to the mother during pregnancy and delivery, implementing recom-mended obstetric interventions, providing additional prophy-laxis to the infant during the first 6 weeks after birth, and avoidance of breast feeding. In the United States, as a result of prenatal and perinatal interventions, the number of vertically acquired AIDS cases declined 83% between 1992 (907 cases) and 2001 (150 cases). Most transmissions that occur involve women who do not receive antiretroviral therapy during pregnancy, either because the infection is undiagnosed or because of lack of prenatal care. Mother-to-child transmission rates continue to be high in resource-limited settings where access to antiretroviral therapy and safe infant formula is infrequent. Worldwide, an estimated 2.3 million children are infected with HIV, most of them in Africa, South and South-east Asia, and parts of South America. In 2006, there were an estimated 530,000 new infections and 380,000 deaths in chil-dren younger than 15 years.

Sexual activity (both heterosexual and homosexual) is the main mode of infection after puberty, with a smaller number of cases resulting from the sharing of contaminated needles. In the United States, seroprevalence rates are highest among gay men and injecting drug users. However, the proportion of new AIDS cases in 2005 acquired by heterosexual contact exceeded the proportion acquired by injecting drug use. Youth (ages 13–24 years) and women of color are dispropor-tionately represented among new cases. In developing nations, heterosexual contact is the most common mode of transmission among adults and the prevalence is slightly higher among women.

As a result of careful donor screening and testing of the donated blood, HIV transmission resulting from blood products is now extremely rare (1:2,000,000 transfusions). Casual, classroom, or household contact with an HIV-infected person poses no risk.

▶ Pathogenesis

Most transmission of HIV occurs via mucosal surfaces. Virus is transported to regional lymph nodes and by approxi-mately 48 hours after infection, replicating virus is found throughout all lymphoid tissues. Nonhuman primate mod-els using a related virus indicate that a massive loss of mature CD4 T-helper lymphocytes occurs during the first days of infection. During acute infection, high levels of HIV are detected in the bloodstream. In adults, the level of viremia declines without therapy concurrent with the appearance of an HIV-specific host immune response, and plasma viremia usually reaches a steady-state level about 6 months after primary infection. The amount of virus present in the plasma at that point and thereafter is predictive of the rate of disease progression for the individual. Despite ongoing virus replication, a period of clinical latency occurs, lasting from 1 year to more than 12 years during which the infected person is asymptomatic. The virus and anti-HIV immune responses are in a steady state, with high levels of virus production and destruction balanced against production and destruction of CD4 lymphocytes. Eventually, the balance favors the virus, and the viral burden increases as the CD4 lymphocyte count declines.

In the pre-antiretroviral treatment era, approximately 30% of infants with vertically acquired HIV infection had virus detectable in the blood at birth, presumed to be infection acquired in utero. In-utero infection represents a larger fraction of vertical infections in populations where interventions to prevent transmission, often initiated during the second trimester or later, are common. Infants who acquire HIV during labor and delivery test negative for HIV at birth but soon have detectable virus, usually by 2–4 weeks. The level of viremia rises steeply, reaching a peak at age 1–2 months. In contrast to adults, infants have a gradual decline in plasma viremia that extends beyond 2 years. Infants generally have plasma virus levels 10 times higher than those in adults. Less is known about the viral dynamics following transmission via breast feeding.

▶ Clinical Findings

A. Symptoms and Signs

The manifestations described in this section are likely to be observed in children with untreated infection or in those unresponsive to therapy. Children given effective antiretroviral therapy usually have few symptoms, most of which stem from use of these medications.

The CDC has developed disease staging criteria for HIV-infected children (see Tables 39–1 and 39–2). The criteria incorporate clinical symptoms ranging from no symptoms to mild, moderate, and severe symptoms (categories N, A, B, and C, respectively) and age-adjusted CD4 lymphocyte counts (immunologic categories 1, 2, or 3, corresponding to none, moderate, or severe immune suppression, respectively). Each child is classified both by CD4 lymphocyte count and by clinical category. Category C diagnoses are the diseases associated with late-stage disease and confer a diagnosis of AIDS.

1. Primary acute infection—The incubation period is 2–4 weeks for primary infection acquired by adults and adolescents through high-risk behavior. Nonspecific symptoms occur in 30–90% of new infections (eg, flu- or mild mono-nucleosis-like illness) but may not be brought to medical attention. In some U.S. cities, anonymous screening of blood samples demonstrates laboratory evidence of acute HIV infection in 1% of emergency department patients. Diagnosis requires a high index of suspicion. Infected persons may present with fever, fatigue, malaise, pharyngitis, enlarged lymph nodes, and hepatosplenomegaly. Less commonly seen signs, but more specific to HIV, are mild oral ulcerations; a diffuse macular, erythematous rash; and mild meningitis or encephalopathy. Occasionally, thrush, *Candida* esophagitis, or genital ulcers are observed. These early symptoms of primary infection resolve spontaneously within 1–2 weeks, although some persons have fatigue and depression for weeks or months.

A primary infection syndrome is rarely recognized following perinatal acquisition. Newborns with perinatal HIV infection are rarely symptomatic at birth. Size and physical features are not different from uninfected neonates. However, 75–95% will demonstrate some sign (mostly nonspecific) by age 1 year.

2. Nonspecific symptoms—These may be observed in early- or late-stage disease. Frequent illness (especially recurrent otitis media or sinusitis) is typical, in addition to poor weight gain, chronic cough, chronic diarrhea, developmental delay, unexplained fevers, night sweats, generalized lymphadenopathy, parotid swelling, or hepatosplenomegaly. Delayed growth may be observed as early as age 4 months in some infants. These common early findings may be present for years in an otherwise well child.

3. Infections related to immunodeficiency—Progressive immune dysfunction in both humoral and cell-mediated responses results in susceptibility to infections. Recurrent or serious bacterial infections are more common in children than in HIV-infected adults. Bouts of bacteremia, especially due to *Streptococcus pneumoniae,* can occur in children without suppressed CD4 T-cell counts. Infections with *Mycobacterium tuberculosis* (usually acquired from adults in the household) may be severe. Primary varicella-zoster virus (VZV) infections may be prolonged or severe. Herpes zoster (shingles), including multiple episodes, is common even in the era of combina-

Table 39–2. Immunologic categories based on age-specific CD4 lymphocyte counts and percentages of total lymphocytes.

Immunologic Category	Age of Child					
	< 12 mo		1–5 y		6–12 y	
	cells/µL	(%)	cells/µL	(%)	cells/µL	(%)
1. No evidence of suppression	≥ 1500	(≥ 25)	≥ 1000	(≥ 25)	≥ 500	(≥ 25)
2. Evidence of moderate suppression	750–1499	(15–24)	500–999	(15–24)	200–499	(15–24)
3. Evidence of severe suppression	< 750	(< 15)	< 500	(< 15)	< 200	(< 15)

Adapted from MMWR Recomm Rep 1994;43(RR-12):4.

tion therapy. Recurrent herpes simplex lesions may be large, painful, and persistent. Likewise, persistent aphthous ulcers may cause significant morbidity. Late-stage immunodeficiency is accompanied by susceptibility to a variety of opportunistic pathogens. Pneumonia caused by *Pneumocystis jiroveci* (formerly *Pneumocystis carinii*) is the most common AIDS-defining diagnosis in children with unrecognized HIV infection. The incidence is highest between ages 2 and 6 months and is often fatal during this period. Symptoms are difficult to distinguish from those of viral or atypical pneumonia. (See Chapter 41.) Persistent candidal mucocutaneous infections (oral, cutaneous, and vaginal) are common. Candidal esophagitis occurs with more advanced disease. In children with severe immunosuppression, cytomegalovirus (CMV) infections may result in disseminated disease, hepatitis, gastroenteritis, retinitis, and encephalitis.

Disseminated infection with *Mycobacterium avium* complex (MAC), presenting with fever, night sweats, weight loss, diarrhea, fatigue, lymphadenopathy, hepatomegaly, anemia, and granulocytopenia, occurs in infected children who have CD4 lymphocyte counts below 50–100/μL. A variety of diarrheal pathogens that cause mild, self-limited symptoms in healthy persons may result in severe, chronic diarrhea in HIV-infected persons. These include rotavirus, *Cryptosporidium parvum, Microsporidia, Cyclospora, Isospora belli, Giardia lamblia,* and bacterial pathogens. Chronic parvovirus infection manifested by anemia can occur. Reactivation of toxoplasmosis occurs rarely in children.

4. Organ system disease—HIV infection may cause a variety of organ system symptoms (encephalopathy, pneumonitis, hepatitis, diarrhea, hematologic suppression, nephropathy, and cardiomyopathy). The more common of these are described in this section. On average, HIV-infected children have lower than normal neuropsychological functioning; higher viral load correlates with more severe abnormalities. In many children, neuropsychological deficits do not normalize when antiretroviral therapy is started despite suppression of viremia. Studies are needed to determine if highly active antiretroviral therapy (HAART) early in life will completely prevent the central nervous system effects of HIV. Without antiretroviral therapy, encephalopathy afflicted 20% or more of HIV-infected children. Symptoms included acquired microcephaly, progressive motor deficit, ataxia, pseudobulbar palsy, and failure to attain (or loss of) developmental milestones. Children who are older may have symptoms similar to those observed in infected adults, such as gradual mental status changes initially affecting attention span and memory.

Lymphoid interstitial pneumonitis is characterized by a diffuse peribronchial and interstitial infiltrate composed of lymphocytes and plasma cells. It may be asymptomatic or associated with dry cough, hypoxemia, dyspnea or wheezing on exertion, and clubbing of the digits. Children with this disorder frequently have enlargement of the parotid glands and generalized lymphadenopathy.

Mild to moderate elevation of liver enzymes is frequently observed, and, more rarely, overt clinical hepatitis occurs due to HIV infection itself. However, patients are often taking medications with potential hepatotoxicity, and superinfection with other pathogens (CMV, Epstein-Barr virus [EBV], MAC, hepatitis C, or hepatitis B) that affect the liver is common. Thus, the diagnosis of HIV hepatitis should be one of exclusion. Chronic diarrhea may occur with HIV infection; however, as with hepatitis, it is commonly associated with other gastrointestinal infections.

5. Malignancy—Children with HIV are at increased risk of malignancy. The most commonly occurring tumors are non-Hodgkin lymphomas. Unlike non-Hodgkin lymphomas in immunocompetent persons, these tumors commonly occur at extranodal sites (central nervous system, bone, gastrointestinal tract, liver, or lungs) and are usually high-grade and of B-cell origin. Cervical infection with human papillomavirus is more likely to progress to neoplasia in adolescent females with HIV infection. Carcinoma due to anal human papillomavirus is also a concern. Kaposi sarcoma, a common malignancy among HIV-infected gay males, rarely occurs in children. There is an increased frequency of leiomyosarcomas.

B. Laboratory Findings

HIV antibody is measured by enzyme-linked immunosorbent assay (ELISA; standard or rapid antibody tests). A confirmatory test, usually a Western blot, must be performed because individuals occasionally have nonviral cross-reacting antibodies, which result in a false-positive ELISA or rapid test. Infants born to HIV-infected mothers will have HIV antibody—regardless of infection status—owing to transplacental passage of maternal antibody. Maternal HIV antibody is lost in all children by 18 months. After that age, HIV antibody testing can be used to make the diagnosis of infection. In the early weeks after acute HIV infection acquired by high-risk behaviors, HIV antibody may be absent. Most patients will seroconvert by 6 weeks, but occasionally seroconversion does not occur for 3–6 months. When acute HIV infection is suspected, tests for circulating virus (see below) should be obtained.

HIV nucleic acid, RNA (in plasma) or DNA (in blood cells), can be detected by several methods, including polymerase chain reaction (PCR), branched DNA chain assay (bDNA), and nucleic acid sequence-based amplification (NASBA). These tests are highly sensitive with a lower limit of detection of 20 copies/mL of plasma. An HIV protein (p24) can also be detected in plasma; the test is less costly, but is less sensitive. Quantitative measures of HIV RNA in plasma are valuable for predicting the rate of disease progression and are a surrogate marker of response to antiretroviral therapy.

Using nucleic acid detection, infants at risk of vertical HIV infection can be diagnosed by age 2–4 months. At birth, approximately 30% of infected infants have detectable HIV RNA and DNA. Infants acquiring HIV in the peripartum period (late gestation, labor, and delivery) will have negative results for HIV RNA and DNA at birth due to low levels of circulating virus, but soon have detectable virus. By age 6 weeks, almost all perinatally infected infants will become positive for HIV nucleic acid. An infant who is not breast feeding and has had at least two negative HIV cultures or nucleic acid detection tests, both performed after age 1 month and at least one performed after age 2–4 months, is very unlikely to be infected. The infant should be followed up for clinical symptoms and tested for HIV antibody at ages 12, 15, and 18 months to confirm reversion to seronegative status, thereby confirming the absence of infection. Breast-fed infants may acquire HIV at any time until they are fully weaned; to confirm absence of HIV infection, HIV nucleic acid tests should be preformed at least 6 weeks after the last exposure.

The hallmark of HIV disease progression is decline in the absolute number and percentage of CD4 T lymphocytes and an increasing percentage of CD8 T lymphocytes. The CD4 T-lymphocyte values are predictive of the child's risk of opportunistic infections. Healthy infants have CD4 T-lymphocyte numbers and percentages much higher than in adults; these gradually decline to adult levels by age 6 years. Hence, age-adjusted values must be used when assessing a child's CD4 T-lymphocyte parameters (see Table 39–2).

Hypergammaglobulinemia of IgG, IgA, and IgM is characteristic and may be observed as early as age 9 months. Late in the disease, some individuals may become hypogammaglobulinemic. Hematologic abnormalities (anemia, neutropenia, and thrombocytopenia) may occur due to effects of HIV disease or, more commonly, due to adverse effects of medications. With brain involvement, the cerebrospinal fluid may either be normal or the protein elevated and a mononuclear pleocytosis present.

C. Imaging

Cerebral imaging can demonstrate atrophy and calcification in the basal ganglia and frontal lobes in patients with encephalopathy. Chest radiographs of children with lymphoid interstitial pneumonitis show diffuse interstitial reticulonodular infiltrates, occasionally with hilar adenopathy. The chest radiograph in *P jiroveci* pneumonia typically demonstrates perihilar infiltrates progressing to bilateral diffuse alveolar disease.

▶ Differential Diagnosis

HIV infection should be in the differential diagnosis for children being evaluated for immunodeficiency. Depending on the degree of immunosuppression, the presentation in HIV infection may be similar to that in B-cell, T-cell, or combined immunodeficiencies, such as hypogammaglobinemia and severe combined immunodeficiency. (See Chapter 31.) HIV infection should also be considered in the evaluation of children with failure to thrive or developmental delay. Children or adolescents with chronic HIV infection may present with generalized lymphadenopathy or hepatosplenomegaly resembling infections with viruses such as EBV or CMV. Because blood tests are definitive for the diagnosis of HIV infection, the diagnosis can be readily established or excluded. The

diagnosis of chronic HIV infection is made with HIV antibody testing in a child older than age 18 months. In younger infants, a negative result usually excludes HIV infection; a positive result must be confirmed by testing for viral nucleic acid. In rare cases, HIV-infected children with hypogammaglobulinemia have falsely negative antibody tests. Any child suspected of having HIV infection whose serologic test results are negative should be tested by a nucleic acid–based test. Absence of maternal risk factors or history of negative test results during pregnancy, particularly if documentation of the results is lacking, should not dissuade the provider from testing for HIV if the patient has signs consistent with the diagnosis.

The symptoms of acute primary infection in the adolescent may be similar to those of mononucleosis caused by EBV or CMV, toxoplasmosis, rubella, secondary syphilis, influenza, enterovirus, or viral hepatitis. In the first weeks of acute infection, HIV antibody tests will be negative. However, the diagnosis can be made by detection of HIV RNA in plasma. Seroconversion occurs over 2–6 weeks in symptomatic patients. Diagnosis of acute HIV infection has important public health implications, because patients are highly infectious during the first months after infection. Studies are ongoing to determine if treatment during early infection improves prognosis. Thus, HIV RNA testing is warranted if the patient has a history of high-risk behavior or an alternative diagnosis is lacking.

▶ Prevention

Vertical transmission can be substantially prevented by giving antiretroviral medications to the mother during pregnancy and to the newborn. Combination therapy that results in viral suppression to less than 1000 copies/mL reduces transmission rates to less than 1%. Therefore, the CDC and the American College of Obstetrics and Gynecology now recommend offering HIV testing, with an option to refuse, as a part of routine prenatal care for all pregnant women irrespective of risk factors. Women who present in labor should be tested for HIV antibody using recently approved rapid tests that give results within 60 minutes. Women found to be infected should be counseled regarding all HIV-related pregnancy care issues, including the benefits and risks of therapy with antiretroviral agents. Women in resource-rich settings generally receive three-drug combination regimens during pregnancy. Zidovudine should be incorporated into the regimen if possible because it has the greatest efficacy and safety of currently available drugs. Antiretroviral therapy begun in the last weeks of pregnancy, during labor, or even within 48 hours after birth, also reduces perinatal infection, although less profoundly. Short-course treatment can reduce transmission by 30–50% in women who are diagnosed late in pregnancy or at delivery.

Elective cesarean delivery reduces the risk of transmission by 50% and should be offered to women who are not receiving antiretroviral therapy or who have viral loads over 1000 copies/mL despite treatment. Women receiving combination therapy that suppresses viral load to below 1000 copies/mL have a very low risk of transmission. For these women, the benefit and risk of cesarean delivery should be considered on an individual basis. Because breast milk can carry the virus, breast feeding by HIV-infected mothers is contraindicated when access to safe formula can be ensured. In developing countries transmission via breast milk remains a major mode of pediatric HIV infection.

The only 100% effective method of avoiding sexual transmission of HIV infection is abstinence or limiting sexual contact to a mutually monogamous partner who is not HIV-infected. However, condoms—used consistently and correctly—are highly effective in preventing transmission between stable, sexually active couples in which only one partner is HIV-infected. In two studies, seroconversions occurred in 0–2% of discordant couples using condoms consistently compared with 10–15% of couples with inconsistent condom use. A third study reported 1.1 seroconversions per 100 person-years of observation among consistent condom users compared with 9.7 seroconversions among inconsistent users. The CDC provides detailed instructions on correct condom use. Prompt treatment of other sexually transmitted diseases, especially those associated with mucosal ulceration, also reduces the risk of sexual transmission.

Postexposure prophylaxis with antiretroviral medications begun as soon as possible is recommended for people with an occupational exposure that carries a risk of HIV transmission. Prophylaxis is also recommended for people with a nonoccupational exposure that is not likely to recur (eg, sexual assault or condom rupture) who present within 72 hours of the exposure. Detailed guidelines regarding assessment of the level of risk and selection of postexposure therapy are published by the CDC.

Horizontal transmission (ie, in the absence of sexual contact or injecting drug use) of HIV is exceedingly rare and is associated with exposure of broken skin or mucous membranes to HIV-infected blood or bloody secretions. Because undiagnosed HIV-infected infants and children might be enrolled, all schools and day care centers should have policies with simple guidelines for using universal precautions to prevent transmission of HIV infection in these settings. Saliva, tears, urine, and stool are not contagious if there is no gross blood in these fluids. A barrier protection (eg, latex or rubber gloves or thick pads of fabric or paper) should be used when possible contact with blood or bloody body fluids may occur. Objects that might be contaminated with blood, such as razors or toothbrushes, should not be shared. No special care is required for dishes, towels, toys, or bedclothes. Blood-soiled clothing may be washed routinely with hot water and detergent. Contaminated surfaces may be disinfected easily with a variety of agents, including household bleach (1:10 dilution), some commercial disinfectants (eg, Lysol), or 70% isopropyl alcohol.

▶ **Treatment**

HIV infection calls for specific antiretroviral treatment to prevent progressive deterioration of the immune system as well as prophylactic measures at late stages of HIV infection to prevent opportunistic infections. Whenever possible, children should be enrolled in collaborative treatment studies. Current information on clinical trials may be obtained at:

http://aidsinfo.nih.gov/clinical_trials

Guidelines for the treatment of HIV developed by a national working group of pediatric HIV specialists are published by the U.S. Public Health System at:

http://aidsinfo.nih.gov/guidelines

The treatment paradigm changes frequently; therefore, prior to initiating treatment, expert consultation should be obtained.

A. Specific Measures

1. Principles of HIV treatment—Treatment of HIV is aimed at suppressing viral replication. The rate of disease progression is directly correlated with the number of HIV copies circulating in plasma. Antiretroviral treatment that reduces HIV replication is associated with increases in CD4 T-lymphocyte counts, reconstitution of immune function, and arrest of disease progression. Children have a remarkable ability to restore normal CD4 T-cell counts, even when treatment is started at an advanced disease stage. However, it is clear that even the most potent regimens fail to eradicate virus. HIV persists in long-lived resting cells and cessation of antiretroviral treatment results in resumption of viremia and decline in CD4 lymphocytes. Therefore, treatment for HIV with currently available modalities must be a lifelong endeavor. Once therapy has been initiated, the patient should be monitored every 3 months for changes in plasma virus copy number, CD4 lymphocyte count, symptoms, and adverse drug effects.

Emergence of drug-resistant HIV during therapy is a major challenge. HIV has a high spontaneous mutation rate, and emergence of drug resistance during treatment is frequent. Many antiretroviral drugs select for resistant mutations in the virus within weeks to a few months when used as monotherapy. Prevention of resistance mutations requires complete suppression such that virus is not replicating and has no opportunity to generate new mutations. Achieving potent viral suppression requires a combination of at least three antiviral agents. Treatment with a combination of drugs with different mechanisms of action provides an additional barrier to resistance as the virus must be resistant to all the drugs in the combination. Finally, strict adherence to the prescribed treatment is critical. Studies demonstrate that more than 95% of the doses must be taken in order to maintain optimal viral suppression. Therefore programs and services that enhance adherence are essential adjuncts of any HAART regimen.

Determining the best time to initiate treatment is a subject of ongoing discussion and research. Once treatment is initiated there are risks of drug toxicity as well as the risk of developing drug resistance if adherence is suboptimal, thereby limiting future treatment options. Some children with HIV live many years without HIV-related symptoms. On the other hand, early treatment may better preserve immune function and foster normal growth and development. Thus it is important to start treatment when the risk of disease progression outweighs the risk of starting the medication. The Department of Health and Human Services publishes guidelines for the use of antiretroviral drugs for patients in the United States at the National Institutes of Health AIDSinfo web site (http://aidsinfo.nih.gov). These guidelines are frequently updated, and the most current online version should be consulted when treatment decisions are made.

At any age, once significant symptoms of HIV are present, the patient is likely to have ongoing disease progression. Therefore treatment is indicated for any child or adolescent with symptoms in category C or B (excluding lymphoid interstitial pneumonia or a single serious bacterial illness; see Table 39–1). For asymptomatic adults and for adolescents the guidelines for antiretroviral treatment initiation are primarily based on CD4 and some clinical conditions. Treatment is recommended for patients with absolute CD4 T-cell counts below 350 cells/mm^3 and may be considered for those with CD4 counts over 350. Treatment is recommended for all patients who are pregnant or have HIV-associated nephropathy, irrespective of CD4 T-cell count.

For infants and children, the relative risk of disease progression and the predictive value of CD4 and viral load for progression vary with age. Age-specific criteria for CD4 count and viral load should be considered in the decision to treat or defer therapy. A high proportion of infants will have rapid progression during the first year of life. It is uncertain whether frequent monitoring of CD4 counts is effective in identifying infants who will have rapid progression. Viral loads do not distinguish rapid versus slow progression for individual infants in the first year of life. Therefore, current guidelines recommend treatment for any infant younger than age 12 months with CD4 levels below 25% and many experts initiate treatment for all infants younger than 12 months.

Children who have survived without treatment beyond age 12 months have a lower risk of progression. Further, at this age, CD4 parameters are more predictive of the level of risk. A large meta-analysis determined that CD4 levels of less than 20% for children aged 1–4 years and less than 15% for those older than age 4 years were associated with a 10% and 5% risk of progression to AIDS and death, respectively. Treatment is recommended for children meeting these age-based CD4 criteria, irrespective of symptoms or viral load. Studies have demonstrated that the estimated 1-year risk of death is two to three times higher in children with a plasma HIV RNA load of 100,000 copies/mL compared with 10,000 copies/mL. As a result the guidelines recommend consideration of treatment for asymptomatic or mildly symptomatic children with an HIV RNA load of 100,000 copies/mL or higher. Likewise, treatment should be considered for CD4

levels of 20–24% in children aged 1–4 years, or 15–24% in children older than 4 years. If a child is asymptomatic and has a CD4 levels above 25% and viral load of less than 100,000 copies/mL, treatment may be deferred with repeated evaluation at 3–4 month intervals.

2. Considerations in selecting antiretroviral medications— The process of selecting a combination of medications for a particular patient has become highly complex. The U.S. Food and Drug Administration (FDA) has approved 21 drugs and several fixed drug combinations from five different drug classes for the treatment of HIV (Table 39–3). The clinician must consider the potency of the drugs, tolerability, simplicity of dosing, drug interactions, prior drug therapy, and viral resistance profiles.

Potency, the intrinsic ability of the regimen to fully suppress viral replication, is foremost because without complete suppression resistant virus will emerge. Tolerability is also critical because regimens that are poorly tolerated fail due to poor adherence. When selecting a tolerable regimen, the circumstances and priorities of each individual patient and family must be considered. Certain side effects that may be acceptable to one person may be intolerable to another. Likewise, the frequency of dosing may have a great effect on adherence of some patients to the drug regimen, whereas others may be satisfied with frequent dosing provided that the number or size of pills is reduced. Over the years, more drugs have become available that can be given once daily and require fewer total pills or liquids.

Drug interactions between different antiretroviral medications, and with other medications, are frequent and must be considered when selecting a combination of drugs. Most of the protease inhibitors and non-nucleoside reverse transcriptase inhibitors are metabolized by cytochrome P-450 (CYP-450) isotypes and therefore can induce or inhibit the metabolism of other drugs that are metabolized by that pathway. Some combinations lead to significant decreases or increases in drug levels, and combined use is contraindicated. On the other hand, the drug interactions can be advantageous, and certain combinations of protease inhibitors can be used so that therapeutic plasma levels can be achieved with lower doses (and fewer pills). Drug absorption and metabolism can vary widely between individuals, especially for the protease inhibitor class. Therefore, therapeutic drug monitoring to determine the level of drug in serum and adjust doses to achieve therapeutic levels is recommended by some experts.

The potential for viral resistance should be evaluated when selecting a combination. Optimally, an initial regimen would select viral resistance mutations that do not confer cross-resistance to a large number of other drugs. This permits an opportunity to use alternative regimens if resistance to the initial regimen develops. The process is aided by laboratory methods (genotyping and phenotyping) to determine the presence of virus with specific drug resistance mutations in the patient.

Table 39–3. Antiretroviral drugs approved by the U.S. Food and Drug Administration.

Drug Class or Drug Name	Potential Adverse Effects[a]	Mechanism of Action
Nucleoside/nucleotide reverse transcriptase inhibitors (NRTI)	Lactic acidosis (rare but potentially fatal)	Chain termination of HIV DNA
Abacavir (ABC; Ziagen)	Hypersensitivity reaction	
Didanosine (ddI; Videx)	Pancreatitis, peripheral neuropathy, nausea, diarrhea	
Emtricitabine (FTC; Emtriva)	Minimal toxicity	
Lamivudine (3TC; Epivir)	Minimal toxicity	
Stavudine (d4T; Zerit)	Peripheral neuropathy, lipodystrophy, pancreatitis	
Tenofovir (TDF; Viread)	Headache, nausea, diarrhea, bone demineralization, renal insufficiency (rare)	
Zidovudine (ZDV, AZT; Retrovir)	Anemia, neutropenia, gastrointestinal intolerance, headache	
Non-nucleoside reverse transcriptase inhibitors (NNRTI)	Rash, rarely Stevens-Johnson syndrome	Synthesis of HIV DNA inhibited
Delavirdine (DLV, Rescriptor)	Increased liver transaminases, headache	
Efavirenz (EFV, Sustiva)	Central nervous system symptoms, increased transaminases, teratogenic in monkeys	
Nevirapine (NVP, Viramune)	Hepatitis	
Protease inhibitors (PI)	Glucose intolerance, risk of bleeding in hemophilics, dyslipidemia, lipodystrophy, transaminase elevation	Production of noninfectious virions
Atazanavir (ATV, Reyataz)	Increased indirect bilirubin	
Darunavir (DRV, Prezista)	Rash (cross-reaction with sulfonamide), gastrointestinal intolerance	
Fosamprenavir (FPV, Lexiva)	Rash, oral paresthesia	
Indinavir (IDV, Crixivan)	Nephrolithiasis, increased indirect bilirubin	
Lopinavir/ritonavir (LPV/r, Kaletra)	Gastrointestinal intolerance	
Nelfinavir (NFV, Viracept)	Diarrhea	
Ritonavir (RTV, Norvir)	Nausea, circumoral paraesthesias, hepatitis, pancreatitis, taste perversion	
Saquinavir hard gel (SQV, Invirase)	Gastrointestinal intolerance	
Tipranavir (TPV, Aptivus)	Hepatic toxicity, rash (cross-reaction with sulfonamide)	
Integrase inhibitor		Integration of viral nucleic acid in host genome prevented
Raltegravir (Isentress)	Diarrhea, nausea, headache, and fever	
Entry inhibitors		Viral entry inhibited
Enfuvirtide (T-20, Fuzeon)	Injection site reactions, increased rate of bacterial pneumonias, hypersensitivity reactions (< 1%)	Fusion inhibited
Maraviroc (Selzentry)	Hepatic toxicity, cardiac events, postural hypotension, cough, fever, upper respiratory infections	CCR5 co-receptor antagonist
Fixed drug combinations		
Abacavir/lamivudine (Epzicom)	See individual drugs	
Tenofovir/emtricitabine (Truvada)	See individual drugs	
Tenofovir/emtricitabine/efavirenz (Atripla)	See individual drugs	
Zidovudine/lamivudine (Combivir)	See individual drugs	
Zidovudine/lamivudine/abacavir (Trizavir)	See individual drugs	

[a]Relative incidence of adverse events depends on specific drug.

3. Specific antiretroviral medications

A. NUCLEOSIDE AND NUCLEOTIDE REVERSE TRANSCRIPTASE INHIBITORS (NRTIs)—The NRTIs act as nucleotide analogues, which are incorporated into HIV DNA during transcription by the HIV reverse transcriptase. The result is chain termination and failure to complete provirus, preventing incorporation of HIV genome into cellular DNA. The human mitochondrial DNA polymerase also has limited affinity for these analogues, the degree varying with the drug. Incorporation of the analogue into mitochondrial DNA is one mechanism thought to lead to adverse effects including pancreatitis, peripheral neuropathy, bone marrow suppression (anemia or neutropenia), and lipodystrophy (loss of peripheral fat and accumulation of visceral fat). Lactic acidosis with hepatic steatosis (fatty liver) is a rare but potentially fatal complication that may result from mitochondrial toxicity.

A hypersensitivity reaction (not related to mitochondrial toxicity) to abacavir occurs in approximately 10% of patients. The reaction, characterized by a flulike syndrome with or without rash, may be fatal with continued treatment or rechallenge.

B. NON-NUCLEOSIDE REVERSE TRANSCRIPTASE INHIBITORS (NNRTIs)—NNRTIs also inhibit HIV DNA synthesis but act at a different site on the viral enzyme so that cross-resistance does not occur with NRTIs. The NNRTIs have potent antiretroviral activity, but single amino acid mutations in the viral reverse transcriptase protein often induce resistance to all three drugs in this class. The most common toxicity is rash, which may be severe. Efavirenz is associated with central nervous system symptoms (ie, dizziness and confusion), which usually resolve after the initial weeks of use. Inflammation of the liver, rarely fatal, may occur with any of the drugs in the class, but is more common with nevirapine.

C. PROTEASE INHIBITORS—Protease inhibitors (PIs) bind the HIV protease and interfere with assembly of infectious virions. Acute adverse effects are mainly gastrointestinal intolerance and rash as well as other effects specific to the particular drug (see Table 39–3). All PIs are associated with a risk of glucose intolerance, elevated transaminases, or bleeding in hemophiliacs. Most are associated with dyslipidemia (elevated cholesterol and triglycerides) and may contribute to lipodystrophy. An exception is atazanavir, which is not associated with changes in serum lipids. These drugs are highly potent and usually require multiple mutations for high-level resistance to develop. Taste and pill burden limit tolerability of these medications. The PIs are metabolized by the hepatic CYP-450 enzymes, resulting in many interactions with other drugs, including other antiretrovirals. Careful attention to drug interactions is necessary when treating a patient taking a PI. Regimens combining two PIs can take advantage of the drug interactions and improve the pharmacokinetic properties of the drugs.

D. INTEGRASE INHIBITOR—Raltegravir is the first of this class to be FDA approved. The drug inhibits the viral integrase enzyme and prevents integration of HIV-1 nucleic acid into the host genome. Studies demonstrate rapid decreases in viral load with this drug.

E. ENTRY INHIBITORS—Enfuvirtide binds to the viral envelope protein and interferes with HIV fusion with the host cell plasma membrane, thereby preventing entry of the virus into the cell. Enfuvirtide must be administered parenterally, and local reactions at the injection site are common. Maraviroc is a chemokine receptor antagonist that binds one of the co-receptor proteins (CCR5) on the host CD4 T cell. This blocks viral binding and prevents cell entry for virus that uses that receptor. The drug is approved for patients who have multi-drug-resistant virus that has been demonstrated by laboratory testing to use the particular co-receptor.

B. General Measures

1. Immunizations—Combined diphtheria-tetanus-acellular pertussis, inactivated poliovirus, conjugated *Haemophilus influenzae* type b, conjugated *Streptococcus pneumoniae*, hepatitis B, and hepatitis A vaccines should be given as recommended for healthy children. (See Chapter 9.) The conjugated meningococcal vaccine and human papillomavirus vaccine are also recommended. Studies evaluating the immunogenicity of these vaccines in HIV-infected children are underway. A dose of 23-valent polysaccharide vaccine at age 2 years and a booster after 3–5 years is recommended in addition to the conjugated pneumococcal vaccine series given in infancy. Infected children and their household contacts should receive inactivated influenza vaccine annually after age 6 months. In general, live virus vaccines should be avoided. However, the risk of measles is considered greater than the potential risk of the vaccine in asymptomatic children; thus measles-mumps-rubella vaccine should be given at age 12 months, with the second dose given 1 month later, provided the child does not have evidence of severe immunosuppression (category C or category 3). Varicella vaccine, also a live virus, should be considered after the potential risks and benefits are weighed, for asymptomatic or mildly symptomatic HIV-infected children older than age 12 months with CD4 T-lymphocyte levels of 15% or more. HIV-infected children receive two doses of varicella vaccine administered 3 months apart.

Because antibody titers to vaccines decline with time and with progression of immune deficiency, prophylaxis with immune globulin for measles exposure and tetanus immune globulin for tetanus-prone wounds should be given regardless of immunization status.

2. Prophylaxis for infections—Children with suppressed CD4 lymphocyte numbers benefit from prophylactic treatment to prevent opportunistic infections. Children who have had their CD4 counts restored to category 1 or 2 for over 2–4 months can be taken off prophylactic treatments. Antibiotic prophylaxis for *P jiroveci* pneumonia has been extremely effective. Because this infection has its highest incidence during the first year of life, *P jiroveci* pneumonia prophylaxis is given to all infants born to HIV-infected mothers beginning at age 4–6 weeks. When tests for HIV DNA or RNA are demonstrated negative at age 3–4 months, prophylaxis may be discontinued. HIV-infected infants should continue on prophylactic drugs until age 12 months, when further treatment is based on assessment of symptoms and age-adjusted CD4 lymphocyte counts every 3 months. Published guidelines from the CDC for *P jiroveci* pneumonia prophylaxis are summarized in Tables 39–4 and 39–5.

Children with hypogammaglobulinemia or a history of serious or multiple bacterial infections may benefit from monthly intravenous immune globulin if they are not receiving trimethoprim–sulfamethoxazole and have not responded well to antiretroviral therapy. Clarithromycin or azithromycin reduces the frequency of disseminated MAC with a survival benefit for children with very low CD4 counts.

Recurrent mucocutaneous candidiasis can be prevented with nystatin, clotrimazole, or fluconazole. Oral antiviral prophylaxis (acyclovir, valacyclovir, or famciclovir) is effective for recurrent severe herpes simplex or VZV infections.

HIV-infected children have a higher risk of progressive *M tuberculosis* infections. Because the child's infection is usually

Table 39–5. Drug regimens for *Pneumocystis jirovaci* prophylaxis for children over age 4 weeks.

Recommended regimen
Trimethoprim-sulfamethoxazole, 150 mg TMP/m²/d plus 750 mg SMX/m²/d, administered orally, divided into two doses per day 3 days a week on consecutive days
Alternative (same total daily dosages):
Single daily dose 3 days a week on consecutive days
Divided twice-daily doses 7 days a week
Divided twice-daily doses 3 days a week on alternate days
Alternative if trimethoprim-sulfamethoxazole is not tolerated[a]
Dapsone, 2 mg/kg/d (not to exceed 100 mg) orally once daily or 4 mg/kg (not to exceed 200 mg) orally once weekly
Aerosolized pentamidine (children over age 5 y), 300 mg via Respirgard II inhaler monthly
Atovaquone, age 1–3 mo and > 24 mos, 30 mg/kg orally once daily; age 4–24 mo, 45 mg/kg orally once daily

[a]If dapsone, aerosolized pentamidine, or atovaquone is not tolerated, some clinicians use intravenous pentamidine, 4 mg/kg every 2–4 wk.
Adapted from 2002 USPHS/IDSA Guidelines for the Prevention of Opportunistic Infections in Persons infected with Human Immunodeficiency Virus. Available at http://www.aidsinfo.nih.gov/guidelines.

Table 39–4. *Pneumocystis jiroveci*[a] pneumonia prophylaxis for HIV-exposed and infected infants by age and HIV infection status.

Age/Infection Status	*P jiroveci* Prophylaxis
Birth to 4–6 wk	No prophylaxis
4–6 wk to 2 mo	Prophylaxis
2–12 mo	
HIV-infected or indeterminate	Prophylaxis
HIV infection reasonably excluded[b]	No prophylaxis
1–5 y, HIV-infected	Prophylaxis if CD4 count < 500/μL or CD4 < 15%[c]
6–12 y, HIV-infected	Prophylaxis if CD4 count < 200/μL or CD4 < 15%[c]

[a]Formerly *Pneumocystis carinii*.
[b]Among children who have had two or more negative HIV cultures or PCR tests, at least one of which is performed after age 1 month and one of which is performed at age 2–4 months or older.
[c]Prophylaxis should be considered on a case-by-case basis for children who might otherwise be at risk for *Pneumocystis* pneumonia, such as those with rapidly declining CD4 counts or percentages or children with category C conditions.
Adapted from 2002 USPHS/IDSA Guidelines for the Prevention of Opportunistic Infections in Persons Infected with Human Immunodeficiency Virus. Available at: http://www.aidsinfo.nih.gov/guidelines.

acquired from adult household contacts, the child and other household members should be skin-tested for tuberculosis yearly if they belong to a population with substantial risk for exposure to *M tuberculosis*.

3. Infections and other conditions—Rates of bacteremia, especially pneumococcal bacteremia, and shingles, are higher among HIV-infected children, even in the absence of severe suppression of CD4 counts. Shingles occurs 10 times more frequently among HIV infected children compared with age-matched healthy children. VZV and herpes simplex virus infections are treated with acyclovir, because symptoms may be prolonged in children with HIV. Short courses of valacyclovir or famciclovir—drugs with good bioavailability—are also effective, although not approved for children. Aphthous ulcers also occur in children, even when on suppressive antiretroviral drug therapy. Symptomatic CMV infection is treated with ganciclovir or foscarnet and requires ongoing secondary prophylaxis if CD4 lymphocyte counts remain low. MAC requires treatment with a multidrug regimen to delay the emergence of resistance. Lymphoid interstitial pneumonitis may respond to corticosteroid therapy. Chronic parvovirus as a cause of anemia should be investigated and can be treated with intravenous immune globulin. Anemia and granulocytopenia, whether drug-induced or HIV-induced, may respond to epoetin alfa (erythropoietin) and filgrastim (granulocyte colony-stimulating factor, G-CSF), respectively. Rarely transfusions are needed; CMV-seronegative blood should be used.

4. General support—Growth failure (weight and height) is one of the earliest and most sensitive markers of disease progression. The cause is a combination of increased metabolic needs related to chronic infection and decreased caloric intake. Supplemental nutrition in the form of oral supplements may be required. Some antiretroviral drugs cause elevated cholesterol and triglycerides. A cross-sectional study found elevated serum cholesterol in 13% of children with HIV compared with 5% of uninfected pediatric controls. Although the long-term consequences of drug-induced hyperlipidemia in HIV-infected children are unknown, diet modification and exercise are recommended. Nutritional evaluation and counseling should be a part of early care and continue throughout the child's care.

Evaluation and support for psychosocial needs of HIV-affected families is imperative. As with other chronic illnesses, HIV infection affects all family members, and it also carries an additional social stigma. Emotional concerns and financial needs are more prominent than medical needs at many stages of the disease process and influence the family's ability to comply with a medical treatment regimen. HIV-infected children often have comorbid mental health conditions. Rates of attention-deficit/hyperactivity disorder range from 20–50% in various studies. Hospital admissions for mental health disorders are more frequent among HIV-infected children. In one study dual diagnosis of HIV and a mental health disorder occurred in 85% of adolescents who acquired HIV infection through high-risk behaviors. Ideally, care should be coordinated by a team of caregivers that is familiar with this disease and the newest therapies, and that has access to community resources.

5. Public health considerations—The infant or child who is well enough to attend day care or school should not be treated differently from other children. The exception may be a toddler with uncontrollable biting behavior or bleeding lesions that cannot be covered adequately; in these situations, the child may be withheld from group day care. Optimally the school health care provider and teacher will be aware of the diagnosis, but there is no legal requirement that any individual at the school or day care center be informed. The parents and child may prefer to keep the diagnosis confidential, because the stigma associated with HIV infection may be difficult to overcome. Adolescents with HIV should receive counseling on the risk of transmission through sexual activity and shared needles. Programs should be made available to encourage use of barrier protection and to develop strategies for disclosure to their partners and other friends.

▶ Prognosis

There is a bimodal presentation of HIV disease progression in vertically infected children. Without treatment, about 20–30% of HIV-infected infants develop an AIDS-defining illness by age 1 year and die before age 2–3 years (considered to be rapid progressors). Mortality among infants born in some developing countries is even higher and may approach 50% in the first years of life. Cohorts of infants with rapid progression have higher median peak and median average levels of viremia over the first year of life than do other HIV-infected children. Other predictors of rapid progression are low absolute counts of CD4 and suppressor-killer T (CD8) lymphocytes in the first 6 months. In the remainder of infants the disease progresses more slowly, with 5% progressing to AIDS or death per year and median survival of 10 years based on studies performed in the United States and Europe. These so-called slow progressors generally have lower levels of viremia and a more gradual decline in CD4 lymphocyte counts. In rare instances children and adults with untreated infection show no evidence of immune suppression for 8–10 years or more. Studies indicate that both viral and host genetic factors, not fully defined, play a role in determining the rate of disease progression.

The initiation of antiretroviral therapy dramatically alters the natural history by slowing disease progression and permitting restoration of most immune function. Plasma viremia and age-adjusted CD4 lymphocyte counts are used to assess the risk of progression and response to antiretroviral treatment. With the introduction of HAART, mortality rates for HIV-infected children in the United States declined 80% between 1994 and 1999. Many children, infected from birth, are entering adolescence and young adulthood. With recognition of the longer survival time in most infected children, this disease is now approached as a chronic, rather than acutely terminal, illness. The complexity of antiretroviral drug therapy requires care from a provider with HIV expertise. Primary care physicians are encouraged to participate in the care of HIV-infected children in collaboration with centers staffed by personnel with expertise in pediatric HIV issues.

REFERENCES

AIDS Institute New York State Department of Health. Supportive Care Issues for Children with HIV Infection, 2001:18-1-18-22. Available at: http://www.hivguidelines.org/public_html/center/clinicalguidelines/ped_adolescent_hiv_guidelines/htmlpeds_supportive_care/pdf/supportive_care.pdf and http://www. hivguidelines.org/GuideLine.aspx?pageID=258&guideLineID=36.

American Academy of Pediatrics, Committee of Pediatric AIDS and Committee on Infectious Diseases: Issues related to human immunodeficiency virus transmission in schools, child care, medical settings, the home, and community. Pediatrics 1999; 104(2 Pt 1):318 [PMID: 10429018].

Bulterys M et al, for the Mother-Infant Rapid Intervention at Delivery (MIRIAD) Study Group: Rapid HIV-1 testing during labor: A multicenter study. JAMA 2004;292:219 [PMID: 15249571].

Centers for Disease Control and Prevention: 1994 Revised classification system for human immunodeficiency virus infection in children less than 13 years of age. MMWR Recomm Rep 1994;43(RR-12):1 [PMID: 7908403].

Fowler MG et al: Reducing the risk of mother-to-child human immunodeficiency virus transmission: Past successes, current progress and challenges, and future directions. Am J Obstet Gynecol 2007;197(3 Suppl):S3 [PMID: 17825648].

Gona P et al: Incidence of opportunistic and other infections in HIV-infected children in the HAART era. JAMA 2006;296:292 [PMID: 16849662].

Havens PL, Waters D: Management of the infant born to a mother with HIV infection Pediatr Clin North Am 2004;51:909 [PMID: 15275981].

HIV Paediatric Prognostic Markers Collaborative Study: Predictive value of absolute CD4 cell count for disease progression in untreated HIV-1-infected children. AIDS 2006;20:1289 [PMID: 16816558].

Leonard EG, McComsey GA: Antiretroviral therapy in HIV-infected children: The metabolic cost of improved survival. Infect Dis Clin North Am 2005;19:713 [PMID: 16102657].

McConnell MS et al, for the Pediatric Spectrum of HIV Disease Consortium: Trends in antiretroviral therapy use and survival rates for a large cohort of HIV-infected children and adolescents in the United States, 1989–2001. J Acquir Immune Defic Syndr 2005;38:488 [PMID: 15764966].

Mellins CA et al: The role of psychosocial and family factors in adherence to antiretroviral treatment in human immunodeficiency virus-infected children. Pediatr Infect Dis J 2004;23:1035 [PMID: 15545859].

Mofenson LM et al: Treating opportunistic infections among HIV exposed and infected children: Recommendations from CDC, the National Institutes of Health, and the Infectious Diseases Society of America. Clin Infect Dis 2005; 40(Suppl 1):S1 [PMID: 15655768].

Nozyce ML et al: A behavioral and cognitive profile of clinically stable HIV-infected children. Pediatrics 2006;117:763 [PMID: 16510656].

Perinatal HIV Guidelines Working Group: Public Health Service Task Force Recommendations for Use of Antiretroviral Drugs in Pregnant HIV-1 Infected Women for Maternal Health and Interventions to Reduce Perinatal HIV-1 Transmission in the United States. October 12, 2006 1-65. Available at: http://aidsinfo.nih.gov/ContentFiles/PerinatalGL.pdf.

Smith et al; U.S. Department of Health and Human Services: Antiretroviral postexposure prophylaxis after sexual, injection-drug use, or other nonoccupational exposure to HIV in the United States: Recommendations from the U.S. Department of Health and Human Services. MMWR Recomm Rep 2005;54(RR-2):1 [PMID: 15660015].

Working Group on Antiretroviral Therapy and Medical Management of HIV-Infected Children: Guidelines for the Use of Antiretroviral Agents in Pediatric HIV Infection. October 26, 2006 1-126. Available at http://aidsinfo.nih.gov/ContentFiles/PediatricGuidelines.pdf.

Zetola NM, Pilcher CD: Diagnosis and management of acute HIV infection. Infect Dis Clin North Am 2007;21:19 [PMID: 17502228].

Infections: Bacterial & Spirochetal

John W. Ogle, MD
Marsha S. Anderson, MD

▼ BACTERIAL INFECTIONS

GROUP A STREPTOCOCCAL INFECTIONS

ESSENTIALS OF DIAGNOSIS
& TYPICAL FEATURES

Streptococcal pharyngitis:

▶ Clinical diagnosis based entirely on symptoms; signs and physical examination unreliable.

▶ Throat culture or rapid antigen detection test positive for group A streptococci.

Impetigo:

▶ Rapidly spreading, highly infectious skin rash.

▶ Erythematous denuded areas and honey-colored crusts.

▶ Group A streptococci are grown in culture from most (not all) cases.

▶ General Considerations

Group A streptococci (GAS) are common gram-positive bacteria producing a wide variety of clinical illnesses, including acute pharyngitis, impetigo, cellulitis, and scarlet fever, the generalized illness caused by strains that elaborate erythrogenic toxin. GAS can also cause pneumonia, septic arthritis, osteomyelitis, meningitis, and other less common infections. GAS infections may also produce nonsuppurative sequelae (rheumatic fever and acute glomerulonephritis).

The cell walls of streptococci contain both carbohydrate and protein antigens. The C-carbohydrate antigen determines the group, and the M- or T-protein antigens determine the specific type. In most strains, the M protein appears to confer virulence, and antibodies developed against the M protein are protective against reinfection with that type.

GAS are almost all β-hemolytic. These organisms may be carried without symptoms on the skin and in the pharynx, rectum, and vagina. Between 10% and 15% of school-aged children in some studies are asymptomatic pharyngeal carriers of GAS. Streptococcal carriers are individuals who do not mount an immune response to the organism and are therefore believed to be at low risk for nonsuppurative sequelae. All GAS are sensitive to penicillin. Resistance to erythromycin is common in some countries and has increased in the United States.

A. Clinical Findings

1. Respiratory infections

A. INFANCY AND EARLY CHILDHOOD (< AGE 3 YEARS)—The onset is insidious, with mild symptoms (low-grade fever, serous nasal discharge, and pallor). Otitis media is common. Exudative pharyngitis and cervical adenitis are uncommon in this age group.

B. CHILDHOOD TYPE—Onset is sudden, with fever and marked malaise and often with repeated vomiting. The pharynx is sore and edematous, and generally there is tonsillar exudate. Anterior cervical lymph nodes are tender and enlarged. Small petechiae are frequently seen on the soft palate. In **scarlet fever,** the skin is diffusely erythematous and appears sunburned and roughened (sandpaper rash). The rash is most intense in the axillae, groin, and on the abdomen and trunk. It blanches except in the skin folds, which do not blanch and are pigmented (Pastia's sign). The rash usually appears 24 hours after the onset of fever and rapidly spreads over the next 1–2 days. Desquamation begins on the face at the end of the first week and becomes generalized by the third week. Early in the course of infection, the surface of the tongue is coated white, with the papillae enlarged and bright red (so-called white strawberry tongue). Subsequently desquamation occurs, and the tongue appears beefy red (strawberry tongue). The face generally shows circumoral pallor. Petechiae may be seen on all mucosal surfaces.

C. ADULT TYPE—The adult type of GAS is characterized by exudative or nonexudative tonsillitis with fewer systemic symptoms, lower fever, and no vomiting. Scarlet fever is uncommon in adults.

2. Impetigo—Streptococcal impetigo begins as a papule that vesiculates and then breaks, leaving a denuded area covered by a honey-colored crust. Both *Staphylococcus aureus* and GAS are isolated in some cases. The lesions spread readily and diffusely. Local lymph nodes may become swollen and inflamed. Although the child often lacks systemic symptoms, a high fever and toxicity may be present. If flaccid bullae are noted, the disease is called bullous impetigo and is caused by an epidermolytic toxin-producing strain of *S aureus*.

3. Cellulitis—The portal of entry is often an insect bite or superficial abrasion. A diffuse, rapidly spreading cellulitis occurs that involves the subcutaneous tissues and extends along the lymphatic pathways with only minimal local suppuration. Local acute lymphadenitis occurs. The child is usually acutely ill, with fever and malaise. In classic erysipelas, the involved area is bright red, swollen, warm, and very tender. The infection may extend rapidly from the lymphatics to the bloodstream.

Streptococcal perianal cellulitis is an entity peculiar to young children. Pain with defecation often leads to constipation, which may be the presenting complaint. The child is afebrile and otherwise well. Perianal erythema, tenderness, and painful rectal examination are the only abnormal physical findings. Scant rectal bleeding with defecation may occur. A perianal swab culture usually yields heavy growth of GAS. A variant of this syndrome is streptococcal vaginitis in prepubertal girls. Symptoms are dysuria and pain; marked erythema and tenderness of the introitus and blood-tinged discharge are seen.

4. Necrotizing fasciitis—This dangerous disease is reported sporadically and may occur as a complication of varicella infection. About 20–40% of cases are due to GAS; 30–40% are due to *S aureus*; and the rest are a result of mixed bacterial infections. The disease is characterized by extensive necrosis of superficial fasciae, undermining of surrounding tissue, and usually systemic toxicity. Initially the skin overlying the infection is tender and pale red without distinct borders, resembling cellulitis. Blisters or bullae may appear. The color deepens to a distinct purple or in some cases becomes pale. Tenderness out of proportion to the clinical appearance, skin anesthesia (due to infarction of superficial nerves), or "woody" induration suggest necrotizing fasciitis. Involved areas may develop mild to massive edema. Early recognition and aggressive debridement of necrotic tissue are essential.

5. Group A streptococcal infections in newborn nurseries—GAS epidemics occur occasionally in nurseries. The organism may be introduced into the nursery from the vaginal tract of a mother or from the throat or nose of a mother or a staff member. The organism then spreads from infant to infant. The umbilical stump is colonized while the infant is in the nursery. Like staphylococcal infections, there may be no or few clinical manifestations while the infant is still in the nursery. Most often, a colonized infant develops a chronic, oozing omphalitis days later. The organism may spread from the infant to other family members. Serious and even fatal infections may develop, including sepsis, meningitis, empyema, septic arthritis, and peritonitis.

6. Streptococcal sepsis—Serious illness from GAS sepsis is now more common both in children and in adults. Rash and scarlet fever may be present. Prostration and shock result in high mortality rates. Pharyngitis is uncommon as an antecedent illness. Underlying disease is a predisposing factor.

7. Streptococcal toxic shock syndrome (STSS)—Toxic shock syndrome caused by GAS has been defined. Like *S aureus*–associated toxic shock, multiorgan system involvement is a prominent part of the illness. The diagnostic criteria include (1) isolation of GAS from a normally sterile site, (2) hypotension or shock, and (3) at least two of the following: renal impairment (creatinine > 2 times the upper limit of normal for age), thrombocytopenia (< 100,000/mm^3), or coagulopathy, liver involvement (transaminases > 2 times normal), acute respiratory distress syndrome, generalized erythematous macular rash or soft tissue necrosis (myositis, necrotizing fasciitis, gangrene). In cases that otherwise meet clinical criteria, isolation of GAS from a nonsterile site (throat, wound, or vagina) is indicative of a probable cause.

B. Laboratory Findings

Leukocytosis with a marked shift to the left is seen early. Eosinophilia regularly appears during convalescence. β-Hemolytic streptococci are cultured from the throat. The organism may be cultured from the skin and by needle aspiration from subcutaneous tissues and other involved sites such as infected nodes. Occasionally blood cultures are positive. Newer rapid antigen detection tests such as optical immunoassays and DNA chemiluminescence probes are very specific, and in some cases are almost as sensitive as traditional throat culture. However, sensitivity varies with the type of test used and the experience level of the laboratory or office. Many experts recommend backup throat culture in patients with negative rapid strep antigen tests. Patients with positive rapid strep antigen tests do not need a confirmation by throat culture, since the specificity of antigen tests are high.

Antistreptolysin O (ASO) titers rise about 150 units within 2 weeks after acute infection. Elevated ASO and anti-DNase B titers are useful in documenting prior throat infections in cases of acute rheumatic fever. The streptozyme test detects antibodies to streptolysin O, hyaluronidase, streptokinase, DNase B, and NADase. It is somewhat more sensitive than the measurement of ASO titers.

Proteinuria, cylindruria, and minimal hematuria may be seen early in children with streptococcal infection. True post-streptococcal glomerulonephritis is seen 1–4 weeks after the respiratory or skin infection.

Differential Diagnosis

Streptococcal infection in early childhood must be differentiated from adenovirus and other respiratory virus infections. The pharyngitis in herpangina (coxsackie A viruses) is vesicular or ulcerative. Herpes simplex also causes ulcerative lesions, which most commonly involve the anterior pharynx, tongue, and gums. In infectious mononucleosis, the pharyngitis is also exudative, but splenomegaly and generalized adenopathy are typical, and laboratory findings are often diagnostic (atypical lymphocytes, elevated liver enzymes, and a positive heterophil or other serologic test for mononucleosis). Uncomplicated streptococcal pharyngitis improves within 24–48 hours if penicillin is given and by 72–96 hours without antimicrobials.

Group G and group C streptococci are uncommon causes of pharyngitis but have been implicated in epidemics of sore throat in college students. Acute rheumatic fever does not occur following group G or group C infection, although acute glomerulonephritis is a complication. *Arcanobacterium hemolyticum* may cause pharyngitis with scarlatina-like or maculopapular truncal rash. In diphtheria, systemic symptoms, vomiting, and fever are less marked; pharyngeal pseudomembrane is confluent and adherent; the throat is less red; and cervical adenopathy is prominent. Pharyngeal tularemia causes white rather than yellow exudate. There is little erythema, and cultures for β-hemolytic streptococci are negative. A history of exposure to rabbits and a failure to respond to antimicrobials may suggest the diagnosis. Leukemia and agranulocytosis may present with pharyngitis and are diagnosed by bone marrow examination.

Scarlet fever must be differentiated from other exanthematous diseases (principally rubella), erythema due to sunburn, drug reactions, Kawasaki disease, toxic shock syndrome, and staphylococcal scalded skin syndrome (see also Table 38–3).

Complications

Suppurative complications of GAS infections include sinusitis, otitis, mastoiditis, cervical lymphadenitis, pneumonia, empyema, septic arthritis, and meningitis. Spread of streptococcal infection from the throat to other sites—principally the skin (impetigo) and vagina—is common and should be considered in every instance of chronic vaginal discharge or chronic skin infection, such as that complicating childhood eczema. Both acute rheumatic fever and acute glomerulonephritis are nonsuppurative complications of GAS infections.

A. Acute Rheumatic Fever (See Chapter 19)

B. Acute Glomerulonephritis

Acute glomerulonephritis (AGN) can follow streptococcal infections of either the pharynx or the skin—in contrast to rheumatic fever, which follows pharyngeal infection only. AGN may occur at any age, even infancy. In most reports of AGN, males predominate by a ratio of 2:1. Rheumatic fever occurs with equal frequency in both sexes. Certain M types are associated strongly with post-streptococcal glomerulonephritis (nephritogenic types). The serotypes producing disease on the skin often differ from those found in the pharynx.

The incidence of AGN after streptococcal infection is variable and has ranged from 0–28%. Several outbreaks of AGN in families have involved 50–75% of siblings of affected patients in 1- to 7-week periods. Second attacks of glomerulonephritis are rare. The median period between infection and the development of glomerulonephritis is 10 days. In contrast, acute rheumatic fever occurs after a median of 18 days.

C. Post-Streptococcal Reactive Arthritis

Following an episode of group A streptococcal pharyngitis, a reactive arthritis develops in some patients. This reactive arthritis is believed to be due to immune complex deposition and is seen about 1–2 weeks following the acute infection. Patients with post-streptococcal reactive arthritis do not have the full constellation of clinical and laboratory criteria needed to fulfill the Jones criteria for a diagnosis of acute rheumatic fever.

Treatment

A. Specific Measures

Treatment is directed toward both eradication of acute infection and prevention of rheumatic fever. In patients with pharyngitis, antibiotics should be started early to relieve symptoms and should be continued for 10 days to prevent rheumatic fever. Although early therapy has not been shown to prevent AGN, it seems advisable to treat impetigo promptly in sibling contacts of patients with post-streptococcal nephritis. Neither sulfonamides nor trimethoprim–sulfamethoxazole is effective in the treatment of streptococcal infections. Although topical therapy for impetigo with antimicrobial ointments (especially mupirocin) is as effective as systemic therapy, it does not eradicate pharyngeal carriage and is less practical for extensive disease.

1. Penicillin—Except for penicillin-allergic patients, penicillin V (phenoxymethyl penicillin) is the drug of choice. Penicillin resistance has never been documented. For children weighing less than 27 kg, the regimen is 250 mg, given orally two or three times a day for 10 days. For heavier children, adolescents, or adults 500 mg two or three times a day is recommended. Giving penicillin V (250 mg) twice daily is as effective as more frequent oral administration or intramuscular therapy. Once-daily oral amoxicillin (750 mg) has been shown, in one study of children 3–18 years of age, to be as effective as penicillin V given three times a day. Another alternative for treatment of pharyngitis and impetigo is a single dose of benzathine penicillin G, given intramuscularly (0.6 million units for children weighing < 60 lb [27.2 kg] and 1.2 million units for children weighing > 60 lb [27.2 kg]). Intramuscular delivery ensures compliance, but is painful. Parenteral therapy is indicated if vomiting or sepsis is present. Mild cellulitis due to GAS may be treated orally or intramuscularly.

Cellulitis requiring hospitalization can be treated with aqueous penicillin G (150,000 units/kg/d, given intravenously in four to six divided doses) or cefazolin (80–100 mg/kg/d, given intravenously in three divided doses) until there is marked improvement. Penicillin V (50 mg/kg/d in four divided doses) or cephalexin (50–75 mg/kg/d in four divided doses), may then be given orally to complete a 10-day course. Acute cervical lymphadenitis may require incision and drainage. Treatment of necrotizing fasciitis requires emergency surgical debridement followed by high-dose parenteral antibiotics appropriate to the organisms cultured.

2. Other antibiotics—For penicillin-allergic patients with pharyngitis or impetigo the following alternative regimens have been used: erythromycin estolate (20–40 mg/kg/d in two to four divided doses) for 10 days; clarithromycin (15 mg/kg/d in two divided doses) for 10 days; and azithromycin (12 mg/kg/d) once daily for 5 days. Erythromycin resistance, although not currently widespread in the United States, was reported in 48% of strains tested in Pittsburgh in 2001. Penicillin-allergic patients from areas with high rates of erythromycin resistance may require an alternative antibiotic. Clindamycin, cephalexin, ceftibuten, cefdinir, cefadroxil, azithromycin, and clarithromycin are other effective oral antimicrobials. Each of these drugs should be given for 10 days, with the exception of azithromycin which is given for 5 days. The dosage of clindamycin is 10–20 mg/kg/d orally in four divided doses. Patients with immediate, anaphylactic hypersensitivity to penicillin should not receive cephalosporins, because up to 15% will also be allergic to cephalosporins. In most studies, bacteriologic failures after cephalosporin therapy are less frequent than failures following penicillin. However, cephalosporins are generally more expensive than penicillin. Additionally, there are few conclusive data on the ability of these agents to prevent rheumatic fever. Therefore, penicillin remains the agent of choice for nonallergic patients. Many strains are resistant to tetracycline.

For infections requiring intravenous therapy, aqueous penicillin G (250,000 units/kg in six divided doses) given intravenously is usually the drug of choice. Cefazolin (100–150 mg/kg/d intravenously or intramuscularly in three divided doses); clindamycin (25–40 mg/kg/d intravenously in four divided doses); and vancomycin (40 mg/kg/d intravenously in four divided doses) are alternatives in penicillin-allergic patients. Clindamycin is preferred by many experts and may be superior to penicillin for necrotizing fasciitis if the organism is susceptible to it. Clindamycin should not be used alone empirically for severe, suspected GAS infections because a small percentage of isolates in the United States are resistant to it. Some physicians use both penicillin and clindamycin in patients with necrotizing fasciitis or STSS.

3. Serious GAS disease—Serious GAS infections, such as pneumonia, osteomyelitis, septic arthritis, sepsis, endocarditis, meningitis, and STSS, require parenteral antimicrobial therapy. Penicillin G is the drug of choice for these invasive infections. Clindamycin, in addition to penicillin G, is advocated by many experts for STSS or necrotizing fasciitis. Necrotizing fasciitis requires prompt surgical debridement. In STSS, volume status and blood pressure should be monitored and patients evaluated for a focus of infection, if not readily apparent. Intravenous immune globulin (in addition to antibiotics) has been used in severe cases.

4. Treatment failure—Even when compliance is perfect, organisms will be found in cultures in 5–15% of children after cessation of therapy. Reculture is indicated only in patients with relapse or recrudescence of pharyngitis or those with a personal or family history of rheumatic fever. Repeat treatment at least once with an oral cephalosporin or clindamycin is indicated in patients with recurrent culture-positive pharyngitis.

5. Prevention of recurrences in rheumatic individuals—The preferred prophylaxis for rheumatic individuals is benzathine penicillin G, 1.2 million units intramuscularly every 4 weeks. If the risk of streptococcal exposure is high, every-3-week dosing is preferred. One of the following alternative oral prophylactic regimens may be used: sulfadiazine, 0.5 g once a day (if < 27 kg) or 1 g once a day (if > 27 kg); penicillin V, 250 mg twice daily; or erythromycin, 250 mg twice daily. Continued prophylaxis is recommended for at least 5 years or until age 21 years (whichever is longer) if carditis is absent. Prophylaxis in these individuals should be continued if the risk of contact with persons with GAS is high (eg, parents of school-aged children, pediatric nurses, and teachers). In the presence of carditis without residual heart or valvular disease, a minimum of 10 years (or well into adulthood, whichever is longer) is the minimum duration. If the patient has residual valvular heart disease, many recommend lifelong prophylaxis. These patients should be at least 10 years from their last episode of rheumatic disease and at least 40 years of age prior to considering discontinuation of prophylaxis. A similar approach to the prevention of recurrences of glomerulonephritis may be indicated during childhood when there is a suspicion that repeated streptococcal infections coincide with flare-ups of glomerulonephritis.

6. Post-streptococcal reactive arthritis—In contrast to rheumatic fever, nonsteroidal agents may not dramatically improve joint symptoms. However, like patients with rheumatic fever, some patients with post-streptococcal reactive arthritis have developed carditis several weeks to months after their arthritis symptoms began. Therefore, some experts recommend antibiotic prophylaxis of these patients for 1 year and monitoring for signs of carditis (see recommendations for prevention of recurrences of rheumatic fever, above). If carditis does not develop, prophylaxis could then be discontinued.

If carditis develops, the patient should be considered to have acute rheumatic fever and prophylaxis continued as described above.

B. General Measures

Acetaminophen is useful for pain or fever. Local treatment of impetigo may promote earlier healing. Crusts should first be soaked off. Areas beneath the crusts should then be washed with soap daily.

C. Treatment of Complications

Rheumatic fever is best prevented by early and adequate penicillin treatment of the streptococcal infection.

D. Treatment of Carriers

Identification and treatment of GAS carriers is difficult. There are no established clinical or serologic criteria for differentiating carriers from the truly infected. Some children receive multiple courses of antimicrobials, with persistence of GAS in the throat, leading to a "streptococcal neurosis" on the part of families.

In certain circumstances, eradication of carriage may be desirable: (1) when a family member has a history of rheumatic fever; (2) when an episode of STSS or necrotizing fasciitis has occurred in a household contact; (3) multiple, recurring, documented episodes of GAS in family members despite adequate therapy; and (4) during an outbreak of rheumatic fever or GAS-associated glomerulonephritis. Clindamycin (20 mg/kg/d, given orally in three divided doses, to a maximum of 150 mg/dose) or a combination of rifampin (20 mg/kg/d, given orally for 4 days) and penicillin in standard dosage given orally has been used to attempt eradication of carriage.

▶ Prognosis

Death is rare except in infants or young children with sepsis or pneumonia. The febrile course is shortened and complications eliminated by early and adequate treatment with penicillin.

Bisno AL et al: Practice guidelines for the diagnosis and management of group A streptococcal pharyngitis. Infectious Diseases Society of America. Clin Infect Dis 2002;35:113 [PMID: 12087516].

Gerber MA: Diagnosis and treatment of pharyngitis in children. Pediatr Clin North Am 2005;52:729 [PMID: 15925660].

Tanz RR. Shulman ST: Chronic pharyngeal carriage of group A streptococci. Pediatr Infect Dis J 2007;26:175 [PMID: 17259882].

Vincent MT et al: Pharyngitis. Am Fam Physician 2004;69:1465 [PMID: 15053411].

Vinh DC, Embil JM: Rapidly progressive soft tissue infections. Lancet Infect Dis 2005;5:501 [PMID: 16048719].

The Working Group on Severe Streptococcal Infections: Defining the group A streptococcal toxic shock syndrome: Rationale and consensus definition. JAMA 1993;269:390 [PMID: 8418347].

GROUP B STREPTOCOCCAL INFECTIONS

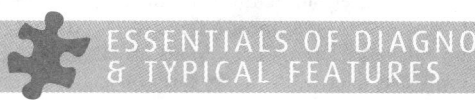

ESSENTIALS OF DIAGNOSIS & TYPICAL FEATURES

Early-onset neonatal infection:

▶ Newborn younger than age 7 days, with rapidly progressing overwhelming sepsis, with or without meningitis.

▶ Pneumonia with respiratory failure is frequent; chest radiograph resembles that seen in hyaline membrane disease.

▶ Leukopenia with a shift to the left.

▶ Blood or cerebrospinal fluid (CSF) cultures growing group B streptococci.

Late-onset Infection:

▶ Meningitis, sepsis, or other focal infection in a child aged 1–16 weeks with blood or CSF cultures growing group B streptococci.

▶ General Considerations

The incidence of perinatal group B streptococci (GBS) disease has declined dramatically since screening of pregnant mothers and provision of intrapartum chemoprophylaxis began. However, neonatal infections due to GBS still occur. Although most patients with GBS disease are infants younger than age 3 months, cases are seen in infants aged 4–5 months. Serious infection also occurs in women with puerperal sepsis, immunocompromised patients, patients with cirrhosis and spontaneous peritonitis, and diabetic patients with cellulitis. Two distinct clinical syndromes distinguished by differing perinatal events, age at onset, and serotype of the infecting strain occur in infants.

Risk factors for early-onset group GBS disease include maternal GBS colonization, gestational age less than 37 weeks, rupture of membranes more than 18 hours prior to presentation, young maternal age, history of a previous infant with invasive GBS disease, African-American or Hispanic ethnic origin, and low or absent maternal GBS anticapsular antibodies.

▶ Clinical Findings

A. Early-Onset Infection

"Early-onset" illness is observed in newborns younger than 7 days old. The onset of symptoms in the majority of these infants occurs in the first 48 hours of life, and most are ill within 6 hours. Apnea is often the first sign. Sepsis, meningitis, apnea, and pneumonia are the most common clinical presentations. There is a high incidence of associated maternal obstetric complications, especially premature labor and prolonged rupture of the membranes. Newborns with early-onset disease are severely ill at the time of diagnosis, and more than 50% die. Although most infants with early-onset infections are full-term, premature infants are at increased risk for the disease. Newborns with early-onset infection acquire GBS in utero as an ascending infection or during passage through the birth canal. When early-onset infection is complicated by meningitis, more than 80% of the bacterial isolates belong to serotype III. Postmortem examination of infants with early-onset disease usually reveals pulmonary inflammatory infiltrates and hyaline membranes containing large numbers of GBS.

B. Late-Onset Infection

"Late-onset" infection occurs in infants between ages 7 days and 4 months (median age at onset, about 4 weeks). Maternal obstetric complications are not usually associated with late-onset infection. These infants are usually not as ill at the time of diagnosis as those with early-onset disease, and the mortality rate is lower. In recent series, about 37% of patients have meningitis and 46% have sepsis. Septic arthritis and osteomyelitis, meningitis, occult bacteremia, otitis media, ethmoiditis, conjunctivitis, cellulitis (particularly of the face or submandibular area), lymphadenitis, breast abscess, empyema, and impetigo have been described. Strains of GBS possessing the capsular type III polysaccharide antigen are isolated from more than 95% of infants with late-onset disease, regardless of clinical manifestations. The exact mode of transmission of the organisms is not well defined.

C. Diagnosis

Culture of GBS from a normally sterile site such as blood, pleural fluid, or CSF provides proof of diagnosis. Frequent false-positive results limit the usefulness of testing for GBS antigen in urine and CSF.

▶ Prevention

Many women of childbearing age possess type-specific circulating antibody to the polysaccharide antigens for GBS. These antibodies are transferred to the newborn via the placental circulation. Carriers delivering healthy infants have significant serum levels of IgG antibody to this antigen. In contrast, women delivering infants who develop either early- or late-onset GBS disease rarely have detectable antibody in their sera.

Monovalent and bivalent vaccines with type II or III polysaccharide antigens have been studied in pregnant women, with 80–90% of vaccine recipients developing fourfold or greater increases in GBS capsular polysaccharide type-specific IgG. These reports suggest that a multivalent vaccine could be developed and given to pregnant women to prevent many cases of early-onset GBS disease.

The Centers for Disease Control and Prevention (CDC) has issued culture-based maternal guidelines for the prevention of early-onset GBS disease.

▶ CDC Recommendations for Prevention of Perinatal GBS Disease

1. All pregnant women should be screened at 35–37 weeks' gestation with a vaginal and rectal culture for GBS. *Exceptions:* Women with known GBS bacteriuria during the current pregnancy or women who have delivered a previous infant with GBS disease do not need screening—all these women need intrapartum prophylaxis.
2. If GBS status is unknown at onset of labor or rupture of membranes, intrapartum chemoprophylaxis should be administered to women with any of the following:

   a. Gestation less than 37 weeks.
   b. Rupture of membranes more than 18 hours.
   c. Intrapartum temperature of greater than 38°C (> 100.4°F)

3. Women with GBS colonization and a planned cesarean delivery done prior to labor and rupture of membranes do not routinely need intrapartum antimicrobial prophylaxis (IAP).
4. IAP recommendations (Table 40–1).
5. Empiric treatment of a neonate whose mother received IAP for prevention of GBS (Figure 40–1).

▶ Treatment

Intravenous ampicillin and an aminoglycoside is the initial regimen of choice for newborns with presumptive invasive GBS disease. For neonates younger than 7 days of age with meningitis, the recommended ampicillin dosage is 200–300 mg/kg/d, given intravenously in three divided doses. For infants older than 7 days of age, the recommended ampicillin dosage is 300 mg/kg/d, given intravenously in four to six divided doses. Penicillin G can be used once GBS is identified and clinical and microbiologic responses have occurred. GBS are less susceptible than other streptococci to penicillin, and high doses are recommended, especially for meningitis. In infants with meningitis, the recommended dosage of penicillin G varies with age: for infants age 7 days or younger, 250,000–450,000 units/kg/d, given intravenously in three divided doses; for infants older than age 7 days, 450,000–500,000 units/kg/d, given intravenously in four to six divided doses.

A second lumbar puncture after 24–48 hours of therapy is recommended by some experts to assess efficacy. Duration of therapy is 2–3 weeks for meningitis; at least 4 weeks for osteomyelitis, cerebritis, ventriculitis, or endocarditis; and 10–14 days for most other infections. Therapy does not eradicate carriage of the organism.

Although streptococci have been universally susceptible to penicillins, increasing minimum inhibitory concentrations (MICs) have been observed in some isolates. In one U.S. study, 10 of 574 rectovaginal isolates obtained from pregnant women in South Carolina were not fully penicillin-susceptible. However, all isolates were vancomycin-susceptible. Resistance of isolates to clindamycin and erythromycin has increased significantly worldwide in the past few years.

Table 40–1. Centers for Disease Control and Prevention recommended regimens for intrapartum prophylaxis for perinatal group B streptococcal (GBS) disease.[a]

Recommended	Penicillin G, 5 million units IV initial dose, then 2.5 million units IV q4h until delivery
Alternative	Ampicillin, 2 g IV initial dose, then 1 g IV q4h until delivery
If penicillin allergic[b]	
Patients not at high risk for anaphylaxis	Cefazolin, 2 g IV initial dose, then 1 g IV q8h until delivery
Patients at high risk for anaphylaxis[c]	
GBS susceptible to clindamycin and erythromycin[d]	Clindamycin, 900 mg IV q8h until delivery
GBS resistant to clindamycin or erythromycin or susceptibility unknown	Vancomycin,[e] 1 g IV q12h until delivery

[a]Broader-spectrum agents, including an agent active against GBS, may be necessary for treatment of chorioamnionitis.
[b]History of penicillin allergy should be assessed to determine whether a high risk for anaphylaxis is present. Penicillin-allergic patients at high risk for anaphylaxis are those who have experienced immediate hypersensitivity to penicillin including a history of penicillin-related anaphylaxis; other high-risk patients are those with asthma or other diseases that would make anaphylaxis more dangerous or difficult to treat, such as persons being treated with β-adrenergic-blocking agents.
[c]If laboratory facilities are adequate, clindamycin and erythromycin susceptibility testing should be performed on prenatal GBS isolates from penicillin-allergic women at high risk for anaphylaxis.
[d]Resistance to erythromycin is often, but not always, associated with clindamycin resistance. If a strain is resistant to erythromycin, but appears susceptible to clindamycin, it may have inducible resistance to clindamycin.
[e]Cefazolin is preferred over vancomycin for women with a history of penicillin allergy other than immediate hypersensitivity reactions, and pharmacologic data suggest it achieves effective intra-amniotic concentrations. Vancomycin should be reserved for penicillin-allergic women at high risk for anaphylaxis.
Reprinted, with permission, from Schrag S et al: Prevention of perinatal Group B streptococcal disease. Revised guidelines from CDC. MMWR Recomm Rep 2002;51(RR-11):1.

Apgar BS, Greenberg G: Prevention of group B streptococcal disease in the newborn. Am Fam Physician 2005;71:903 [PMID: 15768620].

Baker CJ et al: Safety and immunogenicity of a bivalent group B streptococcal conjugate vaccine for serotypes II and III. J Infect Dis 2003;188;66 [PMID: 22708435].

Centers for Disease Control and Prevention: Group B streptococcus. http://www.cdc.gov/groupbstrep/hospitals/hospitals_guidelines.htm

Centers for Disease Control and Prevention (CDC): Perinatal group B streptococcal disease after universal screening recommendations—United States, 2003–2005. MMWR Morb Mortal Wkly Rep 2007;56:701 [PMID: 17637595].

Heath PT, Feldman RG: Vaccination against group B streptococcus. Expert Rev Vaccines 2005;4:207 [PMID:15889994].

Pettersson K: Perinatal infection with group B streptococci. Semin Fetal Neonat Med 2007;12:193 [PMID: 17347062].

Schrag SJ et al: Group B streptococcal disease in the era of intrapartum antibiotic prophylaxis. N Engl J Med 2000;342:15 [PMID: 10620644].

Schrag SJ et al: Prevention of perinatal group B streptococcal disease: Revised recommendations from CDC. MMWR Recomm Rep 2002;51(RR-11):1 [PMID: 12211284].

STREPTOCOCCAL INFECTIONS WITH ORGANISMS OTHER THAN GROUP A OR B

Streptococci of groups other than A and B are part of the normal flora of humans and can occasionally cause disease. Group C or group G organisms occasionally produce pharyngitis (with an ASO rise), but without risk of subsequent rheumatic fever. AGN may occasionally occur. Group D streptococci and *Enterococcus* species are normal inhabitants of the gastrointestinal tract and may produce urinary tract infections, meningitis, and sepsis in the newborn, as well as endocarditis. Nosocomial infections caused by *Enterococcus* are frequent in neonatal and oncology units and in patients with central venous catheters. Nonhemolytic aerobic streptococci and β-hemolytic streptococci are normal flora of the mouth. They are involved in the production of dental plaque and probably dental caries and are the most common cause of subacute infective endocarditis. Finally, there are numerous anaerobic and microaerophilic streptococci, normal flora of the mouth, skin, and gastrointestinal tract, which alone or in combination with other bacteria may cause sinusitis, dental abscesses, brain abscesses, and intra-abdominal or lung abscesses.

▶ Treatment

A. Enterococcal Infections

Enterococcus faecalis and *Enterococcus faecium* are the two most common and most important strains causing human infections. In general, *E faecalis* is more susceptible to antibiotics than *E faecium*, but antibiotic resistance is commonly seen with both species.

1. Infections with ampicillin-susceptible enterococci— Lower tract urinary infections can be treated with oral amoxicillin. Pyelonephritis should be treated intravenously with ampicillin and gentamicin (gentamicin dosing may need to be adjusted for altered renal function). Sepsis or meningitis in the newborn should be treated intravenously with a combination of ampicillin (100–200 mg/kg/ d in three divided doses) and gentamicin (3 mg/kg/d in three divided doses). Peak serum gentamicin levels of 3–5 mcg/mL are adequate as gentamicin is used as a synergistic agent. Endocarditis requires 4–6 weeks of intravenous treatment. Penicillin G (250,000 units/kg/d in six to eight divided doses) plus gentamicin (3 mg/kg/d in three divided doses) is most often used. Cephalosporins are not effective.

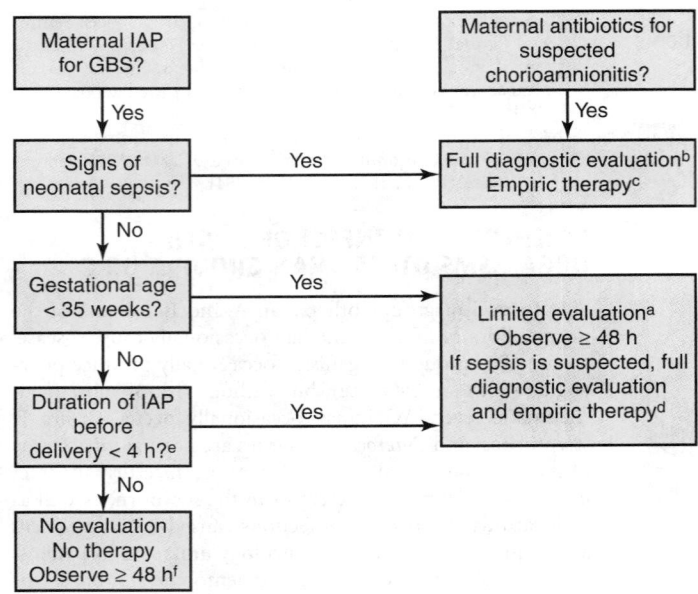

▲ Figure 40–1. Algorithm for treatment of a newborn whose mother received intrapartum antimicrobial prophylaxis (IAP) for prevention of group B streptococci (GBS) or suspected chorio-amnionitis. This algorithm is not an exclusive course of management. Variations that incorporate individual circumstance or institutional preferences may be appropriate. (Reproduced, with permission, from Schrag S et al: Prevention of perinatal group B streptococcal disease, revised guidelines from CDC. MMWR Recomm Rep 2002;51[RR-11]:1.)

ᵃ If no maternal intrapartum prophylaxis for GBS was administered despite an indication being present, data are insufficient on which to recommend a single management strategy.

ᵇ Includes complete blood cell count and differential, blood culture, and chest radiograph if respiratory abnormalities are present. When signs of sepsis are present, a lumbar puncture, if feasible, should be performed.

ᶜ Duration of therapy varies depending on results of blood culture, cerebrospinal fluid findings, if obtained, and the clinical course of the infant. If laboratory results and clinical course do not indicate bacterial infection, duration may be as short as 48 h.

ᵈ CBC with differential and blood culture.

ᵉ Applies only to penicillin, ampicillin, or celazoin and assumes recommended dosing regimens.

ᶠ A healthy-appearing infant who was 38 weeks' gestation at delivery and whose mother received 4 h of intrapartum prophylaxis before delivery may be discharged home after 24 h if other discharge criteria have been met and a person able to comply fully with instructions for home observation will be present. If any one of these conditions is not met, the infant should be observed in the hospital for at least 48 h and until criteria for discharge are achieved.

2. Infections with ampicillin-resistant or vancomycin-resistant enterococci—Ampicillin-resistant enterococci are often susceptible to vancomycin (40–60 mg/kg/d in four divided doses). Vancomycin-resistant enterococci are usually also resistant to ampicillin. Two agents are effective against vancomycin-resistant enterococci and approved for use in adults. Quinupristin–dalfopristin (Synercid) is approved for infections with vancomycin-resistant *E faecium* (not effective against *E faecalis*). Linezolid (Zyvox) is approved for vancomycin-resistant *E faecalis* and *E faecium* infections. Both agents are bacteriostatic against enterococci. Isolates resistant to these newer agents have been reported. Infectious disease consultation is recommended when use of these drugs is entertained or when vancomycin-resistant enterococcal infections are identified.

B. Viridans Streptococcal Infections (Subacute Infective Endocarditis)

It is important to determine the penicillin sensitivity of the infecting strain as early as possible in the treatment of viridans streptococcal endocarditis. Resistant organisms are most commonly seen in patients receiving penicillin prophylaxis for rheumatic heart disease. Strains sensitive to penicillin G (MIC < 0.1 mcg/mL) may be treated for 4 weeks with penicillin, 150,000–200,000 units/kg/d intravenously, with gentamicin (lower "synergy" dose of 1 mg/kg per dose every 8 hours in patients with normal renal function) added during the first 2 weeks. There is considerable experience with 2-week therapy in adult patients using penicillin and gentamicin. Similarly, excellent results have been obtained with ceftriaxone once daily for 4 weeks. If the MIC is 0.5 mcg/mL or higher, longer therapy and higher doses of penicillin G must be used (200,000–300,000 units/kg/d intravenously in combination with gentamicin for 4–6 weeks). If the MIC is 0.1–0.5 mcg/mL, penicillin G at the higher dose for a minimum of 4 weeks is recommended, with gentamicin added for the first 2 weeks. Vancomycin, 40 mg/kg/d, is usually preferred for resistant strains and patients allergic to penicillin.

Butler KM: Enterococcal infection in children. Semin Pediatr Infect Dis 2006;17:128 [PMID: 16934707].

Das I, Gray J: Enterococcal bacteremia in children: A review of seventy five episodes in a pediatric hospital. Pediatr Infect Dis J 1998;17:1154 [PMID: 9877366].

Lomaestro BM: Resistance to linezolid. Are we surprised? How hard should we look? Ann Pharmacother 2003;37:909 [PMID: 12773084].

Mutnick AH et al: Linezolid resistance since 2001: SENTRY Antimicrobial Surveillance Program. Ann Pharmacother 2003; 37:769 [PMID: 12773059].

Torres-Viera C, Embry LM: Approaches to vancomycin resistant enterococci. Curr Opin Infect Dis 2004;17:541 [PMID: 15640708].

Wilson WR et al: Antibiotic treatment of adults with infective endocarditis due to streptococci, enterococci, staphylococci, and HACEK microorganisms. JAMA 1995;274:1706 [PMID: 7474277].

PNEUMOCOCCAL INFECTIONS

ESSENTIALS OF DIAGNOSIS & TYPICAL FEATURES

Bacteremia:

▶ High fever (> 39.4°C).

▶ Leukocytosis (> 15,000/μL).

▶ Age 6–24 months.

Pneumonia:

▶ Fever, leukocytosis, and tachypnea.

▶ Localized chest pain.

▶ Localized or diffuse rales. Chest radiograph may show lobar infiltrate (with effusion).

Meningitis:

▶ Fever, leukocytosis.

▶ Bulging fontanelle, neck stiffness.

▶ Irritability and lethargy.

All types:

▶ Diagnosis confirmed by cultures of blood, CSF, pleural fluid, or other body fluid.

▶ General Considerations

Sepsis, sinusitis, otitis media, pneumonitis, meningitis, osteomyelitis, cellulitis, arthritis, vaginitis, and peritonitis are all part of a spectrum of pneumococcal infection. Clinical findings that correlate with occult bacteremia in ambulatory patients include age (6–24 months), degree of temperature elevation (> 39.4°C), and leukocytosis (> 15,000/μL). Although each of these findings is in itself nonspecific, a combination of them should arouse suspicion. This constellation of findings in a child who has no focus of infection may be an indication for blood cultures and antibiotic therapy. The cause of most of such bacteremic episodes is pneumococci.

Streptococcus pneumoniae is a common cause of acute purulent otitis media and is the organism responsible for most cases of acute bacterial pneumonia in children. The disease is indistinguishable on clinical grounds from other bacterial pneumonias. Effusions are common, although frank empyema is less common. Abscesses also occasionally occur.

The incidence rate of pneumococcal meningitis has decreased since incorporation of the pneumococcal conjugate vaccine into the infant vaccine schedule. However, pneumococcal meningitis is still more common than *Haemophilus influenzae* type b meningitis. Pneumococcal meningitis, sometimes recurrent, may complicate serious head trauma, particularly if there is persistent leakage of CSF. This has led some physicians to recommend the prophylactic administration of penicillin or other antimicrobials in such cases.

Children with sickle cell disease, other hemoglobinopathies, congenital or acquired asplenia, and some immunoglobulin and complement deficiencies are unusually susceptible to pneumococcal sepsis and meningitis. They often have a catastrophic illness with shock and disseminated intravascular coagulation (DIC). Even with excellent supportive care, the mortality rate is 20–50%. The spleen is important in the control of pneumococcal infection by clearing organisms from the blood and producing an opsonin that enhances phagocytosis. Autosplenectomy may explain why children with sickle cell disease are at increased risk of developing serious pneumococcal infections. Children with cochlear implants are at higher risk for pneumococcal meningitis. Children who have, or who are planning to receive, a cochlear implant should receive age-appropriate pneumococcal vaccination (> 2 weeks prior to surgery if possible).

S pneumoniae rarely causes serious disease in the neonate. Although *S pneumoniae* does not normally colonize the vagina, transient colonization does occur. Serious neonatal disease—including pneumonia, sepsis, and meningitis—may occur and clinically is similar to GBS infection.

Since being introduced in clinical medicine, penicillin has been the agent of choice for pneumococcal infections. Many strains are still highly susceptible to penicillin, and in those cases, penicillin is still the drug of choice. However, pneumococci with moderately increased resistance to penicillin are found in most communities, and reports of treatment failure, particularly in meningitis, are common. The prevalence of these relatively penicillin-resistant strains in North America varies geographically. Pneumococci with high-level resistance to penicillin and multiple other drugs are increasingly encountered throughout the United States. Pneumococci from normally sterile body fluids should be routinely tested for susceptibility to penicillin as well as other drugs.

Pneumococci have been classified into 90 serotypes based on capsular polysaccharide antigens. The frequency distribution of serotypes varies at different times, in different geographic areas, and with different sites of infection. Serotypes 4, 6B, 9V, 14, 18C, 19F, and 23F cause about 80–85% of invasive pneumococcal infections in young children. Similar serotypes—6B, 9V, 14, 19A, 19F, and 23F—are responsible for most of the penicillin-resistant isolates. A protein conjugate pneumococcal vaccine (Prevnar) is available for immunization of young children. It includes polysaccharide or oligosaccharide of seven different *S pneumoniae* serotypes conjugated to a protein carrier. The serotypes in the vaccine cause the bulk of pediatric invasive pneumococcal disease. The development of this vaccine is important in the prevention of pneumococcal disease because young children (< age 2 years), who are most at risk for the disease, are unable to immunologically mount a predictable response to the 23-valent polysaccharide vaccine. This vaccine is discussed further in Chapter 9. Recently, a report from Alaska described a rising incidence of invasive pneumococcal disease in Native American children caused by serotypes not represented in the conjugate vaccine. Whether serotype replacement will become more widespread remains to be seen. For older children and adults, the 23-valent pneumococcal vaccine is generally recommended.

Clinical Findings

A. Symptoms and Signs

In pneumococcal sepsis, fever usually appears abruptly, often accompanied by chills. There may be no respiratory symptoms. In pneumococcal sinusitis, mucopurulent nasal discharge may occur. In infants and young children with pneumonia, fever and tachypnea without auscultatory changes are the usual presenting signs. Respiratory distress is manifested by nasal flaring, chest retractions, and tachypnea. Abdominal pain is common. In older children, the adult form of pneumococcal pneumonia with signs of lobar consolidation may occur, but sputum is rarely bloody. Thoracic pain (from pleural involvement) is sometimes present, but is less common in children. With involvement of the right hemidiaphragm, pain may be referred to the right lower quadrant, suggesting appendicitis. Vomiting is common at onset but seldom persists. Convulsions are relatively common at onset in infants.

Meningitis is characterized by fever, irritability, convulsions, and neck stiffness. The most important sign in very young infants is a tense, bulging anterior fontanelle. In older children, fever, chills, headache, and vomiting are common symptoms. Classic signs are nuchal rigidity associated with positive Brudzinski and Kernig signs. With progression of untreated disease, the child may develop opisthotonos, stupor, and coma.

B. Laboratory Findings

Leukocytosis is often pronounced (20,000–45,000/μL), with 80–90% polymorphonuclear neutrophils. Neutropenia may be seen early in very serious infections. The presence of pneumococci in the nasopharynx is not a helpful finding, because up to 40% of normal children carry pneumococci in the upper respiratory tract. Large numbers of organisms are seen on Gram-stained smears of endotracheal aspirates from patients with pneumonia. In meningitis, CSF usually shows an elevated white blood cell (WBC) count of several thousand, chiefly polymorphonuclear neutrophils, with decreased glucose and elevated protein levels. Gram-positive diplococci may be seen on some (but not all) stained smears of CSF sediment. Antigen detection tests are not useful.

Differential Diagnosis

There are many causes of high fever and leukocytosis in young infants; 90% of children presenting with these features have a disease other than pneumococcal bacteremia, such as human herpesvirus 6, enterovirus, or other viral infection; urinary tract infection; unrecognized focal infection elsewhere in the body; or early acute shigellosis.

Infants with upper respiratory tract infection who subsequently develop signs of lower respiratory disease are most likely to be infected with a respiratory virus. Hoarseness or wheezing is often present. A radiograph of the chest typically shows perihilar infiltrates and increased bronchovascular markings. Viral respiratory infection often precedes pneumococcal pneumonia; therefore, the clinical picture may be mixed.

Staphylococcal pneumonia may be indistinguishable early in its course from pneumococcal pneumonia. Later, pulmonary cavitation and empyema occur. Staphylococcal pneumonia is most common in infants.

In primary pulmonary tuberculosis, children do not have a toxic appearance, and radiographs show a primary focus associated with hilar adenopathy and often with pleural involvement. Miliary tuberculosis presents a classic radiographic appearance.

Pneumonia caused by *Mycoplasma pneumoniae* is most common in children aged 5 years and older. Onset is insidious, with infrequent chills, low-grade fever, prominent headache and malaise, cough, and, often, striking radiographic changes. Marked leukocytosis (> 18,000/μL) is unusual.

Pneumococcal meningitis is diagnosed by lumbar puncture. Without a Gram-stained smear and culture of CSF, it is not distinguishable from other types of acute bacterial meningitis.

Complications

Complications of sepsis include meningitis and osteomyelitis; complications of pneumonia include empyema, parapneumonic effusion, and, rarely, lung abscess. Mastoiditis, subdural empyema, and brain abscess may follow untreated pneumococcal otitis media. Both pneumococcal meningitis and peritonitis are more likely to occur independently without coexisting pneumonia. Shock, DIC, and Waterhouse-Friderichsen syndrome resembling meningococcemia are occasionally seen in pneumococcal sepsis, particularly in asplenic patients. Hemolytic-uremic syndrome may occur as a complication of pneumococcal pneumonia or sepsis.

▶ **Treatment**

A. Specific Measures

All *S pneumoniae* isolated from normally sterile sites should be tested for susceptibility to penicillin. Susceptible strains (MIC ≤ 0.06 mcg/mL) can be treated with penicillin, ampicillin, or amoxicillin. Penicillin-intermediate (MIC 0.1–1.0 mcg/mL) or penicillin-resistant strains (MIC ≥ 2.0 mcg/mL) should be tested for susceptibility to cephalosporins, vancomycin, and selected other drugs. Therapy with penicillin, amoxicillin, or cephalosporins will usually succeed in cases of bacteremia or pneumonia due to intermediate-resistant isolates because serum levels in excess of the MIC can be achieved. Therapy of meningitis, empyema, osteomyelitis, and endocarditis due to nonsusceptible *S pneumoniae* is more difficult, because penetration of antimicrobials to these sites is limited. Vancomycin and third-generation cephalosporins are indicated in these and other serious or life-threatening infections pending susceptibility test results.

1. Bacteremia—In studies done prior to immunization of young children with conjugated pneumococcal vaccine, 3–5% of blood cultures in patients younger than 2 years of age yielded *S pneumoniae*. These percentages are expected to decrease now that an effective vaccine is available. However, pneumococcal disease will not disappear, as the vaccine prevents only 85% of invasive disease. Many experts treat suspected bacteremia with ceftriaxone (50 mg/kg, given intramuscularly or intravenously). Compared with oral amoxicillin (80–90 mg/kg/d), ceftriaxone may reduce fever and the need for hospitalization. However, meningitis occurs with the same frequency despite presumptive therapy. All children with blood cultures that grow pneumococci should be reexamined as soon as possible. The child who has a focal infection, such as meningitis, or who appears septic should be admitted to the hospital to receive parenteral antimicrobials. If the child is afebrile and appears well or mildly ill, outpatient management is appropriate. If the physician is confident that close follow-up can be achieved, lumbar puncture is not mandatory. Severely ill children, in whom infection with *S pneumoniae* is suspected, should be treated with vancomycin until the susceptibilities of the organism are known.

2. Pneumonia—For infants (1 month of age or older), severely ill patients, and immunocompromised hosts with susceptible organisms appropriate regimens include aqueous

penicillin G (250,000–400,000 units/kg/d, given intravenously in four to six divided doses), cefotaxime (50 mg/kg every 8 hours), or ceftriaxone (50 mg/kg every 12–24 hours). If susceptibilities are not known and the patient is severely ill, vancomycin (10 mg/kg every 6 hours) should be used as part of the regimen to provide coverage for penicillin- or cephalosporin-resistant pneumococcus. Once results of susceptibility testing are available, the regimen can be tailored. Mild pneumonia may be treated with amoxicillin (80–90 mg/kg/d) for 7–10 days. Alternative regimens include oral macrolides and cephalosporins.

3. Otitis media—Most experts recommend oral amoxicillin (80–90 mg/kg/d, divided in two doses) as first-line therapy. The standard course of therapy is 10 days; however, many physicians have been treating uncomplicated cases in children older than 2 years for 5 days, based on recent studies. Treatment failures may be treated with amoxicillin–clavulanate (80–90 mg/kg/d of the amoxicillin component in the 14:1 formulation), intramuscular ceftriaxone, cefuroxime axetil, or cefdinir. Clarithromycin or azithromycin can also be used.

4. Meningitis—Until bacteriologic confirmation and susceptibility testing are completed, patients should receive vancomycin (60 mg/kg/d, given intravenously in four divided doses) and cefotaxime (300 mg/kg/d intravenously in four divided doses), or vancomycin (see previous dosage) and ceftriaxone (100 mg/kg/d, given intravenously in two divided doses). Corticosteroids (dexamethasone, 0.6 mg/kg/d, in four divided doses for 4 days) are recommended by many experts as adjunctive therapy for pneumococcal meningitis. However, by reducing inflammation of the meninges, steroids may reduce the entry of vancomycin into the CSF. The addition of rifampin (10 mg/kg per dose twice a day, intravenously or orally) is used by some experts if both vancomycin and steroids are given, as it penetrates CSF well and may aid in sterilization (rifampin should never be used alone for treatment of meningitis). A repeat lumbar puncture at 24–48 hours should be considered to ensure sterility of the CSF if dexamethasone is given, if resistant pneumococci are isolated, or if the patient is not demonstrating expected improvement after 24–48 hours on therapy.

If the isolate is determined to be penicillin-susceptible, aqueous penicillin G can be administered (300,000–400,000 units/kg/d, given intravenously in four to six divided doses for 10–14 days). Use of ceftriaxone or cefotaxime is acceptable alternative therapy in penicillin- and cephalosporin-susceptible isolates. Consult an infectious disease specialist or the *Red Book* (American Academy of Pediatrics, 2006) for therapeutic options for isolates that are nonsusceptible to penicillin or cephalosporins.

▶ **Prognosis**

In children, case fatality rates of less than 1% should be achieved except for meningitis, where rates of 5–20% still prevail. The presence of large numbers of organisms without a prominent CSF inflammatory response or meningitis due to a penicillin-resistant strain indicates a poor prognosis. Serious neurologic sequelae, particularly hearing loss, are frequent following pneumococcal meningitis.

Advisory Committee on Immunization Practices: Pneumococcal vaccination for cochlear implant candidates and recipients: Updated recommendations of the Advisory Committee on Immunization Practices. MMWR Morb Mortal Wkly Rep 2003;52:739 [PMID: 12908457].

Advisory Committee on Immunization Practices: Preventing pneumococcal disease among infants and young children. MMWR Morb Mortal Wkly Rep 2000;40:1 [PMID: 11055835].

Kaplan S: Management of pneumococcal meningitis. Pediatr Infect Dis J 2002;21:589 [PMID: 12182395].

Singleton T et al: Invasive pneumococcal disease caused by nonvaccine serotypes among Alaska Native children with high levels of 7-valent pneumococcal conjugate vaccine coverage. JAMA 2007;297:1784 [PMID:17456820].

Toltzis P, Jacobs MR: The epidemiology of childhood pneumococcal disease in the United States in the era of conjugate vaccine use. Infect Dis Clin North Am 2005;19:629 [PMID: 16102653].

Whitney CG et al: Decline in invasive pneumococcal disease after the introduction of protein-polysaccharide conjugate vaccine. N Engl J Med 2003;348:1737 [PMID: 12724479].

STAPHYLOCOCCAL INFECTIONS

Staphylococcal infections are common in childhood. Staphylococcal skin infections range from minor furuncles to the varied syndromes now collectively referred to as scalded skin syndrome. Staphylococci are the major cause of osteomyelitis and of septic arthritis and are an uncommon but important cause of bacterial pneumonia. A toxin produced by certain strains causes staphylococcal food poisoning. Staphylococci are responsible for most infections of artificial heart valves. They cause toxic shock syndrome (see later discussion). Finally, they are found in infections at all ages and in multiple sites, particularly when infection is introduced from the skin or upper respiratory tract or when closed compartments become infected (pericarditis, sinusitis, cervical adenitis, surgical wounds, abscesses in the liver or brain, and abscesses elsewhere in the body).

Staphylococci that do not produce the enzyme coagulase are termed *coagulase-negative* and are seldom speciated in the clinical microbiology laboratory. Most *S aureus* strains produce coagulase. *S aureus* and coagulase-negative staphylococci are normal flora of the skin and respiratory tract. The latter rarely cause disease except in compromised hosts, the newborn, or patients with plastic indwelling lines.

Most strains of *S aureus* elaborate β-lactamase that confers penicillin resistance. This can be overcome in clinical practice by the use of a cephalosporin or a penicillinase-resistant penicillin, such as methicillin, oxacillin, nafcillin, cloxacillin, or dicloxacillin. Methicillin-resistant strains of *S aureus* (MRSA) are found worldwide and are now common in certain hospitals and, increasingly, in community-acquired infections in some areas of the United States. Most MRSA retain β-lactamase production, and many are resistant to other antibiotics as well. MRSA are also resistant in vivo to all of the penicillinase-resistant penicillins and cephalosporins. Strains with intermediate susceptibility to vancomycin are occurring more frequently and occasionally vancomycin-resistant strains are isolated. The existence of such strains is of concern because of the inherent virulence of most strains of *S aureus* and because of the limited choices for therapy. *S aureus* produces a variety of exotoxins, most of which are of uncertain importance. Two toxins are recognized as playing a central role in specific diseases: exfoliatin and staphylococcal enterotoxin. The former is largely responsible for the various clinical presentations of scalded skin syndrome. Most strains that elaborate exfoliatin are of phage group II. Enterotoxin causes staphylococcal food poisoning. The exoprotein toxin most commonly associated with toxic shock syndrome has been termed TSST-1. Panton-Valentine leucocidin (PVL) is an exotoxin produced by less than 5% of clinical isolates of methicillin-susceptible *S aureus* (MSSA) and MRSA strains. PVL is a virulence factor that causes leukocyte destruction and tissue necrosis. PVL-producing *S aureus* strains are often community-acquired, and have most commonly produced boils and abscesses. However, they also have been associated with severe cellulitis, osteomyelitis, and deaths from necrotizing pneumonia in otherwise healthy children and young adults.

▶ Clinical Findings

A. Symptoms and Signs

1. Staphylococcal skin diseases—Dermal infection with *S aureus* causes furuncles or cellulitis. *S aureus* are often found along with streptococci in impetigo. If the strains produce exfoliatin, localized lesions become bullous (bullous impetigo).

Scalded skin syndrome is thought to be a systemic effect of exfoliatin. The initial infection may begin at any site but is in the respiratory tract in most cases. There is a prodromal phase of erythema, often beginning around the mouth, accompanied by fever and irritability. The involved skin becomes tender, and a sick infant will cry when picked up or touched. A day or so later, exfoliation begins, usually around the mouth. The inside of the mouth is red, and a peeling rash is present around the lips, often in a radial pattern. Generalized, painful peeling may follow, involving the limbs and trunk but often sparing the feet. More commonly, peeling is confined to areas around body orifices. If erythematous but unpeeled skin is rubbed sideways, superficial epidermal layers separate from deeper ones and slough (Nikolsky sign). In the newborn, the disease is termed *Ritter disease* and may be fulminant. If there is tender erythema but not exfoliation, the disease is termed *nonstreptococcal scarlet fever*. The scarlatiniform rash is sandpaper-like, but strawberry tongue is not seen, and cultures grow *S aureus* rather than streptococcus.

2. Osteomyelitis and septic arthritis—(See Chapter 24.)

3. Staphylococcal pneumonia—Staphylococcal pneumonia in infancy is characterized by abdominal distention, high fever, respiratory distress, and toxemia. It often occurs without predisposing factors or after minor skin infections. The organism is necrotizing, producing bronchoalveolar destruction. Pneumatoceles, pyopneumothorax, and empyema are frequently encountered. Rapid progression of disease is characteristic. Frequent chest radiographs to monitor the progress of disease are indicated. Presenting symptoms may be typical of paralytic ileus, suggestive of an abdominal catastrophe.

Staphylococcal pneumonia usually is peribronchial, beginning with a focal infiltrative lesion progressing to patchy consolidation. Most often only one lung is involved (80%), more often the right. Purulent pericarditis occurs by direct extension in about 10% of cases, with or without empyema.

4. Staphylococcal food poisoning—Staphylococcal food poisoning is a result of ingestion of enterotoxin produced by staphylococci growing in uncooked and poorly refrigerated food. The disease is characterized by vomiting, prostration, and diarrhea occurring 2–6 hours after ingestion of contaminated foods.

5. Staphylococcal endocarditis—*S aureus* may produce infection of normal heart valves, of valves or endocardium in children with congenital or rheumatic heart disease, or of artificial valves. About 25% of all cases of endocarditis are due to *S aureus*. The great majority of artificial heart valve infections involve either *S aureus* or coagulase-negative staphylococci. Infection usually begins in an extracardiac focus, often the skin. Involvement of the endocardium must be suspected in every case of *S aureus* bacteremia, regardless of initial signs. Suspicion must be highest in the presence of congenital heart disease, particularly ventricular septal defects with aortic insufficiency but also simple ventricular septal defect, patent ductus arteriosus, and tetralogy of Fallot.

The presenting symptoms in staphylococcal endocarditis are fever, weight loss, weakness, muscle pain or diffuse skeletal pain, poor feeding, pallor, and cardiac decompensation. Signs include splenomegaly, cardiomegaly, petechiae, hematuria, and a new or changing murmur. The course of *S aureus* endocarditis is rapid, although subacute disease occurs occasionally. Peripheral septic embolization and uncontrollable cardiac failure are common, even when optimal antibiotic therapy is administered, and may be indications for surgical intervention (see later discussion).

6. Toxic shock syndrome—Toxic shock syndrome (TSS) is characterized by fever, blanching erythroderma, diarrhea, vomiting, myalgia, prostration, hypotension, and multiorgan dysfunction. It is due to *S aureus* focal infection, usually without bacteremia. Large numbers of cases have been described in menstruating adolescents and young women using vaginal tampons. TSS has also been reported in boys and girls with focal staphylococcal infections and in individuals with wound infections due to *S aureus*. Additional clinical features include sudden onset; conjunctival suffusion; mucosal hyperemia; desquamation of skin on the palms, soles, fingers, and toes during convalescence; DIC in severe cases; renal and hepatic functional abnormalities; and myolysis. The mortality rate with early treatment is now about 2%. Recurrences are seen during subsequent menstrual periods in as many as 60% of untreated women who continue to use tampons. Recurrences occur in up to 15% of women given antistaphylococcal antibiotics who stop using tampons. The disease is caused by strains of *S aureus* that produce TSST-1 or one of the related enterotoxins.

7. Coagulase-negative staphylococcal infections—Localized and systemic coagulase-negative staphylococcal infections occur primarily in immunocompromised patients, high-risk newborns, and patients with plastic prostheses or catheters. Coagulase-negative staphylococci are the most common nosocomial pathogen in hospitalized low-birth-weight neonates in the United States. Intravenous administration of lipid emulsions and indwelling central venous catheters are risk factors contributing to coagulase-negative staphylococcal bacteremia in newborn infants. In patients with an artificial heart valve, a Dacron patch, a ventriculoperitoneal shunt, or a central venous catheter, coagulase-negative staphylococci are a common cause of sepsis or catheter infection, often necessitating removal of the foreign material and protracted antibiotic therapy. Because blood cultures are frequently contaminated by this organism, diagnosis of genuine localized or systemic infection is often difficult.

B. Laboratory Findings

Moderate leukocytosis (15,000–20,000/μL) with a shift to the left is occasionally found, although normal counts are common, particularly in infants. The sedimentation rate is elevated. Blood cultures are frequently positive in systemic staphylococcal disease and should always be obtained when it is suspected. Similarly, pus from sites of infection should always be aspirated or obtained surgically, examined with Gram stain, and cultured both aerobically and anaerobically. There are no useful serologic tests for staphylococcal disease.

▶ Differential Diagnosis

Staphylococcal skin disease takes many forms; therefore, the differential list is long. Bullous impetigo must be differentiated from chemical or thermal burns, from drug reactions, and, in the very young, from the various congenital epidermolytic syndromes or even herpes simplex infections. Staphylococcal scalded skin syndrome may resemble scarlet fever, Kawasaki disease, Stevens-Johnson syndrome, erythema multiforme, and other drug reactions. A skin biopsy may be critical in establishing the diagnosis. Varicella lesions may become superinfected with exfoliatin-producing staphylococci and produce a combination of the two diseases (bullous varicella).

Severe, rapidly progressing pneumonia with formation of abscesses, pneumatoceles, and empyemas is typical of *S aureus* infection and GAS but may occasionally be produced by pneumococci, *H influenzae,* and GAS.

Staphylococcal food poisoning is often epidemic. It is differentiated from other common-source gastroenteritis syndromes (*Salmonella, Clostridium perfringens,* and *Vibrio parahaemolyticus*) by the short incubation period (2–6 hours), the prominence of vomiting (as opposed to diarrhea), and the absence of fever.

Endocarditis must be suspected in any instance of *S aureus* bacteremia, particularly when a significant heart murmur or preexisting cardiac disease is present. (See Chapter 19.)

Newborn infections with *S aureus* can resemble infections with streptococci and a variety of gram-negative organisms. Umbilical and respiratory tract colonization occurs with many pathogenic organisms (GBS, *Escherichia coli,* and *Klebsiella*), and both skin and systemic infections occur with virtually all of these organisms.

TSS must be differentiated from Rocky Mountain spotted fever, leptospirosis, Kawasaki disease, drug reactions, adenovirus, and measles (see also Table 38–3).

▶ Treatment

A. Specific Measures

Community-acquired MRSA infections are on the rise. The incidence of community-acquired MRSA isolates varies greatly geographically, but in many communities in the United States MRSA is the most common pathogen isolated from patients with skin and soft tissue infections. If the prevalence of MRSA isolates in the community is high and if the patient is seriously ill, vancomycin should be part of the empiric coverage until culture results and susceptibility data are known. Currently, most community-acquired MRSA strains are susceptible to trimethoprim–sulfamethoxazole (TMP–SMX) and some are susceptible to clindamycin. Less serious infections in nontoxic patients may be initially treated using one of these agents while awaiting cultures and susceptibility data. Knowledge of the community MRSA susceptibility patterns is useful in guiding empiric therapy while awaiting susceptibility test results.

For MSSA strains, a β-lactamase-resistant penicillin is the drug of choice (oxacillin, nafcillin, or methicillin). In serious systemic disease, in osteomyelitis, and in the treatment of large abscesses, intravenous therapy is indicated initially (oxacillin or nafcillin, 100–150 mg/kg/d in four divided doses, or methicillin, 200–300 mg/kg/d in four divided doses). When high doses over a long period are required, it is preferable to avoid use of methicillin, because of the frequency with which interstitial nephritis occurs. In life-threatening illness, an aminoglycoside antibiotic (gentamicin or tobramycin) or rifampin may be used in addition for its possible synergistic action.

Cephalosporins may be considered for MSSA infections in patients with a history of penicillin sensitivity unless there is a history of type 1 hypersensitivity reaction (ie, anaphylaxis, wheezing, edema, and hives). Cefazolin, 100–150 mg/kg/d, given intravenously in three divided doses, or cephalexin, 50–100 mg/kg/d, given orally in four divided doses, can be used once a child is able to take oral antibiotics. The third-generation cephalosporins should not generally be used for staphylococcal infections.

For nonmeningeal, suspected nosocomially acquired MRSA infections, vancomycin (40 mg/kg/d intravenously in three or four divided doses) should be used until results of susceptibility testing are available (frequently clindamycin- and TMP–SMX-resistant). Infections due to MRSA frequently do not respond to cephalosporins despite in-vitro testing that suggests susceptibility. For treatment of meningitis, vancomycin must be given in higher doses (60 mg/kg/d divided into four doses). The addition of rifampin is advocated by some (rifampin should not be used alone to treat this condition).

1. Skin infections—Treatment of skin and soft tissue infections depends, in part, on the extent of the lesion, immunocompetence of the host, and the toxicity of the patient. Afebrile, well-appearing patients with small abscesses may do well with incision and drainage (with or without the addition of oral antimicrobials). More serious infections or infections in immunocompromised patients should be treated more aggressively. Hospitalization and intravenous antibiotics may be required. Culture and susceptibility testing help guide therapy regardless of whether the patient initially is started on antibiotics. Results of these tests facilitate therapeutic decisions in cases in which patients do not respond to initial management or empiric intravenous antibiotic therapy was initiated.

For patients who are not sick enough to require hospitalization or intravenous therapy, selection of the best empiric antimicrobial depends on local rates of MRSA and local susceptibilities. β-Lactam antibiotics, such as penicillins and cephalosporins, can no longer be depended on as single agents for the majority of cases in communities with high MRSA rates. TMP–SMX and clindamycin (depending on local susceptibility patterns) may be used for empiric staphylococcal coverage. However, group A streptococci are generally resistant to TMP–SMX and in a small number of cases may also be resistant to clindamycin. Many clinicians empirically use a combination of TMP–SMX and cefazolin for initial treatment until susceptibilities are known. Linezolid is another option, although the cost of this drug is high.

2. Osteomyelitis and septic arthritis—Treatment should be begun intravenously, with antibiotics selected to cover the most likely organisms (staphylococci in hematogenous osteomyelitis; meningococci, pneumococci, staphylococci in children younger than age 3 years with septic arthritis; staphylococci and gonococci in older children with septic arthritis). Knowledge of local MRSA rates will help guide empiric therapy. Antibiotic levels should be kept high at all times.

In osteomyelitis, clinical studies support the use of intravenous treatment until fever and local symptoms and signs have subsided—usually after at least 3–5 days—followed by oral therapy (for susceptible strains, dicloxacillin, 100–150 mg/kg/d in four divided doses; or cephalexin, 100–150 mg/kg/d in four divided doses) for at least 3 additional weeks. Longer treatment may be required, particularly when radiographs show extensive involvement. Treatment of community-acquired MRSA osteomyelitis should be based on susceptibility results; however, isolates are frequently susceptible to TMP–SMX or clindamycin. Vancomycin can be used as part of an empiric regimen while awaiting susceptibilities in seriously ill patients or in areas where MRSA rates are high. In arthritis, where drug diffusion into synovial fluid is good, intravenous therapy need be given only for a few days, followed by adequate oral therapy for at least 3 weeks. In all instances, oral therapy should be administered with careful attention to compliance, either in the hospital or at home. The erythrocyte sedimentation rate (ESR) is a good indicator of response to therapy. Surgical drainage of osteomyelitis or septic arthritis is often required. (See Chapter 24.)

3. Staphylococcal pneumonia—

In the few areas of the country where MRSA is not prevalent, or if the isolate is known to be MSSA, nafcillin and oxacillin are the usual drugs of choice. For sick patients, vancomycin can be used empirically until results of cultures and susceptibility tests are obtained. Linezolid has recently been reported to be as efficacious as vancomycin for the treatment of resistant gram-positive pneumonia and soft tissue infections (cure rates: 95% linezolid vs 94% vancomycin).

Empyema and pyopneumothorax require drainage. The choice of chest tube versus thoracoscopic drainage depends on the practitioner's experience and skill. If staphylococcal pneumonia is treated promptly and empyema drained, resolution in children often is complete.

4. Staphylococcal food poisoning—

Therapy is supportive and usually not required except in severe cases or for small infants with marked dehydration.

5. Staphylococcal endocarditis—

As outlined earlier, high-dose, prolonged parenteral treatment is indicated. Methicillin-susceptible isolates are often treated with oxacillin or nafcillin. Some experts also recommend addition of gentamicin or rifampin for the first 5 days to 2 weeks. In penicillin-allergic patients (type 1 hypersensitivity or anaphylaxis) or patients with MRSA isolates, vancomycin should be used. Therapy lasts in all instances for at least 6 weeks.

Occasionally, medical treatment fails. Signs of treatment failure are (1) recurrent fever without apparent treatable other cause (eg, thrombophlebitis, respiratory or urinary tract infection, drug fever), (2) persistently positive blood cultures, (3) intractable and progressive congestive heart failure, and (4) recurrent (septic) embolization. In such circumstances—particularly (2), (3), and (4)—valve replacement becomes necessary. Antibiotics are continued for at least another 4 weeks. Persistent or recurrent infection may require a second surgical procedure.

6. Toxic shock syndrome—

Treatment is aimed at expanding blood volume, maintaining perfusion pressure with inotropic agents, ensuring prompt drainage of a focus of infection (or removal of tampons or foreign bodies), and giving intravenous antibiotics.

Vancomycin, in addition to a β-lactam antibiotic (oxacillin or nafcillin), can be used for empiric therapy. Some experts would use vancomycin and clindamycin, since clindamycin is a protein synthesis inhibitor and may turn off toxin production. Clindamycin should not be used empirically as a single agent until susceptibilities (when an isolate grows) are known; some strains of S aureus are clindamycin-resistant.

Intravenous immune globulin has been used as adjunctive therapy. Some experts believe that corticosteroid therapy may be effective if given to patients with severe illness early in the course of their disease. Successful antibiotic treatment reduces risk of recurrence.

7. Vancomycin-resistant *Staphylococcus aureus* infections (VRSA)—

Reports of VRSA isolates are rare but are likely to increase in frequency in the future. Such isolates are sometimes susceptible to clindamycin or TMP–SMX. If not, therapeutic options are limited and include use of quinupristin–dalfopristin, linezolid, and daptomycin. Experience is very limited with daptomycin in pediatric patients. Consultation with an infectious disease specialist is recommended.

8. Coagulase-negative staphylococcal infections—

Bacteremia and other serious coagulase-negative staphylococcal infections are treated initially with vancomycin. Coagulase-negative staphylococci are uncommonly resistant to vancomycin. (See Chapter 37 for dosing.) Strains susceptible to methicillin are treated with methicillin, oxacillin, or cefazolin.

Centers for Disease Control and Prevention (CDC): Vancomycin-resistant *Staphylococcus aureus*—New York, 2004. MMWR Morb Mortal Wkly Rep 2004;53:322 [PMID: 15103297].

Daum RS: Clinical practice. Skin and soft-tissue infections caused by methicillin-resistant Staphylococcus aureus. N Engl J Med 2007;357:380 [PMID: 17652653].

Kaplan SL: Use of linezolid in children. Pediatr Infect Dis J 2002;21:870 [PMID: 12352813].

Lowy FD: *Staphylococcus aureus* infections. N Engl J Med 1998; 339:520 [PMID: 9709046].

Reichert B et al: Severe non-pneumonic necrotising infections in children caused by Panton-Valentine leukocidin producing *Staphylococcus aureus* strains. J Infect 2005;50:438 [PMID: 15907553].

MENINGOCOCCAL INFECTIONS

ESSENTIALS OF DIAGNOSIS & TYPICAL FEATURES

▶ Fever, headache, vomiting, convulsions, shock (meningitis).

▶ Fever, shock, petechial or purpuric skin rash (meningococcemia).

▶ Diagnosis confirmed by culture of normally sterile body fluids.

General Considerations

Meningococci (*Neisseria meningitidis*) may be carried asymptomatically for many months in the upper respiratory tract. Less than 1% of carriers develop disease. Meningitis and sepsis are the two most common forms of illness, but septic arthritis, pericarditis, pneumonia, chronic meningococcemia, otitis media, conjunctivitis, and vaginitis also occur. The incidence of invasive diseases in the United States is about 1.2 cases per 100,000 people. An estimated 2400–3000 cases occur in the United States annually. The highest attack rate for meningococcal meningitis is in the first year of life. There also is an elevated attack rate during the teen years. The development of irreversible shock with multiorgan failure is a significant factor in the fatal outcome of acute meningococcal infections.

Meningococci are gram-negative organisms containing endotoxin in their cell walls. Endotoxins cause capillary vascular injury and leak as well as DIC. Meningococci are classified serologically into groups: A, B, C, Y, and W-135 are the groups most commonly implicated in systemic disease. The serologic groups serve as markers for studying outbreaks and transmission of disease. Currently in the United States, serogroup B accounts for about one third of cases. Serogroups C and Y each cause 25% of cases, and serogroup W-135 is responsible for about 15%. Serogroup A causes periodic epidemics in developing countries, but only occasionally is associated with cases of meningococcal disease in the United States. Sulfonamide resistance is common in non–serotype-A strains. *N meningitidis* with increased MICs to penicillin G are reported from South Africa and Spain. A small number of these isolates are reported in the United States. The resistance in these strains is low-level and not due to β-lactamase. Resistant isolates are susceptible to third-generation cephalosporins. Few isolates are resistant to rifampin.

Children develop immunity from asymptomatic carriage of meningococci (usually nontypeable, nonpathogenic strains) or other cross-reacting bacteria. Patients deficient in one of the late components of complement (C6, C7, C8, or C9) are uniquely susceptible to meningococcal infection, particu-larly group A meningococci. Deficiencies of early and alternate pathway complement components also are associated with increased susceptibility.

Clinical Findings

A. Symptoms and Signs

Many children with clinical meningococcemia also have meningitis, and some have other foci of infection. All children with suspected meningococcemia should have a lumbar puncture.

1. Meningococcemia—A prodrome of upper respiratory infection is followed by high fever, headache, nausea, marked toxicity, and hypotension. Purpura, petechiae, and occasionally bright pink, tender macules or papules over the extremities and trunk are seen. The rash usually progresses rapidly. Occasional cases lack rash. Fulminant meningococcemia (Waterhouse-Friderichsen syndrome) progresses rapidly and is characterized by DIC, massive skin and mucosal hemorrhages, and shock. This syndrome also may be caused by *H influenzae, S pneumoniae*, or other bacteria. Chronic meningococcemia is characterized by periodic bouts of fever, arthralgia or arthritis, and recurrent petechiae. Splenomegaly often is present. Patients may be free of symptoms between bouts. Chronic meningococcemia occurs primarily in adults and mimics Henoch-Schönlein purpura.

2. Meningitis—In many children, meningococcemia is followed within a few hours to several days by symptoms and signs of acute purulent meningitis, with severe headache, stiff neck, nausea, vomiting, and stupor. Children with meningitis generally fare better than children with meningococcemia alone, probably because they have survived long enough to develop clinical signs of meningitis.

B. Laboratory Findings

The peripheral WBC count may be either low or elevated. Thrombocytopenia may be present with or without DIC. (See Chapter 28.) If petechial or hemorrhagic lesions are present, meningococci can sometimes be seen microscopically in tissue fluid expressed from a punctured lesion. CSF is generally cloudy and contains more than 1000 WBCs/μL, with many polymorphonuclear neutrophils and gram-negative intracellular diplococci. A total hemolytic complement assay may reveal absence of late components as an underlying cause.

Differential Diagnosis

The skin lesions of *H influenzae* or pneumococci, enterovirus infection, endocarditis, leptospirosis, Rocky Mountain spotted fever, other rickettsial diseases, Henoch-Schönlein purpura, and blood dyscrasias may be similar to meningococcemia. Other causes of sepsis and meningitis are distinguished by appropriate Gram stain and cultures.

Complications

Meningitis may lead to permanent central nervous system (CNS) damage, with deafness, convulsions, paralysis, or impaired intellectual function. Hydrocephalus may develop and requires ventriculoperitoneal shunt. Subdural collections of fluid are common but usually resolve spontaneously. Extensive skin necrosis, loss of digits or extremities, intestinal hemorrhage, and late adrenal insufficiency may complicate fulminant meningococcemia.

Prevention

A. Chemoprophylaxis

Household contacts, day care center contacts, and hospital personnel directly exposed to the respiratory secretions of patients are at increased risk for developing meningococcal infection and should be given chemoprophylaxis with rifampin. The secondary attack rate among household members is 1–5% during epidemics and less than 1% in nonepidemic situations. Children between the ages of 3 months and 2 years are at greatest risk, presumably because they lack protective antibodies. Secondary cases may occur in day care centers and in classrooms. Hospital personnel are not at increased risk unless they have had contact with a patient's oral secretions, for example, during mouth-to-mouth resuscitation, intubation, or suctioning procedures. Approximately 50% of secondary cases in households have their onset within 24 hours of identification of the index case. Exposed contacts should be notified promptly. If they are febrile, they should be fully evaluated and given high doses of penicillin or another effective antimicrobial pending the results of blood cultures.

All intimate contacts should receive chemoprophylaxis for meningococcal disease. The most commonly used agent is rifampin, given orally in the following dosages twice daily for 2 days: 600 mg for adults; 10 mg/kg for children *older* than 1 month old (maximum dosage 600 mg); and 5 mg/kg for infants *younger* than 1 month. Rifampin may stain a patient's tears (and contact lenses), sweat, and urine orange; it may also affect the reliability of oral contraceptives, and alternative contraceptive measures should therefore be employed when rifampin is administered. Rifampin should not be given to pregnant women. Instead, intramuscular ceftriaxone is the preferred agent: 125 mg given as a single dose if the patient is younger than 15 years; 250 mg given as a single dose if older than 15 years. Penicillin and most other antibiotics (even with parenteral administration) are not effective chemoprophylactic agents, because they do not eradicate upper respiratory tract carriage of meningococci. Ciprofloxacin effectively eradicates nasopharyngeal carriage in adults and children but is not approved for use in children or in pregnant women. Throat cultures to identify carriers are not useful.

B. Vaccine

A quadrivalent polysaccharide vaccine prepared from purified meningococcal polysaccharides (A, C, Y, and W-135) is available in the United States for children older than 2 years of age. This vaccine has been used for controlling outbreaks. A quadrivalent meningococcal conjugate vaccine also is available. (See Chapter 9.) This vaccine is licensed for use in children and adults between the ages of 11 and 55 years, and is preferred over the polysaccharide vaccine in the age groups for which the vaccine is licensed. In general, conjugate vaccines provide longer lasting immunity and a more robust immune response than polysaccharide vaccines. Currently meningococcal conjugate vaccine is recommended for the following people:

1. All children at the age 11–12-year preadolescent visit.
2. All children prior to high school entry if they have not had a previous meningococcal vaccine.
3. College students who will be residing in dormitories for the first time.
4. Patients with functional or anatomic asplenia and patients with complement or properdin deficiency.
5. Travelers to areas where meningococcal disease is endemic.
6. Microbiologists who may be working with meningococcal strains.

Close monitoring for potential adverse events has suggested a possible association between recent meningococcal conjugate vaccine receipt and Guillain-Barré syndrome. Between June 2005, when licensure of the vaccine was granted, and March 2007, 17 cases of Guillain-Barré syndrome with onset 2–33 days after vaccine administration had been reported through the Vaccine Adverse Event Reporting System (VAERS). Researchers calculated the U.S. rate of Guillain-Barré syndrome after meningococcal vaccine administration as compared with a background U.S. incidence rate. This analysis suggested that meningococcal conjugate vaccine recipients may have a slightly higher risk of Guillain-Barré syndrome compared with the general population. However, because Guillain-Barré syndrome is such a rare event, definitive study of the association is difficult. What is known is that meningococcal disease is serious and may be fatal and that the vaccine is highly immunogenic. Thus, the Advisory Committee for Immunization Practices and the American Academy of Pediatrics continue to recommend meningococcal conjugate vaccine because the risk of Guillain-Barré syndrome, if it does exist, is small.

Treatment

Blood cultures should be obtained for all children with fever and purpura or other signs of meningococcemia, and antibiotics should be administered immediately as an emergency procedure. There is a good correlation between survival rates and prompt initiation of antibiotic therapy. Purpura and fever should be considered a medical emergency.

Children with meningococcemia or meningococcal meningitis should be treated as though shock were imminent even if their vital signs are stable when they are first seen. If hypotension already is present, supportive measures should be aggressive, because the prognosis is grave in such situations. Treatment should be started emergently and in an intensive care setting but should not be delayed for the sake of transporting the patient. Shock may worsen following antimicrobial therapy due to endotoxin release. To minimize the risk of nosocomial transmission, patients should be placed in respiratory isolation for the first 24 hours of antibiotic treatment.

A. Specific Measures

Antibiotics should be initiated promptly. Because other bacteria, such as *S pneumoniae, S aureus,* or other gram-negative organisms, can cause identical syndromes, initial therapy should be broad. Vancomycin and cefotaxime (or ceftriaxone) are preferred initial coverage. Once *N meningitidis* has been isolated, penicillin G, cefotaxime, or ceftriaxone intravenously for 7 days are the drugs of choice. Relative penicillin resistance is uncommon but has been reported in the United States.

B. General Measures

Most cases of invasive meningococcal disease are treated with intravenous antibiotics for 7 days.

1. Cardiovascular—(See Chapter 13 for management of septic shock.) Corticosteroids are not beneficial. Sympathetic blockade and topically applied nitroglycerin have been used locally to improve perfusion.

2. Hematologic—Adjunctive therapy with heparin is controversial. Because hypercoagulability is frequently present in patients with meningococcemia, some experts believe heparin should be considered for those with DIC. A loading dose of 50 units/kg is followed by 15 units/kg/h as a continuous infusion. The patient is monitored by following the partial thromboplastin time and heparin assay. Recombinant tissue plasminogen activator, concentrated antithrombin III, and recombinant protein C infusions have been tried experimentally to reverse coagulopathy. (See Chapter 28 for the management of DIC.)

▶ Prognosis

Unfavorable prognostic features include shock, DIC, and extensive skin lesions. The case fatality rate in fulminant meningococcemia is over 30%. In uncomplicated meningococcal meningitis, the fatality rate is much lower (10–20%).

Bilukha OO, Rosenstein N; National Center for Infectious Diseases, Centers for Disease Control and Prevention (CDC): Prevention and control of meningococcal disease. Recommendations of the Advisory Committee on Immunization Practices (ACIP). MMWR Recomm Rep 2005;54(RR-7):1 [PMID: 15917737].

Campos-Outcalt D: Meningococcal vaccine: New product, new recommendations. J Fam Pract 2005;54:324 [PMID: 15833222].
Gardner P: Clinical practice. Prevention of meningococcal disease. N Engl J Med 2006;355:1466 [PMID: 17021322].
Rosenstein NE et al: Meningococcal disease. N Engl J Med 2001;344:1378 [PMID:11333996].

GONOCOCCAL INFECTIONS

ESSENTIALS OF DIAGNOSIS & TYPICAL FEATURES

▶ Purulent urethral discharge with intracellular gram-negative diplococci on smear in male patients (usually adolescents).

▶ Purulent, edematous, sometimes hemorrhagic conjunctivitis with intracellular gram-negative diplococci in 2–4-day-old infants.

▶ Fever, arthritis (often polyarticular) or tenosynovitis, and maculopapular peripheral rash that may be vesiculopustular or hemorrhagic.

▶ Positive culture of blood, pharyngeal, or genital secretions.

▶ General Considerations

Neisseria gonorrhoeae is a gram-negative diplococcus. Although morphologically similar to other neisseriae, it differs in its ability to grow on selective media and to ferment carbohydrates. The cell wall of *N gonorrhoeae* contains endotoxin, which is liberated when the organism dies and is responsible for the production of a cellular exudate. The incubation period is short, usually 2–5 days.

Nearly 340,000 cases of gonorrhea were reported in the United States in 2005. Gonococcal disease in children may be transmitted sexually or nonsexually. Prepubertal gonococcal infection outside the neonatal period should be considered presumptive evidence of sexual contact or child abuse. Prepubertal girls usually manifest gonococcal vulvovaginitis because of the neutral to alkaline pH of the vagina and thin vaginal mucosa.

In the adolescent or adult, the workup of every case of gonorrhea should include a careful and accurate inquiry into the patient's sexual practices, because pharyngeal infection resulting from oral sex must be detected if present and may be difficult to eradicate. Efforts should be made to identify and provide treatment to all sexual contacts. When prepubertal children are infected, epidemiologic investigation should be thorough.

Antimicrobial-resistant gonococci are a serious problem. *N gonorrhoeae* infections resistant to tetracyclines, penicillins, and fluoroquinolones are common. Fluoroquinolone antimicrobials are no longer recommended for therapy in the United States. In some cases, clinicians will have very limited choices for therapy. Many clinical laboratories do not routinely perform antimicrobial susceptibility tests on *N gonorrhoeae*, and many infections are documented by non-culture methods.

▶ Clinical Findings

A. Symptoms and Signs

1. Asymptomatic gonorrhea—The ratio of asymptomatic to symptomatic gonorrheal infections in adolescents and adults is probably 3–4:1 in women and 0.5–1:1 in men. Asymptomatic infections are as infectious as symptomatic ones.

2. Uncomplicated genital gonorrhea

A. MALE WITH URETHRITIS—Urethral discharge is sometimes painful and bloody and may be white, yellow, or green. There may be associated dysuria. The patient usually is afebrile.

B. PREPUBERTAL FEMALE WITH VAGINITIS—The only clinical findings initially may be dysuria and polymorphonuclear neutrophils in the urine. Vulvitis characterized by erythema, edema, and excoriation accompanied by a purulent discharge may follow.

C. POSTPUBERTAL FEMALE WITH CERVICITIS—Symptomatic disease is characterized by a purulent, foul-smelling vaginal discharge, dysuria, and occasionally dyspareunia. Fever and abdominal pain are absent. The cervix is frequently hyperemic and tender when touched. This tenderness is not worsened by moving the cervix, nor are the adnexa tender to palpation.

D. RECTAL GONORRHEA—Rectal gonorrhea often is asymptomatic. There may be purulent discharge, edema, and pain during evacuation.

3. Pharyngeal gonorrhea—Pharyngeal infection usually is asymptomatic. There may be some sore throat and, rarely, acute exudative tonsillitis with bilateral cervical lymphadenopathy and fever.

4. Conjunctivitis and iridocyclitis—Copious, usually purulent exudate is characteristic of gonococcal conjunctivitis. Newborns are symptomatic on days 2–4 of life. In the adolescent or adult, infection probably is spread from infected genital secretions by the fingers.

5. Pelvic inflammatory disease (salpingitis)—The interval between initiation of genital infection and its ascent to the uterine tubes is variable and may range from days to months. Menses frequently are the initiating factor. With the onset of a menstrual period, gonococci invade the endometrium, causing transient endometritis. Subsequently salpingitis may occur, resulting in pyosalpinx or hydrosalpinx. Rarely infection progresses to peritonitis or perihepatitis. Gonococcal salpingitis occurs in an acute, a subacute, or a chronic form. All three forms have in common tenderness on gentle movement of the cervix and bilateral tubal tenderness during pelvic examination.

Gonococci or *Chlamydia trachomatis* are the cause of about 50% of cases of pelvic inflammatory disease. A mixed infection caused by enteric bacilli, *Bacteroides fragilis*, or other anaerobes occur in the other 50%.

6. Gonococcal perihepatitis (Fitz-Hugh and Curtis syndrome)—In the typical clinical pattern, the patient presents with right upper quadrant tenderness in association with signs of acute or subacute salpingitis. Pain may be pleuritic and referred to the shoulder. Hepatic friction rub is a valuable but inconstant sign.

7. Disseminated gonorrhea—Dissemination follows asymptomatic more often than symptomatic genital infection and often results from gonococcal pharyngitis or anorectal gonorrhea. The most common form of disseminated gonorrhea is polyarthritis or polytenosynovitis, with or without dermatitis. Monarticular arthritis is less common, and gonococcal endocarditis and meningitis are fortunately rare.

A. POLYARTHRITIS—Disease usually begins with the simultaneous onset of low-grade fever, polyarthralgia, and malaise. After a day or so, joint symptoms become acute. Swelling, redness, and tenderness occur, frequently over the wrists, ankles, and knees but also in the fingers, feet, and other peripheral joints. Skin lesions may be noted at the same time. Discrete, tender, maculopapular lesions 5–8 mm in diameter appear that may become vesicular, pustular, and then hemorrhagic. They are few in number and noted on the fingers, palms, feet, and other distal surfaces and may be single or multiple. In patients with this form of the disease, blood cultures are often positive, but joint fluid rarely yields organisms. Skin lesions often are positive by Gram stain but rarely by culture. Genital, rectal, and pharyngeal cultures must be performed.

B. MONARTICULAR ARTHRITIS—In this somewhat less common form of disseminated gonorrhea, fever is often absent. Arthritis evolves in a single joint. Dermatitis usually does not occur. Systemic symptoms are minimal. Blood cultures are negative, but joint aspirates may yield gonococci on smear and culture. Genital, rectal, and pharyngeal cultures must be performed.

B. Laboratory Findings

Demonstration of gram-negative, kidney-shaped diplococci in smears of urethral exudate in males is presumptive evidence of gonorrhea. Positive culture confirms the diagnosis. Negative smears do not rule out gonorrhea. Gram-stained smears of cervical or vaginal discharge in girls are more difficult to interpret because of normal gram-negative flora, but they may be useful when technical personnel are experienced. In girls with suspected gonorrhea, both the cervical os and the anus should be cultured. Gonococcal pharyngitis requires culture for diagnosis.

Cultures for *N gonorrhoeae* are plated on a selective chocolate agar containing antibiotics (eg, Thayer-Martin agar) to suppress normal flora. If bacteriologic diagnosis is critical, suspected material should be cultured on chocolate agar as well. Because gonococci are labile, agar plates should be inoculated immediately and placed without delay in an atmosphere containing CO_2 (candle jar). When transport of specimens is necessary, material should be inoculated directly into Transgrow medium prior to shipment to an appropriate laboratory. In cases of possible sexual molestation, notify the laboratory that definite speciation is needed, because nongonococcal *Neisseria* species can grow on the selective media.

Nucleic acid amplification tests on urine or genital specimens now enable detection of *N gonorrhoeae* and *C trachomatis*. These tests have excellent sensitivity and are replacing culture in many laboratories. All children or adolescents with a suspected or established diagnosis of gonorrhea should have serologic tests for syphilis and HIV.

Differential Diagnosis

Urethritis in the male may be gonococcal or nongonococcal (NGU). NGU is a syndrome characterized by discharge (rarely painful), mild dysuria, and a subacute course. The discharge is usually scant or moderate in amount but may be profuse. *C trachomatis* is the only proven cause of NGU. Doxycycline (100 mg orally twice a day for 7 days) is efficacious. Single-dose azithromycin, 1 g orally, may achieve better compliance. *C trachomatis* has been shown to cause epididymitis in males and salpingitis in females.

Vulvovaginitis in a prepubertal female may be due to infection caused by miscellaneous bacteria, including *Shigella* and GAS, *Candida,* and herpes simplex. Discharges may be caused by trichomonads, *Enterobius vermicularis* (pinworm), or foreign bodies. Symptom-free discharge (leukorrhea) normally accompanies rising estrogen levels.

Cervicitis in a postpubertal female, alone or in association with urethritis and involvement of Skene and Bartholin glands, may be due to infection caused by *Candida,* herpes simplex, *Trichomonas,* or discharge resulting from inflammation caused by foreign bodies (usually some form of contraceptive device). Leukorrhea may be associated with birth control pills.

Salpingitis may be due to infection with other organisms. The symptoms must be differentiated from those of appendicitis, urinary tract infection, ectopic pregnancy, endometriosis, or ovarian cysts or torsion.

Disseminated gonorrhea presents a differential diagnosis that includes meningococcemia, acute rheumatic fever, Henoch-Schönlein purpura, juvenile rheumatoid arthritis, lupus erythematosus, leptospirosis, secondary syphilis, certain viral infections (particularly rubella, but also enteroviruses and parvovirus), serum sickness, type B hepatitis (in the prodromal phase), infective endocarditis, and even acute leukemia and other types of cancer. The fully evolved skin lesions of disseminated gonorrhea are remarkably specific, and genital, rectal, or pharyngeal cultures, plus cultures of blood and joint fluid, usually yield gonococci from at least one source.

Prevention

Prevention of gonorrhea is principally a matter of sex education, condom use, and identification and treatment of contacts.

Treatment

A. Uncomplicated Urethral, Endocervical, or Rectal Gonococcal Infections in Adolescents

Ceftriaxone (125 mg intramuscularly in a single dose), cefixime (400 mg orally in a single dose), doxycycline (100 mg orally twice a day for 7 days), or azithromycin (1 g orally in a single dose) is recommended unless *C trachomatis* is ruled out. Ceftizoxime, cefotaxime, and cefotetan parenterally are alternative single-dose therapies. Fluoroquinolones are no longer recommended for therapy due to increasing rates of resistance. Cefpodoxime (400 mg) and cefuroxime (1 g orally) are alternatives.

Tetracyclines should be avoided in pregnancy, and repeated doses may stain the teeth of young children. Erythromycin or amoxicillin is recommended for therapy of *C trachomatis* in pregnant women; azithromycin is an alternative regimen. Repeat testing 3 weeks after completion of therapy is recommended in pregnant women.

Spectinomycin (2 g intramuscularly in a single dose) is used for penicillin- and cephalosporin-allergic patients, but is not currently available in the United States. A repeat culture after completion of therapy is not necessary in asymptomatic adolescents after the ceftriaxone–doxycycline regimen. A repeat culture after completion of therapy should be obtained from infants and children.

B. Pharyngeal Gonococcal Infection

Ceftriaxone (125 mg intramuscularly in a single dose) should be used; neither spectinomycin nor amoxicillin is recommended. A repeat culture is recommended 4–7 days after therapy.

C. Disseminated Gonorrhea

Recommended regimens include ceftriaxone (1 g intramuscularly or intravenously once daily) or cefotaxime (1 g intravenously every 8 hours). Oral therapy may follow parenteral therapy 24–48 hours after improvement. Recommended regimens include cefixime (400 mg), cefpodoxime (400 mg), or cefuroxime (1 g) twice daily to complete 7 days of therapy. Fluoroquinolones are not recommended. If concurrent infection with *Chlamydia* is present or has not been excluded, a course of doxycycline, azithromycin, or erythromycin should also be prescribed.

D. Pelvic Inflammatory Disease

Doxycycline (100 mg twice a day orally) and either cefoxitin (2 g intramuscularly or intravenously every 6 hours) or cefotetan (2 g intramuscularly or intravenously every 12 hours) are given until the patient is clinically improved, then doxycycline is administered by mouth to complete 14 days of therapy. Clindamycin and gentamicin given intravenously until the patient improves clinically may be used rather than cefoxitin. Many other regimens have been used for therapy of pelvic inflammatory disease, although comparative efficacy data are limited.

E. Prepubertal Gonococcal Infections

1. Uncomplicated genitourinary, rectal, or pharyngeal infections—These infections may be treated with ceftriaxone (25–50 mg/kg/d to a maximum of 125 mg intramuscularly in a single dose). Children older than age 8 years should also receive doxycycline (100 mg orally twice daily for 7 days). The physician should evaluate all children for evidence of sexual abuse and coinfection with syphilis, *Chlamydia,* and HIV.

2. Disseminated gonorrhea—This should be treated with ceftriaxone (50 mg/kg once daily parenterally for 7 days).

Centers for Disease Control and Prevention et al: Sexually transmitted diseases treatment guidelines, 2006. MMWR Recomm Rep 2006;55(RR-11):1. [PMID: 16888612].
Centers for Disease Control and Prevention (CDC): Update to CDC's sexually transmitted diseases treatment guidelines 2006: Fluoroquinolones no longer recommended for treatment of gonococcal infections. MMWR Morb Mortal Wkly Rep 2007; 56:332 [PMID: 17431378].

BOTULISM

ESSENTIALS OF DIAGNOSIS & TYPICAL FEATURES

▶ Dry mucous membranes.

▶ Nausea and vomiting.

▶ Diplopia; dilated, unreactive pupils.

▶ Descending paralysis.

▶ Difficulty in swallowing and speech occurring within 12–36 hours after ingestion of toxin-contaminated food.

▶ Multiple cases in a family or group.

▶ Hypotonia and constipation in infants.

▶ Diagnosis by clinical findings and identification of toxin in blood, stool, or implicated food.

▶ General Considerations

Botulism is a paralytic disease caused by *Clostridium botulinum,* an anaerobic, gram-positive, spore-forming bacillus

normally found in soil. The organism produces an extremely potent neurotoxin. Of the seven types of toxin (A–G), types A, B, and E cause most human diseases. The toxin, a polypeptide, is so potent that 0.1 mg is lethal for humans.

Food-borne botulism usually results from ingestion of toxin-containing food. Preformed toxin is absorbed from the gut and produces paralysis by preventing acetylcholine release from cholinergic fibers at myoneural junctions. In the United States, home-canned vegetables are usually the cause. Commercially canned foods rarely are responsible. Virtually any food will support the growth of *C botulinum* spores into vegetative toxin-producing bacilli if an anaerobic, nonacid environment is provided. The food may not appear or taste spoiled. The toxin is heat-labile, but the spores are heat-resistant. Inadequate heating during processing (temperature < 115°C) allows the spores to survive and later resume toxin production. Boiling of foods for 10 minutes or heating at 80°C for 30 minutes before eating will destroy the toxin.

Infant botulism is seen in infants younger than age 6 months (median, 10 weeks). The initial symptoms are usually constipation and progressive, often severe hypotonia. Infants younger than age 2 weeks rarely develop botulism. The toxin appears to be produced by *C botulinum* organisms residing in the gastrointestinal tract. In some instances, honey has been the source of spores. Clinical findings include constipation, weak suck and cry, pooled oral secretions, cranial nerve deficits, generalized weakness, and, on occasion, apnea. The characteristic electromyographic pattern of brief, small, abundant motor-unit action potentials (BSAPs) may help confirm the diagnosis.

Annually, 10–15 cases of wound botulism are reported. Most cases occur in drug abusers with infection in intravenous or intramuscular injection sites.

Botulism, as a result of aerosolization of botulinum toxin, also could occur as the result of a bioterrorism event. Only three such cases of botulism have been reported; the incubation period was not well-defined, but was about 72 hours in the reported cases.

▶ Clinical Findings

A. Symptoms and Signs

The incubation period for food-borne botulism is 8–36 hours. The initial symptoms are lethargy and headache. These are followed by double vision, dilated pupils, ptosis, and, within a few hours, difficulty with swallowing and speech. Pharyngeal paralysis occurs in some cases, and food may be regurgitated. The mucous membranes often are very dry. Descending skeletal muscle paralysis may be seen. Death usually results from respiratory failure.

Botulism patients present with a "classic triad": (1) afebrile; (2) symmetrical, flaccid, descending paralysis with prominent bulbar palsies; and (3) clear sensorium. Recognition of this triad is important in making the clinical diagnosis. Botulism is caused by a toxin, thus there is no fever unless secondary infection (eg, aspiration pneumonia) occurs. Common bulbar palsies seen include dysphonia, dysphagia, dysarthria, and diplopia (4 "Ds").

B. Laboratory Findings

The diagnosis is made by demonstration of *C botulinum* toxin in stool, gastric aspirate or vomitus, or serum. Serum and stool samples can be sent for toxin confirmation (done by toxin neutralization mouse bioassay at CDC or state health departments). Foods that are suspected to be contaminated should be kept refrigerated and given to public health personnel for testing. Laboratory findings, including CSF examination, are usually normal. Electromyography suggests the diagnosis if the characteristic BSAP abnormalities are seen. A nondiagnostic electromyogram does not exclude the diagnosis.

▶ Differential Diagnosis

Guillain-Barré syndrome is characterized by ascending paralysis, sensory deficits, and elevated CSF protein without pleocytosis.

Other illnesses that should be considered include poliomyelitis, postdiphtheritic polyneuritis, certain chemical intoxications, tick paralysis, and myasthenia gravis. The history and elevated CSF protein characterize postdiphtheritic polyneuritis. Tick paralysis presents with a flaccid ascending motor paralysis. An attached tick should be sought. Myasthenia gravis usually occurs in adolescent girls. It is characterized by ocular and bulbar symptoms, normal pupils, fluctuating weakness, absence of other neurologic signs, and clinical response to cholinesterase inhibitors.

▶ Complications

Difficulty in swallowing leads to aspiration pneumonia. Serious respiratory paralysis may be fatal despite assisted ventilation and intensive supportive measures.

▶ Treatment

A. Specific Measures

Early treatment of botulism with antitoxin (food-borne or wound botulism) or passive human botulism immune globulin (infant botulism) is beneficial. Treatment should begin as soon as the clinical diagnosis is made (prior to microbiologic or toxin confirmation).

For suspected wound or food-borne botulism, equine antitoxins are available from the CDC through state health departments. Patients should be treated with the bivalent antitoxin (types A and B) and possibly also the monovalent (type E) antitoxin. The state health department or the CDC ([770] 488-7100) can be contacted for help in obtaining products and for consultation. Both preparations are given by slow intravenous infusion. All patients need to be screened for hypersensitivity to the products prior to initiat-

ing the infusion; small challenge doses are given (see package insert). Patients who have reactions to the challenge doses are desensitized prior to receiving antitoxin infusion. In addition to the antitoxin, 24-hour diagnostic consultation, epidemic assistance, and laboratory testing services are available from the CDC through state health departments.

For treatment of infant botulism, intravenous human botulism immune globulin (Baby-BIG) is approved by the U.S. Food and Drug Administration (FDA) for use. Baby-BIG is a product containing high titers of neutralizing antibodies against type A and B toxin and is made from pooled plasma of adults who were immunized with a botulism toxoid vaccine. Results of a placebo-controlled clinical trial of use in infant botulism showed reduction in the mean hospital stay (2.5 weeks in treated patients vs 5.5 weeks in the placebo group) and decrease in mechanical ventilation time in the Baby-BIG–treated group. Although the cost of the preparation is high ($45,000 in 2007), it still is cost-saving since there is a substantial reduction in hospital days, intensive care unit stay, and ventilator time in treated infants. Baby-BIG is not indicated for use in any form of botulism (wound, food-borne) other than infant botulism. To obtain Baby-BIG (in any state), contact the California Department of Public Health at: (510) 540-2646.

B. General Measures

General and supportive therapy consists of bed rest, ventilatory support (if necessary), fluid therapy, enteral or parenteral nutrition, and administration of purgatives and high enemas. Aminoglycoside antimicrobials and clindamycin may exacerbate neuromuscular blockage and should be avoided.

▶ Prognosis

The mortality rate has declined substantially in recent years and currently is at 6%. In nonfatal cases, symptoms subside over 2–3 months and recovery is usually complete.

Fox CK et al: Recent advances in infant botulism. Pediatr Neurol 2005;32:149 [PMID: 15730893].

Long SS: Infant botulism and treatment with BIG-IV (BabyBIG). Pediatr Infect Dis J 2007;26:261 [PMID: 17484226].

Villar RG et al: Botulism: The many faces of botulinum toxin and its potential for bioterrorism. Infect Dis Clin North Am 2006; 20:313 [PMID: 16762741].

TETANUS

ESSENTIALS OF DIAGNOSIS & TYPICAL FEATURES

▶ Nonimmunized or partially immunized patient.

▶ History of skin wound.

▶ Spasms of jaw muscles (trismus).

► Stiffness of neck, back, and abdominal muscles, with hyperirritability and hyperreflexia.

► Episodic, generalized muscle contractions.

► Diagnosis is based on clinical findings and the immunization history.

► General Considerations

Tetanus is caused by *Clostridium tetani*, an anaerobic, gram-positive bacillus that produces a potent neurotoxin. In unimmunized or incompletely immunized individuals, infection follows contamination of a wound by soil containing clostridial spores from animal manure. The toxin reaches the CNS by retrograde axon transport, is bound to cerebral gangliosides, and appears to increase reflex excitability in neurons of the spinal cord by blocking function of inhibitory synapses. Intense muscle spasms result. Two thirds of cases in the United States follow minor puncture wounds of the hands or feet. In many cases, no history of a wound can be obtained. Injecting substances and drug abuse may be risk factors (in individuals who are not tetanus-immune). In the newborn, usually in underdeveloped countries, infection generally results from contamination of the umbilical cord. The incubation period typically is 4–14 days but may be longer. In the United States, cases in young children are due to failure to immunize. Eighty-five percent of cases occur in adults older than 25 years.

► Clinical Findings

A. Symptoms and Signs

The first symptom often is mild pain at the site of the wound, followed by hypertonicity and spasm of the regional muscles. Characteristically, difficulty in opening the mouth (trismus) is evident within 48 hours. In newborns, the first signs are irritability and inability to nurse. The infant may then develop stiffness of the jaw and neck, increasing dysphagia, and generalized hyperreflexia with rigidity and spasms of all muscles of the abdomen and back (opisthotonos). The facial distortion resembles a grimace (risus sardonicus). Difficulty in swallowing and convulsions triggered by minimal stimuli such as sound, light, or movement may occur. Individual spasms may last seconds or minutes. Recurrent spasms are seen several times each hour, or they may be almost continuous. In most cases, the temperature is normal or only mildly elevated. A high or subnormal temperature is a bad prognostic sign. Patients are fully conscious and lucid. A profound circulatory disturbance associated with sympathetic overactivity may occur on the second to fourth day, which may contribute to the mortality rate. This is characterized by elevated blood pressure, increased cardiac output, tachycardia (> 20 beats/min), and arrhythmia.

B. Laboratory Findings

The diagnosis is made on clinical grounds. There may be a mild polymorphonuclear leukocytosis. The CSF is normal with the exception of mild elevation of opening pressure. Serum muscle enzymes may be elevated. Transient electrocardiographic and electroencephalographic abnormalities may occur. Anaerobic culture and microscopic examination of pus from the wound can be helpful, but *C tetani* is difficult to grow, and the drumstick-shaped gram-positive bacilli often cannot be found.

► Differential Diagnosis

Poliomyelitis is characterized by asymmetrical paralysis in an incompletely immunized child. The history of an animal bite and the absence of trismus may suggest rabies. Local infections of the throat and jaw should be easily recognized. Bacterial meningitis, phenothiazine reactions, decerebrate posturing, narcotic withdrawal, spondylitis, and hypocalcemic tetany may be confused with tetanus.

► Complications

Complications include sepsis, malnutrition, pneumonia, atelectasis, asphyxial spasms, decubitus ulcers, and fractures of the spine due to intense contractions. They can be prevented in part by skilled supportive care.

► Prevention

A. Tetanus Toxoid

Active immunization with tetanus toxoid prevents tetanus. (See Chapter 9.) Immunity is almost always achieved after the third dose of vaccine. A booster at the time of injury is needed if none has been given in the past 10 years—or within 5 years for heavily contaminated wounds. Nearly all cases of tetanus (99%) in the United States are in nonimmunized or incompletely immunized individuals. Many adolescents and adults lack protective antibody.

B. Wound Care and Prophylaxis for Tetanus-Prone Wounds

Wounds that are contaminated with soil, debris, feces, or saliva are at increased risk for tetanus. Puncture wounds or wounds that contain devitalized tissue are at increased risk of infection with *C tetani*. This includes wounds that result from crush injury, frostbite, burns, or avulsion. All wounds should be adequately cleaned, foreign material removed, and debrided if necrotic or devitalized tissue is present or if residual foreign matter is present. The decision to use tetanus toxoid–containing vaccine or human tetanus immune globulin (TIG) depends on the type of injury and the tetanus immunization status of the patient. (See Chapter 9, and Table 9–5.) TIG should be used in children with fewer than three previous tetanus toxoid immunizations (DPT, DPaT, DT, Td, Tdap) who have tetanus-prone wounds, and should be administered to HIV-infected children with tetanus-prone wounds, regardless of their immunization history. When TIG is indicated for wound prophylaxis 250 units are given intramuscularly. If tetanus immunization is incomplete, a dose of age-appropriate vaccine should be given. When both are indicated, tetanus toxoid and TIG should be administered concurrently at different sites using different syringes. (See Chapter 9.)

Prophylactic antimicrobials are useful if the child is unimmunized and TIG is not available.

▶ Treatment

A. Specific Measures

Serotherapy lowers the mortality rate from tetanus, but not dramatically. Human TIG in a single dose of 3000–6000 units, intramuscularly, is given to children and adults. Doses of 500 units have been used in infants. If TIG is indicated, but not available, intravenous immune globulin in a dose of 200–400 mg/kg intravenously can be used. Surgical debridement of wounds is indicated, but more extensive surgery or amputation to eliminate the site of infection is not necessary. Antibiotics are given to attempt to decrease the number of vegetative forms of the bacteria to decrease toxin production: oral metronidazole (30 mg/kg/d in four divided doses; maximum 4 g/d) for 10–14 days is the preferred agent.

B. General Measures

The patient is kept in a quiet room with minimal stimulation. Control of spasms and prevention of hypoxic episodes are crucial. Diazepam or another anxiolytic is useful (0.6–1.2 mg/kg/d intravenously in six divided doses). In the newborn, two or three divided doses should be given. Large doses (up to 25 mg/kg/d) may be required for older children. Diazepam is given intravenously until muscular spasms become infrequent and the generalized muscular rigidity much less prominent. The drug may then be given orally and the dosage reduced as the child improves. Mechanical ventilation and muscle paralysis are necessary in severe cases. Nasogastric or intravenous feedings should be used to limit stimulation of feedings and prevent aspiration.

▶ Prognosis

The fatality rate in newborns and heroin-addicted individuals is high. The overall mortality rate in the United States is 11%. The fatality rate depends on the quality of supportive care, the patient's age, and the patient's vaccination history. Many deaths are due to pneumonia or respiratory failure. If the patient survives 1 week, recovery is likely.

Bunch TJ et al: Respiratory failure in tetanus: Case report and review of a 25-year experience. Chest 2002;122:1488 [PMID: 12377887].

Centers for Disease Control and Prevention: Tetanus. http://www.cdc.gov/vaccines/pubs/pinkbook/downloads/tetanus.pdf

Rhee P et al: Tetanus and trauma: A review and recommendations. J Trauma Injury Infect Crit Care 2005;58:1082 [PMID: 15920431].

GAS GANGRENE

ESSENTIALS OF DIAGNOSIS & TYPICAL FEATURES

▶ Contamination of a wound with soil or feces.

▶ Massive edema, skin discoloration, bleb formation, and pain in an area of trauma.

▶ Serosanguineous exudate from wound.

▶ Crepitation of subcutaneous tissue.

▶ Rapid progression of signs and symptoms.

▶ Clostridia cultured or seen on stained smears.

▶ General Considerations

Gas gangrene (clostridial myonecrosis) is a necrotizing infection that follows trauma or surgery and is caused by several anaerobic, gram-positive, spore-forming bacilli of the genus *Clostridium*. The spores are found in soil, feces, and vaginal secretions. In devitalized tissue, the spores germinate into vegetative bacilli that proliferate and produce toxins, causing thrombosis, hemolysis, and tissue necrosis. *Clostridium perfringens,* the species causing approximately 80% of cases of gas gangrene, produces at least eight such toxins. The areas involved most often are the extremities, abdomen, and uterus. *Clostridium septicum* may also cause myonecrosis and causes septicemia in patients with neutropenia. Nonclostridial infections with gas formation can mimic clostridial infections and are more common. Neutropenia is a risk factor for this severe infection.

▶ Clinical Findings

A. Symptoms and Signs

The onset of gas gangrene usually is sudden, often 1 day after trauma or surgery (mean, 3–4 days), but can be delayed up to 20 days. The skin around the wound becomes discolored, with hemorrhagic bullae, serosanguineous exudate, and crepitation in the subcutaneous tissues. Pain and swelling usually are intense. Systemic illness appears early and progresses rapidly to intravascular hemolysis, jaundice, shock, toxic delirium, and renal failure.

B. Laboratory Findings

Isolation of the organism requires anaerobic culture. Gram-stained smears may demonstrate many gram-positive rods and few inflammatory cells.

C. Imaging

Radiographs may demonstrate gas in tissues, but this is a late finding and is also seen in infections with other gas-forming organisms or may be due to air introduced into tissues during trauma or surgery.

D. Operative Findings

Direct visualization of the muscle at surgery may be necessary to diagnose gas gangrene. Early, the muscle is pale and edematous and does not contract normally; later, the muscle may be frankly gangrenous.

Differential Diagnosis

Gangrene and cellulitis caused by other organisms and clostridial cellulitis (not myonecrosis) must be distinguished. Necrotizing fasciitis may resemble gas gangrene.

Prevention

Gas gangrene can be prevented by the adequate cleansing and debridement of all wounds. It is essential that foreign bodies and dead tissue be removed. A clean wound does not provide a suitable anaerobic environment for the growth of clostridial species.

Treatment

A. Specific Measures

Penicillin G (300,000–400,000 units/kg/d intravenously in six divided doses) should be given, usually combined with clindamycin or metronidazole. Clindamycin, metronidazole, meropenem, and imipenem–cilastatin are alternatives for penicillin-allergic patients. Some experts recommend a combination of penicillin and clindamycin.

B. Surgical Measures

Surgery should be prompt and extensive, with removal of all necrotic tissue.

C. Hyperbaric Oxygen

Hyperbaric oxygen therapy has been shown to be effective, but it is not a substitute for surgery. A patient may be exposed to 2–3 atm in pure oxygen for 1- to 2-hour periods for as many sessions as necessary until clinical remission occurs.

Prognosis

Clostridial myonecrosis is fatal if untreated. With early diagnosis, antibiotics, and surgery, the mortality rate is 20–60%. Involvement of the abdominal wall, leukopenia, intravascular hemolysis, renal failure, and shock are ominous prognostic signs.

Langham M, Arnold L: Clostridial myonecrosis in an adolescent male. Pediatrics 2005;116:e737 [PMID: 16199671].

Smith-Slatas CL et al: Clostridium septicum infections in children: A case report and review of the literature. Pediatrics 2006; 117:e796 [PMID: 16567392].

DIPHTHERIA

ESSENTIALS OF DIAGNOSIS & TYPICAL FEATURES

▶ Gray, adherent pseudomembrane, most often in the pharynx but also in the nasopharynx or trachea.

▶ Sore throat, serosanguineous nasal discharge, hoarseness, and fever in a nonimmunized child.

▶ Peripheral neuritis or myocarditis.

▶ Positive culture.

▶ Treatment should not be withheld pending culture results.

General Considerations

Diphtheria is an acute infection of the upper respiratory tract or skin caused by toxin-producing *Corynebacterium diphtheriae*. Diphtheria in the United States is rare; five cases have been reported since 2000, and only 48 cases were reported from 1980–1997. However, significant numbers of elderly adults and unimmunized children are susceptible to infection. Diphtheria still occurs in epidemics in countries where immunization is not universal. Travelers to these areas may acquire the disease.

Corynebacteria are gram-positive, club-shaped rods with a beaded appearance on Gram stain. The capacity to produce exotoxin is conferred by a lysogenic bacteriophage and is not present in all strains of *C diphtheriae*. In immunized communities, infection probably occurs through spread of the phage among carriers of susceptible bacteria rather than through spread of phage-containing bacteria themselves. Diphtheria toxin kills susceptible cells by irreversible inhibition of protein synthesis.

The toxin is absorbed into the mucous membranes and causes destruction of epithelium and a superficial inflammatory response. The necrotic epithelium becomes embedded in exuding fibrin and red and white blood cells, forming a grayish pseudomembrane over the tonsils, pharynx, or larynx. Any attempt to remove the membrane exposes and tears the capillaries, resulting in bleeding. The diphtheria bacilli within the membrane continue to produce toxin, which is absorbed and may result in toxic injury to heart muscle, liver, kidneys, and adrenals, and is sometimes accompanied by hemorrhage. The toxin also produces neuritis, resulting in paralysis of the soft palate, eye muscles, or extremities. Death may occur as a result of respiratory obstruction or toxemia and circulatory collapse. The patient may succumb after a somewhat longer time as a result of cardiac damage. The incubation period is 2–7 days.

Clinical Findings

A. Symptoms and Signs

1. Pharyngeal diphtheria—Early manifestations of diphtheritic pharyngitis are mild sore throat, moderate fever, and malaise, followed fairly rapidly by prostration and circulatory collapse. The pulse is more rapid than the fever would seem to justify. A pharyngeal membrane forms and may spread into the nasopharynx or the trachea, producing respiratory obstruction. The membrane is tenacious and gray and is surrounded by a narrow zone of erythema and a broader zone of edema. The cervical lymph nodes become swollen, and swelling is associated with brawny edema of the neck (so-called bull neck). Laryngeal diphtheria presents with stridor, which can progress to obstruction of the airway.

2. Other forms—Cutaneous, vaginal, and wound diphtheria account for up to one third of cases and are characterized by ulcerative lesions with membrane formation.

B. Laboratory Findings

Diagnosis is clinical. Direct smears are unreliable. Material is obtained from the nose, throat, or skin lesions, if present, for culture, but specialized culture media are required. Between 16 and 48 hours is required before identification of the organism. A toxigenicity test is then performed. Cultures may be negative in individuals who have received antibiotics. The WBC count usually is normal, but hemolytic anemia and thrombocytopenia are frequent.

▶ Differential Diagnosis

Pharyngeal diphtheria resembles pharyngitis secondary to β-hemolytic streptococcus, Epstein-Barr virus, or other viral respiratory pathogens. A nasal foreign body or purulent sinusitis may mimic nasal diphtheria. Other causes of laryngeal obstruction include epiglottitis and viral croup. Guillain-Barré syndrome, poliomyelitis, or acute poisoning may mimic the neuropathy of diphtheria.

▶ Complications

A. Myocarditis

Diphtheritic myocarditis is characterized by a rapid, thready pulse; indistinct heart sounds, ST-T wave changes, conduction abnormalities, dysrhythmias, or cardiac failure; hepatomegaly; and fluid retention. Myocardial dysfunction may occur from 2–40 days after the onset of pharyngitis.

B. Polyneuritis

Neuritis of the palatal and pharyngeal nerves occurs during the first or second week. Nasal speech and regurgitation of food through the nose are seen. Diplopia and strabismus occur during the third week or later. Neuritis may also involve peripheral nerves supplying the intercostal muscles, diaphragm, and other muscle groups. Generalized paresis usually occurs after the fourth week.

C. Bronchopneumonia

Secondary pneumonia is common in fatal cases.

▶ Prevention

A. Immunization

Immunization with diphtheria toxoid combined with pertussis and tetanus toxoids (DTaP) should be used routinely for infants and children. (See Chapter 9.)

B. Care of Exposed Susceptibles

Children exposed to diphtheria should be examined, and nose and throat cultures obtained. If signs and symptoms of early diphtheria are found, antibiotic treatment should be instituted. Immunized asymptomatic individuals should receive diphtheria toxoid if a booster has not been received within 5 years. Unimmunized close contacts should receive either erythromycin orally (40 mg/kg/d in four divided doses) for 7 days or benzathine penicillin G intramuscularly (25,000 units/kg), active immunization with diphtheria toxoid, and observation daily.

▶ Treatment

A. Specific Measures

1. Antitoxin—To be effective, diphtheria antitoxin should be administered within 48 hours. (See Chapter 9.)

2. Antibiotics—Penicillin G (150,000 units/kg/d intravenously) should be given for 10 days. For penicillin-allergic patients, erythromycin (40 mg/kg/d) is given orally for 10 days.

B. General Measures

Bed rest in the hospital for 10–14 days is usually required. All patients must be strictly isolated for 1–7 days until respiratory secretions are noncontagious. Isolation may be discontinued when three successive nose and throat cultures at 24-hour intervals are negative. These cultures should not be taken until at least 24 hours have elapsed since the cessation of antibiotic treatment.

C. Treatment of Carriers

All carriers should receive treatment. Erythromycin (40 mg/kg/d orally in three or four divided doses), penicillin V potassium (50 mg/kg/d for 10 days), or benzathine penicillin G (600,000–1,200,000 units intramuscularly) should be given. All carriers must be quarantined. Before they can be released, carriers must have three negative cultures of both the nose and the throat taken 24 hours apart and obtained at least 24 hours after the cessation of antibiotic therapy.

▶ Prognosis

Mortality varies from 3–25% and is particularly high in the presence of early myocarditis. Neuritis is reversible; it is fatal only if an intact airway and adequate respiration cannot be maintained. Permanent heart damage from myocarditis occurs rarely.

Centers for Disease Control and Prevention: Diphtheria. http://www.cdc.gov/ncidod/dbmd/diseaseinfo/diphtheria_t.htm

Fatal respiratory diphtheria in a U.S. traveler to Haiti—Pennsylvania, 2003. MMWR Morb Mortal Wkly Rep 2004;52–53:1285 [PMID: 14712177].

Sing A, Heesemann J: Imported cutaneous diphtheria, Germany, 1997–2003. Emerg Infect Dis 2005;11:343 [PMID: 15759338].

INFECTIONS DUE TO ENTEROBACTERIACEAE

ESSENTIALS OF DIAGNOSIS & TYPICAL FEATURES

▶ Diarrhea by several different mechanisms due to *Escherichia coli.*

▶ Hemorrhagic colitis and hemolytic-uremic syndrome.

▶ Neonatal sepsis or meningitis.

▶ Urinary tract infection.

▶ Opportunistic infections.

▶ Diagnosis confirmed by culture.

▶ General Considerations

Enterobacteriaceae are a family of gram-negative bacilli that are normal flora in the gastrointestinal tract and are also found in water and soil. They cause gastroenteritis, urinary tract infections, neonatal sepsis and meningitis, and opportunistic infections. *Escherichia coli* is the organism in this family that most commonly causes infection in children, but *Klebsiella, Morganella, Enterobacter, Serratia, Proteus,* and other genera are also important, particularly in the compromised host. *Shigella* and *Salmonella* are discussed in separate sections.

E coli strains capable of causing diarrhea were originally termed enteropathogenic (EPEC) and were recognized by serotype. It is now known that *E coli* may cause diarrhea by several distinct mechanisms. Classic EPEC strains cause a characteristic histologic injury in the small bowel termed adherence and effacement. Enterotoxigenic *E coli* (ETEC) causes a secretory, watery diarrhea. ETEC adheres to enterocytes and secretes one or more plasmid-encoded enterotoxins. One of these, heat-labile toxin, resembles cholera toxin in structure, function, and mechanism of action. Enteroinvasive *E coli* (EIEC) are very similar to *Shigella* in their pathogenetic mechanisms. Enterohemorrhagic *E coli* (EHEC) cause hemorrhagic colitis and the hemolytic-uremic syndrome. The most common EHEC serotype is O157:H7, although several other serotypes cause the same syndrome. These strains elaborate one of several cytotoxins, closely related to Shiga toxin produced by *Shigella dysenteriae*. Outbreaks of hemolytic-uremic syndrome associated with EHEC have followed consumption of inadequately cooked ground beef. Thorough heating to 68–71°C is necessary. Unpasteurized fruit juice, various uncooked vegetables, and contaminated water also have caused infections and epidemics. The common source for EHEC in all of these foods and water is the feces of cattle. Person-to-person spread including spread in day care centers by the fecal-oral route has been reported.

E coli that aggregate on the surface of hep cells in tissue culture are termed enteroaggregative (EAggEC) *E coli*. EAggEC cause diarrhea by a distinct but unknown mechanism.

Eighty percent of *E coli* strains causing neonatal meningitis possess specific capsular polysaccharide (K1 antigen), which, alone or in association with specific somatic antigens, confers virulence. Approximately 90% of urinary tract infections in children are caused by *E coli. E coli* binds to the uroepithelium by P-fimbriae, which are present in more than 90% of *E coli* that cause pyelonephritis. Other bacterial cell surface structures, such as O and K antigens, and host factors are also important in the pathogenesis of urinary tract infections.

Klebsiella, Enterobacter, Serratia, and *Morganella* are normally found in the gastrointestinal tract and in soil and water. *Klebsiella* may cause a bronchopneumonia with cavity formation. *Klebsiella, Enterobacter,* and *Serratia* are often hospital-acquired opportunists associated with antibiotic usage, debilitated states, and chronic respiratory conditions. They frequently cause urinary tract infection or sepsis. In many newborn nurseries, nosocomial outbreaks caused by antimicrobial-resistant *Klebsiella* or *Enterobacter* species are a major problem.

Many of these infections are difficult to treat because of antibiotic resistance. Antibiotic susceptibility tests are necessary. Parenteral third-generation cephalosporins are usually more active than ampicillin, but resistance due to high-level production of chromosomal cephalosporinase may occur. *Enterobacter* and *Serratia* strains broadly resistant to cephalosporins also cause infections in hospitalized newborns and children. Aminoglycoside antibiotics are usually effective but require monitoring of serum levels to ensure therapeutic and nontoxic levels.

▶ Clinical Findings

A. Symptoms and Signs

1. *E coli* gastroenteritis—*E coli* may cause diarrhea of varying types and severity. ETEC usually produce mild, self-limiting illness without significant fever or systemic toxicity, often known as traveler's diarrhea. However, diarrhea may be severe in newborns and infants, and occasionally an older child or adult will have a cholera-like syndrome. EIEC strains cause a shigellosis-like illness, characterized by fever, systemic symptoms, blood and mucus in the stool, and leukocytosis, but currently are uncommon in the United States. EHEC strains cause hemorrhagic colitis. Diarrhea initially is watery and fever usually is absent.

Abdominal pain and cramping occur; diarrhea progresses to blood streaking or grossly bloody stools. Hemolytic-uremic syndrome occurs within a few days of diarrhea in 2–5% of children and is characterized by microangiopathic hemolytic anemia, thrombocytopenia, and renal failure. (See Chapter 22.)

2. Neonatal sepsis—Findings include jaundice, hepatosplenomegaly, fever, temperature lability, apneic spells, irritability, and poor feeding. Respiratory distress develops when pneumonia occurs; it may appear indistinguishable from respiratory distress syndrome in preterm infants. Meningitis is associated with sepsis in 25–40% of cases. Other metastatic foci of infection may be present, including pneumonia and pyelonephritis. Sepsis may lead to severe metabolic acidosis, shock, DIC, and death.

3. Neonatal meningitis—Findings include high fever, full fontanelles, vomiting, coma, convulsions, pareses or paralyses, poor or absent Moro reflex, opisthotonos, and occasionally hypertonia or hypotonia. Sepsis coexists or precedes meningitis in most cases. Thus, signs of sepsis often accompany those of meningitis. CSF usually shows a cell count of over 1000/µL, mostly polymorphonuclear neutrophils, and bacteria on Gram stain. CSF glucose concentration is low (usually less than half that of blood), and the protein is elevated above the levels normally seen in newborns and premature infants (> 150 mg/dL).

4. Acute urinary tract infection—Symptoms include dysuria, increased urinary frequency, and fever in the older child. Nonspecific symptoms such as anorexia, vomiting, irritability, failure to thrive, and unexplained fever are seen in children younger than age 2 years. Young infants may present with jaundice. As many as 1% of school-aged girls and 0.05% of boys have asymptomatic bacteriuria. Screening for and treatment of asymptomatic bacteriuria is not recommended.

B. Laboratory Findings

Because *E coli* are normal flora in the stool, a positive stool culture alone does not prove that the *E coli* in the stool are causing disease. Serotyping, tests for enterotoxin production or invasiveness, and tests for P-fimbriae are performed in research laboratories. MacConkey agar with sorbitol substituted for lactose (SMAC agar) is useful to screen stool for EHEC. Serotyping and testing for enterotoxin are available at many state health departments. Blood cultures are positive in neonatal sepsis. Cultures of CSF and urine should also be obtained. The diagnosis of urinary tract infections is discussed in Chapter 22.

▶ Differential Diagnosis

The clinical picture of EPEC infection may resemble that of salmonellosis, shigellosis, or viral gastroenteritis. Neonatal sepsis and meningitis caused by *E coli* can be differentiated from other causes of neonatal infection only by blood and CSF culture.

▶ Treatment
A. Specific Measures

1. *E coli* gastroenteritis—Gastroenteritis due to EPEC seldom requires antimicrobial treatment. Fluid and electrolyte therapy, preferably given orally, may be required to avoid dehydration. Bismuth subsalicylate reduces stool volume by about one third in infants with watery diarrhea, probably including ETEC. In nursery outbreaks, *E coli* gastroenteritis has been treated with neomycin (100 mg/kg/d orally in three divided doses for 5 days). Clinical efficacy is not established. Traveler's diarrhea may be treated with TMP–SMX in children and with fluoroquinolones in adults, although resistance to these drugs is increasing. Azithromycin is an alternative. The risk of hemolytic-uremic syndrome may increase following treatment of EHEC colitis, and antimicrobials should be withheld in suspected cases.

2. *E coli* sepsis, pneumonia, or pyelonephritis—The drugs of choice are ampicillin (150–200 mg/kg/d, given intravenously or intramuscularly in divided doses every 4–6 hours), cefotaxime (150–200 mg/kg/d, given intravenously or intramuscularly in divided doses every 6–8 hours), ceftriaxone (50–100 mg/kg/d, given intramuscularly as single dose or in two divided doses), and gentamicin (5.0–7.5 mg/kg/d, given intramuscularly or intravenously in divided doses every 8 hours). Treatment is continued for 10–14 days. Amikacin or tobramycin may be used instead of gentamicin if the strain is susceptible. Third-generation cephalosporins are often an attractive alternative as single-drug therapy and do not require monitoring for toxicity.

3. *E coli* meningitis—Third-generation cephalosporins such as cefotaxime (200 mg/kg/d intravenously in four divided doses) are given for a minimum of 3 weeks. Ampicillin (200–300 mg/kg/d intravenously in four to six divided doses) and gentamicin (5.0–7.5 mg/kg/d intramuscularly or intravenously in three divided doses) also are effective. Treatment with intrathecal and intraventricular aminoglycosides does not improve outcome. Serum levels need to be monitored.

4. Acute urinary tract infection—(See Chapter 22.)

▶ Prognosis

Death due to gastroenteritis leading to dehydration can be prevented by early fluid and electrolyte therapy. Neonatal sepsis with meningitis is still associated with a mortality rate of over 50%. Most children with recurrent urinary tract infections do well if they have no underlying anatomic defects. The mortality rate in opportunistic infections usually depends on the severity of infection and the underlying condition.

Anjay MA et al: Leukocytosis as a predictor for progression to haemolytic uraemic syndrome in Escherichia coli O157:H7 infection. Arch Dis Child 2007;92:820 [PMID: 17715449].

Centers for Disease Control and Prevention: Diarrheagenic Escherichia coli. http://www.cdc.gov/ncidod/dbmd/diseaseinfo/ escherichia coli O157:H7_g.htm

DuPont HL: Therapy for and prevention of traveler's diarrhea. Clin Infect Dis 2007;45(Suppl 1):S78 [PMID: 17582576].

Kanellopoulos TA et al: First urinary tract infection in neonates, infants and young children: A comparative study. Pediatr Nephrol 2006;21:1131 [PMID: 16810514].

Ochoa TJ, Cleary TG: Epidemiology and spectrum of disease of Escherichia coli O157. Curr Opin Infect Dis 2003;16:259 [PMID: 12821818].

Raffaelli RM al: Child care-associated outbreak of Escherichia coli O157:H7 and hemolytic uremic syndrome. Pediatr Infect Dis 2007;26(10):951 [PMID: 17901803].

PSEUDOMONAS INFECTIONS

ESSENTIALS OF DIAGNOSIS & TYPICAL FEATURES

▶ Opportunistic infection.
▶ Confirmed by cultures.

General Considerations

Pseudomonas aeruginosa is an aerobic gram-negative rod with versatile metabolic requirements. The organism may grow in distilled water and in commonly used disinfectants, complicating infection control in medical facilities. *P aeruginosa* is both invasive and destructive to tissue as well as toxigenic due to secreted exotoxins, all factors that contribute to virulence. Other genera previously classified as *Pseudomonas* frequently cause nosocomial infections and infections in immunocompromised children. *Stenotrophomonas maltophilia* (previously *P maltophilia*) and *Burkholderia cepacia* (previously *P cepacia*) are the most frequent.

P aeruginosa is an important cause of infection in children with cystic fibrosis, neoplastic disease, neutropenia, or extensive burns and in those receiving antibiotic therapy. Infections of the urinary and respiratory tracts, ears, mastoids, paranasal sinuses, eyes, skin, meninges, and bones are seen. *Pseudomonas* pneumonia is a common nosocomial infection in patients receiving assisted ventilation.

P aeruginosa sepsis may be accompanied by characteristic peripheral lesions called ecthyma gangrenosum. Ecthyma gangrenosum also may occur by direct invasion through intact skin in the groin, axilla, or other skinfolds. *P aeruginosa* is an infrequent cause of sepsis in previously healthy infants and may be the initial sign of underlying medical problems. *P aeruginosa* osteomyelitis often complicates puncture wounds of the feet. *P aeruginosa* is a frequent cause of malignant external otitis media and of chronic suppurative otitis media. Outbreaks of vesiculopustular skin rash have been associated

with exposure to contaminated water in whirlpool baths and hot tubs.

P aeruginosa infects the tracheobronchial tree of nearly all patients with cystic fibrosis. Mucoid exopolysaccharide, an exuberant capsule, is characteristically overproduced by isolates from patients with cystic fibrosis. Although bacteremia seldom occurs, patients with cystic fibrosis ultimately succumb to chronic lung infection with *P aeruginosa*. Infection due to *B cepacia* has caused a rapidly progressive pulmonary disease in some colonized patients and may be spread by close contact.

Osteomyelitis of the calcaneus or other foot bones occurs after punctures such as stepping on a nail and is commonly due to *P aeruginosa*.

▶ Clinical Findings

The clinical findings depend on the site of infection and the patient's underlying disease. Sepsis with these organisms resembles gram-negative sepsis with other organisms, although the presence of ecthyma gangrenosum suggests the diagnosis. The diagnosis is made by culture. *Pseudomonas* infection should be suspected in neonates and neutropenic patients with clinical sepsis. A severe necrotizing pneumonia occurs in patients on ventilators.

Patients with cystic fibrosis have a persistent bronchitis that progresses to bronchiectasis and ultimately to respiratory failure. During exacerbations of illness, cough and sputum production increase with low-grade fever, malaise, and diminished energy.

The purulent aural drainage without fever in patients with chronic suppurative otitis media is not distinguishable from that due to other causes.

▶ Prevention

A. Infections in Debilitated Patients

Colonization of extensive second- and third-degree burns by *P aeruginosa* can lead to fatal septicemia. Aggressive debridement and topical treatment with 0.5% silver nitrate solution, 10% mafenide cream, or silver sulfadiazine will greatly inhibit *P aeruginosa* contamination of burns. (See Chapter 11 for a discussion of burn wound infections and prevention.)

B. Nosocomial Infections

Faucet aerators, communal soap dispensers, disinfectants, improperly cleaned inhalation therapy equipment, infant incubators, and many other sources that usually are associated with wet or humid conditions all have been associated with *Pseudomonas* epidemics. Infant-to-infant transmission by nursery personnel carrying *Pseudomonas* on the hands is frequent in neonatal units. Careful maintenance of equipment and enforcement of infection control procedures are essential to minimize nosocomial transmission.

C. Patients with Cystic Fibrosis

Chronic infection of the lower respiratory tract occurs in nearly all patients with cystic fibrosis. The infecting organism is seldom cleared from the respiratory tract, even with intensive antimicrobial therapy, and the resultant injury to the lung eventually leads to pulmonary insufficiency. Treatment is aimed at controlling signs and symptoms of the infection.

▶ Treatment

P aeruginosa is inherently resistant to many antimicrobials and may develop resistance during therapy. Mortality rates in hospitalized patients exceed 50%, owing both to the severity of underlying illnesses in patients predisposed to *Pseudomonas* infection and to the limitations of therapy. Antibiotics effective against *Pseudomonas* include the aminoglycosides, ureidopenicillins (ticarcillin and piperacillin), β-lactamase inhibitor with a ureidopenicillin (ticarcillin–clavulanate and piperacillin–tazobactam), expanded-spectrum cephalosporins (ceftazidime and cefepime), imipenem, meropenem, and ciprofloxacin. Antimicrobial susceptibility patterns vary from area to area, and resistance tends to appear as new drugs become popular. Treatment of infections is best guided by clinical response and susceptibility tests.

Gentamicin or tobramycin (5.0–7.5 mg/kg/d, given intramuscularly or intravenously in three divided doses) or amikacin (15–22 mg/kg/d, given in two or three divided doses) in combination with ticarcillin (200–300 mg/kg/d, given intravenously in four to six divided doses) or with another antipseudomonal β-lactam antibiotic is recommended for treatment of serious *Pseudomonas* infections. Ceftazidime (150–200 mg/kg/d, given in four divided doses) or cefepime (150 mg/kg/d, given in three divided doses) has excellent activity against *P aeruginosa*. Treatment should be continued for 10–14 days. Treatment with two active drugs is recommended for all serious infections.

Pseudomonas osteomyelitis due to punctures requires thorough surgical debridement and antimicrobial therapy for 2 weeks. *Pseudomonas* folliculitis does not require antibiotic therapy.

Oral or intravenous ciprofloxacin is also effective against susceptible *P aeruginosa,* but is not approved by the FDA for use in children except in the case of urinary tract infection. Nonetheless, in some circumstances of antimicrobial resistance, or when the benefits clearly outweigh the small risks, ciprofloxacin may be used.

Chronic suppurative otitis media responds to intravenous ceftazidime (150–200 mg/kg/d in three or four divided doses) given until the drainage has ceased for 3 days. Twice-daily ceftazidime with aural debridement and cleaning given on an outpatient basis has also been successful. Swimmer's ear may be caused by *P aeruginosa* and responds well to topical drying agents (alcohol–vinegar mix) and cleansing.

▶ Prognosis

Because debilitated patients are most frequently affected, the mortality rate is high. These infections may have a protracted course, and eradication of the organisms may be difficult.

Iversen BG et al: An outbreak of *Pseudomonas aeruginosa* infection caused by contaminated mouth swabs. Clin Infect Dis 2007;44: 794 [PMID: 17304450].

Korvoca J et al: Bacteraemia due to *Pseudomonas putida* and other *Pseudomonas* non-*aeruginosa* in children J Infect 2005;51:81 [PMID: 15979496].

Lahiri T: Approaches to the treatment of initial *Pseudomonas aeruginosa* infection in children who have cystic fibrosis. Clin Chest Med 2007;28:307 [PMID: 17467550].

Merlo CA et al: Incidence and risk factors for multiple antibiotic-resistant *Pseudomonas aeruginosa* in cystic fibrosis. Chest 2007;132:562 [PMID: 17646236].

Yu Y et al: Hot tub folliculitis or hot hand-foot syndrome caused by *Pseudomonas aeruginosa.* J Am Acad Dermatol 2007;57:596 [PMID: 17658195].

SALMONELLA GASTROENTERITIS

ESSENTIALS OF DIAGNOSIS & TYPICAL FEATURES

- ▶ Nausea, vomiting, headache, meningismus.
- ▶ Fever, diarrhea, abdominal pain.
- ▶ Culture or organism from stool, blood, or other specimens.

▶ General Considerations

Salmonellae are gram-negative rods that frequently cause food-borne gastroenteritis and occasionally bacteremic infection of bone, meninges, and other foci. Three species—*Salmonella typhi, Salmonella choleraesuis,* and *Salmonella enteritidis*—and approximately 2000 serotypes are recognized. *Salmonella typhimurium* is the most frequently isolated serotype in most parts of the world. An estimated 4 million cases of salmonellosis occur yearly in the United States, but only 40,000 are reported.

Salmonellae are able to penetrate the mucin layer of the small bowel and attach to epithelial cells. Organisms penetrate the epithelial cells and multiply in the submucosa. Infection results in fever, vomiting, and watery diarrhea; the diarrhea occasionally includes mucus and polymorphonuclear neutrophils in the stool. Although the small intestine is generally regarded as the principal site of infection, colitis also occurs. *S typhimurium* frequently involves the large bowel.

Salmonella infections in childhood occur in two major forms: (1) gastroenteritis (including food poisoning), which may be complicated by sepsis and focal suppurative complications; and (2) enteric fever (typhoid fever and paratyphoid fever) (see next section). Although the incidence of typhoid fever has decreased in the United States, the incidence of

Salmonella gastroenteritis has greatly increased in the past 15–20 years. The highest attack rates occur in children younger than age 6 years, with a peak in the age group from 6 months to 2 years.

Salmonellae are widespread in nature, infecting domestic and wild animals. Fowl and reptiles have a particularly high carriage rate. Transmission results primarily from ingestion of contaminated food. Transmission from human to human occurs by the fecal-oral route via contaminated food, water, and fomites. Numerous foods, including meats, milk, cheese, ice cream, chocolate, contaminated egg powder, and frozen whole egg preparations used to make ice cream, custards, and mayonnaise are associated with outbreaks. Eggs with contaminated shells that are consumed raw or undercooked have been incriminated in outbreaks and sporadic cases. Animal contact also can be a source for salmonella.

Because salmonellae are susceptible to gastric acidity, the elderly, infants, and patients taking antacids or H_2-blocking drugs are at increased risk for infection. Most cases of *Salmonella* meningitis (80%) and bacteremia occur in infancy. Newborns may acquire the infection from their mothers during delivery and may precipitate outbreaks in nurseries. Newborns are at special risk for developing meningitis.

Epidemiologic studies suggest that 100 mild cases of Salmonella infection occur for each case detected by a positive culture. In 2005, 45,000 cases of Salmonella infection were reported in the United States.

▶ Clinical Findings

A. Symptoms and Signs

There is a very wide range of severity of infection. Infants usually develop fever, vomiting, and diarrhea. The older child also may complain of headache, nausea, and abdominal pain. Stools are often watery or may contain mucus and, in some instances, blood, suggesting shigellosis. Drowsiness and disorientation may be associated with meningismus. Convulsions occur less frequently than with shigellosis. Splenomegaly occasionally occurs. In the usual case, diarrhea is moderate and subsides after 4–5 days, but it may be protracted.

B. Laboratory Findings

Diagnosis is made by isolation of the organism from stool, blood, or, in some cases, from urine, CSF, or pus from a suppurative lesion. The WBC count usually shows a polymorphonuclear leukocytosis but may show leukopenia. *Salmonella* isolates should be reported to public health authorities for epidemiologic purposes. Stool cultures are rarely positive when obtained from children who develop diarrhea after 3 days of hospitalization.

▶ Differential Diagnosis

In staphylococcal food poisoning, the incubation period is shorter (2–4 hours) than in *Salmonella* food poisoning (12–24 hours). Fever is absent, and vomiting rather than diarrhea is the main symptom. In shigellosis, many pus cells usually are seen on a stained smear of stool, and the peripheral WBC count is more likely to slow a marked left shift, although some cases of salmonellosis are indistinguishable from shigellosis. *Campylobacter* gastroenteritis commonly resembles salmonellosis clinically. Culture of the stools is necessary to distinguish the causes of bacterial gastroenteritis.

▶ Complications

Unlike most types of infectious diarrhea, salmonellosis is frequently accompanied by bacteremia, especially in newborns and infants. Septicemia with extraintestinal infection is seen, most commonly with *Salmonella choleraesuis* but also with *S enteritidis, S typhimurium,* and *S paratyphi* B and C. The organism may spread to any tissue and may cause arthritis, osteomyelitis, cholecystitis, endocarditis, meningitis, pericarditis, pneumonia, or pyelonephritis. Patients with sickle cell anemia or other hemoglobinopathies have a predilection for the development of osteomyelitis. Severe dehydration and shock are more likely to occur with shigellosis but may occur with *Salmonella* gastroenteritis.

▶ Prevention

Measures for the prevention of *Salmonella* infections include thorough cooking of foodstuffs derived from contaminated sources, adequate refrigeration, control of infection among domestic animals, and meticulous meat and poultry inspections. Raw and undercooked fresh eggs should be avoided. Food handlers and child care workers with salmonellosis should have three negative stool cultures before resuming work. Asymptomatic children, who have recovered from *Salmonella* infection, do not need exclusion.

▶ Treatment

A. Specific Measures

In uncomplicated *Salmonella* gastroenteritis, antibiotic treatment does not shorten the course of the clinical illness and may prolong convalescent carriage of the organism. Colitis or secretory diarrhea due to *Salmonella* may improve with antibiotic therapy.

Because of the higher risk of sepsis and focal disease, antibiotic treatment is recommended in infants younger than age 3 months, in severely ill children, and in children with sickle cell disease, liver disease, recent gastrointestinal surgery, cancer, depressed immunity, or chronic renal or cardiac disease. Infants younger than age 3 months with positive stool cultures or suspected salmonellosis sepsis should be admitted to the hospital, evaluated for focal infection including cultures of blood and CSF, and given treatment intravenously. A third-generation cephalosporin is recommended due to frequent resistance to ampicillin and TMP–SMX. Older patients developing bacteremia during the course of gastroenteritis should receive parenteral treatment initially, and a careful search should be made for additional foci of infection. After signs and symptoms subside, these patients should receive oral medication. Parenteral and oral treatment should last a total of 7–10 days. Longer treatment is indicated for specific complications. If susceptibility tests indicate resistance to ampicillin, third-generation cephalosporins or TMP–SMX should be given. Fluoroquinolones also are efficacious but are not approved for administration to children. Fluoroquinolones are used for strains resistant to multiple other drugs.

Salmonella meningitis is best treated with ampicillin (200–300 mg/kg/d intravenously in four to six divided doses) and a third-generation cephalosporin (cefotaxime, ceftriaxone) for 3 weeks. If the child improves rapidly and the CSF is sterile, treatment may be completed with a single drug, the choice guided by results of susceptibility tests.

Outbreaks on pediatric wards are difficult to control. Strict hand washing, cohorting of patients and personnel, and ultimately closure of the unit may be necessary.

B. Treatment of the Carrier State

About half of patients may have positive stool cultures after 4 weeks. Infants tend to remain convalescent carriers for up to a year. Antibiotic treatment of carriers is not effective.

C. General Measures

Careful attention must be given to maintaining fluid and electrolyte balance, especially in infants.

▶ Prognosis

In gastroenteritis, the prognosis is good. In sepsis with focal suppurative complications, the prognosis is more guarded. The case fatality rate of *Salmonella* meningitis is high in infants. There is a strong tendency to relapse if treatment is not continued for at least 14–21 days.

Amieva MR: Important bacterial gastrointestinal pathogens in children: A pathogenesis perspective. Pediatr Clin North Am 2005;52:749, vi [PMID: 15925661].

Centers for Disease Control and Prevention: *Salmonella* infection (salmonellosis). http://www.cdc.gov/ncidod/diseases/submenus/sub_salmonella.htm

Preliminary FoodNet Data on the incidence of infection with pathogens transmitted commonly through food—10 states, 2006. MMWR Morb Mortal Wkly Rep 2007;56:336 [PMID: 17431379].

Turtle-associated salmonellosis in humans—United States, 2006–2007. MMWR Morb Mortal Wkly Rep 2007;56:649 [PMID: 17615521].

Zaidi MB et al: Nontyphoidal *Salmonella* from human clinical cases, asymptomatic children, and raw retail meats in Yucatan Mexico. Clin Infect Dis 2006;42:21 [PMID: 16323087].

TYPHOID FEVER & PARATYPHOID FEVER

ESSENTIALS OF DIAGNOSIS & TYPICAL FEATURES

▶ Insidious or acute onset of headache, anorexia, vomiting, constipation or diarrhea, ileus, and high fever.

▶ Meningismus, splenomegaly, and rose spots.

▶ Leukopenia; positive blood, stool, bone marrow, and urine cultures.

▶ General Considerations

Typhoid fever is caused by the gram-negative bacillus *Salmonella typhi*. Paratyphoid fevers, which are usually milder but may be clinically indistinguishable, are caused by *Salmonella paratyphi* A, *Salmonella schottmülleri*, or *Salmonella hirschfeldii* (formerly *Salmonella paratyphi* A, B, and C). Children have a shorter incubation period than do adults (usually 5–8 days instead of 8–14 days). The organism enters the body through the walls of the intestinal tract and, following a transient bacteremia, multiplies in the reticuloendothelial cells of the liver and spleen. Persistent bacteremia and symptoms then follow. Reinfection of the intestine occurs as organisms are excreted in the bile. Bacterial emboli produce the characteristic skin lesions (rose spots). Symptoms in children may be mild or severe, but children younger than age 5 years rarely have severe typhoid fever.

Typhoid fever is transmitted by the fecal-oral route and by contamination of food or water. Unlike other *Salmonella* species, there are no animal reservoirs of *S typhi*; each case is the result of direct or indirect contact with the organism or with an individual who is actively infected or a chronic carrier.

About 250 cases per year are reported in the United States, 80% of which are acquired during foreign travel.

▶ Clinical Findings

A. Symptoms and Signs

In children, the onset of typhoid fever usually is sudden rather than insidious, with malaise, headache, crampy abdominal pains and distention, and sometimes constipation followed within 48 hours by diarrhea, high fever, and toxemia. An encephalopathy may be seen with irritability, confusion, delirium, and stupor. Vomiting and meningismus may be prominent in infants and young children. The classic lengthy three-stage disease seen in adult patients often is shortened in children. The prodrome may last only 2–4 days, the toxic stage only 2–3 days, and the defervescence stage 1–2 weeks.

During the prodromal stage, physical findings may be absent, or there may merely be some abdominal distention and tenderness, meningismus, mild hepatomegaly, and minimal splenomegaly. The typical typhoidal rash (rose spots) is present in 10–15% of children. It appears during the second week of the disease and may erupt in crops for the succeeding 10–14 days. Rose spots are erythematous maculopapular lesions 2–3 mm in diameter that fade on pressure. They are found principally on the trunk and chest and they generally disappear within 3–4 days. The lesions usually number fewer than 20.

B. Laboratory Findings

Typhoid bacilli can be isolated from many sites, including blood, stool, urine, and bone marrow. Blood cultures are positive in 50–80% of cases during the first week and less often later in the illness. Stool cultures are positive in about 50% of cases after the first week. Urine and bone marrow cultures also are valuable. Most patients will have negative cultures (including stool) by the end of a 6-week period. Serologic tests (Widal reaction) are not as useful as cultures because both false-positive and false-negative results occur. Leukopenia is common in the second week of the disease, but in the first week, leukocytosis may be seen. Proteinuria, mild elevation of liver enzymes, thrombocytopenia, and DIC are common.

▶ Differential Diagnosis

Typhoid and paratyphoid fevers must be distinguished from other serious prolonged fevers. These include typhus, brucellosis, malaria, tularemia, miliary tuberculosis, psittacosis, vasculitis, lymphoma, mononucleosis, and Kawasaki disease. The diagnosis of typhoid fever often is made clinically in developing countries, but the accuracy of clinical diagnosis is variable. In developed countries, where typhoid fever is uncommon and physicians are unfamiliar with the clinical picture, the diagnosis often is not suspected until late in the course. Positive cultures confirm the diagnosis.

▶ Complications

The most serious complications of typhoid fever are gastrointestinal hemorrhage (2–10%) and perforation (1–3%). They occur toward the end of the second week or during the third week of the disease.

Intestinal perforation is one of the principal causes of death. The site of perforation generally is the terminal ileum or cecum. The clinical manifestations are indistinguishable from those of acute appendicitis, with pain, tenderness, and rigidity in the right lower quadrant.

Bacterial pneumonia, meningitis, septic arthritis, abscesses, and osteomyelitis are uncommon complications, particularly if specific treatment is given promptly. Shock and electrolyte disturbances may lead to death.

About 1–3% of patients become chronic carriers of *S typhi*. Chronic carriage is defined as excretion of typhoid bacilli for more than a year, but carriage is often lifelong. Adults with underlying biliary or urinary tract disease are much more likely than children to become chronic carriers.

▶ Prevention

Routine typhoid vaccine is not recommended in the United States but should be considered for foreign travel to endemic areas. An attenuated oral typhoid vaccine produced from strain Ty21a has better efficacy and causes minimal side effects but is not approved for children younger than age 6 years. A capsular polysaccharide vaccine (ViCPS) requires one intramuscular injection and may be given to children age 2 years and older. (See Chapter 9.)

▶ Treatment

A. Specific Measures

Third-generation cephalosporins such as cefotaxime (150 mg/kg divided in three doses), azithromycin (10 mg/kg on day 1, followed by 5 mg/kg for 7 days), or a fluoroquinolone are used for presumptive therapy. Antimicrobial susceptibility testing and local experience are used to direct subsequent therapy. Equally effective regimens for susceptible strains include the following: TMP–SMX (10 mg/kg trimethoprim and 50 mg/kg sulfamethoxazole per day orally in two or three divided doses), amoxicillin (100 mg/kg/d orally in four divided doses), and ampicillin (100–200 mg/kg/d intravenously in four divided doses). Aminoglycosides and first- and second-generation cephalosporins are clinically ineffective regardless of in-vitro susceptibility results. Ciprofloxacin or other fluoroquinolones are efficacious but not approved in children, but may be used for multiply resistant strains. Treatment duration is 14–21 days. Patients may remain febrile for 3–5 days even with appropriate therapy.

B. General Measures

General support of the patient is exceedingly important and includes rest, good nutrition, and careful observation, with particular regard to evidence of intestinal bleeding or perforation. Blood transfusions may be needed even in the absence of frank hemorrhage.

▶ Prognosis

A prolonged convalescent carrier stage may occur in children. Three negative cultures after all antibiotics have been stopped are required before contact precautions are stopped. With early antibiotic therapy, the prognosis is excellent, and the mortality rate is less than 1%. Relapse occurs 1–3 weeks later in 10–20% of patients despite appropriate antibiotic treatment.

Bhan MK et al: Typhoid and paratyphoid fever. Lancet 2005;366:749 [PMID: 16125594].

Edino ST et al: Prognostic factors in typhoid ileal perforation: A prospective study of 53 cases. J Natl Med Assoc 2007;99:1042 [PMID: 17913115].

Farrar J: A personal perspective on clinical research in enteric fever. Clin Infect Dis 2007;45(Suppl 1):S9 [PMID: 17582579].

Fraser A et al: Vaccines for preventing typhoid fever. Cochrane Database Syst Rev 2007;(3):CD001261 [PMID: 17636661].

Kumar R et al: Multidrug-resistant typhoid fever. Indian J Pediatr 2007;74:39 [PMID: 17264451].

Parry CM et al: Randomized controlled comparison of ofloxacin, azithromycin, and an ofloxacin-azithromycin combination for treatment of multidrug-resistant and nalidixic acid-resistant typhoid fever. Antimicrob Agents Chemother 2007;51:819 [PMID: 17145784].

Thaver D et al: Fluoroquinolones for treating typhoid and paratyphoid fever (enteric fever). Cochrane Database Syst Rev 2005;(2):CD004530 [PMID: 15846718].

SHIGELLOSIS (BACILLARY DYSENTERY)

ESSENTIALS OF DIAGNOSIS & TYPICAL FEATURES

▶ Cramps and bloody diarrhea.

▶ High fever, malaise, convulsions.

▶ Pus and blood in diarrheal stools examined microscopically.

▶ Diagnosis confirmed by stool culture.

▶ General Considerations

Shigellae are nonmotile gram-negative rods of the family Enterobacteriaceae and are closely related to *E coli*. The genus *Shigella* is divided into four major groups, A–D, representing *Shigella dysenteriae*, *Shigella flexneri*, *Shigella boydii*, and *Shigella sonnei*, respectively. Approximately 30,000 cases of shigellosis are reported each year in the United States. *S sonnei* followed by *S flexneri* are the most common isolates.

S dysenteriae, which causes the most severe diarrhea of all species and the greatest number of extraintestinal complications, accounts for less than 1% of all *Shigella* infections in the United States.

Shigellosis may be a serious disease, particularly in young children, and without supportive treatment an appreciable mortality rate results. In older children and adults, the disease tends to be self-limited and milder. *Shigella* is usually transmitted by the fecal-oral route. Food- and water-borne outbreaks are increasing in occurrence, but are less important overall than person-to-person transmission. The disease is very communicable—as few as 200 bacteria can produce illness in an adult. The secondary attack rate in families is high, and shigellosis is a serious problem in day care centers and custodial institutions. *Shigella* organisms produce disease by invading the colonic mucosa, causing mucosal ulcer-

ations and microabscesses. A plasmid-encoded gene is required for enterotoxin production, chromosomal genes are required for invasiveness, and smooth lipopolysaccharides are required for virulence. An experimental vaccine is under development and is safe and immunogenic in young children.

▶ Clinical Findings

A. Symptoms and Signs

The incubation period of shigellosis is usually 2–4 days. Onset is abrupt, with abdominal cramps, urgency, tenesmus, chills, fever, malaise, and diarrhea. Hallucinations and seizures sometimes accompany high fever. In severe forms, blood and mucus are seen in small stools (dysentery), and meningismus and convulsions may occur. In older children, the disease may be mild and may be characterized by watery diarrhea without blood. In young children, a fever of 39.4–40°C is common. Rarely there is rectal prolapse. Symptoms generally last 3–7 days.

B. Laboratory Findings

The total WBC count varies, but often there is a marked shift to the left. The stool may contain gross blood and mucus, and many neutrophils are seen if mucus from the stool is examined microscopically. Stool cultures are usually positive; however, they may be negative because the organism is somewhat fragile and present in small numbers late in the disease, and because laboratory techniques are suboptimal for the recovery of shigellae.

▶ Differential Diagnosis

Diarrhea due to rotavirus infection is a winter rather than a summer disease. Usually children with rotavirus infection are not as febrile or toxic as those with shigellosis, and in rotavirus infection, stool does not contain gross blood or neutrophils. Intestinal infections caused by *Salmonella* or *Campylobacter* are differentiated by culture. Grossly bloody stools in a patient without fever or stool leukocytes suggest *E coli* O157:H7 infection. Amebic dysentery is diagnosed by microscopic examination of fresh stools or sigmoidoscopy specimens. Intussusception is characterized by an abdominal mass (so-called currant jelly stools) without leukocytes, and by absence of fever. Mild shigellosis is not distinguishable clinically from other forms of infectious diarrhea.

▶ Complications

Dehydration, acidosis, shock, and renal failure are the major complications. In some cases, a chronic form of dysentery occurs, characterized by mucoid stools and poor nutrition. Bacteremia and metastatic infections are rare but serious complications. Febrile seizures are common. Fulminating fatal dysentery and hemolytic-uremic syndrome occur rarely.

Treatment

A. Specific Measures

Resistance to TMP–SMX (10 mg/kg/d trimethoprim and 50 mg/kg/d sulfamethoxazole, given in two divided doses orally for 5 days) is now commonly encountered in many communities and limits the use of this otherwise effective drug combination to cases where results of susceptibility testing are known. Amoxicillin is not effective. Ampicillin (100 mg/kg/d, given in four divided doses) is also efficacious if the strain is sensitive. Parenteral ceftriaxone and oral cefixime are both effective; experience with other third-generation oral cephalosporins is limited. Azithromycin (12 mg/kg/d on day 1, then 6 mg/kg/d for 4 days) was superior to cefixime in one study. Ciprofloxacin (500 mg, given twice daily for 5 days) is efficacious in adults but is not approved for use in children. However, it may be used in children who remain symptomatic and in need of therapy, and when multiply resistant strains limit other preferred choices. Successful treatment reduces the duration of fever, cramping, and diarrhea and terminates fecal excretion of *Shigella*. Tetracycline and chloramphenicol are also effective, but resistance is common. Presumptive therapy should be limited to children with classic shigellosis or known outbreaks. Afebrile children with bloody diarrhea are more commonly infected with EHEC. Antimicrobial therapy of EHEC may increase the likelihood of hemolytic-uremic syndrome.

B. General Measures

In severe cases, immediate rehydration is critical. A mild form of chronic malabsorption syndrome may supervene and require prolonged dietary control.

Prognosis

The prognosis is excellent if vascular collapse is treated promptly by adequate fluid therapy. The mortality rate is high in very young, malnourished infants who do not receive fluid and electrolyte therapy. Convalescent fecal excretion of *Shigella* lasts 1–4 weeks in patients not receiving antimicrobial therapy. Long-term carriers are rare.

Ashkenazi S: *Shigella* infections in children: New insights. Semin Pediatr Infect Dis 2004:15:246 [PMID: 15494948].

Jain SK et al: Antimicrobial-resistant *Shigella sonnei*: Limited antimicrobial treatment options for children and challenges of interpreting in vitro azithromycin susceptibility. Pediatr Infect Dis J 2005;24:494 [PMID: 15933557].

Mandomando I et al: Epidemiology and clinical presentation of shigellosis in children less than five years of age in rural Mozambique. Pediatr Infect Dis J 2007;26:1059 [PMID: 17984817].

Niyogi SK: Increasing antimicrobial resistance—an emerging problem in the treatment of shigellosis. Clin Microbiol Infect 2007;13:1141 [PMID: 17953700].

CHOLERA

ESSENTIALS OF DIAGNOSIS & TYPICAL FEATURES

▶ Sudden onset of severe watery diarrhea.

▶ Persistent vomiting without nausea or fever.

▶ Extreme and rapid dehydration and electrolyte loss, with rapid development of vascular collapse.

▶ Contact with a case of cholera or with shellfish, or the presence of cholera in the community.

▶ Diagnosis confirmed by stool culture.

General Considerations

Cholera is an acute diarrheal disease caused by the gram-negative organism *Vibrio cholerae*. It is transmitted by contaminated water or food, especially contaminated shellfish. Typical disease is generally so dramatic that in endemic areas the diagnosis is obvious. Individuals with mild illness and young children may play an important role in transmission of the infection.

Asymptomatic infection is far more common than clinical disease. In endemic areas, rising titers of vibriocidal antibody are seen with increasing age. Infection occurs in individuals with low titers. The age-specific attack rate is highest in children younger than age 5 years and declines with age. Cholera is unusual in infancy.

Cholera toxin is a protein enterotoxin that is primarily responsible for symptoms. Cholera toxin binds to a regulatory subunit of adenylyl cyclase in enterocytes, causing increased cyclic adenosine monophosphate and an outpouring of NaCl and water into the lumen of the small bowel.

Nutritional status is an important factor determining the severity of the diarrhea. Duration of diarrhea is prolonged in adults and children with severe malnutrition.

Cholera is endemic in India and southern and Southeast Asia and in parts of Africa. The most recent pandemic, caused by the El Tor biotype of *V cholerae* 01, began in 1961 in Indonesia. Epidemic cholera spread in Central and South America, with a total of 1 million cases and 9500 deaths reported through 1994. Cases in the United States occurred in the course of foreign travel or as a result of consumption of contaminated imported food. Cholera is increasingly associated with consumption of shellfish. Interstate shipment of oysters has resulted in cholera in several inland states. Cholera is now rare in the United States with fewer than 10 cases per year reported.

V cholerae is a natural inhabitant of shellfish and copepods in estuarine environments. Seasonal multiplication of *V cholerae* may provide a source of outbreaks in endemic areas. Chronic cholera carriers are rare. The incubation period is short, usually 1–3 days.

Clinical Findings

A. Symptoms and Signs

Many patients infected with *V cholerae* have mild disease, with 1–2% developing severe diarrhea. During severe cholera, there is a sudden onset of massive, frequent, watery stools, generally light gray in color (so-called rice-water stools) and containing some mucus but no pus. Vomiting may be projectile and is not accompanied by nausea. Within 2–3 hours, the tremendous loss of fluids results in life-threatening dehydration, hypochloremia, and hypokalemia, with marked weakness and collapse. Renal failure with uremia and irreversible peripheral vascular collapse will occur if fluid therapy is not administered. The illness lasts 1–7 days and is shortened by appropriate antibiotic therapy.

B. Laboratory Findings

Markedly elevated hemoglobin (20 g/dL) and marked acidosis, hypochloremia, and hyponatremia are seen. Stool sodium concentration may range from 80–120 mEq/L. Cultural confirmation requires specific media and takes 16–18 hours for a presumptive diagnosis and 36–48 hours for a definitive bacteriologic diagnosis.

Prevention

Cholera vaccine is available and provides 50% efficacy. Protection lasts 3–6 months. Cholera vaccine is not generally recommended for travelers. Tourists visiting endemic areas are at little risk if they exercise caution in what they eat and drink and maintain good personal hygiene. In endemic areas, all water and milk must be boiled, food protected from flies, and sanitary precautions observed. Simple filtration of water is highly effective in reducing cases. Thorough cooking of shellfish prevents transmission. All patients with cholera should be isolated.

Chemoprophylaxis is indicated for household and other close contacts of cholera patients. It should be initiated as soon as possible after the onset of the disease in the index patient. Tetracycline (500 mg/d for 5 days) is effective in preventing infection. TMP–SMX may be substituted in children.

Treatment

Physiologic saline or lactated Ringer solution should be administered intravenously in large amounts to restore blood volume and urine output and prevent irreversible shock. Potassium supplements are required. Sodium bicarbonate, given intravenously, also may be needed initially to overcome profound metabolic acidosis from bicarbonate loss in the stool. Moderate dehydration and acidosis can be corrected in 3–6 hours by oral therapy alone, because the active glucose transport system of the small bowel is normally functional. The optimal composition of the oral solution (in mEq/L) is as follows: Na^+, 90; Cl^-, 80; and K^+, 20 (with glucose, 110 mmol/L).

Treatment with tetracycline (50 mg/kg/d orally in four divided doses for 2–5 days) or azithromycin (10 mg/kg/d in one dose for 1–5 days) shortens the duration of the disease in children and prevents clinical relapse but is not as important as fluid and electrolyte therapy. Tetracycline resistance occurs in some regions, and ciprofloxacin may be used depending on local resistance patterns. TMP–SMX should be used in children younger than age 9 years.

Prognosis

With early and rapid replacement of fluids and electrolytes, the case fatality rate is 1–2% in children. If significant symptoms appear and no treatment is given, the mortality rate is over 50%.

Ali M et al: Herd immunity conferred by killed oral cholera vaccines in Bangladesh: A reanalysis. Lancet 2005;366:7 [PMID: 15993232].

Qureshi K et al: Breast milk reduces the risk of illness in children of mothers with cholera: Observations from an epidemic of cholera in Guinea-Bissau. Pediatr Infect Dis J 2006;25:1163 [PMID: 17133163].

Saha D et al: Single-dose azithromycin for the treatment of cholera in adults. N Engl J Med 2006;354:2452 [PMID: 16760445].

CAMPYLOBACTER INFECTION

ESSENTIALS OF DIAGNOSIS & TYPICAL FEATURES

► Fever, vomiting, abdominal pain, diarrhea.
► Presumptive diagnosis by darkfield or phase contrast microscopy of stool wet mount or modified Gram stain.
► Definitive diagnosis by stool culture.

General Considerations

Campylobacter species are small gram-negative, curved or spiral bacilli that are commensals or pathogens in many animals. *Campylobacter jejuni* frequently causes acute enteritis in humans. In the 1990s, *C jejuni* was responsible for 3–11% of cases of acute gastroenteritis in North America and Europe. In many areas, enteritis due to *C jejuni* is more common than that due to *Salmonella* or *Shigella*. *Campylobacter fetus* causes bacteremia and meningitis in immunocompromised patients. *C fetus* may cause maternal fever, abortion, stillbirth, and severe neonatal infection. *Helicobacter pylori* (previously called *Campylobacter pylori*) causes gastritis and peptic ulcer disease in both adults and children. (See Chapter 20.)

Campylobacter colonizes domestic and wild animals, especially poultry. Numerous cases have been associated with sick puppies or other animal contacts. Contaminated food and water, improperly cooked poultry, and person-to-person spread by the fecal-oral route are common routes of transmission. Outbreaks associated with day care centers, contaminated water supplies, and raw milk have been reported. Newborns may acquire the organism from their mothers at delivery.

► Clinical Findings

A. Symptoms and Signs

C jejuni enteritis can be mild or severe. In tropical countries, asymptomatic stool carriage is common. The incubation period is usually 1–7 days. The disease usually begins with sudden onset of high fever, malaise, headache, abdominal cramps, nausea, and vomiting. Diarrhea follows and may be watery or bile-stained, mucoid, and bloody. The illness is self-limiting, lasting 2–7 days, but relapses occur in 15–25% of cases. Without antimicrobial treatment, the organism remains in the stool for 1–6 weeks.

B. Laboratory Findings

The peripheral WBC count generally is elevated, with many band forms. Microscopic examination of stool reveals erythrocytes and pus cells.

Isolation of *C jejuni* from stool is not difficult but requires selective agar, incubation at 42°C rather than 35°C, and incubation in an atmosphere of about 5% oxygen and 5% CO_2 (candle jar is satisfactory).

► Differential Diagnosis

Campylobacter enteritis may resemble viral gastroenteritis, salmonellosis, shigellosis, amebiasis, or other infectious diarrheas. Because it also mimics ulcerative colitis, Crohn disease, intussusception, and appendicitis, mistaken diagnosis can lead to unnecessary surgery.

► Complications

The most common complication is dehydration. Other uncommon complications include erythema nodosum, convulsions, reactive arthritis, bacteremia, urinary tract infection, and cholecystitis. Guillain-Barré syndrome may follow *C jejuni* infection by 1–3 weeks.

► Prevention

No vaccine is available. Hand washing and adherence to basic food sanitation practices help prevent disease. Hand washing and cleaning of kitchen utensils after contact with raw poultry are important.

► Treatment

Treatment of fluid and electrolyte disturbances is important. Antimicrobial treatment with erythromycin in children (30–50 mg/kg/d orally in four divided doses for 5 days), azithromycin for 5 days, or ciprofloxacin terminates fecal excretion. Fluoroquinolone-resistant *C jejuni* are now common world-

wide. Therapy given early in the course of the illness will shorten the duration of symptoms but is unnecessary if given later. Antimicrobials used for shigellosis, such as TMP–SMX and ampicillin, are inactive against *Campylobacter*. Supportive therapy is sufficient in most cases.

► Prognosis

The outlook is excellent if dehydration is corrected and misdiagnosis does not lead to inappropriate diagnostic or surgical procedures.

Centers for Disease Control and Prevention: *Campylobacter* infections. http://www.cdc.gov/ncidod/dbmd/diseaseinfo/campylobacter_g.htm

Nachamkin I et al: Patterns of Guillain-Barre syndrome in children: Results from a Mexican population. Neurology 2007; 69:1665 [PMID: 17898327].

Ternhag A et al: A meta-analysis on the effects of antibiotic treatment on duration of symptoms caused by infection with *Campylobacter* species. Clin Infect Dis 2007;44:696 [PMID: 17278062].

TULAREMIA

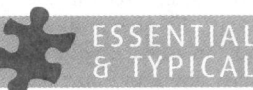

ESSENTIALS OF DIAGNOSIS & TYPICAL FEATURES

- ► A cutaneous or mucous membrane lesion at the site of inoculation and regional lymph node enlargement.
- ► Sudden onset of fever, chills, and prostration.
- ► History of contact with infected animals, principally wild rabbits, or history of tick exposure.
- ► Positive culture or immunofluorescence from mucocutaneous ulcer or regional lymph nodes.
- ► High serum antibody titer.

► General Considerations

Tularemia is caused by *Francisella tularensis*, a gram-negative organism usually acquired directly from infected animals (principally wild rabbits) or by the bite of an infected tick. Occasionally infection is acquired from infected domestic dogs or cats; by contamination of the skin or mucous membranes with infected blood or tissues; by inhalation of infected material; by bites of fleas or deer flies that have been in contact with infected animals; or by ingestion of contaminated meat or water. The incubation period is short, usually 3–7 days, but may vary from 2–25 days.

Ticks are the most important vector of tularemia and rabbits are the classic vector. It is important to seek a history of rabbit hunting, skinning, or food preparation in any patient who has a febrile illness with tender lymphadenopathy, often in the region of a draining skin ulcer.

Clinical Findings

A. Symptoms and Signs

Several clinical types of tularemia occur in children. Sixty percent of infections are of the ulceroglandular form and start as a reddened papule that may be pruritic, quickly ulcerates, and is not very painful. Soon, the regional lymph nodes become large and tender. Fluctuance quickly follows. There may be marked systemic symptoms, including high fever, chills, weakness, and vomiting. Pneumonitis occasionally accompanies the ulceroglandular form or may be seen as the sole manifestation of infection (pneumonic form). A detectable skin lesion may be absent, and localized lymphoid enlargement may exist alone (glandular form). Oculoglandular and oropharyngeal forms also occur. The latter is characterized by tonsillitis, often with membrane formation, cervical adenopathy, and high fever. In the absence of a primary ulcer or localized lymphadenitis, a prolonged febrile disease reminiscent of typhoid fever can occur (typhoidal form). Splenomegaly is common in all forms.

B. Laboratory Findings

F tularensis can be recovered from ulcers, regional lymph nodes, and sputum of patients with the pneumonic form. However, the organism grows only on an enriched medium (blood-cystine-glucose agar), and laboratory handling is dangerous owing to the risk of airborne transmission to laboratory personnel. Immunofluorescent staining of biopsy material or aspirates of involved lymph nodes is diagnostic, although it is not widely available.

The WBC count is not remarkable. Agglutinins are present after the second week of illness, and in the absence of a positive culture their development confirms the diagnosis. An agglutination titer of 1:160 or higher is considered positive.

Differential Diagnosis

The typhoidal form of tularemia may mimic typhoid, brucellosis, miliary tuberculosis, Rocky Mountain spotted fever, and mononucleosis. Pneumonic tularemia resembles atypical or mycotic pneumonitis. The ulceroglandular type of tularemia resembles pyoderma caused by staphylococci or streptococci, plague, anthrax, and cat-scratch fever. The oropharyngeal type must be distinguished from streptococcal or diphtheritic pharyngitis, mononucleosis, herpangina, or other viral pharyngitides.

Prevention

Children should be protected from insect bites, especially those of ticks, fleas, and deer flies, by the use of proper clothing and repellents. Because rabbits are the source of most human infections, the dressing and handling of such game should be performed with great care. If contact occurs, thorough washing with soap and water is indicated.

Treatment

A. Specific Measures

Historically, streptomycin was the drug of choice. Gentamicin and amikacin also are efficacious, more available, and familiar to clinicians. A 10-day course is usually sufficient; although more severe infections may need longer therapy. Doxycycline is effective, but relapse rates are higher. Doxycycline is not usually recommended for children younger than 8 years of age unless benefits of use outweigh the risk of dental staining. Ciprofloxacin also can be used in patients with less severe disease. Ciprofloxacin is not approved for children younger than 18 years, and is not usually recommended in children unless benefits outweigh risks. Failures occur with ceftriaxone.

B. General Measures

Antipyretics and analgesics may be given as necessary. Skin lesions are best left open. Glandular lesions occasionally require incision and drainage.

Prognosis

The prognosis is excellent in cases of tularemia that are recognized early and treated appropriately.

Ellis J et al: Tularemia. Clin Microbiol Rev 2002;15:631 [PMID: 12364373].

Eliasson H et al: Tularemia: Current epidemiology and disease management. Infect Dis Clin North Am 2006;20:289 [PMID: 16762740].

Center for Infectious Disease Research and Policy: Tularemia. http://www.cidrap.umn.edu/cidrap/content/bt/tularemia/biofacts/tularemiafactsheet.html

Parola P, Raoult D: Ticks and tickborne bacterial diseases in humans: An emerging infectious threat. Clin Infect Dis 2001;32:897 [PMID: 11247714].

PLAGUE

ESSENTIALS OF DIAGNOSIS & TYPICAL FEATURES

▶ Sudden onset of fever, chills, and prostration.

▶ Regional lymphadenitis with suppuration of nodes (bubonic form).

▶ Hemorrhage into skin and mucous membranes and shock (septicemia).

▶ Cough, dyspnea, cyanosis, and hemoptysis (pneumonia).

▶ History of exposure to infected animals.

General Considerations

Plague is an extremely serious acute infection caused by a gram-negative bacillus, *Yersinia pestis*. It is a disease of rodents that is transmitted to humans by flea bites. Plague bacilli have been isolated from rodents in 15 of the western states in the United States. Direct contact with rodents, rabbits, or domestic cats may transmit fleas infected with plague bacilli. Most cases occur from June through September. Human plague in the United States appears to occur in cycles that reflect cycles in wild animal reservoirs.

▶ Clinical Findings

A. Symptoms and Signs

Plague assumes several clinical forms; the two most common are bubonic and septicemic. Pneumonic plague, the form that occurs when organisms enter the body through the respiratory tract, is uncommon.

1. Bubonic plague—Bubonic plague begins after an incubation period of 6 days with a sudden onset of high fever, chills, headache, vomiting, and marked delirium or clouding of consciousness. A less severe form also exists, with a less precipitous onset, but with progression over several days to severe symptoms. Although the flea bite is rarely seen, the regional lymph node, usually inguinal and unilateral, is painful and tender, 1–5 cm in diameter. The node usually suppurates and drains spontaneously after 1 week. The plague bacillus produces endotoxin that causes vascular necrosis. Bacilli may overwhelm regional lymph nodes and enter the circulation to produce septicemia. Severe vascular necrosis results in widely disseminated hemorrhage in skin, mucous membranes, liver, and spleen. Myocarditis and circulatory collapse may result from damage by the endotoxin. Plague meningitis or pneumonia may occur following bacteremic spread from an infected lymph node.

2. Septicemic plague—Plague may initially present as septicemia without evidence of lymphadenopathy. In some series, 25% of cases are initially septicemic. Septicemic plague carries a worse prognosis than bubonic plague, largely because it is not recognized and treated early. Patients may present initially with a nonspecific febrile illness characterized by fever, myalgia, chills, and anorexia. Plague is frequently complicated by secondary seeding of the lung causing plague pneumonia.

3. Primary pneumonic plague—Inhalation of *Y pestis* bacilli causes primary plague pneumonia. This form of plague has been transmitted to humans from cats with pneumonic plague and would be the form of plague most likely seen after aerosolized release of *Y pestis* in a bioterrorist incident. After an incubation of 1–6 days, the patient develops fever, cough, shortness of breath, and the production of bloody, watery, or purulent sputum. Gastrointestinal symptoms are sometimes prominent. Because the initial focus of infection is the lung, buboes are usually absent; occasionally cervical buboes may be seen.

B. Laboratory Findings

Aspirate from a bubo contains bipolar-staining gram-negative bacilli. Pus, sputum, and blood all yield the organism. Rapid diagnosis can be made with fluorescent antibody detection or polymerase chain reaction (PCR) on clinical specimens. Confirmation is made by culture or serologic testing. Laboratory infections are common enough to make bacterial isolation dangerous. Cultures are usually positive within 48 hours. Paired acute and convalescent sera may be tested for an antibody rise in those cases with negative cultures.

▶ Differential Diagnosis

The septic phase of the disease may be confused with illnesses such as meningococcemia, sepsis caused by other bacteria, and rickettsioses. The bubonic form resembles tularemia, anthrax, cat-scratch fever, streptococcal adenitis, and cellulitis. Primary gastroenteritis and appendicitis may have to be distinguished.

▶ Prevention

Proper disposal of household and commercial wastes and chemical control of rats are basic elements of plague prevention. Flea control is instituted and maintained with liberal use of insecticides. Children vacationing in remote camping areas should be warned not to handle dead or dying animals. Domestic cats that roam freely in suburban areas may contact infected wild animals and acquire infected fleas. There is no commercially available vaccine for plague.

▶ Treatment

A. Specific Measures

Streptomycin (30 mg/kg/d intramuscularly in two to three divided doses) or gentamicin (7.5 mg/kg/d intravenously in three divided doses) for 7–10 days after defervescence is effective. For patients not requiring parenteral therapy, doxycycline may be given. Doxycycline is not usually recommended for children younger than 8 years of age unless benefits of use outweigh the risk of tooth staining. Plague bacilli that are multiply resistant to antimicrobials are uncommon but of serious concern.

Mortality is extremely high in septicemic and pneumonic plague if specific antibiotic treatment is not started in the first 24 hours of the disease.

Every effort should be made to effect resolution of buboes without surgery. Pus from draining lymph nodes should be handled with gloves.

B. General Measures

Pneumonic plague is highly infectious, and droplet isolation is required until the patient has been on effective antimicrobial therapy for 48 hours. All contacts should receive prophylaxis with oral doxycycline 2.2 mg/kg per dose (maximum dose 100 mg) given twice a day for 7 days. State health officials should be notified immediately about suspected cases of plague.

C. Prophylaxis

Persons who have face-to-face contact or household exposure to a patient with plague should be instructed to closely monitor themselves for fever or other symptoms and to seek medical attention immediately if they develop. Persons who have close personal contact (< 2 m) with a person with pneumonic plague should receive antimicrobial prophylaxis for 7 days. TMP–SMX can be used in children; doxycycline or ciprofloxacin can be used in adults.

▶ Prognosis

The mortality rate in untreated bubonic plague is about 50%. The mortality rate for treated pneumonic plague is 50–60%. Recent mortality rates in New Mexico were 3% for bubonic plague and 71% for the septicemic form.

Centers for Disease Control and Prevention: Plague. http://www.cdc.gov/ncidod/dvbid/plague

Dennis DT, Chow CC: Plague. Pediatr Infect Dis J 2004;23:69 [PMID: 14743050].

Ligon BL: Plague: A review of its history and potential as a biological weapon. Semin Pediatr Infect Dis 2006;17:161 [PMID: 16934711].

Prentice MB, Rahalison L: Plague. Lancet 2007;369:1196 [PMID: 17416264].

HAEMOPHILUS INFLUENZAE TYPE B INFECTIONS

ESSENTIALS OF DIAGNOSIS & TYPICAL FEATURES

▶ Purulent meningitis in children younger than age 4 years with direct smears of CSF showing gram-negative pleomorphic rods.

▶ Acute epiglottitis: high fever, drooling, dysphagia, aphonia, and stridor.

▶ Septic arthritis: fever, local redness, swelling, heat, and pain with active or passive motion of the involved joint in a child 4 months to 4 years of age.

▶ Cellulitis: sudden onset of fever and distinctive cellulitis in an infant, often involving the cheek or periorbital area.

▶ In all cases, a positive culture from the blood, CSF, or aspirated pus confirms the diagnosis.

▶ General Considerations

H influenzae type b (Hib) has become uncommon because of widespread immunization in early infancy. The 99% reduction in incidence seen in many parts of the United States is due to high rates of vaccine coverage and reduced nasopharyngeal carriage after vaccination. Forty percent of cases occur in children younger than 6 months who are too young to have completed a primary immunization series. Hib may cause meningitis, bacteremia, epiglottitis (supraglottic croup), septic arthritis, periorbital and facial cellulitis, pneumonia, and pericarditis.

Disease due to H influenzae types A, C, D, E, F, or unencapsulated strains is rare, but it now accounts for a larger proportion of positive culture results. Third-generation cephalosporins are preferred for initial therapy of Hib infections. Ampicillin is adequate for culture-proved Hib susceptible strains.

Unencapsulated, nontypeable H influenzae frequently colonize the mucous membranes and cause otitis media, sinusitis, bronchitis, and pneumonia in children and adults. Bacteremia is uncommon. Neonatal sepsis similar to early-onset GBS is recognized. Obstetric complications of chorio-amnionitis and bacteremia are usually the source of neonatal cases.

Ampicillin resistance occurs in 25–40% of nontypeable H influenzae.

▶ Clinical Findings

A. Symptoms and Signs

1. Meningitis—Infants usually present with fever, irritability, lethargy, poor feeding with or without vomiting, and a high-pitched cry.

2. Acute epiglottitis—The most useful clinical finding in the early diagnosis of Hib epiglottitis is evidence of dysphagia, characterized by a refusal to eat or swallow saliva and by drooling. This finding, plus the presence of a high fever in a toxic child—even in the absence of a cherry-red epiglottis on direct examination—should strongly suggest the diagnosis and lead to prompt intubation. Stridor is a late sign. (See Chapter 18.)

3. Septic arthritis—Hib is a common cause of septic arthritis in unimmunized children younger than age 4 years in the United States. The child is febrile and refuses to move the involved joint and limb because of pain. Examination reveals swelling, warmth, redness, tenderness on palpation, and severe pain on attempted movement of the joint.

4. Cellulitis—Cellulitis due to Hib occurs almost exclusively in children between the ages of 3 months and 4 years but is now uncommon as a result of immunization. Fever is usually noted at the same time as the cellulitis, and many infants appear toxic. The cheek or periorbital (preseptal) area is usually involved.

B. Laboratory Findings

The WBC count in Hib infections may be high or normal with a shift to the left. Blood culture is frequently positive. Positive culture of aspirated pus or fluid from the involved site proves the diagnosis. In untreated meningitis, CSF smear may show the characteristic pleomorphic gram-negative rods.

C. Imaging

A lateral view of the neck may suggest the diagnosis in suspected acute epiglottitis, but misinterpretation is common. Intubation should not be delayed to obtain radiographs. Haziness of maxillary and ethmoid sinuses occurs with orbital cellulitis.

▶ Differential Diagnosis

A. Meningitis

Meningitis must be differentiated from head injury, brain abscess, tumor, lead encephalopathy, and other forms of meningoencephalitis, including mycobacterial, viral, fungal, and bacterial agents.

B. Acute Epiglottitis

In croup caused by viral agents (parainfluenza 1, 2, and 3, respiratory syncytial virus, influenza A, adenovirus), the child has more definite upper respiratory symptoms, cough, hoarseness, slower progression of obstructive signs, and lower fever. Spasmodic croup usually occurs at night in a child with a history of previous attacks. Sudden onset of choking and paroxysmal coughing suggests foreign body aspiration. Retropharyngeal abscess may have to be differentiated from epiglottitis.

C. Septic Arthritis

Differential diagnosis includes acute osteomyelitis, prepatellar bursitis, cellulitis, rheumatic fever, and fractures and sprains.

D. Cellulitis

Erysipelas, streptococcal cellulitis, insect bites, and trauma (including popsicle panniculitis or other types of freezing injury) may mimic Hib cellulitis. Periorbital cellulitis must be differentiated from paranasal sinus disease without cellulitis, allergic inflammatory disease of the lids, conjunctivitis, and herpes zoster infection.

▶ Complications

A. Meningitis (See Chapter 23)

B. Acute Epiglottitis

The disease may rapidly progress to complete airway obstruction with complications owing to hypoxia. Mediastinal emphysema and pneumothorax may occur.

C. Septic Arthritis

Septic arthritis may result in rapid destruction of cartilage and ankylosis if diagnosis and treatment are delayed. Even with early treatment, the incidence of residual damage and disability after septic arthritis in weight-bearing joints may be as high as 25%.

D. Cellulitis

Bacteremia may lead to meningitis or pyarthrosis.

▶ Prevention

Four separate carbohydrate protein conjugate Hib vaccines are currently available. (See Chapter 9.)

The risk of invasive Hib disease is highest in unimmunized, or partially immunized, household contacts who are younger than 4 years of age. The following situations require rifampin chemoprophylaxis of all household contacts to eradicate potential nasopharyngeal colonization with Hib and limit risk of invasive disease: (1) families where at least one household contact is younger than age 4 years and either unimmunized or incompletely immunized against Hib; (2) an immunocompromised child (of any age or immunization status) resides in the household; or (3) a child younger than age 12 months resides in the home and has not received three doses of the Hib vaccine. Preschool and day care center contacts may need prophylaxis if more than one case has occurred in the center in the previous 60 days (discuss with state health officials). The index case also needs chemoprophylaxis unless treated with ceftriaxone or cefotaxime (both are effective in eradication of Hib from the nasopharynx). Household contacts and index cases younger than 1 month of age who need chemoprophylaxis should be given rifampin, 20 mg/kg per dose (maximum adult dose, 600 mg) orally, once daily for 4 successive days. Infants who are younger than 1 month of age should be given oral rifampin (10 mg/kg per dose once daily for 4 days). Rifampin should not be used in pregnant females.

▶ Treatment

All patients with bacteremic or potentially bacteremic Hib diseases require hospitalization for treatment. The drugs of choice in hospitalized patients are a third-generation cephalosporin (cefotaxime or ceftriaxone) until the sensitivity of the organism is known. Meropenem is an alternative choice.

Persons with invasive Hib disease should be in droplet isolation for 24 hours after initiation of parenteral antibiotic therapy.

A. Meningitis

Therapy is begun as soon as bacterial meningitis has been identified and CSF, blood, and other appropriate cultures have been obtained. Therapy is begun with cefotaxime (50 mg/kg intravenously every 6 hours) or ceftriaxone (50 mg/kg intravenously every 12 hours). If the organism is sensitive to ampicillin, it is the drug of choice. Therapy should preferably be given intravenously for the entire course. Ceftriaxone may be given intramuscularly if venous access becomes difficult.

Duration of therapy is 10 days for uncomplicated meningitis. Longer treatment is reserved for children who respond slowly or in whom complications have occurred.

Dexamethasone given immediately after diagnosis and continued for 4 days may reduce the incidence of hearing loss in children with Hib meningitis. The use of dexamethasone is controversial, but when it is used the dosage is 0.6 mg/kg/d in four divided doses for 4 days. Starting dexamethasone more than 6 hours after antibiotics have been initiated is unlikely to provide benefits.

Repeated lumbar punctures are usually not necessary in Hib meningitis. They should be obtained in the following circumstances: unsatisfactory or questionable clinical response, seizure occurring after several days of therapy, and prolonged (7 days) or recurrent fever if the neurologic examination is abnormal or difficult to evaluate.

B. Acute Epiglottitis (See Chapter 18)

C. Septic Arthritis

Initial therapy should include an effective antistaphylococcal antibiotic and cefotaxime or ceftriaxone (dosage as for meningitis). If the isolate is sensitive to ampicillin, it is given in a dosage of 200–300 mg/kg/d intravenously in four divided doses. If a child is improved following initial intravenous therapy, oral amoxicillin (75–100 mg/kg/d in four divided doses every 6 hours) may be administered under careful supervision to complete a 2-week course. Alternative oral agents for ampicillin-resistant organisms include amoxicillin–clavulanic acid or second- or third-generation cephalosporins. Ideally, susceptibility to these agents should be proved prior to use. Drainage of infected joint fluid is an essential part of treatment. In joints other than the hip, this can often be accomplished by one or more needle aspirations. In hip infections—and in arthritis of other joints when treatment is delayed or clinical response is slow—surgical drainage is advised. The joint should be immobilized.

D. Cellulitis, Including Orbital Cellulitis

Initial therapy should include an agent effective against staphylococci in combination with cefotaxime or ceftriaxone. Ampicillin may be used if the isolate is susceptible. Therapy is given parenterally for 3–7 days, followed by oral treatment as for septic arthritis, and supportive and symptomatic treatment as required. There is usually marked improvement after 72 hours of treatment. Antibiotics should be given for at least 10–14 days.

▶ Prognosis

The case fatality rate for Hib meningitis is less than 5%. Young infants have the highest mortality rate. One of the most common neurologic sequelae, developing in 5–10% of patients with Hib meningitis, is sensorineural hearing loss. Patients with Hib meningitis should have their hearing

checked during the course of the illness or shortly after recovery. Children in whom invasive Hib infection develops despite appropriate immunization should have tests to investigate immune function and to rule out HIV. The case fatality rate in acute epiglottitis is 2–5%. Deaths are associated with bacteremia and the rapid development of airway obstruction. The prognosis for the other diseases requiring hospitalization is good with the institution of early and adequate antibiotic therapy.

Heath PT et al: Non-type b *Haemophilus influenzae* disease: Clinical and epidemiologic characteristics in the *Haemophilus influenzae* type b vaccine era. Pediatr Infect Dis J 2001;20:300 [PMID: 11303834].

Tristram S et al: Antimicrobial resistance in Haemophilus influenzae. Clin Microbiol Rev 2007;20:368 [PMID: 17428889].

PERTUSSIS (WHOOPING COUGH)

ESSENTIALS OF DIAGNOSIS & TYPICAL FEATURES

▶ Prodromal catarrhal stage (1–3 weeks) characterized by mild cough and coryza, but without fever.

▶ Persistent staccato, paroxysmal cough ending with a high-pitched inspiratory "whoop."

▶ Leukocytosis with absolute lymphocytosis.

▶ Diagnosis confirmed by PCR or culture of nasopharyngeal secretions.

▶ General Considerations

Pertussis is an acute, highly communicable infection of the respiratory tract caused by *Bordetella pertussis* and characterized by severe bronchitis. Children usually acquire the disease from symptomatic family contacts. Adults who have mild respiratory illness, not recognized as pertussis, frequently are the source of infection. Asymptomatic carriage of *B pertussis* is not recognized. Infectivity is greatest during the catarrhal and early paroxysmal cough stage (for about 4 weeks after onset).

Pertussis cases have increased in the United States since 1980. In 2004 and 2005, about 20,000 cases were reported. The morbidity and mortality of pertussis is greatest in young children. Fifty percent of children younger than age 1 year with a diagnosis of pertussis are hospitalized.

The duration of active immunity following natural pertussis is not known. Reinfections are usually milder. Immunity following vaccination wanes in 5–10 years. The majority of young adults in the United States are susceptible to pertussis infection, and disease is probably common but unrecognized.

Bordetella parapertussis causes a similar but milder syndrome.

B pertussis organisms attach to the ciliated respiratory epithelium and multiply there; deeper invasion does not occur. Disease is due to several bacterial toxins, the most potent of which is pertussis toxin, which is responsible for lymphocytosis and many of the symptoms of pertussis.

▶ Clinical Findings

A. Symptoms and Signs

The onset of pertussis is insidious, with catarrhal upper respiratory tract symptoms (rhinitis, sneezing, and an irritating cough). Slight fever may be present; temperature greater than 38.3°C suggests bacterial superinfection or another cause of respiratory tract infection. After about 2 weeks, cough becomes paroxysmal, characterized by 10–30 forceful coughs ending with a loud inspiration (the whoop). Infants and adults with otherwise typical severe pertussis often lack characteristic whooping. Vomiting commonly follows a paroxysm. Coughing is accompanied by cyanosis, sweating, prostration, and exhaustion. This stage lasts for 2–4 weeks, with gradual improvement. Cough suggestive of chronic bronchitis lasts for another 2–3 weeks. Paroxysmal coughing may continue for some months and may worsen with intercurrent viral respiratory infection. In adults, older children, and partially immunized individuals, symptoms may consist only of irritating cough lasting 1–2 weeks. Clinical pertussis is milder in immunized children.

B. Laboratory Findings

WBC counts of 20,000–30,000/μL with 70–80% lymphocytes typically appear near the end of the catarrhal stage. Severe pulmonary hypertension and hyperleukocytosis are associated with severe disease and death in young children with pertussis. Many older children and adults with mild infections never demonstrate lymphocytosis. The blood picture may resemble lymphocytic leukemia or leukemoid reactions. Identification of *B pertussis* by culture or PCR from nasopharyngeal swabs or nasal wash specimens proves the diagnosis. The organism may be found in the respiratory tract in diminishing numbers beginning in the catarrhal stage and ending about 2 weeks after the beginning of the paroxysmal stage. After 4–5 weeks of symptoms, cultures are almost always negative. Culture requires specialized media and careful attention to specimen collection and transport. PCR detection is replacing culture in most pediatric centers because of improved sensitivity, decreased time to diagnosis, and cost. Enzyme-linked immunosorbent assays (ELISAs) for detection of antibody to pertussis toxin or filamentous hemagglutinin may be useful for diagnosis but interpretation of antibody titers may be difficult in previously immunized patients. The chest radiograph reveals thickened bronchi and sometimes shows a "shaggy" heart border.

▶ Differential Diagnosis

The differential diagnosis of pertussis includes bacterial, tuberculous, chlamydial, and viral pneumonia. Cystic fibro-sis and foreign body aspiration may be considerations. Adenoviruses and respiratory syncytial virus may cause paroxysmal coughing with an associated elevation of lymphocytes in the peripheral blood, mimicking pertussis.

▶ Complications

Bronchopneumonia due to superinfection is the most common serious complication. It is characterized by abrupt clinical deterioration during the paroxysmal stage, accompanied by high fever and sometimes a striking leukemoid reaction with a shift to predominantly polymorphonuclear neutrophils. Atelectasis is a second common pulmonary complication. Atelectasis may be patchy or extensive and may shift rapidly to involve different areas of lung. Intercurrent viral respiratory infection is also a common complication and may provoke worsening or recurrence of paroxysmal coughing. Otitis media is common. Residual chronic bronchiectasis is infrequent despite the severity of the illness. Apnea and sudden death may occur during a particularly severe paroxysm. Seizures complicate 1.5% of cases, and encephalopathy occurs in 0.1%. The encephalopathy frequently is fatal. Anoxic brain damage, cerebral hemorrhage, or pertussis neurotoxins are hypothesized, but anoxia is most likely the cause. Epistaxis and subconjunctival hemorrhages are common.

▶ Prevention

Active immunization (see Chapter 9) with DTaP vaccine should be given in early infancy. The recent increase in incidence of pertussis is primarily due to increased recognition of disease in adolescents and adults. A booster dose of vaccine in adolescents between the ages of 11 and 18 years is recommended. Subsequent booster doses of Tdap are recommended for adults aged 18–60 years to replace Td boosters.

Chemoprophylaxis with azithromycin or erythromycin should be given to exposed family and hospital contacts, particularly those younger than age 2 years, although data to support the efficacy of such preventive therapy are not strong. Hospitalized children with pertussis should be isolated because of the great risk of transmission to patients and staff. Several large hospital outbreaks have been reported.

▶ Treatment

A. Specific Measures

Antibiotics may ameliorate early infections but have no effect on clinical symptoms in the paroxysmal stage. Erythromycin is the drug of choice because it promptly terminates respiratory tract carriage of *B pertussis*. Resistance to macrolides has been rarely reported. Patients should be given erythromycin estolate (40–50 mg/kg/24 h in four divided doses for 14 days). A recent study suggests that 7 days and 14 days of treatment are equally effective. Treatment with clarithromycin for 7 days and azithromycin for 5 days was equal to erythromycin for 14 days. Ampicillin (100 mg/kg/d in four divided doses) may also be used for erythromycin-intolerant patients. Azithromycin is often preferred due to ease of compliance and decreased gastrointestinal side effects.

Corticosteroids reduce the severity of disease but may mask signs of bacterial superinfection. Albuterol (0.3–0.5 mg/kg/d in four doses) has reduced the severity of illness, but tachycardia is common when the drug is given orally, and aerosol administration may precipitate paroxysms.

B. General Measures

Nutritional support during the paroxysmal phase is important. Frequent small feedings, tube feeding, or parenteral fluid supplementation may be needed. Minimizing stimuli that trigger paroxysms is probably the best way of controlling cough. In general, cough suppressants are of little benefit.

C. Treatment of Complications

Respiratory insufficiency due to pneumonia or other pulmonary complications should be treated with oxygen and assisted ventilation if necessary. Convulsions are treated with oxygen and anticonvulsants. Bacterial pneumonia or otitis media requires additional antibiotics.

▶ Prognosis

The prognosis for patients with pertussis has improved in recent years because of excellent nursing care, treatment of complications, attention to nutrition, and modern intensive care. However, the disease is still very serious in infants younger than age 1 year; most deaths occur in this age group. Children with encephalopathy have a poor prognosis.

Halasa NB et al: Fatal pulmonary hypertension associated with pertussis in infants: Does extracorporeal membrane oxygenation have a role? Pediatrics 2003;112:1274 [PMID: 14654596].

Halperin SA: The control of pertussis—2007 and beyond. N Engl J Med 2007;356:110 [PMID: 17215528].

Rendi-Wagner P et al: Impact of a pertussis booster vaccination program in adolescents and adults on the epidemiology of pertussis in Austria. Pediatr Infect Dis J 2007;26:806 [PMID: 17721375].

Yildirim I et al: Frequency of pertussis in children with prolonged cough. Scand J Infect Dis 2007;Oct 11:1 [Epub ahead of print] [PMID: 17934983].

LISTERIOSIS

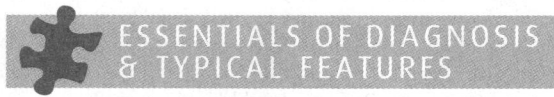

ESSENTIALS OF DIAGNOSIS
& TYPICAL FEATURES

Early-onset neonatal disease:

▶ Signs of sepsis a few hours after birth in an infant born with fetal distress and hepatosplenomegaly; maternal fever.

Late-onset neonatal disease:

▶ Meningitis, sometimes with monocytosis in the CSF and peripheral blood.

▶ Onset at age 9–30 days.

▶ General Considerations

Listeria monocytogenes is a gram-positive, non–spore-forming aerobic rod distributed widely in the animal kingdom and in food, dust, and soil. It causes systemic infections in newborn infants and immunosuppressed older children. In pregnant women, infection is relatively mild, with fever, aches, and chills, but is accompanied by bacteremia and sometimes results in intrauterine or perinatal infection with grave consequences for the fetus or newborn. One fourth of cases occur in pregnant women, and 20% of their pregnancies end in stillbirth or neonatal death. *Listeria* is present in the stool of approximately 10% of the healthy population. Persons in contact with animals are at greater risk. Outbreaks of listeriosis have been traced to contaminated cabbage in coleslaw, soft cheese, hot dogs, luncheon meats, and milk. *Listeria* infections have decreased since the adoption of strict regulations for ready-to-eat foods; fewer than 900 cases were reported in 2005.

Like GBS infections, *Listeria* infections in the newborn can be divided into early and late forms. Early infections are more common, leading to a severe congenital form of infection. Later infections are often characterized by meningitis.

▶ Clinical Findings

A. Symptoms and Signs

In the early neonatal form, symptoms of listeriosis usually appear on the first day of life and always by the third day. Fetal distress is common, and infants frequently have signs of severe disease at birth. Respiratory distress, diarrhea, and fever occur. On examination, hepatosplenomegaly and a papular rash are found. A history of maternal fever is common. Meningitis may accompany the septic course. The late neonatal form usually occurs after age 9 days and can occur as late as 5 weeks. Meningitis is common, characterized by irritability, fever, and poor feeding.

Listeria infections are rare in older children and usually are associated with immunodeficiency. Several recent cases were associated with tumor necrosis factor-α neutralizing agents. Signs and symptoms are those of meningitis, usually with insidious onset.

B. Laboratory Findings

In all patients except those receiving white cell depressant drugs, the WBC count is elevated, with 10–20% monocytes. When meningitis is found, the characteristic CSF cell count is high (> 500/μL) with a predominance of polymorphonuclear neutrophils in 70% of cases. Monocytes may predominate in up to 30% of cases. Gram-stained smears of CSF are usually negative, but short gram-positive rods may be seen. The chief pathologic feature in severe neonatal sepsis is miliary granulomatosis with microabscesses in liver, spleen, CNS, lung, and bowel.

Culture results are frequently positive from multiple sites, including blood from the infant and the mother.

▶ Differential Diagnosis

Early-onset neonatal disease resembles hemolytic disease of the newborn, GBS sepsis or severe cytomegalovirus infection, rubella, or toxoplasmosis. Late-onset disease must be differentiated from meningitis due to echovirus and coxsackievirus, GBS, and gram-negative enteric bacteria.

▶ Prevention

Immunosuppressed, pregnant, and elderly patients can decrease the risk of *Listeria* infection by avoiding soft cheeses, by thoroughly reheating or avoiding delicatessen and ready-to-eat foods, by avoiding raw meat and milk, and by thoroughly washing fresh vegetables.

▶ Treatment

Ampicillin (150–300 mg/kg/d every 6 hours intravenously) is the drug of choice in most cases of listeriosis. Gentamicin (2.5 mg/kg every 8 hours intravenously) has a synergistic effect with ampicillin and should be given in serious infections and to patients with immune deficits. Vancomycin may be substituted for ampicillin when empirically treating meningitis. If ampicillin cannot be used, TMP–SMX also is effective. Cephalosporins are not effective. Treatment of severe disease should continue for at least 2 weeks.

▶ Prognosis

In a recent outbreak of early-onset neonatal disease, the mortality rate was 27% despite aggressive and appropriate management. Meningitis in older infants has a good prognosis. In immunosuppressed children, prognosis depends to a great extent on that of the underlying illness.

Centers for Disease Control and Prevention: Listeriosis. http://www.cdc.gov/ncidod/dbmd/disease info/listeriosis_g.htm

Gottlieb SL et al: Multistate outbreak of listeriosis linked to turkey deli meat and subsequent changes in US regulatory policy. Clin Infect Dis 2006;42:29 [PMID: 16323088].

Varma JK et al: Listeria monocytogenes infection from foods prepared in a commercial establishment: A case-control study of potential sources of sporadic illness in the United States. Clin Infect Dis 2007;44:521 [PMID: 17243054].

Voetsch AC et al: Reduction in the incidence of invasive listeriosis in foodborne diseases active surveillance network sites, 1996–2003. Clin Infect Dis 2007;44:513 [PMID: 17243053].

TUBERCULOSIS

ESSENTIALS OF DIAGNOSIS & TYPICAL FEATURES

▶ All types: positive tuberculin test in patient or members of household, suggestive chest radiograph, history of contact, and demonstration of organism by stain and culture.

▶ Pulmonary: fatigue, irritability, and undernutrition, with or without fever and cough.

▶ Glandular: chronic cervical adenitis.

▶ Miliary: classic snowstorm appearance of chest radiograph.

▶ Meningitis: fever and manifestations of meningeal irritation and increased intracranial pressure. Characteristic CSF.

▶ General Considerations

Tuberculosis is a granulomatous disease caused by *Mycobacterium tuberculosis*. It is a leading cause of death throughout the world. Children younger than age 3 years are most susceptible. Lymphohematogenous dissemination through the lungs to extrapulmonary sites, including the brain and meninges, eyes, bones and joints, lymph nodes, kidneys, intestines, larynx, and skin, is more likely to occur in infants. Increased susceptibility occurs again in adolescence, particularly in girls within 2 years of menarche. Following substantial increases in disease during the 1980s, tuberculosis incidence has decreased since 1992 due to increased control measures. More than 10,000 new cases were reported in 2005. High-risk groups include ethnic minorities, foreign-born persons, prisoners, residents of nursing homes, indigents, migrant workers, and health care providers. However, 50% of cases occurred in U.S.-born persons. HIV infection is an important risk factor for both development and spread of disease. Pediatric tuberculosis incidence mirrors the trends seen in adults.

Exposure to an infected adult is the most common risk factor in children. The primary complex in infancy and childhood consists of a small parenchymal lesion in any area of the lung with caseation of regional nodes and calcification. Post-primary tuberculosis in adolescents and adults commonly occurs in the apices of the lungs and is likely to cause chronic progressive cavitary pulmonary disease with less tendency for hematogenous dissemination. *Mycobacterium bovis* infection is clinically identical to *M tuberculosis*. *M bovis* may be acquired from unpasteurized dairy products obtained outside the United States.

▶ **Clinical Findings**

A. Symptoms and Signs

1. Pulmonary—(See Chapter 18.)

2. Miliary—Diagnosis is usually based on the classic "snow-storm" or "millet seed" appearance of lung fields on radiograph, although early in the course of disseminated tuberculosis the chest radiograph may show no or only subtle abnormalities. Choroidal tubercles are sometimes seen on funduscopic examination. Other lesions may be present and produce osteomyelitis, arthritis, meningitis, tuberculomas of the brain, enteritis, or infection of the kidneys and liver.

3. Meningitis—Symptoms include fever, vomiting, headache, lethargy, and irritability, with signs of meningeal irritation and increased intracranial pressure, cranial nerve palsies, convulsions, and coma.

4. Lymphatic—The primary complex may be associated with a skin lesion drained by regional nodes or chronic cervical node enlargement or infection of the tonsils. Involved nodes may become fixed to the overlying skin, suppurate, and drain.

B. Laboratory Findings

The Mantoux test (0.1 mL of intermediate-strength purified protein derivative [PPD] [5 TU] inoculated intradermally) is positive at 48–72 hours if there is significant induration (Table 40–2). Parental reporting of skin test results is often inaccurate. All tests should be read by professionals trained to interpret Mantoux tests. False-negative results occur in malnourished patients, in those with overwhelming disease, and in 10% of children with isolated pulmonary disease. Temporary suppression of tuberculin reactivity may be seen with viral infections (eg, measles, influenza, varicella, and mumps), after live virus immunization, and during corticosteroid or other immunosuppressive drug therapy. For these reasons, a negative Mantoux test does not exclude the diagnosis of tuberculosis. When tuberculosis is suspected in a child, household members and adult contacts (eg, teachers and caregivers) also should be tested immediately. Multiple puncture tests (tine tests) should not be used because they are associated with false-negative and false-positive reactions, and because standards for interpretation of positive results do not exist. γ-Interferon release assays are approved to replace Mantoux skin tests in adults. These assays have much higher specificity due to less common false-positive results from nontuberculosis mycobacteria and BCG. They are done on blood obtained by venipuncture and are further advantageous in requiring only a single visit; however, these tests are not yet sufficiently studied in children.

The ESR is usually elevated. Cultures of pooled early morning gastric aspirates from three successive days will yield *M tuberculosis* in about 40% of cases. Biopsy may be necessary to establish the diagnosis. Therapy should not be delayed in sus-

Table 40–2. Interpretation of tuberculin skin test reactions.[a]

Degree of Risk	Risk Factors	Positive Reaction
High	Recent close contact with a case of active tuberculosis	≥ 5 mm induration
	Chest radiograph compatible with tuberculosis	
	Immunocompromise	
	HIV infection	
Medium	Current or previous residence in high-prevalence area (Asia, Africa, Latin America)	≥ 10 mm induration
	Skin test converters within past 2 y	
	Intravenous drug use	
	Homelessness or residence in a correctional institution	
	Recent weight loss or malnutrition	
	Leukemia, Hodgkin disease, or diabetes mellitus	
	Age < 4 y	
Low	Children ≥ 4 y without any risk factor	≥ 15 mm induration

[a]Standard intradermal Mantoux test, 5 test units.

pected cases. The CSF in tuberculous meningitis shows slight to moderate pleocytosis (50–300 WBCs/μL, predominantly lymphocytes), decreased glucose, and increased protein.

The direct detection of mycobacteria in body fluids or discharges is best done by staining specimens with auramine-rhodamine and examining them with fluorescence microscopy; this method is superior to the Ziehl-Neelsen method.

C. Imaging

Chest radiograph should be obtained in all children with suspicion of tuberculosis at any site or with a positive skin test. Segmental consolidation with some volume loss and hilar adenopathy are common findings in children. Pleural effusion also occurs with primary infection. Cavities and apical disease are unusual in children but are common in adolescents and adults.

▶ **Differential Diagnosis**

Pulmonary tuberculosis must be differentiated from fungal, parasitic, mycoplasmal, and bacterial pneumonias; lung abscess; foreign body aspiration; lipoid pneumonia; sarcoidosis; and mediastinal cancer. Cervical lymphadenitis is most likely due to streptococcal or staphylococcal infections. Cat-scratch fever and infection with atypical mycobacteria may need to be distinguished from tuberculous lymphadenitis. Viral meningoencephalitis, head trauma (child abuse), lead poisoning, brain abscess, acute bacterial meningitis, brain tumor, and disseminated fungal infections must be excluded in tuberculous meningitis. The skin test in the patient or family contacts is frequently valuable in differentiating these conditions from tuberculosis.

Prevention

A. BCG Vaccine

Bacille Calmette–Guérin (BCG) vaccines are live-attenuated strains of *M bovis*. Although neonatal and childhood administration of BCG is carried out in countries with a high prevalence of tuberculosis, protective efficacy varies greatly with vaccine potency and method of delivery. Because the great majority of children who have received BCG still have negative Mantoux tests, the past history of BCG vaccination should be ignored in interpreting the skin test. In the United States, BCG vaccination is not recommended.

B. Isoniazid Chemoprophylaxis

Daily administration of isoniazid (10 mg/kg/d orally; maximum 300 mg) is advised for children who are exposed by prolonged close or household contact with adolescents or adults with active disease. Isoniazid is given until 2 months after last contact. At the end of this time, a Mantoux test should be done, and therapy should be continued for an additional 7 months if the test is positive.

C. Other Measures

Tuberculosis in infants and young children is evidence of recent exposure to active infection in an adult, usually a family member or household contact. The source contact (index case) should be identified, isolated, and given treatment to prevent other secondary cases. Reporting cases to local health departments is essential for contact tracing. Exposed tuberculin-negative children should usually receive isoniazid chemoprophylaxis. If a repeated skin test is negative 2–3 months following the last exposure, isoniazid may be stopped. Routine tuberculin skin testing is not recommended for children without risk factors who reside in communities with a low incidence of tuberculosis. Children with no personal risk for tuberculosis but who reside in communities with a high incidence of tuberculosis should be given a skin test at school entry and then again at age 11–16 years. Children with a risk factor for acquiring tuberculosis should be tested every 2–3 years. Incarcerated adolescents and children living in a household with HIV-infected persons should have annual skin tests.

Children who immigrate into the United States from a country with a high incidence of infection should receive a skin test on entry to the United States or upon presentation to health care providers. A past history of BCG vaccine should not delay skin testing.

Treatment

A. Specific Measures

Most children with tuberculosis in the United States are hospitalized initially. If the infecting organism has not been isolated from the presumed contact for susceptibility testing, reasonable attempts should be made to obtain it from the child using morning gastric aspirates, sputum, bronchoscopy, thoracentesis, or biopsy when appropriate. Unfortunately, cultures are frequently negative in children, and the risk of these procedures must be weighed against the yield. Therapy is given daily for 14 days and then reduced to 2–3 times per week for the duration of the course. Directly observed administration of all doses of antituberculosis therapy by a trained health care professional is essential to ensure compliance with therapy.

Children with positive skin tests (see Table 40–2) without evidence of active disease have latent tuberculosis and should receive 9 months of isoniazid (10 mg/kg/d orally; maximum 300 mg) therapy. In children with active pulmonary disease, therapy for 6 months using isoniazid (10 mg/kg/d), rifampin (15 mg/kg/d), and pyrazinamide (25–30 mg/kg/d) in a single daily oral dose for 2 months, followed by isoniazid plus rifampin (either in a daily or twice-weekly regimen) for 4 months appears effective for eliminating isoniazid-susceptible organisms. For more severe disease, such as miliary or CNS infection, duration is increased to 12 months or more, and a fourth drug (streptomycin or ethambutol) is added for the first 2 months. In communities with resistance rates greater than 4%, initial therapy should usually include four drugs.

1. Isoniazid—The hepatotoxicity from isoniazid seen in adults and some adolescents is rare in children. Transient elevation of aminotransferases (up to three times normal) may be seen at 6–12 weeks, but therapy is continued unless clinical illness occurs. Routine monitoring of liver function tests is unnecessary unless prior hepatic disease is known or the child is severely ill. Peripheral neuropathy associated with pyridoxine deficiency is rare in children, and it is not necessary to add pyridoxine unless significant malnutrition coexists.

2. Rifampin—Although it is an excellent bactericidal agent, rifampin is never used alone owing to rapid development of resistance. Hepatotoxicity may occur but rarely with recommended doses. The orange discoloration of secretions is benign but may stain contact lenses or clothes.

3. Pyrazinamide—This excellent sterilizing agent is most effective during the first 2 months of therapy. With the recommended duration and dosing, it is well tolerated. Although pyrazinamide elevates the uric acid level, it rarely causes symptoms of hyperuricemia in children. Use of this drug is now common for tuberculous disease in children, and resistance is almost unknown. Oral acceptance and CNS penetration are good.

4. Ethambutol—Because optic neuritis is the major side effect in adults, ethambutol has usually been given only to children whose vision can be reliably tested for loss of color differentiation. Optic neuritis is rare and usually occurs in those receiving more than the recommended dosage of 25 mg/kg/d. Documentation of optic toxicity in children is lacking despite considerable worldwide experience. Therefore, many four-drug regimens for children now include ethambutol.

5. Streptomycin—Streptomycin (20–30 mg/kg/d, given intramuscularly in one or two doses) should be given for 1 or 2 months in severe disease. The child's hearing should be tested periodically during use as ototoxicity is common.

B. Chemotherapy for Drug-Resistant Tuberculosis

The incidence of drug resistance is increasing and reaches 10–20% in some areas of the United States. Transmission of multiply drug-resistant and extensively drug-resistant strains to contacts has occurred in some epidemics. Consultation with local experts in treating tuberculosis is important in these difficult cases. Therapy should continue for 12 months or longer. Often, four to six first- and second-line medications are needed.

C. General Measures

Corticosteroids may be used for suppressing inflammatory reactions in meningeal, pleural, and pericardial tuberculosis and for the relief of bronchial obstruction due to hilar adenopathy. Prednisone is given orally, 1 mg/kg/d for 6–8 weeks, with gradual withdrawal at the end of that time. The use of corticosteroids may mask progression of disease. Accordingly, the clinician needs to be sure that an effective regimen is being used.

▶ Prognosis

If bacteria are sensitive and treatment is completed, most children are cured with minimal sequelae. Repeat treatment is more difficult and less successful. With antituberculosis chemotherapy (especially isoniazid), there should now be nearly 100% recovery in miliary tuberculosis. Without treatment, the mortality rate in both miliary tuberculosis and tuberculous meningitis is almost 100%. In the latter form, about two thirds of patients receiving treatment survive. There may be a high incidence of neurologic abnormalities among survivors if treatment is started late.

American Thoracic Society, CDC, Infectious Diseases Society of America: Treatment of tuberculosis. MMWR Recomm Rep 2003;52(RR-11):1 [PMID: 12836625].

Centers for Disease Control and Prevention (CDC): Trends in tuberculosis incidence, 2006. MMWR Morb Mortal Wkly Rep 2007;56:245 [PMID: 17380106].

Mandalakas AM et al: Predictors of Mycobacterium tuberculosis infection in international adoptees. Pediatrics 2007;120(3):e610 [PMID: 17766501].

Sterling TR et al: Immune function in young children with previous pulmonary or military-meningeal tuberculosis and impact of BCG vaccination. Pediatrics 2007;120(4):e912 [PMID: 17908747].

Taylor Z et al; American Thoracic Society; Centers for Disease Control and Prevention; Infectious Diseases Society of America: Controlling tuberculosis in the United States. Recommendations from the American Thoracic Society, CDC, and the Infectious Diseases Society of America. MMWR Recomm Rep 2005;54(RR-12):1 [PMID: 16267499].

INFECTIONS WITH NONTUBERCULOUS MYCOBACTERIA

ESSENTIALS OF DIAGNOSIS & TYPICAL FEATURES

▶ Chronic unilateral cervical lymphadenitis.

▶ Granulomas of the skin.

▶ Chronic bone lesion with draining sinus (chronic osteomyelitis).

▶ Reaction to PPD-S (standard) of 5–8 mm, negative chest radiograph, and negative history of contact with tuberculosis.

▶ Diagnosis by positive acid-fast stain or culture.

▶ Disseminated infection in patients with AIDS.

▶ General Considerations

Various species of acid-fast mycobacteria other than *M tuberculosis* may cause subclinical infections and occasionally clinical disease resembling tuberculosis. Strains of nontuberculous mycobacteria are common in soil, food, and water. Organisms enter the host by small abrasions in skin, oral mucosa, or gastrointestinal mucosa. Strain cross-reactivity with *M tuberculosis* can be demonstrated by simultaneous skin testing (Mantoux) with PPD-S (standard) and PPD prepared from one of the atypical antigens. Unfortunately, reagents prepared for routine nontuberculosis skin testing are not available to clinicians.

The Runyon classification of mycobacteria includes the following:

Group I. Photochromogens (PPD-Y): (*Mycobacterium kansasii, M marinum*) Yellow color develops on exposure to light in previously white colony grown 2–4 weeks in the dark.

Group II. Scotochromogens (PPD-G): (*Mycobacterium scrofulaceum*) Colonies are definitely yellow-orange after incubation in the dark. Organisms may be found in small numbers in the normal flora of some human saliva and gastric contents. Subclinical infection is widespread in the United States, but clinical disease appears rarely.

Group III. Nonphotochromogens (PPD-B): "Battey avianswine group" grows as small white colonies after incubation in the dark, with no significant development of pigment on exposure to light. Infection with *Mycobacterium* *avium* complex (MAC) is prevalent on the East Coast of the United States, particularly the Southeast, and in patients with AIDS.

Group IV. "Rapid growers": (*Mycobacterium fortuitum, M chelonei*) Within 1 week after inoculation they form colonies closely resembling *M tuberculosis* morphologically.

▶ Clinical Findings

A. Symptoms and Signs

1. Lymphadenitis—In children, the most common form of infection due to mycobacteria other than *M tuberculosis* is cervical lymphadenitis. MAC is the most common organism. A submandibular or cervical node swells slowly and is firm and initially somewhat tender. Low-grade fever may occur. Over time, the node suppurates and may drain chronically. Nodes in other areas of the head and neck and elsewhere are sometimes involved.

2. Pulmonary disease—In the western United States, pulmonary disease is usually due to *M kansasii*. In the eastern United States, it may be due to MAC. In other countries, disease is usually caused by MAC. In adults, there is usually underlying chronic pulmonary disease. Immunologic deficiency may be present. Presentation is clinically indistinguishable from that of tuberculosis. Adolescents with cystic fibrosis may be infected with nontuberculous mycobacteria.

3. Swimming pool granuloma—This is due to *M marinum*. A solitary chronic granulomatous lesion with satellite lesions develops after minor trauma in infected swimming pools. Minor trauma in home aquariums or other aquatic environments also may lead to infection.

4. Chronic osteomyelitis—Osteomyelitis is caused by *M kansasii, M fortuitum,* or other rapid growers. Findings include swelling and pain over a distal extremity, radiolucent defects in bone, fever, and clinical and radiographic evidence of bronchopneumonia. Such cases are rare.

5. Meningitis—Disease is due to *M kansasii* and may be indistinguishable from tuberculous meningitis.

6. Disseminated infection—Rarely, apparently immunologically normal children develop disseminated infection due to nontuberculous mycobacteria. Children are ill, with fever and hepatosplenomegaly, and organisms are demonstrated in bone lesions, lymph nodes, or liver. Chest radiographs are usually normal. Between 60% and 80% of patients with AIDS will acquire MAC infection, characterized by fever, night sweats, weight loss, and diarrhea. Infection usually indicates severe immune dysfunction and is associated with CD4 lymphocyte counts less than 50/μL.

B. Laboratory Findings

In most cases, there is a small reaction (< 10 mm) when Mantoux testing is done. Larger reactions may be seen. The chest radiograph is negative, and there is no history of contact with a case of tuberculosis. Needle aspiration of the node excludes bacterial infection and may yield acid-fast bacilli on stain or culture. Fistulization should not be a problem because total excision is usually recommended for infection due to atypical mycobacteria. Cultures of any normally sterile body site will yield MAC in immunocompromised patients with disseminated disease. Blood cultures are positive, with a large density of bacteria.

▶ Differential Diagnosis

See section on differential diagnosis in the previous discussion of tuberculosis and in Chapter 18.

▶ Treatment

A. Specific Measures

The usual treatment of lymphadenitis is complete surgical excision. Occasionally excision is impossible because of proximity to branches of the facial nerve. Chemotherapy may then be necessary. Response of extensive adenopathy or other forms of infection varies according to the infecting species and susceptibility. Usually, combinations of two to four medications administered for months are required. Isoniazid, rifampin, and ethambutol (depending on sensitivity to isoniazid) will result in a favorable response in almost all patients with *M kansasii* infection. Chemotherapeutic treatment of MAC is much less satisfactory because resistance to isoniazid, rifampin, and pyrazinamide is common. Susceptibility testing is necessary to optimize therapy. Most clinicians favor surgical excision of involved tissue if possible and treatment with at least three drugs to which the organism has been shown to be sensitive. Disseminated disease in patients with AIDS calls for a combination of three or more active drugs. Clarithromycin or azithromycin and ethambutol is started, in addition to one or more of the following drugs: ethionamide, capreomycin, amikacin, rifabutin, or ciprofloxacin. *M fortuitum* and *M chelonei* are usually susceptible to amikacin plus cefoxitin followed by erythromycin, clarithromycin, azithromycin, or doxycycline, and may be successfully treated with such combinations. Swimming pool granuloma due to *M marinum* is usually treated with doxycycline (in children older than age 9 years) or rifampin, plus ethambutol, clarithromycin, or TMP–SMX for a minimum of 3 months. Surgery may also be beneficial.

B. General Measures

Isolation of the patient is usually not necessary. General supportive care is indicated for the child with disseminated disease.

▶ Prognosis

The prognosis is good for patients with localized disease, although fatalities occur in immunocompromised children who have disseminated disease.

Brantley JS et al: Cutaneous infection with *Mycobacterium abscessus* in a child. Pediatr Dermatol 2006;23:128 [PMID: 16650219].

Lindeboom JA et al: Cervicofacial lymphadenitis in children caused by *Mycobacterium haemophilum*. Clin Infect Dis 2005; 41:1569 [PMID: 16267728].

Lindeboom JA et al: Tuberculin skin testing is useful in the screening for nontuberculous mycobacterial cervicofacial lymphadenitis in children. Clin Infect Dis 2006;43:1547 [PMID: 17109286].

Vu TT et al: Nontuberculous mycobacteria in children: A changing pattern. J Otolaryngol 2005;34(Suppl 1):S40 [PMID: 16089239].

LEGIONELLA INFECTION

ESSENTIALS OF DIAGNOSIS & TYPICAL FEATURES

► Severe progressive pneumonia in a child with compromised immunity.

► Diarrhea and neurologic signs are common.

► Positive culture requires buffered charcoal yeast extract media and proves infection.

► Direct fluorescent antibody staining of respiratory secretions proves infection.

General Considerations

Legionella pneumophila is a ubiquitous gram-negative bacillus that causes two distinct clinical syndromes: Legionnaire disease and Pontiac fever. Usually Legionnaire disease is an acute, severe pneumonia that is frequently fatal in immunocompromised patients. Pontiac fever is a mild, flulike illness that spares the lungs and is characterized by fever, headache, myalgia, and arthralgia. The disease is self-limited and is described in outbreaks in otherwise healthy adults.

Over 40 species of *Legionella* have been discovered, but not all cause disease in humans. *L pneumophila* causes most infections. *Legionella* is present in many natural water sources as well as domestic water supplies (faucets and showers). Contaminated cooling towers and heat exchangers have been implicated in several large institutional outbreaks. Person-to-person transmission has not been documented.

Few cases of Legionnaire disease have been reported in children. Most were in children with compromised cellular immunity. In adults, risk factors include smoking, underlying cardiopulmonary or renal disease, alcoholism, and diabetes.

L pneumophila is thought to be acquired by inhalation of a contaminated aerosol. The bacteria are phagocytosed but proliferate within macrophages. Cell-mediated immunity is necessary to activate macrophages to kill intracellular bacteria.

Clinical Findings

A. Symptoms and Signs

Onset of fever, chills, anorexia, and headache is abrupt. Pulmonary symptoms appear within 2–3 days and progress rapidly. The cough is nonproductive early. Purulent sputum occurs late. Hemoptysis, diarrhea, and neurologic signs (including lethargy, irritability, tremors, and delirium) are seen.

B. Laboratory Findings

The WBC count is usually elevated. Chest radiographs show rapidly progressive patchy consolidation. Cavitation and large pleural effusions are uncommon. Cultures from sputum, tracheal aspirates, or bronchoscopic specimens, when grown on specialized media are positive in 70–80% of patients at 3–7 days. Direct fluorescent antibody staining of sputum or other respiratory specimens is only 50–70% sensitive but 95% specific. A negative result on culture or direct fluorescent antibody staining of sputum or tracheal secretions does not rule out disease due to *Legionella*. PCR detection of respiratory secretions for *Legionella* is available at some centers. A urine immunoassay for *Legionella* antigen is more sensitive than the immunoassay using respiratory secretions and is highly specific. Serologic tests are available, but a maximum rise in titer may require 6–8 weeks.

Differential Diagnosis

Legionnaire disease is usually a rapidly progressive pneumonia in a patient who appears very ill with unremitting fevers. Other bacterial pneumonias, viral pneumonias, *Mycoplasma* pneumonia, and fungal disease are all possibilities and may be difficult to differentiate clinically in an immunocompromised patient.

Complications

In sporadic untreated cases, mortality rates are 5–25%. In immunocompromised patients with untreated disease, mortality approaches 80%. Hematogenous dissemination may result in extrapulmonary foci of infection, including pericardium, myocardium, and kidneys. *Legionella* may be the cause of culture-negative endocarditis.

Prevention

No vaccine is available. Hyperchlorination and periodic superheating of water supplies in hospitals have been shown to reduce the number of organisms and the risk of infection.

Treatment

Intravenous azithromycin, 10 mg/kg/d given as a once-daily dose (maximum dose 500 mg), is the drug of choice. Rifampin (20 mg/kg/d divided in two doses) may be added to the regimen in gravely ill patients. Ciprofloxacin and levofloxacin are effective in adults but are not approved for use in children. Duration of therapy is 5–10 days if azithromycin is used; for other antibiotics a 14–21-day course is recommended. Oral therapy may be substituted for intravenous therapy as the patient's condition improves.

Prognosis

Mortality rate is high if treatment is delayed. Malaise, problems with memory, and fatigue are common after recovery.

Fields BS et al: *Legionella* and Legionnaires' disease: 25 years of investigation. Clin Microbiol Rev 2002;15:506 [PMID: 12097254].

Roig J et al: *Legionella* spp.: Community acquired and nosocomial infections. Curr Opin Infect Dis 2003;16:145 [PMID: 12734447].

PSITTACOSIS (ORNITHOSIS) & *CHLAMYDIA PNEUMONIAE* INFECTION

ESSENTIALS OF DIAGNOSIS & TYPICAL FEATURES

▶ Fever, cough, malaise, chills, headache.

▶ Diffuse rales; no consolidation.

▶ Long-lasting radiographic findings of bronchopneumonia.

▶ Isolation of the organism or rising titer of complement-fixing antibodies.

▶ Exposure to infected birds (ornithosis).

General Considerations

Psittacosis is caused by *Chlamydia psittaci*. When the agent is transmitted to humans from psittacine birds (parrots, parakeets, cockatoos, and budgerigars), the disease is called psittacosis or parrot fever. However, other avian genera (eg, pigeons and turkeys) are common sources of infection in the United States, and the general term *ornithosis* often is used. The agent is an obligate intracellular parasite. Human-to-human spread rarely occurs. The incubation period is 5–14 days. The bird from which the disease was transmitted may not be clinically ill.

Chlamydia pneumoniae may cause atypical pneumonia similar to that due to *M pneumoniae*. Transmission is by respiratory spread. Infection appears to be most prevalent during the second decade; half of surveyed adults are seropositive. Only a small percentage of infections result in clinical pneumonia. The disease may be more common than atypical pneumonia due to *M pneumoniae*. Lower respiratory tract infection due to *C pneumoniae* is uncommon in infants and young children.

Clinical Findings

A. Symptoms and Signs

1. *C psittaci*—The disease is extremely variable but tends to be mild in children. The onset is rapid or insidious, with fever, chills, headache, backache, malaise, myalgia, and dry cough. Signs include pneumonitis, altered percussion notes and breath sounds, and rales. Pulmonary findings may be absent early. Dyspnea and cyanosis may occur later. Splenomegaly, epistaxis, prostration, and meningismus are occasionally seen. Delirium, constipation or diarrhea, and abdominal distress may occur.

2. *C pneumoniae*—Clinically, *C pneumoniae* infection is similar to *M pneumoniae* infection. Most patients have mild upper respiratory infections. Lower respiratory tract infection is characterized by fever, sore throat (perhaps more severe with *C pneumoniae*), cough, and bilateral pulmonary findings and infiltrates.

B. Laboratory Findings

1. *C psittaci*—In psittacosis, the WBC count is normal or decreased, often with a shift to the left. Proteinuria is common. *C psittaci* is present in the blood and sputum during the first 2 weeks of illness and can be isolated by inoculation of specimens into mice or embryonated eggs, but culture is available only in research laboratories. A fourfold rise in complement fixation titers in specimens obtained at least 2 weeks apart or a single titer above 1:32 is considered evidence of infection. The titer rise may be blunted or delayed by therapy. Infection with *C pneumoniae* may lead to diagnostic confusion because cross-reactive antibody may cause falsely positive *C psittaci* titers. Microimmunofluorescence and PCR assays are specific but usually not available for *C psittaci*.

2. *C pneumoniae*—A fourfold rise in IgG titer (microimmunofluorescence antibody test) or an IgM titer above 1:16 is evidence of infection. IgG antibody peaks 6–8 weeks after infection. *C pneumoniae* can be isolated from nasal wash or throat swab specimens after inoculation into cell culture. A PCR assay also is available.

C. Imaging

The radiographic findings in psittacosis are those of central pneumonia that later becomes widespread or migratory. Psittacosis is indistinguishable from viral pneumonias by radiograph. Signs of pneumonitis may appear on radiograph in the absence of clinical suspicion of pulmonary involvement.

Differential Diagnosis

Psittacosis can be differentiated from viral or mycoplasmal pneumonias only by the history of contact with potentially infected birds. In severe or prolonged cases with extrapulmonary involvement the differential diagnosis is broad, including typhoid fever, brucellosis, and rheumatic fever.

Complications

Complications of psittacosis include myocarditis, endocarditis, hepatitis, pancreatitis, and secondary bacterial pneumonia. *C pneumoniae* infection may be prolonged or may recur.

Treatment

Doxycycline should be given for 14 days after defervescence to patients older than age 8 years with psittacosis. Alternatively, erythromycin, azithromycin, or clarithromycin may be used in younger children. Supportive oxygen may be needed. The patient should be kept in isolation. *C pneumoniae* responds to macrolides or doxycycline: a 14-day course is recommended.

Compendium of measures to control *Chlamydia psittaci* infection among humans (psittacosis) and pet birds (avian chlamydiosis), 2000. MMWR Recomm Rep 2000;49(RR-8):3 [PMID: 10914931].

Tsai MH et al: Chlamydial pneumonia in children requiring hospitalization: Effect of mixed infection on clinical outcome. J Microbiol Immunol Infect 2005;38:117 [PMID: 15843856].

CAT-SCRATCH DISEASE

ESSENTIALS OF DIAGNOSIS & TYPICAL FEATURES

- ▶ History of a cat scratch or cat contact.
- ▶ Primary lesion (papule, pustule, or conjunctivitis) at site of inoculation.
- ▶ Acute or subacute regional lymphadenopathy.
- ▶ Aspiration of sterile pus from a node.
- ▶ Laboratory studies excluding other causes.
- ▶ Biopsy of node or papule showing histopathologic findings consistent with cat-scratch disease and occasionally characteristic bacilli on Warthin-Starry stain.
- ▶ Positive cat-scratch serology (antibody to *Bartonella henselae*).

General Considerations

The causative agent of cat-scratch disease is *Bartonella henselae,* a gram-negative bacillus that also causes bacillary angiomatosis. Cat-scratch disease is a benign, self-limited form of lymphadenitis. Patients often report a cat scratch (67%) or contact with a cat or kitten (90%). The cat almost invariably is healthy. The clinical picture is that of a regional lymphadenitis associated with an erythematous papular skin lesion without intervening lymphangitis. The disease occurs worldwide and is more common in the fall and winter. It is estimated that more than 20,000 cases per year occur in the United States. The most common systemic complication is encephalitis.

Clinical Findings

A. Symptoms and Signs

About 50% of patients with cat-scratch disease develop a primary lesion at the site of the wound. The lesion usually is a papule or pustule that appears 3–10 days after injury and is located most often on the arm or hand (50%), head or leg (30%), or trunk or neck (10%). The lesion may be conjunctival (10%). Regional lymphadenopathy appears 10–50 days later and may be accompanied by mild malaise, lassitude, headache, and fever. Multiple sites are seen in about 10% of cases. Involved nodes may be hard or soft and 1–6 cm in diameter. They are usually tender, and 10–20% of them suppurate. The overlying skin may be inflamed. Lymphadenopathy usually resolves in about 2 months but may persist for up to 8 months.

Unusual manifestations include erythema nodosum, thrombocytopenic purpura, conjunctivitis (Parinaud oculoglandular fever), parotid swelling, pneumonia, osteolytic lesions, mesenteric and mediastinal adenitis, neuroretinitis, peripheral neuritis, hepatitis, granulomata of the liver and spleen, and encephalitis.

Immunocompetent patients may develop an atypical systemic form of cat-scratch disease. These patients have prolonged fever, fatigue, and malaise. Lymphadenopathy may be present. Hepatosplenomegaly or low-density hepatic or splenic lesions visualized by ultrasound or computed tomography scan are seen in some patients.

Infection in immunocompromised individuals may take the form of bacillary angiomatosis, presenting as vascular tumors of the skin and subcutaneous tissues. Immunocompromised patients may also have bacteremia or infection of the liver (peliosis hepatis).

B. Laboratory Findings

Serologic evidence of *Bartonella* infection by indirect fluorescent antibody or ELISA with a titer above 1:64 is supportive of the diagnosis. PCR assays are available. Cat-scratch skin test antigens are not recommended.

Histopathologic examination of involved tissue may show pyogenic granulomas or bacillary forms demonstrated by Warthin-Starry silver stain. There usually is some elevation in the ESR. In patients with CNS involvement, the CSF is usually normal but may show a slight pleocytosis and modest elevation of protein.

Differential Diagnosis

Cat-scratch disease must be distinguished from pyogenic adenitis, tuberculosis (typical and atypical), tularemia, plague, brucellosis, lymphoma, primary toxoplasmosis, infectious mononucleosis, lymphogranuloma venereum, and fungal infections.

Treatment

Treatment of cat-scratch disease adenopathy is controversial because the disease usually resolves without therapy and the patient is typically not exceedingly ill. Treatment of typical cat-scratch disease with a 5-day course of azithromycin has been shown to speed resolution of lymphadenopathy in some patients. The best therapy is reassurance that the adenopathy is benign and will subside spontaneously with time (mean duration of illness is 14 weeks). In cases of nodal suppuration, needle aspiration under local anesthesia relieves the pain. Excision of the involved node is indicated in cases of chronic adenitis. In some reports, azithromycin, gentamicin, ciprofloxacin, rifampin, or TMP–SMX have been useful. Azithromycin is used by many experts if treatment of adenopathy is desired because it is given once a day, is reasonably priced, and was studied in one randomized placebo-controlled trial. In that trial, lymph node volume decreased faster than placebo by 1 month; there was no difference in long-term resolution in the azithromycin and placebo groups.

Immunocompromised patients with evidence of infection should be treated with antibiotics: long-term therapy (months) in these patients with azithromycin, erythromycin, or doxycycline often is needed to prevent relapses. Immunocompetent patients with more severe disease or evidence of systemic infection should also be treated with antibiotics.

▶ Prognosis

The prognosis is good if complications do not occur.

Bass JW et al: Prospective randomized double blind placebo-controlled evaluation of azithromycin for treatment of cat scratch disease. Pediatr Infect Dis J 1998;17:447 [PMID: 9655532].

English R: Cat-scratch disease. Pediatr Rev 2006;27:123 [PMID: 16581952].

Massei F et al: The expanded spectrum of bartonellosis in children. Infect Dis Clin North Am 2005;19:691 [PMID: 16102656].

Schutze GE: Diagnosis and treatment of *Bartonella henselae* infections. Pediatr Infect Dis J 2000;19:1185 [PMID: 11144381].

▼ SPIROCHETAL INFECTIONS

SYPHILIS

ESSENTIALS OF DIAGNOSIS & TYPICAL FEATURES

Congenital:

▶ All types: history of untreated maternal syphilis, a positive serologic test, and a positive darkfield examination.

▶ Newborn: hepatosplenomegaly, characteristic radiographic bone changes, anemia, increased nucleated red cells, thrombocytopenia, abnormal spinal fluid, jaundice, edema.

▶ Young infant (3–12 weeks): snuffles, maculopapular skin rash, mucocutaneous lesions, pseudoparalysis (in addition to radiographic bone changes).

▶ Children: stigmata of early congenital syphilis, interstitial keratitis, saber shins, gummas of nose and palate.

Acquired:

▶ Chancre of genitals, lip, or anus in child or adolescent.

▶ History of sexual contact.

▶ General Considerations

Syphilis is a chronic, generalized infectious disease caused by a spirochete, *Treponema pallidum*. In the acquired form, the disease is transmitted by sexual contact. Primary syphilis is characterized by the presence of an indurated painless chancre, which heals in 7–10 days. A secondary eruption involving the skin and mucous membranes appears in 4–6 weeks. After a long latency period, late lesions of tertiary syphilis involve the eyes, skin, bones, viscera, CNS, and cardiovascular system.

Congenital syphilis results from transplacental infection. Infection may result in stillbirth or produce illness in the newborn, in early infancy, or later in childhood. Syphilis occurring in the newborn and young infant is comparable to secondary disease in the adult but is more severe and life-threatening. Late congenital syphilis (developing in childhood) is comparable to tertiary disease.

Congenital syphilis is increasing in the United States due to increasing primary and secondary syphilis in women of childbearing age, and perhaps due to inadequate diagnosis and treatment of syphilis in prenatal care programs.

▶ Clinical Findings

A. Symptoms and Signs

1. Congenital Syphilis

A. NEWBORNS—Most newborns with congenital syphilis are asymptomatic. If infection is not detected and treated, symptoms develop within weeks to months. When clinical signs are present, they usually consist of jaundice, anemia with or without thrombocytopenia, increase in nucleated red blood cells, hepatosplenomegaly, and edema. Overt signs of meningitis (bulging fontanelle or opisthotonos) may be present, but subclinical infection with CSF abnormalities is more likely.

B. YOUNG INFANTS (3–12 WEEKS)—The infant may appear normal for the first few weeks of life only to develop mucocutaneous lesions and pseudoparalysis of the arms or legs. Shotty lymphadenopathy may be felt. Hepatomegaly is universal, with splenomegaly in 50% of patients. Other signs of disease similar to those seen in the newborn may be present. Anemia has been reported as the only presenting manifestation of congenital syphilis in this age group. "Snuffles" (syphilitic rhinitis), characterized by a profuse mucopurulent discharge, are present in 25% of patients. A syphilitic rash is common on the palms and soles but may occur anywhere on the body. The rash consists of bright red, raised maculopapular lesions that gradually fade. Moist lesions occur at the mucocutaneous junctions (nose, mouth, anus, and genitals) and lead to fissuring and bleeding.

Syphilis in the young infant may lead to stigmata recognizable in later childhood, such as rhagades (scars) around the mouth or nose, a depressed bridge of the nose (saddle nose), and a high forehead (secondary to mild hydrocephalus associated with low-grade meningitis and frontal periostitis). The permanent upper central incisors may be peg-shaped with a central notch (Hutchinson teeth), and the cusps of the sixth-year molars may have a lobulated mulberry appearance.

C. CHILDREN—Bilateral interstitial keratitis (at age 6–12 years) is characterized by photophobia, increased lacrimation, and vascularization of the cornea associated with exudation. Chorioretinitis and optic atrophy may also be seen. Meningovascular syphilis (at age 2–10 years) is usually slowly progressive, with mental retardation, spasticity, abnormal pupillary response, speech defects, and abnormal CSF. Deafness sometimes occurs. Thickening of the periosteum of the anterior tibias produces saber shins. A bilateral effusion in the knee joints may occur but is not associated with sequelae. Soft inflammatory growths called gummas may develop in the nasal septum, palate, long bones, and subcutaneous tissues.

2. Acquired syphilis—The primary chancre of the genitals, mouth, or anus may occur from genital, anal, or oral sexual contact. If the chancre is missed, signs of secondary syphilis, such as rash, fever, headache, and malaise, may be the first manifestations.

B. Laboratory Findings

1. Darkfield microscopy—Treponemes can be seen in scrapings from a chancre and from moist lesions.

2. Serologic tests for syphilis—There are two general types of serologic tests for syphilis: treponemal and nontreponemal. The latter (Venereal Disease Research Laboratory, or VDRL) is useful for screening and follow-up of known cases. A rapid test (the rapid plasma reagin, or RPR) is useful for screening, but positive sera should be examined further by quantitative nontreponemal and treponemal tests. Positive nontreponemal tests are confirmed with the more specific fluorescent treponemal antibody absorbed (FTA-ABS) test. False-positive FTA-ABS tests are uncommon except with other spirochetal disease.

One or 2 weeks after the onset of primary syphilis (chancre), the FTA-ABS test becomes positive. The VDRL or a similar nontreponemal test usually turns positive a few days later. By the time the secondary stage has been reached, virtually all patients show both positive FTA-ABS and positive nontreponemal tests. During latent and tertiary syphilis, the VDRL may become negative, but the FTA-ABS test usually remains positive. The quantitative VDRL or a similar nontreponemal test should be used to follow-up treated cases (see following discussion).

Positive serologic tests in cord sera may represent passively transferred antibody rather than congenital infection and therefore must be supplemented by a combination of clinical and laboratory data. Elevated total cord IgM is a helpful but nonspecific finding. A specific IgM–FTA-ABS is available, but negative results are not conclusive and should

not be relied on. Demonstration of characteristic treponemes by darkfield examination of material from a moist lesion (skin; nasal or other mucous membranes) is definitive. Serial measurement of quantitative VDRL is also very useful, because passively transferred antibody in the absence of active infection should decay with a normal half-life of about 18 days.

In one study, 15% of infants with congenital syphilis had negative cord blood serology, presumably due to maternal infection late in pregnancy.

C. Imaging

Radiographic abnormalities are present in 90% of infants with symptoms of congenital syphilis and in 20% of asymptomatic infants. Metaphyseal lucent bands, periostitis, and a widened zone of provisional calcification may be present. Bilateral symmetrical osteomyelitis with pathologic fractures of the medial tibial metaphyses (Wimberger sign) is almost pathognomonic.

▶ Differential Diagnosis

A. Congenital Syphilis

1. Newborns—Sepsis, congestive heart failure, congenital rubella, toxoplasmosis, disseminated herpes simplex, cytomegalovirus infection, and hemolytic disease of the newborn have to be differentiated. A positive Coombs test and blood group incompatibility distinguish hemolytic disease.

2. Young infants—Injury to the brachial plexus, poliomyelitis, acute osteomyelitis, and septic arthritis must be differentiated from pseudoparalysis. Coryza due to viral infection often responds to symptomatic treatment. Rash (ammoniacal diaper rash) and scabies may be confused with a syphilitic eruption.

3. Children—Interstitial keratitis and bone lesions of tuberculosis are distinguished by positive tuberculin reaction and chest radiograph. Arthritis associated with syphilis is unaccompanied by systemic signs, and joints are nontender. Mental retardation, spasticity, and hyperactivity are shown to be of syphilitic origin by strongly positive serologic tests.

B. Acquired Syphilis

Herpes genitalis, traumatic lesions, and other venereal diseases must be differentiated.

▶ Prevention

A serologic test for syphilis should be performed at the initiation of prenatal care and repeated at delivery. In mothers at high risk for syphilis, repeated tests may be necessary. Serologic tests may be negative on both the mother and infant at the time of birth if the mother acquires syphilis near term. Adequate treatment of mothers with secondary syphilis before the last month of pregnancy reduces the incidence of congenital syphilis from 90% to less than 2%. Examination and serologic testing of sexual partners and siblings should also be done.

▶ Treatment

A. Specific Measures

Penicillin is the drug of choice for *T pallidum* infection. If the patient is allergic to penicillin, erythromycin or one of the tetracyclines may be used.

1. Congenital syphilis

A. INITIAL EVALUATION AND TREATMENT—Infants born to seropositive mothers require careful examination and quantitative antitreponemal (VDRL, RPR) syphilis testing. The same quantitative antitreponemal test used in evaluating the mother should be used in the infant so the titers can be compared. Maternal records regarding the diagnosis of syphilis, treatment, and follow-up titers should be reviewed. Infants should be further evaluated for congenital syphilis in any of the following circumstances:

- The maternal titer has increased fourfold.
- The infant's titer is at least fourfold greater than the maternal titer.
- Signs of syphilis are found on examination.
- Maternal syphilis was not treated or was inadequately treated during pregnancy.
- Maternal syphilis was treated with a nonpenicillin regimen, or the regimen or dose of medication is undocumented.
- Maternal syphilis was treated during pregnancy, but therapy was completed less than 4 weeks prior to delivery.
- Maternal syphilis was treated appropriately during pregnancy, but without the appropriate decrease in maternal nontreponemal titers after treatment.

The complete evaluation of an infant for possible congenital syphilis includes complete blood count, liver function tests, long bone radiographs, CSF examination (cell counts, glucose, and protein), CSF VDRL, and quantitative serologic tests. In addition, the placenta and umbilical cord should be examined pathologically using fluorescent antitreponemal antibody, if available. An ophthalmologic examination may also be done.

Treatment for congenital syphilis is indicated for infants with physical signs, umbilical cord or placenta positive for DFA-TP staining or darkfield examination, abnormal radiographs, elevated CSF protein or cell counts, reactive CSF VDRL, or serum quantitative nontreponemal titer that is more than fourfold higher than the maternal titer (using same test). Infants with proved or suspected congenital syphilis should receive either (1) aqueous crystalline penicillin G, 50,000 units/kg per dose intravenously every 12 hours (if < 1 week old) or (2) every 8 hours (if 1–4 weeks old) for 10 days. All infants diagnosed after age 4 weeks should receive 50,000–60,000 units/kg per dose aqueous crystalline penicillin intravenously every 6 hours for 10 days.

Additionally, treatment should be given to infants whose mothers have inadequately treated syphilis, to those whose mothers received treatment less than 1 month before delivery, to those whose mothers have undocumented or inadequate serologic response to therapy, and to those whose mothers were given nonpenicillin drugs to treat syphilis. In these instances, if the infant is asymptomatic, has a normal physical examination, normal CSF parameters, nonreactive CSF VDRL, normal bone films, quantitative nontreponemal titer less than fourfold of the mother's titer, and good follow-up is certain, some experts would give a single dose of penicillin G benzathine, 50,000 units/kg intramuscularly. If there is any abnormality in the preceding evaluation or if the CSF testing is not interpretable, the full 10 days of intravenous penicillin should be given. Close clinical and serologic monthly follow-up is necessary.

Asymptomatic, seropositive infants with normal physical examinations born to mothers who received adequate syphilis treatment (completed > 4 weeks prior to delivery) and whose mothers have an appropriate serologic response (fourfold or greater decrease in titer) to treatment may be at lower risk for congenital syphilis. Some experts believe complete laboratory and radiographic evaluation in these infants (CSF and long bone films) is not necessary. Infants who meet the preceding criteria, who have nontreponemal titers less than fourfold higher than maternal titers, and for whom follow-up is certain can be given benzathine penicillin G, 50,000 units/kg, administered intramuscularly in a single dose. Infants should be followed with quantitative serologic tests and physical examinations until the nontreponemal serologic test is negative (see discussion of follow-up, below). Rising titers or clinical signs usually occur within 4 months in infected infants, requiring a full evaluation (including CSF studies and long bone radiographs) and institution of intravenous penicillin therapy.

B. FOLLOW-UP FOR CONGENITAL SYPHILIS—Children treated for congenital syphilis need physical examinations at 1 and 2 months after completion of therapy, and both physical examinations and quantitative VDRL or RPR tests should be performed at 4, 6, and 12 months after the end of therapy or until the tests become nonreactive. Repeat CSF examination, including a CSF VDRL test, every 6 months until normal is indicated for infants with a positive CSF VDRL reaction or with abnormal cell counts or protein in the CSF. A reactive CSF VDRL test at the 6-month interval is an indication for retreatment. Titers decline with treatment and are usually negative by 6 months. Repeat treatment is indicated for children with rising titers or stable titers that do not decline.

2. Acquired syphilis of less than 1 year's duration—

Benzathine penicillin G (50,000 units/kg, given intramuscularly, to a maximum of 2.4 million units) is given to adolescents with primary, secondary, or latent disease of less than 1 year's duration. All children should have a CSF examination (with CSF VDRL) prior to commencing therapy, to exclude neurosyphilis. Adolescents and adults need a CSF examination if clinical signs or symptoms suggest neurologic involvement or if they are HIV-infected.

3. Syphilis of more than 1 year's duration (late latent disease)—Syphilis of more than 1 year's duration (without evidence of neurosyphilis) requires weekly intramuscular benzathine penicillin G therapy for 3 weeks. CSF examination and VDRL test should be done on all children and patients with coexisting HIV infection or neurologic symptoms. In addition, patients who have failed treatment or who were previously treated with an agent other than penicillin need a CSF examination and CSF VDRL.

4. Neurosyphilis—Aqueous crystalline penicillin G is recommended, 200,000–300,000 units/kg/d in four to six divided doses, given intravenously for 10–14 days. The maximum adult dose is 4 million units per dose. This regimen should possibly be followed by an intramuscular course of benzathine G penicillin, 50,000 units/kg given once a week for 3 consecutive weeks, to a maximum dose of 2.4 million units.

B. General Measures

Penicillin treatment of early congenital or secondary syphilis may result in a dramatic systemic febrile illness termed the Jarisch-Herxheimer reaction. Treatment is symptomatic, with careful follow-up. Transfusion may be necessary in infants with severe hemolytic anemia.

Prognosis

Severe disease, if undiagnosed, may be fatal in the newborn. Complete cure can be expected if the young infant is given penicillin. Serologic reversal usually occurs within 1 year. Treatment of primary syphilis with penicillin is curative. Permanent neurologic sequelae may occur in meningovascular syphilis.

Centers for Disease Control and Prevention: Congenital syphilis—United States, 2000. JAMA 2001;286(5):529 [PMID: 11508285].

Chakraborty R, Luck S: Managing congenital syphilis again? The more things change. Curr Opin Infect Dis 2007;20:247 [PMID: 17471033].

Sexually transmitted diseases treatment guidelines—2006. MMWR Recomm Rep 2006;55(RR-11):1 [PMID:16888612].

Walker GJ, Walker DG: Congenital syphilis: A continuing but neglected problem. Semin Fetal Neonat Med 2007;12:198 [PMID: 17336171].

RELAPSING FEVER

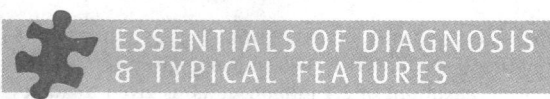

ESSENTIALS OF DIAGNOSIS & TYPICAL FEATURES

► Episodes of fever, chills, malaise.
► Occasional rash, arthritis, cough, hepatosplenomegaly, conjunctivitis.

► Diagnosis confirmed by direct microscopic identification of spirochetes in smears of peripheral blood.

General Considerations

Relapsing fever is a vector-borne disease caused by spirochetes of the genus *Borrelia*. Epidemic relapsing fever is transmitted to humans by body lice (*Pediculus humanus*) and endemic relapsing fever by soft-bodied ticks (genus *Ornithodoros*). Tick-borne relapsing fever is endemic in the western United States. Although several hundred cases are reported per year, substantial underdiagnosis occurs. Transmission usually takes place during the warm months, when ticks are active and recreation or work brings people into contact with *Ornithodoros* ticks. Infection is often acquired in mountain camping areas and cabins. The ticks are nocturnal feeders and remain attached for only 5–20 minutes. Consequently, the patient seldom remembers a tick bite. Rarely, neonatal relapsing fever results from transplacental transmission of *Borrelia*. Both louse-borne and tick-borne relapsing fever may be acquired during foreign travel.

Clinical Findings

A. Symptoms and Signs

The incubation period is 4–18 days. The attack is sudden, with high fever, chills, tachycardia, nausea and vomiting, headache, myalgia, arthralgia, bronchitis, and a dry, nonproductive cough. Hepatomegaly and splenomegaly appear later. Meningeal irritation may be present. An erythematous rash may be seen over the trunk and extremities, and petechiae may be present. After 3–10 days, the fever falls. Jaundice, iritis, conjunctivitis, cranial nerve palsies, and hemorrhage occur more commonly during relapses.

The disease is characterized by relapses at intervals of 1–2 weeks and lasting 3–5 days. The relapses duplicate the initial attack but become progressively less severe. In louse-borne relapsing fever, there is usually a single relapse. In tick-borne infection, two to six relapses occur.

B. Laboratory Findings

During febrile episodes, the patient's urine contains protein, casts, and occasionally erythrocytes; a marked polymorphonuclear leukocytosis is present; and about 25% of patients have a false-positive serologic test for syphilis. Examination of the peripheral blood smear is the diagnostic test of choice. Spirochetes can be found in the peripheral blood by direct microscopy in approximately 70% of cases by darkfield examination or by Wright, Giemsa, or acridine orange staining of thick and thin smears. Spirochetes are not found during afebrile periods. Immunofluorescent antibody (or ELISA confirmed by Western blot) can sometimes help establish the diagnosis serologically. However, high titers of *Borrelia hermsii* can cross-react with *Borrelia burgdorferi* (the agent in Lyme disease) in immunofluorescent antibody assay, ELISA, and Western blots. Serologic specimens can be sent to the Division of Vector-Borne Infectious Diseases, Centers for Disease Control and Prevention, Fort Collins, CO 80522.

Differential Diagnosis

Relapsing fever may be confused with malaria, leptospirosis, dengue, typhus, rat-bite fever, Colorado tick fever, Rocky Mountain spotted fever, collagen-vascular disease, or any fever of unknown origin.

Complications

Complications include facial paralysis, iridocyclitis, optic atrophy, hypochromic anemia, pneumonia, nephritis, myocarditis, endocarditis, and seizures. CNS involvement occurs in 10–30% of patients.

Treatment

For children younger than age 8 years who have tick-borne relapsing fever, standard dosages of penicillin or erythromycin should be given for 10 days. Older children may be given doxycycline. Chloramphenicol is also efficacious and was often used in the past.

Severely ill patients should be hospitalized. Patients may experience a Jarisch-Herxheimer reaction (usually noted in the first few hours after commencing antibiotics). Isolation precautions are not necessary for relapsing fever. Contact precautions are recommended for patients with louse infestations.

Prognosis

The mortality rate in treated cases of relapsing fever is very low, except in debilitated or very young children. With treatment, the initial attack is shortened and relapses prevented. The response to antimicrobial therapy is dramatic.

Cadavid D, Barbour AG: Neuroborreliosis during relapsing fever: Review of the clinical manifestations, pathology, and treatment of infections in humans and experimental animals. Clin Infect Dis 1998;26:151 [PMID: 9455525].

Roscoe C, Epperly T: Tick-borne relapsing fever. Am Fam Physician 2005;72:2046 [PMID: 16342835].

LEPTOSPIROSIS

ESSENTIALS OF DIAGNOSIS & TYPICAL FEATURES

▶ Biphasic course lasting 2–3 weeks.

▶ Initial phase: high fever, headache, myalgia, and conjunctivitis.

▶ Apparent recovery for 2–3 days.

▶ Return of fever associated with meningitis.

▶ Jaundice, hemorrhages, and renal insufficiency (severe cases).

▶ Culture of organism from blood and CSF (early) and from urine (later), or direct microscopy of urine or CSF.

▶ Positive leptospiral agglutination test.

General Considerations

Leptospirosis is a zoonosis caused by many antigenically distinct but morphologically similar spirochetes. The organism enters through the skin or respiratory tract. Classically the severe form (Weil disease), with jaundice and a high mortality rate, was associated with infection with *Leptospira icterohaemorrhagiae* after immersion in water contaminated with rat urine. It is now known that a variety of animals (eg, dogs, rats, and cattle) may serve as reservoirs for pathogenic *Leptospira,* that a given serogroup may have multiple animal species as hosts, and that severe disease may be caused by many different serogroups.

In the United States, leptospirosis usually occurs after contact with dogs. Cattle, swine, or rodents may transmit the organism. Sewer workers, farmers, abattoir workers, animal handlers, and soldiers are at risk for occupational exposure. Outbreaks have resulted from swimming in contaminated streams and harvesting field crops. In the United States, about 100 cases are reported yearly, about one third of them in children.

Clinical Findings

A. Symptoms and Signs

1. Initial phase—The incubation period is 4–19 days (mean, 10 days). Chills, fever, headache, myalgia, conjunctivitis (episcleral injection), photophobia, cervical lymphadenopathy, and pharyngitis commonly occur. The initial leptospiremic phase lasts for 3–7 days.

2. Phase of apparent recovery—Symptoms typically (but not always) subside for 2–3 days.

3. Systemic phase—Fever reappears and is associated with headache, muscular pain and tenderness in the abdomen and back, and nausea and vomiting. Lung, heart, and joint involvement occasionally occurs. These manifestations are due to extensive vasculitis.

A. CENTRAL NERVOUS SYSTEM INVOLVEMENT—The CNS is involved in 50–90% of cases. Severe headache and mild nuchal rigidity are usual, but delirium, coma, and focal neurologic signs may be seen.

B. RENAL AND HEPATIC INVOLVEMENT—In about 50% of cases, the kidney or liver is affected. Gross hematuria and oliguria or anuria is sometimes seen. Jaundice may be associated with an enlarged and tender liver.

c. Gallbladder involvement—Leptospirosis may cause acalculous cholecystitis in children, demonstrable by abdominal ultrasound as a dilated, nonfunctioning gallbladder. Pancreatitis is unusual.

d. Hemorrhage—Petechiae, ecchymoses, and gastrointestinal bleeding may be severe.

e. Rash—A rash is seen in 10–30% of cases. It may be maculopapular and generalized or may be petechial or purpuric. Occasionally erythema nodosum is seen. Peripheral desquamation of the rash may occur. Gangrenous areas are sometimes noted over the distal extremities. In such cases, skin biopsy demonstrates the presence of severe vasculitis involving both the arterial and the venous circulations.

B. Laboratory Findings

Leptospires are present in the blood and CSF only during the first 10 days of illness. They appear in the urine during the second week, where they may persist for 30 days or longer. Culture is difficult and requires specialized media and conditions. The WBC count often is elevated, especially when there is liver involvement. Serum bilirubin levels usually remain below 20 mg/dL. Other liver function tests may be abnormal, although the aspartate transaminase usually is elevated only slightly. An elevated serum creatine kinase is frequently found. CSF shows moderate pleocytosis ($< 500/\mu L$)—predominantly mononuclear cells—increased protein (50–100 mg/dL), and normal glucose. Urine often shows microscopic pyuria, hematuria, and, less often, moderate proteinuria (++ or greater). The ESR is elevated markedly. Chest radiograph may show pneumonitis.

Serologic antibodies measured by enzyme immunoassay may be demonstrated during or after the second week of illness. The serologic test of choice is a microscopic agglutination test using live organisms (performed at the CDC). Leptospiral agglutinins generally reach peak levels by the third to fourth week. A 1:100 titer is considered suspicious; a fourfold or greater rise is diagnostic. A PCR assay may be available at specialized research centers or through the CDC.

Differential Diagnosis

Fever and myalgia associated with the characteristic episcleral injection should suggest leptospirosis. During the prodrome, malaria, typhoid fever, typhus, rheumatoid arthritis, brucellosis, and influenza may be suspected. Later, depending on the organ systems involved, a variety of other diseases need to be distinguished, including encephalitis, viral or tuberculous meningitis, viral hepatitis, glomerulonephritis, viral or bacterial pneumonia, rheumatic fever, subacute infective endocarditis, acute surgical abdomen, and Kawasaki disease (see Table 38–3).

Prevention

Preventive measures include avoidance of contaminated water and soil, rodent control, immunization of dogs and other domestic animals, and good sanitation. Immunization

or antimicrobial prophylaxis with doxycycline may be of value to certain high-risk occupational groups.

Treatment

A. Specific Measures

Aqueous penicillin G (150,000 units/kg/d, given in four to six divided doses intravenously for 7–10 days) should be given when the diagnosis is suspected. Studies in severely ill patients indicate a benefit even if treatment is started 4 days after onset. A Jarisch-Herxheimer reaction may occur. Oral doxycycline may be used for mildly ill patients.

B. General Measures

Symptomatic and supportive care is indicated, particularly for renal and hepatic failure and hemorrhage. Contact isolation is recommended, due to potential transmission from contact with urine.

Prognosis

Leptospirosis is usually self-limiting and not characterized by jaundice. The disease usually lasts 1–3 weeks but may be more prolonged. Relapse may occur. There are usually no permanent sequelae associated with CNS infection, although headache may persist. The mortality rate in the United States is 5%, usually from renal failure. The mortality rate may reach 20% or more in elderly patients who have severe kidney and hepatic involvement.

Bharti AR et al; Peru-United States Leptospirosis Consortium: Leptospirosis: A zoonotic disease of global importance. Lancet Infect Dis 2003;3:757 [PMID: 14652202].

Levett PN: Leptospirosis. Clin Microbiol Rev 2001;14:296 [PMID: 11292640].

Palaniappan RU et al: Leptospirosis: Pathogenesis, immunity, and diagnosis. Curr Opin Infect Dis 2007;20:284 [PMID: 17471039].

LYME DISEASE

ESSENTIALS OF DIAGNOSIS & TYPICAL FEATURES

▶ Characteristic skin lesion (erythema migrans) 3–30 days after tick bite.

▶ Arthritis, usually pauciarticular, occurring about 4 weeks after appearance of skin lesion. Headache, chills, and fever.

▶ Residence or travel in an endemic area during the late spring to early fall.

General Considerations

Lyme disease is a subacute or chronic spirochetal infection caused by *Borrelia burgdorferi* and transmitted by the bite of an infected deer tick (*Ixodes* species). The disease was known in Europe for many years as tick-borne encephalomyelitis, often associated with a characteristic rash (erythema migrans). Discovery of the agent and vector followed investigation of an outbreak of pauciarticular arthritis in Lyme, Connecticut, in 1977.

Although cases are reported from many countries, the most prominent endemic areas in the United States include the Northeast, upper Midwest, and West Coast. The northern European countries also have high rates of infection. More than 20,000 cases were reported in the United States in 2005. The disease is spreading as a result of increased infection in and distribution of the tick vector. Most cases with rash are recognized in spring and summer, when most tick bites occur; however, because the incubation period for joint and neurologic disease may be months, cases may present at any time. *Ixodes* ticks are very small, and their bite often is unrecognized.

▶ Clinical Findings

A. Symptoms and Signs

Erythema chronicum migrans, the most characteristic feature of Lyme disease, develops in 60–80% of patients. Between 3 and 30 days after the bite, a ring of erythema develops at the site and spreads over days. It may attain a diameter of 20 cm. The center of the lesion may clear (resembling tinea corporis), remain red, or become raised (suggesting a chemical or infectious cellulitis). Many patients are otherwise asymptomatic. Some have fever (usually low-grade), headache, and myalgias. Multiple satellite skin lesions, urticaria, or diffuse erythema may occur. Untreated, the rash lasts days to 3 weeks.

In up to 50% of patients, arthritis develops several weeks to months after the bite. Recurrent attacks of migratory, monarticular, or pauciarticular arthritis involving the knees and other large joints occur. Each attack lasts for days to a few weeks. Fever is common and may be high. Complete resolution between attacks is typical. Chronic arthritis develops in less than 10% of patients, more often in those with the DR4 haplotype.

Neurologic manifestations develop in up to 20% of patients and usually consist of Bell palsy, aseptic meningitis (which may be indistinguishable from viral meningitis), or polyradiculitis. Peripheral neuritis, Guillain-Barré syndrome, encephalitis, ataxia, chorea, and other cranial neuropathies are less common. Seizures suggest another diagnosis. Untreated, the neurologic symptoms are usually self-limited but may be chronic or permanent. Although fatigue and nonspecific neurologic symptoms may be prolonged in a few patients, Lyme disease is not a cause of chronic fatigue syndrome. Self-limited heart block or myocardial dysfunction occurs in about 5% of patients.

B. Laboratory Findings

Most patients with only rash have normal laboratory tests. Children with arthritis may have moderately elevated ESRs and WBC counts; the antinuclear antibodies and rheumatoid factor tests are negative or nonspecific; streptococcal antibodies are not elevated. Circulating IgM cryoglobulins may be present. Joint fluid may show up to 100,000 cells with a polymorphonuclear predominance, normal glucose, and elevated protein and immune complexes; Gram stain and culture are negative. In patients with CNS involvement, the CSF may show lymphocytic pleocytosis and elevated protein; the glucose and all cultures and stains are normal or negative. Abnormal nerve conduction may be present with peripheral neuropathy.

C. Diagnosis

Lyme disease is a clinical diagnosis. History, physical examination, and laboratory features are important to consider. The causative organism is difficult to culture. Serologic testing may support the clinical diagnosis. Antibody testing should be performed in experienced laboratories. Serologic diagnosis of Lyme disease is based on a two-test approach: an ELISA and an immunoblot to confirm a positive or indeterminate ELISA. Antibodies may not be detectable until several weeks after infection has occurred; therefore, serologic testing in children with a typical rash is not recommended. Therapy early in disease may blunt antibody titers. Recent studies have shown considerable intralaboratory and interlaboratory variability in titers reported. Overdiagnosis of Lyme disease based on atypical symptoms and positive serology appears to be common. Sera from patients with syphilis, HIV, and leptospirosis may give false-positive results. Patients who receive appropriate treatment for Lyme disease may remain seropositive for years. Diagnosis of CNS disease requires objective abnormalities of the neurologic examination, laboratory or radiographic studies, and consistent positive serology.

▶ Differential Diagnosis

Aside from the disorders already mentioned, the rash may resemble pityriasis, erythema multiforme, a drug eruption, or erythema nodosum. Erythema chronicum migrans is nonscaly, minimally tender or nontender, and persists longer in the same place than many of the more common childhood erythematous rashes. The arthritis may resemble juvenile rheumatoid arthritis, reactive arthritis, septic arthritis, reactive effusion from a contiguous osteomyelitis, rheumatic fever, leukemic arthritis, systemic lupus erythematosus, and Henoch-Schönlein purpura. Spontaneous resolution in a few days to weeks helps differentiate Lyme disease from juvenile rheumatoid arthritis, in which arthritis lasting a minimum of 6 weeks is required for diagnosis. The neurologic signs may suggest idiopathic Bell palsy, viral or parainfectious meningitis or meningoencephalitis, lead poisoning, psychosomatic illness, and many other conditions.

▶ Prevention

Prevention consists of avoidance of endemic areas, wearing long sleeves and pants, frequent checks for ticks, and application of tick repellents. Ticks usually are attached for 24–48 hours before transmission of Lyme disease occurs. Ticks should be removed with a tweezer by pulling gently without twisting or excessive squeezing of the tick. Permethrin sprayed on clothing decreases tick attachment. Repellents containing high concentrations of DEET may be neurotoxic and should be used cautiously and washed off when tick exposure ends. The CDC does not recommend prophylactic antibiotics for tick bites in asymptomatic individuals.

▶ Treatment

Antimicrobial therapy is beneficial in most cases of Lyme disease. It is most effective if started early. Prolonged treatment is important for all forms. Relapses occur in some patients on all regimens.

A. Rash, Early Infections

Amoxicillin, 25–50 mg/kg/d orally in two divided doses (to a maximum of 2 g/d) for 14–21 days can be used for children of all ages. Doxycycline (100 mg orally twice a day) for 14–21 days may be used for children older than age 8 years. Erythromycin (30 mg/kg/d) or cefuroxime is used in penicillin-allergic children, although erythromycin may be less effective than amoxicillin.

B. Arthritis

The amoxicillin or doxycycline regimen (same dosage as for the rash) should be used, but treatment should continue for 4 weeks. Parenteral ceftriaxone (75–100 mg/kg/d) or penicillin G (300,000 units/kg/d, given intravenously in four divided doses for 2–4 weeks) is used for persistent arthritis.

C. Bell Palsy

The same oral drug regimens may be used for 3–4 weeks.

D. Other Neurologic Disease or Cardiac Disease

Parenteral therapy for 2–3 weeks is recommended with either ceftriaxone (75–100 kg/d in one daily dose) or penicillin G (300,000 units/kg/d intravenously in four divided doses).

Arnez M: Antibiotic treatment of children with erythema migrans. Clin Infect Dis 2007;44:1133 [PMIC: 17366464].

Centers for Disease Control and Prevention: Lyme disease. http://www.cdc.gov/ncidod/dvbid/lyme

CDC: Lyme disease—United States, 2003–2005. MMWR Morb Mortal Wkly Rep 2007;56:573 [PMID: 17568368].

Halperin JJ et al: Practice parameter: Treatment of nervous system Lyme disease (an evidence-based review): Report of the Quality Standards Subcommittee of the American Academy of Neurology. Neurology 2007;69:91 [PMID: 17522387].

Infections: Parasitic & Mycotic

Samuel R. Dominguez, MD, PhD

Adriana Weinberg, MD

Myron J. Levin, MD

▼ PARASITIC INFECTIONS

Parasitic diseases are common and may present clinically in a variety of ways (Table 41–1). Although travel to endemic areas suggests particular infections, many are transmitted through fomites or acquired from contact with human carriers and can occur anywhere. Some of the less common parasitic infections and those seen primarily in the developing world are presented in abbreviated form in Table 41–2.

Selection of Patients for Evaluation

The incidence of parasitic infections varies greatly with geographic area. Children who have traveled or lived in areas where parasitic infections are endemic are at risk for infection with a variety of intestinal and tissue parasites. Children who have resided only in developed countries are usually free of tissue parasites (except *Toxoplasma*). Searching for intestinal parasites is expensive for the patient and time-consuming for the laboratory. More than 90% of ova and parasite examinations performed in most hospital laboratories in the United States are negative; many have been ordered inappropriately. An approach to determining which children with diarrhea need such examinations is presented in Figure 41–1. It can be more cost-effective to treat symptomatic U.S. immigrants with albendazole or nitazoxanide, broad-spectrum antiparasitic drugs, and to investigate only those whose symptoms persist.

Immunodeficient children are very susceptible to protozoal intestinal infections. Multiple opportunists are frequently identified, and the threshold for ordering tests should be low for these children.

Specimen Processing

For tissue parasites, contact the laboratory for proper collection procedures. Diarrheal stools may contain trophozoites that die rapidly during transport. The specimen should be either examined immediately or placed in a stool fixative such as polyvinyl alcohol. Fixative vials for home collection of stool are available. They may contain toxic compounds, so they should be stored safely. Fixed specimens are stable at room temperature. Formed stools usually contain cysts that are more stable. It is also best to fix these after collection, although they may be reliably examined after transport at room temperature.

Eosinophilia & Parasitic Infections

Although some parasites commonly cause eosinophilia, in developed countries other causes are much more common and include allergies, drugs, and other infections. Heavy intestinal nematode infections cause eosinophilia; they are easily detected on a single ova and parasite examination. Light nematode infections and common protozoal infections—giardiasis, cryptosporidiosis, and amebiasis—rarely cause eosinophilia. Eosinophilia is also unusual or minimal in more serious infections such as amebic liver abscess and malaria.

The most common parasitic infection in the United States that causes significant eosinophilia with negative stool examination is toxocariasis. In a young child with unexplained eosinophilia and a negative stool examination, a serologic test for *Toxocara* may be the next appropriate test. Trichinosis is a rare cause of marked eosinophilia; strongyloidiasis is a cause of eosinophilia that may be difficult to diagnose with stool examinations. The differential diagnosis of eosinophilia is broad for patients who have been in developing countries (see Table 41–1).

Table 41–1. Signs and symptoms of parasitic infection.

Sign/Symptom	Agent	Comments[a]
Abdominal pain	*Anisakis*	Shortly after raw fish ingestion.
	Ascaris	Heavy infection may obstruct bowel, biliary tract.
	Clonorchis	Heavy, early infection. Hepatomegaly later.
	Entamoeba histolytica	Hematochezia, variable fever, diarrhea.
	Fasciola hepatica	Diarrhea, vomiting.
	Hookworm	Iron deficiency anemia with heavy infection.
	Strongyloides	Eosinophilia, pruritus. May resemble peptic disease.
	Trichinella	Myalgia, periorbital edema, eosinophilia.
	Trichuris	Diarrhea, dysentery with heavy infection.
Cough	*Ascaris*	Wheezing, eosinophilia during migration phase.
	Paragonimus westermani	Hemoptysis; chronic. May mimic tuberculosis.
	Strongyloides	Wheezing, pruritus, eosinophilia during migration or dissemination.
	Toxocara	Affects ages 1–5 y; hepatosplenomegaly; eosinophilia.
	Tropical eosinophilia	Pulmonary infiltrates, eosinophilia.
Diarrhea	*Blastocystis*	Possibly with heavy infection in immunosuppressed or immunocompetent individuals.
	Cyclospora	Watery; severe in immunosuppressed individuals
	Cryptosporidium	Watery; prolonged in normals, chronic in immunosuppressed individuals.
	Dientamoeba fragilis	Only with heavy infection.
	Entamoeba histolytica	Hematochezia, variable fever; no eosinophilia.
	Giardia	Afebrile, chronic; anorexia
	Schistosoma	Chronic; hepatosplenomegaly (some types).
	Strongyloides	Abdominal pain; eosinophilia.
	Trichinella	Myalgia, periorbital edema, eosinophilia.
	Trichuris	With heavy infection.
Dysentery	*Balantidium coli*	Swine contact.
	Entamoeba histolytica	Few to no leukocytes in stool; fever; hematochezia.
	Schistosoma	During acute infection.
	Trichuris	With heavy infection.
Dysuria	*Enterobius*	Usually girls with worms in urethra, bladder; nocturnal, perianal pruritus.
	Schistosoma	Hematuria. Exclude bacteriuria, stones (some types).
Headache (and other cerebral symptoms)	*Angiostrongylus*	Eosinophilic meningitis.
	Naegleria	Fresh-water swimming; rapidly progressive meningoencephalitis.
	Plasmodium	Fever, chills, jaundice, splenomegaly. Cerebral ischemia (with *P falciparum*).
	Taenia solium	Cysticercosis. Focal seizures, deficits; hydrocephalus, aseptic meningitis.
	Toxoplasma	Meningoencephalitis (especially in infants and the immunosuppressed); hydrocephalus in infants.
	Trypanosoma	African forms. Chronic lethargy (sleeping sickness).
Pruritus	*Ancylostoma braziliense*	Creeping eruption; dermal serpiginous burrow.
	Enterobius	Perianal, nocturnal.
	Filaria	Variable; seen in many filarial diseases.
	Hookworm	Local at penetration site in heavy exposure.
	Strongyloides	Diffuse with migration; may be recurrent.
	Trypanosoma	African forms; one of many nonspecific symptoms.

(continued)

Table 41–1. Signs and symptoms of parasitic infection. *(Continued)*

Sign/Symptom	Agent	Comments[a]
Fever	*Entamoeba histolytica*	With acute dysentery or liver abscess.
	Leishmania donovani	Hepatosplenomegaly, anemia, leukopenia.
	Plasmodium	Chills, headache, jaundice; periodic.
	Toxocara	Cough, hepatosplenomegaly, eosinophilia.
	Toxoplasma	Generalized adenopathy; splenomegaly.
	Trichinella	Myalgia, periorbital edema, eosinophilia.
	Trypanosoma	Early stage, African forms; lymphadenopathy.
Anemia	*Diphyllobothrium*	Megaloblastic due to B_{12} deficiency; rare.
	Hookworm	Iron deficiency.
	Leishmania donovani	Fever, hepatosplenomegaly, leukopenia (kala-azar).
	Plasmodium	Hemolysis.
	Trichuris	Heavy infection; due to iron loss.
Eosinophilia	*Angiostrongylus*	Eosinophilic meningitis.
	Fasciola	Abdominal pain.
	Filaria	Microfilariae in blood; lymphadenopathy.
	Onchocerca	Skin nodules, keratitis.
	Schistosoma	Chronic; intestinal or genitourinary symptoms.
	Strongyloides	Abdominal pain, diarrhea.
	Toxocara	Hepatosplenomegaly, cough; affects ages 1–5 y.
	Trichinella	Myalgia, periorbital edema.
	Tropical pulmonary eosinophilia	Cough.
Hematuria	*Schistosoma*	*S haematobium.* Bladder, urethral granulomas. Exclude stones, bacteriuria.
Hemoptysis	*Paragonimus westermani*	Lung fluke. Variable chest pain; chronic.
Hepatomegaly	*Clonorchis*	Heavy infection. Tenderness early; cirrhosis late.
	Echinococcus	Chronic; cysts.
	Entamoeba histolytica	Toxic hepatitis or abscess. No eosinophilia.
	Leishmania donovani	Splenomegaly, fever, pancytopenia.
	Schistosoma	Chronic; hepatic fibrosis, splenomegaly (some types).
	Toxocara	Splenomegaly, eosinophilia, cough; no adenopathy.
Splenomegaly	*Leishmania donovani*	Hepatomegaly, fever, anemia.
	Plasmodium	Fever, chills, jaundice, headache.
	Schistosoma	Hepatomegaly.
	Toxocara	Eosinophilia, hepatomegaly.
	Toxoplasma	Lymphadenopathy, other symptoms.
Lymphadenopathy	Filaria	Inguinal typical; chronic.
	Leishmania donovani	Hepatosplenomegaly, pancytopenia, fever.
	Schistosoma	Acute infection; fever, rash, arthralgia, hepatosplenomegaly.
	Toxoplasma	Cervical common; may involve single site; splenomegaly.
	Trypanosoma	Localized near bite or generalized; hepatosplenomegaly (Chagas disease); generalized (especially posterior cervical) in African forms.

[a]Symptoms usually related to degree of infestation. Infestation with small numbers of organisms is often asymptomatic.

Table 41–2. Some parasitic infections seen less commonly in developed regions.

Agent (Disease)	Geographic Region	Vector	Symptoms and Signs	Laboratory Findings	Diagnosis	Therapy and Comments
Angiostrongylus cantonensis (eosinophilic meningitis)	Hawaii, Asia, Pacific Islands	Snails, slugs	Ingestion (usually inadvertent) followed in 1–4 wk by meningitis of variable severity. Paresthesias.	Eosinophils in CSF and blood	Positive serology. Larvae may be present in CSF.	Fever absent or low. No focal lesions on CNS imaging. No specific therapy. Steroids may be beneficial. Mebendazole may help.
Clonorchis sinensis (liver fluke infection)	Asia	Raw fish	Adult flukes obstruct biliary tree. Acute: hepatomegaly, fever, jaundice, urticaria. Late: cirrhosis, carcinoma.	Variable liver function abnormalities	Ova in feces.	Praziquantel. Advanced disease not treatable. Liver transplant.
Leishmania braziliensis, L mexicana (chiclero ulcer)	South America	Sandfly	Painful mucocutaneous ulcers or granulomas. Nasolabial lesions common.	—	Skin biopsy. Positive skin test, serology.	Same as for *L donovani;* ketoconazole.
Leishmania donovani (kala-azar)	Mideast, India, Mediterranean, South and Central America	Sandfly	Fever, generalized adenopathy, hepatosplenomegaly weeks to months after infection.	Pancytopenia, hypergammaglobulinemia	Organisms in skin biopsy. Positive skin test, serology.	Sodium stibogluconate, meglumine antimonate, pentamidine, amphotericin B.
Leishmania tropica (Oriental sore)	Asia, India, North Africa	Sandfly	Papule at bite site (usually on face, limbs) develops after weeks to months, then ulcerates and scars.	—	Organisms in skin biopsy. Positive skin test, serology.	Same as for *L donovani.*
Paragonimus westermani (lung fluke infection)	Asia, South America, Africa	Raw crabs, crustaceans	Cough, hemoptysis. Rarely seizures, other CNS signs if migration to brain occurs.	—	Large ova in concentrated specimens, feces. Cystic nodular lesions on chest radiograph or CNS imaging.	Resembles pulmonary tuberculosis. Praziquantel very effective.
Trypanosoma brucei (sleeping sickness)	Africa	Tsetse fly	Hepatosplenomegaly, adenopathy. Nodule at bite site (resolves). Recurrent fever, headache, myalgia, progressive encephalitis.	Elevated ESR, anemia, CSF pleocytosis	Organisms in marrow, nodes, spleen. Positive serology.	Suramin, eflornithine, pentamidine, melarsoprol.
Trypanosoma cruzi (Chagas disease)	South and Central America, Mexico	Reduviid bug	Acute: painful red nodule at bite site, conjunctivitis, periorbital edema (Romaña sign), fever, local ± generalized adenitis. Late: myocarditis, megaesophagus, megacolon.	Mononuclear leukocytosis	Organisms in peripheral blood. Positive serology.	Nifurtimox or benznidazole may help early. No therapy for late disease. May be transmitted by blood transfusion or congenitally.
Wuchereria, Brugia (filariasis)	Tropics, subtropics	Mosquito	Chronic adenopathy, often inguinal. Obstructive lymphedema.	Eosinophilia	Concentrated blood smears for larvae. Positive serology.	Diethylcarbamazine kills larvae. Surgery for lymphatic obstruction.

CNS, central nervous system; CSF, cerebrospinal fluid; ESR, erythrocyte sedimentation rate.

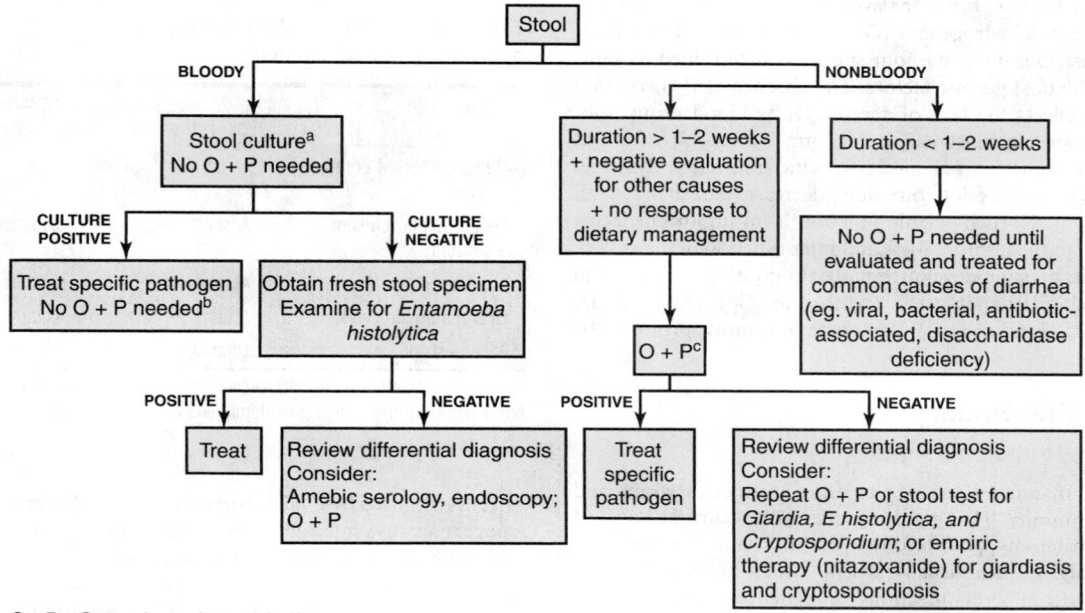

Figure 41–1. Parasitologic evaluation of acute diarrhea.

O + P = Ova and parasite examination.

[a]*Shigella, Salmonella, Campylobacter, E coli (Escherichia coli)* O 157, *Yersinia*: assay for *Clostridium difficile* toxin if recent antimicrobial use.

[b]Unless critically ill, from endemic area for amebiasis, or unresponsive to standard therapy.

[c]Include examination for *Cryptosporidium* and *Cyclospora*; immediate stool fixation needed if stool is diarrheal.

PROTOZOAL INFECTIONS

SYSTEMIC INFECTIONS

1. Malaria

 ESSENTIALS OF DIAGNOSIS & TYPICAL FEATURES

▸ Residence in or travel to an endemic area.

▸ Cyclic paroxysms of chills, fever, and intense sweating.

▸ Headache, backache, cough, abdominal pain, nausea, vomiting, diarrhea.

▸ Coma, seizures.

▸ Splenomegaly, anemia.

▸ Malaria parasites in peripheral blood smear.

▸ General Considerations

Malaria kills a million children worldwide each year and is undergoing a resurgence in areas where it was previously controlled. Approximately 1000 imported cases are diagnosed in the United States each year; local transmission may also occasionally take place from imported cases. The female anopheline mosquito transmits the parasites—*Plasmodium vivax* (most common), *P falciparum* (most virulent), *P ovale* (similar to *P vivax*), and *P malariae*. The gametocytes ingested from an infected human form sporozoites in the mosquito; when these are inoculated into a susceptible host, they infect hepatocytes. The preerythrocytic phase (hepatic) is about 1–2 weeks for all but *P malariae* infection (3–5 weeks), but the initial symptoms may be delayed for up to a year in *P falciparum*, 4 years in *P vivax*, and decades in *P malariae* infections. Merozoites released into the circulation from hepatocytes infect red cells (young cells by *P vivax* and *P ovale*, old cells by *P malariae*, and all cells by *P falciparum*) and begin the synchronous erythrocytic cycles, rupturing the infected cells at regular 48- or 72-hour intervals. Asynchronous cycles causing daily fevers are most common in early stages of infection. Survival is associated with a progressive decrease in intensity of cycles; relapses years later may occur from persistent hepatic infection, which occurs in *P vivax*, *P ovale* and *P malariae* infections. Infection acquired congenitally or from transfusions or needlesticks does not result in a hepatic phase.

Susceptibility varies genetically; certain red cell phenotypes are partially resistant to *P falciparum* infection (hemoglobin S, hemoglobin F, thalassemia, and possibly glucose-6-phosphate dehydrogenase [G6PD] deficiency). The worldwide distribution of the four species is determined to some extent by host genetic factors. The absence of *P vivax* from Africa reflects the lack of specific Duffy blood group substances among most native Africans. Recurrent infections result in some natural species-specific immunity; this does not prevent infection but does decrease parasitemia and symptoms. Normal splenic function is an important factor because of the immunologic and filter function of the spleen. Asplenic persons develop rapidly progressive malaria with many circulating infected erythrocytes (including mature forms of *P falciparum*). Maternal immunity protects the neonate.

▶ Clinical Findings

A. Symptoms and Signs

Clinical manifestations vary according to species, strain, and host immunity. The infant presents with recurrent bouts of fever, irritability, poor feeding, vomiting, jaundice, and splenomegaly. Rash is usually absent, which helps distinguish malaria from viral infections in patients presenting with similar symptoms. In older children, the pathognomonic constellation of headache, backache, chills, myalgia, and fatigue is more easily elicited. Fever may be cyclic (every 48 hours for all but *P malariae* infection, in which it occurs every 72 hours) or irregular (most commonly observed with *P falciparum*). Between attacks, patients may look quite well. If the disease is untreated, relapses cease within a year in *P falciparum* and within several years in *P vivax* infections, but may recur decades later with *P malariae* infection. Infection during pregnancy often causes intrauterine growth restriction or premature delivery, but rarely true fetal infection.

Physical examination in patients with uncomplicated cases may show only mild splenomegaly and anemia.

B. Laboratory Findings

The diagnosis of malaria relies on detection of one or more of the four human plasmodia in blood smears. Most acute infections are caused by *P vivax, P ovale,* or *P falciparum,* although 5–7% are due to multiple species. Giemsa-stained thick smears offer the highest diagnostic accuracy for malaria parasites. Identification of the *Plasmodium* species relies on morphologic criteria (Table 41–3) and requires an experienced observer.

Alternative techniques of similar or higher diagnostic accuracy for *P falciparum* include enzyme-linked immunosorbent assay (ELISA), DNA hybridization, and polymerase chain reaction (PCR). Rapid antigen detection tests (RDTs) have recently been developed and are starting to be used in malaria endemic areas in Africa. A unique feature of the microscopic examination is the semiquantitative estimate of the parasitemia, which is best done on thin smears. This information is particularly useful in the management of

Table 41–3. Differentiation of malaria parasites on blood smears.

	Plasmodium falciparum	*P vivax, P ovale*
Multiple infected erythrocytes	Common	Rare
Mature trophozoites or schizonts	Absent[a]	Common
Schüffner dots	Absent	Common
Enlarged erythrocytes	Absent	Common
Banana-shaped gametocytes	Common	Absent

[a]Usually sequestered in the microcirculation. Rare cases with circulating forms have extremely high parasitemia and a poor prognosis.

infections caused by *P falciparum,* in which high parasitemia (more than 10% infected erythrocytes or more than 500,000 infected erythrocytes/μL) is associated with high morbidity and mortality and requires hospitalization. Treatment response of *P falciparum* and chloroquine-resistant *P vivax* infections is best monitored by daily parasitemia assays. Constant or increased number of infected erythrocytes after 48 hours of treatment or after the second hemolytic crisis suggests an inadequate therapeutic response. Other laboratory findings that reflect the severity of hemolysis include decreased hematocrit, hemoglobin, and haptoglobin levels; increased reticulocyte count; and hyperbilirubinemia and increased lactate dehydrogenase. Thrombocytopenia is common, but the incidence of leukocytosis is variable.

▶ Differential Diagnosis

Relapsing fever may be associated with borreliosis, brucellosis, sequential common infections, Hodgkin disease, juvenile rheumatoid arthritis, rat-bite fever, or one of the idiopathic periodic fevers. Other common causes of high fever and headache include influenza, *Mycoplasma pneumoniae* or enteroviral infection, sinusitis, meningitis, enteric fever, tuberculosis, occult pneumonia, or bacteremia. Fever, headache, and jaundice in a patient returning from tropical areas indicate that leptospirosis and yellow fever should be included in the differential diagnosis. Malaria may also coexist with other diseases.

▶ Complications & Sequelae

Severe complications are limited to *P falciparum* infection and result from microvascular obstruction and tissue ischemia. Impaired consciousness and seizures are the most common complications of malaria in children. In addition, respiratory failure, renal impairment, severe bleeding, and shock are associated with a poor prognosis. Among the laboratory abnormalities, hypoglycemia, acidosis, elevated aminotransferases, and parasitemia greater than 10% characterize severe malaria.

Prevention

Malaria chemoprophylaxis should be instituted 2 weeks (weekly regimens) to 2 days (daily regimens) before traveling to an area of endemic infection to permit changes if the drug is not tolerated. Because the antimalarial drugs recommended for prophylaxis do not kill sporozoites, therapy should be continued for 1 week (atovaquone–proguanil) or 4 weeks (all other regimens) after returning from an endemic area to cover infection acquired at departure.

Chloroquine is the drug of choice for prophylaxis of *P vivax, P ovale, P malariae,* and chloroquine-sensitive *P falciparum* (Table 41–4). Chloroquine is safe for all ages and during pregnancy. Side effects (dizziness, blurred vision, and headache) can be reduced by administering half of the weekly dose twice per week. Effects of chloroquine on heart rhythm are infrequent and are typically associated with rapid intravenous infusion or overdosage. Chloroquine has immunosuppressive properties and has been reported to impair immunization against rabies but not against yellow fever.

For chloroquine-resistant *P falciparum,* the regimens of choice are weekly mefloquine, daily doxycycline, or daily atovaquone–proguanil. The side effects of mefloquine are headache, dizziness, and blurred vision. This drug is now considered safe during pregnancy, but is not used in children weighing less than 5 kg. Daily doxycycline is recommended for patients older than age 8 years who are unable to tolerate mefloquine. Women on prolonged doxycycline therapy tend to develop yeast vaginitis, and it is advisable to supply them with nystatin suppositories. Atovaquone–proguanil is better tolerated than mefloquine. For optimal absorption, this drug should be administered with food or no later than 45 minutes after a meal. Daily primaquine is also effective. Primaquine is also used to prevent relapse of *P vivax* or *P ovale* infections. Primaquine is contraindicated for patients with G6PD deficiency, in whom it induces hemolysis. Less effective alternatives include chloroquine plus proguanil or chloroquine alone, with one therapeutic dose of pyrimethamine–sulfadoxine made available for self-treatment in the advent of potential breakthrough, signaled by fever while in areas where medical attention is not readily available.

No drug regimen guarantees protection against malaria. If fever develops within 1 year (particularly within 2 months) after travel to an endemic area, patients should be advised to seek medical attention. Insect repellents, insecticide-impregnated bed nets, and proper clothing are important adjuncts for malaria prophylaxis.

Treatment

Treatment for malaria includes a variety of supportive strategies in addition to the antimalarial drugs. It is advisable to hospitalize nonimmune patients infected with *P falciparum*

Table 41–4. Chemoprophylaxis of malaria.[a]

Drug	Dosage
Chloroquine-sensitive areas[b]	
Chloroquine	5 mg base/kg/wk up to 300 mg (adult dose)
Chloroquine-resistant areas	
Mefloquine	0.125 tablet (31.25 mg) once a week (5–10 kg)
	0.25 tablet (62.5 mg) once a week (11–20 kg)
	0.5 tablet (125 mg) (21–30 kg)
	0.75 tablet (187.5 mg) (31–45 kg)
	1 tablet (250 mg) (> 45 kg)
Doxycycline	2 mg/kg/daily (age > 8 y) up to 100 mg (adult dose)
Atovaquone–proguanil	11–20 kg: 62.5 mg/25 mg daily (1 pediatric tablet)
	21–30 kg: 125 mg/50 mg daily (2 pediatric tablets)
	31–40 kg: 187.5 mg/75 mg daily (3 pediatric tablets)
	> 40 kg: 250 mg/100 mg (1 adult tablet)
Primaquine	0.6 mg/kg base daily up to 30 mg (adult dose)
Chloroquine Plus	As above
Proguanil	50 mg daily (age < 2 y)
	100 mg (age 2–6 y)
	150 mg (age 7–10 y)
	200 mg (age > 10 y)
Self-presumptive therapy	
Atovaquone–proguanil (carry a course for self-treatment of febrile illness when medical care is not immediately available)	< 5 kg: not indicated
	5–8 kg: 2 pediatric tablets daily × 3 d
	> 8–10 kg: 3 pediatric tablets daily × 3 d
	> 10–20 kg: 1 adult tablet daily × 3 d
	> 20–30 kg: 2 adult tablets daily × 3 d
	> 30–40 kg: 3 adult tablets daily × 3 d
	> 40 kg: 4 adult tablets daily × 3 d
Relapse of *P vivax* or *P ovale*[c]	
Primaquine	0.3 mg base/kg/d up to 15 mg (adult dose) during the last 2 wk of prophylaxis

[a]Updated malaria chemoprophylaxis information may be obtained by calling the Centers for Disease Control and Prevention Hot Line at (404) 332-4555 or on the web at http://www.cdc.gov.
[b]Chloroquine-resistant *Plasmodium falciparum* has not yet been identified in Central America west of the Panama Canal zone, Haiti, Dominican Republic, Mexico, and most of the Middle East.
[c]Optional. Observation and prompt initiation of treatment when relapse occurs is sufficient.

until a decrease in parasitemia is demonstrated, indicating that treatment is effective and severe complications are unlikely to occur.

Partially immune patients with uncomplicated *P falciparum* infection and nonimmune persons infected with *P vivax*, *P ovale*, or *P malariae* can receive treatment as outpatients if follow-up is reliable. For children, hydration and treatment of hypoglycemia are of utmost importance. Anemia, seizures, pulmonary edema, and renal failure require conventional management. Corticosteroids are contraindicated for cerebral malaria because of increased mortality. In severe malaria, exchange transfusion can be lifesaving, particularly in nonimmune persons with parasitemia greater than 15%.

Choice of antimalarial treatment depends on the immune status of the person, plasmodium species, degree of parasitemia, and geographical region of acquisition. An algorithm for the treatment of malaria is shown in Figure 41–2 and a description of the recommended antimalarial drugs available in the United States is provided in Table 41–5. Artemisinin derivatives clear parasites very rapidly and are now widely used as key components in malaria treatment worldwide, but currently they are not available in the United States.

Chen LH et al: Controversies and misconceptions in malaria chemoprophylaxis for travelers. JAMA 2007;297:2251 [PMID: 17519415].

Griffith KS et al: Treatment of malaria in the United States. JAMA 2007;297:2264 [PMID: 17519416].

2. Babesiosis

Babesia microti is a malaria-like protozoan that infects and lyses erythrocytes of wild and domestic animals in North America and Europe. In the United States, human babesiosis has been identified in the coastal areas of New England, northern California and Washington State, and in the lakes region of the upper Midwest. Humans accidentally enter the cycle when bitten by *Ixodes scapularis* (deer tick), one of the intermediate hosts and vectors of *B microti*. After inoculation, the protozoan penetrates the erythrocytes and starts an asynchronous cycle that causes hemolysis.

▶ Clinical Findings

A. Symptoms and Signs

The incubation period is 1–3 weeks but may extend up to 6 weeks. Many times the tick bite is unnoticed. Symptoms are nonspecific and include sustained or cyclic fever up to 40°C, shaking chills, malaise, myalgias, headache, and dark urine. Hepatosplenomegaly is an uncommon finding. The disease is usually self-limited, but severe cases have been described in asplenic patients and immunocompromised hosts. Because they share a common vector, physicians should consider the

possibility of coinfection with *Borrelia burgdorferi* or *Anaplasma phagocytophilum* in any patient diagnosed with *Babesia* infection.

B. Laboratory Findings

The presence of viral infection-like symptoms and identification of babesial parasites in blood by microscopic evaluation of thin or thick blood smears or by PCR amplification of babesial DNA is required to make the diagnosis. *Babesia* parasites are intraerythrocytic organisms that resemble *P falciparum* ring forms. Specific serologic tests are also available through the Centers for Disease Control and Prevention.

▶ Treatment

Clindamycin (7–10 mg/kg, up to 600 mg, every 8 hours) in combination with quinine (8 mg/kg, up to 650 mg, every 8 hours) or azithromycin (10 mg/kg up to 500 mg on the first day, followed by 5 mg/kg up to 250 mg/day) and atovaquone (20 mg/kg, up to 750 mg, twice a day) for 7–10 days is the treatment of choice. Other antimalarial drugs, including chloroquine, have been unsuccessful. Partial or complete RBC exchange transfusion is indicated for persons with severe babesiosis, as indicated by high grade parasitemia (≥ 10%), significant hemolysis, or renal, hepatic, or pulmonary compromise.

Wormser GP et al: The clinical assessment, treatment, and prevention of Lyme disease, human granulocytic anaplasmosis, and babesiosis: Clinical practice guidelines by the Infectious Disease Society of America. Clin Infect Dis 2006;43:1089 [PMID: 17029130].

3. Toxoplasmosis

 ESSENTIALS OF DIAGNOSIS & TYPICAL FEATURES

- ▶ Congenital toxoplasmosis: chorioretinitis, microphthalmia, strabismus, microcephaly, hydrocephaly, convulsions, psychomotor retardation, intracranial calcifications, jaundice, hepatosplenomegaly, abnormal blood cell counts.

- ▶ Acquired toxoplasmosis in an immunocompetent host: lymphadenopathy, hepatosplenomegaly, rash.

- ▶ Acquired or reactivated toxoplasmosis in an immunocompromised host: encephalitis, chorioretinitis, myocarditis, and pneumonitis.

- ▶ Ocular toxoplasmosis: chorioretinitis.

- ▶ Serologic evidence of infection with *Toxoplasma gondii* or demonstration of the agent in tissue or body fluids.

▶ General Considerations

Toxoplasma gondii is a worldwide parasite of animals and birds. Felines, the definitive hosts, excrete oocysts in their

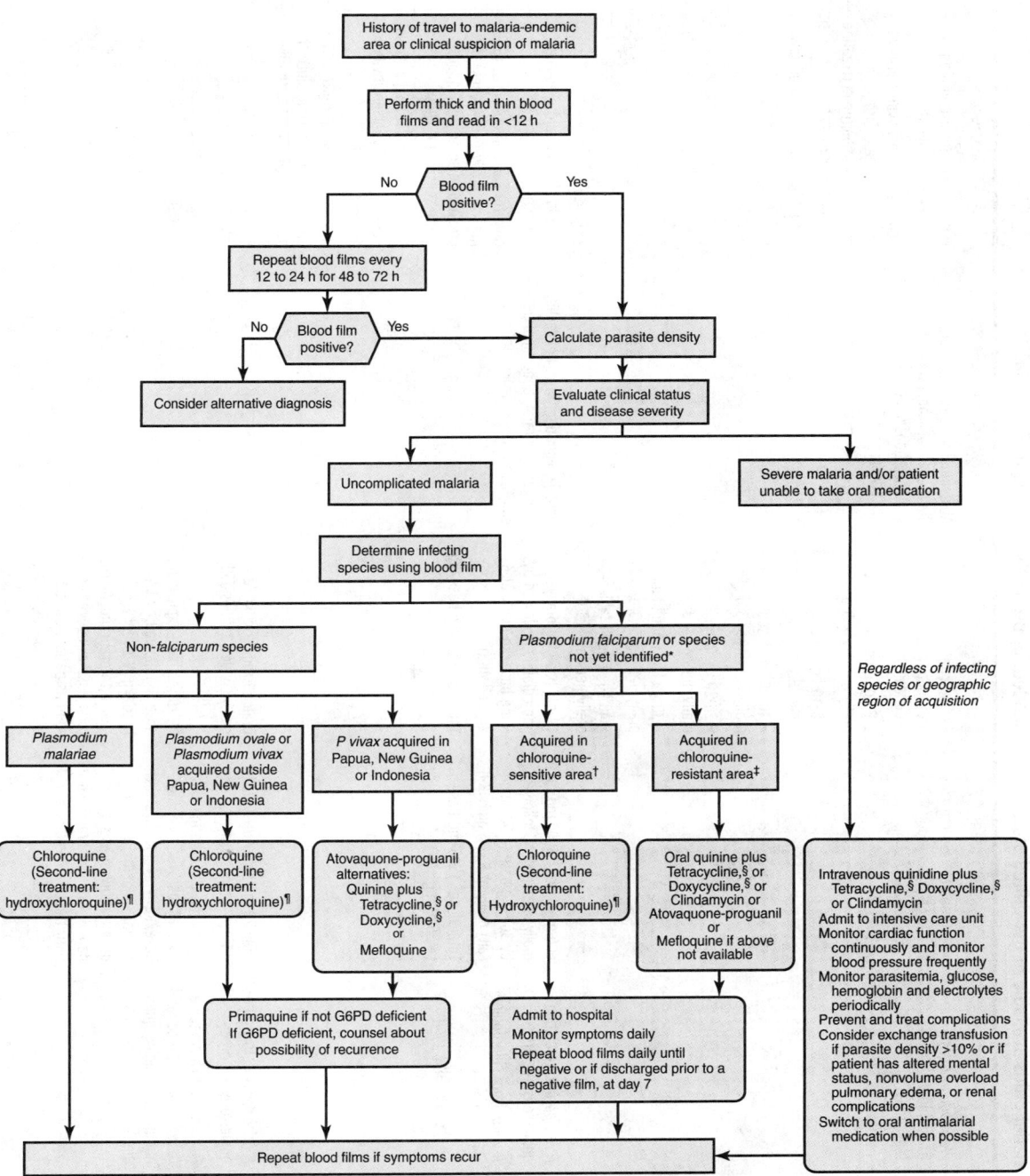

*If species not yet identified is subsequently diagnosed as a non-*falciparum* infection, then complete treatment as per the identified species recommendations. G6PD indicates glucose-6-phosphate dehydrogenase. †Central America west of the Panama Canal, Mexico, Hispaniola, parts of China, and the Middle East. ‡All malaria-endemic countries except those listed in second footnote. §Contraindicated in pregnant women and children younger than 8 years of age. ¶Drug options for chloroquine-resistant *P falciparum* may also be used if chloroquine or hydroxychloroquine cannot be used.

▲ **Figure 41–2.** **Malaria treatment algorithm.** (Reproduced, with permission, from Griffiths KS et al: Treatment of malaria in the United States. JAMA 2007;297:2264–2277. Copyright © 2007, American Medical Association. All rights reserved.)

Table 41–5. Antimalarial drugs available in the United States recommended for use in the treatment of malaria.

Drug	Indication	Adult Dosage	Pediatric Dosage[a]	Potential Adverse Effects	Comments
Atovaquone-proguanil (oral)	Plasmodium falciparum from chloroquine-resistant areas	Adult tablet = 250 mg atovaquone/100 mg proguanil; 4 adult tablets orally per day × 3 d	Pediatric tablet = 62.5 mg atovaquone/25 mg proguanil; 5-8 kg: 2 pediatric tablets orally per day × 3 d; > 8-10 kg: 3 pediatric tablets orally per day × 3 d; > 10-20 kg: 1 adult tablet orally per day × 3 d; > 20-30 kg: 2 adult tablets orally per day × 3 d; > 30-40 kg: 3 adult tablets orally per day × 3 d; > 40 kg: 4 adult tablets orally per day × 3 d	Abdominal pain, nausea, vomiting, diarrhea, headache, rash, mild reversible elevations in liver aminotransferase levels	Not indicated for use in pregnant women due to limited data; Contraindicated if hypersensitivity to atovaquone or proguanil; severe renal impairment (creatine clearance < 30 mL/min); Should be taken with food to increase absorption of atovaquone
Chloroquine phosphate	P falciparum from chloroquine-sensitive areas; P vivax from chloroquine-sensitive areas; All P ovale; all P malariae	600-mg base (= 1000 mg salt) orally immediately, followed by 300-mg base (= 500 mg salt) orally at 5, 24, and 48 h; Total dose: 1500-mg base (= 2500 mg salt)	10-mg base/kg orally immediately, followed by 6-mg base/kg orally at 6, 24, and 48 h; Total dose: 25-mg base/kg	Nausea, vomiting, rash, headache, dizziness, urticaria, abdominal pain, pruritus	Safe in children and pregnant women; Give for chemoprophylaxis (500 mg salt orally every week) in pregnant women with chloroquine-sensitive P vivax; Contraindicated if retinal or visual field change; hypersensitivity to 4-aminoquinolines; Use with caution in those with impaired liver function since the drug is concentrated in the liver
Clindamycin (oral or IV)	P falciparum from chloroquine-resistant areas; P vivax from chloroquine-resistant areas (in combination with quinine-quinidine)	Oral: 20-mg base/kg/d orally divided 3 times daily × 7 d; IV: 10-mg base/kg loading dose IV followed by 5-mg base/kg IV every 8 h; switch to oral clindamycin (oral dose as above) as soon as patient can take oral medication; treatment course = 7 d	Oral: 20-mg base/kg/d orally divided 3 times daily × 7 d; IV: 10-mg base/kg loading dose IV followed by 5-mg base/kg IV every 8 h; switch to oral clindamycin (oral dose as above) as soon as patient can take oral medication; treatment course = 7 d	Diarrhea, nausea, rash	Always use in combination with quinine-quinidine; Safe in children and pregnant women

Drug	Indication	Adult dose	Pediatric dose	Adverse effects	Comments
Doxycycline (oral or IV)	P falciparum from chloroquine-resistant areas P vivax from chloroquine-resistant areas (in combination with quinine-quinidine)	Oral: 100 mg orally twice daily × 7 d IV: 100 mg IV every 12 h and then switch to oral doxycycline (as above) as soon as patient can take oral medication; treatment course = 7 d	Oral: 2.2 mg/kg orally every 12 h × 7 d IV: IV only if patient is not able to take oral medication; for children < 45 kg, give 2.2 mg/kg IV every 12 h and then switch to oral doxycycline (dose as above) as soon as patient can take oral medication; for children ≥ 45 kg, use same dosing as for adults; treatment course = 7 d	Nausea, vomiting, diarrhea, abdominal pain, dizziness, photosensitivity, headache, esophagitis, odynophagia Rarely, hepatotoxicity, pancreatitis, and benign intracranial hypertension seen with tetracycline class of drugs	Always use in combination with quinine-quinidine Contraindicated in children < 8 y, pregnant women, and persons with hypersensitivity to tetracyclines While food, milk, and divalent and trivalent cations decrease the absorption of tetracycline, doxycycline can be taken with food, including milk products, which helps to decrease gastrointestinal disturbances To prevent esophagitis, the tetracyclines should be taken with large amounts of fluids, and patients should not lie down for 1 h after taking the drugs Concurrent treatment with barbiturates, carbamazepine, or phenytoin may cause a reduction in serum concentrations of doxycycline
Hydroxychloroquine (oral)	Second-line alternative for treatment of: P falciparum from chloroquine-sensitive areas P vivax from chloroquine-sensitive areas All P ovale; all P malariae	620-mg base (= 800 mg salt) orally immediately, followed by 310-mg base (= 400 mg salt) orally at 6, 24, and 48 h Total dose: 1550-mg base (= 2000 mg salt)	10-mg base/kg orally immediately, followed by 5-mg base/kg orally at 6, 24, and 48 h Total dose: 25-mg base/kg	Nausea, vomiting, rash, headache, dizziness, urticaria, abdominal pain, pruritus[b]	Safe in children and pregnant women Give for chemoprophylaxis (310-mg base orally every week) in pregnant women with chloroquine-sensitive P vivax Contraindicated if retinal or visual field change; hypersensitivity to 4-aminoquinolines Use with caution in those with impaired liver function

(continued)

Table 41–5. Antimalarial drugs available in the United States recommended for use in the treatment of malaria. (*Continued*)

Drug[c]	Indication	Adult Dosage	Pediatric Dosage[a]	Potential Adverse Effects	Comments
Mefloquine[c]	P falciparum from chloroquine-resistant areas, except Thailand-Burmese and Thailand-Cambodian border regions P vivax from chloroquine-resistant areas	684-mg base (= 750 mg salt) orally as initial dose, followed by 456-mg base (= 500 mg salt) orally given 6–12 h after initial dose Total dose = 1250 mg salt	13.7-mg base/kg (= 15 mg salt/kg) orally as initial dose, followed by 9.1-mg base/kg (= 10 mg salt/kg) orally given 6–12 h after initial dose Total dose = 25 mg salt/kg	Gastrointestinal complaints (nausea, vomiting, diarrhea, abdominal pain); mild neuropsychiatric complaints (dizziness, headache, somnolence, sleep disorders); myalgia, mild skin rash, and fatigue; moderate to severe neuropsychiatric reactions, electrocardiographic changes, including sinus arrhythmia, sinus bradycardia, first degree atrioventricular block, prolongation of QTc interval, and abnormal T waves	Contraindicated if hypersensitive to the drug or to related compounds; cardiac conduction abnormalities; psychiatric disorders; and seizure disorders Do not administer if patient has received related drugs (chloroquine, quinine, quinidine) < 12 h earlier May be used for chemoprophylaxis (250 mg salt orally every week) in pregnant women with chloroquine-resistant P vivax
Primaquine phosphate	Radical cure of P vivax and P ovale (to eliminate hypnozoites)	30-mg base orally per day × 14 d	0.5-mg base/kg orally per day × 14 d	Gastrointestinal disturbances, methemoglobinemia (self-limited), hemolysis in persons with G6PD deficiency	Must screen for G6PD deficiency prior to use Contraindicated in persons with G6PD deficiency; pregnant women Should be taken with food to minimize gastrointestinal adverse effects
Quinine sulfate (oral)	P falciparum from chloroquine-resistant areas P vivax from chloroquine-resistant areas	542-mg base (= 650 mg salt)[d] orally 3 times daily × 3 d (infections acquired outside Southeast Asia) to 7 d (infections acquired in Southeast Asia)	8.3-mg base/kg (= 10 mg salt/kg) orally 3 times daily × 3 d (infections acquired outside Southeast Asia) to 7 d (infections acquired in Southeast Asia)	Cinchonism,[e] sinus arrhythmia, junctional rhythms, atrioventricular block, prolonged QT interval ventricular tachycardia, ventricular tachycardia, ventricular fibrillation (these are rare and more commonly seen with quinidine), hypoglycemia	Combine with tetracycline, doxycycline, or clindamycin, except for P vivax infections in children < 8 y or pregnant women Contraindicated in hypersensitivity including history of blackwater fever, thrombocytopenic purpura, or thrombocytopenia associated with quinine or quinidine use; many cardiac conduction defects and arrhythmias[f]; myasthenia gravis; optic neuritis

Drug	Indication	Adult dosage	Pediatric dosage[a]	Adverse effects	Comments
Quinidine gluconate (IV)	Severe malaria (all species, independently of chloroquine resistance) Patient unable to take oral medication Parasitemia > 10%	6.25-mg base/kg (= 10 mg salt/kg) loading dose IV over 1-2 h, then 0.0125-mg base/kg/min (= 0.02 mg salt/kg/min) continuous infusion for at least 24 h; Alternative regimen: 15-mg base/kg (= 24 mg salt/kg) loading dose IV infused over 4 h, followed by 7.5 mg base/kg (= 12 mg salt/kg) infused over 4 h every 8 h, starting 8 h after the loading dose (see package insert); once parasite density < 1% and patient can take oral medication, complete treatment with oral quinine, dose as above; Quinidine-quinine course = 7 d in Southeast Asia (3 d in Africa or South America)	Same as adult	Cinchonism, tachycardia, prolongation QRS and QTc intervals, flattening of T-wave (effects are often transient) Ventricular arrhythmias, hypotension, hypoglycemia	Combine with tetracycline, doxycycline, or clindamycin Contraindicated in hypersensitivity; thrombocytopenic purpura or thrombocytopenia associated with quinine or quinidine use; many cardiac conduction defects and arrhythmias[g]; myasthenia gravis; optic neuritis
Tetracycline (oral or IV)	P falciparum from chloroquine-resistant areas; P vivax from chloroquine-resistant areas (in combination with quinine-quinidine)	Oral: 250 mg orally 4 times daily × 7 d; IV: dosage same as for oral	25 mg/kg/d orally divided 4 times daily × 7 d; IV: dosage same as for oral	See doxycycline	See doxycycline

[a] Pediatric dosage should never exceed adult dosage.
[b] Extrapolated from chloroquine literature.
[c] Mefloquine should not be used to treat P falciparum infections acquired in the following areas: borders of Thailand with Burma (Myanmar) and Cambodia, western provinces of Cambodia, eastern states of Burma (Myanmar), border between Burma and China, Laos along borders of Laos and Burma (and adjacent parts of Thailand-Cambodia border), and southern Vietnam due to resistant strains.
[d] Quinine sulfate capsule manufactured in the United States is in a 324-mg dose; therefore, 2 capsules should be sufficient for adult dosing.
[e] Nausea, vomiting, headache, tinnitus, deafness, dizziness, and visual disturbances.
[f] Refer to quinine sulfate, package insert (Mutual Pharmaceutical Inc, Philadelphia, Pa, August 2005).
[g] Refer to quinidine gluconate, package insert (Eli Lily Co, Indianapolis, Ind, February 2002).
G6PD, glucose-6-phosphate dehydrogenase; IV, intravenous.

feces. Ingested mature oocysts or tissue cysts lead to tachyzoite invasion of the intestinal cells. Intracellular replication of the tachyzoites causes cell lysis and spread of the infection to adjacent cells or to other tissues via the bloodstream. In chronic infection, *T gondii* appears as bradyzoite-containing tissue cysts that do not trigger an inflammatory reaction. In immunocompromised hosts, tachyzoites are released from the cysts and begin a new cycle of infection.

The two major routes of *Toxoplasma* transmission to humans are oral and congenital. Oocysts survive for up to 18 months in moist soil. Oral infection occurs after ingestion of cysts on contaminated surfaces (including pica) and in undercooked meat or other food products. Oocyst survival is limited in dry, very cold, or very hot conditions, and at high altitude, which probably accounts for the lower incidence of toxoplasmosis in these climatic regions. In the United States, less than 1% of cattle and 25% of sheep and pigs are infected with toxoplasmosis. In humans, depending on geographic area, seropositivity increases with age from nil to 10% in children younger than age 10 years, to 3–70% in adults.

Congenital transmission occurs during acute infection of pregnant women; this occurs in 0.2–1% of all pregnancies in the United States. Rarely, fetal infection has been documented in immunocompromised mothers who have chronic toxoplasmosis. The rate of vertical transmission in patients with untreated toxoplasmosis increases from 10% in the first trimester to 60% in the third. Symptomatic disease, however, is more likely to follow infection in early gestation (20–25%) compared with late gestation (< 11%). Treatment during pregnancy decreases transmission by 60%.

▶ Clinical Findings

A. Congenital Toxoplasmosis

Congenital toxoplasmosis has a variety of manifestations, including miscarriage, prematurity, and stillbirth. Most frequently, symptomatic infants present with a combination of fever, microcephaly or hydrocephaly, hepatosplenomegaly, jaundice, chorioretinitis, convulsions, abnormal cerebrospinal fluid (xanthochromia and mononuclear pleocytosis), and cerebral calcifications. Other findings include strabismus, eye palsy, maculopapular rash, pneumonitis, myocarditis, thrombocytopenia, lymphocytosis and monocytosis, and an erythroblastosis-like syndrome. The overall mortality rate for congenital toxoplasmosis, which is approximately 10%, is higher in neonates who are symptomatic at birth.

B. Acquired *Toxoplasma* Infection in the Immunocompetent Host

Only 10–20% of acute *Toxoplasma* infections produce symptoms. Patients usually present with lymphadenopathy without fever. The nodes are discrete, variably tender, and do not suppurate. Cervical lymph nodes are most frequently involved, but any nodes may be enlarged. Less common findings include fever, malaise, myalgias, fatigue, hepatosplenomegaly, low lymphocyte counts (usually < 10%), and liver enzyme elevations. Unilateral chorioretinitis may occur. The disease is self-limited, although lymph node enlargement may persist or may wax and wane for a few months to 1 or even more years. Rarely, an apparently healthy child may develop severe disseminated disease associated with myocarditis, pneumonitis, or encephalitis.

Toxoplasmic lymphadenitis must be distinguished from other causes of infectious mononucleosis-like syndromes (< 1% are caused by *Toxoplasma*).

C. Acute Toxoplasmosis in the Immunodeficient Host

Patients infected with human immunodeficiency virus (HIV), and those with lymphoma, leukemia, or transplantation, are at high risk for developing severe disease (encephalitis, chorioretinitis, myocarditis, or pneumonitis) following acute infection or reactivation. Children born to HIV- and *Toxoplasma*-infected mothers may acquire both pathogens in utero.

D. Ocular Toxoplasmosis

In active congenital toxoplasmosis, chorioretinitis is usually bilateral and shows acute inflammatory foci on funduscopic examination. This generally resolves, leaving depigmented scars of the retina surrounded by areas of hyperpigmentation. Chorioretinitis may reactivate in a single eye later in life. The appearance of the ocular lesion is not specific and mimics other granulomatous ocular diseases.

E. Diagnostic Findings

Active infection is diagnosed by demonstration of *T gondii* or its DNA in blood or body fluids; by visualization of tachyzoites in histologic sections or cytology preparations, or cysts in placenta or fetal tissues; by characteristic lymph node histology; or serologically (most commonly used). IgG antibodies, measured by the Sabin-Feldman dye test, immunofluorescence, ELISA, or particle agglutination, become detectable 1–2 weeks after infection, peak at 1–2 months, and after decreasing at variable speed, persist for life. IgM antibodies, measured by ELISA or particle agglutination, appear earlier and decline faster than IgG antibodies. Absence of both serum IgG and IgM virtually rules out the diagnosis of toxoplasmosis. Acute toxoplasmosis in an immunocompetent host is best documented by analyzing IgG and IgM in paired blood samples drawn 3 weeks apart. Because high antibody titers (IgM or IgG) can persist for several months after acute infection, a single high-titer determination is nonspecific. However, seroconversion or a fourfold increase in titer confirms the diagnosis. In the immunocompromised host, serologic tests are not sensitive, and active infection is documented by PCR or finding tachyzoites by histologic examination.

Patients with *Toxoplasma* chorioretinitis typically have low levels of specific IgG and absent IgM. The diagnosis can be confirmed by demonstrating high antibody titers in aqueous fluid.

Congenital infection is documented by anti-*Toxoplasma* IgM or IgA antibodies in the blood of the neonate. Prenatal diagnosis of congenital infection requires a combination of ultrasonography (to detect ventricle enlargement) and amniotic fluid PCR or cord blood serology. Amniotic fluid PCR is highly sensitive and carries fewer risks than cord puncture.

▶ Differential Diagnosis

Congenital toxoplasmosis must be differentiated from cytomegalovirus infection, rubella, herpes simplex infection, syphilis, Lyme disease, listeriosis, erythroblastosis, and the encephalopathies that accompany degenerative diseases. Acquired infection mimics viral, bacterial, or lymphoproliferative disorders.

▶ Prevention

Pregnant women and immunocompromised patients should wash hands thoroughly after handling raw meat, cook meat to 66°C or greater, wash fruits and vegetables before consumption, and avoid contact with cat feces. Serologic screening of pregnant women is warranted in areas of high prevalence. A first test should be performed by 10–12 weeks of pregnancy. Seronegative patients should be retested at 20–22 weeks' gestation and near term. Seroconverters require specific therapy.

▶ Treatment

Treatment does not reverse central nervous system (CNS) damage in neonates, but does markedly decrease late sequelae. A year of treatment is recommended for all congenitally infected infants; symptomatic patients receive 6 months of pyrimethamine and sulfadiazine, followed by alternating spiramycin and pyrimethamine–sulfadiazine monthly for the next 6 months. Subclinical infection is treated with pyrimethamine and sulfadiazine for 6 weeks, followed by alternating spiramycin for 6 weeks with pyrimethamine–sulfadiazine for 4 weeks.

Oral pyrimethamine at 1 mg/kg/d (maximum, 25 mg) causes gastrointestinal upset, leukopenia, thrombocytopenia, and rarely, agranulocytosis. Frequent blood counts should be performed to guide therapy. Leucovorin calcium (folinic acid), 5 mg given intramuscularly every 3 days, decreases myelotoxicity. The dosage of sulfadiazine is 40–45 mg/kg twice a day orally (maximum, 8 g/d). Clindamycin can be substituted for sulfadiazine in patients who cannot tolerate sulfonamides. Spiramycin and trimethoprim–sulfamethoxazole are less active.

Since acquired infection is usually self-limited, the potentially toxic therapy should be prescribed with discretion when the illness is uncomplicated.

In chorioretinitis, antimicrobial therapy (pyrimethamine and sulfadiazine) is used for 4 weeks. A course of corticosteroids (prednisone, 1.5 mg/kg up to 75 mg) is recommended when lesions involve the macula or the optic nerve. Lesions tend to improve after 10 days of therapy.

In primary infection during pregnancy, spiramycin is started immediately. Pyrimethamine plus sulfadiazine, alternating every 3 weeks with spiramycin, are used when fetal infection has been documented.

Montoya JG et al: Diagnosis and management of toxoplasmosis. Clin Perinatol 2005;32:705 [PMID: 16085028].
Petersen E: Toxoplasmosis. Semin Fetal Neonatal Med 2007; 12:214 [PMID: 17321812].

GASTROINTESTINAL INFECTIONS

1. Amebiasis

ESSENTIALS OF DIAGNOSIS & TYPICAL FEATURES

▶ Acute dysentery: diarrhea with blood and mucus, abdominal pain, tenesmus.

or

▶ Chronic nondysenteric diarrhea.

or

▶ Hepatic abscess.

▶ Amebas or cysts in stool or abscesses; amebic antigen in stool.

▶ Serologic evidence of amebic infection.

▶ General Considerations

Amebiasis, caused by *Entamoeba histolytica,* is a common problem in areas with poor sanitation. An estimated 10% of the world's population is infected with *E histolytica* or *Entamoeba dispar,* and an estimated 100,000 people die of amebic infection each year. Amebiasis should be suspected in patients with a history of travel to, or contact with individuals who may be asymptomatic carriers from, endemic areas. In the United States, amebiasis may occur in homes for the handicapped, where poor hygiene fosters the spread of enteric pathogens. *E histolytica* has been found in the stools of as many as 30% of homosexual men. Individuals of any age may be infected. Transmission is usually fecal-oral, often from asymptomatic carriers who pass cysts. Trophozoites are killed by stomach acid and are not infectious. Infection with *E dispar,* which is morphologically identical to *E histolytica* but results only in asymptomatic carriage, is ten times more common than infection with *E histolytica.* Furthermore, only 10% of *E histolytica* infections result in gastrointestinal or other symptoms.

Clinical Findings

A. Symptoms and Signs

Patients with intestinal amebiasis can have asymptomatic cyst passage, or be symptomatic with acute amebic proctocolitis, chronic nondysenteric colitis, or ameboma. Because all *E dispar* infections and up to 90% of *E histolytica* infections are asymptomatic, carriage is the most common manifestation of amebiasis. Patients with acute amebic colitis typically have a 1- to 2-week history of watery stools containing blood and mucus, abdominal pain, and tenesmus. A minority of patients are febrile or dehydrated. Abdominal examination may reveal pain over the lower abdominal quadrants. Fulminant colitis is an unusual complication of amebic dysentery and is associated with a grave prognosis (> 50% mortality). Patients with fulminant colitis present with severe bloody diarrhea, fever, and diffuse abdominal pain. Children younger than age 2 years appear to be at increased risk for this condition. Chronic amebic colitis is clinically indistinguishable from idiopathic inflammatory bowel disease; patients present with recurrent episodes of bloody diarrhea over a period of years. Ameboma is a localized amebic infection, usually in the cecum or ascending colon, which presents as a painful abdominal mass.

The most common complication of intestinal amebiasis is intestinal perforation and peritonitis. Perianal ulcers, a less common complication, are painful, punched-out lesions that usually respond to medical therapy. Infrequently, colonic strictures may develop following colitis.

Extraintestinal amebiasis can result in liver, lung, and cerebral abscesses, and rarely genitourinary disease. Patients with amebic liver abscess, the most common form of extraintestinal amebiasis, present with recent-onset fever and right upper quadrant tenderness. The pain may be dull or pleuritic or referred to the right shoulder. Physical examination reveals liver enlargement in less than 50% of affected patients. Some patients have a subacute presentation lasting 2 weeks to 6 months. In these patients, hepatomegaly, anemia, and weight loss are common findings, and fever is less common. Jaundice and diarrhea are rarely associated with an amebic liver abscess.

The most common complication of amebic liver abscess is pleuropulmonary amebiasis due to rupture of a right liver lobe. Lung abscesses may occur from hematogenous spread. Cough, dyspnea, and pleuritic pain can also be caused by the serous pleural effusions and atelectasis that frequently accompany amebic liver abscesses. Rupture of hepatic abscesses can lead to peritonitis and more rarely to pericarditis. Cerebral amebiasis is an infrequent manifestation. Genitourinary amebiasis, which is also uncommon, results from rupture of a liver abscess, hematogenous dissemination, or lymphatic spread.

B. Diagnostic Findings

Intestinal amebiasis is diagnosed by detecting the parasite on stool examination or mucosal biopsy. The clinical differential diagnosis of acute amebic colitis includes bacillary diarrhea and perhaps infection with *Balantidium coli* and *Dientamoeba fragilis,* which have occasionally been associated with acute diarrhea, but whose pathogenic role remains controversial. Chronic amebic colitis has to be distinguished from inflammatory bowel disease, *Cyclospora,* and perhaps *B coli.* Occult blood is present in virtually all cases of amebic colitis and can be used as an inexpensive screening test. Fecal leukocytes are uncommon. The presence of hematophagous trophozoites in feces indicates pathogenic *E histolytica* infection.

Ideally, a wet mount preparation of the stool should be examined within 20 minutes after collection to detect motile trophozoites. Otherwise, specimens should be fixed with polyvinyl alcohol or refrigerated to avoid disintegration of the trophozoites. Examination of three separate stool specimens has 90% sensitivity for the diagnosis of amebic dysentery. However, infection of the ascending colon, amebomas, and extraintestinal infections frequently yield negative stool examinations. The antigen detection test for stool is very sensitive and more specific, because it detects *E histolytica*–specific antigens that do not cross-react with *E dispar.* Colonoscopy and biopsy are most helpful in diagnosing amebic colitis when stool samples lack ova or parasites. Barium studies are contraindicated for patients with suspected acute amebic colitis because of the risk of perforation.

The presence of antibodies against *E histolytica* can differentiate *E histolytica* from *E dispar* infections. The antibody response follows both intestinal and extraintestinal invasive amebiasis and can be used for diagnostic purposes. ELISA and indirect hemagglutination assays are positive in 85–95% of invasive *E histolytica* colitis or amebic abscess. However, these antibodies persist for years, and a positive result does not distinguish between acute and past infection. Noninvasive imaging studies have greatly improved the diagnosis of hepatic abscesses. Ultrasonographic examination and computed tomography (CT) are sensitive techniques that can guide fine-needle aspiration to obtain specimens for definitive diagnosis. Because an amebic abscess may take up to 2 years to completely resolve on CT scans, imaging techniques are not recommended for therapeutic evaluation.

Prevention & Treatment

Travelers to endemic areas need to follow the precautions for preventing enteric infections—drink bottled or boiled water and eat cooked or peeled vegetables and fruits.

Treatment of amebic infection is complex because different agents are required for eradicating the parasite from the bowel or tissue (Table 41–6). Whether treatment of asymptomatic cyst passers is indicated is a controversial issue. The prevalent opinion is that asymptomatic infection with *E histolytica,* as evidenced by amebic cysts in the stool and a positive serologic test, should be treated in nonendemic areas. If serologic tests are negative, the cysts are more likely to represent infection with the nonpathogenic *E dispar,* which does not require treatment. Noninvasive infections

Table 41–6. Treatment of amebiasis.

Type of Infection	Drug of Choice	Dosage
Asymptomatic	Paromomycin	25–35 mg/kg/d in three doses for 7 d
	or	
	Iodoquinol	30–40 mg/kg/d (maximum, 2 g) in 3 doses for 20 days
	or	
	Diloxanide furoate[a]	20 mg/kg/d up to 1.5 g/d in three doses for 10 d
Intestinal disease and hepatic abscess[b]	Metronidazole	35–50 mg/kg/d up to 2.25 g/d in three doses for 10 d
	or	
	Tinidazole[c]	50 or 60 mg/kg up to 2 g/d for 3 d

[a]Diloxanide furoate is available from the CDC Drug Service: (404) 639-3670.
[b]Treatment should be followed by iodoquinol or another intraluminal cysticidal agent.
[c]Not marketed in the United States; higher dosage is for hepatic abscess.

may be treated with paromomycin. Paromomycin, a nonabsorbable aminoglycoside, can be used safely during pregnancy and has only mild intestinal side effects, including flatulence and increased number of stools. Diloxanide furoate is relatively nontoxic and used widely outside the United States. The treatment of invasive amebiasis requires metronidazole. Metronidazole has a disulfiram-like effect and should be avoided in patients receiving ethanol-containing medications. Tinidazole, a more potent nitroimidazole against amebic infection, can be used for shorter treatment courses and is well tolerated in children.

In patients who cannot tolerate metronidazole or tinidazole, erythromycin and tetracycline are active against intestinal trophozoites, but are inactive against trophozoites in liver abscesses. Conversely, chloroquine is active only against hepatic amebiasis. Treatment of invasive amebiasis should always be followed with an intraluminal cysticidal agent, even if the stool examination is negative. Metronidazole and paromomycin should not be given concurrently, because the diarrhea that is a common side effect of paromomycin may make it difficult to assess response to therapy. Patients with large, thin-walled hepatic abscesses may need therapeutic aspiration to avoid abscess rupture. Patients with amebiasis should be placed under enteric precautions.

Haque R et al: Amebiasis. N Engl J Med 2003;348:16 [PMID: 12700377].
Tanyuksel M et al: Comparison of two methods (microscopy and enzyme-linked immunosorbent assay) for the diagnosis of amebiasis. Exp Parasitol 2005;110:322 [PMID: 15955332].

Thielman NM et al: Acute infectious diarrhea. N Engl J Med 2004;350:38 [PMID: 14702426].

2. Giardiasis

ESSENTIALS OF DIAGNOSIS & TYPICAL FEATURES

▶ Chronic relapsing diarrhea, flatulence, bloating, anorexia, poor weight gain.

▶ Absence of fever and hematochezia.

▶ Detection of trophozoites, cysts, or *Giardia* antigens in stool.

General Considerations

Giardiasis, caused by *Giardia lamblia,* is the most common intestinal protozoal infection in children in the United States and in most of the world. Endemic worldwide, the infection is classically associated with drinking contaminated water, either in rural areas or in areas with faulty purification systems. But even ostensibly clean urban water supplies can be contaminated intermittently. Persons have acquired the infection in swimming pools. Fecal-oral contamination allows person-to-person spread. Day care centers have become a major source of infection, with an incidence of up to 50% reported in some centers. No symptoms occur in 25% of infected persons, facilitating spread to household contacts. Food-borne outbreaks also occur. Although infection is rare in neonates, giardiasis may occur at any age.

Clinical Findings

A. Symptoms and Signs

Giardia infection is followed by asymptomatic cyst passage, acute self-limited diarrhea, or a chronic syndrome of diarrhea, malabsorption, and weight loss. Acute diarrhea occurs 1–2 weeks after infection and is characterized by abrupt onset of diarrhea with greasy, malodorous stools; malaise; flatulence; bloating; and nausea. Fever and vomiting occur in a minority of patients. Urticaria, reactive arthritis, biliary tract disease, gastric infection, and constipation have occasionally been reported. The disease has a protracted course (> 1 week) and frequently leads to weight loss. Patients who develop chronic diarrhea complain of profound malaise, lassitude, headache, and diffuse abdominal pain in association with bouts of diarrhea—most typically foul-smelling, greasy stools—intercalated with periods of constipation or normal bowel habits. This syndrome can persist for months until specific therapy is administered or until it subsides spontaneously. Chronic diarrhea frequently leads to malabsorption, steatorrhea, vitamin A and vitamin B_{12} deficiencies, and disaccharidase depletion. Lactose intolerance, which develops in 20–40% of patients, can persist for several weeks after treatment and needs to be differentiated from relapsing giardiasis or reinfection.

B. Laboratory Findings

The diagnosis of giardiasis relies on finding the parasite in stool or duodenal aspirates or detecting *Giardia* antigen in feces. For ova and parasite examination, a fresh stool provides the best results. Liquid stools have the highest yield of trophozoites, which are more readily found on wet mounts. With semiformed stools, the examiner should look for cysts in fresh or fixed specimens, preferably using a concentration technique. When these techniques are applied carefully, one examination has a sensitivity of 50–70%; three examinations increase the sensitivity to 90%. *Giardia* antigen detection by means of immunofluorescence ELISAs, nonenzymatic immunoassays, and direct fluorescence antibody tests are becoming the standard diagnostic tests in the United States. They are comparable in cost to a stool ova and parasite examination, have a more rapid return of results, and are 85–90% sensitive and 95–100% specific. With a careful stool ova and parasite examination or with the use of a new antigen test, direct sampling of the duodenal contents should be restricted to particularly difficult cases. Three methods are currently available: the string test (Entero-Test), duodenal aspiration, and duodenal biopsy.

▶ Prevention

The prevention of giardiasis requires proper treatment of water supplies and interruption of person-to-person transmission. Travelers to developing countries or wilderness areas should halogenate or boil (for over 10 minutes) drinking water and avoid uncooked foods that might have been washed with contaminated water. Sexual transmission is prevented by avoiding oral-anal and oral-genital sex. Interrupting fecal-oral transmission requires strict hand washing. However, outbreaks of diarrhea in day care centers might be particularly difficult to eradicate, and reinforcing hand-washing and treating the disease in both symptomatic and asymptomatic carriers may be necessary.

▶ Treatment

Metronidazole, tinidazole, and nitazoxanide are the drugs of choice for treatment of giardiasis. When given at 5 mg/kg (up to 250 mg) three times a day for 5 days, metronidazole has 80–95% efficacy. The drug is well tolerated in children. It has a disulfiram-like effect and should be avoided in patients receiving ethanol-containing medication. Metronidazole can be administered safely during pregnancy. Tinidazole has an efficacy approaching 90% when given as a single dose of 50 mg/kg (up to 2 g). Nitazoxanide is available in liquid formulation and requires only 3 days of treatment. Recommended doses are 100 mg (5 mL) every 12 hours for children 12–47 months of age and 200 mg (10 mL) for 4- to 11-year-olds. Furazolidone is sometimes used in children because it is available in suspension. Administered at 1.5 mg/kg (up to 100 mg) four times daily for 7–10 days, it has only 80% efficacy. Furazolidone may cause gastrointestinal side effects, turn urine red, and cause mild hemolysis in patients with G6PD deficiency. For patients who do not respond to therapy, or who suffer relapse, a second course with the same drug or switching to another drug is equally effective. In cases of repeated treatment failure, albendazole (400 mg/d for 5–10 days), although not specifically recommended in the United States for the treatment of giardiasis, is an effective option.

Huang DB et al: An updated review on Cryptosporidium and Giardia. Gastroenterol Clin North Am 2006;35:291 [PMID: 16880067].

3. Cryptosporidiosis

Cryptosporidium parvum is an intracellular protozoan that has gained importance because it causes severe diarrhea in patients with acquired immunodeficiency syndrome (AIDS) and in other immunodeficient persons. The parasite is ubiquitous and infects and reproduces in the epithelial cell lining of the digestive and respiratory tracts of humans and most other vertebrate animals. Humans acquire the infection from contaminated water supplies, including swimming pools and lake water, or from close contact with infected humans or animals.

▶ Clinical Findings

A. Symptoms and Signs

Immunocompetent persons infected with *Cryptosporidium* usually develop self-limited diarrhea (2–26 days) with or without abdominal cramps. Diarrhea is intermittent and scant or continuous, watery, and voluminous. Low-grade fever, nausea, vomiting, loss of appetite, and malaise may accompany the diarrhea. Children younger than age 2 years appear more susceptible to infection than older children. Immunocompromised patients (either cellular or humoral deficiency) tend to develop prolonged disease, which usually subsides only after the immunodeficiency is corrected. Other clinical manifestations associated with cryptosporidiosis in immunocompromised hosts include cholecystitis, pancreatitis, hepatitis, and respiratory symptoms.

B. Laboratory Findings

Cryptosporidiosis has no characteristic laboratory features other than identification of the microorganism in feces or on biopsy. ELISA and PCR tests are more sensitive than staining of stool specimens or concentrates.

▶ Prevention & Treatment

Prevention of *Cryptosporidium* infection is limited by oocyst resistance to some of the standard water purification procedures and to common disinfectants. Enteric precautions are recommended for infected persons. Boiled or bottled drinking water may be considered for those at high risk for developing chronic infection (eg, inadequately treated patients with AIDS).

Immunocompetent patients and those with temporary immunodeficiencies respond to treatment with nitazoxanide, antidiarrheal agents, and hydration. Immunocompromised patients usually require more intense supportive care with parenteral nutrition in addition to hydration and nonspecific antidiarrheal agents. Octreotide acetate, a synthetic analogue of somatostatin that inhibits secretory diarrhea, has been associated with symptomatic improvement, but not with parasitologic cure. Among the antiparasitic agents, nitazoxanide, paromomycin–azithromycin, rifabutin, and hyperimmune bovine colostrum, in that order, have met with success. For patients with AIDS, institution of effective antiretroviral therapy eliminates symptomatic cryptosporidiosis.

Chen X et al: Cryptosporidiosis. N Engl J Med 2002;346:1723 [PMID: 12037153].

Huang DB et al: An updated review on Cryptosporidium and Giardia. Gastroenterol Clin North Am 2006;35:291 [PMID: 16880067].

4. Cyclosporiasis

Cyclospora is a coccidian that infects both humans and animals with worldwide distribution. It causes food-associated outbreaks, characterized by an incubation period of 2–11 days followed by watery diarrhea in relapsing patterns, sometimes alternating with constipation. Other symptoms include profound fatigue, vomiting, and myalgias. The infection can be unusually severe in immunocompromised patients. Although the illness is self-limited, it may last for several weeks. Diagnosis is based on finding oocysts 8–10 mm in diameter on examination of stool specimens stained with acid-fast stain. The treatment of choice is trimethoprim–sulfamethoxazole for 7 days.

Lewthwaite P: Gastrointestinal parasites in the immunocompromised. Curr Opin Infect Dis 18:427 [PMID: 16148530].

5. Free-Living Amebas

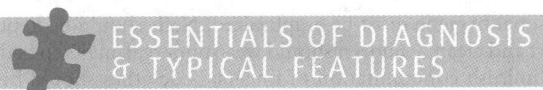

ESSENTIALS OF DIAGNOSIS & TYPICAL FEATURES

- ▶ Acute meningoencephalitis: fever, headache, meningismus, acute mental deterioration.
- ▶ Swimming in warm, fresh water in an endemic area.
- ▶ Chronic granulomatous encephalitis: insidious onset of focal neurologic deficits.
- ▶ Keratitis: pain, photophobia, conjunctivitis, blurred vision.

▶ General Considerations

Infections with free-living amebas are uncommon. *Naegleria* species, *Acanthamoeba* species, and *Balamuthia* (previously called leptomyxid) amebas have been associated with human disease.

Acute meningoencephalitis, caused by *Naegleria fowleri*, occurs mostly in children and young adults. Patients present with abrupt fever, headache, nausea and vomiting, meningismus, and decreased mental status a few days to 2 weeks after swimming in warm freshwater lakes. Swimming history may be absent. CNS invasion occurs after nasal inoculation of *N fowleri*. The disease is rapidly progressive, and death ensues within 1 week of onset.

Chronic granulomatous encephalitis, caused by *Acanthamoeba* or *Balamuthia,* occurs most commonly in patients who are immunocompromised from corticosteroid use, chemotherapy, or AIDS. There is no association with freshwater swimming. This disease has an insidious onset of focal neurologic deficits, and approximately 50% of patients present with headache. Skin, sinus, or lung infections with *Acanthamoeba* precede many of the CNS infections and may still be present at the onset of neurologic disease. The granulomatous encephalitis progresses to fatal outcome over a period of weeks to months (average 6 weeks).

Acanthamoeba keratitis is a corneal infection associated with minor trauma or use of soft contact lenses in otherwise healthy persons. Frequently misdiagnosed as herpes simplex or bacterial keratitis, *Acanthamoeba* keratitis has a characteristic dendritiform epithelial pattern that suggests the diagnosis.

▶ Clinical Findings & Differential Diagnosis

Amebic encephalitis should be included in the differential diagnosis of acute meningoencephalitis in children with a history of recent freshwater swimming. The cerebrospinal fluid (CSF) is usually hemorrhagic, with leukocyte counts that may be normal early in the disease, but later range from 400–2600/μL with neutrophil predominance, low to normal glucose, and elevated protein. The etiologic diagnosis relies on finding trophozoites on a wet mount of the CSF.

Granulomatous encephalitis is diagnosed by brain biopsy of CT-identified nonenhancing lucent areas. The CSF of these patients is usually nondiagnostic with intermediate white blood cell counts, elevated protein, and decreased glucose. *Acanthamoeba* or leptomyxid amebas have not been found in the CSF; however, they can be visualized in biopsies or grown from brain or other infected tissues.

Acanthamoeba keratitis is diagnosed by finding the trophozoites in corneal scrapings or by isolating the parasite from corneal specimens or contact lens cultures.

▶ Prevention

Because primary amebic meningitis occurs infrequently, active surveillance of lakes for *N fowleri* is not warranted.

However, in the presence of a documented case, it is advisable to close the implicated lake to swimming. *Acanthamoeba* keratitis can be prevented by heat disinfection of contact lenses, by storage of lenses in sterile solutions, and by not wearing lenses when swimming in fresh water.

▶ Treatment

The few patients who have survived acute amebic meningoencephalitis received high-dose intravenous and intrathecal amphotericin B, accompanied by miconazole, rifampin, and sulfisoxazole in some cases. The first two cases of successful treatment of *Balamuthia* encephalitis were reported after combination therapy with flucytosine, pentamidine, fluconazole, sulfadiazine, and a macrolide.

Acanthamoeba keratitis responds well to surgical debridement followed by 3–4 weeks of topical 1% miconazole; 0.1% propamidine isethionate; and polymyxin B sulfate, neomycin, and bacitracin (Neosporin).

Deetz TR et al: Successful treatment of *Balamuthia* amoebic encephalitis: Presentation of two cases. Clin Infect Dis 2003; 37:1304 [PMID: 14583863].

Khan NA: Acanthamoeba: Biology and increasing importance in human health. FEMS Microbiol Rev 2006;30:564 [PMID: 16774587].

TRICHOMONIASIS

Trichomonas vaginalis infection is discussed in Chapter 42.

METAZOAL INFECTIONS

NEMATODE INFECTIONS

1. Enterobiasis (Pinworms)

ESSENTIALS OF DIAGNOSIS & TYPICAL FEATURES

▶ Anal pruritus.
▶ Worms in the stool or eggs on perianal *skin*.

▶ General Considerations

This worldwide infection is caused by *Enterobius vermicularis*. The adult worms are about 5–10 mm long and lives in the colon; females deposit eggs on the perianal area, primarily at night, which cause intense pruritus. Scratching contaminates the fingers and allows transmission back to the host (autoinfection) or to contacts.

▶ Clinical Findings

A. Symptoms and Signs

Although blamed for myriad symptoms, pinworms are definitely associated only with localized pruritus. Adult worms may migrate within the colon or up the urethra or vagina in girls. They can be found within the bowel wall, in the lumen of the appendix (usually an incidental finding by the pathologist), in the bladder, and even in the peritoneal cavity of girls. The granulomatous reaction that may be present around these ectopic worms is usually asymptomatic. Worm eradication may correspond with the cure of recurrent urinary tract infections in some young girls.

B. Laboratory Findings

The usual diagnostic test consists of pressing a piece of transparent tape on the child's anus in the morning prior to bathing, then placing it on a drop of xylene on a slide. Microscopic examination under low power usually demonstrates the ova. Occasionally eggs or adult worms are seen in fecal specimens. Parents may also notice adult worms.

▶ Differential Diagnosis

Nonspecific irritation or vaginitis, streptococcal perianal cellulitis (usually painful with marked erythema), and vaginal or urinary bacterial infections may at times resemble pinworm infection, although the symptoms of pinworms are often so suggestive that a therapeutic trial is justified without a confirmed diagnosis.

▶ Treatment

A. Specific Measures

Treat all household members at the same time to prevent reinfections. Because the drugs are not active against the eggs, therapy should be repeated after 2 weeks to kill the recently hatched adults.

Pyrantel pamoate is given as a single dose (11 mg/kg; maximum, 1 g); it is safe and very effective. Mebendazole (100 mg) and albendazole (400 mg) in a single dose are highly effective for this infection at all ages.

B. General Measures

Personal hygiene must be emphasized. Nails should be kept short and clean. Children should wear undergarments to bed to diminish contamination of fingers; bedclothes should be laundered frequently. Although eggs may be widely dispersed in the house and multiple family members infected, the disease is mild and treatable.

Brown MD: Enterobius vermicularis. N Engl J Med 2006;354:e12 [PMID: 16571876].

St Georgiev V: Chemotherapy of enterobiasis (oxyuriasis). Expert Opin Pharmacother 2001;2:267 [PMID: 11336585].

2. Ascariasis

▶ Abdominal cramps and discomfort.

▶ Large, white or reddish, round worms, or ova in the feces.

▶ General Considerations

Together with the whipworm and hookworms (see below), *Ascaris* comprises the group of so-called "soil-transmitted helminths." This group of parasites causes human infection through contact with eggs or larvae that thrive in the moist soil of the tropics and subtropics. Worldwide more than a billion people are infected with one species of these parasites, and especially in less developed countries, it is not uncommon for children to be chronically infected with all three worms. Children infected with these worms are at increased risk for malnutrition, stunted growth, intellectual retardation, and cognitive and education deficits. Together, the soil-transmitted helminths are one of the world's most important causes of physical and intellectual growth retardation.

Ascaris lumbricoides is a worldwide human parasite. Ova passed by carriers may remain viable for months under the proper soil conditions. The ova contaminate food or fingers and are subsequently ingested by a new host. The larvae hatch, penetrate the intestinal wall, enter the venous system, reach the alveoli, are coughed up, and return to the small intestine, where they mature. The female lays thousands of eggs daily.

▶ Clinical Findings

A. Symptoms and Signs

Infections usually remain asymptomatic; severe cases, however, can be associated with pain, weight loss, anorexia, diarrhea, or vomiting. Adult worms may be seen in feces or vomitus. Rarely, they perforate or obstruct the small bowel, biliary system, or appendix. Large numbers of larvae migrating through the lungs may cause an acute, transient eosinophilic pneumonia (Löffler syndrome).

B. Laboratory Findings

The diagnosis is made by observing the large roundworms (1.5–4 cm) in the stool or by microscopic detection of the ova.

▶ Treatment

Because the adult worms live less than a year, asymptomatic infection need not be treated. Mebendazole (100 mg twice a day for 3 days or 500 mg once), pyrantel pamoate (a single dose of 11 mg/kg; maximum, 1 g), and albendazole (400 mg

in a single dose, or 200 mg in children 1–2 years of age) are highly and equally effective. In cases of intestinal or biliary obstruction, piperazine (150 mg/kg initially, followed by six doses of 65 mg/kg every 12 hours by nasogastric tube) is recommended because it narcotizes the worms and helps relieve obstruction. However, surgical removal is occasionally required.

Bethony J et al: Soil-transmitted helminth infections: Ascariasis, trichuriasis, and hookworm. Lancet 2006;367:1521 [PMID: 16679166].

3. Trichuriasis (Whipworm)

Trichuris trichiura is a widespread human and animal parasite common in children living in warm, humid areas conducive to survival of the ova. The adult worms live in the cecum and colon; the ova are passed and become infectious after several weeks in the soil. Ingested infective eggs hatch in the upper small intestine. Unlike *Ascaris*, *Trichuris* does not have a migratory tissue phase. Symptoms are not present unless the infection is severe, in which case pain, diarrhea, and mild abdominal distention are present. Massive infections may also cause rectal prolapse and dysentery. Detection of the characteristic barrel-shaped ova in the feces confirms the diagnosis. Adult worms may be seen in the prolapsed rectum or at proctoscopy; their thin heads are buried in the mucosa, and the thicker posterior portions protrude. Mild to moderate eosinophilia may be present.

Mebendazole (100 mg orally twice a day for 3 days or 500 mg once) or albendazole (400 mg in a single dose for 3 days, or 200 mg in children 1–2 years of age) improves gastrointestinal symptoms and terminates constitutional symptoms.

Bethony J et al: Soil-transmitted helminth infections: Ascariasis, trichuriasis, and hookworm. Lancet 2006;367:1521 [PMID: 16679166].

4. Hookworm

▶ Iron deficiency anemia.

▶ Abdominal discomfort, weight loss.

▶ Ova in the feces.

▶ General Considerations

The common human hookworms are *Ancylostoma duodenale* and *Necator americanus*. Both are widespread in the tropics and subtropics. The larger *A duodenale* is more pathogenic because it consumes more blood, up to 0.5 mL per worm per day.

The adults live in the jejunum. Eggs are passed in the feces and develop and hatch into infective larvae in warm, damp soil within 2 weeks. The larvae penetrate human skin on contact, enter the blood, reach the alveoli, are coughed up and swallowed, and develop into adults in the intestine. The adult worms attach with their mouth parts to the mucosa, from which they suck blood. Blood loss is the major sequela of infection. Infection rates reach 90% in areas without sanitation.

A separate species, *A braziliense* (dog or cat hookworm), causes creeping eruption (cutaneous larva migrans). This disease occurs mainly on the warm-water American coasts.

▶ Clinical Findings

A. Symptoms and Signs

The larvae usually penetrate the skin of the feet and cause intense local itching (ground itch). This subsides as the larvae continue their migration. Löffler syndrome may supervene during lung migration. In creeping eruption, the nonhuman *Ancylostoma* larvae migrate blindly in the skin before dying, creating serpiginous burrows.

Mild intestinal infections produce no symptoms. Severe infections cause iron deficiency anemia and malnutrition. Occasionally abdominal pain and diarrhea may be observed.

B. Laboratory Findings

The large ova of both species of hookworm are found in feces and are indistinguishable. Microcytic anemia, hypoalbuminemia, eosinophilia, and hematochezia occur in severe cases.

▶ Prevention

Fecal contamination of soil and skin contact with potentially contaminated soil should be avoided.

▶ Treatment

A. Specific Measures

Albendazole (400 mg orally in a single dose, or 200 mg in children 1–2 years of age), mebendazole (100 mg orally twice a day for 3 days), and pyrantel pamoate (11 mg/kg, to a maximum of 1 g, daily for 3 days) are the drugs of choice. Topical thiabendazole or albendazole or oral thiabendazole are useful for creeping eruption.

B. General Measures

Iron therapy may be as important as worm eradication.

▶ Prognosis

The outcome is usually excellent.

Bethony J et al: Soil-transmitted helminth infections: Ascariasis, trichuriasis, and hookworm. Lancet 2006;367:1521 [PMID: 16679166].

5. Strongyloidiasis

ESSENTIALS OF DIAGNOSIS & TYPICAL FEATURES

▶ Abdominal pain, diarrhea.
▶ Eosinophilia.
▶ Larvae in stools and duodenal aspirates.
▶ Serum antibodies.

▶ General Considerations

Strongyloides stercoralis is unique in having both parasitic and free-living forms; the latter can survive in the soil for several generations. The parasite is found in most tropical and subtropical regions of the world. The adults live in the submucosal tissue of the duodenum and occasionally elsewhere in the intestines. Eggs deposited in the mucosa hatch rapidly; the first-stage (rhabditiform) larvae, therefore, are the predominant form found in duodenal aspirates and feces. The larvae mature rapidly to the tissue-penetrating filariform stage and initiate internal autoinfection. The filariform larvae also inhabit the soil and can penetrate the skin of another host, subsequently migrating into veins and pulmonary alveoli, reaching the intestine when coughed up and swallowed.

Older children and adults are infected more often than are young children. Even low worm burden can result in significant clinical symptoms. Infestations due to poor sanitation and hygiene are noteworthy. Immunosuppressed patients may develop fatal disseminated strongyloidiasis, known as the hyperinfection syndrome.

▶ Clinical Findings

A. Symptoms and Signs

At the site of skin penetration, a pruritic rash may occur. Large numbers of migrating larvae can cause wheezing, cough, and hemoptysis. Although one third of intestinal infections are asymptomatic, the most prominent features of strongyloidiasis include abdominal pain, distention, diarrhea, vomiting, and occasionally malabsorption.

Patients with cellular immunodeficiencies and those on corticosteroid therapy may develop disseminated infection involving the intestine, the lungs, and the meninges. Gram-negative sepsis may complicate disseminated strongyloidiasis.

B. Laboratory Findings

Finding larvae in the feces, in duodenal aspirates, on a string test (Entero-Test), or in sputum is diagnostic. IgG antibodies measured by ELISA or immunoblot are sensitive and specific for *Strongyloides*. These persist after successful therapy. Marked eosinophilia is common.

Differential Diagnosis

Strongyloidiasis should be differentiated from peptic disease, celiac disease, regional or tuberculous enteritis, hookworm infection, and other causes of intestinal symptoms or malabsorption. The pulmonary phase may mimic asthma or bronchopneumonia. Patients with severe infection can present with an acute abdomen.

Prevention & Treatment

Thiabendazole (50 mg/kg/d in two doses for 2 days; maximum, 3 g/d) and ivermectin (0.2 mg/kg/d for 1 or 2 days) are the drugs of choice. Relapses are common. In the hyperinfection syndrome, 2–3 weeks of therapy may be necessary. Patients from endemic areas should be tested for specific antibodies and receive treatment before undergoing immunosuppression.

Keiser PB et al: *Strongyloides stercoralis* in the immunocompromised population. Clin Microbiol Rev 2004;17:208 [PMID: 14726461].

6. Visceral Larva Migrans (Toxocariasis)

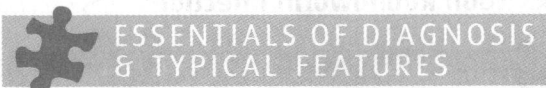

ESSENTIALS OF DIAGNOSIS & TYPICAL FEATURES

► Visceral involvement including hepatomegaly, marked eosinophilia, and anemia.
► Posterior or peripheral ocular inflammatory mass.
► Elevated antibody titers in serum or aqueous fluid; demonstration of *Toxocara* larvae in biopsy specimen.

General Considerations

Visceral larva migrans is a worldwide disease. The agent is the cosmopolitan intestinal ascarid of dogs and cats, *Toxocara canis* or *Toxocara cati*. The eggs passed by infected animals contaminate parks and other areas that young children frequent. Children with pica are at increased risk. In the United States, seropositivity ranges from 2.8% in unselected populations to 23% in southern states to 54% in rural areas. Ingested eggs hatch and penetrate the intestinal wall, then migrate to the liver, lungs, eyes, and other organs, where they die and incite a granulomatous inflammatory reaction.

Clinical Findings

A. Visceral Larva Migrans

Toxocariasis is usually asymptomatic, but young children (aged 1–5 years) sometimes present with anorexia, fever, fatigue, pallor, abdominal distention, abdominal pain, nausea, vomiting, and cough. Hepatomegaly is common, sple-nomegaly is unusual, and adenopathy is absent. Lung involvement, usually asymptomatic, can be demonstrated readily by radiologic examination. Seizures are common, but more severe neurologic abnormalities are infrequent. Eosinophilia with leukocytosis, anemia, and elevated liver function tests are typical laboratory findings. ELISA is sensitive, specific, and useful in confirming the clinical diagnosis. Most patients recover spontaneously, but disease may last up to 6 months.

B. Ocular Larva Migrans

This condition occurs in older children and adults who present with a unilateral posterior or peripheral inflammatory mass. History of visceral larva migrans and eosinophilia are typically absent. Anti-*Toxocara* antibody titers are low in the serum and high in vitreous and aqueous fluids.

C. Diagnostic Findings

Hypergammaglobulinemia and elevated isohemagglutinins sometimes result from cross-reactivity between *Toxocara* antigens and human group A and B blood antigens. The diagnosis is confirmed by finding larvae in granulomatous lesions. Positive serology in high titers and the exclusion of other causes of hypereosinophilia allow a presumptive diagnosis to be made in typical cases.

Differential Diagnosis

Diseases associated with hypereosinophilia must be considered. These include trichinosis (enlarged liver not common; muscle tenderness common), eosinophilic leukemia (rare in children; eosinophils are abnormal in appearance), collagen-vascular disease (those associated with eosinophilia are rare in young children), strongyloidiasis (no organomegaly; enteric symptoms are common), early ascariasis, tropical eosinophilia (occurring mainly in India), allergies, and hypersensitivity syndromes.

Prevention & Treatment

A. Specific Measures

The clinical benefit of specific anthelmintic therapy is not defined. Treatment with albendazole (400 mg twice a day for 5 days) or mebendazole (100–200 mg twice a day for 5 days) is indicated for severe complications of brain, lung, or heart.

B. General Measures

Treating any cause of pica, such as iron deficiency, is important. Corticosteroids are used to treat marked inflammation of lung, eye, or other organs. Pets should be dewormed routinely. Other children in the household may be infected. Mild eosinophilia and positive serologic tests may be the only clue to their infection. Therapy is not necessary for these individuals.

7. Trichinosis

▶ Vomiting, diarrhea, and pain within 1 week of eating infected meat.
▶ Fever, periorbital edema, myalgia, and marked eosinophilia.

General Considerations

Trichinella spiralis is a small roundworm that inhabits hogs and several other meat-eating animals. The human cycle begins with ingestion of viable larvae in undercooked meat. In the intestine, the larvae develop into adult worms that mate and produce hundreds of larvae. The larvae enter the bloodstream and migrate to the striated muscle where they continue to grow and eventually encyst. Symptoms are caused by the inflammatory response in the intestines or muscle.

Clinical Findings

A. Symptoms and Signs

Most infections are asymptomatic. The initial bowel penetration may cause nausea, vomiting, diarrhea, and cramps within 1 week after ingestion of contaminated meat. This may progress to the classic myopathic form, which consists of fever, periorbital edema, myalgia, and weakness. Many organs may be infected by the migrating larvae: diaphragm, heart, lungs, kidneys, spleen, skin, and brain. Severe cerebral involvement may be fatal. Myocarditis may also be severe or fatal. Symptoms usually peak after 2–3 weeks, but may last months. Children typically have milder clinical and laboratory findings than adults.

B. Laboratory Findings

Marked eosinophilia is the rule. Serology confirms the diagnosis. Muscle biopsy is rarely necessary.

Differential Diagnosis

The classic symptoms are pathognomonic if one is aware of this disease. It has to be distinguished from dermatomyositis, typhoid fever, sinusitis, influenza with myopathy, and angioneurotic edema.

Prevention

Because a microscopic examination must be performed, meat in the United States is not inspected for trichinosis. Although all states require the cooking of hog swill, hog-to-hog or hog-to-rat cycles may continue. All pork and sylvatic meat (eg, bear or walrus) should be heated to at least 65°C. Freezing meat to at least –15°C for 3 weeks may also prevent transmission. Animals used for food should not be fed or allowed access to raw meat.

Treatment

Mebendazole has activity against the intestinal, circulating, and tissue stages of infection. The adult dose is 200–400 mg three times a day for 3 days followed by 400–500 mg three times a day for 10 days. Pediatric dosing has not been standardized and recommendations range from 5–25 mg/kg/d divided in three doses for 14 days. Concurrent corticosteroids are used in an attempt to prevent the Herxheimer reaction associated with treatment.

Prognosis

Death may occur within the first weeks, but most infections are self-limited.

Ozdemir D et al: Acute trichinellosis in children compared with adults. Pediatr Infect Dis J 2005:24:897 [PMID: 16220088].

8. Raccoon Roundworm Infections

▶ Eosinophilic meningoencephalitis or encephalopathy.
▶ Ocular larva migrans.
▶ Contact with raccoons or raccoon feces.

General Considerations

Human infections with *Baylisascaris procyonis,* the raccoon roundworm, have been increasingly recognized, particularly in children. The definitive host of this ascarid is the raccoon. Humans who ingest the eggs excreted in raccoon feces become intermediate hosts when the larvae penetrate the gut and disseminate via the bloodstream to the brain, eyes, viscera, and muscles. Young age, pica, and exposure to raccoon feces (eg, while camping) represent the main risk factors for this infection. Most of the infections are asymptomatic, but cases of severe encephalitis (neural larva migrans) and endophthalmitis (ocular larva migrans) occur. Symptoms typically begin 2–4 weeks after inoculation. CNS infections characteristically present as acute, rapidly progressive encephalitis with eosinophilic pleocytosis of the CSF. Both CNS and ocular infections resemble other larva migrans infections such as toxocariasis; therefore *B procyonis* should be considered in the differential diagnosis of these infections when *Toxocara* serology is negative. The diagnosis of *B procyonis* is established by observing the larvae on examination of tissue biopsies or by serology. Treatment consists of anthelmintics and corticosteroid anti-inflammatory drugs. Prognosis is reserved, since complete resolution of symptoms has not been achieved thus far.

Gavin PJ et al: Baylisascariasis. Clin Microbiol Rev 2005;18:703 [PMID: 16223954].

CESTODE INFECTIONS (FLUKES)

1. Taeniasis & Cysticercosis

ESSENTIALS OF DIAGNOSIS & TYPICAL FEATURES

▶ Mild abdominal pain; passage of worm segments (taeniasis).

▶ Focal seizures, headaches (neurocysticercosis).

▶ Cysticerci present in biopsy specimens, on plain films (as calcified masses), or on CT scan or magnetic resonance imaging.

▶ Proglottids and eggs in feces; specific antibodies in serum or CSF.

▶ General Considerations

Both the beef tapeworm (*Taenia saginata*) and the pork tapeworm (*Taenia solium*) cause taeniasis. The adults live in the intestines of humans; the egg-laden distal segments, or proglottids, break off and are passed in feces, disintegrating and releasing the ova in the soil. After ingestion in food or water by cattle or pigs, the eggs hatch and the larvae migrate to and encyst in skeletal muscle. Encysted larvae in meat ingested by humans mature into adult tapeworms.

Humans can be an intermediate host for *T solium* (but not *T saginata*), and the larvae released from ingested eggs encyst in a variety of tissues, especially muscle and brain. Full larval maturation occurs in 2 months, but the cysts cause little inflammation until they die months to years later. Inflammatory edema ensues with calcification or disappearance of the cyst. A slowly expanding mass of sterile cysts at the base of the brain may cause obstructive hydrocephalus (racemose cysticercosis).

Both parasites are distributed worldwide. Contamination of foods by eggs in human feces allows infection without exposure to meat or travel to endemic areas. Asymptomatic cases are common, but neurocysticercosis is a leading cause of seizures in endemic areas.

Person-to-person spread may occur, resulting in infection of individuals with no exposure to infected meat.

▶ Clinical Findings

A. Symptoms and Signs

1. Taeniasis—In most tapeworm infections, the only clinical manifestation is the passage of fecal proglottids, which are white, motile bodies 1–2 cm in size. They occasionally crawl out onto the skin and down the leg, especially the larger *T saginata*. Children may harbor the adult worm for years and complain of abdominal pain, anorexia, and diarrhea.

2. Cysticercosis—Most cases are asymptomatic. Subcutaneous nodules of 1–2 cm may be the only sign. After several years, the cysticerci calcify and appear as radiographic opacities. Brain cysts may remain silent or cause seizures, headache, hydrocephalus, and basilar meningitis. Rarely, the spinal cord is involved. Neurocysticercosis manifests an average of 5 years after exposure, but may cause symptoms in the first year of life. In the eye, cysts cause bleeding, retinal detachment, and uveitis. Definitive diagnosis requires histologic demonstration of larvae or cyst membrane. Presumptive diagnosis is often made by the characteristics of the cysts seen on CT scan or magnetic resonance imaging; the differential diagnosis may include tuberculoma, brain abscess, arachnoid cyst, and tumor. The presence of *T solium* eggs in feces is uncommon, but supports the diagnosis.

B. Laboratory Findings

Eggs or proglottids may be found in feces or on the perianal skin (using the tape method employed for pinworms). Eggs of both *Taenia* species are identical. The species are identified by examination of proglottids.

Peripheral eosinophilia is minimal or absent. CSF eosinophilia is seen in 10–75% of cases of neurocysticercosis; its presence supports an otherwise presumptive diagnosis.

ELISA antibody titers are eventually positive in up to 98% of serum specimens and over 75% of CSF specimens from patients with neurocysticercosis. Solitary cysts are associated with seropositivity less often than are multiple cysts. High titers tend to correlate with more severe disease. CSF titers are higher if cysts are near the meninges.

▶ Treatment

A. Taeniasis

Praziquantel (5–10 mg/kg once) and albendazole are equally effective. Feces free of segments or ova for 3 months suggest cure.

B. Cysticercosis

Specific treatment is reserved for patients with meningitis, or enhancing or cystic parenchymal lesions. In contrast, those with inactive disease require only symptomatic treatment (anticonvulsants). Albendazole, 15 mg/kg/d (maximum, 800 mg) divided in two doses daily for 8 days, is the treatment of choice. Larval death may result in clinical worsening because of inflammatory edema. A short course of dexamethasone may decrease these symptoms. Giant subarachnoidal cysts may require more than one cycle of therapy or surgery (or both). Follow-up scans every several months help assess the response to therapy. Treatment of patients with calcified lesions and seizure disorder results in a decrease of generalized seizures.

Prevention

The incidence in the United States is low because beef and pork are inspected for taeniasis. Prevention requires proper cooking of meat, careful washing of raw vegetables and fruits, treatment of intestinal carriers, avoiding the use of human excrement for fertilizer, and providing proper sanitary facilities.

Prognosis

The prognosis is good in intestinal taeniasis. Symptoms associated with a few cerebral cysts may disappear in a few months; heavy brain infections may cause death or chronic neurologic impairment.

Del Brutto OH et al: Meta-analysis: Cysticidal drugs for neurocysticercosis: Albendazole and praziquantel. Ann Intern Med 2006; 145:43 [PMID: 16818928].

Garcia HH et al: A trial of antiparasitic treatment to reduce the rate of seizures due to cerebral cysticercosis. N Engl J Med 2004; 350:249 [PMID: 14724304].

Nash TE et al: Treatment of neurocysticercosis: Current status and future research needs. Neurology 2006;67:1120 [PMID: 17030744].

2. Hymenolepiasis

Hymenolepis nana, the cosmopolitan human tapeworm, is a common parasite of children; *Hymenolepis diminuta,* the rat tapeworm, is rare. The former is capable of causing autoinfection. Larvae hatched from ingested eggs penetrate the intestinal wall and then reenter the lumen to mature into adults. Their eggs are immediately infectious for the same or a new host. The adult is only a few centimeters long. Finding the characteristic eggs in feces is diagnostic.

H diminuta has an intermediate stage in rat fleas and other insects; children are infected when they ingest these insects.

Light infections with either tapeworm are usually asymptomatic; heavy infection can cause diarrhea and abdominal pain. Therapy is with praziquantel (25 mg/kg once).

3. Echinococcosis

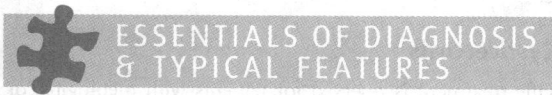
ESSENTIALS OF DIAGNOSIS
& TYPICAL FEATURES

▶ Cystic tumors of liver, lung, kidney, bone, brain, and other organs.
▶ Eosinophilia.

▶ Urticaria and pruritus if cysts rupture.
▶ Protoscoleces or daughter cysts in the primary cyst.
▶ Positive serology.
▶ Epidemiologic evidence of exposure

General Considerations

Dogs, cats, and other carnivores are the hosts for *Echinococcus granulosus.* Cystic and alveolar echinococcosis (hydatid disease) cause significant morbidity and mortality worldwide. Endemic areas include Australia, New Zealand, and the southwestern United States, including Native American reservations where shepherding is practiced. The adult tapeworm lives in sheep intestines, and eggs are passed in the feces. When ingested by humans, the eggs hatch, and the larvae penetrate the intestinal mucosa and disseminate in the bloodstream to produce cysts; the primary sites of involvement are the liver (60–70%) and the lungs (20–25%). A unilocular cyst is most common. Over years, the cyst may reach 25 cm in diameter, although most are much smaller. The cysts of *Echinococcus multilocularis* are multilocular and demonstrate more rapid growth.

Clinical Findings

A. Symptoms and Signs

Clinical disease is due to pressure from the enlarging cysts, vessel erosion, and sensitization to cyst or worm antigens. Liver cysts present as slowly expanding tumors that may cause biliary obstruction. Most are in the right lobe and extend inferiorly; 25% are on the upper surface and may be asymptomatic for years. Omental torsion or hemorrhage from vessel erosion may occur.

Rupture of a pulmonary cyst causes coughing, dyspnea, wheezing, urticaria, chest pain, and hemoptysis; cyst and worm remnants are found in sputum. Brain cysts may cause focal neurologic signs and convulsions; renal cysts cause pain and hematuria; bone cysts cause pain.

B. Laboratory Findings

Presumptive diagnosis is made by a combination of radiographic or ultrasonographic and serologic findings. ELISA, which is the method most widely used for antibody testing, is highly sensitive, but has limited specificity.

Confirmation may be obtained by ultrasonography-guided fine-needle aspiration coupled with parasitologic examination for protoscoleces, rostellar hooks, antigens, or DNA. Eosinophilia is variable and may be absent. Serologic tests are useful for diagnosis and follow-up of therapy.

C. Imaging

Pulmonary or bone cysts may be visible on plain films. Other imaging techniques are preferred for cysts in other organs. Visualization of daughter cysts is highly suggestive of echinococcosis.

Differential Diagnosis

Tumors, bacterial or amebic abscess, and tuberculosis (pulmonary) must be considered.

Complications

Sudden cyst rupture with anaphylaxis and death is the worst complication. If the patient survives, secondary infections from seeding of daughter cysts may occur. Segmental lung collapse, secondary bacterial infections, effects of increased intracranial pressure, and severe renal damage due to renal cysts are other potential complications.

Treatment

Definitive therapy of *E multilocularis* requires meticulous surgical removal of the cysts, preceded by careful injection of the cyst with formalin, iodine, or 95% alcohol solution to sterilize infectious protoscoleces, freezing the cyst wall and injecting silver nitrate prior to its removal, or puncture-aspiration/injection-reaspiration technique, which is best suited for treatment of multiple cysts. A surgeon familiar with this disease should be consulted. Medical therapy may be of additional benefit, particularly in disseminated disease. Albendazole (15 mg/kg/d for 28 days with repeat courses as necessary following a 14-day rest period) is effective in many cases of *E granulosus* infection (hydatid disease). If the cyst leaks or ruptures, the allergic symptoms must be managed immediately.

Prognosis

Patients with large liver cysts may be asymptomatic for years. Surgery is often curative for lung and liver cysts, but not always for cysts in other locations. Secondary disease has a much worse prognosis; about 15% of patients with this disease die.

Craig PS: Prevention and control of cystic echinococcosis. Lancet Infect Dis 2007;7:385 [PMID: 17521591].

TREMATODE INFECTIONS

Schistosomiasis

ESSENTIALS OF DIAGNOSIS & TYPICAL FEATURES

▶ Transient pruritic rash after exposure to fresh water.

▶ Fever, urticaria, arthralgias, cough, lymphadenitis, and eosinophilia.

▶ Weight loss, anorexia, hepatosplenomegaly.

▶ Hematuria, dysuria.

▶ Eggs in stool, urine, or rectal biopsy specimens.

General Considerations

One of the most common serious parasitic diseases, schistosomiasis, is caused by several species of *Schistosoma* flukes. *Schistosoma japonicum*, *S mekongi*, and *S mansoni* involve the intestines and *S haematobium*, the urinary tract. The first two species are found in eastern and southeastern Asia; *S mansoni* in tropical Africa, the Caribbean, and parts of South America; and *S haematobium* in northern Africa.

Infection is caused by free-swimming larvae (cercariae), which emerge from the intermediate hosts, certain species of freshwater snails. The cercariae penetrate human skin, migrate to the liver, and mature into adults, which then migrate through the portal vein to lodge in the bladder veins (*S haematobium*), superior mesenteric veins (*S mekongi* and *S japonicum*), or inferior mesenteric veins (*S mansoni*). Clinical disease results primarily from inflammation caused by the many eggs that are laid in the perivascular tissues or that embolize to the liver. Escape of ova into bowel or bladder lumen allows microscopic visualization and diagnosis from stool or urine specimens, as well as contamination of fresh water and infection of the snail hosts that ingest them.

Clinical Findings

Much of the population in endemic areas is infected but asymptomatic. Only heavy infections produce symptoms.

A. Symptoms and Signs

The cercarial penetration may cause a pruritic rash; larval migration may cause fever, urticaria, and cough; the maturation phase may cause tender hepatosplenomegaly followed by days to weeks of fever and malaise as the worms migrate to their final destination. Bladder infection results in dysuria, hematuria, reflux, stones, and incontinence. Secondary pyelonephritis and ureteral obstruction may occur. Intestinal infection is usually asymptomatic. The final stages of disease caused by the parasite in mesenteric veins are characterized by hepatic fibrosis, portal hypertension, splenomegaly, ascites, and bleeding from esophageal varices. The chronic inflammation in the urinary tract associated with *S haematobium* infections may result in obstructive uropathy, stones, infection, bladder cancer, fistulas, and anemia due to chronic hematuria. Spinal cord granulomas and paraplegia due to egg embolization into the Batson plexus have been reported.

B. Laboratory Findings

The diagnosis is made by finding the species-specific eggs in feces (*S japonicum*, *S mekongi*, *S mansoni*, and occasionally *S haematobium*) or urine (*S haematobium* and occasionally *S mansoni*). If no eggs are found, concentration methods should be used. A rectal biopsy may reveal *S mansoni* and should be done if other specimens are negative. Peripheral eosinophilia is common, and eosinophils may be seen in urine.

Prevention

The best prevention is to avoid contact with contaminated fresh water in endemic areas. Efforts to destroy the snail hosts have been successful in areas of accelerated economic development.

Treatment

A. Specific Measures

Praziquantel is the treatment of choice for schistosomiasis. A dosage of 40 mg/kg/d in two divided doses (*S mansoni* or *S haematobium*) or 20 mg/kg three times in 1 day (*S japonicum* or *S mekongi*) is very effective and nontoxic. Praziquantel has no effect on eggs and immature worms and therefore a repeat dose 4–6 weeks later is sometimes needed. Oxamniquine (20 mg/kg/d in two doses once per day) is an alternative regimen for treatment of *S mansoni* infection. Artemether (6 mg/kg every 3 weeks) may prevent new infections or reinfection after curative treatment.

B. General Measures

Therapy of nutritional deficiency or secondary bacterial infections may be needed. The patient's urinary tract should be

evaluated carefully in *S haematobium* infection; reconstructive surgery may be needed. Hepatic fibrosis requires careful evaluation of the portal venous system and surgical management of portal hypertension when appropriate.

Prognosis

Therapy decreases the worm burden and liver size, despite continued exposure in endemic areas. Early disease responds well to therapy, but once significant scarring or severe inflammation has occurred, eradication of the parasites is of little benefit.

Gryseels B et al: Human schistosomiasis. Lancet 2006;368:1106 [PMID: 16997665].

MYCOTIC INFECTIONS

Fungi can be classified as yeasts, which are unicellular and reproduce by budding; as molds, which are multicellular and consist of tubular structures (hyphae) and grow by elongation and branching; or as dimorphic fungi, which can exist either as yeasts or molds depending on environmental conditions. Fungal infections can be categorized as shown in Table 41–7.

Table 41–7. Pediatric fungal infections.

Type	Agents	Incidence	Diagnosis	Diagnostic Tests	Therapy	Prognosis
Superficial	*Candida* Dermatophytes *Malassezia*	Very common	Simple	KOH prep	Topical	Good
Subcutaneous	*Sporothrix*[a]	Uncommon	Simple[b]	Culture	Oral	Good
Systemic: normal host	*Coccidioides* *Histoplasma* *Blastomyces*	Common: regional	Often presumptive	Chest radiograph; serology, antigen detection (histoplasmosis; blastomycosis); histology; culture of body fluids or tissue	None[c] or systemic	Good
Systemic: opportunistic infection	*Candida*[a] *Pneumocystis*[d] *Aspergillus* Mucorales *Malassezia* *Pseudallescheria* *Cryptococcus*	Uncommon	Difficult[e]	Tissue biopsy, culture, antigen detection (cryptococcosis)	Systemic, prolonged	Poor if therapy is delayed and in severely immunocompromised patients

[a]*Candida* and *Sporothrix* in immunocompromised patients may cause severe, rapidly progressive disease and require systemic therapy.
[b]Sporotrichosis may require biopsy for diagnosis.
[c]Often self-limited in normal host.
[d]Now reclassified as a fungus. Asymptomatically infects many normal hosts.
[e]Except *Cryptococcus*, which is often diagnosed by antigen detection.
KOH, potassium hydroxide.

In the United States, systemic disease in normal hosts is commonly caused by three organisms—*Coccidioides, Histoplasma,* and *Blastomyces*—which are restricted to certain geographic areas. Prior residence in or travel to these areas, even for a brief time, is a prerequisite for inclusion in a differential diagnosis. Of these three, *Histoplasma* most often relapses years later in patients who are immunosuppressed.

Immunosuppression, foreign bodies (eg, central catheters), ulceration of gastrointestinal and respiratory mucosa, broad-spectrum antimicrobial therapy, malnutrition, HIV infection, and neutrophil defects or depletion are major risk factors for opportunistic fungal disease.

Laboratory diagnosis may be difficult because of the small number of fungi present in some lesions, slow growth of some organisms, and difficulty in distinguishing normal colonization of mucosal surfaces from infection. A tissue biopsy with fungal stains and culture is the best method for diagnosing systemic disease with some fungi. Repeat blood cultures may be negative even in the presence of intravascular infections. Serologic tests are useful for diagnosing coccidioidomycosis and histoplasmosis, and antigen detection is useful for diagnosing histoplasmosis and cryptococcosis.

The common superficial fungal infections of the hair and skin are discussed in Chapter 14.

BLASTOMYCOSIS

ESSENTIALS OF DIAGNOSIS & TYPICAL FEATURES

▶ Residence in or travel to an endemic area.

▶ In immunocompetent patients, most often a self-limited flulike illness; acute pneumonia occurs in a minority of cases.

▶ Complications include progressive pneumonia and disseminated disease (CNS, skin, bone and joints, genitourinary tract).

▶ Diagnosis by culture of specimens from bronchoscopy, skin, or other tissue.

▶ General Considerations

The causative fungus, *Blastomyces dermatitidis,* is found in soil primarily in the Mississippi and Ohio River valleys, additional southeastern and south central states, and the states bordering the Great Lakes. Transmission is by inhalation of spores. Subclinical disease is common. Severe disease is much more common in adults and males. In children, infection rates are similar in both sexes.

▶ Clinical Findings

A. Symptoms and Signs

Primary infection is unrecognized or produces pneumonia. Acute symptoms include cough, chest pain, headache, weight loss, and fever occurring several weeks to months after inoculation. Infection is usually self-limited in immunocompetent patients. In some patients an indolent progressive pulmonary disease occurs after an incubation period of 30–45 days. Cutaneous lesions usually represent disseminated disease; local primary inoculation is rare. Slowly progressive ulcerating lesions with a sharp, heaped-up border or verrucous lesions occur. Bone disease resembles other forms of chronic osteomyelitis. Lytic skull lesions in children are typical, but long bones, vertebrae, and the pelvis may be involved. Extrapulmonary disease occurs in 25–40% of patients with progressive disease. A total body radiographic examination is advisable when blastomycosis is diagnosed in the skin or another nonpulmonary site. The genitourinary tract involvement characteristic of dissemination in adults is rare in prepubertal children. Lymph nodes, brain, and kidneys may be involved.

B. Laboratory Findings

Diagnosis requires isolation or visualization of the fungus. Pulmonary specimens (sputum, tracheal aspirates, or lung biopsy) may be positive with conventional stains or fungal cell wall stains. An initial suppurative response is followed by an increase in the number of mononuclear cells, and then formation of noncaseating granulomas. The budding yeasts are thick-walled, have refractile walls, and are very large and distinctive. Sputum specimens are positive in 50–80% of cases and skin lesions are positive in 80–100%. The fungus can be grown readily in most laboratories, but 1–2 weeks are required. Serologic tests are generally not helpful for diagnosis. An ELISA antigen detection method, similar to that used for histoplasmosis, is useful for detecting *Blastomyces* antigen in urine and other body fluids.

C. Imaging

Radiographic consolidation and fibronodular interstitial and alveolar infiltrates are typical; effusions, hilar nodes, and cavities are less common. The paucity of cavitation distinguishes acute blastomycosis from histoplasmosis and tuberculosis. Miliary patterns also occur with acute infection. Chronic disease can develop in the upper lobes, with cavities and fibronodular infiltrations similar to those seen in tuberculosis, but unlike in tuberculosis or histoplasmosis, these lesions rarely caseate or calcify.

▶ Differential Diagnosis

Primary pulmonary infection resembles acute viral, bacterial, or mycoplasmal infections. Blastomycosis should be considered when a significant pulmonary infection in an endemic area fails to respond to antibiotic therapy. Subacute infection mimics tuberculosis, histoplasmosis, and coccidioidomycosis. Chronic pulmonary or disseminated disease must be differentiated from cancer, tuberculosis, or other fungal infections.

Treatment

Mild pulmonary blastomycosis does not require treatment; indeed, it is rarely recognized. Recommended therapy for life-threatening (especially in the immunocompromised patient) or CNS infections is amphotericin B (0.7–1.0 mg/kg intravenously for a total of 1.5–2.0 g). Itraconazole (6–8 mg/kg/d for 6 months) is preferred for other forms of blastomycosis. Bone disease may require a full year of itraconazole therapy. Surgical debridement is required for devitalized bone, drainage of large abscesses, and pulmonary lesions not responding to medical therapy.

Kaufman CA: Endemic mycoses: Blastomycosis, histoplasmosis, and sporotrichosis. Infect Dis Clin North Am 2006;20:645 [PMID: 16984873].

Mongkolrattanothai K et al: Urine antigen detection of blastomycosis in pediatric patients. Pediatr Infect Dis J 2006;25:1076 [PMID: 17072135].

CANDIDIASIS

ESSENTIALS OF DIAGNOSIS & TYPICAL FEATURES

► In normal or immunosuppressed individuals: superficial infections (oral thrush or ulcerations; vulvovaginitis; erythematous intertriginous rash with satellite lesions); fungemia related to intravascular devices.

► In immunosuppressed individuals: systemic infections (renal, hepatic, splenic, pulmonary, or cerebral abscesses); cotton-wool retinal lesions; cutaneous nodules.

► In either patient population: budding yeast and pseudo-hyphae are seen in biopsy specimens, body fluids, or scrapings of lesions; positive culture.

General Considerations

Disease due to *Candida* is caused by *Candida albicans* in 60–80% of cases; similar systemic infection may be due to *C tropicalis, C parapsilosis, C glabrata,* and a few other *Candida* species. Speciation is important because of differences in pathogenicity and response to azole therapy. In tissue, pseudohyphae or budding yeast (or both) are seen. *Candida* grows on routine media more slowly than bacteria; growth is usually evident on agar after 2–3 days and in blood culture media in 2–7 days.

C albicans is ubiquitous and often present in small numbers on skin, mucous membranes, or in the intestinal tract. Normal bacterial flora, intact epithelial barriers, neutrophils and macrophages in conjunction with antibody and complement, and normal lymphocyte function by skin test reactivity are factors in preventing invasion. Disseminated infection is almost always preceded by prolonged broad-spectrum antibiotic therapy, instrumentation (including intravascular catheters), or immunosuppression. Patients with diabetes mellitus are especially prone to superficial *Candida* infection; thrush and vaginitis are most common. *Candida* is the third most common blood isolate in hospitals in the United States and is a common cause of catheter-related urinary tract infection.

Clinical Findings

A. Symptoms and Signs

1. Oral candidiasis (thrush)—Adherent creamy white plaques on the buccal, gingival, or lingual mucosa are seen. These may be painful. Lesions may be few and asymptomatic, or they may be extensive, extending into the esophagus. Thrush is very common in otherwise normal infants in the first weeks of life; it may last weeks despite topical therapy. Spontaneous thrush in older children is unusual unless they have recently received antimicrobials. Corticosteroid inhalation for asthma predisposes patients to thrush. HIV infection should be considered if there is no other reason for oral thrush, or if it is persistent or recurrent. Angular cheilitis is the name given to painful erythematous fissures caused by *Candida* at the corners of the mouth, often in association with a vitamin or iron deficiency.

2. Vaginal infection—Vulvovaginitis occurs in sexually active girls, in diabetic patients, and in girls receiving antibiotics. Thick, odorless, cheesy discharge with intense pruritus is typical. The vagina and labia are usually erythematous and swollen. Outbreaks are more frequent before menses.

3. Skin infection

A. DIAPER DERMATITIS—Diaper dermatitis is often due entirely or partly to *Candida*. Pronounced erythema with a sharply defined margin and satellite lesions is typical. Pustules, vesicles, papules, or scales may be seen. Weeping, eroded lesions with a scalloped border are common. Any moist area, such as axillae or neck folds, may be involved.

B. CONGENITAL SKIN LESIONS—These lesions may be seen in infants born to women with *Candida* amnionitis. A red maculopapular or pustular rash is seen. Dissemination may occur in premature infants, or in term infants after prolonged rupture of membranes.

C. SCATTERED RED PAPULES OR NODULES—Such findings may represent cutaneous dissemination.

D. PARONYCHIA AND ONYCHOMYCOSIS—These conditions occur in immunocompetent children but are often associated with immunosuppression, hypoparathyroidism, or adrenal insufficiency (*Candida* endocrinopathy syndrome). The selective absence of specific T-cell responses to *Candida* can lead to marked, chronic skin and nail infections called chronic mucocutaneous candidiasis.

E. CHRONIC DRAINING OTITIS MEDIA—This problem may occur in patients who have received multiple courses of antibiotics and are superinfected with *Candida*.

4. Enteric infection—Esophageal involvement in immunosuppressed patients is the most common enteric manifestation. It is manifested by substernal pain, dysphagia, painful swallowing, and anorexia. Nausea and vomiting are common in young children. Most patients do not have thrush. Stomach or intestinal ulcers also occur. A syndrome of mild diarrhea in normal individuals who have predominant *Candida* on stool culture has also been described, although *Candida* is not considered a true enteric pathogen. Its presence more often reflects recent antimicrobial therapy.

5. Pulmonary infection—Because the organism frequently colonizes the respiratory tract, it is commonly isolated from respiratory secretions. Thus demonstration of tissue invasion is needed to diagnose *Candida* pneumonia or tracheitis. It is rare, being seen in immunosuppressed patients and patients intubated for long periods, usually while taking antibiotics. The infection may cause fever, cough, abscesses, nodular infiltrates, and effusion.

6. Renal infection—Candiduria may be the only manifestation of disseminated disease. More often, candiduria is associated with instrumentation, an indwelling catheter, or anatomic abnormality of the urinary tract. Symptoms of cystitis may be present. Masses of *Candida* may obstruct ureters and cause obstructive nephropathy. *Candida* casts in the urine suggest renal tissue infection.

7. Other infections—Endocarditis, myocarditis, meningitis, and osteomyelitis usually occur only in immunocompromised patients or neonates.

8. Disseminated candidiasis—Skin and mucosal colonization precedes, but does not predict dissemination. Too often, dissemination is confused with bacterial sepsis. This occurs in neonates—especially premature infants—in an intensive care unit setting, and is recognized when the infant fails to respond to antibiotics or when candidemia is documented. These infants often have unexplained feeding intolerance, cardiovascular instability, apnea, new or worsening respiratory failure, glucose intolerance, thrombocytopenia, or hyperbilirubinemia. A careful search should be carried out for lesions suggestive of disseminated *Candida* (retinal cotton-wool spots or nodular dermal abscesses). If these findings are absent, diagnosis is often based presumptively on the presence of a compatible illness in an immunocompromised patient, a burn patient, or a patient with prolonged postsurgical or intensive care unit course who has no other cause for the symptoms; who fails to respond to antimicrobials; and who usually has *Candida* colonization of mucosal surfaces. Treatment for presumptive infection is often undertaken because candidemia is not identified antemortem in many such patients.

Hepatosplenic candidiasis occurs in immunosuppressed patients. The typical case consists of a severely neutropenic patient who develops chronic fever, variable abdominal pain, and abnormal liver function tests. No bacteria are isolated, and there is no response to antimicrobials. Symptoms persist even when neutrophils return. Ultrasound or CT scan of the liver and spleen demonstrates multiple round lesions. Biopsy is needed to confirm the diagnosis.

B. Laboratory Findings

Budding yeast cells are easily seen in scrapings or other samples. A wet mount preparation of vaginal secretions is 40–50% sensitive; this is increased to 50–70% with the addition of 10% potassium hydroxide. The use of a Gram-stained smear is 70–100% sensitive. The presence of pseudohyphae suggests tissue invasion. Culture is definitive. Ninety-five percent of positive blood cultures will be detected within 3 days, but cultures may remain negative (10–40%) even with disseminated disease or endocarditis. *Candida* should never be considered a contaminant in cultures from normally sterile sites. *Candida* in any number in appropriately collected urine suggests true infection. Antigen tests are not sensitive or specific enough for clinical use. Antibody tests are not useful. The ability of yeast to form germ tubes when incubated in human serum gives a presumptive speciation for *C albicans*.

▶ Differential Diagnosis

Thrush may resemble formula (which can be easily wiped away with a tongue blade or swab, revealing normal mucosa without underlying erythema or erosion), other types of ulcers (including herpes), burns, or oral changes induced by chemotherapy. Skin lesions may resemble contact, allergic, chemical, or bacterial dermatitis; miliaria; folliculitis; or eczema. Candidemia and systemic infection should be considered in any seriously ill patient with the risk factors previously mentioned.

▶ Complications

Failure to recognize disseminated disease early is the greatest complication. Arthritis and meningitis occur more often in neonates than in older children. Blindness from retinitis, massive emboli from large vegetations of endocarditis, and abscesses in any organ are other complications; the greater the length or degree of immunosuppression and the longer the delay before therapy, the more complications are seen.

▶ Treatment
A. Oral Candidiasis

In infants, oral nystatin suspension (100,000 units four to six times a day in the buccal fold after feeding until resolution) usually suffices. Nystatin must come in contact with the lesions because it is not absorbed systemically. Older children may use it as a mouthwash (200,000–500,000 units four times a day), although it is poorly tolerated because of its taste. Clotrimazole troches (10 mg) four times a day are an alternative in older children. Prolonged therapy with either agent or more frequent dosing may be needed. Painting the lesions with a cotton swab dipped in gentian violet (0.5–1%) is visually dramatic and messy, but may help refractory cases. Eradication of *Candida* from pacifiers, bottle nipples, toys, or the mother's breasts (if the infant is breast feeding and there is candidal infection of the nipples) may be helpful.

Oral azoles, such as fluconazole (6 mg/kg/d), are effective in older children with candidal infection refractory to nystatin. Discontinuation of antibiotics or corticosteroids is advised when possible.

B. Skin Infection

Cutaneous infection usually responds to a cream or lotion containing nystatin, amphotericin B, or an azole. Associated inflammation, such as severe diaper dermatitis, is also helped by concurrent use of a topical mild corticosteroid cream, such as 1% hydrocortisone. One approach is to keep the involved area dry; a heat lamp and nystatin powder may be used. Suppression of intestinal *Candida* with nystatin and eradicating thrush may speed recovery and prevent recurrence of the diaper dermatitis.

C. Vaginal Infections

Vulvovaginal candidiasis (see Chapter 42) is treated with clotrimazole, miconazole, triazoles, or nystatin (cheapest if generic is used) suppositories or creams, usually applied once nightly for 3–7 days. In general, nystatin is less effective and longer therapy is required. A high-dose clotrimazole formulation need be given for only a single night. *Candida* balanitis in sexual partners should be treated. Oral azole therapy is equally effective. A single 150-mg oral dose of fluconazole is effective for vaginitis. It is more expensive, but very convenient. No controlled study has shown that treating colonization of male sexual partners prevents recurrence in females. Frequent recurrent infections may require elimination of risk factors, the use of oral therapy, or some prophylactic antifungal therapy, such as a single dose of fluconazole weekly.

D. Renal Infection

Candiduria is treated with a 7- to 14-day course of fluconazole, which is concentrated in the urine. Renal abscesses or ureteral fungus balls require intravenous antifungal therapy. Surgical debridement may be required. Removal of an indwelling catheter is imperative. Amphotericin B may improve poor renal function caused by renal candidiasis, even though the drug is nephrotoxic.

E. Systemic Infection

Systemic infection is dangerous and resistant to therapy. Surgical drainage of abscesses and removal of all infected tissue (eg, a heart valve) are required for cure. Hepatosplenic candidiasis should be treated until all lesions have disappeared or are calcified on imaging studies. Treatment of systemic infection has traditionally utilized amphotericin B. Lipid forms of amphotericin B retain the antifungal potency of the free drug, but are much better tolerated. Although they are much more expensive than amphotericin B, they are indicated for patients who are intolerant of conventional therapy and for those whose infection is refractory to treatment or who have a high likelihood of developing renal toxicity from such therapy. Fluconazole and the newer azole drugs, such as itraconazole (best absorbed from the liquid solution), voriconazole, and a new class of drugs, echinocandins, are used interchangeably with amphotericin; in general these are less toxic. These new drugs also are often effective against fluconazole-resistant candidal infection.

Correction of predisposing factors is important (eg, discontinuing antibiotics and immunosuppressives, and improving control of diabetes). Flucytosine (50–75 mg/kg/d orally in four doses; keep serum levels below 75 mcg/mL) may be additive or synergistic to amphotericin B. Flucytosine is frequently added to treat neonatal infections, but clinical outcome seems to be similar when amphotericin B is used alone. Unlike amphotericin B, flucytosine penetrates tissues well. It should not be used as a single agent in serious infections because resistance develops rapidly.

Fluconazole, itraconazole, and voriconazole are acceptable alternatives for serious *C albicans* infections in nonneutropenic patients and are often effective as first-line therapy in immunocompromised patients. The decision to use systemic azole therapy should include consideration of the local experience with azole-resistant *Candida*. Susceptibility testing for *Candida* species is now available to guide this decision. *C glabrata* and *C krusei* are common isolates that may be resistant to fluconazole; these are often susceptible to the newer azoles and echinocandins. Infected central venous lines must be removed immediately; this alone often is curative. Persistent fever and candidemia suggest infected thrombus, endocarditis, or tissue infection. If the infection is considered limited to the line and environs, a 14-day course (after the last positive culture) of a systemic antifungal agent following line removal is recommended for immunocompromised patients. Systemic azole therapy should also be considered for immunocompetent patients with candidemia, because of the late occurrence of focal *Candida* infection in some cases.

Fluconazole is well absorbed (oral and intravenous therapy are equivalent), reasonably nontoxic, and effective for a variety of *Candida* infections. Fluconazole dosage is 8–12 mg/kg/d in a single daily dose for initial therapy of severely ill children. Selected patients with prolonged immunosuppression (eg, after bone marrow transplantation) should receive fluconazole, itraconazole, or intermittent amphotericin B prophylaxis. These drugs are less expensive than the lipid formulations of amphotericin.

Prognosis

Superficial disease in normal hosts has a good prognosis; in abnormal hosts, it may be refractory to therapy. Early therapy of systemic disease is often curative if the underlying immune response is adequate. The outcome is poor when therapy is delayed or when host response is inadequate.

Kalfa VC et al: The syndrome of chronic mucocutaneous candidiasis with selective antibody deficiency. Ann Allergy Asthma Immunol 2003;90:259 [PMID: 12602677].

Segal E: Candida, still number one—what do we know and where are we going from there? Mycoses 2005;48(Suppl 1):3 [PMID: 15887329].

Spellberg BJ et al: Current treatment strategies for disseminated candidiasis. Clin Infect Dis 2006;42:244 [PMID: 16355336].

Wiley JM et al: Efficacy and safety of amphotericin B lipid complex in 548 children and adolescents with invasive fungal infections. Pediatr Infect Dis J 2005;24:167 [PMID: 15702047].

Zaoutis T, Walsh TJ: Antifungal therapy for neonatal candidiasis. Curr Opin Infect Dis 2007;20:592 [PMID: 17975409].

COCCIDIOIDOMYCOSIS

ESSENTIALS OF DIAGNOSIS & TYPICAL FEATURES

► Residence in or travel to an endemic area.

► Primary pulmonary form: fever, chest pain, cough, anorexia, weight loss, and often a macular rash or erythema nodosum or multiforme.

► Primary cutaneous form: skin trauma followed in 1–3 weeks by an ulcer and regional adenopathy.

► Spherules seen in pus, sputum, CSF, joint fluid; positive culture.

► Appearance of precipitating (early) and complement-fixing antibodies (late).

General Considerations

Coccidioidomycosis is caused by the dimorphic fungus *Coccidioides immitis,* which is endemic in the Sonoran Desert areas of western parts of Texas, southern New Mexico and Arizona, southern California, northern Mexico, and South America. Infection results from inhalation or inoculation of arthrospores (highly contagious and readily airborne in the dry climate). Even brief travel in or through an endemic area, especially during windy seasons, may allow infection. Human-to-human transmission does not occur. More than half of all infections are asymptomatic, and less than 5–10% are associated with significant pulmonary disease. Chronic pulmonary disease or dissemination occurs in less than 1% of cases.

Clinical Findings

A. Symptoms and Signs

1. Primary disease—The incubation period is 10–16 days (range, 7–28 days). Symptoms vary from those of a mild fever and arthralgia to severe influenza-like illness with high fever, nonproductive cough, pleurisy, myalgias, arthralgias, headache, night sweats, and anorexia. Upper respiratory tract signs are not common. Severe pleuritic chest pain suggests this diagnosis. Signs vary from none to rash, rales, pleural rubs, and signs of pulmonary consolidation. Weight loss may occur.

2. Skin disease—Up to 10% of children develop erythema nodosum or multiforme. These manifestations imply a favorable host response to the organism. Less specific maculopapular eruptions occur in a larger number of children. Skin lesions can occur following fungemia. Primary skin inoculation sites develop indurated ulcers with local adenopathy. Contiguous involvement of skin from deep infection in nodes or bone also occurs. The presence of chronic skin lesions with this fungus should lead to a search for other areas of infection (eg, lung).

3. Chronic pulmonary disease—This is uncommon in children. Chronic disease is manifested by chronic cough (occasionally with hemoptysis), weight loss, pulmonary consolidation, effusion, cavitation, or pneumothorax.

4. Disseminated disease—This is less common in children than adults. It is more common in infants, neonates, pregnant women (especially during the third trimester), blacks, Filipinos, American Indians, and patients with HIV or other types of immunosuppression. One or more organs may be involved. The most common sites involved are bone or joint (usually a single bone or joint; subacute or chronic swelling, pain, redness), nodes, meninges (slowly progressive meningeal signs, ataxia, vomiting, headache, and cranial neuropathies), and kidney (dysuria and urinary frequency). As with most fungal diseases, the evolution of the illness is usually slow.

B. Laboratory Findings

Direct examination of respiratory secretions, pus, CSF, or tissue may reveal large spherules (30–60 μm) containing endospores. These are the product of coccidioidal spores germinating in tissue. Phase-contrast microscopy is useful for demonstrating these refractile bodies; Gram or methylene blue stains are not helpful, but periodic acid–Schiff reagent, methenamine silver, and calcofluor stains are. Fluffy, gray-white colonies grow within 2–5 days on routine fungal and many other media. CSF cultures are often negative.

Routine laboratory tests are nonspecific. The sedimentation rate is usually elevated. Eosinophilia may occur, particularly prior to dissemination, and is more common in coccidioidomycosis than in many other conditions with similar symptoms. Meningitis causes a mononuclear pleocytosis (70% with eosinophils) with elevated protein and mild hypoglycorrhachia.

Within 2–21 days, most patients develop a delayed hypersensitivity reaction to coccidioidin skin test antigen (Spherulin, 0.1 mL intradermally, should produce 5-mm induration at 48 hours). Erythema nodosum predicts strong reactivity; when this reaction is present the antigen should be diluted 10–100 times before use. The skin test may be negative in immunocompromised patients or in those with disseminated disease. Positive reactions may remain for years and do not prove active infection.

Antibodies consist of precipitins (usually measurable by 2–3 weeks in 90% of cases and gone by 12 weeks) and complement-fixing antibodies (delayed for several weeks; appear as the precipitins are falling and disappear by 8 months, unless dissemination or chronic infection occurs). The extent of the complement-fixing antibody response reflects the severity of infection. Persistent high levels suggest dissemination. Serum precipitins usually indicate acute infection. Excellent ELISA assays are now available to detect IgM and IgG antibodies against the precipitin and complement-fixing antigens. The presence of antibody in CSF indicates CNS infection.

C. Imaging

Approximately half of symptomatic infections are associated with abnormal chest radiographs—usually infiltrates with hilar adenopathy. Pulmonary consolidation, effusion, and thin-walled cavities may be seen. About 5% of infected patients have asymptomatic nodules or cysts after recovery. Unlike reactivation tuberculosis, apical disease is not prominent. Bone infection causes osteolysis that enhances with technetium. Cerebral imaging may show hydrocephalus and meningitis; intracranial abscesses and calcifications are unusual. Radiographic evolution of all lesions is slow.

▶ Differential Diagnosis

Primary pulmonary infection resembles acute viral, bacterial, or mycoplasmal infections; subacute presentation mimics tuberculosis, histoplasmosis, and blastomycosis. Chronic pulmonary or disseminated disease must be differentiated from cancer, tuberculosis, or other fungal infections.

▶ Complications

Dissemination of primary pulmonary disease is associated with ethnic background, prolonged fever (> 1 month), a negative skin test, high complement-fixation antibody titer, and marked hilar adenopathy. Local pulmonary complications include effusion, empyema, and pneumothorax. Cerebral infection can cause noncommunicating hydrocephalus due to basilar meningitis.

▶ Treatment

A. Specific Measures

Mild pulmonary infections in most normal hosts require no therapy. These patients should be assessed for 1–2 years to document resolution and to identify any complications. Antifungal therapy is used for prolonged fever, weight loss (> 10%), prolonged duration of night sweats, severe pneumonitis (especially if persisting for 4–6 weeks), or any form of disseminated disease. Neonates, pregnant women, and patients with high antibody titer also receive treatment. Therapy is often utilized for pregnant women and subjects with high-risk racial origins.

Amphotericin B is used to treat severe disease (1 mg/kg/d until improvement, then reduce dose; total duration, 2–3 months). Lipid formulations are used at 2–5 mg/kg/d. In general, the more rapidly progressive the infection, the more compelling the case for amphotericin B therapy. However, posaconazole and voriconazole appear to be effective and their role as first-line therapy is being determined. For less severe disease and for meningeal disease, fluconazole or itraconazole are preferred (duration of therapy is > 6 months, and is indefinite for meningeal disease). Measurement of serum levels is suggested to monitor therapy. Chronic fibrocavitary pneumonia is treated for at least 12 months. Lifelong suppressive therapy is recommended after treating coccidioidal meningitis. Itraconazole may be superior to fluconazole. Refractory meningitis may require prolonged intrathecal or intraventricular amphotericin B therapy. Pregnant patients should not receive azoles.

B. General Measures

Most pulmonary infections require only symptomatic therapy, self-limited activity, and good nutrition. They are not contagious.

C. Surgical Measures

Excision of chronic pulmonary cavities or abscesses may be needed. Infected nodes, sinus tracts, and bone are other operable lesions. Azole therapy should be given prior to surgery to prevent dissemination, and should be continued for 4 weeks arbitrarily or until other criteria for cure are met.

▶ Prognosis

Most patients recover. Even with amphotericin B, however, disseminated disease may be fatal, especially in those racially predisposed to severe disease. Reversion of the skin test to negative or a rising complement-fixing antibody titer are ominous signs. Individuals who later in life undergo immunosuppressive therapy or develop HIV may experience reactivation of dormant disease. Thus, some transplant and oncology programs determine prior infection by serology and either provide prophylaxis or observe patients closely during periods of intense immune suppression.

Anstead GM, Graybill JR: Coccidioidomycosis. Infect Dis Clin North Am 2006;20:621 [PMID: 16984872].

Catanzaro A et al: Safety, tolerance, and efficacy of posaconazole therapy in patients with nonmeningeal disseminated or chronic pulmonary coccidioidomycosis. Clin Infect Dis 2007;45:562 [PMID: 17682989].

Saubolle MA et al. Epidemiologic, clinical, and diagnostic aspects of coccidioidomycosis. J Clin Microbiol 2007;45:26 [PMID: 17108067].

CRYPTOCOCCOSIS

ESSENTIALS OF DIAGNOSIS & TYPICAL FEATURES

▶ Acute pneumonitis in immunocompetent individuals.

▶ Immunosuppressed patients especially vulnerable to CNS infection (headache, vomiting, cranial nerve palsies, meningeal signs; mononuclear cell pleocytosis).

▶ Cryptococcal antigen detected in CSF; also in serum and urine in some patients.

▶ Readily isolated on routine media.

▶ General Considerations

Cryptococcus neoformans is a ubiquitous soil yeast. It appears to survive better in soil contaminated with bird excrement, especially that of pigeons. However, most infections in humans are not associated with a history of significant contact with birds. Inhalation is the presumed route of inoculation. Infections in children are rare, even in heavily immunocompromised patients such as those with HIV infection. Immunocompetent individuals can also be infected. Asymptomatic carriage does not occur.

▶ Clinical Findings

A. Symptoms and Signs

1. Pulmonary disease—Pulmonary infection precedes dissemination to other organs. It is frequently asymptomatic (ie, many older children and adults have serologic evidence of prior infection) and less often clinically apparent than cryptococcal meningitis. Pneumonia is the primary manifestation in one third of patients and CNS disease in 50%; cryptococcal pneumonia may coexist with cerebral involvement. Symptoms are nonspecific and subacute—cough, weight loss, and fatigue.

2. Meningitis—The most common clinical disease is meningitis, which follows hematogenous spread from a pulmonary focus. Symptoms of headache, vomiting, and fever occur over days to months. Meningeal signs and papilledema are common. Cranial nerve dysfunction and seizures may occur.

3. Other forms—Cutaneous forms are usually secondary to dissemination. Papules, pustules, and ulcerating nodules are typical. Bones (rarely joints) may be infected; osteolytic areas are seen, and the process may resemble osteosarcoma. Many other organs, especially the eye, can be involved with dissemination.

B. Laboratory Findings

The CSF usually has a lymphocytic pleocytosis; it may be completely normal in immunosuppressed patients who have cryptococcal meningitis. Direct microscopy may reveal organisms in sputum, CSF, or other specimens. The capsular antigen can be detected by latex agglutination or ELISA, which are both sensitive (> 90%) and specific. Serum, CSF, and urine may be tested. The serum may be negative if the only organ infected is the lung. False-negative CSF tests have been reported. The organism grows well after several days on many routine media; for optimal culture, collecting and concentrating a large amount of CSF (10 mL) is recommended, because the number of organisms may be low.

C. Imaging

Radiographic findings are usually lower lobe infiltrates or nodular densities; less often effusions; and rarely cavitation, hilar adenopathy, or calcification. Single or multiple focal mass lesions (cryptococcoma) may be detected in the CNS on CT or magnetic resonance imaging scan.

▶ Differential Diagnosis

Cryptococcal meningitis may mimic tuberculosis, viral meningoencephalitis, meningitis due to other fungi, or a space-occupying CNS lesion. Lung infection is difficult to differentiate from many causes of pneumonia.

▶ Complications

Hydrocephalus may be caused by chronic basilar meningitis. Symptomatic intracranial hypertension is common. Significant pulmonary or osseous disease may accompany the primary infection or dissemination.

▶ Treatment

Patients with symptomatic pulmonary disease should receive fluconazole for 3–6 months. All immunocompromised patients should have a lumbar puncture to rule out CNS infection; this should also be done for immunocompetent patients with cryptococcal antigen in the serum. Severely ill patients should receive amphotericin B (0.7 mg/kg/d). Meningitis is treated with amphotericin B and flucytosine (100 mg/kg/d). This combination is synergistic and allows lower doses of amphotericin B to be used. Therapy is usually 6 weeks for CNS infections (or for 1 month after sterilization) and 8 weeks for osteomyelitis. An alternative is to substitute fluconazole after 2 weeks of the combination therapy and continue fluconazole alone for 8–10 weeks. Fluconazole is the preferred maintenance therapy to prevent relapses in high-risk (HIV) patients. CSF antigen levels should be checked after 2 weeks of therapy. Intracranial hypertension is treated by frequent spinal taps or a lumbar drain.

Prognosis

Treatment failure, including death, is common in immunosuppressed patients, especially those with AIDS. Lifelong maintenance therapy may be required in these patients. Poor prognostic signs are the presence of extrameningeal disease; fewer than 20 cells/μL of initial CSF; and initial CSF antigen titer greater than 1:32.

Chayakulkeeree M, Perfect JR: Cryptococcosis. Infect Dis Clin North Am 2006;20:507 [PMID: 16984867].

Lindell RM et al: Pulmonary cryptococcosis. CT findings in immunocompetent patients. Radiology 2005;236:326 [PMID: 15987984].

Pappas PG: Managing cryptococcal meningitis is about handling the pressure. Clin Infect Dis 2005;40:480 [PMID: 15668875].

Subramanian S, Mathai D: Clinical manifestations and management of cryptococcal infection. J Postgrad Med 2005;51(Suppl 1):S21 [PMID: 16519251].

HISTOPLASMOSIS

ESSENTIALS OF DIAGNOSIS & TYPICAL FEATURES

- ▶ Residence in or travel to an endemic area.
- ▶ Pneumonia with flulike illness.
- ▶ Hepatosplenomegaly, anemia, leukopenia if disseminated.
- ▶ Histoplasmal antigen in urine, blood, or CSF.
- ▶ Detection of the organism in smears or tissue or by culture.

General Considerations

The dimorphic fungus *Histoplasma capsulatum* is found in the central and eastern United States (Ohio and Mississippi River valleys), Mexico, and most of South America. Soil contamination is enhanced by the presence of bat or bird feces. The small yeast form (2–4 μm) is seen in tissue, especially within macrophages. Infection is acquired by inhaling spores that transform into the pathogenic yeast phase. Infections in endemic areas are very common at all ages and are usually asymptomatic. Over two thirds of children are infected in these areas. Reactivation is very rare in children; it may occur years later, usually owing to significant immunosuppression. Reinfection also occurs.

The extent of symptoms with primary or reinfection is influenced by the size of the infecting inoculum.

Clinical Findings

Because human-to-human transmission does not occur, infection requires exposure in the endemic area—usually within prior weeks or months. Congenital infection does not occur.

A. Symptoms and Signs

1. Asymptomatic infection (90% of infections)— Asymptomatic histoplasmosis is usually diagnosed by the presence of scattered calcifications in lungs or spleen and a positive skin test. The calcification may resemble that caused by tuberculosis but may be more extensive than the usual Ghon complex.

2. Pneumonia—Approximately 5% of patients have mild to moderate disease. Most of these patients are not recognized as having a histoplasmal infection. Acute pulmonary disease may resemble influenza, with fever, myalgia, arthralgia, and cough occurring 1–3 weeks after exposure; the subacute form resembles infections such as tuberculosis, with cough, weight loss, night sweats, and pleurisy. Chronic disease is unusual in children. Physical examination may be normal, or rales may be heard. A small number of patients may have immune-mediated signs such as arthritis, pericarditis, and erythema nodosum. The usual duration of the disease is less than 2 weeks, followed by complete resolution. Symptoms may last several months and still resolve without antifungal therapy.

3. Disseminated infection (5% of infections)— Fungemia during primary infection probably occurs in the first 2 weeks of all infections, including those with minimal symptoms. Transient hepatosplenomegaly may occur, but resolution is the rule in immunocompetent individuals. Heavy exposure, severe underlying pulmonary disease, and immunosuppression are risk factors for progressive reticuloendothelial cell infection, with anemia, fever, weight loss, organomegaly, bone marrow involvement, and death. Dissemination may occur in otherwise immunocompetent children; usually they are younger than age 2 years.

4. Other forms—Ocular involvement consists of multifocal choroiditis. This usually occurs in immunocompetent adults who exhibit other evidence of disseminated disease. Brain, pericardium, intestine, and skin (oral ulcers and nodules) are other involved sites. Adrenal gland involvement is common with systemic disease.

B. Laboratory Findings

Routine tests are normal or nonspecific in the benign forms. Pancytopenia is present in many patients with disseminated disease. The diagnosis can be made by demonstrating the organism by histology or culture. Tissue yeast forms are small and may be mistaken for artifact. They are usually found in macrophages, occasionally in peripheral blood leukocytes in severe disease, but rarely in sputum, urine, or CSF. Cultures of infected fluids or tissues may yield the organism after 1–6 weeks of incubation on fungal media, but even cultures of bronchoalveolar lavage or transbronchial biopsy specimens in immunocompromised patients are often negative (15%). Thus bone marrow and tissue specimens are needed. Detection of histoplasmal antigen in blood, urine, CSF, and bronchoalveolar lavage fluid is the most sensitive diagnostic test (90% positive in the urine with disseminated disease; 75% positive with acute pneumonia). The level of antigen correlates with the extent of the infection, and antigen levels can be used to follow the response to therapy and to indicate low-grade infection persisting after completion of therapy (eg, in a child with HIV infection).

Antibodies may be detected by immunodiffusion and complement fixation; the latter rises in the first 2–6 weeks of illness and fall unless dissemination occurs. Cross-reactions occur with some other endemic fungi. A single high titer or rising titer indicates a high likelihood of disease. Antigen detection has replaced serology as a rapid diagnostic test.

C. Imaging

Scattered pulmonary calcifications in a well child are typical of past infection. Bronchopneumonia (focal midlung infiltrates) occurs with acute disease, often with hilar and mediastinal adenopathy, occasionally with nodules, but seldom with effusion. Apical cavitation occurs with chronic infection, often on the background of preexisting pulmonary infection.

▶ Differential Diagnosis

Pulmonary disease resembles viral infection, tuberculosis, coccidioidomycosis, and blastomycosis. Systemic disease resembles disseminated fungal or mycobacterial infection, leukemia, histiocytosis, or cancer.

▶ Treatment

Mild infections do not require therapy. Treatment is indicated for severe pulmonary disease (diffuse radiographic involvement); disseminated disease; when endovascular, CNS, or chronic pulmonary disease is present; and for children younger than age 1 year. Treatment should also be considered for patients who do not improve after 1 month. Disseminated disease in infants may respond to as few as 10 days of amphotericin B, although 4–6 weeks (or 30 mg/kg total dosage) is usually recommended. Amphotericin B is the preferred therapy for moderately severe forms of the disease. Patients with severe disease may benefit from a short course of corticosteroid therapy (see also later section on *Pneumocystis jiroveci*). Surgical excision of chronic pulmonary lesions is rarely required. Itraconazole (3–5 mg/kg/d for 6–12 weeks;

achieve peak serum level of >1.0 mcg/mL) appears to be equivalent to amphotericin B therapy for mild disease and can be substituted for amphotericin B in severe disease after a favorable initial response. With chronic pulmonary, CNS, or disseminated disease, prolonged therapy may be required.

Quantitation of fungal antigen is useful for directing therapy. Histoplasmosis can reactivate in previously infected individuals who subsequently become immunosuppressed. Chronically immunosuppressed patients (eg, those with HIV) may require lifelong maintenance therapy with an azole.

▶ Prognosis

Patients with mild and moderately severe infections have a good prognosis. With early diagnosis and treatment, infants with disseminated disease usually recover; the prognosis worsens if the immune response is poor.

Silveira F, Paterson DL: Pulmonary fungal infections. Curr Opin Pulm Med 2005;11:242 [PMID: 15818187].
Wheat LJ et al: Clinical practice guidelines for the management of patients with histoplasmosis: 2007 update by the Infectious Diseases Society of America. Clin Infect Dis 2007;45:807 [PMID: 17806045].

SPOROTRICHOSIS

ESSENTIALS OF DIAGNOSIS & TYPICAL FEATURES

- ▶ Subacute cutaneous ulcers.
- ▶ New lesions appearing proximal to existing lesions along a draining lymphatic.
- ▶ Absence of systemic symptoms.
- ▶ Isolation of *Sporothrix schenckii* from wound drainage or biopsy.

▶ General Considerations

Sporotrichosis is caused by *Sporothrix schenckii*, a dimorphic fungus present as a mold in soil, plants, and plant products from most areas of North and South America. Spores of the fungus can cause infection when they breach the skin at areas of minor trauma. Sporotrichosis has been transmitted from cutaneous lesions of pets.

▶ Clinical Findings

Cutaneous disease is by far the most common manifestation. Typically at the site of inapparent skin injury an initial papular lesion will slowly become nodular and ulcerate. Subsequent new lesions develop in a similar fashion proximally along lymphatics draining the primary lesion. This sequence of developing painless, chronic ulcers in a linear pattern is strongly suggestive of the diagnosis. Solitary lesions may exist and some lesions may develop a verrucous character. Systemic symptoms are absent and laboratory evaluations are normal, except for acute phase reactants. The fungus rarely disseminates in immunocompetent hosts, but bone and joint infections have been described. Cavitary pneumonia is an uncommon manifestation when patients inhale the spores. Immunocompromised patients, especially those with HIV infection, may develop disseminated skin lesions and multiorgan disease with extensive pneumonia.

▶ Differential Diagnosis

The differential diagnosis of nodular lymphangitis (sporotrichoid infection) includes other endemic fungi and some bacteria, especially atypical mycobacteria. Diagnosis is made by culture. Biopsy of skin lesions will demonstrate a suppurative response with granulomas and provides the best source for laboratory isolation. Occasionally the characteristic yeast will be seen in the biopsy.

▶ Treatment & Prognosis

Treatment is with itraconazole (100 mg/d or 5 mg/kg/d) for 3–6 months. Prognosis is excellent with lymphocutaneous disease in immunocompetent children. Pulmonary or osteo-articular disease, especially in immunocompromised individuals, requires longer therapy, and surgical debridement may be required.

Bonifaz A et al: Sporotrichosis in childhood: Clinical and therapeutic experience in 25 patients. Pediatr Dermatol 2007;24:369 [PMID: 17845157].
Kauffmann CA et al: Clinical practice guidelines for the management of sporotrichosis. Clin Infect Dis 2007;45:1255 [PMID: 17968818].

OPPORTUNISTIC FUNGAL INFECTIONS

These infections occur most commonly when patients are treated with corticosteroids, antineoplastic drugs, or radiation, thereby reducing the number or function of neutrophils and competent lymphocytes. Inborn errors in immune function (combined immune deficiency or chronic granulomatous disease) may also be complicated by these fungal infections. Infection is also facilitated by altering the normal flora with antibiotics and by disruption of mucous membranes with antineoplastic therapy or skin and with indwelling lines and tubes.

Table 41–8 indicates that filamentous fungi are prominent causes of severe systemic fungal disease in immunocompromised patients. *Aspergillus* species (usually *fumigatus*) and Zygomycetes (usually Mucorales) cause subacute pneumonia and sinusitis and should be considered when these conditions do not respond to antibiotics in immunocompromised patients. *Aspergillus* species are common invasive organisms in patients with chronic granulomatous disease. Mucormycosis is especially likely to produce severe sinusitis in patients with chronic acidosis, usually because of poorly controlled diabetes.

This fungus may invade the orbit and cause brain infection. Mucormycosis also occurs in patients receiving iron chelation therapy. These fungal infections may disseminate widely. Imaging procedures may suggest the etiology, but they are best diagnosed by aspiration or biopsy of infected tissues. *Cryptococcus*, which can cause disease in the immunocompetent host, is more likely to be clinically apparent and severe in immunocompromised patients. This yeast causes pneumonia and is a prominent cause of fungal meningitis. *Candida* species in these patients cause fungemia and multiorgan disease, with lung, esophagus, liver, and spleen frequently affected.

Malassezia furfur is a yeast that normally causes the superficial skin infection known as tinea versicolor (see Chapter 14). This organism is considered an opportunist when it is associated with prolonged intravenous therapy, especially central lines used for hyperalimentation. The yeast, which requires skin lipids for its growth, can infect lines when lipids are present in the infusate. Some species will grow in the absence of lipids. Unexplained fever and thrombocytopenia are common. Pulmonary infiltrates may be present. The diagnosis is facilitated by alerting the bacteriology laboratory to add olive oil to culture media. The infection will respond to removal of the line or the lipid supplement. Amphotericin B may hasten resolution.

Opportunistic fungal infections are always included in the differential diagnosis for immunocompromised patients with unexplained fever or pulmonary infiltrates. These pathogens should be aggressively pursued with imaging studies and with tissue sampling when clues are available. These infections are difficult to treat. Amphotericin B and appropriate triazole drugs are usually indicated. The echinocandins and voriconazole are now used to treat *Candida* and *Aspergillus* infections. Combinations of current antifungal drugs are being tested to improve the outcome. Many children who will have depressed phagocytic and T-cell–mediated immune function for long periods should receive antifungal prophylaxis, most often itraconazole.

Maschmeyer G et al: Invasive aspergillosis: Epidemiology, diagnosis and management in immunocompromised patients. Drugs 2007;67:1567 [PMID: 17661528].
Silveira FP, Hussain S: Fungal infections in solid organ transplantation. Med Mycol 2007;45:305 [PMID: 17510855].
Spellberg B et al: Novel perspectives on mucormycosis: Pathophysiology, presentation, and management. Clin Microbiol Rev 2005;18:556 [PMID: 16020690].

PNEUMOCYSTIS JIROVECI INFECTION

ESSENTIALS OF DIAGNOSIS & TYPICAL FEATURES

- ▶ Significant immunosuppression.
- ▶ Fever, tachypnea, cough, dyspnea.
- ▶ Hypoxemia; diffuse interstitial infiltrates.

Table 41–8. Unusual fungal infections in children.

Organism	Predisposing Factors	Route of Infection	Clinical Disease	Diagnostic Tests	Therapy and Comments
Aspergillus species	None	Inhalation of spores	Allergic bronchopulmonary aspergillosis; wheezing, cough, migratory infiltrates, eosinophilia.	Organisms in sputum; positive skin test; specific IgE antibody; elevated IgE levels.	Hypersensitivity to fungal antigens. Use steroids. Antifungals may not be needed.
	Immunosuppression	Inhalation of spores	Progressive pulmonary disease: consolidation, nodules, abscesses. Sinusitis. Disseminated disease: usually lung, brain; occasionally intestine, kidney, heart, bone. Invades blood vessels.	Demonstrate fungus in tissues by stain or culture; septate hyphae branching at 45-degree angle.	Amphotericin B, voriconazole, and oral caspofungin are equally effective; these can be used in combination.
Malassezia furfur, M pachydermatis	Central venous catheter, usually lipid infusion (can occur in the absence of lipid)	Line infection from skin colonization	Sepsis; pneumonitis, thrombocytopenia.	Culture of catheter or blood on lipid-enriched media (for *M furfur; M pachydermatis* does not need lipid). Fungus may be seen in buffy coat.	Discontinuation of lipid may be sufficient. Remove catheter. Short-term amphotericin B may be added. Organism ubiquitous on normal skin; requires long-chain fatty acids for growth.
Mucorales (*Mucor, Rhizopus, Absidia*)	Immunosuppression, diabetic acidosis, iron chelation therapy	Inhalation, mucosal colonization	Rhinocerebral: sinus, nose, necrotizing vasculitis; central nervous system spread. Pulmonary. Disseminated: any organ.	Broad aseptate hyphae branching at 90-degree angles demonstrates fungus in tissues by stain. Culture: rapidly growing, fluffy fungus.	Amphotericin B, surgical debridement; voriconazole and posaconazole may also be effective or can be used as a second agent for combined therapy. Poor prognosis.
Pseudallescheria boydii	Immunosuppression	Inhalation	Disseminated abscesses (lung, brain, liver, spleen, other).	Culture of pus or tissue.	Surgical drainage; voriconazole or caspofungin.
	Minor trauma	Cutaneous	Mycetoma (most common).	Yellow-white granules in pus. Culture.	Aggressive surgery. Amputation may be needed.
Sporothrix schenckii	Minor trauma (thorns, splinters)	Cutaneous	Chronic skin ulcers, subcutaneous nodules along lymphatics. Rarely pneumonia, osteomyelitis, arthritis in immunocompromised host.	Gram or fungal stain of pus or tissue may show "hockey stick" organisms. Culture of pus, tissue.	Itraconazole, drainage, débridement.

▶ General Considerations

Although classified as a fungus on the basis of structural and nucleic acid characteristics, *Pneumocystis* responds readily to antiprotozoal drugs and antifols. It is a ubiquitous pathogen. Initial infection is presumed to occur asymptomatically via inhalation, usually in early childhood, and to become a clinical problem upon reactivation during immune suppression. There is evidence that person-to-person transmission may contribute to symptomatic disease. Nevertheless, it appears that in the normal host clinical disease rarely occurs. A syndrome of afebrile pneumonia similar to that caused by *Chlamydia trachomatis* in normal infants has been described, but its etiology is rarely appreciated. Whether by reactivation or new exposure, severe signs and symptoms occur chiefly in patients with abnormal T-cell function such as occurs with HIV infection, hematologic malignancies, and organ transplantation. Prolonged, high-dose corticosteroid therapy for any condition is a risk factor; onset of illness as steroids are tapered is a typical presentation. Severely malnourished infants with no underlying illness may also develop this infection, as can those with congenital humoral or cellular immunodeficiency. The incubation period is usually at least 1 month after onset of immunosuppression.

Pneumocystis pneumonia is a common complication of advanced HIV infection and is one of the diseases that defines AIDS. Prophylaxis usually prevents this infection (see Chapter 39).

Infection is generally limited to the lower respiratory tract. In advanced disease, spread to other organs occurs.

▶ Clinical Findings

A. Symptoms and Signs

In most patients, a gradual onset of fever, tachypnea, dyspnea, and mild, nonproductive cough occurs over 1–4 weeks. Initially the chest is clear, although retractions and nasal flaring are present. At this stage the illness is nonspecific. Hypoxemia out of proportion to the clinical and radiographic signs is an early finding; however, even minimally decreased arterial oxygen pressure values should suggest this diagnosis in immunosuppressed children. Tachypnea, nonproductive cough, and dyspnea progress. Respiratory failure and death occur without treatment. In some children with AIDS or severe immunosuppression from chemotherapy or organ transplantation, the onset may be abrupt and progression more rapid. Acute dyspnea with pleuritic pain may indicate the related complication of pneumothorax.

The general examination is unremarkable except for tachypnea and tachycardia; rales may be absent. There are no upper respiratory signs, conjunctivitis, organomegaly, enanthem, or rash.

B. Laboratory Findings

Laboratory findings reflect the individual child's underlying illness and are not specific. Serum lactate dehydrogenase levels may be elevated markedly as a result of pulmonary damage. In moderately severe cases, the arterial oxygen pressure is less than 70 mm Hg or the alveolar-arterial gradient is less than 35 mm Hg.

C. Imaging

Early chest radiographs are normal. The classic pattern in later films is that of bilateral, interstitial, lower lobe alveolar disease starting in the perihilar regions, without effusion, consolidation, or hilar adenopathy. High-resolution CT scanning may reveal extensive ground-glass attenuation or cystic lesions. Older HIV-infected patients present with other patterns, including nodular infiltrates, lobar pneumonia, cavities, and upper lobe infiltrates.

D. Diagnostic Findings

Diagnosis requires finding characteristic round (6–8 mm) cysts in a lung biopsy specimen, bronchial brushings, alveolar washings, induced sputum, or tracheal aspirates. The latter specimens are less sensitive but are more rapidly and easily obtained. They are more often negative in children with leukemia compared with those with HIV infection; presumably, greater immunosuppression results in larger numbers of organisms. Because pneumonia in immunosuppressed patients may have many causes, negative results from tracheal secretions should prompt more aggressive diagnostic attempts. Bronchial washing using fiberoptic bronchoscopy is usually well tolerated and rapidly performed.

Several rapid stains—as well as the standard methenamine silver stain—are useful. The indirect fluorescent antibody method is most sensitive. These methods require competent laboratory evaluation, because few organisms may be present and many artifacts may be found.

▶ Differential Diagnosis

In immunocompetent infants, *C trachomatis* pneumonia is the most common cause of the afebrile pneumonia syndrome described for *Pneumocystis*. In older immunocompromised children, the differential diagnosis includes influenza, respiratory syncytial virus, cytomegalovirus, adenovirus, and other viral infections; bacterial and fungal pneumonia; pulmonary emboli or hemorrhage; congestive heart failure; and *Chlamydia pneumoniae* and *Mycoplasma pneumoniae* infections. Lymphoid interstitial pneumonitis, which occurs in older infants with HIV infection, is more indolent and the patient's lactate dehydrogenase level is normal (see Chapter 39). *Pneumocystis* pneumonia is uncommon in children who are complying with prophylactic regimens.

▶ Prevention

Children at high risk for developing *Pneumocystis* infection should receive prophylactic therapy. Children at risk include those with hematologic malignancies, children who for other reasons are receiving intensive chemotherapy or high-dose corticosteroids, and children with organ transplants or advanced HIV infection. All children born to HIV-infected mothers should receive prophylaxis against *Pneumocystis* starting at age 6 weeks until HIV infection has been ruled out, or if the infant is infected, until the patient's immunologic status has been clarified (see Chapter 39). The prophylaxis of choice is trimethoprim–sulfamethoxazole (150 mg/m^2/d of trimethoprim and 750 mg/m^2/d of sulfamethoxazole) for 3 consecutive days of each week. Alternatives to this prophylaxis regimen are described in Chapter 39.

► Treatment

A. General Measures

Supplemental oxygen and nutritional support may be needed. The patient should be in respiratory isolation.

B. Specific Measures

Trimethoprim–sulfamethoxazole (20 mg/kg/d of trimethoprim and 100 mg/kg/d of sulfamethoxazole in four divided doses intravenously or orally if well tolerated) is the treatment of choice. Improvement may not be seen for 3–5 days. Duration of treatment is 3 weeks in HIV-infected children. Methylprednisolone (2–4 mg/kg/d in four divided doses intravenously) should also be given to HIV-infected patients with moderate to severe infection (partial oxygen pressure < 70 mm Hg or alveolar-arterial gradient > 35) for the first 5 days of treatment. The dosage is reduced 50% for the next 5 days, and further reduced by 50% until antibiotic treatment is completed. If trimethoprim–sulfamethoxazole is not tolerated or there is no clinical response in 5 days, pentamidine isethionate (4 mg/kg once daily by slow intravenous infusion) should be given. There is growing concern that antimicrobial resistance may be developing in some locations. Clinical efficacy is similar with pentamidine, but adverse reactions are more common. These reactions include dysglycemia, pancreatitis, nephrotoxicity, and leukopenia. Other effective alternatives in adults include atovaquone, trimethoprim plus dapsone, and primaquine plus clindamycin.

► Prognosis

The mortality rate is high in immunosuppressed patients who receive treatment late in the illness.

Hidalgo A et al: Accuracy of high-resolution CT in distinguishing between *Pneumocystis carinii* pneumonia and non-*Pneumocystis carinii* pneumonia in AIDS patients. Eur Radiol 2003;13: 1179 [PMID: 12695843].

LaRocque RC et al: The utility of sputum induction for diagnosis of *Pneumocystis* pneumonia in immunocompromised patients without human immunodeficiency virus. Clin Infect Dis 2003;37:1380 [PMID: 1453873].

Mahindra AD, Grossman SA: *Pneumocystis carinii* pneumonia in HIV negative patients with primary brain tumors. J Neurooncol 2003;63:263 [PMID: 12892232].

Shankar SM, Nania JJ: Management of *Pneumocystis jiroveci* pneumonia in children receiving chemotherapy. Paediatr Drugs 2007;9:310 [PMID: 17927302].

REFERENCES

Blyth CC et al: Antifungal therapy in children with invasive fungal infections: A systematic review. Pediatrics 2007;119:772 [PMID: 17403849].

Hotez PJ et al: Control of neglected tropical diseases. N Engl J Med 2007;357:1018 [PMID: 17804846].

Petrikkos G, Skiada A: Recent advances in antifungal therapy. Inter J Antimicrob Agents 2007;30:108 [PMID: 17524625].

Reddy M et al: Oral drug therapy for multiple neglected tropical diseases. JAMA 2007;298:1911 [PMID: 17954542].

Ryan ET et al: Illness after international travel. N Engl J Med 2002;347:505 [PMID: 12181406].

Sexually Transmitted Infections

Ann-Christine Nyquist, MD, MSPH
Eric J. Sigel, MD

The rate of sexually transmitted infections (STIs) acquired during adolescence remains high despite widespread educational programs and increased access to health care. The highest age-specific rates for gonorrhea, chlamydia, and human papillomavirus (HPV) infection occur in adolescents and young adults. By age 18 years, half of youth will have had sexual intercourse. One quarter of those having intercourse will develop an STI—an estimated 3 million teenagers per year. Adolescents contract STIs at a higher rate than adults because of sexual risk-taking, age-related biologic factors, and barriers to health care access. Providers need to comply with state-sanctioned confidentiality laws covering STI-related services, while recognizing the importance of confidentiality to adolescents. Except in a few states, adolescents can provide consent for the diagnosis and confidential treatment of STIs without parental consent or knowledge. In many states, adolescents can also provide consent for human immunodeficiency virus (HIV) counseling and testing.

Providers should screen sexually experienced adolescents for STIs and use this opportunity to discuss risk reduction. Health education counseling should be nonjudgmental and appropriate for the developmental level, yet sufficiently thorough to identify risk behaviors because many adolescents may not readily acknowledge engaging in these behaviors.

ADOLESCENT SEXUALITY

The spectrum of sexual behavior includes holding hands and kissing; touching, expanding to mutual masturbation; oral-genital contact; and vaginal and anal intercourse. Each has its associated risks. A small, but statistically significant, trend has occurred in the epidemiology of sexual risk-taking toward less sexual involvement and later onset of vaginal intercourse. The most recent Youth Risk Behavior Survey (2005) reports that 47% of high school students have had vaginal intercourse during their lifetime; unchanged from the 2003 survey. Six percent of teenagers have initiated sex by age 13. Significant racial and gender differences exist, with 16% of black students

(27% of males and 7% of females), 7% of Hispanics, and 4% of whites initiating sex by age 13. Thirty-four percent of students have had sex in the prior 3 months—49% of twelfth-graders and 22% of ninth-graders. Condom use has increased, with 63% of youth reporting that either they or their partner had used a condom during their last sexual intercourse, compared with 42% in 1999. Paradoxically, condom use decreases with age—75% of ninth-graders report condom use at last intercourse compared with 55% of twelfth-graders.

Oral sex has not been as well studied. A recent study reports that 38% of boys and 42% of girls in the tenth grade engaged in oral sex, with only 17% using any protection. A significant number of teenagers exhibit higher-risk sexual behavior; 14% overall have had four or more sexual partners in their lifetime—21% of high school seniors and 9% of freshman. Racial and ethnic differences exist as well: having four or more sexual partners is more common among black males (39%) than among Hispanic males (22%) or white males (12%). One million teenagers become pregnant annually. Almost 8% of students have been physically forced to have sexual intercourse when they did not want to—10% of females and 5% of males. Anal intercourse occurs in both heterosexual and homosexual populations.

Adolescents may not yet identify themselves as gay, lesbian, or bisexual, but continue to question and to engage in high-risk behaviors with multiple partners. Anywhere from 10% to 30% of males experiment with same-sex partners in some fashion, with 4–10% practicing anal sex. Frequently teenage males have their first same-sex experience with partners who are significantly older, which puts them at higher risk for STIs. Lesbians often experiment with male partners during their teen years as they sort out their sexual orientation, placing them at increased risk for pregnancy and STIs.

Impaired judgment related to alcohol or drug use creates an environment for unsafe sexual experimentation. Eighty-two percent of high school students have experimented with alcohol; 50% of high school senior boys have been drunk in the last 30 days. Nationwide, among students who were currently having sexual intercourse, 25% used alcohol or drugs the last time they had sex. This additional barrier to decision-making results in decreased condom use and an increased incidence of forced sex.

RISK FACTORS

Certain behaviors and experiences put the adolescent at higher risk for developing STIs. These include early age at sexual debut, lack of condom use, multiple partners, prior STI, history of STI in a partner, and sex with a partner who is 3 or more years older. The type of sex affects risk as well, with intercourse being riskier than oral sex. Other risk-taking behaviors associated with STIs in adolescents are smoking, alcohol use, drug use, dropping out of school, pregnancy, and watching X-rated movies.

The adolescent female is especially predisposed to chlamydia, gonorrhea, and HPV infection because the cervix during adolescence has an exposed squamocolumnar junction. The rapidly dividing cells in this area are especially susceptible to microorganism attachment and infection. During early to mid puberty this junction slowly invaginates as the uterus and cervix mature, and by the late teens to early 20s the squamocolumnar junction is inside the cervix.

Datta SD et al: Gonorrhea and chlamydia in the United States among persons 14 to 39 years of age, 1999 to 2002. Ann Intern Med 2007;147:89 [PMID: 17638719].

DiClemente RJ, Crosby RA: Preventing sexually transmitted infections among adolescents: 'The glass is half full'. Curr Opin Infect Dis 2006;19:39 [PMID: 16374216].

Duncan P et al: Childhood and adolescent sexuality. Pediatr Clin North Am 2003;50:765 [PMID: 12964693].

Eaton DK et al: Youth risk behavior surveillance—United States, 2005. MMWR Surveill Summ 2006;55(SS-5):1 [PMID: 16760893].

Halpern-Flesher BL et al: Oral versus vaginal sex among adolescents: Perceptions, attitudes, and behavior. Pediatrics 2005;115:845 [PMID: 15805354].

Prinstein MJ et al: Adolescent oral sex, peer popularity, and perceptions of best friend's sexual behavior. J Pediatr Psychol 2003;28:243 [PMID: 22616299].

Rietmeijer CA: Risk reduction counseling for prevention of sexually transmitted infections: How it works and how to make it work. Sex Transm Infect 2007;83:2 [PMID: 17283359].

Risser WL et al: The epidemiology of sexually transmitted infections in adolescents. Semin Pediatr Infect Dis 2005;16:160 [PMID: 16044389].

PREVENTION OF SEXUALLY TRANSMITTED INFECTIONS

Efforts to reduce STI risk behavior should begin before the onset of sexual experimentation: first by helping youth personalize their risk for STIs and encouraging positive behaviors that minimize these risks, and then by enhancing communication skills with sexual partners about STI prevention, abstinence, and condom use.

Primary prevention focuses largely on education and risk-reduction techniques. It is essential to recognize that a key task

of adolescence is developing sexual identity. Teenagers are sexual beings and will decide if, when, and how they are going to initiate sexual involvement. Health care providers should routinely address sexuality as part of well adolescent checkups. Being open and frank about the risks and benefits of each specific type of sexual activity will help youth think about their decision and the consequences. Although more than 90% of students have been taught about HIV infection and other STIs in school, adolescents still have a difficult time personalizing risk. Discussing prevalence, symptoms, and sequelae of STIs can raise awareness and help teenagers make informed decisions about initiating sexual activity and the use of safer sex techniques. Making condoms available reiterates the message that safer sex is vital to health. Discussing condoms, dental dams, and the proper use of lubrication also facilitates safer sex practices. Condoms prevent infections with HIV, HPV, gonorrhea, *Chlamydia,* and herpes simplex virus (HSV). They are probably effective in preventing other STIs as well.

Secondary prevention requires identifying and treating STIs (see next section on Screening) before infected individuals transmit infection to others. Access to medical care is critical to this objective. Identifying and treating STIs in partners are essential in limiting the spread of these infections. Cooperation with the state or county health department is valuable, because these agencies assume the responsibility for locating the contacts of infected persons and ensuring appropriate treatment.

Tertiary prevention is directed toward complications of a specific illness. Examples of tertiary prevention would be treating pelvic inflammatory disease (PID) before infertility develops; following the serologic response to syphilis to prevent late-stage syphilis; treating cervicitis to prevent PID; or treating a chlamydial infection before epididymitis ensues.

Finally, preexposure vaccination against hepatitis B or hepatitis A reduces the risk for these preventable STIs. All adolescents should have prior or current immunization against hepatitis B. (See Chapter 9.) However, because hepatitis B infection is frequently sexually transmitted, this vaccine is especially critical for all unvaccinated patients being evaluated for an STI. Hepatitis A vaccination is recommended for males who have sex with men and for injection drug users. Preexposure vaccination for HPV in females can decrease risk for cervical dysplasia and cervical cancer as well as decrease risk for genital warts. (See Chapter 9.)

DiClemente RJ et al: A programmatic and methodologic review and synthesis of clinic-based risk-reduction interventions for sexually transmitted infections: Research and practice implications. Semin Pediatr Infect Dis 2005;16:199 [PMID: 16044394].

SCREENING FOR SEXUALLY TRANSMITTED INFECTIONS

An essential part of screening is by history. Teenagers should be asked open-ended questions about their sexual experiences to assess their risk for STIs. The ability of the health care provider to obtain an accurate sexual history is crucial in prevention and control efforts. Questions must be explicit and understandable to the youth. If the adolescent has ever engaged in sexual activity, the provider needs to determine what kind of sexual activity (mutual masturbation or oral, anal, or vaginal sex); whether it has been heterosexual, homosexual, or both; whether birth control and condoms were used; and whether it has been consensual or forced. During the interview the clinician should take the opportunity to discuss risk-reduction techniques regardless of the history obtained from the youth. Importantly, female health care providers are twice as likely as male providers to screen female teenagers for STIs, so male health care providers need to better use screening opportunities.

A routine laboratory screening process is warranted if the patient has engaged in intercourse, presents with STI symptoms, or reports a partner with an STI. The availability of nucleic acid amplification tests (NAATs), primarily for *Chlamydia* and *Neisseria gonorrhoeae,* has changed the nature of STI screening and intervention. These amplification tests are more than 95% sensitive and more than 99% specific, using either urine or cervical/urethral swabs. Annual screening of all sexually active females aged 25 years or younger is recommended for *Chlamydia trachomatis*. Routine chlamydial testing should be considered for all adolescent males and, in particular, males who have sex with men, have new or multiple sex partners, or are in correctional facilities.

Initial screening for urethritis in males begins with a physical examination. A first-catch urine sample (the first 10–40 mL of voided urine collected after not voiding for 2 hours) should be sent for *Chlamydia* and *N gonorrhoeae* testing if there are no signs (urethral discharge or lesions) or symptoms. With signs or symptoms, a urethral swab should be sent to test for both *N gonorrhoeae* and *Chlamydia*. A wet mount preparation should then be done on a spun urine sample or from urethral discharge, evaluating for the presence of *Trichomonas vaginalis*.

Screening asymptomatic females has become more complicated because a variety of approaches are available. Generally, either a first-void urine specimen or a cervical swab is used to screen for *Chlamydia* and *N gonorrhoeae* by NAAT. When screening for *N gonorrhoeae*, it is important to recognize that certain NAATs are less sensitive when using urine compared with a cervical swab and may not be approved for urine screening. A wet preparation of the vaginal secretions should be performed annually to check for bacterial vaginosis and trichomoniasis, and a potassium hydroxide (KOH) preparation done to screen for yeast infections. The Papanicolaou (Pap) smear serves to evaluate the cervix for the presence of HPV. The first Pap smear should be performed 3 years after the initiation of sexual intercourse, and then annually. HPV typing is no longer recommended.

For both sexes if high-risk behavior is present (three or more partners in the last 6 months or more than two partners per year for several years), then screening for hepatitis B

surface antigen is warranted if the individual was not fully immunized prior to initiation of sexual intercourse. The presence of hepatitis B surface antigen indicates either the carrier state or active infection. Presence of only hepatitis B surface antibody identifies vaccinated individuals, whereas presence of hepatitis B core antibody and hepatitis B surface antibody identifies individuals with past infection (see Chapter 21).

In urban areas with a relatively high rate of syphilis or in males who have sex with men, an RPR/VDRL (rapid plasma reagin/Venereal Disease Research Laboratory) test should be drawn yearly. RPR and HIV antibody tests should be done in all individuals in whom a concomitant STI is present.

Fortenberry JD: Sexually transmitted infections. Screening and diagnosis guidelines for primary care pediatricians. Pediatr Ann 2005;34:803 [PMID: 16285634].

Gaydos CA: Nucleic acid amplification tests for gonorrhea and chlamydia: Practice and applications. Infect Dis Clin North Am 2005;19:367 [PMID: 15963877].

Olshen E, Shrier LA: Diagnostic tests for chlamydial and gonorrheal infections. Semin Pediatr Infect Dis 2005;16:192 [PMID: 16044393].

SIGNS & SYMPTOMS

For males, the most common symptoms are dysuria and penile discharge resulting from urethral inflammation. Less common symptoms are scrotal pain, hematuria, proctitis, and pruritus in the pubic region. Signs include epididymitis, orchitis, and urethral discharge. Rarely do males develop systemic symptoms. For females, the most common symptoms are vaginal discharge and dysuria. Vaginal itching and irregular menses or spotting are also common. Abdominal pain, fever, and vomiting, although less common, are signs of PID. Pain in the genital region and dyspareunia may be present.

Signs that can be found in both males and females with an STI include genital ulcerations, adenopathy, and genital warts.

THE MOST COMMON ANTIBIOTIC-RESPONSIVE SEXUALLY TRANSMITTED INFECTIONS

C trachomatis and *N gonorrhoeae* are STIs that are epidemic in the United States and are readily treated when appropriate antibiotics are administered in a timely fashion.

CHLAMYDIA TRACHOMATIS INFECTION

▶ General Considerations

C trachomatis is the most common bacterial cause of STIs in the United States. Three million cases are estimated to occur annually in adolescents and young adults. *C trachomatis* is an obligate intracellular bacterium that replicates within the cytoplasm of host cells. Destruction of *Chlamydia*-infected cells is mediated by host immune responses.

▶ Clinical Findings

A. Symptoms and Signs

Clinical infection in females manifests as dysuria, urethritis, vaginal discharge, cervicitis, or PID. The presence of mucopus at the cervical os (mucopurulent cervicitis) is a sign of *Chlamydia* infection or gonorrhea. *Chlamydia* infection is asymptomatic in 75% of females.

Chlamydial infection may be asymptomatic in 70% of males or manifest as dysuria, urethritis, or epididymitis. Some patients complain of urethral discharge. On clinical examination a clear white discharge may be found after milking the penis. Proctitis or proctocolitis from *Chlamydia* may occur in adolescents practicing receptive anal intercourse.

B. Laboratory Findings

NAAT (polymerase or ligase chain reaction) is the most sensitive (92–99%) way to detect *Chlamydia*. Enzyme-linked immunosorbent assay or direct fluorescent antibody tests are less sensitive, but may be the only testing option in some centers. Culture is mandated for sexual abuse cases.

A cervical swab, using the manufacturer's swab provided with the specific test, or first-void urine specimen should be obtained. Often a single swab can be used to collect both the *Chlamydia* and *N gonorrhoeae* specimen. To optimize detection of *Chlamydia* from the cervix, columnar cells need to be collected by inserting the swab in the os and rotating it 360 degrees. If rectal symptoms are present, a rectal specimen should be obtained.

The first-void urine test for leukocyte esterase was previously used for screening asymptomatic, sexually active males. Due to the high false-positive rate this screening technique is now less commonly used. In symptomatic males, examination of the urine sediment for white blood cells (WBCs) can provide evidence of urethritis, although it is often impractical to perform in a clinical setting. In general, a first-void urine sample, or urethral swab for NAAT should be obtained at least annually. Some studies suggest that more frequent screenings—every 6 months—in higher-prevalence populations can decrease the rate of chlamydial infection. Evaluation of the symptomatic male patient or an asymptomatic contact for *Chlamydia* is the same.

For both males and females, testing urine allows for more frequent screening and simplifies screening in settings such as schools and correctional facilities, or among the military and other groups.

▶ Complications

Epididymitis is a complication in males. Reiter syndrome occurs in association with chlamydial urethritis. This should be suspected in male patients who are sexually active and present with low back pain (sacroiliitis), arthritis (polyarticular), characteristic mucocutaneous lesions, and conjunctivitis. PID is an important complication in females.

▶ Treatment

Infected patients and their contacts, regardless of the extent of signs or symptoms, need to receive treatment (Table 42–1). Because adolescents have a high risk of acquiring a repeat *Chlamydia* infection within several months of the first infection, all infected females should be retested 3–4 months after treatment. Retesting for *Chlamydia* in males previously infected 3 months after treatment is suggested although there is limited evidence as to the benefit.

Geisler WM: Management of uncomplicated *Chlamydia trachomatis* infections in adolescents and adults: Evidence reviewed for the 2006 Centers for Disease Control and Prevention sexually transmitted diseases treatment guidelines. Clin Infect Dis 2007;44:S77 [PMID: 17342671].

Meyers DS et al: Screening for chlamydial infection: An evidence update for the U.S. Preventive Services Task Force. Ann Intern Med 2007;147:135 [PMID: 17576995].

NEISSERIA GONORRHOEAE INFECTION

▶ General Considerations

Gonorrhea is the second most prevalent bacterial STI in the United States, where an estimated 600,000 new *N gonorrhoeae* infections occur each year. In the United States the rate of reported gonorrhea was 115.6 cases per 100,000 population in 2005, representing the first increase in this rate since 1999. Gonorrhea rates continued to be highest among adolescents and young adults. The overall gonorrhea rate was highest for 20- to 24-year-olds (506.8), which is over four times higher than the national gonorrhea rate. Among females in 2005, 15- to 19-year-olds and 20- to 24-year-olds had the highest rates of gonorrhea (624.7 and 581.2, respectively); among males, 20- to 24-year-olds had the highest rate (436.8).

Sites of infection include the cervix, urethra, rectum, and pharynx. In addition, gonorrhea is a cause of PID. Humans are the natural reservoir. Gonococci are present in the exudate and secretions of infected mucous membranes.

▶ Clinical Findings

A. Symptoms and Signs

In uncomplicated gonococcal cervicitis, females may be symptomatic 23–57% of the time, presenting with vaginal discharge and dysuria. Urethritis and pyuria may also be present. Mucopurulent cervicitis with a yellowish discharge may be found, and the cervix may be edematous and friable. Other symptoms include abnormal menstrual periods and dyspareunia. Approximately 15% of females with endocervical gonorrhea have signs of involvement of the upper genital tract. Compared with *Chlamydia* infection, pelvic inflammation with gonorrhea often has a shorter duration, but an increased intensity of symptoms, and is more often associated with fever. Symptomatic males usually have a yellowish-green urethral discharge and burning on urination, but most

Table 42–1. Treatment regimens for sexually transmitted infections.

	Recommended Regimens	Pregnancy[a] [Category]
Pelvic inflammatory disease (PID)		
Parenteral therapy regimen A	Cefotetan, 2 g IV q 12 h	Safe [B]
Note: Therapy should be continued for 24–48 h after patient has improved; therapy can then be switched to either oral regimen to complete a 14-d course.	or	
	Cefoxitin, 2 g IV q 6 h	Safe [B]
	plus	
	Doxycycline, 100 mg IV or PO q 12 h	Contraindicated [D]
Parenteral therapy regimen B	Clindamycin, 900 mg IV q 8 h	Safe [B]
Note: Once clinically improved for 48 h, patients can continue doxycycline, 100 mg PO bid for 14 d total.[b]	plus	
	Gentamicin, 2 mg/kg IV loading dose, then 1.5 mg/kg IV q 8 h	Safe [B]
Alternative parenteral regimens	Ampicillin/sulbactam, 3 g IV q 6 h	Safe [A]
	plus	
	Doxycycline, 100 mg IV or PO q 12 h	Contraindicated [D]
Recommended oral regimen	Ceftriaxone, 250 mg IM once	Safe [B]
Note: Pregnant patients with PID and women with tubo-ovarian abscesses should be hospitalized and given parenteral antibiotics.[b]	plus	
	Doxycycline, 100 mg, PO bid for 14 d with or without	Contraindicated [D]
	Metronidazole, 500 mg PO bid for 14 d	Safe [B]
	or	
	Cefoxitin, 2 g IM once plus probenecid, 1 g PO	Safe [B]
	plus	
	Doxycycline, 100 mg, PO bid for 14 d with or without	Contraindicated [D]
	Metronidazole, 500 mg PO bid for 14 d	Safe [B]
	or	
	Other parenteral third-generation cephalosporin (eg, ceftizoxime or cefotaxime)	Safe [B]
	plus	
	Doxycycline, 100 mg, PO bid for 14 d with or without	Contraindicated [D]
	Metronidazole, 500 mg PO bid for 14 d	Safe [B]
Cervicitis		
	Azithromycin, 1 g PO as single dose	Safe [B]
	or	
	Doxycycline, 100 mg PO bid for 7 d	Contraindicated [D]
Gonorrhea, uncomplicated		
Cervicitis, urethritis, rectal	Ceftriaxone, 125 mg IM as single dose	Safe [B]
Note: Empiric treatment for *Chlamydia trachomatis* with azithromycin or doxycycline is recommended due to coexisting infection in 20–40% of patients with gonorrhea infection if chlamydial infection is not ruled out.[c]	or	
	Cefixime, 400 mg PO as single dose	Safe [B]
Alternative regimen	Spectinomycin, 2 g in a single IM dose	Safe [B]
	or	
	Cephalosporins single-dose regimens[c]	Safe [B]
Pharyngitis	Ceftriaxone, 125 mg IM once	Safe [B]
Gonorrhea, disseminated		
Note: Treat IV until clinically improved (usually 48 h; then switch to PO); complete at least a 7-d course.[d]	Ceftriaxone, 1 g IV or IM q 24 h	Safe [B]

(continued)

Table 42–1. Treatment regimens for sexually transmitted infections. *(Continued)*

	Recommended Regimens	Pregnancy[a] [Category]
Alternative regimens	Cefotaxime, 1 g IV q 8 h	Safe [B]
	or	
	Ceftizoxime, 1 g IV q 8 h	Safe [B]
	or	
	Spectinomycin, 2 g IM q 12 h	Safe [B]
Oral regimen[d]	Cefixime, 400 mg PO bid	Safe [B]
	or	
	Cefixime suspension, 400 mg by suspension (200 mg/5 mL) PO bid	Safe [B]
	or	
	Cefpodoxime, 400 mg PO bid	Safe [B]
Nongonococcal, nonchlamydial urethritis		
	Azithromycin, 1 g PO as single dose	Safe [B]
	or	
	Doxycycline, 100 mg PO bid for 7 d	Contraindicated [D]
Alternative regimens	Erythromycin base, 500 mg PO qid for 7 d	Safe [B]
	or	
	Erythromycin ethylsuccinate, 800 mg PO qid for 7 d	Safe [B]
	or	
	Ofloxacin, 300 mg PO bid for 7 d[d]	Contraindicated [C]
	or	
	Levofloxacin, 500 mg PO once daily for 7 d[d]	Contraindicated [C]
Recurrent or persistent urethritis	Metronidazole, 2 g PO as single dose	Safe [B]
	or	
	Tinidazole, 2 g PO as single dose	Contraindicated [C]
	plus	
	Azithromycin, 1 g PO as single dose (if not used for initial episode)	Safe [B]
Proctitis, proctocolitis, and enteritis		
	Ceftriaxone 125 mg IM	Safe [B]
	plus	
	Doxycycline, 100 mg PO bid for 7 d	Contraindicated [D]
***Trichomonas vaginalis* vaginitis or urethritis**		
	Metronidazole, 2 g PO as single dose	Safe [B]
	or	
	Tinidazole, 2 g PO as single dose	Contraindicated [C]
Alternative regimen	Metronidazole, 500 mg PO bid for 7d	Safe [B]
Bacterial vaginosis		
	Metronidazole, 500 mg PO bid for 7 d	Safe [B]
	or	
	Metronidazole, 0.75% gel, 5 g intravaginally once daily for 5 d	Safe [B]
	or	
	Clindamycin cream, 2%, one applicator intravaginally at bedtime for 7 d	Safe [B]
Alternative regimen	Clindamycin, 300 mg PO bid for 7 d	Safe [B]
	or	
	Clindamycin ovule, 100 mg intravaginally once at bedtime for 3 d	Safe [B]

(continued)

Table 42–1. Treatment regimens for sexually transmitted infections. *(Continued)*

	Recommended Regimens	Pregnancy[a] [Category]
Vulvovaginal candidiasis		
	Butoconazole, clotrimazole, miconazole, terconazole or tioconazole, intravaginally for 1, 3, or 7 d	Safe [B]
	or	
	Butoconazole sustained-release, 5 g once intravaginally	Safe [B]
	or	
	Fluconazole, 150 mg oral tablet, in single dose	Contraindicated [C]
Syphilis		
Early (primary, secondary, or latent < 1 y)	Benzathine penicillin G, 2.4 million units IM (for patients > 40 kg)	Safe [B]
	or	
	Benzathine penicillin G, 50,000 units/kg IM (for patients < 40 kg); up to 2.4 million units in one dose	Safe [B]
	or	
	Doxycycline, 100 mg PO bid for 14 d	Contraindicated [D]
Late (> 1 y duration or of unknown duration)	Benzathine penicillin G, 7.2 million units total, administered as 3 doses of 2.4 million units IM each at 1-week intervals	Safe [B]
	or	
	Benzathine penicillin G, 50,000 units/kg IM (for patients < 40 kg) once a week for 3 consecutive weeks; up to 2.4 million units in one dose	Safe [B]
	or	
	Doxycycline, 100 mg PO bid for 28 d	Contraindicated [D]
Neurosyphilis		
	Aqueous crystalline penicillin G, 18–24 million units/d, administered as 3–4 million units IV q 4 h or continuous infusion for 10–14 d	Safe [B]
Alternative regimen (if compliance can be assured)	Procaine penicillin, 2.4 million units IM once daily	Safe [B]
	plus	
	Probenicid, 500 mg PO qid for 10–14 d	Safe [B]
Epididymitis		
Most likely caused by gonococcal or chlamydial infection	Ceftriaxone, 250 mg IM as single dose	
	plus	
	Doxycycline, 100 mg PO bid for 10 d	
Most likely caused by enteric organisms; patient older than 35 y or allergies to cephalosporins or tetracyclines (or both)	Ofloxacin, 300 mg PO bid for 10 d	
	or	
	Levofloxacin, 500 mg PO once daily for 10 d	
***Chlamydia trachomatis* infection**		
Cervicitis or urethritis	Azithromycin, 1 g PO as single dose	Safe [B]
	or	
	Doxycycline, 100 mg PO bid for 7d	Contraindicated [D]
Alternative regimen[b]	Erythromycin, 500 mg PO qid for 7 d	Safe [B]
	or	
	Erythromycin ethylsuccinate, 800 mg PO qid for 7 d	Safe [B]
	or	
	Ofloxacin, 300 mg PO bid for 7 d	Contraindicated [C]
	or	
	Levofloxacin 500 mg PO once daily for 7 d	Contraindicated [C]

Table 42–1. Treatment regimens for sexually transmitted infections. (*Continued*)

	Recommended Regimens	Pregnancy[a] [Category]
Granuloma inguinale		
	Doxycycline, 100 mg PO bid for 3 weeks or longer	Contraindicated [D]
Alternative regimen	Ciprofloxacin, 750 mg PO bid for at least 3 weeks	Contraindicated [C]
	or	
	Erythromycin base, 500 mg PO qid for at least 3 weeks	Safe [B]
	or	
	Azithromycin, 1 g PO once per week for at least 3 weeks	Safe [B]
	or	
	Trimethoprim-sulfamethoxazole, one double-strength tablet PO bid for 3 weeks or longer	Contraindicated [C]
Lymphogranuloma venereum		
	Doxycycline, 100 mg PO bid for 21 d	Contraindicated [C]
Alternative regimen	Erythromycin, 500 mg PO qid for 21 d	Safe [B]
Herpes simplex infection		
First episode, genital	Acyclovir, 400 mg PO tid for 7–10 d	Safe [B]
	or	
	Famciclovir, 250 mg PO tid for 7–10 d	Safe [B]
	or	
	Valacyclovir, 1 g PO bid for 7–10 d	Safe [B]
Episodic therapy for recurrent genital herpes	Acyclovir, 400 mg PO tid for 5 d	Safe [B]
	or	
	Acyclovir, 800 mg PO bid for 5 d	Safe [B]
	or	
	Acyclovir, 800 mg PO tid for 2 d	Safe [B]
	or	
	Famciclovir, 125 mg PO bid for 5 d	Safe [B]
	or	
	Famciclovir, 1000 mg PO bid for 1 d	Safe [B]
	or	
	Valacyclovir, 500 mg PO bid for 3 d	Safe [B]
	or	
	Valacyclovir, 1 g PO once daily for 5 d	Safe [B]
Suppressive therapy for recurrent genital herpes	Acyclovir, 400 mg PO bid	Safe [B]
	or	
	Famciclovir, 250 mg PO bid	Safe [B]
	or	
	Valacyclovir, 500 mg PO daily (if < 10 recurrences per year; if ≥ 10 recurrences use 1 g daily)	Safe [B]
Chancroid		
	Azithromycin, 1 g PO as single dose	Safe [B]
	or	
	Ceftriaxone 250 mg IM once	Safe [B]
	or	
	Ciprofloxacin, 500 mg PO bid for 3 d	Contraindicated [D]
	or	
	Erythromycin base, 500 mg PO tid for 7 d	Safe [B]

(continued)

Table 42–1. Treatment regimens for sexually transmitted infections. *(Continued)*

	Recommended Regimens	Pregnancy[a] [Category]
Human papillomavirus infection		
External lesions	Podophyllin, 25% in benzoin tincture applied directly to warts; wash off in 1–4 h [contraindicated for urethral or intravaginal lesions]	Contraindicated [X]
Note: Topical therapies usually require weekly treatments for 4 consecutive weeks	or	
	Trichloroacetic acid (85%); apply directly to warts; wash off in 6–8 h	Safe
	or	
	Podofilox, 0.5% solution; apply bid for 3 d; used by patient at home; practitioner needs to demonstrate how compound is applied (to be used only on external lesions)	Contraindicated [C]
	or	
	Imiquimod 5% cream, applied 3 times per week overnight (maximum of 16 weeks)	Contraindicated [C]
	or	
	Cryotherapy: liquid nitrogen, cryoprobe Safe Laser surgery	Safe
Ectoparasitic infections		
Pubic lice[e]	Permethrin 1% creme rinse: wash off after 10 min	Safe [B]
	or	
	Pyrethins with piperonyl butoxide: apply, wash off after 10 min	Safe [B]
Alternative regimen	Malathion 0.5% lotion: wash off after 8-12 h	Safe [B]
	or	
	Ivermectin, 250 mcg/kg repeated in 2 weeks	Contraindicated [C]
Scabies	Permethrin cream 5%: apply to entire body from the neck down, wash off after 8–14 h	Safe [B]
	or	
	Ivermectin, 200 mcg/kg PO, repeat in 2 weeks	Contraindicated [C]
Alternative regimen	Lindane (1%): apply to entire body from neck down, wash off after 8 h	Contraindicated [C]

[a]FDA use in pregnancy ratings: [A] *Controlled studies show no risk.* Adequate, well-controlled studies in pregnant women have failed to demonstrate a risk to the fetus in any trimester of pregnancy. [B] *No evidence of risk in humans.* Adequate, well-controlled studies in pregnant women have not shown increased risk of fetal abnormalities despite adverse findings in animals, in the absence of adequate human studies, animal studies show no fetal risk. The chance of fetal harm is remote but remains a possibility. [C] *Risk cannot be ruled out.* Adequate, well-controlled human studies are lacking, and animal studies have shown a risk to the fetus or are lacking as well. There is a chance of fetal harm if the drug is administered during pregnancy; but the potential benefits outweigh the potential risk. [D] *Positive evidence of risk.* Studies in humans, or investigational or postmarketing data, have demonstrated fetal risk. Nevertheless, potential benefits from the use of the drug may outweigh the potential risk. For example, the drug may be acceptable if needed in a life-threatening situation or serious disease for which safer drugs cannot be used or are ineffective. [X] *Contraindicated in pregnancy.* Studies in animals or humans, or despite adverse findings in animals, or investigational or postmarketing reports have demonstrated positive evidence of fetal abnormalities or risk that clearly outweighs any possible benefit to the patient.

[b]Doxycycline is contraindicated in pregnancy. Alternative therapies during pregnancy which include erythromycin, azithromycin, and amoxicillin are not as effective, but are clinically useful if the recommended regimens cannot be used due to allergy or pregnancy.

[c]Single-dose cephalosporin regimens include ceftizoxime (500 mg IM) or cefoxitin (2 g IM) administered with probenecid (1 g PO) or cefotaxime (500 mg IM). Some evidence indicates that cefpodoxime (400 mg) and cefuroxime axetil (1 g) might be oral alternatives.

[d]If parenteral cephalosporin therapy is not feasible, use of fluoroquinolones (levofloxacin, 500 mg PO once daily, or ofloxacin, 400 mg PO bid for 14 d) with or without metronidazole (500 mg PO bid for 14 d) may be considered if community prevalence and individual risk of gonorrhea is low. Tests for gonorrhea must be performed prior to instituting therapy and if NAAT test is positive, parenteral cephalosporin is recommended. If culture for gonorrhea is positive, treatment should be based on results of antimicrobial susceptibility.

[e]Bedding and clothing need to be decontaminated by washing in hot water or by dry cleaning. Regimen may be repeated in 1 week if complete response is not achieved.

bid, twice daily; IM, intramuscular; IV, intravenous; NAAT, nucleic acid amplification test; PO, orally (by mouth); qid, 4 times daily; tid, 3 times daily.

males (55–67%) with *N gonorrhoeae* are asymptomatic. Both males and females can develop gonococcal proctitis and pharyngitis after appropriate exposure.

B. Laboratory Findings

A cervical swab from females should be sent for NAAT or cultured on Thayer-Martin agar. Obtaining specimens from the rectum or pharynx when clinically indicated will increase the likelihood of positive results. Pharyngeal infection requires more intensive therapy. Nongonococcal *Neisseria* species reside in the vagina, thereby negating the value of the Gram stain in a female. NAAT screening of female urine can be used; however, polymerase chain reaction (PCR) testing is less sensitive (83%) compared with ligase chain reaction (99%).

Culture or NAAT for *N gonorrhoeae* in males can be achieved with a swab of the urethra or first-void urine. Urethral culture is less sensitive (85%) compared with the 95–99% sensitivity using NAAT methods on either urethral or urine specimens. Gram stain of urethral discharge showing gram-negative intracellular diplococci indicates gonorrhea in a male.

If proctitis is present, appropriate cultures should be obtained and treatment for both gonorrhea and *Chlamydia* infection given. If oral exposure to gonorrhea is suspected, cultures should be taken and the patient given empiric treatment.

Differential Diagnosis

Gonococcal pharyngitis needs to be differentiated from streptococcal infection, herpes simplex pharyngitis, and infectious mononucleosis. *Chlamydia* infection needs to be differentiated from gonococcal infection.

Complications

Disseminated gonococcal infection occurs in a minority (0.5–3%) of patients with untreated gonorrhea. Hematogenous spread most commonly causes arthritis and dermatitis. The joints most frequently involved are the wrist, metacarpophalangeal joints, knee, and ankle. Skin lesions are typically tender, with hemorrhagic or necrotic pustules or bullae on an erythematous base occurring on the distal extremities. Disseminated disease occurs more frequently in females than in males. Risk factors include pregnancy and gonococcal pharyngitis. Gonorrhea is complicated occasionally by perihepatitis and very rarely by endocarditis or meningitis.

Treatment

Historically, patients diagnosed with gonorrhea were treated for chlamydia as well. As chlamydia testing has become more sensitive, the Centers for Disease Control and Prevention suggests that treatment for coinfection is not necessary if testing for chlamydia has been done by NAAT. Their guidelines also state that *N gonorrhoeae* and *C trachomatis* do not require tests of cure when they are treated with first-line

medications, unless the patient remains symptomatic. If retesting is indicated it should be delayed for 1 month after completion of therapy if NAATs are used to document a test of cure. Retesting might also be considered for sexually active adolescents likely to be reinfected. Patients should be advised to abstain from sexual intercourse until both they and their partners have completed a course of treatment. Treatment for disseminated disease may require hospitalization (see Table 42–1). Quinolones should no longer be used to treat gonorrhea due to high levels of quinolone resistance in all populations in the United States. Failure of initial treatment should prompt reevaluation of the patient and consideration of retreatment with ceftriaxone.

Centers for Disease Control and Prevention: Update to CDC's sexually transmitted diseases treatment guidelines, 2006: Fluoroquinolones no longer recommended for treatment of gonococcal infections. MMWR Morb Mortal Wkly Rep 2007;56:332 [PMID: 17431378].

Newman LM et al: Update on the management of gonorrhea in adults in the United States. Clin Infect D 2007;44:S84 [PMID: 17342672].

THE SPECTRUM OF SEXUALLY TRANSMITTED INFECTIONS

The patient presenting with an STI usually has one or more of the signs or symptoms described in this section. Management considerations for STIs include assessing the patient's adherence to therapy and ensuring follow-up, treating STIs in partners, and determining pregnancy risk. Treatment of each STI is detailed in Table 42–1.

CERVICITIS

General Considerations

Cervicitis is caused by *C trachomatis* or *N gonorrhoeae* approximately 30% of the time. HSV, *T vaginalis,* and *Mycoplasma genitalium* are less common causes. Bacterial vaginosis has emerged as a new condition associated with cervicitis. Cervicitis can also be present without an STI.

Clinical Findings

A. Symptoms and Signs

Cervicitis is often asymptomatic, but many females have an abnormal vaginal discharge or postcoital bleeding. Purulent or mucopurulent endocervical exudate visible in the endocervical canal or on an endocervical swab specimen is characteristic of cervicitis. The cervix is often friable with easily induced bleeding.

B. Laboratory Findings

Although endocervical Gram stain may show an increased number of polymorphonuclear leukocytes, this finding has a low positive predictive value and is not recommended for diagnosis. Patients with cervicitis should be tested for *C trachomatis*, *N gonorrhoeae*, and trichomoniasis by using the most sensitive and specific tests available at the site.

► Complications

Persistent cervicitis is difficult to manage and requires reassessment of the initial diagnosis. Cervicitis can persist despite repeated courses of antimicrobial therapy. Presence of a large ectropion can contribute to persistent cervicitis.

► Treatment

Empiric treatment for both gonorrhea and chlamydial infection is recommended when the prospect of follow-up is questionable or the patient is part of a high-risk population. If the patient is asymptomatic except for cervicitis, then treatment may wait until diagnostic test results are available (see Table 42–1). Follow-up is recommended if symptoms persist. Patients should be instructed to abstain from sexual intercourse until they and their sex partners are cured and treatment is completed.

Marrazzo JM, Martin DH: Management of women with cervicitis. Clin Infect D 2007;44:S102 [PMID: 17342663].

PELVIC INFLAMMATORY DISEASE

► General Considerations

Pelvic inflammatory disease (PID) is defined as inflammation of the upper female genital tract and may include endometritis, salpingitis, tubo-ovarian abscess, and pelvic peritonitis. It is the most common gynecologic disorder necessitating hospitalization for female patients of reproductive age in the United States. Over 1 million females develop PID annually, and 275,000 are hospitalized. The incidence is highest in the teen population. Teenage girls who are sexually active have a high risk (1 in 8) of developing PID, whereas women in their 20s have one-tenth the risk. Predisposing risk factors include multiple sexual partners, younger age of initiating sexual intercourse, prior history of PID, and lack of condom use. Lack of protective antibody from previous exposure to sexually transmitted organisms and cervical ectopy contribute to the development of PID. Many adolescents with subacute or asymptomatic disease are never identified.

PID is a polymicrobial infection. Causative agents include *N gonorrhoeae*, *Chlamydia*, anaerobic bacteria that reside in the vagina, and genital mycoplasmas. Vaginal douching and other mechanical factors such as an intrauterine device or prior gynecologic surgery increase the risk of PID by providing access of lower genital tract organisms to pelvic organs. Recent menses and bacterial vaginosis have been associated with the development of PID.

► Clinical Findings

A. Symptoms and Signs

Acute PID is difficult to diagnose because of the wide variation in the symptoms and signs. No single historical, clinical, or laboratory finding has both high sensitivity and specificity for the diagnosis. Diagnosis of PID is usually made clinically (Table 42–2). Typical patients have lower abdominal pain, nausea, vomiting, and fever. However, the patient may be afebrile. Vaginal discharge is variable. Cervical motion tenderness, uterine or adnexal tenderness, or signs of peritonitis are often present. Mucopurulent cervicitis is present in 50% of patients. Tubo-ovarian abscesses can often be detected by careful physical examination (feeling a mass or fullness in the adnexa).

B. Laboratory Findings

Laboratory findings include elevated WBCs with a left shift and elevated acute phase reactants (erythrocyte sedimentation rate or C-reactive protein). A positive test for *N gonorrhoeae* or *C trachomatis* is supportive, although 25% of the time neither of these bacteria is detected. Pregnancy needs to be ruled out, because patients with an ectopic pregnancy can present with abdominal pain. All female patients with acute PID should be offered HIV testing.

C. Diagnostic Studies

Laparoscopy is the gold standard for detecting salpingitis; it can be used if the diagnosis is in question or to help differen-

Table 42–2. Diagnostic criteria for pelvic inflammatory disease (PID).

Minimum criteria
Empiric treatment of PID should be initiated in sexually active young women and others at risk for sexually transmitted infections if one or more of the following minimum criteria are present:
• They are experiencing pelvic or lower abdominal pain and no other cause(s) for the illness can be identified
• Cervical motion tenderness or uterine tenderness or adnexal tenderness
Additional supportive criteria
Oral temperature > 38.3°C (101°F)
Abnormal cervical or vaginal mucopurulent discharge
Presence of white blood cells on saline microscopy of vaginal secretions
Elevated erythrocyte sedimentation rate or elevated C-reactive protein
Laboratory documentation of infection with *Neisseria gonorrhoeae* or *Chlamydia trachomatis*
Definitive criteria (selected cases)
Histopathologic evidence of endometritis on endometrial biopsy
Tubo-ovarian abscess on sonography or other radiologic tests
Laparoscopic abnormalities consistent with PID

Adapted, with permission, from Centers for Disease Control and Prevention. Sexually transmitted diseases treatment guidelines 2006. MMWR Recomm Rep 2006;55(RR-11).

tiate PID from an ectopic pregnancy, ovarian cysts, or adnexal torsion. The clinical diagnosis of PID has a positive predictive value for salpingitis of 65–90% in comparison with laparoscopy. Pelvic ultrasonography also is helpful in detecting tubo-ovarian abscesses, which are found in almost 20% of teens with PID. Transvaginal ultrasound is more sensitive than abdominal ultrasound.

Differential Diagnosis

Differential diagnosis includes other gynecologic illnesses (ectopic pregnancy, threatened or septic abortion, adnexal torsion, ruptured and hemorrhagic ovarian cysts, dysmenorrhea, endometriosis, or mittelschmerz); gastrointestinal illnesses (appendicitis, cholecystitis, hepatitis, gastroenteritis, or inflammatory bowel disease); and genitourinary illnesses (cystitis, pyelonephritis, or urinary calculi).

Complications

Scarring of the fallopian tubes is one of the major sequelae of PID. After one episode of PID, 17% of patients become infertile, 17% develop chronic pelvic pain, and 10% will have an ectopic pregnancy. Infertility rates increase with each episode of PID; three episodes of PID result in a 73% infertility rate. Duration of symptoms appears to be the largest determinant of infertility. Fitz-Hugh-Curtis syndrome is inflammation of the liver capsule (perihepatitis) from either hematogenous or lymphatic spread of organisms from the fallopian tubes. This results in right upper quadrant pain and elevation of liver function tests.

Treatment

The objective of treatment is both to achieve a clinical cure and to prevent long-term sequelae. Recent data have demonstrated no differences in short-term and long-term clinical and microbiologic response rates between parenteral and oral therapy. PID is frequently managed at the outpatient level, although some clinicians argue that all adolescents with PID should be hospitalized because of the rate of complications. Severe systemic symptoms and toxicity, signs of peritonitis, inability to take fluids, pregnancy, nonresponse or intolerance of oral antimicrobial therapy, and tubo-ovarian abscess support hospitalization. In addition, if the health care provider believes that the patient will not adhere to treatment, hospitalization is warranted. Surgical drainage may be required to ensure adequate treatment of tubo-ovarian abscesses.

The treatment regimens described in Table 42–1 are broad spectrum to cover the numerous microorganisms associated with PID. All treatment regimens should be effective against *N gonorrhoeae* and *C trachomatis* because negative endocervical screening tests do not rule out upper reproductive tract infection with these organisms. Outpatient treatment should be reserved for compliant patients who have classic signs of PID without systemic symptoms. Patients with PID who

receive outpatient treatment should be reexamined within 24–48 hours, with phone contact in the interim, to detect persistent disease or treatment failure. Patients should have substantial improvement within 48–72 hours. An adolescent should be reexamined 7–10 days after the completion of therapy to ensure the resolution of symptoms.

Banikarim C, Chacko MR: Pelvic inflammatory disease in adolescents. Semin Pediatr Infect Dis 2005;16:175 [PMID: 16044391].
Gray-Swain MR, Peipert JF: Pelvic inflammatory disease in adolescents. Curr Opin Obstet Gynecol 2006;18:503 [PMID: 16932044].
Haggerty CL, Ness RB: Newest approaches to treatment of pelvic inflammatory disease: A review of recent randomized clinical trials. Clin Infect Dis 2007;44:953 [PMID: 17342647].
Ness RB et al: Effectiveness of treatment strategies of some women with pelvic inflammatory disease: A randomized trial. Obstet Gynecol 2005;106:573 [PMID: 16135590].
Walker CK, Wiesenfeld HC: Antibiotic therapy for acute pelvic inflammatory disease: The 2006 Centers for Disease Control and Prevention sexually transmitted diseases treatment guidelines. Clin Infect Dis 2007;44:S111 [PMID: 17342664].

URETHRITIS

General Considerations

The most common bacterial causes of urethritis in males are *N gonorrhoeae* and *C trachomatis*. Additionally, *T vaginalis*, HSV, *Ureaplasma urealyticum*, and *M genitalium* cause urethritis. Approximately 20% of nongonococcal, nonchlamydial urethritis can be attributed both to *M genitalium* and *U urealyticum*. Coliforms may cause urethritis in males practicing insertive anal intercourse. Mechanical manipulation or contact with irritants can also cause transient urethritis. It is important to recognize that urethritis in both males and females is frequently asymptomatic.

Females often present with symptoms of a urinary tract infection from which no enteric bacterial pathogens are isolated, and often have urethritis caused by the organisms just described.

Clinical Findings

A. Symptoms and Signs

If symptomatic, males present most commonly with a clear or purulent discharge from the urethra, dysuria, or urethral pruritus. Hematuria and inguinal adenopathy can occur. Most infections caused by *C trachomatis* and *T vaginalis* are asymptomatic, while 70% of males with *M genitalium* and 23–90% with gonococcal urethritis are symptomatic.

B. Laboratory Findings

In a symptomatic male a positive leukocyte esterase test on first-void urine, or microscopic examination of first-void urine demonstrating more than 10 WBCs per high-power field, is suggestive of urethritis. Gram stain of urethral secretions demonstrating more than 5 WBCs per high-power field is also suggestive. Gonococcal urethritis is established by documenting the presence of WBCs containing intracellular gram-negative diplococci. Urethral swab or first-void urine for culture or NAAT should be sent to the laboratory to detect *N gonorrhoeae* and *C trachomatis*. Evaluation for *T vaginalis* by a wet preparation of either urethral discharge or spun urine should be considered when the other test results are negative. Additionally, PCR testing is more sensitive for *T vaginalis* than culture or direct microscopy. Specific PCR testing of urine is available for *Mycoplasma* and *Ureaplasma*, though it is not often clinically utilized.

Complications

Complications include recurrent or persistent urethritis, epididymitis, prostatitis, or Reiter syndrome.

Treatment

See Table 42–1 for treatment recommendations. Patients with objective evidence of urethritis should receive empiric treatment for gonorrhea and *Chlamydia* infection, ideally directly observed in the office. If the infection is unresponsive to initial treatment, and the infection is NAAT-negative, trichomoniasis should be ruled out, and nongonococcal, nonchlamydial urethritis should be suspected and treated appropriately. Patients should be instructed to return for evaluation if symptoms persist or recur after completion of initial empiric therapy. Symptoms alone, without documentation of signs or laboratory evidence of urethral inflammation, are not a sufficient basis for retreatment (see Table 42–1). Sexual partners should either be evaluated or treated as well for gonorrhea and *Chlamydia* infection.

Falk L et al: Symptomatic urethritis is more prevalent in men infected with *Mycoplasma genitalium* than with *Chlamydia trachomatis*. Sexually Transm Infect 2004;80:289 [PMID: 15295128].
Simpson T, Oh MK: Urethritis and cervicitis in adolescents. Adolesc Med Clin 2004;15:253 [PMID: 15449844].

EPIDIDYMITIS

General Considerations

Epididymitis is most often caused by *C trachomatis* or *N gonorrhoeae*. Epididymitis caused by *Escherichia coli* occurs among males who are the insertive partners during anal intercourse and in males who have urinary tract abnormalities.

Clinical Findings

A. Symptoms and Signs

Epididymitis is associated with unilateral testicular pain and tenderness. Palpable, tender swelling of the epididymis is usually present. The spermatic cord may also be tender and swollen. Often these symptoms are accompanied by asymptomatic urethritis.

B. Laboratory and Diagnostic Studies

Diagnosis is generally made clinically. Color Doppler ultrasound can help make the diagnosis. Although often not available, radionuclide scanning of the scrotum is the most accurate method of diagnosis. Laboratory evaluation is identical to evaluation for suspected urethritis.

Differential Diagnosis

Acute epididymitis associated with sexual activity must be distinguished from orchitis due to infarct, testicular torsion, viral infection, testicular cancer, tuberculosis, or fungal infection.

Complications

Infertility is rare, and chronic local pain is uncommon.

Treatment

Empiric therapy is indicated before culture results are available. As an adjunct to therapy, bed rest, scrotal elevation, and analgesics are recommended until fever and local inflammation subside. Lack of improvement of swelling and tenderness within 3 days requires reevaluation of both the diagnosis and therapy (see Table 42–1). Sex partners should be evaluated and treated as well for gonorrhea and *Chlamydia* infections.

PROCTITIS, PROCTOCOLITIS, & ENTERITIS

General Considerations

Proctitis occurs predominantly among persons who participate in anal intercourse. Enteritis occurs among those whose sexual practices include oral-fecal contact. Proctocolitis can be acquired by either route depending on the pathogen. Common sexually transmitted pathogens causing proctitis or proctocolitis include *C trachomatis* (including lymphogranuloma venereum serovars), *Treponema pallidum*, HSV, *N gonorrhoeae*, *Giardia lamblia*, and enteric organisms.

Clinical Findings

A. Symptoms and Signs

Proctitis, defined as inflammation limited to the distal 10–12 cm of the rectum, is associated with anorectal pain, tenesmus, and rectal discharge. Acute proctitis among persons who have recently practiced receptive anal intercourse is most often sexually transmitted. The symptoms of proctocolitis combine those of proctitis, plus diarrhea or abdominal cramps (or both), because of inflamed colonic mucosa more than 12 cm from the anus. Enteritis usually results in diarrhea and abdominal cramping without signs of proctitis or proctocolitis.

B. Laboratory and Diagnostic Studies

Evaluation may include anoscopy or sigmoidoscopy, stool examination, culture for appropriate organisms, and serology for syphilis.

Treatment

Management will be determined by the etiologic agent. (See Table 42–1 and Chapter 40). Reinfection may be difficult to distinguish from treatment failure.

Hamlyn E, Taylor C: Sexually transmitted proctitis. Postgrad Med J 2006;82:733 [PMID:17099092].

VAGINAL DISCHARGE

Adolescent girls may have a normal physiologic leukorrhea, secondary to turnover of vaginal epithelium. Infectious causes of discharge include *T vaginalis, C trachomatis, N gonorrhoeae,* and bacterial vaginosis pathogens. Candidiasis is a yeast infection that produces vaginal discharge, but is not usually sexually transmitted. Vaginitis is characterized by vaginal discharge, vulvar itching, and irritation, and by possible vaginal odor. Discharge may be white, gray, or yellow. Physiologic leukorrhea is usually white, homogeneous, and not associated with itching, irritation, or foul odor. Mechanical, chemical, allergic, or other noninfectious irritants of the vagina may cause vaginal discharge.

1. Bacterial Vaginosis

General Considerations

Bacterial vaginosis is a polymicrobial infection of the vagina caused by an imbalance of the normal bacterial vaginal flora. The altered flora has a paucity of hydrogen peroxide–producing lactobacilli and increased concentrations of *Mycoplasma hominis* and anaerobes, such as *Gardnerella vaginalis* and *Mobiluncus*. It is unclear whether bacterial vaginosis is sexually transmitted, but it is associated with having multiple sex partners.

Clinical Findings

A. Symptoms and Signs

The most common symptom is a heavy, malodorous, homogeneous gray-white vaginal discharge. Patients may report vaginal itching or dysuria. The fishy odor may be more noticeable after intercourse or during menses, when the high pH of blood or semen volatilizes the amines.

B. Laboratory Findings

Bacterial vaginosis is most often diagnosed by the use of clinical criteria, which include (1) presence of gray-white discharge, (2) fishy (amine) odor before or after the addition of 10% KOH (whiff test), (3) pH of vaginal fluid greater than 4.5 determined with narrow-range pH paper, and (4) presence of "clue cells" on microscopic examination. Clue cells are squamous epithelial cells that have multiple bacteria adhering to them, making their borders irregular and giving them a speckled appearance. Diagnosis requires three out of four criteria, although many female patients who fulfill these criteria have no discharge or other symptoms.

Complications

Bacterial vaginosis during pregnancy is associated with adverse outcomes such as premature labor, preterm delivery, intra-amniotic infection, and postpartum endometritis. In the nonpregnant individual, it may be associated with PID and urinary tract infections.

Treatment

All female patients who have symptomatic disease should receive treatment to relieve vaginal symptoms and signs of infection (see Table 42–1). Pregnant patients should receive treatment to prevent adverse outcomes of pregnancy. Treatment for patients who do not complain of vaginal discharge or itching, but who demonstrate bacterial vaginosis on routine pelvic examination, is unclear. Because some studies associate bacterial vaginosis and PID, the recommendation is to have a low threshold for treating asymptomatic bacterial vaginosis. Follow-up visits are unnecessary if symptoms resolve. Recurrence of bacterial vaginosis is not unusual. Follow-up examination 1 month after treatment for high-risk pregnant patients is recommended.

Males do not develop infection equivalent to bacterial vaginosis. Treatment of male partners has no effect on the course of infection in females.

Brotman RM et al: Findings associated with recurrence of bacterial vaginosis among adolescents attending sexually transmitted diseases clinics. J Pediatr Adolesc Gynecol 2007;20:225 [PMID: 17673134].
O'Brien RF: Bacterial vaginosis: many questions—any answers? Curr Opin Pediatr 2005;17:473 [PMID: 16012258].
Walker CK, Wiesenfeld HC: Antibiotic therapy for acute pelvic inflammatory disease: The 2006 Centers for Disease Control and Prevention sexually transmitted diseases treatment guidelines. Clin Infect D 2007;44: S111 [PMID: 17342664].

2. Trichomoniasis

General Considerations

Trichomoniasis is caused by *T vaginalis*, a flagellated protozoan that infects 5–7 million people annually in the United States.

Clinical Findings

A. Symptoms and Signs

Fifty percent of females with trichomoniasis develop a symptomatic vaginitis with vaginal itching, a green-gray malodorous frothy discharge, and dysuria. Occasionally postcoital bleeding and dyspareunia may be present. The vulva may be erythematous and the cervix friable.

B. Laboratory Findings

Mixing the discharge with normal saline facilitates detection of the flagellated protozoan on microscopic examination (wet preparation). The infection may be detected by the pathologist when reviewing the Pap smear. Culture and PCR testing are available when the diagnosis is unclear. PCR tests are sensitive, but expensive and not readily available. Two FDA-approved, point-of-care antigen-based detection assays for *T vaginalis* are now available. Both are performed on vaginal secretions and have a sensitivity greater than 83.3% and a specificity greater than 97%. Trichomonal urethritis frequently causes a positive urine leukocyte esterase test and WBCs on urethral smear.

▶ Complications

Male partners of females diagnosed with trichomoniasis have a 22% chance of having trichomoniasis. Half of males with trichomoniasis will have urethritis. *Trichomonas* infection in females has been associated with adverse pregnancy outcomes.

▶ Treatment

See Table 42–1 for treatment recommendations.

Schwebke JR, Burgess D: Trichomoniasis. Clin Microbiol Rev 2004;17:794 [PMID: 15489349].

3. Vulvovaginal Candidiasis

▶ General Considerations

Vulvovaginal candidiasis is caused by *Candida albicans* in 85–90% of cases. Most females will have at least one episode of vulvovaginal candidiasis in their lifetime, and almost half will have two or more episodes. The highest incidence is between ages 16 and 30 years. Predisposing factors include recent use of antibiotics, diabetes, pregnancy, and HIV. Risk factors include vaginal intercourse, use of oral contraceptives, and use of spermicide. This is rarely a sexually transmitted infection. Recurrences generally reflect reactivation of colonization.

▶ Clinical Findings

A. Symptoms and Signs

Typical symptoms include pruritus and a white, cottage cheese–like vaginal discharge without odor. The itching is more common midcycle and shortly after menses. Other symptoms include vaginal soreness, vulvar burning, vulvar edema and redness, dyspareunia, and dysuria (especially after intercourse).

B. Laboratory Findings

The diagnosis is usually made by visualizing yeast or pseudo-hyphae with 10% KOH (90% sensitive) or Gram stain (77% sensitive) in the vaginal discharge. Fungal culture can be used if symptoms and microscopy are not definitive or if disease is unresponsive or recurrent. However, culture is not very specific as colonization is common in asymptomatic females. Vaginal pH is normal with yeast infections.

▶ Complications

The only complication of vulvovaginal candidiasis is recurrent infections (ie, four or more episodes annually). Most females with recurrent infection have no apparent predisposing or underlying conditions.

▶ Treatment

Short-course topical formulations effectively treat uncomplicated vaginal yeast infections (see Table 42–1). The topically applied azole drugs are more effective than nystatin. Treatment with azoles results in relief of symptoms and negative cultures in 80–90% of patients who complete therapy. Oral fluconazole as a one-time dose is an effective oral medication. Patients should be instructed to return for follow-up visits only if symptoms persist or recur. Six-month prophylaxis regimens have been effective in many female patients with persistent or recurrent yeast infection. Recurrent disease is usually due to *C albicans* that remains susceptible to azoles, and should be treated for 14 days with oral azoles. Some non-albicans *Candida* will respond to itraconazole or boric acid gelatin capsules (600 mg daily for 14 days) intravaginally. Treatment of sex partners is not recommended, but may be considered for females who have recurrent infection.

GENITAL ULCERATIONS

In the United States, young, sexually active patients who have genital ulcers have genital herpes, syphilis, or chancroid. The relative frequency of each disease differs by geographic area and patient population; however, in most areas, genital herpes is the most prevalent of these diseases. More than one of these diseases could be present in a patient with genital ulcers. All ulcerative diseases are associated with an increased risk for HIV infection. The acute retroviral syndrome of HIV infection may be accompanied by oral and genital ulcers.

Ulcers are vaginal, vulvar, or cervical in females, and on any part of the penis in males. Oral lesions may occur concomitantly with genital ulcerations in HSV infection and syphilis. Each etiologic agent has specific characteristics that are described in the following sections. Lesion pain, inguinal lymphadenopathy, and urethritis may be found in association with the ulcers.

1. Herpes Simplex Virus Infection

▶ General Considerations

HSV is the most common cause of visible genital ulcers. At least 50 million people are infected with genital herpes in the United States. Approximately 0.5–1.5 million new cases occur each year. Approximately 30% of primary herpetic genital lesions are caused by HSV type 1 (HSV-1), and the rest by type 2 (HSV-2). As with oral HSV infections, many primary genital infections are asymptomatic (60–80%) or not recognized as herpetic in origin.

Clinical Findings

A. Symptoms and Signs

Symptomatic initial HSV infection causes vesicles of the vulva, vagina, cervix, penis, rectum, or urethra, which are quickly followed by shallow, painful ulcerations. Atypical presentation of HSV infection includes vulvar erythema and fissures. Urethritis may occur. Initial infection can be severe, lasting up to 3 weeks, and be associated with fever and malaise, as well as localized tender adenopathy. The pain and dysuria can be extremely uncomfortable, requiring sitz baths, topical anesthetics, and occasionally catheterization for urinary retention.

Symptoms tend to be more severe in females. Recurrence in the genital area with HSV-2 is likely (65–90%). Recurrent genital herpes is of shorter duration (5–7 days), with fewer lesions and usually no systemic symptoms. Prodromal pain in the genital, buttock, or pelvic region is common prior to recurrences. First-episode genital herpes infection caused by HSV-1 is usually the consequence of oral-genital sex. Primary HSV-1 infection is as severe as HSV-2 infection, and treatment is the same. Recurrence of HSV-1 happens in less than 50% of patients, and the frequency of recurrences is much less than in those patients with prior HSV-2 infection.

B. Laboratory Findings

Diagnosis of genital HSV infection is often made presumptively, but in one large series this diagnosis was incorrect for 20% of cases. Culture or antigen testing of the vesicles can confirm the diagnosis, but sensitivity decreases with advancing age of the ulcer. Several serologic tests with sensitivities between 80% and 90% are available and can distinguish between HSV-1 and HSV-2, which is important for prognosis. Recurrent genital ulceration is suggestive of HSV infection.

Differential Diagnosis

Any genital ulcer should be cultured for HSV and differentiated from syphilis and chancroid ulcers. The character of the ulcers and inguinal nodes differs in these diseases. (See next sections on Syphilis and Chancroid.)

Complications

Complications, usually with the first episode of genital HSV infection, include viral meningitis, urinary retention, transmission to newborns at birth, and pharyngitis. Infection with genital HSV, whether active or not, greatly increases the likelihood of transmitting or acquiring HIV infection within couples discordant for HIV.

Prevention

All patients with active lesions should be counseled to abstain from sexual contact. Almost all patients have very frequent periodic asymptomatic shedding of HSV, and most cases of genital HSV infection re transmitted by persons who are unaware that they have the infection or are asymptomatic when transmission occurs. Reactivation can occur in individuals who never had symptomatic disease. Individuals with prior HSV infection should be encouraged to always use condoms to protect susceptible partners. Antiviral prophylaxis of infected individuals reduces shedding and significantly reduces the chance of transmission to their sexual partners.

Treatment

Antiviral drugs administered within the first 5 days of primary infection decrease the duration and severity of HSV infection (see Table 42–1). The effect of antivirals on the severity or duration of recurrent disease is limited. For best results, therapy should be started with the prodrome or during the first day of the attack. Patients should have a prescription at home to initiate treatment. If recurrences are frequent and cause significant physical or emotional discomfort, patients may elect to take antiviral prophylaxis on a daily basis to reduce the frequency (70–80% decrease) and duration of recurrences. Treatment of first or subsequent attacks will not prevent future attacks, but recurrence frequency decreases in many individuals over time.

Auslander BA et al: Genital herpes in adolescents. Semin Pediatr Infect Dis 2005;16:24 [15685146].

Patel R et al: Managing patients with genital herpes and their sexual partners. Infect Dis Clin N Am 2005;19:427 [PMID:15963881].

2. Syphilis

General Considerations

Syphilis is an acute and chronic STI caused by infection with *T pallidum*. The national rate of syphilis has increased annually after reaching an all time low in 2000. Increases have been observed in both genders, but predominantly in males who have sex with men. In 2005, the rate of syphilis was highest among women in the 20- to 24-year-old age group (3.0 cases per 100,000 population) and among men in the 35- to 39-year-old age group (13.2 cases per 100,000 population).

Clinical Findings

A. Symptoms and Signs

Skin and mucous membrane lesions characterize the acute phase of primary and secondary syphilis. Lesions of the bone, viscera, aorta, and central nervous system predominate in the chronic phase (tertiary syphilis) (see Chapter 40). Prevention of syphilis is also important because syphilitic mucosal lesions facilitate transmission of HIV.

Primary syphilis usually presents as a solitary chancre—a painless ulcer with an indurated base and associated nontender, firm adenopathy. The chancre appears 10–90 days after exposure and resolves spontaneously 4–8 weeks later. Because it is painless, it may go undetected, especially if the lesion is within the vagina. Chancres may occur on the genitalia, lips, or anus. Secondary syphilis occurs 4–10 weeks after the chancre appears, with generalized malaise, adenopathy, and a nonpruritic maculopapular rash that often includes the palms and soles. Secondary syphilis resolves in 1–3 months, but can recur. Verrucous lesions known as condylomata lata may develop on the genitalia. These must be distinguished from genital warts.

B. Laboratory Findings

If the patient has a suspect primary lesion, is at high risk, is a contact, or may have secondary syphilis, a nontreponemal serum screen—either RPR or VDRL—should be performed. If the nontreponemal test is positive, then a specific treponemal test, a fluorescent treponemal antibody-absorbed (FTA-ABS) or microhemagglutination–*Treponema pallidum* (MHA-TP) test, is done to confirm the diagnosis. An additional diagnostic tool is darkfield microscopy, which can be used to detect spirochetes in scrapings of the chancre base. Darkfield examinations and direct fluorescent antibody tests of lesion exudate or tissue are the definitive methods for diagnosing early syphilis.

If a patient is engaging in high-risk sexual behavior or is living in an area in which syphilis is endemic, RPRs should be drawn yearly to screen for asymptomatic infection. Syphilis is reportable to state health departments, and all contacts need to be evaluated. Patients also need to be evaluated for other STIs, especially HIV, because HIV-infected patients have increased rates of failure with some treatment regimens.

▶ Complications

Untreated syphilis can lead to tertiary complications with serious multiorgan involvement, including aortitis and neurosyphilis. Transmission to the fetus can occur from an untreated pregnant individual (see Chapters 1 and 40).

▶ Treatment

See Table 42–1 for treatment recommendations. Patients should be reexamined clinically and serologically with nontreponemal tests at 6 and 12 months after treatment. If signs or symptoms persist or recur, or patients do not have a fourfold decrease in their nontreponemal test titer, they should be considered to have failed treatment or be reinfected and need retreatment.

French P: Syphilis. BMJ 2007;334:143 [PMID:17235095].
Stoner BP: Current controversies in the management of adult syphilis. Clin Infect Dis 2007;44:S130 [PMID:17342666].

3. Chancroid

▶ General Considerations

Chancroid is caused by *Haemophilus ducreyi*. It is relatively rare, but is endemic in some urban areas, and has been associated with HIV infection, drug use, and prostitution. Ten percent of patients with chancroid acquired in the United States are coinfected with HSV or syphilis.

▶ Clinical Findings

A. Symptoms and Signs

The typical lesion begins as a papule that erodes after 24–48 hours into an ulcer. The ulcer has ragged, sharply demarcated edges and a purulent base, is painful (unlike syphilis), solitary, and somewhat deeper than HSV infection. Tender, fluctuant (unlike syphilis and HSV) inguinal adenopathy is present in one third of patients. A painful ulcer in combination with suppurative inguinal adenopathy is very often chancroid.

B. Laboratory Findings

Gram stain shows gram-positive cocci arranged in a boxcar formation. Culture, which has a sensitivity of less than 80%, can be performed on a special medium that is available in academic centers. Some clinical laboratories have developed their own PCR testing.

▶ Differential Diagnosis

Chancroid is distinguished from syphilis by the painful nature of the ulcer and the associated tender suppurative adenopathy. HSV vesicles often produce painful ulcers, but these are multiple, smaller, and shallower than chancroid ulcers. Adenopathy associated with initial HSV infection does not suppurate. A presumptive diagnosis of chancroid should be considered in a patient with typical painful genital ulcers and regional adenopathy, if the test results for syphilis and HSV are negative.

▶ Treatment

Symptoms improve within 3 days after therapy (see Table 42–1). Most ulcers resolve in 7 days, although large ulcers may take 2 weeks to heal. All sexual contacts need to be examined and given treatment, even if asymptomatic.

Lewis DA: Chancroid: Clinical manifestations, diagnosis, and management. Sex Transm Infect 2003;79:68 [PMID: 12576620].

4. Other Ulcerations

Lymphogranuloma venereum (LGV), caused by *Chlamydia trachomatis* serovars L1, L2, or L3, is rare in the United States, with the exception of communities of males who have sex with men where prevalence of LGV is increasing. Patients with LGV present with a painless vesicle or ulcer that heals spontaneously, followed by development of tender adenopathy, either unilateral or bilateral. A classic finding is the groove sign—an inguinal crease created by concomitant involvement of inguinal and femoral nodes. These nodes become matted and fluctuant and may rupture. LGV can cause proctocolitis with rectal ulceration, purulent anal discharge, fever, tenesmus, and lower abdominal pain, primarily in communities of males who have sex with men. Diagnosis can be made by culturing a node aspirate for *Chlamydia* or by serology. Differential diagnosis during the adenopathy phase includes bacterial adenitis, lymphoma, and cat-scratch disease. Differential diagnosis during the ulcerative phase encompasses all causes of genital ulcers. See Table 42–1 for treatment recommendations.

Granuloma inguinale, or donovanosis, is caused by *Klebsiella granulomatis*, a gram-negative bacillus that is rare in the United States. An indurated subcutaneous nodule erodes to form a painless, friable ulcer with granulation tissue. Diagnosis is based on clinical suspicion and supported by a Wright or Giemsa stain of the granulation tissue that reveals intracytoplasmic rods (Donovan bodies) in mononuclear cells. See Table 42–1 for treatment recommendations.

Herring A, Richens J: Lymphogranuloma venereum. Sex Transm Infect 2006;82(Suppl 4):iv23 [PMID: 17151048].

Pathela P et al: Lymphogranuloma venereum: Old pathogen, new story. Curr Infect Dis Rep 2007;9:143 [PMID: 17324352].

Richardson D, Goldmeier D: Lymphogranuloma venereum: An emerging cause of proctitis in men who have sex with men. Int J STD AIDS 2007;18:11 [PMID: 17326855].

GENITAL WARTS & HUMAN PAPILLOMAVIRUS

▶ General Considerations

Condylomata acuminata, or genital warts, are caused by HPV, which can also cause cervical dysplasia and cervical cancer. An estimated 20 million people are infected annually with HPV, including approximately more than 9 million sexually active adolescents and young adults 15–24 years of age. The majority (74%) of new HPV infections occurs among those 15–24 years of age; in females younger than age 25 years, the prevalence ranges between 28% and 46%. Estimates suggest that 32–50% of adolescent females having sexual intercourse in the United States have HPV infections, though only 1% may have visible lesions. HPV is transmitted sexually: 30–60% of males whose partners have HPV have evidence of condylomata on examination. An estimated 1 million new cases of genital warts occur every year in the United States.

Up to 100 serotypes of HPV have been identified. HPV types 6 and 11 cause approximately 90% of genital warts, whereas HPV types 16 and 18 cause more than 70% of cervical dysplasia. The infection is more common in persons with multiple partners and in those who initiate sexual intercourse at an early age.

The American Cancer Society indicates that there is little risk of missing an important cervical lesion until 3–5 years after initiation of intercourse. Pap smears should be obtained after this time or by age 21. Thereafter, annual cervical screening should be performed using conventional Pap smears.

▶ Clinical Findings

A. Symptoms and Signs

For males, verrucous lesions are found on the shaft or corona of the penis. Lesions also may develop in the urethra or rectum. Lesions do not produce discomfort. They may be single or found in clusters. Females develop verrucous lesions on any genital mucosal surface, either internally or externally.

B. Laboratory Findings

External, visible lesions have unique characteristics that make the diagnosis straightforward. Condylomata acuminata can be distinguished from condylomata lata (syphilis), skin tags, and molluscum contagiosum by application of 5% acetic acid solution. Acetowhitening is used to indicate the extent of cervical infection.

Pap smears detect cervical abnormalities. HPV infection is the most frequent cause of an abnormal smear. Pap smear findings are graded by the atypical nature of the cervical cells. These changes range from atypical squamous cells of undetermined significance (ASCUS) to low-grade squamous intraepithelial lesions (LSIL) and high-grade squamous intraepithelial lesions (HSIL). LSIL encompasses cellular changes associated with HPV and mild dysplasia. HSIL includes moderate dysplasia, severe dysplasia, and carcinoma in situ.

Follow-up for ASCUS is controversial, as only 25% progress to dysplasia, and the remainder are unchanged or regress. If ASCUS is present, options for follow-up management include (1) immediate colposcopy, (2) repeat Pap smears at 6-month intervals for three intervals, or (3) an HPV DNA test for oncogenic HPV types. If high-risk HPV DNA is positive or if HSIL is found, colposcopy should be performed. If LSIL is detected, colposcopy is not needed, but a repeat Pap smear should be done in 1 year and if LSIL or HSIL are subsequently detected, the patient should be referred for colposcopy for direct visualization or biopsy of the cervix (or both). If a Pap smear shows signs of inflammation only, and concomitant infection such as vaginitis or cervicitis is present, the smear should be repeated after the infection has cleared.

▶ Differential Diagnosis

The differential diagnosis includes normal anatomic structures (pearly penile papules, vestibular papillae, and sebaceous glands), molluscum contagiosum, seborrheic keratosis, and syphilis.

▶ Complications

Because genital warts can proliferate and become friable during pregnancy, many experts advocate their removal during pregnancy. HPV types 6 and 11 can cause laryngeal papillomatosis in infants and children. Complications of appropriate treatment include scarring with changes in skin pigmentation or chronic pain at the treatment site. Cervical cancer is the most common and important sequel of HPV.

Prevention

The use of condoms may reduce, but does not eliminate, the risk for transmission to uninfected partners. The quadrivalent HPV vaccine is 96–100% effective in preventing HPV 6 and 11–related genital warts and HPV 16 and 18–related cervical dysplasia. It is recommended for girls and women aged 9–26 years. (See Chapter 9.)

Treatment

All penile and external vaginal or vulvar lesions can be treated topically. Treatment may need to occur weekly for 4–6 weeks. An experienced practitioner should treat internal and cervical lesions (see Table 42–1). Treatment may clear the visible lesions but may not reduce the presence of virus, nor is it clear whether transmission of HPV is reduced.

Warts may resolve or remain unchanged if left untreated or they may increase in size or number. Treatment can induce wart-free periods in most patients. Most recurrences occur within the 3 months following completion of a treatment regimen. Appropriate follow-up of abnormal Pap smears is essential to detect any progression to malignancy.

Barr E. Tamms G: Quadrivalent human papillomavirus vaccine. Clin Infect Dis 2007;45:609 [PMID: 17682997].

Centers for Disease Control and Prevention: Quadrivalent human papillomavirus vaccine: Recommendations of the Advisory Committee on Immunization Practices (ACIP). MMWR Morb Mortal Wkly Rep 2007;56:1[PMID:17380109].

Dunne EF, Markowitz LE: Genital human papillomavirus infection. Clin Infect Dis 2006;43:624 [PMID:16886157].

Gravitt PE, Jamshidi R: Diagnosis and management of oncogenic cervical human papillomavirus infection. Infect Dis Clin North Am 2005;19:439 [PMID: 15963882].

Lacey CJ: Therapy for genital human papillomavirus-related disease. J Clin Virol 2005;32(Suppl 1):S82 [PMID: 15753016].

O'Mahony C. Genital warts: Current and future management options Am J Clin Dermatol 2005;6:239 [PMID:16060711].

ASCCP Consensus Guidelines for Management of Abnormal Cervical Cytology http://www.asccp.org/consensus/cytological.shtml

OTHER VIRAL INFECTIONS

1. Hepatitis (See also Chapter 21)

General Considerations

Hepatitis B and hepatitis C are often STIs. Hepatitis B is at least 10 times more common than HIV in the adolescent population. Since 1998, sexual transmission has accounted for approximately 50% of the estimated 181,000 new hepatitis B infections that occur annually in the United States. Heterosexuals who have unprotected sex with multiple partners and males who have sex with men are the groups at highest risk for sexual transmission.

Hepatitis C generally is transmitted through blood products and shared intravenous needles, although about 10% of hepatitis C infections have been linked to sexual transmission. Hepatitis C needs to be considered in teenagers who are symptomatic and engage in high-risk sexual behavior or intravenous drug use. Outbreaks of sexually transmitted hepatitis A infection have occurred among males who have sex with men, although the efficiency of sexual transmission is low.

2. Human Immunodeficiency Virus (See also Chapter 39)

General Considerations

Half of the 40,000 new HIV-infected cases occurring yearly in the United Status are in youth and young adults aged 13–24 years. Because of the long latency period between infection with HIV and progression to AIDS, it is felt that many HIV-positive young adults contracted HIV during adolescence. The number of females who become HIV-positive has increased dramatically, representing almost half of teenagers with HIV infection.

Risk factors for contracting HIV include a prior STI, infrequent condom use, practicing insertive or receptive anal sex (both males and females), prior genital HSV infection, practicing survival sex (ie, trading sex for money or drugs), intravenous drug or crack cocaine use, crystal methamphetamine use, homelessness, and being the victim of sexual abuse (males). HIV infection should be considered in all sexually active youth, whether they have sex with males, females or both.

Clinical Findings

A. Symptoms and Signs

Adolescents may be asymptomatic with recent HIV infection or may present with the acute retroviral syndrome, which is evident 2–6 weeks after exposure. Fever, malaise, lymphadenopathy, rash, upper respiratory symptoms, oral and genital ulcerations, aseptic meningitis, and thrush may occur. If HIV infection is suspected, diagnosis is made in the acute period (before seroconversion) by HIV RNA PCR testing or HIV p24 antigen detection.

B. Laboratory Findings

All persons with an STI should be screened for HIV by serology. Adolescents may also present to the office requesting an HIV test. In either case, a careful history of sexual behavior should be obtained to assess risk and intervene with risk-reduction counseling. It is also necessary to determine how teens may respond to being told they are HIV-positive and what support systems they have in place. If an adolescent is homeless; does not have emotional support from family, friends, or a counselor; or threatens suicide or homicide in response to the idea of being HIV-positive, then testing should be deferred until the health care provider is confident that the youth will be safe if the test result is positive.

Treatment

Many experts recommend aggressive antiretroviral treatment of patients diagnosed with acute retroviral syndrome.

DeLaMora P et al: Caring for adolescents with HIV. Curr HIV/AIDS Rep 2006;3:74 [PMID:16608663].

Futterman DC: HIV and AIDS in adolescents. Adolesc Med Clin 2004;15:369 [PMID: 15449850].

National Institutes of Health–sponsored AIDS information site: http://aidsinfo.nih.gov/

3. HIV Post–Sexual Exposure Prophylaxis

The risk of acquiring HIV infection through sexual assault or abuse is low but present. The risk for HIV transmission per episode of receptive penile-anal sexual exposure is estimated at 0.5–3%; the risk per episode of receptive vaginal exposure is estimated at less than 0.1–0.2%. HIV transmission also occurs from receptive oral exposure, but the risk is unknown. Specific circumstances of an assault might increase risk for HIV transmission (eg, trauma, including bleeding) with vaginal, anal, or oral penetration; site of exposure to ejaculate; HIV viral load in ejaculate; duration of HIV infection in the assailant; and presence of an STI, prior genital HSV infection, or genital lesions in the assailant or survivor.

Health care providers who consider offering postexposure therapy should take into account the likelihood that exposure to HIV occurred, the potential benefits and risks of such therapy, and the interval between the exposure and initiation of therapy. It will be helpful to know the HIV status of the sexual contact. In general, postexposure therapy is not recommended when more than 72 hours has passed since exposure. If the patient decides to take postexposure therapy, clinical management should be implemented according to published Centers for Disease Control and Prevention guidelines.

Centers for Disease Control and Prevention: Antiretroviral postexposure prophylaxis after sexual, injection-drug use, or other nonoccupational exposure to HIV in the United States: Recommendations from the U.S. Department of Health and Human Services. MMWR Recomm Rep 2005;54(RR-2) [PMID: 15660015].

Fajman N, Wright R: Use of antiretroviral HIV post-exposure prophylaxis in sexually abused children and adolescents treated in an inner-city pediatric emergency department. Child Abuse Negl 2006;30:919 [PMID: 16939690].

Havens PL et al: Postexposure prophylaxis in children and adolescents for nonoccupational exposure to human immunodeficiency virus. Pediatrics 2003;111:1475 [PMID: 22662832].

Olshen E et al: Postexposure prophylaxis: An intervention to prevent human immunodeficiency virus infection in adolescents. Curr Opin Pediatr 2003;15:379 [PMID: 12891049].

ECTOPARASITIC INFECTIONS

1. Pubic Lice

Pthirus pubis, the pubic louse, lives in pubic hair. The louse or the nits can be transmitted by close contact from person to person. Patients complain of itching and they may report having seen the insect. Examination of the pubic hair may reveal the louse crawling around or attached to the hair. Closer inspection may reveal the nit or sac of eggs, which is a gelatinous material (1–2 mm) stuck to the hair shaft. See Table 42–1 for treatment recommendations.

2. Scabies

Sarcoptes scabiei, the causative organism in scabies, is smaller than the louse. It can be identified by the classic burrow, which is created by the organism laying eggs and traveling just below the skin surface. Scabies can be sexually transmitted by close skin-to-skin contact and can be found in the pubic region, groin, lower abdomen, or upper thighs. The rash is intensely pruritic, especially at night, erythematous, and scaly.

See Table 42–1 for treatment options. Ivermectin represents a new oral therapeutic option for scabies and may hold particular promise in the treatment of severe infestations or in epidemic situations. When treating with lotion or shampoo, the entire area needs to be covered for the time specified by the manufacturer. One treatment usually clears the infestation, although a second treatment may be necessary. Bed sheets and clothes must be washed in hot water. Both sexual and close personal or household contacts within the preceding month should be examined and treated.

Leone PA: Scabies and pediculosis pubis: An update of treatment regimens and general review. Clin Infect Dis 2007;44:S153 [PMID: 17342668].

EVALUATION OF SEXUALLY TRANSMITTED INFECTIONS IN SEXUAL ABUSE & ASSAULT

Sexual abuse and sexual violence are common. Half of rape victims are younger than age 18 years. Rape is both a medical and a psychological emergency. Evaluation and treatment after sexual abuse or assault depends on the patient's age, his or her ability to communicate what occurred, and the timing of the abuse.

Teenagers usually can describe the kind of abuse (eg, oral, anal, vaginal; receptive or insertive), and evaluation needs to be directed accordingly. If the abuse has occurred in the preceding 72 hours, most states require for legal purposes that a rape kit be used. All practitioners should have access to a rape kit, which guides the practitioner through a stepwise collection of evidence and cultures. A thorough physical examination is indicated to evaluate for other signs of trauma.

Beyond 72 hours, evaluation is tailored to the history provided. The involved orifices should be cultured for *N gonorrhoeae* and *C trachomatis* (NAAT is not admissible in court), and vaginal secretions evaluated for *Trichomonas.* RPR, hepatitis B, and HIV serology should be drawn at baseline and repeated in 2–3 months. Pregnancy testing should be done as indicated.

Trichomoniasis, bacterial vaginosis, chlamydia, and gonorrhea are the most frequently diagnosed infections among women and girls who have been sexually assaulted. Because the prevalence of these STIs is substantial among sexually experienced females, their presence after an assault does not necessarily signify acquisition during the assault.

Prophylactic therapy using ceftriaxone (125 mg IM in a single dose), metronidazole (2 g orally in a single dose), and either azithromycin (1 g orally in a single dose) or doxycycline (100 mg orally twice a day for 7 days) should be offered when patients present for evaluation. Hepatitis B vaccination should be administered to patients if they have not been previously vaccinated. No effective prophylaxis is available for hepatitis C. Evaluating the perpetrator for STI, if possible, can help determine risk exposure and guide prophylaxis. HIV prophylaxis should be considered in certain circumstances (discussed earlier). Emergency contraception should be given if the abuse occurred within 72 hours. Psychological assessment at the time of presentation, as well as over the next several months, is a top priority. Any suspected abuse must be reported to the local authorities.

All younger children should be referred to child abuse multidisciplinary teams, which can help with the psychological aspects of the abuse and are well versed in helping children communicate what may have occurred. Colposcopic examination is critical in determining the extent of the damage and provides documentation for the legal system.

Although it is often difficult for persons to comply with follow-up examinations weeks after an assault, such examinations are essential to detect new infections, complete immunization with hepatitis B vaccination if needed, and continue psychological support.

American Academy of Pediatrics: Committee on Adolescence: Care of the adolescent sexual assault victim. Pediatrics 2001;107:1476 [PMID: 21293379].

REFERENCES

Burstein GR, Workowski KA: Sexually transmitted disease treatment guidelines. Curr Opin Pediatr 2003;15:391 [PMID: 12891051].

Centers for Disease Control and Prevention: Sexually transmitted diseases treatment guidelines 2006. MMWR Recomm Rep 2006;55(RR-11):1 [PMID: 16888612]. Available at: http://www.cdc.gov/std/treatment/

Workowski KA, Berman SA: Centers for Disease Control and Prevention sexually transmitted diseases treatment guidelines. Clin Infect Dis 2007;44(Suppl 3):S73 [PMID: 17342670].

Fluid, Electrolyte, & Acid-Base Disorders & Therapy

Douglas M. Ford, MD

REGULATION OF BODY FLUIDS, ELECTROLYTES, & TONICITY

Total body water (TBW) constitutes 50–75% of the total body mass, depending on age, sex, and fat content. After an initial postnatal diuresis, the TBW slowly decreases to the adult range near puberty (Figure 43–1). TBW is divided into the intracellular and extracellular spaces. Intracellular fluid (ICF) accounts for two thirds of the TBW and extracellular fluid (ECF), for one third. The ECF is further compartmentalized into plasma (intravascular) volume and interstitial fluid (ISF).

The principal constituents of plasma are sodium, chloride, bicarbonate, and protein (primarily albumin). The ISF is similar to plasma but lacks significant amounts of protein (Figure 43–2). Conversely, the ICF is rich in potassium, magnesium, phosphates, sulfates, and protein.

An understanding of osmotic shifts between the ECF and ICF is fundamental to understanding disorders of fluid balance. Iso-osmolality is generally maintained between fluid compartments. Because the cell membrane is water-permeable, abnormal fluid shifts occur if the concentration of solutes that cannot permeate the cell membrane in the ECF does not equal the concentration of such solutes in the ICF. Thus NaCl, mannitol, and glucose (in the setting of hyperglycemia) remain restricted to the ECF space and contribute effective osmoles by obligating water to remain in the ECF compartment. In contrast, a freely permeable solute such as urea does not contribute effective osmoles because it is not restricted to the ECF and readily crosses cell membranes. Tonicity, or effective osmolality, differs from measured osmolality in that it accounts only for osmotically active impermeable solutes rather than all osmotically active solutes, including those that are permeable to cell membranes. Osmolality may be estimated by the following formula:

$$mOsm/kg = 2\left(Na^+, mEq/L\right) + \frac{Glucose, mg/dL}{18} + \frac{BUN, mg/dL}{2.8}$$

Although osmolality and osmolarity differ, the former being an expression of osmotic activity per weight (kg) and the latter per volume (L) of solution, for clinical purposes they are similar and occasionally used interchangeably. Oncotic pressure represents the osmotic activity of macromolecular constituents such as albumin in the plasma and body fluids.

The principal mechanisms that regulate ECF volume and tonicity are antidiuretic hormone (ADH), thirst, aldosterone, and atrial natriuretic factor (ANF).

Antidiuretic Hormone

In the kidney, ADH increases water reabsorption in the cortical and medullary collecting ducts, leading to formation of concentrated urine. In the absence of ADH, dilute urine is produced. Under normal conditions, ADH secretion is regulated by the tonicity of body fluids rather than the fluid volume and becomes detectable at a plasma osmolality of 280 mOsm/kg or greater. However, tonicity may be sacrificed to preserve ECF volume, as in the case of hyponatremic dehydration, wherein ADH secretion and renal water retention are maximal.

Thirst

Water intake is commonly determined by cultural factors rather than by thirst. Thirst is not physiologically stimulated until plasma osmolality reaches 290 mOsm/kg, a level at which ADH levels are sufficient to induce maximal antidiuresis. Thirst provides control over a wide range of fluid volumes and can even be a response to an absence of or lack of responsiveness to ADH, with attendant production of copious and dilute urine, as in diabetes insipidus. One who cannot perceive thirst develops profound problems with fluid balance.

Aldosterone

Aldosterone—released from the adrenal cortex in response to decreased effective circulating volume and stimulation of the renin-angiotensin-aldosterone axis or in response to

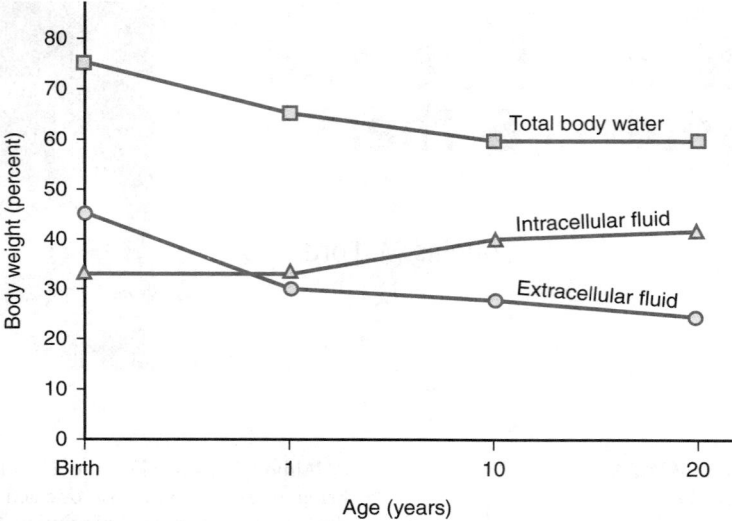

▲ **Figure 43–1.** Body water compartments related to age. (Modified, with permission, from Friis-Hansen B: Body water compartments in children: Changes during growth and related changes in body composition. Pediatrics 1961;28:169.)

increasing plasma K^+—enhances renal tubular reabsorption of Na^+ in exchange for K^+ and to a lesser degree, H^+. At a constant osmolality, retention of Na^+ leads to expansion of ECF volume and suppression of aldosterone release.

Atrial Natriuretic Factor

ANF, a polypeptide hormone secreted principally by the cardiac atria in response to atrial dilation, plays an important role in regulation of blood volume and blood pressure. ANF inhibits renin secretion and aldosterone synthesis and causes an increase in glomerular filtration rate and renal sodium excretion. ANF also guards against excessive plasma volume expansion in the face of increased ECF volume by shifting fluid from the vascular to the interstitial compartment. ANF inhibits angiotensin II- and norepinephrine-induced vasoconstriction and acts in the brain to decrease the desire for salt and inhibit the release of ADH. Thus the net effect of ANF is a decrease in blood volume and blood pressure associated with natriuresis and diuresis.

ACID-BASE BALANCE

The pH of arterial blood is maintained between 7.38 and 7.42 to ensure that pH-sensitive enzyme systems function normally. Acid-base balance is maintained by interaction of the lungs, kidneys, and systemic buffering systems. Over 50% of the blood's buffering capacity is provided by the carbonic acid–bicarbonate system, roughly 30% by hemoglobin, and the remainder by phosphates and ammonium. The carbonic acid–bicarbonate system, depicted chemically as:

$$CO_2 + H_2O \leftrightarrow H_2CO_3 \leftrightarrow H^+ + HCO_3$$

interacts with the lungs, kidneys, and nonbicarbonate systems to stabilize systemic pH. The concentration of dissolved CO_2 in blood is established by the respiratory system and that of HCO_3^- by the kidneys. Disturbances in acid-base balance are initially stabilized by chemical buffering, compensated for by pulmonary or renal regulation of CO_2 or HCO_3^-, and ultimately corrected when the primary cause of the acid-base disturbance is eliminated.

Renal regulation of acid-base balance is accomplished by the reabsorption of filtered HCO_3^- and the excretion of H^+ or HCO_3^- to match the net input of acid or base. When urine is alkalinized, HCO_3^- enters the kidney and is ultimately lost in the urine. Alkalinization of the urine may occur when an absolute or relative excess of bicarbonate exists. However, urinary alkalinization will not occur if there is a deficiency of Na^+ or K^+, because HCO_3^- must also be retained to maintain electroneutrality. In contrast, the urine may be acidified if an absolute or relative decrease occurs in systemic HCO_3^-. In this setting, proximal tubular HCO_3^- reabsorption and distal tubular H^+ excretion are maximal. A "paradoxical aciduria" with low urinary pH may also be seen in the setting of hypokalemic metabolic alkalosis and systemic K^+ depletion when H^+ is exchanged in preference to K^+ in response to mineralocorticoid. Some of the processes involved in acid-base regulation are shown in Figure 43–3.

▼ FLUID & ELECTROLYTE MANAGEMENT

Therapy of fluid and electrolyte disorders is directed toward providing maintenance fluid and electrolyte requirements, replenishing prior losses, and replacing persistent abnormal

▲ **Figure 43–2.** Composition of body fluids. ECF, extracellular fluid; ICF, intracellular fluid; ISF, interstitial fluid.

losses. Therapy should be phased to (1) rapidly expand the ECF volume and restore tissue perfusion, (2) replenish fluid and electrolyte deficits while correcting attendant acid-base abnormalities, (3) meet the patient's nutritional needs, and (4) replace ongoing losses.

The cornerstone of therapy involves an understanding of maintenance fluid and electrolyte requirements. Maintenance requirements call for provision of enough water, glucose, and electrolytes to prevent deterioration of body stores. During short-term parenteral therapy, sufficient glucose is provided to prevent ketosis and limit protein catabolism, although this is usually little more than 20% of the patient's true caloric needs. Prior to the administration of maintenance fluids, it is important to consider the patient's volume status and to determine whether intravenous fluids are needed at all.

Various models have been devised to facilitate calculation of maintenance requirements based on body surface area, weight, and caloric expenditure. A system based on caloric expenditure is most helpful, because 1 mL of water is needed for each kilocalorie expended. The system presented in Table 43–1 is based on caloric needs and is applicable to children weighing more than 3 kg.

As depicted in Table 43–1, a child weighing 30 kg would need 1700 kcal and 1700 mL of water daily. If the child received parenteral fluids for 2 days, the fluid would usually contain 5% glucose, which would provide 340 kcal/d, or 20% of the maintenance caloric needs. Maintenance fluid requirements take into account normal insensible water losses and water lost in sweat, urine, and stool, and assume the patient to

be afebrile and relatively inactive. Thus if excessive losses occur standard "maintenance fluids" will be inadequate. In contrast, if losses are reduced for any reason standard "maintenance fluid" administration would be excessive. Maintenance requirements are greater for low-birth-weight and preterm infants. Table 43–2 lists other factors that commonly alter fluid and caloric needs.

Electrolyte losses occur primarily through the urinary tract and to a lesser degree via the skin and stool. Although maintenance electrolyte estimates vary, reasonable approximations for maintenance needs are 3 mEq Na^+/100 kcal and 2 mEq K^+/100 kcal or 30 mEq Na^+/L and 20 mEq K^+/L, respectively, of intravenous fluid.

It is helpful to monitor the patient's daily weight, urinary output, fluid input, and urine specific gravity. If fluid or electrolyte balance is abnormal, serial determination of electrolyte concentrations, blood urea nitrogen, and creatinine may be necessary. In patients with significant burns, anuria, oliguria, or persistent abnormal losses (eg, from a stoma, or polyuria secondary to a renal concentrating defect), it is important to measure output, and if needed its components, so appropriate replacement can be provided.

DEHYDRATION

Depletion of body fluids is one of the most commonly encountered problems in clinical pediatrics. Children have a high incidence of gastrointestinal diseases, including gastroenteritis, and may demonstrate gastrointestinal symptoms in

$$pH \, \alpha \, \frac{[HCO_3^-]}{Pco_2}$$

▲ **Figure 43–3.** Maintaining metabolic stability via compensatory mechanisms.

nongastrointestinal conditions. Infants and young children often decrease their oral intake when ill, and their high ratio of surface area to weight promotes significant evaporative losses. Renal concentrating mechanisms do not maximally conserve water in early life, and fever may significantly increase fluid needs. Dehydration decreases ECF volume, leading to decreased tissue perfusion, impaired renal function, compensatory tachycardia, and lactic acidosis. The clinical effects of dehydration relate to the degree of dehydration and to the relative amounts of salt and water lost. Caregivers must be particularly aware of dehydration occurring in breast-fed newborn infants who go home soon after birth and whose mothers fail to produce enough milk. This problem is more common in the hot summer months and has been associated with severe dehydration, brain damage, and death.

The clinical evaluation of a child with dehydration should focus on the composition and volume of fluid intake; the frequency and amount of vomiting, diarrhea, and urine output; the degree and duration of fever; the nature of any administered medications; and the existence of underlying medical conditions. A recently recorded weight, if known, can be very helpful in calculating the magnitude of dehydration. Important clinical features in estimating the degree of dehydration include the capillary refill time, postural blood pressure, and heart rate changes; dryness of the lips and mucous membranes; lack of tears; lack of external jugular venous filling when supine; a sunken fontanelle in an infant;

Table 43–1. Caloric and water needs per unit of body weight.

Body Weight (kg)	kcal/kg	mL of Water/kg
3–10	100	100
11–20	1000 kcal + 50 kcal/kg for each kg > 10 kg	1000 mL + 50 mL/kg for each kg > 10 kg
> 20	1500 kcal + 20 kcal/kg for each kg > 20 kg	1500 mL + 20 mL/kg for each kg > 20 kg

Data from Holliday MA, Segar WE: The maintenance need for water in parenteral fluid therapy. Pediatrics 1957;19:823.

oliguria; and altered mental status (Table 43–3). Children generally respond to a decrease in circulating volume with a compensatory increase in pulse rate and may maintain their blood pressure in the face of severe dehydration. A low or falling blood pressure is, therefore, a late sign of shock in children, and when present should prompt emergent treatment. Salient laboratory parameters include a high urine specific gravity (in the absence of an underlying renal concentrating defect), a relatively greater elevation in blood urea nitrogen than in creatinine, a low urinary [Na$^+$] excretion (< 15 mEq/L), and an elevated hematocrit or serum albumin level secondary to hemoconcentration.

Emergent intravenous therapy is indicated when there is evidence of compromised perfusion (inadequate capillary refill, tachycardia, poor color, oliguria, or hypotension). The initial goal is to rapidly expand the plasma volume and to prevent circulatory collapse. A 20 mL/kg bolus of isotonic fluid should be given intravenously as rapidly as possible. Either colloid (5% albumin) or crystalloid (normal saline or Ringer lactate) may be used. Colloid is particularly useful in hypernatremic patients in shock, in malnourished infants, and in neonates. If no intravenous site is available, fluid may be administered intraosseously through the marrow row space of the tibia. If there is no response to the first fluid bolus, a second bolus may be given. When adequate tissue

Table 43–2. Alterations of maintenance fluid requirements.

Factor	Altered Requirement
Fever	12% per degree C[a]
Hyperventilation	10–60 mL/100 kcal
Sweating	10–25 mL/100 kcal
Hyperthyroidism	Variable: 25–50%
Gastrointestinal loss and renal disease	Monitor and analyze output. Adjust therapy accordingly.

[a]Do not correct for 38°C; correct 24% for 39°C.

Table 43–3. Clinical manifestations of dehydration.

Clinical Signs	Degree of Dehydration		
	Mild	Moderate	Severe
Decrease in body weight	3–5%	6–10%	11–15%
Skin			
Turgor	Normal ±	Decreased	Markedly decreased
Color	Normal	Pale	Markedly decreased
Mucous membranes	Dry ⟶		Mottled or gray; parched
Hemodynamic signs			
Pulse	Normal	Slight increase	Tachycardia
Capillary refill	2–3 s	3–4 s	> 4 s
Blood pressure	Normal ⟶		Low
Perfusion	Normal ⟶		Circulatory collapse
Fluid loss			
Urinary output	Mild oliguria	Oliguria	Anuria
Tears	Decreased ⟶		Absent
Urinary indices			
Specific gravity	> 1.020 ⟶		Anuria
Urine [Na⁺]	< 20 mEq/L ⟶		Anuria

perfusion is demonstrated by improved capillary refill, decreased pulse rate and urine output, and improved mental status, deficit replacement may be instituted. If adequate perfusion is not restored after 40 mL/kg of isotonic fluids, other pathologic processes must be considered such as sepsis, occult hemorrhage, or cardiogenic shock. Isotonic dehydration may be treated by providing half of the remaining fluid deficit over 8 hours and the second half over the ensuing 16 hours in the form of 5% dextrose with 0.2–0.45% saline containing 20 mEq/L KCl. In the presence of metabolic acidosis, potassium acetate may be considered. Maintenance fluids and replacement of ongoing losses should also be provided. Typical electrolyte compositions of various body fluids are depicted in Table 43–4, although it may be necessary to measure the specific constituents of a patient's fluid losses to guide therapy. If the patient is unable to eat for a prolonged period, nutritional needs must be met through hyperalimentation or enteral tube feedings.

Oral rehydration may be provided to children with mild to moderate dehydration. Clear liquid beverages found in the home, such as broth, soda, juice, and tea, are inappropriate for the treatment of dehydration. Commercially available solutions provide 45–75 mEq/L of Na⁺, 20–25 mEq/L of K⁺, 30–34 mEq/L of citrate or bicarbonate, and 2–2.5% glucose. Frequent small aliquots (5–15 mL) should be given to provide approximately 50 mL/kg over 4 hours for mild dehydration and up to 100 mL/kg over 6 hours for moderate dehydration. Oral rehydration is contraindicated in children with altered levels of consciousness or respiratory distress who cannot drink freely; in children suspected of having an acute surgical abdomen; in infants with greater than 10% volume depletion; in children with hemodynamic instability; and in the setting of severe hyponatremia ([Na⁺] < 120 mEq/L) or hypernatremia ([Na⁺] > 160 mEq/L). Failure of oral rehydration due to persistent vomiting or inability to keep up with losses mandates intravenous therapy. Successful oral rehydration requires explicit instructions to caregivers.

The type of dehydration is characterized by the serum [Na⁺]. If relatively more solute is lost than water, the [Na⁺] falls, and hyponatremic dehydration ([Na⁺] < 130 mEq/L) ensues. This is important clinically because hypotonicity of the plasma contributes to further volume loss from the ECF

Table 43–4. Typical electrolyte compositions of various body fluids.

	Na⁺ (mEq/L)	K⁺ (mEq/L)	HCO₃⁻ (mEq/L)
Diarrhea	10–90	10–80	40
Gastric	20–80	5–20	0
Small intestine	100–140	5–15	40
Ileostomy	45–135	3–15	40

Adapted, with permission, from Winters RW: *Principles of Pediatric Fluid Therapy.* Little, Brown, 1973.

into the intracellular space. Thus tissue perfusion is more significantly impaired for a given degree of hyponatremic dehydration than for a comparable degree of isotonic or hypertonic dehydration. It is important to note, however, that significant solute losses also occur in hypernatremic dehydration. Furthermore, because plasma volume is somewhat protected in hypernatremic dehydration, it poses the risk of underestimating the severity of dehydration. Typical fluid and electrolyte losses associated with each form of dehydration are shown in Table 43–5.

HYPONATREMIA

Hyponatremia may be factitious in the presence of high plasma lipids or proteins, which decrease the percentage of plasma volume that is water. Hyponatremia in the absence of hypotonicity also occurs when an osmotically active solute, such as glucose or mannitol, is added to the ECF. Water drawn from the ICF dilutes the serum [Na$^+$] despite isotonicity or hypertonicity.

Patients with hyponatremic dehydration generally demonstrate typical signs and symptoms of dehydration (see Table 43–3), because the vascular space is compromised as water leaves the ECF to maintain osmotic neutrality. The treatment of hyponatremic dehydration is fairly straightforward. The magnitude of the sodium deficit may be calculated by the following formula:

$$Na^+ deficit =$$
$$\left(Na^+ desired - Na^+ observed\right) \times$$
$$Bodyweight\ (kg) \times 0.6$$

Half of the deficit is replenished in the first 8 hours of therapy, and the remainder is given over the following 16 hours. Maintenance and replacement fluids should also be provided. The deficit plus maintenance calculations generally approximate 5% dextrose with 0.45% saline. The rise in serum [Na$^+$] should not exceed 2 mEq/L/h. The dangers of too rapid correction of hyponatremia include cerebral dehydration and injury due to fluid shifts from the ICF compartment.

Hypovolemic hyponatremia also occurs in cerebral salt wasting associated with central nervous system (CNS) insults,

a condition characterized by high urine output and elevated urinary [Na$^+$] (> 80 mEq/L) due to an increase in ANF. This must be distinguished from the syndrome of inappropriate secretion of ADH (SIADH), which may also become manifest in CNS conditions and certain pulmonary disorders. In contrast to cerebral salt wasting, SIADH is characterized by euvolemia or mild volume expansion and relatively low urine output due to ADH-induced water retention. Urinary [Na$^+$] is high in both conditions, though generally not as high as in SIADH. It is important to distinguish between these two conditions, because the treatment of the former involves replacement of urinary salt and water losses, whereas the treatment of SIADH involves water restriction.

In cases of severe hyponatremia (serum [Na$^+$] < 120 mEq/L) with CNS symptoms, intravenous 3% NaCl may be given over 1 hour to raise the [Na$^+$] to 120 mEq/L, to alleviate CNS manifestations and sequelae. In general, 6 mL/kg of 3% NaCl will raise the serum [Na$^+$] by 5 mEq/L. If 3% NaCl is administered, estimated Na$^+$ and fluid deficits should be adjusted accordingly. Further correction should proceed slowly, as outlined earlier.

Hypervolemic hyponatremia may occur in edematous disorders such as nephrotic syndrome, congestive heart failure, and cirrhosis, wherein water is retained in excess of salt. Treatment involves restriction of Na$^+$ and water and correction of the underlying disorder. Hypervolemic hyponatremia due to water intoxication is characterized by a maximally dilute urine (specific gravity < 1.003) and is also treated with water restriction.

HYPERNATREMIA

Although diarrhea is commonly associated with hyponatremic or isonatremic dehydration, hypernatremia may develop in the presence of persistent fever or decreased fluid intake or in response to improperly mixed rehydration solutions. Extreme care is required to treat hypernatremic dehydration appropriately. If the serum [Na$^+$] falls precipitously, the osmolality of the ECF drops more rapidly than that of the CNS. Water shifts from the ECF compartment into the CNS to maintain osmotic neutrality. If hypertonicity is corrected too rapidly (a drop in [Na$^+$] of greater than 0.5–1 mEq/L/h), cerebral edema, seizures, and CNS injury may occur. Thus following the initial restoration of adequate tissue perfusion using isotonic fluids, a gradual decrease in serum [Na$^+$] is desired (10–15 mEq/L/d). This is commonly achieved using 5% dextrose with 0.2% saline to replace the calculated fluid deficit over 48 hours. Maintenance and replacement fluids should also be provided. If the serum [Na$^+$] is not correcting appropriately, the free water deficit may be estimated as 4 mL/kg of free water for each milliequivalent of serum [Na$^+$] above 145 and provided as 5% dextrose over 48 hours. If metabolic acidosis is also present, it must be corrected slowly to avoid CNS irritability. Potassium is provided as indicated—as the acetate salt if necessary. Electrolyte concentra-

Table 43–5. Estimated water and electrolyte deficits in dehydration (moderate to severe).

Type of Dehydration	H$_2$O (mL/kg)	Na$^+$ (mEq/kg)	K$^+$ (mEq/kg)	Cl$^-$ and HCO$_3^-$ (mEq/kg)
Isotonic	100–150	8–10	8–10	16–20
Hypotonic	50–100	10–14	10–14	20–28
Hypertonic	120–180	2–5	2–5	4–10

Adapted, with permission, from Winters RW: *Principles of Pediatric Fluid Therapy*. Little, Brown, 1982.

tions should be assessed every 2 hours in order to control the decline in serum [Na$^+$]. Elevations of blood glucose and blood urea nitrogen may worsen the hyperosmolar state in hypernatremic dehydration and should also be monitored closely. Hyperglycemia is often associated with hypernatremic dehydration and may necessitate lower intravenous glucose concentrations (eg, 2.5%).

Patients with diabetes insipidus, whether nephrogenic or central in origin, are prone to develop profound hypernatremic dehydration as a result of unremitting urinary free water losses (urine specific gravity < 1.010), particularly during superimposed gastrointestinal illnesses associated with vomiting or diarrhea. Treatment involves restoration of fluid and electrolyte deficits as described earlier as well as replacement of excessive water losses, with subsequent water deprivation testing during daylight hours to distinguish responsiveness to ADH. The evaluation and treatment of nephrogenic and central diabetes insipidus are discussed in detail in Chapters 22 and 32, respectively.

Hypervolemic hypernatremia (salt poisoning), associated with excess total body salt and water, may occur as a consequence of providing improperly mixed formula, excessive NaCl or NaHCO$_3$ administration, or as a feature of primary hyperaldosteronism. Treatment includes the use of diuretics, and potentially, concomitant water replacement or even dialysis.

POTASSIUM DISORDERS

The predominantly intracellular distribution of potassium is maintained by the actions of Na$^+$-K$^+$-ATPase in the cell membranes. Potassium is shifted into the ECF and plasma by acidemia and into the ICF in the setting of alkalosis, hypochloremia, or in conjunction with insulin-induced cellular glucose uptake. The ratio of intracellular to extracellular K$^+$ is the major determinant of the cellular resting membrane potential and contributes to the action potential in neural and muscular tissue. Abnormalities of K$^+$ balance are potentially life-threatening. In the kidney, K$^+$ is filtered at the glomerulus, reabsorbed in the proximal tubule, and excreted in the distal tubule. Distal tubular K$^+$ excretion is regulated primarily by aldosterone. Renal K$^+$ excretion continues for significant periods even after the intake of K$^+$ is decreased. Thus by the time urinary [K$^+$] decreases, the systemic K$^+$ pool has been depleted significantly.

The causes of net K$^+$ loss are primarily renal in origin. Gastrointestinal losses through nasogastric suction or vomiting reduce total body K$^+$ to some degree. However, the attendant volume depletion results in an increase in plasma aldosterone, promoting renal excretion of K$^+$ in exchange for Na$^+$. Diuretics (especially thiazides), mineralocorticoids, and intrinsic renal tubular diseases (eg, Bartter syndrome) enhance the renal excretion of K$^+$. Clinically, hypokalemia is associated with neuromuscular excitability, decreased peristalsis or ileus, hyporeflexia, paralysis, rhabdomyolysis, and arrhythmias. Electrocardiographic changes include flattened T waves, a shortened PR interval, and the appearance of U waves. Arrhythmias associated with hypokalemia include premature ventricular contractions; atrial, nodal, or ventricular tachycardia; and ventricular fibrillation. Hypokalemia increases responsiveness to digitalis and may precipitate overt digitalis toxicity. In the presence of arrhythmias, extreme muscle weakness, or respiratory compromise, intravenous K$^+$ should be given. If the patient is hypophosphatemic ([PO$_4$$^{-3}$] < 2 mg/dL), a phosphate salt may be used. The first priority in the treatment of hypokalemia is the restoration of an adequate serum [K$^+$]. Providing maintenance amounts of K$^+$ is usually sufficient; however, when the serum [K$^+$] is dangerously low and K$^+$ must be administered intravenously, it is imperative that the patient have a cardiac monitor. Intravenous K$^+$ should generally not be given faster than at a rate of 0.5 mEq/kg/h. Oral K$^+$ supplements may be needed for weeks to replenish depleted body stores.

Hyperkalemia—due to decreased renal K$^+$ excretion, mineralocorticoid deficiency or unresponsiveness, or K$^+$ release from the ICF compartment—is characterized by muscle weakness, paresthesias, and tetany; ascending paralysis; and arrhythmias. Electrocardiographic changes associated with hyperkalemia include peaked T waves, widening of the QRS complex, and arrhythmias such as sinus bradycardia or sinus arrest, atrioventricular block, nodal or idioventricular rhythms, and ventricular tachycardia or fibrillation. The severity of hyperkalemia depends on the electrocardiographic changes, the status of the other electrolytes, and the stability of the underlying disorder. A rhythm strip should be obtained when significant hyperkalemia is suspected. If the serum [K$^+$] is less than 6.5 mEq/L, discontinuing K$^+$ supplementation is usually sufficient. If the serum [K$^+$] is greater than 7 mEq/L or if potentiating factors such as hyponatremia, digitalis toxicity, and renal failure are present, more aggressive therapy is needed. If electrocardiographic changes or arrhythmias are present, treatment must be initiated promptly. Intravenous 10% calcium gluconate (0.2–0.5 mL/kg over 2–10 minutes) will rapidly ameliorate depolarization and may be repeated after 5 minutes if electrocardiographic changes persist. Calcium should be given only with a cardiac monitor in place and should be discontinued if bradycardia develops. The intravenous administration of a diuretic that acts in the loop of Henle, such as furosemide (1–2 mg/kg), will augment renal K$^+$ excretion and can be very helpful in lowering serum and total body [K$^+$]. Administering Na$^+$ and increasing systemic pH with bicarbonate therapy (1–2 mEq/kg) will shift K$^+$ from the ECF to the ICF compartment, as will therapy with a β-agonist such as albuterol. In nondiabetic patients, 0.5 g/kg of glucose over 1–2 hours will enhance endogenous insulin secretion, lowering serum [K$^+$] 1–2 mEq/L. Administration of intravenous glucose and insulin may be needed as a simultaneous drip (0.5–1 g/kg glucose and 0.3 units of regular insulin per gram of glucose) given over 2 hours with monitoring of the serum glucose level every 15 minutes.

The therapies outlined above provide transient benefits. Ultimately, K^+ must be reduced to normal levels by reestablishing adequate renal excretion using diuretics or optimizing urinary flow, using ion exchange resins such as sodium polystyrene sulfonate orally or as a retention enema (0.2–0.5 g/kg orally or 1 g/kg as an enema), or by dialysis.

ACID-BASE DISTURBANCES

When evaluating a disturbance in acid-base balance, the systemic pH, partial carbon dioxide pressure (PCO_2), serum [HCO_3^-], and anion gap must be considered. The anion gap, $Na^+ - (Cl^- + HCO_3^-)$, is an expression of the unmeasured anions in the plasma and is normally 12 ± 4 mEq/L. An increase above normal suggests the presence of an unmeasured anion, such as occurs in diabetic ketoacidosis, lactic acidosis, salicylate intoxication, and so on. Although the base excess (or deficit) is also used clinically, it is important to recall that this expression of acid-base balance is influenced by the renal response to respiratory disorders and cannot be interpreted independently (as in a compensated respiratory acidosis, wherein the base excess may be quite large). Recently, there has been greater interest in the Stewart approach to acid-base disturbances and the calculation of the "strong ion difference," which is beyond the scope of the present discussion. The interested reader is referred to the review by Gunnerson and Kellum listed in the references at the end of this chapter.

METABOLIC ACIDOSIS

Metabolic acidosis is characterized by a primary decrease in serum [HCO_3^-] and systemic pH due to the loss of HCO_3^- from the kidneys or gastrointestinal tract, the addition of an acid (from external sources or via altered metabolic processes), or the rapid dilution of the ECF with non-bicarbonate–containing solution (usually normal saline). When HCO_3^- is lost through the kidneys or gastrointestinal tract, Cl^- must be reabsorbed with Na^+ disproportionately, resulting in a hyperchloremic acidosis with a normal anion gap. Thus a normal anion gap acidosis in the absence of diarrhea or other bicarbonate-rich gastrointestinal losses suggests the possibility of renal tubular acidosis and should be evaluated appropriately. (See Chapter 22.) In contrast, acidosis that results from addition of an unmeasured acid is associated with a widened anion gap. Examples are diabetic ketoacidosis, lactic acidosis, starvation, uremia, toxin ingestion (salicylates, ethylene glycol, or methanol), and certain inborn errors of organic or amino acid metabolism. Dehydration may also result in a widened anion gap acidosis as a result of inadequate tissue perfusion, decreased O_2 delivery, and subsequent lactic and keto acid production. Respiratory compensation is accomplished through an increase in minute ventilation and a decrease in PCO_2. The patient's history, physical findings, and laboratory features should lead to the appropriate diagnosis.

The ingestion of unknown toxins or the possibility of an inborn error of metabolism (see Chapter 34) must be considered in children without an obvious cause for a widened anion gap acidosis. Unfortunately, some hospital laboratories fail to include ethylene glycol or methanol in their standard toxicology screens, so that these toxins must be requested specifically. This is of critical importance when therapy with fomepizole (4-methylpyrazole) must be considered for either ingestion—and instituted quickly to head off profound toxicity. Ethylene glycol (eg, antifreeze) is particularly worrisome because of its sweet taste and accounts for a significant number of toxin ingestions. Screening by fluorescence of urine under a Wood's lamp is relatively simple but does not replace specific laboratory assessment. Salicylate intoxication has a stimulatory effect on the respiratory center of the CNS; thus patients may initially present with respiratory alkalosis or mixed respiratory alkalosis and widened anion gap acidosis.

Most types of metabolic acidosis will resolve with correction of the underlying disorder, improved renal perfusion, and acid excretion. Intravenous $NaHCO_3$ administration may be considered in the setting of metabolic acidosis when the pH is less than 7.0 or the [HCO_3^-] is less than 5 mEq/L, but only if adequate ventilation is ensured. The dose (in milliequivalents) of $NaHCO_3$ may be calculated as:

$$\text{Weight (kg)} \times \text{Base deficit} \times 0.3$$

and given as a continuous infusion over 1 hour. The effect of $NaHCO_3$ in lowering serum potassium and ionized calcium concentrations must also be considered and monitored.

METABOLIC ALKALOSIS

Metabolic alkalosis is characterized by a primary increase in [HCO_3^-] and pH resulting from a loss of strong acid or gain of buffer base. The most common cause for a metabolic alkalosis is the loss of gastric juice via nasogastric suction or vomiting. This results in a Cl^--responsive alkalosis, characterized by a low urinary [Cl^-] (< 20 mEq/L) indicative of a volume-contracted state that will be responsive to the provision of adequate Cl^- salt (usually in the form of normal saline). Cystic fibrosis may also be associated with a Cl^--responsive alkalosis due to the high losses of NaCl through the sweat, whereas congenital Cl^--losing diarrhea is a rare cause of Cl^--responsive alkalosis. Chloride-resistant alkaloses are characterized by a urinary [Cl^-] greater than 20 mEq/L and include Bartter syndrome, Cushing syndrome, and primary hyperaldosteronism, conditions associated with primary increases in urinary [Cl^-], or volume-expanded states lacking stimuli for Cl^- reabsorption. Thus the urinary [Cl^-] is helpful in distinguishing the nature of a metabolic alkalosis, but must be specifically requested in many laboratories because it is not routinely included in urine electrolyte screens. The serum [K^+] is also low in these settings (hypokalemic metabolic alkalosis) owing to a combination of increased mineralocorticoid activity associated with volume contraction, the shift of K^+ to the ICF compartment, preferential reabsorption of Na^+ rather than K^+ to preserve intravascular volume, or primary mineralocorticoid excess.

RESPIRATORY ACIDOSIS

Respiratory acidosis develops when alveolar ventilation is decreased, increasing PCO_2 and lowering systemic pH. The kidneys compensate for respiratory acidosis by increasing HCO_3^- reabsorption, a process that takes several days to manifest. Patients with acute respiratory acidoses frequently demonstrate air hunger with retractions and the use of accessory respiratory muscles. Respiratory acidoses occur in upper or lower airway obstruction, ventilation-perfusion disturbances, CNS depression, and neuromuscular defects. Hypercapnia is not as detrimental as the hypoxia that usually accompanies these disorders. The goal of therapy is to correct or compensate for the underlying pathologic process, to improve alveolar ventilation. Bicarbonate therapy is not indicated in a pure respiratory acidosis, because it will worsen the acidosis by shifting the equilibrium of the carbonic acid–bicarbonate buffer system to increase PCO_2.

RESPIRATORY ALKALOSIS

Respiratory alkalosis occurs when hyperventilation results in a decrease in PCO_2 and an increase in pH. Patients may experience tingling, paresthesias, dizziness, palpitations, syncope, or even tetany and seizures due to the associated decrease in ionized calcium. Causes of respiratory alkalosis include psychobehavioral disturbances, CNS irritation from meningitis or encephalitis, and salicylate intoxication. Therapy is directed toward the causal process. Rebreathing into a paper bag will decrease the severity of symptoms in acute hyperventilation.

REFERENCES

Adrogue JA, Madias NE: Management of life-threatening acid–base disorders: Parts 1 and 2. N Engl J Med 1998;338:26, 107 [PMID: 9414329].

Avner ED: Clinical disorders of water metabolism: Hyponatremia and hypernatremia. Pediatr Ann 1995;24:23 [PMID: 7715960].

Fall PJ: A stepwise approach to acid-base disorders. Practical patient evaluation for metabolic acidosis and other conditions. Postgraduate Med 2000;107:249 [PMID: 10728149].

Finberg L et al: Water and Electrolytes in Pediatrics: Physiology, Pathophysiology and Treatment, 2nd ed. WB Saunders, 1993.

Gunnerson KJ, Kellum JA: Acid-base and electrolyte analysis in critically ill patients: Are we ready for the new millennium? Curr Opin Crit Care 2003;9:468 [PMID:14639065].

Hellerstein S: Fluids and electrolytes: Physiology. Pediatr Rev 1993;14:70 [PMID: 8493184].

Jospe N, Forbes G: Fluids and electrolytes: Clinical aspects. Pediatr Rev 1996;17:395 [PMID: 8937172].

Kappy MS, Ganong CA: Cerebral salt wasting in children: The role of atrial natriuretic hormone. Adv Pediatr 1996;43:271 [PMID: 8794180].

Liebelt EL: Clinical and laboratory evaluation and management of children with vomiting, diarrhea, and dehydration. Curr Opin Pediatr 1998;10:461 [PMID: 9818241].

McDonald RA: Disorders of potassium balance. Pediatr Ann 1995;24:31 [PMID: 7715961].

Roberts KB: Fluid and electrolytes: parenteral fluid therapy. Pediatr Rev 2001;22:380 [PMID: 11691948].

Watkins SL: The basics of fluid and electrolyte therapy. Pediatr Ann 1995;24:16 [PMID: 7715959].

White ML, Liebelt: Update on antidotes for pediatric poisoning. Pediatr Emerg Care 2006;22:740 [PMID:17110870].

Pediatric Laboratory Medicine & Reference Ranges

Georgette Siparsky, PhD
Frank J. Accurso, MD

Laboratory tests provide valuable information necessary to evaluate a patient's condition and to monitor recommended treatment. Chemistry and hematology test results are compared with those of healthy individuals or those undergoing similar therapeutic treatment to determine clinical status and progress. In the past, the term *normal ranges* relayed some ambiguity because statistically, the term *normal* also implied a specific (gaussian or normal) distribution and epidemiologically it implied the state of the majority, which is not necessarily the desirable or targeted population. This is most apparent in cholesterol levels, where values greater than 200 mg/dL are common, but not desirable. Use of the term *reference range* or *reference interval* is therefore recommended by the International Federation of Clinical Chemistry (IFCC) and the Clinical and Laboratory Standards Institute (CLSI, formerly the National Committee for Clinical Laboratory Standards, NCCLS) to indicate that the values relate to a reference population and clinical condition.

Reference ranges are established for a specific age (eg, α-fetoprotein), sex, and sexual maturity (eg, luteinizing hormone and testosterone); they are also defined for a specific pharmacologic status (eg, taking cyclosporine), dietary restrictions (eg, phenylalanine) and stimulation protocol (eg, growth hormone). Similarly, diurnal variation is a factor (eg, cortisol), as is degree of obesity (eg, insulin). Some reference ranges are particularly meaningful when combined with other results (eg, parathyroid hormone and calcium), or when an entire set of analytes is evaluated (eg, lipid profile: triglyceride, cholesterol, high-density lipoprotein, and low-density lipoprotein).

Laboratory tests are becoming more specific and measure much lower concentrations than ever before. Therefore reference ranges should reflect the analytical procedure, as well as reagents and instrumentation used for a specific analysis. As test methodology continues to evolve, reference ranges are modified and updated.

CHALLENGES IN DETERMINING & INTERPRETING PEDIATRIC REFERENCE INTERVALS

The pediatric environment is particularly challenging for the determination of reference intervals since growth and developmental stages do not have a distinct and finite boundary by which test results can be tabulated. Reference ranges may overlap and, in many cases, complicate diagnosis and treatment. Collection and allocation of test results by age for the purpose of establishing a reference range is a convenient and manageable way to report them, but caution is needed in their interpretation and clinical correlation.

A particular difficulty lies in establishing reference ranges for analytes whose levels are changed under scheduled stimulation conditions. The common glucose tolerance test is such an example, but more complex endocrinology tests (eg, stimulation by clonidine and cosyntropin) require skill and extensive experience to interpret. Reference ranges for these serial tests are established over a long period of time and are not easily transferable between test methodologies. Changing analytical technologies adds a new dimension to the challenges of establishing pediatric reference ranges.

GUIDELINES FOR USE OF DATA IN A REFERENCE RANGE STUDY

The College of American Pathologists provides guidelines for the adoption of reference ranges used in hospitals and commercial clinical laboratories. It recognizes the enormous task of establishing a laboratory's own reference ranges, and recommends alternatives to the process. A laboratory may acquire reference ranges by:

1. Conducting its own study to evaluate a statistically significant number of "healthy" volunteers. It is a monumental task for a laboratory to develop its own pediatric reference ranges, because parental consent and

procedural approval by review boards need to be addressed. The numerous age categories to be evaluated also add to the complexity and size of the study.

2. Adopting ranges established by the manufacturer of a particular analytical instrument. The laboratory must validate the data by analyzing a sample of 20 "reference" subjects (patients representing that specific population) to confirm that the adopted range is truly representative of that group.

3. Using reference data in the general medical literature and conferring with physicians to make sure the data agree with their clinical experience. A validation study is also recommended.

4. Analyzing hospital patient data. Laboratory test results from hospital patients have been used to compute reference ranges provided they fulfill stated clinical criteria. Patient records need to indicate that the patient's specific medical condition does not influence the analyte whose reference range is being determined. For example, a child undergoing surgery for bone fracture repair is expected to have normal electrolytes and thyroid function, whereas a child examined for precocious puberty should not be included in a reference range study for luteinizing hormone. In the REALAB Project, Grossi et al chose the "inclusion criterion," whereby tests that have a single laboratory measurement were used; justification was based on the fact that persons with repeated testing had a higher probability of being diseased and their results should be excluded from the study.

Statistically, the sample size of a hospital patient study should be considerably larger than that of a healthy group. A study from a healthy population may require 20 subjects to be statistically significant, whereas a hospital population should evaluate a minimum of 120 patients. At Children's Hospital in Denver, the free thyroxine reference range was recently established using 1480 clinic and hospital patient results in this manner.

STATISTICAL COMPUTATION OF REFERENCE INTERVALS

The establishment of reference intervals is based on a statistical distribution of test results obtained from a representative population. The CLSI recommendation for data collection and statistical analysis provides guidelines for managing the data. For clinicians, it is not important that they can reproduce the calculation. It is far more critical to understand the benefits and restrictions provided by the described statistical approaches, and to evaluate patient results with these limitations in mind.

In reviewing the statistics, 95% of all results will be inherently included in the reference range. Note that 5% of that population will have "abnormal" results, when in fact they are "healthy" and an integral part of the reference group

study. Similarly an equivalent 5% of the "ill" population will have laboratory results within the reference range. These are inherent features of the statistical computation. Taking that analysis one step further, the probability of a healthy patient having a test result within a calculated reference range is

$$P = 0.95$$

When multiple tests or panels of tests are used, the combined probability of all the test results falling in their respective reference ranges drops dramatically. For example, the probability of all results from 10 tests in the complete metabolic panel being in the reference range is

$$P = (0.95)^{10} = 0.60$$

Therefore, about one third of healthy patients will have one test result in the panel that is outside the reference range.

A. Parametric Method of Computation

The parametric method of establishing reference intervals is simple, though not always representative, since it is based on the assumption that the data have a gaussian distribution. A mean (x) and standard deviation (s) are calculated; test results of 95% of that specific population will fall within the mean ± 1.96s, as shown in Figure 44–1.

Where the distribution is not gaussian, a mathematical manipulation of the values (eg, plotting the log of the value, instead of the value itself) may give a gaussian distribution. The mean and standard deviation are then converted back to give a usable reference range.

B. Nonparametric Method of Computation

The nonparametric method of establishing reference ranges is currently recommended by CLSI since it defines outliers as those in the extreme 2.5 percentile of the upper and lower limits of data respectively. The number of data points excluded at the limits depends on the skew of the curve, and

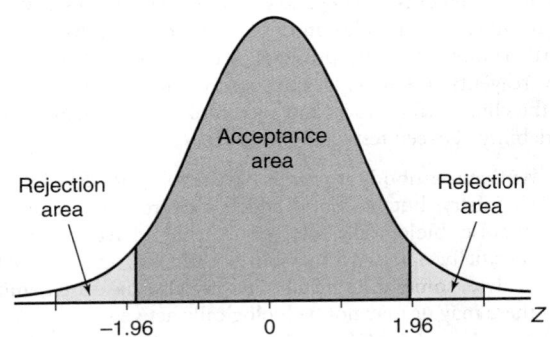

▲ **Figure 44–1.** Gaussian distribution and parametric calculation using x ± 1.96s to define the range.

▲ **Figure 44–2.** Histogram of free thyroxine (FT4) using clinic and hospital patients at Children's Hospital in Denver.

so the computation accommodates a nongaussian distribution. A histogram depicting the nongaussian distribution of data from a free thyroxine reference range study conducted at Children's Hospital in Denver is shown in Figure 44–2.

WHY REFERENCE INTERVALS VARY

Recent modifications to reference ranges are due to the introduction of new and improved analytical procedures, advanced automated instrumentation, and standardization of reagents and reference materials. Reference ranges are also affected by preanalytical variations that can occur during sample collection, processing, and storage.

Preanalytical variations of biological origin can occur when specimens are drawn in the morning versus in the evening, or from hospitalized recumbent patients versus ambulatory outpatients. Variations may also be caused by metabolic and hemodynamic factors. Preanalytical factors may be a product of the socioeconomic environment or ethnic background (eg, genetic or dietary).

Analytical variations are caused by differences in analytical measurements and depend on the analytical tools as well as an inherent variability in obtaining a quantitative value. Furthermore, scientific progress is constantly introducing new reagents, instruments, and improved testing procedures to the clinical laboratory, and each tool adds an element of variability between tests.

1. **Antigen–antibody reactions** have revolutionized clinical chemistry, but have also added a degree of variability because biologically derived reagents have different specificity and sensitivity. In addition to the targeted analyte, some of its metabolites are also measured, and these may or may not be biologically active.
2. **Reference materials** continue to be reviewed and evaluated by organizations such as the World Health Organization and the National Institute for Standards and

Technology. A new standard was recently established for troponin I, and reference ranges were modified to reflect the new standard.

3. **Analytical instrumentation** with advanced electronics and robotics has improved accuracy of results and increased throughput. However, they have added an element of variability between instruments from different manufacturers.
4. **Analytical detection methods** have also made big strides as they have expanded from simple ultraviolet–visible spectrophotometry, to fluorescence, nephelometry, radio-immunoassay, and chemiluminescence. For example, the third-generation thyroid-stimulating hormone assays can now measure concentrations as low as 0.001 µIU/mL, and the reference range was recently modified to reflect the improved sensitivity of the assay.

SENSITIVITY & SPECIFICITY

Despite its statistical derivation, a reference interval does not necessarily provide a finite and clear-cut guideline as to whether a patient has a disease. There will always be a segment of the population with test values that fall within the reference interval, but clinical manifestations that indicate disease is present. Similarly, a segment of the population will have test values outside the reference interval, but no clinical signs of disease. The ability of a test and corresponding reference interval to detect individuals with disease is defined by the diagnostic sensitivity of the test. Similarly, the ability of a test to detect individuals without disease is described by the diagnostic specificity. These characteristics are governed by the analytical quality of the test, as well as the numerical parameters (reference interval) that define the presence of disease. The tolerance level for the desired sensitivity and specificity of a test requires significant input from clinicians.

Generally, specificity increases as sensitivity decreases. A typical reference range frequency distribution, shown in Figure 44–3 (solid line), provides information on the test results of a number of healthy subjects, or individuals without the disease. A second curve (dashed line) shows test results for individuals with the disease. As with most tests, there is an overlap area. A patient with a test result of 1 is likely healthy, and the result indicates a true negative (TN) for the presence of disease. A patient with a test result of 9 is likely to have the disease and the test result is a true positive (TP). There is a small, but significant population with a test result of 2–5 in whom the test is not 100% conclusive. A statistical analysis may determine the most likely cutoff for healthy individuals, but the clinically acceptable cutoff depends on the test as well as clinical correlation. Where the treatment is aggressive and has serious side effects, a clinician may choose to err on the side of caution and hold treatment for anyone with a test value of less than 6.

▲ Figure 44–3. Frequency distribution of test results for patients with and without disease. FN, false negative; FP, false positive; TN, true negative; TP, true positive.

If cutoff values for the reference interval are such that a test result indicates that a healthy patient has the disease, the result is a false positive (FP). Conversely if a test result indicates that a patient is well when in fact he or she has the disease, the result is a false negative (FN). To define the ability of the test and reference interval to identify a disease state, the diagnostic sensitivity and specificity are measured.

$$\text{Diagnostic sensitivity} = \frac{TP}{(TP + FN)}$$

$$\text{Diagnostic specificity} = \frac{TN}{(TN + FP)}$$

In the example shown in Figure 44–3, a reference interval of 0.5–3 will provide more TN results and minimize FP results. Alternatively, a reference interval of 0.5–4 will increase the rate of FN. Thus an increase in sensitivity leads to a decrease in specificity. A medical condition that requires aggressive treatment may necessitate a test and corresponding reference interval with a high sensitivity, which is a measure of the TP rate. This is accomplished at the expense of lowering specificity.

A reference interval is a statistical representation of test results from a finite population, but it is by no means inclusive of every member of the group. It is merely one component in the measure of a patient's status, to be viewed in relation to the sensitivity and specificity of the test.

Clinical laboratory data are frequently interpreted using a dynamic approach rather than from the perspective of a static state, so that each value is compared with another, instead of a strict reference range. In this case, time series analysis of relative values may provide more important information than comparison against a reference range. Examples include the evaluation of enzyme activity over time and various stimulation studies for endocrine assessment. Drug monitoring is also a dynamic process.

PEDIATRIC REFERENCE INTERVALS

The establishment of reference ranges is a complex process. Assumptions are made in the management of data processes, regardless of whether "healthy" individuals or hospital patients are used for the accumulation of test results. Analytical instrument manufacturers conduct large studies to identify reference intervals for each specific analyte, and pediatric values have always been the most challenging. Some of the manufacturers' recommended reference intervals are listed in Table 44–1 for general chemistry, Table 44–2 for endocrinology, and Table 44–3 for hematology. The interpretation of chemistry and hematology laboratory results is equally complex and forms a continuous challenge for physicians and the medical community at large.

Table 44–1. General chemistry.

Analyte, Units, Specimen Type	Age	Male Range	Female Range
Albumin (g/dL) S, P	1–7 d	2.4–3.9	1.9–4.0
	8–30 d	2.1–4.5	1.9–4.4
	31–90 d	2.1–4.8	2.0–4.2
	3–6 mo	2.2–4.9	2.3–4.4
	6 mo–1 y	2.2–4.7	2.3–4.7
	1–3 y	3.5–4.2	3.5–4.7
	4–6 y	3.6–5.2	3.6–5.2
	7 y–Adult	3.8–5.6	3.8–5.6

(continued)

Table 44–1. General chemistry. *(Continued)*

Analyte, Units, Specimen Type	Age	Male Range	Female Range
Alkaline phosphatase (U/L) S, P	1–7 d	121–351	107–357
	8–30 d	138–486	107–474
	31–90 d	101–467	125–547
	4–6 mo	94–425	125–449
	7–12 mo	101–394	101–431
	1–3 y	185–383	185–383
	4–6 y	191–450	191–450
	7–9 y	218–499	218–499
	10–11 y	174–624	169–657
	12–13 y	245–584	141–499
	14–15 y	169–618	103–283
	16–19 y	98–317	82–169
Alanine aminotransferase (U/L) S, P	1–7 d	20–54	21–54
	8–30 d	24–54	22–46
	1–3 mo	27–54	26–61
	4–6 mo	26–55	26–51
	7–12 mo	26–59	26–55
	1–3 y	19–59	24–59
	4–6 y	24–49	24–49
	10–11 y	24–49	24–44
	12–13 y	24–68	24–44
	14–15 y	24–59	19–44
	16–19 y	24–54	19–49
Ammonia (μmol/L)	All Ages	< 51	< 51
Amylase (U/L) S, P	1–30 d	< 18	< 18
	31–182 d	< 43	< 43
	183–365 d	< 81	< 81
	1 y–Adult	< 106	< 106
Aspartate aminotransferase (U/L) S, P	1–7 d	26–98	20–93
	8–30 d	16–67	20–69
	1–3 mo	16–60	16–61
	4–6 mo	16–62	16–60
	7–12 mo	16–52	16–60
	1–3 y	16–57	16–57
	5–6 y	10–47	10–47
	7–9 y	10–36	5–36
	12–13 y	10–36	5–26
	16–19 y	10–41	0–26
Blood urea nitrogen (mg/dL) S, P	0–4 d	3–19	3–19
	5 d–2 y	6–17	6–17
	3–12 y	8–18	8–18
	13–18 y	9–21	9–21
C3 (mg/dL) S	0–6 mo	38–100	39–91
	6 mo–3 y	58–119	49–109
	4–6 y	68–127	65–122
	7–9 y	78–140	70–124

(continued)

Table 44–1. General chemistry. *(Continued)*

Analyte, Units, Specimen Type	Age	Male Range	Female Range
	10–12 y	75–107	74–127
	13–15 y	66–134	75–118
	16–18 y	77–125	62–120
C4 (mg/dL)	0–6 mo	13–30	14–28
S	6 mo–3 y	17–48	17–43
	4–6 y	23–47	21–42
	7–9 y	21–37	20–42
	10–12 y	21–38	18–47
	13–15 y	21–51	20–38
	16–18 y	21–39	15–41
Calcium (mg/dL)	0–7 d	7.6–11.3	7.8–11.2
S, P	8–30 d	8.8–11.6	8.6–11.8
	31–90 d	8.7–11.2	8.2–11.0
	91–180 d	8.5–11.3	8.0–11.4
	181–365 d	8.0–10.9	8.1–11.0
	1–3 y	8.9–9.9	8.9–9.9
	4–11 y	9.0–10.1	9.0–10.1
	12–13 y	9.0–10.6	9.0–10.6
	14 y–Adult	9.3–10.7	9.3–10.7
Chloride (mmol/L)	0–6 mo	97–108	97–108
S, P	6 mo–1 y	97–106	97–106
	> 1 y	97–107	97–107
Cholesterol (mg/dL)	0–1 mo	38–174	56–195
S, P	2–6 mo	53–194	59–216
	7–12 mo	83–205	68–216
	1–3 y	37–178	37–178
	4–6 y	103–184	103–184
	7–9 y	107–245	107–245
	10–11 y	120–228	122–242
	12–13 y	122–228	120–211
	14–15 y	101–222	125–211
	16–18 y	105–218	101–215
Creatine kinase	0–90 d	29–303	43–474
(U/L)	3–12 mo	25–172	27–242
S, P	13–24 mo	28–162	25–177
	2–10 y	31–152	25–177
	11–14 y	31–152	31–172
	15–18 y	34–147	28–142
Cardiac troponin I (ng/mL)	0–30 d	0–8.4	0–8.4
S, P	31–90 d	0–0.7	0–0.7
	3–6 mo	0–0.5	0–0.5
	7–12 mo	0–0.3	0–0.3
	1–18 y	< 0.1	< 0.1
Creatinine (mg/dL)	0–7 d	0.7–1.2	0.7–1.2
S, P	7 d–1 mo	0.3–0.8	0.3–0.8
	1 mo–1 y	0.2–0.5	0.2–0.5

(continued)

Table 44-1. General chemistry. *(Continued)*

Analyte, Units, Specimen Type	Age	Male Range	Female Range
	1–3 y	0.2–0.8	0.2–0.8
	10–12 y	0.5–1.1	0.5–1.1
γ-Glutamyl transferase (U/L) S, P	1–7 d	25–168	18–148
	8–30 d	23–174	16–140
	1–3 mo	16–147	16–140
	4–6 mo	5–93	13–123
	7–12 mo	8–38	8–59
	1–3 y	2–15	2–15
	4–6 y	5–17	5–17
	7–9 y	9–20	9–20
	10–11 y	12–25	12–23
	12–13 y	12–39	10–20
	14–15 y	8–29	10–22
	16–19 y	6–30	6–23
Glucose (mg/dL) S, P	0–1 d	36–110	36–89
	1–7 d	47–110	47–110
	> 7 d	54–117	54–117
Glucose–CSF (mg/dL)	Neonate	41–84	41–84
	16 y	41–84	41–84
Glucose–urine (mg/dL)	Neonate	6–19	6–19
High-density lipoprotein cholesterol (mg/dL) S, P	0–< 2 y	12–60	12–60
	2–< 7 y	26–68	16–62
	7–< 12 y	28–76	26–77
	12–15 y	22–73	28–79
	16–19 y	28–72	24–74
IgA (mg/dL) S, P	1–30 d	0–11	0–10
	31–182 d	0–40	0–42
	183–365 d	1–82	6–68
	1–3 y	9–137	15–111
	4–6 y	44–187	33–166
	7–9 y	58–204	28–180
	10–12 y	46–218	55–193
	13–15 y	29–251	62–241
	16–18 y	68–259	69–262
IgG (mg/dL) S, P	1–30 d	197–833	162–872
	31–182 d	140–533	311–664
	183–365 d	130–156	325–647
	1–3 y	413–1112	451–1202
	4–6 y	468–1328	560–1319
	7–9 y	582–1441	485–1473
	10–12 y	685–1620	586–1609
	13–15 y	590–1600	749–1640
	16–18 y	522–1703	804–1817

(continued)

Table 44–1. General chemistry. *(Continued)*

Analyte, Units, Specimen Type	Age	Male Range	Female Range
IgM (mg/dL) S, P	1–30 d	0–65	1–57
	31–182 d	6–84	0–127
	183–365 d	15–117	0–130
	1–3 y	30–146	35–184
	4–6 y	31–151	42–184
	7–9 y	21–140	30–165
	10–12 y	27–151	42–211
	13–15 y	26–184	34–225
	16–18 y	18–179	45–224
Iron (mcg/dL) S, P		Males and females (5–11 AM)	Males and females (5–11 PM)
	0–24 mo	20–105	20–140
	2–9 y	20–105	20–145
	10–Adult	20–100	20–145
Lactate dehydrogenase (U/L)	1–30 d	178–629	187–600
	1–3 mo	158–373	452–353
S, P	4–6 mo	135–376	158–353
	7–12 mo	129–367	152–327
	1–3 y	164–286	164–286
	4–6 y	155–280	155–280
	7–9 y	141–237	141–237
	10–11 y	141–231	129–222
	12–13 y	141–231	129–205
	16–19 y	117–217	117–213
Magnesium (mg/dL) S, P	7–30 d	1.3–2.7	1.3–2.7
	1 mo–1 y	1.7–2.7	1.7–2.7
	1–3 y	1.6–2.5	1.6–2.5
	4–6 y	1.7–2.4	1.7–2.4
	13–15 y	1.6–2.4	1.6–2.3
Potassium (µmol/L)	0–7 d	3.2–5.7	3.2–5.7
	7–30 d	3.4–6.2	3.4–6.2
S, P	1–6 mo	3.5–5.8	3.5–5.8
	6 mo–1 y	3.5–6.3	3.5–6.3
	> 1 y	3.3–4.7	3.3–4.7
Prealbumin (mg/dL) S, P	0–5 d	8.6–23.2	8.6–23.2
	6 d–1 y	9.6–32.0	9.6–32.0
	2–5 y	16.4–32.0	16.4–32.0
	6–9 y	17.3–34.9	17.3–34.9
	10–13 y	22.2–37.8	22.2–37.8
	14–19 y	24.2–46.6	24.2–46.6
Phosphorus (mg/dL) S, P	0–30 d	2.8–7.0	3.1–7.7
	31–90 d	3.1–6.6	3.1–7.2
	3–12 mo	3.1–6.6	3.1–6.8
	13–24 mo	3.1–6.2	3.1–6.3
	2–12 y	3.1–5.9	3.1–5.9
	13–15 y	3.1–5.3	3.1–5.5
	16–18 y	3.1–5.1	3.1–4.8

(continued)

Table 44–1. General chemistry. *(Continued)*

Analyte, Units, Specimen Type	Age	Male Range	Female Range
Protein–CSF (mg/dL)	0–14 d	15–100	15–153
	15–30 d	15–96	15–100
	31–90 d	15–48	15–93
	3–5 mo	15–48	15–44
	7–24 mo	15–50	15–48
	2–7 y	15–45	15–45
	8–19 y	15–40	15–45
Sodium (μmol/L)	0–7 d	131–144	131–144
S, P	7–31 d	132–142	132–142
	1 mo–1 y	131–140	131–140
	> 1 y	132–141	132–141
Total bilirubin (mg/dL)	0–1 d	< 5.1	< 5.1
S, P	1–2 d	< 7.2	< 7.2
	3–5 d	< 10.3	< 10.3
	1 mo–Adult	< 0.8	< 0.8
Thyroxine (mcg/dL)	1–30 d	3.4–14.5	3.5–13.5
S, P	1–12 mo	5.6–16.4	5.0–13.5
	1–5 y	5.9–11.6	6.7–12.9
	6–10 y	5.7–10.8	5.6–11.0
	11–15 y	4.9–10.5	5.3–10.2
	16–18 y	5.2–9.1	5.5–10.2
Total protein (g/dL)	1–60 d	4.0–7.6	3.6–7.0
S, P	61–180 d	4.0–7.0	4.0–7.6
	181 d–1 y	4.2–7.9	4.6–7.8
	1–3 y	6.0–8.0	6.0–7.8
	7–9 y	6.3–8.1	6.3–8.1
	10–19 y	6.4–8.6	6.4–8.6
Triglycerides (mg/dL)	0–7 d	19–174	26–159
S, P	8–30 d	37–279	33–270
	31–90 d	42–279	34–340
	1–3 y	25–119	25–119
	4–6 y	30–110	30–110
	7–9 y	26–123	26–123
	10–11 y	22–131	37–134
	2–13 y	22–138	35–124
	14–15 y	32–158	36–129
	16–19 y	32–134	35–134
Total carbon dioxide (μmol/L)	0–7 d	13–21	13–21
S, P	7 d–1 mo	13–22	13–22
	1–6 mo	13–23	13–23
	6 mo–1 y	14–23	14–23
	> 1 y	16–25	16–25
Uric acid (mg/dL)	0–15 y	2.2–7.0	2.2–7.0
S, P	16 y–Adult	4.0–8.7	2.4–6.8

B, whole blood; CSF, cerebrospinal fluid; P, plasma; S, serum; U, urine.
All data reproduced, with permission, from Ghoshal AK, Soldin SJ: Evaluation of the Dade Behring Dimension RxL: Integrated chemistry system–pediatric reference ranges. Clin Chim Acta 2003;331:135.

Table 44–2. Endocrine chemistry.

Analyte, Units, Specimen Type	Age	Methodology	Male Range	Female Range
Cortisol (mcg/dL)	< 2 y	DPC Immulite	1.1–33.0	1.1–29.0
S	2–11 y		1.1–31.9	1.1–23.2
	11–18 y		1.1–27.2	1.1–20.3
Estradiol (ng/mL)	Prepuberty	Esoterix	< 1.5	< 1.5
S	Tanner I		0.5–1.1	0.5–2.0
	Tanner II		0.5–1.6	1.0–2.4
	Tanner III		0.5–2.5	0.7–6.0
	Tanner IV		1.0–3.6	2.1–8.5
	Tanner V		1.0–3.6	3.4–17
Follicle-stimulating hormone (mIU/mL)	0–2 y	DPC Immulite	0.1–0.8	0.1–5.9
S	2–5 y		0.1–0.4	10.1–3.6
	6–10 y		0.1–0.3	0.1–1.7
	11–18 y		0.1–7.5	0.1–7.4
	Tanner I		0.16–3.5	0.38–3.6
	Tanner II		0.44–6.0	1.25–8.9
	Tanner III		0.44–6.0	1.25–8.9
	Tanner IV		1.40–11.8	1.65–9.1
	Tanner V		1.28–14.9	1.20–12.3
Growth hormone (ng/mL)	Tanner I	DPC Immulite	0.12–2.8	0.24–5.4
S	Tanner II		0.10–5.7	0.13–8.5
	Tanner III		0.10–5.7	0.13–8.5
	Tanner IV		0.07–7.9	0.14–13.4
	Tanner V		0.10–15.1	0.24–9.9
Insulin-like growth factor-1 (ng/mL)	0–7 d	DPC Immulite	1–26	1–26
S, P	8–15 d		11–41	11–41
	16 d–1 y		55–327	55–327
	1 y		55–327	55–327
	2 y		51–303	51–303
	3 y		49–289	49–289
	4 y		49–283	49–283
	5 y		50–286	50–286
	6 y		52–297	52–297
	7 y		57–316	57–316
	8 y		64–345	64–345
	9 y		74–388	74–388
	10 y		88–452	88–452
	11 y		111–551	111–551
	12 y		143–693	143–693
	13 y		183–850	183–850
	14 y		220–972	220–972
	15 y		237–996	237–996
	16 y		226–903	226–903
	17 y		193–731	193–731
	18 y		163–584	163–584
	19 y		141–483	141–483
	20 y		127–424	127–424

(continued)

Table 44–2. Endocrine chemistry. *(Continued)*

Analyte, Units, Specimen Type	Age	Methodology	Male Range	Female Range
Insulin-like growth factor-binding protein 3 (mcg/mL) S, P	0–7 d	DPC Immulite	0.1–0.7	0.1–0.7
	8–15 d		0.5–1.4	0.5–1.4
	16 d–1 y		0.7–3.6	0.7–3.6
	1 y		0.7–3.6	0.7–3.6
	2 y		0.8–3.9	0.8–3.9
	3 y		0.9–4.3	0.9–4.3
	4 y		1.0–4.7	1.0–4.7
	5 y		1.1–5.2	1.1–5.2
	6 y		1.3–5.6	1.3–5.6
	7 y		1.4–6.1	1.4–6.1
	8 y		1.6–6.5	1.6–6.5
	9 y		1.8–7.1	1.8–7.1
	10 y		2.1–7.7	2.1–7.7
	11 y		2.4–8.4	2.4–8.4
	12 y		2.7–8.9	2.7–8.9
	13 y		3.1–9.5	3.1–9.5
	14 y		3.3–10	3.3–10
	15 y		3.5–10	3.5–10
	16 y		3.4–9.5	3.4–9.5
	17 y		3.2–8.7	3.2–8.7
	18 y		3.1–7.9	3.1–7.9
	19 y		2.9–7.3	2.9–7.3
	20 y		2.9–7.2	2.9–7.2
Luteinizing hormone (mIU/mL) S	0.1–1.5 y	DPC Immulite	ND–4.1	ND–2.3
	1.6–9 y		ND–3.8	ND–1.3
	Tanner I		0.7–1.2	0.7–2.0
	Tanner II		0.3–4.4	0.4–11
	Tanner III		0.3–4.4	0.4–11
	Tanner IV		0.5–4.7	0.9–13
	Tanner V		0.7–10.6	1.1–19
Free thyroxine (ng/dL) S[a]	0–1 d	DPC Immulite	0.8–1.9	0.8–1.9
	1–7 d		1.2–2.5	1.2–2.5
	8 d–Adult		0.8–1.7	0.8–1.7
Thyroid-stimulating hormone (μIU/mL) S	1 y	DPC Immulite	0.40–8.6	0.40–8.6
	2 y		0.36–7.6	0.36–7.6
	3 y		0.33–6.7	0.33–6.7
	4 y		0.33–6.3	0.33–6.3
	5 y		0.34–6.1	0.34–6.1
	6 y		0.34–6.0	0.34–6.0
	7 y		0.35–5.8	0.35–5.8
	8–12 y		0.35–5.7	0.35–5.7
	9 y		0.35–5.6	0.35–5.6
	10 y		0.36–5.5	0.36–5.5
	11 y		0.36–5.5	0.36–5.5
	12 y		0.36–5.4	0.36–5.4

(continued)

Table 44–2. Endocrine chemistry. *(Continued)*

Analyte, Units, Specimen Type	Age	Methodology	Male Range	Female Range
Total testosterone (ng/dL)	Premature	DPC Immulite	37–198	5–22
S	Newborn		75–400	20–64
	Prepubertal		2–30	1–20
	Tanner I		2–23	2–10
	Tanner II		5–70	5–30
	Tanner III		15–280	10–30
	Tanner IV		105–545	15–40
	Tanner V		265–800	10–40

B, whole blood; CSF, cerebrospinal fluid; P, plasma; RBC, red blood cells; S serum; U, urine.
[a]Data from Children's Hospital, Denver, Colorado.
All other data reproduced, with permission, from Soldin SJ et al: Pediatric Reference Ranges, 4th ed. American Association for Clinical Chemistry Press, 2003; and Van Krieken L: Immulite Reproductive Hormone Assays. Available at: http://www.medical.siemens.com/siemens/en_GLOBAL/gg_diag_FBAs/files/news_views/spring00/techreports/zb157-d_www.pdf.

Table 44–3. Hematology.

Analyte, Units, Specimen Type	Age	Male Range	Female Range
White blood cells ($\times 10^9$/L) EDTA whole blood	Newborn	9.0–32.0	9.0–32.0
	1–24 mo	5–13.0	5–13.0
	2–10 y	4–12.0	4–12.0
	10–17 y	4–10.5	4–10.5
	Adult	4–10.5	4–10.5
Red blood cells ($\times 10^{12}$/L) EDTA whole blood	Newborn	4.6–6.7	4.6–6.7
	1–24 mo	3.8–5.4	3.8–5.4
	2–10 y	4.0–5.3	4.0–5.3
	10–17 y	4.2–5.6	4.2–5.6
	Adult	4.7–6.0	4.2–5.4
Hemoglobin (g/dL) EDTA whole blood	Newborn	13–22	13–22
	1–24 mo	9.5–14.0	9.5–14.0
	2–10 y	11.5–14.5	11.5–14.5
	10–17 y	12.5–16.1	12–15
	Adult	13.5–18	12.5–16.0
Hematocrit (%) EDTA whole blood	Newborn	42–70	42–70
	1–24 mo	30–41	30–41
	2–10 y	33–43	33–43
	10–17 y	36–47	35–45
	Adult	42–52	37–47
Mean corpuscular volume (fL) EDTA whole blood	Newborn	90–115	90–115
	1–24 mo	70–90	70–90
	2–10 y	76–90	76–90
	10–17 y	78–95	78–95
	Adult	78–100	78–100

(continued)

Table 44–3. Hematology. *(Continued)*

Analyte, Units, Specimen Type	Age	Male Range	Female Range
Polymorphonuclear leukocytes (absolute) EDTA whole blood	Newborn	6–23.5	6–23.5
	1–24 mo	1.1–6.6	1.1–6.6
	2–10 y	1.4–6.6	1.4–6.6
	10–17 y	1.5–6.6	1.5–6.6
	Adult	1.5–6.1	1.5–6.6
Band cells (absolute) EDTA whole blood	Newborn	< 3.5	< 3.5
	1–24 mo	< 1.0	< 1.0
	2–10 y	< 1.0	< 1.0
	Adult	< 1.0	< 1.0
Lymphocytes (absolute) EDTA whole blood	Newborn	2.5–10.5	2.5–10.5
	1–24 mo	1.8–9.0	1.8–9.0
	2–10 y	1.0–5.5	1.0–5.5
	10–17 y	1.0–3.5	1.0–3.5
	Adult	1.5–3.5	1.5–3.5
Monocytes (absolute) EDTA whole blood	Newborn	< 2.0	< 2.0
	1 mo–Adult	< 1.0	< 1.0
Eosinophils (absolute) EDTA whole blood	Newborn	< 2.0	< 2.0
	1–24 mo	< 0.7	< 0.7
	2–10 y	< 0.7	< 0.3
	10–17 y	< 0.3	< 0.3
	Adult	< 0.3	< 0.7
Basophils (absolute) EDTA whole blood	Newborn	< 0.4	< 0.4
	1–24 mo	< 0.1	< 0.1
Platelets ($\times 10^9$/L) EDTA whole blood	Newborn	150–500	150–500
	1–24 mo	150–500	150–500
	2–10 y	150–500	150–500
	10–17 y	150–500	150–500
	Adult	150–500	150–500

All data reproduced, with permission, from Oski N: *Hematology of Infancy and Childhood.* Saunders, 1987.

REFERENCES

Bishop M et al: *Clinical Chemistry, Principles and Procedures,* 5th ed. Lippincott Williams and Wilkins, 2005.

Burtis CA et al (editors): *Tietz Fundamentals of Clinical Chemistry.* Saunders, 2007.

Clinical and Laboratories Standards Institute (CLSI), (formerly National Committee for Clinical Laboratory Standards): How to Define and Determine Reference Intervals in the Clinical Laboratory. Approved Guidelines, 2nd ed. NCCLS Document C28-A2, June 2000. Available at: http://www.clsi.org/es/source/orders.

College of American Pathology Commission of Laboratory Accreditation: Laboratory Accreditation Program. Chemistry and Toxicology Checklist, March 30, 2005. Available at: http://www.cap.org/apps/docs/laboratory_accreditation/checklists/chemistry_and_toxicology_march2005.pdf.

Cornell University: Clinical Pathology Laboratory–Reference Intervals. Available at: http://www.diaglab.vet.cornell.edu/clinpath/reference/.

Frazer CG: *Biological Variations from Principles to Practice.* American Association for Clinical Chemistry Press, 2001.

Ghoshal AK, Soldin SJ: Evaluation of the Dade Behring Dimension RxL: Integrated chemistry systems–pediatric reference ranges. Clin Chim Acta 2003;331:135 [PMID: 12691874].

Grossi E et al: The REALAB Project: A new method for the formulation of reference intervals based on current data. Clin Chem 2005;51:1232 [PMID: 15919879].

International Federation of Clinical Chemistry and Laboratory Medicine. Available at: http://www.ifcc.org/ifcc.asp.

Kairisto V: Reference Values and Clinical Interpretation of Laboratory Data. Prepared for Internet Publication by Veli Kairisto, University of Turku, Department of Clinical Chemistry. Available at: http://www.med.utu.fi/clinchem/tempus/dl/lessons.htm.

National Institute of Standards and Technology: Standard for Human Cardiac Troponin Complex. Available at: https://srmors.nist.gov/view_detail.cfm?srm=2921.

Oski N: *Hematology of Infancy and Childhood.* Saunders, 1987.

Soldberg H: Using a hospitalized population to establish reference intervals. Pros and cons. Clin Chem 1994;40:2205 [PMID: 7988005].

Soldin SJ et al: *Pediatric Reference Ranges,* 4th ed. American Association of Clinical Chemistry Press, 2003.

Spencer CA et al: Thyrotropin (TSH)-releasing hormone stimu-lation test responses employing third and fourth generation TSH assays. J Clin Endocrinol Metab 1993;76:494 [PMID: 8432796].

Van Krieken L: Immulite Reproductive Hormone Assays. Available at: http://www.medical.siemens.com/siemens/en_GLOBAL/gg_diag_FBAs/files/news_views/spring00/techreports/zb157-d_www.pdf.

Index

NOTE: A *t* following a page number indicates tabular material, and *f* following a page number indicates a figure. Drugs are listed under their generic names. When a drug trade name is listed, the reader is referred to the generic name.